FIFTH EDITION

Rehabilitation of Musculoskeletal Injuries

Peggy A. Houglum, PhD

Kristine L. Boyle-Walker, MPT, OCS, ATC, CHT

Daniel E. Houglum, MSPT, ATC, PRC

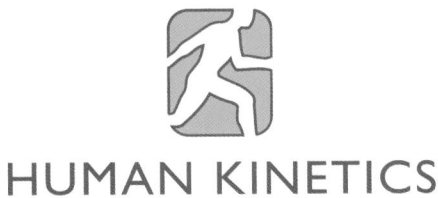

HUMAN KINETICS

Library of Congress Cataloging-in-Publication Data

Names: Houglum, Peggy A., 1948- author. | Boyle-Walker, Kristine L., 1966- author. | Houglum, Daniel E., 1975- author.
Title: Rehabilitation of musculoskeletal injuries / Peggy A. Houglum, Kristine L. Boyle-Walker, Daniel E. Houglum.
Other titles: Therapeutic exercise for musculoskeletal injuries
Description: Fifth edition. | Champaign, IL : Human Kinetics, [2023] | Preceded by Therapeutic exercise for musculoskeletal injuries / Peggy A. Houglum. Fourth edition. 2016. | Includes bibliographical references and index.
Identifiers: LCCN 2021053785 (print) | LCCN 2021053786 (ebook) | ISBN 9781718203150 (hardcover) | ISBN 9781718203167 (epub) | ISBN 9781718203174 (PDF)
Subjects: MESH: Musculoskeletal System--injuries | Rehabilitation--methods | Musculoskeletal Diseases--rehabilitation | Exercise Therapy--methods | Recovery of Function | Athletic Injuries--rehabilitation
Classification: LCC RD97 (print) | LCC RD97 (ebook) | NLM WE 140 | DDC 617.4/7044--dc23/eng/20220801
LC record available at https://lccn.loc.gov/2021053785
LC ebook record available at https://lccn.loc.gov/2021053786

ISBN: 978-1-7182-0315-0 (print)

Acquisitions Editor: Jolynn Gower; **Managing Editor:** Anne E. Mrozek; **Copyeditor:** Kevin Campbell; **Proofreader:** Leigh Keylock; **Editorial Assistant:** Ian Fricker; **Indexer:** Ferreira Indexing; **Permissions Manager:** Dalene Reeder; **Senior Graphic Designer:** Nancy Rasmus; **Cover Designer:** Keri Evans; **Cover Design Specialist:** Susan Rothermel Allen; **Photograph (cover):** bob_bosewell/E+/Getty Images; **Photographs (interior):** © Human Kinetics, unless otherwise noted; **Photo Asset Manager:** Laura Fitch; **Photo Production Specialist:** Amy M. Rose; **Photo Production Manager:** Jason Allen; **Senior Art Manager:** Kelly Hendren; **Illustrations:** © Human Kinetics, unless otherwise noted; **Printer:** Walsworth

Printed in the United States of America   10 9 8 7 6 5 4 3 2 1

The paper in this book was manufactured using responsible forestry methods.

Human Kinetics
1607 N. Market Street
Champaign, IL 61820
USA

United States and International
Website: **US.HumanKinetics.com**
Email: info@hkusa.com
Phone: 1-800-747-4457

Canada
Website: **Canada.HumanKinetics.com**
Email: info@hkcanada.com

E8284

Tell us what you think!
Human Kinetics would love to hear what we can do to improve the customer experience. Use this QR code to take our brief survey.

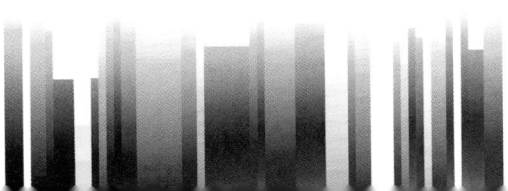

This edition is dedicated to my siblings, Joel, Pam, Joan, Deanna, and Larry. We have always been a close family as kids and remain even closer today as adults. We are siblings by birth and friends by choice. Each one is loved, cherished and special beyond words to me.

—P.A.H.

To my mom and dad, who instilled strength, perseverance, integrity, kindness, and compassion.

To Neil, Tyler, and Brian, who have filled my life with unconditional love, support, and perpetual laughter.

With special thanks to Darwin (in memory), Carol, Pam, Daisy, Abraham, and Cooper, who have provided support, friendship, laughter, and love.

—K.B.W.

To my wife and best friend, Becki, and my wonderful children, Ella and Tyler, for their support, patience, and understanding.

To my parents, Joel and Rita, for their example of how to be a husband and parent.

To my aunt, Peggy, for her consistent example of professionalism and lifelong learning. It is an honor to have worked on this project with you.

—D.E.H.

CONTENTS

PREFACE

This fifth edition is as similar to previous editions of this textbook as it is different from them. There are many changes and many unchanged parts to this new edition.

The New and the Tried-and-True

One of the greatest differences in this edition is the addition of other authors. I am pleased and most thankful to Kris Boyle-Walker, MPT, OCS, ATC, CHT, and Dan Houglum, MSPT, ATC, PRC, for their invaluable contributions. Each of them is an outstanding clinician and educator. They have taken time from their own busy work schedules and other commitments to work with me to create this fifth edition. I am excited to have them on board, and I am sure you will agree with me that they have made important and significant contributions to the textbook. It has been a pleasure for me to work with them and share this experience with them. This textbook is a true collaboration.

In addition to the welcome addition of Dan and Kris, the information contained in this edition includes several revisions worth noting. New and updated information that expands on previous editions, along with additional references, have been included to make this edition even more of an evidence-based textbook than it has been in the past. It has been written with the entry-level master's degree student in mind, but it may also serve practicing clinicians as a reference in their daily patient care. Since most health care organizations, including the National Athletic Trainers' Association, have adopted the World Health Organization's (WHO) International Classification of Function (ICF) model, we present information on this disablement model so our future professionals will work toward the WHO goals, which include using universal definitions to communicate with other health care professionals and caring for patients as individuals with individual needs.

Other new additions to this fifth edition include a section on joint manipulation in chapter 11, the manual therapy chapter. Education paves the way for forward-looking professions; although many states do not yet have manipulation in their practice acts, we feel that it is better to light the way than to wait for it to arrive. Many in the profession already have lit their lamps and can see what is obviously before us, so we are joining them in moving the profession forward.

Chapter 8 is a new chapter for this edition. It includes topics that new professionals face with their patients, but it is information that is not generally taught. New professionals must instruct patients on how to adapt to being temporarily disabled after an injury: how to don a coat with your arm in a sling, how to pick something up from the floor when you've just had back surgery, and so on. This is not a chapter that you commonly see in a textbook, but it contains information that students will find most useful the first time they have to help a patient to problem-solve personal hygiene matters.

Chapter 9 is also new to this edition. It contains abbreviated information on modalities. We have assumed that students have already received most of their information on therapeutic modalities in previous coursework. In this chapter we remind students that modality interventions are part of the overall picture of rehabilitation programs. This chapter also provides bullet points for some of the more important considerations when choosing modalities for a rehabilitation program.

In part IV of the textbook, we have included reference tables of special tests that clinicians can use as examination tools before establishing a rehabilitation program. Some will argue that examination is not part of rehabilitation, but without an examination, one cannot design a rehabilitation program. Examination and rehabilitation go hand-in-hand like a camera and a photograph—you cannot have the latter without the former. Rehabilitation programs are designed for specific injuries or conditions; they must be preceded by a diagnosis. Special tests play an important role when it comes to making an accurate clinical diagnosis. Some of those tests are more accurate than others, and students should know how accurate they are when selecting which ones to use. Therefore, the sensitivity and specificity of these special tests are presented to remind students of the importance of having an accurate diagnosis before designing a rehabilitation program.

You may have noticed that the title of this edition has changed. The name change more aptly reflects the contents of the book; it is a book on rehabilitation, not just therapeutic exercise. To that end, the presentation takes a more medical-model-based approach.

Athletic training education in the past has focused on investigation, identification, and understanding of each element of health care diagnosis and treatment, then putting the components together, primarily through experiential learning to develop a full understanding of injury and its management. Although this is a common educational method, the medical model has been used successfully for many years not only in physician education but also in the allied health professions. The medical model focuses on patient complaints and history along with physical examination and special tests to develop a diagnosis and a treatment plan for specific conditions. Once the basic elements are learned, students are presented with challenges to improve critical thinking and problem-solving so they will try to look at all factors before developing a plan of action and a treatment regimen that will succeed. The medical model allows students to apply their previous knowledge to the task of developing critical thinking skills in a safe and monitored environment where they can gain confidence and self-reliance as they deepen their experience.

The medical model focuses on a specific problem with a view toward management and treatment to resolve the issue. Rather than looking at each element separately, the medical model incorporates all of them so that the student can understand how each element is used not only to identify the patient's problem but to solve it as well.

In presenting this medical model, we assume that students have accumulated basic knowledge and comprehension of core topics such as anatomy, injury, examination, and exercise by the time they are ready for this text. Since these topics are covered in earlier coursework, this edition has eliminated much of the basic science and anatomy and biomechanics information that was in previous editions. The information on these topics that remains is to provide additional background or clarification on the rehabilitation topics. Those topics have been covered in earlier coursework, so students are now prepared to move from those foundations to higher-order skills through the assimilation of their acquired knowledge and critical thinking abilities.

Besides all of these improvements, we have retained many of the previous edition's tried-and-true features. Because most athletic training students are visual learners, the textbook again contains hundreds of photos, drawings, figures, and tables. There are also accompanying videos that may be accessed online. This textbook remains an evidence-based teaching tool, with over 50 pages of references. We have also retained the Evidence in Rehabilitation inserts. These inserts provide the latest evidence on a topic related to the chapter. They are included not only to make the reader aware of new investigations on the horizon but also to tweak the reader's interest in new topics or new twists on a topic.

The Clinical Tips feature has also been retained to give students an important point to recall or a quick summary of a clinically applicable tip. The first part of the textbook deals with the basics of rehabilitation. Then we provide specific applications of techniques for specific body segments and injuries.

The Case Studies feature has also been retained. Each case study has been based on a patient one of us has treated in our careers. We continue to include them since some students may find them not only interesting but also potential learning tools to advance their own understanding of specific injuries and possible interventions.

Additional learning tools at the end of each chapter have remained: Learning Aids, Critical Thinking Questions, and Lab Activities are all included to advance the student to the next step of learning—applying the basic concepts

to practical situations or learning how to use or adapt clinical techniques. Learning Aids are basic applications of information within the chapter, and Critical Thinking Questions take the learner to the next step of expanding those concepts and adapting them to different situations. The Lab Activities are suggestions for hands-on learning that both teach students to apply specific techniques and encourage them to discover how they work.

All chapters throughout the text have undergone significant updating of the information that appeared in the previous edition. Most chapters also now have additional information on previously omitted topics. With changes that have been made for this edition and the strengths we have held onto in this fifth edition, it is our hope that students will continue to find this text an interesting book from which to learn about the theory and practical applications of rehabilitation as much as their instructors will enjoy teaching from it.

Structure and Organization

This text is divided into four parts. Each later part builds on the information presented in previous parts. Part I deals with the basic concepts: what is important in a rehabilitation program, what factors affect a program, and the components involved. It also addresses what happens physiologically to an injury site, the healing process that occurs after an injury, and how injury affects the rehabilitation process. This part also includes disablement models, clinical outcomes assessment, the influence of age on rehabilitation, and evidence-based practice.

Part II presents examination and assessment as they influence rehabilitation. Issues that are integral to rehabilitation include examination and assessment of posture, gait, and neuromotor functions. Unique to this part and to the book is chapter 8. It deals with common activities patients face when required to perform activities with splints or braces. This chapter is unique in that it provides the reader with instructions on how to teach the patient to perform these simple but confounding activities that often bring complication and frustration to a patient's daily routine. No other sports medicine rehabilitation textbook to our knowledge provides this important information.

Part III contains information on rehabilitation tools. These chapters cover topics that are fundamental to every rehabilitation program, including modalities, manual therapy, range of motion, strength, neuromotor control, and performance exercises. A new chapter in this part of the book combines the rehabilitation clinician's roles as detective, problem solver, innovator, and educator to assemble a rehabilitation template that may be used to develop any rehabilitation program for any patient a clinician may encounter. It includes information tidbits that add strength to the framework which becomes the clinician's rehabilitation program. This part familiarizes you with clinical tools that are applied to specific parts of the body in the last section of the book, part IV.

Rehabilitation techniques and progressions are presented for each area of the body in these final chapters of part IV, with special attention given to problems or programs common or unique to specific body segments. Additions that have been made to these chapters include special tests with their sensitivity and specificity ratings for each body segment presented. Since examination is such a vital part of rehabilitation, the examination must be accurate if the rehab program is to be appropriate. Providing the clinician with these data allows the clinician to select special tests which will be reliable in providing the most accurate information.

Terminology

As health care professionals, we should be familiar with terms that are commonly used in the context of identifying, treating, and managing musculoskeletal injuries. The terms that appear in this text use the terminology recommended by the *Board of Certification (BOC)* for athletic trainers. Whether our patients are athletes, industrial workers, or computer programmers, as long they are under medical care, they are considered patients first. Therefore, people needing rehabilitation are referred to as *patients.* Some health care professionals refer to patients as *clients.* We have difficulties with this term since it implies that the clinician is working chiefly to obtain a fee for a service rather than being a professional who provides a service. We should be concerned primarily with the person's health care, not what we may be paid, so *patient* better reflects what should be our priority—improving that person's function and quality of life. As health care professionals, athletic trainers provide myriad services. Athletic trainers are well-rounded clinicians with education and skills in all aspects of patient care from the prevention of injury through immediate care and rehabilitation of that injury. No other allied health care professional has this range of education and training. Since this textbook deals with rehabilitation, the athletic trainer who offers this intervention is referred to as a *rehabilitation clinician* or *clinician.*

Treatment is offered in a *clinic.* The clinic may be an athletic training room, an outpatient clinic, a conditioning facility, a health care facility, or an industrial clinic; wherever the health care professional provides rehabilitation for a patient, the facility is a clinic.

Purpose

This text is a compilation of the authors' almost 100 years of combined clinical experience in rehabilitation and employment in orthopedic, physical therapy, and sports medicine clinics and hospitals. It provides what we believe is comprehensive information about rehabilitation for musculoskeletal injuries. It is meant to be an educational tool for students and a reference text for the practicing rehabilitation clinician. It is meant to offer both time-tested and new information and to challenge both the neophyte and the experienced rehabilitation clinician to provide a new level of insight and information about rehabilitation and our health care professions.

This text does *not* take a cookbook approach to rehabilitation. Instead it provides the background, knowledge, and tools you need to develop the skills to determine what to use for each patient you encounter. It provides the instruments you will need to decide the best course of action, as well as the knowledge about why you are using them; it tells you what to expect when you use a technique and explains the dangers and advantages of various applications, the proper progressions, and ways to apply the knowledge and techniques to specific injuries. Each patient is different and responds differently to injury and treatment; therefore it is neither fair to the patient nor realistic for you to believe that a cookbook approach would be helpful to either of you. The best course of action for you as a rehabilitation clinician is to provide the best program you can with your knowledge, skills, understanding, and appreciation of the whats, whys, and hows of rehabilitation. If you have these assets, you won't need or want a cookbook. This text offers you the tools to develop your own rehabilitation programs for your patients. It is your responsibility to use those tools and your own imagination to provide a sound program that is fun for both you and your patient.

Student Resources

The fifth edition of this text is accompanied by 47 videos in HK*Propel* demonstrating rehabilitation techniques. These demonstrations include how to find the resting position for joint mobilization, joint manipulation techniques, how to use the weight scale for exercises, muscle energy techniques for the sacroiliac joint, core muscle recruitment in exercise, tendon gliding exercises, patient demonstrations for functional activities during times of disability, and many more practical applications.

See the card at the front of the print book for your unique HK*Propel* access code. For ebook users, refer to the HK*Propel* access code instructions on the page immediately following the book cover.

Instructor Resources

Several ancillaries are available to instructors using this text in their courses.

- **Presentation package and image bank:** The presentation package offers instructors detailed lecture notes. The image bank contains most of the art, photos, tables, and typeset figures from the text, which can be used to create custom presentations.

- **Instructor guide:** The instructor guide includes chapter and suggested lecture outlines as well as student activities for the classroom.
- **Test package:** The test bank includes 30 questions for each chapter that can be used to create or supplement tests and quizzes.

- **Chapter quizzes:** Ten auto-gradable quiz questions are provided for each chapter and will be offered in the instructor pack to download and print or to incorporate into your learning management system.

In addition, instructors have access to 47 videos of rehabilitation techniques. Instructors can access all of the ancillary materials by going to HK*Propel*.

ACCESSING THE ONLINE VIDEO

New to this fifth edition are 11 additional high-definition online streaming videos. The 47 total videos can be accessed by visiting HK*Propel*. If you purchased a new print book, follow the directions included on the card attached inside the front of your book. That page includes access steps and the unique key code that you'll need the first time you access the *Rehabilitation of Musculoskeletal Injuries* online resource in HK*Propel*. For ebook users, reference the HK*Propel* access code instructions on the page immediately following the book cover.

Once you have accessed the *Rehabilitation of Musculoskeletal Injuries* online resource in HK*Propel*, you will find links for the 9 chapters that feature video. Once you select a chapter link, you'll see a video player. Scroll through the list of clips until you find the clip you want to watch. Select that clip and the full video will play.

Throughout the book, you'll see cross-references like this pointing you to an online video clip:

 Go to HK*Propel* and watch video 11.1, which demonstrates finding and treating subscapularis trigger points.

Here are the videos you'll find in HK*Propel*:

ACKNOWLEDGMENTS

Writing a textbook is no small feat and involves many individuals, some taking a direct role and others providing behind-the-scenes assistance that is no less important than those working directly in the process. The names you see on the inside cover are those people who have played an active role in making this textbook a reality. Their titles are important but do not reflect the time, effort, and heart that each of them devoted to making this textbook a success. Look at their names and realize that these names represent real people who gave a part of their lives to bringing the book you have before you to life. At its most basic, the book started out as an idea, but it became a reality because of their efforts.

The professionals listed on the inside cover of this textbook are people the three of us have worked with; they are real people with real concerns and a genuine dedication to produce an outstanding book. These people are important to us for several reasons, and we want to recognize them for their outstanding dedication and contributions they each have made to this book. Each of them is experienced in what they do. The tasks they perform for any book are accomplishments unto themselves; however, it must be realized that with the extraordinary size of this textbook, the tasks they normally engage in for a book become dramatically multiplied by the size of this book. The extra workload that is heaped upon them because of the size of the book is difficult to imagine and yet the product they produce is one we are very proud to be a part of; for these reasons, they require special recognition. Jolynn Gower, Acquisitions Editor, is an author's editor. She is well-acquainted with and well-experienced in the book publishing world and did a yeoman's job of melding the publishing company's goals with the authors' ideas to formulate a finished product before the process was even begun. Her insight, foresight, support, and straight-forward approach have been blessings for each of us. Anne Mrozek has the patience of a saint and the persistence of a bulldog. She is a star on our team, and we have been fortunate to have her as our managing editor to see that we stay in line and get the job done! She sees the detail errors we've missed and provides us with wonderful and meaningful suggestions to fix our mistakes. Video/audio/photo production specialist Amy Rose is a hidden gem among the stars at HK. She managed our photo and video shoot, located items we needed like a magician pulling objects out of a magic hat, and saw to it that whatever we needed was there when we needed it. She is reliable beyond measure. Our photographer, Jason Allen, and our videographer, Gregg Henness,

provided a professional's eye to the photos and videos that we needed for this edition. Their expertise was invaluable in adding to the quality achieved and impressions desired from the photos and videos. Jarid Johnson and Sarah Williams volunteered to serve as the models for these photos and videos. Their patience throughout the days of filming and shooting was admirable. The contortionist positions we sometimes had them move into were performed by these well-seasoned models who understood exactly what was being requested. As the medical illustrator for this edition, Heidi Richter attended the photo shoot to gain additional understanding of what we wanted her to achieve with the overdrawings she was to add to some of the photographs. Such willingness to meet with the authors to assure that her artwork would be accurate speaks of a true professional's desire to provide the best art she can to not only reflect the authors' points but add to the quality of the book. Enough cannot be said about the work extraordinaire of the copyeditor, Kevin Campbell. This is the second edition of this book that Kevin has copyedited. This task involves a lot of work for a normal sized text, but one this size magnifies the tasks exponentially. My hat goes off to Kevin for the excellent work he has done to find errors and inconsistencies that we had overlooked. His willingness to copyedit a book this size twice must be a sign of either foolishness or sainthood; I know that Kevin is no fool.

Beyond the people who are listed with their contributions are the other people who provide support without expectations of being recognized. These people are the life-support system for us authors. Without them, we could not do what we set out to do. Some of these people provide their professional services which add to the quality, depth, and understanding of the topics covered within the textbook. Others lend personal assistance, professional advice, hard truths, kind support, valuable insights, and contrary perspectives that enrich the book's content to make it an invaluable resource.

I am foremost indebted to Dan Houglum and Kris Boyle-Walker for their willingness to undertake this enormous task with me. They have each shown themselves to be a professional's professional who is devoted to quality patient care and sharing their knowledge and wisdom with future professionals. The demands they each make upon themselves as professionals should be the gold standard for each of us. Putting your professional prowess on paper is a difficult undertaking; I am both pleased and proud of their sterling success in accomplishing this charge. They have added new perspective, new flavor, and new ideas that move this textbook to a wonderful new level. I am pleased to be riding on their coattails. It has been a pleasure for me to be a part of this textbook with them.

I am once again indebted to Carole Panas, Librarian at Duquesne University, who was my "right hand man" in providing me with ILLIAD resources and references that I asked her to obtain for me. Without her, I would have been at a loss for references from the very start. Carole and the library were made available to me after I retired from Duquesne University because of a generous and supportive university administration. They provided me with special access to the library so that I could accumulate the references I needed to make this edition complete. The university's care and concern for its present and past faculty, staff, and student family are easily reflected in this act. I am grateful to the Administration, Computing and Technology Services, Gumberg Library, and Carole Panas for their generosity and support.

Throughout all of my endeavors, even the crazy ones, my siblings have always been my support and my anchor. They are the ones who keep me focused on the things that are most important in this life. They are the ones who are with me in all matters. They are the ones who keep me afloat. They have always encouraged me to pursue my dreams, even when they didn't understand why it was important to me. By being all of these things for me, they have been the platform of strength from which I have been able to pursue unknown territories, knowing I had them to lean on. Whatever happened, they would remain standing with me, holding me up.

Over the years I have realized that you do nothing by yourself. You need the help of others and you must work together to create an optimal outcome. Those groups of people you learn to rely on vary according to the task to be accomplished, but there must be others to share the load so the task does not become overwhelming or impossible. For this reason, although it may take a village to raise a child, the number of devoted contributors required to produce a textbook is fewer but no less important. It has been my honor and privilege to be a part of a very distinguished, talented, and caring group of personal and professional family members who are the real people responsible for this textbook.

—PAH

I echo Peg's eloquent acknowledgment of our HK family. Jolynn Gower and Anne Mrozek are not only a delight to work with, they are both also consummate professionals who care deeply about their work. I appreciate their guidance, attention to detail, support, and patience throughout this project. Amy Rose is truly a gem. We needed it, she got it. In her words, "the procurement of the shoulder sling will go down as one of my career highlights." We are fortunate

that she was on our book detail! Jason Allen and Gregg Henness were a delight to work with during the photo and video shoot. Their expertise shines through in the photos and videos that you see in this book. Their guidance and patience were much appreciated throughout the weekend of the shoot. Models Jarid Johnson and Sarah Williams are seasoned professionals and truly delivered throughout the days of filming and shooting. I am sure they have a whole new respect for crutches, slings, and braces! Heidi Richter is a medical illustrator who is passionate about her work. We are beyond fortunate to have her gift of illustration for this edition. As Peg mentioned, enough cannot be said about the work extraordinaire of the copyeditor, Kevin Campbell. His attention to detail is unmatched! His keen eye is amazing and much appreciated!

I am grateful to have worked on this project with Peg Houglum and Dan Houglum. I am fortunate to have Peg as a mentor. She has always pushed me to accomplish more than I ever thought I could. I am grateful for her guidance, encouragement, insights, and criticisms. All were necessary for me to complete this undertaking. I am truly blessed to call her my friend. Dan is a great professional with a knowledge base that is endless. It was my great pleasure to have the opportunity to work with him. Peg and Dan, it was an honor to work with you both on this book.

S. John Miller, PhD, PT, ATC, has provided me with the in-depth information that you will find in the manipulation section of the manual therapy chapter. He is the expert I go to when I have questions related to manual therapy. I am fortunate to have him as my colleague and even more fortunate to call him friend.

I am blessed with many colleagues who are phenomenal teachers. Sara Brown, MS, ATC; Tricia Kasamatsu, PhD, ATC; Melissa Montgomery, PhD, ATC; Shane Stecyk, PhD, ATC, CSCS; Cris Stickley, PhD, ATC, CSCS; and Bret Freemyer, PhD, ATC, are my "go to" people for curricular content and CAATE Standards integration into the classroom. Their collective experience and insights have enriched this edition.

Katrina Parsons, MPT, OCS, and Erin Carraway, BA, have provided support and encouragement throughout my writing journey. Katrina assisted me with my research for the ROM and flexibility chapter and offered valuable insight and conclusions which have strengthened the chapter. Each of them, without their knowing it, continually serves as a source of strength and inspiration.

My family has been a source of encouragement and support. I appreciate the sacrifices they have made and the space that they have given me to "write." They are in part contributors to this textbook. I can't imagine life without them. Thank you for believing in me.

—KBW

I've always found a behind-the-scenes process to be very interesting, and this book was no exception. This was an educational journey and, like Peg and Kris, I am indebted to the Human Kinetics team for all of their work and assistance. The entire group was beyond helpful and truly professional. Jolynn Gower and Anne Mrozek have been equal parts supportive and encouraging during this process. I am particularly grateful to Amy Rose. She had my back and, without exaggeration, saved the day. Amy, thank you very much for everything you did for me and us. Jason Allen and Gregg Henness were exceptional. Their attention to detail and timely advice were consistently spot-on. Jarid Johnson and Sarah Williams were very patient with us. Their energy level, preparedness, and professionalism are a testament to them and their craft. Heidi Richter is able to take an idea that is in our heads, and make it come to life on the page. And Kevin Campbell makes his job appear to be much easier than it is. It is impossible to express my level of gratitude to the HK family.

Peg Houglum has been a professional mentor of mine for my entire career, but to be able to work on this project with my aunt has been one of the most wonderful experiences of my life. I feel very fortunate to have been able to share this experience with her. How special our professional and personal relationship is to each other is not lost on either one of us, and working on this book together was truly amazing. Over the years, Peg has introduced me to several of her friends and colleagues, and many of them are among the best in the profession. Kris Boyle-Walker is no exception. Her breadth of knowledge and expertise is matched only by her attention to detail and professionalism. It has been a joy working with Kris on this book.

Peg is one of the reasons I am in this wonderful profession and she has been there to help me along this journey. I've been very fortunate to work with and be influenced by many exceptional teachers and colleagues. Jim Booher, PhD, PT, ATC, helped me get on the right path and guided me both professionally and educationally. Ron Hruska, MPA, PT, has been very generous with his time and energy. His mentorship has helped guide my professional growth, and I am grateful to call him a friend. Lisa Mangino, PT, DPT, PCS, C/NDT, PRC; Louise Kelley, DPT, PTC; Robert George, DC, PRC; Jesse Ham, PT, CMP, PRC; and Donna Parise-Byrne, PT, NCPT, PRC, have all mentored, helped, and pushed me to improve, learn, and grow. I am very thankful to Roger Chams, MD, for the guidance, expertise, and friendship he has shown me and my family. He provided me opportunities for professional growth that proved to be instrumental in my career development. There have been countless patients and other professionals who believed in me and provided opportunities for me to grow and prove myself, and for that, I am eternally grateful.

Thank you to my parents for their love and leadership. Thank you to my siblings and their families for their support. Thank you to my wife and kids for their patience and belief in me not only during this process, but in my career. I am humbled by their sacrifices and understanding. They make me better in all things.

—DEH

PART I

Healing and Other Factors Related to Rehabilitation Decisions

I keep six honest serving men
(They taught me all I knew)
Their names are What and Why and When
And How and Where and Who.

Rudyard Kipling, 1865-1936, author

What, why, when, how, where, and *who* are questions that are continually asked in health care. Knowing the answers to them is not always easy or even possible. Understanding them can be even more difficult. Trying to know and understand the answers, however, is the goal of health care professionals. Knowing and understanding these whats, whys, whens, hows, wheres, and whos of health care define the differences between technicians and professionals.

It is one thing to merely do something, and another to understand why something is done. To be a true health care professional, you must not only know how to perform the techniques and skills that are a part of the profession, but even more importantly, you must have the knowledge to appreciate why a technique or skill is used and understand the impact of its application. The challenge does not lie in applying a weight to an ankle but in knowing *why* it is done, *when* it should be done, and *what* impact this action has on the body. In a speech delivered in 1985, Diane Ravitch said, "The person who knows 'how' will always have a job. The person who knows 'why' will always be his boss." The technician knows how; the health care professional knows why. A technician can apply the technique, but a professional knows, appreciates, and understands the impact of its application.

To develop as a professional and gain this knowledge, appreciation, and understanding of rehabilitation, you must first establish a foundation. Once this foundation is established, the larger concepts of rehabilitation can be addressed. This foundation includes the theories and fundamentals of rehabilitation.

The fundamentals on which rehabilitation is based include the principles, goals, and objectives of rehabilitation; legal and ethical levels of clinical practice; levels of evidence and the importance of basing clinical practice on sound evidence; how to communicate with other colleagues around the world; and the importance of restoring patients to an acceptable level of function in the society in which they live, work, and play. These building blocks of rehabilitation interventions are covered in chapter 1.

In chapter 2, rehabilitation foundations are expanded as you are introduced to what happens within the body when an injury occurs. Starting an activity or procedure before the healing tissue can tolerate the stress can be very detrimental, so it is vital that you understand aspects of healing from its nuances to its complexities. As you administer a rehabilitation program, you must be continually aware of the healing progression if your program is to succeed.

Rehabilitation can be applied in many ways. Simply changing a patient's position from side-lying to supine can significantly change the stress of an exercise or the impact of a treatment. In chapter 3 you are introduced to the intimate relationship between healing and rehabilitation. The first part of the chapter looks at that relationship from a healing perspective, while the last part of the chapter takes the perspective of rehabilitation and how it is driven by recovery and healing.

How can you determine what a patient's body can tolerate orthopedically and physiologically? Before you can determine how to treat a patient, you must consider the patient's age. Age must be a consideration in designing a rehabilitation program and establishing its constraints. Chapter 4 discusses the differences in physical and physiological responses to rehabilitation that occur based on age. There are limits and abilities in all age groups; the clinician must understand these and use that understanding to establish expectations and goals for each patient.

Once these basic factors have been established, we can move on to other critical elements of a comprehensive rehabilitation program. We will explore therapeutic interventions, techniques, and applications. First, however, as you read through part I, think of patients you have seen or rehabilitation processes with which you have been involved. When you do, you will begin to realize that these foundational models, constructs, theories, and rationales play a vital role in any clinician's daily work. It is imperative that you understand and appreciate these basic concepts if you are to create and administer a successful rehabilitation program.

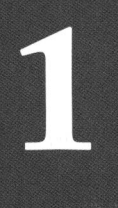

Introduction to Rehabilitation

Objectives

After completing this chapter, you should be able to do the following:

1. Indicate the personal issues that the rehabilitation clinician must keep in mind when treating a patient.
2. Define rehabilitation.
3. Discuss how examination of a patient is related to rehabilitation of that patient.
4. Describe the components of a rehabilitation program.
5. Identify the phases of rehabilitation.
6. Explain what disablement models are and why they are important in rehabilitation.
7. Outline the importance of evidence-based practice and outcomes-based rehabilitation.

Amanda had been in her first athletic training position for three weeks. She felt good about her position as assistant athletic trainer at the Division I university and was excited about being the athletic department's first rehabilitation coordinator. Until now, the athletic trainers had delivered rehabilitation to patients in a casual, inconsistent manner. It was Amanda's job to organize and ensure optimal, efficient, and cooperative rehabilitation programs for all patients. She understood and appreciated the importance of the World Health Organization's model for treating her patients as individuals and looking at them not just as patients with an injury but as whole persons.

Amanda's first real challenge came early in the football season when the first-string quarterback, Tony "Fast Gun" Johns, underwent a surgical reconstruction of his anterior cruciate ligament (ACL). Tony was a promising athlete whose football future depended on a good outcome of his knee rehabilitation program. Amanda felt a lot of pressure and mistrust from the coaching staff, Tony's parents, and Tony himself. Amanda wasn't sure whether their anxiety was because of the injury, the history of the department's care for these types of injuries, or her own limited experience. Amanda felt the best way to gain their trust was to manage Tony's case well. She knew that she must do a good job not only of rehabilitating Tony's knee, but also of rehabilitating him as a person whose needs, expectations, and goals were specific to him and to the demands he must confront both at the start of his rehabilitation program and after he completed it.

The best interest of the patient is the only interest to be considered, and in order that the sick may have the benefit of advancing knowledge, union of forces is necessary.

Dr. William Mayo, 1861-1939, physician and surgeon and one of seven founders of the Mayo Clinic

The preceding quote from Dr. Will Mayo reminds us of the importance of putting our patients first and working together with other health care providers to achieve the common goal of optimal treatment outcomes for every patient who comes to us for help. This chapter provides an overview of rehabilitation and describes what it means to provide rehabilitation to a patient, what the components of rehabilitation include, and how they fit together in a progression as the patient improves. This chapter also introduces aspects of clinical practice that are relevant to health care providers around the world, and it describes what evidence-based practice means and why outcomes matter in today's health care environment. Although the topics in this chapter are varied, they all form the foundation for a rehabilitation program, and clinicians must understand them.

Definition of Rehabilitation

Before we can begin an in-depth discussion of rehabilitation, we must define it. Then we can identify the elements and determine how to design our own programs.

According to *Taber's Cyclopedic Medical Dictionary*,[1] **rehabilitation** is "the process of treatment and education that help disabled individuals to attain maximum function, a sense of well-being, and a personally satisfying level of independence." This definition of rehabilitation is very different than it was even a few years ago, when rehabili-

tation was defined as "the restoration of an individual or a part to normal or near normal function."[2] The differences between these two definitions may seem modest, but they are in fact profound.

One of the main influences on this change in the definition has been the work of the World Health Organization (WHO). Headquartered in Geneva, Switzerland, the WHO is an agency of the United Nations whose primary concerns include the advancement of international public health and the reduction of disease worldwide. The WHO is responsible for creating norms and setting standards by which countries can provide optimal health care to their citizens. The organization monitors and provides support for implementing these standards and also leads in the shaping of research agendas to address world health concerns.[3]

Over the years, the WHO has been a key player in health-related activities around the world. Because of the common language, definitions, and systems the WHO has put in place, it has become easier for professionals around the world to communicate with accuracy and precision. One of the definitions created to reflect the worldwide medical community's perspective on rehabilitation was created in 2011; the WHO defines rehabilitation as "a set of measures that assist individuals who experience, or are likely to experience, disability to achieve and maintain optimal functioning in interaction with their environments."[4]

This definition has changed not only the way rehabilitation is defined in this country, but also how it is performed and what it includes. One thing to notice in the WHO definition is that there is a compounded element of concern for the patient. The definition not only includes whether or not the patient can perform a specific function, but it also identifies how that patient is able to function in the environment and society in which he or she is expected to engage. The "old" definition had no regard for the person's social environment; it only addressed what the person could do in spite of an injury or illness. We will discuss this in more detail when we look at clinical practice and how decisions are made in daily patient care.

CLINICAL TIPS

Given the ever-changing discoveries and advances in health care, after you graduate you will continue to learn new and different ways of treating your patients. It is important to maintain an active interest in your profession and to keep current with changes in its practices and values. Even the terminology can change, and your performance systems can be left in the dust if you fail to keep current.

Personal Issues

Rehabilitation in the orthopedic and sports arena includes several personal issues for our patients. Clinicians must keep these personal issues in mind, for they influence how we proceed as professionals when dealing one-on-one with patients. These issues are important enough that they are presented before the elements of rehabilitation are presented, for without an awareness of what the patient expects and how that patient reacts to what you do, your efforts are handicapped before you begin.

Patients seek you out because they need specific care to resolve their injuries, and they believe you can solve the health problems that prevent them from performing as they should. It is your responsibility to treat them with a professional attitude and to use your knowledge and skills to the best of your ability. However, before you begin your treatment, you must bear in mind the facets of patient care that follow.

Consent

Rehabilitation clinicians use their professional skills, knowledge, and best professional judgment to design what they feel is the best course of rehabilitation for a patient. Sometimes the patient may not wish to follow that course of treatment. Or the patient may refuse to perform a particular activity. You can try to convince the patient that the activity is appropriate for a variety of reasons, but if the patient refuses, you cannot force him or her to do it. For example, if a gymnast who suffered an ankle sprain refused to do the non-weight-bearing pool therapy that you recommended, you would probably explain why it would be beneficial for her to go into the water. If she continued to refuse, you could not force her into the pool. It would be up to you to find an alternative program for her. Likewise, if you wanted a basketball player with a subluxating shoulder to start doing medicine-ball work, but he refused because he lacked confidence that his shoulder could tolerate the exercise, the same policy would apply. You could explain why this was an important activity and reassure him that

your professional skills, knowledge, experience, and observation of his performance tell you that his shoulder was ready. If he still refused, you would have to use a different type of exercise that was less threatening to him yet still accomplished the same goal. You could reintroduce the activity later in the program when the patient's confidence had grown.

The patient always has the last say on what is or is not done with or to his or her body. Patients give consent for treatment by doing what is asked during the rehabilitation program, but they can always say no. The patient's consent is assumed to be given in the treatment process until it is taken away. As a rehabilitation clinician, you must always respect the patient's right to consent to or refuse treatment. Generally, your knowledge, skill, experience, and self-confidence earn the patient's confidence and trust, so compliance with your program is ongoing. However, on occasions where the patient refuses any aspect of treatment for any reason, you must respect that refusal. The best way to prevent this type of situation is to have the knowledge to create an appropriate rehabilitation program, confidence in your professional skills, and an ability to create the same confidence in your patients.

Touch

Rehabilitation usually involves touching the patient. We palpate injuries on a daily basis, feel for spasm and temperature, and touch painful and swollen areas routinely. For this reason, touch becomes something we often do not think about, yet we must always be sensitive to the patient's perception of our touch.

Touching a patient should always be done for a specific reason and with a goal in mind. For example, if you touch the thigh of a patient who has suffered a contusion to the quadriceps, the pressure applied and the area palpated should be appropriate. Casual touch is never condoned.

Touching is an integral and necessary part of a rehabilitation clinician's duties, but a patient may not be accustomed to the intimacy of touch in this context. Before you place your hands on a patient or perform a specific task, you must always explain to the patient what you intend to do and why. Presenting yourself in a professional manner, being deliberate in how you touch, demonstrating respect for the patient, and having sensitivity for the patient's situation can help to reassure the patient and enable you to perform your tasks appropriately.

If you are not sure how a patient will respond to your touch, it is best to have another professional present. If you are dealing with a patient whose cultural rituals and restrictions are not familiar to you, ask the patient's permission before you place your hands on him or her. In today's litigious environment, touch—even when it is purely professional and necessary—can be questioned. If you work with athletes, you will find that most injured athletes are treated in an athletic training clinic where other people are around. However, if you find yourself in an isolated situation or if you think that questions may arise later, you should take precautions. Have another professional or someone else present in the room during your patient encounter, keep the treatment room door open, or provide the treatment in a common room where others are present. It is often wise to listen to your instincts; if you have an uneasy feeling about a situation, be cautious.

CLINICAL TIPS

Be considerate of the patient by explaining that you are about to touch the patient and what you intend to do before you proceed. Do not assume that the patient knows and approves of what you intend to do without first informing the patient.

Personal Response

Everyone responds differently to an injury and to the subsequent rehabilitation program. Expecting a patient to progress in the same way as the last patient you had with a similar injury can prove to be frustrating for both of you. It is no more realistic to compare one patient to another than it is for a parent to compare one child to his sibling. Individual physiological and biochemical differences can profoundly affect a patient's responses to an injury.[5, 6] Other nonphysical variables can also influence a patient's recovery, including outside support from friends, teammates, and family; the patient's psychological makeup and response to the injury; the degree and types of outside pressures the patient may feel; and the goals and rewards the patient may want to achieve. The program should be guided and designed based on the responses of each patient.

Personal Needs

In addition to having different responses to an injury and its treatment, patients will also have different needs that must be met if they are to be fully rehabilitated. For example, if you have two patients, Sam and Joe, who work in the same factory, and they each have an ankle sprain, the rehabilitation requirements will be different for Sam, who must jump on and off a forklift and drive it, than for Joe, whose job it is to maintain the assembly line.

Patients have other needs that must be considered. Although two patients may be on the same sport team, they may have different social environments that dictate different needs. You must assess each patient as a whole person, not as just a sprained ankle or a dislocated shoulder. These personal variations should always be a consideration when you design the patient's rehabilitation program. For example, you may be treating two college swimmers with elbow tendinopathy; one lives on campus in a dorm and the other lives at home and helps his father milk cows twice a day. They will have entirely different needs that must be addressed if their rehabilitation programs are to succeed.

Objectives

Objectives are the desired outcomes of our rehabilitation efforts. There are three basic objectives for any rehabilitation program. The first is related directly to the principle of treating the whole patient; it is to prevent deconditioning of uninjured areas. The second objective is to rehabilitate the injured part in a safe, efficient, and effective manner. The third objective is to return the patient to an optimal degree of function within the environment in which he or she is to perform.

Prevent Deconditioning

Preventing deconditioning includes considering the total patient by providing exercises for the cardiovascular system, the uninvolved areas of the injured extremity or segment, and the uninvolved extremities. For example, if the patient has a knee injury that prevents weight bearing on that limb, the patient can maintain cardiovascular conditioning by performing pool exercises or working out on an upper-body ergometer. The patient can also maintain good strength and range of motion of the trunk, upper body, and uninvolved lower extremity by using weights and other exercises for these segments. Exercises for the involved extremity's hip and ankle can also be used to prevent deconditioning of those areas without applying undue stress to the injured knee.

Because of the nature of the injury or the medical restrictions involved, it may sometimes take some imagination to develop exercises that challenge the uninjured parts while not harming the injured area. Still, it is important for you to design programs that include maintaining current conditioning levels as much as possible.

Rehabilitate the Injured Part

Good knowledge of the injury, the healing process, and methods of rehabilitation is paramount in achieving the objective of rehabilitating the injured part. You must use good judgment along with this knowledge to enable the patient to progress safely and effectively through the rehabilitation program. You must be able to explain any decision made; combining evidence-based information with common sense will enable you to make the best choices. Evidence-based practice is presented later in this chapter.

Rehabilitation treatments can enhance and promote recovery, but they can also be harmful and ineffective if used incorrectly. It is your responsibility to know the appropriate use of this highly effective yet potentially dangerous therapy.

Returning to Optimal Function as a Contributing Member

For athletes, this means returning them to a level of athletic function which makes them valuable team players. For employees it means that once they have completed their rehabilitation program, they are able to return to jobs and lives as contributing members of their work and home environments.

It is important for injured patients to be able to return to their lives and resume the roles they had prior to their injuries. When the clinician designs a rehabilitation program, these issues of what is expected of the patient when he or she returns to their work and home environments must be included in the overall plan if full rehabilitation is to be provided.

When the main objectives are achieved, the patient can return to his or her optimal level of function in a manner that is safe yet quick, effective yet efficient, and assertive yet cautious. This means that you must use all the tools available to promote healing, restore the functions that were lost to injury, and help the patient to regain confidence that he or she can return with at least the same level of competence as before the injury. This should be done in the minimum amount of time needed for optimal healing without excessive time away from the patient's desired activities.

There is often a fine line between going too slowly and going too quickly. The program should stress the patient just enough to provide gains, not losses, with regular progression. Visualize the following image to grasp this concept: During each treatment session, every treatment you provide moves the patient up a hill toward its peak, which is your treatment session's goal. Therefore, you must provide enough stress in a treatment session to produce as much forward and upward gain as possible. At the same time, it is very important to avoid pushing so far that the patient goes over the top and down the other side (applying so much stress that it causes deleterious effects). Likewise, if the patient is not sufficiently stressed in his or her treatment sessions, the ultimate goal will take longer to achieve. As the patient progresses, each day's peak advances to a different level until the final peak, completion of the rehabilitation program, is achieved.

Elements of Rehabilitation

The elements of a rehabilitation program include all activities related to the care and treatment of orthopedic or sports-related injuries. Each of these components will be introduced here and discussed in detail in later chapters. It is important to present an overview here so that you may understand how these elements fit together. Each is important to the entire program; if one is missing, the program is incomplete.

Examination

Rehabilitation programs are based on a problem-solving approach to the patient's injury, deficiencies, and goals.[7] Before you can establish a rehabilitation program, you must first perform an examination to identify the patient's

injury and to discover any deficiencies that prevent the patient from achieving his or her goals. An **examination** is the process by which the clinician gathers subjective and objective information to identify the patient's injury and define deficiencies so that an appropriate rehabilitation program can be designed.

The examination is the starting point for any rehabilitation program. Clinicians continually examine and reexamine their patients throughout the rehabilitation program. An examination enables you to determine whether your treatment is beneficial or not. For example, if your goal is to increase range of motion, then goniometric measurements before and after a treatment will enable you to gauge its effectiveness. If you record motion gains, then you know your treatment selection is appropriate. If you want to reduce a patient's pain, you need to ask the patient before you treat him what his pain level is and then ask again after the treatment what his pain level is; if it hasn't changed, then you need to change your treatment regimen to achieve the goals you have established.

Examination is intimately connected to all aspects of rehabilitation. The only way to establish goals is to examine the patient so you can determine the patient's current condition. How much swelling is present? How much range of motion is lost? What is the status of the injured area's strength? These and other questions are assessed on the first day of rehabilitation. They are also reexamined regularly throughout the rehabilitation program.

Without an examination you can neither identify what treatment the patient needs nor can you determine if the treatment program you are providing is effective. Examination and rehabilitation are so closely interwoven that one serves no purpose without the other. You must continually examine and assess the patient's condition to assure both yourself and the patient that your program is achieving its goals. This fact cannot be overstated. Since examination is performed often and throughout the rehab process, it is covered in more depth in chapter 5.

CLINICAL TIPS

Basic to *any* rehabilitation program is an examination. After the first time a patient is seen, the clinician *must* examine the patient before each treatment session begins and before and after each treatment provided within that session. This step is particularly important for determining whether the selected treatments are beneficial and whether the patient is making appropriate progress. The best outcomes are achieved when the clinician is faithful in determining what applications are most appropriate and which treatments provide the best results.

There are two elements that must be included to make the examination complete. These are assessment (evaluation) and testing. Each of them will be addressed here.

Assessment

An **assessment** is sometimes also referred to as an **evaluation** and is defined as the use of the clinician's judgment and abilities to assimilate the information from the examination, the medical record, and the patient's signs and symptoms to reach a clinical diagnosis. Once the examination is completed and the clinician assimilates the information gathered into an evaluation or assessment, the rehabilitation program can be created.

In a sense, the clinician is a scientist who is on a mission to identify the patient's problem so the rehabilitation program can be designed. Throughout the examination, the clinician looks for clues, starting with the patient's complaints. Those complaints include signs and symptoms. To those complaints the clinician adds any relevant medical history, such as tests or X-rays that have been performed. Once the clinician has accumulated all of the information about the patient's condition, she then organizes her data so she can create a list of hypotheses, or possible diagnoses. She then tests her hypotheses to either eliminate or confirm those potential clinical diagnoses; this list of potential diagnoses is sometimes referred to as rule-out diagnoses. A **rule-out diagnosis** or **differential diagnosis** refers to a list of the most likely injuries or conditions based on the information gathered.[8] To narrow the list of potential diagnoses to the *actual* one, the clinician may perform a variety of special tests that will either confirm or eliminate each diagnosis. After elimination of all but one hypothesis through these tests, the remaining diagnosis is revealed as *the* clinical diagnosis.

CLINICAL TIPS

Several different diagnoses may have similar or overlapping signs and symptoms. The clinician uses his knowledge of those groupings, skills in testing, and ability to define and identify the correct diagnosis from his accumulated data.

Part of the assessment includes determining the severity of the patient's signs and symptoms. It is common for signs and symptoms caused by orthopedic and sports injuries to interfere with the patient's ability to begin an active recovery process. These interfering limitations must be treated before exercises can begin. For example, if a patient's muscle spasm following a low back sprain is so severe that he cannot move without pain, that spasm and pain must be treated first.

An examination and assessment are not only performed at the time of the patient's first treatment session but also at each subsequent treatment session. Before a clinician can provide an appropriate treatment, he must first examine and assess the patient. Has the patient's condition worsened or improved since the last treatment? Have other signs or symptoms developed that were not present before? Can the patient perform different activities today, or can you discontinue certain types of treatment because she has improved enough that she no longer benefits from treatments you provided during the last session? The only way you can answer these questions and others that may occur is to examine the patient and assess her condition before you begin your treatment.

You also must identify whether specific steps of the treatment session are producing the desired results. You can only do this by assessing the patient before and after the treatment. For example, if you provide joint mobilization to increase knee flexion, you must assess the amount of knee flexion your patient has before you perform joint mobilization and then again after you've completed the treatment to note the changes. If you have not made gains, either it is the wrong treatment or your technique is ineffective. You must decide why your treatment was unsuccessful and determine what else you can offer that may produce better results. The only way you can provide optimal treatment is to assess the effects of each treatment you provide and assess the overall effects of every treatment session.

Tests

An examination is only as good as the accuracy of the diagnostic tests used in that examination.[9, 10] These tests are used to narrow the differential diagnoses list down to the clinical diagnosis for which the patient will be treated. Therefore, the clinical tests a clinician uses in an examination must be accurate in their ability to predict a positive or a negative result if the patient either does or does not have the condition for which the test is used. However, before the predictive value of a diagnostic test can be identified, the test must first have reliability and validity. **Reliability** of a test is how often the test will produce consistent results under the same conditions.[11]

There are two types of reliability that determine the consistency and usefulness of a test. The person who observes or measures the test is called a *rater*. Clinically, this person is usually the clinician who performs the test. One type of reliability tells how consistent it is when the same clinician uses the test more than once and on different patients and has the same results (intrarater reliability). The other type of reliability occurs when a group of clinicians uses the same diagnostic test on the same patients and has the same results (interrater reliability). Reliability measures are expressed either as κ (kappa) or ICC (intraclass correlation coefficient). When the reliability is close to 1.0 in either κ or ICC, it means that the diagnostic test is more reliable than a test that has a reliability score farther from 1.0. Clinical tests have a wide range of reliability scores and generally do not reach 1.0 because the human element of both the patient and the clinician make it very difficult to be either consistent or perfectly reliable all the time. In research where the diagnostic tests clinicians perform are investigated for their reliability, levels of reliability measures must reach a minimum ICC or κ before a test may be considered consistent enough for clinicians to rely on for its results. These standard acceptable measures of reliability are:[12]

- ICCs that are greater than 0.90 are indicative of excellent reliability.
- ICCs that are between 0.75 and 0.9 are indicative of good reliability.
- ICCs that are between 0.5 and 0.75 are indicative of moderate reliability.
- ICCs that are less than 0.5 are indicative of poor reliability.

In addition to a diagnostic test's having to show accurate results when it is used, it must also be able to test what it is supposed to test. **Validity** is the degree to which a test measures what it is intended to measure.[11] Clinicians generally do not validate a test or equipment used in an examination; that task is performed by clinical researchers. For example, clinicians commonly accept that a goniometer is a valid instrument for measuring joint range of motion (ROM) since it was long ago determined to be a valid instrument for ROM tests.[13, 14] On the other hand, some tests have been introduced more recently, and they have not yet withstood enough examinations to be fully recognized as reliable. For example, although many investigators have verified that the Star Excursion Balance Test (SEBT) may be used to both test and rehabilitate dynamic balance in patients,[15-18] other investigators have not yet agreed with such findings.[19, 20] In these cases when the validity is not so clear-cut, it is your responsibility as your patient's clinician to read and compare the investigations and decide for yourself whether a particular diagnostic test or rehabilitation exercise may be beneficial for your patient.

The validity of a test refers to how well that test can accurately assess the presence or absence of the condition in the patient. If you use the Neer test on a patient who may have a subacromial impingement, you need to know if that test will give you a positive sign if subacromial impingement is present or a negative sign if it is not. The terms used to define these situations are *sensitivity* and *specificity*. **Sensitivity** is defined as the test's ability to produce a positive result when the condition being tested for really is present. In other words, that test has sensitivity when its results are positive. The quantitative sensitivity of a specific diagnostic test has been determined through research investigations that have compared the results of that test with a test that has been established as the gold standard of diagnostics for a particular condition. A **gold standard** is the criterion measure or test that is the best at

producing the most accurate results, and it is the standard by which all other measures or tests that propose to produce the same outcome are assessed. Sensitivity is also referred to as *true positive*. A **true positive** means that if the patient demonstrates a positive sign when the diagnostic test is performed on him, he has the condition.[11] If the clinical test has a lower sensitivity, the test may show a positive result when the patient does not have the condition; this is known as a **false positive**. For example, if a special test that examines the presence of an anterior cruciate ligament injury has a sensitivity of 40%, it means that the test will be correct 40% of the time, and 60% of the time the test results will show that a patient has the condition when she does not really have it.

Specificity is at the other end of the validity spectrum. **Specificity** is defined as a diagnostic test's ability to produce a negative result when the patient really does not have the condition.[11] This is also referred to as **true negative**. A diagnostic test that has a high specificity will not test positive when the test is administered to a patient who does not have the condition. Therefore, when you use a test with a high specificity on a patient who does not have the condition, you can expect that the patient will have a negative test result. If a clinical test has a low specificity, it may be more likely to show a negative result when the patient actually has the condition; this is referred to as a **false negative**. For example, if a test for a peroneal subluxation has a specificity of 35%, it means that 35% of the time that test will show a negative test result when the person does not have the condition, and 65% of the time the test will produce a negative sign when the patient actually has the condition.

Therefore, you have four possible outcomes when you administer a diagnostic test. These outcomes are presented here in table 1.1.

The closer the specificity and sensitivity ratings are to 1.0, or 100%, the more reliable they are for producing the correct results. In other words, if a test's specificity is 1.0, it will always produce a negative result when the condition is not present. If the test's specificity is 95%, its result will be accurate in demonstrating that the person does not have the condition in 95 out of 100 people, and in 5 out of 100 people the test will show a negative result when the person does have the condition. This same rule applies for sensitivity results of a test; results are based on the frequency of positive outcomes relative to the percent of time it is accurate in demonstrating a positive result when the patient has the condition.

In most cases, high sensitivity and high specificity are at opposite ends of a diagnostic spectrum. If a test has a high sensitivity, it is highly likely that the condition is present if the person's test result is positive. On the other hand, if a test with a high specificity is used and its results are negative, it is highly likely that the person does not have

TABLE 1.1　Specificity and Sensitivity of Test Results

	DIAGNOSTIC TEST RESULTS	
	Injury or disease *is* present	**Injury or disease is *not* present**
Positive clinical test	**True positives** The test produces a positive result when the patient actually does have the condition. **High sensitivity** **SpPin**	**False positives** The test produces a positive result when the patient does not have the condition. **Low sensitivity**
Negative clinical test	**False negatives** The test produces a negative result when the patient actually does have the condition. **Low specificity**	**True negatives** The test produces a negative result when the patient does not have the condition. **High sensitivity** **SnNout**

the condition. Two mnemonics can help you remember these differences. **SnNout** (high **S**ensitivity, **N**egative result means rule **out** the condition), and **SpPin** (high **Sp**ecificity, **P**ositive result means rule **in** the condition).

Tests that have high sensitivity are important when you want to rule out a condition. For example, if you perform the Neer test to assess whether your patient has a rotator cuff tear and you know that this test has a sensitivity of 85%,[21] you realize that 85% of the time a negative outcome to this test will accurately indicate no rotator cuff tear and 15% of the time a negative outcome will be a false negative. Those conditions that can be costly in terms of life, time, or expense, such as a displaced or nondisplaced fracture, would most especially benefit from tests with a high sensitivity.

A clinical test may be sensitive but not specific—that is, it may produce a positive result without necessarily creating a clear picture of a patient's condition. Tests that have a high sensitivity are less stringent in their testing criteria.[11, 22] Therefore, these types of tests will have fewer erroneous results; however, they may not be able to focus on a precise diagnosis. For example, if we look closely at the Neer test, we see that its sensitivity for identifying the existence of a rotator cuff tear is 85%, so if we get a positive sign in a patient, we can suspect a rotator cuff tear. As it turns out, the Neer test has a low specificity when it is compared to the gold standard, arthroscopic findings.[21] In other words, the patient may have a positive test result but not a rotator cuff tear.

Therefore, it is best to use a combination of clinical tests that have high sensitivity and high specificity in a patient examination. When your patient shows positive results in the highly sensitive tests you use, demonstrating the likelihood of having the condition for which you are testing, you should then also use tests with high specificity to correctly identify false positive results you may have obtained in the highly sensitive tests.[23] You can then more assuredly make a correct diagnosis.

Some tests will have published sensitivity and specificity results, while others are published with positive and negative predictive values. Some tests may be new enough that neither type of measure is currently available. When measures are available, it is your responsibility as a clinician to investigate what is published so you know what is current about the tests. You also use your own experiences to assess for yourself how well a specific test works for you in your clinical environment. In part IV of this textbook, you will find some of the published results for the special tests to help you determine which tests may be the most beneficial for you to use in your clinical practice.

Problems and Goals

Following an examination and assessment of a patient's injury or illness, the clinician creates a list of problems that should be addressed in the treatment program. This list is recorded with the greatest problems or most significant deficiencies listed first, with the other problems following in descending order of importance. This problem list serves as a guide to setting goals for resolving those issues. There should be a goal for every problem identified.

Likewise, for every specified goal, there should be a treatment plan for achieving that goal. Goals are the results a person strives to achieve. The ultimate goal of a rehabilitation program is to restore the patient to an optimal level of function within the environment to which the patient will return. Usually, although not always, this optimal level means complete recovery—that is, a return to the functions and abilities the patient had before the injury. In addition to this ultimate goal, other goals are usually included as desired outcomes of a rehabilitation program. The elements of the rehabilitation program are selected to satisfy those goals, so identifying them is an important step in the rehabilitation process.

These additional goals may be divided into long-term goals and short-term goals. **Long-term goals** are those goals that are to be achieved at the end of the rehabilitation

CLINICAL TIPS

It is important to know which special tests have a high sensitivity (SnNout) to rule out a condition and which special tests have a high specificity (SpPin) to tell you that it is likely that the patient has a condition. It is good to perform more than one test to obtain accurate results from your examination.

Typically, clinical tests are created by practicing clinicians who see a need to identify the presence of a specific condition. These special tests are often presented to the clinical world before a gold standard for the test is developed. When a gold standard is not available, a test is assessed for its accuracy by looking at predictive values.[24] A **positive predictive value (PPV)** is the likelihood that a patient whose test result is positive really has the condition. A **negative predictive value (NPV)** is the likelihood that a patient whose test result is negative does not have the condition. These values are related to the test's

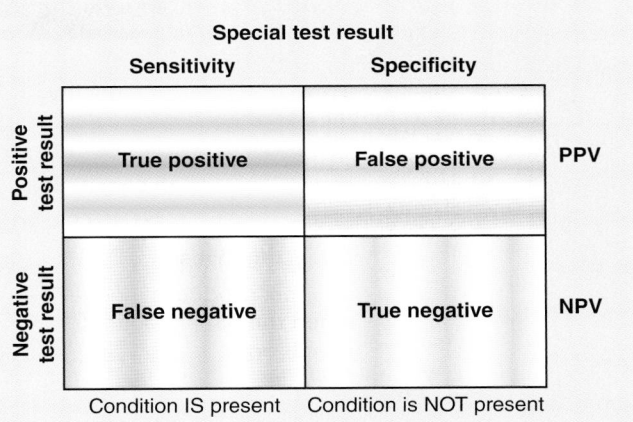

sensitivity and specificity in that the PPV and NPV are calculated by dividing the true number of true results by the sum of the number of true and false results. In other words, researchers determine a test's PPV by dividing the number of true positive results by the sum of the true positive and false positive test results. Likewise, investigators determine a test's NPV by dividing the number of true negative results by the sum of the true negative and false negative results they have seen in their research on that special test. By comparing the accurate results with all of the accurate and inaccurate test outcomes, we can get an idea of how well the test can truly identify either the presence or the absence of the condition for which it is testing. Because sensitivity and specificity are related to positive and negative predictive values, respectively, if a test has a high specificity and a high NPV, it is unlikely that the patient has the condition. On the other hand, a test that has a high sensitivity and a high positive predictive value is very likely to produce a positive outcome when the patient has the condition and is unlikely to produce a positive outcome when the patient does not have the condition. In other words, if a test has a high negative predictive value, it is likely that if the patient's test result is negative, he does not have the condition for which the test is given; however, if a test has a high positive predictive value, it is likely that if the patient's test result is positive, he has the condition for which the test is given. See the illustration for a graphic representation of these concepts.

process, while **short-term goals** are those that are achieved before the long-term goals; they serve as stepping-stones, or points of progression, toward the final goals. We often find that if we look at everything we must achieve to reach our ultimate goals, we get overwhelmed and do not know where to begin. However, if we break those big goals into smaller, step-by-step goals, we can focus on these smaller goals and move in a direction to accomplish all our goals. It is also easier to recognize progress when we focus on short-term goals.

Rehabilitation goals are set by the patient and clinician working together. Both parties must agree if the rehabilitation program is to succeed. Establishing these goals fulfills a number of useful purposes. Goals can help guide the patient's treatment, they can provide a way to measure changes in the patient's condition, and they can motivate the patient throughout the rehabilitation process.[25, 26, 27] Once we identify the deficiencies a patient has as a result of an injury, surgery, or illness and establish a list of problems that are preventing the patient from functioning optimally, the goals that must be achieved to remove those problems and restore the patient to either premorbid or

optimal function come into focus. Goals and problem lists are presented in more detail in chapter 5.

Once the short-term and long-term goals are established, a plan of treatment to achieve those goals is created. Each rehabilitation technique in the patient's program is intended to achieve at least one of the goals. As a clinician, you should always have the treatment goals in mind, and you should remain focused on achieving those goals with each element you include in your program. You should be able to justify every aspect of your rehabilitation program.

CLINICAL TIPS

Clinical examination, a problem list, and a goal list are all integral parts of the rehabilitation program; without them, a rehabilitation program cannot be created. Goals are created from the list of problems a patient has as a result of an injury. Only after the clinician has examined the patient to identify the problems and created goals to resolve those problems can a rehabilitation program be designed to achieve those goals.

Components of Rehabilitation

By the time the patient's examination and assessment, lists of problems and goals, and treatment plan have been established, the rehabilitation program is well underway. As integral segments of the rehabilitation process, these elements are the foundation upon which the rehabilitation program progresses. As the patient improves, the problem and goal lists change to reflect the changes seen in the patient that are gleaned from the clinician's reexaminations and re-assessments. From this foundation, the rehabilitation program follows a specific sequence of treatments that are progressive and coincide with the healing process that occurs following an injury or surgery. The treatments follow a sequence because each one is based on the previous component's successful completion, much like a pyramid (figure 1.1), in which blocks are placed one on another, layer by layer, until the structure is complete. This concept will become clearer as we discuss each component in this section.

A rehabilitation program is more understandable when it is divided into units or phases. However, the body never works in such clearly delineated phases. There is always overlap between the phases. For example, during the phase when flexibility is emphasized, some strengthening may also occur. Likewise, when strength is the main focus in the next phase, several exercises may be included for motion gains and for more aggressive stresses. The clinician must realize where in the healing process the patient is, what levels of stress may be safely applied, and what problems need to be addressed at any time within the rehabilitation

program. These considerations are realized by the clinician before any exercise or activity is added to the patient's program.

Reduce Signs and Symptoms of Inflammation and Correct Deviations

In accordance with the problems and goals that have been established, the treatment begins by reducing signs and symptoms of inflammation. Inflammation is discussed in detail in chapter 2. It is important to realize that inflammation is a necessary part of the healing process. However, inflammation produces unwanted signs and symptoms such as pain, swelling, muscle spasm, and reduced function of the injured segment. These signs and symptoms must be treated before other factors, such as loss of motion and weakness, are addressed.

Additional factors may also be addressed during this early time of rehabilitation. Along with the injury and its consequences, the patient's problems may include a structural or functional deviation that might have contributed to the injury. For example, if a patient has hip pain, perhaps a leg length discrepancy is contributing to the problem. Or perhaps a patient with shoulder impingement has poor posture that has led to the impingement. In these cases, the clinician can reduce the abnormal stresses caused by these structural or functional deviations by correcting or reducing the defect during this time in the rehabilitation program.

Flexibility and Range of Motion

Once the injury site is past the inflammation phase of healing and the side effects that accompany this phase are subsiding with the treatment techniques the clinician uses, the rehabilitation priority advances to the next priority, restoring mobility and flexibility. Achieving flexibility early in the rehabilitation program is important for two reasons. First, it serves as a foundation for the other factors that will be achieved in later stages of rehabilitation. To make this point clear, consider the example of an injured hurdler with restricted mobility of the hamstrings; strength and coordination would be of little importance if the hurdler lacked the flexibility needed to extend the limb over the hurdle.

The second reason to emphasize range of motion restoration at this point in the therapeutic exercise portion of the rehabilitation program is the effect that the healing process has on injured tissue. As injured tissue heals, scar tissue forms. As scar tissue continues to progress in its healing timeline, it contracts to make the scar smaller, and the longer the healing continues, the more resilient and permanent the tissue becomes. These effects are important in eventually minimizing the scar, but they can also be detrimental because as the tissue forms, contracts,

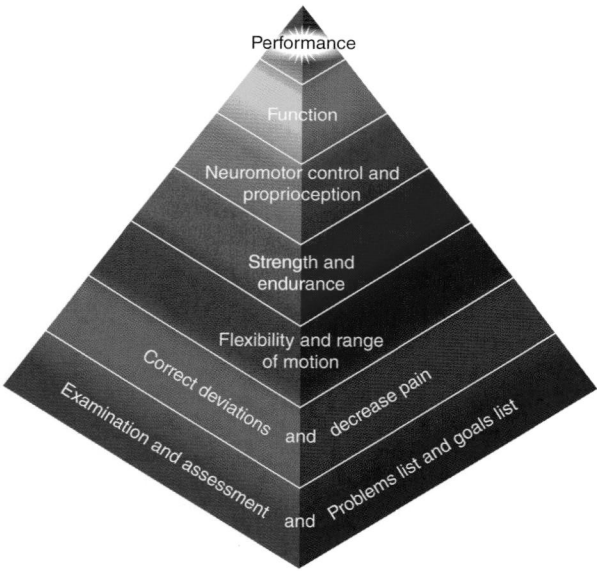

Figure 1.1   Pyramid demonstrating the components and progression of a rehabilitation program, one component advancing from the foundation set by the previous component.

and matures, it attaches to and pulls on adjacent tissue and establishes stronger adhesive bonds as it matures. If tissue mobility and flexibility are not addressed while the scar tissue is young and immature, soft-tissue adhesions in the area will restrict joint motion and mobility in an extremity.

As we will learn in chapter 2, there is a window of opportunity during the healing process in which scar tissue mobility can be influenced and changed. Once that time frame has passed, the likelihood of achieving full range of motion is diminished considerably. Although restoration of other parameters is also sought during this stage of rehabilitation, flexibility must be the primary emphasis. More detail about elements involved in mobility, flexibility, and range of motion are provided in chapter 12.

Strength and Muscle Endurance

As an injured site's healing and mobility progress and healing tissue matures to tolerate additional stresses, achieving normal strength and muscular endurance becomes the priority of the next progression in rehabilitation. With any injury, some strength is lost. The amount of strength and muscle endurance lost depends on the area injured, the extent of the injury, and the amount of time the patient has been disabled by the injury.

Of all the parameters of rehabilitation, strength is probably the most obvious and most often restored after an injury. A weightlifter with a sprained knee obviously cannot return to competition until full knee strength is restored. An auto mechanic must have normal shoulder strength to return to work after suffering a dislocation.

However, the need for muscle endurance and the relationship between muscle strength and endurance are sometimes not considered. If a baseball pitcher has good rotator cuff strength but no endurance beyond 10 repetitions, how will he be able to pitch more than a couple of innings in a game? If a UPS driver can leg press 225 kg (496 lb) but can climb only one flight of stairs, will she be able to deliver heavy packages for an entire shift?

Muscular strength and endurance are two dimensions within a continuum of muscle resistance. Essential concepts of muscle strength and endurance are presented in chapter 13.

Neuromotor Control

Since we need neuromotor control over all of our movements, it cannot be ignored when it comes to returning a patient to his or her optimal level of function. This is the focus in the next level of progression in the rehabilitation program. Impairment of the neuromotor system often accompanies orthopedic injuries, either because the neuromotor elements themselves are injured or because lack of use or restricted use causes performance to decline. In either case, neuromotor training must be incorporated into the rehabilitation program to restore what has been lost.

Both the central nervous system and the peripheral nervous system need reeducation to restore neuromotor performance. The peripheral receptors may have been damaged at the time of injury. Both muscles and joints have proprioceptors that provide the body with feedback about where it is in space at any given time, and these may be injured when muscles and joint structures are injured.[28, 29] The information provided by these nerves, especially in the lower extremities, is important for balance.

How well the body functions mechanically is directly dependent upon the health of muscle, nerves, and joints. The neuromechanical function of the body combines the status of the biomechanical system and the neural system; when they are healthy, they can work together to perform as desired.[30]

In the early phases of rehabilitation, the clinician may focus on the injured body segment, but the clinician must not forget that the whole person must be treated throughout the rehabilitation program. The patient usually expects to return to former levels of function. Therefore, the focus of rehabilitation must be on the whole person, not just on the injury site. The body is a complex chain of interacting systems that merge to create smooth, desirable, and expected movements of the entire body.[31] Restoring the person so that he or she can perform at preinjury levels within the environment to which he or she will return is the ultimate goal of rehabilitation. The details on how neuromotor elements are rehabilitated are presented in chapter 14.

Function and Performance

Function and performance are the two final phases of rehabilitation before the patient is released from the rehabilitation program. Functional activities precede performance activities. Accurate execution of function- and performance-specific skills requires attainment of all previous parameters first. Sometimes it is difficult to determine when neuromotor activities end and functional exercises begin. This is because some neuromotor exercises could be considered functional exercises. Likewise, some functional exercises could be thought of as performance-specific exercises for some sports or job tasks. For example, a neuromotor exercise may be jumping side to side over hurdles or cones, but that could also be a functional exercise for someone who is a soccer goalie or a football defender. Jumping side to side may also be a performance-specific exercise for a tennis player. How these exercises are labeled is based primarily on when in the program they occur and what the goal is for the specific exercise. If the goal is to increase speed of motion, then it is likely a neuromotor exercise, but if the goal is to improve lateral motion accuracy, it is likely a functional exercise. It becomes a performance-specific exercise if the patient is on the field or court and performing a specific sport skill that involves side-to-side movement.

There is an evolution of exercises in the last half of the rehabilitation program that moves from an emphasis on neuromotor reeducation to an ability to execute normal drills that mimic the patient's typical activities. The last step before returning to normal activities involves the execution of performance-specific exercises. In this final stage, patients regain the confidence they need to perform at their previous activity level. Concepts and examples for this phase of rehabilitation are discussed in chapter 15. When the patient can achieve specific goals established for these activities, the rehabilitation clinician can be assured that the final long-term goal of fully rehabilitating the patient has been achieved.

CLINICAL TIPS

The different types of therapeutic exercise within a rehabilitation program must address the following physiological parameters in proper order: first, flexibility and range of motion; second, muscle strength and endurance; third, neuromotor control, including balance, coordination, and agility; fourth, functional performance; and fifth, performance-specific activities.

Phases of Rehabilitation

Patients usually seek treatment from orthopedic health care professionals because of pain related to an injury. Unfortunately, this pain is usually accompanied by other problems that need to be addressed before the patient can be restored to an optimal level of function. The rehabilitation program targets these problems.

A rehabilitation program can be divided into four phases or stages: (1) inactive, (2) active, (3) resistive, and (4) advanced phases. These phases coincide with the healing progression from the time immediately after an injury when healing tissue is treated with caution to the end of the healing process when heavy stresses may be safely applied to tissue. This is illustrated in figure 1.2. Each rehabilitation phase overlaps with the phase on either side of it. These four phases are presented in more detail below.

Inactive Phase

This first phase of rehabilitation occurs during the inflammation phase in the early days of healing. The injury is painful and edematous, and the patient is reluctant or unable to use the injured part normally. During this time the recently damaged region is vulnerable, for it is weak and at risk of additional injury if inappropriately managed. The inflammatory phase of the healing process is well underway, so the typical signs of injury and subsequent inflammation are readily apparent. This is a time of relative inactivity for the injured segment, when treatment is focused on relieving the immediate problems that occur from injury and insult to surrounding tissue. If these factors are controlled and healing is encouraged in an optimal environment, advancement to the remaining healing phases occurs on schedule. The clinician treats these signs and symptoms while taking care to avoid additional damage. Stress to damaged tissue is avoided during this phase.

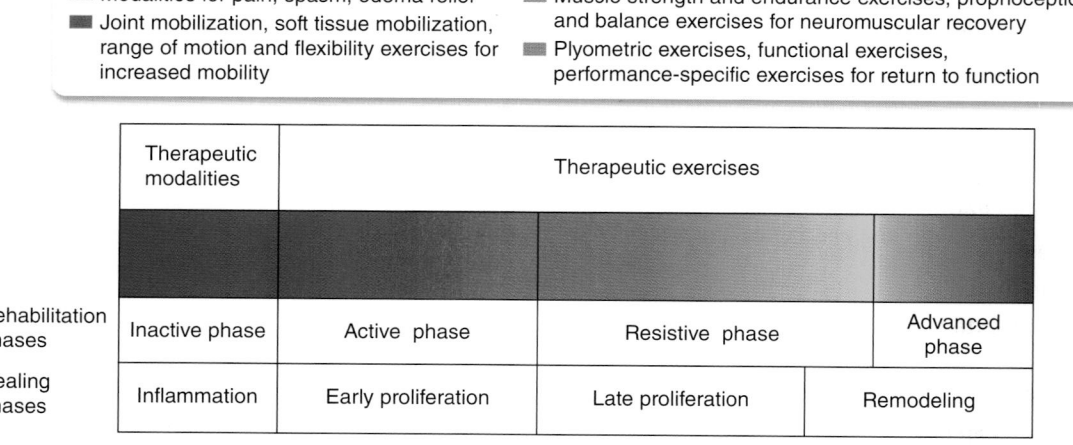

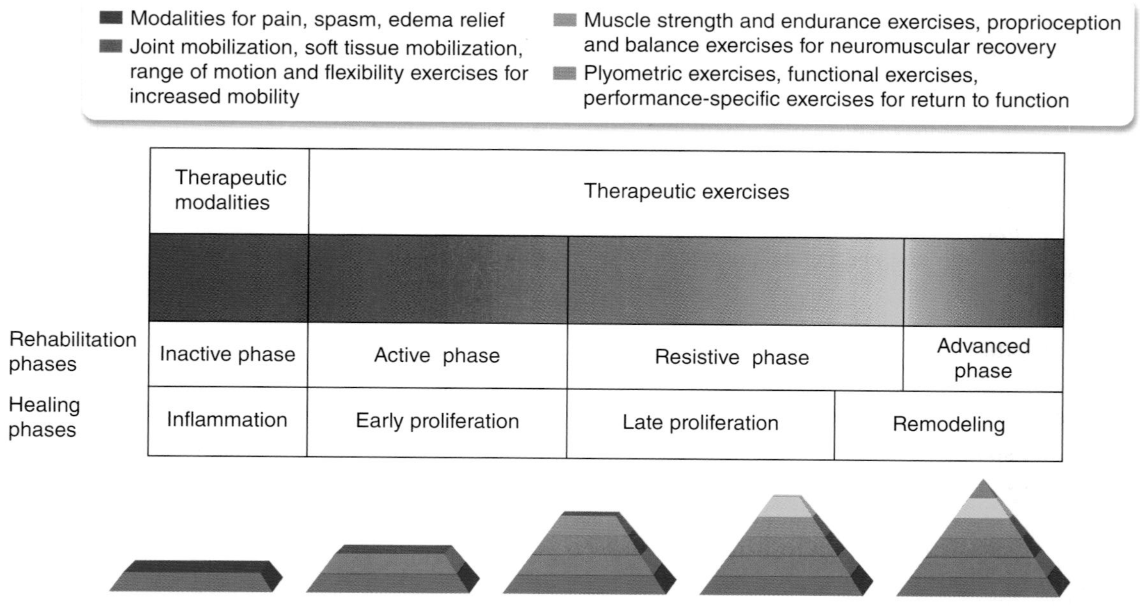

Figure 1.2   Phases of rehabilitation coincide with healing phases.

Refer to figure 1.2 to see that this phase is timed with the first phase of healing.

The goals of this phase are to *relieve* pain, edema, and muscle spasm. An additional goal is to maintain proper conditioning in the unaffected body segments and the cardiovascular system. Because the injured segment is in the inflammation phase of healing, caution is an important aspect of the treatment protocol during this time. Aggravating the injury site is contraindicated.

The inactive phase is a time when pharmacological and therapeutic modalities are important to effective rehabilitation.[32] Although rehabilitation clinicians cannot prescribe medications, the goals of this phase may be achieved with the use of a number of modalities, such as thermal and electrical modalities, massage, and other manual therapies that focus on reducing pain, spasm, and swelling. Motion and exercise are usually not performed during this phase to avoid putting stress on fragile healing tissue.

Modalities

Therapeutic modalities are used early in the rehabilitation program primarily to reduce pain, edema, and muscle spasm and to promote healing.[32, 33] There are a number of modalities that have been tested, verified, and commonly used to effectively treat orthopedic injuries. The selection of which to use depends on a number of factors. These factors include the modalities' availability; the treatment goals; the treatment area; modality indications and efficacy based on research; the patient's age, perspective, and experience; time, cost, and risk; and the clinician's experience, confidence in the modality, and personal preferences. Modalities can be classified according to the type of energy they produce or use in treatments of acute, subacute, and chronic injuries: thermal (heat and cold), electrical (stimulation or facilitation), electromagnetic (lasers), acoustical (ultrasound or shock wave), or mechanical (traction, compression, or manual).

Some of these modalities have similar effects, even though their energy sources are different. Each of these modalities has been investigated in laboratories throughout the world to determine their therapeutic efficacy, benefits, and uses for various injuries and conditions. Table 1.2 presents a summary of the effects of these modality categories. Information on the most commonly used modalities and their specific uses and roles in rehabilitation is provided in chapter 9.

Exercises

As previously mentioned, exercise that involves the injured part is contraindicated during the early days of healing. However, it is important to treat the whole patient. This means that the unaffected body segments should be exercised to maintain the level of function they had before the injury. It is just as important to keep the mobility, strength

TABLE 1.2 Modality Groups and Their Overall Effects in Rehabilitation Treatments of Orthopedic Injuries

Modality effects	Cold	Heat	Ultrasound	Laser	Elec stim	Shock wave	Traction	Compression	Manual therapy
Accelerate healing	X	X	X	X	X	X			
Reduce inflammation symptoms	X		X	X		X		X	
Reduce pain	X	X	X	X	X	X	X	X	X
Reduce edema	X		X	X	X			X	X
Reduce blood flow	X								
Increase blood flow		X	X	X		X			X
Reduce metabolism	X								
Increase metabolism		X							
Reduce tissue extensibility	X								
Increase tissue extensibility		X	X				X		X
Reduce muscle spasm	X	X	X		X		X		X
Promote healing			X	X		X			
Transport compounds			X		X				
Facilitate muscle activity and function					X		X		X

Based on Malanga, Yan, and Stark (2015); Anwer et al. (2018); Bialosky et al. (2009); Cheng, Hsu, and Lin (2020); Cotler et al. (2015); Dedes et al. (2018); Ennis et al. (2016); Kloth (2014); Miller, Smith, Bailey et al. (2012); Speed (2001).[32, 34-42]

and endurance, coordination, and agility of the uninjured segments at preinjury levels as it is to promote the healing of the injured segment.[43] Exercising the uninjured segments may improve patients' psychological outlook and improve patient compliance during the rehabilitation program, shifting their attention from an uncertain future to recovery and return to function.[44]

Additionally, the injured segment may benefit from the exercises and activities of its uninjured counterpart.[45, 46] Although the injured part is not exercising, there is evidence that neural adaptations occur to provide some level of strength maintenance in the unexercised contralateral segment.[45] This concept was first demonstrated in the 1800s[47] and serves to remind us that we can influence even rigidly immobilized segments in a positive manner.

The inactive phase of rehabilitation occurs during the inflammation phase of healing. In severe injuries and after surgeries, the inactive phase of rehabilitation may extend beyond the period of inflammation and into the early days of proliferation. Depending on the injury's severity, location, and onset; the patient's age and health; and other factors, early range-of-motion activities may be initiated at the end of the inactive phase.

Active Phase

Phase II of the rehabilitation program begins once the injured segment's healing has progressed from inflammation to the proliferation phase. The phases of healing are described in more detail in chapter 2; for now, note that tissue strength through collagen fiber development is gradually increasing during this phase, and structures are becoming resilient enough to tolerate some stress. Therefore, mild activity of the injured segment may be permitted. Although pain, edema, and muscle spasm are resolving, they may be minor but not entirely resolved, so some therapeutic modalities may continue into this phase. It should be anticipated, however, that these problems are resolved and eliminated before the end of phase II.

Goals during phase II are to improve mobility through gains in range of motion and flexibility and to resolve any remaining problems from inflammation. In addition to therapeutic modalities that may be necessary for symptomatic relief, treatment in this phase includes range-of-motion exercises and may include mobility techniques such as joint and soft-tissue mobilization. For severe injuries and postoperative conditions, remaining edema may show evidence of changing from pitting edema to brawny edema; in these cases, manual techniques must be used to soften the tissue to permit mobility of the surrounding soft tissue. If any exercises were started during late inflammation, range of motion was likely the only exercise at that time. Because of the tissue's gains in increased stability during the active phase, early strength and proprioception exercises may begin, but this decision is based on a number

of factors, such as the type of tissue that was injured, the location of the injury, and the patient's age. The closer to the inflammation phase the injury is, the more cautious the clinician should be with the amount of stress applied to newly developing tissue. In some cases, exercises may not be permitted until 3 to 4 weeks after injury;[48-50] waiting much longer than this time to allow movement of the segment can result in serious and permanent changes in the injured site's mobility.[51, 52]

Modalities

Therapeutic modalities will be used during this phase to relieve any of the continued signs and symptoms of inflammation. These signs and symptoms may include prolonged swelling and residual pain. Assuming that the patient is not experiencing new swelling and that what remains is only from the original injury, cryotherapy will be of little value in further reducing the old edema. Cryotherapy treatments for the reduction of edema are applied for 3 to 5 days post-injury or postoperatively.[53, 54] However, if pain is still an issue for the patient, cryotherapy may still be beneficial for pain reduction after it is no longer effective for reducing swelling.[55]

Other manual modalities may be incorporated into the rehabilitation program during this phase. As mentioned, soft-tissue pitting edema that occurs in an orthopedic injury may result in local lymphedema which delays or complicates the removal of that edema.[56] In these cases, heat along with manual treatments such as massage, soft-tissue mobilization, and compression with elevation may help to open blocked lymphatic and venous return.[57]

Depending on the degree of muscle weakness that has been affected by the injury or surgery, it may be necessary to use electrical modalities to facilitate muscle activity. Electrical modalities for muscle facilitation can be initiated either in this phase or in the first rehabilitation phase. This decision is determined by the extent of the injury or surgery, the specific muscle involved, the patient's abilities, and the physician's preference.

Exercises

Because the healing process has continued, making the damaged tissues stronger, the site can now withstand early active movements without risking injury to newly forming tissue. The injured site cannot yet withstand resistive forces, but active motion without resistance may now be used in the rehabilitation program.

Range of motion and flexibility are important factors to restore during the active phase and are the primary therapeutic exercises used in this phase. Along with joint and soft-tissue mobilization techniques, passive, active-assistive, and active exercises can be used to improve motion; however, the type of tissue, the injury's severity, and the location of the injury will dictate the specific motion type permitted. For example, active exercises are generally used before passive motion exercises in the hand,[58] but passive motion activities are initiated before active exercises after musculotendinous injuries of other segments such as the knee or shoulder.[59, 60]

Strengthening exercises are not usually included in this phase. The tissue involved, type of injury, patient issues, and physician preference are some factors that determine whether strength exercises begin in phase II. If strengthening is initiated during this phase, it will be toward the end of this phase; early strengthening exercises will likely include isometrics and easy concentric, concentric–eccentric, or eccentric exercises. Isometric exercises are often performed at either multiple angles, midrange, or in an anatomic position, depending on mobility and medical restrictions for motion.

Resistive Phase

By the time the patient progresses to the resistive phase, range of motion is nearly or completely normal.

Modalities

Since edema and pain are no longer issues to be resolved, modalities are not needed during this phase. Occasionally, a patient may feel more comfortable having ice or cryotherapy applied to the injured site after the completion of exercises at this time; however, there is no physiological reason this treatment is needed, assuming that there is no new insult to the injured site because of the treatment provided.

As stated, the patient's mobility and motion are normal or close to it by the time this phase begins. In cases where normal mobility is not yet achieved for some reason, it may be necessary to apply a heat modality before efforts begin to increase the range of motion or mobility of the affected tissue. The selection of a superficial or a deep heat depends on the depth of the problem tissue, the specific site, the patient's age and physical condition, and the availability of modalities to the clinician.

Exercises

In cases where strengthening exercises were begun in the active phase, muscle strength and endurance may have improved somewhat by the start of the resistive phase, but they may still be quite deficient. This phase is called the resistive phase because our primary goal includes using resistance exercises to completely restore any deficiencies in strength, agility, and endurance. During the resistive phase, tensile strength is significantly greater than in earlier healing phases, so the clinician and patient can focus on resolving the remaining deficiencies. The early part of this phase deals with factors at the third and fourth tiers of the rehabilitation pyramid (figure 1.1).

Strength exercises are initially performed in a straight plane and progress to diagonal or functional positions when the patient has enough strength in straight-plane movement to control the extremity correctly through a single-plane motion. By using straight-plane activities early during the strengthening phase, the clinician and patient focus on those muscles that are weak and need to be isolated so that stronger muscles do not overpower them in their responsibility to perform the specific motion for which they were designed. It is recommended that strength exercises early in this phase begin with high repetitions and low resistance.[61] This reduces stress on joints and newly formed soft-tissue structures that may not yet be strong enough to tolerate the shear or overload forces produced by heavy resistance. Neuromotor exercises also begin at a simple level and progress as healing continues through this phase.

Phase III begins anywhere from the end of the proliferation phase into the remodeling phase of healing. The point at which this rehabilitation phase begins depends on the specific injury, physician preference for progression, and the patient's response to the program. Most of the time, intensive resistance begins during later proliferation. The resistive phase is often delayed when rehabilitation involves structures with delayed healing or containing tenuous tissue. Goals during phase III include maintaining the parameters that have been restored and restoring the patient's strength, muscle endurance, and agility to normal levels.

As healing continues, exercises that are incorporated later in this phase include more aggressive strength and muscle endurance exercises than were used at the beginning of the phase. Additionally, more aggressive neuromotor exercises that progress from simple to complicated activities are included. It is during the last half of this phase that the fifth tier of rehabilitation, agility, is addressed.

Even if motion is normal, flexibility exercises should continue in this phase to prevent a loss of motion—wound contraction continues because of the myofibril activity during the ongoing healing process. If flexibility is not yet normal, more assertive stretching exercises occur during this phase.

The goals of this phase are the restoration of range of motion and mobility, strength and muscle endurance, and neuromotor performance. Strength exercises in the latter half of this phase are in transition. Resistive exercises advance from single-plane to diagonal or multiplanar activities and finally into more functional movement patterns. This advancement is possible because the muscle strength and neuromotor control are now at levels that allow the patient to maintain extremity control by accurately recruiting the appropriate muscles to move the segment to produce the desired result. Therefore, neuromotor activities also become more complex by the end of this phase. These exercises may include multiple task activities, and the aim is to help prepare the patient for the stresses of functional activities in the next phase.

Advanced Phase

Once the goals established for phase III are achieved, the patient moves into the final phase of rehabilitation, the advanced phase. It is during this phase that the sixth, and final, tier of the rehabilitation pyramid is addressed. This phase is called the *advanced phase* because exercises during this part of the rehabilitation program mimic all the stresses that the patient will encounter when he or she returns to normal activities. By the time the patient reaches this final phase, flexibility, strength, and muscle endurance are all at normal or near-normal levels, so the patient is ready for more advanced, normal activities that further stress the injured area in preparation for a return to his or her customary functions.

Modalities

During this final phase there is no need for any type of therapeutic modality. If any modality is required as part of the rehabilitation program at this time, the patient is not ready for this phase.

Exercises

At this point, the only real deficit lies in the patient's functional and performance abilities, so exercises during this phase are designed to restore these abilities. Flexibility and strength activities are now at maintenance levels, and the major emphasis is on finely tuning the patient's performance for a smooth transition and a return to normal participation in a normal environment. Function- and performance-specific exercises are vital in this final phase and must always be part of a rehabilitation program.

The goals in this phase are to restore the patient's functional abilities and to use performance-specific exercises that will permit the patient to resume all preinjury participation in a normal environment. Functional activities evolve to performance-specific exercises. Functional activities begin at reduced levels of stress, speed, force, and distance, and these parameters are continually increased as the patient's body adjusts to the stresses, eventually enabling the patient to perform normal functions. Once the patient's functional exercise performance achieves normal levels, the transition is made to performance-specific exercises. A patient who demonstrates normal performance in these activities has achieved the final goals of the rehabilitation program and is discharged.

Progression of Rehabilitation Phases

You may have noticed by now that, like the examination and assessment process, the rehabilitation program and its progression follow a systematic and methodical regimen. A good rehabilitation program progresses in a challenging yet safe manner for the patient. The progression rate is in accordance with the severity of the injury, the type of injury, and the patient's response to the injury and its treatment. A good rehabilitation progression matches the patient's healing rate and challenges the patient without causing deleterious effects such as increased pain or swelling or decreased ability to perform. The rehabilitation progression is presented in image form in figure 1.3. A general rehabilitation program is presented to provide you with an idea of an overall progression. Regardless of the injury or body segment affected, a rehabilitation program will follow this general outline for progression from one phase to another and from one type of treatment, whether it is modalities or exercises, to another. The concept and specifics of exercise progression are presented in more detail in chapter 13.

Within each treatment session the clinician performs an evaluation of the patient's status before and during treatment. An examination is performed not only to identify how the patient reacted to the previous treatment but also to confirm that healing is occurring as expected. As the patient moves through the rehabilitation program and healing moves from the inflammation phase to the proliferation phase, evidence of inflammation subsides. Pain, edema, and reduced function become less evident as healing establishes a more permanent and healthy structure. If the patient's inflammatory signs and symptoms persist, the clinician must identify the reasons for this delay in healing. As long as the injured segment remains in the inflammatory phase, the patient cannot advance in the rehabilitation program. The healing phases are presented in chapter 2. Clinicians must be aware of the normal progression of healing so that, when it does not occur as anticipated, they can intervene to prevent delayed rehabilitation outcomes.

Clinical Practice

Clinical practice is affected by many considerations. These variables include laws at the state level and ethics at the national level, and other factors lie at an international level. The remainder of this chapter looks at these factors and how they will affect how you perform within your own clinical practice.

Laws and Ethics

There is so much more to clinical practice than just being able to put together a patient's rehabilitation program. As health care professionals, clinicians have a responsibility not only to themselves and their patients, but to their employers, fellow professionals, and their profession to act in a consistently honorable and professional manner, respecting others and following the legal and ethical standards established by their profession and the lawmakers of the states in which they work.

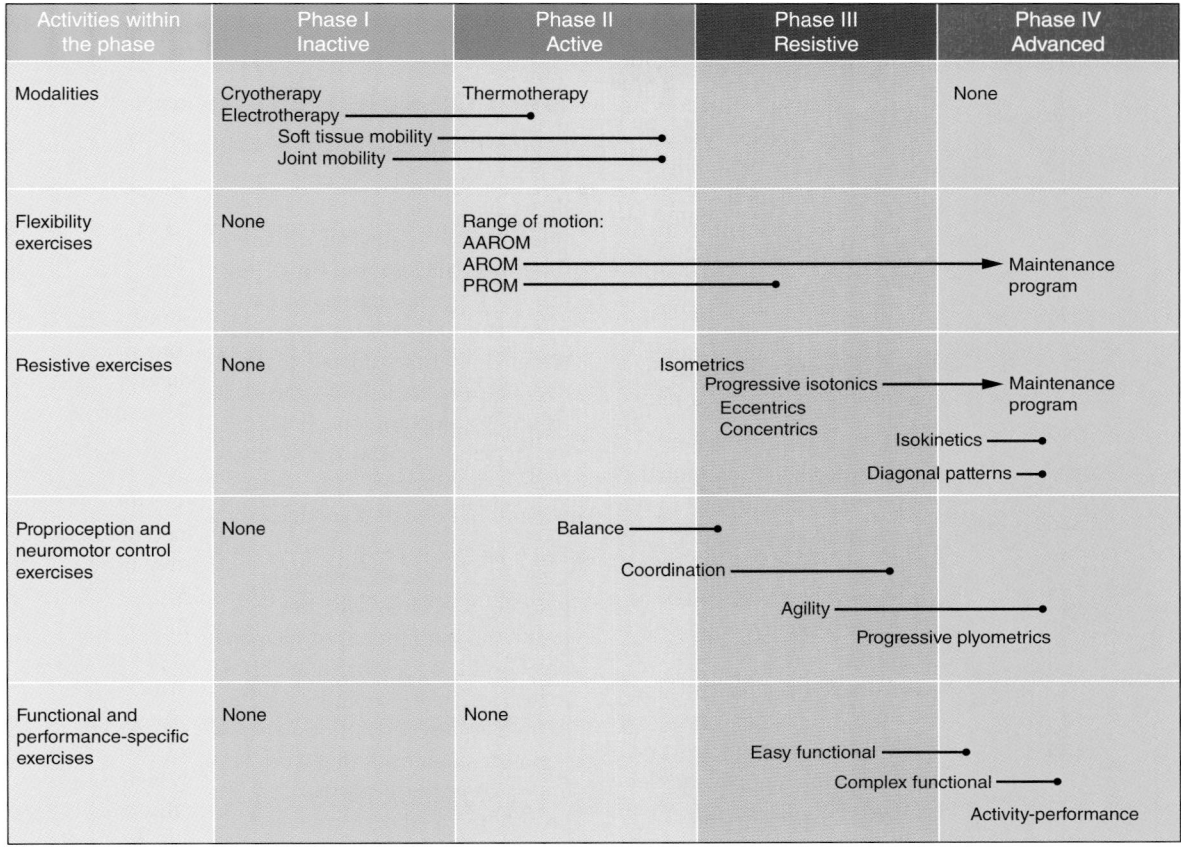

Activities within the phase	Phase I Inactive	Phase II Active	Phase III Resistive	Phase IV Advanced
Modalities	Cryotherapy Electrotherapy ——————— Soft tissue mobility ———————— Joint mobility ————————	Thermotherapy		None
Flexibility exercises	None	Range of motion: AAROM AROM ————————————— PROM —————————————		→ Maintenance program
Resistive exercises	None		Isometrics Progressive isotonics ——————— Eccentrics Concentrics Isokinetics ——— Diagonal patterns —●	→ Maintenance program
Proprioception and neuromotor control exercises	None	Balance ———————— Coordination ——————— Agility ——————— Progressive plyometrics		
Functional and performance-specific exercises	None	None	Easy functional ———————— Complex functional ——— Activity-performance	

Figure 1.3 The rehabilitation progression. Modality and exercise application continuum within a rehabilitation program. The progression within each phase is based on the tissue's healing status and ability to withstand applied stresses.

State Regulation

Each state has its own legal guidelines that determine the parameters within which clinicians must operate. It is your responsibility to know and operate within the regulations of the state in which you practice.

Ethics

In addition to legal obligations that guide a professional's conduct, ethical codes of conduct are no less important in guiding our actions as health care professionals. A **code of ethics** is defined as "a summary of a profession's values and standards of conduct."[1] Health care providers must act in accordance with both the laws of the state and the code of ethics of the profession. Each health care profession has a code of ethics that establishes honorable values by which practitioners are to deliver health care to their patients, regard other professionals within and outside of their own profession, and promote and demonstrate best practices with integrity and reliability.

Founders of health care professions realize the importance of providing guidelines for standards of behavior and for ensuring high-quality, principled care for patients. A code of ethics is often one of the earliest documents any health care profession creates for its members. Once established, the document may be periodically revised to keep in stride with current societal norms and issues, but the primary precepts remain the same. A health care professional is well advised to be familiar with the profession's code of ethics and to abide by its established codes of behavior.

Disablement Models

Laws and ethics are important for protecting patients and for improving patient outcomes. They ensure that the professional providing care is qualified. In addition to laws and ethics, there are other professional tools used to improve patient outcomes. Our goal in rehabilitation has been to return the patient to his or her optimal level of function. Usually that means returning the patient to a former level of ability and performance. However, over the past 20 years or so, the way in which we define and assess a patient's ability and performance has changed. Instead of focusing on an injury, disease, or illness, we consider how an injury, disease, or illness affects the person as an individual and as a member of a group or society. How that person is affected by the injury helps determine how we plan our treatment. This method of treatment is referred to as patient-centered care, or patient-oriented evidence that matters (POEM).[62-64] This change in focus now puts the patient at the center, not the provider or the injury, disease, or illness. Patients' concerns, what is important to them, and how they are affected by the condition determine the plan and treatment approach.

This new way of looking at patients and the problems we treat is based on what is called disablement models. Disablement models are used in both clinical and research fields of rehabilitation. A **disablement model** for the rehabilitation clinician is a conceptual model that helps us create a plan of treatment that addresses the individual.[65] Although an ankle sprain is a common occurrence in the sports world, each person who suffers an ankle sprain is unique and has unique expectations and needs. If we do not consider the person and look only at the ankle sprain, we may fall short of the patient's expectations and fail to adequately address his or her needs.

Although disablement models have been around since the 1960s, it has only been within the last 20 years that health care professions have started to move to a universal system of disability management. Disablement models are useful to health care professionals in helping them determine appropriate clinical outcome tools and advance evidence-based practice within the profession.[65] When pathology occurs, it often causes either temporary or permanent changes in people's daily functions. In addition to the physical or physiological ways disease or injury intrudes on individual lives, those pathologies also have social, psychological, and environmental effects. Likewise, those social, psychological, and environmental factors can change the impact of pathology on individuals.[66] Therefore, a disablement model may be defined as a system that provides common terminology by which an individual's disability based on clinical diagnosis, rehabilitation, laws, limitations, impairments, and societal function may be identified. Because of how they look at the effect of injury or disease on an individual, disablement models ultimately force health care professionals to treat patients as individuals rather than just as injuries and to identify problems the rehabilitation program must address to guide each person to an optimal recovery. Since everyone has different social, environmental, and psychological makeups, the health care provider cannot pigeonhole patients with an ankle sprain or a shoulder dislocation and classify the impact such an injury will have on any patient; a patient's ability to function after an injury depends on much more than just the type and severity of the injury. We will look at two commonly accepted disablement models to give us a better

idea of how to approach an injury from a person-centered rather than an injury-centered perspective.

Nagi Disablement Model

During the 1960s, an American sociologist established a framework of concepts surrounding the relationship between disability and how rehabilitation of illness and injury creates a system of care and treatment. Until this time there had been a lot of inconsistency in the use of terminology among health care professionals and in the understanding of what constituted impairment and functional limitations related to disability.[67] Nagi's model of disablement took into consideration four components: pathology, impairments, functional limitations, and disability. His model looked at how any pathology such as disease, illness, or injury affects a person and how that changes the person. In effect, his model indicated that in the presence of any pathology, a domino effect occurred within the individual to create a disability. Nagi explained that when pathology occurs, whether it is illness or injury, it can lead to an impairment of the person's normal anatomical, physiological, or structural abilities. This impairment may in turn lead to one or more functional limitations, which he defined as any restriction in a person's physical or mental actions and abilities that would interfere with the person's ability to perform normal tasks or responsibilities.[68] This level of reduced performance he labeled *disability*, and he defined it as the pattern of behavior that is impaired or less than normal and occurs as a result of functional limitations imposed upon the person.[67] The Nagi disablement model is illustrated in figure 1.4.

Nagi recognized that disability started with pathology at the cellular level. Any number of pathological causes, from acute trauma to degenerative changes to diseases, can interrupt normal cellular function. Secondary effects of these interruptions in the body's homeostasis affect the body system or segment that has been disturbed by the injury or illness and prevent it from performing normally; this is the impairment segment of Nagi's disablement model. From this diminished performance of the body system or segment, limitations occur that restrict the patient's ability to perform specific functions. Depending on what has been injured and the specific segment that has been affected, the patient may have difficulty walking, bearing weight, or using an extremity. These functional limitations are disabilities. Nagi identified an individual's disability based on what a person could do when functional changes occurred because of injury or disease and compared the person's function to what the person was expected to do in his or her social or physical environment. Because the patient's environment must be included in the definition of disability, disability for one person is not always a disability

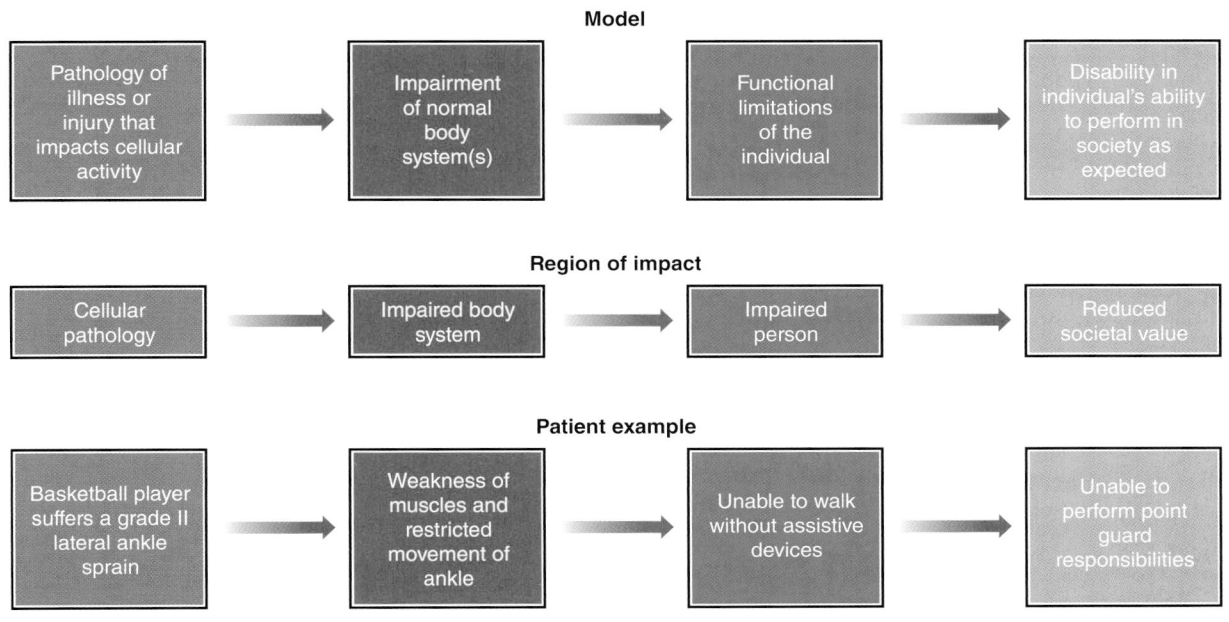

Figure 1.4 Nagi disablement model. Cellular pathology leads to impairment of normal system function, which leads to limitations of the individual, ultimately leading to the individual's inability to perform as expected within the society or environment.

Based on Nagi (1965).[67]

for another person with the same physical limitation in a different environment. For example, an inability to raise the arm overhead because of a muscle strain may be considered a disability for a spiker on a volleyball team, but it may not be a disability for a retired computer programmer who never raises his hands higher than his shoulders.

Nagi's goal in rehabilitation was to reverse the course of the disability by reducing the functional limitations and guiding the patient to an optimal level of function, restoring the person to a useful role in society.[67] It was his contention that a disability does not define the person but is a relative concept that is based on the person's interaction with his or her society and environment, and that person's ability is not necessarily limited by a pathology.[69] There are other factors that must be considered and are equally meaningful in defining one's abilities and restrictions. Rather than putting people with a specific condition or injury into a box, Nagi contended that what matters is how well they can function in society and meet society's expectations of them. Just because a person suffers a rupture of the anterior cruciate ligament does not mean that he or she is defined by that injury; Nagi contends that each person's disability should be defined according to how well that person performs his or her duties and responsibilities in spite of the injury. The individual is defined by ability rather than by the disability.[70] In essence, Nagi was saying that the presence of an injury or impairment does not mean that one has a functional limitation, and if there is no functional limitation, there is no disability.[71]

Nagi recognized that each person is different and responds to illness or injury differently. He called these differences "external modifiers" and identified them as factors that affect how an injury or illness affects the person's reaction to it and how it may affect the person's movement. He acknowledged that there are individual physiological, anatomical, and mental health differences along with differences in education, life experiences, habits, social support, and coping strategies that determine how a person reacts to his or her level of disability. Of course, Nagi also recognized other factors such as the patient's age, overall health, the presence of comorbidities, and the degree of illness or injury and the role they also play in determining one's degree of disability. All of these factors must be considered to come to a conclusion of an individual's level of disability.

Under such a patient-centered program, rehabilitation plans take into consideration the specific goals of the patient. What the patient wants to achieve from a rehabilitation program becomes the central focus of intervention. The clinician must communicate with the patient to understand what is important to him or her and then establish a rehabilitation program that achieves those goals.

WHO International Classification of Functioning

The World Health Organization (WHO) is an agency within the United Nations. It focuses on the promotion of health around the world; it promotes the advancement of and access to primary health care, especially for the underserved; and it serves to identify, mitigate, and manage health emergencies throughout the world.[72] Part of its role is to encourage better and more consistent communication and sharing of information between health care providers around the world by advancing the use of a universal language and definitions, regardless of settings or environments.[73] By developing a universal language, the WHO has made it possible not only for clinical communications to develop internationally but also for research to be more consistent and relevant to health care providers worldwide.

ICD-10

One of the items the WHO developed to create a universal language was what has become known as the International Classification of Diseases Tenth Revision, ICD-10. It is a data system that classifies causes of morbidity and mortality. Once the WHO authorized countries to use this system, the United States National Center for Health Statistics (NCHS) was charged with adapting the ICD-10 into the American health care system.[74] What eventually came out of the NCHS work is known as the International Classification of Diseases, Tenth Revision, Clinical Modification (ICD-10-CM). This document has been in use within the United States since October 1, 2015. These codes classify not only diseases, illnesses, and injuries but their severity and complexity as well. In the case of injuries, it also identifies how and where the injury occurred.

The ICD-10-CM codes include a combination of alpha and numeric characters and are anywhere from three to nine characters long, and they begin with a letter.[75] The letter indicates the type of body structure that is affected by the diagnosis, or what type of condition is diagnosed. These are called chapters or categories. A dot follows if more than three characters are used. That dot is followed by anywhere from four to six additional characters that are used to provide more specific details about the diagnosis, such as the cause of the injury or illness, anatomic site, severity of the injury or illness, and any other clinical details that further describe the diagnosis.[75] Table 1.3 provides a list of these chapters. As can be seen from table 1.3, most diagnostic ICD-10-CM codes that rehabilitation clinicians will deal with are in chapter 13, which is a list of diseases of the musculoskeletal system and connective tissue, and these will have diagnosis codes beginning with M. Table 1.3 provides a few examples of codes for some of the different musculoskeletal and connective tissue diagnoses.

Health care professionals usually refer to these codes as ICD-10 codes. However, there are actually three differ-

ent codes that are referred to in this manner. The ICD-10 codes are those developed by the WHO. The ICD-10-CM (Clinical Modification) codes are based on the ICD-10 codes that were modified by the NCHS and accepted by the WHO; these codes are used in outpatient facilities in the United States. The ICD-10 and ICD-10-CM are similar, but there are more ICD-10-CM codes than there are ICD-10 codes. The ICD-10-PCS (Procedure Classification System) are not based on the WHO system but were developed by the Department of Health and Human Services' Center for Medicare and Medicaid Services (CMS); these codes concern only inpatient hospital services. For most rehabilitation clinicians who deal with non-hospitalized patients, the ICD-10-PCS codes are not relevant.

Because of the work of the WHO to develop a common language for communication within the health care world, ICDs have become a universal system of disease, illness, injury, and death classifications. This system has helped clinicians in several different functions, allowed for comparisons of health care services and systems, and advanced medical research.[74] These codes are used by physicians, health care workers, public health agencies, researchers, and insurance companies around the world to track diseases and deaths and to compile world health statistics. They are used to determine payment of services, identify health care needs within communities, and compile data about health, disease, and death worldwide. The ICD-10 and the document presented in the next section, ICF, are meant to complement each other; the ICD-10 identifies diseases, injuries, and illnesses while the ICF clarifies how well an individual functions with the condition identified in the ICD-10.

ICF

In the first decade of this century, the World Health Organization expanded on Nagi's patient-centered idea of health care and focused on expanding the list of factors that influence perceptions and definitions of health and disability.[76] In its most recent disablement model, the WHO advocated that all countries treat people with disabilities equally by passing laws that recognize them as contributing members of society rather than drains on society.

The WHO encourages us to realize that a disability is a relationship between a person's condition and his or her environment, and it is that relationship which determines the extent of the person's disability. For example, if Sam lives in an environment where there are no elevators and he is confined to a wheelchair, he has a greater disability and makes more limited contributions to his society than Joe, who is also confined to a wheelchair but lives in an environment that has elevators. Sam and Joe may both have the same physical condition, but Sam is considered disabled because his mobility is restricted, not by his physical condition but by his environment.

TABLE 1.3 ICD-10-CM Categories

Chapter	Description	Codes
1	Certain infectious and parasitic diseases	A00–B99
2	Neoplasms	C00–D49
3	Diseases of the blood and blood-forming organs and certain disorders involving the immune mechanism	D50–D89
4	Endocrine, nutritional, and metabolic diseases	E00–E89
5	Mental, behavioral, and neurodevelopmental disorders	F01–F99
6	Diseases of the nervous system	G00–G99
7	Diseases of the eye and adnexa	H00–H59
8	Diseases of the ear and mastoid process	H60–H95
9	Diseases of the circulatory system	I00–I99
10	Diseases of the respiratory system	J00–J99
11	Diseases of the digestive system	K00–K95
12	Diseases of the skin and subcutaneous tissue	L00–L99
13	Diseases of the musculoskeletal system and connective tissue **Examples of some M code blocks:** M15–M19 = osteoarthritis M60–M63 = disorders of muscle M65–M67 = disorders of synovium and tendon M70–M79 = other soft-tissue disorders M80–M85 = disorders of bone density and structure M91–M94 = chondropathies	M00–M99
14	Diseases of the genitourinary system	N00–N99
15	Pregnancy, childbirth, and the puerperium	O00–O9A
16	Certain conditions originating in the perinatal period	P00–P96
17	Congenital malformations, deformations, and chromosomal abnormalities	Q00–Q99
18	Symptoms, signs, and abnormal clinical and laboratory findings not elsewhere classified	R00–R99
19	Injury, poisoning, and certain other consequences of external causes	S00–T88
20	External causes of morbidity	V00–Y99
21	Factors influencing health status and contact with health services	Z00–Z99

Based on ICD10Data.com.[75]

In its discussion of disability, the WHO also recognized the existence of other factors that add to the total definition of one's disability. Some of these factors are socioeconomic. Socioeconomic factors include a person's education level, wealth, class or acceptability within a society, and rural or urban residential setting; each of these factors can impact the extent to which one is defined as disabled. Personal factors such as age, sex, ethnicity, religion, intellect, height, weight, mental abilities, and other physical factors can also either exaggerate or minimize the definition of a person's disability.

With these factors in mind, the World Health Organization developed another classification system for disability. This system is known as the International Classification of Functioning, Disability and Health (ICF). While the ICD provides a universal system of identifying and defining diagnoses, the ICF is the universal system that serves to identify health and disability as they relate to individuals.

The World Health Organization uses a standard language and model by which one's health is defined by the environmental and personal factors that limit one's ability to function within his or her society.[77] In other words, a person's disability is not a medical problem but a result of how the person's impairment interacts with the environment.[73]

Figure 1.5 provides a diagrammatic view of the WHO's ICF model. We can see in this model that there are a number of factors that go into identifying disability. These elements factor into the concept of disability: the impairments of the body and its functions, the limitations of an individual's activity that are influenced by that impairment as well as the contextual factors of the environment and personality factors, and the participation restrictions. Table 1.4 contains a list of the WHO definitions of terms used in the ICF model. Functioning, disability, and impairment are terms that are often used in disablement models. They identify a person's ability to function at personal and societal levels. In addition to referring to the patient's body functions and structures, activities, and participation, **functioning** is the term the WHO uses to identify a neutral or a positive interaction between an individual's health condition and his or her personal and societal context.[76] On the other hand, **disability** refers to impairments of body functions and structures, activity limitations, and participation restrictions; it denotes the negative interaction between a person's health condition and his or her context.[76] **Impairments** are changes in the body's functions or structures that result in either mental or physical pathology. These changes can be caused by injury, illness, disease, or genetics and usually involve a pathological condition. These conditions can be either temporary or permanent. Impairments can occur in either the body's functions, which include the physiological functions of the body's systems, or in the body's structures, which include the organs and limbs.

Figure 1.6 indicates that the interaction between the patient's body functions and structures, personal activity level, and societal participation can be either improved or hampered by contextual factors. The combinations of these factors and how they interact with each other define that person's level of disability. The more positive the effects of those factors on the patient's functioning, the less disability the patient has. The opposite is true as well: The more negative the influence of contextual factors on the patient's functioning, the greater is his disability. Disability can apply to any functioning classification—that is, dysfunction can affect a patient's body structures and function, activity level, or participation in society.[3, 76] The ICF, then, identifies one's ability to function on three different levels. The first level is the body structure or system that has been affected by an injury, disease, or other factor that creates dysfunction of that body structure or system. The second

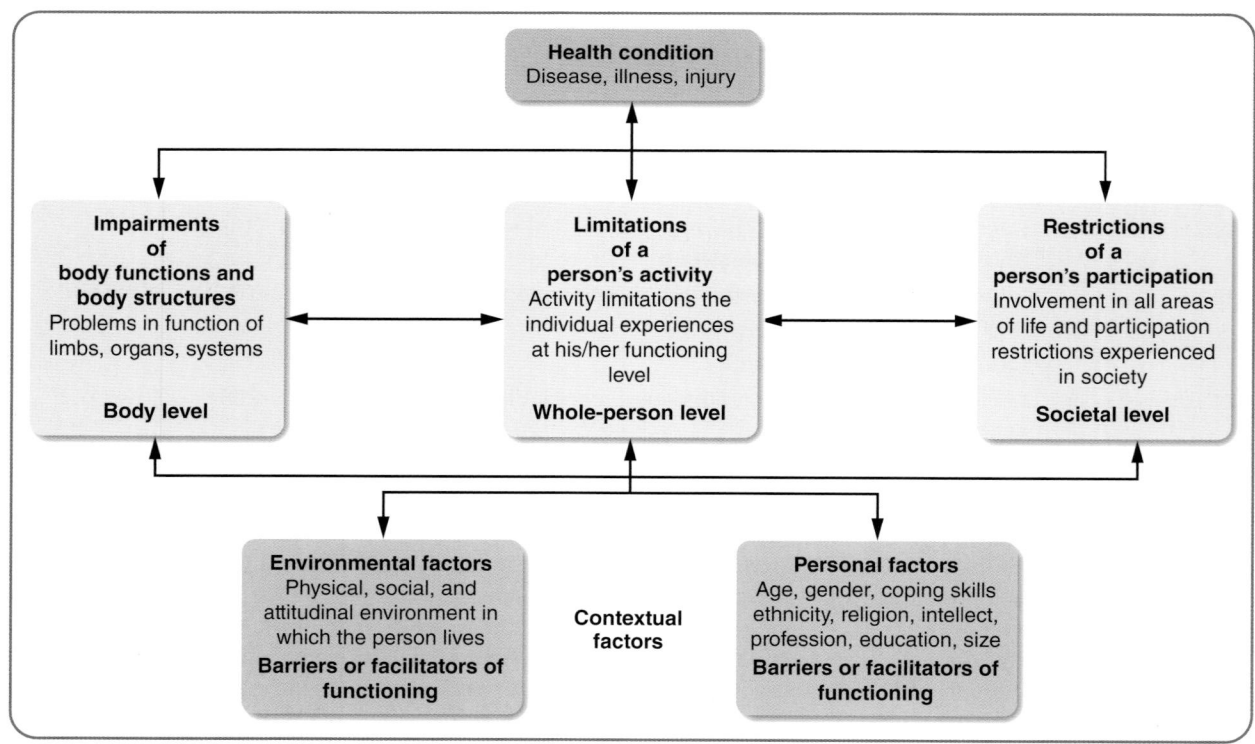

Figure 1.5 World Health Organization disablement model: International Classification of Functioning.

Adapted from World Health Organization (2001).[3]

TABLE 1.4   World Health Organization Terminology in the ICF Model

Term	Definition
Activity	Execution or performance of a task by an individual. Within the ICF, it often refers to the ability to perform self-care, domestic life, and activities of daily living.
Activity limitations	Difficulties one has or may have in performing an activity.
Body functions	Physiological or psychological systems of the body.
Body structures	Anatomical segments, including organs, extremities, and their components.
Capacity qualifier	Identifies what people actually do in the environment in which they live and how they function without accommodation or assistance. This qualifier identifies the amount of independence one has in the personal activity domain. In coding, this qualifier is referred to as the second qualifier.
Contextual factors	Factors that include aspects of one's environment, life experiences, and personal qualities that may influence one's response to and experience with the health condition.
Disability	An umbrella term that refers to an impairment, limitation, or restriction a person experiences in personal or social situations. It denotes the negative impact that contextual factors have on one's abilities.
Domains	The three levels of human functioning: (1) body segment or body parts, (2) the whole person, and (3) the person living in his or her social environment.
Environmental factors	The physical, social, and attitudinal environment in which an individual lives. These factors include items such as products and technology; climate and terrain where the person lives; alterations made to the person's environment; supportive relationships; and available systems, services, and policies. The factors can be either barriers or facilitators of one's functioning.
Health conditions	Diseases, disorders, illness, and injuries.
Impairment	Problems in body functions or structures that affect normal function.
Functioning	An umbrella term for body functions and structures, activities, and participation. It denotes either a positive or a neutral impact that contextual factors have on one's abilities.
Participation	The involvement one is able to have in life situations.
Participation restrictions	The problems one experiences in life situations.
Performance qualifier	Identifies or estimates the optimal level of function a person is able to perform in his or her environment without any accommodations or assistance; in other words, this qualifier identifies the amount of restriction a person experiences on his or her own. In coding, this is referred to as the first qualifier.
Personal factors	The qualities, characteristics, and background of an individual that include but are not limited to intellect, age, sex, size, ethnicity, religion, education, and marital status. These factors have an impact on how a person interprets and experiences disability. These have not yet been classified, so they are not included in the ICF model or coding system.
Qualifiers	Factors that identify the presence of a decrease in functioning in each domain (body function and structure, activity, or participation). In the body function and structure domain, qualifiers use a point system to record and identify the degree or severity of impairment. In activity and performance domains, qualifiers indicate how well an individual performs a task or the potential to perform a task.

Based on World Health Organization (2001).[3]

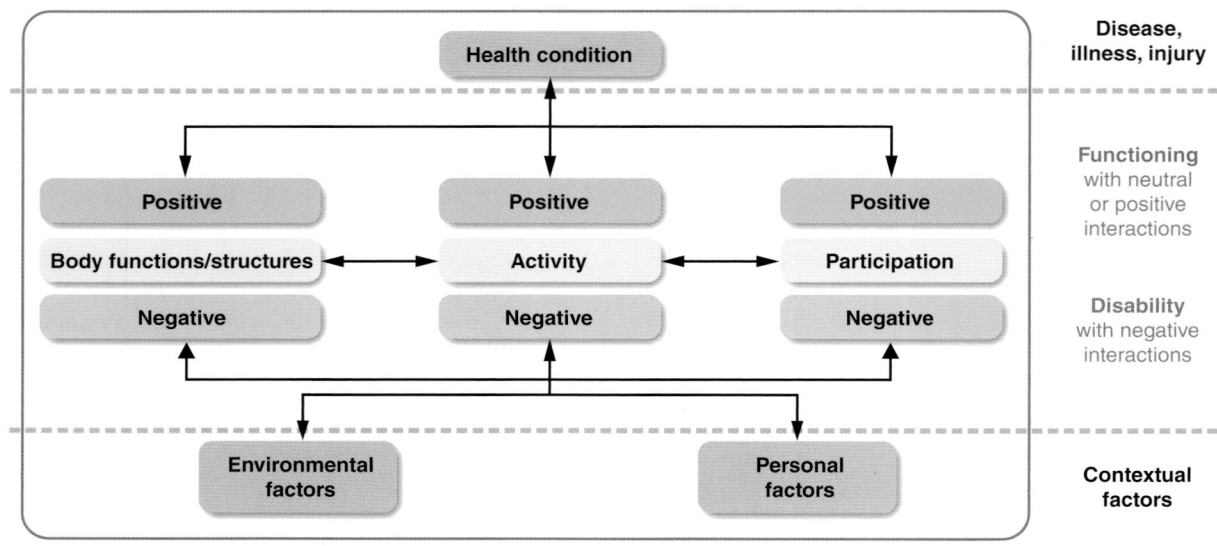

Figure 1.6   World Health Organization disablement model: functioning and disability.

level is how well a person can perform necessary activities for self-care, domestic life, and activities of daily living. The third level is a person's contribution to society; how well can he or she perform the activities that are expected of a contributing member of society?

The WHO developed this system of International Classification of Functioning, Disability and Health with the intention of focusing on a person's positive aspects and the contributions someone with a disability can make rather than on their limitations. Rather than classify people, the ICF functions to describe an individual and how he or she functions at a personal and societal level in his or her environment within the context of health.

The system that the WHO has developed to identify levels of functioning uses numerical and letter codes that identify each element that affects a person's ability to function as an individual and as a member of society. The classification system is broken down into two parts: Part 1 is Functioning and Disability, and it includes body functions and structures, activities, and participation. Part 2 is Contextual Factors and includes the environmental factors and personal factors (see figure 1.7).[3] These two parts represent the interaction between a person's health and the personal and environmental factors that directly affect her. Those parts are further divided into components, which are identified by letters. As seen in table 1.5 and figure 1.7, body functions are labeled "b"; body structures are "s"; activities and participation have the "d" label; and environmental factors have the "e" label. Components are divided into constructs and qualifiers. The first level of these divisions is called a chapter; this level is a single digit that indicates 1 of the 8 chapters where the various body functions and structures are listed. The second level has

two digits while third and fourth levels each have one digit. There may be one to four qualifiers after the domain letter.

It may be easiest to use an example to see how this system works. Let us take an example of a track and field discus thrower who suffered a strain of his right deltoid during a practice session. The injury would be classified as "s" because it is an injury that affects a body structure. The first letter of the code is the prefix or the component, and it is followed by a series of numbers, each representing a level of information. The chapter is s7 because the injury involves a movement-related structure (see table 1.5). From there, each chapter has different levels that further identify and define the problem. These levels are categorized numerically beginning with the second level, then the third level, then the fourth, and so on; the chapter is the first level in the domain. Each of these levels has descriptions for each sublevel. Figure 1.8 shows how the ICF system is laid out in its hierarchical structure.

Continuing with the shoulder injury example, the second level under the s7 category involves structures. These structures are divided into nine possible selections. These selections include:

s710 Structure of the head and neck region

s720 Structure of the shoulder region

s730 Structure of the upper extremity

s740 Structure of the pelvic region

s750 Structure of the lower extremity

s760 Structure of the trunk

s770 Additional musculoskeletal structures related to movement

TABLE 1.5   ICF Domains and Subdomains and Their Labels

Domain label	Domain	Subdomain label	Subdomains or chapters
b	Body functions	b1	Mental functions
b	Body functions	b2	Sensory functions and pain
b	Body functions	b3	Voice and speech functions
b	Body functions	b4	Cardiovascular, hematological, immunological, and respiratory systems
b	Body functions	b5	Digestive, metabolic, and endocrine systems
b	Body functions	b6	Genitourinary and reproductive functions
b	Body functions	b7	Neuromusculoskeletal and movement-related functions
b	Body functions	b8	Skin and related structural functions
s	Body structures	s1	Nervous system structures
s	Body structures	s2	Eye, ear, and related structures
s	Body structures	s3	Voice, speech, and related structures
s	Body structures	s4	Cardiovascular, immunological, and respiratory structures
s	Body structures	s5	Digestive, metabolic, and endocrine structures
s	Body structures	s6	Genitourinary and reproductive structures
s	Body structures	s7	Movement-related structures
s	Body structures	s8	Skin and related structures
d	Activities and participation	d1	Learning and applying knowledge
d	Activities and participation	d2	General tasks and demands
d	Activities and participation	d3	Communication
d	Activities and participation	d4	Mobility
d	Activities and participation	d5	Self-care
d	Activities and participation	d6	Domestic life
d	Activities and participation	d7	Interpersonal interactions and relationships
d	Activities and participation	d8	Major life areas
d	Activities and participation	d9	Community, social, and civic life
e	Environmental factors	e1	Products and technology
e	Environmental factors	e2	Natural environment and human-made changes to environment
e	Environmental factors	e3	Support and relationships
e	Environmental factors	e4	Attitudes
e	Environmental factors	e5	Services, systems, and policies

Based on World Health Organization (2001).[3]

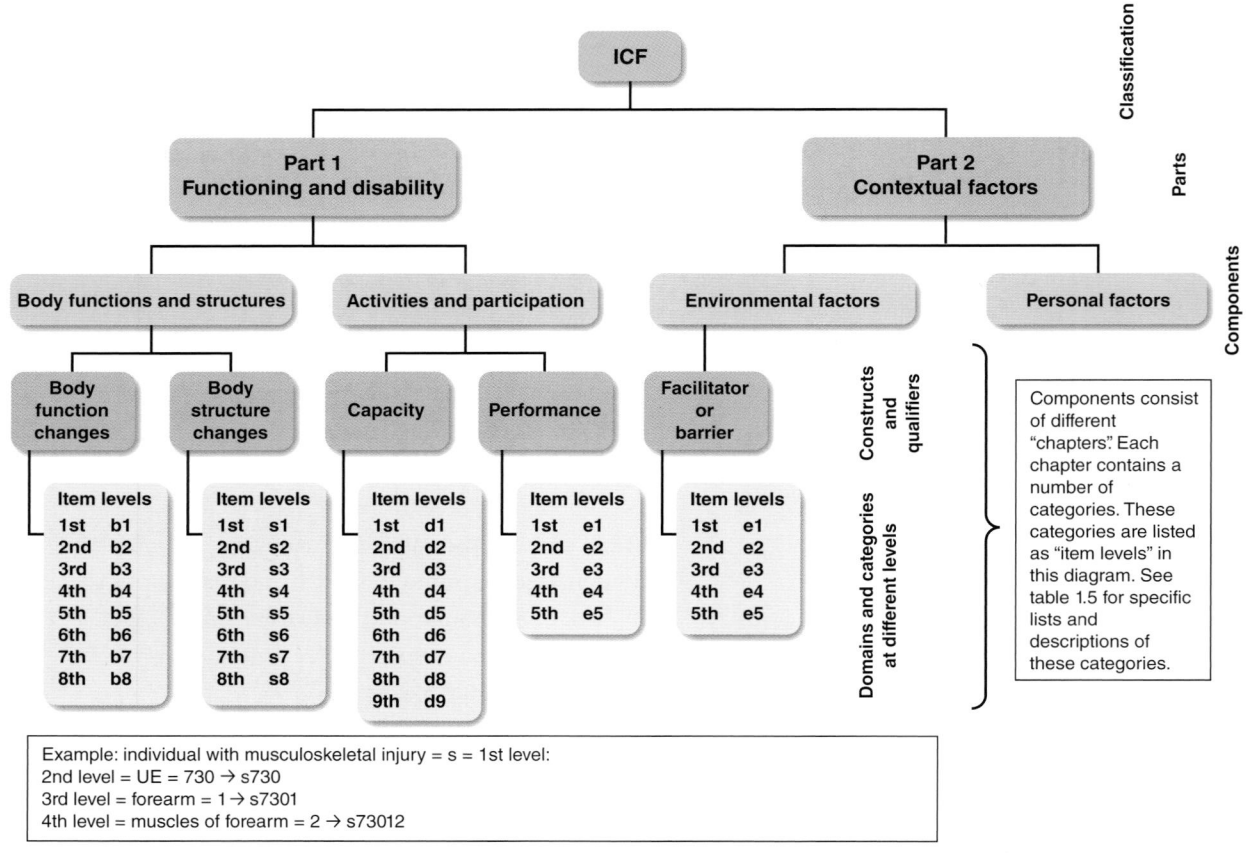

Figure 1.7   WHO ICF structure and coding.

Adapted by permission from WHO, *How to Use the ICF: A Practical Manual for Using the International Classification of Functioning, Disability and Health* (Geneva, Switzerland: WHO, 2013), 18.

Body functions	Body structures	Activities and participation	Environmental factors	Domain
b	s	d	e	Domain codes
b1 – b8	s1 – s8	d1 – d9	e1 – e5	Chapter codes
b110 – b899	s110 – s899	d110 – d999	e110 – e599	2nd level codes
b1100 – b7809 b11420 – b54509	s1100 – s7809 s11420 – s54509	d1150 – d9309	e1100 – e5959	3rd level codes 4th level codes

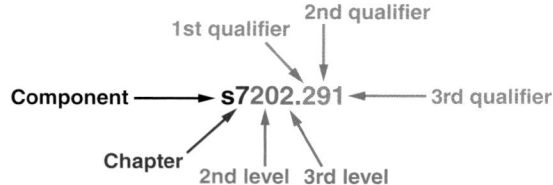

Figure 1.8   Hierarchical design of the ICF categories and their codes.

s780 Structures related to movement, other specified

s790 Structures related to movement, unspecified[78]

From the list, we see that the most appropriate selection is s720. The third and fourth levels move into more and more specific categories of detail. The second level in the shoulder includes these selections:

s7200 Bones of the shoulder region

s7201 Joints of the shoulder region

s7202 Muscles of the shoulder region

s7203 Ligaments and fascia of the shoulder region

s7208 Structure of the shoulder region, other specified

s7209 Structure of the shoulder region, unspecified[78]

Because the patient suffered an injury to the rotator cuff, the code now advances to s7202. Once the code is identified, qualifiers are added to provide the code with meaning.[78] The qualifiers indicate the severity or extensiveness, location, and nature of the injury or disease. The decimal point ends the code and qualifiers follow the decimal point. Qualifiers include at least one number. The first qualifier number indicates the extent of the injury or impairment; the second number identifies whether there is any change in the structure, or the nature of the impairment. The third number identifies the location of the injury or impairment. Table 1.6 provides a list of the coding for the first, second, and third qualifiers.

If we continue with our discus thrower's injury, we know that the deltoid strain was a grade 2 strain (first qualifier),

but there were no changes in the appearance or nature of the structure (second qualifier), and it was an injury to the right shoulder (third qualifier). Therefore, this patient's ICF code is s7202.291. Anyone around the world who knows these codes would understand the extent, nature, location, and identification of this patient's injury.

There are many advantages to using the ICF disablement model. When all the data are input into the ICF, a profile of the individual and how injury or disease affects that person's quality of life and performance is created. It also provides a record of progress as a person's functioning improves with treatment. The ICF, as a tool to guide treatment, complements the ICD as a tool for diagnosis. Because the ICF is a universal tool, comparisons across clinical practices around the world are possible. The tool's most obvious benefit is to the patient, for its focus is on the patient and how the injury or disease affects not only the body segment but perhaps more importantly, how it affects the patient's quality of life and ability to contribute to society.

Evidence-Based Practice and Outcomes-Based Practice

Of the factors that reflect today's clinical practice across all health professions, two of the most important are evidence-based practice and outcome-based practice. The former deals with what has been demonstrated to produce the best results in practice while the latter deals with the treatment results and the patient's interpretation of those

TABLE 1.6   Codes for Qualifiers

First qualifier: extent of injury or illness	Second qualifier: nature of impairment	Third qualifier: location of impairment
0 No impairment (0-4%)	0 No change in structure	0 More than one region
1 Mild impairment (5-24%)	1 Total absence	1 Right
2 Moderate impairment (25-49%)	2 Partial absence	2 Left
3 Severe impairment (50-95%)	3 Additional part	3 Both sides
4 Complete impairment (96-100%)	4 Aberrant dimensions	4 Front
8 Not specified	5 Discontinuity	5 Back
9 Not applicable	6 Deviating position	6 Proximal
	7 Qualitative changes in structure	7 Distal
	8 Not specified	8 Not specified
	9 Not applicable	9 Not applicable

Based on World Health Organization (2001).[3]

results. Both factors are important, not only for guiding patient care; they also serve to assure all those affected by a patient's treatment, including employers and coaches, physicians and clinicians, payers and investors, and most obviously the patient and family members, that the care offered has the best opportunity to succeed in returning the patient to optimal function. In other words, all those individuals who are concerned about the results of a patient's treatment are assured that their investment, whether it is in money, time, energy, effort, or emotion, will see their desired effect.

Evidence-Based Practice

Evidence-based practice is the application of information gleaned from current, quality research that is combined with the clinician's skills and experience, along with the patient's needs, goals, and priorities, to provide the patient with the best and most appropriate level of care.[79] These elements of evidence-based practice are not necessarily equal, but each is an important part of providing optimal patient care. Figure 1.9 is probably a whimsical schematic, but it nevertheless presents the three parts that create the best evidence-based practice. As the image portrays, not all of these elements receive equal consideration in what determines evidence-based practice. Unlike the image, sometimes the clinician's experience and skills are more important than the other two, and at other times the research evidence is the strongest consideration in determining what practice is the best evidence-based practice in a particular situation with a specific patient. In situations where there is little research on a specific treatment, the clinician will rely on the experience of past uses with former patients, and research will play a small role. If a patient's main concern is being able to climb three floors to her third-floor walkup apartment with crutches before she improves the status of her injured knee, then the best practice the clinician should

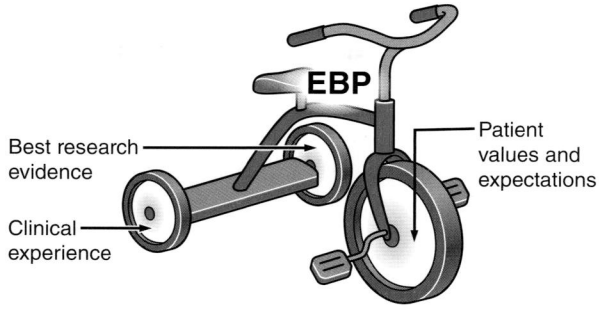

Figure 1.9 The elements of evidence-based practice. Evidence-based practice is based on the patient's personal values and expectations of what will be achieved in rehabilitation, the clinician's experience and skills, and the best current research available. These elements do not hold equivalent values nor are they given the same value all the time; depending on specific circumstances, any of the three elements may become the largest wheel.

deliver is treatment that will provide her with the ability to get home first.

The goal of every health care professional should be the delivery of quality care to patients. Over the past 20 years, there has been astronomical growth in medical and health care research;[65] this growth is important because research is the foundation for evidence-based practice.

The research element of evidence-based practice is not just any research, but research that exhibits quality in its questions, design, methods, and outcomes, which lead to reliable health care answers. The clinician cannot assume that because a research study is published in a reviewed journal, the content can be considered gospel. It is the clinician's responsibility to critically review and assess the investigation for its quality. If other investigations on the same topic have revealed different results, then the clinician needs to understand why the differences exist. Are different populations or groups used? Are the methods different, and if so, are they different in ways that could create different results? Did the methods narrow the focus of each study to eliminate unwanted variables that could alter the results? Did the data analysis in the studies differ enough to prevent both studies from producing similar results? Did the studies have sufficient power to produce reliable results? Did the investigators eliminate as many control variables and limitations as possible to provide reliable results? The clinician must read professional articles to maintain a current knowledge of clinical applications, but critical eye is needed to understand the quality of research.

Clinical investigations whose results conflict often present young clinicians with a difficult decision: whether to use the technique studied in their clinical practice. This is where the second part of the definition of evidence-based practice becomes important and often becomes the deciding factor for more experienced clinicians, especially when empirical scientific information is lacking. In addition to empirical evidence, evidence-based practice relies on the clinician's anecdotal evidence. The clinician's anecdotal evidence is obtained either from his or her own experience or the experience of others in using a clinical technique or application and then assessing those results. Clinicians who find success using certain skills or techniques are likely to use them with subsequent patients and to continue to assess the results until they are convinced of the treatment's effectiveness. As neophyte professionals, new clinicians with problem-solving skills may also experiment with various unproven techniques and evaluate their usefulness in their own practice. The use of anecdotal evidence is important not only in creating good results for patients but also in raising questions for additional research. For example, several years ago Jenny McConnell devised taping techniques for patellofemoral pain syndrome.[80] She indicated that her taping techniques reduced pain by realigning the patella.[80] Her technique spurred a number of empirical studies that demonstrated that pain was significantly reduced but that the tape did not essentially realign the patella.[81-83] Although theories have evolved, investigators are still working to identify how this technique relieves pain while clinicians continue to use it for pain relief in their patients.

Finally, the third element of evidence-based practice must be considered by the clinician if he or she is to provide optimal treatment: Satisfy the patient's own needs, goals, priorities, and expectations. Rather than letting the clinician's goals guide the treatment plan, the clinician must identify what the patient wants and needs. For example, if the patient is not interested in resuming running after a severe lower-extremity injury but only wants to be able to walk and climb stairs, then the clinician is obligated to design the treatment program to reach those goals, regardless of the fact that the clinician's best-practice knowledge and skills would allow full restoration of the patient's running performance level.

Evidence-based practice is the expected level of performance for any clinician. Performing at any level less than that is irresponsible and unethical, and it places the goals of the treatment program at risk. The clinician decides what rehabilitation techniques and applications to use based on three factors: empirical evidence, his or her own clinical experience or that of others, and the goals, needs, and desires of the patient. Designing a rehabilitation program based on all three elements of evidence-based practice is sound clinical practice.

Outcomes-Based Practice

As the health care world has moved from a disease-centered perspective to a patient-centered perspective, more focus has been placed on health care delivery from the view of the patient. To a significant degree, the disablement models and evidence-based practice that have already been presented have the patient at their center. One way to measure the attitude and perspective patients have about the health care they receive is by simply asking them. This is most commonly done using what is known as outcomes-based instruments. These tools serve multiple purposes; beyond helping clinicians assess the outcomes of their clinical practice, they are also important in health care record keeping. Not only can they help the clinician in providing useful information about patient perceptions of treatment quality and effectiveness, but they can be especially valuable when clinicians bill for their services; third-party providers often require evidence of outcomes for reimbursement.[84, 85]

Outcomes are important to the understanding, use, and justification of programs used to treat patients. In today's health care world, outcomes have become important to many stakeholders.[86] Outcomes can be based on various criteria, including clinician or patient perspectives. *Clinician-based outcomes* deal more with objective criteria such as changes in range of motion, strength, and coordination,[87] while *patient-based outcomes* are based on the patients' perceptions of how well they meet their own requirements for living.[87] Other outcomes are based on the varied interests of other stakeholders, such as employers who are concerned with the employee returning to work or insurance companies whose primary interest is in cost-effective outcomes.[88] As various outcomes instruments have evolved, it has become clear that one of the most crucial parameters is the patient's perspective of his or her ability to return to a previous level of function and thus to achieve an optimal quality of life.[86] Because of the focus on patient-centered care, current outcomes instruments rate the success of treatment programs mainly on the basis of the patient's satisfaction.[89]

An *outcomes tool* is usually a questionnaire that is given before the start of the treatment or rehabilitation program, at some time during the program, and at its conclusion. Questions often relate to the patient's interpretation of his or her condition before and after treatment and to the patient's perception of different aspects of the treatment, including quality of care, professional attitudes, and effectiveness of the program in achieving optimal return-to-function goals. Input from the clinician providing the treatment program is also often obtained. Final results are then compiled and statistically analyzed to provide information to today's medical providers, patients, and payers. Figure 1.10 shows the Lower-Extremity Functional Scale (LEFS), an example of a specific outcomes questionnaire.

Outcomes tools are divided into two categories—general health status measurement tools and region-specific measurement tools. A generic status measurement tool is used to assess a patient's physical, social, and emotional health and is used for a variety of illnesses and treatment environments. The gold standard for the generic health status tool is the SF-36, originally advanced by John E. Ware, Jr.[91, 92] Although it has been demonstrated to be a reliable and valid tool, it is time consuming to administer and

Evidence in Rehabilitation

Using the three most important elements (patient expectations and goals, your own clinical experience, and empirical clinical evidence) to guide your rehabilitation programs is the means by which you are most likely to achieve successful outcomes in the programs you design and execute for and with your patients. These elements provide sound reasoning for treatment decisions and are the basis upon which decisions are made throughout the rehabilitation process.

LOWER-EXTREMITY FUNCTION

It will be useful in your rehabilitation program to know if you are having difficulty with any specific activities at this time. Please indicate your ability for each activity by circling the appropriate number. Your selected number should reflect what you feel you are able to do today.

Activity	Unable to perform	I can perform but with great difficulty	I can perform with moderate difficulty	I can perform with a little difficulty	I can perform without difficulty	This is something I do not do regularly
Any of your usual work, housework, or school activities	0	1	2	3	4	5
Your usual recreational activities	0	1	2	3	4	5
Your usual hobbies	0	1	2	3	4	5
Getting into the bath	0	1	2	3	4	5
Getting out of the bath	0	1	2	3	4	5
Walking in the house	0	1	2	3	4	5
Putting on shoes and socks	0	1	2	3	4	5
Lifting objects such as a grocery bag	0	1	2	3	4	5
Performing light activities at home	0	1	2	3	4	5
Performing heavy activities at home	0	1	2	3	4	5
Getting in and out of the car	0	1	2	3	4	5
Walking more than 15 minutes	0	1	2	3	4	5
Walking less than 15 minutes	0	1	2	3	4	5
Going up or down 1 flight of stairs	0	1	2	3	4	5
Standing more than 15 minutes	0	1	2	3	4	5
Standing more than 1 hour	0	1	2	3	4	5
Running on flat ground	0	1	2	3	4	5
Running on hills	0	1	2	3	4	5
Hopping/jumping	0	1	2	3	4	5
Getting out of bed	0	1	2	3	4	5

Figure 1.10 Sample outcomes assessment tool.
Data from Binkley et al. (1999).[90]

was not designed as a tool with which to make treatment decisions for individual patients.[93] Other instruments have been developed with fewer questions to obtain the desired information.[92] A variety of condition-specific outcomes tools have been created over the past several years to more accurately examine and assess items that are related to specific injuries or illnesses and reveal improvements in patient conditions with treatment applications. Tools specific for patient outcomes related to low-back pain,[88, 94] hip,[95, 96] knee,[95, 97-100] ankle,[95, 101, 102] and upper extremity

Evidence in Rehabilitation

Here are examples of outcomes instruments for various lower-extremity injuries:

- Crown WH, Henk HJ, Vanness DJ. Some cautions on the use of instrumental variables estimators in outcomes research: How bias in instrumental variables estimators is affected by instrument strength, instrument contamination, and sample size. *Value Health.* 14:1078-0184;2011.[119]

- Griffin DR, Parson N, Mohtadi NG, et al. A short version of the International Hip Outcome Tool (iHOT-12) for use in routine clinical practice. *Arthroscopy.* 28:611-616;2012.[120]

- Hung M, Nickisch F, Beals TC, et al. New paradigm for patient-reported outcomes assessment in foot & ankle research: computerized adaptive testing. *Foot Ankle Int.* 33:621-626;2012.[102]

- Niki H, Tatsunami S, Haraguchi N, et al. Development of the patient-based outcome instrument for foot and ankle: Part 2: Results from the second field survey: Validity of the Outcome Instrument for the foot and ankle version 2. *J Orthop Sci.* 16:556-564;2011.[121]

- Peer MA, Lane J. The knee injury and osteoarthritis outcome score (KOOS): a review of its psychometric properties in people undergoing total knee arthroplasty. *J Orthop Sports Phys Ther.* 43:20-28;2013.[97]

- Rodriguez-Merchan EC. Knee instruments and rating scales designed to measure outcomes. *J Orthop Traumatol.* 13:1-6;2012.[100]

---

have been developed and published.[103, 104] There are even patient-outcome instruments for anterior cruciate ligament injuries.[100, 105, 106] Within the last few years there have also been a number of outcomes instruments that have been investigated or validated for use within the athletic population.[107-113]

For many conditions there are few patient-outcomes instruments available,[93] but these instruments cannot be interchanged. For example, a tool that measures patellofemoral injury treatment or rehabilitation outcomes is not a reliable tool to measure outcomes of treatment or rehabilitation for a shoulder dislocation, and a tool designed to measure treatment outcomes on a teenaged student may not be applicable to measuring treatment outcomes on a middle-aged laborer. They may all come under the category of outcomes assessment instruments, but they have their specific uses, and one cannot be substituted for the other. It would be similar to using a hammer to drive a screw into a piece of wood; you could do it, but your results would not be good.

Outcomes are important in many fields of health care and medicine. They are used in physicians' offices, outpatient clinics, and hospitals. They are used to modify treatment, justify treatment, evaluate the effectiveness of protocols, judge treatment responses, and assist in the authorization of payment. An outcomes assessment tool can be provided by an outside agency, which analyzes the results from many treatment providers around the country, or it can be devised and analyzed by a single facility.

A couple of the more commonly used outcome research tools in rehabilitation are the Functional Independence Measure (FIM),[114] a tool used primarily for inpatient rehabilitation facilities, and Focus on Therapeutic Outcomes (FOTO), a tool for outpatient rehabilitation facilities.[115]

Different users of an assessment tool evaluate their results differently, depending on their perspective. For example, an insurance company may use outcomes research results to decide what is usual and customary for the expected duration and cost to treat a specific injury. A patient may use outcomes research results to see whether the treatment program meets his or her needs. Health care providers may look at the outcomes study results to assess whether the programs being used to treat specific injuries and individual patients in their facility are effective, cost efficient, and achieve the goals of the professional administering the treatment.

There are occasions, however, when outcomes assessments are used incorrectly to generalize results to a larger population or a different situation. Inappropriate inferences should be avoided, for they are misleading, unfair, and erroneous. Most clinicians are interested in whether the outcomes demonstrate how the patient perceives the benefits of care in terms of how well he or she can perform normal activities.[65, 99, 116]

Regardless of the reason for using an outcomes-based instrument, it should accurately reflect the patient's perceptions of care and demonstrate the treatment or rehabilitation program's effectiveness accurately.

Figure 1.10 provides an example of a general lower-extremity function assessment tool that delves into questions that focus mainly on the activities of daily living. As you can see, it is designed to identify patients' perceptions of how they function in a variety of common daily tasks. Since it does not ask specific questions about athletic performance, it would not be an accurate tool to use with an athlete who is more interested in being able to perform his normal sports activities. It does, however, provide a nice example of a grading scale, and it also shows that when a tool is designed, questions included must be pertinent to the patient's daily activities and demands.

Figure 1.10 is in contrast to figure 1.11, which not only includes queries about the patient's ability to perform activities of daily living but also specific athletic performance questions. This instrument is used specifically for patients who have suffered ankle and foot injuries and has been shown to be a reliable tool for both athletes and nonathletes.[117, 118]

Because rehabilitation programs must be as effective and efficient as possible in treating patients and returning them to optimal function, clinicians are concerned with outcomes. Clinicians who practice in an athletic training clinic or industrial setting may not think outcomes are important for them since they are not paid a fee for service like providers in outpatient clinics or hospitals. However, as systems of health care and payment continue to change, all rehabilitation venues, and therefore all rehabilitation clinicians, will eventually have to deal with outcomes assessments more formally than they typically do now. Better clinicians are proactive rather than reactive, and this is especially true in the realm of outcomes.

Summary

Health care has evolved from being a disease- and injury-focused system to a patient-centered system. The rehabilitation of orthopedic and sports injuries now focuses on how it affects the patient and the patient's ability to perform both at a personal level and within that patient's group or society. This chapter offers an overview of rehabilitation and includes the definition of what it means to provide rehabilitation to a patient, what the components of rehabilitation include, and how they fit together and provide a progression as the patient improves. This chapter also introduces aspects of clinical practice that are relevant to health care providers around the world and presents some of the important points about evidence-based practice and why outcomes matter in today's health care environment. Although this chapter includes varied topics, they all form the foundation for a rehabilitation program—a program that works for the patient and is successful in achieving the patient's goals and expectations. As the rehabilitation clinician, you must understand the concepts that have been presented in this chapter, for they provide the basis for health care delivery today.

	No difficulty	Slight difficulty	Moderate difficulty	Extreme difficulty	Unable to do	N/A
Standing	☐	☐	☐	☐	☐	☐
Walking on even ground	☐	☐	☐	☐	☐	☐
Walking on even ground without shoes	☐	☐	☐	☐	☐	☐
Walking up hills	☐	☐	☐	☐	☐	☐
Walking down hills	☐	☐	☐	☐	☐	☐
Going up stairs	☐	☐	☐	☐	☐	☐
Going down stairs	☐	☐	☐	☐	☐	☐
Walking on uneven ground	☐	☐	☐	☐	☐	☐
Stepping up and down curbs	☐	☐	☐	☐	☐	☐
Squatting	☐	☐	☐	☐	☐	☐
Coming up on your toes	☐	☐	☐	☐	☐	☐
Walking initially	☐	☐	☐	☐	☐	☐
Walking 5 minutes or less	☐	☐	☐	☐	☐	☐
Walking approximately 10 min	☐	☐	☐	☐	☐	☐
Walking 15 minutes or more	☐	☐	☐	☐	☐	☐

Figure 1.11   Foot and Ankle Ability Measure (FAAM). Activities of Daily Living Subscale*

From Martin et al. (2005)[117]

Because of your foot and ankle, how much difficulty do you have with:

	No difficulty at all	Slight difficulty	Moderate difficulty	Extreme difficulty	Unable to do	N/A
Home responsibilities	☐	☐	☐	☐	☐	☐
Activities of daily living	☐	☐	☐	☐	☐	☐
Personal care	☐	☐	☐	☐	☐	☐
Light to moderate work (standing, walking)	☐	☐	☐	☐	☐	☐
Heavy work (push/pulling, climbing, carrying)	☐	☐	☐	☐	☐	☐
Recreational activities	☐	☐	☐	☐	☐	☐

How would you rate your current level of function during your usual activities of daily living from 0 to 100, with 100 being your level of function prior to your foot or ankle problem and 0 being the inability to perform any of your usual daily activities?

__ __ __.0 %

Sports Subscale

Because of your foot and ankle, how much difficulty do you have with:

	No difficulty at all	Slight difficulty	Moderate difficulty	Extreme difficulty	Unable to do	N/A
Running	☐	☐	☐	☐	☐	☐
Jumping	☐	☐	☐	☐	☐	☐
Landing	☐	☐	☐	☐	☐	☐
Starting and stopping quickly	☐	☐	☐	☐	☐	☐
Cutting/lateral movements	☐	☐	☐	☐	☐	☐
Low impact activities	☐	☐	☐	☐	☐	☐
Ability to perform activity with your normal technique	☐	☐	☐	☐	☐	☐
Ability to participate in your desired sport as long as you would like	☐	☐	☐	☐	☐	☐

How would you rate your current level of function during your sports related activities from 0 to 100, with 100 being your level of function prior to your foot or ankle problem and 0 being the inability to perform any of your usual daily activities?

__ __ __.0 %

Overall, how would you rate your current level of function?

__ Normal   __Nearly normal   __Abnormal   __Severely abnormal

Figure 1.11   >*continued*

LEARNING AIDS ▬ ▬ ▬   ▬▬▬▬▬▬▬▬▬ ▬ ▬   ▬▬▬▬▬▬▬▬ ▬ ▬ ▬   ▬▬▬ ▬

Key Concepts and Review

1. Indicate the personal issues that the rehabilitation clinician must keep in mind when treating a patient.

The rehabilitation clinician must consider and respect the patient throughout the rehabilitation process. The patient must consent to all aspects of treatment; if the patient refuses any aspect of treatment, the clinician must respect the patient's wishes. Touch is a personal issue; the clinician must obtain permission before touching a patient, and the patient can withdraw that permission at any time. Each person responds differently to an injury and to the subsequent rehabilitation program, and the clinician must realize that patients cannot be compared and should not be treated identically. Finally, patients will also have different needs that must be met if they are to be fully rehabilitated in the most appropriate manner.

2. Define rehabilitation.

Rehabilitation is the process of treatment and education that help disabled individuals attain their maximum function, a sense of well-being, and a personally satisfying level of independence. Rehabilitation is about improving a person's abilities to an optimal level of function that allows that person to be a productive member of his or her social unit.

3. Discuss how examination of a patient is related to rehabilitation.

Before a rehabilitation program is established, an examination is performed to identify the patient's injury and discover what deficiencies exist that are preventing the patient from achieving his or her goals. An examination is the process by which the clinician gathers subjective and objective information to identify the patient's injury and define deficiencies so that an appropriate rehabilitation program may be designed. The examination is the starting point for any rehabilitation program.

4. Describe the components of a rehabilitation program.

The first component is the examination and assessment. Next is the correction of any deviations that may be contributing to the patient's current complaints. At first this involves addressing the inflammatory signs and symptoms that may be interfering with the patient's ability to function. Once these are treated, the clinician's focus shifts to regaining range of motion and flexibility, strength and endurance, neuromotor functions, and finally the function- and performance-specific restorations that will allow the patient to resume his or her former level of activity.

5. Identify the phases of rehabilitation.

A rehabilitation program can be divided into four phases or stages: (1) inactive, (2) active, (3) resistive, and (4) advanced phases. These phases correlate with the healing progression from the time immediately following an injury all the way to the point where heavy stresses may be safely applied to tissue toward the end of the healing process.

6. Explain what disablement models are and why they are important in rehabilitation.

Disablement models are conceptual models that help clinicians to create a plan of treatment that addresses the individual. Because of how they look at the effect of injury or disease on an individual, disablement models force health care professionals to view and treat patients as individuals rather than just injuries and to identify specific problems the rehabilitation program must address to restore a person to his or her optimal recovery status.

7. Outline the importance of evidence-based practice and outcomes-based rehabilitation.

Clinical practice is centered on providing a patient with the best care possible. Best care is centered on evidence-based practice, which means the clinician uses current evidence in the literature that demonstrates best care, incorporates anecdotal results when empirical evidence demonstrating appropriate results is lacking, and incorporates the patient's desires, needs, and goals in an effort to provide the patient with the best possible outcome.

Outcomes-based assessment involves determining whether a program that you design for a patient produces the expected response and whether the program meets expectations and goals. The most recent outcomes instruments have moved from a clinician-based outcome to a patient-based outcome; they focus more on the patient's interpretation of the success of treatment.

Critical Thinking Questions

1. How would you handle an ethical and perhaps legal situation in which a newly graduated clinician with whom you worked did not properly complete the requirements established by the profession's certification and examination board to sit for the qualifying examination but was able to get his university program's director to sign off on the required documents anyway? Would you report him to the licensing board or the profession's ethics council, discuss it with him or your supervisor, or ignore it? Or something else?

2. If you were treating a patient whose injury was severe enough to doubt whether she would return to full sport participation at her preinjury level, how would you deal with her if she stated that it was her goal to return to her sport and resume her starting role on the team? Would you tell her in the beginning that returning to her prior level of participation was questionable? Would you let the patient discover the reality herself? Would you ease the patient into that reality? What other options would you consider?

3. If you were Amanda in the chapter's opening scenario, what would be some of the policies you would develop for rehabilitation programs for the department? How would you go about creating rehabilitation protocols; what things would you consider? What would be some of the things you would think about as you put together the quarterback's rehabilitation program?

Lab Activities

1. Find online an outcomes tool that can be used with athletes who have suffered anterior cruciate ligament (ACL) tears.
   • Identify what type of athlete this instrument is most appropriate for (male, female; preteen, adult; soccer, basketball).
   • Find another lower extremity outcomes tool and compare this one to the ACL tool for athletes. Identify how they are different and the groups the two tools could be used with and what groups would not be appropriate for each tool.

2. Role-play a situation where you and your lab partner are the clinician and a patient. The patient is a 60-year-old who suffered a stroke about 8 months ago that has affected his balance. The patient recently sprained his left ankle when he tripped on a step, but he remains intent on resuming his ability to play tennis. Role-play how the clinician and patient work out realistic goals for the patient's rehabilitation program.

2

Concepts of Healing

Objectives

After completing this chapter, you should be able to do the following:

1. Explain the differences between primary and secondary healing.
2. Identify the healing phases.
3. Describe the primary processes of each healing phase.
4. Discuss the causes for the signs of inflammation.
5. Explain the influence of growth factors in healing.
6. Discuss the differences between acute and chronic inflammation.
7. Discuss the healing characteristics of specific tissues.
8. Identify the relevance of tensile strength.
9. Discuss factors that can modify the healing process.
10. Explain the role NSAIDs play in inflammation.

||||||||||||||||||||||||||||||||||||||||||||||||||||||||||||||||||||||||||||||||||||||||||||||||||||||||||||||||||||||||||||

Daniel Edds has been assigned to work with gymnast Becki Gumble, who underwent an Achilles tendon repair 7 d ago and is now in the clinic for her first day of rehabilitation. Daniel's knowledge of healing allows him to judge where in the healing process such an injury should be and what rehabilitation techniques can be safely applied to the Achilles tendon at this time. He understands the tendon's tensile strength and the precautions that apply for repairs such as Becki's. He also understands the status of the healing connective tissue and the biochemical and anatomical reparative processes that are now underway.

However, Daniel suspects that Becki has poor eating habits. Before applying rehabilitation techniques, Daniel decides to discuss the importance of proper nutrition and the role proteins, vitamins, and minerals play in tissue healing.

Healing is an inside job.

B.J. Palmer, 1882-1961, son of Daniel David Palmer, founder of chiropractic, who developed the chiropractic profession and education program his father had created.

Mr. Palmer's knowledge of healing at the time he practiced and taught was far less than what we know today. The entire healing process is still not fully understood, but we do know that understanding as much as we can is important to creating safe and effective rehabilitation programs for our patients. As a professional who rehabilitates orthopedic and sport injuries, you have a duty to stay current in your knowledge of healing, and you must understand the impact your rehabilitation techniques may have on the healing process. A wealth of information about healing has appeared in recent years, but there remain many aspects that are still unknown, even to experts. What is presented here is the most current information we have on the body's response to injury and the process it undergoes in an effort to return to normal.

Contrary to Mr. Palmer's statement that healing occurs from the inside, some of the more recent studies on healing involve investigations into external manipulations of the healing process to either make healing more efficient[1] or modify the process to actually regenerate tissue using tissue engineering[2] and stem cell applications.[3] As you move through this chapter you will see occasional mention made of these newer restorative and engineering advances, but anything more than a brief introduction to these emerging topics is beyond the scope of this chapter. The purpose of this chapter is to provide you with the most current information we have on the body's normal healing process.

Healing in human beings usually results in scarring. Although there are occasions when the body replaces damaged tissue with normal tissue, it is more common with sport and orthopedic injuries for scar tissue to be the end result of the healing process. This chapter covers the elements of the healing process that are involved in scar tissue formation after injury.

Despite all that has been written and investigated on healing, much still eludes us. The information presented in this chapter comes from the research of many people, groups, and institutions. It is an introductory presentation to a complex topic and addresses what clinicians should know to safely apply their rehabilitation techniques.

This chapter introduces many terms that may be new and unfamiliar to you. Table 2.1 defines the terms that appear in boldface in this chapter and describes their most common function or their significance in the healing process. You can also find these terms in the glossary at the end of this text, but they are placed here in a table for your convenience and quick reference.

Primary and Secondary Healing
||||||||||||||||||||||||||||||||||||||||||||||||||||||||||||||||||||||||||||||||||

There are many ways to classify injuries. Some refer to the type of injury as either primary (direct) or secondary (inflammatory), while others discuss injuries as either acute (from direct trauma) or chronic (from overuse), and still others may choose to use superficial (involving the epidermis or dermis) or deep (involving deeper structures).

Regardless of the term used to classify an injury, when an injury occurs, the healing process that follows depends on the extent of the injury and the approximation of the wound site's stump ends. If the separation of tissue is small, a bridge of cells binds the ends together. This is called healing by **primary intention**. This type of healing commonly occurs in minor wounds. It also occurs in surgical incisions where the stump ends are sutured together.

In more severe wounds where the stump ends are farther apart and cannot be bridged by single cells, the wound heals by producing cells from the bottom and sides of the wound to fill in the space created by the wound. This is called healing by **secondary intention**. This type of healing occurs, for example, in second-degree sprains where injured ligament tissue is separated by distance and is not surgically repaired. Healing by secondary intention usually takes longer and results in a larger scar.

CLINICAL TIPS

Healing by primary intention occurs through a small bridge of tissue when the wound separation is small. Healing by secondary intention occurs by filling in the wound with new tissue from the sides and bottom when the separation is large. Scars are usually larger when healing occurs by secondary intention. If it is a dermal wound, it is at greater risk of infection because the time it remains open and the time it takes to heal are longer.

TABLE 2.1 Terminology of Wound Healing

Term	Definition	Significance or function
Acetylcholine	An organic chemical that serves as a neurotransmitter at the neuromuscular junction of striated muscles.	Causes vasodilation.
Adrenaline	See *Epinephrine*.	
Anabolic state	One of two states of the human body throughout the day. The building up of the body's complex chemical compounds from simpler compounds. Energy is usually required. See *Catabolic state*.	Protein synthesis during healing is important for the immune system and for restoration and maintenance of tissues that play a role in wound repair.
Angiogenesis	Formation of blood vessels.	Provides for normal healing events and subsequent scar tissue formations that follow.
Antihemophilic factor A	A protein in normal plasma. Lacking in individuals with hemophilia A. Factor VIII.	Essential for normal blood clotting.
Antihemophilic factor B	Also known as Christmas factor, it is a plasma protein. Individuals without it have hemophilia B. Called Christmas factor because it was first discovered in a boy whose last name was Christmas. Factor IX.	Necessary for blood clotting; without it, bleeding is difficult to control.
Arachidonic acid	An unsaturated essential fatty acid.	A precursor in the production of leukotrienes, prostaglandins, and thromboxanes.
Basophil	A white blood cell in the subgroup of polymorphonuclear leukocytes (PMNs).	See *Granular leukocytes*.
Biomarkers	Biological markers are molecules whose identification within the body is rated according to what is normal in either quantity or quality.	The amount or presence of specific biomarkers may indicate or predict the presence or outcome of disease or healing. For example, increased protease levels are seen in chronic wounds.
Bradykinin	A local tissue hormone that is activated by the interaction of proteases with the Hageman factor.	A very potent local vasodilator. It increases vascular permeability and stimulates local pain receptors.
Callus	Fibrous matrix formed at a bone fracture site.	Immobilizes the bone fragments and serves as the foundation for eventual bone replacement.
Catabolic state	One of two states of the human body throughout the day. The breakdown of the body's complex chemical compounds into simpler compounds. Energy is usually released. See also *Anabolic state*.	Protein depletion impairs healing, delaying the healing process by prolonging the inflammatory process and impairing collagen synthesis and proteoglycan production.
Chemokines	Chemotactic cytokines that are secreted by a number of cells in a wound such as endothelium, fibroblasts, keratinocytes, neutrophils, and macrophages.	Primarily involved in preventing angiogenesis during clot formation and remodeling phases but promoting angiogenesis during inflammation and proliferation phases.
Chemotactic factor	A chemical gradient. Also referred to as a *chemotactin* or *chemo-attractant*.	See *Chemotactin*.
Chemotactin	An agent that facilitates chemotaxis.	Must be present and must function properly to promote the healing process.
Chemotaxis	Movement or orientation of cells in response to a chemical stimulus after an injury, which occurs through complex and incompletely understood processes.	Cells either become oriented along a chemical concentration gradient or move in the direction of that gradient. For example, chemicals attract platelets, red blood cells, and PMNs into an injured area.

>continued

TABLE 2.1 >*continued*

Term	Definition	Significance or function
Clotting factors	Proteins in the blood. They are referred to by either Roman numerals or their name: Factor I = Fibrinogen Factor II* = Prothrombin Factor III = Thromboplastin, or tissue factor Factor IV = Ionized calcium Factor V = Proaccelerin, or labile factor Factor VII* = Proconvertin, or stable factor Factor VIII = Antihemophilic factor A, or antihemophilic globulin Factor IX* = Plasma thromboplastin component, Christmas factor Factor X* = Stuart-Prower factor Factor XI = Plasma thromboplastin antecedent, Hemophilia C, or Rosenthal syndrome Factor XII = Hageman factor Factor XIII = Fibrin stabilizing factor, or Laki-Lorand factor	They are involved in the coagulation cascade and are released at the time of injury to control bleeding.
Collagen	Major type of protein in the body. There are about 30 types of collagen, but the most common types include these five: I is most abundant, high in tensile strength, and found in dermis, fascia, bone, ligaments, tendon, and scar tissue. II is found in cartilage. III is found in blood vessels, embryonic connective tissue, and granulation tissue of recent wounds. IV is found in basement membranes. V is found in interstitial tissue and placenta.	Forms inelastic bundles to provide structure, integrity, and tensile strength to tissues.
Collagenase	An enzyme produced by newly formed epithelial cells and fibroblasts.	Involved in degradation of collagen during tissue repair. Important in controlling collagen content in a wound.
Common pathway	This is the third pathway in the coagulation cascade. Also known as the thrombin pathway.	Completes the blood clotting cascade to form the fibrin plug.
Complement system	Various proteins found in serum.	Act as chemotactic factors for neutrophils and phagocytes.
Cytokines	Substances (mostly proteins) are released by certain cells. Cytokines regulate the immune response and mediate intercellular communication. It has been discovered that many growth factors and cytokines can have similar functions, so the terms are sometimes used interchangeably when the case is appropriate.	The release of cytokines throughout the healing process will either facilitate or inhibit activity.
Drug interaction	When one drug enhances or reduces the effectiveness of other drugs also being taken.	It is important to know what drugs a person takes so that the drugs do not render each other either harmful or ineffective.
Duration of drug action	Amount of time the blood level of the drug is above the level needed to obtain a minimum therapeutic effect.	Determined by the drug's half-life.

Term	Definition	Significance or function
Elastin	An essential protein of connective tissue's elastic structures. Arranged in a wavy orientation.	Its wavy arrangement allows tissue to change shape when stress is applied and resume normal conditions after stress is removed. It plays an, as yet, unknown role in the remodeling phase.
Endothelial cells	Large, flat cells that line blood and lymphatic vessels.	Are restored during angiogenesis.
Endothelial leukocytes	Large white blood cells that circulate in the bloodstream and tissues.	Act as phagocytes to remove debris from an injured area.
Enzymes	These substances are most often proteins that work as catalysts to increase the rate of chemical reactions within cells.	Many enzymes are involved throughout the healing process, turning anatomical and physiological procedures on and off at appropriate times to either form scar tissue or regenerate new tissue.
Eosinophil	A white blood cell in the subgroup of polymorphonuclear leukocytes (PMNs).	Promote hemostasis and tissue repair in healing. See *Granular leukocytes*.
Epidermal growth factor (EGF)	Growth factor produced by platelets during early inflammation and proliferation phases.	In early inflammation, EGF signals the start of a cascade to enhance cell mobility. During early proliferation, it increases the epithelialization rate, and during later proliferation it prevents excessive scarring.
Epinephrine	A hormone. Also called adrenaline.	A potent stimulator of the sympathetic nervous system and a powerful vasopressor. Increases blood pressure, stimulates the heart muscle, accelerates heart rate, increases cardiac output, and increases metabolic activities such as glycogenolysis and glucose release.
Erythrocyte	An element of blood. Also known as *red blood cell (RBC)* or *corpuscle*.	Used for oxygen transport.
Extracellular matrix	The basic material from which tissue develops. Produced by fibroblasts in wounds. Composed of fibers and ground substance.	Serves as a foundation on which new tissue is formed by providing mechanical cell support, binding growth factors, and regulating cellular processes.
Extrinsic pathway	Blood clotting that occurs when plasma comes in contact with an extrinsic trigger to start the blood clotting cascade. Involves factors III, VII, and X. See also *Intrinsic pathway*.	This is the normal mechanism that begins hemostasis following trauma. Tissue factor is exposed and comes in contact with plasma to begin the clotting process that will ultimately form the fibrin plug.
Exudate	Material that escapes from blood vessels after an injury. Contains high concentrations of protein, cells, and other materials from injured cells.	As PMNs die and decompose, exudate may resemble pus, although no infection is present.
Fibrillogenesis	Development of fine fibers.	Early development of collagen fibers seen during the proliferation healing phase.
Fibrin	Insoluble fibrous protein formed by fibrinogen.	Important in clotting.
Fibrinogen	An enzyme present in plasma.	Converts to fibrin to form a plug in early healing at the injury site.
Fibrinolysin	An enzyme in plasma released in later healing.	Converts fibrin into a soluble substance to unplug the lymphatic system at the injury site.
Fibrinolysis	The process of normal breakdown of clots.	Occurs about 3 days after injury to remove the fibrin clot formed during hemostasis.

> continued

TABLE 2.1 >continued

Term	Definition	Significance or function
Fibrin stabilizing factor	A proenzyme in the circulating blood that is activated by thrombin. Factor XIII.	It binds to the fibrin clot to stabilize the wound site's hemostasis.
Fibroblast	A connective tissue cell that differentiates into chondroblasts, osteoblasts, and collagenoblasts.	Forms the fibrous tissues that support and bind a variety of tissues.
Fibroblast growth factor (FGF)	Growth factor produced by endothelial cells, vascular smooth muscle cells, neural cells, and keratinocytes.	Stimulates the proliferation and migration of endothelial cells, fibroblasts, chondrocytes, and myoblasts. Also stimulates production of fibronectin, proteoglycans, and collagen as well as cell migration, granulation tissue formation, and neovascularization during proliferation.
Fibrocyte	An inactive fibroblast.	See Fibroblast.
Fibronectin	An adhesive glycoprotein found in most body tissues and serum.	Cross-links to collagen in connective tissue, thereby playing a role in the adhesion of fibroblasts to fibrin. Also involved in the collection of platelets in an injured area and the enhancement of myofibroblast activity. Fibronectin is plentiful in early granulation tissue formation but gradually disappears during the remodeling phase.
Glycoprotein	A protein–carbohydrate compound and an element of ground substance. Includes fibronectin.	Probably cross-links with collagen so tissue can withstand pressure or stress.
Glycosaminoglycans (GAGs)	Compounds that occur mostly in proteoglycans. Nonfibrous elements of ground substance in the extracellular matrix. Examples: hyaluronic acid, proteoglycans.	Different GAGs have different functions: stimulate fibroblast proliferation, promote collagen synthesis and maturation, contribute to tissue resilience, and regulate cell function.
Granuloma	Hard mass of fibrous tissue.	Occurs in chronic inflammatory conditions when the body produces collagen around a foreign substance to protect itself from that substance.
Granular leukocytes	White blood cells (WBCs) that are divided into three groups of polymorphonuclear leukocytes (PMNs): neutrophils, eosinophils, and basophils.	Among their functions, they are chemotactic and phagocytic and release histamine and serotonin to produce vasoactive reactions after injury.
Granulation tissue	Newly formed, highly vascular tissue that is produced during wound healing. Consists of fibroblasts, macrophages, and neovascular cells within a connective tissue matrix of collagen, hyaluronic acid, and fibronectin.	Eventually forms the scar of the wound. Has a beefy-red appearance with small, red, velvety nodular masses (new blood vessel formations) seen in newly forming tissue.
Ground substance	Gel-like material in which connective tissue cells and fibers are imbedded. Part of the connective tissue or extracellular matrix.	Reduces friction between the connective tissue fibers when forces are applied to the structure. Adds to the area's density.
Growth factor	Usually a protein that binds to receptors on cell surfaces. Growth factors have a number of sources, including platelets, lymphocytes, epithelial cells, and macrophages. Many growth factors and cytokines can have similar functions, so the terms are sometimes used interchangeably when the case is appropriate. Also referred to as growth hormone factor.	Performs numerous complex roles, stimulates re-epithelialization, and is chemotactic for macrophages, monocytes, and neutrophils. Its role is not thoroughly understood, but it is believed to play important roles throughout tissue repair.
Hageman factor	A plasma protein that is activated by negatively charged surfaces.	Initiates the blood coagulation process in the intrinsic pathway.

Term	Definition	Significance or function
Half-life	Amount of time it takes for the level of a drug in the bloodstream to diminish by one-half.	Determines the frequency with which a medication is taken.
Hemostasis	This is the body's immediate response to injury, stopping or arresting bleeding. It is the first phase in the healing process.	Circulating platelets and clotting factors in the bloodstream move to the site of injury. They attract other chemicals and cells at the very start of healing.
High molecular weight kininogen factor (HMWK)	A circulating plasma protein. Is inactive in the bloodstream until it adheres to binding proteins of injured endothelium. Factor XV.	Initiates blood coagulation in the intrinsic pathway.
Histamine	A local tissue hormone released by mast cells and granulocytes.	Increases vascular permeability to release proteins and fibronectin to the injury site.
Hyaluronic acid	A major component of early granulation tissue.	Promotes cell movement and migration during repair. Stimulates fibroblast proliferation. Produces edema by absorbing large amounts of water to increase fibroblast migration. Greatest amounts are seen in a wound during the first 4–5 days. See also *Glycosaminoglycan (GAG)*.
Insulin-like growth factor (IGF)	Important growth factor in healing and tissue repair.	Regulates general tissue growth, development, and repair. Also plays an important role in muscle tissue repair and reinnervation.
Intrinsic pathway	Blood clotting mechanism that occurs without adding an extrinsic factor. The Hageman factor begins the intrinsic pathway and is activated in the bloodstream when it encounters negatively charged molecules. Involves factors XII, XI, IX, VIII, X, and V. See also *Extrinsic pathway*.	This process starts within the bloodstream and is triggered by internal damage to the blood vessel wall. It is considered the "workhorse" of the clotting cascade because this is where more activations occur.
Kallikrein	A proteolytic enzyme found in blood plasma, lymph, and other exocrine secretions.	Forms kinins and activates plasminogen, a precursor of plasmin. Increases vascular permeability and vasodilation. Activated by the Hageman factor.
Keloid	An exaggerated scar that usually occurs on the dermis after injury.	Keloid scars are hyperplastic and painful. They are disfiguring and can severely restrict joint motion if they cross a joint. They are more prevalent in individuals with darker skin color. They contain excessive irregular collagen bands.
Kinin	A generic term for polypeptides that are related to bradykinin. A potent local tissue hormone found in injured tissue, released from plasma proteins. Examples: bradykinin, kallidin.	Mediates the classic signs of inflammation. Acts like histamine and serotonin on the microvascular system in the early inflammation phase to cause increased microvascular permeability.
Leukocytes	*White blood cells (WBCs)* or *corpuscles*. Different types include polymorphonuclear leukocytes and mononuclear cells.	Have phagocytic properties to remove debris from an injury site.
Leukotriene	A compound formed from arachidonic acid.	Regulates inflammatory reactions. Some leukotrienes stimulate the movements of leukocytes into the area of an injury.
Lipid	A heterogeneous group of fats and fatlike substances, including fatty acids and steroids.	Serves as a source of fuel and is important to the structure and makeup of cells.
Lymphocytes	Nonphagocytic mononuclear leukocytes found in blood and lymph.	Serve as important structures in the body's immune system by producing antibodies.

> continued

TABLE 2.1 *>continued*

Term	Definition	Significance or function
Macrophages	Mononuclear phagocytes that arise from stem cells in bone marrow.	Considered to be among the regulators of the repair process. Serve to phagocytize injury areas of debris, kill microorganisms, and secrete substances into an injury site, including enzymes, fibronectin, and coagulation factors. Play a role in keeping the inflammatory process localized; enhance collagen deposition and fibroblast proliferation.
Mast cells	Connective tissue cells. Also referred to as mastocytes and labrocytes.	Store and produce various mediators of inflammation. Through their release of histamine, enzymes, and other mediators, mast cells increase local blood flow, attract immune cells, stimulate cell production of fibroblasts and endothelial cells, and promote and control remodeling of extracellular matrix.
Matrix	Substance of a tissue. This term can refer to either intracellular or extracellular structure.	Forms the basis from which a structure develops.
Mediator	An umbrella term that identifies any intermediary substance or cell that interacts with or transmits information with chemicals or cells.	Their interactions and transmissions initiate or provide for the series of events and progression throughout the healing cycle.
Monocytes	Mononuclear phagocytic leukocytes.	Remove debris from an injury site. Formed in the bone marrow and transported to tissues where they become macrophages.
Mononuclear phagocyte	Any cell capable of ingesting particulate matter. The term usually refers to macrophages (polymorphonuclear leukocytes) and monocytes (mononuclear phagocytes).	Migrate to areas of injured or infected tissue and develop into macrophages to ingest microorganisms and debride an injury site. They defend the body against many organisms and are among the last cells to leave an area of inflammation.
Myoblast	A cell formed from myogenic cells in muscle.	Forms myotubes, which eventually evolve into muscle fiber.
Myofibroblasts	Fibroblasts that have a combination of the ultrastructural features of a fibroblast and the qualities of a smooth muscle cell.	Responsible for wound contraction. Results in a smaller scar.
Myogenic cells	Cells arising from muscle that later become myoblasts.	See *Myoblast.*
Neurotransmitters	Hormones such as norepinephrine, epinephrine, and acetylcholine, which are found in capillary, arteriole, and artery walls.	Released at the injury site to enhance platelet and leukocyte adherence to the vessel surface. They play an important role in the regulation of inflammation and angiogenesis.
Neutrophil	White blood cell in the polymorphonuclear leukocyte group of WBCs.	Contain toxic chemicals that bind to microorganisms to kill them. See also *Polymorphonuclear leukocyte.*
Norepinephrine	A hormone.	Acts as a powerful vasoconstrictor at the immediate onset of injury. Its effects may last from a few seconds to a few minutes.
Osteoblasts	Osteogenic cells from periosteum.	Lay down the callus of fractured bone. Convert later to chondrocytes.
Osteoclasts	Large multinuclear cells.	Resorb dead, necrotic bone tissue.
Osteocytes	Cells characteristic of adult bone.	Maintain new bone mineralization.

Term	Definition	Significance or function
Platelet-derived growth factor (PDGF)	Substance found in platelets.	Essential for the growth of connective tissue cells. Stimulates the migration of polymorphonuclear leukocytes.
PGE$_1$	See *Prostaglandin*.	Increases vascular permeability by causing vasodilation.
PGE$_2$	See *Prostaglandin*.	Is chemotactic to attract leukocytes to the area of an injury.
Phagocyte	Category of white blood cells. See *Mononuclear phagocyte* and *Polymorphonuclear leukocyte (PMN)*.	Engulf and absorb bacteria, debris, and other particles. Protect the body against infections and remove dead cells and debris from injured or infected sites.
Phospholipids	Lipids that contain phosphoric acid.	Stimulate the clotting mechanism. Found in all cells and in layers of plasma membranes.
Plasma thromboplastin antecedent	A protein that aids in blood coagulation. Persons with a deficiency have hemophilia C, which is most often revealed by frequent nosebleeds or following tooth extractions. Factor XI.	Contributes to blood clot formation by activating factor IX
Plasmin	An enzyme that occurs in plasma as plasminogen.	Converts fibrin to soluble substances. It is activated by kallikrein and other activators.
Plasminogen activator	See *Fibrinolysin*.	Blocks other proteins to promote dissolution of the fibrin clot.
Platelets	Irregular cell fragments found in blood.	The first cells seen at an injury site and considered among the regulatory cells of healing. Release growth factors. Form a plug at the injury to stop bleeding. Their unique and specialized ability to adhere to damaged endothelial cells promotes both clotting and repair at the injury site.
Polymorphonuclear leukocyte (PMN)	A type of white blood cell with more than one nucleus. One of the granular leukocytes. Also referred to as a *neutrophil*.	Chemotactic and phagocytic in the healing process.
Prekallikrein	A protease that combines with HMWK. It is the precursor of plasma kallikrein. Factor XIV.	Cleaved by the Hageman factor to produce kallikrein in the initial phase of the intrinsic pathway.
Primary hemostasis	The body's immediate and first response to injury as it attempts to stop bleeding that results from the injury.	Platelets immediately merge into the area to plug the injury site.
Primary intention	Healing that occurs with minor wounds or surgical wounds.	Re-epithelialization closes the wound within 48 h. Scarring is minimal when healing by primary intention occurs.
Proaccelerin	A protein made in the liver. Factor V.	Helps convert prothrombin to thrombin.
Proconvertin	A protein. Factor VII.	Initiates the coagulation cascade in conjunction with tissue factor.
Proenzyme	The inactive form of an enzyme within a cell. It usually becomes active once it leaves the cell. Also known as zymogen.	Many proenzymes are involved in blood coagulation following injury. They are converted from inactive to active enzymes and form the clotting cascade.

> continued

TABLE 2.1 >continued

Term	Definition	Significance or function
Prothrombin	The inactive version of thrombin that normally flows within the blood. Factor II.	Becomes activated by factor X to become IIa, or thrombin.
Prostaglandin (PG)	Hormone formed primarily from arachidonic acid when a cell membrane is damaged. Its release requires the complement system and follows kinin formation. Specific PG compounds are designated by adding a letter, A through I, and a subscript number, 1 through 3, to designate the number of hydrocarbon bonds. Examples: PGE_1 and PGE_2.	Mediates cell migration during inflammation and modulates serotonin and histamine. Some PGs increase pain sensitivity, induce fever, and suppress lymphocyte transformation, thereby inhibiting the inflammatory reaction. Mediates myofibroblasts, initiates early phases of injury repair, and plays a role in later stages of inflammation.
Protease	An enzyme.	Acts as a catalyst to split interior peptide bonds in protein. Activates kallikrein to release bradykinin, ultimately causing increased vascular permeability and an increase in concentration of proteins and cells in the wound spaces.
Proteoglycan	Substance found in tissues, including synovial fluid and connective tissue matrix. Proteoglycan solutions are very viscous lubricants and are sulfated GAGs. See also *Glycosaminoglycan*.	Provides a resilient matrix to inhibit cell migration. Regulates cell function and proliferation and regulates collagen fibrillogenesis.
Reactive oxygen species (ROS)	Unstable molecule containing oxygen.	ROSs are generated in response to cytokines and bacterial invasions to kill bacteria. They serve as regulators of inflammatory signaling.
Reticulin	Collagen-like fiber. Some consider it *Type III collagen fiber*.	Forms the early framework for collagen deposition in a wound.
Satellite cells	Stem cells present in muscle that lie within muscle in a normally dormant state.	These cells become activated at an injury and regenerate new muscle tissue. They also regulate fibroblast presence and activity during healing.
Secondary intention	Healing that occurs in large wounds associated with soft-tissue loss. The wound heals with granulation tissue from the bottom and sides of the wound. Epithelial tissue does not form until granulation tissue has filled the wound.	Larger scar formation occurs with healing by secondary intention. Wound contraction is evident with this healing.
Serotonin	A hormone released by mast cells and platelets.	Produces vasoconstriction in small vessels after norepinephrine activity is complete; occurs only when blood vessel endothelial walls are damaged. In later phases, initiates reactions leading to collagen cross-linking. Also involved in granuloma formation.
Steady state of a drug	Occurs when the average level of a drug remains constant in the blood, and the amount of drug leaving the body is equal to the amount being absorbed.	On average, occurs after about 5 doses; equals the drug's half-life.
Stem cell	A cell with the ability to become a specialized cell type in the body and perform specialized functions.	Starts as a generic cell and then develops into special cells with unique responsibilities, becoming mature skin, bone, blood, nerves, etc. Science may eventually use them to replace damaged cells and tissues throughout the body. Currently, they are used most often in dermal wounds.

Term	Definition	Significance or function
Stuart-Prower factor	An enzyme that is produced in the liver and requires vitamin K for its production. It is the first factor in the common pathway. Factor X.	It cleaves to prothrombin to produce thrombin.
Tenocyte	Tendon cell.	Converts to fibroblasts during tendon healing.
Tensile strength	Maximal amount of stress or force that a structure can withstand before tissue failure occurs.	Varies as tissue healing occurs; must be taken into account when determining appropriate stress application during rehabilitation.
Thrombin	An enzyme.	Converts fibrinogen to fibrin to form a fibrin plug early in the inflammation phase. In later inflammation, it stimulates fibronectin production and fibroblast proliferation.
Thromboxane	A compound that is produced by platelets and is unstable. Its half-life is 30 s. Related to prostaglandins.	Acts as a vasoconstrictor and is a potent inducer of platelet aggregation.
Tissue factor (TF)	A protein that is present in subendothelial tissue and in leukocytes. Factor III.	When cells are damaged, TF from within the cells is exposed and comes in contact with plasma, triggering the extrinsic pathway for blood clotting.
Transforming growth factor-alpha (TGF-⊠)	Growth factor produced in macrophages, brain cells, and keratinocytes.	Important in promoting angiogenesis.
Transforming growth factor-beta (TGF-⊠)	Growth factor produced in platelets, macrophages, lymphocytes, fibroblasts, bone cells, and keratinocytes.	Attracts inflammatory cells to the injury site. Stimulates fibroblasts to produce fibronectin and collagen to ultimately create the extracellular matrix.
Vascular endothelial growth factor (VEGF)	Growth factor produced by endothelial cells, macrophages, lymphocytes, granulocytes, monocytes, megakaryocytes, and smooth muscle cells.	Forms granulation tissue. Stimulates endothelial migration for enhanced angiogenesis.
Von Willebrand factor	This is a protein that helps form a blood clot. Factor XVI.	It binds to cells, molecules, and other proteins, especially factor VIII, and is important in platelet adhesion to wound sites.
White blood cells (WBCs)	Cells in the blood. There are subgroups of WBCs such as polymorphonuclear (PMN) leukocytes (multiple nuclei) and mononuclear leukocytes (one nucleus). Within the PMN subgroup are further divisions of WBCs: neutrophils, basophils, and eosinophils. Within the mononuclear subgroup there are two groups: monocytes and lymphocytes.	They fight infection and play an active role in wound healing.

*The liver must use vitamin K to produce these factors.

Healing Phases

Whether the body heals by secondary or primary intention, the process through which it proceeds is consistent and predictable in most situations. We do not yet entirely understand the process, but we can determine the outcomes of each phase.

Most of the research on various aspects of healing involve injuries that have occurred to dermal tissue;[4-8] although there may be some differences in the timing and other factors, the essential elements presented here occur in any tissue injury the rehabilitation clinician treats. Healing is a continually changing continuum of events. To clarify the process, researchers and clinicians divide the events into three[9, 10] or four[11, 12] different phases. Keep in mind, however, that as far as the body is concerned, the process is ongoing, without clear-cut delineations. The body merely continues the process until the end is achieved. These are the four phases designated by researchers and clinicians:

1. Hemostasis phase
2. Inflammation phase
3. Proliferation, or fibroplastic, phase
4. Remodeling, or maturation, phase

Healing is extremely complex from beginning to end. It starts the instant the body is injured and in some cases takes more than a year to complete. The body functions like a well-trained army to protect itself from invaders and injury, but once the body's condition is disrupted, it works as quickly as possible to restore the status quo. How the body recognizes when it is injured, how it recruits cells and chemicals, how it turns those factors off when it is appropriate, and how it moves through each process so efficiently and effectively are questions that have yet to be fully answered. Healing is a far more complex process than we can relay beyond the cursory explanation in this chapter. Table 2.2 presents a simplified version of the four stages of healing with the primary events that occur within each stage. For each of the events to occur within each of these phases, several elements, including cytokines, **chemokines**, **mediators**, growth factors, and cells may be needed. Each of these elements perform specific events at specific times throughout the healing process to ultimately resolve an injury by either healing it with scar tissue or resolving it with regenerated tissue.[13] Some of these interactions cause other substances to enter the site of injury, while other interactions change a process, reduce levels of substances, or transform structures. Oftentimes chemicals affect cells by attaching to **receptor sites** on the cells; these chemicals can then enter the cell to stimulate or change the cell's functions or alter the cell in some way.

Healing is a sophisticated process the body performs exceptionally well in most cases. In other cases, such as chronic wounds or **keloid** scars, the body doesn't perform as well. Fortunately, these are the exceptions rather than the rule. Let us look briefly at each healing phase to gain an appreciation of the body's normal healing process.

Hemostasis Phase

The advent of abundant new information on the initial reaction at an injury site has resulted in the addition of a category to the healing process, **hemostasis**. With any injury, local blood vessels are also damaged. It is this damage to the vasculature that actually initiates the body's response. Hemostasis involves the process of stopping blood flow into the injury site from these locally damaged vessels. This is the shortest healing phase but one of the more necessary ones since the others do not occur until hemostasis takes place.

When blood and lymph vessel walls suffer damage, an immediate local vasoconstriction occurs in the small vessels as the result of vasospasm.[14] This is the first of three steps in the hemostasis phase.[15] Vasoconstriction is shortly followed by vasodilation. You may have observed this when you suffered a laceration or other skin injury. At first there is no bleeding, but within less than a minute the wound starts to bleed. The second and third steps in hemostasis then occur rapidly and concurrently because the second step, primary hemostasis, is intimately connected to the third step, secondary hemostasis.[15] As **platelets** normally moving throughout the bloodstream flow out of the damaged vessel wall come in contact with the vessel wall's damaged endothelial cells; this contact with exposed collagen activates the platelets to form aggregates.[10] Platelets play a very important role in hemostasis; in fact, they provide a number of functions, among which are adhesion and activation.[16] Their first role, as mentioned, is to create a blood clot through an aggregate formation by adhering

TABLE 2.2   Summary of Healing Phases and Primary Activities Within Each One

Hemostasis phase	Inflammation phase	Proliferation phase	Remodeling phase
Vasoconstriction	Vasodilation	Fibroblast infiltration	Collagen remodeling to Type I
Platelet activation	Vascular permeability	Re-epithelialization	Scar tissue maturation
Platelet plug formation	Neutrophil infiltration	Angiogenesis	Microvascular regression
Coagulation cascade	Macrophage infiltration	Extracellular matrix formation	Tensile strength increase
Fibrin plug formation	Lymphocyte infiltration	Type III collagen formation	
	Debridement	Wound contraction by myofibroblasts	

to collagen and other platelets. This initial clot that is formed is weak, consisting of those platelets that adhere to the collagen ends with some support coming from **von Willebrand factor**. The initial clot forms the **primary hemostasis** that creates a "dam" to stop the "river" of blood flow caused by the injury.[16, 17]

When platelets make contact with injured collagen ends and the injured cells' extracellular matrix, they are stimulated to release a number of important elements. These substances released by platelets include clotting factors, growth factors, and cytokines.[12] As more platelets move into the area and add to the dam, a clot forms.[16] This platelet-based formation serves as the base onto which a stronger formation will attach. In a short time, clotting factors go through a cascade of events to form a more stable fibrin-based plug.[14] This coagulation cascade is the process by which the body develops the final hemostasis step, secondary hemostasis.

This clotting process is sometimes referred to as the blood clotting cascade or the coagulation cascade[14, 18, 19] because once the process is in motion, a series of events occurs in rapid succession, each step facilitated by the previous one, to create the fibrin clot, or fibrin plug. Several years ago Davie and Ratnoff[20] and MacFarlane[21] compared the sequence of events that occurs during blood clot formation to a waterfall. They explained that protein-clotting factors affect other protein factors by behaving like enzymes to activate specific factors, and this follows a specific sequence of events until a fibrin clot is formed.[20] Although it was not well understood at the time, they knew that one clotting factor could activate another. We now know that when a clotting factor is activated, it changes from its inactive protein form to its activated enzyme form.

Clotting factors have been long identified by Roman numerals, ordered in the sequence in which they were discovered.[22] Rather than renaming the clotting factor once it became activated, it was decided to add an *a* to the Roman numeral. For example, factor II became factor IIa when it was activated; in this example, factor II is also known as prothrombin, but when it becomes activated it converts to thrombin. See table 2.3 for a list of the clotting factors, their Roman numeral assignments, the names by which they were known before the Roman numeral system became established, and their functions in hemostasis. Normally, these clotting factors flow through the bloodstream in their inactive forms. When an injury occurs, endothelial cells that make up the inner lining of the blood vessel wall become damaged and release tissue factor (III). Tissue factor then triggers the series of events that Davie and Ratnoff[20] termed a "waterfall sequence," which later evolved to become known as the "coagulation cascade" or the "blood clotting cascade."

The coagulation system is generally divided into three different pathways: extrinsic, intrinsic, and common.[23] The **extrinsic pathway** is sometimes referred to as the tissue factor pathway or TF pathway because the protein that attaches to cell surfaces is named **tissue factor**. This pathway requires the plasma that carries this protein to come into contact with something extrinsic—outside the blood serum—to trigger the blood clotting mechanism.[14, 19] The **intrinsic pathway** is also referred to as the contact pathway because it can be triggered without adding an outside factor to the blood serum.[14, 19] The final pathway, the **common pathway**, consists of the cascade of activation of clotting factors that ultimately cleave thrombin from prothrombin to form a stable clot.[14, 19] Figure 2.1 provides an illustration of the three cascade pathways involved in hemostasis and identifies the clotting factors for each of the pathways.

The fibrin mesh that results from the coagulation cascade binds together in a cross-link arrangement with the exposed collagen and platelets that formed the initial hemostatic plug; this forms a lattice-like complex that further reinforces the platelet plug and forms the fibrin plug. This plug is stronger than the primary plug and results in what is known as the **secondary hemostasis**. This secondary plug is temporary, and although it is stronger than the platelet plug, it is still relatively fragile. In these early hours it provides the wound's only **tensile strength**.[24] Tensile strength is the maximal stress or force a structure is able to withstand before that structure fails. As healing progresses, this weak plug is replaced by stronger Type III collagen.

In addition to blood vessels, the more fragile lymph vessels are also damaged at the time of injury. Leakage from these vessels is also halted by the fibrin plug formation. Once fluid accumulates in the extracellular spaces, as it does after an injury, the only way this edema can be removed is through the lymph system. Unfortunately, because the lymph vessels are blocked by the fibrin plug, their ability to reduce the area's swelling is compromised. Once the injured site becomes stable, **fibrinolysin** is released. Fibrinolysin is a plasma-derived enzyme that converts fibrin from an insoluble to a soluble protein to promote the absorption of the fibrin plug, and it allows the lymph vessels to perform their normal function, draining the area of edema (excess fluid).[25] This process, fibrinolysis, occurs during the inflammation phase at about day 3.[25]

Inflammation Phase

Inflammation often has negative connotations. In reality, it is an important and necessary step in the healing process. Without inflammation, the body would be unable to completely heal after injury. If inflammation did not occur, proliferation, maturation, and final resolution would not

TABLE 2.3 Clotting Factors

Clotting factor Roman numeral and its conversion numeral	Clotting factor name	Additional names	Functions	Clotting pathway
I → Ia	Fibrinogen		Converts fibrinogen to fibrin to form a clot	Common
II → IIa	Prothrombin		Converts to thrombin	Common
III → IIIa	Tissue factor	TF	Triggers blood clotting through the extrinsic mechanism	Extrinsic
IV → IVa	Calcium	Ca++	Binds to phospholipids to facilitate clotting	All three
V → Va	Proaccelerin	Labile factor		Extrinsic and intrinsic
VI → VIa	No longer exists		Thought to be identical to factor V	None
VII → VIIa	Proconvertin	Stable factor	Initiates the coagulation cascade with tissue factor	Extrinsic
VIII → VIIIa	Antihemophilic factor A		Essential for blood clotting	Intrinsic
IX → IXa	Antihemophilic factor B	Christmas factor	Essential for blood clotting	Intrinsic
X → Xa	Stuart-Power factor		Combines with prothrombin to create thrombin in the final pathway	Extrinsic and intrinsic
XI → XIa	Plasma thromboplastin antecedent	Hemophilia C or Rosenthal syndrome	Helps generate thrombin to form the fibrin clot	Intrinsic
XII → XIIa	Hageman factor		Initiates the blood clotting cascade of the intrinsic pathway	Intrinsic
XIII → XIIIa	Fibrin stabilizing factor	Laki-Lorand factor	Stabilizes the fibrin clot by enabling cross-links within the fibrin strands	Common
XIV → XIVa	Prekallikrein	PK or F Fletcher	Cleaved by the Hageman factor to produce kallikrein	Intrinsic
XV → XVa	High molecular weight kininogen	HMWK or F Fitzgerald	Initiates blood coagulation	Intrinsic
XVI → XVIa	von Willebrand factor	vWf	Important in platelet adhesion at wounds; binds to other proteins	Intrinsic
XVII → XVIIa	Antithrombin III			Anticoagulant
XVIII → XVIIIa	Heparin cofactor II			Anticoagulant
XIX → XIXa	Protein C		Prevents coagulation by inactivating factors V and VIII	Anticoagulant
XX → XXa	Protein S		Prevents coagulation by inactivating factors V and VIII	Anticoagulant

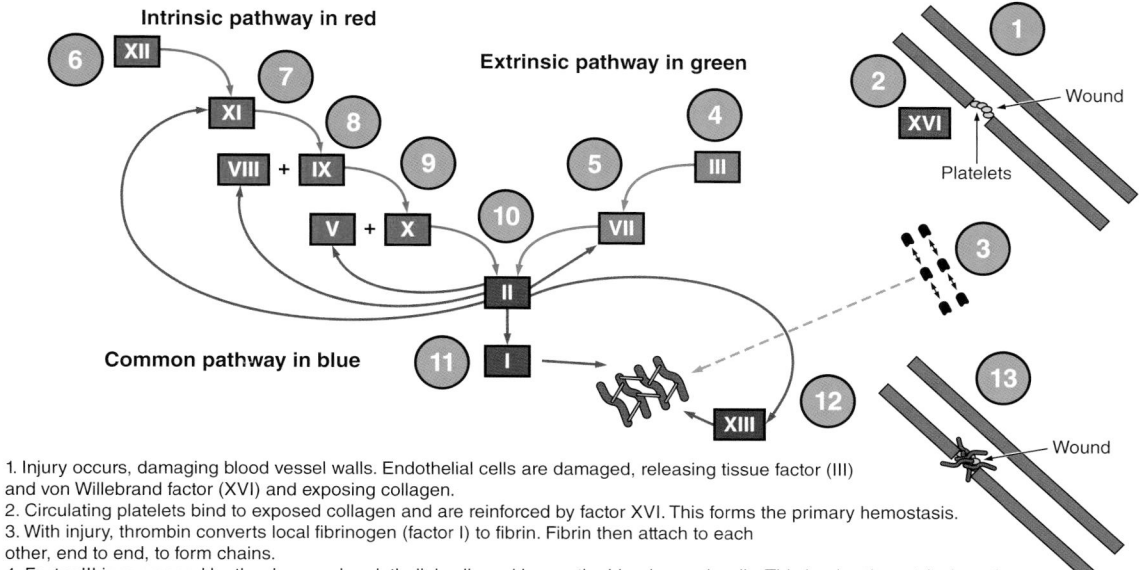

Intrinsic pathway in red

Extrinsic pathway in green

Common pathway in blue

1. Injury occurs, damaging blood vessel walls. Endothelial cells are damaged, releasing tissue factor (III) and von Willebrand factor (XVI) and exposing collagen.
2. Circulating platelets bind to exposed collagen and are reinforced by factor XVI. This forms the primary hemostasis.
3. With injury, thrombin converts local fibrinogen (factor I) to fibrin. Fibrin then attach to each other, end to end, to form chains.
4. Factor III is expressed by the damaged endothelial cells making up the blood vessel walls. This begins the extrinsic pathway.
5. Factor IIIa activates factor VII to become VIIa.
6. Hageman factor (XII) becomes activated with exposure to endothelial collagen from the damaged blood vessel walls and becomes XIIa.
7. Factor XIIa activates factor XI to become XIa.
8. Factor XIa activates IX to become IXa.
9. Factor IXa activates factor X (Stuart-Prower) into factor Xa.
10. In the intrinsic pathway, factor Xa activates factor II (prothrombin). In the extrinsic pathway, factor III also activates factor II. At this point the intrinsic and extrinsic pathways merge to become the common pathway. The activated version of prothrombin is thrombin.
11. Thrombin performs a number of activities: It activates factors V, VII, VIII, XI, and XIII to convert each of them to their active form (Va, VIIa, VIIIa, XIa, and XIIIa, respectively). It also activates fibrinogen to convert it from I to Ia (fibrin). NOTE: Factors V and VIII are co-factors that must work with factors X and IX, respectively, in order for those factors to function as they should.
12. Factor XIII activates to form the cross bridges between the fibrin strands to form a fibrin mesh.
13. The fibrin mesh holds the platelet plug together and forms the stronger secondary hemostasis.

Figure 2.1   Cascade of coagulation events involving clotting factors following an injury, leading to hemostasis via the fibrin plug formation. In each step, each factor is a proenzyme that becomes activated by a prior catalyst, and it in turn activates the next factor until the cascade becomes complete with the clot formation. The brown circled numbers are the sequential steps in this cascade of events.

take place. On the other hand, inflammation becomes harmful when it is prolonged beyond the normal healing time.

The goal of rehabilitation clinicians is to allow inflammation to occur but to minimize its secondary effects of localized edema, pain, redness, warmth, and reduced function. This is done at the time of injury by applying initial first aid: ice, compression, elevation, and rest.

As the injury's status changes over the first few days, the clinician minimizes inflammation and encourages healing to continue along its normal path by using various treatment modalities.[26] To make appropriate decisions about when to use therapeutic modalities and therapeutic exercise techniques in the rehabilitation program, the clinician must understand the healing process. Let us examine the series of events involved in the second phase of healing, the inflammation phase.

Once a clot forms, the inflammation phase begins.[27] As the platelets adhere to collagen and other extracellular matrix structures, they activate to change shape.[16] Platelets, along with other substances present in the region, stimulate the mobilization of chemicals and cells into the injured area.[28] These extremely complex processes take 2 to 3 d and sometimes up to a week to 10 d to complete.[9] A simplified version of hemostasis and the inflammation phases is presented in figure 2.2. The injured area is an extremely busy site during this time as the body tries to protect the site and begin the process of returning to the status quo as well as possible.

CLINICAL TIPS

The four phases of healing are hemostasis, inflammation, proliferation, and remodeling. During hemostasis, the injury is contained and stabilized by clot formation. During inflammation, debris is removed in preparation for recovery. During proliferation, the presence and activity of fibroblasts, myofibroblasts, and collagen peak to begin granulation tissue formation and angiogenesis. During remodeling, wound contraction is well underway, and Type III collagen converts to Type I collagen to stabilize and restore the injury site.

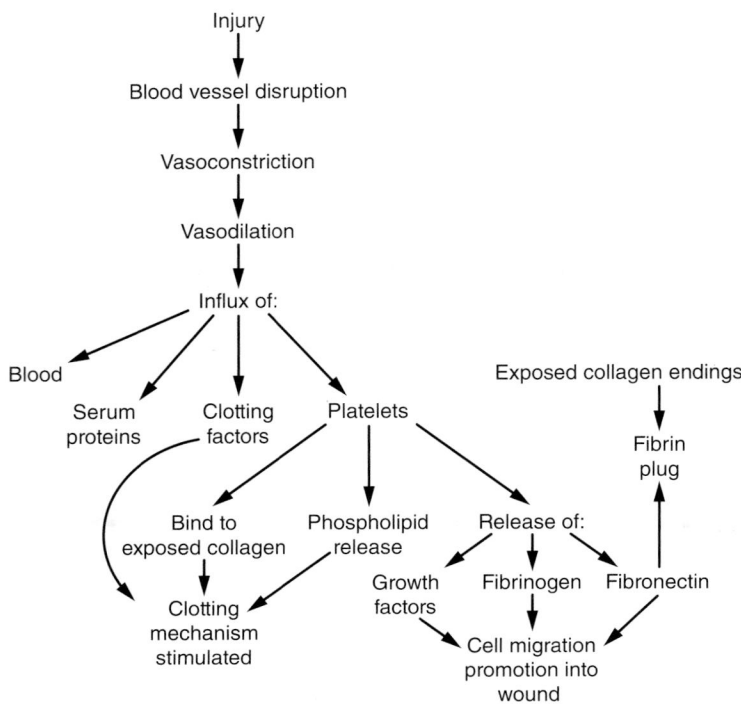

Figure 2.2   Immediate injury response.

Cellular Reactions

As during the hemostasis phase, several cells enter the injured site at the start of injury and continue to migrate throughout the inflammation phase. Platelets and other cells that formed the fibrin clot continue to work in other ways during the early days of inflammation, releasing chemicals that attract other cells and chemicals into the area, including additional platelets, leukocytes, and fibroblasts.[10] Cytokines and growth factors play important roles throughout the healing process. **Cytokines** are proteins that are produced by various cells, especially white blood cells. They also are produced by platelets and endothelium. Examples of cytokines include interleukins (IL), interferons (IF), and tumor necrosis factors (TNF). These cytokines have a variety of responsibilities, such as expressing growth hormones; attracting macrophages, fibroblasts, and neutrophils; and stimulating neovascularization.[29] Figure 2.3 is a schematic presentation of this process. As these products accumulate in the injury, chemicals are released, and other cells are attracted into the area. Platelets release other important substances, such as **fibronectin**, **growth factors**, and **fibrinogen**.[28] The growth factors released by platelets include platelet-derived growth factor (PDGF), fibroblast growth factor (FGF), transforming growth factor alpha (TGF-α), and transforming growth factor beta (TFG-β).[10, 12] Each of these substances is important in the healing process. Table 2.4 summarizes

their actions and those of other growth factors that are active during the healing process.

During early inflammation within the first few hours of injury, the body tries to remove debris from the site. This process is started within 5 or 6 h of injury by **neutrophils**, or **polymorphonuclear leukocytes (PMNs)**. These PMNs contain toxic chemicals that allow them to bind to microorganisms and destroy them. The inflammation phase is named after these cells. Neutrophils are the most plentiful white blood cells in the body, and they migrate into the wound in great numbers, but their presence is short-lived. Other white blood cells in the granular leukocyte family include eosinophils and basophils; these white blood cells play a larger role in immune and allergic responses than they do in tissue healing after injury.[35, 36]

The cells that replace the neutrophils are the **mononuclear phagocytes**: **monocytes** and **macrophages**. These cells become the predominant cells at the injury site within 24 to 48 h. Both PMNs and macrophages act as **phagocytes** to remove debris and dead tissue from the area.[37, 38] Macrophages perform a number of tasks in addition to phagocytosis. They are now thought to be important regulators in the wound-healing response in addition to removing debris; other activities of macrophages include assisting in the fight against infections, promoting the inflammation phase as well as ending it, and secreting cytokines and growth factors that either recruit or activate

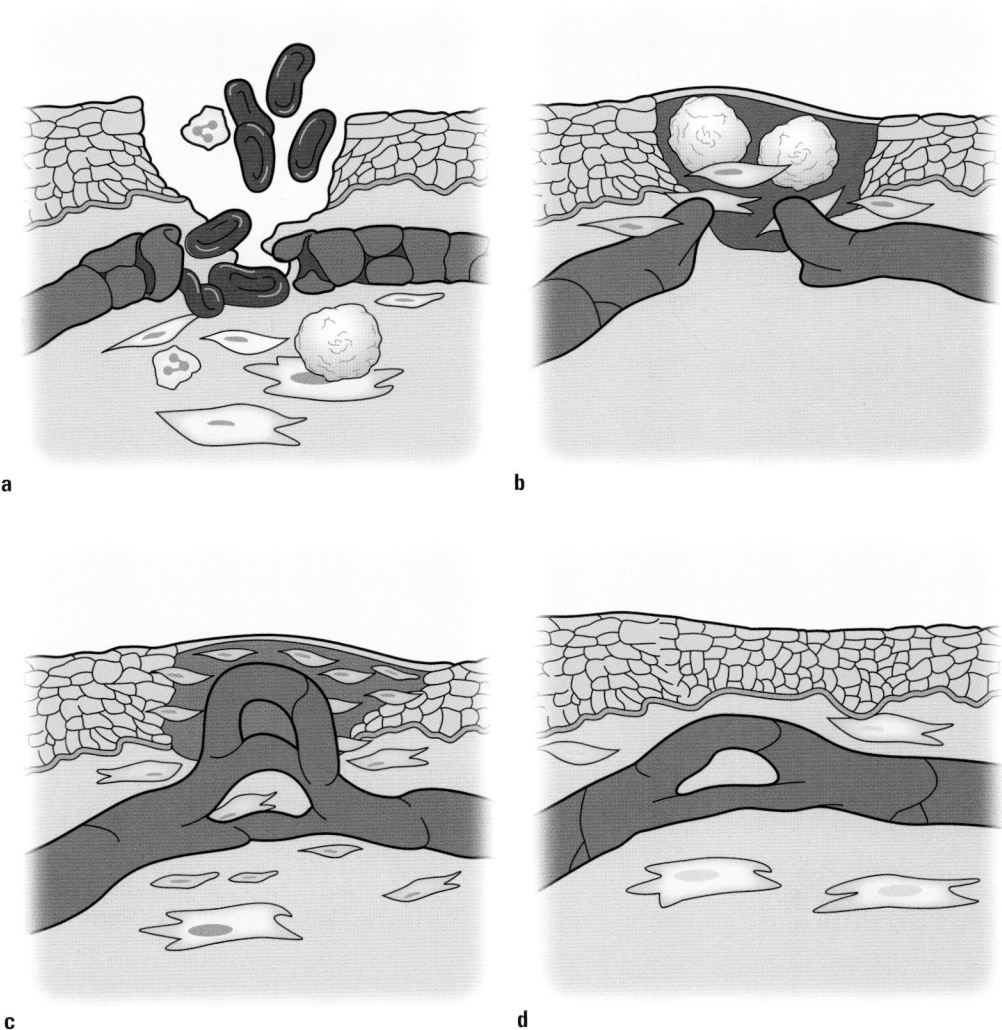

Figure 2.3   Epidermal wound healing. *(a)* Release of blood and blood products at time of injury. *(b)* Macrophages and fibroblasts in the area with capillary buds apparent. *(c)* Angiogenesis has caused anastomosis with new capillary growth. Fibroblasts are present in large numbers. *(d)* Re-epithelialization has occurred. Regression of earlier established capillaries is noted.

other cells that play a role in the repair process.[39] As we move through the healing process, these additional tasks of macrophages will be noted when they occur.

As the inflammatory process proceeds, an inflammatory **exudate** is formed from the fluid escaping from the local vessels, dead tissue as a result of the injury, and dying PMNs as their short life spans (about 24 h)[40] end. Inflammatory exudate is commonly whitish and differs from the exudate seen in an infection, which contains bacteria and has a yellow, brown, or green tint to the discharge. Although normally produced exudate is often referred to as pus, Peacock[41] feels that this is a misnomer and prefers to refer to this uninfected substance as *cell aggregation centers,* not pus.

Debridement (removal of debris) is necessary for healing to continue. Before the subsequent healing phases can occur, the injury site must be cleared of excess fluid and other waste materials that have accumulated. Much like remodeling a room or rebuilding an engine, all of the old and useless materials must be removed before new construction can begin. For this reason alone, macrophages are vital to the healing process, but they perform other important functions as well. Once at the injury site, they recruit and activate other macrophages to assist in debridement. Macrophages also release growth factors and may trigger the termination of tissue growth when the healing process is complete.[12]

TABLE 2.4   Growth Factors That Influence Healing

Growth factor	Source	Target	Cell proliferation and chemotactic activity
Epidermal growth factor (EGF)	Epithelial cells Macrophages Monocytes Platelets	Fibroblasts Epithelium Endothelium	Signals the start of the cascade of chemical events that enhance cell mobility. Increases epithelialization rate. Prevents excessive scarring.
Transforming growth factor alpha (TGF-α)	Platelets Macrophages Epithelium	Endothelial cells Fibroblasts Epithelial cells	Similar functions to EGF but is a stronger angiogenesis factor. Is chemotactic for and stimulates production of keratinocytes and fibroblasts.
Transforming growth factor beta (TGF-β)	Macrophages Platelets Mast cells Epithelium	Endothelium Fibroblasts Epithelial cells Lymphocytes Epithelium Monocytes	Attracts inflammatory cells to the site. Stimulates extracellular matrix production. Stimulates fibroblasts to produce fibronectin and collagen.
Fibroblast growth factor (FGF)	Macrophages Monocytes Endothelial cells Keratinocytes Fibroblasts Smooth muscle cells Mast cells Chondrocytes	Fibroblasts Endothelium Keratinocytes	Stimulates proliferation and migration of endothelial cells, fibroblasts, chondrocytes, and myoblasts. Stimulates production of fibronectin, proteoglycans, and collagen. Stimulates cell migration, granulation tissue formation, and neovascularization.
Platelet-derived growth factor (PDGF)	Platelets Macrophages Monocytes Endothelial cells Epithelial cells	Fibroblasts	Attracts neutrophils and macrophages to the site. Increases production of other growth factors. Increases fibroblast production of collagenase.
Insulin-like growth factor (IGF)	Fibroblasts Macrophages Endothelial cells	Fibroblasts Keratinocytes	Regulates tissue growth, development, and repair. Affects muscle tissue repair and reinnervation by increasing protein production, cell proliferation, and cell migration. Improves wound strength.
Vascular endothelial growth factor (VEGF)	Endothelial cells Macrophages Lymphocytes Granulocytes Monocytes Megakaryocytes Smooth muscle cells	Endothelial cells	Forms granulation tissue. Stimulates endothelial migration for enhanced angiogenesis.
Keratinocyte growth factor (KGF)	Fibroblasts	Keratinocytes	Stimulates migration, differentiation, and proliferation of keratinocytes in skin wounds.

Based on Falabella and Falanga (2001); Diegelmann and Evans (2004); Alfaro et al. (2013); Koria (2012); Demidova-Rice, Hamblin, and Herman (2012); Pandit, Ashar, and Feldman (1999); Steenfos (1994).[10, 12, 30-34]

Chemical Reactions

There is an intimate interaction between cells and chemicals throughout healing. A cascade of events occurs because of their interacting stimuli.[28] Some cells stimulate the production of chemicals, and certain chemicals at the injury site stimulate the arrival or production of specific cells in the area. This process of attraction or stimulation is called **chemotaxis**.

A good example of chemotaxis is the series of events that causes vascular permeability. Vascular permeability is a crucial event that initiates the inflammation phase. It allows cells and chemicals that normally remain in the bloodstream to enter the injury site and perform their healing functions so that the area's structures can return as nearly as possible to normal. Vascular permeability is initially caused by **histamine** in the injured site. Histamine is released by cells such as platelets, PMNs, and **mast cells** that enter the area. Histamine is a **chemotactic factor** for **leukocytes**, or white blood cells, causing them to enter the injury site. Histamine is a short-lived, local hormone whose function of vascular permeability is continued by **serotonin** and **kinins**, which enter the area as histamine quantities recede.[9] Serotonin is released by mast cells and platelets, and kinins are released by plasma.[16, 42, 43]

The presence of kinins in the injury site is short term; they are followed by **prostaglandin (PG)** formation. Once kinins are released and a **complement system** is formed from serum proteins, PGs are discharged by damaged cells. This stimulation of proteins that are normally inactive until they enter the area of injury is also referred to as a **complement cascade** because of the surge of events that follow the activation of this system. These proteins are important to the healing process.[28] They are stimulated to release cytokines; the end result increases phagocytosis to clear damaged cells, foreign substances, and other debris from the injury site.[44]

There are two PGs that are most evident and perform important functions: PGE_1 and PGE_2. The functions of PGE_1 include local vasodilation[45, 46] and increasing vascular permeability.[47] PGE_2 is responsible for accelerating the completion of platelet aggregation.[48] In addition to the roles played in wound healing, there is also consistent evidence to demonstrate that both PGE_1 and PGE_2 are vital in the body's immune system defenses.[49] As healing progresses, they both appear to stimulate repair of the damaged area and permit advancement to the proliferative phase. They also seem to have a role in continuing inflammation at the same time.[50] It is these compounds that are influenced by anti-inflammatory drugs, discussed later in this chapter.

During all of this continuous activity, additional chemical reactions are also occurring. **Hageman factor**, also known as **factor XII**, is area plasma protein that becomes activated. In its activated state as an enzyme, it stimulates the production of **kallikrein**, which increases vascular permeability and vasodilation.[41]

Signs of Inflammation

Many complex events are ongoing during the inflammation phase. The injured area undergoes intense activity during this time. We see evidence of the degree of activity as common signs of inflammation, including localized redness, edema, pain, increased temperature, and loss of normal function. Edema is caused by the leakage of fluid, cells, and chemicals into the area because of the local vasodilation and increased vascular permeability. The increase in local cellular and chemical activity increases local temperature. Histamine and other released hormones along with vasodilation cause redness. Edema is also the result of more substances in the area and of the blockage of lymph vessels whose normal function of drainage is constrained by the newly formed fibrin plug. Chemical substances that are released at the site, including histamine, prostaglandins, and **bradykinin**,[51] make the local nerve endings hypersensitive and irritable, causing pain. Pressure from edema on nerve endings also causes pain. Pain causes a withdrawal reflex, which reduces the function of surrounding structures, limiting the patient's normal functional ability. Direct damage to tissues also prevents them from functioning normally. These signs and their primary causes are illustrated in figure 2.4.

Proliferation Phase

As previously mentioned, there is an overlap of phases as the injury site heals. Figure 2.5 demonstrates that there is no clear-cut delineation between one phase and another. Rather, as the body steadily accomplishes the tasks in one phase, the next phase evolves. The proliferation phase begins 3 to 4 d after the injury and continues for 2 to 4 weeks.[52]

Although many cells and chemicals are involved during the inflammation phase, the macrophages (monocytes) are most responsible for removing debris and dead tissue from the area. As this task is accomplished and reaching its end, the development and growth of new blood vessels and **granulation tissue** begins. This transition from debridement to **angiogenesis** and formation of granulation tissue marks the beginning of the proliferation phase. Angiogenesis occurs at a rapid rate during this phase. This process is important, for scar tissue formation requires vascular production and supply if subsequent events of healing are to follow.

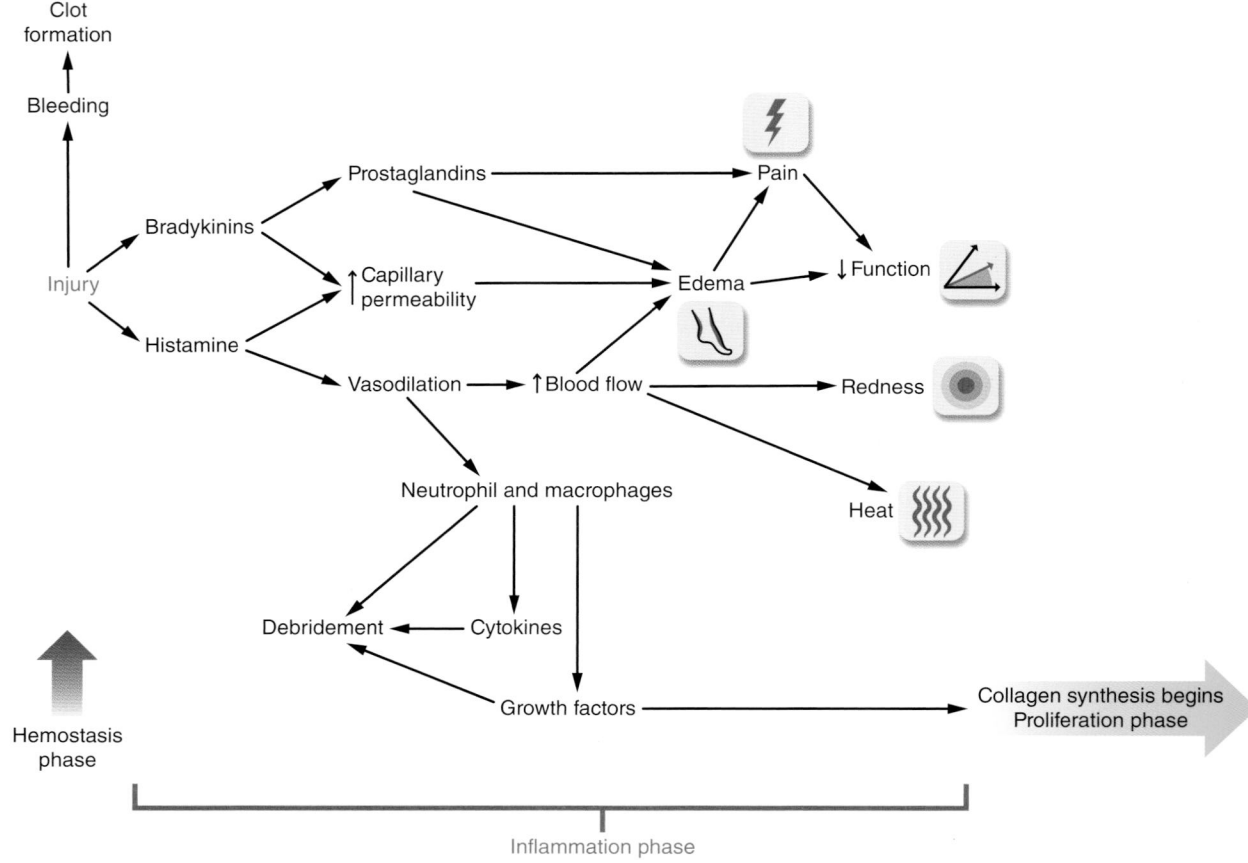

Figure 2.4 The inflammation phase of healing immediately follows the hemostatic phase and leads into the proliferation phase. A number of activities, including the release of mediators such as compounds and growth factors resulting in cellular reactions and various infiltrations, lead to the signature signs of inflammation: pain, edema, redness, warmth, and reduced functional level of the injured segment.

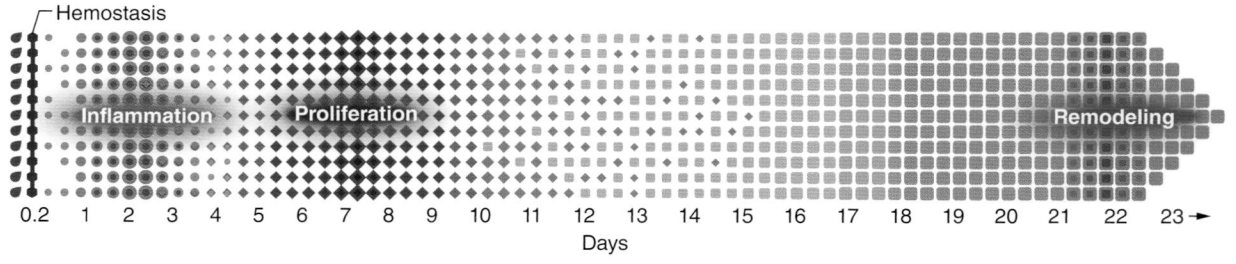

Figure 2.5 Tissue healing phases. Note the overlap of these phases and the increase in predominance of the phases over time before the next phase evolves.

The cells largely responsible for production of this new growth are **fibroblasts**. Fibroblasts are seen in greatly increased numbers 3 to 5 d after injury. This significant increase in fibroblasts and a decrease to minimal or non-existent levels of PMNs are the hallmarks of the wound site's transition from inflammation to proliferation. Other activities that indicate that the injury is transitioning into the proliferation phase include a significant increase in extracellular collagen production, increased **proteoglycans**, and epithelial cell mitosis. The duration of the proliferation phase depends on factors such as the size and site of the injury and the tissue type involved. Generally, the proliferation phase is thought to last 2 to 4 weeks.[41]

As is true during the inflammation phase, there is an interactive response among cells and chemicals in the area throughout the proliferation phase. Additional growth factors, for example, enter into the area because of chemotaxis produced by platelets and macrophages. In turn, these growth factors are responsible for the local migration and proliferation of **endothelial cells**, fibroblasts, and conversion of some fibroblasts to **myofibroblasts**.[9, 30, 53]

Growth factors and cytokines mediate new blood vessel development.[54, 55] Another important factor in angiogenesis is the oxygen pressure gradient between the wound edges and wound bed.[56, 57] Low oxygen levels in the area facilitate an influx of cells and growth factors to increase angiogenesis.[58, 59] In addition to growth factors, migration of fibroblasts is also important during proliferation because these are cells that are primarily responsible for new capillary and **extracellular matrix (ECM)** formation. Although the initially formed matrix is not very strong, it holds the wound together and helps protect it from infection and stress.[4, 60] This wound matrix is eventually replaced by a collagen matrix that is stronger and protects the new blood vessels that are forming during this time. Fibroblasts produce substances that will eventually make up this matrix. These substances, which include collagen, proteoglycans, and elastin, are needed for ultimate scar tissue formation and maturation.[28]

Granulation tissue is the combination of the matrix and newly formed capillary buds. Granulation tissue is typically a bright, beefy red color. This is because the new capillary buds make up a significant part of the granulation tissue.[61, 62] Endothelial cells, the most important cells in the formation of these capillaries, contain a **plasminogen activator**.[63, 64] The plasminogen activator breaks down and removes the fibrin network that was formed during the inflammation phase so that lymphatic flow for removing local excess fluid can be restored.

The extracellular matrix has two components: fibrous and nonfibrous elements. The nonfibrous element is **ground substance**. This is a gel-like substance composed of **glycosaminoglycan (GAG)**, proteoglycans, and **glycoproteins**. The ground substance fills in the spaces between the fibrous elements of the ECM and reduces friction between the fibers when stress is applied to the tissue.

Fibrous elements of the ECM include collagen, **reticulin**, and **elastin**. Collagen and reticulin are inelastic, while elastin has elastic qualities. The combination of these types of fibers provides both tensile strength and some resilience to stresses that are applied to the tissue.

During the early proliferation phase, in the first 5 to 7 d after injury, the fibroblasts produce these elements of the extracellular matrix.[65, 66] They form the ground substance and rapidly lay down collagen. The activity during this phase is the result of new capillary growth by the fibroblasts. Capillary growth is followed by epithelial development across the granulating wound.[57] As the epithelium progresses across the wound, epithelial cells and fibroblasts stimulated by the epithelial cells both release **collagenase**.[67] Collagenase is an enzyme that prevents overproduction of collagen in a wound. This is an important process in normal tissue healing. An example of uncontrolled collagen production is keloid formations (excessive scar tissue formations), a condition sometimes seen in dermal injuries.[68]

Collagen produced in these early days of healing is Type III collagen. It is seen as early as 48 to 72 h after the injury occurs.[12] The fiber structure of Type III collagen is weak and thin. Although it is relatively weak, it is the substance that provides the wound's primary tensile strength in the early stages of healing. Type III collagen is laid down in a haphazard manner, without organized arrangement, further reducing the injury site's tensile strength. It is later replaced by Type I collagen, a stronger and more durable collagen.

Tensile strength is directly related to the amount, type, and arrangement of collagen.[69] By day 7 there is a significant amount of collagen in the area. By the second week, immature Type III collagen begins to be replaced by the stronger Type I collagen, and cross-links between the collagen fibers develop.[70] Both of these occurrences add significant strength to the injury site.

While these processes are occurring, a GAG known as **hyaluronic acid**, a part of the extracellular matrix, is present and also contributes to the healing process. Hyaluronic acid is a gel-like substance that draws water into the area and holds it there.[71] This provides additional room for the proliferating fibroblasts in the wound site.

Although the proliferation phase generally occurs from 5 d after the injury to around day 21,[41] this timeline can vary.[65] The type of tissue damaged and the extent of the injury are factors that make this timeline variable. In slower-healing tissue with extensive injury, proliferation is known to take much longer than 3 weeks.

External signs seen in this phase demonstrate the ongoing healing activity that cannot be seen. The combination of increased capillaries present and additional water volume accounts for the redness and swelling in the area. Pressure-sensitive nerve endings cause the site to be sensitive to the area's increased volumetric pressure just as the tension-sensitive nerve endings make the area painful when it is stretched.

Remodeling Phase

During the remodeling phase, the wound matures and converts to permanent scar tissue. There is much yet to be understood about this phase, for it has not been as well studied as other healing phases.[10] Some of the activities that began during the proliferation phase continue into the remodeling phase. One example of this is wound contraction. Myofibroblasts are responsible for this activity. These cells have been observed in wounds by the fifth day and have been seen more than 2 months after the injury.[72, 73] Some of the fibroblasts convert to myofibroblasts that migrate to the wound's periphery and pull the wound edges toward the center to reduce the wound's size.[73] The entire mechanism and function of myofibroblasts is very complex. With additional understanding of myoblasts' role and functions in healing, investigators have used these knowledge advances to alter tissue engineering techniques to improve skin graft properties.[74] In spite of the advances in our understanding of myofibroblasts, there is much we must learn before we can fully comprehend their unique functions. Wound contraction also occurs with continued remodeling because of collagen production, collagen cross-linking, and adhesions between collagen and adjacent tissues.[75]

Wound contraction makes the scar smaller. This is advantageous, but it can be detrimental when joints are affected. If an injury occurs across or near a joint, scar tissue contraction and adhesions can limit motion at that joint. Indirect effects of wound contraction may also occur if the wound is large and impacts adjacent areas. Some investigators are finding that the introduction of growth factors into healing tissue may reduce wound contraction.[76] The clinical importance of preventing the adverse effects of scar tissue contraction is discussed later in this chapter in the section "Factors That Affect Healing."

Another activity that begins during the proliferation phase and continues into the remodeling phase is collagen transition. As Type I collagen is synthesized, Type III collagen is destroyed. When the construction rate of Type I fibers equals the destruction rate of Type III fibers, the healing process advances to the final and longest phase, remodeling. This phase is generally about 12 months long, but it may range from 6 months to 18 months.[68, 77]

A number of activities diminish as the area becomes more stable and more permanent in its cellular and structural arrangement.[10] The large number of capillaries created during the proliferation phase to promote tissue growth is no longer needed and recedes. The extra capillaries will eventually disappear entirely.[41] Glycoproteins, GAGs, and the cells responsible for them—fibroblasts—in the extracellular matrix decrease significantly. Myofibroblasts also diminish.

With these cellular changes, visible changes can also be seen. These observable changes include the loss of the granulation tissue's red color with progressive color changes, first to whitish, and eventually to more normal skin tones as scar tissue completes its maturation. With the loss of extracellular matrix substances, swelling diminishes. Wound sensitivity also lessens.

As collagen converts to predominantly Type I, the tissue becomes more resilient and more resistant to stress and destruction. As fluid content becomes less, the collagen fibers develop more cross-links with each other, further strengthening the scar's structure. This collagen cross-linking becomes the primary source of the scar's tensile strength.[78]

The primary activity during the remodeling phase is the change that occurs in the wound's collagen structure and arrangement; hence its name. Tensile strength becomes enhanced with changes in its collagen fiber arrangement. When collagen fibers align in an organized, parallel fashion, collagen is able to form its greatest number of cross-links and thereby possess optimal strength. The greatest degree of function and mobility occurs when collagen has this organized arrangement.[41] External forces properly applied to tissue can influence and enhance this arrangement.[79]

Table 2.5 summarizes in chronological order the phases of healing and identifies the primary activities and their timeline. Figure 2.6 presents the healing phases with their primary cells and important functions for each of the phases highlighted in boxes.

Growth Factors

Growth factors are proteins that serve many functions. They interact with each other and with other substances to promote the healing process. Growth factors are in the cytokine classification.[80] Not all cytokines are growth factors, but because there are many similarities between them, the terms are often used interchangeably,[80] although such usage is not always accurate. Their complete role in healing is complex and not yet fully understood. One reason their function is difficult to understand is that their action *in vitro* is different than it is *in vivo*, so what is observed in the laboratory is not necessarily what occurs in the body.[81, 82] Another complication is that what they do and how they perform in laboratory animals is not necessarily what occurs in humans.

CLINICAL TIPS

A number of growth factors are important for normal healing. If they are not present, healing is delayed or prevented.[12] Recent studies demonstrate accelerated healing with applications of these growth factors.[83]

TABLE 2.5   Chronology of Wound Healing

Phase	Time	Activity	Purpose or result
Hemostasis	Immediate	Vascular contraction followed by vasodilation and infiltration and activation of platelets Enzymatic cascade	Platelets adhere to collagen stump ends to create an initial blood clot; platelets also release chemicals that attract other substances into the area to begin inflammation. Fibrinogen converts to fibrin to aid in sealing damaged vessels by forming a fibrin mesh that intertwines with the initial clot formed by platelets to establish a stronger fibrin clot.
Inflammation	1 d	Platelets continuing to activate Growth factors present Neutrophil migration	Chemoattractant for inflammatory cells, macrophages, and neutrophils. Fight contamination. Release growth factors and biologically reactive substances, secrete cytokines to attract monocytes and other specialized cells. Macrophages engulf debris to clean area in preparation for healing.
Inflammation	1–2 d	→ Monocyte migration	Phagocytose bacteria. Area is warm, red, tender, swollen.
Inflammation	2 d	Growth factors present	Attract fibroblasts to produce collagen, proteoglycans, fibronectin, elastin.
Inflammation	2–3 d	Fibroblasts producing Type III collagen	Provide more strength than fibrin clot.
Proliferation	3–4 d	→ Rapid increase in fibroblasts Increased epithelial cell mitosis Increased synthesis of extracellular collagen Increased proteoglycans	Extracellular matrix is formed via granulation tissue development. Platelets and macrophages release angiogenic factors secondary to low oxygen tension to stimulate vascular bud production on damaged capillary ends.
Proliferation	5 d	→ Myofibroblast production	Wound contraction.
Proliferation	5–7 d	Collagen synthesis very active	Increased production of Type III collagen.
Remodeling	5–9 d	Reduction in fibroblasts Reduction in macrophages Reduction in wound vascularity → Reduction in fibronectin in proportion to the amount of Type I collagen formed	Reduces redness.
Remodeling	10 d	Myofibroblasts present	Wound contraction continues.
Remodeling	12 d	→ Type III collagen converting to Type I	Increased strength of structure.
Remodeling	6–18 wk	→ Reduction in capillaries	Reduced fluid content, increased scar density.
Remodeling	6–18 mo	Collagenase, gelatinase, stromelysins stimulated via growth factors Completion of all healing	Breakdown of cellular matrix and progressive slowdown of tissue synthesis to end repair process.

Note: → = Key activities of each phase

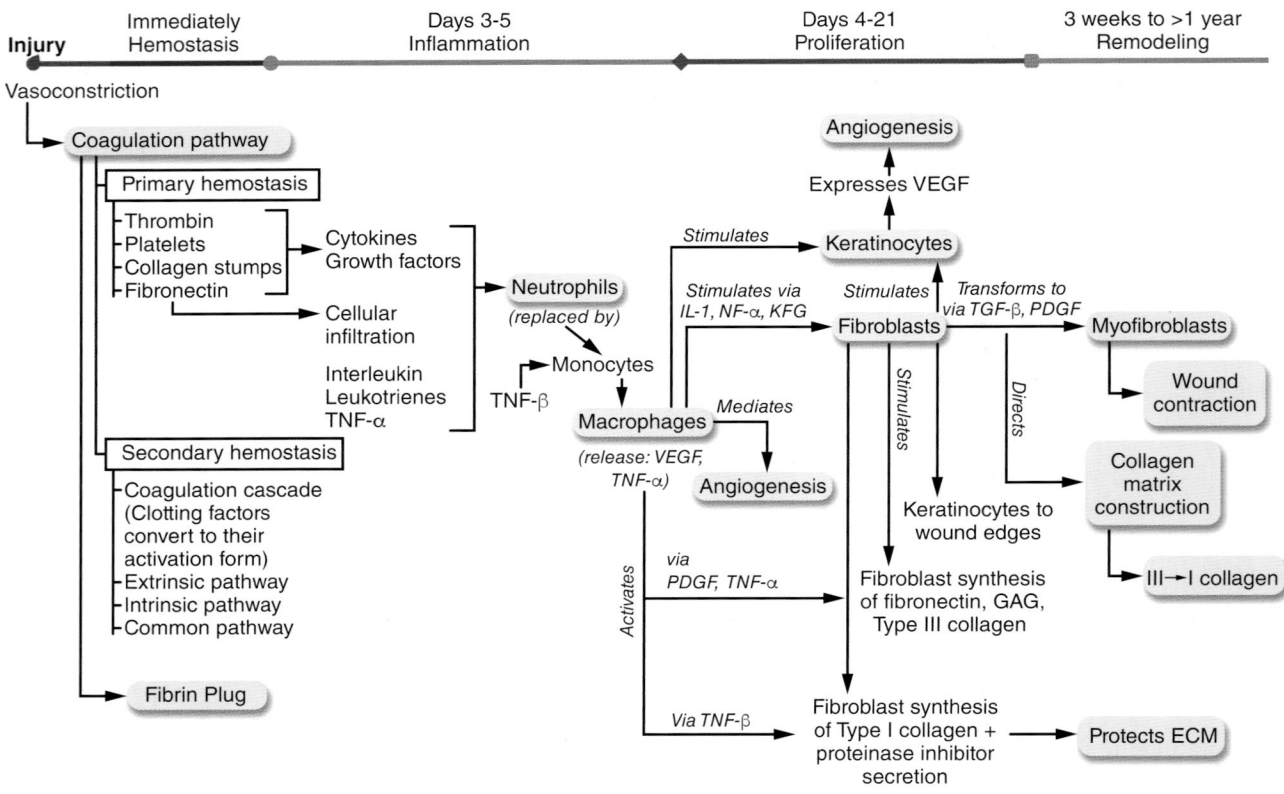

Figure 2.6   Healing begins at the moment of injury. Hemostasis occurs immediately, followed quickly by inflammation, then proliferation, and finally remodeling. Each phase includes unique activities that mark the progression from one phase to another. The primary cells and activities of each phase are highlighted in boxes throughout the healing process.

Specific growth factors perform specific tasks that affect specific cells in order to speed or enhance the healing process. Growth factors are named for the target cells they affect, for their source, or for their behavior. For example, the growth factor affecting the epidermis is called epidermal growth factor (EGF), the growth factor derived from platelets is called **platelet-derived growth factor (PDGF)**, and transforming growth factors (TGFs) transform, or change, other substances. Many growth factors work together to cause desired healing outcomes. Some growth factors are chemotactic, and others stimulate cell production.

Growth factors play a vital role in several key activities throughout healing.[30-32, 84-86] They control the migration and proliferation of cells that are vital to wound healing, including fibroblasts, macrophages, epithelial cells, and endothelial cells.[12, 56] Some growth factors are important in the early hours of inflammation, acting as stimulators of vasoconstriction and vasodilation.[54] Growth factors also affect the formation of the fibrin plug.[12, 64] Others play a role in controlling macrophages and prevent the phagocytization of healthy cells.[70] In the proliferation phase, some growth factors assist and coordinate the capillary endothelial production.[55, 87-89] Several growth factors are responsible for angiogenesis and for granulation tissue and collagen production.[30, 67, 70, 90] Growth factors in the remodeling phase stimulate the degradation of Type III collagen and the synthesis of Type I collagen.[10]

A few growth factors stand out as primary players in healing and are worth identifying. One group is the EGFs. They stimulate the production of a number of cells, including epithelial cells, endothelial cells, and fibroblasts. EGFs also draw epithelial cells into the damaged area and stimulate fibroblasts to produce GAG.[6, 86, 91, 92]

Another important group of growth factors is the fibroblast growth factors (FGFs). They are believed to be primarily responsible for the formation of new vascular and granulation tissue after injury.[93] They promote angiogenesis by stimulating fibroblasts and capillary endothelial cell proliferation. They also stimulate the production of chondrocytes (cartilage cells), keratinocytes (keratin-producing epidermal cells), and myoblasts.[6, 86, 90, 91, 94]

Platelets in a wound excrete a number of growth factors that aid in the healing process.[12, 54, 70, 91, 95] These growth factors include platelet-derived growth factor (PDGF) and the transforming growth factors, factor-alpha (TGF-α) and factor-beta (TGF-β). There is evidence that PDGF may stimulate events during the proliferation phase and may encourage healing of chronic ulcers.[4, 12, 96]

The primary TGF in wound healing is TGF-β. This growth factor has a number of responsibilities. Research has demonstrated that TGF-β stimulates healing during the inflammation and angiogenesis phases by increasing macrophage activity and stimulating epithelialization.[12, 33, 70] It is involved in stimulating extracellular matrix production and coordinating the process of neovascularization (angiogenesis).[54, 90] TGF-β also coordinates the actions of other growth factors to regulate the healing process.[34] Either directly or indirectly, TGF-β is responsible for causing the events that lead to granulation tissue formation.

The PDGF group is a family of growth factors that facilitate the production of collagenase by stimulating fibroblast activity.[90] The PDGFs are particularly active during the remodeling phase, when they prepare the extracellular matrix.[12, 82] They are produced by a variety of cells besides platelets, including macrophages, fibroblasts, epithelial cells, and vascular endothelial cells.[12]

Many other growth factors play roles in wound healing. Their function is not entirely understood, but their presence is vital if healing is to occur. Table 2.4 summarizes some of the most common growth factors in the healing process.

In open wounds, the persistence of foreign substances, such as bacteria, causes continued inflammation. If an insoluble, non-phagocytizable foreign substance, such as a sand grain or unabsorbed extracellular blood, is the cause of chronic inflammation, the area's response is the formation of a **granuloma**. Macrophages become chemotactic for fibroblasts, recruiting them to invade the area. The foreign substance then becomes surrounded by the collagen that these fibroblasts produce to isolate the substance and form a granuloma.

It has been shown that chronic wounds have deficient growth factor levels.[4, 32, 60, 96, 99] The experimental introduction of growth factors such as PDGF, TGF-β, IGF-1, and others has improved healing.[99, 100] According to Hom[99] and Schultz and Wysocki,[4] studies have also revealed that **protease** occurs at higher levels in chronic wounds. Protease degrades growth factors to prevent their presence in the wound. The studies that have investigated chronic wounds and growth factors have looked at several different effects, causes, and preventions and have all come up with one conclusion: Growth factors are necessary for proper healing; when they are not present, healing is impaired or prevented.[6, 32, 60, 85, 96]

Although not technically a chronic wound condition, overuse injuries are often so classified. Overuse and overload activities lead to cumulative trauma that exceeds the tissue's stress tolerance. An injury of this nature is actually a continual reinjury, not a chronic wound.

Healing of Specific Tissues

Specific types and compositions of tissue show specific differences in the timing of each healing phase, although each tissue type proceeds from inflammation through proliferation to remodeling in the generalized timeline we

Chronic Inflammation

Normal healing of tissue occurs in the sequence just described. Occasionally, the injury does not progress along this normal timeline. It gets stuck in the inflammation phase and cannot advance into the other healing phases. This condition is referred to as *chronic inflammation*. Recall that in acute inflammation, the large number of granular leukocytes that initially invades the injured area is replaced with mononuclear phagocytes. The cells are transformed into larger macrophages and giant cells to debride the area. As the area is cleared of waste and foreign matter, these cells normally diminish in number, but in chronic inflammations their higher numbers persist at the site.

Although we have much to learn about chronic inflammation, some substances have been identified as primary perpetrators of inflammation. It is known that large numbers of neutrophils are present in chronic inflammations.[12, 51] It is thought that since they release enzymes like collagenase, they destroy collagen and prevent the matrix from developing.[12, 51] Persistent inflammation has been observed in wounds with macrophages and pro-inflammatory cytokines.[13, 97] Cytokines and growth factors are crucial to the normal inflammatory phase of healing, for they are chemotactic for other chemicals and cells that are needed for healing. However, for some reason the sequential distribution of anti-inflammatory cytokines that should be released by immune cells such as local neutrophils, monocytes, mast cells, and T cells are suppressed.[13] It may be that the overabundance and activation of neutrophils and macrophages in the wound results in excessive production of reactive oxygen species (ROS), a type of unstable molecule (because of its unmated electron) that damages and causes cell death by damaging its DNA and proteins. This may perpetuate the need for anti-inflammatory cytokines and growth factors.[13] Since ROS serve to regulate inflammatory signaling,[98] their continued presence may help perpetuate the inflammatory process.

have discussed. Given structural, cellular, and chemical differences, however, it is not reasonable to expect muscle tissue, for example, to follow the same recovery timeline that bone or ligament follows. Let's take a look at some of the differences in tissues that we commonly see after orthopedic and athletic injuries. Because the hemostasis phase is similar in onset, activity, and duration for all injuries, it is omitted in this section; however, bear in mind that hemostasis occurs immediately before the inflammation phase for each of these tissues.

Recent research has involved tissue engineering and acceleration of healing through altered mechanisms. Efforts to alter normal and problem healing of various tissues have included investigations into ligament and tendon,[101-103] articular cartilage,[2] and bone and cartilage.[3, 104] An in-depth presentation of how these engineering investigations might change the way we deal with orthopedic and sports injuries in the future is beyond the scope of this chapter. Occasional tidbits of information related to tissue engineering may dot this chapter, but only to make you aware of potential future changes. It is most important for current students of allied health care to understand the routine courses of healing commonly dealt with in rehabilitation.

Ligaments

When a ligament is torn, frayed stump ends are present where the ligament separated. The ligament undergoes the expected inflammation process, including local edema formation. The injured ligament stumps become engulfed in fluid, causing the ends to become friable, or fragile, and easily degraded. Local vascular permeability increases and permits the normal inflammatory products, including PMNs and **lymphocytes**, to invade the area. **Erythrocytes** and other cells accumulate to fill the gap between the stump ends. Within the first 24 to 48 h, macrophages and monocytes enter the area to begin debridement.[105] Macrophages also begin to secrete growth factors that begin epithelial growth and granulation tissue formation. Table 2.6 summarizes the timeline of ligamentous tissue healing.

Although it depends upon the size of the ligament injury, the specific ligament, the amount of edema, and other individual factors, the proliferation phase usually begins within 48 to 72 h after the injury with extracellular matrix development and proceeds through the production of collagen and ground substance by the fibroblasts.[105] Platelets in the area release a number of growth factors, such as PDGF, TGF-β, and EGF. Macrophages are also producing PDGF, TGF-β, and FGF. These growth factors are chemotactic for cells (including fibroblasts) that produce collagen. This phase continues for up to 6 weeks.[105] Other routine processes occur during this phase, including the formation of capillary buds that will eventually join with existing vessels. Phagocytosis also continues during

CLINICAL TIPS

Although all tissues follow the same general steps in healing, the specific timing of healing in different tissues—such as ligaments, tendons, muscles, cartilage, and bone—varies and involves events that are specific to the tissue. The clinician must be aware of these timing variations because healing is one of the key factors that guides the progression of rehabilitation.

this time. The quantity of collagen being synthesized is greater than the amount being degraded, so there is a net increase in collagen during proliferation.

Several weeks later, the remodeling phase is heralded by the conversion of Type III collagen to Type I collagen and an increase in the number of collagen cross-links.[106] There is also a reduction of edema, fibroblasts, and macrophages, and the area takes on a more normal appearance. This final stage may take 18 months to 2 years to complete.[107-109]

Tendons

Tendon healing is characterized by the inflammation phase taking days, the proliferation phase taking weeks, and the remodeling phase taking months.[110] Tendons vary in their healing rate, depending on the magnitude, duration, and location of the injury and the age of the patient.[111-113] This section deals with acute injuries to tendons and not to tendinopathies.

Although most of the research on tendons and tendon injuries has been performed on animals, it is generally believed that most human tendon ruptures have been preceded by some degree of tendon degeneration.[114] Often this preinjury degradation is asymptomatic and goes undetected.[113]

As with ligaments, the tendon inflammatory phase is from about 3 d[115] to 7 to 8 d[114, 116] long, depending on the specific tendon injured. Tendons have support from local structures that aid in the initial healing process.[117] These structures include the periosteum of underlying bone, the synovial sheath, the epitenon, and the endotenon. These structures provide the vascular supply and fibroblasts that are needed for healing. The epitenon and endotenon provide macrophage-like cells and fibroblasts to begin debridement. Table 2.7 summarizes the tendon healing timeline.

Following the hematoma formation during hemostasis, the inflammatory process begins with the presence of neutrophils, macrophages, and platelets that release cytokines and growth factors.[114]

The proliferation phase follows the inflammation phase and continues until about the 21st day after the injury's onset,[114] although the precise duration of this phase depends

TABLE 2.6   Ligament Healing Timeline

Phase	Time	Activity
Inflammation	First few hours	The injury site fills with erythrocytes, leukocytes, and lymphocytes. The ligament stumps become progressively more friable with the accumulation of serous fluid in the area.
	24 h	Monocytes and macrophages infiltrate the area. Fibroblasts begin to appear and eventually become significant in number.
	48–72 h	Fibroblasts produce the extracellular matrix.
Proliferation	3–21 d	Proliferation begins.
	1–2 wk	Fibrocytes and macrophages are numerous. Random collagen fibers and abundant ground substance are seen. Fragile vascular granulation tissue is seen at the injury site. The extracellular matrix continues to be synthesized by fibroblasts. Macrophages, mast cells, and fibroblasts continue to predominate. Vascular buds appear in the wound to communicate with existing capillaries. Elastin is seen in the area.
	2 d–6 wk	Proliferation phase occurs, during which cellular and matrix structures replace the blood clot formed during inflammation.
Remodeling	14–21 d	Remodeling begins.
	6 wk–12 mo	Macrophages and fibroblasts diminish.
	8 wk	Revascularization is complete.
	Up to 12 mo	Collagen concentration stabilizes, with Type I collagen replacing Type III and collagen cross-links increasing in number. Ligament becomes more normal.
	40–50 wk	Near-normal tensile strength is restored.
	1–2 yr	Healing is complete.

on a variety of factors, including age, comorbidities, activity level, size of injury, and surgical repair technique used.[118, 119] After the first week or so after an acute tendon injury, collagen synthesis begins and continues at a rapid rate for the first 4 weeks.[115, 116] Cell proliferation and migration of tenocytes into the wound area and angiogenesis also occur during this proliferation phase.[114] During the second week, the collagen starts becoming more organized, so that by as soon as the end of the second week the cells are beginning to align themselves in the direction of applied stress.[115] Collagen synthesis continues until day 35.[41] Granulation tissue produced by fibroblasts migrating from surrounding connective tissue and from the tendon sheath is also present as early as day 13, and afterward it appears in rapidly forming quantities.[62] Mediators during this time stimulate the recruitment of fibroblasts from local endotenon, epitenon, and paratenon structures to aid in the healing process.[114] By day 28, collagen and active fibroblasts producing the collagen are clearly aligned along the tendon's long axis.[41] This alignment helps the remaining collagen to form in a proper orientation.

As mentioned, during the first 3 weeks, the area undergoes a significant revascularization. With revascularization, it is possible to begin mobilization of a surgically repaired tendon after day 21.[120-122] Immobilization before

this time allows for reconstruction and restoration of local circulation. Thus, immobilization is necessary not for the tendon to reconnect, but for the local vascularity to be restored.[115, 116]

By the end of 3 weeks, the synovial sheath is also reconstituted.[115] Although the synovial sheath has not been presented in this discussion, note that not all tendons have sheaths, but those that do may develop postinjury complications of adhesion formations between the tendon and its sheath if these structures are not properly managed early on. All tendons have an endotenon. An **endotenon** is a continuous mesh of loose connective tissue that surrounds tendon fascicles, or bundles of tendon fibers, within an entire tendon. This structure contains blood and lymph vessels and nerves and allows the fascicles to slide against each other as the tendon changes shape during muscle contraction. This endotenon is continuous with the epitenon. The **epitenon** is the connective tissue structure that surrounds the entire tendon. On the other hand, a **tendon sheath** is fibrous tissue whose purpose is to reduce friction between the tendon and the adjacent structure. A tendon sheath has two layers, an inner synovial layer and an outer parietal layer that are continuous with each other.[123]

It is important to mention these structures because they determine how a tendon is going to heal after injury. There

TABLE 2.7 Tendon Healing Timeline

Phase	Time	Activity
Inflammation	First 3 d	Cells that originate from extrinsic peritendinous tissue and from intrinsic tissue from the epitenon and endotenon are active.
	5 d	Wound gap is filled by phagocytes.
	1 wk	Collagen synthesis is initiated, with new collagen fibers placed in a random and disorganized way.
Proliferation	10 d	Collagen synthesis is maximal.
	2 wk	Extracellular matrix develops and fills the defect area, providing support for cells to migrate into the wound.
	3 wk	The endotenon produces significant fibroblast proliferation in the injury site. Significant revascularization occurs. The synovial sheath is rebuilt, and a smooth gliding surface develops. Fibroblasts start becoming oriented in line with the tendon's axis.
	4 wk	Fibroblasts predominate in the healing area. Collagen content increases. Collagen is fully oriented with the tendon's long axis.
	35 d	Collagen synthesis is completed.
	42 d	Fibroblasts that have proliferated from the endotenon are the primary cells, simultaneously synthesizing collagen while contributing to collagen resorption.
Remodeling	6–10 wk	Healing changes from cellular activity to fibrous repair.
	2 mo	Collagen is mature and realigned along the tendon's axis.
	112 d	Fibroblasts have reverted to tenocytes, Type III collagen has been replaced by Type I, and maturation is complete.
	40–50 wk	Strength is 85% to 95% normal.

are two types of tendon healing, intrinsic and extrinsic. Intrinsic healing occurs when the tendon heals as a result of the production and proliferation of tenocytes from the tendon's injured epitenon and endotenon, while extrinsic healing occurs when the source of healing is from a migration of cells originating from the synovial tendon sheath.[124] Those tendons that heal through the intrinsic system seem to recover with improved biomechanics and fewer complications.[125] On the other hand, extrinsic tendon healing can result in adhesions of the tendon to its surrounding sheath, disrupting the tendon's normal gliding abilities within the tendon sheath.[124, 126] It is for this reason that the hand's flexor tendons, which are enclosed in tendon sheaths throughout the length of the hand and wrist, have been extensively investigated. New repair procedures that have advanced from these investigations incorporate early movement protocols whose outcomes have led to the achievement of successful hand rehabilitation outcomes.[127]

As tendon healing progresses, the injury moves to the remodeling phase. During this phase, the injury site becomes less cellular and the amount of glycosaminoglycan in the area is reduced.[128] This phase can last several months. It is during this time that the restorative alignment of what is to become scar tissue occurs; the collagen bundles that are forming are oriented along the longitudinal axis of the tendon.[129] The Type I collagen that is developing has more cross-links and greater tensile strength than the Type III collagen it is replacing. This increase in tensile strength as a result of the collagen realignment and maturation starts about 6 to 8 weeks after injury.[130] Throughout this phase, the injured site transitions from being primarily cellular to being predominantly fibrous tissue.[129] When Type I collagen replaces Type III collagen and the fibroblasts revert to their original status as **tenocytes**, the remodeling phase is finished. This occurs by day 112.[115]

When a tendon is surgically repaired, the tendon and the surrounding soft tissue, including blood vessels, fascia, and skin, all become one wound. The area fills with edema that quickly becomes a sticky gel. This gel is viscous and can become a thick, dense scar. The dense scar will limit the gliding of the tendon and thereby impede function of the tendon's muscle, ultimately limiting the success of rehabilitation.[116] For normal function to be restored, abnormal scar tissue adhesions must be kept to a minimum and must not be allowed to bind together structures that are normally separated. The tendon should glide within its sheath, the skin should move freely from subcutaneous structures, and the blood vessels and nerves should have normal mobility. One major factor determining the success of this separation of subcutaneous structures is duration of immobilization.

Evidence in Rehabilitation

As scientific investigations advance our knowledge and understanding of cell development, repair, and manipulation, inquiries into how the healing process may be improved through tissue engineering also emerge. A recent update on the latest developments in the progression of tendon healing has revealed some interesting new concepts. Zhu and colleagues[131] report that efforts at reducing the risk of repaired tendon failure have focused on encouraging the development of an extracellular matrix (ECM). Since the ECM is vital to tendon healing but needs time to fill the gap between tendon stumps, investigations are ongoing on ways to reduce ECM development time. A lot of research focuses on inserting a collagen scaffold into the healing site; early studies have shown that this scaffold both increases the amount of tissue formation and improves the quality of the new tissue. Other studies are investigating the results of embedding additional tissue, such as stem cells, into the scaffold before it is inserted in the wound site. Although the studies reported by Zhu and colleagues are still in the animal phase of research, the results are promising for future investigations using human subjects.

It may be possible in the future to significantly improve healing after tendon rupture. Changes in the healing rate of tendon tissue will require rehabilitation clinicians to change their rehabilitation programs. Perhaps patients will someday be able to resume normal activities after a much shorter time than they do now.

The effects of immobilization are discussed in further detail in chapter 12. Tendon gliding is addressed in more detail in chapter 23.

Tendons are susceptible to chronic inflammatory conditions. It is known that fibroblasts are stimulated during tendon activity, and these fibroblasts increase prostaglandin production, thereby creating an inflammatory condition.[50] Tendinopathy will be presented in more detail in chapter 3.

Muscles

Although muscle tissue may heal like the tissues previously discussed and may follow the same three phases to ultimately produce scar tissue, muscle also contains unique structures that permit it to regenerate. These structures are **satellite cells**. Satellite cells are muscle stem cells.[132] These cells fuse with adjacent myofibers to repair and regenerate muscle tissue.[133] It is believed that some destruction of muscle tissue occurs daily in routine activities. This destruction also occurs during regular exercises, especially eccentric exercise.[132] The satellite cells restore and replace muscle cells routinely damaged during activity.[43, 132, 133] When a small muscle injury is revascularized and reinnervated and occurs in a muscle type that can regenerate, satellite cells replace injured muscle tissue with new muscle tissue.[43] Larger injuries, however, such as ruptures or severe lacerations, heal with scar tissue. With scar tissue formation, overproduction of the extracellular matrix occurs at 2 weeks and accelerates for up to 4 weeks postinjury; this process, known as fibrosis, inhibits skeletal muscle regeneration.[134] Table 2.8 summarizes the muscle's healing timeline.

In the early hours of healing, injured muscle tissue appears to follow the same sequence as other tissue. Neutrophils are among the first cells to arrive at the site of injury, and they are seen as soon as an hour from the onset of injury.[43] They continue to accumulate until they reach their peak numbers about 12 to 24 h after the injury's onset.[135] Phagocytes, primarily macrophages, invade the site within 6 h after an injury. As neutrophils perform their functions and die, usually within a few hours,[136] the macrophages become the predominant cells in the area for the next 10 d as they debride the area.

Macrophages continue to play an important role after muscle injury throughout each of the steps of muscle tissue regeneration.[137] They not only play a role in both facilitating and resolving the inflammatory phase, but they also serve as the main source of cytokines, chemokines, and growth factors that guide muscle repair and regeneration.[137]

Angiogenesis begins at day 3 once the injury moves from inflammation to proliferation and peaks at day 5.[83] In the proliferation phase, muscle tissue regeneration occurs between postinjury days 7 to 10 and peaks at 2 weeks.[83] Regeneration occurs when **myogenic cells** are activated. These cells evolve into **myoblasts**, which fuse together to form myotubes. Myotubes are seen in the injury site by day 13. Through a complex progression of events, these myotubes become muscle fibers and are apparent in the area by day 18. Macrophages play a role in helping to differentiate the myogenic cells as well as promoting myotube formations.[132, 138] The final muscle regeneration step is completed with the development of the neural part of the neuromuscular structure. When the process is complete, satellite cell levels return to normal and resume their daily function of less intensive, ongoing muscle tissue replacement.[134] Overall, the regeneration process for injured muscle tissue generally begins during the first 4 to 5 d after an injury and peaks at 2 weeks; following this time of peak activity, regeneration then undergoes a gradual decline in activity until it is completed by 3 to 4 weeks after the injury.[139]

Certain conditions must exist for muscle regeneration to occur. These include (1) a source of myoblasts, (2)

TABLE 2.8   Muscle Healing Timeline (Regeneration)

Phase	Time	Activity
Inflammation	6 h	Fragmentation of injured muscle fibers begins. Macrophages appear.
	1–4 d	Fibroblasts appear.
	1 wk	Ability to produce muscle tension is progressively reduced.
		Muscle regeneration of minor injury begins through activation of satellite cells.
		Muscle is able to produce near-normal tension.
	2–3 wk	Fibrosis begins.
		Scar tissue is seen in more significant muscle injuries.
Proliferation	7–11 d	Tensile strength reaches near normal.
	10 d	Large number of phagocytes, primarily macrophages, are seen at the injury site.
	13 d	Regenerating myotubes are seen.
	18 d	Cross-striated muscle fibers appear.
Remodeling	6 wk–6 mo	Contraction ability is 90% normal.

adequate blood supply, (3) adequate innervation, (4) the presence of an extracellular matrix, and (5) limited stress across the wound while it is healing.[122] If one of these conditions is lacking, the muscle injury heals by scar formation and not by regeneration.[122] When a muscle heals with scar tissue rather than new muscle tissue, strength is lost because normal muscle generates force, but scar tissue can only transfer force.[140] In cases of larger muscle injuries, several of the essential factors needed for tissue regeneration are interrupted, so the injury site will try to regenerate, but the regeneration process will be overtaken by fibrosis; that is, it will be overridden by scar tissue.[134] When the mass of damaged muscle is larger than 3 g (0.1 oz),[134] or a few millimeters in length,[141] the muscle heals via the scarring process and goes through the sequence of healing we have discussed with the formation of Type III collagen that then evolves into Type I collagen as scar tissue matures. Unfortunately, most muscle strains health professionals treat are these larger injuries.

Articular Cartilage

Although there are many types of collagen and cartilage, the ones clinicians have the greatest concern for when it comes to joints are articular cartilage, hyaline cartilage, fibrocartilage, and elastic collagen. Hyaline cartilage dissipates loads applied to joints. Commonly referred to as articular cartilage, it lines the surfaces of diarthroidal, or synovial, joints. On the other hand, fibrocartilage transfers loads between the tendons and ligaments and the bone. Examples of fibrocartilage are found in the intervertebral discs and the temporomandibular joint. A third structure, elastic collagen, provides a flexible support to external structures and is similar to hyaline cartilage.

Although articular cartilage contains eight different types of collagen, it is composed primarily of Type II collagen.[142] When articular cartilage heals, Type I collagen is the primary result. Cartilage does have some regenerative capability; the problem is that articular cartilage regenerates more slowly than scar tissue is deposited.[143] Fibrocartilage seems to have a better capacity to regenerate than articular cartilage.[144]

The differences between Type I and Type II cartilage are key factors in how an injured site manages stress after healing. Articular cartilage is composed of 60% to 80% water, and 80% of its dry weight is Type II cartilage.[145] Its extracellular matrix holds a lot of water because of the proteoglycans it contains. There is more water and there are fewer collagen fibers at the surface of articular cartilage; the reverse is true closer to the subchondral bone, where the articular cartilage attaches.[146] When a person bears weight on a joint, the articular cartilage provides a dual system to protect the joint.[147, 148] When a joint first accepts a compression force, such as body weight when a person rises to stand, the articular cartilage releases the water within the extracellular matrix to accept that force.[149] This is called *fluid phase acceptance* (figure 2.7). If weight bearing continues, as in prolonged standing, the fluid dissipates so that the lower layers of articular cartilage, where denser collagen is present, provide for continued protection of the joint.[149] This secondary compression phase is called *solid phase acceptance*. In very prolonged standing, articular cartilage may suffer dehydration.[149] Fibrocartilage does not have this structural arrangement, so it cannot offer the same protection to joints that hyaline cartilage does.

Whether or not an articular cartilage injury heals depends on three variables: the depth of the defect, the

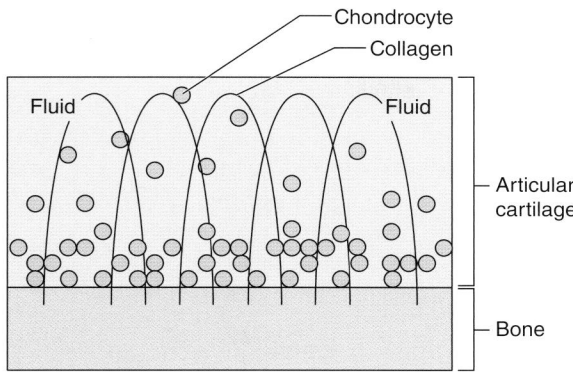

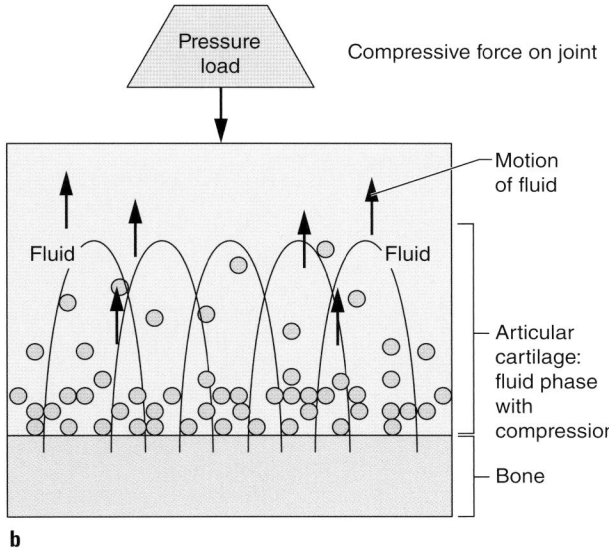

Figure 2.7 Schematic demonstrating the fluid phase of articular cartilage. *(a)* At rest without a load applied to cartilage. *(b)* Fluid phase of articular cartilage when a load is applied; there is a local increase in interstitial fluid pressure which causes the fluid to flow out of the extracellular matrix, providing a cushion-like protection. Modeled after a schematic from Rheumaportal.com.

maturity of the cartilage, and the location of the defect.[144, 150] Small, full-thickness defects repair with fibrocartilage via the blood supply in the bone adjacent to the lesion, but partial-thickness defects do not repair.[151] Partial-thickness lesions degenerate and do not heal because there is no vascular supply available.[152]

In full-thickness lesions, the healing course of articular cartilage, as with most other tissue healing, follows a sequence of events initiated with macrophages and fibrin plug formation. Bone adjacent to the full-thickness articular cartilage lesion bleeds into the area.[151] Fibroblasts appear in the area to perform their rebuilding tasks. As the site advances into the remodeling phase, collagen becomes the prevalent structure. See table 2.9 for a general outline of the sequence of events in cartilage healing.

Partial-thickness articular cartilage lesions are a source of concern for surgeons because many people experience these types of injuries. Partial-thickness articular cartilage injuries often become necrotic and lead to osteoarthritis because they lack any blood supply to heal.[152]

Various surgical repairs are used to delay this degenerative process. Most of these procedures have been to the knee because articular injuries are very common in this joint.[153, 154] The surgical techniques are classified into three types: cleaning the joint, repairing the joint, and restoring the joint.[142] They all provide the patient with additional time before joint replacement might be needed. The first, cleaning, involves ridding the joint of structures that produce pain in the joint; these surgical techniques are not reparative or restorative for the joint. These procedures include lavage and debridement. The goals of these procedures are to clean the joint and improve function by reducing the patient's pain. They are the easiest for the surgeon to perform, and they require the fewest precautions in postoperative rehabilitation.

Reparative procedures include abrasion arthroplasty, drilling, and microfractures. These surgical procedures are performed through an arthroscope. Abrasion arthroplasty, as the name implies, superficially abrades the articular

TABLE 2.9 Articular Cartilage Healing Timeline

Phase	Time	Activity
Inflammation	48 h	Fibrin clot is formed to fill the defect.
	5 d	Fibroblasts are in the area and combine with collagen fibers to replace the clot.
Proliferation	2 wk	Fibroblasts differentiate, and islands of chondrocytes appear.
	1 mo	Fibroblasts have been completely differentiated.
Remodeling	2 mo	Satisfactory repair has occurred, with the defect resembling cartilage in appearance. The majority of collagen present, however, is Type I.
	6 mo	A combination of Type I and Type II calcified cartilage has a normal appearance.

surface without going down to subchondral bone to promote a healing response from the cells within the joint.[155] Drilling and microfracture techniques repair the area of damaged articular cartilage by causing stem cells from the subchondral bone's marrow to migrate into the site via the bleeding that occurs with these techniques. A primary difference between these two techniques is the size and depth of the drill holes made in the subchondral bone to facilitate a bone marrow reaction. Microfracture repair features less chondral destruction and has produced better results, so it is often the preferred reparative procedure.[156, 157]

Results of the reparative procedures, especially the microfracture process, initially show evidence of pseudonormal articular cartilage in the lesion sites.[152] Articular cartilage develops very slowly and becomes quickly overrun by fibrocartilage because of its more rapid formation and development.[152] Fibrocartilage is less able to withstand stresses than articular cartilage because it has a higher friction coefficient.[158] Hence, until more refined surgical procedures are developed, reparative procedures will relieve pain and delay the patient's need for additional surgery but will not regenerate articular cartilage. These reparative procedures will likely provide for a longer period of pain-free and improved function postoperatively than the cleaning procedures. There is some evidence to suggest that children may recover from articular cartilage injuries better than adults since children continue to produce articular cartilage during their growth years, especially if they are active.[159]

Two relatively new techniques that serve as restorative procedures include osteochondral plug implantation and autologous chondrocyte transplantation.[160] The osteochondral implantations use either the patient's healthy, non-weight-bearing bone and cartilage or a cadaver donation. An **allogenic graft** is one that is taken from another person; it is also referred to as a *cadaver graft, homogeneous graft,* or *homograft*. An **autologous graft** of articular cartilage and bone is taken from the patient from the same joint as the damaged cartilage, but it is removed from a part of the joint that does not bear weight; this transfer can be either as one to three plugs that are inserted into the defective site or as a larger group of plugs inserted into a large site. The transfer of one to three osteochondral plugs into the defective site is called an *osteochondral autologous transfer system (OATS)*.[161] When several more plugs are used to repair the injury, it is called a *mosaicplasty* because it has a mosaic appearance[162] (figure 2.8). Since these are relatively new procedures, long-term results are not yet available, but early indications reveal good outcomes.[162] A recent study looking at results almost 5 years post-repair demonstrate good clinical results for both the osteochondral plug harvested sites and the implanted sites.[163] A procedure to replace articular cartilage with homogeneous cartilage, known as *autologous chondrocyte transplanta-*

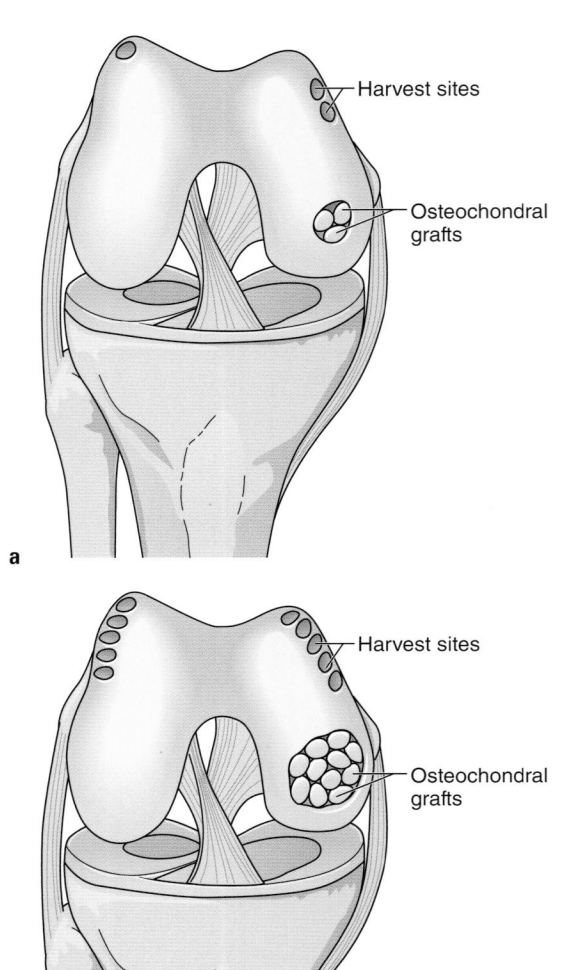

Figure 2.8 Osteochondral autologous transfer system (OATS). *(a)* Single osteochondral transfer for small lesions. *(b)* Mosaicplasty osteochondral transfers are for larger lesions.

tion, was reported by Brittberg and colleagues[164] from the University of Göteborg, Sweden. Autologous chondrocyte implantation is an expensive, complex process that involves at least two surgical procedures. The first surgery extracts healthy chondrocytes from the patient. The cells are then cultured in a lab for up to 21 d until a sufficient number of cells have replicated to fill the defect. The patient undergoes another surgery where the cultured cells are injected into the articular defect, and the defect is covered with a periosteal patch that is taken from the distal tibia.[164] Since Brittberg and colleagues' initial report, investigations have occurred into the use of natural and synthetic scaffolds to develop chondrocyte transplant methods; initial success is promising in both short-term and medium-term studies.[165]

For regeneration of articular cartilage to occur, the following conditions must be present:[166]

- Cells that will proliferate and differentiate into chondrocytes must be located in or migrate to the wound site.
- A mechanical stimulus that enhances articular cartilage formation must be present.
- Protection from excessive loads must be sufficient to allow cartilage repair without causing damage.
- Normal joint conformation must be maintained or restored.

These elements must be considered during the rehabilitation of chondral surgeries. Rehabilitation procedures for chondral surgeries are discussed in chapter 19.

Bone

As with other tissues, hemostasis is the first healing phase. This is when the damaged blood vessels provide for an influx of stem cells into the fracture site.[128] Growth factors released by platelets are chemotactic for macrophages. Once hemostasis is complete, injured bone tissue undergoes its inflammation phase that lasts from 3 to 5 d[167] up to about 1 week;[128] it is during this time that fibroblast and macrophage numbers reach their peak. The necrotic ends of the fractured bone and metabolic wastes are debrided to clear the way and set the stage for the next phase.

During this next phase, the proliferative phase, the bone demonstrates its ability to regenerate. **Osteoblasts**, bone-generating cells, invade the area via the periosteum. As these cells go to work, a **callus** is formed at the site of each bone fragment end. This soft callus, whose formation takes 3 to 4 weeks, is a fibrous **matrix** of collagen that eventually becomes bone. Osteoblasts gradually replace this temporary formation with endochondral bone, which becomes the hard callus.[27] The callus has an internal component and an external component. The external callus immobilizes the fragment ends, eventually bridges the two fragments, and allows stress to be applied to the bone without harming the fracture site before it completely heals. The initial endochondral bone consists of immature woven bone but is eventually converted into lamellar bone so the region's strength and stability are restored.[168] By the third week, the bony ends are united. It takes 7 to 40 d after injury for the fracture site to become mechanically stable with a soft callus.[167] Table 2.10 demonstrates the healing timeline of bone.

As the osteoblasts move along the stump ends and farther away from the blood supply, they convert to chondrocytes, which produce a layer of cartilage. Osteogenic cells cover the chondrocytes. A fibrous layer covers these cells. This process occurs simultaneously on the external and internal layers in the bone's marrow cavity. The soft callus matures into a hard callus as the fibrous matrix converts into spongy bone. In a not fully understood process, the spongy bone converts to normal compact bone over time. In the long bones of adults, this routinely takes 3 to 4 months.[169]

During the remodeling phase, the callus size is reduced, the medullary canal is reestablished, the conversion to bone tissue is finalized, and normal oxygen and cellular alignment are restored (provided appropriate stresses are applied, via the application of Wolff's law), so the end product is as strong as or stronger than the original bone.[167]

Tensile Strength During Healing

As defined earlier, **tensile strength** is the maximal amount of stress or force that a structure can withstand before

TABLE 2.10 Bone Healing Timeline

Phase	Time	Activity
Inflammation	Immediately	PMNs, plasma, and lymphocytes appear.
	First few hours	Fibroblasts invade the area.
	3–4 d	Hematoma forms. Fractured edges become necrotic. Mast cells occur at the site. Macrophages remove debris. Osteoclasts mobilize in the area.
Proliferation	Up to 4 wk	Hard callus develops. Osteoclasts continue to remove dead bone. Endosteal blood supply continues to develop.
	3–4 wk	Hard callus develops. Osteoclasts continue to remove dead bone. Endosteal blood supply continues to develop.
	4–6 wk	External blood supply dominates.
Remodeling	6–10 wk	Medullary circulation is reestablished.
	3–4 mo	Fracture is healed, but remodeling continues.
	12 wk	Near-normal strength is attained.

tissue failure occurs. In other words, tensile strength is the amount of outside force that can be applied to a muscle, tendon, ligament, or bone before it tears or breaks. Healthy tissue withstands high amounts of tensile force. Once injured, however, investigators agree that the tissue's tensile strength seldom returns to 100% of its prior level; they do not agree, however, on what the new level of the tissue's tensile strength is.[122]

The idea that injured tissue's tensile strength never returns to normal is about the only fact on which researchers agree. Disagreements arise because of various differences between investigation methods, including research technique variations, different animals and specific structures investigated, and different degrees of injury. Some investigations are *in vitro* and others are *in vivo*. It is difficult to extrapolate animal research findings to humans, and it is even more difficult to find people who are willing to suffer intentional injuries in order to study tensile strength after injury. Studies often investigate only one structure or tissue type that is isolated in a lab. Results of these tensile strength studies are, by necessity, narrow, but because they do not take into consideration the contributions of surrounding tissues to a region's overall strength through their own framework, function, configuration, or attachment, actual tensile strength of an injured segment is difficult to determine accurately.

The contributing strength of surrounding tissues may explain why athletes often return to full competition 6 months after reconstructive surgery without becoming reinjured, even though the healing tissue does not regain its full tensile strength for 1 year or more after injury. There are many unanswered questions about the tensile strength of healing and healed tissue; nevertheless, clinicians must be aware of current knowledge, incomplete though it may be.

During the inflammation phase, normal tensile strength of injured tissues declines rapidly to around 50%.[115] Depending on the specific tissue involved, this decline occurs in 24 to 48 h. In the very early stage of healing, the injured site's strength derives from the fibrin clot, which cannot withstand much stress. Tensile strength is at its lowest during this time.[79] Around day 5, tensile strength begins to increase. Lacking significant collagen, the injured tissue relies on other structures in the area, including the granulation tissue and ground substance, for this increase in strength.

As collagen becomes more plentiful and cross-links develop, the area's tensile strength increases. Collagen conversion from Type III to Type I and the increased number of cross-links are the main reasons for tensile strength development.

Studies have demonstrated that the amount of time needed to develop tensile strength in muscle tissue varies, depending on the animal investigated. Rat studies show that by 6 weeks after injury, 90% of normal tensile

strength is achieved, and in the cat, it takes 6 months.[133] Bone strength is the exception to the rule of not returning to normal strength; its strength returns to 83% of normal 12 weeks after injury[170] and to at least normal eventually, albeit months to years after injury.[167] Ligaments and tendons vary in the time they need to achieve near-normal strength, depending on the specific structure.[122] These tissues approach near-normal levels anywhere from 17 to 50 weeks after injury.[171]

Researchers agree that once an injury occurs, the injured soft-tissue structure never regains full tensile strength.[122] Tensile strength initially increases rapidly after the inflammation phase, then slows and even regresses as Type III collagen degrades and is replaced with Type I collagen.[172] Depending on the structure, it may take a year or more for an injured part to regain maximal tensile strength.

Factors That Affect Healing

A number of outside influences can profoundly or subtly affect the healing process. Some of these factors have a negative impact, while others have a positive impact. Some of them can be manipulated while others cannot. This section provides a brief look at the more common issues that must be realized in rehabilitation.

CLINICAL TIPS

Factors that affect healing include drugs, surgical repairs, and personal factors such as the patient's age, systemic diseases, nutrition, the size of the injury, infection, and the depth and breadth of spasm, pain, dysfunction, and swelling caused by the injury. The clinician can influence some of these factors, such as spasm, pain, dysfunction, and swelling; can work to prevent infection; can encourage the patient to eat nutritionally; and can urge the patient to maintain optimal health in the presence of systemic diseases. Since drugs can affect healing, the clinician should be aware of all medications the patient is taking, including prescription and non-prescription as well as illegal or social drugs, and the effect they may have on the healing process. Additional influences the rehabilitation clinician may have on healing by using rehabilitation techniques will be addressed in chapter 3.

Oxygen

Tissues need oxygen to survive. When an injury occurs, not only is the oxygen supply locally disrupted but the metabolically active cells need increased levels of oxygen.[11] Because of these factors, temporary hypoxia occurs at the wound site. This condition signals cytokines and growth factors to move into the area to introduce macrophages and fibroblasts.[173] If this hypoxia persists, the wound does not heal.[11] Oxygen is important for energy production in the ATP cycle, cell metabolism, and proper wound healing.[59] A person whose vascular status is compromised may develop chronic, unhealed wounds. Chronic hypoxia leads to acidosis and inadequate ATP production, which prevent the wound from advancing in the normal healing process.[59] Following initial episodes of hypoxia, oxygenation is needed throughout all healing phases. For this reason, factors that cause vasoconstriction, such as smoking, stress, and diabetes, delay or restrict normal wound healing.[59] Various dressings and barometric chambers continue to be investigated as possible means by which to encourage proper healing.

Drugs

Patients often consult with a rehabilitation clinician for information about the drugs that have been prescribed after injury. Therefore, the clinician should have a basic understanding of medications, be aware of his or her own limited knowledge, and readily refer the patient to either the physician or a pharmacist for additional information.

Clinicians should remember certain general rules of thumb about medications. All drugs, even vitamins, have the potential to produce undesirable side effects. Any drug should be used with caution and taken according to recommendations of the physician, pharmacist, or manufacturer of over-the-counter (OTC) medications. If undesirable side effects occur, the physician should be contacted for instructions to either discontinue the medication or change its administration. All drugs have a **duration of action**, the length of time that the amount of drug in the blood is above the level needed to obtain a minimal therapeutic effect. This length of time is determined by the half-life of the drug. A drug's **half-life** is the amount of time it takes for the level of the drug in the bloodstream to diminish by half. The frequency with which the drug is administered is based on its half-life. The shorter the half-life, the more often the drug must be administered to obtain a minimal therapeutic effect. The example given in Houglum and colleagues[174] demonstrates this concept: Naproxen, with a half-life of about 14 h, is administered twice a day, whereas ibuprofen, with a half-life of around 2 h, is administered three to four times a day.

A goal of drug administration is to achieve a steady state. A **steady state** occurs when the average level of drug remains constant in the blood; a steady state exists when the amount absorbed into the blood equals the amount removed through metabolism or excretion. After the first few administrations of the drug, the amount of drug in the bloodstream increases until this steady state is achieved. As a rule of thumb, a steady state is achieved after the dosing of the drug has continued for a time equal to 4 to 5 half-lives.[174] For example, using 5 half-lives to calculate the time needed to reach steady state, if a drug has a half-life of 12 h and is given twice a day, a steady state is achieved by the middle of the third day (5 × 12 h). If a drug has a half-life of 2 h and is administered every 6 h, a steady state occurs after the third dose (5 × 2 h) because the first dose is at time 0, the second is at 6 h, the third at 12 h, and so on. The difference between 4 and 5 half-lives is nominal: After 4 half-lives, a steady state of 94% is reached, and it increases to 97% after 5 half-lives.[174] Therefore, a patient's compliance in taking medication is important for achieving a steady state and producing the desired results. If a patient fails to take prescribed medication, the intended results may not be achieved. By the same token, taking more than the prescribed dosage may not produce better results faster. In fact, it can be deleterious. "More is better" does not apply to drug dosages. Taking higher or more frequent doses of a drug results in higher concentrations that may produce toxic side effects. Taking two different anti-inflammatory drugs, whether they are prescription or OTC medications, should also be avoided because it is equivalent to increasing the dosage and can be dangerous. These precautions should be explained to patients for any medications they take.

Most drugs taken by mouth are absorbed in the small intestine. If medication is taken with liquid, a full glass of liquid is advisable, not just a swallow. The liquid helps dissolve the medication and also increases the speed with which the drug moves from the stomach to the small intestine. If a drug is to be taken with food, it is absorbed at a slower rate, and the food may reduce otherwise irritating effects the drug may have on the stomach.

Exercise immediately after ingestion can alter drug absorption because blood that is normally allotted to the gastrointestinal tract is shunted to working muscles. With delayed movement of medication from the stomach to the small intestine, stomach lining irritation may increase.[174] For this reason, it may not be a good idea to take an anti-inflammatory medication immediately before exercise, especially when the stomach is empty.

NSAIDs

Anti-inflammatory drugs are among the drugs most commonly purchased by athletes today, either by prescription or over-the-counter (OTC).[175, 176] The most often used of these are the nonsteroidal anti-inflammatory drugs (NSAIDs). Recent investigations have revealed that there are no detrimental effects from using NSAIDs after injury except in the case of fractures and chronic inflammations.[177-179] The NSAIDs are used to reduce pain and promote healing by minimizing inflammation in acute injuries. In the short term, NSAIDs may be more beneficial than other pain-relieving drugs such as opioids, which may become habit forming.[180]

NSAIDs reduce inflammation by inhibiting the enzymes cyclooxygenase-1 (COX-1) and cyclooxygenase-2 (COX-

2). The primary reason for NSAID use in sport injury therapy is to reduce pain by inhibiting prostaglandin (PG) production. Prostaglandins stimulate local nociceptors (pain-receptive nerve endings) and enhance edema formation by increasing vascular permeability. By limiting PG production, NSAIDs can encourage healing progression from the inflammation phase to the proliferation phase. By reducing edema and pain, range-of-motion and other therapeutic exercises can begin sooner to promote recovery.

Several prescription and OTC NSAIDs are available. Refer to table 2.11 for a list of commonly used NSAIDs. People respond differently to each of these drugs. As a rule, the amount of NSAID in the OTC dosage is half the equivalent prescription medication. One person may find better results from aspirin, whereas another may find aspirin ineffective but have great relief from ibuprofen. Another person may find that naproxen upsets the stomach but tolmetin causes no problems. Physicians commonly try a different NSAID if a patient does not respond appropriately to the first. Because each person responds differently, trial and error is often used to discover the medication that is most effective in achieving desired therapy goals.

Because NSAIDs inhibit PG production through changes in **arachidonic acid** metabolism, other physiological functions are also affected. Besides affecting the inflammation phase of local injuries, PGs play an important role in protecting the stomach lining. Therefore, one of the most common side effects of NSAIDs is stomach upset. For this reason, people with a history of ulcers or allergy to aspirin should not use NSAIDs. Stomach upset, nausea, and vomiting are possible side effects and may discourage a patient from continuing to use NSAIDs. Generally, the tendency for stomach upset and ulcers to occur increases the longer a person uses NSAIDs.

NSAIDs may also be harmful to kidney and cardiac functions. Arachidonic acid plays an important role in renal physiology, so people with renal disease may not be able to use NSAIDs. Because of the heart's relationship to renal function, people with congestive heart failure should avoid NSAIDs.

Like most other drugs, NSAIDs should be avoided by women who are pregnant or who are nursing infants since NSAIDs may be harmful to the fetus or infant.

TABLE 2.11 NSAIDs

Generic name	Brand name	Doses/d	Maximum daily adult dose (mg)[a]
NONSELECTIVE COX INHIBITORS			
Aspirin[b]	many	4	4000
Fenoprofen	Nalfon	3–4	3200
Flurbiprofen	Ansaid	2–4	300
Ibuprofen[b]	Advil	3–4	3200
Indomethacin	Indocin	2–4	200
Ketoprofen[b]	Actron	3–4	300
Naproxen Na[b]	Aleve	2	1650
Piroxicam	Feldene	1	20
Sulindac	Clinoril	2	400
Tolmetin Na	Tolectin	3	1800
Diclofenac	Voltaren	2–4	200
Oxaprozin	Daypro	1	1800
SELECTIVE COX-2 INHIBITORS			
Celecoxib	Celebrex	1–2	400
SLIGHTLY SELECTIVE COX-2 INHIBITORS			
Etodolac	Lodine	2–3	1000
Meloxicam	Mobic	1	15
Nabumetone	Relafen	1–2	2000

[a]Typical daily dose may be considerably less.

[b]Available without prescription.

Adapted by permission from J.E. Houglum, "Pharmacologic Considerations in the Treatment of Injured Athletes with Nonsteroidal Anti-Inflammatory Drugs," *Journal of Athletic Training* 33 (1998): 259-263.[181]

A family of NSAIDs was approved by the FDA in the late 1990s. These drugs primarily inhibit COX-2 by their influence on arachidonic acid metabolism. The more traditional NSAIDs are nonselective and affect both COX-1 and COX-2 to varying degrees. The COX-1 enzyme is involved in many homeostatic processes in the body such as renal function, bronchial tone, platelet aggregation, temperature regulation, and gastric mucosa protection.[182] On the other hand, the selective COX-2 medications function primarily in the inflammation process. While the nonspecific NSAIDs inhibit both COX-1 and COX-2, the selective COX-2 inhibitors isolate their activity to the inflammation-producing activity of COX-2, so these newer NSAIDs reduce inflammation with less impact on gastric and kidney cells and other normal essential functions dependent upon COX-1.[182] Unfortunately, selective COX-2 inhibitors have been found to increase the risk of stroke and heart attack in some people taking them, especially those at increased risk for cardiovascular disease.[183, 184] Although at one time there were several brands of COX-2 inhibitors on the market, since 2011 Celebrex (celecoxib) is the only remaining COX-2 inhibitor; the others have been removed from the market by their manufacturers. A group of NSAIDs known as slightly selective COX-2 inhibitors have subsequently been developed. These drugs are not as selective as celecoxib, so while they are not as inclined to reduce stomach upset as the selective COX-2 inhibitor NSAIDs, they are less likely to produce stomach upset as frequently as the non-selective NSAIDs.[185]

Steroid medication is also used to control inflammation, but its use is currently limited because of its severe side effects. It is usually prescribed in large doses for a short amount of time. Administration is closely monitored by the prescribing physician because of the possible severe side effects.[186]

Drug Interactions

Any drug can interact with other drugs also being taken to either enhance or reduce their effectiveness. This is known as **drug interaction**. For example, NSAIDs increase blood-clotting time by affecting the role of arachidonic acid in platelet aggregation, and therefore they magnify the effects of drugs used in anticoagulant therapy. NSAIDs may also decrease the effectiveness of other drugs such as diuretics (medication to increase urine excretion, usually administered to relieve systemic swelling), beta blockers (medication that slows heart rate), angiotensin-converting enzyme inhibitors (medication used to lower blood pressure), and oral hypoglycemic agents (medication taken orally to control type 2 diabetes). Antacids delay the rate at which an NSAID is absorbed.

Other Drugs

Some medications may delay the healing process. Antibiotics, antineoplastic drugs, heparin, nicotine, and corticosteroids can all delay healing. The rehabilitation clinician should be aware of any medication the patient is taking in order to consider when the normal healing process may be affected because of the medications.

Individualized Modifying Factors

A number of other factors affect healing, including the performance of the surgeon in cases of surgical wounds or the patient's personal factors. The patient's personal factors can include issues that existed before the injury and issues that are secondary to the injury. Each person's situation will be unique, and progress will depend on these individualized factors. Some of these factors are inherent; the clinician may not have much influence over them but should be aware of them and the impact they may have on the patient's injury. Factors over which the clinician has no control include surgical repairs, the patient's age, systemic diseases from which the patient suffers, and wound size. Other factors such as infection, spasm, and swelling can be reduced with appropriate and timely treatment. Nutrition can be influenced through instruction and advice to the patient.

Surgical Repairs

The physician's surgical and sterile techniques have a direct effect on the healing of injuries that are repaired surgically. Infection complicates and delays the healing process. The quality of the surgeon's repair technique and follow-up care directly influences when rehabilitation can be started. If a surgeon's technique results in increased rather than decreased postoperative edema, tissue repair is delayed. If a surgeon immobilizes an injury for 3 months rather than 3 weeks, rehabilitation progress will be slower.

Age

Age can be a factor that alters healing.[187] A good blood supply is crucial for any injury to heal properly. A poor blood supply delays or prevents an injury from healing properly. Blood supply is often impaired with age.[188, 189] Diseases associated with age also can affect healing.

Disease

Certain systemic diseases can impede healing. If a patient has diabetes or other endocrine disease, HIV, arthritis, connective tissue disease, carcinoma, or other systemic diseases, extra care should be taken with healing wounds. Additionally, conditions not often seen in athletes that can delay healing include renal, hepatic, cardiovascular, and autoimmune diseases. If a patient has any of these conditions, the clinician is wise to be especially cautious.

Wound Size

Generally, the more extensive the injury, the more time needed for healing to occur. If a patient suffers a first-degree ankle sprain, he or she may be able to participate in practice the next day. However, if a patient has a second-degree ankle sprain, he or she may be unable to return to practice for a week or more.

The larger the destruction of tissue and the greater the separation between tissue ends, the longer it will take for the body to debride the area and connect the stump ends. Similarly, the greater the injury, the greater the resulting scar tissue formation. Scar tissue can impede rehabilitation, depending on where the scar tissue is and how long the injured site is immobilized before exercises begin. For example, scar tissue extending across a joint may restrict that joint's mobility as the scar tissue matures, especially when it is undergoing scar minimization as myofibroblasts work to shrink the scar. The duration of immobilization has a significant impact on the scar's effects on function; as a scar advances in its collagen aggregation and maturation processes, it becomes less responsive to clinicians' efforts to alter its impact on mobility and function.

Infection

Infection is a possibility any time an open wound remains open, whether it is an abrasion, a surgical wound, or a needle stick. Precautions should always be taken to prevent infection, regardless of the source or size of the wound. Infection always delays healing.[190] When an infection occurs, the wound site develops a greater scar than it would otherwise have had.

Nutrition

Nutrition plays an important part in healing.[191] The clinician should encourage the patient to have good nutrition through well-balanced meals to enhance healing. Diets lacking in protein, carbohydrates, vitamins (especially A and C), or minerals (especially the trace minerals zinc and copper) make healing more difficult.[192]

Muscle Spasm

Spasm is a reflex that occurs with injury as the body tries to minimize the injury by immobilizing the affected area. Pain and muscle inhibition combine to diminish function. Spasms result in ischemia by contracting muscles and compressing blood vessels, restricting blood flow. Applying immediate first aid to the area is important in reducing spasm and ultimately improving the rate of tissue healing and the function of the injured part.

Swelling

The amount of swelling that occurs for persons with similar injuries varies. As a rule, however, the more severe the injury, the greater the swelling. Swelling is caused by fluid moving from its normal location within cells and the bloodstream into the interstitial spaces and can include blood, watery fluid from damaged cells, and plasma fluids.[193] The body interprets extracellular blood as a foreign substance and recruits the immune system to fight it, further adding to the amount of fluid and cells in the area. This edema formation also puts pressure on sensitive nerve endings, causes reflex muscular inhibition, and negatively affects nutrient exchange at the site of injury.[194] These factors ultimately increase pain, reduce function, and slow healing. The greater the amount of accumulated extravascular blood and fluid, the greater the symptoms of inflammation and the longer it will take the body to progress from inflammation to proliferation. It is therefore crucial for the clinician to apply immediate treatment to minimize the edema and thereby promote healing. Minimizing edema also reduces inflammation, pain, and loss of function.

Advances in Investigation

Over the past several years, a plethora of research has been conducted about healing and how to advance healing, both in specific tissues and in the generic realm of tissue healing. This section presents a brief summary of current investigations of these topics.

Stem Cells

Stem cells are unique, nonspecific cells that can differentiate, or change, into different cell types that become specialized in their appearance and function. When stem cells divide, they can either become new stem cells or differentiate into specialized cells such as bone cells, muscle cells, nerve cells, or blood cells. Only stem cells have the ability to replicate themselves into more stem cells or become different types of cells. Stem cells can divide and replicate themselves many times and remain unspecialized, but specialized cells such as nerve cells or blood cells cannot reproduce themselves. When we say stem cells are unspecialized, this means there is no specific tissue structure that allows them to perform specific functions like nerve or muscle cells do. All human cells start as stem cells, but as they continue to divide and mature under the right conditions, they differentiate into specific kinds of cells to perform specific functions.

Although there are different ways to categorize stem cells, there are basically two types of stem cells from which all categories of stem cells come: embryonic stem cells and adult stem cells. Embryonic stem cells originate from embryos. Adult stem cells are present throughout a person's body. They are found in various tissues and organs and are thought to exist in these tissues to repair and maintain the tissue in which they are located.[195] Because of the ethical concerns that arise from using embryonic stem cells in research, adult stem cells, sometimes called somatic stem cells, are harvested and reprogrammed in laboratory settings, allowing those cells to develop into different types of cells.[196] Future uses in stem cell applications to healing go beyond scar tissue healing and involve actual regeneration of new tissue; this is the exciting prospect of stem cell therapy for injuries and disease.

Currently in the clinical world, the most common use of stem cells appears to be for dermal wounds such as chronic wounds and burns.[1, 197-199] Other avenues of stem cell use are also being investigated with promising initial results. Tissues such as bone,[3] muscle,[83, 139] tendons,[200] and ligaments[201] are all being identified as structures that will benefit from stem cell therapy after injury. The future of stem cell therapy appears bright.

Tissue Engineering

According to the National Institute of Biomedical Imaging and Bioengineering,[202] tissue engineering is defined as "an interdisciplinary and multidisciplinary field that aims at the development of biological substitutes that restore, maintain, or improve tissue function." A variety of substances are used in tissue engineering in addition to the body's cells, including plastic and other polymers and proteins.[203] Polymers used in tissue engineering can be synthetic inorganic materials,[204] but they are more often composed of organic molecules that have been synthesized by living organisms.[205] These polymers are called biopolymers and come from plants in the form of starches, cellulose, and natural rubber; animals in the form of collagen and hyaluronic acid; and smaller animal and plant forms such as bacteria, algae, and fungi.[205] As part of the engineering process, these polymers are used to build scaffolds that create an environment that is conducive to new tissue formation. Cells from the body are inserted into these porous, mesh-like scaffolds, which produce interactions with other cells and ultimately form new tissue.[206]

The challenge in today's world of tissue engineering is to mimic normal tissue's development and functions.[207] The extracellular matrix (ECM) provides the optimal scaffold in normal, healthy tissue; however, ECM is impossible to replicate with our current creative systems and abilities.[204] Scaffolds are necessary in tissue repair, for they are the bed from which new tissue grows.

There are many research avenues currently investigating scaffold development through tissue engineering. Studies of ways to restore tissue of injured muscle,[131] tendon,[102] bone,[3] articular cartilage,[208] and intervertebral discs[204] are well underway. Though tissue engineering and scaffold design and development have progressed by leaps and bounds in the past few years, there is more yet to be known and accomplished before tissue repair using these advances becomes commonplace.[209-211] Many problems have yet to be solved; among the most important is improving vascularization strategies and developing a desirable matrix around the newly forming microvasculature.[207] New and ongoing investigations into scaffolds and their means of providing a consistent and beneficial environment for all biophysiological and biochemical elements needed for tissue regeneration will reveal interesting and exciting information in the years to come.

Summary

There are four phases of healing. Although healing proceeds moment by moment without clear delineations between its phases, these phases give health care providers a system to better understand and appreciate the healing process and the progression that must occur to complete it. Outside factors such as growth factors, diet, age, and injury severity will influence healing. There are new revelations on the horizon in the world of healing that are being identified through investigations into stem cell and tissue engineering. Although advances in these topics have been significant over the past few years, science is just beginning to open this world to us and to show us the potential it contains for the future.

LEARNING AIDS

Key Concepts and Review

1. Explain the differences between primary and secondary healing.

Primary healing produces a minimal scar and occurs when the damaged edges of a wound are close to each other, whereas secondary healing produces a bigger scar because the wound must heal by filling in tissue from the bottom and sides of the wound.

2. Identify the healing phases.

The body follows a very complex and not fully understood process of healing, going through four phases: hemostasis, inflammation, proliferation, and remodeling.

3. Describe the primary processes of each healing phase.

During the shortest healing phase, hemostasis, there is a brief vasoconstriction followed by vasodilation. Platelets become activated to stimulate the infiltration of inflammatory products and growth factors. During inflammation, platelets combine with collagen and other structures to form a fibrin plug. Neutrophil migration begins the inflammation process, fibrin plug production prevents fluid and blood from escaping, monocyte migration rids the area of debris, angiogenesis restores blood flow, and Type III collagen is produced. Proliferation occurs when fibroblasts, myofibroblasts, and collagen synthesis are at their peak. During remodeling, healing slows, wound contraction is well underway, and Type III collagen is converted to Type I collagen.

4. Discuss the causes for the signs of inflammation.

Redness, localized warmth, swelling, pain, and dysfunction are all signs of inflammation. Redness occurs because of increased circulation and released chemicals, localized warmth and swelling are caused by interstitial fluid leakage and increased metabolic activity in the area, and pain is caused by pressure on nerve endings from edema and damage to nerves in the area. Dysfunction occurs because of the physical restrictions of swelling, damage to structures, and the muscular inhibition from the pain.

5. Explain the influence of growth factors in healing.

Growth factors play an important role throughout tissue healing. Several growth factors influence the healing process. They assist in causing cell proliferation and chemotactic activity that are vital to healing.

6. Discuss the differences between acute and chronic inflammation.

Acute inflammation occurs through a systematic progression of chemical and cellular activity. Chronic inflammation occurs when the injury site cannot proceed from the inflammatory phase to the proliferation phase because leukocytes remain in the area and granulocytes cannot fully debride the area, so mononuclear cells persist.

7. Discuss the healing characteristics of specific tissues.

Ligaments, tendons, muscle, bone, and cartilage all follow the general healing process, but their healing also has aspects unique to their own cellular makeup. For example, muscle has myogenic cells that can regenerate muscle tissue, bone has osteoblasts, and tendons have tenocytes.

8. Identify the relevance of tensile strength.

Tensile strength enables a structure to withstand stresses. Once an area is damaged, its tensile strength will never be restored to 100% of normal except in bone. In spite of this, a patient can safely return to normal participation if the injury has properly healed and a proper rehabilitation program has been followed.

9. Discuss factors that can modify the healing process.

Healing of any tissue is influenced by a number of factors. These include the use of medications (especially anti-inflammatory drugs), the application of first aid, edema and pain, infection, and nutrition. Other factors over which the clinician has no control include the physician's surgical technique and the patient's age and general health.

10. Explain the role NSAIDs play in inflammation.

NSAIDs reduce the effects of inflammation by altering chemical production or the impact of specific chemicals on the healing process in soft tissues. If administered correctly, they can reduce the inflammation phase to promote healing. They have a deleterious effect, however, on healing bone.

Critical Thinking Questions

1. If you were Daniel in the opening scenario, how would you approach Becki to discuss whether or not she has anorexia? How could anorexia affect Becki's healing process? What could you do to counteract her anorexia? What precautions should you take to "do no harm"?

2. A patient who undergoes an outpatient surgical repair of the elbow comes to you 3 d after the surgery to begin rehabilitation. Where in the healing process do you estimate this patient to be, and what healing activities are occurring?

3. A patient with a second-degree ankle sprain that occurred 4 d ago comes to you for rehabilitation. The patient is 50 years old, has diabetes, severe swelling, and cramps in the calf muscles, is taking Coumadin and an oral hypoglycemic medication, and has been taking oral anti-inflammatories for the past 3 d. What precautions must you consider? How would your treatment be different for a patient who is 22 years old, has severe swelling and cramps in the calf muscles, has been taking oral anti-inflammatories for the past 3 d, and is in otherwise good health?

Lab Activities

1. Identify three reliable websites to which you can refer for additional information on general tissue healing, the stages of healing, or the healing of specific tissues.

2. Identify three medications kept in your own home, and list what influence, if any, they may have on healing.

3. Investigate the influences three growth hormones have on healing. Where are they produced in the body, how are they attracted to an injury site, and during what stage of healing would you expect them to be most evident? Why?

3

Impact of Healing on Rehabilitation

Objectives

After completing this chapter, you should be able to do the following:

1. Identify the three Rs of rehabilitation, and explain how they relate to healing.
2. Discuss the timing of treatment with the various stages of healing.
3. Provide a rationale for why only modalities are used during the first and second phases of healing.
4. Identify the actions a clinician should take if a returning patient reports increased pain and swelling as a result of the previous treatment session.
5. Compare and contrast the treatments provided in the first phase of healing and the last phase of healing, and provide a rationale for why they are different.

Reetah Scholls is Joel Eddy's first new patient of the day. He knows that she recently underwent a rotator cuff repair and is coming to the clinic today for her initial examination before beginning her rehabilitation program. Joel knows that one of the first things he must identify is the specific date of her surgery since the amount of time that has passed since the surgery will have a direct impact on how he will treat her surgical repair today.

A mind, once stretched by a new idea, never regains its original dimensions.

Author Unknown

You know from chapter 2 what occurs when a person suffers an injury. This chapter expands on that information and challenges you to stretch your own mind to apply what you learned in chapter 2 to the creation of a rehabilitation program. As a professional who rehabilitates orthopedic and sport injuries, you have a duty to understand healing and how rehabilitation affects healing, as well as how the healing timeline dictates the progression of rehabilitation. This chapter correlates the timing of rehabilitation steps with the timeline of healing to help you produce optimal results for both healing and rehabilitation.

The first half of this chapter describes rehabilitation's impact on the results of healing. As the tissues undergo healing, changes are observed in signs and symptoms and in how those tissue structures function. Each of these changes is addressed in rehabilitation so that the end result can be a fully functioning, normally operating person who can return to previous levels of activity.

The second half of this chapter looks at the stages of healing and what rehabilitation techniques are used at each stage. This part of the chapter presents the rationale for decisions about what to include or exclude in rehabilitation at a given healing stage to obtain optimal outcomes.

Figure 3.1 provides a graphic representation of what is discussed in the first half of this chapter. This figure presents the three Rs of rehabilitation that coincide with

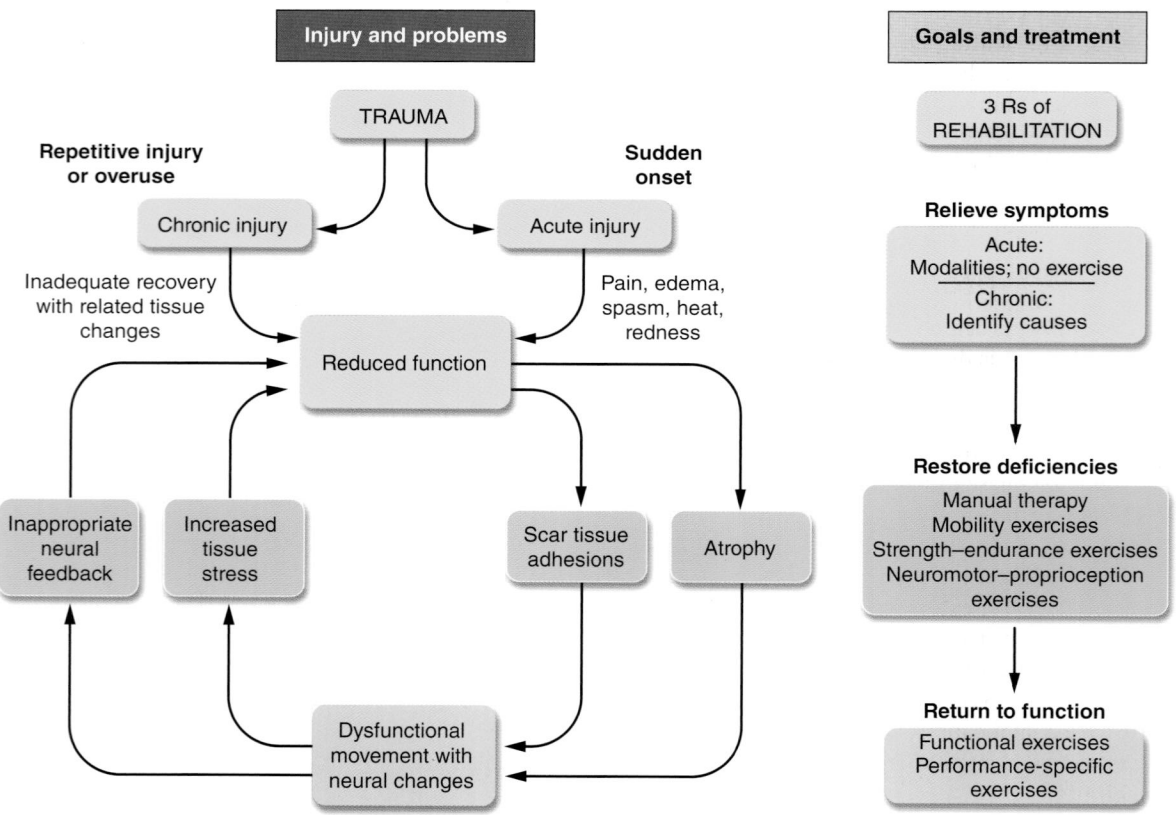

Figure 3.1 The physical changes that result from the healing process and the three Rs of rehabilitation that are used as these changes occur. As the injury's status changes, rehabilitation treatment and goals must change to meet new abilities and make new demands.

the body's responses throughout the healing process. The three Rs include the treatment and goals that coincide with the healing tissue's changing status. They serve as a quick review of what occurs from either a physiological or a physical standpoint after an injury, and they indicate how clinicians can have a positive impact on an injury's outcome. Clinicians must know appropriate techniques that positively influence the healing process.

The clinician can have a positive or a negative influence on healing, depending on the specific treatment and when it is applied. Knowledge plays a vital part in the delivery of treatment. Knowing how to apply a treatment is the easy part; knowing when to apply it, at what intensity, and to what effect is more difficult.

There are many ways to define rehabilitation and to develop a rehabilitation program. Regardless of how rehabilitation is defined or how the clinician outlines a plan of care, the ultimate goal of any program is an optimal outcome for the patient. Before we create a rehabilitation progression, we must first identify how healing affects elements of the rehabilitation program and guides your plan of care.

The Three Rs of Rehabilitation

Clinicians must correlate rehabilitation with what is going on during healing. Based on the changes that occur throughout the healing process, we can divide a rehabilitation program's plan of care into three segments. To make it easy to remember, we call these divisions the three Rs of rehabilitation: (1) *relieve* symptoms, (2) *restore* deficiencies, and (3) *return* to function. Each R will be presented here.

Relieve Symptoms

Rehabilitation efforts begin at the time of injury during the hemostasis phase. It is during the hemostasis and inflammation phases that the first R occurs. During this time, the rehabilitation clinician's first efforts are to relieve the signs and symptoms produced by the injury itself and by the inflammation phase of healing that follows.

This initial treatment is commonly known as first aid, and the type and quality of treatment provided at the time of injury have a direct impact on the problems that must be addressed later. For example, if efforts are not made to stop bleeding and reduce edema, the later rehabilitation plan must include treatments to address any complications that may arise from excessive ecchymosis and edema formation. These complications can include delayed healing and increased pain, impairment, functional limitations, and disability.[1, 2]

Recall from chapter 2 that the hemostasis phase is followed immediately by the inflammation phase. It is during the inflammation phase that swelling increases as chemokines, cells, and growth factors stream into the injury

site because of increased capillary permeability. Even when hemostasis has been achieved, swelling continues because of the activities of these chemicals and cells, which are required as part of the healing process. Generally, the greater the degree of injury, the greater will be the swelling that ensues.

The only substance holding the injury site together and preventing additional bleeding for the first several days following injury is the fibrin clot. This structure is weak and easily disrupted. Therefore, the clinician must be cautious in managing the injury during this time.

The symptoms that clinicians are concerned about during this early rehabilitation phase include edema, pain, localized temperature increase, and muscle spasm. Although the injury site may be too fragile and painful to begin rehabilitation exercises, there is a need to address these debilitating signs and symptoms, which are the effects of inflammation.

Therapeutic Modalities

Although immediate treatment at the time of an injury is considered first aid, it is really the first step in rehabilitation. The effectiveness of this first aid determines how complex the early care in the inflammation phase must be. At the outset of an injury there is damage to the blood vessels, causing bleeding into the wound area. Immediate-care goals include minimizing blood and fluid loss.

Treatments used from the time of the injury's onset through the next few days include various modalities to restore hemostasis and minimize the signs and symptoms of inflammation. Among the most widely used of these modalities are cryotherapy, compression, and elevation.[3] Although the combined effect of these treatments has not been clinically validated through experimental investigation, investigations have shown that these are each individually effective treatments immediately after injury.[3] Bouts of compression and elevation for 15 to 20 min, repeated each hour for 6 h, have demonstrated beneficial effects in reducing bleeding and tissue damage.[4] Cryotherapy has a direct impact on the amount of postinjury edema and is an important modality in these early days.[4, 5]

Additional beneficial modalities may also be used to resolve the physiological effects of injury as the inflammation phase progresses. The modalities most often used during this time, in addition to the continued use of cryotherapy and compression,[6, 7] include electrical stimulation[8] and ultrasound.[9] These modalities will be briefly presented here, but a more thorough review of them may be found in chapter 9.

Cryotherapy   **Cryotherapy** is an umbrella term for any cold modality. Some of the most common cryotherapy methods used for orthopedic and sports injuries include ice bags, cold-water immersion, and commercial cold packs. We have already briefly discussed cryotherapy as an immediate treatment during the clot-forming phase that begins the healing process, but it is also a useful modality during the inflammation phase of healing. Cryotherapy is used during this second phase to reduce the signs and symptoms of inflammation.[10, 11] Although cryotherapy will not affect existing edema, it can reduce newly formed edema.[12]

Cryotherapy also helps reduce the patient's pain[13, 14] and muscle spasm.[15, 16] As muscles relax, pain subsides. As pain subsides, there is general relaxation that allows for a better night's sleep.[17] Quality sleep is a requirement for essential healing.[18] Therefore, the use of ice or other cryotherapy applications during early inflammation when pain and muscle spasm are most acute can not only relieve those symptoms but also aid in the healing process.

Electrical Stimulation   Electrical stimulation applied during the first week after a ligamentous injury enhances protein synthesis to help promote healing.[10] Because tendon and ligament structures are similar,[19-21] electrical stimulation may also have the same effects when applied to tendons.

Electrical stimulation applied to muscles may relax muscle spasm.[10] When facilitating muscle contraction, electrical stimulation may also help to relieve local edema by pumping this excessive extracellular fluid into the lymph system.[22] Reducing edema reduces pressure on local nerve receptors, thereby reducing pain. As the pain subsides, the patient may move the part more willingly and may thus have more function of the injured segment.

Therapeutic Exercise

Exercise is not advised during the inflammation phase. The strongest element protecting the injured microvessels is the tenuous fibrin clot. This structure is easily damaged by forces applied to it.[23] Any new bleeding restarts the inflammation process from the beginning, ultimately adding to the healing time. Exercise stress applied to the damaged tissues during this time exacerbates the injury, resulting in additional tissue damage. This new tissue insult also adds to the effects of inflammation—pain, edema, spasm, and reduced function—to make exercise difficult and add to the patient's pain.

There is one exception to this construct: continuous passive motion (CPM) machines are sometimes used immediately after surgery.[24] These machines provide minimal stress to the surgical site and have been shown to minimize postoperative signs and symptoms.[25] Continuous passive motion machines are used immediately after some but not all orthopedic surgeries. Their use is beneficial primarily in surgical cases that include rotator cuff repair,[23] articular cartilage repair,[26] total knee arthroplasty,[27] and ankle fixations.[28]

Restore Deficiencies

Once the injury advances from the inflammation phase to the proliferation phase, angiogenesis occurs, fibroblasts become predominant, and tissue development and restoration begins. Injured tissues start their recovery and can now tolerate a bit more stress than they could withstand during the inflammation phase. New capillary formation supports collagen deposits that strengthen the new structures as tissues grow and develop. Myoblasts also enter the area to begin scar tissue contraction. During this time, modality treatments can continue to be helpful, as can certain types of therapeutic exercises.

Therapeutic Modalities

As the inflammation phase wanes and the proliferation phase progresses, the rehabilitation clinician has a wider selection of modalities from which to choose. These may include a variety of cryotherapy techniques, electrical stimulation, and low-power laser.[29-31]

Cryotherapy   There are no sharp transitions from one healing phase to the next; factors such as the severity and type of injury, the location of the injury, and the patient's age, general health, and size can affect the rate of healing. The timelines provided are averages, so individual healing rates may vary from those averages. Therefore, some clinicians continue treatments with cryotherapy beyond the inflammation phase and extend its use into the early proliferation phase. Such a practice is common and acceptable.

The physiological effects of cryotherapy can lead to reductions in pain, muscle spasm, inflammation, and edema.[32] Cryotherapy modalities used during the early proliferation phase may include those that were used during the inflammation phase; these modalities include ice packs, cold-water immersion, and commercial cold packs.

It can sometimes be difficult to determine how long to continue using cryotherapy treatments following an acute injury. Guidelines have been published that aid the clinician in making this decision. These guidelines are identified by Starkey[33] and include identifying answers to these seven questions:

1. Is the swelling still increasing from day to day?
2. Does more swelling occur with any type of activity?
3. Is motion of the injured part limited because pain occurs with movement?
4. Based on your assessment, do you think the injury is still in the inflammation phase?
5. Does your light or moderate touch of the injury site still produce complaints of pain?
6. Does the patient seem to improve when you apply cryotherapy?
7. Is the injury site still warm to your touch?

If the answer to all of these questions is no, then heat may be used to treat the injury.[33] The questions are listed not in Starkey's original order but in the order that our experience indicates is from the most to the least important indication of continued inflammation. If only a few of the answers are yes, then the clinician can decide whether to continue cryotherapy or convert to thermotherapy based on which questions were answered yes; the first few questions are more important indicators of continued inflammation than the last few.

In addition to reducing the negative signs and symptoms of inflammation, cryotherapy applications also reduce blood flow and cellular metabolism.[32] These effects are advantageous during hemostasis and inflammation because they help diminish blood loss from damaged blood vessels and reduce the oxygen needs of local tissue; however, once bleeding has stopped, the next healing progression is tissue development. For this development to occur, there must be adequate oxygen and blood flow to local tissues so that necessary metabolites, cells, and nutrients are available for angiogenesis and cellular growth.

Thermotherapy   **Thermotherapy** is the application of therapeutic heat[34] to create a desired outcome. Those desired outcomes are related to the physiological effects of the application of different heat therapies to the injured segment.

There are common physiological effects of thermotherapy that generally apply to most heat therapies. These effects include pain reduction, muscle spasm relief, and increased blood flow.[15] In addition, because heat modalities improve blood flow, they encourage healing and promote the delivery of oxygen and nutrients to healing tissues.[32] There is also evidence that heat therapy promotes angiogenesis.[35] Such physiological effects are desirable during the third phase of healing, which depends on new blood vessel development and an inflow of nutrients and oxygen for tissue growth. An additional effect of heat application is improved connective tissue extensibility.[15] Since muscle, tendons, ligaments, and fascia contain connective tissue, their flexibility, ability to elongate, and ability to undergo plastic deformation are improved with heat therapy.[15, 36, 37]

Once the injury site is past the inflammation phase, the clinician advances the patient from cryotherapy to thermotherapy for these beneficial effects. Cold and heat both provide pain and muscle spasm relief. The additional benefits of heat that cannot be delivered by cold are important, and they justify clinician decisions to convert to thermotherapy during mid- and late proliferation.

After the inflammatory phase, heat can be beneficial when applied before passive exercise. It can increase circulation to encourage healing and a better exchange of nutrients and waste products.[15] It can also relax muscles to permit better exercise execution with less pain, and it can reduce tissue viscosity to make an area more pliable for stretching.[10]

As with cryotherapy, there is a variety of thermotherapy modalities from which the clinician may choose to appropriately treat the patient. The modalities chosen depend on the clinician's preference, modality availability, the patient's age, the specific injury and location, and the depth and extent of injury.

Deep Heats: Ultrasound and Diathermy   In addition to the superficial thermotherapy modalities, deeper heat modalities are also available to be used during the proliferation phase of healing. It is believed that ultrasound and diathermy may speed healing and enhance the effects of exercise by improving motion with less pain.[10]

Ultrasound has the benefit of producing thermal as well as mechanical effects. As a source of deep heat, ultrasound may be a useful prestretch application for small-area tendon and capsular adhesions that lie deeper than superficial heat can reach effectively.[38]

Electrical Stimulation   Just as cryotherapy often carries over into the proliferation phase, electrical stimulation is another modality that may extend from the inflammation phase into this healing phase. Additionally, other applications beyond muscle spasm relief may be helpful as the patient moves into mid- and late proliferation.

On those occasions when pain and muscle spasm continue into the early proliferation phase, electrical stimulation for muscle relaxation and pain relief is still appropriate. However, once muscle spasm is resolved, electrical stimulation may be continued to enhance healing.[39]

During the later proliferation phase, electrical stimulation may also be used to retard muscle atrophy, which can be a secondary effect of injury or prolonged inactivity.[40] Electrical stimulation is used to facilitate muscle contraction and encourage reactivation and recruitment of dormant fibers.[10] During short-term denervation, it may facilitate muscle contraction until nerve function is restored. Electrical stimulation may also be used to reduce or relieve muscle spasm.[10]

The rehabilitation clinician should know what treatment results to pursue and should choose modalities that are most likely to produce those results. The modalities presented here are just examples of those that may be selected to achieve rehabilitation goals. They are not a complete inventory of modalities that clinicians may have available. A more focused presentation of modalities is presented in chapter 9.

Therapeutic Exercise

Until the injury enters the proliferation phase of healing, the injured site is too fragile to risk either active or passive exercises, which can place undesirable stress on the injured tissues. However, local tissue strength changes once angiogenesis and collagen formation begin. In the proliferation phase, growth and development occur in a rapidly changing environment with the advance of new blood vessel formation and collagen fibers creating a supportive and stable framework. This phase is the beginning of a progression of strength gains and tissue maturity that constantly improves regional tissue resiliency until the final, permanent structure is completed.

When tissues are well into the proliferation phase, exercise treatments begin in earnest. These exercises include exercise and activity selections that are focused on improving flexibility, strength, and neuromotor control. Since the structure is now stronger, more rigorous stretching exercises may be included if the patient's mobility or range of motion remains deficient. Strength exercises are begun after mobility exercises and begin with easier exercises that progress in association with continued healing; as tissue strength improves, greater resistance is offered to the healing structures. The same approach is used for neuromotor exercises; resistance, stress, and complexity begin at low levels and increase in step with the tissue's healing process.

As tissues advance along the healing continuum, additional stresses are applied to coincide with the strength and resilience gains that result from healing. If the clinician misjudges either the amount of stress applied by an activity or the tissue's ability to withstand that stress, the patient will report increased pain or swelling from that rehabilitation session. This judgment error occurs to even the most experienced clinicians, but its outcome serves as an important tool for providing an indication of how much stress the tissues can tolerate. The clinician now has a more accurate idea of the healing structure's limits and can more accurately predict when to retry this previously harmful activity. When increased pain and swelling occur, it is appropriate to apply cryotherapy to reduce the new edema and relieve the pain; within a day or two, this modality is discontinued when the issue's inflammatory response is resolved.

Throughout the proliferation phase, therapeutic exercises are progressive in their intensity, complexity, and rigor as the injured segment becomes stronger and more resilient. As the patient approaches the end of the proliferation phase and moves closer to the remodeling phase, the elements (i.e., flexibility and ROM, strength, muscle endurance, and neuromotor control) that were deficient at the beginning of this phase should be approaching normal levels.

Return to Function

As the healing process continues into the later proliferation phase and early remodeling phase, new tissues continue to become stronger and develop a more permanent structure. Coinciding with this healing progression, the rehabilitation program moves from an earlier treatment combination of therapeutic modalities and therapeutic exercise to its final focus of returning the patient to his or her former level of function.

Therapeutic Modalities

As the patient's rehabilitation program progresses into this final healing phase, fewer modalities are needed because the injured area is more closely approaching normal function and the injury is either healed or well on its way to being healed. As the patient enters the final stages of rehabilitation, ice is no longer needed after exercise. In fact, if the patient continues to have new swelling or increased pain that requires cryotherapy after therapeutic exercises when in the remodeling phase, an examination is required because these symptoms should not occur this late in the healing process.

By the time the patient enters the later proliferation and early remodeling phase, there is no evidence of inflammation. Thus, there is no additional need for modalities, either heat or cold. However, it is common for patients to request cryotherapy after they finish their therapeutic exercise sessions. They have likely become accustomed to receiving cryotherapy after treatment, and it has become part of the ritual, even though it is no longer needed. The clinician can decide to either continue with the post-exercise habit or try to educate the patient about why it is not needed. It does no harm to provide the cryotherapy, nor does it provide any physiological benefit.

Therapeutic Exercise

Minimal deficiencies may remain during the last part of the proliferation phase in muscle strength and endurance, proprioception, and neuromotor control. As the patient begins to prepare for a return to normal activities, these variables should progress to normal or near-normal status before the patient advances to the final exercises in the rehabilitation treatments.

As was true with exercises during the proliferation phase, therapeutic exercises become progressive in their intensity, complexity, and rigor as the injured segment becomes more resilient, stronger, and more durable during the remodeling phase.

Once the patient's strength and basic neuromotor control return to normal or near-normal, the clinician modifies the rehabilitation program in preparation for the patient's return to normal activities. It is during this time that the clinician includes treatment activities that mimic the demands of normal activities and even includes specific tasks required of those activities. This progression not only re-educates and refines the patient's neuromotor pathways, but it also allows the patient to realize that the healed body segment can perform at preinjury activity levels.

As with other exercises throughout the rehabilitation program, performance goals are established in incremental steps for these functional and performance-specific exercises. As the patient achieves each goal, new goals are established until the patient attains the final goal and demonstrates normal performance of all the skills and tasks required of him or her by the sport or job to which the patient intends to return.

Timing of Rehabilitation Through the Healing Phases

This part of the chapter relates to the specific factors within the healing phases that need to be considered when designing a rehabilitation program. Instead of focusing mainly on the results of the healing phases, we look more closely at each phase to further understand the clinical decisions that must be made as the rehabilitation program progresses.

Table 3.1 identifies those aspects of rehabilitation that are coordinated with the healing timeline. A rehabilitation progression is always determined by where the injury is in its healing process. The clinician's knowledge of the healing process and appreciation of where the patient's injury is within that process throughout the rehabilitation program is vital to the program's successful outcome.

Because a rehabilitation program is designed around an injury's healing sequence, clinicians must understand both the general aspects of healing and the specific modifications involved in the healing of different tissues. They must also be aware of any modifying factors that may alter the normal healing time. For example, children and elderly patients do not heal at the same rate as young adults,[41] and patients who smoke or take illicit drugs may experience delayed healing.[42, 43] Any number of factors may interfere with normal healing, so it is important to obtain an accurate and thorough history at the time of the initial examination.

The question then becomes, Since I cannot see the physical status of the internal injury, how do I know when to progress a patient in the rehabilitation program? The answer was essentially addressed in chapter 1 in the discussion on evidence-based practice (EBP). Recall that EBP includes three elements: empirical knowledge from evidence obtained through research and investigation, the clinician's experience and skill, and the patient's needs and goals. In the early stages of healing, the most important elements are the first two; later in the healing process, all three elements are important for the clinician. So EBP should guide decision-making throughout the rehabilitation program.

The information in chapter 2 is based on research from hundreds of investigators on the topic of healing. This knowledge serves as the foundation for the clinician as the patient moves through the healing process. Additionally, the clinician's skills of history taking, observation, palpation, examination, and assessment provide him or her with information about the patient's current status. In subsequent follow-up examinations, current results are compared with previous results. A number of factors are identified, assessed, and compared to previous examinations: What tissue was involved in the injury? How long ago did the injury occur? How much swelling, pain, and dysfunction did the patient have initially? How have the injured site's local temperature and pain changed? Is muscle spasm still present? Is the edema changing? How is soft-tissue mobility changing? Are joint mobility and range of motion changing? Can the patient take off her jacket more easily? The clinician obtains information from the empirical evidence, patient self-reports, and the clinician's own clinical skills and experience to identify where in the healing process the patient is each time the patient returns for treatment. Answers to these questions and all pertinent information are gathered to guide the clinician's treatment decisions.

As mentioned earlier, the three Rs—relieve symptoms, restore deficiencies, and return to function—form a general framework that defines rehabilitation in terms of these three major goals. We now look at the specific stages of healing rather than the goals of treatment and discuss the rationale for decisions about what to include in rehabilitation during each healing phase to optimize healing outcomes. Some of the information may seem redundant to you, but as you continue reading, differences will become apparent. Refer to table 3.1 as you go through the next few pages to obtain a summary of the details in the text.

Hemostasis Phase

We know that hemostasis begins immediately when the injury occurs. We also know that this is the quickest and shortest phase of healing. It begins immediately and ceases once the blood clot and then the fibrin plug form.

Damaged blood vessels result in an outpouring of blood that must be stopped. As mentioned earlier, a combination of cryotherapy, elevation, and compression is the most commonly used and accepted form of treatment. The goal is to stop the bleeding by encouraging clot and fibrin plug formation. Once this has occurred, the hemostasis phase is over.

Since the only treatment provided in this phase is aimed at minimizing the injury effects by reducing bleeding and loss of fluids from the injured tissues, cryotherapy is the only modality of choice. Elevation and compression are

TABLE 3.1   Coordinating Rehabilitation Program Activities With the Healing Timeline

Healing phase	Timeline	Healing characteristics	Rehabilitation interventions	Goals for rehabilitation
Hemostasis	Day 0	Bleeding initiates blood clot and then fibrin plug formation.	Cryotherapy: Ice pack, ice cup, cryobath, cold pack	Promote blood clot and fibrin plug formation. Minimize bleeding.
Inflammation	Days 1–3	Pain, edema, muscle spasm, elevated local temperature, loss of function.	Cryotherapy: Ice pack, ice cup, cryobath, cold pack	Relieve pain, relieve swelling, reduce local temperature.
			Electrical stimulation	Relieve spasm, relieve pain.
			Compression	Reduce swelling.
			Elevation	Reduce swelling.
			Low-power laser	Relieve pain.
			Exercise for non-affected parts	Maintain uninjured CV and strength, etc.
Early proliferation	Days 2–10	Less muscle spasm. May have some level of continued pain; elevated local temperature and loss of function begin to subside. Type III collagen begins to form. Angiogenesis begins.	Cryotherapy: Ice pack, ice cup, cryobath, cold pack if inflammation remains apparent	Relieve pain, relieve swelling as indicated.
			Electrical stimulation	Relieve spasm, relieve pain, encourage healing.
			Low-power laser	Relieve pain, encourage healing.
			ROM activities	Gain motion, relieve pain, relieve spasm, reduce edema.
			Joint mobilization, grades I–II	Relieve pain.
			Cryotherapy post-treatment only if indicated	Reduce possible inflammatory effects from overly aggressive treatment.
Late proliferation	Days 7–21	Inflammation signs and symptoms are gone. Oxygen demands increase and need for increased blood flow occurs because of increased angiogenesis and Type III collagen formation. Some Type III collagen begins conversion to Type I collagen.	Thermotherapy modalities	Encourage circulation, prepare tissue for other treatments.
			High-voltage electrical stimulation	Reduce edema, reestablish lymphatic flow.
			Russian or interferential electrical stimulation	Muscle reeducation, muscle contraction facilitation.
			Joint mobilization, grades I–II	Relieve pain.
			Selected massage techniques	Relieve swelling, reestablish lymph flow.
			Cryotherapy only if needed	Reduce possible inflammatory effects from overly aggressive treatment.

Healing phase	Timeline	Healing characteristics	Rehabilitation interventions	Goals for rehabilitation
Early remodeling	Days 14–48	Type III collagen being replaced with Type I collagen. Scar tissue becoming more permanent. Tensile strength increases with collagen maturation. Function continues to improve. No inflammatory signs or symptoms are present.	Superficial or deep heat modalities during first week. Cardiovascular exercises for warm-up after first week of early remodeling as modalities are discontinued.	Warm superficial and deep tissues in preparation for rehabilitation exercises.
			ROM activities	Restore and maintain motion.
			Joint mobilization, grades I–IV	Relieve pain, restore mobility.
			Strength, endurance, and neuromotor control activities	Restore lost physical parameters.
			Cryotherapy only if needed	Reduce possible inflammatory effects from overly aggressive treatment.
Late remodeling	Day 42 to 18 months	Scar tissue is mature. Cells and chemicals of proliferation are gone. Tensile strength is optimized.	ROM maintenance activities	Maintain normal range of motion and mobility.
			Neuromotor control activities that mimic normal functions	Prepare patient for return to normal activities.

usually also applied to further enhance the effect of minimizing blood loss, edema formation, and pain. Immobilization or limiting the use of the injured segment provides for reduced pain and minimized risk of additional injury.

Heat modalities are not used during this phase since thermotherapy increases cellular metabolism, vasodilation, and capillary permeability, none of which is desirable at this time. Exercise or movement of the injured segment is also contraindicated at this time since it will easily disrupt blood clot formation and will only exacerbate the injury.

Inflammation Phase

Even before the hemostasis phase is finished, the inflammation phase is well underway. Care must be taken not to disturb the newly formed, tenuous fibrin plug, which provides the injured site's primary stability and strength. Recall from chapter 2 that during the first 3 d after injury, much physiological activity is occurring at the injury site. Among other activities, macrophages are trying to clear the area's debris so fibroblasts can start their rebuilding tasks. We know that undue stress to the injury during this time reinjures the site, disrupts the fibrin clot, and produces additional edema. For these reasons, exercise is usually contraindicated during the inflammation phase. In addition

to the pain that makes it difficult to exercise, the fragility of the injured site makes it too vulnerable to risk re-injury during this time.

Modalities are used during the inflammation phase to relieve the signs and symptoms associated with inflammation. Any heat modality is contraindicated because its effects on blood flow and viscosity encourage bleeding rather than control it.[32] Modalities used during inflammation primarily include the cryotherapy modalities whose effects reduce pain, edema, and local temperature. Some clinicians also use electrical stimulation to reduce pain and muscle spasm.[44] Other clinicians have also found effective pain relief with the use of low-level laser therapy.[45]

The most important point to remember during the inflammation phase is that heat modalities and therapeutic exercise are not used. With few exceptions, they are contraindicated because their application during this time will have deleterious effects on the healing process.

Although the injury site itself cannot tolerate stresses, even patients with recent surgical repairs can work toward one rehabilitation goal (discussed in chapter 1): maintaining the conditioning status of uninjured parts and the cardiovascular system. For example, if a patient underwent right knee surgery, he or she could maintain cardiovascular conditioning by performing activities such as one-legged cycling or upper-body cardiovascular activities. Upper-body weightlifting and left lower-extremity resistance exercises could also be included at this time. Some evidence indicates that exercising the contralateral limb provides some gains in strength in the involved extremity.[46-48]

Early Proliferation Phase

By the end of the first week, the injured site is well into the early proliferation phase. Type I collagen is forming, allowing the area to become stronger and able to withstand more stress compared to its ability during the first few post-injury days. The site of injury is still very weak compared to normal tissue, but it can tolerate some controlled stress. At this time, depending on the injury and the specific tissue involved, flexibility exercises and, in some instances, very early strengthening activities may be initiated. There are, however, some exceptions to this general rule.

Tendon repair is one exception. Some surgeons permit range-of-motion exercises but no strengthening exercises until the third week.[49] Others prefer to wait 6 weeks or longer before beginning strength activities.[50] Some surgeons allow strengthening exercises after 1 week because collagen fibers are being synthesized rapidly and reach their maximum levels by day 10. These surgeons feel that the collagen is strong enough at this time to start mild resistive exercises, often in the form of isometrics. Other surgeons prefer to wait 3 weeks because by then the synovial sheath has been rebuilt to provide a smooth gliding surface for the tendon. Physicians who wait 6 weeks presumably do so because by then the new collagen is fairly mature and the risk of rupture is significantly less. The risk of waiting too long to initiate motion after surgery is that the tendons become bound down by scar tissue adhesions. It is important to know the physician's preferred protocol for the initiation of rehabilitation.

Range-of-motion and flexibility exercises begin during the early proliferation phase. By the end of the first week of healing, collagen is forming, and some fibers may even begin their transformation from weak Type III to stronger, permanent Type I collagen. Cross-link formations strengthen collagen bonds, providing additional strength to the overall structure.[51]

Although new tissue is not strong enough to tolerate resistive exercises at this time, as a general rule, range of motion activities may be initiated. The most effective gains in range of motion are made during the first 3 to 8 weeks after injury.[52] Changes in motion can be made relatively easily with new scar tissue because its higher water content and greater amount of glycosaminoglycans (GAG) restrict cross-link formations in the earlier stages of Type I collagen formation. This structural arrangement allows a stretch force to have a more effective impact on tissue lengthening during this time. It is mechanically easier to change new scar tissue than it is to affect the length of older scar tissue.[53] As scar tissue becomes more mature with the passage of time, it becomes more resistant to change by external forces applied to it because of its reduced fluid and GAG content and its more numerous collagen cross-links.[54] Because scar tissue's strength and response to external forces change with its maturity, different techniques for achieving flexibility are used at different times in the rehabilitation process.[3] In other words, specific flexibility techniques that will be effective depend on the scar tissue's maturity.

Strength exercises are occasionally included toward the end of the early proliferation phase, but only if it is safe to do so. Depending on the severity and type of injury and the patient's status, early strength exercises may include only isometrics. The clinician must be aware of the tissue stresses that occur with strength activities. Care must always be taken to stress the tissues enough to provide the desired results without overstressing them and causing damage.

If damage occurs because rehabilitation activities overly stressed newly forming tissues, new signs and symptoms of inflammation will occur. These cases must be treated as new injuries: Ice, compression, and elevation are immediately applied as the injured site goes through this new inflammation phase. Strength activities are contraindicated during the inflammation phase.

Even though the injured site is stronger during the proliferation phase, it still remains much weaker than normal tissue, so care must be taken and EBP must be incorporated to determine the types and intensity of exercises used during this phase. This is the time when collagen is converting from Type III to Type I, becoming stronger but not yet nearly as strong as it will become; tendons and ligaments are particularly vulnerable in this phase.

Because the early proliferation phase immediately follows the inflammation phase, and the healing phases do not abruptly end but merge with each subsequent phase, there are usually some remaining signs and symptoms of inflammation during the early proliferation phase. For this reason, it is common that modalities used to relieve inflammation are continued into the early proliferation phase.

In summary, any remaining signs and symptoms that carry over from the inflammation phase into the proliferation phase receive continued treatment with the modalities used to treat them during the inflammation phase. Thermotherapies are applied during this time both to satisfy the demands of newly forming tissues and to resolve remaining inflammation signs and symptoms. Exercises are often initiated during this time. These exercises are primarily flexibility and range-of-motion exercises since the window of opportunity in which motion gains may be made is limited; the more developed scar tissue becomes, the less likely flexibility exercises will affect it. Strength exercises, if they begin in this phase, are often limited to isometric exercises. Caution must be taken to limit stresses applied to newly forming tissues since they remain weak and easily vulnerable to injury with even low-level stresses.

Late Proliferation Phase

As the injury site enters the later proliferation phase, anywhere from 1 to 3 weeks after the injury, those chemicals and cells that were active during inflammation have evacuated the wound site. There may be a few lymphocytes in the area continuing to clean up stray debris, but the main elements present are those dealing with localized reconstruction and scar tissue production: fibroblasts and collagen.

It is during this time that a heat modality, or thermotherapy, often replaces cryotherapy. During this phase, the fibrin clot has been replaced by stronger structures: collagen. With all of the new tissue construction underway during this phase, there is a need for improved local circulation; tissue growth and development require more nutrition and oxygen. Therefore, once inflammatory signs and symptoms are gone, the cryotherapy is no longer needed.

Thermotherapy may also be used to prepare the tissues for other rehabilitation treatments. For example, there is evidence that the results of manual therapy can be improved when it is preceded by thermotherapy.[55] Although some clinicians continue to apply heat for extended treatment sessions before exercise, active exercise is more effective than a heat modality to warm-up and increase blood flow of tissues during the later proliferation phases.[33]

Other modalities are also used during the later proliferation phase. These modalities are selected to achieve specific goals within the rehabilitation program. For example, high-voltage electrical stimulation (HVES) may be used if edema continues to be a problem.[56] HVES effectively reestablishes lymphatic flow.[57] The body interprets interstitial edema as a foreign substance because that excess fluid should not be there. The only way this "foreign substance" is transported from the area is through the lymphatic system.

Biofeedback and other forms of electrical stimulation may also be used during this phase to facilitate the desired response from atrophied muscles or from muscles that do not respond appropriately because of neuromotor deficiencies. For example, if a long-term shoulder injury has created pathological recruitment of scapular muscles, biofeedback treatments are beneficial in restoring proper muscle timing activation.[58]

The electrical stimulation used to strengthen muscle can be categorized as either neuromuscular electrical stimulation (NMES) or interferential stimulation (IFS). An alternating current (AC) is used with either system. Both systems also make use of high-frequency waveforms, although the IFS modalities incorporate low-frequency waves as well. Russian stimulation is a type of NMES. The evidence for the use of NMES is conflicting; some investigators have found positive benefits for strength with its application while others have not.[40, 59-61]

Sometimes IFS is referred to as interferential currents (IFC). This modality uses two electrical waves; one has a constant high frequency and the other has a changing, or variable, lower frequency. These two waves interfere with one another inside the body to affect muscle contraction. Research investigations demonstrate that IFS improves range of motion and pain,[62] and it also has good results when used for strength gains.[63]

Although several biomechanical and histochemical changes occur during this time, the newly forming tissues still cannot tolerate significant stresses. It's only been about 2 weeks since the injury, so the clinician must continue to respect the healing process and be cautious about the forces applied to the injured structures. Because collagen continues to form and mature during this part of the proliferation phase, stresses sufficient to improve range of motion and mobility may be increased as the tissues progress through proliferation, but the clinician should remain vigilant to avoid overstressing tissues.

Joint mobilizations may advance from grades used to reduce pain to those that will improve the mobility of soft tissue surrounding the joints. Mild capsular stretches may be initiated during this time to promote range of motion and to improve mobility within the joint. In addition to using joint mobilization for synovial joint capsule mobility, other manual techniques can also be used during this time to reduce restrictions that may exist within other soft-tissue structures. For example, massage and myofascial release may be appropriate if the clinician identifies through manual palpation that soft-tissue adhesions are hampering mobility. It may be necessary to use massage to either relax tense muscles or reduce edema that may persist in this phase. Trigger points or tender points in the affected area may require manual techniques to relieve these painful points.

Range-of-motion exercises continue to grow in importance during this latter part of the proliferation phase. Depending on the tissues affected and location of the injury, flexibility exercises during this time may include passive (PROM) or active (AROM) range-of-motion exercises. Since newly forming tissues are relatively young and immature, the need for prolonged stretches to improve mobility is highly unlikely. Because tissue remains immature, active and passive stretches should be sufficient to improve motion and mobility. These types of exercises are addressed in chapter 12.

Early Remodeling Phase

This is the time when tissues remodel to become more permanent structures. A substantial increase in collagen cross-links creates a stronger structure that tolerates additional stress. The collagen seen during this time is Type I collagen, which will be the permanent collagen that becomes the scar. Along with these structural modifications, the patient's ability to perform more activities improves. There is no inflammatory healing going on in this phase. Each day brings the patient closer to complete healing.

Once again, it is possible for a clinician to provide an exercise or activity that is too stressful for the healing part. The clinician is cognizant of this risk and looks for new signs of inflammation, especially when an exercise progresses from one level to the next. It is not always easy to determine how much stress a recovering injury can tolerate, but that is what the clinician must do. The exercise intensity should correlate with the tissue's ability to withstand those stress levels in accordance with its healing timeline. Results of those applied stresses are continually assessed to ensure optimal rehabilitation. This assessment includes observations and simple questions addressed to the patient to ascertain the results of the last treatment. Increased edema, increased pain, and diminished function are signs that the exercises were too severe for the injury. Questions may include, "Did your knee have more swelling last night?" "Was there more pain in your shoulder after you left the clinic yesterday?" or "Was it easier or more difficult to walk on one crutch after the last treatment?" If you determine that an exercise produced undesirable effects, the appropriate action is to retreat to a previous exercise level until the injured segment can tolerate the increased stress. If no deleterious effects occur, the current course of treatment is appropriate.

As you would expect, as the scar tissue becomes more resilient and stable, the injury can tolerate more stress. Because of the tissue's improved resilience in this phase, this is the time when resistive exercises are added into the rehabilitation program. The injury site is stronger but is not yet normal, so caution and observation continue to play important roles in the rehabilitation progression.

The clinician uses skills of observation and investigative evidence combined with past patient experiences to determine the stresses that a patient may tolerate. The clinician combines his or her knowledge of the healing process with information gained from those past successful patient experiences to determine the most appropriate time to introduce specific resistance exercises. In addition, the clinician's observation of the individual patient helps to reveal not only when the patient is physically and psychologically ready for this progression but also what the patient's physical and emotional reactions will be to those exercises. Knowing when to add these exercises and how to read the outcome of their effects are important clinical skills.

As the patient enters early remodeling, the injured site's mobility is approaching normal. The clinician continues to restore the last elements of joint and soft-tissue motion but also begins to place more emphasis on progressive muscle strength and endurance activities. These exercises begin with low resistance and higher repetitions and then advance to increased resistance as the healing segment continues in its healing progression. Details and rationale for strength exercises and their progression are presented in chapter 13.

Neuromotor control and proprioception restoration activities are also begun during this phase. These activities include a range of exercises that provide gains in balance, agility, speed, and coordination. Like the strength exercises, these exercises are progressive and become more advanced until the patient transitions to functional activities that stress specific segments and tissues in preparation for advancement to performance-specific exercises.

Sometimes heat modalities are indicated during the early remodeling phase. If deep scar tissue interferes with the patient's function or makes it difficult for the patient to have full motion or produces pain with activity, scar tissue adhesions must be treated to relieve these issues. A heat modality is indicated if reduced tissue viscosity and relaxation for easier manipulation or mobilization of the tissue are desired.[33] Depending on how deep the tissue is, the clinician will select a modality such as diathermy and ultrasound for deeper structures or a modality such as a hot pack or whirlpool for more superficial tissues before applying manual techniques.

Manual therapy techniques applied during this phase may vary depending on the problems that must be addressed. Manual therapy includes soft tissue and joint mobilization and manipulation techniques. Manual therapy is often used for pain relief, joint mobility gains, soft-tissue mobility gains, and scar tissue adhesion releases.[64-69] Included under the umbrella of manual therapy are a number of techniques and applications. Treatments in this manual therapy category include joint mobilization, massage, trigger point therapy, and muscle energy, to name just a few. The specific choice of technique is determined by the specific problem, the availability of tools if needed for the task, and the clinician's skill level and experience. Chapter 11 provides information on manual therapy and the most common techniques and practices.

By the end of this phase, the patient should have normal motion, and any restricted mobility should be resolved. If this is not the case, it may be necessary to use more assertive techniques to achieve the desired range of motion or to assess other segments that might be contributing to the restriction. For example, a patient's inability to elevate the shoulder to its end ranges may be secondary to costovertebral joint restrictions. Since tissue contraction will continue as the injured site continues to heal, the clinician should provide the patient with a maintenance program of flexibility activities so any motion gained is not lost because the patient stopped performing the stretching exercises.

Late Remodeling Phase

By the time the injury reaches the late remodeling phase, substantial strength is present throughout the formerly injured site. The region begins to function in a manner that approaches normal. There is no pain, edema, or restriction to motion. The injured site is now at a point where the final steps to total recovery occur.

It is during this phase that modalities are not needed. The injury site is stable, and heat or cold modalities are not needed to facilitate the progress of rehabilitation. What is needed at this point is a variety of exercises that will restore performance ability and return the patient safely to previous activities.

Exercises for range of motion and mobility by this time are at a maintenance level. Injured joints and soft-tissue structures that lost flexibility or mobility have had those deficiencies addressed during earlier rehabilitation phases so optimal mobility is present by the time the patient moves to this final rehabilitation phase. Ongoing scar contraction may occur during this phase as collagen continues to reorganize and create new cross-links, so the clinician should provide the patient with flexibility activities that maintain mobility.[70, 71]

If necessary, exercises designed to achieve the final gains in muscle endurance and strength and neuromotor control and proprioception are continued in this phase. Beyond those activities, exercises that are more activity-specific are the emphasis of this last phase of the rehabilitation program. These activities prepare the patient to return to his or her former level of function in the personal and social environment in which he or she resides.

These functional and activity-specific exercises not only allow the injured segment to adapt to the normal stresses that it will encounter once the patient returns to normal activities, but they also help the patient realize that the injury is resolved and the injured segment is able to perform at its optimal functioning level. Patients often lack confidence in their ability to return to previous activities; fear of reinjury is common.[72] Fear of reinjury can have a negative impact on the patient's performance, especially as the patient nears the end of the program.[73] This is another reason why it is important for the clinician to prepare the patient for a confident return to work or sport participation. The clinician instills confidence by having the patient perform specific skills to demonstrate his or her restored competence; the patient sees by his or her own performance that there is no reason to question the integrity of the formerly injured segment. This demonstration occurs through a progression of functional and performance-specific exercises that mimic the demands the patient will face when he or she returns to work or sport.

If the exercise demands are meant to satisfy the patient's performance expectations, the clinician must know exactly what those demands are. If the clinician does not know what specific skills are required, then he or she must gather information from the patient, a colleague, or a coach or supervisor to design exercises for this phase of the program. The exercises begin at a basic skill level and advance as the patient's performance improves and each level's goals are met. Much like the other exercises throughout the rehabilitation program, the complexity and difficulty of the activity-specific exercises are increased as the patient learns, adapts, and performs to the level expected, achieving the goals that have been set before advancement to the next level of difficulty occurs.

Once all the goals have been met and results are confirmed through reevaluation, the rehabilitation program is complete. When all goals are met, the patient can safely and confidently return to full, active participation in the sport or work environment.

Timing of Treatment Response

Patients often ask, "How long before I can start running?" or "How long will it be before I can play ball again?" or "When can I go back to work?" There are many factors that can make these questions impossible to answer, especially at the first treatment session. Some of the more obvious factors include the severity of injury, the type of tissue involved, whether surgery is needed, the age and sex of the patient, the sport or work or environment to which the patient is returning, the physician or surgeon's perspective, complications or other health factors of the patient, the number of previous injuries to the body segment, the competitive level of the athlete, and the person's physiological, psychological, and emotional makeup.

It is easier to estimate the durations for some program segments than for others, but they all depend on the severity of the injury, the secondary effects resulting from the injury, patient compliance, and the body part involved. For example, if acute injury effects such as spasm, edema, and pain are optimally treated at the time of injury, they may result in minimal postinjury effects, so during the rehabilitation phase they may be easily managed. Although spasm, edema, and pain are treated first in a rehabilitation program and are more quickly treated than other factors such as loss of motion, strength, and function, it is not always easy to predict when they will be resolved. It is wise not to predict when they will be resolved unless the clinician can make an accurate judgment.

Most rehabilitation protocols for specific injuries have an estimated duration and course of treatment. You will find throughout part IV of this text several different exercise protocols for various conditions; each has an estimated timeline of events and exercise sequencing that provides a guide for the clinician. For example, you will find that an average time for recovery from a shoulder labral repair surgery is about 5 to 6 months, but several factors can make this estimation either too short or too long. For example, it may take longer if the patient also had a biceps tendon injury that was repaired, or recovery may require less time if the labral repair required only one suture and was in a non-stressed segment of the joint. Additionally, if the patient is compliant with the rehabilitation program, improvements may occur sooner than if he isn't compliant; if he has a systemic disease that affects healing, the program may be delayed; if the patient's surgeon wants to follow a conservative treatment protocol, the program may be prolonged; if the patient stresses the surgical site more than he is instructed, he may reinjure the part, delaying the program; or if there is more swelling or spasm than normal so it takes longer than usual to remove these factors, the program may take longer than average.

Severe injuries or conditions involving prolonged disability or immobilization produce muscle atrophy. This topic is discussed in more detail in chapter 13, but for now it is important to realize that when a muscle does not perform its normal functions, it loses first strength, then size. The longer a muscle is restricted from performing normal function, the more strength and size it loses;[74] these factors may be restored during rehabilitation programs.

Once a rehabilitation program begins, the clinician must be aware of the responses typically seen and normally expected in patients. The strength responses that occur are dependent upon the same factors we have already discussed. When strength exercises begin, there is usually a rapid increase in strength early in the program.[75] This is the result of neuromuscular reeducation or motor learning.[76] The neuromuscular element is "reawakened," if you will, relearning what it has lost from injury, surgery, or disuse. Fortunately, this system is a quick learner, so the patient and clinician are usually very pleased with the early outcomes of rehabilitation. This rapid gain is demonstrated in figure 3.2.

Actual changes in muscle size are not seen for 6 weeks after strengthening therapeutic exercises are initiated.[74] These changes occur much more slowly than the initial rapid strength changes (figure 3.2) because of the physiological alterations required for a change in muscle size to become evident. As a result, after the first several weeks of rehabilitation, slower strength gains are seen in the rehabilitation program. In some cases when rehabilitation is extensive and prolonged, gains may even stagnate, with very minimal changes noted in the patient's strength progression. This slower response to exercise can be a time when the patient feels discouraged. The clinician must be aware that this process is normal and must be able to explain to the patient that with continued activity

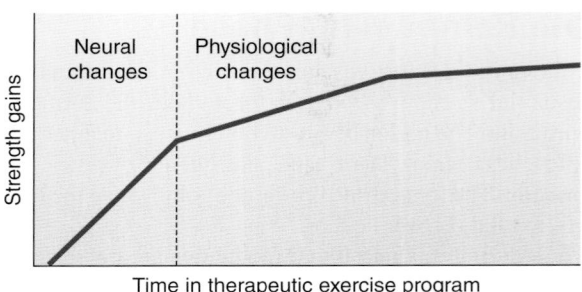

Figure 3.2   Clinical observations of normal strength progression in a therapeutic exercise program. Progression occurs quickly in the early stage as neuromuscular reeducation occurs. Strength gains slow as the patient progresses and physiological changes in the muscle occur.

and perseverance in the program, the patient will see not only gains in strength but changes in muscle size. Often this period of little or no change is suddenly replaced by a spurt of increased strength gains. In cases where there has been prolonged immobilization or inactivity with profound weakness and atrophy, this cycle may occur more than once during the course of the rehabilitation program. Fortunately, the more common case is that the cycle occurs only once throughout an extended rehabilitation program.

Summary

Rehabilitation clinicians must have a good understanding of the healing process because it plays a crucial role in a rehabilitation program. This chapter presents two different perspectives on a rehabilitation program's development. First we consider rehabilitation in terms of its major goals, the three Rs of rehabilitation, and second, we consider rehabilitation in terms of what the patient needs based on where the injury is within the timeline of healing. The rehabilitation clinician's treatment choices and their success will depend mainly on the clinician's ability to accurately identify where the patient is in the healing process. During the hemostatic phase, only cryotherapy modalities along with compression, elevation, and rest are appropriate to minimize the injury's effects. The inflammation phase is where modalities are applied for pain, edema, and spasm relief. Once the injury enters the proliferation phase, exercise begins with range of motion. From this point, the patient progresses to strength and muscle endurance, neuromotor control and proprioception, and then into functional and performance-specific exercises before being tested to assess his or her ability to return to normal activities.

LEARNING AIDS

Key Concepts and Review

1. Identify the three Rs of rehabilitation, and explain how they relate to healing.

The first R is *relieve symptoms*. The goal here is to minimize the injury by applying cryotherapy, elevation, and compression to control bleeding and swelling. It is also important to address the secondary effects that result from the injury: swelling, pain, spasm, redness, and reduced function. Reducing the patient's use of the injured part will also protect it from reinjury.

The second R is *restore deficiencies*. The goal here is to restore those physical and physiological functions that have been impaired because of the injury: range of motion and mobility, strength and muscle endurance, and neuromotor control and proprioception.

The third R is *return to function*. The goal of this last R is to optimize the patient's functioning so that he or she may return to a former level of activity.

2. Discuss the timing of treatment with the various stages of healing.

Treatments are incorporated into the rehabilitation program according to the injury site's healing status. During the hemostasis phase, the clinician uses cryotherapy modalities along with compression and elevation to reduce the loss of fluids and blood from the injured site. Immobilizing the injured area will also protect it from further insult and damage.

During the inflammation phase, the clinician uses cryotherapy, electrical stimulation, and laser to reduce the secondary effects of inflammation. Effects such as pain, swelling, muscle spasm, and limited function will respond to these modalities.

During the proliferation phase, there is less use of modalities except to relieve any remaining fragments from inflammation. This phase is when exercises begin, but because the injured site remains weak, exercises must be applied cautiously. These exercises are primarily range-of-motion and mobility activities. Toward the end of proliferation, some strength exercises may be incorporated.

During the remodeling phase, strength and neuromotor building exercises and activities are added until the patient approaches normal levels in these parameters. As the injury site gains normal mobility, strength, and coordination, performance-specific exercises are added to the rehabilitation program. These final exercises mimic whatever activities the patient must perform after discharge from rehabilitation.

3. Provide a rationale for why only modalities are used during the first and second phases of healing.

Modalities are used to relieve the secondary effects of injury. They help bring about a reduction in pain and swelling so that the patient's recovery can move from a level of minimal function toward a more functional result. Exercises are contraindicated because the fragile structure stabilizing the injury site is easily damaged; exercises would damage the fibrin plug and result in re-injury.

4. Identify the actions a clinician should take if a returning patient reports increased pain and swelling as a result of the previous treatment session.

The pain and swelling occur because something in the previous treatment was more than the injured site could tolerate. The clinician should treat it as a new injury, applying cryotherapy, compression, and elevation, and should assess the severity of the deleterious reaction. Returning to the previous level of treatment and reassessing each day before the treatment session to determine how the injury is responding is advised. The clinician should wait until the site has recovered from this most recent episode and perhaps reduce the amount of increase the next time a treatment's stress level is advanced.

5. Compare and contrast the treatments provided in the first phase of healing and the last phase of healing, and provide a rationale for why they are different.

At the time of the first phase, hemostasis, the most important goal is to reduce the bleeding and swelling. Treatment is limited to cryotherapy modalities along with elevation and compression. Exercises are contraindicated. During the last phase, later remodeling, the tissues are well on their way toward the final aspects of healing. There is no need for modalities at this time. Mobility, strength, and neuromotor control are all approaching normal levels, so the emphasis is on preparing the patient physically and emotionally to return to normal activities. Exercises to maintain what has been achieved are used along with activity-specific exercises that mimic the stresses to which the patient will return.

Critical Thinking Questions

1. As Joel in the opening scenario, you find out that Reetah's surgery was 3 weeks ago. What does this tell you in terms of where she is in the healing process? Besides the date of her surgery, what other factors must Joel consider to determine what her initial treatments will include? What would you anticipate will be her problems today as Joel evaluates her?

2. If a patient presents to you with a grade II pectoralis major strain that occurred 2 weeks ago, at what healing phase would you estimate the injury to be? What would be your criteria for determining your answer in addition to the time since the injury's onset?

3. A patient who undergoes an outpatient surgical repair of the elbow comes to you 3 d after the surgery to begin rehabilitation. Where in the healing process do you estimate this patient to be, and what healing activities are occurring? What would you do for treatment in the first 3 d of your treatment program? What would you do for treatment in the first 3 weeks of your treatment program? What factors would you consider to determine when to change the treatment program?

4. A patient with a second-degree ankle sprain that occurred 4 d ago comes to you for rehabilitation. If the patient is 50 years old; has diabetes, severe swelling, and cramps in the calf muscles; is on Coumadin and an oral hypoglycemic medication; and has been taking oral anti-inflammatories for the past 3 d, what would your treatment program include? How would your treatment be different if the patient is 22 years old, has no chronic medical condition but has severe swelling and cramps in the calf muscles, and has been taking oral anti-inflammatories for the past 3 d?

Lab Activities

1. Identify three reliable websites to which you can refer for additional information on the timing of a rehabilitation progression for an acute patellar dislocation.

2. List the types of rehabilitation techniques you could use within each phase of healing. Create your list for a specific injury and specific patient (e.g., age, occupation or sport, and so on).

3. Identify three criteria and list them in order of their importance in deciding how long to continue using cryotherapy to treat an acute injury. Explain why these criteria are used to determine whether to continue with cryotherapy.

4

Age Considerations in Rehabilitation Plan and Program Design

Objectives

After completing this chapter, you should be able to do the following:

1. Describe why there are more people involved in sport and recreation today and therefore more who incur musculoskeletal injuries.
2. Discuss why little is known about sport injuries in the very young and the very old.
3. Explain why it is important to know how to manage musculoskeletal injuries of preadolescent and older people.
4. Provide an outline of growth and development based on the Tanner system, and explain how boys and girls vary in the process.
5. Identify the problems associated with an anterior cruciate ligament reconstruction for a younger person.
6. Explain the precautions that one should take when providing a rehabilitation program to an older patient.
7. Identify the progression of osteoarthritis.
8. Discuss the secondary factors that add to debilitation when osteoarthritis occurs.

During his career, Tyler Dean has worked in athletic training clinics for high schools and universities. His new job at a sport clinic has a varied clientele, including age groups from 10 years old to patients in their 80s. This is the first time Tyler has worked with anyone over the age of 35. Although he has not been at this clinic long, he is surprised to realize how much he enjoys working with older patients. One of his favorites is a 70-year-old tennis player, Carol. She has played tennis since high school. Tyler is treating her because she suffered a moderate ankle sprain when she ran to the net for a ball and rolled over on her ankle. She is eager to get back to playing tennis, but Tyler is hesitant to push her as hard as he does his 20-year-old patients. He realizes that there are physical and physiological considerations he must think about as he progresses Carol in her rehabilitation program.

Physical fitness is not only one of the most important keys to a healthy body, it is the basis of dynamic and creative intellectual activity.

John F. Kennedy, 1917-1963,
35th president of the United States

This chapter deals with conditions that affect the entire body throughout a lifetime. At the top of that list is age; as you will find after reading this chapter, members of different age groups require different considerations when it comes to dealing with their injuries. Preteen and teen-aged patients are not small adults, just as patients who are middle-aged and older do not have 25-year-old bodies. Therefore, we address the considerations that are unique to different age groups.

Activity Levels, Stages of Life, and Health Care

Much has changed in the past half century in the worlds of sport and leisure activity. First, there is more of both, and second, many more people participate in both sport and leisure activity than ever before. Along with sport participation comes the risk of incurring an injury. The Centers for Disease Control and Prevention (CDC) reports that in 2019, just under 3 million children and adolescents were injured in organized sport and recreational activity. Twice as many males as females incurred sports-related injuries.[1] As you would expect, collision or contact sports have higher injury rates; football, basketball, baseball, and soccer accounted for nearly 80% of all sports-related emergency room visits for children between the ages of 5 and 14 years.[1] Clubs and interscholastic competitions for most sports are available for millions of teens and preteen athletes around the country.

Physicians across the United States advocate exercise for both children and older adults to promote individual health. With higher expectations of longevity, there are now more organized sport activities for older adults than in the past. Senior adults have many opportunities for competitive events. Not only are there municipally organized and club-related events and competitions such as races and tournaments, there are also national and international competitive events such as Senior Olympics for older adults.

From birth to death, the body is continually changing. Some changes are for the good, some are for maintenance, and some are not so good, but they happen in all of us as we grow, develop, and age. The natural progression is from a stage of growth and development in youth to one of maturation and adaptation in the young adult stage and then to the final stage of regression in ability and function. In youth, the body learns functions that become automatic such as balance, standing, walking, and tossing a ball. Throughout this time, nerves, muscles, and bones change as they adapt to the stresses applied to them during growth and performance. In the young adult stage, the body continues to develop and adjust to the new skills being learned by becoming more refined and modified for more sophisticated movements and activities. These can be activities that seemed complicated at first but quickly become automatic, such as dancing, driving a car, solving physics equations, or juggling. However, in the advance to older years, some of the activities that were once simple are no longer so easy. It becomes more difficult to respond as quickly to a stimulus as before. Falling becomes more frequent because strength diminishes, and reactions are slower. It isn't possible to hit a golf ball as far down the fairway as it was in the younger years. Catching and throwing a ball become challenging. Stretching the hamstrings after running is more difficult. Some people move through these maturation stages slowly and others more quickly, and some spend more time in one stage than another, but everyone moves through these stages during the progression from birth to old age.

It is these varied stages that the rehabilitation clinician must consider for each patient. How old is the patient? Where in the maturation process is the patient? Does the patient have any comorbidities? How will this influence the rehabilitation program for this patient? What accommodations are needed because of this patient's age and health status? In dealing with athletes, why is it necessary to think about a patient's age? These are some of the questions this chapter answers.

With the explosion of youth leagues for all sports, and with more baby boomers remaining active in recreational and leisure activities who are either approaching or well into retirement age, there is perhaps a wider range of ages than ever before of people who suffer activity-related musculoskeletal injuries. As clinicians in outpatient clinics, we also see several types of work-related injuries in patients over age 30. Although we realize that each person is unique, we often do not take into consideration how age influences a body's response to the demands therapeutic interventions impose on it. The body's reaction to those demands can be a direct result of the person's age. That is why this topic appears at this point in the book. Once you have learned about it in this chapter, remember that when you develop a therapeutic rehabilitation program, your patient's age must be considered in the program's design.

Trends in Work and Leisure Time

It wasn't long ago that work consumed most people's waking hours. Within the last half century, after many industrial and technological advances, people now live lives that are more consumed with leisure time than with work time.

This slow but steady evolution from long workdays to more leisure time has led to an increase in the number and types of leisure activity and the number of people participating in them. People of both sexes and varying economic backgrounds, differing skill levels, and varying degrees of commitment participate in such regular activities as dancing, golf, tennis, cycling, baseball, softball, swimming, racquetball, basketball, soccer, aerobics, weightlifting, tai chi, and rowing, as well as various other types of recreational, league, and competitive pursuits.

Impact on Injury and Health Care

Health services are affected by the fact that people are living longer; health services are also among the types of services most often used by consumers of all ages.[2, 3] Health professions are called on to help not only those who are living longer but also those who have yet to enter the workforce—preadolescents and adolescents.[2, 4] Among those who participate in athletics, the young and the old are populations that we know little about in terms of injury epidemiology, but we do know that if they participate in sports, injuries will occur. We also know that both younger and older athletes differ from early-adult athletes, who are the ones we most commonly consider when addressing the treatment and rehabilitation of musculoskeletal injuries. These differences are important because they affect the patient's response to injury and to recovery. It is our responsibility as rehabilitation clinicians to know these differences and to understand how they influence the patients we treat in the age groups at either end of the life spectrum.

Physical Activity Throughout Life

Our sport rehabilitation practices are based on studies that usually involve subjects in their early adult years. Since many of the studies are performed on university campuses, the age range of subjects is commonly from 18 to 25. These subjects are in the physical prime of their lives, having passed through puberty and having yet to enter their declining years. There have been relatively few studies of sport injuries in either older age groups or younger populations. However, there has been an abundance of research on both the progression of physical development and the regression of physical ability associated with aging. The next section deals with the preteen and teen years of puberty when physical change is most evident. It is also during these years that people come to rehabilitation clinicians with first-time sport injuries.

Pediatric Considerations

From the perspective of the medical community, the pediatric population includes anyone from the time before birth to the completion of puberty, usually by age 21.[5] The years 18 to 21 are considered a transition time during which medical care switches from pediatric-care to adult-care health care professionals.[6] Before computer technology, children were more engaged in free play than in organized sport. The current generation of children engages in a variety of activities from physical education classes to community-based team sports and some free play, but most of their sport participation is through organized athletics.[7-9] There is a recent trend toward early sport specialization.[7, 10] Koester[9] contends that with the decline of free play, youngsters begin sport activities without first establishing a physical conditioning base that protects them from injury. There is growing concern that early sport participation, especially sport specialization, may lead to adverse health effects and increased risk of injury.[7, 10, 11] With the growing incidence of pediatric injuries, what must rehabilitation clinicians consider as they treat these patients?

General Physiological Considerations

Most of the physiological considerations for pediatric patients have to do with the developmental stage and the structure injured. The severity of the injury and the way in which the patient responds to the injury and the recovery process are elements that we must also consider.

Kids Are Not Short Adults

People under age 21 are not adults in either their physiological or their physical maturity. Likewise, they cannot be treated as adults in their rehabilitation programs. Adjustments must be made for the patient's physical and physiological maturity if the clinician is to ensure a safe and appropriate progression of injury care and rehabilitation.

Growth and Development

Before we distinguish the unique features of a rehabilitation program and a progression for this group, we must identify the growth and development factors that affect the program. Although there are several systems for categorizing maturation in youth, one of the more commonly used systems is the Tanner growth chart, presented in table 4.1.[12] This is a staging system that was first developed during the early 1960s and later updated to reflect changes in the development rate of children.[13, 14] The Tanner system identifies developmental stages for secondary sexual characteristics, rate of height changes, and muscle development.[14] A typical pubertal growth pattern begins with a phase of acceleration, which is followed by a phase of deceleration before growth ceases.[15] Growth stops when the epiphyses close, at approximately 18 years in girls and 20 years in boys.[16] Girls begin this growth pattern earlier and end it earlier, usually about 2 years ahead of their male counterparts throughout the process. Although the exact age when puberty begins varies from one person to another, the average starting age for girls is 9 years and for boys is 11 years.[15]

Before puberty, boys do better in physical fitness tests of aerobic fitness, strength, speed, and agility, while girls do better in balance and flexibility tests.[17-19] Once children enter puberty and become preadolescents and adolescents and their bodies take on more mature external physical appearances, they still have internal physical qualities that vary greatly from those of adults. The following discussion focuses on some important considerations for rehabilitation clinicians.

Bone Factors   Children's bones grow until the end of puberty. Longitudinal bone growth occurs at the growth plate, called the physis. A **physis**, or **growth plate**, is a complex cartilaginous matrix that lies near the end of the longitudinal bone and forms new bone, providing for growth of the long bone. The epiphysis sits on the distal end of the physis and forms the joint end of the bone (figure 4.1). Salter and Harris[20] developed an injury classification method for the various degrees of physis injuries. Their classification system is presented in table 4.2. Another segment of the bone that is not present in mature bones is the growth site of an apophysis. An **apophysis** is a protrusion of bone where a tendon or ligament attaches (figure 4.2). Until a bone matures, physis and apophysis sites are susceptible to excessive shear or compressive forces. Compressive stress to a physis can result in fractures that damage the bone's growth center, stopping bone growth. Shear stresses to an apophyseal plate can cause the tendon to pull away from its bone attachment.

Young bones are more resilient and elastic than adult bones, so young bones can tolerate greater stresses before

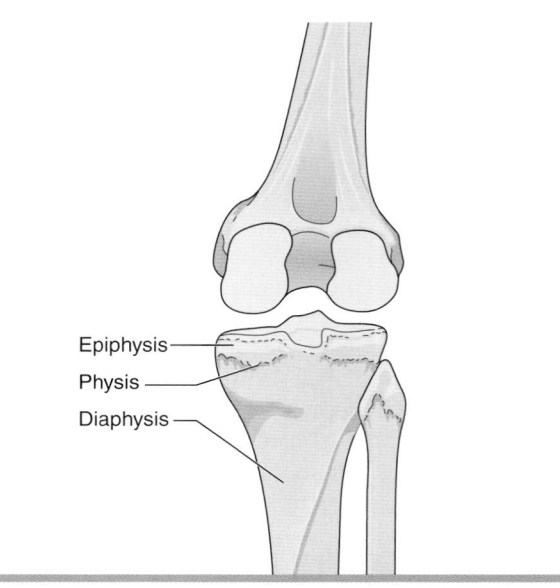

Epiphysis
Physis
Diaphysis

Figure 4.1   Long bone growth areas. The physis is the cartilaginous section of long bones that creates greater length of the bone.

TABLE 4.1   Tanner Stages of Development

Tanner stage	Adolescence level	Male characteristics	Female characteristics
I	Preadolescence	No pubic hair	No pubic hair, flat breasts
II	Early adolescence	Darkening of pubic hair; enlargement of testes	Sparse pubic hair; small, raised breasts
III	Middle adolescence	Coarsening and curling of pubic hair; increased penis size	Coarsening and curling of pubic hair; enlargement and raising of breasts
IV	Middle adolescence	Continued penis growth	Formation of areola and nipple contour separate from breast development
V	End of adolescence	Presence of adult genitalia	Presence of adult genitalia

Based on Tanner (1962).[12]

TABLE 4.2   Salter-Harris Epiphyseal Fracture Classifications

	Classification	Characteristics	Cause	Notations
Type I	I	Separation of the cartilage from the bone without any bone fracture	Avulsion or shearing force	A common epiphyseal injury during the early years. It has the best outcome.
Type II	II	A fracture that extends through the physis and into the metaphysis but not the epiphysis	Shearing or avulsion; occurs in children over 10 years old	Most common epiphyseal plate injury. The growing cartilage cells remain intact, so growth still occurs.
Type III	III	A fracture through the physis and epiphysis	Intra-articular shearing force	Not a common injury. May require surgery. Prognosis is good as long as circulation to the epiphysis remains intact.
Type IV	IV	Intra-articular fracture from the epiphysis through the physis and into the metaphysis	Impact or torsional stress	A complete split is present. ORIF (open reduction and internal fixation) is necessary to realign epiphyseal plate and prevent growth stoppage.

>continued

TABLE 4.2 >*continued*

	Classification	Characteristics	Cause	Notations
Type V	V	Compression fracture of the epiphyseal plate	A crushing force during a lateral motion or stress resulting in displacement of the epiphysis; occurs in uniplanar joints	These injuries are commonly dismissed as sprains. Although weight bearing is restricted for 3 weeks, prognosis is poor.

Data from Salter and Harris (1963).[20]

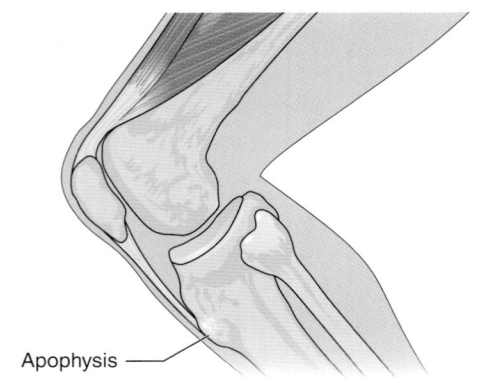

Figure 4.2 An apophysis is an outgrowth of bone to which a tendon or ligament attaches. Until its growth center closes during the later teen years, it is susceptible to tension and shear stress injuries to the tendon that attaches to the apophysis.

Apophysis

a fracture occurs. Because of this bone elasticity and resilience, fractures in youth are different from fractures in adults. Immature bones may suffer a "greenstick fracture," or partial fracture, in which one side of the bone is broken and the opposite side is only bent. When a fracture involves the epiphysis or physis, bone growth or alignment (or both) may be affected. For this reason, additional care is taken with these fractures.

Articular Cartilage Factors The articular cartilage of children and adolescents is similar to physis in its construction and tolerance to stress, especially shearing forces.[21, 22] In other words, it is a structure that is subject to injury. However, there is evidence that articular cartilage in these age groups may heal better than in adults and has an ability to regenerate that is not seen in adults. What is important is that these injuries be detected immediately and that the care provided after the diagnosis offer enough stress to encourage proper healing but not so much as to

cause deterioration of healing tissues. Articular cartilage defects in the knee can develop into osteoarthritis in later years. There is evidence to indicate that healthy articular cartilage volume increases in children who are active and involved in vigorous activity compared to those who are sedentary; active children gain twice as much articular cartilage as sedentary children.[23, 24] This suggests that perhaps children who are active may be less likely to develop osteoarthritis in later years.[23]

Muscle Factors Girls and boys have essentially equivalent muscle proportion and strength before puberty. Once children enter puberty, however, muscle size and strength become greater in boys than in girls. The males' greater testosterone levels are primarily responsible for these developing differences. Both groups, however, have the potential for greater muscle strength than bone strength during their growth spurts.[25, 26] It is during this time that apophyseal injuries may occur, especially if the child participates in sports. One reason for the occurrence of these injuries is that bone growth is stimulated by muscle growth,[25-28] so bone growth spurts lag behind muscle growth spurts.

There has been a dispute for several years about whether preadolescent children should engage in strengthening activities. People who argue against such activities are inclined to believe that strength exercises during the preadolescent years place the person at risk for epiphyseal injuries secondary to unnecessary loading and shear stresses. However, a policy statement published by the American Academy of Pediatrics (AAP)[29] indicates that strength-training programs do not have a detrimental effect on young athletes, although precautions should be taken when skeletally immature persons participate in weight training. The following is a summary of the AAP strength-training recommendations for preadolescents and adolescents.

1. Proper resistance techniques and safety precautions should be followed so that strength-training programs for preadolescents and adolescents are safe and effective. Whether it is necessary or appropriate to start such a program and which level of proficiency the youngster already has attained in his or her sport activity should be determined before a strength-training program is started.

2. Preadolescents and adolescents should avoid powerlifting, bodybuilding, and maximal lifts until they reach physical and skeletal maturity.

3. Athletes should not use performance-enhancing substances or anabolic steroids. Athletes who participate in strength-training programs should be educated about the risks associated with the use of such substances.

4. When pediatricians are asked to recommend or evaluate strength-training programs for children and adolescents, the following issues should be considered:

   - Before beginning a formal strength-training program, a medical evaluation should be performed by a pediatrician or family physician. Youth with uncontrolled hypertension, seizure disorders, or a history of childhood cancer and chemotherapy should be withheld from participation until additional treatment or evaluation. When indicated, a referral may be made to a pediatric or family physician sports medicine specialist who is familiar with various strength-training methods as well as risks and benefits for preadolescents.

   - Children with complex congenital cardiac disease (cardiomyopathy, pulmonary artery hypertension, or Marfan syndrome) should have a consultation with a pediatric cardiologist before beginning a strength-training program.

   - Aerobic conditioning should be coupled with resistance training if general health benefits are the goal.

   - Strength-training programs should include a 10 to 15 min warm-up and a cool-down.

   - Athletes should have an adequate intake of fluids and proper nutrition because both are vital in the maintenance of muscle energy stores, recovery, and performance.

   - Specific strength-training exercises should be learned initially with no load (no resistance). Once the exercise technique has been mastered, incremental loads can be added using either body weight or other forms of resistance. Strength training should involve 2 to 3 sets of higher repetitions (8 to 15) 2 to 3 times per week and should be at least 8 weeks in duration.

   - A general strengthening program should address all major muscle groups. It should include the core, and exercises should be performed through the complete range of motion. More sport-specific areas may be addressed subsequently.

   - Any sign of injury or illness from strength training should be evaluated fully before allowing the athlete to resume the exercise program.

   - Instructors or personal trainers should have certifications that include specific qualifications in pediatric strength training.

   - Proper technique and strict supervision by a qualified instructor are critical safety components in any strength-training program involving preadolescents and adolescents.

Tendon Factors   Because bone lengthening lags behind muscle lengthening, during growth spurts the muscle's tendon applies increasing tension on the apophyseal attachments. The bony growth site is less resilient than muscle tissue, so the apophyseal plate is usually the site of injury after repetitive-stress occurrences. An additional fact is that with lagging bony lengthening during muscle growth spurts, inherent tension is applied to the apophyseal plate as tension is transmitted from the muscle along the tendon to its insertion. Some common apophyseal plates in which we see these types of injuries are the calcaneus with Sever's disease, medial humeral epicondyle with Little League elbow, and tibial tubercle with Osgood-Schlatter disease.[9, 27, 30, 31]

Neurological Factors   The neurological system controls the muscular system with respect to strength, performance, and skill execution. Skill execution is assessed as the ability to perform accurately and efficiently. Accuracy and efficiency are achieved through repetition of the activity; the skill is corrected and refined as it becomes ingrained within the neuromuscular system.[32, 33] Strength gains occur in prepubescent children but not because of an increase in muscle size as in adults. Essentially, neural changes and improved neuromuscular recruitment are responsible for strength gains in children before puberty.[34]

Thermoregulatory Factors   Since prepubescent children do not have the sweat mechanisms that adults have, their ability to release heat is different. Prepubescent children have a higher convection rate than adults.[35, 36] This means that their blood is diverted to the surface to reduce heat buildup within the body, as evidenced by increased skin coloration during exercise in this age group.

Children expend more energy per body mass in heat than adults.[34] Greater energy expenditure translates to greater heat output. If a child and an adult are running at the same speed, the child will expend 20% more body heat per kilogram than the adult.[35, 36]

Sweating is a primary means of evaporative heat dissipation. Although children older than 2 years have as many sweat glands as adults, this does not mean that they can produce sweat as well as adults. Heat dissipation through sweat production depends on how soon the sweat response occurs and the amount of sweat produced. Children produce a little more than half the amount of sweat that adults produce.[35, 36] Boys sweat more than girls, and postpubertal youngsters sweat more than either pre- or midpubertal youngsters. Given the importance of sweating in heat dissipation, prepubertal and midpubertal youngsters have a disadvantage under hot environmental conditions. Children lose more fluid than electrolytes while sweating in high temperatures,[37, 38] so it is important to take frequent breaks to replace these lost fluids.

Considerations in Rehabilitation

The prepubescent, midpubescent, and postpubescent age groups vary greatly in physical and psychological maturity. Rehabilitation clinicians must be aware of these variations in order to provide the best possible rehabilitation programs for people in all age groups. Given the brief discussion in the preceding sections, you can see that many changes occur in the body between the beginning of middle school and the end of high school, the time when we often see these patients' first-time injuries. How we treat these patients and their injuries may have a profound impact on them both physically and emotionally.

Sport Injuries in School-Aged Patients

It has been estimated that nearly 60 million children between the ages of 6 and 18 participate in some form of organized sport,[30, 39] with an estimated 44 million participating in more than one sport.[30] Most of the musculoskeletal injuries seen in pediatric patients in emergency departments in the United States occur as a result of sport participation.[40, 41] With the profound increase in organized sport for younger athletes, it is likely that rehabilitation clinicians will treat younger patients with athletic injuries since more injuries occur during organized sport than in free-play activities.[4, 42] More schools are employing certified athletic trainers who not only will treat these young patients but also will likely see the injuries occur.[43, 44]

Anyone participating in sports is at risk for injury. Youngsters whose bones are not yet mature and whose skill levels are not fully developed are at even greater risk of injury.[45] Each year approximately 3.5 million children who are 14 years old and younger receive medical care from emergency departments for sports-related injuries. Another 5 million youth are seen by their primary care physicians or a sports medicine clinic for sports-related injuries.

Sever's disease, stress fractures, Osgood-Schlatter disease, jumper's knee, apophysitis, and tendinopathies are common repetitive-induced conditions.[27, 30, 46] Often, these injuries occur when bones or soft tissues are stressed excessively during growth spurts,[27, 30, 46] or because of poor technique, or both. Most fractures in early adolescence are Salter-Harris type II fractures; these occur primarily from a combination of rapid growth and physis weakness.[47, 48]

Regardless of the cause, the young patient's injury complaints are similar to those of an adult. Treatment progression, however, is complicated by the fact that the youngster may still be growing, and the injury site is not mature, so it cannot tolerate the same level of stresses as its adult counterpart can or receive the same treatments to manage it.

Acute sprains may be severe enough to indicate surgical repair. Anterior cruciate ligament ruptures are occurring with more regularity in teens and preteens.[49-52] These skeletally immature patients require unique considerations. One of the primary concerns with this injury is avoiding the epiphyseal growth plate when the surgical graft is implanted. The surgeon must know the patient's physiological age to prevent growth plate damage. As indicated in figure 4.3, Kocher and Tucker[52] vary their anterior cruciate ligament (ACL) reconstruction procedure according to the patient's physiological age, classified into one of three groups:

- Prepubescent: Either no surgery is performed and a functional brace is used for protection, or a physeal-sparing and combined intra-articular and extra-articular reconstruction is performed using an autogenous iliotibial band graft.

- Adolescent with significant growth remaining: Surgery features a transphyseal ACL reconstruction using autogenous hamstring tendons with fixation away from the physes.

- Older adolescent approaching skeletal maturity: Surgery is a conventional adult ACL reconstruction with interference screw fixation using either autogenous central-third patellar tendon or autogenous hamstrings.

Rehabilitation Considerations for Sport Injuries of School-Aged Patients

Just as surgeons must adapt their surgical techniques to accommodate growth and developmental stages, rehabilitation clinicians must make adjustments in their rehabilitation programs. Not only do we have the physiological and physical immaturity issues to consider, but it also can be challenging to maintain a young patient's interest in and focus on rehabilitation exercises. Young patients often do not realize the importance of performing exercises correctly; instead their priority is completing them as quickly as possible. With these patients, clinicians need to use their imaginations to make exercises fun while accomplishing the program's goals. Additionally, clinicians must use different cues depending on the patients' developmental

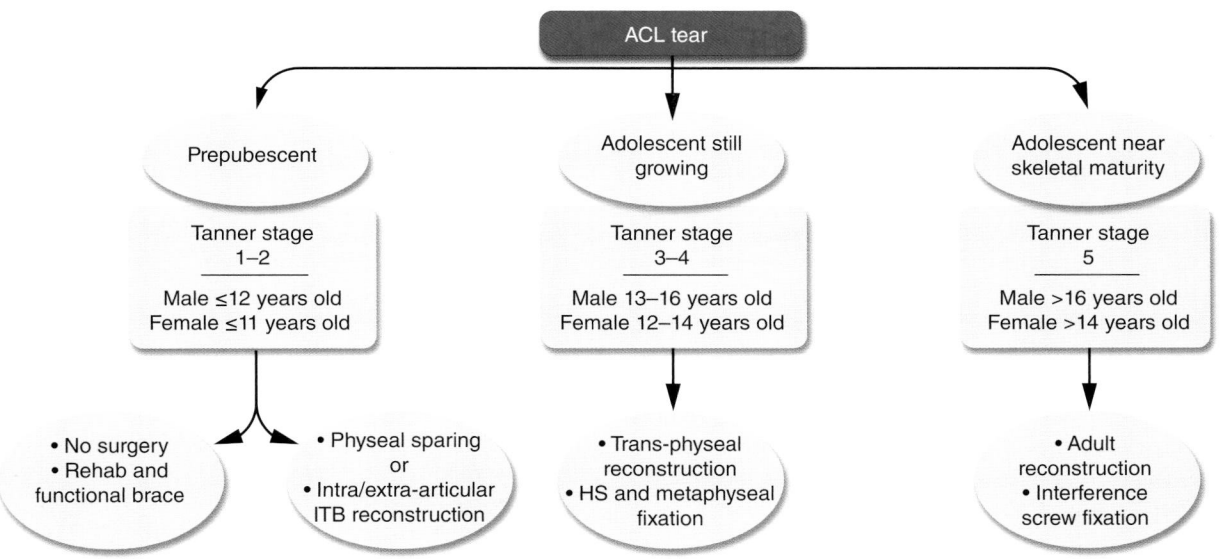

Figure 4.3 Surgical decision-making for anterior cruciate ligament injuries in skeletally immature patients.

stage. Exercises must be carefully monitored throughout the program for correct execution and proper compliance.

Proper care provided as soon as possible is a key factor in successful treatment and future good health. It is during the school-age years that genetic and acquired postural deviations are often discovered. Sometimes these deviations result in an athletic injury. The rehabilitation clinician should assess each young patient for postural deviations as part of a routine rehabilitation examination. Immediate care involves the use of modalities such as ice and electrical stimulation to relieve inflammation, pain, and edema. Several modalities are contraindicated for this age group, especially when applied over immature bones; the clinician must be aware of these contraindications and avoid them. Range-of-motion exercises to restore flexibility begin after reduction of pain and swelling. Strengthening exercises with primary emphasis on endurance activities are the next part of the progression. The final phase in a youngster's rehabilitation program involves the restoration of proprioception, balance, and agility before sport-specific activities.

Preparation and planning for a youth's rehabilitation program must account for the physical variations between younger patients and adults. Those factors have already been outlined; next we see how they need to be considered in relation to rehabilitation.

Bone and Articular Cartilage Factors   When we manage injuries to bone, epiphysis, physis, or articular cartilage, the primary concern is preventing additional damage to these structures. Bone heals quickly in young patients, but if the growth regions of bone are injured, one must be careful to avoid activities that cause pain, which is a key sign that stresses are excessive. Rehabilitation is gradual and progressive. Most epiphyseal injuries have

good outcomes if managed appropriately.[20, 50, 53, 54] Most fractures are immobilized in either a cast or a splint. A common site of injury and restriction after immobilization is the elbow joint. Although many fractures in children need little postinjury rehabilitation, elbow joint immobilization often requires post-immobilization treatment. This treatment includes joint mobilizations and mobility exercises to restore full motion since the elbow joint often loses its mobility quickly after immobilization, and it is difficult for the patient to restore full motion without help. It may take several months to restore full elbow motion.[55, 56]

After any immobilization, the clinician's initial goals are to reduce inflammation and restore motion. Active range-of-motion exercises are often enough to restore motion when a program is begun shortly after immobilization. When necessary, assistive motion exercises and other types of activities to facilitate motion gains are used. If the joint is stable and demonstrates a capsular motion restriction, joint mobilization may also be used to restore full motion. Grade II joint mobilization is often used early in rehabilitation to help increase joint fluid mobility and reduce pain. When pain is diminished, grade III joint mobilization can be used to increase joint mobility.

Muscle and Tendon Factors   Individuals of any age benefit from strengthening exercises. It is important, however, that exercises for prepubescent children and young adolescents involve two factors: supervision and endurance. Instead of heavy weights, patients in these age groups benefit more from high-repetition, low-resistance bouts. It is recommended that any youngster below the Tanner stage V level begin with a resistance less than maximal.[26, 57] The number of repetitions should be eight at a minimum and should not lead to severe muscle fatigue. It is better to increase repetitions before increasing resistance when progressing in rehabilitation.[26, 57] Our usual routine for preadolescent patients who are motivated is sets of up to 20 or even 30 repetitions before increasing resistance. A rest of 1 to 2 min between exercises should be incorporated into the program. The clinician must give the patient instructions and cautions about the proper execution of the exercises before having him or her perform any exercise with weights. The clinician then monitors the patient and provides input as needed to ensure correct performance.

Both manual resistance and resistance to the opposite extremity are useful exercises for young injured patients. There is evidence to demonstrate that exercising one extremity helps to strengthen the contralateral extremity. Manual resistance can be an engaging activity for the young patient who may prefer to make a game out of the exercise, trying to "conquer" the clinician and "win."

Neurological and Thermoregulatory Factors

Recall that prepubescent patients will not increase their muscle bulk but will make strength gains. As these patients continue with repetitions, their accuracy also improves because the repetitions create an engram within the neuromuscular pathways.[58, 59] This becomes important as the patient begins the last phase of the rehabilitation program, working on functional and sport-specific activities. Begin the sport-specific activities with exercises that the patient can perform. As patients improve, the exercises advance to become more challenging.

Because of the thermoregulatory factors mentioned previously, children often look red-faced during a workout. This is normal, but on hot, humid days there should be more rest breaks and frequent water breaks. Because a young person's thermal regulation is not as efficient as an adult's, careful observation throughout an exercise program is warranted. Adolescent patients have a more efficient sweating mechanism than prepubescent patients, but care should always be taken when anyone exercises in high heat and humidity.

Geriatric Considerations

The body continues to mature through the adolescent years and reaches its peak potential for physical conditioning in the 20s and early 30s. The reversal of this process begins so slowly that it is not until many years later that a decline in abilities is noticed. This is the normal aging process. Perhaps it is slow to allow people time to mentally adjust to these physical changes. Before clinicians can safely treat older patients, we must understand the changes their bodies undergo and realize that our performance expectations cannot be the same as for our younger patients.

More people in this older population remain active well into their 70s and 80s. As with other age groups, with participation in sports and vigorous activities comes the risk of injury.[60, 61] We encounter older patients seeking treatment in our clinical practices; therefore, we must be aware of the physiological changes that naturally occur with the aging process, for these changes directly affect rehabilitation.[60, 62, 63] Those older patients who want to remain active after injury will need additional consideration. Physiological changes that occur with aging are presented in this section.

General Physiological Considerations

It was Bette Davis who said, "Old age ain't no place for sissies!" She was likely referring to the fact that with age, the body changes in ways that are not always desirable. Older patients deserve as much care and attention as the younger people we treat in our clinical practices. Although these older patients have often lived many more years than those of us who treat them, inside they still feel young and even energetic.[64-66]

Body Changes With Age

Moving into the 20s and 30s, the human body begins a decline that proceeds slowly into old age. Assuming that the body hits its peak at age 20 and has a 1% functional loss per year, it takes 50 to 60 years to decline by about 40% at age 75.[67, 68] Some systems move through this aging process much more slowly than others, but all body systems decline during aging. This section reviews the systems pertinent to orthopedic functions. The systems of primary concern are the muscular, skeletal, and neural systems. Generally, connective tissue becomes stiffer.[60, 69] This affects muscles, tendons, joints, and other structures surrounded by or composed of connective tissue. Flexibility is reduced, and the risk of injuries such as sprains and strains increases since increased stiffness changes the stress–strain curve of connective tissue structures.[69] Muscular strength and speed of contraction decline with aging.[70, 71] The decline of the muscular and neural systems can have a profound effect on balance control. One out of four older people falls each year.[72] One out of five falls causes a serious injury, such as a broken bone or a head injury. Additionally, comorbidities are common among aging adults.[73]

Comorbidity is defined as the simultaneous presence of two or more **morbid** conditions or diseases in the same person. Multiple comorbidities can affect health and well-being.[73] As the body ages, there are many factors that a rehab clinician must consider when designing a rehabilitation program.

Muscular Factors   Aging is a complex process that is associated with changes in muscle mass, strength, and function. The muscular system declines about 40% overall from age 20 to age 80.[74, 75] **Sarcopenia** is a decrease in muscle mass secondary to aging. Sarcopenia involves a reduction in both the size and number of muscle fibers, similar to the reductions that occur with muscle disuse.

Intramuscular fat infiltration increases with age.[76, 77] These conditions will negatively affect muscle function. After age 25, the number of the body's muscle fibers begins to diminish.[75, 78] Accompanying the reduction in muscle size is a decrease in muscle strength and power. There are fewer functioning myosin heads, which diminishes the number of possible bonds between the actin and myosin during muscle activity, resulting in less strength. Muscle strength is reduced by 15% each decade up to age 70 and by 30% each decade after that.[70]

The speed of muscle contraction also declines with age, and the point of peak muscle output is more delayed as the body ages.[71, 78, 79] The faster Type II muscle fibers decline at a faster rate than the Type I fibers. This appears to be more prevalent in the lower extremities.[71, 75] In the quadriceps, the fast-twitch fibers diminish about 20% more readily than the slow-twitch fibers during the third and fourth decades.[78] There is also some evidence that the normally reduced output levels of hormones related to aging may have an effect on muscle strength.[80]

Muscle endurance declines with age as well. This reduced muscle endurance may be the result of reduced contractile function and diminished metabolic activity within the muscle.[78] Capillary density diminishes during aging; this capillary reduction may be secondary to a decline in muscle fibers.[81] In turn, diminished muscle endurance and naturally reduced blood flow may result from this reduced capillary density, and these effects, along with fewer mitochondria in muscle fibers, all diminish glucose availability and result in a less efficient phosphocreatine reconversion mechanism.[75, 82]

On the other hand, older people can benefit from exercise through improved muscle performance. Evidence consistently demonstrates that muscle strength and endurance can improve with exercise in older adults.[60, 63, 71, 78, 83, 84] Muscle size, speed, and coordination also increase with exercise in this age group, and this has been shown to improve function and quality of life.[63, 80]

Skeletal Factors We include both bones and joints when we consider the skeletal system. The body's synovial joints are made up of fibrocartilaginous ligaments and capsules, while the joint surfaces are covered with articular cartilage that is nourished by its subchondral bone and the joint's synovia. The synovial fluid also provides lubrication for the joint. Remember from the discussion in chapter 2 on articular cartilage that proteoglycan aggregates, enmeshed within the Type II collagen, bind with the water in articular cartilage to provide protection from compressive forces on joints. As the body ages, the aggregates become shorter, and less proteoglycan is produced.[85-87] These changes result in less water within the articular cartilage and lead to increased joint surface stress. Unfortunately, the thickness of articular cartilage also diminishes with age.[77, 85, 88-90] Eventually, degenerative disease of the joints, characterized by cartilage degradation, osteophyte formation, joint

inflammation, and decreased function occur.[77, 88] Of people aged 18 to 44 years, 7.1% reported physician-diagnosed arthritis.[91] This increased to 29.3% in people aged 45 to 64 years and 49.6% in people aged 65 years and older.[91]

Osteoarthritis is the most common form of arthritis and one of the leading causes of disability.[85, 91] It is often the result of primary or secondary trauma to a joint that occurred at an earlier age. As the person ages, evidence of fraying and thinning of articular cartilage appears, eventually producing degeneration of the joint's articular surface. Because osteoarthritis is a degenerative condition of the joint, it is also called degenerative joint disease or DJD. Once the articular cartilage is worn, the bone itself has no protection. Since articular cartilage has no pain receptors but bone does, the patient gradually begins to have progressively worsening pain as the osteoarthritic joint continues to degenerate. Eventually, the degeneration and accompanying pain compromise daily activities—in the case of lower-extremity joints, making it hard even to walk. Upper-extremity joint osteoarthritis is also debilitating; overhead and functional activities become difficult if not impossible to perform. Figure 4.4 illustrates a healthy joint and an osteoarthritic joint.

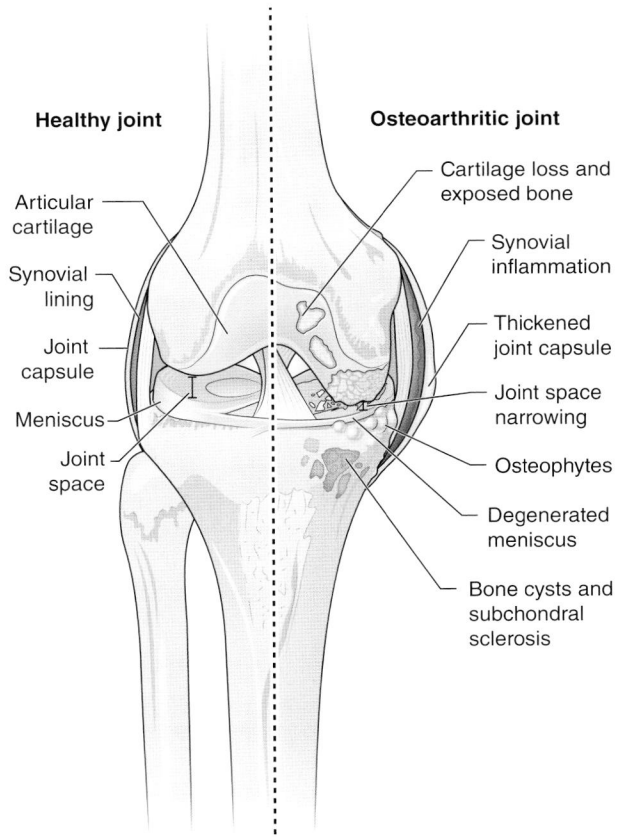

Figure 4.4 Healthy joint and osteoarthritic joint. Note the degeneration of the meniscus, the thinning of articular cartilage, the degradation of the articular surface, osteophyte formations, and synovial inflammation.

Evidence of Rehabilitation

Osteoarthritis (OA) is a very common disabling condition and is a leading cause of pain and disability.[85] Osteoarthritis of the knee alone affects 250 million people worldwide.[85] Because of the prevalence of osteoarthritis among adults, research in recent years has investigated not only the epidemiology but also associated risk factors, including joint injury or overuse, nutrition, weight, bone density, and smoking.[92, 95] Additionally, joint alignment studies note an increased risk of OA that is especially evident in the knees of people with genu valgus.[96] Injury to a joint is also a major factor leading to osteoarthritis, especially in the knee.[85] Previous knee injuries have been shown to accelerate the OA process.[85, 95] Given this information, it is very likely that clinicians will treat osteoarthritis patients throughout their careers. Knowledge of this disease and its effects is crucial to providing optimal care for these patients.

Osteoarthritis affects more than 30 million Americans.[92] It is estimated that by 2030, over 67 million Americans will suffer from some form of osteoarthritis.[93] The end result of osteoarthritis typically involves a joint arthroplasty (replacement). In 2010, 2.5 million Americans had a total hip replacement and 4.7 million Americans had a total knee replacement.[94] With the aging of the baby boomer generation, it is estimated that 11 million Americans will have a total hip or knee replacement in 2030.[94] Many people who suffer joint injuries today will be the patients undergoing joint replacement surgery 20 years from now. Total joint replacement should always be considered a last-resort treatment, but when pain and functional limitations interfere with quality of life, joint replacement is usually the best option.

Whether an upper- or a lower-extremity joint has osteoarthritis, the entire extremity's function is affected. For example, if the elbow is osteoarthritic, the shoulder and wrist will be weak and may even have reduced motion because the elbow is too painful to use normally. The same is true in the lower extremity; if the ankle is affected, both the hip and the knee will also demonstrate weakness and even loss of normal motion. Therefore, the entire extremity must be examined for motion and strength changes during rehabilitation.

It is well known that after the onset of menopause, women become more susceptible to osteopenia and osteoporosis. **Osteopenia** is a mild to moderate loss of bone density that places women at risk for advancing to osteoporosis. **Osteoporosis** is marked loss of bone density. People with osteoporosis are at risk for fractures. Both conditions are related to calcium deficiency or bone demineralization. See figure 4.5.

Bone accretion occurs from birth through adolescence with approximately 90% of bone mass acquired by age 20.[97] Loss of bone mass is a naturally occurring event in both men and women. Bones are at their strongest when we are in our 20s.[97, 98] When women reach their late 30s and men their early 40s, bone mineral density starts to decline, and this persists throughout life.[77, 97] The decline begins slowly at first, but the process speeds up as women enter postmenopausal ages.[77, 88, 97, 99] At this time, bone mass declines because osteoblasts cannot replace calcium at the

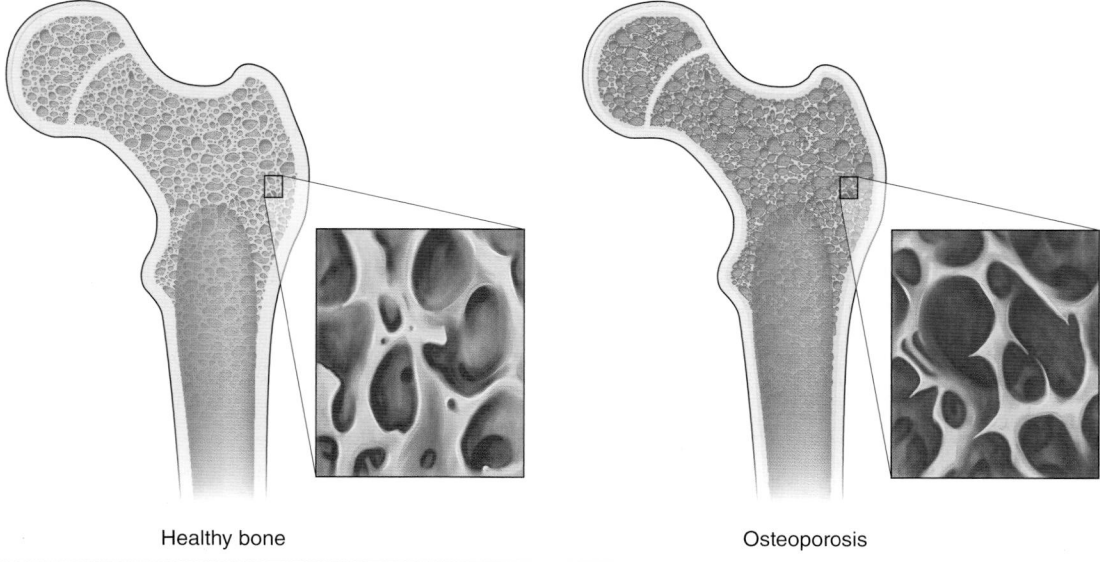

Healthy bone   Osteoporosis

Figure 4.5   Healthy bone and osteoporotic bone. Note the thinning, porous appearance of the osteoporotic bone.

same pace at which it is reabsorbed. Osteoporosis is the most prevalent bone disorder.[97]

Exercise, however, positively affects bones and joints. Bone strength improves with weight-bearing activities.[97, 98, 100] Exercise also influences bone health by preserving bone mass and preventing the death of bone cells.[77, 88, 97, 98, 101]

Neural Factors   Nerves and their excitation change with age.[102] Changes in the neural system affect proprioception, motion sense, and joint position.[103] These, in turn, influence balance and coordination. Autonomic reflexes, including neuromotor reflexes, become less sensitive, and reaction times become longer from stimulus to response.[60, 104] Another aspect of neuromuscular decline is the reduced speed of neural stimuli transmission from sensory receptors to the muscle fibers.[78, 104, 105] These changes make it more difficult for older people to react to sudden changes in position. In summary, balance and speed of movement are impaired with aging. These neural changes accompanied by diminished muscle strength and function associated with aging place the individual at greater risk for falls.

When dealing with older patients, we must consider other neurological factors that prevent them from reacting to their environment as they did when they were younger. These factors involve sensory systems other than the proprioceptive system. Loss of hearing is a natural decline in most people.[106] Because of slower neural transmission mechanisms, it takes longer for older people to grasp what they hear than it does for younger persons. You may have been told by an older person that he or she has difficulty understanding you because you speak too fast. Moreover, since memory also declines with age, even healthy older people may forget oral instructions.

Additional existing neurological pathologies make it difficult for an aged person to respond to a clinician's instructions in the same way as a younger patient. For example, for someone who has reduced sensation secondary to conditions such as diabetic neuropathy or cardiovascular compromise, standing or walking on an unstable surface may be too challenging. If older patients have reduced vision because of cataracts or other ophthalmological pathologies, they may find it difficult to read instructions on home exercise programs. If patients have difficulty hearing, they may not hear instructions properly.

Comorbidities   Comorbidity is associated with decreased functional outcomes and more complex clinical management. We have already discussed some comorbidities that occur with aging. Chronic illnesses and pathology such as arthritis, osteoporosis, heart disease, hypertension, diabetes, peripheral neuropathy, cancer, and elevated BMI (body mass index) can reduce people's physical function, independence, and quality of life.[107, 108] In general, activity becomes more limited as we age, and

this trend significantly increases for each decade after age 65.[107] The presence of comorbidities can profoundly affect a patient's function and ability to participate in a rehabilitation program.

Chronic illnesses are often managed with medications. Blood thinners can be used to treat heart disease. The Agency for Healthcare Research and Quality recommends that high-impact activities be avoided when patients are taking blood thinners. A stationary bike or walking would be preferred over a road or mountain bike and jogging. Heavy weights and aggressive manual therapy techniques should also be avoided when a patient is taking blood thinners. Beta-blockers and alpha-blockers are often used to treat heart disease and hypertension. These medications will lead to an altered heart rate–workload relationship and may affect exercise training intensity.[109] Angiotensin-converting enzyme (ACE) inhibitors may be used to treat heart disease, hypertension, and diabetes. The side effects of ACE inhibitors can include weakness, headaches, and dizziness. Statins can be used to treat heart disease, diabetes, and hyperlipidemia. Myopathy with exercise training has been associated with the use of statins.[110] It is important to understand the relationship of medications to exercise and to be aware of any contraindications that are associated with the use of specific medications. Table 4.3 provides a quick reference to commonly used drugs in older adults.[109-113]

Type 2 diabetes patients are often sedentary older people who are overweight and have a lower capacity for exercise.[109] Exercise therapy must be closely monitored in these patients. In addition, exercise should be postponed when a hypoglycemic episode has occurred during the last 24 h.[109] A higher BMI is correlated with aging.[95, 108] An elevated BMI is also associated with slower gait speed, decreased strength, limited mobility, and decreased physical function.[108] As rehabilitation clinicians, we must consider patient comorbidities when designing rehabilitation programs, and we must make modifications as needed to ensure patient safety and realistic outcomes. For patients in this group, progressive exercise training adaptations, changes in the type of aerobic exercise training, and the inclusion of low-weight-bearing exercise is recommended.[109]

Rehabilitation Considerations for Injuries in Older Patients

A significant amount of evidence demonstrates that exercise has a positive influence on the aging process.[60, 68, 71, 78, 83, 101, 114] For this reason older adults who exercise regularly may show less regression than is typical of their age group. Exercise improves many physiological and physical parameters in older adults; cardiovascular function, muscle strength, balance and coordination, flexibility, and endurance all increase with regular exercise.[115-118]

TABLE 4.3 Commonly Administered Drugs in Older Adults

Drug	Indications	Side effects
Blood thinners (e.g., warfarin, Coumadin, heparin)	Prevent blood clots in heart disease	Bleeding, dizziness, weakness
Beta-blockers (e.g., Lopressor, Tenormin, Inderal)	Heart disease, hypertension	Dizziness, fatigue
Alpha-blockers (e.g., Doxazosin, Prazosin, Terazosin)	Heart disease, hypertension	Dizziness, headache, weakness, fatigue
ACE inhibitors (e.g., Lotensin, Lisinopril, Perindopril)	Heart disease, hypertension, diabetes	Dizziness, headache, weakness, drowsiness
Statins (e.g., Lipitor, Torvast, Lescol)	Heart disease, hyperlipidemia, diabetes	Myopathy with exercise

Based on Agency for Healthcare Research and Quality (2018)[111]; Deichmann et al. (2015)[110]; Hansen et al. (2018)[109]; Ogbru[112]; Merck[113]

Research has also demonstrated that muscle mass increases in older subjects who undergo a strengthening program, albeit at a slower and lesser rate than in younger adults.[83, 116] Furthermore, older persons engaged in a regular exercise program demonstrate less risk of falling than nonexercising older subjects.[60, 119, 120]

The benefits of a regular exercise program and the importance of older Americans' engagement in regular exercise prompted the American College of Sports Medicine (ACSM) to establish a position on and recommendations for exercise regimens for older adults in 1998[101] and then to update its recommendations in 2009.[121] Since this text deals with rehabilitation, not conditioning, the ACSM program is not included here. Guidelines for such things as strength progression and heart rate during exercise are presented, however, since these and other physical concerns must be considered when creating and implementing a rehabilitation program for an older patient.

Cardiovascular System Because the cardiovascular system of an older adult cannot tolerate the same stresses as that of a younger person, the clinician should be aware of the patient's heart rate, especially during endurance activities. Until the clinician knows the patient's physiological response to exercise, it may be necessary to monitor heart rate and blood pressure. The American Heart Association's recommendation[122] for older people is to establish a heart rate maximum for exercise by subtracting the person's age from 220, then multiplying that number by 50% to 85%; this is the maximum target heart rate for that person. Although there is some dispute about the accuracy of using such a formula to determine target heart rate,[123] no other methods have been developed as a reliable replacement; hence, it remains a commonly used formula for determining target heart rate for all ages. Table 4.4 provides a quick reference for target heart rate for various adult ages and

TABLE 4.4 Target Heart Rates for Various Ages

Age	Maximum heart rate (MHR)	Target heart rate at 50% MHR	Target heart rate at 55% MHR	Target heart rate at 60% MHR	Target heart rate at 65% MHR	Target heart rate at 70% MHR	Target heart rate at 75% MHR	Target heart rate at 80% MHR	Target heart rate at 85% MHR
40	180	90	99	108	117	126	135	144	153
45	175	88	97	105	114	123	131	140	149
50	170	85	94	102	111	119	128	136	145
55	165	83	91	99	107	116	124	132	141
60	160	80	88	96	104	113	120	128	136
65	155	78	86	93	101	110	116	124	132
70	150	75	83	90	98	105	113	120	128
75	145	73	80	87	94	102	109	116	123
80	140	70	77	84	91	98	105	112	119
85	135	68	74	81	88	95	101	108	115

Based on formula 220 − age × ___% = target HR.

intensity levels. A person's overall health status, specific complaints, and activity history are important factors in determining the level of maximum heart rate. For example, if you work with an older adult who has not exercised for a while, 50% of the maximum heart rate may be a good starting point in his early rehabilitation phases. It is likely that older athletes know their normal exercise heart rate and will be able to inform you of this target. As the patient's condition improves, a gradual increase to the normal target heart rate may be indicated.

Neuromuscular System Muscles in older patients can gain size, strength, and power in response to exercise, although the muscles respond more slowly to exercise than do those of younger patients.[116, 124] The tendons of older patients also regain some of their stiffness and strength with exercise.[125] These studies seem to indicate that exercise can alleviate aging factors to some degree.

CLINICAL TIPS

Target heart rate for older adults will vary according to age and physical abilities. The target heart rate formula (220 − age × ___%) may be used only as a guideline, but specific changes from the calculated target heart rate may be needed, depending on the person's overall health and history of exercise and activity level.

Muscles atrophy and lose strength after injury. This change occurs at all ages. The strength and muscle changes related to old age are similar to the changes seen after injury or immobilization.[71, 78, 126] Given that older adults can improve their strength and muscle function, and given that the changes seen in muscle during inactivity and during aging are similar, it seems clear that strengthening exercises in a rehabilitation program can produce strength gains in older patients. Therefore, strength training is advocated for older patients.[83, 115, 116, 127, 128]

Although strength gains can be made in older patients, these gains occur more slowly than in younger patients.[129] In fact, the speed with which gains occur in many muscular parameters is slower in older patients. This includes the rate at which endurance improves. It also includes the speed of muscle contraction, so agility exercises are performed more slowly than with younger patients.[119]

Proprioception plays a large part in balance, coordination, and agility. Young people perform better on balance tests than older people do.[130] Springer and colleagues developed normative data for a timed single-leg stand balance test.[131] With the eyes open, subjects aged 18 to 39 averaged 43.3 s, 40 to 49 averaged 40.3 s, 50 to 59 averaged 37.0 s, 60 to 69 averaged 26.9 s, 70 to 79 averaged 15.0 s, and 80 to 99 averaged 6.2 s. Table 4.5 provides a quick reference

TABLE 4.5 Rehabilitation Expectations in Performing Single-Leg Stand Balance With Eyes Open

Age group (years)	Time (seconds)
18-49	40
50-59	35
60-69	25
70-79	15
80-99	5

Based on Springer et al. (2007).[131]

for rehabilitation expectations in the performance of a single-leg stand balance with eyes open.[131]

Younger people can balance for a longer time than older people can. Injury can reduce one's ability to perform balance activities, so it is logical to assume that an older injured person will have more profound deficiencies in balance than a younger injured person.

CLINICAL TIPS

If one part of an extremity is not used normally because of persistent pain or ongoing injury, the entire extremity is not used normally; therefore, disuse of one part of that extremity extends the deleterious effects of disuse to the entire extremity. This is true for any body part, regardless of the cause of the injury, the age of the patient, or preinjury status.

Considerations in Designing a Rehabilitation Program

Some of the factors we should consider when designing a rehabilitation program for an older patient have already been mentioned, and we have alluded to others. This section summarizes these necessary considerations.

Older patients may move more slowly than younger patients, so additional time may be needed for an initial examination and assessment. Since hearing difficulties and slower comprehension may both be issues for the patient, it is important to speak slowly and clearly. A low-pitched voice is usually easier to hear than a high-pitched voice, so make a conscious effort to speak in a lowered pitch, especially if you are female. Remember that vision can be a problem with older patients. If you give patients exercises to do at home, it may be beneficial to use larger-font handouts with diagrams to accompany your verbal instructions. This will help patients to remember the exercises you provide.

Older patients may have compromised vascular systems, so it may take them longer than younger patients to heal after an injury. As with any patient, the older patient's response to your program is a useful guide to progression. If the patient reports increased pain or swelling, the program may be progressing too quickly for his or her body to adjust. Remind the patient that good nutrition and adequate water intake are both important for optimal healing.

Older patients may have limited flexibility. Hamstring flexibility is usually less in older patients than in younger patients, and men generally have less flexibility than women. Given that muscle tissue and tendon tissue are weaker in older patients, overstretching should be avoided. Stretching exercises, however, should be used with patients who lack normal flexibility. Ballistic flexibility exercises are not recommended for older patients due to aging-related changes that occur in the neuromuscular system. The size and number of muscle fibers decrease, muscles become weaker, and the speed of muscle contraction declines with aging. The bouncing, repetitive manner of ballistic stretching may be too aggressive for these age-related changes. Both static stretching and dynamic stretching have been shown to improve flexibility in older people.[132, 133]

Strengthening exercises will be a part of an older patient's rehabilitation program. Recommendations for sets and repetitions in strengthening programs for all healthy populations, including the elderly, have been established by ACSM and other professional groups. However, there are no recommendations for elderly persons with orthopedic and sport-related injuries. Lacking any research evidence in this area, we have devised a protocol based on our own experiences and existing related evidence.

It has already been mentioned that older people normally have diminished muscle strength, muscle endurance, and muscle mass. Because of an age-related thinning of articular cartilage that occurs along with these muscle changes, it seems that the best way to improve muscle strength is not to overstress joints and body support with heavy weights but rather to improve muscle function through muscle endurance exercises. Such exercises will improve strength and muscle endurance and will build muscle tissue without overstressing the joints. Avoidance of heavy weights will also prevent falls caused by the patient's inability to balance the added weight. Our preference is to start with two sets of 12 to 15 repetitions and progress to three sets of 12 to 15 repetitions before moving to three sets of 20 to 25 repetitions. When an older patient can lift a specific weight for the sets and repetitions that have been set as the goal for up to three consecutive treatments, then the resistance is increased. The number of visits using a particular goal before the weight is increased will depend on a variety of factors, including the patient's age, fitness level, and long-term goals.

Light weights are recommended; adjustments will depend on the patient's response to the weight initially used. If the patient completes sets and repetitions beyond the goal or even expresses a desire to use more weight with the first attempt, then rapid adjustments can be made. Lower-extremity closed-chain exercises involving multiple joints and muscles allow greater resistance to be used than when one muscle is isolated in an open-chain exercise. For example, a smaller weight such as 5 lb (about 2 kg) may be as much as a patient can manage in an open-chain knee extension exercise, but the same patient may be able to perform a half squat with half the body weight on each lower extremity because the ankle and hip muscles assist in the activity. The loss of bone mass that naturally occurs with aging has been shown to benefit from light-weight resistance exercise.

Reflexes and reactions to body position changes do not occur as quickly in older patients as in younger patients.[103] When you use a new exercise that requires balance, it is prudent for you to spot the patient for protection from possible falls. A slower-than-normal progression may also be beneficial to ensure that the patient can manage a new exercise with less risk of falling. For example, if the patient has been working on a single-leg stance on the floor, it may be better to advance to a foam rubber pad before advancing to a more unstable surface than the pad. Using small increments between the progressions will help to prevent falls and will also give patients confidence in their own abilities. Remember that although some 70-year-old patients may be able to achieve 30 s, the average single-limb balance goal for this age group is 15 s. Progression in balance will be slower than with younger patients. As with strengthening, it is beneficial to have a patient remain at a given level for up to three sessions before advancing to a new, more difficult level.

Warm-up and cool-down are important aspects of an exercise program. Keeping in mind the target heart rates in table 4.4 and the patient's conditioning level, a warm-up activity such as a 10 min stationary bike or elliptical exercise may be more appropriate for an older patient than walking or jogging on a treadmill.[103] A cool-down should involve dynamic activities performed at a low to moderate metabolic intensity to increase blood flow and should involve exercise that is preferred by the patient.[134]

CLINICAL TIPS

When dealing with older patients, keep these factors in mind: Speak a little more loudly and more slowly with a deeper voice, provide home exercise handouts with images and larger print, and allow more than the normal length of time for the patient evaluation.

Summary

This chapter describes different elements that affect the body throughout a lifetime. Age must be a consideration when treating injured people. Individuals at a wide range of ages participate in sport and lifelong exercise. Because they are active, everyone from youngsters to senior-aged adults is at risk for injury. When people suffer injuries at any age, they turn to clinicians for treatment. Clinicians must therefore understand the impact age has on both recovery and rehabilitation progression. Although young people may heal faster than older people, they are at risk for joint injuries that may affect their growth. Older people who suffer injuries similar to those of younger people will neither heal nor progress in their rehabilitation programs at the same rate as their younger counterparts. This chapter addresses the important distinctions relevant to injuries and rehabilitation in these groups compared to the young adult population.

LEARNING AIDS

Key Concepts and Review

1. Describe why there are more people involved in sport and recreation today and therefore more who incur musculoskeletal injuries.

There are more youth leagues and more organized sports than in previous generations. In addition, people are living longer, and the baby boomer generation is more involved in athletic activities throughout their adult years and into their retirement years than were previous generations.

2. Discuss why little is known about sport injuries in the very young and the very old.

Our sport rehabilitation practices are based on information obtained from studies that usually involve subjects in their early adult years. Because many of the studies are performed on university campuses, the subjects' age range is 18 to 25. These subjects are in the physical prime of their lives; they have passed through puberty and have not yet entered their declining years. Relatively few studies have investigated sport injuries in either older or younger populations.

3. Explain why it is important to know how to manage musculoskeletal injuries of preadolescent and older people.

National statistics on the employment of certified athletic trainers in the United States indicate that approximately half of this group and over one-third of physical therapists work in outpatient clinics. These are the settings in which younger and older people are treated for their orthopedic and sport injuries. These two groups are growing in number, so there will be a growing number of injuries seen in outpatient clinics. Rehabilitation clinicians must know how to treat these groups if they are to provide safe and successful rehabilitation programs.

4. Provide an outline of growth and development based on the Tanner system, and explain how boys and girls vary in the process.

The Tanner system identifies developmental stages for secondary sexual characteristics, rate of height changes, and muscle development. A typical pubertal growth pattern begins with a phase of acceleration; this is followed by a phase of deceleration before growth ceases. Growth stops when the epiphyses close, at approximately 18 years in girls and 20 years in boys. Girls begin this growth pattern earlier and end it earlier, usually about two years ahead of their male counterparts in each case. Although the exact age when puberty begins varies from one person to another, the average starting age for girls is 9 years and for boys is 11 years.

5. Identify the problems associated with an anterior cruciate ligament reconstruction for a younger person.

Because the patient's physis remains open, reconstruction must avoid damaging the still-growing bone. Instability of the joint because of either ACL injury or injury to the meniscus is likely to result in premature osteoarthritis. Care must be taken both during the surgery and in rehabilitation to ensure optimal healing without damage to articular cartilage or the epiphyseal plate.

6. Explain the precautions that one should take when providing a rehabilitation program to an older patient.

Instructions should be given slowly and the voice should be low in pitch if the patient has difficulty hearing. Visual instructions with larger-than-normal print and images are advisable for all older patients, especially those with vision problems. Flexibility exercises may be included as with other age groups, although ballistic stretching should be avoided. Strength exercises should begin with a low resistance for 12 to 15 repetitions and should progress slowly to three sets of 20 to 25 repetitions. The progression should allow for a few days at one level before the patient advances to the next weight. Balance and coordination exercises should begin at a low level and progress with small increments from one level to the next. Adequate warm-up and cool-down are recommended for each session. Consider patient comorbidities when designing a rehabilitation program, and make necessary modifications to ensure patient safety and realistic outcomes.

7. Identify the progression of osteoarthritis.
Osteoarthritis is often the result of trauma to a joint at an earlier age. Since articular cartilage does not have a blood supply, it gradually degenerates rather than heals. As the person gets older, evidence of fraying and thinning of articular cartilage appears, eventually causing a degeneration of the joint surface. In the absence of injury, as we age, articular cartilage changes its composition and loses some of its hydration, all of which make it susceptible to wear and tear through its normal functions during compression and weight bearing. Once the articular cartilage is worn, the bone surface has no protection. Since articular cartilage has no pain receptors but bone does, the patient gradually begins to have progressively worsening episodes of pain with use or with weight bearing on the osteoarthritic joint.

8. Discuss the secondary factors that add to debilitation when osteoarthritis occurs.
Pain and reduced function secondary to the pain produce muscle weakness and declining mobility. Muscle weakness and motion loss then add more stress to already weakened joints. As the muscles weaken and the joint deteriorates, deformity becomes more evident. Gait patterns deviate, muscles atrophy, and pain causes a loss of normal function and of the ability to perform daily activities.

Critical Thinking Questions

1. An 11-year-old competitive cheerleader comes to you with a diagnosis of Sever's disease, with more pain in the left heel than in the right. Her mother indicates that the patient is very competitive at the national level and wants to compete in the upcoming season, which starts in 2 months. Your examination demonstrates extreme tenderness on the left heel and moderate tenderness on the right heel. She cannot jump because of pain. How will you explain this condition to the patient and her mother? What will you do for her rehabilitation program? What precautions must you consider? What will you tell the patient and her mother about the upcoming competitive season?

2. A 65-year-old patient is diagnosed with osteoarthritis in his hip. He has associated pain and dysfunction. He has type 2 diabetes and peripheral vascular disease. Today is his first time in outpatient rehabilitation. It is his goal to return to golfing, an activity he performs at least twice a week on a league team. You have just completed your examination of him and his abilities. He has limited mobility and decreased strength, and he walks with an antalgic gait pattern. What will your treatment today include? What interventions will you include in his rehab program? List the precautions you must remember relative to his age.

3. A 70-year-old patient comes to you with a diagnosis of distal radius fracture. Her cast was just removed. In your examination you find that she fractured her radius secondary to a fall. In fact, she has a history of four falls in the last 6 months. What will your rehab program include? What precautions must you consider?

Lab Activities

1. Find X-rays of joints of teenagers and older adults. Compare the X-rays, and identify how they differ and how they are the same.

2. Look up the ACSM recommendations for both the youth and the older adult populations' exercise programs. Create a table with two columns (youth and older adult), and place a listing of these recommendations for each of the groups in their respective columns. Identify the similarities and differences between the two. How do you explain these differences and similarities? Do you think you could use any of the recommendations in a rehabilitation program?

3. Create a table with three columns (preadolescent, young adult-25, older adult-65+) and three rows (skeletal, muscular, neural). Outline the skeletal, muscular, and neural factors for each age group. How might these factors affect a rehabilitation program?

4. Make a list of common comorbidities associated with older adults. How will each comorbidity affect a rehabilitation program? What precautions must you take with each comorbidity?

PART II

Examination and Assessment

The body is a sacred garment. It's your first and last garment; it is what you enter life in and what you depart life with, and it should be treated with honor.

Martha Graham, 1894-1991, American modern dancer and choreographer

As you progress through part II of this text, you should continue to grow in your knowledge of rehabilitation and your appreciation of the complexity, expanse, and intricacy of the information you should have as a rehabilitation clinician. Part I presented an overview of the general concepts of rehabilitation. This part moves into some specific factors that are important to every rehabilitation program you will design.

At their most basic, these factors involve skills of observation and comprehension. You will not only put what you learned in part I into common practice, but you will also see how examination, and assessment based on that examination, create both a profile of problems and a path for treatment. These concepts of observation, examination, and combining the results will serve as the foundational elements when you move into part IV.

Chapter 5 introduces you to the parts of a rehabilitation examination. Examinations enable clinicians to discover patient problems and deficiencies. These discoveries enable the clinician to create a plan of rehabilitation to correct those deficiencies and to move the patient toward optimal recovery. Without an examination, there can be no rehabilitation plan. The chapter provides you with information on how to put together all you have learned from the examination in a way that provides you with a road map for a rehabilitation program. This chapter ends with vitally important legal information on record keeping.

Chapter 6 presents information about posture. It is common to find that postural abnormalities, the ways that people use their bodies in physical activity, and muscle imbalances all contribute to an injury or to the body's failure to respond to treatment. Static posture in standing and sitting are presented. These postures are "ideal" in that they serve as a reference point from which you can examine a patient and create a correction program for pathologies.

Chapter 7 presents an overview of normal walking and running. It presents you with the elements you will need to examine a patient's gait before performing your detailed examination. Gait analysis gives you insights into potential problems and causes of pathology you will see in your examinations. Chapter 7 also discusses ambulation with assistive devices and the correct way to use them. You will also read about how to teach patients to use assistive devices correctly, a critical topic for ambulation safety.

Chapter 8 is a new chapter on function. This is an important chapter because it deals with topics that will be significant to you as a clinician but are not often found in textbooks. This chapter deals with problems faced by patients with short-term disability, especially surgical patients, and how to deal with them. You will often be the one they go to for answers. Rather than leaving you stranded, we have offered a number of examples with solutions for many of these common problems. There are also accompanying photographs and online videos that may help you to help patients address their concerns.

Once you have completed this part, you will be a step closer to putting together rehabilitation programs. As you proceed through these chapters, continue to use your deductive reasoning skills, the knowledge that you have already acquired, and your common sense to see if you can anticipate the information presented in each chapter.

5

Overall Progression of Examination Procedures for Rehabilitation

Objectives

After completing this chapter, you should be able to do the following:

1. Discuss the primary elements of a subjective examination.
2. Outline an objective examination procedure that includes all primary elements.
3. Outline the process of determining a clinical diagnosis.
4. Explain how a plan of care is designed and on what factors it is based.
5. Discuss the importance of documentation in the rehabilitation process.
6. Define the SOAP note, and explain its significance to rehabilitation.
7. Identify two additional medical records used in rehabilitation, and demonstrate their importance.

|||||||||||||||||||||||||||||||||||||||||||||||||||||||||||||||||||||||||||||||||||||||||||||||||||||||||||||||||||||||||||||||||||||||||||||||||||||||||||

Erin was fulfilling her observation hours in an outpatient clinic. She noticed that Katrina, her clinical instructor, would follow the same procedure when she would examine a new patient. However, she also noticed that some of the testing procedures varied during the examination. Perplexed, Erin asked Katrina about patient examination. Katrina outlined the procedures for a rehabilitation examination, explained the differential diagnosis process, explained how to identify the patient's problems in terms of impairments and functional limitations, described how to establish rehabilitation goals from those problems, and explained how to develop a plan of care based on both the patient's problems and the rehabilitation goals.

Erin had been exposed to record keeping for initial injuries; however, she was not familiar with the record-keeping procedures for rehabilitation. She had seen SOAP notes and progress reports during her observation, but she did not understand what these notes meant or their relevance.

A doctor who cannot take a good history and a patient who cannot give one are in danger of giving and receiving bad treatment.

Anonymous

The examination and assessment process for an injury serve as the foundation for a rehabilitation program. Patients must first be examined to determine their functional limitations and clinical diagnoses. During the initial examination, the clinician determines what deficiencies exist, the extent of the injury, how the injury affects the patient's function and quality of life, and what other factors may affect the rehabilitation program. From this information, the rehabilitation clinician decides what should or should not be incorporated into designing the rehabilitation program.

The examination is an ongoing process. The initial examination is needed to determine a baseline and to obtain a clinical diagnosis of the injury. Once that has been determined, the examination process continues through all phases of the patient's rehabilitation program. The effectiveness of the treatment is based on the ongoing reexamination of the patient's functional status. As the patient's functional status changes, so too must the plan of care to ensure that the patient's rehabilitation goals are being met and that function and quality of life are improving.

In short, an examination must precede an assessment, and both are needed, not only at the beginning and end of a rehabilitation program, but throughout the program as well. The only way to determine what treatment is indicated is to perform an examination and assessment; likewise, the only way to know whether the chosen treatment is producing the desired results is to examine and assess before and after the treatment. Examination, assessment, and treatment are so closely interwoven that one serves no purpose without the other.

Because examination and assessment are so vital to putting together a rehabilitation program, this chapter will show you how to develop an assessment based on the patient's examination, how to create a list of potential diagnoses from that assessment, and how to follow the steps that lead from that list of diagnoses to your ultimate goal, the rehabilitation plan. The chapter is divided into three parts. The first part deals with the subjective and objective aspects of an examination. The second part discusses clinical decision making, including formulating an assessment and developing a clinical diagnosis, a patient problem list, rehabilitation goals, and a plan of care. The third part introduces medical records that should be kept throughout the rehabilitation process. This is not a textbook on how to conduct examinations, so the examination process will be only briefly covered with an emphasis on identifying the elements that are important for developing a rehabilitation program.

CLINICAL TIPS

Examination is an important part of the rehabilitation program; you cannot create a rehabilitation program without first performing one. Subjective and objective examinations are needed to develop a list of potential diagnoses. The patient's problem list, plan of care, and rehabilitation program are then developed.

Subjective and Objective Examination: Making a Profile

||||||||||||||||||||||||||||||||||||||||||||||||||||||||||||||||||||||||||||||||||||||||||||||||||||||||||||||||||||||||||||||||||||||||||

The first part of performing an initial examination is determining the patient's functional limitations and the extent and involvement of the injury. This is done by performing a subjective examination (also known as taking a history) and an objective examination.

In the examination, the clinician seeks information on the severity, irritability, nature, and stage of a patient's injury.[1] The examination is composed of subjective and objective elements. The **subjective examination** includes the history of the injury and the patient's experience of pain and other symptoms. It also involves gathering information about the patient's past medical history and current health status. It is usually obtained from the patient and serves to guide the objective portion of the examination. Information may also be obtained from a medical record, family member, or other medical professional. The patient often provides clues that may be missed if the clinician fails to listen carefully. Like the anonymous author of the chapter's opening quote suggests, the treatment can only be as good as the information obtained from the examination. The subjective portion of the examination provides the clinician with a lot of valuable information and, to a great extent, guides the objective portion of the examination process.

The **objective examination** reveals the observable signs and effects of the injury and involves inspecting, testing, and palpating the injury. The information gathered in the subjective and objective examinations enables the rehabilitation clinician to formulate an assessment of the patient's injury and determine the most appropriate interventions for achieving the rehabilitation goals that have been established for the patient.

Subjective Examination

The subjective examination is conducted to obtain general information about the patient, a history of the present condition, the patient's past medical history, personal reports of pain and other symptoms, and current functional limitations. The subjective examination helps you to determine the extent of the injury, how the injury affects the patient's function and quality of life, what you should include in the objective examination, and how aggressively you can perform the objective examination. The specific questions to ask during the history vary depending on a variety of factors, such as the area injured and the severity and nature of the injury.

Because it is important to have an accurate and complete history before conducting the objective examination, your ability to listen to the patient is as fundamental as asking the right questions. Sir William Osler, MD, who is regarded as the father of modern medicine, famously said, "Listen to the patient, he is telling you the diagnosis." Along with listening, the history you take is only as good as the questions you ask. If you expect a thorough and accurate history from the patient, you must ask questions that will reveal all that is needed to obtain a complete picture. Although patients have the information, they may not provide it without prompting since they may not realize how important it may be. So you must ask questions to get all the information you need to effectively complete your examination.

One of the main reasons good questions and listening skills are important is that the information you obtain from the subjective examination guides your objective examination. For example, in your subjective examination you may determine that one of the patient's functional limitations is an inability to reach overhead into her cupboards.

In the objective examination, you must determine what impairment(s) are causing that functional limitation: Is it pain in one of the upper extremity joints, back, or hip? Lack of mobility of the shoulder, elbow, or hand joints? Myofascial restriction anywhere in the upper extremity or trunk? Weakness of the shoulder, scapula, elbow, or wrist? Muscle spasm present somewhere in the chain? Or any combination of these factors? The better the information you obtain from the subjective examination, the better you will be able to focus your objective examination to include the tests you will need to narrow your list of differential diagnoses to your final clinical diagnosis.

To obtain a thorough and accurate history, it is best to ask open-ended questions that avoid simple yes-or-no answers. For example, rather than ask, "Is it painful to walk?" a better question is "What activities cause you more pain?" The questions should be simple and straightforward. They should be presented in a logical and systematic sequence. Although there are specific questions that must be asked, each patient's history is different, and the line of questioning should be unique to each situation. In the subjective examination, the idea is to develop an overall patient profile. Refer to figure 5.1 for an overview of the subjective examination.

General Information

General information about the patient is useful in completing an accurate profile, which should include prior level of function and expectations of the rehabilitation program. The patient's age is important for identifying certain injuries and for deciding what treatment to apply. For example, ultrasound is not a treatment option for a 13-year-old's knee injury because of the knee's immature epiphyseal plates at that age, but it may be an appropriate choice for an adult.

The patient's normal activity level and the activities the patient wishes to resume after rehabilitation give you an idea of her expectations and goals and the physical abilities she will need in order to meet those expectations. See figure 5.1 for specific examples of general information to obtain.

Medical History

Getting a medical history of previous injury is important. If there has been a previous injury, the treatment that was rendered at that time and the outcome of rehabilitation can provide important information for your planning of the objective examination, assessment, and treatment. For example, recurring ankle sprains can produce additional scar tissue in or around the joint, restrict soft-tissue mobility, reduce strength and proprioceptive abilities, or increase laxity and instability of the joint. Repeated muscle strains may cause tendinopathy. Recurring knee meniscus lesions may lead to chronic synovitis. Repetitive injuries to a joint may eventually cause osteoarthritis. A history of ankle sprains may be the reason the patient is

---

OVERVIEW OF SUBJECTIVE EXAMINATION

General Information
Age

Occupation, sport (position)

Recreational activities

Limb dominance

Medical History
Prior history of injury, treatment, disposition

Comorbidities

Medications

Mental status

History of the Present Condition
Mechanism and date of injury

Patient's primary complaints

Patient functional limitations and their impact on ADLs, occupation, sport

Pain Profile
Location, type, severity

Aggravating and easing factors

Pattern relative to ADLs, occupation, sport, time of day

Additional Information
Other symptoms

Prior treatment

Diagnostic tests

Patient-based outcome tools

Figure 5.1 Overview of subjective exam.

now complaining of knee, hip, or back pain. Knowing this provides important baseline information not only for planning the examination but also for planning the rehabilitation program.

Questions about the general health of the patient and whether the patient is taking any medications can reveal information that influences your understanding of the injury as well as your treatment plan. The patient may have comorbidities that could affect treatment, such as diabetes, asthma, or cardiovascular disease. It is important to know about such conditions before designing a rehabilitation program. You would need to closely monitor such a patient if you planned to use aerobic exercise as an intervention. Similarly, it is important to identify medications the patient may be taking. Certain medications can affect the healing process as well as the patient's performance in the rehabilitation program. The patient's general mental status must also be determined in the subjective examination. Is the patient oriented to person, place, time, and situation? If your patient has dementia or a recent traumatic brain injury (TBI), this will certainly affect not only your treatment plan but also your implementation of the rehabilitation program.

History of the Present Condition

Allow the patient to explain in his or her own words how the injury occurred. There may not always be a specific injury; the symptoms may have had an insidious onset. In an acute injury, knowing the mechanism of injury provides vital information about the extent of the injury

and the tissues involved. In a chronic injury, the symptoms are more likely to result from a change in physical stress that has been brought on by a change in behavior, such as a change in posture, a new work assignment, a new training routine, or a change in training equipment. The patient can generally identify the specific change or occurrence that has created his or her primary complaint; this cause must be identified. Along with identifying why the patient is turning to you for help, it is important to identify the functional limitations that have resulted from this injury and the impact these limitations have on the patient's ability to perform sport or work activities and ADLs. The goal of your subjective investigation is to get an idea of the tissues involved, the extent of that involvement, and the disability that has occurred because of the patient's injury.

Pain Profile

A profile of the patient's pain helps determine the nature and severity of the injury and what you should include in your objective examination and initial treatment plan.

The location, type, and severity of pain should be qualified and quantified. Two commonly used scales to quantify the intensity of pain are the visual analogue scale (VAS)[2,3] and the Numeric Pain Rating Scale (NPRS).[4] These scales are also useful for measuring pain intensity before and after treatment. The McGill Pain Questionnaire (MPQ)[5] is a self-reporting tool used for patients with complex pain or multiple diagnoses. It measures both quality and intensity of pain.

Obtaining additional information beyond the pain's intensity helps you design the rehabilitation program. For example, if you know that sitting aggravates a patient's back pain, then your rehabilitation program will not include seated exercises in the early rehabilitation phase. The type of pain is important to know, for it helps you identify the diagnosis. For example, aching pain is more inflammation-based, pain during movement is likely a musculoskeletal-based pain, and sharp pain is more indicative of an acute injury. Likewise, the location of the pain is important; your knowledge of anatomy will help you identify the nature of the injury. The anatomic structures present in a specific location narrow the possibilities of injured tissue types. Along with the information you have gathered, you can narrow the list of potential diagnoses as you continue your subjective examination.

Additional Information

Additional information in your subjective examination is helpful as you complete the patient history and profile. Knowledge of other symptoms helps identify symptom generators. For example, symptoms of numbness and tingling typically indicate nerve involvement. The presence of these symptoms requires the rehabilitation clinician to complete neurological tests in the objective portion of the examination.

In addition, knowledge of treatments provided, either self-administered or provided by others, help you determine the severity of the injury and the tissue type involved. Knowing whether ice or heat has been applied may change your impression of the injury. The involved area may be very swollen because no treatment was given, heat was applied, or the patient swells easily.

Also, knowledge of any medications the patient has taken is important. If the patient has taken medication, it may mask pain or change the results of the tests you perform. Furthermore, knowing what diagnostic tests have been performed, such as X-rays or MRI, can help you further rule out or confirm a clinical diagnosis.

Patient-Based Outcome Tool

A patient-based outcome tool is completed by the patient. This document provides information about the patient's perception of how well he performs in society and his own life requirements. Patient-based outcomes are obtained from the patient via self-report questionnaires or surveys.[6] They cover many facets of health status, including symptoms, physical functioning, and psychological and social well-being as perceived by the patient. Self-report measures are used to evaluate the patient's status at any point: initial examination, reassessment, and discharge. They are also used to evaluate changes in the patient's status over time as a result of the rehabilitation program.[6] Refer to figure 1.10 in chapter 1 for an example of the Lower Extremity Functional Scale (LEFS).

CLINICAL TIPS

Most patients consult with clinicians to relieve pain, so obtaining an accurate profile of the patient's pain is important. Such a profile should include questions that deal not only with the location, description, and intensity of pain but also with how it changes during a 24 h period, including relative to ADLs, occupation, or sport. Determining which activities aggravate or relieve pain is important as well.

Objective Examination

Once you complete your subjective examination, it is time to perform your objective examination. From the subjective examination, you will have formulated a list of differential diagnoses. Your goal in the objective examination is to determine the exact structures involved and the extent of the injury's effects so that you can identify the clinical diagnosis from your list of differential diagnoses and then design your course of treatment.

You already have a lot of information about the injury even before you begin your physical examination. This information guides your objective examination. From your subjective examination, you have an idea of the nature of the problem, the severity and irritability of the injury, how aggressive or cautious you should be in performing your objective examination, which special tests to use to either rule in or out your differential diagnoses, and which contraindications to consider. Although you may expect certain findings from your objective examination, keep an open mind, and look at all possibilities for the injury and the tissues involved. Do not assume that you know what the diagnosis is until you have a complete picture based on the accumulated information from both the subjective and objective segments. Narrowing your scope of vision may lead you to an inaccurate conclusion and cause you to create an inappropriate rehabilitation program.

If an injury is irritable, your objective examination should be brief, relatively gentle, and minimally stressful to the injury. On the other hand, if an injury is not irritable, your examination can be more aggressive. Consider lateral ankle symptoms that began 2 d ago following an inversion ankle injury; there is now significant swelling and persistent pain that increases with weight bearing or with any active or passive motion. This is considered irritable and needs only a gentle, brief examination. Your differential diagnoses will likely include lateral ankle strain, lateral ankle sprain, and ankle fracture. Once you determine your clinical diagnosis, you can then provide initial treatment. At a later stage when the injury is less irritable, a more aggressive and complete examination can be performed. Now, however, your evaluation goal is to determine what treatment will best reduce the current symptoms so that the injury becomes less irritable and you can begin an effective rehabilitation process. If a patient can walk without pain and has minimal edema, your objective examination can be more aggressive and more thorough so that you can determine the extent of the injury, the tissues involved, and the treatment approach that will most effectively and efficiently return the patient to normal activity.

A **comparable sign** is an active or passive movement that reproduces the patient's pain symptom.[7] Although it is not always easy to find a comparable sign in an objective examination, the rehabilitation clinician usually tries to produce one. A comparable sign is then used during reexaminations to determine the effectiveness of the treatments rendered. Refer to figure 5.2 for an overview of the objective examination.

Visual Inspection

Your visual inspection starts the moment you see the patient enter your facility. An observation of general movement, posture, and gait will provide information about the patient's function. For example, is the patient guarded with his or her posture and movements, walking with a limp, protecting an upper extremity against the body, or moving comfortably? This will give you some details about the severity and irritability of the symptoms as well as insight into the patient's movement patterns. Your visual inspection of the injured area includes noting any abnormalities that need closer examination.

Joint and Muscle Function

Range of motion (ROM), accessory motion, and manual muscle testing (MMT) provide objective data for evaluating joint and muscle function. A patient's sex, age, occupation, and sport influence joint mobility;[8-10] therefore, these fac-

tors must be considered when a patient's joint mobility is measured. For example, normal knee range of motion will be different for a 50-year-old male jogger than it will be for a 20-year-old female gymnast, just as the amount of normal accessory motion of a 23-year-old professional pitcher's shoulder will differ from a 25-year-old truck driver's.

Active Range of Motion   Active range of motion (AROM) is joint motion that is produced when the patient voluntarily contracts the muscles that cross the joint (figure 5.3). The clinician examines both the quality and quantity of active motion the patient produces. For AROM to be considered normal, full motion must occur, and it should be smooth and unobstructed throughout the entire motion.

The quality and quantity of AROM will depend on different factors. For example, AROM differs with the presence or absence of pain during active movement of the part. The quality and quantity of AROM also depend on the patient's willingness and ability to move it, the strength of the muscles moving the joint, the available range of motion of the joint, and the **arthrokinematics** of the joint. For example, the tibia must slide anteriorly on the femur to extend the knee; when the joint's accessory mobility is restricted because of capsular tightness, normal arthrokinematics cannot occur, so the knee's motion is not normal.

Limited accessory movement is not the only factor that can cause restricted joint motion. There are other potential causes that the clinician must investigate when motion is abnormal. These additional factors include the presence of edema, ligament restrictions, muscle inflexibility, muscle weakness, and mechanical blockage from a loose body or osteophyte. All of these, alone or in combination, can prevent a patient from achieving full range of motion. As

---

OVERVIEW OF OBJECTIVE EXAMINATION

Visual Inspection
General movement observation

Posture

Gait

Deformity, swelling, discoloration

Open wounds, abrasions, scars

Joint and Muscle Function
Range of motion (active and passive)

Accessory motion

Manual muscle testing

Special Tests

Neurologic Tests
Sensory

Motor

Reflex

Palpation
Point tenderness

Deformity

Temperature

Texture

Tissue quality (tone, edema, spasm)

Functional Testing
Neuromotor control and proprioception

Movement screens

Figure 5.2   Overview of objective examination.

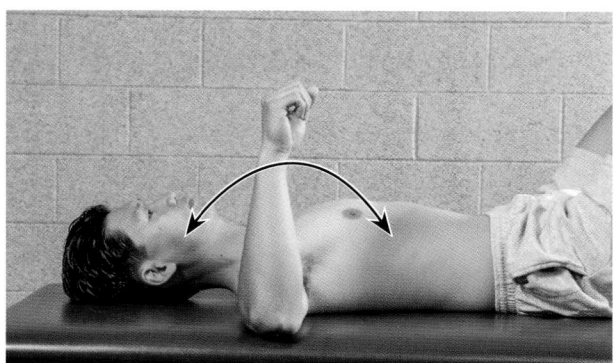

Figure 5.3   Active range of motion results from the patient's own effort without assistance from anyone or anything else.

your examination proceeds with the various tests you have selected, the cause or causes should be identified.

The quantity of movement should be objectively measured and documented. It is also important to observe and record the quality of movement. Is the movement full and fluid, or is it irregular, hesitant, or jerking? Does motion occur through substitution by other muscles? If active motion causes pain, where in the motion does it occur? Is the pain in the midrange of an arc of motion? Midmotion pain often indicates an irritated structure, such as the shoulder's supraspinatus tendon during shoulder elevation.[11]

Information about the patient's ability to move helps you determine what to include in your rehabilitation program. How well the patient moves the injured part also provides insight into which special tests you should include in your examination and the aggressiveness with which you can perform them.

Passive Range of Motion   Passive range of motion **(PROM)** is the amount of movement produced without any active participation by the patient; the clinician or another external force moves the joint through the available ROM (figure 5.4). Again, it is important to observe and feel the quantity and quality of movement. Before you passively

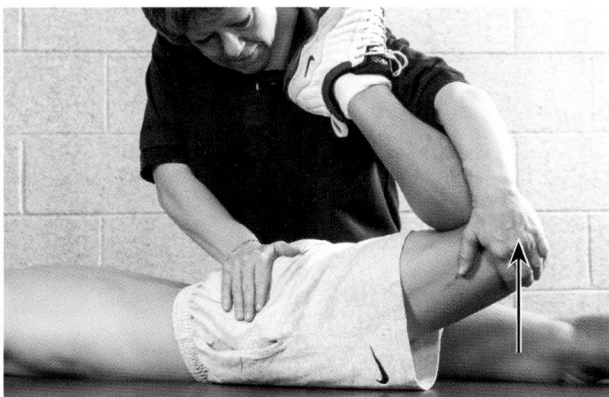

Figure 5.4   Passive range of motion occurs through an outside force without any active involvement of the patient.

move the joint through its motion, instruct the patient to tell you if pain occurs in the motion and if so, where in the motion it occurs. Observe the patient's facial expressions, which also may indicate pain. Move the joint through the range of motion as far into the pain as the patient tolerates so you can obtain an accurate impression of the amount of motion possible. If the patient's pain prevents you from moving to the end of the joint's available motion, you will know because you will not feel a physical end of movement. You should document the reason for not achieving full motion. Passive-motion pain likely occurs because either inert structures (ligaments and capsules) or active structures (muscles) are stretched.

As you move a joint through its motion, it is also important to note its end-feel. If the patient's symptoms are not too irritable, apply **overpressure** at the end of the joint's PROM to assess its end-feel. The **end-feel** is the nature of the resistance at the end of a joint's range of movement. The end-feel can be normal or pathological, depending on the joint and its range of motion compared to what is typically expected. For example, a shoulder joint's end-feel should be similar from one shoulder to another for the same sex and age group, but it will differ from the end-feel of an ankle joint for that same group of people. Several authors have identified and described various end-feels.[12, 13] Regardless of its description, an abnormal end-feel is usually also painful, while a normal end-feel is not painful. The combination of pain with an abnormal end-feel aids in the identification of pathology in a joint. Cyriax[12] and Kaltenborn[13] both use simple systems to identify end-feels. Table 5.1 lists the Cyriax and Kaltenborn end-feel classifications. To truly consider a joint to be normal, firm overpressure must produce a painless and full range of motion.[7]

As a clinician, you must recognize normal joint end-feel. A normal muscular end-feel is generally soft and a little rubbery; for example, when you flex a patient's hip with the knee in full extension to assess hamstring flexibility, you feel the hamstring stopping your passive motion. On the other hand, a normal bony end-feel is hard. This end-feel is felt when you move an elbow passively into full extension. A capsular end-feel is a firm, leathery sensation that occurs when you bring a joint to the end of its motion.[12] It is firm but not hard. If you move a normal, uninjured shoulder into full lateral rotation you will feel a firm, leathery end-feel.

When you palpate an end-feel that is not expected for that joint, the joint is likely pathologic. For example, a capsular end-feel can also be felt in a pathologic joint, such as a knee that has no edema or inflammation but does have joint capsular restriction before its normal end motion.

Accessory Motion   Accessory joint motion is motion that cannot be produced actively by the patient but is needed for full, normal motion of a joint. For example, the

TABLE 5.1   End-Feel Classifications

System	Normal end-feels	Abnormal end-feels
Cyriax[12]	Capsular	Capsular in abnormal point in motion
	Bone-to-bone	Bone-to-bone in abnormal point in motion
	Tissue approximation	Springy block
		Spasm
		Empty
Kaltenborn[13]	Soft	Any end-feel that either is of an abnormal quality for a joint or occurs at an abnormal point in the joint's range of motion
	Firm	
	Hard	

clavicle must rotate posteriorly for full shoulder flexion to occur. Another good example of accessory joint motion is distraction and medial-lateral rotation of a finger's metacarpophalangeal joint (figure 5.5). It is not a motion that the patient can produce voluntarily, but the clinician can distract and rotate the phalanx easily by grasping, pulling, and rotating the proximal phalanx on its metacarpal. This accessory rotation must be present for full, active finger flexion and extension to occur.

Accessory joint motion must be examined to determine overall joint mobility using joint play. A gliding or distracting stress is applied to assess capsular mobility. Remember, this must be compared bilaterally.

The mobility of a joint can be normal, **hypermobile** (excessive), or **hypomobile** (less than normal). Keep in mind that athletes may demonstrate mobility patterns that fall outside the normal expected ranges. For example, baseball players tend to have a decreased amount of glenohumeral internal rotation in their throwing shoulder,[14] and gymnasts tend to demonstrate an excessive amount of joint mobility.[15]

Joints that are hypomobile may be so because of either muscle spasms or capsular restrictions. Capsular restrictions can occur after injury, surgery, or immobilization. If a joint lacks full capsular mobility, your treatment plan should include joint mobilization techniques. Joint mobilization techniques are discussed in chapter 11.

When a joint's capsule loses mobility because of scar tissue adhesions, a capsular pattern develops. A **capsular pattern** is a characteristic pattern of loss of motion secondary to shortening or adhesions of the joint capsule. Each synovial joint has a specific capsular pattern.[12] Full joint motion cannot occur if there is capsular restriction. You must know what normal joint end-feel is for each joint so you will recognize when a true restriction exists.

Manual Muscle Testing   An examination of muscles surrounding the injured area involves investigating their strength and endurance in addition to their motion. A number of procedures are available to examine muscular strength and endurance. The most commonly used clinical technique is **manual muscle testing (MMT)** or isometric strength testing (figure 5.6).[16] Other techniques can be used and are discussed in chapter 13. Table 5.2 lists the muscle strength grades used in a manual muscle test. A more extensive table can be found in chapter 13.

A muscle's MMT result will dictate how you begin strengthening that specific muscle. For example, if you grade the gluteus medius at 2/5, you will begin strength

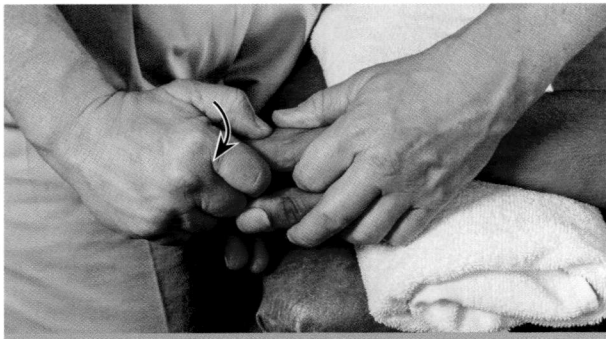

Figure 5.5   Accessory joint mobility, such as rotation of the proximal phalanx on its metacarpal, cannot be performed actively but is needed for full active joint motion to occur.

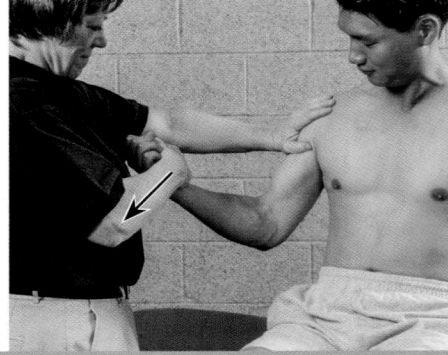

Figure 5.6   Muscular strength testing may be performed a number of ways, but the most commonly used technique is manual muscle testing. Muscle strength testing techniques are presented in chapter 13.

TABLE 5.2   Muscle Strength Grades

Numerical grade	Qualitative grade	Definition
5	Normal (N)	Able to resist maximum force throughout a full range of motion in a gravity-dependent position.
4	Good (G)	Able to resist some force throughout a full range of motion in a gravity-dependent position.
3	Fair (F)	Able to move the segment through a full range of motion against gravity but with no resistance.
2	Poor (P)	Able to move the segment through a full range of motion but with gravity eliminated.
1	Trace (T)	Palpation reveals a contraction of the muscle, but no limb motion occurs.
0	Zero (0)	No perceptible contraction is present.

exercises for the muscle in a gravity-eliminated position. In this example, supine hip abduction exercises are more appropriate than standing or side-lying hip abduction exercises.

Special Tests

Special tests are specific procedures applied to anatomic structures intended to reproduce the patient's symptoms or to create a comparable sign. Examples of special tests include the Lachman test for ACL integrity and the Whipple test for supraspinatus tear. These tests are usually compared bilaterally and reported as being positive or negative. Special tests correlated with specific diagnoses will be presented throughout part IV of this text.

Neurological Tests

Neurological testing includes examination of sensory, motor, and reflex parameters. These testing procedures are used if you suspect nerve root impingement, peripheral nerve entrapment, nerve compression syndromes, or central nervous system damage. Neurological testing is performed if the patient experiences radicular symptoms extending into the upper or lower extremities or complains of numbness or tingling.

Palpation

Palpation is the process of using the sense of touch to evaluate tissue damage or pathology. Palpation of the injury site is typically performed last because palpation can irritate the tissues and can also lead to inaccurate conclusions, especially if the patient is apprehensive or guarded.

Several structures are examined at a site with palpation. Skin and subcutaneous tissue are examined by light touch for temperature, tissue quality, texture, mobility, and point tenderness. Light passive movement of the skin and subcutaneous tissue against underlying structures is performed to reveal any tissue adhesions, as is commonly seen after immobilization, excessive edema with immobilization, or healing scars. Reduced tissue mobility results when adhesions develop between the subcutaneous tissue and underlying structures. Deficiencies like these warrant soft-tissue mobilization techniques as part of the treatment plan.

Palpation of fascia, muscles, ligaments, and tendons for tenderness, trigger points, deformity, and texture is important in examining causes of pain, motion restriction, and irritability. Examination of an area starts with light palpation of superficial structures; if the tissue's irritability permits, palpation pressure then increases to permit palpation of deeper structures. Palpation of deeper structures requires a sensitive touch, not heavy pressure. Just as areas of restriction are detected through palpation, so too are areas of tenderness. Areas of spasm, crepitus, nodules, and scar tissue are also palpated. Palpation is used to locate specific sites of tenderness and to identify the specific tissue involved.

CLINICAL TIPS

Information from the patient about the history of the injury, subjective symptoms, and how the injury affects the patient's function is gathered during the subjective examination. The objective examination involves inspecting, palpating, and testing to determine the extent and severity of the injury. Once the subjective and objective examinations are completed, the clinician interprets the information gained from these examinations to form an assessment and a clinical diagnosis. A list of patient problems in terms of impairments and functional limitations is developed from which rehabilitation goals are then created. The rehabilitation program is designed to resolve the patient problems and achieve the rehabilitation goals. Ultimately, the rehabilitation program is designed to improve patient function and quality of life.

Functional Testing

Functional tests are not always performed at the time of the initial examination. The point at which they are included in the examination varies. The irritability and severity of the injury dictate when these tests are appropriate. A functional test is used to determine whether a specific activity produces pain, to determine the injured part's ability to perform an activity, and to identify the quality of movement during the activity. Balance, coordination, agility, and proprioception play key roles in a patient's ability to perform functional tasks. Function will be discussed further in chapter 8.

Interpreting Results and Designing a Rehabilitation Program

Once the subjective and objective examinations are complete, you interpret the information you have accumulated and formulate an assessment. An **assessment** is a conclusion based on the information gathered. In the assessment, you use your clinical judgment and abilities to assimilate the information you have obtained from the examination, the medical record, and the patient's signs, symptoms, and impairments to identify a clinical diagnosis. From the assessment, you develop the patient's problem list, which is based on the patient's impairments and functional limitations. The problem list serves as a guide to setting rehabilitation goals; for every problem, you establish a goal. You then develop a plan of care that will resolve those problems and achieve those goals. The plan includes the prognosis, which is your best judgment of how well the patient will recover from the injury and return to optimal function.

Quality patient care is based on the clinician's ability to make sound clinical judgments. Clinical decision making involves understanding a patient problem, making judgments, developing a plan, implementing interventions, and evaluating outcomes.[17-19] All clinical decisions in patient care must be based on the unique needs of each patient. You are most likely to succeed if you design your rehabilitation programs using the three elements of evidence-based practice: patient expectations and goals, your own clinical experience, and current empirical clinical evidence.[20] These elements provide the basis for decision making throughout the rehabilitation process. The rehabilitation program's ultimate goal is to return the patient to his or her optimal level of function. See figure 5.7 for a patient-centered care model of patient management.

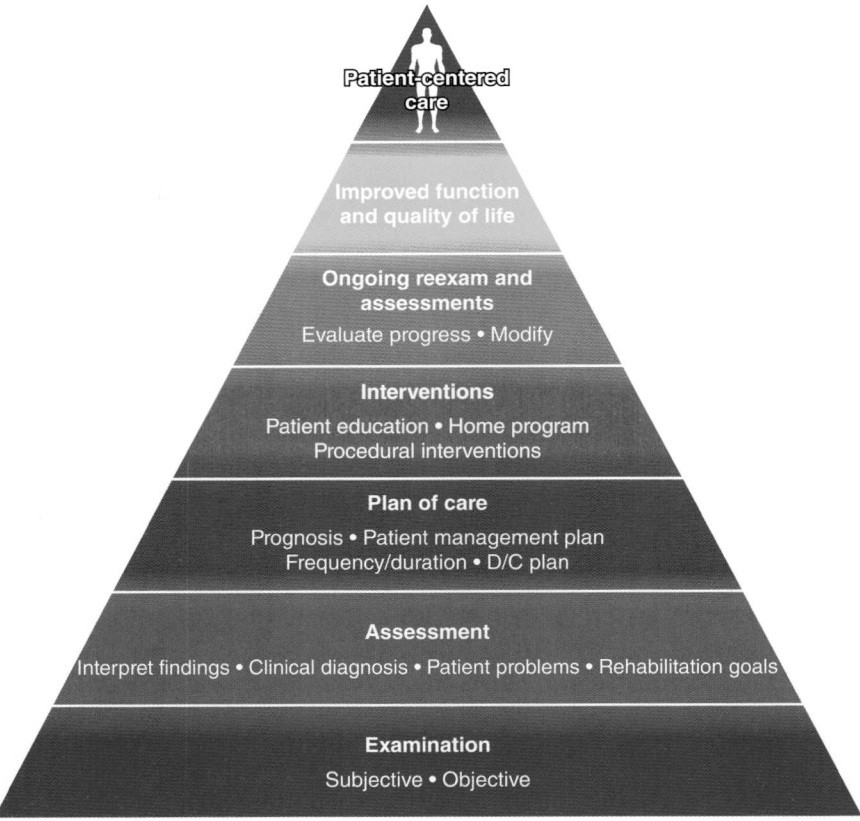

Figure 5.7 Patient-centered care model of patient management.

Assessment

One of the primary tasks in the assessment is determining the clinical diagnosis. Before the clinical diagnosis is identified, a list of possible diagnoses is made. This is known as the list of differential diagnoses, or rule-out diagnoses. A list of patient problems is also included in the assessment. Once the patient problems are identified, each problem is given a rehabilitation goal: What does the patient want to accomplish in addressing the problem? The rehabilitation goals serve as checkpoints for determining the success of the rehabilitation program.

Differential Diagnosis and Clinical Diagnosis

Differential diagnosis is a potential diagnosis from which the patient is suffering. A list of differential diagnoses is created by the clinician, based on the information obtained from the patient's subjective examination. The clinician narrows that list using results from the objective examination to identify the patient's clinical diagnosis. Developing a differential diagnosis list is crucial during the subjective examination because it determines which tests are used in the objective examination. The clinician uses his or her ability to recognize patterns of signs and symptoms, along with deductive reasoning and problem-solving skills, to group the patient's findings and thereby identify the most accurate clinical diagnosis.[21]

The process of determining differential diagnoses involves problem solving and critical thinking. It requires the ability to compare information obtained from the patient's objective and subjective examinations with known profiles of standard injuries.[22] Therefore, to be a good diagnostician you must be able to: (1) recognize signs, symptoms, and causes of various diagnoses, (2) compare the patient's signs, symptoms, and history with those of known conditions, and (3) use deductive reasoning to identify the correct diagnosis. In essence, differential diagnosis is a good example of the art and science involved in medicine: the science of knowing injury and disease profiles and the art of creating a patient profile and performing the tests to identify the correct diagnosis.

When and how do you use differential diagnosis in the rehabilitation examination and assessment process? The "when" question is easy to answer: You create an initial differential diagnosis list when you have completed the subjective examination. With each answer the patient provides, more data are provided to change the possibilities of diagnosis. Some diagnoses are added to your mental list while others are removed. For example, if a patient tells you that he is having pain in his left shoulder and down his arm, you may think he likely has a rotator cuff injury, but if he adds that he is 40 years old and has a family history of heart disease, you may expand your differential diagnosis list to include myocardial infarction. If he also states that he is left-handed and recently increased his tennis playing from 2 to 4 d per week, you may add tendinopathy to your differential diagnosis list.

By the time you have completed the subjective portion of your examination, you should have a differential diagnosis list on which you can base the objective examination. If we continue with our 40-year-old with left shoulder pain, you now have a list of diagnoses that likely includes rotator cuff tear, myocardial infarction, and tendinopathy. After you complete the visual inspection, you notice that he has a forward head posture with rounded shoulders, which is consistent with his daily 8 h desk job that he mentioned to you in his history. You know that such a posture is associated with glenohumeral impingement, so this diagnosis is added to your list. Using a visual analogue scale, he rates his pain as 4 out of 10 in intensity. In addition to palpation and range-of-motion and strength tests, you also take his vital signs and find them to be normal. You note his shoulder ROM is limited to 150° of flexion and internal rotation is limited to 20°. Both movements provoke his pain. When you performed his strength tests, you identified 4/5 weakness in his left supraspinatus and scapular rotator muscles. He also complained of pain during the strength testing of the rotator cuff. Because of these test results, you are ruling out myocardial infarction as a diagnosis but keeping rotator cuff injury, tendinopathy, and glenohumeral impingement on your differential diagnosis list. Based on your current list of diagnoses, you will perform special tests that will either confirm a diagnosis or rule out a condition from your differential diagnosis list.

By the time you begin the assessment portion of the examination, the list can sometimes be narrowed down to one clinical diagnosis, but there will be times when it cannot. This can occur when you do not have enough testing equipment or facilities at your disposal to further discriminate between diagnoses. If we continue with our 40-year-old, the special tests may prove positive for tendinopathy, rotator cuff injury, and glenohumeral impingement. An X-ray or MRI can diagnostically confirm one of these diagnoses, but these techniques are not at your disposal. However, you must still identify the correct diagnosis, so you use deductive reasoning to compare the patient's findings with known sequelae of your differential diagnosis list. In our example, you can likely eliminate rotator cuff tear because he did not report any specific incident where he suffered an acute injury, and he is relatively young for degenerative rotator cuff pathology. You also know that he has poor posture that has weakened the scapular muscles and placed chronic stress on the rotator cuff, conditions seen in glenohumeral impingement. He may have a rotator cuff tendinopathy, but this condition is similar in many ways to glenohumeral impingement and is also treated similarly. Because of your objective test results and the fact that his pain has a recent onset, you conclude that his condition is more likely glenohumeral impingement than rotator cuff tendinopathy.

A differential diagnosis evolves throughout the examination, with the list changing as additional information is gathered. It is much like putting a jigsaw puzzle together. First, you put the pieces together that match in color or image; so, too, with differential diagnosis, you group subjective and objective results into diagnostic categories that match your findings. Next, you continue to put puzzle pieces together as you identify more specific matches and find that they are creating an image; likewise, with differential diagnosis, as you add information, you add and remove different diagnoses and narrow the options, creating a clearer picture of the patient's diagnosis. Finally, you place all the pieces into their logical order so you can see the picture clearly, both in the jigsaw puzzle and in clinical diagnosis.

Patient Problems

Once the clinical diagnosis is identified, the rehabilitation clinician creates a list of problems that the patient must overcome to return to normal function. These problems can be divided into three categories: (1) physical impairment, (2) functional limitations, and (3) disability.[23] A physical impairment is a physiological, anatomical, or biomechanical loss that reduces the body's normal abilities. Functional limitations restrict the patient's ability to perform normal daily pursuits. A disability is an inability or limitation of the ability to do what is expected of a typical member of a society, group, or team.

The problems are usually listed in order of severity. The most pressing problem is listed first, with the other problems listed thereafter. Following the most pressing problem, the remaining problems are listed either in order of their severity and impact or by when they will be resolved relative to the other problems. Disability-level problems are usually listed last because we must reduce impairment and improve function before we can address disability. If we use our 40-year-old tennis player as an example, we could list his problems as: (1) 4/10 pain, (2) poor posture, (3) 4/5 supraspinatus and scapular muscle weakness, (4) difficulty reaching overhead, and (5) reduced level of function—inability to play tennis. The physical impairments would be pain, faulty posture, and muscle weakness. Difficulty reaching overhead is a functional limitation. His disability is his inability to play tennis. It may be argued that it is better to place his muscle weakness before his posture, but since his posture is likely causing his weakness and pain, it is placed before muscle weakness. Pain is placed first because this is the main reason he seeks treatment, and it must be treated before the other problems can be addressed. As the acuity of pain is decreased, interventions for posture, muscle weakness, and function are initiated.

Treatment Goals

This part of the assessment includes creating a list of treatment goals. The American Physical Therapy Association *Guide to Physical Therapist Practice* defines treatment goals as "the intended impact on function as a result of implementing a plan of care."[24] Treatment goals address patient problems, and the problems are based on the findings of the examination. The long-term goals include returning the patient to an optimal level of function. For every problem listed, there should be a long-term goal to address it. Short-term goals are intermediary steps toward achieving a long-term goal. The goals should be patient-centered, that is, meaningful to the patient. In addition, they must be specific, measurable, functionally driven, and time limited.[24]

It is important for the patient to help you in setting goals because it brings in his or her values and also improves the likelihood of compliance with the rehabilitation program. Furthermore, it will ensure that the patient has realistic expectations about the rehabilitation process. In the case of our 40-year-old tennis player, his long-term goals would include (1) shoulder flexion to 180° to enable him to reach into overhead cabinets without pain—6 weeks and (2) full pain-free return to playing tennis—6 weeks. Notice that the first long-term goal addresses resolution of the patient's functional limitation and the second goal addresses resolution of his disability.

The short-term goals would address pain, posture, and muscle weakness; these problems involve his physical impairments. A common duration for a short-term goal is 2 weeks. You should estimate how far you expect the patient to progress in the next 2 weeks of your rehabilitation program and base your treatment on those goals. After these 2 weeks, you assess the patient's progress and identify whether the goals you set have been achieved. If they have, then you establish new short-term goals for the next 2 weeks. If a goal you set has not been achieved, you should identify why it has not been met. Was your goal unrealistic, did the patient not work as hard as you had anticipated, or were there unforeseen obstacles that prevented the progress you had anticipated? Every 2 weeks, the short-term goals are reestablished until the final short-term goals are equivalent to the long-term goals that were set at the time of the initial examination. Once all of the long-term goals are achieved, the rehabilitation program is complete.

CLINICAL TIPS

For every patient problem listed, there must be a long-term goal to address and resolve it. A long-term goal should not be listed if a problem associated with it has not been identified. Sometimes one problem may have more than one long-term goal.

Plan of Care

After you have completed the initial examination, evaluated the data, made a clinical diagnosis, and determined the patient problems and treatment goals, a plan of care is developed. The plan of care is where you will express your opinions about the patient's prognosis, or potential for attaining an optimal level of function. Many factors will influence the patient's prognosis. Some of these are age, comorbidities, the severity and complexity of the injury, and the patient's motivation. Considering our 40-year-old tennis player, his impairments are relatively minor with 4/10 pain, 4/5 muscle weakness, mild range-of-motion deficits, and faulty posture. He is motivated to return to playing tennis. His functional limitations are minimal with difficulty reaching overhead. His disability is his difficulty playing tennis. He has a relatively low comorbidity status; his cardiovascular disease is controlled with medications. Given these factors, his prognosis for rehabilitation is good. With an appropriately designed rehabilitation program, we expect that he will return to an optimal level of function that includes tennis.

In the plan of care, you also develop the patient's management plan. For example, the plan of care may also involve referral to specialists or additional medical screening. The frequency and duration of the rehabilitation program and specific discharge plans are also included in the plan of care.

Interventions

Intervention refers to the rehabilitation clinician's purposeful interactions directly related to the patient's care.[24] Your interventions with the patient include not only rehabilitation techniques and applications, but also patient education and instructions.

Patient Education and Instructions

Patient education is arguably the most important intervention you have with your patient. It is a critical component of the rehabilitation program. Education begins during your initial contact with the patient. Educate the patient about the examination process. Explaining what you do as you move through the examination will put the patient at ease and will also build trust in your competence. Educating the patient about the clinical diagnosis, prognosis, and plan of care will facilitate an understanding of the prescribed therapeutic interventions. When you help patients make the connection between their pathology, impairments, functional limitations, and disability, you can ensure better compliance with your program.[25]

Instructions go beyond simply telling patients how to perform an exercise; the clinician watches the patient's performance and makes corrections to ensure the correct execution of all exercises. Beyond exercises, patient instructions may also involve telling them how to move into and maintain proper posture, incorporate correct body mechanics, use assistive devices, reduce edema, improve ergonomics, or lift properly. Provide your patients with written materials and illustrations to reinforce verbal instructions. As a rehabilitation clinician, it is your responsibility to teach your patients how they can get better and improve their function.

Procedural Interventions

Procedural interventions refer to the specific procedures used during rehabilitation. For example, modalities, manual therapy, stretching exercises, strengthening exercises, balance activities, functional training, and plyometrics may be selected for your patient's program. Many interventions are available for rehabilitation programs; which ones you use will depend on the patient's problems and goals. The interventions you select will also depend on such other factors as the specific injury, physician preferences, equipment availability, research evidence, and your own clinical experience and skill. For example, if your goals include relieving swelling and pain, then you will select modalities or manual therapy techniques to reduce swelling and pain.

Evidence-based clinical practice guidelines have been developed for the management of specific musculoskeletal conditions.[26] Clinical practice guidelines are based on systematic review of meta-analyses of the best available data on a topic. The Institute of Medicine defines a clinical practice guideline as a "systematically developed statement to assist practitioner and patient decisions about appropriate healthcare for specific clinical circumstances."[27] Clinical practice guidelines have been developed for patellofemoral pain,[28] heel pain,[29] knee pain and sprains,[30, 31] low back pain,[32] Achilles pain,[33] and ankle pain and sprains.[34] If the patient presents with the noted specific set of clinical circumstances, then the appropriate clinical practice guideline can help the clinician to provide an evidence-based rehabilitation program to optimize patient outcomes.

In summary, a good rehabilitation program changes as the patient's problems decline and his or her status improves. As short-term goals are achieved, new short-term goals are set. To meet those goals, new treatment techniques and interventions are used. Short-term goals are re-established in 2-week bouts as the patient makes progress. Ultimately, the final short-term goals are equivalent to the long-term goals that were initially set when the patient began the rehabilitation program.

Routine Reexaminations and Assessment

A brief examination and assessment take place before each treatment session, then again before a specific intervention within the session, after that intervention, and sometimes periodically throughout treatment to determine whether a specific technique is achieving its goals. For example, before applying a modality, you perform an examination to determine the extent of muscle spasm that is present. You do another examination after the modality intervention to assess the efficacy of the treatment. Similarly, you perform an examination before applying a joint mobilization technique to determine the amount of joint restriction. An examination during the treatment determines whether joint mobility is improving as the mobilization technique is applied. An examination after the joint mobilization technique determines its effectiveness: Did your treatment achieve the improvements in pain reduction, range of motion, and joint mobility that you expected? How much more motion is there?

The only way to assess whether the treatment produces the desired effects is to examine the injury's status before and after the treatment to determine if it made a difference. Examination and assessment are also performed after therapeutic exercise. Sometimes the exercise effects are determined immediately: Was the patient able to perform the exercise correctly? Could the patient have tolerated a higher resistance or more repetitions? Did the patient favor the injured extremity during the exercise? At other times, the effectiveness and appropriateness of exercise are determined at the next treatment session: Did the patient suffer any unwanted side effects, such as more pain or edema after the last treatment? Was there any muscle soreness without pain and edema? Your presession findings determine your rehabilitation program for the day. These findings also indicate whether your program is appropriate or what program changes are needed to achieve your goals and desired results.

The routine reexaminations do not have to be complex or time-consuming. It may be as simple as asking the patient how he feels. There may be occasions when more involved pretreatment reexaminations are required, such as repeating a specific test or measure before treatment begins. The most important reason for performing these examinations is so the clinician knows whether or not each treatment produces the desired results.

Record Keeping and Documentation

Documentation in health care is a crucial part of rehabilitation. It sometimes can seem boring, tedious, and overwhelming to health care professionals, but communication and documentation are critical to ensuring that people receive appropriate, high-quality, comprehensive, patient-centered rehabilitation services.[35, 36] Through documentation you report the patient's impairments, functional limitations and disability; her examination findings and rehabilitation goals; the treatment rendered and its effects; and the final outcomes of a rehabilitation program.

For a number of reasons, you should keep thorough but concise medical records. They can be referred to later to determine progress; they can be used to facilitate communication with other rehabilitation clinicians to provide consistent patient care; they are legal documents and can be used to demonstrate compliance with all applicable regulations; they may be used by payors to assess the appropriateness of care and reimbursement; and they may also be used for research and outcomes analysis.[35-37] Documentation can be in the form of paper charts or electronic records. There are many electronic documentation systems available commercially in the medical field. Larger facilities and college health centers typically use such systems. An electronic medical record (EMR) is a digital version of a patient's paper chart.[37] Regardless of the system used, documentation standards remain the same.

Because medical records are legal documents, all records that are not typed must be recorded clearly and legibly in pen, not pencil. Recorded items should not be erased, blacked out, or covered with correction fluid or tape; an error should be corrected with one line drawn through it and your initials and the date next to it, indicating that you have altered the record. You should always sign or initial and date the record after completing documentation. Ideally, all documentation should occur during or immediately after the patient encounter to ensure accuracy and to ensure timely communication with other health care professionals involved in the patient's care. Ultimately, it is your professional responsibility to comply with medical industry standards and statutory regulations of record keeping.[37]

Recording the Examination

Many different forms and formats can be used to record the examination. Most health care facilities develop their own forms. Preprinted forms are easy to use and provide for consistency and thoroughness in examinations. Electronic documentation systems have templates for examinations. Although forms and systems may differ, the completed documentation should include all the necessary information discussed in this chapter.

The examination record should include information from the patient's subjective examination, including the current injury's history, mechanism, and date of occurrence; functional limitations and their impact on ADLs, work tasks, or sport activities; pain profile; medical history and comorbidities; history of previous injuries and treatments; results of patient-based outcome tools; and if the patient is an athlete, the patient's sport and position. Any tests that have been ordered and their results should be included as well.

The objective portion of the record should include observations and visual inspections. The physical examination findings on range of motion, muscle strength, joint stability, soft-tissue mobility, and neurological tests are also included. Palpation and special test results are included in this section as well. If any functional tests are included in the objective examination, they are reported in this section too.

In the assessment section of the examination record you will document your interpretation of the subjective and objective findings. Here is where your clinical diagnosis, patient problem list, and rehabilitation goals are inserted.

The final portion of the examination record is the plan of care. This section should include the patient prognosis, patient management plan, frequency and duration of patient care, and a discharge plan. A copy of the examination is usually forwarded to the physician as a professional courtesy. It also completes the physician's records and is a means of communication and coordination between the rehabilitation clinician and the physician.

Recording Treatment Sessions

Recording your treatment session is as important as recording your examination. A common method of treatment session record keeping is the SOAP (subjective, objective, assessment, and plan) note, which is thoroughly described in Gateley and Borcherding.[38] SOAP notes are the most universally used system of problem-oriented record keeping in the medical profession. SOAP notes are popular because they are clear, concise, easily understood, and provide a plan of action for subsequent treatment. The next section outlines information that is included in SOAP notes.

S: Subjective

Subjective notes are what the patient says. Direct quotes with quotation marks can be used. A common mistake is to put the clinician's impressions or assessments in this category. For example, a statement such as *"The patient seems depressed"* is incorrect. A more correct statement would be, *"The patient states that he feels depressed,"* or *"The patient states that he is having trouble sleeping, has lost his appetite, and doesn't feel like working on his rehabilitation program,"* or *"I am feeling depressed about my progress."*

O: Objective

Objective notes record what is done in the treatment session that day. They also include any objective measurements or examination and test results. Specific exercises can be noted, including weights and reps, or an exercise record sheet or grid can be used where that information is included. For example:

1. *Manual therapy L knee: Pétrissage to quad, ITB, distal adductors. Patellofemoral joint mobs, all directions – grade III. PROM knee flex and ext.*

2. *Ther ex per grid: increased reps and added leg press.*

3. *Ice L knee × 15min*

4. *Home program: added body weight squats to 90deg. × 10, 4 times a day.*

5. *L knee ROM = 0-115°*

You notice that if a home exercise program is given to a patient, it is included in the objective portion of the SOAP note since it is something that was performed or given during that day's treatment session. In addition, any objective measures that are made during this treatment session are placed in the objective portion of the SOAP note.

Many organizations use an exercise record sheet (figure 5.8) as part of their objective reporting. This is particularly useful in rehabilitation, where many exercises are included from one treatment session to the next. It saves time by reducing paperwork and needless repetition, yet still provides an accurate record of treatment.

A: Assessment

Just as in the initial rehabilitation examination, the assessment recorded for the treatment session is your interpretation of the problems being addressed and how the patient and the injury responded to the treatment that day. Here are some examples without the use of standard medical abbreviations that would normally be used:

A: *Patient continues to walk with an antalgic gait secondary to pain in the medial knee joint.*

A: *His range of motion and strength are improving but remain deficient.*

A: *He seems to be depressed about the injury but was willing to perform all activities in the treatment session.*

P: Plan

This is the near-future treatment plan. What will you do with the patient at the next treatment session? The treatment session plan should change from one session to the next, and it may not always be adhered to during the succeeding treatment session, depending on the patient's response to the previous treatment. For example, the clinician may have recorded in the previous treatment's plan: *"P: Begin jogging activities next treatment,"* but if the patient reports that the injury has been more painful since the last treatment, the clinician may choose to defer jogging activities and tend to the issue causing the increased pain first. Depending on the specific objectives of treatment and the patient's response to it, the plan may include a variety of statements. Here are some examples without the use of standard medical abbreviations that would normally be used:

P: *Add early proprioceptive activities with single-leg stance and balance pad next treatment.*

P: *If pain persists, use electrical stimulation to reduce pain.*

EXERCISES

Name: _Brian Fredness_   DX: _L Bicipital Rupture_

MD: _Dr. Abraham_   Precautions: _DOI 4-01-2020_

Date	5/20/2020	5/22/2020	5/24/2020	5/27/2020	5/29/2020	6/1/2020	6/3/2020					
Exercise	Reps / Wt	Reps / Wt	Reps / Wt	Reps / Wt	Reps / Wt	Reps / Wt	Reps / Wt	Reps / Wt	Reps / Wt	Reps / Wt	Reps / Wt	Reps / Wt
Biceps curl	2×15 / 15#	2×20 / 20#	2×12 / 20#	15, 12 / 20#	2×15 / 20#	20, 15 / 20#	2×20 / 20#					
French curl	2×10 / 8#	2×12 / 8#	15, 12 / 8#	2×15 / 8#	20, 15 / 8#	20, 17 / 8#	20, 19 / 8#					
Wall pushup	→		2×20 / 0	3×15 / 0	3×15 / 0	2×20, 15 / 0	3×20 / 0					
Military press-up	→			15, 12 / 15#	2×15 / 15#	2×15 / 15#	20, 18 / 15#					
Supination	→					2×12 / 4#	17, 15 / 4#					
Pronation	→					2×12 / 8#	18, 16 / 8#					

Figure 5.8   Exercise record sheet.

P: *Continue strengthening program progression as tolerated, add weight to heel raise, and increase repetitions on leg press.*

P: *Progress note - Patient to see ortho next Monday.*

Additional Records

Additional records help to form a complete synopsis of treatment and progression for a patient. They provide a well-rounded perspective of progress, a summary of overall

Evidence in Rehabilitation

An article published on medical record management points out a number of reasons why records are essential for every health care professional. In their article, Bali and colleagues[39] indicate that "Medical records are the one most important aspect on which practically every medico-legal battle is won or lost." They contend that maintaining records of patient care is the only way one can prove that treatment was provided properly. They strongly advocate that "all clinicians improve the standard of maintenance and preservation of medical records." Anyone involved in providing health care should keep accurate records of any and all treatment rendered.

results, and a reference in the event of future injury. They are kept in the patient's file along with the initial examination and treatment session records.

Reexaminations

When the patient is seen for physician follow-up visits, a reexamination or progress report should be sent with the patient or sent in advance, and a copy is kept in the patient's medical records as well. The progress note provides the physician with a summary of the rehabilitation program and the patient's progress. It also allows communication between the rehabilitation clinician and the physician and helps to ensure that both are on common ground in the patient's care.

Additionally, the progress note gives you and other clinicians who may work with the patient a regular summary of the changes in the patient's condition. Objective and subjective changes that occur over time are sometimes difficult to assess when you work with a patient regularly, but they are easily seen with a glance at your reexamination notes. When you use progress notes, you can judge more easily whether the patient is progressing appropriately.

Documentation of reexamination includes data from repeated or new examination elements; it is used to evaluate progress and to modify or redirect intervention.[40] The reexamination report should include selected components of the subjective and objective examination to update the patient's functioning or disability status.[40] Any patient-based outcome tools that were completed at the time of the initial examination or prior reexaminations should be redone and documented. The number of treatment sessions is noted in the report. Your interpretation of the reexamination findings and progress toward treatment goals is included. If the treatment goals need revision, it can be done at the time of the reexamination. Finally, your recommendation of continued care or discharge is made. If you are recommending continuing care, you must include an updated plan of care that includes proposed interventions, treatment goal revisions, and the frequency and duration of further rehabilitation.

Discharge Summary

When the patient achieves the long-term goals of the rehabilitation program and is discharged from care, a brief discharge summary is completed; one copy is sent to the physician, and another is kept in the patient's medical record. A discharge summary is important because it confirms that the patient completed the rehabilitation program. It includes the patient's function at the time of discharge and summarizes the rehabilitation program and its duration. Information such as the patient's diagnosis, number of treatment sessions, start and end dates of care, patient-based outcome scores, progress toward rehabilitation goals, and discharge plan are commonly included in the discharge summary. If the patient suffers another injury to the same area at a later date, the discharge summary also provides a quick reference to the patient's response to treatments, willingness to work in a therapeutic exercise program, and status at the time he completed the rehabilitation program; it could provide insight, especially if a different clinician is working with the patient, into expectations or issues that may need to be addressed with this new injury and treatment course.

CLINICAL TIPS

Record keeping is essential for judging the treatment's effectiveness and program progression, communicating with other caregivers, serving as a reference in the event of reinjury, and verifying patient compliance. Records also function as legal documents.

Summary

The examination serves as the starting point from which a rehabilitation program is designed. The clinician is an investigator who works to identify the source of the patient's problem. This investigation includes a systematic process by which the patient's history, pain profile, impairments, and functional limitations are determined. Then, in the objective segment of the examination, baseline measurements of observation, joint and muscle function, neurologic status, functional capacity, and special test results are obtained. From these elements the clinician can assemble a complete picture of the patient's condition. Once the assessment is completed and the differential diagnosis list has been whittled down to one clinical diagnosis, the clinician can identify the patient's problems and propose a plan of care. Both long- and short-term goals are established by the patient and the clinician to outline a planned approach to achieve an optimal recovery. Accurate record keeping is critical and includes records of examinations, progress, treatments, and discharge summaries.

LEARNING AIDS

Key Concepts and Review

1. Discuss the primary elements of a subjective examination.

The subjective portion of the examination should include a history of the injury, a pain profile, a medical history, general patient information, patient-based outcome tools, and additional questions about factors that may affect the injury.

2. Outline an objective examination procedure that includes all primary elements.

The objective portion of the examination includes observation and visual inspection, examining joint and muscle function, special tests, neurological tests, palpation, and functional tests if appropriate.

3. Outline the process of determining a clinical diagnosis.

A list of differential diagnoses is determined based on the information obtained from the subjective examination. The clinician uses the objective examination to narrow the list and identify the clinical diagnosis.

4. Explain how a plan of care is designed and on what factors it is based.

A plan of care is developed after an assessment is made of the results of the examination. A list of patient problems based on the findings dictates a list of treatment interventions to relieve those problems.

5. Discuss the importance of documentation in the rehabilitation process.

Documentation is critical to ensure that patients receive appropriate, high-quality, comprehensive, patient-centered care. Documentation also serves a legal purpose to demonstrate compliance with all applicable regulations.

6. Define the SOAP note, and explain its significance to rehabilitation.

A SOAP note is a common method of record keeping. It includes subjective reports from the patient, objective treatment provided, assessment of the results of and tolerance to the treatment, and plan of treatment for the next session. It provides a record of progress and facilitates consistency of treatment.

7. Identify two additional medical records used in rehabilitation, and demonstrate their importance.

A reexamination or progress note to the physician, written when the patient returns to the physician for follow-up visits, and a discharge summary when the patient resumes normal activities are common rehabilitation records. They are important because they outline progress in patient function.

Critical Thinking Questions

1. Describe the difference between an examination that occurs at the time of an injury and one that occurs before a rehabilitation program is started. Why are these differences important? What information may be different from one evaluation to the other?

2. Since pain is often the dominant complaint, an accurate pain profile provides you with a good idea of its source and how to proceed in your treatment program. Can you identify the most common types of pain and what they classically indicate? How does duration or intensity of pain influence the treatment you provide?

3. Your objective examination is based on the results of the subjective examination. How would your objective examination of a patient who reports severe pain most of the time compare with an examination of a patient who has minimal pain most of the time with occasional severe pain? If the patient's pain prevents you from performing all the tests you would like, what should your objective examination include, and what do you do for treatment?

4. Is it possible to have a rehabilitation goal without a patient problem? Is it possible to have a patient problem without a rehabilitation goal? How are these two factors related? If the rehabilitation goals change, does that mean the patient problem has changed?

5. You have been newly hired at a university that has not kept medical records beyond the initial injury incident report and daily clinic visitation record. How would you change the system to make

it more compliant with record-keeping standards for medical facilities? What forms would you develop to make the process as simple as possible? What minimum record-keeping requirements would you put into place? What are the justifications for these changes?

Lab Activities

1. Indicate which of the following statements are S statements, which are O statements, which are A statements, and which are P statements:

   A. Pt c/o L wrist pain.

   B. Pt will demonstrate a normal gait pattern 95% of the time within 3 wk.

   C. Flexion in lying reproduces pt's worst R LE pain.

   D. Pulsed US @ 1.5-2.0 W/cm² to R upper trap for 5 min.

   E. States onset of pain was in July 2019.

   F. AROM: WNL bilat LEs.

   G. ↑ AROM R shoulder to WNL within 2 mo.

   H. Will inquire if pt can be referred to orthopedist.

   I. Pt was too groggy after pain medication and could not follow instructions well.

2. Write the 2-week goals for each of the following scenarios:

   Scenario A:

   Dx: Fx R tibial plateau. Long leg cast was applied 1 week ago.

   S: "I am afraid I'll fall if I try to walk with this cast on my leg."

   O: Amb: Not attempted; MD wants pt to begin with crutches, NWB R LE.

   A: Pt has difficulty with standing; this may be a slow process based on pt's initial reaction to treatment.

   P: Long-term goal: Indep amb c̄ crutches for unlimited distances on level surfaces & stairs within 1 mo.

   Short-term goal: _____

   Hint: You estimate that the patient will be able to ambulate 100 ft × 2 on level surfaces and require minimal assistance on stairs in 1 week.

   Scenario B:

   Dx: Neck strain

   S: c/o neck pain of an intensity of 9/10 with any movement of the neck.

   O: AROM: 0-5° cervical rotation L & R.

   A: May have neck pain for a few weeks.

   P: Long-term goal: ↑ neck AROM to WNL & pain free within 1 mo.

   Short-term goal: _____

   Hint: You judge that the patient will be able to move her head to ~10° of rotation to either side in 2 d.

3. Read the following report and convert it into a SOAP note:

   When I saw the patient this morning, he reported that he didn't sleep well after his last treatment session. He reported that the pain in his right shoulder was more intense than it usually was after the treatment, going from a 3 to a 6 on the 10-point scale, and he thinks that it might be because of the new strength exercise that was added last time. Since he was sorer today, I decided not to continue with the overhead lat pulldown exercise with 60 lb we started last time and to keep his shoulder exercises at no higher elevation than 90°. I started out with ultrasound to the supraspinatus tendon at 1.5 W/cm² for 5 min. The ultrasound was followed by some joint mobilization, grade II for glenohumeral distraction, then grade III for anterior-posterior glides and inferior glides for about 5 min, and then I finished with more grade II distractions. After the mobilization he did his stretching exercises. The stretching exercises included stretches for 30 s each to his shoulder lateral rotators, flexors, abductors, and horizontal abductors. The strengthening exercises I had him do today included wall push-ups for 2 sets of 20, shoulder medial rotation in side-lying on his right side with 7 lb for 3 sets of 15, shoulder lateral rotation in side-lying on his left side with 5 lb for 3 sets of 15, shoulder abduction with him standing using 5 lb and going to only 45° for 3 sets of 20. I finished his treatment today with ice to the shoulder for 15 min. I instructed him to do only his usual range-of-motion exercises for flexion, abduction, lateral rotation, and horizontal adduction for his home program until the pain subsides to where it was before the last treatment. I also told him to put ice on the shoulder for 15 min at home if the pain increases again. He said he felt better after today's treatment and thought he would sleep better tonight. Next time I'll see how he feels before we start his program. If he is better, I will try the lat pulldown exercise again but with less weight. If he still has more pain, I think I should probably refer him to the physician.

4. For 2 weeks you have been treating a soccer player with an old hamstring strain that has not resolved. At the end of the 2 weeks, you want to examine how he has progressed with the treatments you have performed.

   A. What tests will you perform?

   B. How will you know if your treatment program has been effective?

   C. What soccer activities will you have him perform as part of his functional activities?

5. Three days ago a gymnast suffered a left grade II ankle sprain. You are going to start her on rehabilitation today.

   A. What will your examination include before you begin her program?

   B. What will be the determining factors in what to include in your treatment program today?

   C. How will you know if you have provided an appropriate program for her?

6. A 65-year-old patient is reporting that she has pain in her right knee but that she doesn't remember injuring it recently. What questions would you ask her? What is your reason for asking each question?

7. With your lab partner lying on the treatment table, go to the end range of the following motions and describe what you feel for each end-range position:

   A. Elbow extension

   B. Elbow flexion

   C. Knee extension

   D. Knee flexion

   E. Subtalar inversion

   F. Shoulder flexion

   G. #2 MCP extension

6

Posture

Objectives

After completing this chapter, you should be able to do the following:

1. Identify the primary elements of proper alignment in standing from anterior, posterior, and side views.
2. Discuss common postural faults of the spine, upper extremities, and lower extremities.
3. Recognize the relationship between abnormal posture and muscle imbalances.
4. Outline corrective exercises for common postural faults.

Dan Maki was hired by the local furniture manufacturing company to rehabilitate the company's injured employees. Dan has provided the employees with in-service training on proper lifting mechanics, and injuries have decreased as a result. Nonetheless, some injuries still occur.

His most recent patient, Dee, is about to begin performance activities before returning to her workstation at full duty. Dee injured her back about 3 weeks ago when she lifted a box incorrectly. At the time of the initial examination, Dan noticed that Dee's posture in both sitting and standing was poor, so he corrected her posture very early in the program. Because Dan wants to be sure that Dee can avoid another injury, he implements an initial rehabilitation program to improve her sitting and standing posture before progressing to more advanced and work-specific activities.

A good stance and posture reflect a proper state of mind.

Morihei Ueshiba, 1883-1969,
Japanese martial artist,
founder of aikido

This chapter opens the door on the topic of posture. If you are to improve a person's posture, you must first identify what is normal. This chapter deals with normal standing and sitting posture, common causes and effects of pathological posture, and correct body mechanics. Body mechanics, as discussed here, relates to daily activities, sport activities, and activities that you as a rehabilitation clinician perform during your treatment session with patients.

Once you have an appreciation for proper posture, it will become easier for you to examine injuries, especially chronic injuries, and develop the appropriate rehabilitation programs. You, as the rehabilitation clinician, should use proper posture to conserve energy, avoid injuries, and provide efficient and effective manual therapy and manual resistance applications for your patients.

Posture

Posture is the relative alignment of the body segments with one another. When a person has good posture, the body's alignment is balanced so that stress on the body segments is minimal. Poor posture puts the body's alignment out of balance, causing exaggerated stresses to various body segments.[1] Over time, this continual stress, even at relatively low levels, causes anatomical adaptations. These changes alter one's ability to perform and affect the body's overall efficiency.

Clinicians can anticipate problems that will need to be addressed in a patient's rehabilitation program by observing the patient's posture.[2] You must be able to identify normal posture to understand the causes of pathological posture. As you learned in chapter 5, the examination is an important part of the rehabilitation program. Examination identifies the patient's deficiencies and problems that need to be addressed, and it also provides the basis upon which

to judge whether treatments are effective. Examining the patient's problem before and after a treatment is the only way to make these determinations. Therefore, as you learn the treatment techniques in this text, you also need to review and, in some cases, learn the examination procedures that go hand in hand with any good clinician's treatment practices. For this reason, standing posture is briefly reviewed before pathological conditions are presented.

Static standing posture is used as the reference for posture evaluation. Although people seldom stand completely still, static posture can reveal abnormalities in relative balance and alignment of body parts that can affect structure and function during motion. Before we can discuss improper posture, we must identify normal posture.

Correct Normal Symmetrical Standing Posture

Standing posture is assessed in three planes: sagittal, frontal, and transverse. A plumb line is used as the reference point in a symmetrical standing posture examination. This term is derived from the Latin word, *plumbum,* meaning "lead." A **plumb line** is a string with a weight (formerly a lead weight, but any slightly heavy object will do) at the end. When suspended, the string forms a vertical line. The patient stands behind the plumb line as posture is assessed.

Anterior View

From the anterior, or front, view, the plumb line bisects the body into symmetrical left and right sides (figure 6.1). The patient stands so that the feet are equidistant from the plumb line. The arms are relaxed with the palms of the hands facing the lateral thighs. In a symmetrical standing posture, the line bisects the nose and mouth and runs through the central portion of the sternum, umbilicus, and pubic bones. The earlobes are level with one another, as are the shoulders, fingertip ends, nipples, iliac crests, patellae, and medial malleoli. The patellae point straight ahead with the feet straight or turned slightly outward. The knees and ankles are in line with each other, with the knees angled neither inward nor outward.

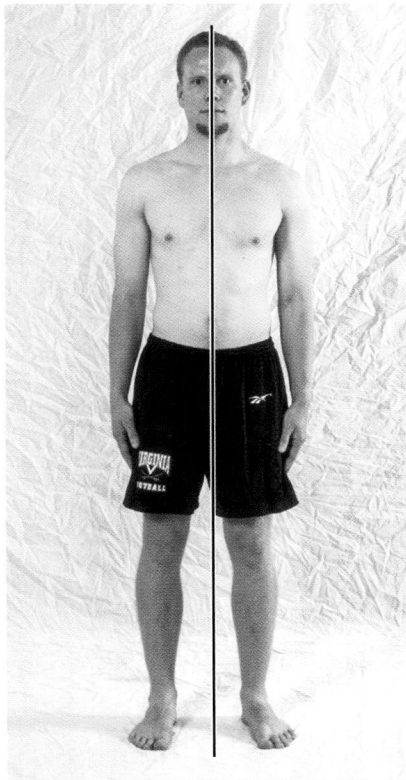

Figure 6.1 Frontal posture view.

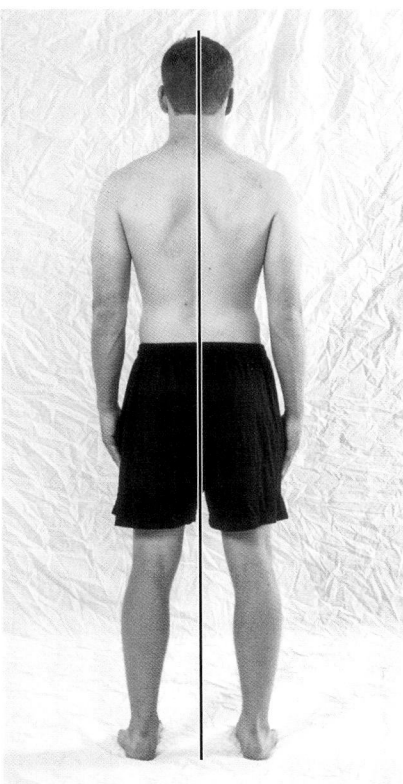

Figure 6.2 Posterior posture view.

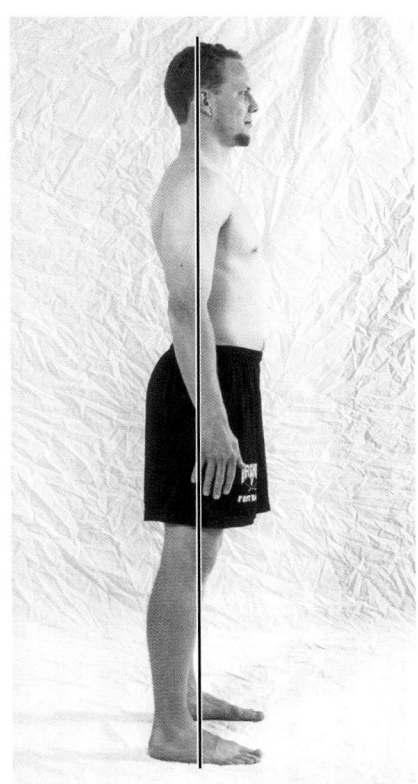

Figure 6.3 Lateral posture view.

Posterior View

The posterior, or back, view demonstrates alignment similar to that observed from the anterior view (figure 6.2). In a symmetrical standing posture, the plumb line bisects the head and follows the spinous processes from the cervical through the lumbar spine. The earlobes, shoulders, scapulae, hips, posterior superior iliac spine, gluteal fold, posterior knee creases, and medial malleoli appear level from left to right. The scapulae lie against the rib cage between the second and seventh ribs and about 5 cm (2 in.) from the spinous processes. Each calcaneus is erect, with a line that is perpendicular to the floor bisecting the calcaneus vertically. Trunk muscles appear balanced with symmetrical development. The shoulders are relaxed with the gap between the elbows and lateral trunk equal from left to right. Body weight appears equally distributed over the two feet.

Lateral View

From a lateral or side view, the patient stands with the plumb line slightly anterior to the lateral malleolus (figure 6.3). When the patient is positioned with the plumb line referenced at the ankle, observe the lateral alignment from the head down. In symmetrical standing posture, the plumb line passes posterior to the external auditory meatus, the earlobe, and the bodies of the cervical vertebrae. The plumb line passes through the center of the shoulder joint and the greater trochanter. It also runs midway between the back and chest and the back and abdomen, just posterior to the hip joint, and slightly anterior to the center of the knee just behind the patella. A horizontal line connects the anterior superior iliac spine (ASIS) and posterior superior iliac spine (PSIS). The patient remains relaxed with the body's weight balanced between the heel and the forefoot, with slightly more weight perceived through the heels. The knees are straight but not locked. The chin is slightly tucked, and the chest is held slightly up and forward. There is a mild curve inward in the low-back and neck regions, with a slight curve backward in the thoracic region.

Correct Sitting Alignment

As in standing, correct sitting posture is a relatively passive event. Students in high school and college and many people in the workforce spend much of their day in chairs. Incorrect sitting posture can aggravate an existing injury, and prolonged sitting with poor posture can make the person susceptible to injury.

In a correct alignment, the chair seat height allows the person's feet to rest comfortably on the floor with the knees and hips at least at 90°. The knees should be at least the same height as the hips, but preferably slightly higher. If the person is short, placing the feet on an object to allow these knee and hip angles is an acceptable alternative. The chair seat depth should be such that the edge of the seat does not press against the back of the person's knees. The chair back supports the lumbar and thoracic spine and is high enough to reach the inferior scapular border. Higher-backed executive chairs provide full thoracic support and permit the person to lean back comfortably. If the chair has arms, they should be at a level that provides for shoulder relaxation and permits the forearms to rest comfortably with the elbows at 90° (figure 6.4). Due to the normal 30° to 40° of thoracic kyphosis, the scapulae should have little to no pressure on them while sitting.

If the person is sitting at a desk, the chair height should be such that the person's forearms rest comfortably on the desk with the shoulders relaxed. If the chair height must be increased to achieve a correct position, a footrest may be needed to maintain proper knee and hip positions and still keep the feet flat. When the person uses a computer keyboard, the forearms are at 90° or slightly less (0° is full extension), and the wrists are in a neutral position with the fingers resting on the keyboard.

Normal Human Spinal Position

As mentioned previously, one must understand what is normal, or neutral, before one can assess dysfunction. The normal, neutral position of the sacral base averages 30° of sacral nutation (anterior rotation);[3] the average position of the lumbar lordosis is 33° with neutral lumbar lordosis ranging from 25° to 40°;[4] neutral position of the thoracic

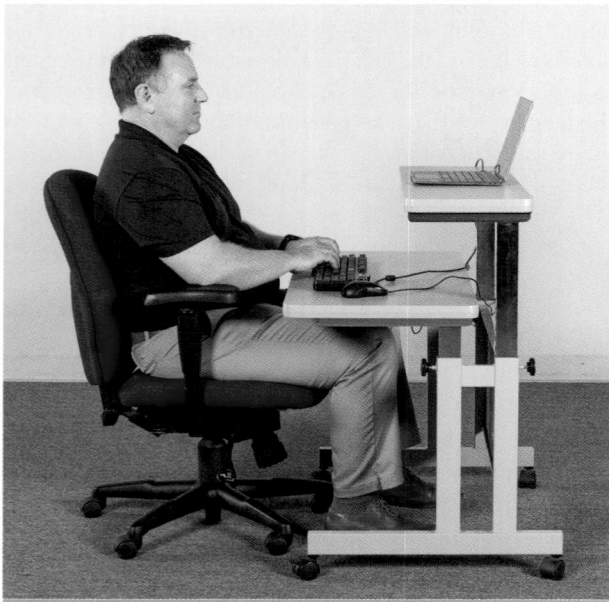

Figure 6.4   Correct alignment in sitting. The feet rest comfortably on the floor with the hips and knees at 90° to 110°. If the chair has arms, their height allows the elbows to rest at 90°, and a computer keyboard is at a height where the wrists are in neutral.

spine is 27° to 40° of kyphosis;[5] neutral position of the cervical spine is 31° to 40° of cervical lordosis.[6] These values are considered neutral, or "zero," because these are positions where the spinal curves are in good alignment and in the strongest position for the sacrum and spine. Figure 6.5 provides a visual image of these spinal curves. Deviation from these sagittal plane values places the spine segment in either flexion or extension, and deviation at one spinal level will affect the adjacent spinal levels. For example, a decrease in normal thoracic kyphosis (flat back posture) will result in increased lumbar spine lordosis. Abnormal posture alters the mechanics and increases stress on these and adjacent structures. Therefore, postural change in one region of the body may result in pain elsewhere. For this reason, the rehabilitation clinician who is presented with a patient who has abnormal posture must be aware of the possibility that the patient's dysfunction may actually be located at another segment rather than at the site of pain.

Pathological Alignment

Good posture allows us to use our bodies efficiently and effectively. Bad posture, however, places abnormal stresses on the body and increases the demands on it during performance.[7] Over time, bad posture habits develop, causing shortening of some structures and lengthening of opposing structures with secondary weakness of both shortened and lengthened structures. These changes can impair one's efficiency of movement. Inefficient movement burdens an already stressed area during performance and, over time, can lead to pain or injury.[8] For this reason, the rehabilitation clinician should know the common pathological postures. This knowledge can help in the development of appropriate corrective therapeutic exercise programs.

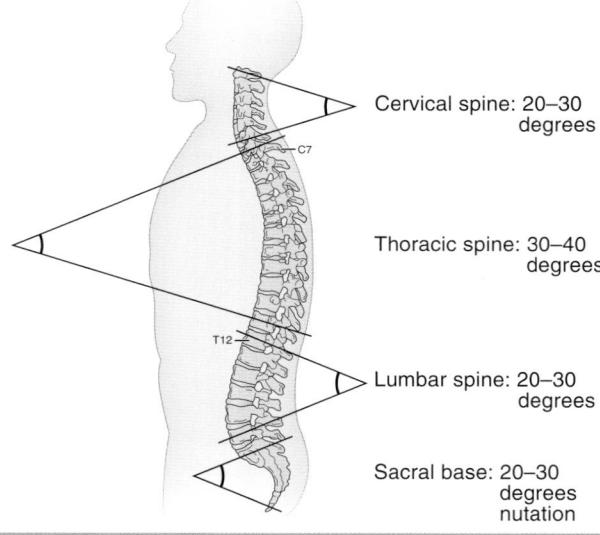

Figure 6.5   Neutral spine position. Each spinal segment has a position in which the least stress occurs for that segment.

Abnormal alignment is usually clinically recorded in relative terms. Rather than precise measurement, terms such as "mild," "moderate," and "severe" are used to describe abnormal alignment. For example, a swimmer may have a mild forward-head posture, or a gymnast may have a severe lumbar lordosis. Accurate spinal measures are only obtained using an X-ray.

Pelvis and Lumbar Area

Common posture faults in the pelvis and lumbar area include excessive lumbar lordosis and scoliosis. Scoliosis is discussed in the section Thoracic Area. An anterior pelvic tilt is associated with lumbar lordosis, while a posterior pelvic tilt is seen with a reduction of lumbar lordosis. Often associated with an increase or a decrease in lumbar lordosis is an anterior pelvic tilt or posterior pelvic tilt, respectively.

A normal lumbar curve is approximately 25° to 40° of lordosis,[4] but a lumbar curve greater than that places undue stress on the lumbar spine and other segments (figure 6.6). An excessive lumbar **lordosis**, also referred to as "sway-back" in lay terms, is accompanied by an anterior pelvic tilt in which the ASIS is rotated down in relation to the PSIS. This posture can be caused by overactive hip flexors and overactive low back extensors pulling on the lumbar spine, resulting in weak abdominal muscles, especially lower abdominals, weak gluteals, weak hamstrings, and increasing difficulty in performing diaphragm inhalation.[9] Over time, this abnormal postural alignment can result in tightness of lumbar fascia, increased stress on the spine's anterior longitudinal ligament, a narrowing of the vertebral disc spaces that leads to a narrowing of the intervertebral foramen, and approximation of the vertebral articular facets. These changes can result in nerve root compression, sciatica, joint inflammation, degenerative disc, and

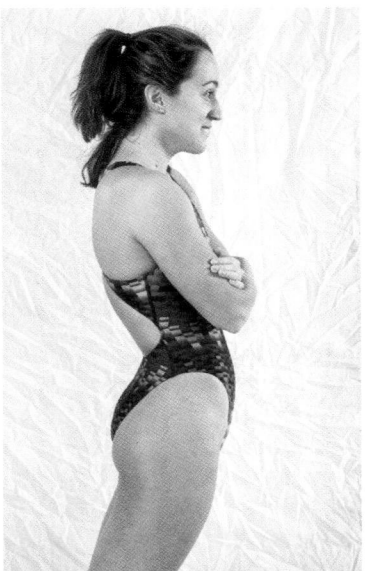

Figure 6.6 Excessive lumbar lordosis.

vertebral changes.[10-13] This posture is associated with a concomitant reduction of normal thoracic kyphosis and a reduction of normal cervical lordosis.

Thoracic Area

For a variety of reasons, one of the common postural faults the human body lapses into is spinal extension; in the midback region, this translates to a flattening of the upper back, or a reduction of the thoracic curve. This flattening is characterized by an "at-attention" posture that includes retracted scapulae in either an elevated or depressed position and flat neck characterized by a decrease in cervical lordosis.[14] This posture results in hyperactivity in the thoracic erector spinae and scapular retractors; at the same time, secondary weakness of the scapular protractors and anterior thoracic muscles develops due to their lengthened state. The scapular retractors and posterior rotator cuff often present with weakness because of their hyperactivity. This posture increases soft-tissue compression between the first rib and clavicle, which can generate thoracic outlet syndrome.[15]

A flattened thoracic kyphosis results in compensation from the adjacent spinal sections; therefore, the clinician will also observe an increase in lumbar lordosis, anteriorly tipped pelvis, flexion of the midcervical region resulting in a reduction of cervical lordosis with forward head posture, and a plethora of cranial, scapular, humeral, femoral, tibial, and calcaneal compensations as the body tries to perform normal life tasks in this posture.[9, 16, 17]

A spinal column that functions in its normal sagittal-plane curves is 10 times stronger than a spine that becomes extended and loses its normal sagittal-plane curvature.[3] When the body can easily attain its proper sagittal curves throughout the spine, the body moves appropriately. For the remainder of this chapter, a "neutral spine" is in reference to a spinal column that can attain and function in its sagittal-plane curvature as shown in figure 6.5.

An analogy, or comparable visual image, for normal sagittal spinal alignment is that of a spiral staircase, or a single helix that is visualized as a two-dimensional structure (figure 6.7). This structure permits movement in all three planes of motion. Such a structure can also absorb pressure and permit changes of direction. From top to bottom, the spine has a gradual progression from lordosis to kyphosis and returning to lordosis. In this analogy, if two or three stairs are set in the same position, that specific curve of the spiral staircase is no longer harmonious, stable, or balanced in its three-dimensional function. Likewise, if the adjacent vertebrae do not align in their two-dimensional helix-like arrangement, individual spinal segments become "stuck" in their three-dimensional movements. Although the example is viewed from a two-dimensional model for simplification, the effects of a pathological position of one vertebra impact three-dimensional movement of the spine.

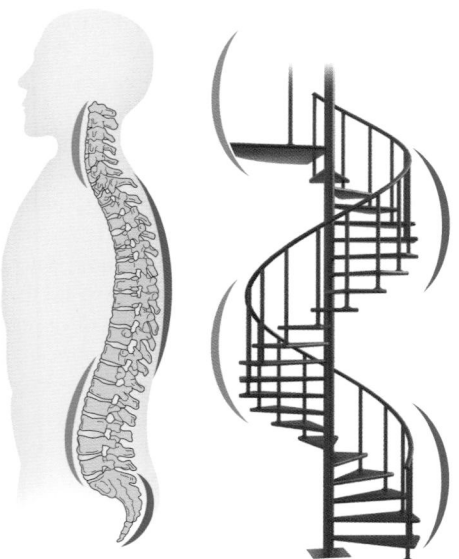

Figure 6.7   The spinal segments in the sagittal plane are similar to the two-dimensional image of a spiral staircase. Each segment gradually changes its angle relative to the stair above and below it to create a strong, flexible structure.

Spiral staircase used in illustration: Image by Jazella from Pixabay

In this normal progressively curved alignment, the spine permits ease of frontal plane motions such as crawling, walking, standing, or running, where the body's center of mass must shift side to side. Mechanical engineers and architects use rounded forms when appropriate because a curved structure handles and distributes stress more easily than a straight structure. The human body is no different; the spine must maintain its inherent curves to be stable, reduce stresses, and permit smooth frontal plane movement.

Because each spinal segment moves, the natural spinal curves are modified as the spine adapts to those stresses that are applied to it. The thoracic region can become excessively rounded, thus influencing the positions of the adjacent lumbar or cervical segments. A mild kyphosis in the thoracic spine is normal, but an excessive **thoracic kyphosis**, or excessive rounding of the thoracic area, is not (figure 6.8). This pathological presentation occurs in response to an increase in lumbar lordosis or a decrease in cervical lordosis.

In excessive thoracic kyphosis, chest muscles, including the intercostals and pectoralis major and minor, are usually in a shortened position and are counterbalanced by lengthened thoracic erector spinae, rhomboids, and trapezius muscles. An exaggerated thoracic kyphosis is typically associated with a round-shoulder posture. The scapulae are also protracted, resulting in more than the normal 5 cm (2 in.) distance between the medial scapula border and the vertebral spinous processes.

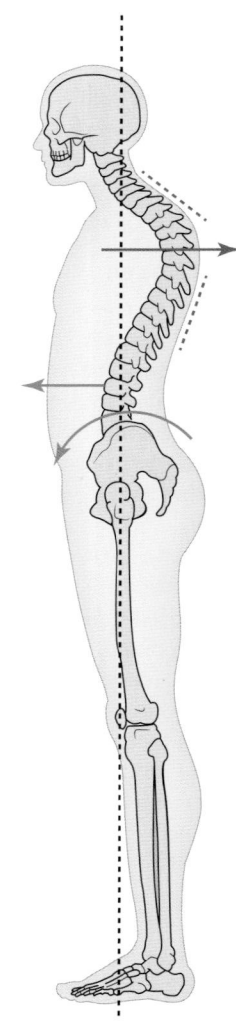

Figure 6.8   Increased thoracic kyphosis with associated extension (or absence of normal kyphosis/flexion) of the thoracic spine segments above and below the hyperkyphotic thoracic segment. The cervical spine's decreased lordosis and the lumbar spine's increased lordosis meet at the hyperkyphotic segment.

An increase in thoracic kyphosis can lead to **thoracic outlet syndrome**.[18] Secondary cervical problems can result from excessive pressure placed on the cervical area by malalignment of the thoracic spine. People such as swimmers who place high demands on rhomboid and trapezius muscle groups[19] can experience fatigue in these groups because of these muscles' concomitant lengthened and weakened status.

Although an X-ray is the gold standard for determining if a spine truly presents with a scoliotic curve, a spinal curve, if present, may be noted during the observation portion of an examination. Scoliosis is usually seen in either the thoracic or the lumbar spine, but it usually affects both areas to some degree. Scoliosis is seen more often in the thoracic region than in other spinal sections, however.[20] **Scoliosis** is a lateral curve of the normally straight spine and is classified as either a C-curve or an S-curve. A C-curve is indicated as either right or left C-curve according to its side of convexity. A C-curve with a compensating secondary curve is called an S-curve (figure 6.9). In an attempt to keep the head level, the body compensates for a C-curve by developing a counterbalancing lesser lateral curve that results in an S-curve. Scoliosis usually also includes a rotation of the vertebrae. If this occurs in the thoracic spine, an asymmetry of rib position is observed from an anterior or posterior view, with one side of the rib cage more anterior than the contralateral side. Pelvic landmarks are usually not level, and shoulders are often not level in scoliosis as well.

Although idiopathic scoliosis is the most common form of scoliosis,[21] some of the known causes for scoliosis include congenital deformities of the spine, congenital leg-length differences, and asymmetrical postural and activity preferences. For example, tennis players may develop a scoliosis because of their participation in a unilateral sport.[22] Tight soft-tissue structures occur on the side of the concavity, while lengthened structures are on the convex side of the scoliosis curve.

Scoliosis can cause muscle fatigue and increased ligamentous stress on the convex side because of weakness and lengthening of those structures. Impingement of nerve roots with secondary nerve root pain occurs on the concave side. If the scoliosis is caused by a congenital leg-length discrepancy, the foot of the longer leg has a lower longitudinal arch as the body tries to compensate for the leg length difference.[23]

A scoliosis should not be confused with a lateral shift of the thoracic or lumbar spine. A shift is present when the pelvis and shoulders do not lie in the same frontal plane. Either the pelvis or the shoulders are shifted to the left or right of the midline of the body (figure 6.10). This shift is caused by muscle spasm or pain from an impinged nerve root as the body tries to move away from the source of pain.[24] Pain associated with a shift is usually a temporary condition that is relieved when the cause is eliminated.

Head and Cervical Area

In response to the abnormal lumbar and thoracic alignment, the cervical spine develops a compensatory alignment. The cervical spine can also develop abnormal pathological alignment with chronically poor posture.[25] For example, sitting with the chin resting on a hand supported by the elbow on a desk or table or keeping the head forward of the body while at a computer will both tend to create exaggerated cervical curves. When the head is positioned forward of the spine, the lower cervical spine flattens, and the upper cervical spine has an excessive extension. Therefore, a loss of normal cervical lordosis, also known as forward head posture, or FHP, usually involves an increased flexion of the lower cervical spine and an increased extension of the upper cervical spine (figure 6.11).

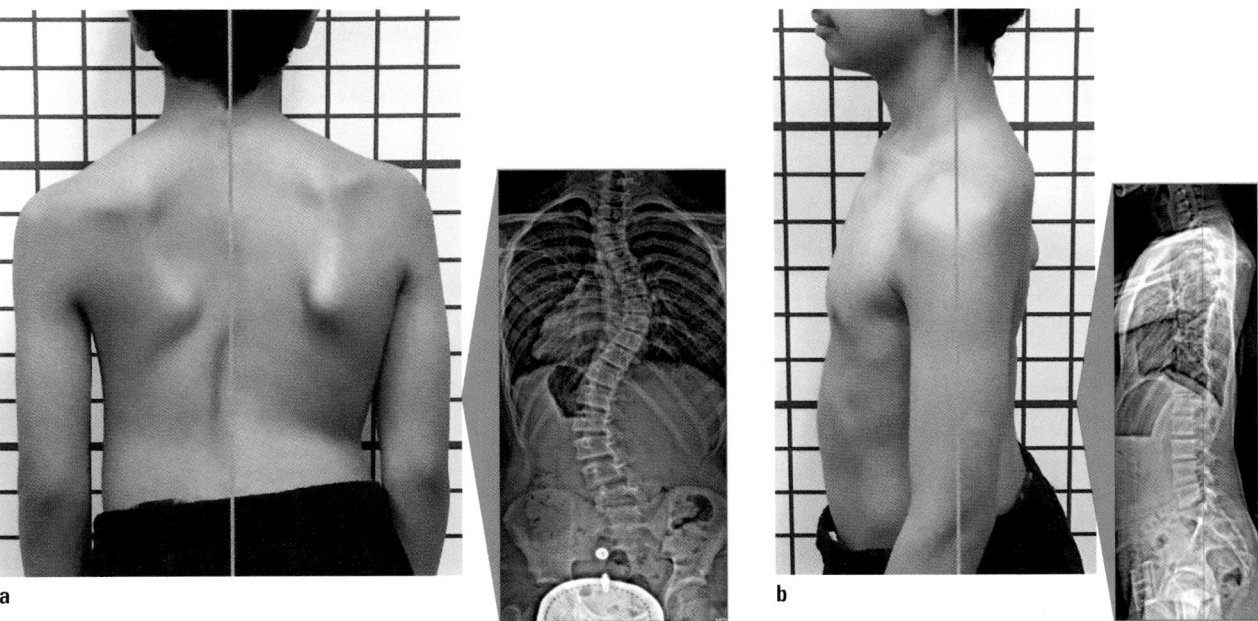

a   b

Figure 6.9 Scoliosis. Notice the uneven hips, unequal arm hang (right scapula is more abducted from the midline compared to the left) and unequal shoulder and scapula heights.

Courtesy of Lisa Mangino, PT, DPT, PCS, C/NDT, PRC, SBS-C2.

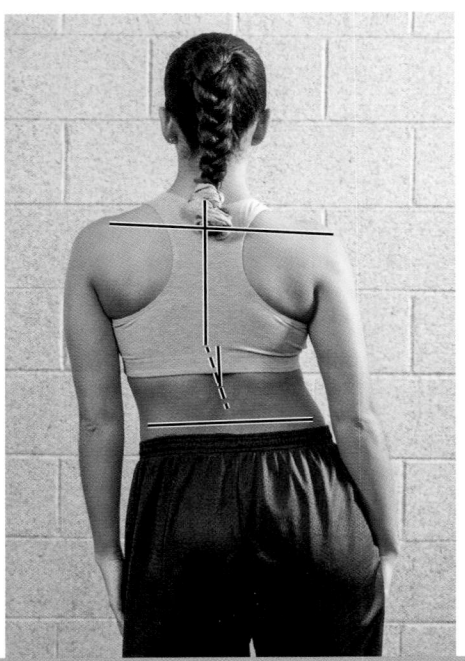

Figure 6.10 Lateral shift. Notice the uneven hips with a shift of the trunk to the left. The shoulders are uneven and are not stacked over the pelvis as they normally are, and rather than a gradual curve that is seen in scoliosis, a straighter alignment in a shift of the vertebrae (toward the left in this case) is observed.

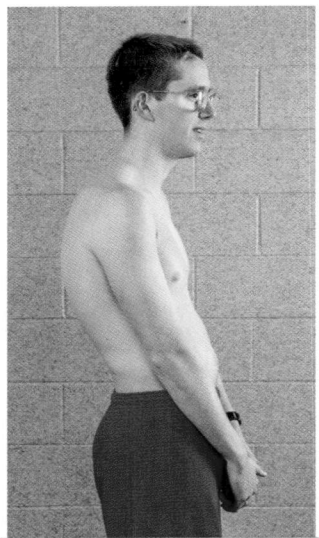

Figure 6.11 A reduction of cervical lordosis is often accompanied by increased thoracic kyphosis and lumbar lordosis as seen in this individual. See the similarities among figures 6.6, 6.8, and 6.11. Each figure presents pathologic curves of different spinal levels, but each also demonstrates pathological changes at other levels.

Muscle weakness of the lower cervical, upper thoracic erector spinae, and anterior neck regions is overpowered by the shortness of upper cervical muscles, including the levator scapulae, sternocleidomastoid, scalenes, suboccip-

itals, and upper trapezii. This muscle imbalance encourages and perpetuates abnormal cervical posture.

Many problems can result from prolonged poor cervical posture.[26] Both pathologically long and short muscles experience weakness and fatigue (see chapter 13). The exaggerated cervical position also increases cervical disc pressure, adds irritation to cervical facet joints, increases nerve root pressure, and impinges on neurovascular bundles to increase the risk of thoracic outlet syndrome.[27, 28] This prolonged abnormal positioning also increases the stresses applied to the cervical spine's posterior and anterior longitudinal ligaments. Scholastic and collegiate athletes who spend their days in the classroom often sit with their elbows on the desk and their chins in their hands, and people in the workforce spend their days at a computer sitting in a rounded-back and forward-head position, the most common positions that place increased stress on the cervical spine.[29] Long-term posterior longitudinal ligament stress creates a "dowager's hump" at the base of the cervical spine in persons with chronic forward-head posture along with a flat thoracic spine. In addition, temporomandibular joint stress can be exaggerated by abnormal cervical posture, leading to temporomandibular joint disorders.[30]

Lower Extremities

Lower-extremity malalignment in the feet, knees, or hips is often the result of compensation from other structures along the closed kinetic chain, or it can be the source of pathology within that closed kinetic chain. Common postural faults in the lower extremities include excessive flexion or extension, excessive abduction or adduction, and excessive medial or lateral rotation. The normal angle between the femoral neck and the femoral shaft in adults is 120° to 125° (figure 6.12). This angle is larger in infants and children, decreasing from 150° in a newborn to 133° in a teenager until it reaches 120° to 125° in the adult years.[31] An abnormally larger angle is referred to as **coxa valga**, and a smaller-than-normal angle is called **coxa vara**. As the neck–shaft angle increases with a coxa valga, there is an apparent lengthening of the limb. The opposite is true with a coxa vara, in which the limb shortens as the neck–shaft angle decreases. People with coxa valga have a higher propensity for eventual hip joint arthritis,[32] whereas those with coxa vara are more prone to femoral neck fractures.[33, 34]

In the transverse plane of the femur, there is a normal forward projection of the femoral neck relative to the position of the femoral condyles. This angle decreases with age during developmental years. A newborn's femoral neck–condyle angle is around 30°, whereas in adults it is 8° to 15° (figure 6.13). **Anteversion**, an increased angle, results in greater hip medial rotation and causes squinting patellae and toeing-in during standing. A decreased angle, called **retroversion**, produces greater hip lateral rotation, so in standing, the feet rotate outward. Anteversion decreases hip stability and places the hip at risk for dislocation, whereas retroversion increases the joint's stability.

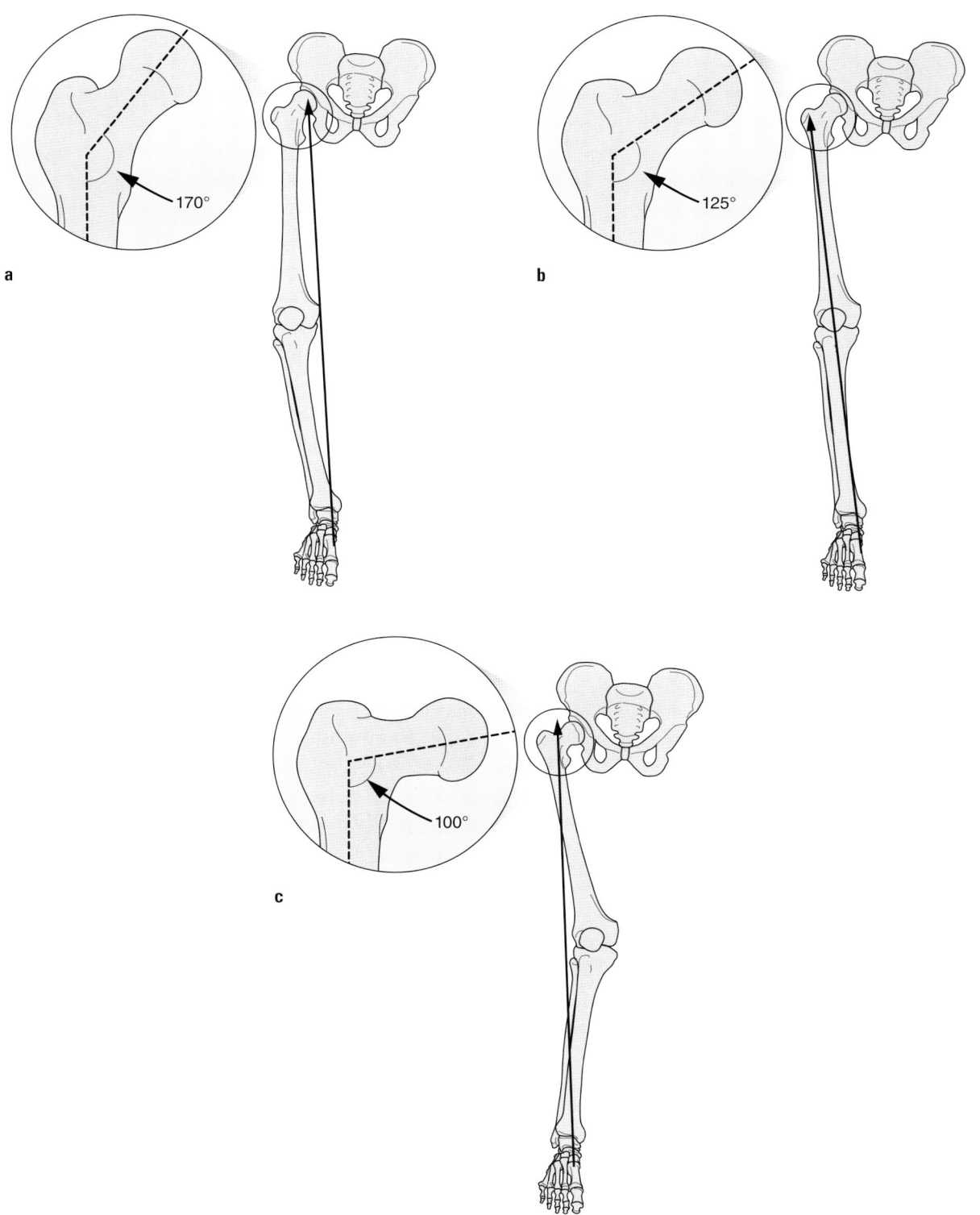

Figure 6.12 Femoral neck–shaft angles: *(a)* coxa valga causes increased femoral-joint pressure during single-leg stance with the more vertical alignment of forces delivered into the joint, *(b)* normal position, *(c)* coxa vara produces increased stress on the femoral neck during single-leg stance because of the lengthened moment arm.

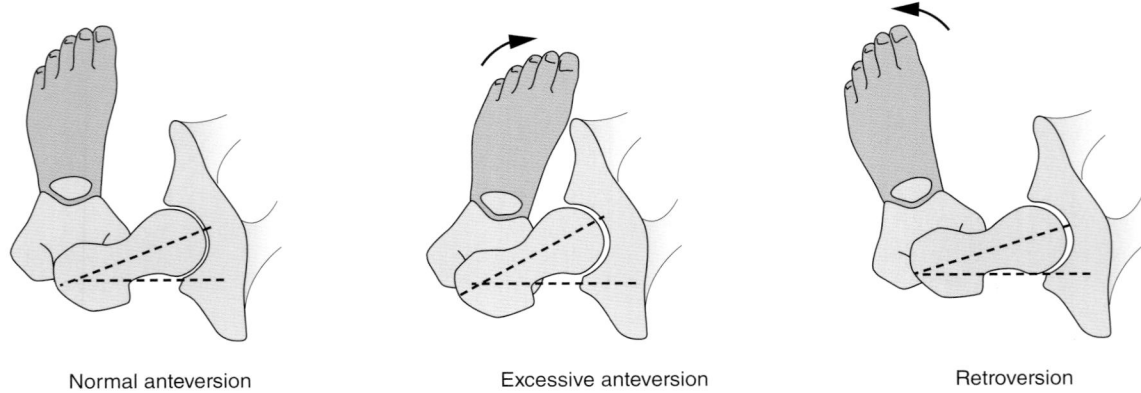

Normal anteversion   Excessive anteversion   Retroversion

Figure 6.13   Relative position of the femoral neck and femoral condyles. Normal anteversion in an adult is 8° to 15°.

The normal sagittal alignment of the femur and tibia at the knee is straight; an angling of the knees toward each another is **genu valgus** or **genu valgum**. A bowing outward of the knees is **genu varus** or **genu varum** (figure 6.14). These malalignments have a variety of causes. If they occur on one side, unilateral pelvic rotation is likely the cause. Quadriceps disuse can produce genu valgus. Genu valgus deformities can be the cause or source of excessive foot pronation, and varus deformities can be related to high arches.

In normal standing, the patellae face forward with the feet positioned forward or slightly outward. The condition in which the patellae face toward each other is referred to as **squinting patellae** and may be related to medial hip rotation, hip anteversion, medial tibial rotation, or adduction of

the feet (figure 6.15). The condition in which the patellae angle away from each other is referred to as **frog's eye** or **grasshopper eye**. This condition is often the result of lateral hip rotation or tibial rotation; the feet are positioned in abduction. Patellar and femur position are linked,[35] and femur position is linked to pelvic position.[36] For every 5° of pelvic rotation, there is 1.2° to 1.6° of femoral rotation.[36] Therefore, in your examination it is important to properly assess pelvic orientation and determine the cause of pathological alignment.

In a side view, the knee is straight but not locked in a proper alignment. If the line of gravity falls in front of the patella, the knee is hyperextended, a condition referred to as **genu recurvatum** (figure 6.16). Excessive stress is placed on the knee's ligamentous structures in this position.

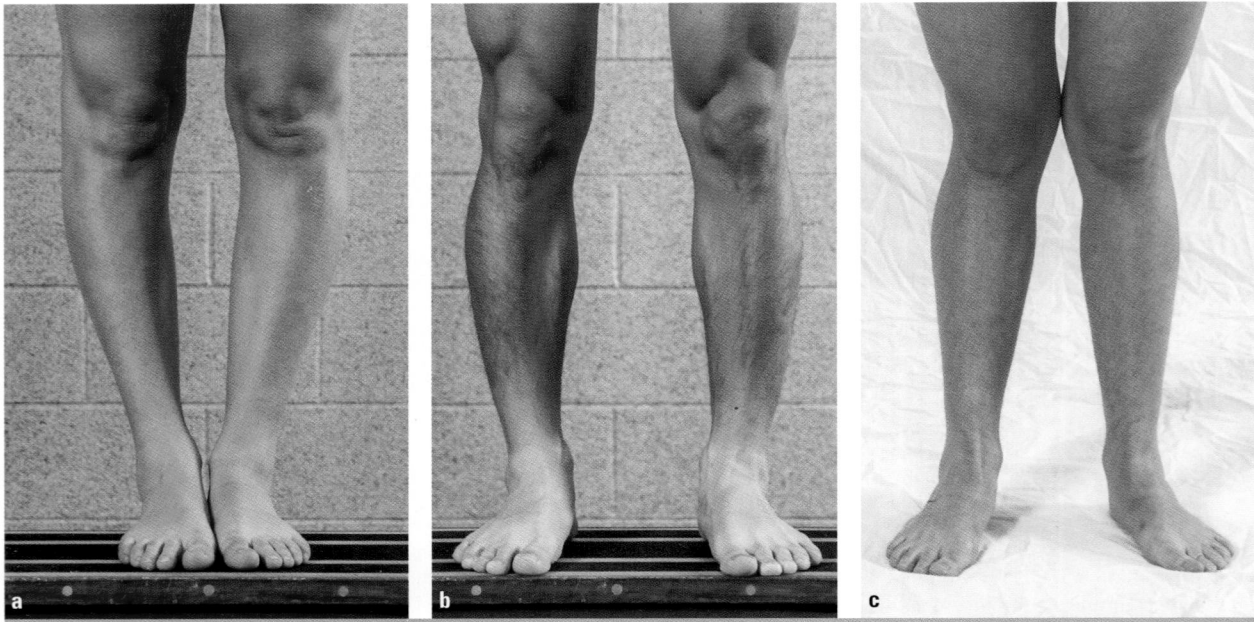

Figure 6.14   Knee alignment in the sagittal plane: *(a)* genu varus, *(b)* normal, *(c)* genu valgus.

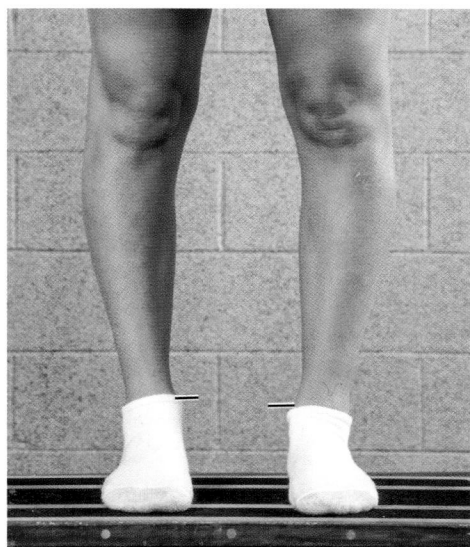

Figure 6.15 Left squinting patella. Notice the different heights of the medial malleoli and the relative position differences between the anterior tibial crests.

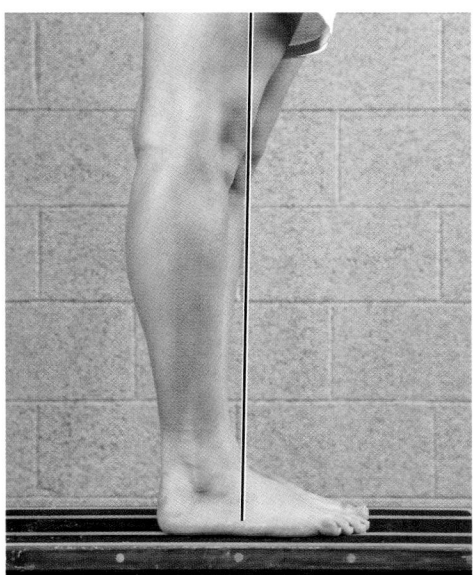

Figure 6.16 Genu recurvatum.

Genu recurvatum is commonly accompanied by excessive lumbar lordosis and anterior pelvic rotation.

Tibial torsion is present when the leg appears rotated relative to the thigh. This is most evident when looking at the patellar positions relative to the positions of the feet. In an adult, the feet normally toe out slightly from the sagittal axis of the body[37] (figure 6.17). In newborns, this angle is as small as 2°, but by age 5 to 7 years most of the leg's lateral rotation is achieved.[38] Excessive tibial torsion

is usually a lateral torsion and is correlated with feet facing laterally when the knees face forward; when the feet point forward, the knees are medially rotated. There are many ways to measure tibial torsion.[39-43] One of the commonly used methods to measure tibial torsion is to place the patient supine with the patellae facing directly upward. A line bisecting the medial and lateral malleoli creates an angle with the horizontal plane of the tabletop; this is the tibial torsion measurement (figure 6.18). Normal values are less than 20° to 25°.[8] Excessive lateral tibial torsion can increase patellofemoral stresses and lead to instability and fat-pad entrapment.[44]

Medial tibial torsion is associated with genu varum, and lateral tibial torsion is associated with genu valgum. These conditions can appear with habitual use of poor sitting postures, especially in children, as seen in figure 6.19.

Foot position can influence knee, hip, and pelvic positions, and the converse is true as well. One method

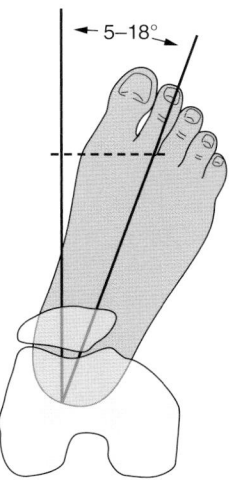

Figure 6.17 Normal adult foot position in weight bearing.

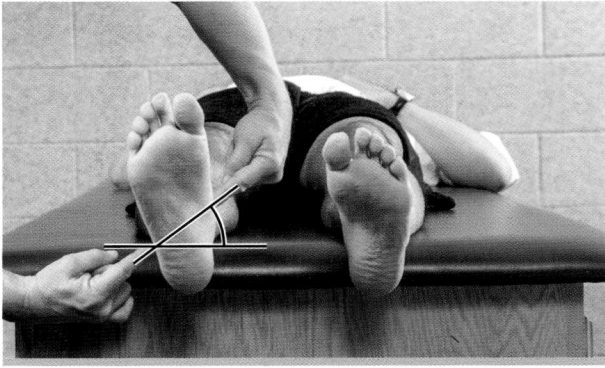

Figure 6.18 With the patella facing the ceiling, a line between the medial and lateral malleolus forms an angle with a line parallel to the tabletop for identifying the individual's tibial torsion.

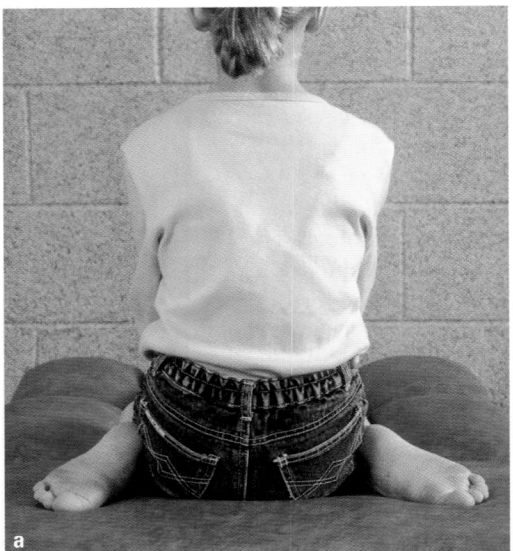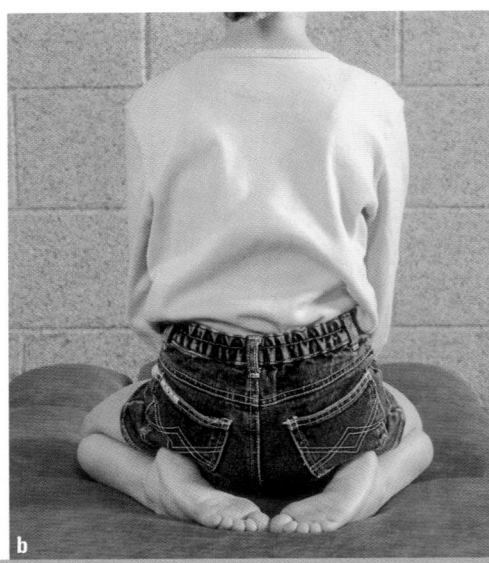

Figure 6.19 How youngsters sit on their legs has an influence on their tibial alignment: *(a)* sitting with knees in full flexion and tibias laterally rotated encourages lateral tibial torsion; *(b)* sitting on legs with knees in full flexion and tibias medially rotated encourages medial tibial torsion.

of analyzing foot position is measuring the foot's medial longitudinal arch. Although there are various techniques for measuring medial longitudinal arch height, a common way involves drawing a line from the distal aspect of the medial malleolus to the weight-bearing surface of the first metatarsophalangeal joint. In both weight bearing and non–weight bearing, the navicular tuberosity should be on the line[45] (figure 6.20). If the navicular tuberosity falls below the line, the arch is abnormally low; if it falls above the line, the arch is abnormally high. A very high arch is **pes cavus**. A very low arch, **pes planus**, can be associated with excessive foot pronation and calcaneal eversion, and it can be accompanied by genu valgum or femoral anteversion.[46] A pes planus foot is usually hypermobile, allowing for

excessive rearfoot and forefoot motion during gait. This type of foot structure may not have the stability to create a strong platform for propulsion, and it places excessive stresses on soft-tissue structures and adjacent joints as the patient tries to perform power and agility activities. The greater the foot's hypermobility, the greater is its loss of stability. Increased stress on foot and ankle structures, especially when combined with restricted motion, can lead to overuse injuries such as plantar fasciitis and Achilles tendinopathy.[47]

Calcaneal eversion with increased forefoot pronation is observed from a posterior view of the ankle. In this position, the Achilles tendon appears to be at less than a 90° angle to the floor, and the calcaneus is everted (figure 6.21).

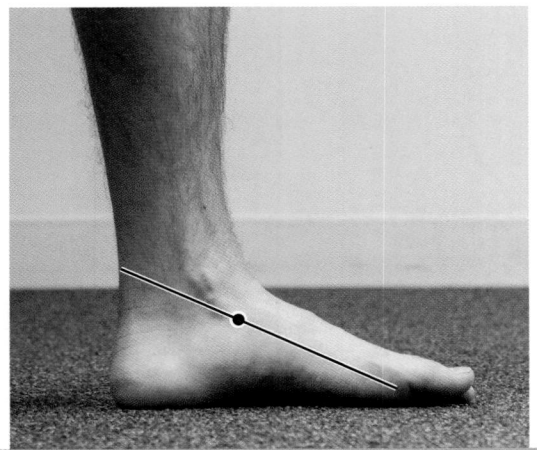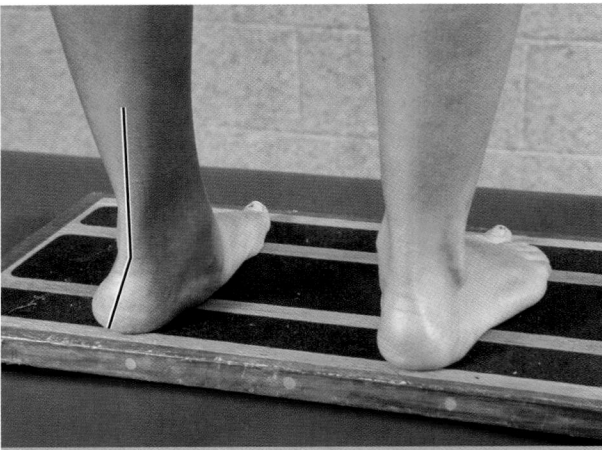

Figure 6.20 Normal alignment of the navicular on Feiss's line.

Figure 6.21 Pronation. Notice the everted position of the left calcaneus.

Pes cavus, a higher-than-normal arch, is associated with a more rigid foot structure and produces less mobility of the joints of the rearfoot and forefoot. This type of foot has a reduced ability to absorb stress and is thus more prone to stress fractures.[48] With reduced flexibility and associated diminution of stress-absorption capacity, increased stress is imposed on the lower extremity. A high arch is also often associated with hammertoes or claw toes and can be related to femoral retroversion.

Toes are normally straight. A positioning of the great toe laterally toward the other toes is called **hallux valgus**. A common cause of hallux valgus is hypermobility of the foot. Over time, this additional stress on the first metatarsophalangeal joint during terminal gait causes it to become deformed[49] (figure 6.22).

Toes that become flexed or hyperextended at their metatarsophalangeal and interphalangeal joints are known as claw toes or hammertoes. **Claw toes** are hyperextended at the metatarsophalangeal joint, flexed at the proximal interphalangeal joint, and straight at the distal interphalangeal joint; **hammertoes** are hyperextended at the metatarsophalangeal joint, flexed at the proximal interphalangeal joint, and hyperextended at the distal interphalangeal joint. These toe alignments are usually accompanied by a high longitudinal arch and a rigid foot. Corns and calluses on the toes develop secondary to abnormal pressures as the elevated portion of the toes rubs against the inside of the shoe's toe box.

Upper Extremities

The areas mainly affected by bad posture in the upper extremity are the shoulders and scapulae. If a person has a poor thoracic posture with rounded shoulders, the scapulae protract forward and rotate downward and anteriorly on the rib cage; this shoulder complex alignment can occur either unilaterally or bilaterally, depending on the cause of the pathology. This malalignment presents itself as an anterior position of the glenohumeral joint with the dorsal hands facing forward, resting on the anterior thigh rather than at the lateral thigh as they should be (figure 6.23).

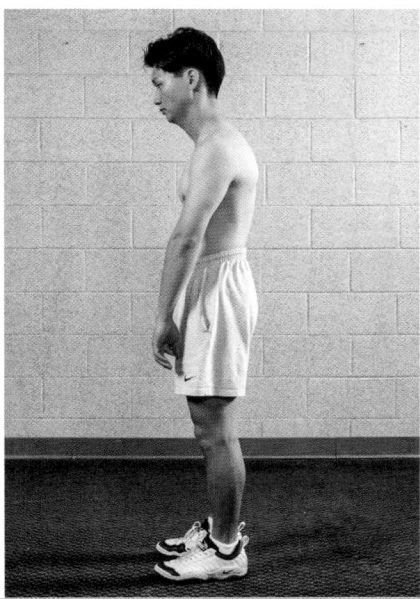

Figure 6.23 Upper-extremity posture deviation is most noticeable by the placement of the hands on the anterior thighs rather than the lateral thighs. Note the cervical and thoracic spine alignments that are producing the shoulder and arm positions.

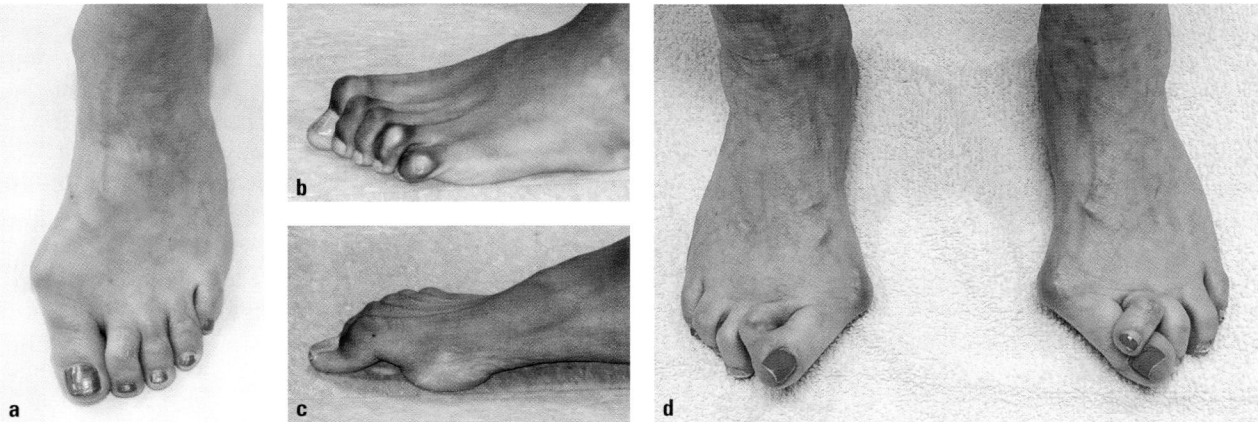

Figure 6.22 Toe deformities: *(a)* hallux valgus, *(b)* claw toes, *(c)* hammertoes, *(d)* overriding and underriding toes.
© Peggy Houglum

This malalignment can lead to glenohumeral impingement, weak over-lengthened scapular rotators, and shortened anterior shoulder girdle muscles. The secondary soft-tissue changes that result can cause inefficient use and increased stresses on the shoulder complex during upper-extremity activities, placing the person at risk for upper-extremity injuries.

Muscle Imbalances

Muscle imbalances often are both a cause and a result of poor posture. To correct a patient's posture, the clinician must first be able to identify the specific muscle imbalances and then determine whether they are the cause or the result of poor posture.

Causes

Poor posture results from an abnormal relationship between the forces that act on an area. Normal posture occurs when there is a balance of forces acting on bones and joints. Normal posture permits an efficient and effective use of the body to produce the desired motions.

When a body is in bad posture, the joints and muscles are already under stress, and any activity increases that stress. In bad posture, muscles must work harder to produce desired motions because they, too, are out of their optimal functional alignments and are not as efficient or as effective in producing those motions. This muscle alignment results in incorrect timing and movement during performance.[50] In other words, bad posture prevents optimal muscle performance. For example, a freestyle swimmer with rounded shoulders has difficulty getting enough shoulder lateral rotation and abduction on the recovery phase of the stroke, so either hand entry into the water is premature, or the swimmer has to compensate with an exaggerated body roll. The swimmer will eventually suffer a subacromial impingement injury because the scapula does not upwardly rotate and retract as it should. If this swimmer were to come to you with a rotator cuff tendinopathy and you did not correct the posture and muscle imbalances, your treatment success would be short-lived, for the injury would recur.

Sometimes pain in an area is the result of poor posture or muscle imbalances in another area. The site of pain is not always the source of the problem. For example, a gymnast who complains of back pain and demonstrates an increase in lumbar lordosis may in fact be having back pain because of hip flexor overactivity.

Commonly, the source of muscle imbalance is a loss of motion or flexibility in a muscle or muscle group and a lengthening and weakness from prolonged or sustained stretch of the opposing muscle or muscle group.[50] If a muscle actively shortens or poor posture passively positions it in a shortened state, its opposing muscle is passively lengthened and inhibited via the neurological reciprocal innervation system.[51] It is this reciprocal system that allows us to feed ourselves, walk, and perform most activities. For example, when you perform a biceps curl, the biceps shorten and the triceps relax to lengthen; or when you're prone and bend your knee, the hamstrings shorten and the quadriceps relaxes to lengthen.

There is, however, a significant difference between neurological length changes during normal activity and prolonged changes in a muscle's resting length due to abnormal posture.[52] Sustained passive or active shortening of one muscle because of poor posture causes a loss of both flexibility and strength in that shortened muscle. Likewise, the sustained passive lengthening of the opposite muscle causes a loss of strength and tone in this lengthened muscle. In chapter 13 you will learn this concept in more detail. For now, it is important to realize that a muscle performs best when it is at its optimal length; once it assumes either a lengthened or shortened position, regardless of whether its positioning is active or passive, that muscle cannot function optimally.

Additionally, changes in fascia length accompany muscle tissue length changes when the changes occur over time.[53] One can compare the results of sustained lengthening to what occurs when a weight is hung on the end of a rubber band for an extended period. When the weight is removed, the rubber band has less tone than before, and less spring. So too, a muscle that is positionally lengthened loses its tone and becomes weaker. If a patient performed only flexibility exercises to restore balance, he or she would not restore deficient muscle strength, but would only increase muscle length.

Some activities are more likely to cause postural deviations than others are. For example, participants in sports that emphasize muscle activity of anterior more than posterior body regions, such as swimming and boxing, are more likely to develop postural deviations. Unilateral activities such as racket sports encourage muscle imbalance from left to right and can cause postural deviations such as lateral spinal curvatures.[54]

As the body ages, postural deviations become more pronounced.[55] Without treatment or correction, a mild forward-head posture in a young adult becomes a moderate forward-head posture in the middle-aged adult and becomes even more severe as the person continues to age. These changes occur because as muscles naturally weaken with age, it is increasingly difficult for them to oppose their tight opposing structures, so pathological postures become even more apparent as people age—further increasing joint and muscle stresses.

Muscle imbalance can also result from joint abnormalities. These abnormalities run the spectrum from hypermobility to hypomobility.[56] When joints are hypermobile, the muscles must work harder to provide stability. This is true for both uniplanar and multiplanar joints. Joints that lack normal mobility—hypomobile joints—have less-than-normal motion and place additional stresses on both muscles and joints. Hypermobility and hypomobility can also add stresses to other body segments. For example, the person who has foot-joint hypermobility causing excessive pronation may develop patellar tendinopathy.[57] Foot pronation rotates the tibia medially to move the patellar tendon's tibial tuberosity insertion, so malalignment stresses are applied to the tendon.

Injuries can also cause muscle imbalances. Scar tissue adhesions after an injury can cause a joint to become hypomobile, especially if the joint was either injured or immobilized immediately after the injury. The deleterious effects of immobilization are discussed in chapter 12.

Another cause of imbalances is muscle strains. If the injured muscle is not properly rehabilitated or if unwanted adhesions within the muscle occur, the site can either be weaker than it was before the injury or it can lose mobility, resulting in increased stress to the site or adjacent areas.

Chapter 17 includes a more detailed discussion of muscle imbalances as they affect posture. Chapter 17 identifies the muscle imbalances that occur, the posture that results from these imbalances, and how they should be treated by the rehabilitation clinician to both resolve neck, back, and trunk problems and prevent their recurrence.

Treatment

It is important in any injury examination to assess the patient's posture and look for muscle imbalances that may either have contributed to the injury or resulted from the injury. You should also look at the entire body, not merely the injured site, because postural deviations from other locations may have contributed to the pain or injury.

Postural deviations should be corrected, not only to address the patient's current injury, but also to prevent recurrence. If a postural deviation is either the primary source of an injury or a contributing factor, you must correct it as part of the rehabilitation program if you are to prevent a recurrence of the injury.

In correcting postural deviations, the rehabilitation clinician must first identify the reason(s) why a structure is tight and its opposing structure is overstretched. He or she can then give the patient exercises to correct the muscle imbalance—that is, lengthen the short or tight structures and improve stiffness (strength) of the opposing lengthened (weak) structures. For example, if the freestyle swimmer's posture is a rounded-shoulder position, examination will show that the anterior chest muscles are tight; the downward scapular rotators are tight; and the upper-back muscles, scapular retractors, and upward scapular rotator groups are lengthened, having less tone and stiffness.

The treatment program should include lengthening exercises for the pectoralis minor, anterior deltoid, and pectoralis major, and strengthening activities for the lower trapezius, middle trapezius, rhomboids, and posterior deltoid. It should also include activities that will recruit and retrain muscles to produce the desired activity correctly. It is useful to provide reminders that will facilitate correct postural alignment—for example, a visual cue such as a colored dot on the face of the patient's watch or on a fingernail can be used to remind the patient to think about and correct his or her posture. An example of a more direct reminder is tape applied between the shoulder blades to help the patient remember to keep the shoulders in correct alignment (figure 6.24). Stretchable pre-tape provides feed-

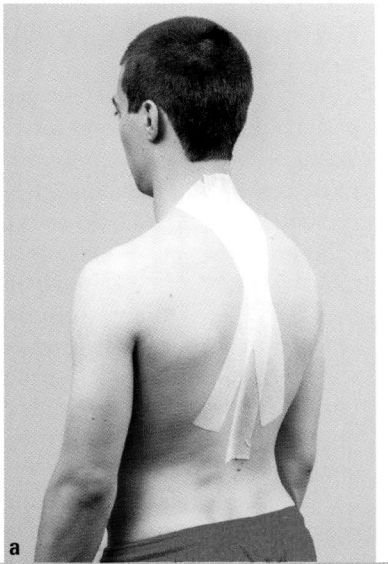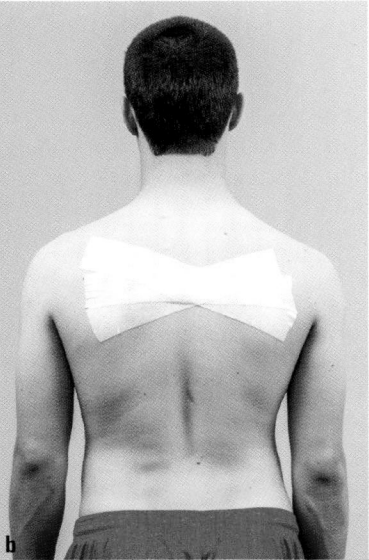

Figure 6.24 *(a)* For a tactile reminder of proper cervical posture, tape is applied to the posterior neck and thoracic back while the patient stands in proper posture. *(b)* For tactile reminders to correct rounded shoulders, the patient retracts and depresses the shoulders into proper alignment, and stretch pre-tape such as Cover-Roll (BSN Medical, Hamburg, Germany) is applied between the scapulae.

back if the patient strays from a properly aligned postural position. The tape provides the patient with feedback when he or she moves out of proper posture. The tape may be worn for 24 hours, if tolerated. The tape may be applied if the patient needs reminders to maintain a proper posture, but it should not be applied until the muscles have gained enough strength to maintain a proper position. If muscle fatigue occurs while the tape is worn, the tape should be removed.

A person who wishes to change her posture must take steps to correct it. The patient must become aware of the abnormal posture and then make a deliberate effort to change it; without this conscious effort, posture does not change. As the patient continues to improve muscle balance through corrective exercises and works to maintain a proper posture more and more often, the posture eventually improves with less conscious effort.

It is more difficult in the initial stages than it will be later for the patient to change posture, for two primary reasons. The first reason is habit. Habit, whether good or bad, is easy and comfortable and thus difficult for anyone to change. The second reason is the relationship between the lengthened and tight muscles. The tight muscles overpower the lengthened muscles, making it difficult for the patient to maintain a proper posture when attempting correction. As the muscle imbalance lessens, posture correction becomes easier.

Posture- and Muscle-Imbalance-Related Injuries

To illustrate the muscle imbalance and postural change process, let's look at a couple of examples of injuries and the relationship between improper posture and muscle imbalance.

Lower Extremity

Iliotibial band (ITB) friction syndrome often occurs in athletes, particularly in runners. The pain occurs along the ITB and is typically located along the superior-lateral aspect of the knee or toward the hip. The patient reports that the pain worsens with hill running. The examination reveals a tight ITB, and the patient stands with the leg in more medial rotation than normal. Muscle testing demonstrates weakness of the quadriceps and hip abductors and lateral hip rotators, and likely weakness of the gluteus maximus as well.[58, 59] Examination of the soft tissue along the ITB reveals tenderness in areas of soft-tissue thickness and restricted soft-tissue mobility.

Treatment includes softening the ITB-restrictive areas with deep-friction massage, along with stretching and strengthening exercises for the tight ITB. These exercises strengthen the hamstrings so the pelvis can move from an anteriorly tipped position toward a posterior pelvic tilt,[60, 61] strengthen the previously short and weak gluteus maximus, and strengthen the previously short posterior gluteus medius. As the pelvic and lumbar positions are restored, retraining the quadriceps is the final phase in the restoration of posture and muscle balance. Instructions to the patient include conscious positional correction.

Upper Extremity

A common upper-extremity problem in patients who participate in upper-extremity sports such as tennis, golf, swimming, and gymnastics is secondary subacromial impingement. This problem often appears as rotator cuff tendinopathy, and the patient complains of pain with movements such as shoulder elevation, putting the hand behind the back, and resisted shoulder activities. He or she experiences pain through the middle arc of shoulder elevation range of motion, and the impingement tests produce positive signs. The rotator cuff tendons are tender to palpation at their insertion on the greater tubercle. Examination of muscles reveals tightness of the pectoralis minor, anterior deltoid, latissimus, and pectoralis major. The rhomboids and levator scapulae may also be tight. Weakness is apparent in the lower and middle trapezii, serratus anterior, infraspinatus, and teres minor. The glenohumeral joint capsule may have areas of restriction secondary to reduced muscle mobility. The scapula may not rotate fully into an upward and retracted position because of its position on the rib cage; the result is pain and weakness of the upward rotators and tightness and weakness of the downward rotators.

Effective treatment of this condition must include correcting the faulty posture, strengthening weak muscles, and stretching and strengthening tight muscles. Optimal balance between muscle length and strength of opposing muscle groups is the goal that will lead to reduced impingement in the shoulder.

It is important to make the patient aware of the proper posture of the shoulder and cervical and thoracic spine so that he or she can work at improving posture and alignment. Exercises should include stretches for pectoralis minor, pectoralis major, and latissimus dorsi muscles. Strengthening exercises should include appropriate exercises for the serratus anterior, lower and middle trapezius, infraspinatus, and teres minor. Restoring the balance between scapular upward and downward rotators, protractors and retractors, and elevators and depressors must be part of the rehabilitation program. Because weakness and improper timing of the lengthened posterior scapular muscles is one of the sources of shoulder impingement, retraining the scapular depressors, retractors, and upward rotators to provide the appropriate movement of the scapula during glenohumeral movement is vital to reducing impingement of the rotator cuff.

A Challenging Example

Let's look at one more example so you can outline an appropriate corrective program. A basketball player comes to you with complaints of pain around the patella, especially when jumping for a rebound. He also has pain going down stairs, and in the weight room he has pain on the knee extension and squat machines. When he stands in front of you, the patellae face forward and the feet are in laterally rotated positions. In weight bearing, the longitudinal arches are low. When he performs a step-down exercise, you notice that he lacks full control of the knee and that there is a medial–lateral knee wobble as he lowers himself. Flexibility testing shows tightness of the ITB, but range of motion of the knee is normal. Strength testing indicates weakness of the quadriceps, and you can see some atrophy of the vastus medialis oblique (VMO) compared to that of the contralateral knee. There is also weakness in the gluteus maximus and gluteus medius. With the patient in long sitting, the patella sits on the anterior femur with its medial side higher than the lateral side. When he contracts the quadriceps, you observe that the patella primarily tracks laterally. What is the cause of this person's pain, and what treatment plan would you provide for him? Think for a moment before you read on to identify the source of his problem and the types of corrective exercises and the progression you would recommend to resolve this problem.

The cause of the patient's pain is a malalignment and maltracking of the patella. This malalignment, in turn, is caused by a combination of weakness of the VMO, tightness of the ITB, and malalignment of the feet. Lower-than-normal arches can either result from or lead to medial tibial rotation, which increases stresses on the patella. Weakness in his gluteal muscles causes the knee to wobble when he lowers himself from a step; this instability adds to the stress of the patellofemoral joint. The patella is not tracking normally because his pelvis is in anterior

rotation. This pelvic position places his femur in a medially rotated position, which causes gluteus muscle weakness and fatigue as it continually works to laterally rotate the femur. The effect of these stresses is weakness of the VMO and tightness of the ITB, which overpowers the weakened VMO's medial pull on the patella. There may also be an imbalance between the vastus lateralis and the VMO that would add to the lateral tracking problem. Tightness of the ITB can also be responsible for the lateral tilt of the patella.

Treatment for this patient should include stretching exercises for the hip and ITB, and repositioning the pelvis by strengthening the proximal hamstrings. Progressive strengthening exercises for the VMO, such as terminal knee-extension exercises, squats, step exercises, and lunges are added later to the rehabilitation program; these exercises should be pain free and should increase in intensity, repetitions, and number of sets as the patient's strength increases. Strengthening the gluteus maximus and gluteus medius is also necessary. For example, exercises may include resisted hip lateral rotation and hip abduction, clam exercises, and side-lying bridges. If inspection of the feet reveals excessive pronation, taping the arch and limiting rearfoot motion may be beneficial; orthotics may provide a more permanent solution.

The exercises you select should be designed to increase the flexibility and strength of the short muscles and increase the strength of the lengthened muscles so muscle balance is restored. If modalities are the only treatment technique used or if flexibility is the only type of exercise included, the rehabilitation program will provide temporary relief from pain but will not provide long-term relief of the patient's complaints or permit a full return to sport participation and normal activity.

Summary

Since poor posture can have an impact on injury and injury recovery, patient posture is evaluated as part of the rehabilitation evaluation. A postural examination can reveal any pathology that needs to be confirmed during the objective testing procedures. Posture examination includes evaluation of static posture from anterior, posterior, and lateral views, and looking for abnormalities in alignment from the head down to the toes. Pathological skeletal and joint positions and muscle imbalances, which either account for or are signs and symptoms of many postural deviations, must be corrected if a rehabilitation program is to have a lasting positive outcome.

LEARNING AIDS

Key Concepts and Review

1. Identify the primary elements of proper alignment in standing from anterior, posterior, and side views.

In an anterior position, a plumb line bisects the nose and mouth and runs through the central portion of the sternum, umbilicus, and pubic symphysis. In a symmetrical standing posture, the earlobes are level with one another, as are the shoulders, fingertip ends, nipples, iliac crests, patellae, and medial malleoli. The patellae point straight ahead, with the feet facing forward or turned slightly outward. The knees and ankles are in line with each other with the knees angled neither inward nor outward in relation to each other.

From a side view, the plumb line passes through the external auditory meatus, the earlobe, the bodies of the cervical vertebrae, the center of the shoulder joint, and the greater trochanter. The plumb line runs midway between the back and chest as well as between the back and abdomen, slightly posterior to the hip joint, and slightly anterior to the center of the knee just behind the patella. A horizontal line connects the ASIS and PSIS. The patient remains relaxed, with the body's weight balanced between the heel and the forefoot. The knees are straight but not locked. The chin is not tucked. There is a mild curve inward of the low back and neck regions, and a slight curve backward in the thoracic region.

In the posterior view, a plumb line bisects the head and follows the spinous processes from the cervical through the lumbar spine. The earlobes, shoulders, scapulae, hips, PSIS, gluteal fold, posterior knee creases, and medial malleoli each appear level left to right. The scapulae lie against the rib cage between the second and seventh ribs and about 5 cm (2 in.) from the spinous processes; each calcaneus is erect with the calcaneal tendon perpendicular to the floor. Trunk muscles appear balanced, with symmetrical development. The shoulders are positioned down and relaxed. Body weight appears equally distributed over both feet.

2. Discuss common postural faults of the spine, upper extremities, and lower extremities.

Common postural faults of the spine include lateral or anterior–posterior spinal deformities such as a slight lateral spinal curve, scoliosis, increased lumbar lordosis, flat thoracic spine, increased kyphosis, and forward head posture. Common postural faults of the upper extremities include scapular protraction, resulting in the dorsum of the hand facing forward with the palms on the anterior thighs. Common postural faults of the lower extremities include hip anteversion and retroversion; winking or frog-eye patellae; genu recurvatum; genu and ankle varus and valgus; pes cavus and pes planus; and hammertoes, claw toes, and bunions.

3. Recognize the relationship between abnormal posture and muscle imbalances.

A muscle strength imbalance or shortening of a muscle or muscle group can be caused by common postural faults. These changes usually occur over time. In poor posture, muscles must work harder to produce desired motions because they too are out of their optimal functional positions and are not as efficient or as effective in producing those motions. This faulty muscle alignment results in muscle performance with incorrect timing and strength. In other words, poor posture due to malpositioned bones and joints prevents optimal muscle performance.

4. Outline corrective exercises for common postural faults.

Once the cause of the fault has been determined, corrective exercises are used to reduce or relieve the fault. In most cases, normal spinal curves are restored by strengthening elongated muscles and stretching and strengthening short structures; instruction in corrective muscle firing is fundamental and vital to correction. The person must also make a conscious effort to correct postural faults in order to stop practicing poor habits and establish new, correct ones.

Critical Thinking Questions

1. A shoulder patient you are treating has poor upper-back and cervical posture. You feel that this is complicating the shoulder injury and that you must correct the patient's posture before you can effectively treat the shoulder. How can the thoracic and cervical posture affect the shoulder? What will you do to improve this posture? What cues and instructions will you provide the patient whenever you see him display poor posture?

2. The secretary for your department spends most of her day at the computer and on the phone. She is complaining about upper-back and neck pain and has asked you to help her. On what areas will your examination be focused? What is the probable cause for her complaints, and what can she do to alleviate the problem?

3. A patient with plantar fasciitis has some postural deviations in the lower extremities. In addition to excessively pronated feet, she also has tibial torsion and squinting patellae. What other deviations in the hips would you expect, given these abnormalities?

4. Based on the opening scenario for this chapter, what instructions would you give Dee to improve her standing posture? What instructions would you give to improve her standing posture if you noticed she had a flat thoracic kyphosis? What exercises would you give her?

Lab Activities

1. Perform a posture analysis on a lab partner. Identify all areas of malalignment or deviations from normal posture. Evaluate his or her posture from all three positions. Identify whether there are any corrective causes for these postural deviations by investigating those body segments you see as potential sources of your partner's postural deviations. What exercises would you provide to correct or reduce these deviations?

2. Take photos with your phone of your friends or family members who have postural deviations. There are several posture apps that apply a plumb bob or posture grid to your pictures. Identify which deviations each has and if the deviation is mild, moderate, or severe.

3. In a group of three or four classmates, go around campus and take pictures of as many postural deviations as you can find. After a specific time established by your instructor, report (along with the other teams) the types and numbers of postural deviations you have captured. The team that records the greatest number of types of postural deviations and correctly identifies them is the winner.

7

Gait Cycle and Ambulation Aids

Objectives

After completing this chapter, you should be able to do the following:

1. Discuss the general concepts of gait.
2. Identify the range-of-motion changes during the gait cycle.
3. Explain the lower-extremity muscle activity involved in the gait cycle.
4. Describe the general mechanical differences between walking and running.
5. Discuss one abnormal gait pattern commonly seen after a musculoskeletal injury.
6. Outline the various types of gaits that are used with assistive devices.
7. Explain the technique involved in stair climbing with assistive devices.
8. Identify the safety measures involved in ambulating with assistive devices.

When Michelle, a 38-year-old competitive soccer player, first injured her ankle, she could not walk on it. Her second-degree sprain was conservatively treated with a cast for 2 weeks and then placed in a splint for 4 weeks. By the time veteran clinician Drew Williams first examined Michelle, the splint was off the ankle and she was not using crutches, but she was still unable to walk normally. Drew analyzed her gait to evaluate for deficiencies in range of motion and strength before performing specific motion and strength tests so he could establish a rehabilitation plan. Although he would not have her run today because she was not walking normally, he knew that one day he would analyze her running gait as well.

Since Michelle was still limping severely, he instructed her in walking with one crutch. She had been using two crutches and had become tired of them, so she was resistant to using even one crutch. Drew explained that because of her current gait dysfunction, she needed some assistance, and her best options were either a cane or one crutch. Michelle didn't have access to a cane, but she understood the value of one crutch until she could walk normally without it. Drew was careful to provide her with precautions about using one crutch, and he would not allow her to use it on her own until she demonstrated proper use on the floor, carpet, and stairs.

Walking is breathing; breathing is walking.

Ron Hruska, 1955-,
clinician and founder of the
Postural Restoration Institute

Once static posture is investigated, watching how a patient moves during ambulation, from the feet all the way up to the head, can yield important information about patient pathology. You must first understand what normal gait is before you can determine if a patient is ambulating normally. Since normal gait is a goal of rehabilitation, the clinician must know which deficiencies exist before a patient's gait can be corrected. Also, before you can teach a patient to use assistive devices during ambulation, you must first understand the mechanics of those assistive devices and the desired gait with the devices.

Ambulation is a normal activity that most of us perform every day without thinking about what it involves or how we do it. We just do it. Walking is a neuromechanical event that we usually learn very early in life, and it quickly becomes an activity we easily perform automatically. When something like an injury prevents normal ambulation, walking suddenly becomes difficult and energy consuming. We no longer take it for granted, and it is no longer automatic. However, because the body is so adept at neuromechanical compensation, we quickly establish dysfunctional gait patterns when the need arises, sometimes without conscious awareness of the dysfunction. These gait dysfunctions can cause overuse syndromes secondary to additional stresses that result from the abnormal gait.

As Mr. Hruska implies in the opening quote, there is more to the act of walking than just leg activity. This chapter introduces the musculoskeletal mechanics of not only the lower limbs but also the upper body and trunk during walking and introduces differences between walking and running.

After we present details involved in understanding gait and knowing what to look for in an analysis of walking and running gait, some of the more common orthopedically based pathological gaits are discussed. The chapter concludes with instructions in ambulation with assistive devices.

It is important to know what causes a dysfunctional gait: What makes the patient ambulate like she does? A patient's gait is analyzed not only to correct a deviant gait but also to identify potential physical problems that may be associated with the patient's injury or pain. When dealing with orthopedic patients, most pathological gait occurs because of a mechanical deficiency or pain; there may be joint restriction, muscle inflexibility, or weakness of a muscle or group; any of these pathologies may cause an abnormal gait.[1] After the clinician recognizes the patient's gait deviations and includes the appropriate rehabilitation treatment to resolve these problems, changes to a normal gait occur as the issues resolve.

At the end of the chapter we examine assistive devices in gait. If the patient cannot ambulate normally, assistive devices are indicated; they should be used until the patient demonstrates normal gait. The rehabilitation clinician should instruct the patient in their proper use; therefore, the mechanics of using assistive devices, various gaits with different types of assistive devices on different surfaces, and methods of selecting assistive devices for the patient are described in this chapter. These topics form a vital part of a rehabilitation program, especially programs for lower-extremity injuries.

Normal Gait

Ambulation, or walking, is the method we use to move our bodies from one place to another. The way we walk is called *gait*. Although each person's gait is slightly different from everyone else's, all normal gaits have basic similarities. In fact, considering how many body types and sizes there are among human beings, it is surprising how little normal gait varies from one person to the next. Even so, it is interesting to note how well you can recognize your friend in the distance as he or she walks across campus, based solely on his or her gait. Major differences commonly result from postural variations, weaknesses, structural abnormalities, abnormal joint positions, and soft-tissue length alterations, some of which are discussed in chapter 6.

Knowledge of normal gait is essential to the rehabilitation clinician so that he or she can correct abnormal gait after injury and can understand how to instruct in the use of assistive devices when they are indicated. The ability to perform an accurate gait analysis is important in identifying specific pathologies that can be treated in the rehabilitation program. It is difficult to separate gait assessment from rehabilitation since the rehabilitation clinician must continually assess the patient's progress throughout rehabilitation. Gait reflects a patient's deficiencies, so the rehabilitation clinician assesses a patient's gait whenever the patient walks.[2] Just as the rehabilitation clinician assesses and corrects the incorrect performance of an exercise to achieve desired goals, he or she must also assess and correct improper gait to restore normal ambulation. Because it is so important for the rehabilitation clinician to know, understand, and recognize normal gait, we review it in detail in this chapter.

Before we begin an in-depth discussion of gait, note that it is difficult to locate a substantial body of research into the roles of the shoulder complex and thorax during the gait cycle. Some of the research on the contribution of the shoulder and thorax to the gait cycle is presented, but keep in mind that there is little information available on the upper body's function during gait.

Gait Terminology

Investigations of how people walk began 300 years ago.[3] Since then, gait terminology has continued to evolve as our knowledge has grown. One **gait cycle** is the time from the point at which the heel of one foot touches the ground to the time it touches the ground again. A gait cycle is divided into two phases, the stance phase and the swing phase. An early investigator during the mid-1900s was Vern Inman; he and colleagues observed in a publication that there was little use in dividing the gait cycle beyond these two.[4] However, this opinion was abandoned as people learned more about gait. It is easier to discuss gait details if we divide the gait cycle into subsections.

Since there are two commonly used terminology systems in use today, both are presented here. The first system we will present is referred to as clinical terminology.[5] The **stance phase** occurs when the foot is in contact with the floor and the extremity is bearing partial or total body weight. (*Stance phase* is used in both terminology systems.) The stance phase is subdivided into three parts. **Heel strike**, or **foot strike**, occurs when the heel or foot first comes into contact with the floor. **Foot flat**, as the term implies, occurs when the foot is flat on the floor. In runners and in some pathological gaits, the heel may not be the first part of the foot to strike the ground, so "foot strike" is more

appropriate than "heel strike." By the same reasoning, some believe that the term "foot flat" should be replaced with the term "reversal of fore shear to aft shear" since the foot may not achieve a flat position in some pathological gaits.[6]

The **midstance** phase occurs when the foot is directly under the body's weight and the entire plantar foot is in contact with the floor. Because the body weight transfers entirely to the one supporting leg and the other leg is in the middle of its swing phase, this is also referred to as **single-leg support** or single-limb support. **Heel-off** occurs when the weight begins to transfer to the front of the foot and the heel lifts off the floor. Partial weight remains on the extremity as the contralateral extremity is now in contact with the floor again. **Toe-off** occurs when the foot comes off the floor. From that point, the swing phase begins. The toe-off phase is also referred to as *push-off,* since the extremity now propels the body forward and the limb continues into the second phase of gait. The term *push-off,* however, is controversial. The controversy is whether the limb actually pushes off the ground or if the limb is propelled forward by momentum of the mass.[7, 8]

The second gait phase, **swing phase**, occurs when the foot is not in contact with the floor and no weight is borne on the extremity. The swing phase begins immediately after toe-off and is divided into early, mid-, and late swing phases. Immediately after toe-off, the leg begins its early swing, or **acceleration phase**, as momentum increases from the force obtained at toe-off and propels the extremity forward; only a fraction of the energy consumed during walking is used during the swing phase because of this momentum.[9] As the limb moves from midswing and into late swing, or **deceleration phase**, the limb slows its forward movement to make smooth contact with the floor to begin a new gait cycle.

An alternative terminology system also commonly used today came out of the Rancho Los Amigos Rehabilitation Center's Gait and Motion Analysis Laboratory in Los Angeles County as a result of extensive investigations on gait, both normal and pathological.[10] The person most responsible for this laboratory's gait terminology is Jacquelin Perry.[10] In this nomenclature, initial heel (foot) strike with the floor is termed **initial contact**, and as the foot progresses to increased weight bearing, it goes from initial contact to **loading response** (foot flat), then **midstance** (single-leg support). Using this terminology system, heel-off is **terminal stance**, which progresses to **preswing** (toe-off). The swing phase begins after preswing and is divided into **initial swing** (early swing, or acceleration), **midswing** (midswing), and **terminal swing** (late swing, or deceleration). Some clinicians and researchers prefer this terminology because the terms are more descriptive in discussions of gait.[11] Table 7.1 compares the two terminology systems for easy reference. Either terminology system is acceptable. Personal and regional preferences are likely the most common reasons for using one or the other.

TABLE 7.1   Comparison of Rancho Los Amigos Terminology and Clinical Terminology Identifying Subphases of Gait

Rancho Los Amigos terminology	Clinical terminology	Description
Initial contact	Heel strike	Foot first contacts the ground.
Loading response	Foot flat	The entire foot contacts the ground.
Midstance	Midstance	All body weight is borne on the limb, and the center of mass is directly over the limb.
Terminal stance	Heel-off	Center of mass moves forward of the limb.
Preswing	Toe-off	The time from when the heel moves off the ground to the point right before the foot loses contact with the ground.
Initial swing	Early swing	Beginning of the non-weight-bearing phase of stance.
Midswing	Midswing	Middle of the swing phase as the leg is perpendicular to the ground.
Terminal swing	Late swing	Last section of the non-weight-bearing phase when the limb begins to prepare for weight acceptance and contact with the ground.

If one gait cycle from the beginning of stance phase to the end of swing phase is 100%, stance phase is 62% (usually rounded off to 60%) of the gait cycle. Within stance, heel strike (initial contact) to foot flat (loading response) covers 0% to 12% of the gait cycle; single-leg support (midstance) occurs over the next 12% to 30%; heel-off (terminal stance) begins at 30% and continues to 50% of the gait cycle until toe-off (preswing), which covers the last 12% of the cycle in stance phase.[10] The swing phase then occurs through to complete the remaining percentage (38%) of the gait cycle (figure 7.1). Notice that the stance phases are not equally divided within the time frame; seg-

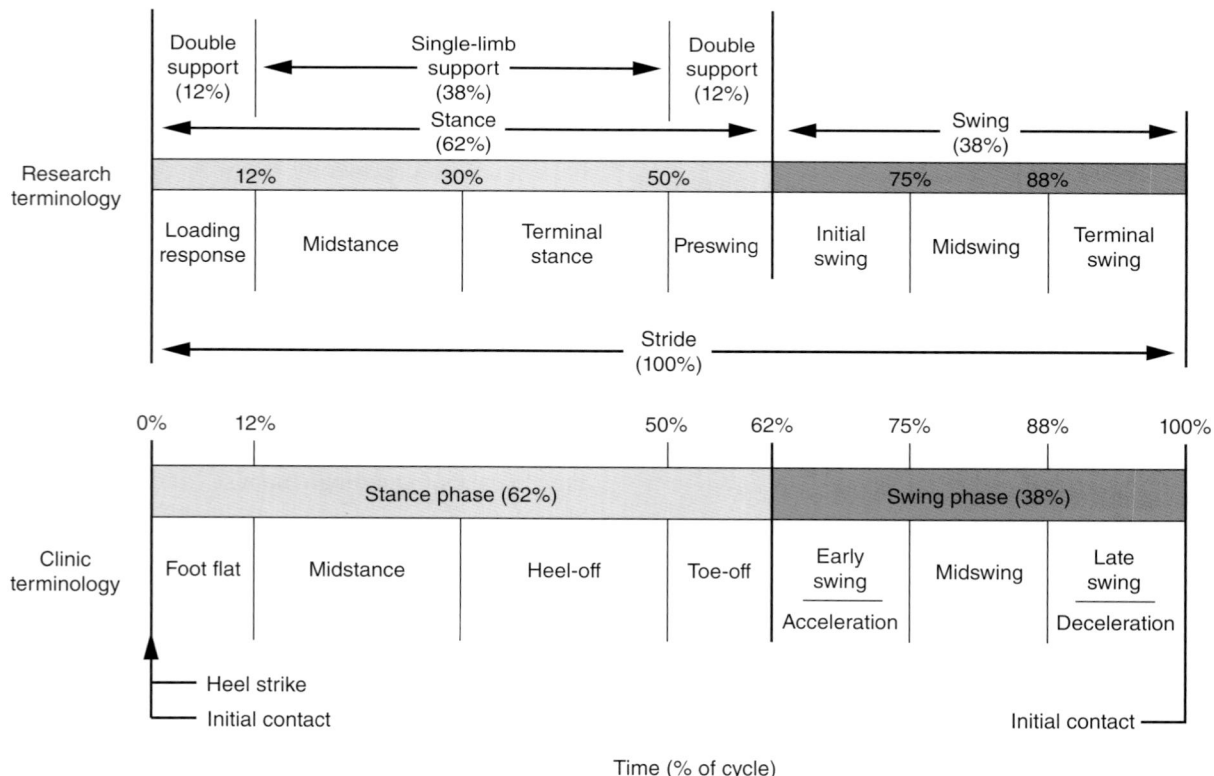

Figure 7.1   *(a)* Single-leg gait cycle and *(b)* double-leg gait cycle.

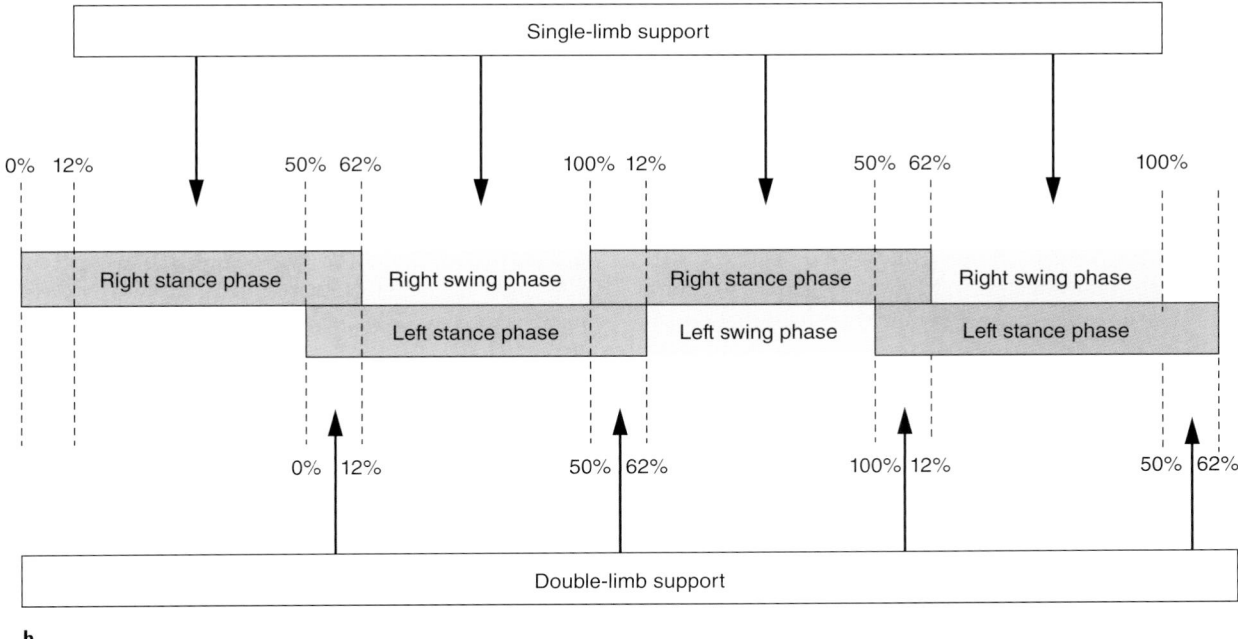

b

Figure 7.1 *>continued*

ments such as initial contact occur instantaneously, while other segments, such as midstance, last for almost 20% of the stance phase. The remaining 38% (usually rounded off to 40%) of the gait cycle is the swing phase. The swing phase segments are close to equivalent, dividing the 40% of non-weight-bearing time (swing phase) into approximate thirds.[10] As the speed of the gait increases, the percentages between the stance and swing phases become more equal. In running, the percentage becomes greater for the swing phase than for the stance phase.

As seen in figure 7.1b, during the first and last 10% of stance in a gait cycle, the body is supported by both lower extremities.[12] These segments of bilateral weight bearing occur at the beginning of the stance phase during heel strike for one limb and at the end of the stance phase, just before toe-off, for the other. This segment of the stance phase is referred to as **double-limb support**.

In addition to terminology for the phases of gait, specific terminology defines other aspects of gait. These other aspects are called spatial characteristics and temporal characteristics. Spatial characteristics include the aspects of gait that can be easily observed by looking at the path taken by the feet as the person walks, that is, the space the body uses during walking. These spatial characteristics include stride length, step length, and step width.

Stride length is the distance from the heel strike of one foot to the heel strike of the same foot in one gait cycle. **Step length** is the distance from the heel strike of one foot to the heel strike of the other foot in one gait cycle. Although stride length depends on the person's height, an average stride length is 156 cm (61 in.).[13] Usually a person's stride length is close to equal between the right and left limbs, but if the person walks fast, the dominant leg may produce greater propulsion to cause a slightly longer step length.[14]

The body's side-to-side movement as weight shifts from one lower extremity to the other is **stride width** (figure 7.2). It is the distance between the midline of one foot at

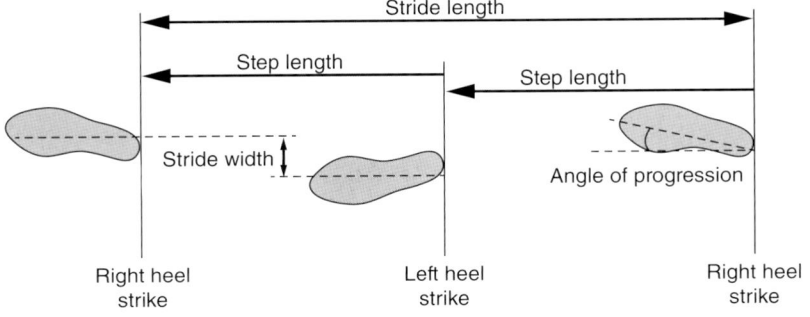

Figure 7.2 Spatial characteristics of gait.

midstance and the midline of the other foot at midstance. Stride width also has individual determining factors such as body size and weight, but the average stride width ranges from 5 cm (about 2 in.)[6] to 8 cm (about 3 in.) ± 3.5 cm.[13]

As a person walks in a straight line, the feet usually are angled slightly from this straight line. The foot is slightly rotated laterally so it does not point in the direction the person is walking. This angle is called the **angle of progression**; it is created by the angle formed between the straight line of the direction in which the person is walking and the line bisecting the foot from the heel to the middle of the forefoot, between the second and third toes.[15] Although it is greater in children, in adults this angle is about 7°.[15]

Temporal characteristics are those factors that relate to time. In gait, they include the rate, or speed, and cadence. There is wide variation in the rate at which people walk. Reports of what is normal walking speed vary. The range is from just under 60 strides per minute[13, 16] to 101 to 122 steps per minute.[17] An average walking speed for adults is about 3 mph, or about 80 m/min.[4, 10] Cadence is the rate and rhythm of gait—not only how fast a person walks but also the sound of his or her gait: Does the rate of the person's gait sound equal on the left and right? Is there a regular rhythm so the limbs sound the same as they strike the ground with the same amount of time between steps? Stance and swing phases are directly influenced as cadence increases from walking to jogging, to running, and to sprinting speeds. We consider the mechanics of running in the section Normal Running Gait later in this chapter. Irregular cadence occurs when pathology affects either the speed or the rhythm of gait. Pathological gaits are presented later in this chapter as well.

Center-of-Mass Pathway

The body's center of mass propels forward and also moves up and down and side to side in all three planes of motion during ambulation. Its relative position changes because of the associated changes in position of the joints and extremities during ambulation.

As the body advances forward in ambulation, it does so very efficiently. Short of the lower extremities being wheels instead of legs, a multijoint system is the most efficient way to propel the body forward. Although a wheel system would move the body most efficiently over flat surfaces, movement over uneven surfaces would become quite difficult. Using a number of joints from the thorax to the first ray, the body optimizes center-of-gravity pathway changes by changing the position of the joints as the body moves, and it simultaneously allows for adjustment to varying types of surfaces and terrain.

For propulsion to be smooth and efficient, the body must produce enough force to move forward but also control its triplanar movements and momentum so it remains stable over its base of support as its position changes.[18] It must

also absorb the impact shock of moving weight from one leg to the other. The loss of one of these elements can result in high stresses applied to other segments, poor quality of movement, high energy requirements, or injury.[19]

Since the body does not move on wheels, its bipedal system causes a sinusoidal motion of its center of mass, which rises and falls an average of about 4 cm (1.6 in.) through a gait cycle.[6] Moving the body's center of mass in a wavelike fashion minimizes the amount of total **excursion**, or distance the center of mass moves, which is a goal in conservative gait[20] (figure 7.3).

Determinants of Gait

The body's center of mass moves through a sinusoidal pattern in vertical and lateral directions during locomotion. This sinusoidal pattern was originally thought to be produced through what Saunders and colleagues[21] identified as six determinants of gait. Their theory stated that energy expenditure requirements during gait were minimized by minimal changes in the body's center of mass. Although more recent investigations have disproved their theory, the concepts presented in their original theory help to identify how the cooperative efforts of the trunk, pelvis, and extremities provide an efficient system of gait.[22-26] Some investigators have put forth the theory that rather than reducing the trajectory of the body's center of mass, some of the determinants absorb mechanical forces generated during heel strike and weight transfer.[27, 28] Since determinants of gait are important for identifying how body segments work together,[28] these concepts are briefly presented here.

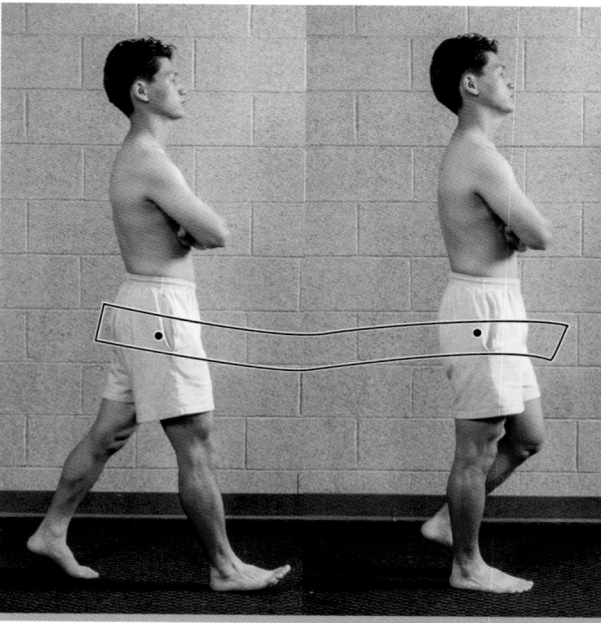

Figure 7.3 Sinusoidal motion of the body's center of mass occurs during normal walking.

Pelvic Rotation

Pelvic rotation occurs around a vertical axis in the transverse plane. As one leg swings forward, that side of the pelvis rotates forward to increase the length of the step. The pelvis attains its maximum rotation on one side, 4°, at the point of double-leg support.[21] With lengthening of the leg, the center of mass does not have to drop as far as it otherwise would (figure 7.4). As the pelvis on the side of the forward swinging leg rotates forward, the pelvis on the opposite side rotates 4° backward; this causes the posterior limb to "lengthen" as well, increasing the stride length. The total pelvic forward–backward rotation is 8°, or 4° on each side.

Pelvic Tilt

During midstance, the pelvis tilts downward on an anterior–posterior axis from the stance leg so the hip on the swing-leg side is slightly lower than on the stance-leg side (figure 7.5). The hip abductors of the stance leg eccentrically control this movement.[10] The body's center of mass is centered over the midfoot during this time, and it moves downward as the swing leg is lowered. In effect, the center of mass lowers by 5° and reduces the vertical displacement of the center of gravity by 4.77 mm (3/16 in.) during midstance.[21] Additionally, there is limited research that demonstrates some assistance comes from the weight-bearing side's lateral abdominal muscles to

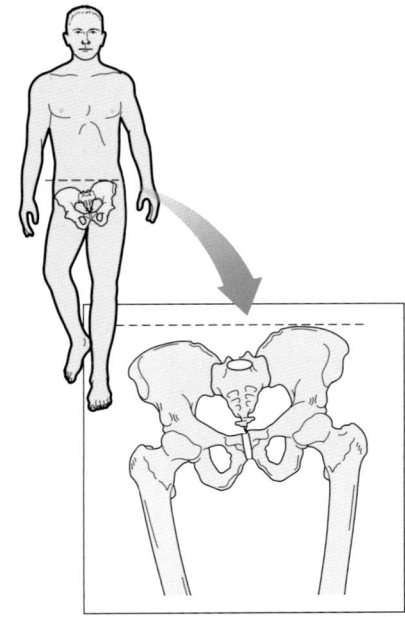

Figure 7.5 Pelvic tilt decreases vertical displacement of the center of mass.

facilitate lateral thoracic side-bending to reduce the laterally directed downward movement of the contralateral, non-weight-bearing limb during midstance.[29]

Knee Flexion at Midstance

At heel strike, the knee is in extension, but immediately afterward, it begins to flex until it flexes to 15° by midstance[30] (figure 7.6). This knee flexion lowers the center of mass when it is at its highest point of the sinusoidal motion curve.

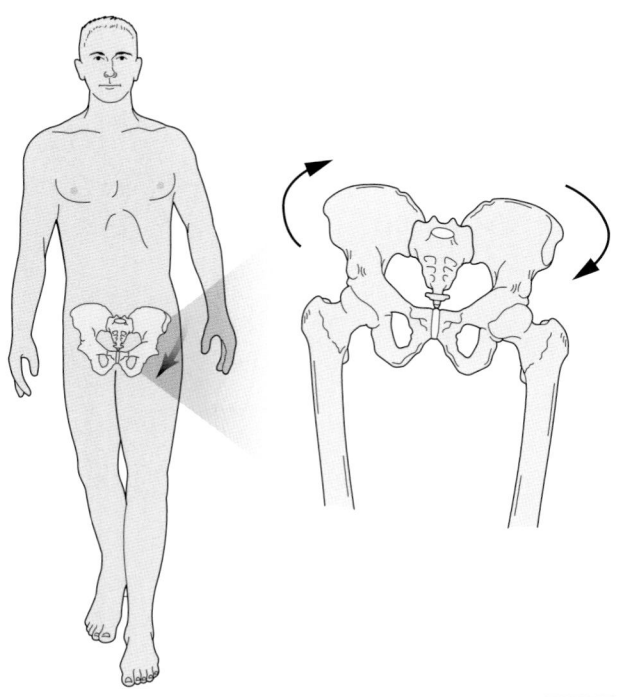

Figure 7.4 Pelvic rotation causes an increase in the length of the leg's step to lower vertical displacement of the body's center of mass and increase the stride length.

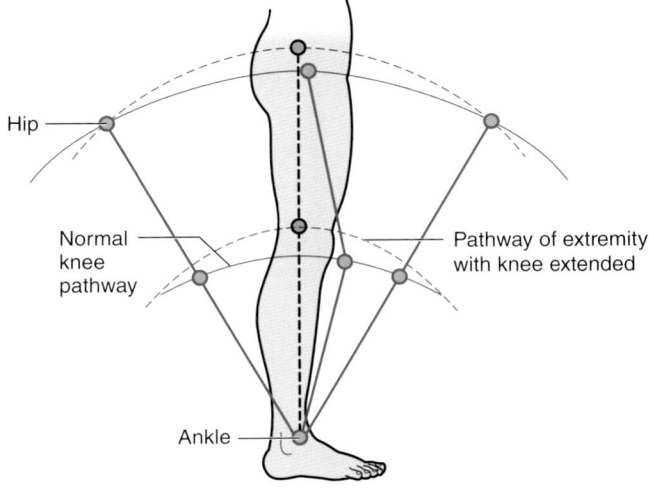

Hip

Normal knee pathway

Pathway of extremity with knee extended

Ankle

Figure 7.6 Knee flexion at midstance decreases vertical displacement of the center of mass at midstance.

Ankle Motion

The center of mass of the ankle joint is highest at heel strike and toe-off and lowest at midstance. This is the opposite of what happens with the knee joint, as seen in figure 7.7. These combined opposing elevations and depressions at the knee and ankle help reduce the vertical excursion of the center of gravity and smooth out its sinusoidal curve throughout the stance phase.

Although the theory set forth by Saunders and colleagues[21] that efficiency in gait was the result of these combined efforts was not challenged for 40 years, we now realize that although these motions occur, they are not what determine efficiency in gait.[31] Indeed, while some of the combined effects of pelvic rotation, pelvic tilt, and knee and ankle motions during stance may minimize the body's vertical displacement, other motions increase it.[31]

Lateral Motion of Pelvis

In order for a person to stand with stability, the body's center of mass must be within its base of support, the feet. When we stand on two feet, the center of mass falls between the feet. To stand on one leg, the body's center of mass must shift so that it is over the supporting leg. If the thighs were arranged in a parallel fashion, a maximum shift of 15 cm (6 in.) of the pelvis would be needed to transfer the center of mass from one supporting leg to the other during single-limb support (figure 7.8).[21] Fortunately, the

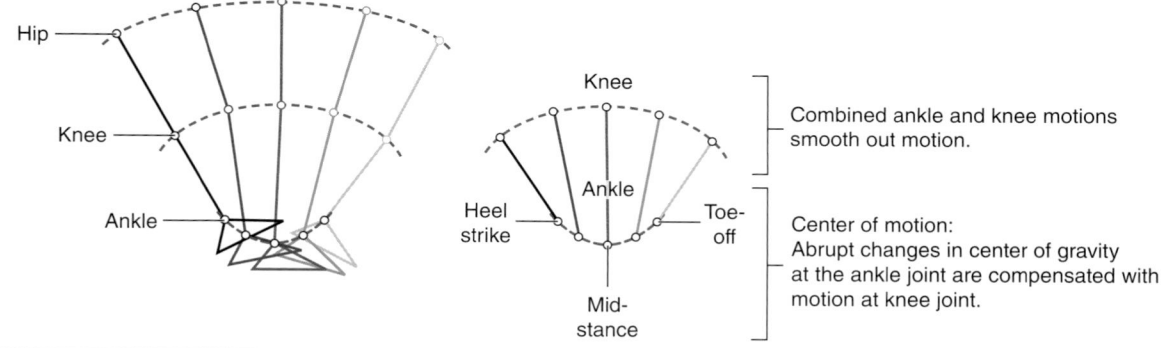

Figure 7.7   Knee and ankle motions in gait. The opposite motions occurring at the ankle and knee reduce vertical excursion of the center of gravity.

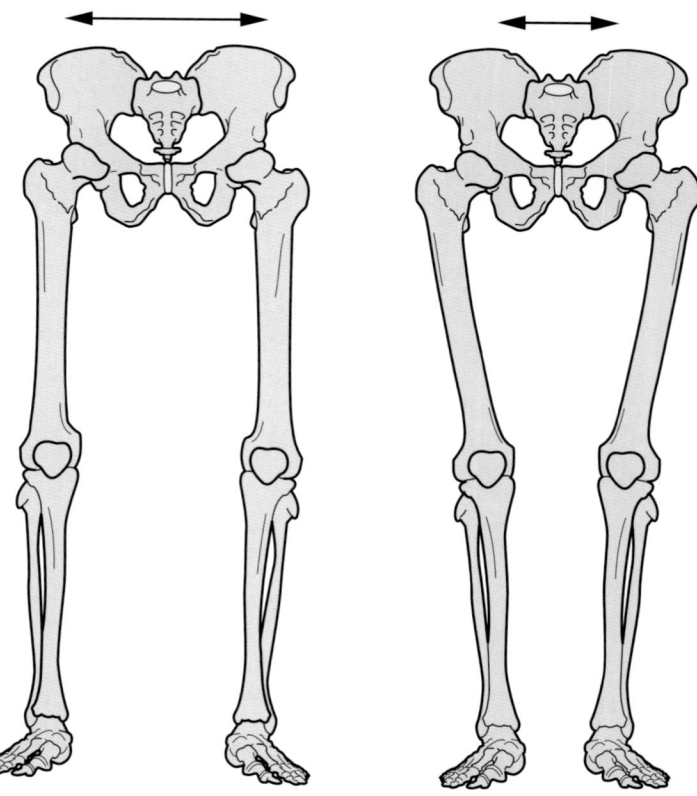

Figure 7.8   Hip and knee alignment in lateral pelvic shift. Adducted thigh alignment reduces lateral sway during gait. *(a)* If the thighs were parallel, it would require a lateral movement of 15 cm during ambulation. *(b)* Normal hip angulation minimizes lateral pelvic motion during ambulation.

a

b

femurs are not straight but are angled medially because of the femoral neck's angle of inclination, so the knees are in a slight valgus position.

The normal stride width for men is 8.1 cm[16] and for women is 7.1 cm.[32] This approximately 3 in., rather than 6 in., lateral sway is also a sinusoidal curve but in a lateral direction, making for smooth movement as the body shifts weight from one leg to the other during ambulation.

The body during gait has often been compared to an inverted pendulum.[31] As seen in figure 7.9, while the pubis may shift laterally only a few inches during the body's lateral sway, the sternum's lateral shift is often greater than 7.6 cm (3 in.).

The maximal position of the left-to-right center of mass curve occurs during midstance of each lower extremity and moves to the body's midline during double-limb support. The maximal height of the sinusoidal curve in vertical displacement also occurs during midstance of each leg and is at its lowest point during double-limb support.

Gait Kinematics

The sinusoidal curves of motion that occur during ambulation are caused by changes in the joints' ranges of motion. Some of these changes are not large but are important for smooth motion. Movement during walking occurs in the sagittal, frontal, and transverse planes within each segment. If movement in one plane is restricted in even one segment, smooth gait will not occur. When normal gait does not occur because of restricted motion or muscle weakness, normal efficiency in walking is lost; energy requirements increase because other segments must work more to compensate for the impaired segments.[23, 37-39] Therefore, the rehabilitation clinician must understand the sequence, degree, and timing of joint motion so that when deficiencies exist, he or she can correct them.

When we think of gait, we most often think in terms of movement occurring in the sagittal plane. This is probably because not only does most motion occur in this plane, but

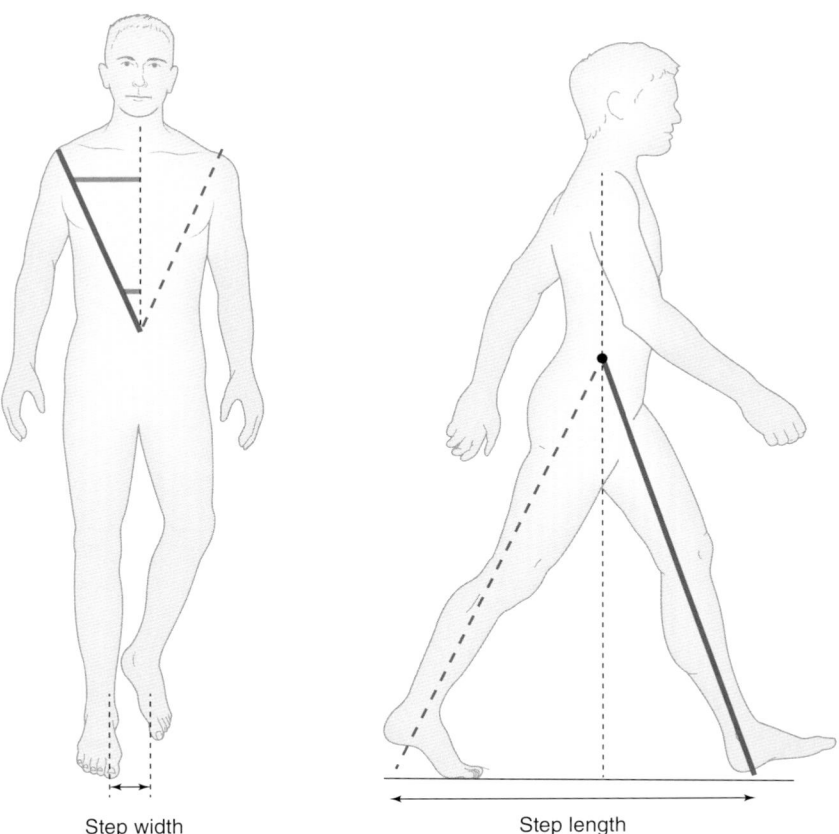

Step width   Step length

Figure 7.9 The human body is often referred to as an inverted pendulum in both the frontal and sagittal planes during ambulation. Such an arrangement causes the more distal segments from the source of the pendulum to have more sway as weight is transferred from left to right and from front to back.

it is most easily observed in this plane. However, we must remember that motion occurs in the frontal and transverse planes as well. As we discuss each of the body segments and their motions, we will include information about all three planes of motion to the degree that it is known. In recent years, transverse plane motion during gait has been identified and quantified because of improved instrumentation in gait laboratories. As techniques and equipment improve, we will learn more about all three planes of motion.

Trunk and Upper Extremities

Throughout all cycles of normal gait, the shoulders, thoracic spine, and rib cage play a role in gait[40, 41] and likely help to keep the body's center of mass within its base of support. Trunk motion coordinates with pelvic motion throughout the gait cycle; as the pelvis rotates in one direction, the trunk rotates in the opposite direction (figure 7.10). In fact, if normal trunk and arm motions do not occur during the gait cycle, pelvis and lower-extremity movements are hindered.[42] Normal arm swing momentum assists the trunk in its rotation; trunk motion is less than arm motion.[42] This coordinated reciprocating movement between the pelvis, trunk, and upper extremities helps make the gait smooth and stable.[43, 44]

Upper Trunk Rotation During the gait cycle, the upper trunk moves to assist other body segments. The descriptions provided here only discuss one side of the body, but the opposite side of the body is performing opposite motions as reciprocating movements. The use of "left" and "right" is for clarity. Figure 7.11 is based on data provided by Romkes and Bracht-Schweizer[45] and provides a visual image of shoulder and thoracic spine motion during ambulation.

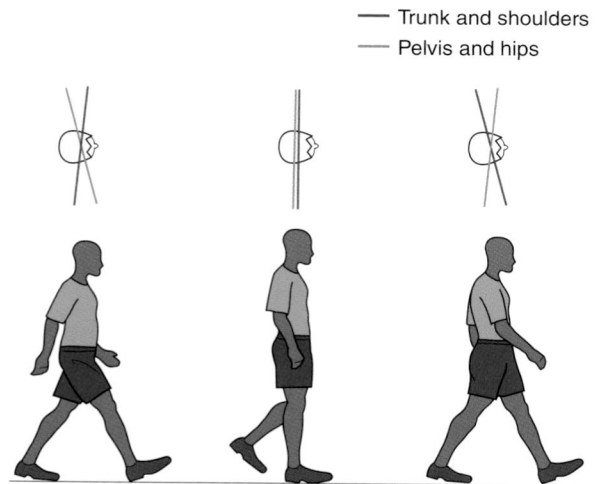

Figure 7.10 Trunk and pelvic rotation using the right lower extremity and right pelvis as the reference extremity.

Adapted from Murray, Drought, and Kory (1964).[16]

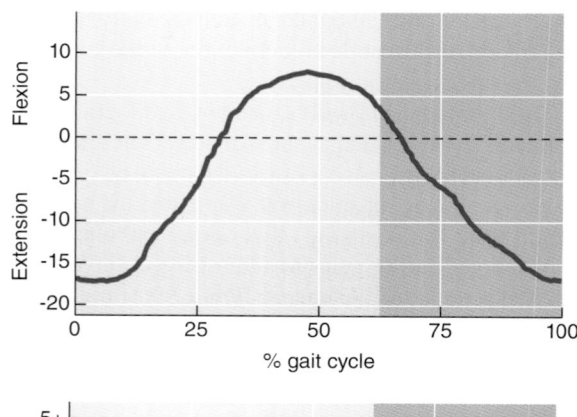

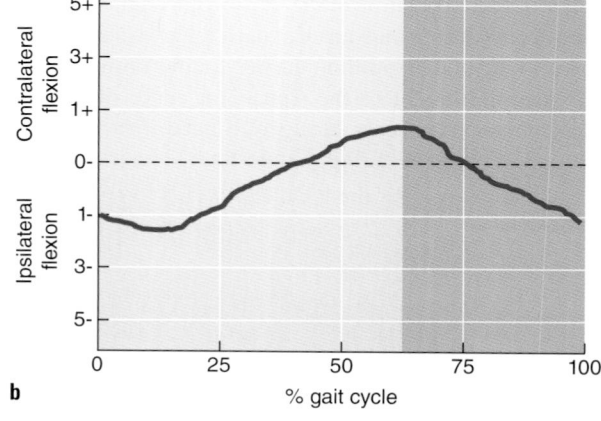

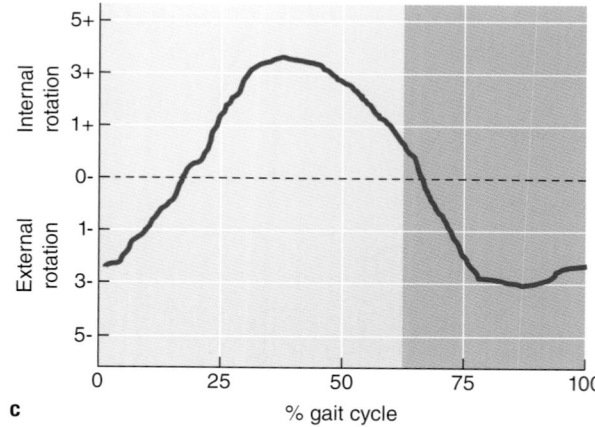

Figure 7.11 Shoulder and thorax range of motion throughout the gait cycle at a subject-determined comfortable speed. *(a)* Shoulder ROM; *(b)* lateral flexion ROM of the thoracic spine; *(c)* rotation ROM of the thoracic spine.

Based on Romkes and Bracht-Schweizer (2017).[45]

• *Heel Strike to Midstance.* The upper trunk begins its work as the body's weight shifts and load acceptance occurs during heel strike and midstance.[29] At right heel strike, the right thorax moves into a position of right trunk rotation and lateral flexion.[45]

Evidence in Rehabilitation

Although the determinants of gait (pelvic rotation, pelvic tilt, midstance knee flexion, ankle motion, foot and knee mechanisms, and hip adduction) are no longer considered methods by which the body improves gait efficiency, as was originally put forth by Saunders and colleagues,[21] they are important for other reasons. When combined, they promote a smooth, flowing movement of the body's center of mass during walking. Using three-dimensional analysis technology that was not available to Saunders and his group when he investigated the determinants of gait, more recent investigators analyzed center-of-mass motion and these determinants and found (1) hip flexion and midstance knee flexion with ankle motion are major contributors to sagittal plane motion, (2) hip adduction and pelvic tilt contribute the most to changes in the frontal plane, and (3) pelvic rotation and pelvic tilt are most responsible for transverse plane movement.[33-35] Other investigators indicate that determinants of gait play a role in absorbing forces during heel strike and weight transfer.[27, 28] It is apparent that we have yet to identify the full role these factors play in gait.[21, 36]

• *Midstance to Toe-Off.* Once the body reaches the middle of right midstance, the upper trunk moves toward left rotation and right lateral flexion. This reversal of direction in the thorax is in preparation for heel strike on the left side.

• *Early Swing.* As the right side begins swing phase, the upper trunk is in left rotation and left lateral flexion. This position promotes a shift of the center of mass to the left side.

• *Late Swing.* Over the course of swing phase on the right side, the trunk will rotate and laterally flex to the right in preparation for heel strike on the right side. This frontal plane and transverse plane motion of the thorax during swing phase helps prepare the body to accept the center of mass onto the right side during the upcoming heel strike.[43]

Scapular and Humeral Motion While humeral motion is linked to thoracic and scapular movement, research indicates that humeral motion has both active and passive contributions during gait.[46-48] Research has shown humeral motion in gait to be mostly passive,[48] and other research has shown that while most of the arm swing is passive, the active portion of arm swing appears to be eccentric deltoid activity.[46] Arm swing helps us maintain our balance[48] and reduces energy expenditure[49-52] during walking. Shoulder and elbow motion have been shown to vary depending on the person's age[53] and walking speed.[45]

• *Heel Strike to Midstance.* At right heel strike, the right scapula is in a position of retraction and begins to move toward protraction and scapular depression.[29, 45, 54, 55] During right midstance, the right scapula will appear to be lower in the frontal plane than the left scapula due to right trunk lateral flexion in this phase. At the same time, the right humerus is at its end-extension position behind the body's midline in 17° of extension and begins its forward motion to its position of near-neutral sagittal plane alignment by midstance.[45] Humeral motion occurs as a result of the momentum the shoulder receives from the movements of the legs, pelvis, and trunk.[46, 48]

• *Midstance to Toe-Off.* As the body moves from right midstance and prepares to transfer its weight to the left lower extremity, the right scapula completes its movement into protraction and elevation. At toe-off, the right scapula appears elevated in the frontal plane when compared to the left scapulae due to left lateral flexion of the trunk in this phase. The right humerus also completes its forward motion into 9° of shoulder flexion[45] to complement the aforementioned right scapular protraction and left trunk rotation.

• *Early Swing.* At the beginning of swing phase, the right scapula is moving toward retraction as the right humerus moves toward shoulder extension. At this point of the gait cycle, the right humerus is in 5° of shoulder flexion and moving toward more shoulder extension.[45] This motion coincides with left trunk rotation. In this phase, the right scapula appears higher in the frontal plane than the left scapula due to left thoracic flexion.

• *Late Swing.* During this phase, the body is preparing for right heel strike. The right scapula continues to move toward retraction as the right humerus moves into 17° of shoulder extension, coinciding with right trunk rotation. In this phase, the right scapula appears lower in the frontal plane than the left scapula due to right trunk lateral flexion.

Pelvis

Pelvic motion is most easily discussed using iliac crest movement as the reference. Overall, there is little iliac crest motion throughout gait, primarily because the pelvis provides a stable base upon which the head, arms, and trunk move and is the structure through which they transfer their contributions to ambulation. Although pelvis movement is defined and measured in terms of iliac crest motion, your clinical visual assessment will use the ASIS (anterior superior iliac spine) and PSIS (posterior superior iliac spine) to identify dysfunctional gait patterns. Forward rotation of the iliac crest produces an anterior pelvic tilt, and backward rotation produces a posterior pelvic tilt. Pelvic motion in the frontal, sagittal, and transverse planes is graphed in figure 7.12.

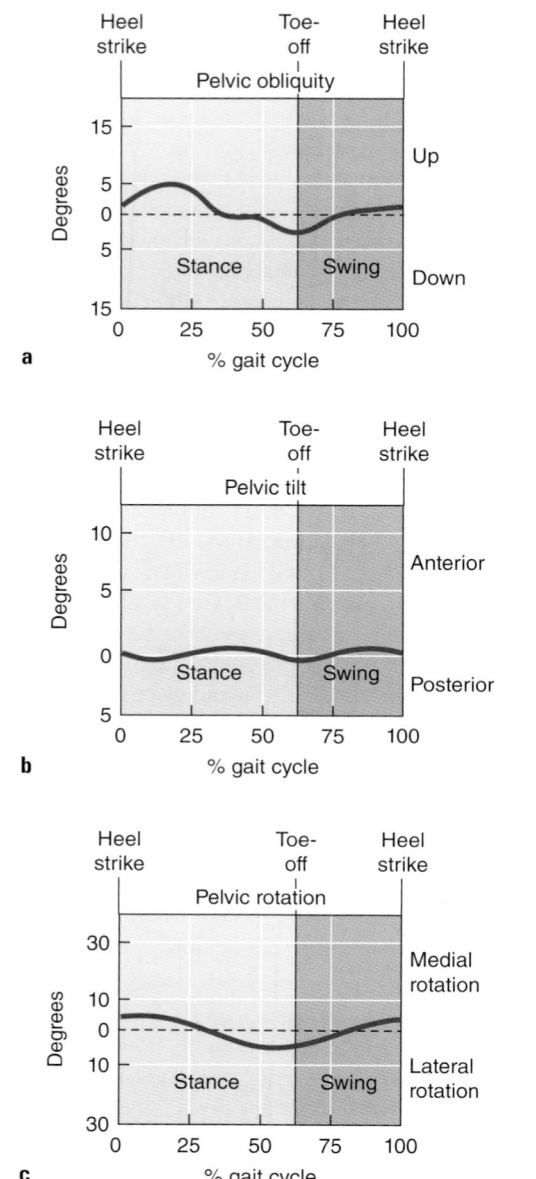

Figure 7.12   Pelvic motion is a triplanar event. Pelvic motion in (a) frontal plane, (b) sagittal plane, (c) transverse plane.

Pelvic motion is necessary during normal gait; however, it is often difficult to precisely identify clinically. Researchers find great differences in their ranges of pelvic motion during ambulation.[56] As with discrepancies found in comparisons of other research on human activity, these differences are not unusual because there is great variation in the selection of subject pools, measurement techniques, walking speeds, and analytical systems. Also, the amount of pelvic motion that occurs during gait is affected by several factors, such as walking speed, sex, and age.[37] The main point to keep in mind as we discuss the measurements on pelvic motion during gait is that motion must occur

in the pelvis,[57] and if motion in any plane is restricted, it affects not only the other motions of the pelvis, but other joint motions in the kinetic chain as well.[58, 59]

Reports of the total motions of the pelvis during a gait cycle vary from one investigator to another. Based on the works of MacWilliams and colleagues,[60] Thurston and Harris,[61] Murray and colleagues,[16] Romkes and Bracht-Schweitzer,[45] and others,[10, 56, 62, 63] total pelvic motion during gait may exist in the ranges these investigators have identified: approximately 4° to 7° of anterior–posterior tilt in the sagittal plane, 7° to 10° of lateral tilt in the frontal plane, and 8° to 15° of rotation in the transverse plane. Much of the pelvic motion coincides with hip motion to optimize that joint's movement. The pelvis is important for upper-body stabilization, especially during single-limb stance, and for transmitting forces from these upper-body segments to the lower extremities, adding to the optimization of walking.[10]

Heel Strike to Midstance   As the heel hits the ground at heel strike, the pelvis remains level and is rotated 5° forward in the sagittal plane (anterior tilt);[4] as the body progresses toward midstance, the pelvis reduces its anterior tilt.[56] In the frontal plane, it is elevated 4° on the stance limb at heel strike and begins to drop after initial contact has been made.[10] As the limb goes from heel strike to midstance, the ipsilateral pelvis medially rotates 4°.[10]

Midstance to Toe-Off   By the time the limb reaches the end-of-stance phase, the stance-side pelvis has moved into a posterior rotation position (posterior tilt) of about 5° in the sagittal plane. In the frontal plane during midstance to toe-off, the pelvis continues to drop until it reaches a total of 8° of lateral movement.[16] During the final moments of stance phase, the ipsilateral pelvis rotates laterally, from the initial position of medial rotation to an ending position of lateral rotation, all in the transverse plane.

Early Swing   In early swing, the pelvis is level and in 5° of posterior rotation, moving toward anterior rotation in the sagittal plane. In the frontal plane, it begins to move from a downward position toward the maximally elevated position it will achieve in late swing. Rotation in the transverse plane is gradual but rhythmic, moving from lateral rotation to medial rotation by late swing.

Late Swing   The pelvis continues its smooth sequence of minimal but vital motion throughout the gait cycle, moving in the sagittal plane from an anterior position at the middle of swing to a posterior position by the end of late swing. Frontal plane movement continues from its maximum downward position during early swing on its way toward an elevated position so that it is slightly elevated by the end of swing. Transverse plane rotation also continues to progress in a medial direction as swing phase is terminated.

Hip

Hip motion also occurs in three planes of movement: frontal, sagittal, and transverse (figure 7.13).

Heel Strike to Midstance At heel strike, the hip is in 25° to 30° of flexion, slight adduction of 2° to 6°, and near-neutral rotation at 5°.[64] As the leg progresses through the stance phase, the hip becomes less flexed and adducted and goes from slight medial rotation to slight lateral rotation by the time the limb is in terminal stance.

Midstance to Toe-Off In the last half of the stance phase, the hip goes from 10° of extension at heel-off to about 5° to 0° extension at toe-off. The hip is at neutral in the frontal plane at heel-off and moves into 4° of abduction at toe-off.[64] After midstance, the hip moves in the transverse plane from medial rotation to neutral at heel-off until it

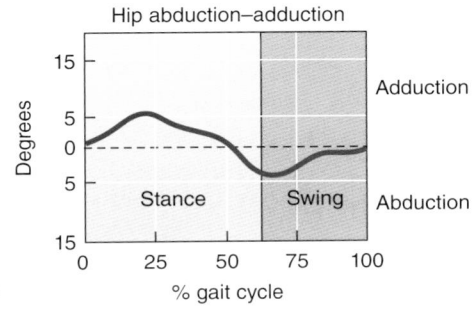

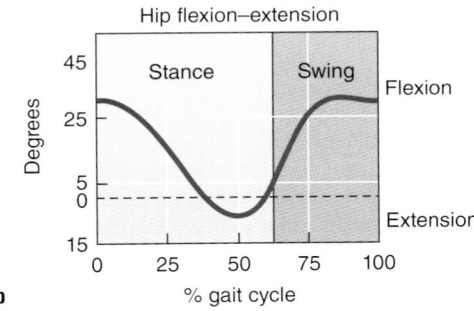

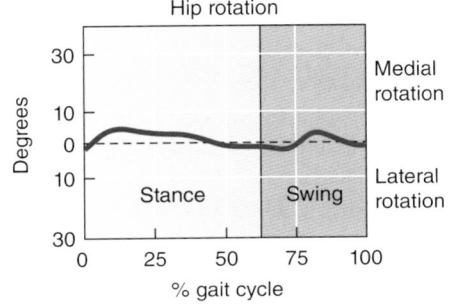

Figure 7.13 Hip motion is triplanar, with the greatest movement occurring in the sagittal plane and the least occurring in the transverse plane. Hip motion in the *(a)* frontal plane, *(b)* sagittal plane, *(c)* transverse plane.

reaches 4° of lateral rotation at toe-off. Part of the apparent hip extension that occurs from midstance to toe-off is the result of a posterior pelvic tilt in the sagittal plane.

Early Swing In its initial swing, the hip continues to flex to 15° to 20° in the sagittal plane, reaches its maximum abduction of an average of 5° in the frontal plane, and continues to have slight lateral rotation in the transverse plane.[33, 65, 66]

Late Swing Sagittal plane movement continues to advance to about 30° just before the end of swing. Frontal plane movement continues to advance from maximal abduction just after the start of early swing toward the midline until a neutral position occurs just before heel strike. Transverse plane movement oscillates throughout swing from medial to neutral to lateral rotation and then back to slight medial rotation just before heel strike.

Total hip motions occurring during the gait cycle include about 40° in the sagittal plane from flexion to extension,[64] 13° of abduction–adduction in the frontal plane, and 8° of rotation in the transverse plane.[10]

Knee

The knee undergoes its greatest amount of motion during the swing phase of the gait cycle. Transverse plane rotation of the knee occurs throughout the gait cycle. Knee rotation is most likely affected by a combination of tibial rotation and hip rotation occurring synchronously.

Heel Strike to Midstance At heel strike, the knee is at or close to full extension in the sagittal plane.[67] The tibia is laterally rotated about 3° in the transverse plane at heel strike. As weight acceptance on the leg increases, the knee flexes from about 12°[68] to 20°.[67] As weight bearing progresses toward midstance, tibial rotation advances medially into midstance (figure 7.14).

Midstance to Toe-Off By the time the extremity reaches midstance, the knee has achieved its maximum stance-phase flexion (about 20°)[10] and now begins to move into full extension at heel-off.[68] After maximal tibial medial rotation occurs just before midstance, a return to lateral rotation occurs during the latter half of stance until maximal lateral rotation occurs immediately before toe-off.[68] Immediately before toe-off, the knee is passively flexed to about 30° by the active movement of the ankle as it goes into plantar flexion, forcing the weight-bearing knee to flex.[69]

Early Swing The knee continues to progress to a maximum of 60° of flexion; this occurs so that the foot clears the ground during the swing phase.[10] In the body's attempt to conserve energy, foot clearance from the ground during swing is a mere 0.87 cm (0.3 in.).[70] That small clearance leaves little room for error. It is no wonder that fatigue or limited knee flexion will increase the likelihood of

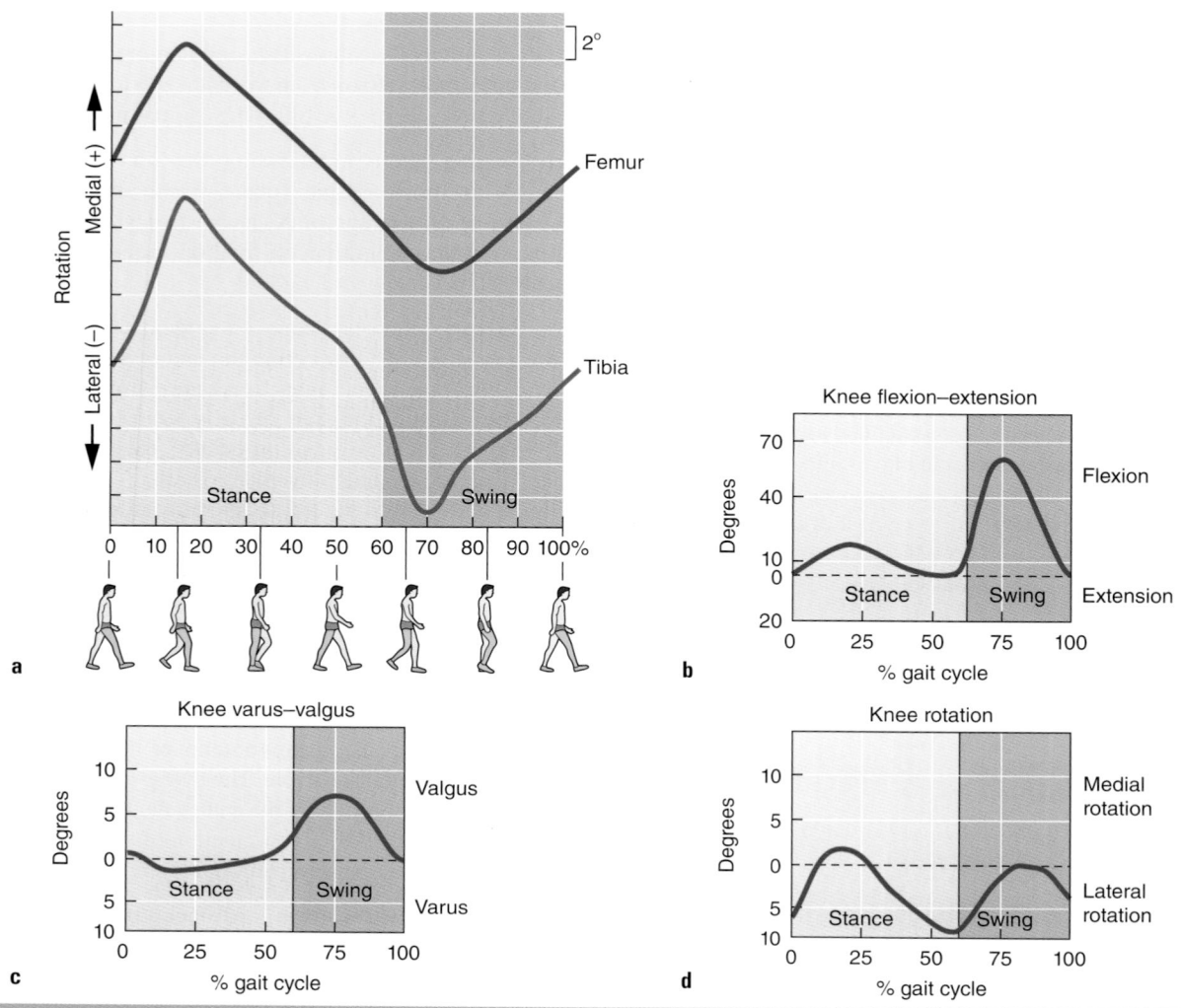

Figure 7.14 Limb rotation and knee motion. *(a)* Maximum medial rotation of femur and hip occur prior to midstance, and maximum lateral rotation occurs at the end of stance and into early swing phase. *(b)* In the sagittal plane, maximum knee extension occurs after midstance, whereas maximum knee flexion occurs in swing phase. *(c)* In the frontal plane, maximum adduction of the knee occurs in the first half of stance, while maximum abduction occurs during midswing. *(d)* In the transverse plane, medial and lateral rotation motions of the knee oscillate throughout the gait cycle, with medial rotation mainly during the first half of stance and movement in that direction occurring during the first half of swing.

stubbing the toe when the foot is moving off the ground. The tibia begins moving from its most laterally rotated position during toe-off toward medial rotation without ever achieving a position in medial rotation; the knee continues to maintain some degree of lateral rotation throughout most of the swing.

Late Swing   After achieving around 60° of flexion in the first half of swing, the knee moves progressively and steadily toward extension during late swing. This progression toward extension continues throughout this phase until it reaches nearly 0° just before heel strike.

Total knee range of motion throughout the gait cycle in the sagittal plane is around 60°, and tibial rotation in the transverse plane is 18°. Maximum knee flexion during the stance phase occurs during midstance, and maximum knee flexion during the swing phase occurs during midswing. Maximum knee medial rotation occurs between heel

strike and midstance in what researchers call the loading response, while maximum lateral rotation occurs at toe-off.

Ankle

The ankle and foot work together during gait and provide balance that is needed as the body moves over uneven ground.[71] The ankle joint is responsible for forward motion and stability, and the foot joints are responsible for medial and lateral adjustments. The foot and ankle work together as a complex, coordinated structure and demonstrate highly variable adaptability and function. As with other measurements throughout this chapter, the values given are averages.

Heel Strike to Midstance   At heel strike, the ankle and toes are in neutral (figure 7.15). The ankle moves into 15° of plantar flexion before midstance as more weight is borne by the extremity.[10] As the body absorbs the forces moving

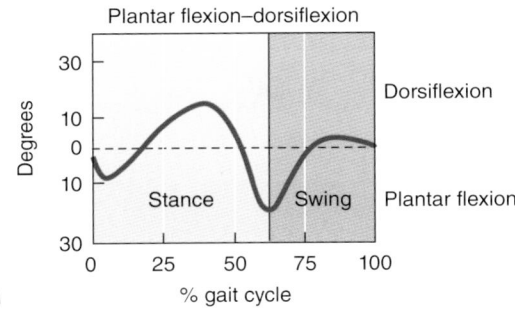

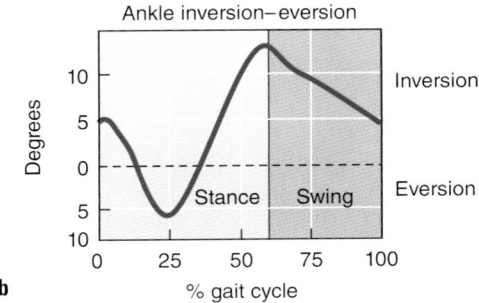

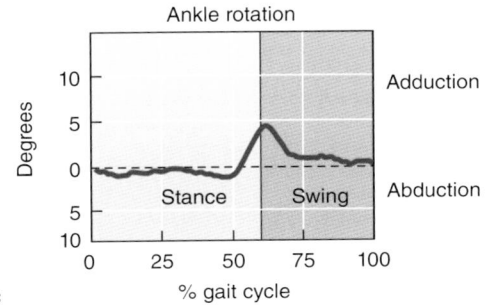

Figure 7.15 Ankle motions during walking. *(a)* Motion in the sagittal plane, *(b)* motion in the frontal plane, and *(c)* motion in the transverse plane.

from heel strike to foot flat, the foot plantar flexes another 5° to 6° and rolls medially.[72] The subtalar joint moves into pronation to accept the impact forces of weight bearing. The toes remain in a neutral position through midstance.

As the limb moves into midstance, the tibia moves from 5° of plantar flexion into 5° of dorsiflexion. This transition from plantar flexion to dorsiflexion permits a smooth glide of the limb as the body moves over its base of support.[10] Immediately after heel strike, the calcaneus everts in the frontal plane to cause subtalar pronation during foot flat. This pronation permits the midtarsal area to remain flexible and adapt to varying terrains. Pronation also allows the foot to act as a shock absorber, reducing the impact stresses that occur at heel strike. The subtalar joint remains in pronation briefly until just before midstance, when it begins to supinate. The longitudinal arch passively lengthens from heel strike until it reaches its maximum length at midstance.[73] At heel strike, the foot makes contact with the ground on

the heel's posterior aspect, slightly lateral to the midline. As the body moves forward and more weight is borne on the single limb, the weight is transmitted from the heel to the midtarsal foot.

Midstance to Toe-Off Following midstance, the ankle moves quickly through 25° of motion from 10° of dorsiflexion to about 15° of plantar flexion by the time of toe-off.[10] The calcaneus inverts in the frontal plane and causes the subtalar joint to move into supination so the foot becomes stable for propulsion at toe-off. The longitudinal arch begins to shorten, and the metatarsophalangeal joints extend to 30° after midstance until reaching maximum hyperextension of about 60° at toe-off.[74] Throughout the swing phase, the metatarsophalangeal joints maintain about 30° of hyperextension to clear the toes from the floor.[75] The interphalangeal joints remain in neutral throughout the stance and swing phases of gait. As stance progresses, the body's weight advances forward on the foot (figure 7.16). At midstance, it is located just behind the metatarsal heads, and at toe-off the weight is primarily over the first and second metatarsophalangeal joints.

Early Swing Once toe-off occurs, the ankle immediately begins movement toward dorsiflexion until it reaches a neutral position. By midswing, the ankle and toes are in a neutral position.

Late Swing The ankle and toes remain close to neutral throughout the remaining part of the swing phase. The subtalar joint also remains close to neutral through the swing phase until late swing, when it starts to move into slight inversion in preparation for ground contact.

Total movement from plantar flexion to dorsiflexion in the sagittal plane is 30°, with both extremes of plantar flexion and dorsiflexion occurring during the stance phase. The extremes of subtalar motion occur with about 5° of eversion during foot flat to somewhere between 8° and 11° of inversion at toe-off.[76, 77] A great deal of motion

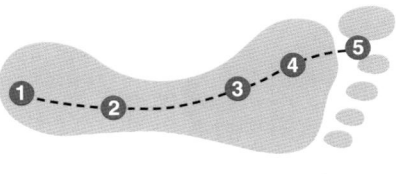

1 = Initial contact (heel strike)
2 = Loading response (foot flat)
3 = Midstance
4 = Terminal stance (heel-off)
5 = Preswing (toe-off)

Figure 7.16 Weight transmission during walking. Initial contact at heel strike occurs in the posterior-lateral heel and advances forward on the foot through the stance phase. At midstance, the body's weight is just behind the metatarsal heads, and at toe-off the weight is primarily over the first and second metatarsal heads.

in the lower extremities occurs during one stride. Figure 7.17 presents a summary of the joints' motions during ambulation. Table 7.2 presents a summary of the amount of motion required in each joint for normal walking; this is important information for rehabilitation clinicians to know since patients often ask when they can start walking without assistive devices. As long as motion is lacking for normal walking, assistive devices will be needed.

Normal Gait

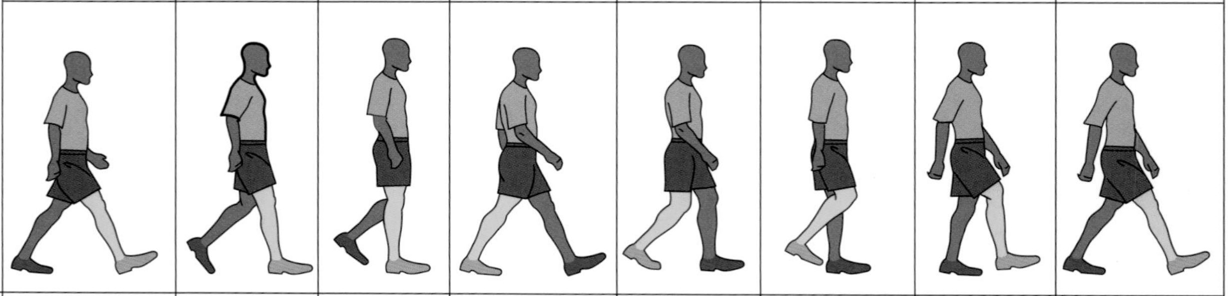

	Stance 60%					Swing 40%		
	Heel strike (initial contact)	Foot flat (loading response)	Midstance	Heel-off (terminal stance)	Toe-off (preswing)	Early swing (initial)	Midswing	Late swing (terminal)
Trunk	Erect Neutral	Erect Neutral	Erect Neutral	Erect Neutral	Erect Neutral	Erect Neutral	Erect Neutral	Erect Neutral
Pelvis	Level in sagittal plane 4° posterior tilt 10° forward rotation in transverse plane Frontal plane downward rotation	Sagittal plane level 5° forward rotation in transverse plane Frontal plane upward rotation	Sagittal plane level Opposite pelvis tilts down 8° in frontal plane Neutral in transverse plane	Sagittal plane level with slight anterior tilt Frontal plane moving to neutral Transverse plane in 5° backward rotation	Sagittal plane level Backward rotation in transverse plane Frontal plane downward rotation	Sagittal plane level Transverse plane in posterior rotation moving forward Frontal plane moving downward	Sagittal plane level Transverse plane moving anterior Frontal plane moving downward	Sagittal plane level 5° forward rotation in transverse plane Frontal plane upward rotation
Hip	30° flexion 10° adduction Near-neutral rotation	30° flexion Slightly more adduction Slight rotation	Extends 15° adduction Slight medial rotation	10° hyper-extension Slight abduction	5° neutral extension Slight medial rotation 4° abduction	20° flexion Slight lateral rotation 5° abduction	Flexing Lateral rotation	30° flexion Mild lateral rotation going to medial rotation
Knee	0° to 5° extension Tibia in lateral rotation Slight abduction	15° to 20° flexion Tibia in medial rotation 3° abduction	Moves toward extension	Full extension	35° flexion	Continue to 60° flexion Tibial lateral rotation	Begin to move to 30° flexion Tibial lateral rotation 8° adduction	Continue to extend
Ankle	Neutral	15° plantar flexion Pronation	10° dorsi-flexion Starts to supinate	Moving into plantar flexion Supination	20° plantar flexion	Moving to neutral	Neutral	Neutral
Toes	Neutral	Neutral	Neutral	MTP: 30° extension IP: Neutral	MTP: 60° extension IP: Neutral	Neutral	Neutral	Neutral

Figure 7.17 Summary of kinetics and kinematics for the hip, knee, and ankle in the sagittal plane through the gait cycle. Walking consists of a continuous flowing change in joint ranges of motion throughout the gait cycle.

Hip

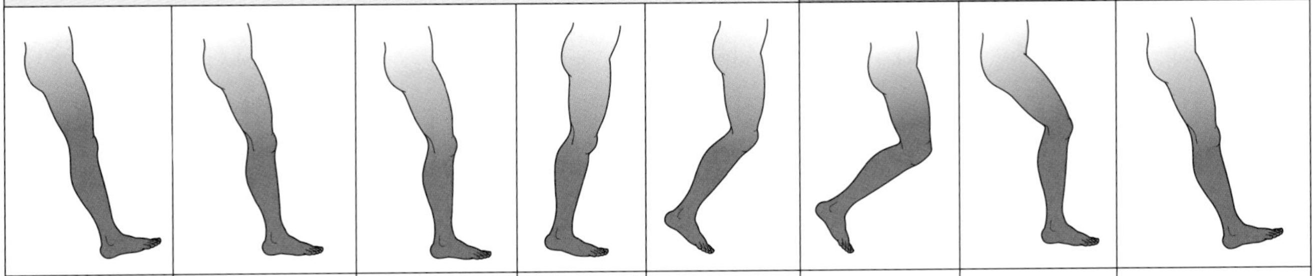

	Stance phase				Swing phase		
Initial contact/ Heel strike	Loading response/ Foot flat	Midstance/ Single-leg support	Terminal stance/ Heel-off	Preswing/ Toe-off	Initial swing/ Early swing	Midswing/ Swing-through	Terminal swing/ Late swing
0%	0–15%	15–40%	40–50%	50–60%	60–75%	75–85%	85–100%
ROM Flexion $30°$ Neutral abduction, adduction, and rotation	$30°$ flexion	Full extension	$10°$ hyper-extension	Neutral extension	$20°$ flexion	Flexion from $20°$ to $30°$	$30°$ flexion
Muscle activity Gluteus maximus, medius, tensor fasciae latae, and hamstrings	Gluteus maximus, gluteus medius, tensor fasciae latae, and hamstrings	Gluteus medius, tensor fasciae latae	Hip flexors to prevent further extension	Hip flexors to initiate swing	Hip flexors	Hip flexors	Hamstrings to decelerate hip

Knee

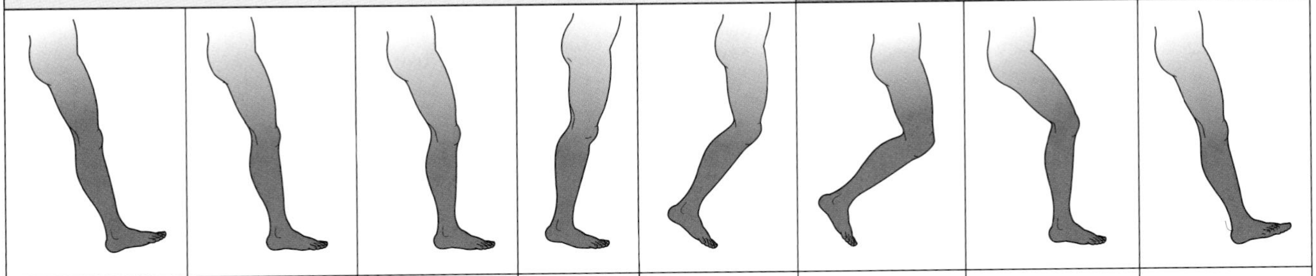

	Stance phase				Swing phase		
Initial contact/ Heel strike	Loading response/ Foot flat	Midstance/ Single-leg support	Terminal stance/ Heel-off	Preswing/ Toe-off	Initial swing/ Early swing	Midswing	Terminal swing/ Late swing
0%	0–15%	15–40%	40–50%	50–60%	60–75%	75–85%	85–100%
ROM Full extension Slight abduction (valgus) $8°$ lateral rotation	$15°$ flexion moving toward medial rotation	Moving toward full extension, abduction, and into lateral rotation	Full extension	$35°$ flexion moving into more abduction	$60°$ flexion About $8°$ abduction occurs by midswing Neutral frontal plane alignment	From $60°$ to $30°$ flexion Moves towards adduction (varus) and from medial to lateral rotation in last half of swing	Extension to $0°$
Muscle activity Quadriceps	Highest point of quadriceps activity Hamstrings active as hip extensors	Quadriceps first half of midstance Once knee is extended, quadriceps silent	None	None	Short head of biceps, sartorius gracilis	None	Quadriceps and hamstrings decelerate the lower extremity

Figure 7.17 >continued

Ankle

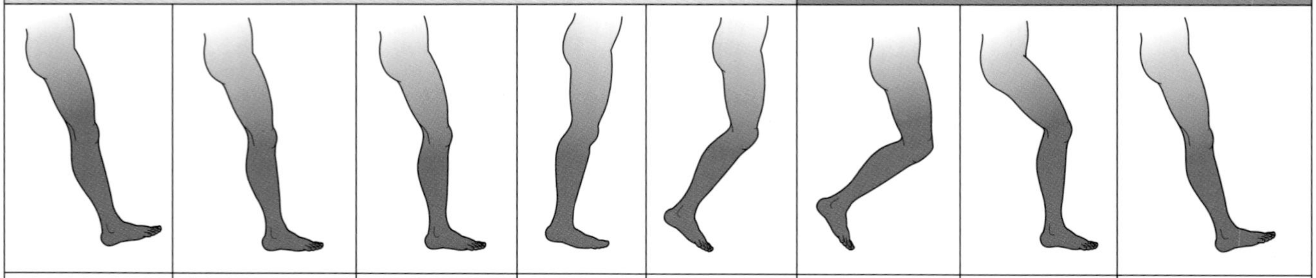

	Stance phase				Swing phase		
Initial contact/ Heel strike	Loading response/ Foot flat	Midstance/ Single-leg support	Terminal stance/ Heel-off	Preswing/ Toe-off	Initial swing/ Early swing	Midswing/ Swing-through	Terminal swing/ Late swing
0%	0–15%	15–40%	40–50%	50–60%	60–75%	75–85%	85–100%
ROM Neutral Sagittal and transverse planes, 5° inversion	15° plantar flexion moving toward eversion	Neutral to 10° dorsiflexion Maximum eversion early then moves toward slight inversion, slight abduction	Heel-off is prior to heel contact Opposite foot moves into plantar flexion after contact Continues inverting	20° plantar flexion maximum inversion approaching maximum adduction	10° plantar flexion moving to neutral Moving towards frontal plane neutral and neutral rotation	Neutral Dorsiflexion–plantar flexion and abduction–adduction progressing toward 5° inversion	Neutral
Muscle activity Dorsiflexors maintain neutral position	Dorsiflexors control rate of plantar flexion, prevent foot slap	Plantar flexors control advance of tibia	Plantar flexors control tibia, restrict dorsiflexion	Dorsiflexors begin activity	Dorsiflexors active for toe clearance	Dorsiflexors maintain neutral position	Dorsiflexors maintain neutral position

Figure 7.17 *>continued*

TABLE 7.2   Summary of Average Required Motion of Each Joint for Normal Walking

Joint	Sagittal plane motion	Frontal plane motion	Transverse plane motion
Pelvis	9° anterior–posterior tilt	16° upward–downward tilt	15° forward–backward rotation
Hip	30° flexion, 10° hyperextension	5° abduction, 15° adduction	10°–15° medial–lateral rotation
Knee	60° flexion 0° extension	3° abduction 8° adduction	20° medial–lateral rotation
Ankle and foot	10° dorsiflexion 20° plantar flexion	5° eversion 11° inversion	2° abduction 7° adduction
1st metatarsophalangeal	60° dorsiflexion	Unknown	Unknown

CLINICAL TIPS

Forces are necessary for ambulation. Muscles act as shock absorbers or decelerators eccentrically, as stabilizers isometrically, or as accelerators concentrically. Some muscles perform only one type of activity, while others perform more than one during gait. Muscles have periods of activity and periods of relative rest so that a person can walk normally for prolonged periods without needing to rest and recover. Motion of the body forward, as in walking, occurs because of active forces produced by muscle as well as passive forces created by the position of the body's center of mass relative to the foot's point of contact with the ground.

Gait Kinetics

Movements that occur during ambulation result from forces acting on the body. These forces (kinetics) include primarily those produced by the muscles, ground reaction forces, gravity, and momentum. Before we look at ground reaction forces, we will see how the muscles work to create ambulation.

Muscle Actions: General Functions in Gait

In gait, the muscles perform one of three actions: acceleration, deceleration, or shock absorption. Muscles also work as stabilizers to secure the body or its segments during movement. Acceleration propels the body or segment forward. Acceleration is generally the result of concentric muscle activity. Deceleration slows down a segment's or body's movement to produce a smooth, controlled motion during ambulation. Deceleration occurs from eccentric activity. Like deceleration, shock absorption is primarily an eccentric activity. Shock absorption occurs primarily during early contact with the ground to reduce impact forces on the body. Since deceleration and shock absorption are both eccentric activities and occur either in preparation for stance or on impact with the ground, separation between these two activities is often not acknowledged, but keep in mind that they are separate tasks. Stabilizer muscles act as guy wires to hold a segment stable during movement. Isometric activity often produces stabilization. Some muscles may act as accelerators during gait and as decelerators at other times, while other muscles are primarily stabilizers throughout the gait cycle.

Obviously, not all muscles are active all the time during gait. The cyclic activity of a muscle in gait provides periods of rest for that muscle. Brief periods of peak muscle activity followed by less activity and rest periods give muscles enough recovery time so an activity like walking can con-

tinue for extended durations, if necessary. Because walking is the means by which we move our bodies from one location to another, it matters quite a bit that locomotion does not need any single muscle to perform continuously.

Muscles need the greatest amount of energy during the stance phase; less energy is needed during the swing phase. The periods of greatest muscle activity are the last 10% of the stance phase and the last 10% of the swing phase. In other words, the greatest muscle activity occurs during periods of acceleration (final stance phase) and deceleration (final swing phase).[78] Periods of relative inactivity occur during midstance and the swing phase. The swing phase is a relatively quiet time for muscle activity because the momentum produced during the final stages of stance propels the lower extremity forward.

Let's take a brief look at the specific muscles that produce ambulation. Once you know what muscles are important for gait, it becomes easier to instruct patients in corrective gait training and to provide therapeutic exercises to correct gait deficiencies.

An easy way to look at gait muscles is to divide them into categories according to their functions. These categories include shock absorbers and decelerators, stabilizers, and accelerators. Some categories overlap because, for example, shock absorption requires deceleration. It is helpful to further divide categories according to the various body segments the muscles influence. Refer to figure 7.18 for a summary of the muscle activity described in the following sections.

Shock Absorbers and Decelerators Eccentric motion produces both shock absorption and deceleration. Not always, but sometimes, a muscle that absorbs shock is also decelerating the limb; it can be difficult at times to determine whether a muscle is acting as a shock absorber or a decelerator. The best way to determine the muscle's action is to identify what the limb is doing when the muscle performs its task. During the first 15% of stance from initial contact to loading response, the quadriceps work as shock absorbers to reduce impact forces. These forces are based on the impact of the body contacting the ground and the ground pushing back in reaction to the body's impact (ground reaction force, or GRF). This principle is based on Newton's third law of motion regarding action–reaction. Depending on the speed of gait, the ground reaction force can be anywhere from 110% at normal walking speed[10] to well over 700% of the body's weight.[80] Muscles absorb these forces by eccentrically moving the lower-extremity joints. At initial contact, the ankle dorsiflexors work as decelerators to prevent the foot from slapping onto the ground. The quadriceps group decelerates knee flexion and controls the amount of knee flexion that occurs during the first 15% of the gait cycle. At the instant the heel makes contact with the floor, the ankle dorsiflexors are at their peak output as they work first isometrically to keep the forefoot off the floor, then immediately act both as decelerators to lower the forefoot and as shock absorbers to absorb impact forces so that the movement is smooth.[10, 81]

During swing phase, the hamstrings work as decelerators of the knee to control the swing of the leg so initial contact occurs smoothly. The hamstrings also act as accelerators in the early portion of stance phase to bring the body's center of mass forward onto the weight-bearing limb.

Stabilizers The hip and torso muscles act as stabilizers to keep the trunk erect as the weight transfers from one leg to the other, preventing excessive side tilting of the pelvis or trunk. The hamstrings stabilize the pelvis to prevent the trunk from leaning forward during weight bearing and during weight transfer from side to side;[35, 82, 83] the gluteus medius, gluteus minimus, and adductor magnus (ischiocondylar adductor) stabilize the pelvis on the femur in the frontal plane;[82, 84] and the internal obliques, external obliques, serratus anterior, upper trapezius, and lower trapezius balance the head, arms, and trunk (HAT) on the pelvis.[29, 46, 79, 85, 86] These groups reach their peak levels of activity in normal gait during the beginning and late stages of stance when weight is transferred from one leg to the

other.[29, 48, 79] The tensor fasciae latae also works during initial swing phase to stabilize the pelvis.[87]

Accelerators Accelerators in the leg and thigh have peak outputs at various times during gait. The posterior calf accelerators exhibit peak activity during the end of stance phase as they propel the leg forward, providing a push-off to produce an accelerated passive momentum of the extremity forward during swing phase.[88] The posterior calf muscles begin to act during the middle portion of the weight-bearing phase as they provide control and balance during weight bearing. This is especially true of the lateral leg muscles, the ankle inverters and evertors.[10] These lateral leg muscles assist with foot stability and balance.[89]

During swing, the foot and toe dorsiflexors lift the foot and toes to clear the floor and position the foot as the limb prepares for heel strike. The thigh accelerators work primarily in the early and middle stages of swing to increase hip flexion so the foot clears the ground.[10] The psoas activity peaks during swing phase, providing motions of hip flexion, femoral lateral rotation, and contralateral lumbar rotation to help keep the body's center of mass over the stance leg.[90]

Muscle Actions Specific to Phases of Gait

Now that we have an idea of how muscles work in gait, let us take a look at each phase of gait to identify how muscles

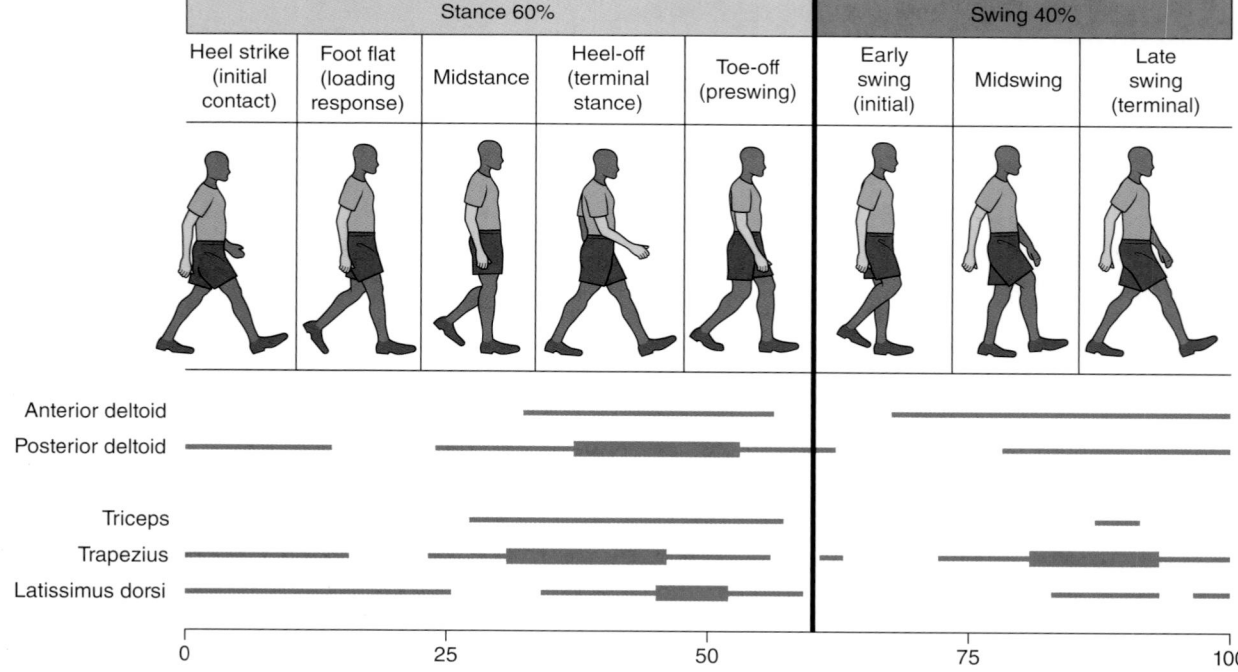

Figure 7.18 Muscle activity during the gait cycle. *(a)* Upper extremity muscle activity. A thicker bar indicates periods of greatest activity. *(b)* Lower-extremity muscle activity. Peaks indicate periods of greatest activity.

Figure 7.18a based on Kuhtz-Buschbeck et al. (2008)[79]; Romkes and Bracht-Schweizer (2017)[45]; Van de Walle et al. (2018)[53]. Figure 7.18b based on data from Perry and Burnfield (2010)[10].

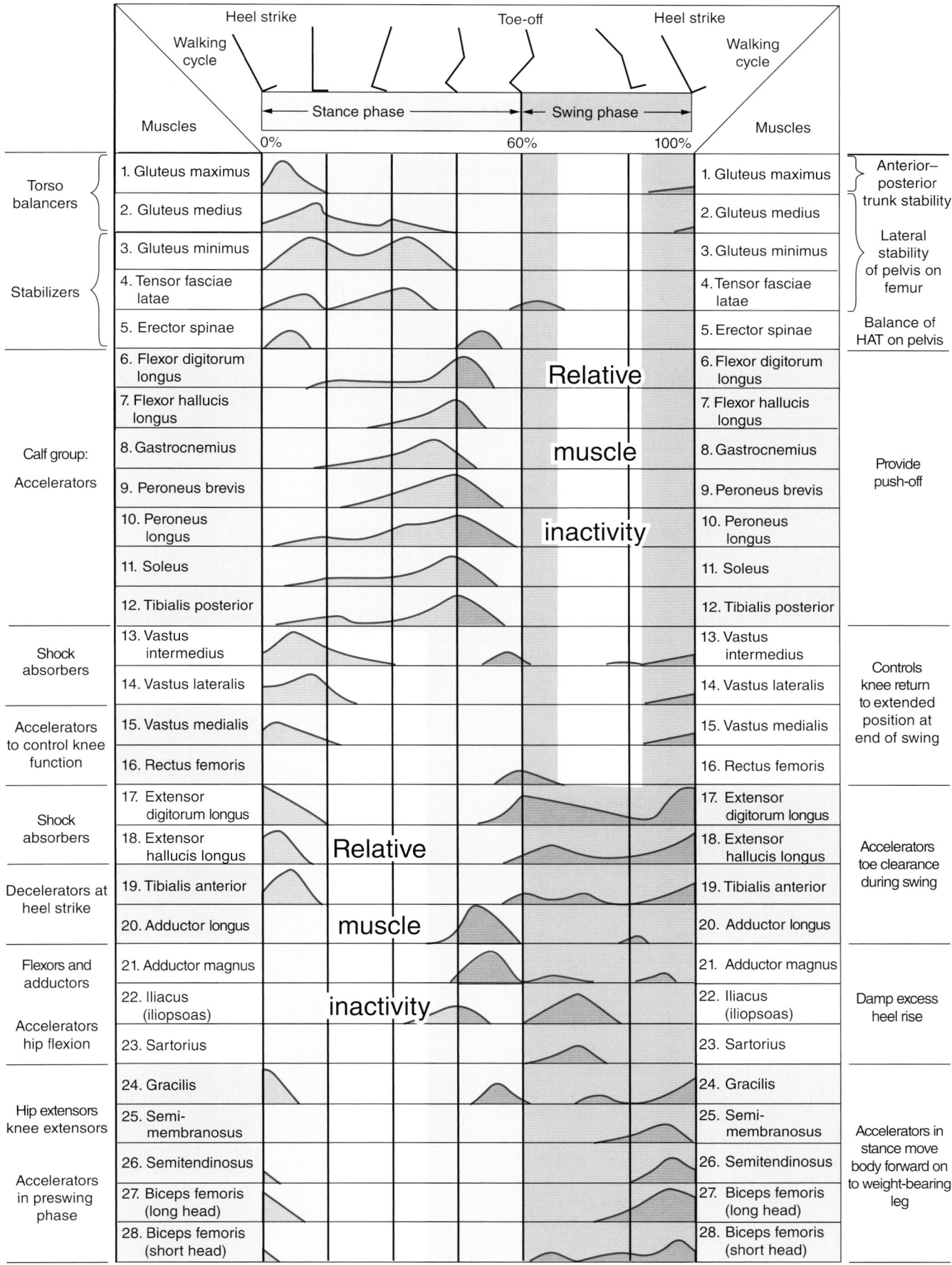

Figure 7.18 *>continued*

work together during walking. Each aspect of the gait cycle is presented in this section. To view how each body segment functions, refer to the images in figure 7.17 as you read through the muscle activities within each phase of gait. Following are the gait cycles using the Rancho Los Amigos terminology with the clinical terminology in parentheses.

Initial Contact (Heel Strike) The limb's rate of speed during the swing phase is rapid, especially in the tibia where normal walking speed creates tibial swing at 350°/s.[10] In moving from this rate to essentially stopping when the limb contacts the ground, stabilization is vital, and it is the primary activity that occurs during initial contact. The erect position of the trunk and the hip-flexed position are stabilized through efforts of the biceps femoris[83] as the limb makes sudden contact with the ground.

The hamstrings complete their task at the knee that began in terminal swing, decelerating the knee in preparation for ground contact. Knee stabilization occurs through passive forces; with the knee anterior to the body's center of mass and posterior to the heel's contact with the ground, the downward vector force stabilizes knee extension.[10]

In the thorax, the posterior deltoid, trapezius, and latissimus dorsi are active in humeral extension and thorax rotation to the same side.[47, 79] These muscles stabilize the humerus and thorax during weight acceptance of the ipsilateral lower extremity. The ipsilateral internal obliques and transversus abdominis and the contralateral external obliques also help stabilize our center of mass over the stance leg.[29]

Loading Response (Foot Flat) The gluteus medius, adductor magnus (ischiocondylar adductor), and hamstring muscles continue to provide trunk stabilization to maintain an erect position as muscles of the more distal limb absorb forces from the impact.[82-84, 91] As the limb begins to accept the body's weight, the gluteus medius limits the contralateral hip's drop in the frontal plane. The tensor fasciae latae also controls the hip and helps stabilize the knee in the frontal plane.[36] With the hip in flexion and the foot now anchored to the ground, an additional forward torque tends to move the body's center of mass forward; however, the ipsilateral internal obliques assist the low traps and hamstrings in maintaining the trunk's upright position.[29, 48, 83, 92] As the knee starts to flex to absorb impact forces, the quadriceps eccentrically controls the rate and amount of knee flexion. Because the tibia is moving forward from its anchor site at the ankle as the ankle dorsiflexors contract and the knee flexes slightly via eccentric quadriceps contraction, the hamstrings contract to counteract these cumulative stresses that are being placed on the anterior cruciate ligament.[10] The ankle continues to absorb impact stresses via the eccentric activity of the anterior muscles through the first half of the loading response.[10] The subtalar joint moves into supination via concentric effort of the tibialis posterior. Peroneal muscles assist in stabilizing the ankle along with the tibialis posterior.[93]

The ankle plantar flexors begin to help stabilize the ankle as the body's center of mass continues to move forward. Ankle frontal plane motion involves moving the subtalar joint into eversion, primarily through the eccentric efforts of the tibialis anterior with some assistance from the tibialis posterior. Subtalar eversion with subsequent pronation causes medial rotation of the tibia and subsequently also the femur; this rotation is limited by the efforts of the biceps femoris to counteract the semimembranosus and subtalar forces.[10]

Midstance (Midstance) During this phase, this limb is the only weight-bearing extremity, so as you may guess, medial–lateral stability and continued progression forward are most important. Midstance is also when the body's center of mass moves from behind the weight-bearing ankle to directly over it and then ahead of the ankle in the last moments of midstance. Gluteus medius and minimus muscles, along with the tensor fasciae latae, provide lateral hip stability and control the amount of contralateral hip drop during this time of single-leg support. Until the center of mass moves over the foot, the quadriceps are controlling knee flexion so the hamstring can perform hip extension to pull the body forward over the anchored limb.[35, 83] Once the center of mass moves over the foot and forward of it, the quadriceps are no longer needed to control knee extension; gravity's vector force between the body's center of mass and the foot on the ground provide passive extension of the knee. A gradual increase in activity of the posterior calf muscles occurs from late loading response and into the remaining aspects of stance.

As the body's center of mass moves over the anchored foot, the posterior muscles control the body's forward progression and then, when the center of mass is forward of the foot, they are responsible for moving the limb forward, controlling knee flexion and managing ankle plantar flexion. The soleus provides stability for the ankle. The gastrocnemius controls knee motion eccentrically to make for a smooth transition from knee flexion to extension. The foot's intrinsic muscles also activate during this single-leg stance phase to help convert the foot to a progressively more rigid structure to prepare for the end of the stance phase.[94]

During this phase of gait, there is significant upper extremity muscle activity. The anterior and posterior deltoids, triceps, trapezius, and latissimus dorsi are all active; of these muscles, the posterior deltoid and trapezius demonstrate the most activity.[79] Some of these muscles are working as accelerators, while others are decelerating.

To date, evidence for the upper body's role during the gait cycle is inconclusive. This may be, at least in part, because arm swing is different at different walking speeds,[45] and some studies had specific walking speeds while others used subject-selected speeds. Also, the relative amount of muscle activity in the upper body is minimal; Kuhtz-Buschbeck and Jing[47] found that the average muscle activity throughout the gait cycle for these muscles was well below 5% of their maximum voluntary isometric contraction (MVIC). Some investigators concluded that the purpose of upper-body activity is to assist the lower body,[47, 48] while others asserted that the upper body's role is to reduce head and neck overactivity,[46] and still others determined that upper-body activity reduces joint reaction forces in the spine.[43] Additional investigations with more consistent methods are needed to enable us to understand the full importance of upper-body contributions to gait.

Terminal Stance (Heel-Off)   Now that the body's center of mass is ahead of the foot on the ground, forces between the center of mass and the foot allow passive extension of the hip and knee, so little muscle effort is needed for these segments. The heel rises passively as the limb moves forward of the foot; during this time, the soleus provides stability for the more proximal joints, and the gastrocnemius controls ankle stability.[10] As the heel continues to rise, the peroneals and tibialis posterior continue their work, stabilizing the ankle in the frontal plane and placing the subtalar joint into supination. The intrinsic foot muscles contract isometrically in this phase to add to the foot's stability as the body's forward momentum moves the foot from foot flat to heel-off.[95]

Preswing (Toe-Off or Push-Off)   It is during this phase that the contralateral limb makes contact with the ground, so the contralateral pelvis begins to elevate as the limb begins to accept body weight. The erector spinae help the hamstrings to maintain an erect trunk,[96] while the hip abductors and adductors stabilize lateral motion during initiation of double-limb support.[10] Hip movement toward flexion and pelvic motion begins with concentric effort from the psoas, iliacus, gluteus maximus, piriformis, and adductor magnus, and continues with activity from the rectus femoris.[36, 97] Knee flexion occurs passively from the combined motions of hip flexion and ankle plantar flexion. The ankle achieves its maximum plantar flexion as the foot leaves the ground.[36] The posterior calf muscles are responsible for propulsion during preswing,[98] but their activity ceases before the end of this phase when the anterior ankle muscles contract concentrically to dorsiflex the ankle in preparation for swing.[99]

The arm is now in shoulder flexion and helps transfer the body's center of mass toward the opposite side as the body prepares to move its weight onto the other lower extremity.[48] The posterior deltoid, trapezius, and latissimus dorsi demonstrate the most activity of the upper extremity muscles working at this time.[79]

Initial Swing (Early Swing)   During this short phase, the stance leg becomes the swing leg and begins its advance forward. The hip continues to flex by concentric contraction of the psoas and iliacus. Ankle and toe extensor muscles continue to work concentrically to maintain ankle dorsiflexion so the foot clears the ground during swing. Most other lower-extremity muscles are relatively inactive during this phase since the limb's momentum, which accumulated from force production during weight bearing, is released as the limb is propelled forward. This is an efficient mechanism that is effective during bipedal motion.[100]

Midswing (Midswing)   Toward the end of this phase, the tibia becomes perpendicular with the ground. The most important actions in this phase are toe and foot clearance from the ground and continued forward progression of the limb. Hip flexor muscle activity begins to diminish. Hamstrings begin to activate as decelerators at the very end of midswing, while knee motion continues to be passively produced. Toe and ankle dorsiflexors continue their isometric contraction to maintain foot clearance from the floor during swing.

While the leg is in midswing, the ipsilateral shoulder moves toward shoulder extension. This upper extremity movement promotes upper trunk rotation in the opposite direction from pelvic rotation (as the upper extremity and trunk rotate in a posterior direction, the ipsilateral hip and pelvis rotate in a forward direction), allowing the head to maintain a forward-looking position and creating normal walking mechanics.[45]

The upper body muscle most active in this phase is the trapezius.[79] Although the relative motions are small, researchers suggest that arm swing and thorax rotation during this phase of gait are important because they add to overall stability and enhance lower-extremity function.[43, 47, 48, 85]

Terminal Swing (Late Swing)   During this phase, the limb is preparing to come once again into contact with the ground. Hamstrings, especially the medial hamstrings, slow the forward swing of the hip and prepare for weight acceptance.[78] The hamstrings are simultaneously slowing the forward swing of the tibia, preventing hyperextension of the knee, and performing posterior pelvic rotation in late swing, all in preparation for initial contact.[35] Toward the end of this phase, the quadriceps activate to stabilize the knee for initial contact.[12] The ankle and foot dorsiflexors prepare the foot for contact as well; the subtalar joint inverts, and the foot and ankle are in neutral dorsiflexion.[101]

Immediately before initial contact, the shoulder concludes its movement into maximum extension with scapular retraction to help the body's center of mass move toward the new stance limb.[85, 86] While the ipsilateral trapezius and the deltoids are most active,[79] the ipsilateral internal obliques and transversus abdominis are also active to help shift the center of mass to prepare for heel strike.[29]

Ground Reaction Forces

Ground reaction forces (GRF) are the forces exerted between the body and the ground during ambulation. Since we move and live in three dimensions, the ground produces reaction forces in three planes. Two are shearing forces that are parallel to the ground, and the third is an impact force that is perpendicular to the ground (y-axis). Shear forces occur in a fore–aft direction (x-axis) and a lateral–medial direction (z-axis). At initial contact, the fore–aft shear force is a forward force between the ground and the foot as the forward-moving foot contacts the ground. During preswing, a backward GRF is produced when the foot pushes into the ground as it moves off the ground and into swing. If you step on ice and lose your footing at initial contact, the forward force causes your extremity to slip forward, so you may land on your backside if you fall. The reverse is true if you lose your footing during preswing; your foot slips backward, causing your body to move forward, so you may land on your outstretched arms, protecting your face and head as you fall.

Shortening stride length reduces fore–aft shear forces but increases vertical forces (figure 7.19). This is why it is safer to walk on ice with a shortened stride length: There is less forward force to slip the foot forward at initial contact and less backward force to slip the foot backward during preswing. Also, with a shortened stride, more of the foot surface is in contact at both the start and the end of stance, so forces are distributed over a larger area.

Fore–aft, or anteroposterior, forces are indicative of the deceleration forces that slow the body during initial contact and the acceleration forces that speed up the body's forward motion before preswing. The medial–lateral shear force is predominantly a medial shear force during initial contact; since the foot hits the ground on the lateral heel, the force produced moves from lateral to medial, or is

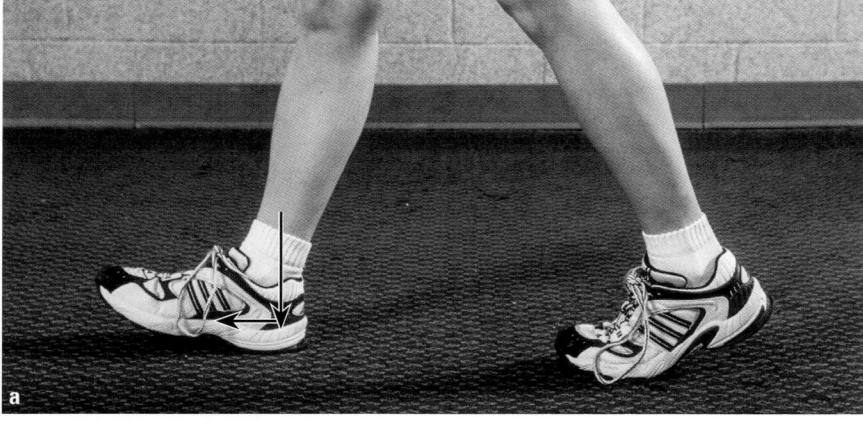

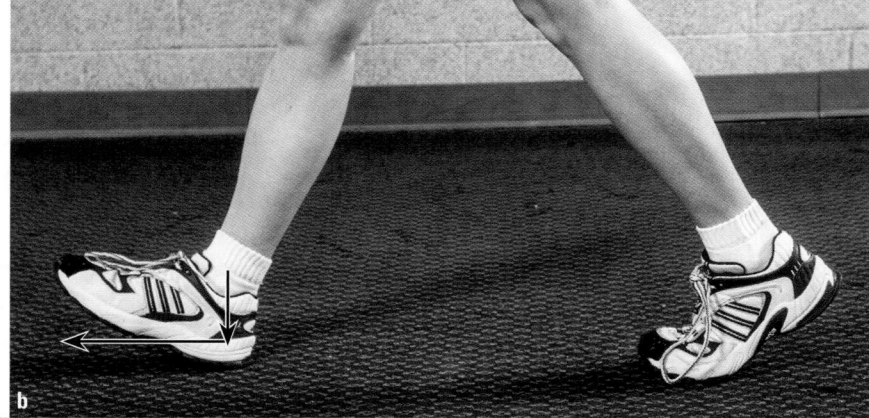

Figure 7.19   Shortened stride reduces fore–aft shear force. *(a)* Shortened stride produces a greater perpendicular force vector than fore–aft force vector. *(b)* A longer stride produces a greater fore–aft force vector than perpendicular force vector.

directed medially. As the entire foot contacts the ground and the subtalar joint pronates, the force becomes a lateral shear force. Although there is slight wavering of the medial–lateral force as the foot moves from a heel-off to a toe-off position, the force remains slightly lateral through the completion of the stance phase.

Vertical forces applied during stance are the effects of several factors, including the body's weight, stride length, cadence, impact style, footwear, and ground surface.[102] The amount of vertical force varies through the gait cycle and reflects the changing forces from shock absorption and deceleration during heel strike to acceleration as the extremity propels forward and moves into the swing phase. The greatest vertical force occurs during push-off as acceleration for forward propulsion occurs.

As you would expect, vertical forces are at minimal levels when the body weight is shared with the other lower extremity during double-limb support (figure 7.20).

It is important to be aware of ground reaction forces while examining for gait and musculoskeletal injuries. Some of the greatest forces applied to the foot occur during acceleration.[103] This can be crucial information when you are treating a patient who is a runner or participates in any activity in which ground reaction forces affect performance. For example, a pitcher who has first metatarsophalangeal joint pain will have difficulty at ball release and will need treatment of the great toe, since ground reaction forces applied to the painful joint significantly affect the pitcher's follow-through.

Clinical Gait Analysis

Now that you know the muscle and joint activity during gait, investigating a patient's gait is a matter of comparing these factors with the patient's presentation. To avoid forgetting something during the examination, it is best to establish a routine for yourself. Have the patient in shorts, and a female patient in a sports bra and a male patient

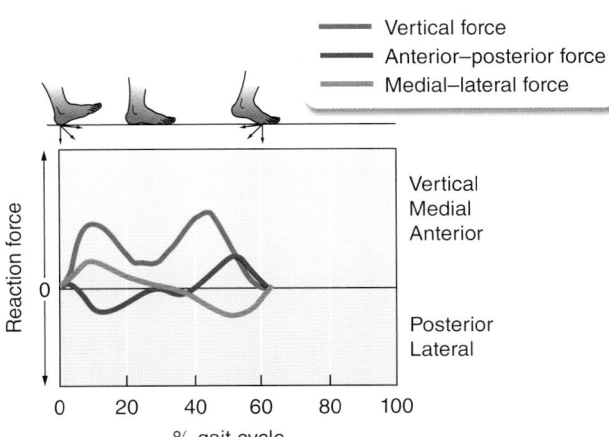

Figure 7.20   Ground reaction forces in walking in all three planes of motion.

shirtless so you can observe the entire body during your analysis. Watch the patient walk in shoes in which they spend most of their day; that will give you an idea of how he or she walks most of the time.

The average cadence range is 60 to 90 steps per minute.[104] Therefore, one step lasts less than 1 s, so joint motion is usually rapid. Because of this rapid cadence, some motions are difficult to detect visually without a video camera, smartphone, or similar device that can slow the motion. If visual recording devices are not available, it is useful to have the patient walk on a treadmill at a comfortable pace while you observe the gait from anterior, lateral, and posterior views. Although gait mechanics are slightly different on a treadmill when compared to walking on the ground,[105-107] for clinical purposes, a treadmill can be very useful.

It is best to take an overall perspective first and notice any gross abnormalities in stride-length differences right to left, stride width, and cadence. Listen to the cadence. Is it even and rhythmic, or is there disparity between the left and right foot sounds?

Next, look at gross movements. See how the body is carried and how it moves. Does the gait appear smooth, or is it halting? Do the shoulders rotate in a direction opposite to the hips, and do both segments rotate through an appropriate degree of motion and equally, left to right? Uneven or restricted trunk motion could indicate back pathology. Are the strides even? An unequal stride may be from an unequal leg length or soft-tissue restrictions on one side. Does one heel leave the floor sooner than the other? Is the arm swing relaxed and equal? Does the arm swing come from the shoulders or the elbows? Do the trunk and neck sit erect on top of the pelvis? Is the step width about 5 to 10 cm (2 to 4 in.) during gait?

After making an overall assessment, begin a joint-by-joint examination while the patient continues walking. Look from anterior, posterior, and lateral views to obtain the best information. You may start from either the feet or the head, but remain consistent with whichever system you choose so you do not forget any segment. You may also look at each segment from posterior, anterior, and lateral views, or if you find it easier, you may choose to look at a segment from all views, then go on to the other segments in the same manner. If the patient's endurance is limited, it may be better to obtain all information from one view before moving to another view since it will take less time to approach the examination in this manner. Observations are outlined in table 7.3. It may be helpful for the novice rehabilitation clinician to develop a form that includes these items so nothing is missed in the gait evaluation.

Pathological Gait

Dysfunctional, or pathological, gait usually occurs because of either neurological or musculoskeletal pathology. Most

TABLE 7.3 Observations in Clinical Gait Analysis

View	Body segment	Observation
Posterior	Head, shoulders, arms, and trunk	Head and neck are laterally flexed in the opposite direction from that of the stance leg. The stance-side shoulder blade looks lower and protracted, while the swing-side shoulder blade is retracted and elevated. Arms remain in the sagittal plane, and may adduct to the midline. The stance-side pelvis appears visibly higher than the swing-side pelvis. Thoracolumbar skin crease is seen on the stance side, indicating thoracic abduction to the stance side.
	Hips	Gluteal size and definition are equal L to R. Hip drops only slightly in frontal plane during swing phase. Medial rotation of thigh occurs in last portion of stance with lateral rotation in swing. Thigh size is equal L to R.
	Knees	Popliteal fossa faces posteriorly throughout gait cycle. Knee creases are at same level L to R throughout the cycle.
	Ankles and feet	Same number of toes are visible in stance on each foot. Same amount of plantar foot is seen on each foot during swing. Each heel strikes the ground on its posterolateral aspect. At heel strike the calcaneus everts, at foot flat the foot pronates, then at midstance the calcaneus moves to an erect position. The heel stays on the ground until the swing limb moves ahead of the stance limb. Calf size is equal L to R.
Anterior	Head, shoulders, arms, and trunk	Many of the observations performed from a posterior perspective are repeated in the anterior view. The navel may turn slightly toward the stance leg. Head remains facing forward, and ears are level L to R. Arm swing forward, or slightly medially toward midline, is more easily seen in this view. Shoulders appear relaxed. Skin creases during shoulder, thorax, and pelvis frontal plane movement are similar L to R.
	Hips	Similar to the posterior perspective, only with a slight frontal plane drop on the swing leg during midstance. Posterior pelvis transverse rotation and posterior tilt occur during initial contact, and anterior pelvis rotation in transverse plane with anterior tilt occurs during last section of stance.
	Knees	Patellae face forward throughout the gait cycle. Note the frontal plane alignment of the knee relative to the rest of the extremity. Quadriceps and VMO should be observed for size symmetry.
	Ankles and feet	Contact with the ground occurs in the same location on each foot. Each forefoot is pointing straight ahead or slightly laterally abducted. Toes on L and R dorsiflex similarly and clear the floor similarly. Longitudinal arches appear similar L to R. Size symmetry of anterior leg muscles should be observed.
Lateral	Head, shoulders, arms, and trunk	Head, shoulders, and trunk remain erect throughout the gait cycle. Head remains over shoulders; as shoulders flex and extend, scapulae move into protraction and retraction, respectively. Arm swings are the same excursion, so each hand reaches the same forward and backward points in space.
	Hips	The hip's greatest flexion is during swing. Thighs should appear equal as they lift upward. The hip is in 0° at midstance and in slight hyperextension at the end of stance. The pelvis remains level throughout the gait cycle.
	Knees	Knee is in extension or near extension at initial contact. As the foot moves to weight acceptance, the knee moves into flexion. As the center of mass moves past the ankle, the knee passively extends, then starts to flex in preswing. There should be about 60° of knee flexion during swing.
	Ankles and feet	Each foot strikes the ground at the heel at the same distance from the center of the body. Each ankle should move smoothly through its range of motion throughout the stance phase. Each heel lifts off the ground as the contralateral foot swings forward of the standing foot. The toes of each foot leave the ground at the same corresponding distance from the body. The tibialis anterior should be seen firing as the foot comes off the ground.

orthopedic patients will have abnormal gait secondary to musculoskeletal problems. For this reason, this section focuses on pathological gait as it relates to orthopedic, or musculoskeletal, injuries. Orthopedic-based pathological gait results when injury, weakness, loss of mobility, or pain prevents a segment from moving as it should during ambulation. The body continues to ambulate, but it must make adjustments to accommodate for the loss of normal function. This compensation places stress on other segments and promotes weakness. If the situation persists, it can cause additional injury. Here we consider a few of the more common pathological gaits resulting from musculoskeletal injuries. Table 7.4 summarizes these pathological gaits.

Trendelenburg Gait

If someone sustains an injury that necessitates prolonged non–weight bearing with an extremity, or if he or she directly injures the hip, the gluteus medius becomes weak. Once the patient resumes full weight bearing, the gluteus medius is too weak to control the pelvis during single-limb stance. The result is either an excessive lateral lean of the trunk to the involved side or a drop of the pelvis on the uninvolved side during single-leg stance on the involved limb. This contralateral pelvic-drop gait is known as a **Trendelenburg gait**.

When the gluteus medius is weak, the pelvis drops excessively on the contralateral, non-weight-bearing side because the strength of the weight-bearing gluteus medius is insufficient to hold the pelvis level (figure 7.21*b*). Consequently, the weight of the pelvis is greater than the strength of the gluteus medius, so the pelvis drops noticeably on the opposite side. To compensate for this, a patient may move the trunk laterally over the weak hip (figure 7.21*c*). This

movement forces the contralateral quadratus lumborum to contract and lift the pelvis. This compensation also reduces the strength required of the gluteus medius by shortening the moment arm length of the pelvis.

Quadriceps Gait

Surgery or severe injury to the knee or quadriceps can leave the quadriceps very weak and unable to function properly during ambulation. Even after strengthening the quadriceps, the patient can continue to ambulate with a pathological gait because of bad habits established during ambulation when the muscle was too weak to be used or properly assisted. With a quadriceps gait, the patient keeps the knee extended at heel strike and throughout the stance phase. If the quadriceps are very weak, immediately after heel strike the patient's trunk leans forward just enough to passively maintain knee extension by positioning the knee so the body's center of mass is ahead of the knee and the foot on the ground is behind the knee. The hamstrings and gastrocnemius then stabilize the knee to keep it locked after heel strike.[108] This style of gait can eventually result in knee hyperextension during standing and walking.

Restricted Knee Motion Gait

Occasionally after surgery, a patient's knee is restricted from achieving full motion. In poorly managed cases or if the patient develops excessive scar tissue, the knee becomes restricted, unable to achieve full range of motion. This is especially problematic when the knee lacks full extension. Rather than moving into near extension at initial contact and then full extension after midstance, the knee remains flexed throughout stance (figure 7.22). This gait may result in an early heel rise during midstance, a shortened stride

TABLE 7.4 Common Musculocutaneous Gait Pathologies, Common Causes, and Examination to Confirm Causes

Gait pathology	Common causes	Examination to confirm
Trendelenburg gait	Weak gluteus medius	Test muscle strength of standing limb's gluteus medius.
Quadriceps gait	Weak quadriceps	Test quadriceps strength.
Restricted knee motion gait	Tightness in knee joint, muscles, or regional soft tissue	Assess joint mobility, muscle flexibility, and scar tissue mobility around injured area.
Ankle lurch gait	Restricted ankle motion	Assess joint mobility, muscle flexibility, and scar tissue mobility around ankle and into distal leg.
Shortened step length	Lack of confidence, instability, restricted joint motion, weakness, pain	Assess balance, strength, joint motion, and joint mobility; special tests for joint integrity; use pain diagram and questions for pain analysis; any segment from the back to the foot may be the location of the cause.
Antalgic gait	Pain	Locate area of pain and identify cause of pain: joint inflammation, tendinopathy, increased joint stresses.

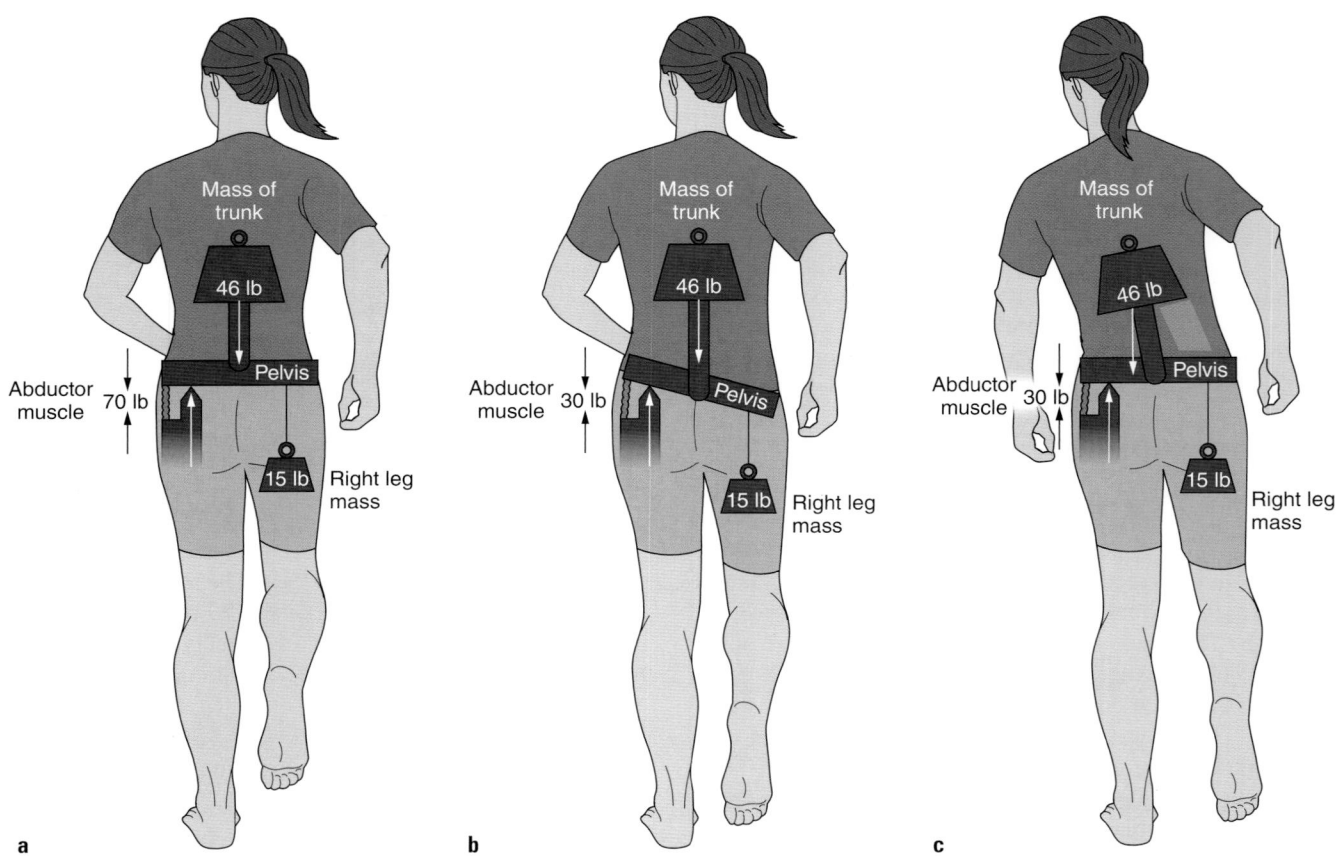

Figure 7.21   Trendelenburg gait occurs because of weakness of the stance leg abductor muscles, resulting in either the non-weight-bearing hip dropping in the frontal plane or the upper body leaning excessively toward the stance limb. *(a)* Normal single-leg stance with level pelvis. *(b)* Trendelenburg gait with dropped pelvis on the swing leg. *(c)* Compensation by the patient, who uses lateral trunk movement over the stance leg to shorten the moment arm of the body's weight and uses the erector spinae and quadratus lumborum on the contralateral side to lift the pelvis.

length with asymmetrical cadence, initial contact at the midfoot, lack of toe-off, and foot lift rather than toe-off.

It is also common for a stiff knee to lack full flexion motion, which affects gait during the swing phase. Three common gait pathologies may be observed as a result of inadequate knee flexion. One pathological pattern recruits the quadratus lumborum to hike the hip so the foot clears the floor during swing since there is insufficient knee flexion to perform the task. If additional clearance is needed during swing, the other substitution patterns are used: The patient may increase hip flexion or circumduct the hip to move the limb in slight abduction so the toes clear the floor.

With restricted mobility, the knee never achieves full extension, so it may appear as if the quadriceps has enough strength to control the knee during the loading response; however, the restricted scar tissue, not the quadriceps, is creating knee stability. Reduced knee motion necessitates a shortened step length with initial contact occurring more toward the midfoot than the heel.

Ankle Lurch Gait

If a person sustains an ankle sprain and subsequently suffers a loss of ankle motion, a pathological gait develops. During midstance when the ankle should move suddenly from plantar flexion to dorsiflexion, the person lurches forward over the foot, has increased knee extension, and moves quickly toward heel-off in an attempt to shorten the time needed for dorsiflexion.

If the patient cannot dorsiflex the ankle to neutral, there will be a rapid movement from initial contact to loading response in which the ankle plantar flexes. Additionally, the patient may use strategies such as ipsilateral hip hiking, increasing knee and hip flexion, or circumducting the hip to clear the toes from the floor during the swing phase.

On the other hand, if the patient lacks sufficient plantar flexion, the sudden lurch occurs during the sections of the stance phase when plantar flexion is required for normal gait: Loading response, the last half of terminal stance, and preswing. In this scenario, the body moves abruptly over

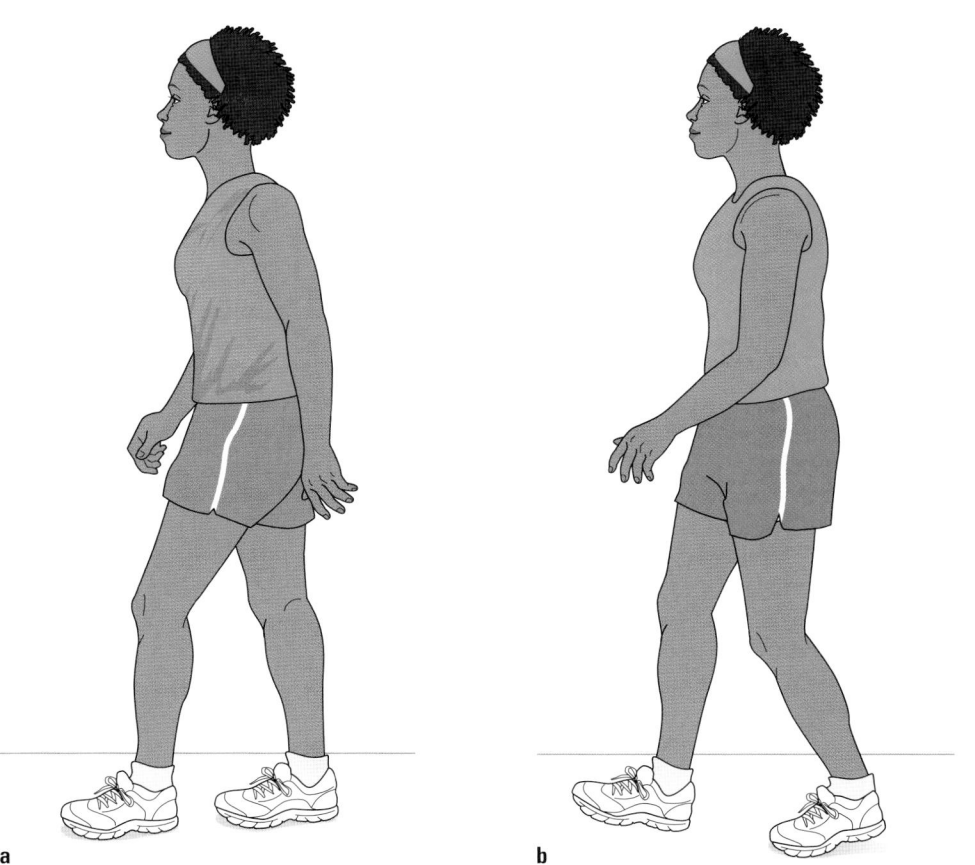

a   b

Figure 7.22   Restricted knee motion. *(a)* Notice the shortened stride length with the left leg and the amount of knee flexion at initial contact. Initial contact occurs not at the heel but more toward the midfoot. *(b)* At terminal stance, the left knee remains flexed, heel-off is premature, and toe-off appears as a foot lift rather than a progressive roll from heel to toes.

the foot after initial contact to reduce the amount of plantar flexion required, and the step length is usually shortened to reduce the amount of plantar flexion required at the start and end of the stance. This shortened step length is seen as the patient makes initial contact more distal on the foot than the heel.

No Weight-Bearing Transfer

Another strategy commonly found in pathological orthopedic gait is to never permit the body's center of mass to shift onto the involved extremity. This strategy may be used with any lower extremity orthopedic injury. The hip remains in abduction as it moves into circumduction during swing phase, and it continues in this alignment during weight bearing when it is used like a bicycle kickstand. Minimal weight is placed onto the involved limb throughout the stance phase, and hip, knee, and ankle motion are dramatically reduced; the result is reduced muscle activity of the entire lower extremity. Because the body's center of mass never shifts onto the involved limb, an asymmetrical cadence occurs with a shortened stride length and swing

phase but longer weight bearing time on the unaffected limb. Although the unaffected limb moves through its swing phase, that phase is very short because the body's center of mass remains on the unaffected side, which requires the patient to sort of "hop" off the unaffected limb to advance it. In addition to the affected limb remaining in an abducted position, there is usually an accompanying lateral trunk lean away from the affected limb. This gait is very similar to the antalgic gait (described below) in the sense that the patient does not want to bear weight on the affected limb; however, the antalgic gait occurs because of pain, while this no-weight-bearing transfer gait occurs because of bad habit, muscle weakness, or lack of confidence in the affected limb's ability to support the patient.

Shortened Step Length

When a patient reduces the step length of one limb but not the other, a change in arm swing is also noted. The contralateral arm swings at a reduced distance to move in time with the shortened step length of the involved lower extremity. Initial contact occurs more forward of the foot than the heel, and the affected limb's progression past midstance may not occur until the other limb is in contact with the ground. There are many reasons for the patient to take a shorter step with the involved limb. Pain, lack of confidence that the limb will support the patient, fear of falling, reduced hip flexion or extension, reduced knee extension, reduced ankle motion, or weakness in any segment may cause a reduced step length.

With such an array of possibilities, the rehabilitation clinician must watch for other signals that could provide insight into the cause of a shortened step length. For example, if the patient fears falling or instability, a wider base with increased step width will be apparent. Reduced motion in any joint will become apparent when the patient is examined on the treatment table for range of motion. Mobility examination of surrounding tissue is compared with muscle flexibility examination to determine if motion loss is the result of tightness in the muscles, restricted joint capsular mobility, or other factors such as scar tissue or fascial restriction. If pain is the cause of an uneven step length, then there are other distinguishing factors that accompany a painful gait; these are presented in the next description of pathological gait.

Antalgic Gait

When a person suffers pain in any joint, muscle, or tendon, you can observe a typical, obvious pathological gait. Facial expressions may also provide a clue. Because the patient reduces the time spent on the painful extremity to minimize the stresses placed on it during gait, the limb's stride length is altered and the cadence is asymmetrical; the auditory result will be apparent. An antalgic gait also presents with the "kickstand" position of the involved extremity, as mentioned previously.

Initial contact is not heel strike but occurs in the middle to distal foot to minimize impact stress. If the knee is the painful region, stance and swing phases are affected,

depending on when pain occurs. If pain occurs during weight bearing, knee flexion during midstance may be exaggerated, especially if the knee has increased edema. If pain occurs during non–weight bearing, knee motion is minimized during the swing phase. To compensate for diminished motion during the swing phase, the patient hikes the hip, goes up on the toes of the uninvolved leg during midstance, or uses hip abduction to create a circum-duction swing of the limb to clear the foot from the floor. If the hip is the site of pain, the hip is usually kept in some abduction, lateral rotation, and about 30° of flexion since the joint is least irritated by weight-bearing pressures in this position. Weight bearing usually occurs on the midfoot to forefoot to relieve joint impact pressures at the ankle during ambulation.

CLINICAL TIPS

Pathological gait is a reflection of injury, weakness, loss of mobility, or pain. To correct a pathological gait, the clinician must first assess the patient's gait, observing for specific deficiencies in the gait pattern, and then perform tests during the examination to determine the causes of the patient's pathological gait.

Normal Running Gait

Running and walking differ, just as running varies at different speeds. Running differs from walking in that the stance phase is shortened, the swing phase is lengthened, there is no time of double support, and there is a nonsupport phase in which neither leg is weight bearing. The nonsupport phase in running, also referred to as the **double-float** phase, occurs during the initial swing phase of one leg and the end of swing phase for the other leg (figure 7.23). Since

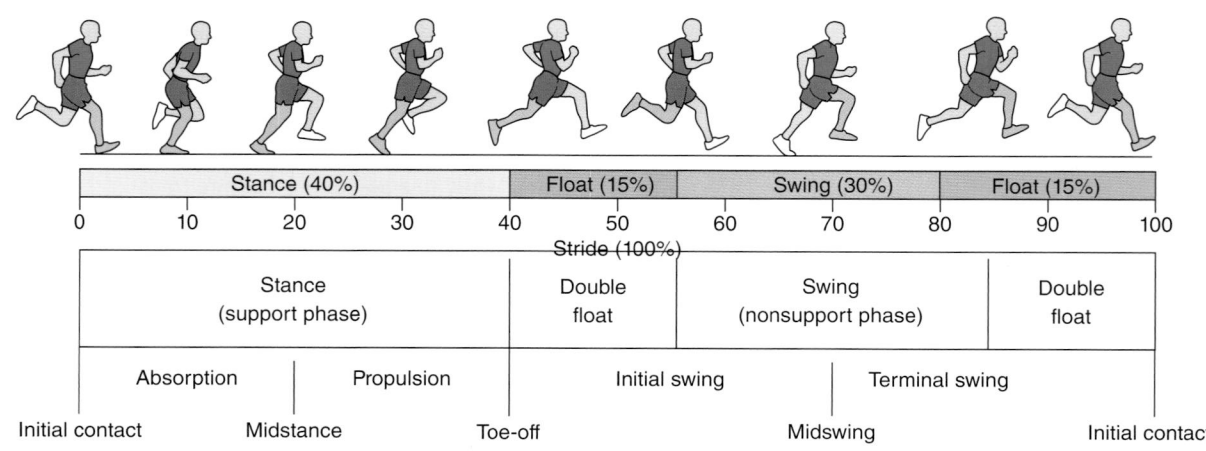

Figure 7.23 Model of one running stride: Double float is unique to running and occurs when there is nonsupport of either extremity.

gait characteristics also change with a change in running speed, categories of running must be defined.

A variety of factors affect running mechanics, including speed, age, somatotype, fatigue, surface, footwear, and skill level. Researchers who compare running speeds vary considerably in their categorizations. In one study, for example, slow runners are defined as those who run 4 m/s (4.4 yd/s) or can run a mile in 6:42 (6 min, 42 s); a fast runner is defined as one who runs 8 m/s (8.7 yd/s) or 91 m (100 yd) in 11.4 s; and a sprinter can run 10 m/s or 100 yd in 9.1 s.[109] In another study, a runner is defined as someone moving at 19.3 km/h (12 mph; about a 5 min mile), and a sprinter is one who can run 27.6 km/h (17.1 mph; 109 m in 12.2 s).[7] Whereas the average walking speed is approximately 1.4 m/s (1.5 yd/s) or about 3 mph, ranges in running speeds vary from 2 to 5.5 times the speed of walking.[110] These variations make running analysis and comparison of results difficult at best.

In most cases, the gait terminology used for running is the same as for walking. A few additional terms are used for running, however. A **running stride** is usually discussed beginning with the non-weight-bearing, or nonsupport, phase rather than the weight-bearing, or support, phase, so it is from toe-off of one foot to toe-off of the opposite foot, and one **running cycle** consists of two running strides. Because runners do not always strike the ground at the heel, initial contact is called **foot strike** rather than heel strike. **Cycle time**, or *stride time*, is the amount of time it takes to perform one step length, or running stride. **Stride rate** is the inverse of stride time. As mentioned previously, the nonsupport phase is the time when there is no weight bearing. The stance phase is sometimes referred to as the *support phase* for consistency with the term "nonsupport phase." Each phase of the running cycle is divided into two subphases that are delineated at the midportion of each phase. The support subphase includes absorption and propulsion, while the nonsupport subphase includes initial swing and terminal swing.

Stride Length and Stride Rate

Although researchers differ in their definitions of running speeds, the information available on running yields several basic observations. Stride length and cadence increase with an increase in velocity.[111, 112] Cycle time decreases with an increase in speed. After about 7 m/s (7.7 yd/s), stride length does not increase markedly, but stride rate does (figure 7.24).[113] As a person's speed increases, the time spent in stance decreases and the time spent in swing increases. One study reported that a runner moving at 5.0 m/s spends 30% of the time in stance and 70% of the time in swing, while a sprinter moving at 9.0 m/s spends 20% of the time in stance and 80% of the time in swing.[114]

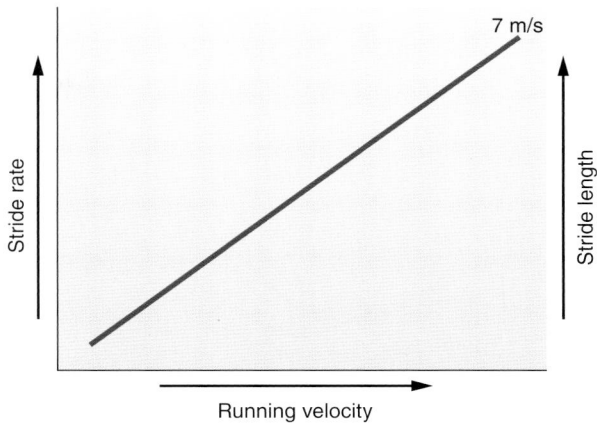

Figure 7.24 Relationships between stride length, stride rate, and running speed. As speed increases, stride length and stride rate also increase until speed is about 7 m/s, beyond which stride length does not change significantly but stride rate continues its increase.

Joint Motions

Generally, as speed increases, the body tends to move its center of mass lower by increasing hip flexion, knee flexion, and ankle dorsiflexion during the early stages of the stance phase.

Trunk and Pelvis

As a person's speed increases, the body's center of mass is lowered. The trunk leans slightly forward during running and more forward during sprinting. The amount of trunk lean increases from 4° to 7° in runners at speeds up to 7 m/s (7.7 yd/s) and to 11.6° in sprinters running at 9.2 m/s (10.1 yd/s).[80] The pelvis also changes position, moving into an anterior tilt as running speed increases. These two motions encourage acceleration forward because the ground reaction force on the body is ahead of the body's center of mass.[115] The anterior pelvic tilt increases running stride length.[80] As running speed increases, there is little change in the amount of anterior pelvic tilt.[116] Although the pelvis moves posteriorly when initial ground contact occurs, the pelvis remains in a relatively anterior position and immediately rotates anteriorly after initial contact, never moving past neutral throughout the running phase.[116] Maximum anterior tilt up to 20° occurs immediately after the foot leaves the ground.[116]

Hip

The hip increases its flexion during midswing with increases in speed, but hip position changes little with speed variations during weight bearing except in sprinting, when the hip never reaches full extension. Generally, hip motion increases as speed increases (figure 7.25).

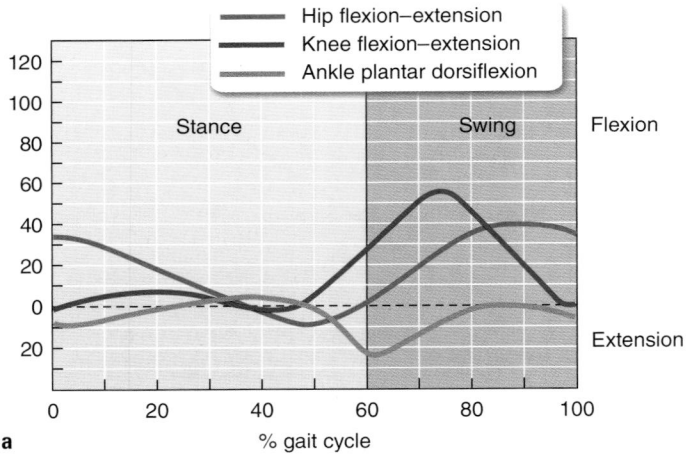

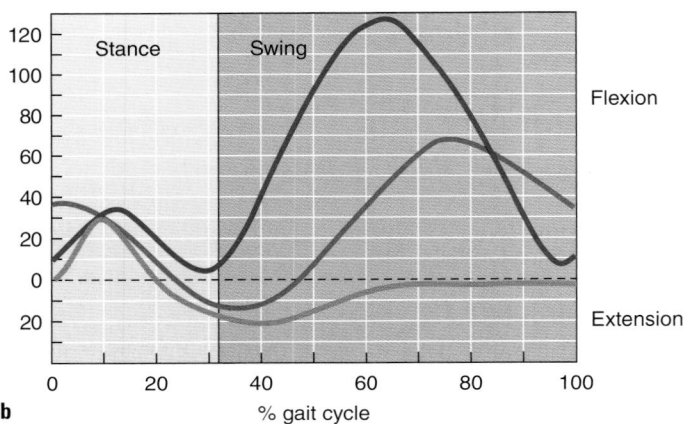

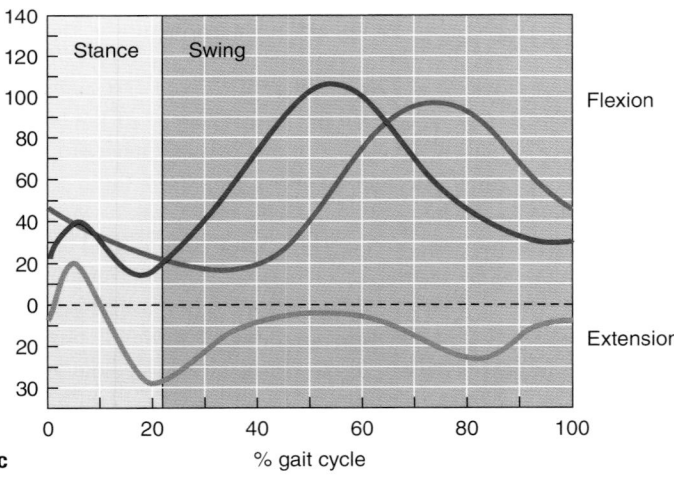

Figure 7.25   Sagittal plane ranges of motion during gait when *(a)* walking, *(b)* running, and *(c)* sprinting. As speed increases, the swing phase (nonsupport phase) time increases, and joint ranges of motion change.

Depending on running speed and individual style, hip motion can range from 11° of extension to 65° of flexion.[116] Maximum hip extension occurs when the foot leaves the ground during walking, but as running speed increases, hip extension decreases.[117] The hip abducts during swing and adducts during weight bearing. Adduction occurs because single-leg stance requires the limb to move more medially, under the body's center of mass. Abduction occurs during swing because of pelvic rotation.[118]

Knee

Knee motion also changes with changes in speed. As with the hip, there are greater degrees of knee flexion and there is less extension with greater speeds. During sprinting, the knee does not extend; it continues throughout the running cycle in varying degrees of flexion. When the foot contacts the ground, knee flexion motion ranges from 20° to 25° to absorb impact stresses, and the knee continues to flex to about 45° by the time the limb reaches the middle of stance.[115] Evidence indicates that at higher speeds the trend is toward extension at toe-off, although full extension is not achieved; the closest the knee gets to full extension is between 10° and 20° from extension.[80, 117] During the swing phase, knee flexion has been recorded between 95° and 120°.[115, 119] Increased knee flexion provides for additional shock absorption, but it also requires greater quadriceps output. This topic is discussed later in the section Kinetics.

Ankle and Foot

Ankle plantar flexion at toe-off has been recorded in ranges between 59° and 75°.[80] Which part of the foot makes initial contact with the ground depends on the angles of the hip, knee, and ankle. Runners usually land on the midfoot.[120] As a rule, faster runners tend to land at the midfoot, and slower runners land at the rearfoot.[118] Unlike walking, when the ankle moves into plantar flexion after contacting the ground, in running, the ankle dorsiflexes to its maximum, allowing the subtalar joint to pronate.[115] Less maximum dorsiflexion during early stance occurs in sprinting than in running because the sprinter's ankle is positioned more toward plantar flexion at initial contact; likewise, in the latter aspect of stance, the sprinter's plantar flexion is greater as he provides the explosive power to push off.[115] Ankle dorsiflexion during swing is least in sprinting and reduced somewhat in running compared to walking; greater hip and knee flexion provides enough lift for the foot to clear the ground.[115] Maximum sagittal plane ankle motion for runners is about 30° of dorsiflexion to

20° of plantar flexion, while sprinters need approximately 20° of dorsiflexion but 30° of plantar flexion.[115]

Supination and pronation are important motions during running.[121] The subtalar joint's ability to pronate, converting the foot to a flexible structure so it can absorb impact stresses when it strikes the ground, is an important element in running.[122] Likewise, as the foot prepares to push off the ground, the subtalar joint moves into supination, locking the foot so it serves as a rigid lever for propulsion of the body forward. Without this ability to convert the foot's alignment in such a manner, not only would running be less efficient, but the risk of injury would substantially increase. Immediately before initial contact, the subtalar joint is in 6° to 8° of inversion, but when contact is made with the ground, the subtalar joint moves to 6° to 8° of eversion.[11]

Ground Reaction Forces

As running speed and stride length increase, ground reaction forces also increase.[122] In running and walking, ground reaction forces reach two peaks in the sagittal plane. The largest sagittal forces occur at the subtalar joint and the knee.[123] Because, as we will see in the next section, the gastrocnemius–soleus complex and the quadriceps provide significant forces in running, this finding is perhaps not surprising. The first GRF peak is at impact during initial contact and involves a sort of braking of the limb. This peak, which occurs very quickly with running, is referred to as the impact peak.[80] The second peak occurs during the last half of support and is referred to as an action peak because of the muscles' influences on it during acceleration, or propulsion, before toe-off (figure 7.26).[80] These impact forces are up to three times body weight.[124]

The ground reaction forces applied in a fore–aft direction coincide with braking in the first 25% of ground contact and with propulsion in the last 25% of ground contact.[124] Because the foot lands ahead of the body's center of mass, initial ground reaction forces are posterior to the limb's anterior force, while the later increase in these forces is anterior to the limb's posterior push off the ground. Of the three planes of motion, the medial–lateral ground reaction forces show the most variability not only between investigations, but also between subjects within those investigations.[12, 80, 123] Because there is no time of double support in running or sprinting, the foot lands with a medially directed force as the limb moves centrally to provide the body's sole base of support. Additionally, the subtalar joint makes initial contact with the ground in supination, adding to the medial forces; the foot goes immediately into pronation to create a laterally directed force.

In the last half of stance, the foot supinates in preparation for push-off, so the forces once again become more medially directed. The variations in medial–lateral ground reaction forces in runners and sprinters may be the result of pelvis width, shoe style, or extent or limitation of supi-

nation and pronation; variations can also result when the runner is a heel, midfoot, or forefoot striker. Of the three planes of ground reaction forces, the medial–lateral plane has the lowest ground reaction forces applied.[115]

Vertical impact forces encountered during running are mathematically combined with joint positions to determine joint moments. Joint moments are the stresses applied to the joints. During running, the knee encounters flexor moments 7.7 times greater than those encountered during walking.[80] The hip and ankle flexion demands during running are double those during walking.[110]

Body weight, surfaces, shoes, speed, and where on the foot the runner lands all influence the peak forces of impact.[121] Softer surfaces can eliminate the impact peak. A good running shoe or one that is not worn out has a lower impact peak than a poorly constructed or worn-out shoe. Runners who land on the midfoot or forefoot have a significantly reduced impact peak compared to those who land on the rearfoot; runners who land on the rearfoot have a single peak, whereas runners who land on the midfoot have a biphasic peak impact.[80] Faster runners have greater ground reaction forces than slower runners.

Kinetics

Specific activity varies greatly, depending on running speeds and the investigation, but a general conclusion is that muscle activity increases with increased running speeds,[125] as seen in figure 7.27. The primary goal of muscles involved in any type of gait is forward movement. This forward movement during running becomes the primary responsibility of the hip flexors and knee extensors during swing.[126] Hip extensors and ankle plantar flexors, especially

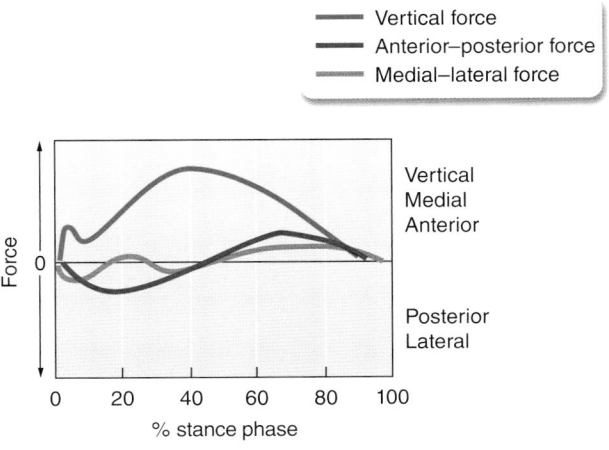

Figure 7.26 Ground reaction forces in running and walking. Vertical GRF in running is shown in red. Notice that the impact ground reaction force in running occurs very quickly. Of these planes of GRF, the most variable in both timing and intensity are the medial–lateral forces seen here in orange.

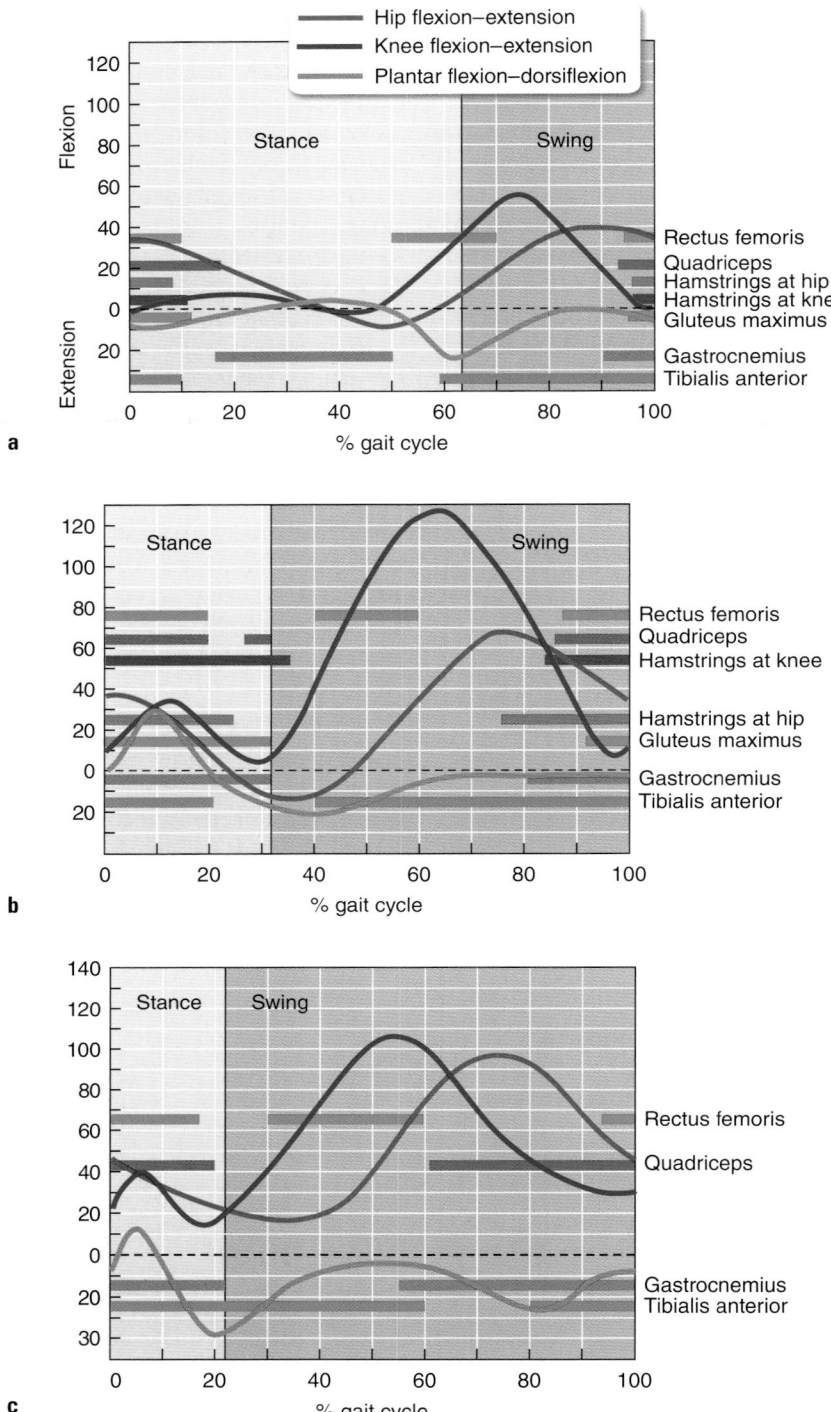

Figure 7.27 Muscle activity with sagittal plane range of motion during *(a)* walk, *(b)* run, and *(c)* sprint.

those muscles that are biarticular, also play important roles in power during running and sprinting.[127] Although the ankle muscles play the largest role in forward progression during walking, the knee muscles do so in running, and the hip muscles are the key power providers during sprinting.[127]

Trunk and Upper Extremities

Core muscles of the trunk serve as the foundation for pelvis and lower-extremity movement during running.[121] Trunk muscles provide rotation of the shoulder and pelvic girdles during running. Upper trunk muscles also aid in respiration. When the foot contacts the ground, the trunk is minimally flexed, but as the foot progresses in the stance phase, the trunk continues to flex until it reaches its maximum flexion of about 13° before the foot leaves the ground.[116] In the frontal plane, the trunk tilts laterally up to 20° toward the stance-leg side.[121] Erector spinae muscles eccentrically control forward trunk flexion while they are assisted by the quadratus lumborum and abdominals during lateral tilting.[121]

Arms help to improve the efficiency of the running gait.[128] Arm swing is believed to be primarily the result of lower-extremity motion whose purpose is to stabilize the upper body by reducing the amount of head and trunk rotation.[46] It has also been demonstrated that arm swing during running reduces energy expenditure.[128] Arm swing also helps the lower extremities to generate forward momentum during running, especially during sprinting.[121]

Hip

The most active time for the gluteus maximus and hamstrings occurs during the last half of swing and into the first part of stance.[125] These muscles act eccentrically both to control trunk lean and to slow the forward progression of the hip to prepare for and to absorb impact forces. In the second half of stance, these two muscles work concentrically to provide powerful hip extension for propulsion forward and to move the trunk over the limb.[124] The semimembranosus is at a particular advantage to provide hip extensor force since it is 1.4 times larger than the biceps femoris.[110] The hamstrings also play a stabilizing role during trunk lean.[110] The gluteus medius is active during stance to stabilize the hip in the frontal plane, similar to its responsibility during walking. Hip adductors are active throughout the running cycle. During stance they co-contract with the hip abductors to stabilize the body over the stance limb and counteract pelvis rotation that occurs as the contralateral leg swings past the stance leg.[121] During early swing, the hip adductors stabilize the limb against the abduction movement that occurs with pelvic rotation, and in the last half of swing they work to adduct the extremity in preparation for initial contact with the ground.[129] The rectus femoris is more active at foot strike to stabilize the hip and knee. The rectus femoris is active concentrically during hip flexion in the early swing phase to lift the extremity during swing, and it plays more of a role at the hip than it does at the knee.[130]

Knee

The quadriceps, especially the vastus lateralis and vastus medialis, are extremely active at foot strike; they continue to be active along with the rectus femoris during the early portion of support during running, while in sprinting, they are active throughout 80% of stance.[131] High demands are placed on the quadriceps muscles during most of the stance phase as they act eccentrically in the beginning to control knee flexion and absorb impact forces and then concentrically toward the end to extend the knee for propulsion.[12] Their activity diminishes as the limb continues through the support phase until the last portion of support, when the knee moves toward extension. The rectus femoris acts eccentrically in early swing to prevent excessive flexion of the knee.[115] During swing, the quadriceps group is inactive until just before foot strike as it prepares for the impact-loading response. As running speeds increase, the amount of time the quadriceps is active in both the stance and swing phases increases.[115]

The hamstrings begin their aggressive activity in the last half of swing phase to prepare the knee to land in the stance phase.[115] The hamstrings continue their activity halfway through stance and may be an active restraint against anterior tibial shear.[115] During the last half of stance, the hamstrings and quadriceps co-contract, presumably either for additional knee support[132] or as a strategy to increase the hip extension function of the hamstrings.[35]

It has been noted that biarticular muscles increase their activity with increases in running speeds.[125] Of particular interest are the biceps femoris and rectus femoris. Activity of the rectus femoris increases significantly, twice in running as speed increases. The first significant increase occurs from the very end of swing into initial contact, when it is used to control the knee, and the second increase occurs at the start of swing when it contributes to hip flexion.[125] Activity of the biceps femoris also increases at two points within the running phase as speed increases: at the last half of swing and at the first portion of stance.[125] It is thought that this muscle contributes to the hip's extension force, using its force to propel the body forward.[133]

Ankle and Foot

A plantar flexion force occurs at the ankle throughout the running gait.[127] At foot strike, the ankle's dorsiflexion is controlled by the body's weight transfer onto the stance leg.[127] The tibialis anterior and triceps surae group co-contract to stabilize the foot at impact. The contraction of the posterior muscle group through most of the stance phase provides tibial stability for improved quadriceps function.[125] If the runner's foot strike occurs at the heel, the tibialis anterior immediately contracts eccentrically to control foot pronation.[110] Unlike most muscles, the tibialis anterior remains active throughout the entire running gait, and its output intensity increases with increased running speed.[134] One study found that its activity ranged from 20% to 85% of its MVIC, which is a level of sustained activity sufficient to increase the risk of injury to the muscle.[134] The triceps surae concentrically contracts to provide thrust for propulsion of the body from the second half of stance into the nonsupport phase.[127] It seems to do this through its ability to transfer power generated by the quadriceps at the knee to the ankle.[135] This is especially true for faster speeds.[80]

The foot everts during the initial portion of stance and then inverts during the later phase of stance.[136] Which muscles are responsible for these actions is disputed among investigators.[136] Since the tibialis posterior is the primary inverter of the foot,[137] it is likely that it controls pronation during early stance through eccentric contraction and then concentrically contracts during the last half of stance to roll the foot into supination so it can serve as a lever for forward propulsion.[123] The tibialis posterior may receive additional help from the gastrocnemius and soleus, especially during the eccentric lowering of the foot into pronation.[70]

Coupling

Coupling is a relatively recent term used in the examination of running mechanics. The term is based on the fact that the timing of peak planes of motion for specific joints is related or coupled.[138] This is not a particularly new idea, but the term is relatively new. Researchers have long appreciated the relative timing of motion between joints. For example, because of past investigations, we know that the rearfoot and knee motions are linked through the subtalar joint.[139] There are several examples of coupling seen in the lower extremity during running: When the rearfoot everts, the tibia medially rotates, moving the knee into medial rotation, adduction, and flexion;[140] ankle plantar flexion couples with knee extension during propulsion before the nonsupport phase;[141] and knee extension couples with hip extension to provide sprinters with peak angular velocity to accelerate.[142]

Investigations of coupling are motivated by the idea that a person might risk injury when the timing of these coupling movements is off—that is, when they are asynchronous.[138] For example, researchers have found that subjects with excessive pronation also have greater knee motion while running, and they conclude that excessive pronation may lead to disrupted kinematic interaction between the

subtalar joint and the knee.[140] It has been demonstrated that those with less rearfoot eversion are at increased risk for foot injuries,[143] while those with greater rearfoot eversion are at increased risk of knee injuries.[144] Investigations of coupling have consistently found that asynchronous coupling occurs in runners with injuries involving the iliotibial band, patellofemoral joint, and rearfoot pronation.[140, 145, 146] In view of these discoveries, it is important for rehabilitation clinicians to understand walking and running gait so that when a patient demonstrates asynchronous coupling or has any of these pathologies, the deficiencies will be easy to identify and correct.

Mechanics of Ambulation With Assistive Devices

Now that you understand normal gait mechanics, you can more easily appreciate the intricacies of ambulation with assistive devices. Assistive devices are used either to provide additional stability during ambulation or to reduce or eliminate weight bearing on a lower extremity. They allow the patient to walk safely without assistance by others. Assistive devices are used when a person cannot walk normally, usually after an injury or surgery. Assistive devices can prevent abnormal gait from causing additional injury and can help patients to avoid poor gait patterns.

Types of Assistive Devices

Several types of assistive devices are available to aid ambulation. Selection depends on several factors, such as the patient's age and size, physical ability and coordination, balance, specific injury, weight-bearing status, and comfort level. Table 7.5 includes a list of the assistive devices commonly used in rehabilitation.

Weight-Bearing Limitations

To a great extent, the type of gait pattern the patient uses is determined not only by the patient's age, balance,

CLINICAL TIPS

The rehabilitation clinician must be aware of weight-bearing limits the physician places on the patient. As the patient's weight-bearing status progresses, the rehabilitation clinician must also instruct the patient in proper gait so bad patterns do not develop. If the patient cannot ambulate properly with either more weight or fewer assistive devices, depending on the weight-bearing allowances, the rehabilitation clinician must not progress the patient until he or she demonstrates proper ambulation technique; it is important that the patient ambulate without a pathological gait pattern.

TABLE 7.5   Assistive Devices Used in Gait

Assistive device	Types available	Weight-bearing (WB) status	Selection criteria	Correct fitting	Notes
Walker	Pick-up Front-wheeled Four-wheeled	PWB NWB extremity FWB or PWB	Needs balance assistance Poor proprioception Older patient	Height is at patient's wrist with arms hanging at their sides in standing. With the hands on the walker's handles, the elbows are flexed 20°-30°.	Unless a patient has multiple injuries, walkers are not usually used. Stairs can be difficult with a walker, but a walker provides the greatest stability of any assistive device.
Cane	Walker cane Large-base quad cane Small-base quad cane Single-ended cane (straight or curved)	PWB FWB	A cane can improve balance by expanding the individual's base of support. It also reduces pain during gait by reducing forces applied to the affected lower extremity. The walker cane may be used by a hemiplegic patient who lacks the use of one upper extremity. The four-prong canes (large/small base) offer greater stability. Patients who need some support but have good to fair balance may use a single-ended cane.	The top of the cane should be at the level of the wrist with the arm relaxed at the side. If it is the correct length, there is a 20°-30° bend at the elbow when used.	Single assistive devices such as canes are used in the contralateral hand to the side of the injured LE. The cane reduces weight-bearing stress on contralateral weak stance muscles. A cane reduces forces on the contralateral lower extremity by up to 25%.[147] Patients may progress from two crutches to one crutch or to a cane as balance, strength, and WB status improve.
Crutches	Underarm Forearm (Lofstrand and Canadian crutches are two different styles of forearm crutches)	NWB PWB	Underarm crutches are used by patients who have good balance. Forearm crutches are used by patients who must remain on crutches throughout their lives or for extended times.	There is a 2- to 3-finger-width space between the top of the underarm crutch and the patient's axilla. The handgrip is measured the same as for other assistive devices for all styles of crutches. The forearm band of any forearm crutch is distal to the elbow.	Crutches offer more mobility than a walker but less stability. They can be used on stairs, ramps, and inclines more easily than a walker. Patients can ambulate faster with crutches than with a walker. Crutches can be treacherous in ice, snow, and rain when surfaces are slippery. Crutches are used most often with younger and more agile patients. Forearm crutches allow the patient's hands to be free without releasing the crutches while standing.

coordination, and strength but also by the weight-bearing limitations placed on the patient by the injury and the physician. Often the choice of assistive device is dictated by the weight-bearing restrictions required for optimal recovery after an injury or surgery. Table 7.6 provides some examples of the most commonly seen weight-bearing limitations in orthopedic injuries and the assistive devices most likely to be used in athletic populations.

Fitting Assistive Devices

Before a patient can use any assistive device, the device must be properly fitted to the person's height. Axillary, or underarm, crutches are measured with the crutch tips flat on the ground and approximately 15 cm (6 in.) lateral to and 15 cm in front of the foot (figure 7.28), so they are at about a 45° angle from the foot.[148] There should be a two- to three-finger space between the top of the axillary pad and the patient's axilla.[148] The handgrip should be at wrist level, such that there is a 20° to 30° bend in the elbow with the crutch at the correct length as the patient stands with the crutches 15 cm laterally and 15 cm anterior to the feet.[148]

Forearm crutches are adjusted so that the handgrip is at the level of the wrist with the arm hanging at the side, and the forearm cuff is just distal to the elbow so it does not interfere with the bend of the elbow. This handgrip height should provide for about a 30° elbow bend during weight bearing. Cane measurements are made with the arm in a relaxed resting position at the side and the cane next to the lower extremity. The top of the cane handle should be at wrist level.

TABLE 7.6   Weight-Bearing Limitations

Weight-bearing status	Weight-bearing status abbreviation	Definition	Assistive device likely used
Non–weight bearing	NWB	No weight is permitted on the lower extremity.	Two crutches. A walker is used if the patient has difficulty with balance or coordination.
Partial weight bearing	PWB	A general term used when no specific restriction is placed on weight bearing. Limitation is usually to the patient's comfort without evidence of pain or increased stress to the injured segment.	Two crutches. A walker is used if the patient has difficulty with balance or coordination. Sometimes the physician may order specific weight-bearing restrictions such as 50% PWB.
Toe-touch weight bearing Touch-down weight bearing	TTWB TDWB	The terms are equivalent. This is a form of partial weight bearing with the permitted amount being limited to only a touch of the foot, usually the toe, on the ground. Sometimes the physician may indicate a specific percentage of weight to be borne on the involved extremity (e.g., 10% TTWB).	Two crutches. A walker is used if the patient has difficulty with balance or coordination.
Weight bearing as tolerated	WBAT	There are no restrictions on the patient's weight-bearing status. The patient is usually transitioning from using crutches to being able to walk normally without them. The clinician must work with the patient to ensure a normal gait during progression from assistive to no assistive devices.	Two crutches, transitioning to one crutch or cane before walking without any assistive devices.
Full weight bearing	FWB	There are no restrictions in the patient's ability to bear weight on the injured limb; he or she can walk normally.	None

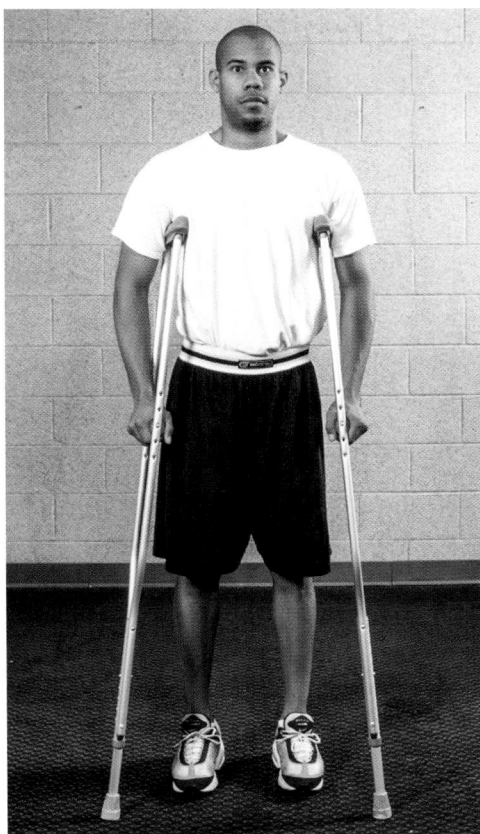

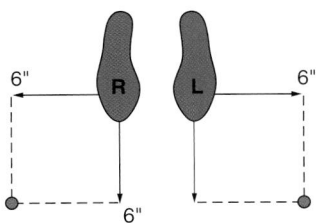

Figure 7.28 With the crutches 15 cm (6 in.) lateral and anterior to the feet, and the shoulders relaxed, proper crutch height should allow two to three fingers between the axilla and axillary pad. Elbows should be flexed 20° to 30°.

Gait Patterns With Crutches

A basic concept in the use of assistive devices is to keep the body's center of mass within the base of support. A person is more stable when using assistive devices because the base of support is larger (figure 7.29). Gait patterns are designated according to the number of support points in contact with the floor. These contacts include the assistive devices and the feet.

Two-Point Gait

There are two variations of this type of gait. In either variation, a two-point gait is used when weight bearing is allowed on the involved extremity but some assistance is needed with weight bearing, balance support, or pain reduction. In some cases, a two-point gait is used when both lower extremities need assistance during walking. In either variation of this gait, the injured leg moves forward with the crutch so the crutch and the involved leg advance simultaneously (figure 7.30). If only one lower extremity is affected, the patient may need either two crutches or only one crutch. In either case, the assistive device or devices move simultaneously with the involved leg. When only one assistive device is needed, the patient may elect to use a cane rather than a crutch. Since the limb and crutch move together in a two-point gait, the limb and assistive device are considered one point and the other lower extremity is considered the other point.

Three-Point Gait

A three-point gait is so termed because there are three points of contact with the floor—two made by the assistive device and one made by the uninvolved extremity's foot. This gait is used when the patient cannot bear weight on one extremity. It is also called a right (or left) non-weight-bearing (NWB) gait. For young, healthy people who have been injured, underarm crutches are the preferred assistive devices. Forearm crutches or a walker can also be used in a three-point gait.

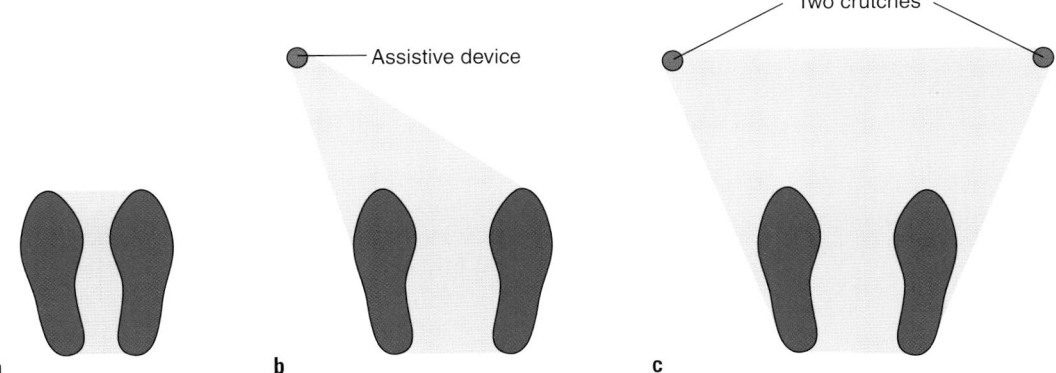

Figure 7.29 Base of support with (a) no assistive devices, (b) one cane or crutch, and (c) two crutches. The base of support increases when assistive devices are used. As long as the patient's center of gravity falls within the base of support, the patient is stable.

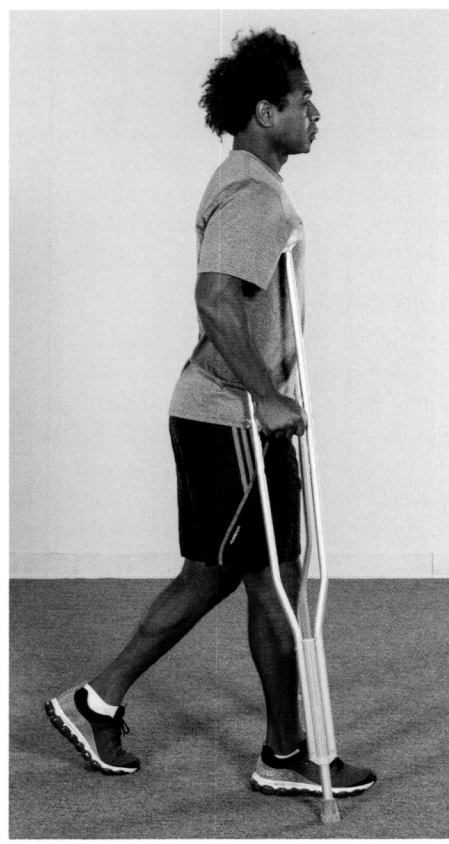

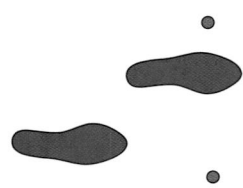

Figure 7.30   A two-point gait is used when a crutch moves simultaneously with the contralateral limb. A two-point gait can be used when either one lower extremity or both lower extremities need assistive devices. In cases where both lower extremities need assistance from crutches, the left crutch moves simultaneously with the right lower extremity and the right crutch moves with the left lower extremity. As with the patient in this photo, since two crutches are used, both crutches move simultaneously with the one involved limb.

In a three-point gait, the patient advances the crutches simultaneously forward along with the NWB extremity; he or she then bears weight on the crutch handles and lifts the weight-bearing leg by pushing down on the crutch handgrips to move the weight-bearing extremity either up to or past the crutches (figure 7.31). This gait is considered a three-point gait because each crutch is one point and the weight-bearing limb is the third point.

When the person swings the weight-bearing leg to the crutches it is called a **swing-to gait**. If the weight-bearing leg is advanced beyond the plane of the crutches, the gait is a swing-through gait. The **swing-through gait** is more difficult and requires more self-confidence and balance than the swing-to gait does. A patient who is hesitant about using the crutches uses a swing-to gait initially; as the person gains confidence and it is safe to do so, he or she advances to a swing-through gait. The swing-through gait allows the patient to walk faster than does the swing-to gait, but it requires more balance and control. The swing-through gait is the fastest gait with assistive devices.

Four-Point Gait

A four-point gait is used by patients who have bilateral lower-extremity involvement and lack sufficient stability for a two-point gait. This gait involves advancing one crutch forward, followed by the contralateral lower extremity and then the other crutch forward followed by its contralateral extremity. For example, the left crutch advances before the right leg and the right crutch moves before the left leg. The difference between this gait and the two-point gait for bilateral lower extremity involvement is that the assistive device is advanced and positioned before the contralateral extremity moves, not simultaneously with it. This type of gait is not used if only one extremity is involved. This gait provides maximum stability for the patient but is the slowest gait using assistive devices.

Single Support

When a single device, either a cane or a crutch, is used, it is placed in the hand contralateral to the leg injury, and a two-point gait is used. Single devices are used primarily for stability, not weight-bearing support, because only about 25% of the body's weight can be borne on a cane or on one crutch.[13, 147]

Single support is essentially a second-class lever system. It is designed to be efficient, so minimal force from the upper extremity is needed to produce the desired support for the involved lower extremity. The injured lower extremity's hip is the fulcrum from which the cane or crutch leverage is applied. The head, arms, and trunk (HAT) create the resistance force that is positioned between the fulcrum (hip) and the cane or crutch (figure 7.32). If the cane or crutch is placed in the hand on the same side as the injured leg, it is a first-class lever with a lot more force on the resistance side (center of mass) of the fulcrum than on the force side (cane) of the fulcrum; therefore, the cane in the ipsilateral hand cannot provide the necessary assistance for the involved extremity. The patient must lean laterally over the involved leg to place the HAT weight (center of mass) over the hip (fulcrum), reducing the body's moment arm to lessen stress on the injured leg. During a proper gait

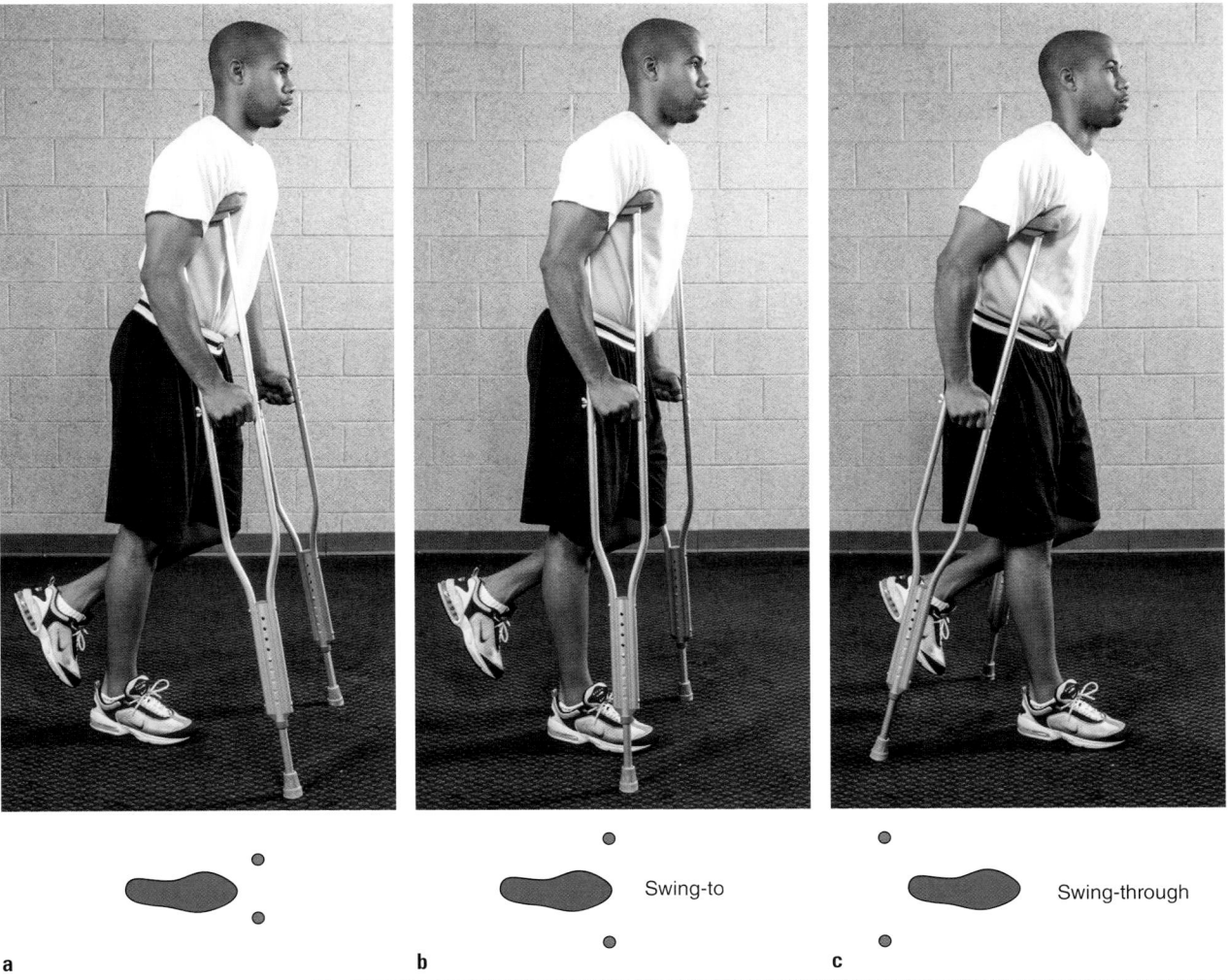

Figure 7.31 In a three-point gait, the patient *(a)* places the crutches in front of the body along with the non-weight-bearing limb and *(b)* advances the weight-bearing leg either to the crutches (swing-to gait) or *(c)* ahead of the crutches (swing-through gait). Weight is borne entirely by the hands during the swing-to or swing-through phase of this gait.

sequence, as the injured leg advances forward, the patient moves the assistive device forward with the contralateral arm, pushing down on the handle with only as much force as is needed to provide enough assistance to the involved lower extremity to create a smooth gait.

Assistive Devices on Various Surfaces

Patients will be ambulating with assistive devices on varying surfaces such as stairs and ramps, so they need instruction before they can safely use the assistive devices without supervision. The risk of injury and falling is significant until the patient demonstrates an ability to be safe on all surface types.

Stairs

When maneuvering stairs with a railing, the patient should use the handrail. A railing provides greater safety since it is more stable than crutches when climbing stairs. When using two crutches on stairs, both are placed in the same hand, the hand farthest from the railing. If the stairs have a handrail on each side, it is easiest if the patient places the hand contralateral to the involved side on the railing when going up or down the stairs.

There are two important points to remember in stair climbing. One is that the uninvolved leg advances up the stairs first and the involved leg advances down the stairs first. This can be confusing, so you can use a simple reminder. "The good go up to heaven and the bad go down to hell" is a reminder that most patients find easy to recall.

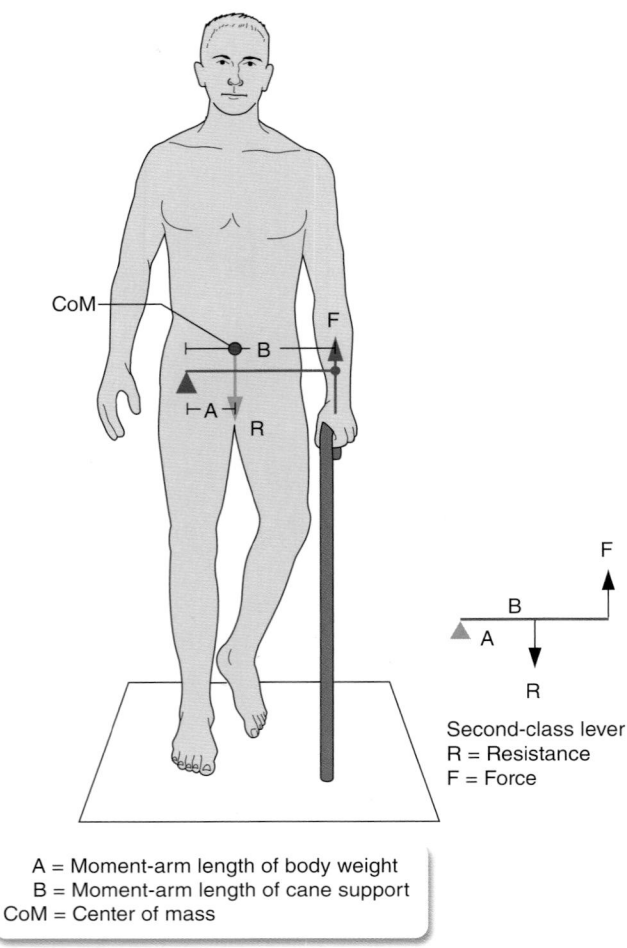

A = Moment-arm length of body weight
B = Moment-arm length of cane support
CoM = Center of mass

Second-class lever
R = Resistance
F = Force

Figure 7.32 Ambulation with single support allows reduced force to be applied to the involved lower extremity when the assistive device is placed in the contralateral hand because it acts as an efficient and effective second-class lever.

The second point is that the assistive device always goes on the same step as the injured extremity. For example, when descending stairs, the patient grasps the railing with one hand and holds both crutches in the opposite hand (figure 7.33*a*). The crutches advance down a stair step (figure 7.33*b*); then the involved extremity is lowered to the same stair step before the uninvolved extremity (figure 7.33*c*). If weight bearing is permitted on the involved lower extremity, the patient bears weight on the hands and involved leg while advancing the uninvolved leg to the same stair step. For ascending stairs, the process is the reverse: the uninvolved leg advances up the stairs first (figure 7.33*d*), and then the crutches and involved leg are raised to the same stair step.

If the stairs do not have a railing, the patient must use the crutches in each hand in lieu of a railing. This is less safe and requires more concentration, especially in the first few attempts; but navigation is feasible using the same concepts as with a railing. Curbs are essentially stairs without railings and are managed the same way (figure 7.34).

Ramps

Ramps may have varying degrees of incline, but the principle for ambulating on them with assistive devices is the same in any case. The most important concept on ramps is that, as with stairs, the crutches and involved leg move together. Another important concept is that the person must take shorter steps going up and down a ramp than when on a flat surface. The tendency is to take larger steps going down a ramp, but this can be dangerous and lead to falls. The patient should also remember to maintain an upright posture going down ramps since the natural pattern is to lean forward. A forward-leaning posture can put the body's center of mass ahead of its base of support, causing the person to fall; reminders to take shorter steps can reduce this risk.

Transfers Into and Out of a Chair

Getting up and down from a chair when using assistive devices can be treacherous. The correct technique will promote safety. When using crutches, the patient places both crutches in the hand on the involved side. The patient grasps the handgrips with the hand and places the crutches in a vertical position near the chair but in front of it and to its side. The other hand is placed on the arm of the chair or on the seat if there are no chair arms. The patient pushes from the crutch handgrips and chair simultaneously to gain assistance to stand. He or she then places a crutch under each arm before proceeding. This technique is used with two crutches, one crutch, or a cane. The steps are reversed to move from standing to sitting. Before sitting down, the patient positions himself or herself so the seat of the chair is felt by the posterior knees. Both crutches are placed in one hand, and the other hand reaches back for the chair's arm. Not until then does the patient sit down.

Safety Instructions and Precautions

Walking with assistive devices can be energy consuming and poses a risk of falling, especially if the activity is performed incorrectly or with faulty equipment. Precautions should be taken at the outset to minimize these risks.

Equipment

Crutch tips, handgrips, and axillary pads should be inspected to make sure that they are not worn or damaged. Lack of tread on a crutch or cane tip can cause the device to slip when weight is applied to it. Cracked or damaged handgrips and axillary pads can cause the pads to become loosened during use and put the patient at risk of falling.

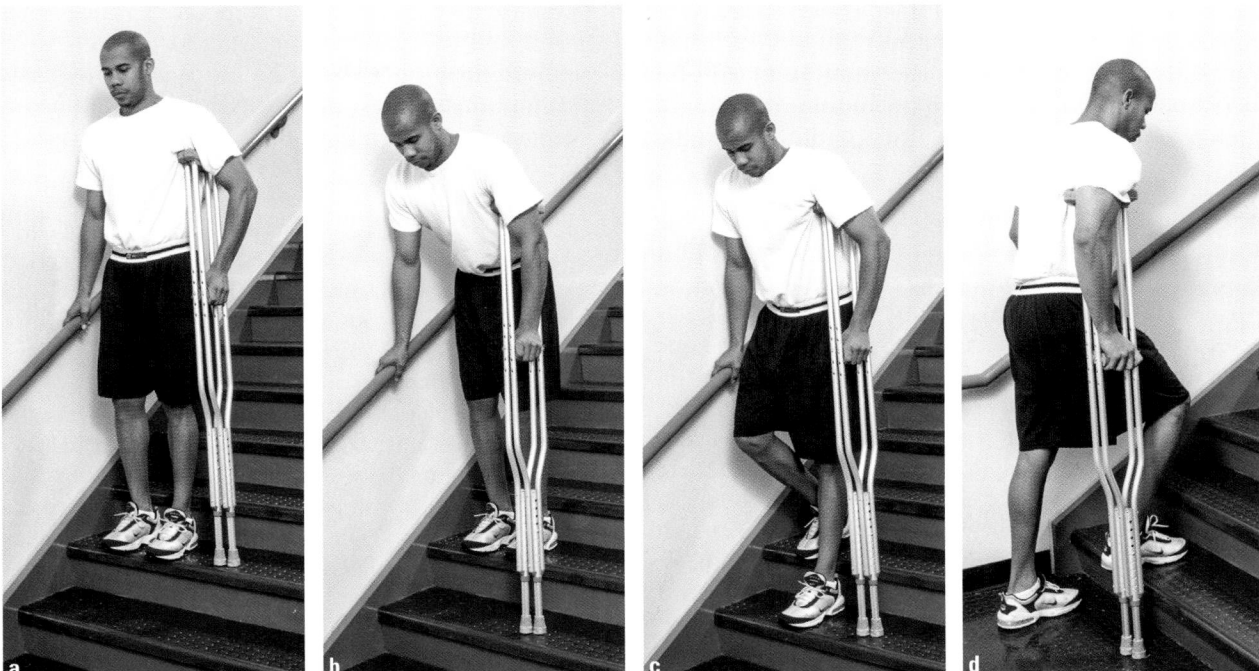

Figure 7.33   How to ambulate on stairs with crutches: *(a)* Use the handrail if one is present, and place both crutches in the ipsilateral hand to the involved LE. *(b)* Advance the crutches to the lower step and move the rail hand to keep the hands even. *(c)* Lower the body to the step, bearing weight on the hands as the involved leg is lowered before the uninvolved leg. *(d)* When going up stairs, the uninvolved leg leads, and the crutches remain on the lower step with the involved leg until the uninvolved leg is secure on the higher step.

Environmental Factors

Throw rugs are among the environmental factors that pose a risk to people using assistive devices. The patient must take care not to trip when walking on rugs of this type. They should be removed until the person can ambulate without assistive devices.

Extra caution must be taken in rain, ice, and snow. A slippery surface increases the patient's risk for falling. Instruct the patient to ambulate more slowly and use smaller steps. If the crutches are placed too far forward, the fore–aft shear force discussed earlier has a greater forward than downward component, causing the crutch to slip forward and putting the person at risk for falling.

To prevent another person from accidentally tripping over or kicking the assistive device, the patient should keep the crutches or cane to his or her side rather than too far in front. An exaggerated outward position also places too much pressure on the patient's sides if axillary crutches are being used. The devices should be advanced far enough forward to provide for an economical gait but not so far that they endanger the patient's balance and increase the risk of falling or endangering another person.

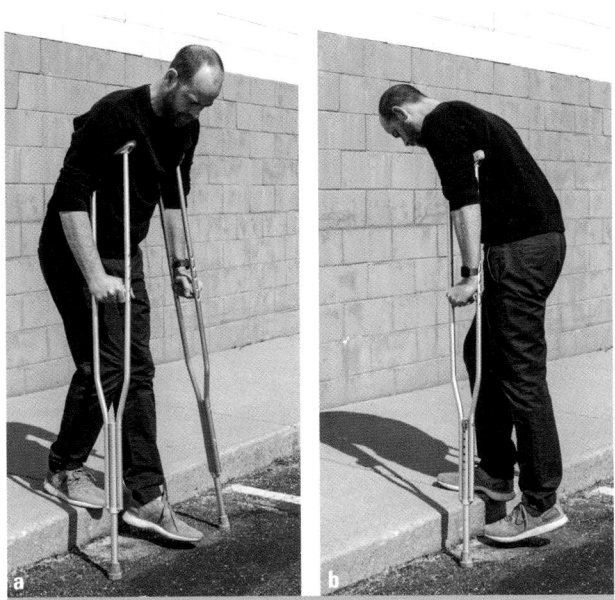

Figure 7.34   Traversing curbs with crutches: *(a)* Stepping down from the curb, the crutches and affected limb go first; *(b)* stepping up onto the curb, the uninvolved limb goes first.

If the crutches are adjusted with screws, the screws should be secured and in working order. Wing nuts should be checked to ensure that they are firmly secured.

Axillary Crutches

The patient should be instructed in the proper use of axillary crutches. The purpose of the axillary pad is not to allow the patient to rest the axilla on it but rather to serve as a cushioning contact against the lateral chest wall so that the crutch does not slip out from under the arm. Resting the axillae on these pads poses a risk of radial nerve damage from pressure on the nerve as it runs through the axilla. The patient's weight should be borne through the hands, not the axillae.

Summary

Abnormal gait occurs after lower-extremity injury; gait assessment is an integral part of rehabilitation since it is involved not only in examination but also treatment of an injury. Before we can assess pathological gait, we must understand normal gait. There are two phases of gait, the stance (62%) and swing phases (38%). Each of these phases is further divided to allow us to analyze gait. The stance phase is divided into initial contact (heel strike), foot flat (loading response), midstance, terminal stance (heel-off), and preswing (toe-off). The swing phase is divided into early swing (acceleration), midswing, and late swing (deceleration).

Determinants of normal gait provide for a sinusoidal motion of the body to make ambulation efficient. Each joint moves through specific ranges of motion in a normal gait. As the gait speed increases, the joint angles also increase.

Lower-extremity muscles that provide force for ambulation act as accelerators, decelerators, and shock absorbers, or stabilizers. Upper-body mechanics also contribute to ambulation and complement lower-body mechanics to create an efficient gait. Ground reaction force occurs because of the impact of the foot on the ground at initial contact and the foot pushing away from the ground at preswing. Depending on the size of the stride, the forces applied in the three planes of motion will vary. There is a brief period of double stance during normal walking, but running has no such period. Running has a float phase when neither foot is in contact with the ground. Muscle activity and forces change from walking to running to sprinting.

Ambulation with assistive devices is necessary when the injured extremity must be protected from full weight bearing. Depending on the weight-bearing restriction, partial or no weight bearing on the extremity may be indicated. In the case of non–weight bearing, crutches or a walker will be used for ambulation. In the case of partial weight bearing, a walker, one or two crutches, or a cane may be used. Specific sequences are used for the various devices and weight-bearing requirements for ambulation on a flat surface, stairs, and hills or ramps. The patient should be measured to ensure that the assistive device is a correct fit, and the patient should be instructed in proper ambulation using these devices before independent use is allowed.

LEARNING AIDS

Key Concepts and Review

1. Discuss the general concepts of gait.

The gait cycle is divided into two phases, stance and swing. The stance phase is divided into initial contact, or heel strike; loading response, or foot flat; midstance; heel-off, or terminal stance; and preswing, or toe-off. The swing phase is divided into initial, or early swing; midswing; and late, or terminal swing. In normal walking, the stance phase constitutes about 60% of the gait cycle. Double support occurs during the initial contact loading response and the preswing-terminal swing.

2. Identify the range-of-motion changes during the gait cycle.

At initial contact, the hip is at about 30° flexion, the knee is at or close to full extension, and the ankle is in neutral. By midstance the hip is extending, the knee has moved from 15° flexion toward extension, and the ankle has moved from 15° plantar flexion to 10° dorsiflexion. At toe-off the hip has moved from 10° extension to neutral, the knee is in 35° flexion, and the ankle is in about 20° plantar flexion. During swing, the hip moves from 20° to 30° flexion, the knee moves into about 60° flexion and progresses to full extension, and the ankle remains in neutral.

3. Explain the lower-extremity muscle activity involved in the gait cycle.

Lower-extremity muscles are divided into groups: accelerators, decelerators and shock absorbers, and stabilizers. Muscles acting as shock absorbers and decelerators usually work eccentrically, muscles acting as accelerators function concentrically, and stabilizer muscles work isometrically. Muscles act in a cyclic fashion, with the greatest activity occurring during early and late stance and early and late swing as muscles prepare to change activity.

4. Describe the general mechanical differences between walking and running.

In running, there is a double-float portion in the gait cycle during which neither lower extremity is in contact with the ground. The stance phase is divided into initial contact, midstance, and toe-off. The swing phase becomes longer than the stance phase, the stride length increases in a curvilinear (nearly linear) fashion in relation to running speed, and ranges of motion for all joints increase with increased running speeds.

5. Discuss one abnormal gait pattern commonly seen after a musculoskeletal injury.

Prolonged knee extension is an example of a common gait after a knee injury with subsequent quadriceps weakness. It occurs because the quadriceps lack control of the knee, and keeping the knee locked relies on ligaments to maintain knee extension and prevents the knee from buckling during weight bearing.

6. Outline the various types of gaits that are used with assistive devices.

A four-point gait is used when both lower extremities need an assistive device during ambulation and the patient lacks good control or balance. A three-point gait is used with two crutches when the involved extremity cannot bear weight. Swing-to and swing-through gaits are variations of three-point gaits. A two-point gait is used when partial weight bearing on the involved extremity is permitted or when both extremities are involved and two crutches are needed, but the patient has enough balance and control to use each assistive device simultaneously with each contralateral lower extremity. In the event that only one lower extremity is involved, the involved extremity and the crutch or cane are advanced simultaneously and the uninvolved limb then advances. When a cane or single crutch is used, it is placed in the hand opposite the involved extremity to minimize forces on the involved lower extremity.

7. Explain the technique involved in stair climbing with assistive devices.

When going up stairs, the patient places the uninvolved extremity on the upper stair, places weight on the crutches only or on the crutches (on the lower stair step) and handrail, and hops up. The crutches and involved extremity then are raised to the stair step. Going down stairs, the patient places the involved extremity and crutches on the lower stair before lowering the uninvolved leg.

8. Identify the safety measures involved in ambulating with assistive devices.

The assistive device should be adjusted for proper fit; crutch tips, pads, and grips should be inspected for wear before use. Proper instruction in the use of assistive devices on various surfaces and in proper transfer techniques should be provided before the patient is permitted independent use. Instructions should include ambulating on slippery surfaces, avoiding axillary pressure with crutches, and proper weight bearing on the involved extremity. Throw rugs should be removed from the patient's environment, and the person should receive instruction about keeping the assistive device close to the body to avoid tripping or falling.

Critical Thinking Questions

1. If the patient you are treating has limited range of motion in dorsiflexion and plantar flexion, what kind of gait deviation would you expect to see? How would it change the timing of the knee and ankle motions? Would the patient have normal knee motion during weight bearing? If not, why not? What possible substitutions might the patient use to compensate for the loss of ankle motion?

2. If a patient has weak quads, there will be full knee extension during midstance. Why will this occur? What must be done before normal knee flexion in midstance occurs?

3. If hip flexors are overactive, what changes in gait will occur? What changes in pelvic rotation can occur? Will overactive hip flexors cause an apparent short-leg syndrome? Why?

4. If the hip abductors are weak, what type of abnormal gait would you expect to see? Identify what can be used to correct this type of gait, and explain the mechanics of how the correction works.

5. You are developing a handout for instructions on gait with crutches. Assuming that the instructions will be for conditions that are non–weight bearing on one extremity, what instructions will you include? What precautions will you include? What surfaces will you deal with in your instructions?

6. Based on the chapter's opening scenario, what instructions should Drew give Michelle for ambulation with one crutch? What precautions should he include? What criteria should he use to determine when Michelle can begin running?

Lab Activities

1. In groups of three or four students, evaluate each person's gait. Evaluate gait from anterior, lateral, and posterior views. Identify any gait deviations for each person. List the deficiencies that are

causing the gait deviations, and identify corrective exercises for each one. Confirm your findings in your gait evaluation with assessment of the suspected deficiencies using other tests. How did your gait assessment results fare when compared with your other examination results?

2. In the same group, go to the campus mall or student union and watch people walking. How many gait deviations can you identify? Is there a common one, or are there various gait abnormalities? Can you identify the source of each gait deviation? Assuming your observations are correct, what exercises would you include to correct the gait deviations you identified? How did findings of other members in your group compare to yours?

3. Measure your lab partner for axillary crutches. Measure your partner for a cane. Instruct him or her in a gait with the crutches with NWB on one leg. Instruct him or her in a gait using PWB on one leg. Practice rising from and lowering into a chair and ambulating on a flat surface, up and down ramps, and up and down stairs.

4. Using a three-point gait, walk around campus with crutches for 15 min. What were the most difficult aspects of walking around campus with crutches? What surprised you the most? How did you find people around you responding to your crutches? What precautions did you take or fears did you feel?

8

Functional Adaptations in Rehabilitation

Objectives

After completing this chapter, you should be able to do the following:

1. Identify one strategy for sleep position and bed mobility for patients after an injury or surgery to the lower extremities, axial skeleton, and upper extremities.

2. Discuss differences in sit-to-stand strategies after an injury to the axial skeleton compared with an injury or surgery to the lower extremities.

3. Explain two unique challenges a patient will face when performing basic hygiene tasks after an injury or surgery.

4. Describe the process for a patient to don a shoulder sling with abduction pillow independently.

5. Discuss two different challenges a patient will face during self-dressing tasks after a lower-extremity injury or surgery compared with an upper-extremity injury or surgery.

6. Define two potential ramifications of lengthy meal preparation for any patient after an injury or surgery.

Ella is in a sling after sustaining a fracture to the greater tubercle and neck of her right humerus. Ella thinks she needs a better story about how she broke her humerus because the actual story is embarrassing. She was riding her bike with some friends on a challenging trail, and she fell off her bike—not on the trail, but at the stoplight by her house when she was coming home. She reached for the crosswalk button and missed the stoplight post altogether. She fell on her outstretched right arm, and she could tell immediately that she had a problem.

Ella's friends took her to the immediate care facility around the corner from her house where she was examined by the physician assistant, Rebecca. After her evaluation, which included several X-rays, Rebecca determined that while Ella had two fractures, surgery wasn't needed. She gave Ella a sling with an abduction pillow and a prescription to begin rehabilitation next week.

Ella decided to go to a rehabilitation clinic on the recommendation of one of her riding buddies, where she met Tyler, her rehabilitation clinician. Tyler is an experienced clinician who understands how frustrating it can be to have an injury to the right shoulder. Since Ella is right-handed, several of her daily tasks will require new strategies. In addition to the range-of-motion, pain management, and strength objectives of her rehabilitation program, there are other daily activities that Ella is struggling to perform without pain in the injured shoulder. While she is still trying to come up with a better story for her injury, Ella's foremost challenge at this point is improving her ability to perform basic daily tasks.

We cannot change the cards we are dealt, just how we play the hand.

Randy Pausch, 1960-2008,
American educator

A rehabilitation clinician must often wear many hats over the course of the rehabilitation process. However, different patients may require the rehabilitation clinician to wear different hats for similar experiences. In addition to physical rehabilitation, the rehabilitation clinician may need to offer emotional assistance as well.[1] Emotional assistance can take many forms;[2] just listening to your patient is a powerful tool in recovery, as is encouragement, respect, and motivation.[1]

This chapter provides the rehabilitation clinician with tools to help patients with those daily activities that we often don't think about until we suffer an injury. In his quote, Mr. Pausch makes reference to the idea that once an event occurs, how we move forward from that event is what matters. In our opening scenario, after Ella's fall and subsequent right humeral fracture, many of her normal daily functions will be affected for the next several weeks because she cannot use her dominant arm as usual. These common activities that we perform during our normal daily routines are called **activities of daily living** (ADLs). These are basic things that most people do without thinking about them. ADLs are performed independently as self-care skills and include activities such as dressing, bathing, eating, and moving from one location to another. Other ADLs may include activities such as cooking, shopping, driving, stair climbing, and any other activity that is routinely performed each day.

The type of function discussed in this chapter is different than return to sport or work activities, which are also called functional activities in other parts of this book. Those tasks are functional with respect to returning to a previous level of performance. Putting on a pair of pants before leaving the house is also a functional task, and Ella must regain her proficiency with that activity before she can return to her previous level of function. This essential level of function is also known as self-care or household tasks. Recovery of these functional activities is especially urgent for someone like Ella, who has temporarily lost the function of her dominant arm. She needs to learn how to get dressed, prepare food, and perform hygiene tasks independently, without help from other people, and without the use of her right arm.

Ella's first visit with Ty will undoubtedly include instruction in how to perform ADLs without suffering additional stress that could jeopardize the healing process in her right arm. Patients often present for their first visit knowing that the injury or surgery has turned their lives upside down, and many formerly easy and mindless ADLs are now very difficult to perform without help and pain.

The hats the clinician must wear in this scenario are those of encourager, confidant, and advisor. As a rehabilitation clinician, you will have professional experience in helping others deal with these ADL issues, or you may have had personal experience with a similar situation after an injury to yourself or a family member. Your personal and professional experience is what the patient will find very useful in this phase of the rehabilitation process.

This chapter presents suggestions for how to perform basic functional ADLs after injury or surgery to various body segments. The functional tasks discussed include sleep and bed mobility, sit to stand, general personal hygiene, donning and doffing a shoulder sling, self-dressing, and meal preparation. The use of assistive devices during gait is discussed in chapter 7, and proper lifting techniques are presented in chapter 17.

Specific ADL Considerations

A number of considerations must be mentioned before specific ADL issues are discussed. The first and most obvious consideration is what segment of the body is affected by injury or surgery. The act of getting out of bed will be different for a spinal surgery patient than for a patient who had shoulder surgery. The second consideration is the type of surgery or injury to that region. Ligament reconstruction of the lateral ankle comes with different functional considerations than a grade II ankle sprain. Similarly, shoulder surgery and hand surgery present different obstacles to the patient's ability to perform ADLs. Likewise, it makes a difference if the injury or surgery occurs to the dominant or nondominant arm. The third consideration is the amount of assistance the patient has at home. If the patient has enough help from friends and family, the stress of performing ADLs is lowered. However, many patients do not have help at home, or help is only available on a part-time basis. It may be uncomfortable for a patient to rely on a friend or neighbor for assistance, especially in self-care tasks. Some older or more disabled patients need assistance to perform most basic functional tasks; in these cases, in-home nursing care may be the best option, or a short time in a rehabilitation facility may be warranted.

Most patients prefer to be as independent as possible after surgery or injury. Therefore, the purpose of this chapter is to give the rehabilitation clinician a few ideas and techniques for instructing patients on how to perform basic functional tasks on their own. An often-overlooked aspect to performing ADLs without help is how much time they will require. Patients should be advised that previously quick, simple tasks can become arduous and can take minutes rather than moments to perform. The patient may experience fatigue, frustration, and possibly anger during the time when the injured segment must remain inactive to allow healing.[3]

When patients feel that their independence is threatened, which it certainly will be after most severe injuries or surgeries, emotional distress is common.[1, 3] The hat the clinician will likely wear during this time is one of encourager. It is difficult for patients to see an end to their situation while they are struggling to perform simple ADLs. The clinician can play a significant role in reducing patients' frustration by teaching them to perform ADLs independently and without irritating the healing structures.

One of the primary objectives in the inactive and early active phases of rehabilitation is to protect the injured area to promote healing. If the patient is in a sling or a brace and is using the involved extremity too often, healing will be slowed.[4] During your career as a rehabilitation clini-

cian, you will see many patients unwittingly, often very creatively, putting their injured segments in harm's way during functional tasks.

CLINICAL TIPS

Patients need the rehabilitation clinician to play different roles at different stages of the rehabilitation process. The roles, or hats, vary depending on the patient and the injury. The hats a rehabilitation clinician wears for one patient may not be the same hats he or she wears for another. The hats may include encourager, motivator, advisor, and confidant. Emotional guidance is often needed to help with physical recovery.[1]

During the early phases of healing, reducing the stress to the involved area allows the body to progress through the inflammatory and early proliferation phases more smoothly, which allows the entire process to follow a more predictable recovery time frame.[5, 6] The hat the rehabilitation clinician wears at this point is advisor as you offer the patient ideas of how to reduce inflammation and stress to the injured region during basic functional tasks. This results in reduction of the patient's pain, discomfort, and swelling, which helps the patient to rest and sleep, and these are all important factors in healing.

As an example, after shoulder surgery, the patient is instructed to wear a sling for a time to allow the repaired tissue to heal before stress is applied to the shoulder. The patient is not to use the shoulder because active muscle contraction during the inactive phase of rehabilitation is counterproductive. Patients may know that they should not use the injured arm to cut a piece of steak, but they may not know that using the injured arm to hold a fork in the steak to keep it still while cutting it with the other arm is also counterproductive. When patients are told not to use a body segment, they often are not aware when they are actually using it. In this example, rehabilitation clinicians know that the shoulder muscles work to stabilize the shoulder when the patient is actively holding the arm still to prevent movement. But the patient may think that as long as he does not move the shoulder away from his body, he is not using the shoulder muscles. This is a common mistake. Therefore, rehabilitation clinicians should take the time to instruct and guide patients on proper adaptations and functional ways to perform their ADLs without endangering their healing tissues.

Specific ADL Modifications

This section includes six of the more common functional ADLs. It is clearly not an all-inclusive list. Nor are the suggestions provided the only alternative ways to perform these ADLs. They serve only to present a few ideas to make rehabilitation clinicians more aware of ways to modify tasks that are often taken for granted until they become difficult to perform. There are few research studies that specifically investigated the best ways to perform ADLs after an injury or surgery. Most of the recommendations in this chapter are based on anecdotal information and years of clinical experience with input from many patients and several clinicians. Over the course of your career, you will no doubt discover other functional tasks that may be unique to one patient but will require your expertise to safely modify. Or you may discover better ways to manage one of the ADLs we present here. Consider this chapter to be a starting point for you that stimulates further thought and conversation on this topic.

Sleep and Bed Mobility

A good night's sleep is an overlooked necessity in the healing process.[7-10] Pain medication after an injury or surgery is recommended for several reasons, and one of them is to help patients sleep better.[11] There are a variety of ways the body can be positioned during sleep in order to reduce stress on the healing member; it depends on the person and on the injury or surgical procedure. There are also a number of ways for the patient to get out of bed without risk to the healing member.

Body Position During Sleep

In the discussion that follows, we place ADL modifications into three categories: lower-extremity injury or surgery, spinal injury or surgery, and upper-extremity injury or surgery. Ideas and examples are provided for sleep positions that may permit quality sleep and promote healing. It is nearly impossible to account for all the ways our patients might move while they are asleep, but they have the most control over how they position themselves at bedtime so that they can most easily fall asleep. Patients can't stay asleep if they can't get to sleep in the first place.

Most people have a sleeping preference and find it most comfortable and easiest to fall asleep in that position: side-lying, supine, or prone. Research indicates supine and side sleeping are linked to less pain in the back and neck than prone sleeping.[12] Anecdotally, if the patient's preference before injury or surgery was prone sleeping, trying to change that sleep position after injury or surgery can be more challenging than changing the sleep position of someone whose preference is either supine or side-lying.

Lower-Extremity Injury or Surgery   Positioning the body during sleep after a lower-extremity injury or surgery is largely dictated by whether a brace is used. If the patient must sleep in a walking boot or knee brace locked at 0° of extension, the better position to sleep in is supine with

the involved extremity elevated. If the patient is in bed, propping both legs up on several pillows may be more comfortable for the patient's low back and the involved lower extremity. If the patient finds that the legs do not remain on the pillows during sleep, placing a suitcase between the mattress and the box springs to elevate the foot of the bed may be useful. If the patient is sleeping in a recliner or in a reclined position, supporting the involved extremity may be all that is needed.

If the patient is in a walking boot, he or she may feel more comfortable sleeping on the uninvolved side. In this position, the limb on top, which is the involved extremity, should be supported with pillows between the knees and feet. This is as much for the uninvolved extremity as it is for the involved one. Without pillows between the knees and feet, the bottom foot and ankle will eventually become sore from lying beneath the weight of the rigid walking boot.

Sometimes, the patient can sleep on the involved side. This position is not necessarily problematic, provided the involved foot or ankle doesn't experience increased soreness from this position. Some patients will use the bottom leg to initiate a change of position during the night or to get out of bed, which can increase soreness in the involved limb. Again, pillows should be used between the foot and knee to cushion the top leg so it doesn't rest on the walking boot.

If the patient has a knee immobilizer, sleeping supine is usually preferred. If the patient has a hinged knee brace and the hinges are unlocked, there can be more variability in sleep positions. If the knee brace is permitted to be unlocked slightly during sleep, the supine position or a reclined position still may be preferred. However, sleeping on the uninvolved side may be an option. Positioning the involved limb with pillows is a necessity, and more pillows may be needed with a knee brace than with a walking boot. Sleeping on the involved side with a knee immobilizer is usually avoided because it is too uncomfortable for most patients.

Once the patient is allowed to sleep without the walking boot or knee immobilizer, positioning often becomes more of a concern because the boot or brace is no longer there to protect the injured segment during sleep, which is an activity that requires movement.[13] Without the orthotic device, it can be a challenge to properly position the patient so he or she can sleep with minimal disruption.

Sleeping in a recliner or in a reclined position may still be preferred because it reduces stress on the low back and also limits the opportunity to roll from one side to the other. Many patients prefer sleeping in a recliner immediately after surgery because of the potential of lingering nausea during recovery from anesthesia. Rolling from side to side can often be painful in the early stages of healing, particularly during sleep. If the patient doesn't have a recliner, sleeping in bed either supine with pillows under both lower extremities as described earlier, or sleeping on the uninvolved side may be an option. In either position, pillows should be used to support the involved extremity to reduce stress and discomfort on the healing structures so the patient can fall asleep.

Spinal Injury or Surgery   Finding a comfortable position in which to fall asleep is often the most challenging task for patients after spinal injury or surgery. Patients who have had an injury or surgery of this type often complain of difficulty sleeping; pain medications are often prescribed to aid in sleep and to relieve postinjury or postoperative pain. Finding a comfortable sleeping position can be exceptionally challenging for this patient population. Once they find that position, patients may begin to reduce their reliance on medication to fall asleep.

Most patients who have had lumbar spine surgery don't wish to sleep supine given the location of the surgical incision. Side-lying in some manner is often preferred, either on the left or the right side, whichever offers less discomfort. Side-lying with pillows between the knees and feet is often the most comfortable position for these patients. Patients may be encouraged to purchase a long body pillow that will fit between the knees and feet at the same time and will help to keep them in a side-lying position.

Another suggestion for spinal support is to place a small folded towel on the bed so when the patient lies on it, the towel is located between the top of the iliac crest and the bottom of the rib cage, as seen in figure 8.1. Slight elevation in this section of the spine can help reduce side-bending of the spine toward the bed. This side-bending can occur if the bed is too soft or too firm, depending on the patient's body type. For some patients, side-bending toward the bed can be painful and can prevent them from falling asleep or staying asleep. The clinician can encourage the patient to experiment with the size and location of the folded towel so it provides support rather than discomfort.

After lumbar spine surgery, some patients prefer to sleep in a recliner. This position with the feet elevated and the body in a reclined position, while technically supine, can sometimes provide a nearly zero-gravity position that some patients find pain-relieving. It is possible for a patient to be uncomfortable sleeping supine but comfortable sleeping in a reclined position.

Cervical spine surgery poses a different set of issues; sometimes the issue isn't getting to sleep, but rather getting into and out of the desired sleep position. Depending on the type of injury incurred or surgery performed, the patient may be required to wear a hard cervical collar for several weeks. If this is the case, the patient will probably feel better trying to sleep in a reclined position rather than supine or side-lying. If a hard cervical collar isn't needed, sleeping in a side-lying position is usually more comfortable. In this position, it is often most comfortable for the patient to sleep with enough support under the neck and head so that he or she perceives the head to be tipped slightly upward. Usually, the head is not actually tipped upward—the patient only perceives it to be so. This position is either neutral or places the neck into a position of slight upward lateral flexion. Another recommendation for this patient may be to lie on a folded towel between the pelvis and rib cage. This slight additional support reduces the pressure felt in the neck when in a side-lying position. An additional suggestion is to place a small towel roll under the neck to support and help maintain the cervical spine in neutral while lying supine or on the side.

Upper-Extremity Injury or Surgery   If the patient has an injury or surgery to the elbow, wrist, hand, or fingers, finding a comfortable sleeping position is typically less challenging than with an injury or surgery to the shoulder or upper humerus. After an injury or surgery to the distal upper extremity, sleeping supine or on the uninvolved side is recommended. When supine, place a pillow under the humerus of the involved upper extremity and an additional pillow on the patient's abdomen to support the wrist and hand. The patient may find that placing pillows under the knees provides slight hip and knee flexion that relaxes the lumbar spine. Should the patient prefer side sleeping, the involved upper extremity should be supported in front of the body with a pillow so the involved hand and wrist do not rest on the bed. In this position, the patient may find sleeping with pillows between the knees and feet to be comfortable as well.

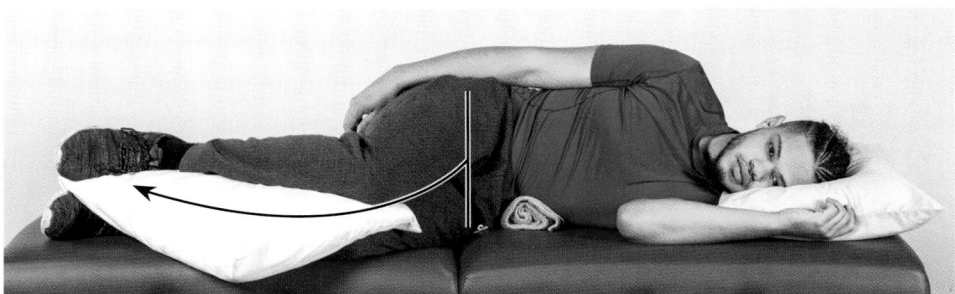

Figure 8.1   Side sleeping with a pillow between the knees and feet while lying on a folded towel to support the lumbar spine.

After an injury or surgery to the shoulder, a sling is typically worn both day and night to protect the healing region. After surgery or serious injury, the sling of choice is usually one with an abduction pillow between the patient's arm and body. This position is more comfortable because it places the shoulder joint in a loose-pack position and reduces tension on the rotator cuff muscles.[14] If the patient must sleep with a sling without an abduction pillow, sleeping in a recliner is the best option to protect the healing tissue and to reduce strain on the cervical region.

Finding a comfortable sleeping position while wearing a sling with an abduction pillow can be a significant challenge. Immediately after shoulder surgery, the patient will usually feel more comfortable sleeping in a reclined or semireclined position. It is also easier for the patient to apply ice or use an ice-water compression device while in this position.

A patient who prefers to sleep in bed may find it easier to fall asleep in a supine or semireclined position with pillows under his or her knees to reduce stress on the lumbar spine. The patient should also consider using an additional pillow under the scapula and humerus to the elbow so the arm doesn't fall back toward the bed, placing strain on the shoulder. Shoulder extension is painful and can be detrimental to the healing tissues.

While it is not impossible to sleep on the uninvolved side while wearing a sling with an abduction pillow, it can be challenging. If the patient is a side-sleeper, several pillows are used to support the upper extremity in the sling and to position the patient without allowing the involved humerus to fall forward into flexion or backward into extension.

Sleeping in a bed, even in a supine position, immediately after shoulder injury or surgery is often uncomfortable for the patient. When possible, sleeping in a recliner after shoulder surgery is usually the most comfortable position. It is also the easiest position to sleep in because the patient doesn't move as much and the shoulder and arm positions are supported.

Bed Mobility

If the patient decides sleeping in bed is the best option, getting into and out of bed can present unique challenges. Your goal in this situation is to provide the patient with the best advice you can to help him or her get into bed, find a good sleeping position, and get out of bed with the least amount of detrimental soreness to the healing structures.

Lower-Extremity Injury or Surgery   Getting into and out of bed and changing positions in bed are usually not too difficult after a lower-extremity injury or surgery. In the best case, when getting into bed, the patient should sit at the edge of the bed with his involved extremity closer to the foot of the bed. Depending on the patient's abilities, balance, and strength in the uninvolved lower extremity, he may need upper-extremity assistance to come to a sitting position. If so, he can use the assistive device he uses for ambulation (figure 8.2). The patient should not put his hands on the bed behind him to slow his descent onto the bed because he could fall if his hands slip. Even if the bed is manufactured with edge support, it is often too forgiving to be used to support the arms.

If patients must wear a boot or knee immobilizer while sleeping, they usually have little difficulty swinging the involved extremity into and out of bed. Should the limb need assistance, patients may use their arms to lift it while the uninvolved limb remains secured on the floor.

After hip surgery, it is common for the involved limb to need assistance from the arms to get it into and out of bed, especially within the first week or two after surgery. In these cases, the patient must secure the foot of the uninvolved lower extremity on the floor while moving the other extremity into or out of bed. Once both lower extremities are in bed, the patient may need to use the upper extremities to scoot away from the edge of the bed and move into a supine position with pillows under his or her knees.

Getting out of bed with a lower-extremity injury or surgical wound requires the use of the uninvolved lower

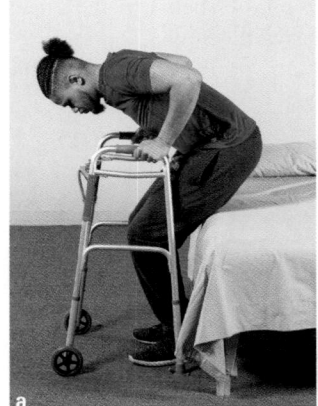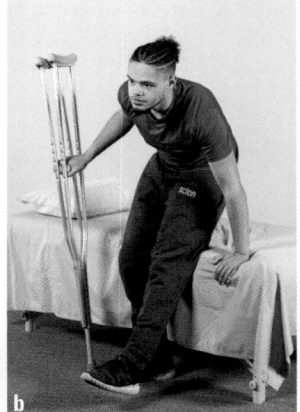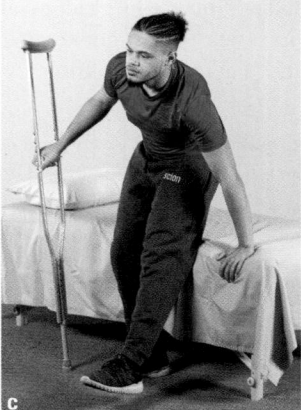

Figure 8.2   Sit to stand from the bed using an assistive device: *(a)* a walker, *(b)* two crutches, and *(c)* one crutch.

extremity and potentially both arms. The patient may need to scoot toward the edge of the bed with the use of his arms so he can move the uninvolved lower extremity off the bed and onto the floor. From this position, the arms can be used to help move the involved lower extremity from the bed to the floor. Once both feet are on the floor, the patient can move to a standing position, either weight bearing or non–weight bearing on the involved extremity, depending on the injury or surgery restrictions.

Spinal Injury or Surgery   It is common for any movement to be painful and challenging after an injury or surgery to the axial skeleton, including getting into and out of bed. Getting into bed often requires the use of both upper and lower extremities. If the patient's involved region is the lumbar spine, lowering herself to the bed is typically slow and is guided by both upper and lower extremities. The patient may use her arms to push down on the back of a chair placed beside the bed to help her get into and out of the bed. If the patient is going to sleep in bed after an injury or surgery to the lumbar spine, using the arms in this way reduces stress on the lumbar region.[15]

After an injury or surgery to the cervical spine, sitting on and standing from the edge of the bed are usually not difficult. This patient population often is challenged by the transitions from sitting to lying and return to sitting. The patient should use the upper extremities to control the descent from sitting and then moving onto the side as the lower extremities are raised toward the bed while the patient lies down (figure 8.3). Once the patient is side-lying, he or she should pause for as long as needed to become comfortable in that position. If the patient does not become comfortable in side-lying, reclining may be a better sleeping position. However, once the patient becomes comfortable in side-lying without nausea or dizziness, he or she can use the upper and lower extremities to slowly scoot away from the side of the bed. Similarly, the patient

should use the arms to slowly push the trunk up from a side-lying position as the legs are simultaneously moving off the edge of the bed toward the floor. Once the patient is in a sitting position, he or she should pause and allow any nausea or dizziness to pass before standing.

This style of upper extremity use with lower-extremity counterbalance to get into and out of bed is also recommended for any patient after a lumbar spine injury or surgery. Moving the lower extremities at the same time and as a counterbalance to the upper body movement is more important for reducing soreness in the lumbar region than in the cervical region; by moving in this way, the body remains as straight as possible and avoids lumbar spine rotation or side-bending, two motions that increase lumbar strain.

Rolling over in bed is sometimes unavoidable. After spinal injury or surgery, rolling over in bed requires some thought in order to avoid unnecessary strain to the spine. When patients roll from left side-lying to right side-lying (figure 8.4), instruct them to straighten the right leg and flex the left hip and knee to approximately 60°. Once they are in that position, instruct them to push the lateral aspect of the left thigh and knee into the bed as the right shoulder performs extension so the right hand can feel the bed. Using the left leg and arm to initiate the rolling motion, and the neuromotor guidance of the right arm, allows the patient to roll supine as a unit. The patient may need a pause in this position to allow any nausea or dizziness to pass. Keeping the left hip and knee flexed so the left foot is flat on the bed and the right knee straight, the patient continues to reach across the body with the left arm and pushes with the left foot down into the bed to roll the upper body and lower body as a unit toward the right side. This concept is called "log rolling" because the intent is to roll the axial skeleton as a unit and avoid unnecessary twisting by using the arms and legs to perform the movement.

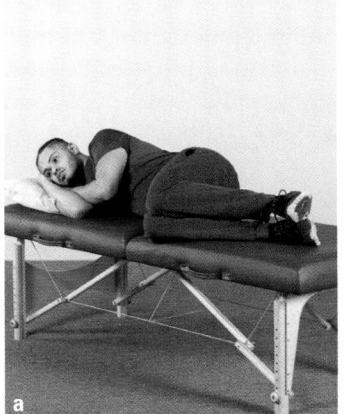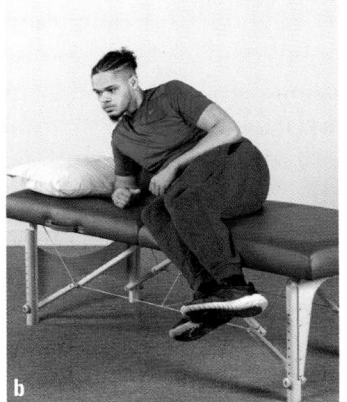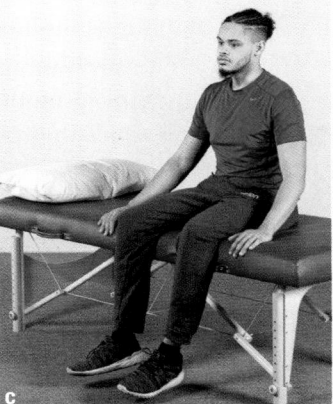

Figure 8.3   Getting into and out of bed using the upper extremities and moving the body as a unit : *(a)* side-lying, *(b)* pushing off, and *(c)* sitting upright. The lower extremities serve as a counterbalance to upper torso movement to prevent rotation and side-bending of the spine.

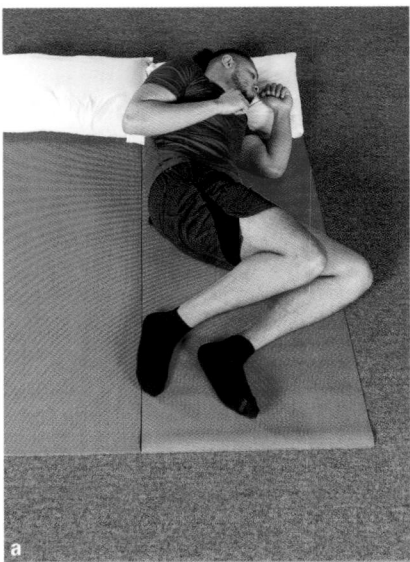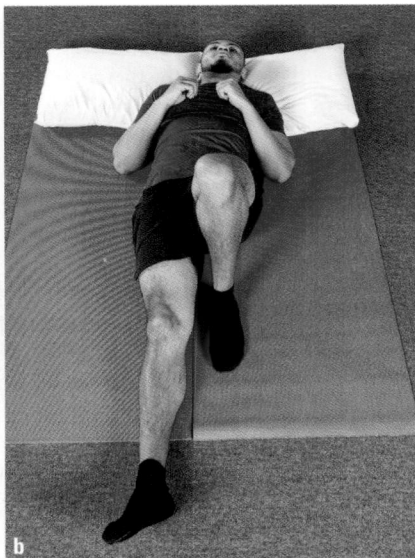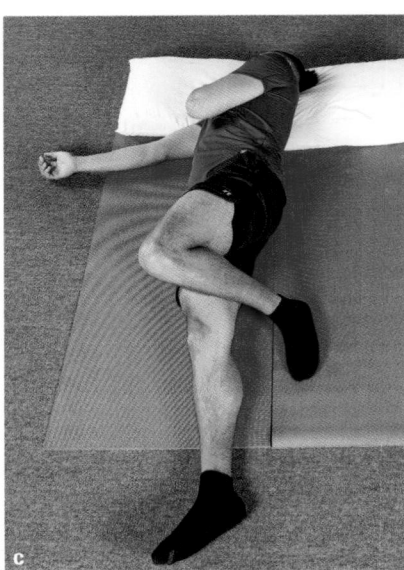

Figure 8.4   Log rolling onto the right side without rotation or side-bending the spine : *(a)* reach the right arm backwards as the right knee is straightened; *(b)* keep the left knee flexed and use it to push the pelvis to roll towards the left as the left arm is reaching across the body; and *(c)* lay on the right side without spinal rotation.

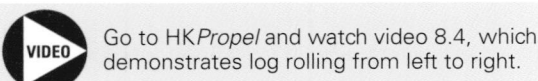 Go to HK*Propel* and watch video 8.4, which demonstrates log rolling from left to right.

Upper-Extremity Injury or Surgery   Bed mobility is usually not a challenge after an upper-extremity injury or surgery. Because the patient's legs are uninvolved, sitting on the edge of the bed and standing again are not difficult. Bed mobility, such as rolling over in bed, is not advised if the patient is wearing a sling, particularly a sling with an abduction pillow. As long as the patient is experiencing soreness while trying to sleep, wearing a sling is recommended. Patients are usually eager to remove the sling as soon as possible after a shoulder injury or surgery. However, removing a sling at night prematurely can lead to reinjury.

Sit to Stand

The sit-to-stand motion is the activity of moving from sitting to standing and back to sitting. This movement is very similar to a squat. Squatting mechanics are discussed in chapter 17; however, this section presents instructions to a patient on how to perform this activity independently when normal movement patterns are impaired after an injury or surgery. Because sit to stand involves the lower extremities, performance of this task after an injury or surgery to the upper extremities will not be covered in this section.

Lower-Extremity Injury or Surgery

The sit-to-stand motion is one that we perform many times over the course of a day, and we do it without conscious awareness until it becomes difficult. When patients cannot use both legs normally, they need instruction to perform

this task. Regardless of the type or location of injury or surgery, the patient should have just slightly more body weight through the heels than through the balls of the feet while moving from sitting to standing. Anecdotally, a 60% to 40% division of body weight between the heel and the forefoot is recommended. Since the patient must lean forward to perform this activity, there is a greater risk of falling if the patient puts more weight on the forefoot than on the heels because of altered use of leg musculature[16] with increased demand on the involved paraspinal musculature.[17] Placing just a little more weight on the heels can reduce the risk of falling forward.

If the patient must wear a walking boot or knee immobilizer or is NWB on the involved extremity, minimal to no weight is placed on this limb during the transfer from sitting to standing. Obviously then, the uninvolved lower extremity becomes the primary mover. If the patient's uninvolved lower extremity is not strong enough to perform sit to stand independently, the upper extremities must assist with the movement (figure 8.5). If a walking boot or knee immobilizer is worn, the involved lower extremity is abducted away from midline and the center of mass is shifted to the uninvolved lower extremity. To rise from sitting, the patient first scoots toward the front third of the chair and flexes the knee so the foot is underneath him to give the uninvolved lower extremity the leverage needed to perform this motion. If this extremity is strong enough, sit to stand can be performed from this position. In cases where the uninvolved lower extremity lacks sufficient strength, the upper extremities provide the assistance to complete this task. Hands may be placed on the chair seat, chair arms, assistive ambulation devices, the back of another nearby

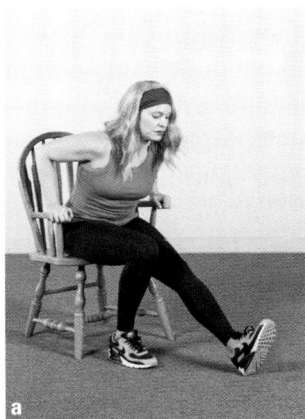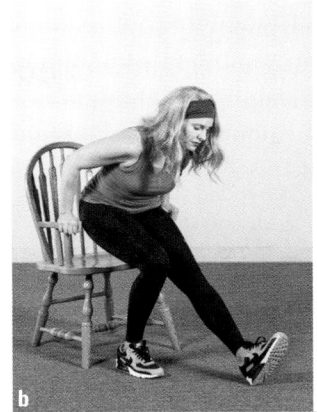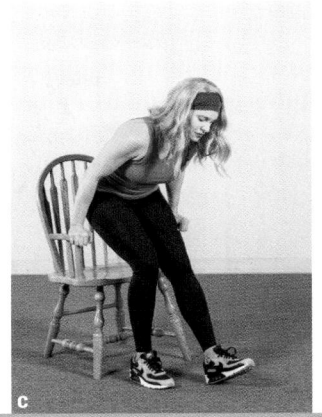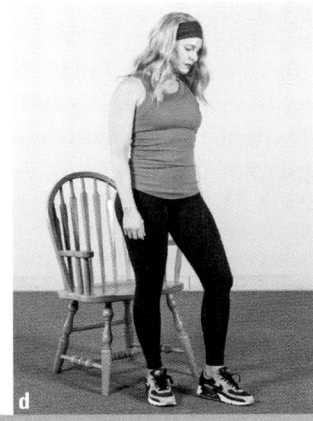

Figure 8.5 Sit to stand using the uninvolved lower extremity and upper extremities: *(a)* lean forward and use the uninvolved right leg and the arms to prepare to stand; *(b)* push up with the right leg and arms without using the left leg; *(c)* continue to use the right leg and arms to stand up without using the left leg; and (d) finish the process while using the uninvolved right leg for standing.

chair, or any nearby sturdy object. Oftentimes, the arms are used merely to start the motion to overcome inertia so the lower extremity can take over and complete the activity. If the patient uses crutches for assistance, care must be taken to prevent them from falling backward and throwing the patient off balance. Similarly, patients who use a cane in sit to stand should be made aware that the cane may tip sideways, causing them to fall.

Patients who are PWB on the involved extremity can use that limb to assist in sit to stand, and the upper-extremity effort diminishes or is eliminated, according to the patient's abilities and needs. When orthotic devices are removed or a hinged knee immobilizer is unlocked and there are no weight-bearing restrictions, the involved lower extremity is used during the sit-to-stand activity.

Once FWB is permitted on the involved extremity, the patient should use both lower extremities equally in the sit-to-stand activity. Patients who have just returned to FWB status are often reluctant to bear weight on the involved extremity at first, so the rehabilitation clinician must watch and correct patients who shift their center of mass toward the uninvolved extremity rather than keeping it between the two. During sit to stand, if the feet are flat but one foot is slightly ahead of the other, the leg of the posteriorly positioned foot will need to work harder.[18]

Once the patient is FWB on the injured extremity, the sit-to-stand activity can be used as a strengthening exercise by changing the way it is performed. One way to do this is to change foot placement. During a normal sit-to-stand activity, the feet are flat on the floor and relatively even with each other. To increase the resistance to the involved extremity and use the activity as an exercise, instruct the patient to place the uninvolved extremity's foot ahead of the involved extremity's foot; during sit to stand, the involved limb must then bear more of the body weight. The farther forward the uninvolved limb's foot is on the floor, the less it is recruited, and the more body weight the involved

limb must lift. Another method of exercise progression incorporates a step stool or block placed under the uninvolved limb's foot; this device shifts the body weight to the involved limb and forces the patient to use that extremity to a greater degree to perform sit to stand. Conversely, when the patient is NWB or PWB on the injured extremity, the farther forward the involved limb's foot is on the floor, the less it is recruited, and the more body weight the uninvolved limb must lift (figure 8.6).

Spinal Injury or Surgery

As described earlier, movement can be painful during the early days of rehabilitation following an axial skeletal injury or surgery. Sit to stand with this patient population is slightly different from patients with lower-extremity injuries. The objective with these patients is to use the legs symmetrically so spinal rotation or side-bending are avoided. The rehabilitation clinician instructs the patient to scoot to the front third of the chair and comfortably place both feet flat on the floor. Patients who must use the upper

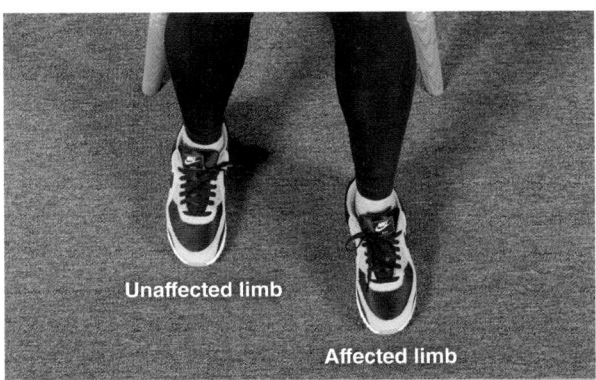

Figure 8.6 Position of the feet in a staggered stance during sit to stand with the involved limb farther forward. This foot position promotes greater use of the uninvolved lower extremity and places less force on the involved limb.

extremities to assist them are instructed to place their hands on a sturdy surface, such as the chair arms or a nearby table. The patient is instructed to lean forward from the hips and not from the back to reduce strain on healing tissue. From this position, the patient uses the lower extremities to stand with slightly more weight on the heels as described previously. This is important for this patient population because the paraspinal muscles are often weak or have a delayed neuromotor response, resulting in an increased tendency to fall forward during sit-to-stand activity. Additionally, pushing with slightly more emphasis through the heels promotes additional activity from the extenders of the hip and knee,[19] reducing stress on the extenders of the trunk.[18]

Verbal cues can be helpful. Asking the patient to lean forward using a "nose over toes" cue can help the patient learn to perform hip hinging without undue lumbar movement. "Push through your heels" can be a useful cue to help the patient to remember to use the legs to stand.

Performing a stand-to-sit task may require the clinician to cue patients to stand so that they can feel the chair behind their legs, perform a hip hinge so the pelvis shifts backward as the upper body leans forward in a "nose over toes" motion, and slowly lower the body with the legs to the seat of the chair. These actions help reduce potential jarring of the spine as the body returns to a seated position.

General Personal Hygiene

This section provides examples for instructing patients in ways to perform some personal hygiene tasks. Some tasks, such as brushing teeth and using eating utensils with the nondominant extremity, are learned by simply performing the task and acquiring neuromotor control. If they know in advance that surgery will be followed by a time of restricted mobility and use of the dominant arm, rehabilitation clinicians should encourage patients to practice performing tasks beforehand with their nondominant arm. Suggest that they place their dominant arm inside their shirt and tuck it to the side so they cannot use it. This will help them understand how basic activities will be affected, and it will give them an opportunity to practice dominant-extremity activities with the nondominant arm.

Lower-Extremity Injury or Surgery

Two of the more difficult hygiene tasks after an injury or surgery to the lower extremity are bathing and toileting. Taking a shower in a walk-in shower is an easier bathing task than taking a bath or shower that requires the patient to get into and out of a bathtub. Whether the patient's bathing facility is a walk-in shower or a bathtub, instruct the patient to put a chair of some kind in the shower. Shower chairs or stools are readily available in many stores as well as online, or the patient can use any chair or seat in the shower provided it is sturdy, waterproof, and not too low for them to comfortably perform sit-to-stand tasks.

Getting into and out of a bathtub for showering is similar to sit to stand. Patients who are NWB on the involved lower extremity use the uninvolved lower extremity and upper extremities to lower themselves to a sitting position on the edge of the bathtub. They then step into the bathtub with the uninvolved lower extremity and use their arms as needed to help move the involved lower extremity into the tub. Using the uninvolved lower extremity and pushing with the upper extremities on the edge of the bathtub, the patient moves onto the shower chair.

If the patient is strong enough and the involved lower extremity doesn't need much assistance from the arms for movement, an alternate method can be considered. The patient sits on the edge of the bathtub and moves the uninvolved lower extremity into the bathtub while the involved lower extremity remains out of it. The patient uses the uninvolved lower extremity and both hands on the edge of the bathtub to push up into a standing position, then uses the bath chair for balance and moves the involved lower extremity into the bathtub.

Before the patient resumes bathing activities, advise him or her to purchase waterproof bandage or an alternative occlusive dressing[20] to keep extra moisture out while protecting and maintaining an appropriately moisturized wound field. Although they may need assistance the first few times bathing is attempted, the task becomes easier as the patient learns, uses the technique, and can also use the involved extremity more as the injury continues to heal.

The challenge of toileting after an injury or surgery to the lower extremity is partly due to the fact that the toilet is often lower than a standard chair. This can be problematic since the lower the seat, the more difficult it is to perform a sit-to-stand activity. The necessary steps in toileting include pulling down pants and undergarments, sitting down, wiping, standing up, pulling up the undergarments and pants, flushing, and handwashing. If the patient wears a walking boot, this process is often not difficult. It is more challenging if the patient must use an immobilizer for the knee (figure 8.7).

If the patient is wearing the knee immobilizer or hinged brace outside of the pants and cannot pull the undergarments and pants down far enough to perform toileting tasks, the patient begins by using both arms to maintain stability on crutches or rails as most, if not all, of the body weight is borne on the uninvolved leg. The patient then removes the knee immobilizer and lowers the pants and undergarments while standing. If the patient cannot bend the involved knee, the patient then must sit down without using or bending the involved lower limb. As described in sit to stand, patients may need the use of their arms to sit on the toilet. Upon completion, the patient performs sit to stand with the use of the uninvolved limb and the upper extremities as needed. While standing on the uninvolved lower extremity, the patient pulls up the undergarments and pants.

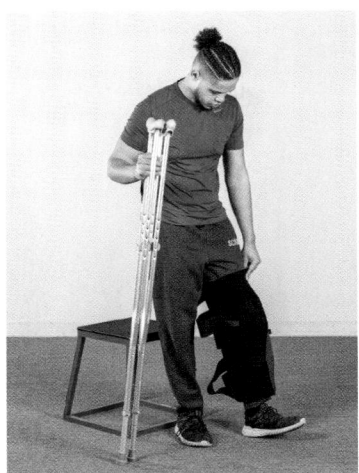

Figure 8.7 Sit to stand from a toilet-height seat while wearing a knee immobilizer.

The patient reapplies the knee immobilizer, which may require the patient to sit on the toilet to do so. After the patient flushes the toilet and washes his or her hands, the patient should also use a cleaning wipe of some kind to wipe the clasps and straps of the immobilizer.

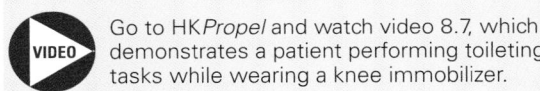

Go to HK*Propel* and watch video 8.7, which demonstrates a patient performing toileting tasks while wearing a knee immobilizer.

In the interest of efficiency, the patient should avoid allowing the pants and undergarments to fall to the floor. If they do happen to fall to the floor, the patient must bend over to pick them up from a standing or seated position, which requires enough trunk flexibility to perform this task repeatedly. If the patient doesn't have adequate trunk flexibility while standing, a grabber or reaching device may be needed. This type of device is described later in this chapter. If the patient can use the involved limb, toileting tasks become much easier and more closely resemble sit-to-stand activities.

Some patients may find the sit-to-stand task from a low toilet seat to be too challenging, even with the use of both upper extremities. In this case, a seat riser may be an option. This device raises the height of the toilet seat so that sit to stand is easier. Following a total knee arthroplasty or a total hip arthroplasty, a portable commode that is higher than a standard toilet may be warranted. Both of these assistive devices can be found online, in a medical supply store, or in some pharmacies.

Other personal hygiene tasks such as applying and removing makeup, brushing teeth, shaving, or hair care and styling may be difficult for lower-extremity patients, especially if they are NWB on the involved extremity. They are likely to find that it is more comfortable to sit to perform these activities than to stand on one lower extremity.

Spinal Injury or Surgery

In this chapter, we assume that the patient has insufficient help at home and must perform ADLs alone. Without assistance, it can be difficult for the patient to cover healing surgical wounds of the spine. Traditionally, the standard of practice is to protect an open incision from shower or bathwater during the initial stages of healing. Since shower or bathwater can introduce bacteria into a healing wound, a sponge bath is often the best temporary form of self-cleansing for these patients. This is often done while sitting rather than standing since prolonged standing can be difficult for patients after spinal injury or surgery. Once the wound is healed, sitting while using the shower is recommended. A shower chair is recommended for patients with other spinal injuries in which wound protection isn't a concern. Interestingly, research has emerged indicating it is unnecessary to protect a fresh surgical incision from shower water because the incident rate of infection is identical whether the incision is protected with an occlusive dressing or not.[21-25]

After wounds are healed, or if they were not a concern, the use of a shower chair is often recommended because the hot water and standing with eyes closed may be problematic for some patients. Cervical spine patients may have difficulty washing their hair because of the cervical and upper-extremity motions required. Depending on the length and thickness of their hair, some patients may opt to wait until the neck is into the later proliferation phase of healing before trying to wash their hair without assistance.

Toileting strategies after lumbar injury or surgery may require a change in how patients wipe themselves. Other than that, the issue of sit to stand is similar to what we have previously discussed. Patients may need to use their arms to perform sit to stand due to the height of the toilet. An elevated toilet seat may benefit this patient population as well.

Other personal hygiene tasks such as toothbrushing, application of contact lenses, and application and removal of makeup may require the patient to sit because it is difficult to stand for extended periods. After an injury or surgery to the cervical region, a patient may respond favorably to the use of an electric toothbrush because it requires less stability and movement from the neck. In severe cases, the patient may find it more comfortable to sit with the head supported against the back of the chair to reduce cervical strain when toothbrushing or flossing. Because mandibular opening is linked to the cranium, C1, and C2,[26-29] the patient may experience cervical soreness from holding his or her mouth open for an extended period. Consequently, sitting with the head supported and taking short breaks while toothbrushing and flossing may reduce cervical soreness.

After a spinal injury or surgery, A patient may find that standing or sitting erect for toothbrushing is less stressful than bending over. If the patient can stand without dizziness or nausea, placing one foot on a small stool while standing at the sink decreases lumbosacral stress. Also, placing one hand on the counter for support while toothbrushing reduces spinal loading.

Upper-Extremity Injury or Surgery

When a patient is in the shower, most surgeons recommend keeping the surgical incisions as clean and dry as possible. After surgery to the hand or wrist, this goal is easily achieved by placing a plastic bag around the involved hand and securing it with a rubber band above the wrist and any surgical incisions. If the surgery involves the forearm, elbow, upper arm, or shoulder, the use of waterproof bandages or similar occlusive dressing can be used to keep the surgical incisions dry.[20] The use of injured fingers, hand, wrist, forearm, or elbow may be contraindicated during showering tasks. This restriction can become particularly tricky if the involved segment is the patient's dominant arm. With the exception of the axilla region of the uninvolved upper extremity, cleaning the rest of the body can be performed with one hand with relative ease. A suggestion for washing the uninvolved axilla is to use a soapy washcloth or loofa. Many patients have the shoulder mobility to use that object to reach the ipsilateral axilla and somewhat wash that region. If the patient's shoulder isn't mobile enough, the patient can use the uninvolved hand to swing the washcloth or loofa toward the axilla of the same arm and adduct the arm to pin the soapy washcloth or loofa between the humerus and rib cage in the axilla region. After showering, patients may struggle at first to dry themselves with one hand, but with repetition they soon become more proficient.

When the forearm or hand is the affected segment, showering is easier than it is with an injury to the upper arm or shoulder. When the involved region is the elbow or distal to the elbow, the extremity's shoulder can still be used for reaching and general movement. When the involved region is the upper arm or shoulder, the involved upper extremity must remain at the patient's side and cannot be used in showering activities. To reduce the risk of soreness, pain, and reinjury, showering tasks are performed only with the uninvolved upper extremity.

When washing the axilla region with upper arm or shoulder involvement, the patient is instructed to bend at the waist and allow both arms to dangle and hang freely in front of the body (figure 8.8). Each axilla region may be cleansed in this position since the involved shoulder is passively hanging and is not actively engaged in moving the arm away from the body. The patient can cleanse each axilla using elbow flexion to reach the axilla region of the opposite arm as demonstrated in video 8.8 in HK*Propel*. This position can also be used to apply antiperspirant and

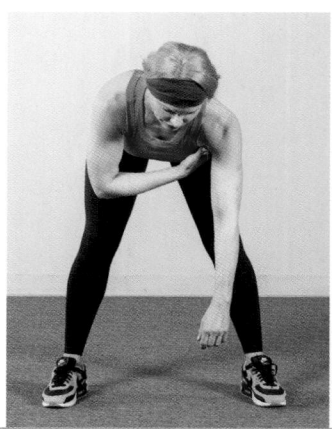

Figure 8.8   Washing the axilla of the involved upper extremity when active motion is not permitted. This position can be used to clean the area and apply antiperspirant and deodorant.

deodorant to the axillae. Cleanliness of the involved axilla is important, especially if the involved upper extremity must remain in a sling throughout the day.

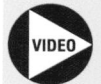 Go to HK*Propel* and watch video 8.8, which demonstrates a patient washing under the uninvolved and involved axilla after shoulder injury or surgery.

Toileting tasks are to be performed with one hand. Some of these tasks require practice and repetition to improve proficiency, while others are not as difficult. It is beneficial to caution the patient to avoid dropping his or her pants and undergarments below the knees because it is easier to pull them back up with one hand if those garments are knee high rather than on the floor. Sometimes it is unavoidable, and the garments fall to the floor. The clinician should be proactive and warn the patient that if he finds himself in this situation it is easier to pull the garments up to his knees with one hand while sitting on the toilet rather than trying to pull them up while standing.

If this patient population finds it too difficult to perform other hygiene and self-care activities such as shaving or applying makeup with the nondominant hand, it may be best to point out that these activities can be postponed to a later date when the dominant hand can perform these tasks. Toothbrushing, although awkward, is often manageable when performed by the nondominant hand because it requires less precision than shaving or applying makeup. Patients with long hair may be unable to style their hair with the use of only one upper extremity. In this case they may be better served to ask for help from a family member, friend, or coworker.

Don and Doff a Shoulder Sling With Abduction Pillow

After an injury or surgery to the shoulder region, the patient must often use a sling with a Velcro-attached abduction pillow. As part of the patient's daily routine during this time, she must be able to put on and remove the sling independently, so you should instruct her in this activity.

During the initial rehabilitation session, the sling must be properly fitted and adjusted to provide comfort with minimal stress to the patient and especially to the injured segment (figure 8.9). Evaluate the position and fit of the sling and abduction pillow. The elbow should sit in the back and bottom of the sling. If the patient cannot feel his or her olecranon process being supported by the sling, shoulder and neck pain are possible. Check the size of the sling to make sure that the patient feels it supporting the humerus and not the forearm or wrist. Sometimes the patient's forearm is too slender or the humerus is too short for the sling. It can be helpful in such cases to fold a small hand towel or washcloth and place it in the pocket of the sling where the elbow's olecranon process should rest. Packing the back of the sling with a comfortable cloth in this way will help the patient to feel the sling's support of the humerus.

The next objective is to ensure that the patient's hand is higher than the elbow. If the hand is lower than the elbow, the shoulder will be supported by the forearm or wrist region; in such a position, the humerus is poorly supported, and this will result in shoulder soreness and neck pain. Once the patient feels comfortable with the sling supporting the distal humerus with slight elevation of the hand relative to the elbow, you can be assured that the sling is performing its intended function. The sling will now hold the humerus and forearm against gravity, allowing for passive support rather than allowing the wrist to actively push the forearm into the sling to support the humerus. This position also uses gravity to reduce edema in the wrist and hand.

The top of the abduction pillow is positioned under the pectoralis muscle. The humerus should be sitting in a comfortable degree of slight shoulder flexion and abduction; some researchers advocate for slight medial humeral rotation,[14] others for neutral to slight lateral humeral rotation,[30, 31] depending on the type of surgery. The position of the abduction pillow helps the humerus to remain in this position of rest to promote healing and reduce soreness.[14, 30, 31] Adjustments to the sling and abduction pillow are made using the pillow support straps around the patient's torso and neck. The strap around the patient's torso should be snug without being tight. This strap prevents the abduction pillow from sliding out of position. Another Velcro strap wraps around the posterior aspect of the patient's involved shoulder and the contralateral aspect of the neck. This strap shouldn't require significant tension if the sling and abduction pillow are positioned correctly, but it shouldn't be loose either. Proper fit and placement of the bolster and sling are important to help keep the hand and elbow supported and the patient comfortable. If the patient feels his neck is providing most of the support for his shoulder, the sling and abduction pillow are not properly adjusted and should be refit.

The shoulder sling with abduction pillow is used after rotator cuff repair,[14] SLAP lesion repair,[31] and total shoulder arthroplasty.[30] Anecdotally, a shoulder sling with abduction pillow can also be used for patients after a fracture to the proximal humerus or a shoulder dislocation, but shoulder slings without abduction pillows are used more often in those cases. In general, if the patient is using a sling without an abduction pillow, the implication is that the patient can use the involved shoulder, provided pain and soreness do not increase. In such cases, patients can don and doff the shoulder sling much more easily than when surgery requires them not to use the shoulder at all. Following are some suggestions on how to advise a patient to independently don and doff a shoulder sling with connected abduction pillow in cases where the involved upper extremity is not to be used.

The patient will often need advice about how to don (put on) and doff (take off) the shoulder sling and abduction pillow independently without the use of the involved upper extremity (figure 8.10). To don the sling, the patient starts

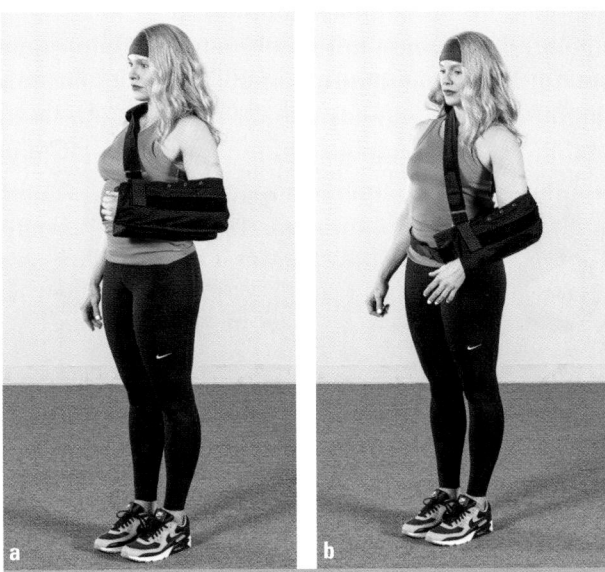

Figure 8.9 Proper sling position. The position of the shoulder in the sling should be abduction, slight flexion, and neutral rotation. The bottom of the sling should be felt by the elbow. The hand should be at least as high as the elbow, preferably higher. The abduction pillow should be under the pectoralis major muscle. *(a)* Correct upper-extremity placement within a sling. *(b)* Incorrect sling position: The sling is too far anterior and the hand is below the elbow, placing strain on the patient's neck.

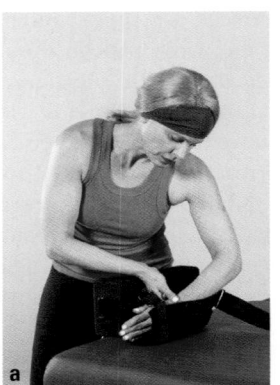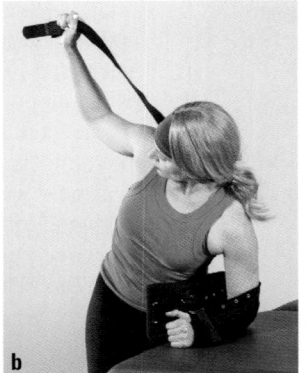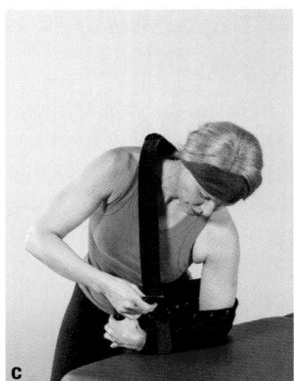

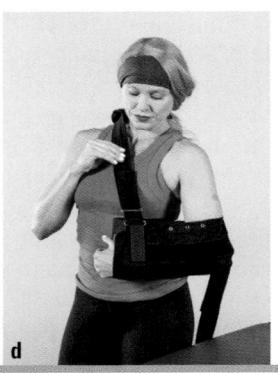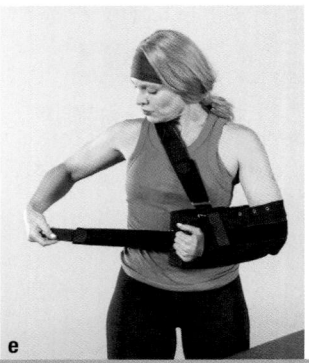

Figure 8.10 Suggested sequence for independently donning a shoulder sling with abduction pillow: *(a)* place the sling on a surface and use the uninvolved hand to guide the involved hand and elbow into the sling; *(b)* squat down slightly to keep the involved arm in the sling as the upper strap is guided around the neck; *(c)* attach the upper strap to the sling; *(d)* stand up, properly position the abduction pillow on the rib cage, and secure the upper strap; and *(e)* attach the torso strap to the sling and secure it to the body.

by placing the sling and connected abduction pillow on a surface such as a table, desk, or countertop. The patient uses the uninvolved upper extremity to ensure that the sling is open and positioned properly. The patient then supports the involved upper extremity with the uninvolved upper extremity, maintaining relaxation of the involved limb. He or she uses the uninvolved upper extremity to move the involved arm passively into the sling envelope.

Depending on the patient's height and the height of the surface on which the sling is positioned, he or she may have to squat down slightly to help the involved limb remain passive during this process. The patient will feel the bottom and back of the sling's envelope, or folded towel if one is necessary, with the olecranon of the distal humerus. The patient then ensures the abduction pillow is snug against his or her body and is high enough that it is next to the ribs and under the pectoralis muscle. Before the patient stands upright and while the arm is still supported by the countertop or desk surface, the patient closes the top of the sling and clips the strap around the neck into place so the sling and abduction pillow remain still when the patient stands upright. Upon standing, the patient clips the strap around his or her torso. If the abduction pillow and sling are properly positioned, the neck strap will feel

as if it has nominal tension on it. The placement of a washcloth in the axilla of the involved upper extremity before donning the sling and abduction pillow provides skin protection and moisture absorption if necessary.

 Go to HK*Propel* and watch video 8.10, which demonstrates a patient independently donning a shoulder sling with abduction pillow without the use of the involved upper extremity.

Independent donning of a shoulder sling with abduction pillow is more challenging than doffing. The involved upper extremity should remain as passive as possible during the doffing process, particularly during the initial inactive phase of healing, in order to reduce stress in the healing structures. As long as the patient performs the process slowly and supports the passive involved upper limb, removing the sling is not complicated. Instruct the patient to squat down or bend over so the involved upper extremity is supported by an elevated surface, such as a countertop or table. The involved upper limb remains relaxed as the uninvolved upper extremity unfastens the torso and cervical straps and opens the top of the sling. While the uninvolved upper extremity is holding the involved upper limb, the patient stands up and leaves the sling and connected abduction pillow on the surface. The patient can then slowly allow the passive involved upper extremity to hang at the side in a relaxed state. The fitting process and learning to don and doff the sling and abduction pillow independently will take some practice, but it is an important step during the patient's initial session, because reducing stress on the healing tissues has long-range benefits in the rehabilitation process.[4]

Self-Dressing

Patients usually cannot schedule an injury or surgery at the most convenient times for recovery. There may be snow on the ground when they need to use crutches, and they may need to put on a coat to go outside while wearing a shoulder sling. Generally, warm weather makes it easier to dress oneself after an injury or surgery. Shorts are easier than jeans. Short-sleeved shirts are easier than long-sleeved shirts. Donning and doffing a jacket with a sling is challenging, not to mention getting around in the ice, snow, and slippery conditions. The proper use of a knee immobilizer and shoulder sling may require temporary fashion adjustments.

One of the main objectives during the inactive phase of rehabilitation is to avoid aggravating or reinjuring the injured segment. If the patient repeatedly becomes sore from self-dressing, the rest of the rehabilitation process could be more difficult and have a poorer outcome.[4]

It is difficult for some patients to be seen in public with baggy pants, shorts, ill-fitting shirts, or other clothing that they don't normally wear. Rehabilitation clinicians can remind their patients that such fashion compromises are temporary, and they can point out that easier dressing makes for less strain on the injured tissues. Temporary fashion sacrifices are often recommended in the interest of healing. It is a fair assumption that most employers, supervisors, coworkers, and peers will be forgiving of fashion faux pas during this stage of recovery.

Lower-Extremity Injury or Surgery

As with other personal hygiene tasks, self-dressing is easiest to do while sitting when the patient has an injury or surgery to a lower extremity. This patient population usually has no difficulty performing self-dressing tasks for the upper body in the seated position. However, they may need some guidance for putting on undergarments, pants, socks, and shoes. For patients with enough trunk flexibility to bend over and don these items on both lower limbs, self-dressing is more inconvenient than difficult. Patients who are NWB on the injured lower extremity may still be able to sit and bend at the hips and trunk to don undergarments, pants, and socks. An alternative strategy is, while sitting, to don the undergarment only on the uninvolved lower extremity and let it remain at ankle level. The patient

then performs sit to stand and places the involved lower extremity into the leg of the undergarment. The patient then sits again and bends at the hips and trunk to pull the undergarment up toward the knees. A similar process is performed for donning pants (figure 8.11).

 Go to HK*Propel* and watch video 8.11, which demonstrates a patient donning pants with NWB involved lower extremity.

However, if the patient lacks the requisite trunk flexibility, a "grabber" may be recommended (figure 8.12). A grabber or "reacher" is any tool that helps the patient to grasp or hold items. These tools can have varying lengths and may be adjustable. The distal end of a grabber is usually a hinged clasp with movement similar to the thumb and index finger, and at the proximal handheld end there is a trigger that the patient uses to open and close the distal clasp. The distal end can also be a hook designed to snag items.

The device is used to increase the patient's ability to reach and grab objects without bending over or climbing onto a stepstool. When used in self-dressing, this tool can be used to grab a sock, undergarment, or pants and pull these items up toward the patient's waist to the point where the patient can complete the task with the hands. Grabbers can be used to dress at the start of the day or to help pull undergarments and pants up after toileting. If the patient is not permitted to flex the involved hip or knee at all, it is difficult to get dressed unless a person has either adequate trunk flexibility or a grabber. When bending and reaching are difficult, it may be easiest for the patient to wear baggy pants and slip-on shoes.

While loose-fitting shoes are not recommended when ambulating with crutches or a knee immobilizer, they may be the only option available to the patient. In this

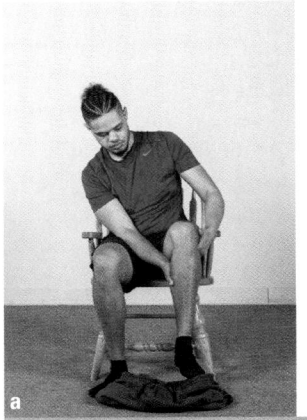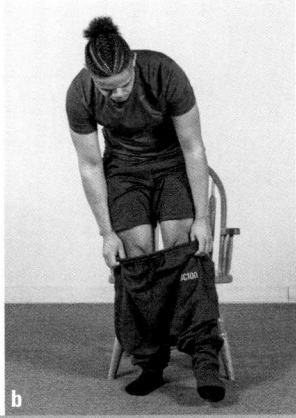

Figure 8.11 Donning pants with NWB involved lower extremity: *(a)* use the arms to place the involved left leg into the pant leg, and *(b)* use the uninvolved right leg to stand up, using the hands to pull the pants up, while not putting weight on the involved left leg.

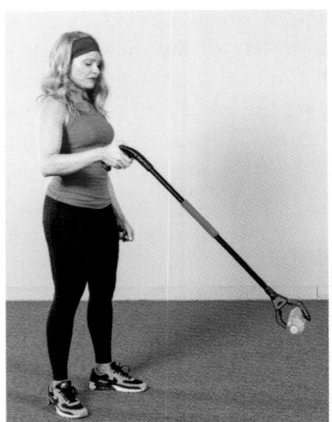

Figure 8.12   Example of a grabber and its use.

case, patients should be warned of the potential fall risk this type of footwear poses, and they must understand that these shoes require them to be more acutely aware of their surroundings during ambulation. As patients progress, they may be able to tolerate standing and putting one foot on the seat of a chair or similar surface to reach and tie shoelaces before being able to tolerate shoe tying from a seated position. For obvious reasons, a wedge or high heel shoe is not recommended during this phase of rehabilitation. Remember, the more the patient can flex the hip and knee and use the involved lower extremity, the easier self-dressing becomes.

In some cases, the physician or surgeon will recommend the patient wear the knee immobilizer or hinged brace on the skin. If a brace can be worn over pants, self-dressing and toileting tasks are as described previously. If the recommendation is to wear it against the skin, the patient may need to modify a few tasks. The patient will probably need to wear baggy athletic or workout pants to slide over the immobilizer or brace. With toileting, the patient allows the pants to drop to the floor and takes the involved lower extremity out of the leg of the pants before pulling down the undergarment. The height of the immobilizer or brace on the patient's involved leg will determine if the patient must remove it before toileting. In most cases, once the involved lower extremity is removed from the leg of the pants, the undergarment can be slid down far enough, preferably not below the uninvolved knee joint, to permit toileting without removal of the immobilizer or brace. However, if the top of it is close to the hip joint, the immobilizer or brace may need to be removed for successful toileting. Once toileting is complete, and the patient has reapplied the immobilizer or brace if removal was necessary, the patient uses the uninvolved lower extremity and upper extremities as needed to stand up. The undergarment is pulled up and the involved lower extremity is placed into the leg of the pants. The patient's trunk mobility determines if the patient

can bend over to the floor and pull the pants up, or if the patient needs a grabber for assistance.

Spinal Injury or Surgery

The advantage this patient population usually has is that he or she should have full or nearly full use of the upper and lower extremities. Therefore, self-dressing is typically easier, but the patient may fatigue quickly. Sitting is usually the easiest position in which to perform most self-dressing and personal hygiene tasks. Patients in this population may experience dizziness and fatigue from standing for even a short time, particularly in the first few days after spinal surgery. Once the patient has performed the requisite personal hygiene tasks while seated, dressing the upper body is typically uneventful. Dressing the lower body may require hip and trunk mobility beyond the patient's current capabilities, resulting in the necessity of a grabber. Or the patient may be able to stand and lean on an object for assistance during lower-extremity dressing. Sometimes leaning with the back against a wall provides enough stability to allow appropriate hip flexion to don undergarments, pants, and socks.

After a cervical spine injury or surgery, repetitive forward bending from a seated or standing position can generate dizziness, nausea, or pain, even if the patient has enough trunk mobility to perform the tasks. A grabber is an option for these patients, as is standing with wall support.

Shoe tying can be difficult for these patients. Most patients can stand and put one foot onto the seat of a chair or something similar; it is usually tolerable to bend forward to tie shoes from this position, even if the patient has had a recent lumbar or cervical surgery. If this position or the activity itself is not tolerated in any position, the patient may need to wear slip-on shoes or sandals until the position and activity are tolerated. As previously indicated, while slip-on shoes are not optimal, they may be the patient's only option. Throw rugs and other obstacles in the house that may cause the patient to fall should be removed in these situations.

Upper-Extremity Injury or Surgery

Self-dressing tasks with a sling and abduction pillow usually also require fashion compromises, particularly in the early stages of the inactive rehabilitation phase. While a sling is not required to be on skin, it shouldn't be applied over several layers of clothes either. After an injury or surgery to the shoulder or upper humerus, baggy clothes may be the best option to make dressing an easier task. Provided the patient has adequate hip and trunk flexibility to bend toward the floor, self-dressing the lower body usually consists of dropping the undergarment on the floor, stepping into the leg holes, and bending at the waist to allow the involved upper extremity to hang completely relaxed while the uninvolved upper extremity pulls the garment up to the waist. The process is repeated for the pants. It is much easier to pull up loose-fitting garments than tight-fitting garments with only one hand. If the patient lacks enough hip and trunk flexion to bend this far, a grabber may be used to pull the garment up enough for the uninvolved upper extremity to finish the task. Alternatively, the patient sits and uses a similar method to that described for standing by placing the garments on the floor and stepping into the legs. Some patients find it challenging to keep the involved upper extremity passive and unused while sitting to dress themselves. If this is the case, the patient should dress the upper body first, apply the sling, and then dress the lower body while sitting.

Socks are very difficult to don with one hand, particularly the foot on the same side as the involved upper extremity. A grabber will probably be needed. Similarly, shoe tying is not possible with one hand. Therefore, these patients commonly default to the use of slip-on shoes or sandals to avoid having to don socks and tie shoes. An alternate position that may work for some patients is to sit in a figure-4 position to don and doff shoes and socks. This position requires hip and trunk flexibility, so it may not work for all patients, but it may be an option worth exploring.

After an injury or surgery to the fingers, hand, wrist, forearm, or elbow, the process is similar to that described for the shoulder, with the exception that the involved upper extremity need not hang passively toward the floor. Since the involved structure is not the shoulder, the primary concern is restricting the movement of the more distal structures. Patients who must protect the elbow, forearm, wrist, hand, or fingers can sit or stand, whichever they prefer. A grabber may still need to be used, depending on the patient's hip and trunk flexibility. Even though the upper-extremity injury or surgery involves a different segment, the process of placing the garment on the floor and the recommendation of loose-fitting garments remains the same.

Self-dressing for the upper body is more challenging when the injury or surgery is to the patient's shoulder. As with lower-body clothing, the shirt should be baggy since it is easier to don and doff. Similar to self-dressing the lower body, the patient bends at the waist slightly, enough to permit the involved upper extremity to hang freely away from the trunk (figure 8.13). The amount of required trunk movement is considerably less than for self-dressing the lower body; the involved upper limb must only move away from the trunk slightly. This event should again be passive so the involved shoulder can be uninvolved in the process. The patient threads the involved limb into the open sleeve and begins to pull the shirt up toward the head. Once the involved limb is in the sleeve, the shirt is pulled over the head as the patient stands upright. The uninvolved limb then reaches up and through the open sleeve to complete the process. The looser the shirt, the easier this process is to perform with a passive involved upper extremity.

If the patient's injury or surgery is below the humerus in the fingers, hand, wrist, forearm, or elbow, the process is far easier since the shoulder of the involved limb can actively participate in putting the arm in the sleeve. Care must be taken to avoid snagging the involved segment on the clothing on the way in and out of the sleeve; this is especially important if the patient is wearing an orthotic, cage, or other protective device.

Should the patient be required to don a buttoned-up shirt, the process is similar, but easier. In the case of a shoulder injury, the patient again bends forward to allow the involved limb to hang passively as the uninvolved limb passes the sleeve onto the involved limb. The patient then stands upright with the involved arm hanging passively as the uninvolved limb moves behind the back to reach into its sleeve. As with overhead shirts, this process of donning a buttoned shirt is much easier when the injury or surgery involves the distal aspect of the upper extremity. It is challenging, but certainly possible, to use one hand to secure all the buttons on a button-up shirt. It is easier to start from

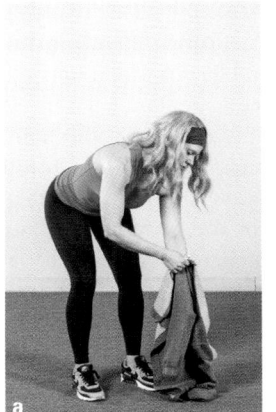 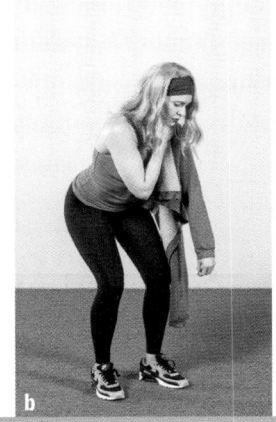 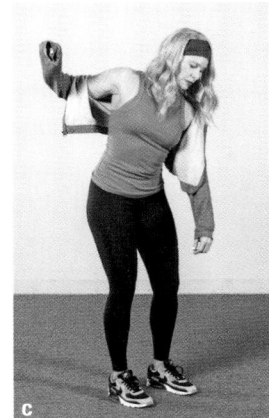

Figure 8.13 Self-dressing without the use of the involved upper extremity: *(a)* bend at the waist to allow the involved left arm to hang passively while the right arm is sliding the sleeve onto the left arm; *(b)* start to stand up while sliding the jacket over the involved limb; and *(c)* while keeping the involved arm passive, slide the uninvolved arm into the sleeve.

the top down rather than from the bottom up. Once the process is completed, the patient dons the shoulder sling and abduction pillow independently.

Female patients often choose to avoid donning and doffing a brassiere in the initial inactive phase of rehabilitation. As the patient becomes more comfortable with the process of self-dressing, donning and doffing a brassiere becomes an increasingly possible task. It is often easier to clasp the brassiere in front of the body using the uninvolved upper extremity to secure the clasp while the involved upper extremity anchors the garment between the humerus and ribs. After rotating the bra around to face the correct direction, the patient again leans over to allow the involved upper extremity to passively hang forward and uses the uninvolved upper limb to pass the brassiere strap around the involved arm and shoulder. The strap for the uninvolved upper extremity then follows suit. Due to the tighter fit of a sports bra, most patients need more time to pass in the healing process before they try to wear that item of clothing.

Meal Preparation

Preparing food after an injury or surgery can be time consuming and inconvenient. Generally, patients prefer to avoid spending a lot of time upright after injury or surgery because the effect of gravity on the healing structures can be a challenging and uncomfortable force to oppose. This is one of the main reasons that meal preparation should be as simple as possible. Most patients during this time have no desire to spend a lot of time in meal preparation and planning. Simple meal preparation requires less time to perform and is encouraged in these early days of rehabilitation. However, being active for short periods during the day does assist the body's overall function,[32] which is why independent ADLs, although time consuming and fatiguing, provide benefits to other aspects of physical and mental recovery.

It is not the purpose of this section to recommend a diet for this patient population. However, rehabilitation clinicians should make their patients aware of the importance of hydration and caloric intake to healing, and meals should be balanced and healthy. Many online resources are available that provide detailed dietary recommendations during the initial phases of healing.

Lower-Extremity Injury or Surgery

Meal preparation without the ability to stand for lengthy periods usually requires one of two solutions: sitting or leaning. If the patient can sit during meal preparation, that is recommended. Even sitting for short periods, such as while waiting for the microwave to finish, is beneficial. If meals can be prepared while sitting, meal preparation can be slightly more complex. However, a patient who needs to use crutches or a walker cannot carry a pan to the stove. The size of the patient's kitchen area is often a determining

factor in how complex meal preparation can be, even if the patient can sit for most of it.

Leaning on the uninvolved lower extremity using a wall, counter, or crutch can be helpful for short periods. Fatigue in the uninvolved limb is a limiting factor, and with fatigue comes an increased risk of falling. Although meal preparation usually requires more work from the upper extremities than from the lower extremities, lower-extremity injuries are stressed during prolonged standing or walking in the early days of rehabilitation, so the patient should be cautioned to avoid increasing soreness in the involved limb. Sitting and leaning on the uninvolved lower extremity are the best options for meal preparation; lower-extremity stress is reduced and upper extremities may be freely used. Patients should be cautioned to plan ahead and think through the meal preparation to accurately determine how stressful the activity will be before they begin an endeavor they cannot finish.

Spinal Injury or Surgery

As was mentioned previously, a patient with an injury or surgery to the axial skeleton still has full or nearly full use of the upper and lower extremities. Because one of the primary issues is fatigue and discomfort from standing for extended periods, the patient should take frequent breaks and sit as needed during meal preparation. There is no advantage in trying to push to the point of fatigue or pain. Fatigue is the body's way of telling us that it is time to rest and reduce stress on the healing structures. If the patient is taught to listen to and to properly interpret the warning signs, a functional task such as meal preparation should not add stress to healing structures.

If the patient must wear a rigid cervical collar, eating will require some adaptations. The higher the collar is on the patient's neck and the more the collar restricts mandibular movement, the more challenging eating becomes. The patient typically will have received dietary suggestions from the physician or surgeon's team. In the event that the patient has not received dietary advice, the clinician's first step would be to contact the referring physician to identify specific restrictions relative to mandibular movement.

The general recommendation for eating is to use a straw. Given that the patient may not be able to chew foods well due to the rigid cervical collar, one of the better delivery systems for nutrients and calories is through smoothies and shakes. Even a basic online search uncovers many recipes and variations for smoothies or similar meals the patient can easily prepare independently and that provide good nutrition to enhance tissue healing. Depending on the surgeon and surgery, the patient may be permitted to remove the rigid collar to eat, while the meal is prepared while wearing the cervical collar. In this scenario, the patient will need to sit up very straight and restrict head and neck movement while eating. It is challenging to remember to look down only with the eyes to see the food and to lift the utensil to the mouth without moving the head and neck for an entire meal. However, as with most every activity described in this chapter, repetition and practice improve proficiency, and these scenarios are temporary.

Upper-Extremity Injury or Surgery

The use of only one upper extremity during meal preparation limits the patient's options. Independent meal preparation takes more time; the process may take even longer if the involved upper extremity is the dominant arm. The less complex meal preparation is, the easier it is for the involved upper extremity to remain passive and relaxed.

It is easier to perform meal preparation and to eat with one upper extremity if these activities don't require the use of both upper extremities at the same time. For example, the patient cannot use a knife to cut food with only one upper extremity. If cutting food is unavoidable, the patient will be better served by asking someone else to do it.

Patients who have the advantage of having surgery scheduled and who can make preparations before surgery should be advised to prepare and freeze meals in advance. It is much easier to pull food from the freezer and to thaw and cook it in a microwave or on a stovetop than it is to make a meal from scratch with the use of only one upper extremity.

Summary

Basic functional tasks, or activities of daily living (ADLs), are important tasks that most patients have to perform every day. If patients don't have adequate assistance at home, guidance from a rehabilitation clinician can be crucial to their ability to maintain an independent lifestyle while recovering from injury. One of the primary objectives in the inactive phase of rehabilitation is for the patient to progress through the stages of healing without reinjury or pain. This means that patients must perform daily activities such as sleeping, getting into and out of bed, dressing themselves, sitting and standing, donning and doffing a sling, performing general hygiene tasks, and preparing a meal without irritating healing structures and without the help of others. Many functional tasks are made more challenging after injury or surgery to any body segment. The role of the rehabilitation clinician may include being an advisor and encourager. Patients often need to be reminded that frustration with basic functional tasks is common but temporary, and it can serve as a noticeable benchmark of improvement. Timely and helpful advice from the clinician can ease the emotional and physical distress that often results from faulty performance of ADLs.

LEARNING AIDS

Key Concepts and Review

1. Identify one strategy for sleep position and bed mobility for patients after an injury or surgery to the lower extremities, axial skeleton, and upper extremities.

Most patients tend to find a reclined position to be comfortable after an injury or surgery because it can reduce strain on the low back and reduce unconscious positional changes during sleep. If the patient is going to sleep in a bed, a supine position with pillows under the knees is recommended. While side sleeping is not recommended if the patient is wearing a shoulder sling, it can be comfortable after an injury or surgery to the lower extremity or axial skeleton, as well as to distal segments of the upper extremity. The use of a pillow between the knees and feet and a folded towel positioned underneath between the rib cage and pelvis often helps the patient to fall asleep. Most patients should use the uninvolved lower and upper extremities to get into and out of bed, as well as to move in bed. It is not recommended that patients support their body weight by pushing on the edge of the bed. However, they can use their arms on a stable object for assistance.

2. Discuss differences in sit-to-stand strategies after an injury to the axial skeleton compared with an injury or surgery to the lower extremities.

After an injury or surgery to a lower extremity, sit-to-stand activities will require extensive use of the uninvolved lower extremity. Should the uninvolved lower limb be unable to provide the requisite force to perform the task, the upper extremities should be used for assistance. As the involved lower extremity begins to gain strength, it should be progressively used more. After a spinal injury or surgery, the patient will have to lean forward to shift his or her center of mass enough to perform sit to stand. However, the patient must feel his or her heels on the ground during this activity to avoid falling forward. This patient population may also benefit from using the arms to help with this task.

3. Explain two unique challenges a patient will face when performing basic hygiene tasks after an injury or surgery.

Personal hygiene challenges vary depending on which region of the body is involved. The challenge for a patient after an injury or surgery to a lower extremity is the inability to stand on the involved lower limb. In addition, toileting activities will require modifications until the involved lower limb can be used. The challenge for a patient after spinal injury or surgery is the inability to move his or her neck or spine well during personal hygiene tasks. Despite the upper and lower extremities generally being uninvolved, fatigue can be a significant factor for these patients. The challenge for a patient after an injury or surgery to an upper extremity is finding a way to become proficient in these tasks while using only one upper limb. This can be a significant challenge if the dominant upper extremity is the involved limb.

4. Describe the process for a patient to don a shoulder sling with abduction pillow independently.

This process is easier if the sling has already been properly fitted by a rehabilitation clinician. First, place the sling on an elevated surface, such as a table or countertop and use the uninvolved hand to guide the involved arm, hand, and elbow into the sling. Second, squat down slightly to keep the involved arm in the sling as the upper strap is guided around the neck. Third, attach the upper strap to the sling with the uninvolved hand. Fourth, stand up, properly position the abduction pillow on the rib cage, and secure the upper strap. Fifth, attach the torso strap to the sling and secure it to the body. Check to be sure the sling is sitting in a neutral position on the side of the body with the hand slightly higher than the elbow.

5. Discuss two different challenges a patient will face during self-dressing tasks after a lower-extremity injury or surgery compared with an upper-extremity injury or surgery.

If the patient does not demonstrate adequate trunk mobility to perform self-dressing tasks, the use of a grabber may be needed after an injury or surgery to a lower extremity. For this patient population, self-dressing tasks are often performed while sitting. This is especially helpful for performing lower-body self-dressing tasks; upper-body tasks are generally much less challenging. Donning undergarments, pants, socks, and shoes may be challenging for patients with an involved lower extremity. Patients who have incurred an upper-extremity injury or surgery may need suggestions about how to perform self-dressing using one upper limb. The challenges for this patient population are that self-dressing tasks require more effort because only one arm can be used. Patients may need to be reminded that extra time will be needed each day to dress themselves and that temporary fashion sacrifices will be necessary.

6. Define two potential ramifications of lengthy meal preparation for any patient after an injury or surgery.

For any patient after an injury or surgery, the longer he or she is upright and walking around, the more fatigue and soreness are likely. While meal preparation often provides a sense of normalcy, it can prove detrimental to the patient's rehabilitation progress if he or she cannot safely complete the necessary tasks. Proper planning and simpler meal preparation are recommended.

Critical Thinking Questions

1. In the scenario presented at the beginning of the chapter, what basic functional activities will Ella encounter in the next 24 h? What should Tyler suggest to Ella to help her better perform self-dressing tasks? How should he instruct her to don her shoulder sling? How would Tyler's self-dressing recommendations change if Ella's accident resulted in hand and wrist injury or surgery? How would his personal hygiene recommendations change if she had sustained wrist and hand injury or surgery?

2. Your first patient of the day is a high school athlete who has had ACL reconstruction in the right knee. The patient's surgery was yesterday, so the knee immobilizer is locked in full extension. What sit-to-stand procedure would you recommend? What advice would you provide the patient for general personal hygiene tasks? Self-dressing? Sleep positioning?

3. Upon checking your caseload for next week, you notice a new patient on your schedule with the diagnosis of C5-C7 fusion. Which basic functional tasks do you suspect this patient may be struggling to perform? Not struggling to perform? Why? Would the tasks you suspect to be a challenge for this patient be the same tasks you would suspect to be a challenge after L4-S1 fusion?

Lab Activities

1. Position your lab partner in a side-lying sleeping position, as if he or she had a spinal injury or surgery. Compare the comfort level in the lumbar and cervical regions when the pillow is removed from between your lab partner's knees. Can your lab partner discern a difference in body weight distribution if he or she lies on a folded towel positioned above the pelvis and below the rib cage? How thick does the folded towed need to be before a change is noted? Can the folded towel be too thick? Instruct your lab partner to roll from one side to the other using log rolling.

2. Instruct your lab partner in a sit-to-stand process without the use of one leg. Does he or she need assistance from the upper extremities? Can your lab partner feel a difference in lower extremity use if one foot is positioned farther back than the other? Can your lab partner perform sit to stand while keeping his or her heels on the floor?

3. This evening, you and your lab partner are not going to use one of your arms at home; instead you will slide one of your arms into your shirtsleeve and leave it there for a few hours. How challenging is it to perform meal preparation? Toileting? Brushing your teeth? Self-dressing? Tomorrow morning, take a shower, dry off, perform your normal personal hygiene routine, and get dressed with one arm only. Which tasks were more challenging and which were less challenging than others? How much longer did it take you to perform these tasks? Compare your findings.

PART III

Rehabilitation Tools

*The whole is more than the
sum of its parts.*

Aristotle,
384 BC-322 BC, Greek philosopher

The next eight chapters delve into specific rehabilitation techniques of applying therapeutic modalities and aquatic therapy as well as using other therapeutic interventions to restore range of motion and flexibility, muscular strength and endurance, coordination and agility, soft-tissue and joint mobility, and functional and performance-specific abilities. Each of these tools can be used to advance a patient from disability to optimal, if not normal, function.

Recall from parts I and II that rehabilitation parameters are observed in a logical, cumulative sequence throughout the rehabilitation program. Part I introduced the concepts that help you understand what is important both during and after rehabilitation. Part II presented the first steps in the rehabilitation process, using your skills of observation, examination, and assessment to identify problems and design programs to correct them. Part III introduces the next essential step: incorporating the tools for rehabilitative intervention. Chapter 9 is a new chapter. It is a review for you; it offers reminders from previous coursework about modalities. The purpose of this chapter is to bring back into focus for you the factors that should be considered when you select modalities, based on the patient's problems and goals. The chapter also provides you with some instruments that you may find easier to use in the process of choosing modalities.

Chapter 10 describes aquatic exercises that are often used in rehabilitation. It provides many images and moves through the progression of exercises in a manner that is easy to follow. Aquatic activities have many advantages in rehabilitation, and they may be a convenient way to begin exercises early in the program.

Chapter 11 deals with all aspects of manual therapy. New information on the topic of joint manipulation has been added. The chapter also includes new information on instrument-assisted soft-tissue mobilization. Because joint mobilization techniques are such an integral part of treating orthopedic and sports injuries, this topic is introduced in this chapter, but specific applications are presented later in part IV.

Chapter 12 is where range of motion and flexibility are discussed—what normal joint motion is, and how to achieve it. Chapter 13 gives you a brief review of muscle anatomy, physiology, and neurophysiology to help you recall how the neural and muscle systems "talk" to each other to create neuromotor function. Methods of improving muscle strength are presented, along with various types of strengthening techniques, program progressions, and precautions.

Chapters 14 and 15 follow with the final segments of a rehabilitation program. Chapter 14 includes information on proprioception, neuromotor control, and the elements that it influences: balance, coordination, and agility. Progression from a static to a dynamic program is also explained. Chapter 15 begins with plyometrics—activities that require flexibility, strength, endurance, and proprioception. Although plyometrics is not always included in a rehabilitation program, it is important to know for those patients who are candidates for it. Plyometric exercises are added toward the end of a rehabilitation program but before performance-specific exercises. The last part of chapter 15 includes concepts of functional exercise and performance-specific exercises. Functional and performance-specific exercises make up the final stage in the progression of a rehabilitation program. To help you to create this final aspect of a rehabilitation progression, examples of an upper-extremity and a lower-extremity program are provided. Information on how to determine the patient's readiness to return to normal activities is also included.

The last chapter, chapter 16, is a new chapter. It puts all that has been presented in the textbook thus far into the final objective: How to put together a rehabilitation program for your patient. This chapter serves as an instruction on how to establish the framework for any rehabilitation program you will design for any patient you are treating. It also provides some important insights and keys that give you additional tidbits to create sound, justifiable programs.

The words of Aristotle apply to this part of the text. As you read through these chapters, the relevance of the information presented in parts I and II will become clearer. By the time you complete this section, you will have the knowledge of the when and a deeper understanding of the how needed for part IV. Parts I and II provided you with the how and why of practical rehabilitation program concepts and applications. When combined with part III, they will provide you with the knowledge, understanding, and insight you will need to become a practicing clinician. By the time you have completed this book, you will be able to apply what you have learned to develop your own rehabilitation programs and become the clinician you want to be.

9

Modalities

Objectives

After completing this chapter, you should be able to do the following:

1. Explain why superficial heat is contraindicated during the inflammation phase of healing.
2. Identify the main differences between superficial heat and cryotherapy.
3. Discuss the differences between treatment effects of ultrasound at 1 MHz and 3 MHz.
4. Identify contraindications for ultrasound.
5. Outline TENS treatment options that may be used to relieve pain.
6. List another type of electrical stimulation that may be used to relieve pain in addition to TENS, and explain how it is different than TENS.
7. Present examples of electrical stimulation that may be used in the first half of a rehabilitation program and what the reason might be for using them.

Joan Reeney is a certified athletic trainer working in a local sports medicine clinic for the past 2 years. Stephen Barrels is a right-handed 62-year-old who directs the city's orchestra. One of his leisure activities includes playing in amateur tennis tournaments throughout the city and state when he has the time. About 3 months ago, he ruptured his right supraspinatus tendon when he was practicing his tennis serve. He underwent a rotator cuff repair after which his right shoulder was placed in a bolster sling for 3 weeks. He told his surgeon that he was taking the orchestra on a 3-week performance tour in Europe and would perform shoulder exercises on his own during the tour.

Stephen has now returned from the orchestra's overseas trip and is seeking treatment from Joan for his right shoulder. Her examination reveals not only weakness throughout the shoulder complex but a frozen shoulder that is painful whenever he tries to elevate the arm. She realizes that she is going to have to deal with the frozen shoulder before she moves on to the rotator cuff repair. She has some options from which to choose to begin her treatment with Stephen today.

Diagnosis is not the end, but the beginning of practice.

Martin H. Fischer, 1879-1962,
German-born American physician and writer

Clinicians understand that a total rehabilitation program includes two main avenues: therapeutic modalities and therapeutic exercises. As we have discussed in previous chapters, modalities are used mainly as a passive form of treatment to achieve a variety of goals, such as reducing pain, relaxing muscle spasm, reducing edema, and promoting healing. Modalities are generally applied during the first half of a rehabilitation program when secondary effects after injury or surgery are most evident and in need of treatment.[1]

An in-depth discussion of modalities is beyond the scope of this textbook. However, we present a brief overview of a few of the more commonly used modalities to illustrate the decisions the rehabilitation clinician makes in designing a patient's program. For more thorough descriptions and information on therapeutic modalities, see the references for this chapter; there are also a number of modality textbooks and articles in professional journals you can consult.

The references cited throughout this chapter support or demonstrate advantageous results with the use of specific modalities; however, it should be noted that modality research evidence is often in conflict, some finding support and justification for their use while others find no benefit or improvement when compared with other treatment selections. The purpose of this chapter is to include brief information on commonly used modalities to provide you with an understanding of how, why, and where these modalities fit into the total rehabilitation program. As a clinician, it is up to you to determine, based on the evidence, your experience, and individual patient parameters, what works best for you and each of your patients in your clinical practice.

Modality Decisions in Rehabilitation

Clinicians create rehabilitation programs to address deficiencies affecting their patients' performance and to return them to an optimal level of performance, whether that optimal level is the patient's former level or a new and different level of function. A patient's performance may be impeded by an injury that occurred suddenly or by one that has developed over time. A patient seeks the clinician when he or she cannot resolve the problems independently. Sometimes the deficiency causes several significant impediments and sometimes it is a rather minor disorder.

Regardless of the injury's severity, type, or cause, the clinician must deal with the problem in a manner that helps the patient. Each rehabilitation tool should have a reason for being included in the program; whether it is a modality, manual technique, or exercise, the clinician must have a specific goal or objective and a plan for its use that is based on the patient's problem list. Such an approach requires the clinician to first evaluate the injury. As Dr. Fischer said in the opening quote, we are best able to treat the patient when we have an accurate diagnosis. Therefore, the clinician's examination becomes an important first step on the way to successful treatment and rehabilitation of the patient's condition.

As was mentioned in chapter 1, the WHO prefers that clinicians identify a patient's abilities not only from the perspective of their medical deficiencies but also on how well they can perform within their own environment. As health care professionals who deal with the entire patient, rehabilitation clinicians come by this perspective easily. During the examination, we identify the patient's limitations and abilities and develop a treatment plan based on where the patient is and what has to be achieved to attain the goals that have been mutually established between patient and clinician. Usually the specific rehabilitation goals lie within the umbrella goal of restoring the patient's status as an active and contributing member of the world in which he or she lives and functions. The specific goals for each patient depend on the abilities and limitations with which the patient presents initially and the progress that occurs as the patient works through the rehabilitation program.

The rehabilitation clinician's contributions to the patient's well-being include not only identifying the correct diagnosis, but also knowing how to resolve the problems that accompany that diagnosis. For example, a tennis player who rolled over on his ankle and subsequently tore the anterior tibiofibular and talofibular ligaments is diagnosed with an ankle sprain. However, before the clinician can rehabilitate the ankle sprain, she must first deal with the problems that resulted from that sprain: pain, swelling, muscle spasm, ecchymosis, and reduced function. If the clinician doesn't see the patient until 2 d after the ankle sprain occurs and finds that it is significantly edematous with ecchymosis present from the toes to the distal leg, the clinician's modality selection will be based on goals that include reducing the swelling and the ecchymosis and ensuring that additional edema does not develop. Since the patient also has pain, the modality that is selected should also reduce pain, or the clinician may choose to use another modality to deal with the patient's pain.

Appropriate modality selection relies on the clinician's knowledge, experience, and skill. Recall from chapter 1 that the components of evidence-based practice (EBP) include not only research evidence for the efficacy of treatment techniques, but also both what is appropriate for each patient and the experience and knowledge the clinician brings from previous patient encounters. The clinician relies on all of these factors to choose the modality whose effects will best achieve the patient's rehabilitation goals.[1]

Just as the clinician knows when specific modalities are most appropriate to include in a rehabilitation program and which ones will best help to achieve the patient's treatment goals, so too the clinician can determine when those modalities are no longer useful. Clinicians know that a modality's use is based on specific needs and goals that are established based on those needs. Clinicians must also identify how to best optimize rehabilitation treatments. Once a modality's goals have been accomplished, there is no need to continue using it. Just as we eliminate early strength exercises in a rehabilitation program once that exercise has achieved the goal for which it was included, a modality is also eliminated from the program once the purpose for its use has been achieved.

Some of the most important decisions involved in using modalities include knowing when to use them, when to use them cautiously, and when to avoid using them altogether. These provisions are called indications, precautions, and contraindications. The difference between precautions and contraindications is most easily explained by identifying contraindications first. If a condition or situation is a **con-**traindication, it means that under no circumstances is the use of a specific treatment or modality acceptable or safe.

Precautions, on the other hand, are situations or conditions in which questions about safety or appropriateness lie in gray areas rather than black-and-white. In other words, the use of a modality could be either beneficial or harmful, depending on specific circumstances that exist with a specific patient. Precautions require the clinician to use common sense and good judgment to decide whether or how to use a modality. For example, impaired circulation is a precaution for the use of superficial heat modalities. Perhaps if a clinician is treating a patient who has impaired circulation in the leg to the point that the extremity from the knee to the toes appears discolored, the clinician may not want to apply a 176°F hot pack but will decide that a 100° whirlpool is appropriate to achieve the goal of improving circulation without overstressing the vascular system. Or if a clinician is treating a patient whose impaired circulation has resulted in not only discoloration of the limb but excessive swelling as well, the clinician may opt not to apply any heat modality and will use active exercise with elevation to reduce the edema.

In other words, precautions are essentially relative contraindications. They require the clinician to understand why a specific condition or situation must be given special consideration and the impact specific modalities will have on those conditions or situations. Each situation must be individually evaluated; for some patients it will be easy to decide if a modality should be contraindicated or used with caution, while for others it will be more difficult to determine. If there is ever a question whether a modality should be used and you cannot decide, it is more prudent to avoid using it; "do no harm" is the most important rule when it comes to making decisions on patient treatment selections.

Indications are those specific signs, symptoms, conditions, or situations that will most likely respond best to a modality or treatment. A benefit will occur if this specific modality is correctly applied to this specific problem. As we discuss some modalities throughout this chapter, the indications, precautions, and contraindications most often associated with each of them is presented. You should become familiar with these, if you are not already, so you can make good treatment decisions for your patients.

Modality Categories in Rehabilitation

We have already learned from previous chapters that modalities play an important role at the injury's onset to minimize the effects and trauma associated with an orthopedic or sport injury. In addition to the initial effects that occur with the application of cryotherapy, there are several other effects that other modalities have on tissues when applied appropriately. This section presents information on the categories of modalities that are available to help the rehabilitation clinician optimize the results of treatment after a patient's injury. The three categories of modalities presented in this chapter include superficial, deep, and electrical modalities. In each of these categories, the most common modalities used in rehabilitation are briefly discussed.

This chapter serves only as a quick review of the essential elements of these modalities. As previously mentioned, an in-depth presentation of modalities is beyond the scope of this book, but the information presented here demonstrates how modalities are an important element of the rehabilitation program. Rehabilitation clinicians must have an acceptable knowledge of them and should be confident in their ability to make fundamental decisions on the most appropriate use of modalities for each patient they serve.

Superficial Heat and Cold

We have already presented some information on this category of modalities. We know that they come under the heading of superficial modalities and are commonly placed into two groups, thermotherapy in the case of heat modalities and cryotherapy in the case of cold modalities. Some examples of thermotherapy modalities include hot packs, infrared lamps, paraffin, fluidotherapy, and hot whirlpools. Examples of cryotherapy modalities include cold packs, ice packs, ice massage, ice baths, cold whirlpools, and vapocoolant sprays. Each modality provides superficial effects since they are applied to the skin and do not cause significant temperature changes in deeper structures. Although both groups are superficial modalities, the effects that cryotherapy and thermotherapy have on a local area are very different.

Before we discuss cryotherapy, we must point out that although there are several research and review articles that promote the benefits and uses of cryotherapy,[2] some authors agree that more high-quality investigations are needed to improve the evidence for cryotherapy's effectiveness.[2-5] That is not to say that there are no benefits to using cryotherapy or that cold therapy is not effective. A plethora of published articles demonstrate the physiological effects of cryotherapy; however, specific studies that look at how effective cold treatments are, especially when compared to other modalities and applied to specific conditions, need additional, stronger studies to demonstrate better evidence than what is currently available. Suffice it to say that many existing studies may be weak but are currently recognized and relied upon for their evidence in the world of allied health professionals. Until stronger studies produce evidence to contradict what is now accepted, the current evidence on cryotherapy will be used to make clinical decisions. In other words, until better evidence exists, the current best practice recommendations have only the existing evidence on which to base clinical decisions.

Physiological Effects of Superficial Heat and Cold

Cryotherapy and thermotherapy may be in the same family of modalities, but because their physiological effects differ, they are used for different purposes. For this reason, delivering the wrong modality at the wrong time in the healing process can lead to problems. Therefore, the clinician must have a good working knowledge of each of these categories.

Although thermotherapy may be delivered to an injury site in different ways (conduction, convection, radiation, or conversion), cryotherapy is usually delivered using conduction, or direct contact, with the treated body part. When conduction is used in either hot or cold application, the direct contact of the modality with the body results in the warmer object transferring its temperature (energy) to the cooler object; therefore, if cryotherapy is applied to the body, then the body's heat moves to the cold object. In the example of an ice pack, the ice melts because the warmth of the injured segment on which it is applied is drawn away from the body and applied to the ice, melting it. On the other hand, when a conductive superficial heat modality, such as a heat pack, is applied to a body segment, heat moves to the cooler body segment to heat up the local tissues to which it is applied; as the body segment's temperature increases, the modality cools.

Regardless of the energy transfer method used by a modality and regardless of the specific modality selected by the clinician, effects that occur with their application will be the same; the superficial heat modalities will all have the same effect. Likewise, all of the superficial cold modalities will provide the same effects, no matter what type of cryotherapy is used to treat the patient. Some of the effects of these cold and heat modalities will be similar to each other, but most of the effects of these two superficial modality groups will be opposite. Tables 9.1 and 9.2 list the most common differences and similarities between the two groups.

Perhaps one of the best known differences between superficial heat and cold modalities is their effects on blood flow: cryotherapy reduces blood flow[6] while thermotherapy increases it.[7] Related to changes in blood flow are vasodilation and vasoconstriction of blood vessels. Local heat application increases vasodilation,[8] while local cold application results in vasoconstriction.[9] When thermotherapy modalities increase local blood vessel diameters, not only does the amount of blood flowing into the area increase but the exchange of oxygen and nutrients with waste is also enhanced.[10] On the other hand, the application of cryotherapy reduces the amount of blood entering a local area; less blood flow diminishes the exchange process.

TABLE 9.1 Superficial Heat and Cold Modalities Have Opposite Effects on Tissue and Function

Function affected	Superficial heat effects	Superficial cold effects
Blood flow	↑	↓
Capillary permeability	↑	↓
Cell metabolism	↑	↓
Local waste removal	↑	↓
Chemical activity	↑	↓
Cellular activity	↑	↓
Oxygen uptake	↑	↓
Tissue viscosity	↓	↓
Tissue elasticity	↑	↓
Inflammation	↑	↓
Edema formation	↑	↓

TABLE 9.2 Similar Effects of Superficial Heat and Cold Applications

Function affected	Superficial heat effects	Superficial cold effects
Pain	↓	↓
Muscle spasm	↓	↓
Muscle strength	↓	↓
Nerve conduction velocity	↓	↓

There are times when an increase in local blood flow is beneficial and other times when it is detrimental. The end of the inflammation phase of healing, when the need for oxygen and nutrients and the accumulation of debris are great, is a time when increased blood flow is beneficial. On the other hand, if a body segment has just been injured and is going through the early inflammation phase, vasodilation would exaggerate the injury's impact; at that point, the more desirable effect would be vasoconstriction with the use of cryotherapy.

Cryotherapy reduces the rate of nerve conduction.[11] Associated with this is a diminished sensation of pain. Pain perception may eventually be reduced to the point of numbness with the application of cryotherapy; this effect may benefit a patient suffering an acute injury or painful condition.

Nerve conduction is also affected when thermotherapy is used, but rather than a numbness, an analgesia results. There may be different reasons that analgesia occurs with the use of heat modalities.[12] One hypothesis is that analgesia is the result of the local increased blood flow that removes painful inflammatory substances from the injury site.[13] Another perspective is based on evidence that indicates that hyperthermia reduces nerve conduction velocity, which leads to a reduction in afferent pain signals.[14] It has also been demonstrated that thermotherapy elevates the patient's pain threshold level;[15] such effects may encour-

age the clinician to apply heat modalities before manual activities such as joint mobilization or passive stretching techniques.

Aside from pain, superficial cold and heat modalities have additional effects on the neural system as it integrates with the muscular system, both directly and indirectly. Both cryotherapy and thermotherapy directly reduce muscle spasm by decreasing the firing rate of the type II afferent nerves.[16, 17] They also both indirectly affect muscle spasm by reducing pain, which will reduce the spasm-pain cycle.[18]

Beyond muscle spasm, superficial cold and hot modalities can also affect the neuromotor system in another way: In research projects using 30 min treatment durations, it was found that the application of either cold or heat reduced muscle strength in the treated body segment.[19, 20] Fortunately, the strength changes are not long-lasting; however, the clinician must keep these effects in mind when planning a patient's treatment program and determining whether modalities would be beneficial or not before exercise.

Cryotherapy and thermotherapy modalities have an impact on connective tissue. Muscles, tendons, ligaments, and scar tissue are examples of tissues that contain connective tissue. When an injury occurs, clinicians know that the patient may be either passively restricted because of the need to stabilize the injury or reluctant to move the injured segment because of pain. We also know that scar tissue develops during the healing process. This combination of scar tissue formation and restricted movement can result in a loss of mobility, increased adhesions, and connective tissue shortening. These factors collectively result in reduced range of motion and function and occur because of the same effect: changes in viscoelasticity of the affected structures because of scar tissue formation.[21] Scar tissue is stiffer than normal tissue; this means that scar tissue has more viscosity and less elasticity than the normal tissue it replaces.

Unfortunately, cryotherapy increases tissue viscosity.[22] However, thermotherapy has been shown to increase tissue elasticity[2] and also to have beneficial effects on plasticity when applied with stretch forces of low, prolonged loads;[23] when this technique is used, plastic deformation occurs, so a permanent change in tissue length is seen.[24] Therefore, if the goal is to create a permanent change in tissue length with flexibility exercises, stretches, or mobilization, application of a heat modality before the exercise or manual therapy treatment would be beneficial.[25]

There are a number of contrasting effects between applications of cold and heat regarding cellular and chemical activity. These effects are particularly important to remember during the first two phases of tissue healing. Both chemical activity and the metabolic rate of tissue will increase with the application of thermotherapy, and along with these increases comes an increase in oxygen uptake;[26] as a result of the increased activity in the local area, the oxygen needs of the tissues also increase. The good news to healing tissue is that associated with these changes is an increase in area nutrients, which combines with the increased oxygen to provide an environment that encourages tissue healing. However, this becomes bad news if the area is still within the inflammation phase of healing; increased metabolic activity and its associated effects place demands on tissue that cannot fulfill those needs; the result is that additional injury occurs with increased swelling, pain, and dysfunction.

On the other hand, because the effects of cold include a reduction in chemical and metabolic activity and oxygen uptake, cryotherapy is the modality of choice during an injury's inflammation and hemostasis phases. When blood supply to tissue is compromised, as it is when an injury occurs, there is less oxygen available to be delivered to the injured area, so the area is at risk of suffering hypoxia. Hypoxia causes oxidative stress to the cells and can result in cell death.[27] Cold modalities that are applied to the injury site reduce the cells' need for oxygen and prevent additional cellular injury that could occur because of hypoxia.[28]

Indications, Precautions, and Contraindications

Because the physiological effects are both different and similar between superficial heat and cold modalities, some of the indications are the same, while others are different for each of the groups. Cryotherapy is indicated in the presence of acute injury, inflammation, pain, and muscle spasm.[29] Cryotherapy is also beneficial in reducing the local metabolic rate, spasticity, and fever. It is also effective in the treatment of chronic conditions such as tendinopathy and bursopathy.[22]

On the other hand, superficial heat is best used after the first 72 h following an acute injury when the risk of continued bleeding is minimal. In other words, after the inflammation phase of healing has passed and the tissue is into the proliferation phase, heat modalities may be beneficial in promoting activities such as opening lymph flow to reduce edema, improving blood flow to encourage oxygen and nutrient exchange with waste products, and increasing cellular activity, oxygen uptake, and cell permeability to facilitate healing. Heat modalities are also indicated to reduce pain and muscle spasm in subacute injuries, and they may be beneficial for chronic inflammations. Table 9.3 provides a quick reference for superficial heat and cold modality indications, precautions, and contraindications for their use.

Therapeutic Ultrasound

Just as there are different modalities under the category of superficial heat, there are also several modalities under the classification of deep heat. Of these deep heat modalities, ultrasound is arguably the most commonly used in rehabilitation.

Physiological Effects of Therapeutic Ultrasound

Although ultrasound is generally considered a deep heat therapy, it may also be applied with minimal heat effects. This is referred to as nonthermal ultrasound, or pulsed ultrasound. It must be realized, however, that although it is called nonthermal, there will be some heat delivered to the tissues because of the interaction between the ultrasound waves and tissues.[30]

Many aspects of therapeutic ultrasound are not addressed here. As stated at the beginning of this chapter, this presentation serves only as an overview of concepts taught in other courses and serves only to highlight some of the more important aspects of modalities to consider when deciding whether to include them in your patient's rehabilitation program. Although various ultrasound applications are used in medicine, this section is limited to therapeutic ultrasound.

In simplest terms, ultrasound, or acoustic, waves are either absorbed or scattered. If the waves are absorbed, they are converted to heat energy.[31] The scattered waves create the nonthermal effects in tissues.[32] The thermal effects on tissue physiology include improvements in blood flow and nerve conduction velocity, increased connective tissue extensibility and cellular membrane permeability,

TABLE 9.3 Indications, Precautions, and Contraindications for Superficial Heat and Cold Modalities

Indications, precautions, and contraindications	Cold	Superficial heat
DESIRED EFFECTS		
Reduce pain	●	●
Relieve spasm	●	●
Prevent or reduce edema formation	●	●
Increase blood flow	●	●
Neuromotor performance	●	
Reduce viscosity	●	●
Promote wound healing	○	●
Resolve subacute inflammation	●	●
CONDITIONS		
Acute inflammation	●	●
Chronic inflammation	●	●
Tendon injuries	●	●
Deep vein thrombosis	●	●
Open wounds	○	●
Cold sensitivity	●	●
Raynaud's disease or urticaria	●	●
Myofascial pain syndrome	●	●
Impaired circulation or peripheral vascular disease	○	○
Impaired sensation	○	○
Malignancy or radiation therapy	●	●
Pregnancy	●	○
Skin diseases	●	●
Hypertension	○	○
Stiffness	●	●
Electronic implants	●	●
Metal implants	●	●
Fever	●	●
BODY SEGMENTS		
Open epiphysis	●	●
Regenerating nerves	●	●
Reproductive organs	●	●
Eyes	○	○
Carotid sinus; ant. neck	●	○
Chest, heart	●	●
Head	●	●

● Indicated. In the presence of specific conditions it is safe to apply the modality, or when specific effects are desired, the modality may be effectively applied.

○ Precaution. This is a relative contraindication. In some instances the modality will be contraindicated, and in others it may be applied with caution.

● Contraindicated. These are absolute conditions or locations where the modality should not be applied.

Note: Precautions are essentially relative contraindications; therefore, in the event that you are unsure whether you should use that modality, err on the side of caution and consider that modality a contraindication for the condition you are treating.

and increases in pain threshold and enzymatic activity.[33, 34] The thermal effects of therapeutic ultrasound are essentially similar to those seen with superficial heat except they occur at a deeper level.

The primary difference between superficial heat modalities and ultrasound is the depth to which heat affects tissues. Continuous ultrasound at 1 MHz can heat tissues to a depth of 5 cm (2 in.), much deeper than any superficial heat modality.[35] Tissues with greater collagen content absorb more ultrasound energy, so tissues such as tendons, ligaments, scar tissue, and fascia will be more affected by the modality's heat effects.[36] Since tendons have less vascularity than muscle, they cannot shunt the heat away, and they will retain heat for a longer time.[37] On the other hand, tissue with higher water content allows ultrasonic waves to pass through it. Therefore, tissues such as articular sacs and fat are not affected.[38] Additionally, subcutaneous fat does not impede ultrasound heating like it does other heating modalities, so it is a good way to heat deeper tissues without affecting more superficial tissues.[39] Figure 9.1 shows the various tissues and their relative ability to absorb ultrasound waves. Those tissues that contain more water allow the waves to pass through them without becoming heated, and those tissues with more protein absorb the waves and are directly affected by ultrasound. Although cartilage and bone contain high amounts of protein, their density causes ultrasound waves to be reflected rather than absorbed. Therefore, cartilage and bone will not benefit from ultrasound like other protein-based structures such as tendons, ligaments, joint capsules, scar tissue, and fascia.[40-44]

Therapeutic ultrasound also provides other biophysical effects in addition to its heating effects. These effects result from the nonthermal impact of ultrasound waves. Nonthermal and thermal effects occur with both continuous and pulsed ultrasound; however, the thermal effects of pulsed ultrasound are significantly less than those of continuous ultrasound.[30, 45] Nonthermal effects are generally identified with pulsed ultrasound, but they occur whenever therapeutic ultrasound is used.

In fact, the term *nonthermal* is used to describe pulsed ultrasound, although, as mentioned, the treatment is not entirely void of heat. The term refers to the fact that there is no relevant heating of tissue occurring. Some authors have replaced the term "nonthermal effect" with "microthermal effect."[46] Nonthermal ultrasound is administered using either a pulsed ultrasound at the same treatment intensities as thermal ultrasound or a continuous ultrasound at reduced intensity levels. Continuous ultrasound delivered at lowered outputs is referred to as low-intensity pulsed ultrasound (LIPUS).

Many researchers have looked at the impact of nonthermal ultrasound during the various healing phases. Although they all agree that ultrasound is contraindicated immediately after an injury when bleeding occurs (hemostasis phase), they do not all agree when the optimal effects of ultrasound occur during the other phases of healing. Some investigators advocate using nonthermal ultrasound during the inflammation phase of acute healing once the bleeding has stopped.[46] Evidence exists to indicate that this treatment is beneficial because ultrasound simulates mast cells and facilitates the inflammatory process to optimize healing results.[33, 47, 48] Other investigators' findings demonstrate that more beneficial effects on healing occur with the application of ultrasound during the proliferation phase.[49-51] During this time, nonthermal ultrasound can encourage the healing process by affecting fibroblasts, myofibroblasts, and endothelial cell formation.[42, 47, 52, 53] Other researchers have found that because of ultrasound's effects on collagen fibers, a good time to use nonthermal ultrasound is during the early remodeling phase.[40, 54, 55] Evidence indicates that the ultrasound realigns collagen fibers and by so doing, improves the tensile strength of healing structures.[51, 56] This modality can also improve scar tissue mobility by increasing the tissue's length;[42] ultrasound appears to do this through its influence on scar tissue's elasticity, cross-link bonds, and collagen alignment.[42, 57]

Overall, there is a lot of evidence upon which researchers can agree that nonthermal ultrasound affects tissue healing. This fact is most notable in fracture healing. Evi-

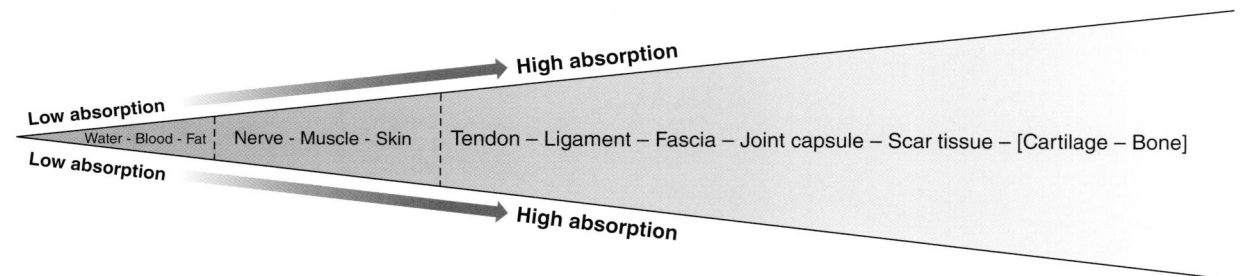

Figure 9.1 Body substances and tissue's ability to absorb ultrasound. Tissues with higher collagen (or other protein) content absorb ultrasonic energy more readily while tissues with high water content allow ultrasonic waves to pass through them.

dence indicates that ultrasound speeds fracture healing by accelerating the production of osteoclasts and angiogenesis and stimulating bone metabolism.[58-60] Increasing the rate of fracture healing has been shown to improve the patient's quality of life since less time is spent recovering from the injury and the return to normal activities is quicker.[61] Based on the evidence available, using nonthermal ultrasound in cases of normal healing would improve the efficiency of the repair phases throughout healing, and in cases of compromised healing, nonthermal ultrasound would boost tissue repair.[46]

Another way ultrasound affects healing is by its influence on cell proliferation. Cell proliferation is important in any tissue repair. During proliferation, cells migrate to the injured site; these cells are responsible for activities such as angiogenesis, extracellular matrix production, and development of what will become permanent tissue. Studies have shown that tendon cell proliferation occurs with either continuous or pulsed ultrasound treatments.[62]

Because ultrasound affects protein-containing cells and substances, nonthermal ultrasound influences many aspects of the healing process. If we identify several of the cells and substances that play a role in healing, it soon becomes apparent how ultrasound can influence healing. Growth factors are proteins, so those infiltrating the injury site will be affected by ultrasound, as will many other cells and substances that invade the area during the inflammation and proliferation healing phases. Table 9.4 is based on information in Johns, 2002.[33] It lists some of the more commonly recognized healing substances and indicates how nonthermal ultrasound treatments affect their normal function.

In summary, the thermal effects of ultrasound are the same as those of other thermal modalities, including increased blood flow, increased tissue viscosity or extensibility, increased nerve conduction velocity, reduced muscle spasm, and reduced pain and other inflammation signs and symptoms. The advantage of ultrasound as a heating agent is that it can heat deeper structures while superficial thermal modalities cannot. A disadvantage of ultrasound is that it heats only small areas. Nonthermal ultrasound effects primarily include healing advancement: cellular permeability, protein synthesis, and increased blood flow.

CLINICAL TIPS

Regardless of the frequency used in therapeutic ultrasound, the nonthermal effects will always be delivered to the targeted tissue, as will some amount of heat. The closer to 100% duty cycle the treatment is set, the greater will be the heat delivered.

Treatment Parameters of Therapeutic Ultrasound

Ultrasound treatment parameters, whether thermal or nonthermal, must be selected before applying the treatment. These parameters include dose, depth and heating desired, duration, duty cycle, and number of treatments. Each of these parameters can vary, and there is no standardized or substantiated recommendation for any of them.[67] The amount of energy delivered to the tissues is the dose, and it is measured in W/cm²; the output of energy emitted by the sound head (watts, abbreviated W) is divided by area of the sound head (cm²).

Ultrasonic heating occurs deeper with 1 MHz than it does with 3 MHz. However, the 1 MHz heating is not as great in tissues or delivered as quickly to the deeper structures, nor do those tissues retain the heat as long.[35, 37] If deeper structures are to be heated effectively, they should receive longer treatment times.[68] It is commonly accepted that 3 MHz treats tissues that are less than 2.5 cm (<1 in.)

TABLE 9.4 Effects of Nonthermal Ultrasound Treatments

Proteins and functions	Healing process affected by changes in proteins and functions
PROTEINS AFFECTED	
Fibroblast growth factor	Endothelial cells migrate and proliferate at the injury site
Collagen	Increases healing rate
Interleukin-1β	Enhances mediation of inflammation phase
Interleukin-2	Enhances T cell growth rate
Interleukin-8	Endothelial cells migrate and proliferate in bone fracture site
Vascular endothelial growth factor	Endothelial cells migrate and proliferate
CELL FUNCTIONS AFFECTED	
Cell proliferation	Increases rate of healing of injured tissues
Lymphocyte adhesion	Promotes angiogenesis of injured region
Vasodilation	Increases blood flow to injury site

Reher et al.[63]; Doan et al.[64]; Johns[33]; Maxwell[47]; Maxwell et al.[65]; Steffen et al.[66]

deep, and 1 MHz treats deeper tissues that are up to 5 cm (2 in.) deep.[35]

Not only do the depth and intensity of heating determine the amount of temperature increase in the treated tissues, but the duration of treatment is also a significant factor. Figure 9.2 is based on the research of Draper et al., 1995.[35] It shows that tissue temperature increases occur at a rate roughly three times faster with ultrasound at 3 MHz than is seen at 1 MHz.

Table 9.5 is a display in specific numbers of the data Draper et al.[35] obtained from the research results shown in figure 9.2. Temperature change measurements occurred at

2.5 cm (1 in.) and 5 cm (2 in.) tissue depths for 1 MHz and at 0.8 cm (0.3 in.) and 1.6 cm (0.6 in.) for 3 MHz. In other words, the more "superficial" ultrasound (3 MHz) heats down to approximately 1/3 in. to 2/3 in., while the deeper ultrasound (1 MHz) treatment reaches between 1 and 2 in., regardless of the intensities used. These results are often used as a guide to determine the duration of therapeutic ultrasound treatment durations; the treatment duration is based on the temperature increase desired and the intensity selected. According to Lehmann and De Lateur[69] and Draper,[70] tissue heating is qualified as mild, moderate, or vigorous heating and is quantified as 1 °C, 2 to 3 °C, and ¾

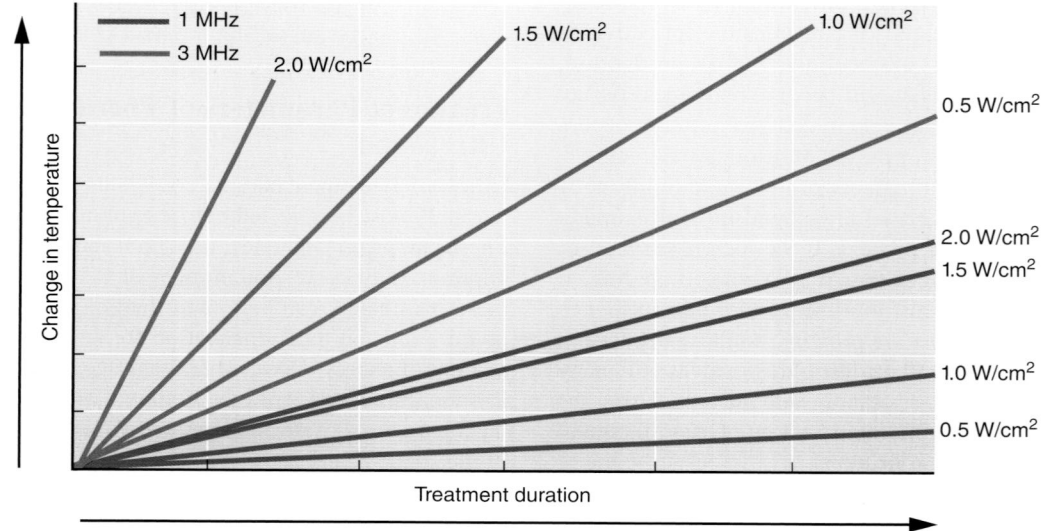

Figure 9.2   Tissue temperature changes over time with ultrasound application.* Notice that tissue temperature increases are much lower and slower with the deeper penetrating ultrasound waves at all intensities.

*Based on Draper et al. (1995).[35]

TABLE 9.5   Heating Rate and Depth of Ultrasound at 1 MHz and 3 MHz

Intensity of ultrasound (W/cm²)	1 MHZ DEEP HEATING		3 MHZ LESS DEEP HEATING	
	Heating depth (cm)	Heating rate increase (°/min)	Heating depth (cm)	Heating rate increase (°/min)
0.5	2.5	.04	0.8	.30
0.5	5.0	.06	1.6	.31
1.0	2.5	.16	0.8	.58
1.0	5.0	.16	1.6	.58
1.5	2.5	.34	0.8	.82
1.5	5.0	.31	1.6	.96
2.0	2.5	.40	.08	1.5
2.0	5.0	.34	1.6	1.3

Based on Draper et al. (1995).[35]

°C increase, respectively. Table 9.6 describes the changes in internal temperatures for the different levels of heating. An example may make it easier to see how this table's information may be used: If you want to increase the tissue temperature of a muscle that was 5 cm (2 in.) deep to a moderate level and used 2.0 W/cm², you would apply the 1 MHz ultrasound treatment for about 7.5 min to achieve your goal of increased tissue temperature by 2 to 3 °C.

As can be seen in figure 9.2, the longer the treatment is applied, the greater are the temperature changes in the treated tissues. So how long is an appropriate treatment? Once again, there are no clear-cut rules. It is advised to treat for 10 to 12 min when 1 MHz ultrasound is used and 3 to 4 min when 2 MHz is used to produce a deep heat treatment;[71] however, total treatment time depends on these factors: the frequency (MHz), dose (W/cm²), time required to heat the tissue to the desired increase (minutes), and your goals for treatment (amount of temperature increase in the tissue). The rate of heating is used to determine the amount of time ultrasound is applied. The general rates are visualized in figure 9.2, but the more precise rates and the depths to which ultrasound reaches, as determined by Draper et al.,[35] are provided in table 9.5.

The duty cycle of ultrasound is the time when ultrasound waves are being delivered to tissues. When ultrasound is continuous, the duty cycle, or amount of time the sound waves are delivered, is 100%. Pulsed ultrasound never has a duty cycle of 100% but has a duty cycle that is a fraction, or percentage, of the total duty cycle. A duty cycle that is not 100% is a pulsed ultrasound wave; the ultrasound wave is alternately delivered and not delivered in a cyclic manner. The amount of pulsed ultrasound delivered can be adjusted as a percentage or ratio. For example, if the duty cycle is set to a 1:1 ratio, 5 s on and 5 s off, the duty cycle is 50%: one cycle is 5 s on plus 5 s off, so 5 s/10 s = 50%. If the pulse ratio is set at 1:2 so the ultrasound wave is on for 5 s and off for 10 s, the duty cycle is 33% (one cycle is 5 s on plus 10 s off for a total of 15 s, and 5 s is 1/3 of 15 s). Table 9.7 provides a quick glance at duty cycles for different ratios of ultrasound on and off cycles.

It may be assumed that if a 100% duty cycle delivers heat to tissue, then the closer to 100% the duty cycle is set, the greater the thermal effects will be; conversely, the lower the duty cycle is set, the less thermal effect the treated tissue will receive. Most researchers seem to set their duty cycle parameters at 10%, 20%, or 50%.[45, 72, 73]

TABLE 9.6 Levels of Temperature Increases and Associated Effects Using Therapeutic Ultrasound

Temperature increase in Celsius	Temperature increase in Fahrenheit	Level of heating	Associated effects	Indications in rehabilitation
1°	33.8°	Mild	Accelerates metabolism.	Subacute injuries Hematomas Edema
2°-3°	35.6°-37.4°	Moderate	Reduces muscle spasm and chronic inflammation. Increases local blood flow.	Pain Chronic inflammations Active trigger points
3-4°	3-39.2°	Vigorous	Increases collagen extensibility. Inhibits sympathetic activity.	Stretch restricted scar tissue, joint capsules, tendons, and ligaments.

Note: The average body internal temperature is about 37.5 °C (99.5 °F).

Based on Lehmann and De Lateur (1990)[69]; Draper (2014).[70]

TABLE 9.7 Ultrasound Pulse Ratios and Duty Cycles

Mode	Pulse ratio	Ratio example	Total time	Duty cycle
Continuous	---	---	---	100%
Pulsed	1:1	5 s on: 5 s off	10 s	50%
Pulsed	1:2	5 s on: 10 s off	15 s	33%
Pulsed	1:3	5 s on: 15 s off	20 s	25%
Pulsed	1:4	5 s on: 20 s off	25 s	20%
Pulsed	1:9	5 s on: 45 s off	50 s	10%

As with treatment administration parameters, it is difficult to determine how long ultrasound treatments should last, and no specific guidelines have been established. A rule of thumb is that 9 to 12 treatments of ultrasound are sufficient.[74] The clinician must obviously watch for outcomes based on the ultrasound treatment; if benefits are apparent, then treatments continue, but if no change occurs in the patient's condition, the clinician should discontinue the ultrasound treatment.

Indications, Precautions, and Contraindications of Ultrasound

As with any rehabilitation treatment, therapeutic ultrasound has its indications, precautions, and contraindications. These are briefly presented here. Ultrasound indications, precautions, and contraindications are summarized in table 9.8.

Because ultrasound can provide heat to deeper structures, when an injury involves structures that are deeper than can be affected by superficial heat and involves a small area, ultrasound is probably the most effective modality to use. Various injuries and conditions respond well to ultrasound. Tendinopathies are conditions that respond well to ultrasound. It is thought that the "itises" respond well because ultrasound not only improves cell permeability to encourage migration and proliferation of healing agents, but it also facilitates transforming growth factor-β, which is important in tendon and ligament healing.[75-77]

Both continuous and pulsed ultrasound provide the nonthermal effects of ultrasound. For this reason, when you take a close look at table 9.8, you realize that the indications, precautions, and contraindications for continuous and pulsed ultrasound are essentially the same. The main difference in their uses has to do with the application of heat to tissues. If heat application for a specific condition is contraindicated, then continuous ultrasound will also be contraindicated, but nonthermal ultrasound will not be contraindicated. On the other hand, if the nonthermal effects of ultrasound are contraindicated, then neither continuous nor nonthermal ultrasound should be used.

Therapeutic ultrasound has been found to break up scar tissue,[78] improve healing and the healing rate of bone and ligaments,[40, 61] and improve the healing of open wounds.[42] Myofascial pain has demonstrated beneficial effects with the application of ultrasound,[79] as have acute and chronic tendon injuries.[80, 81] It is safe to apply therapeutic ultrasound over metal implants since the heat dissipates before it has a chance to build up in the surrounding tissues.[82]

Most of the contraindications listed for therapeutic ultrasound also apply to the use of superficial heat modalities, and usually they are contraindicated because of the deleterious effects of heat rather than because of the nonthermal effects of ultrasound. Those contraindications that are listed because of nonthermal ultrasonic effects are conditions or body segments that are generally avoided with most modalities because either the effects are unknown or it may be too risky to apply modalities there.

Many of the precautionary conditions or effects indicated in table 9.8 for therapeutic ultrasound are listed in other sources as contraindications. Recommendations vary because precautions are relative contraindications; in some cases they will be absolute contraindications and in others the modality may be applied with caution. Precautions

Evidence in Rehabilitation

One modality that is not commonly used in rehabilitation clinics but may be in the future is vibration therapy. This modality is applied to either a local area or to the whole body. Vibration therapy uses a wide range of vibration frequencies ranging from a few to 50 Hz for total body applications to 300 to 500 Hz for local applications.[83, 84] When astronauts spend time in space, they suffer bone loss, muscle strength loss, and reduced circulation and lymphatic effectiveness; however, when Russian cosmonauts started using vibration therapy during their prolonged space flights, they were not only able to stay in space for periods several times longer than their American counterparts, these physical and physiological problems were significantly reduced.[85]

Although not widely used in health care at this point, vibration therapy has the potential to be an appealing modality, especially in long-term rehabilitation situations. Some of the postinjury effects that have been demonstrated with vibration therapy include improved restoration of muscle size and function after injury,[86-88] improved balance in subjects with chronic ankle instability,[89] and reduced injury recovery time.[90] Vibration therapy has also demonstrated encouraging results for conditions such as Parkinson's disease and other neurological disorders.[91, 92] There is evidence to show that this modality may be beneficial in that it decreases the amount of muscle and bone loss that normally occurs during immobilization.[93, 94]

There are many issues regarding vibration therapy that are still unknown. Because of its relatively new use in rehabilitation, there are many theories about how it works; one prevalent theory is that the vibrations stimulate muscle spindles and α-motor neurons, which in turn cause muscle contraction.[95] As with any new idea, there seems to be a number of proponents who defend[83, 92, 93, 96, 97] and skeptics who challenge[86, 98, 99] the value of vibration therapy in rehabilitation. Until researchers can provide clinicians with evidence of its effectiveness and optimal parameters of application, clinicians will use their best judgments in using it with their patients.

Chapter 9 • Modalities **237**

TABLE 9.8 Indications, Precautions, and Contraindications of Ultrasound

Indications, precautions, and contraindications	ULTRASOUND	
	Thermal	**Nonthermal**
DESIRED EFFECTS		
Pain reduction	●	●
Relieve spasm	●	●
Increase blood flow	●	●
Reduce viscosity	●	
Promote wound healing	●	●
Reduce scar tissue formation	●	●
Resolve subacute inflammation	●	●
CONDITIONS		
Acute inflammation	●	●
Chronic inflammation	●	●
Tendon injuries	●	●
DVT	●	●
Open wounds		●
Cold sensitivity	●	●
Raynaud's disease or urticaria	●	●
Myofascial pain syndrome	●	●
Impaired circulation or PVD	●	◐
Impaired sensation	●	◐
Malignancy or radiation therapy	●	●
Pregnancy	●	●
Skin diseases	●	◐
Hypertension	●	●
Stiffness	●	●
Electronic implants	●	●
Metal implants	●	●
BODY SEGMENTS		
Open epiphysis	●	●
Regenerating nerves	◐	◐
Reproductive organs	●	●
Eyes	●	●
Carotid sinus; ant. neck	●	●
Chest, heart	●	●
Head	●	●

● Indicated. In the presence of specific conditions it is safe to apply the modality, or when specific effects are desired, the modality may be effectively applied.

◐ Precaution. This is a relative contraindication. In some instances the modality will be contraindicated, and in others it may be applied with caution.

● Contraindicated. These are absolute conditions or locations where the modality should not be applied.

Note: Precautions are relative contraindications and require the best judgment of the clinician to determine whether ultrasound is indicated or contraindicated in specific situations.

are always dependent upon the professional's experience, confidence, and knowledge and the patient's condition and underlying comorbidities. Caution is always needed when a modality is listed in the precaution category and in situations where the clinician is unsure whether to use a modality. If ever in doubt as to a modality's use, the best choice is to refrain from using a modality.

Therapeutic Electrical Stimulation

Electricity flows either in one direction or back and forth from one direction to another. The unidirected current is known as a direct current (DC), while the current that flows back and forth between two poles in a cyclic manner is known as an alternating current (AC). An extensive discussion of the biophysics of therapeutic electrical stimulation (ES) will not be included here except to relate it to how a rehabilitation clinician should decide which type of ES to use with a patient. This discussion, however, will be a cursory account rather than an in-depth presentation of electrophysiology since this topic is sufficiently covered in other healthcare sources and coursework.

Electrical stimulation is used to facilitate a response in a nerve or muscle. Four types of electrical stimulation are used most often in orthopedic and sports rehabilitation. These include transcutaneous electrical nerve stimulation (TENS), interferential current (IFC), high-voltage pulsed stimulation (HVPS), and neuromuscular electrical stimulation (NMES). Each has specific purposes (table 9.9) and features (table 9.10).

Although each of these electrical stimulation modalities has its own dedicated machine, many manufacturers also offer units that feature a selection of electrical modalities in one unit. Electrotherapy units applied to orthopedic and sports injuries usually use cutaneous electrodes in treatment. These are usually self-adhering, disposable electrodes and come in a variety of sizes to fit the varying needs of patients.

Physiological Effects of Therapeutic Electrical Stimulation

Since each of these electrical modalities function using different means and modes of stimulation, they will operate a little differently. The four types of electrical stimulation will be dealt with separately with comparisons when appropriate.

Transcutaneous Electrical Nerve Stimulation

Transcutaneous electrical nerve stimulator (TENS) units are usually small enough to fit into a pocket or clip on a belt so that a patient may use and wear it throughout the day while performing almost any activity. TENS units are primarily used to produce pain relief, especially for chronic pain patients. Although there are several different modes, TENS is usually used to treat pain via one of three different systems: conventional, acupuncture-like, and intense TENS. Each system, or mode, provides pain relief by adjusting pulse frequency, pulse duration, and current intensity, which affect different noxious nerve transmissions. Table 9.11 provides a comparison of the three primary types of TENS used for pain relief.

Selection of the specific TENS unit settings for a patient is based on the type of pain the patient has and the goals of treatment. Table 9.11 provides a quick reference guide for these parameters. When a TENS unit is applied, there are several electrode placement options that may prove advantageous to the patient. Since each patient's pain and response to pain are different, what electrode arrangement is most successful with different patients will also vary. Some of the more commonly used arrangements include the following:

1. Dermatomal placement: The electrodes are placed around the painful site. When more than one electrode is used, they are on either side of the painful site in the application of dual electrodes, or the site is surrounded by the electrodes when quadripolar electrodes are used.

TABLE 9.9 Types of Electrical Stimulation and Their Functions

Type of electrical stimulation	Pain control	Relieve muscle spasm	Edema reduction	Muscle re-ed	Muscle strengthening	Wound healing
Transcutaneous electrical nerve stimulation (TENS)	✓	✓	—	—	—	—
Interferential current (IFC)	✓	✓	✓	—	—	—
High-voltage pulsed stimulation (HVPS)	✓	✓	✓	✓	—	✓
Neuromuscular electrical stimulation (NMES)	—	—	✓	✓	✓	—

TABLE 9.10   Types of Electrotherapy and Their Features

Electrical stimulation	Waveform	Depolarization	Most common electrode arrangement	Effects	Notes
TENS	Biphasic Monophasic Pulsatile	Sensory, motor, and noxious nerve fibers	Bipolar Quadripolar	Stimulates sensory nerves to either block pain or overstimulate pain receptors.	High TENS: Sensory –> A-beta Low TENS: Sensory –> A-delta Burst: Sensory –> A-delta Brief intense: Sensory –> C
IFC	2 interfering sinusoidal currents: - High frequency - Variable frequency	Motor and sensory nerve fibers	Quadripolar Bipolar is premodulated	Asynchronous waves interfere with each other to reduce pain. Stimulates muscle pumping to reduce edema and spasm.	Sweep: Frequency range = 80-150 Hz Fixed: You set frequency. Able to affect deeper tissues than TENS.
HVPS	Twin-peak, monophasic, pulsed current	Motor and sensory nerve fibers	Bipolar	High intensity, short duration, pulsed current facilitates an increase in electrical charges within tissue.	Used more for wounds, edema, and muscle spasm than for pain control or muscle weakness.
NMES	Biphasic symmetrical	Muscle: Type II fibers first	Bipolar Quadripolar	Activates muscle to strengthen it.	Interrelated with Russian stim and functional electrical stimulation (FES).

TABLE 9.11   Commonly Used TENS and Their Parameters

Parameters	Conventional TENS	Acupuncture-like TENS	Intense TENS
Other names	Low-intensity TENS Sensory TENS	High-intensity TENS Motor TENS Rhythmical TENS	Brief-intense TENS Noxious TENS
Intensity	Low amplitude	High amplitude	High amplitude to uncomfortable level
Pulse frequency	High: >100 pps	Low: 2-4 pps	Variable: 2-7 pps or 100-150 pps
Pulse duration	50-100 µs	150-300 µs	>1 ms
Target nerve	A-beta fibers: Large-diameter non-noxious afferent nerves to produce segmental analgesia	A-delta fibers: Small-diameter cutaneous and motor afferents to produce extra-segmental analgesia	C fibers: Small-diameter cutaneous afferents to produce counterirritation. A-delta will also be stimulated.
Pain relief mechanism	Encephalins released in dorsal horn	Opiates released through stimulation of descending pathways	Opiates released through stimulation of descending pathways
Type of pain treated	Although any pain may benefit, it is best used with acute pain or postoperative pain	Subacute pain Trigger point pain	Chronic pain that interferes with normal daily functions Myofascial-related pain Muscle spasm

> continued

TABLE 9.11 >*continued*

Parameters	Conventional TENS	Acupuncture-like TENS	Intense TENS
Onset of pain relief	Rapid onset (<30 min)	Delayed onset (>30 min)	Rapid onset (<30 min)
Duration of pain relief after treatment	Rapid decline (<30 min)	Delayed decline (>1 h)	Delayed decline (>1 h)
Patient sensation	Comfortable	Strong but comfortable muscle contraction	Uncomfortable but tolerable with some muscle contraction
Treatment duration	Whenever in pain	20-30 min treatments	5-15 min treatments

2. Referral point placement: If acupuncture points or referred trigger points are treated, the electrodes are placed directly over these locations to treat the pain where it originates rather than where the patient reports it.

3. Paraspinal placement: Electrodes are placed on the skin over the dorsal horn of the spinal cord segment that integrates the painful site.

4. Contralateral placement: Electrodes are placed on the opposite extremity that is contralateral to the site of pain.

In addition to the different electrode placements, there are also different electrode configurations that are used with pain-relieving stimulation. Most of the time, TENS uses either monopolar or bipolar configurations. Either of these configurations may be used with either monophasic or biphasic currents. Monopolar configurations often have two unequal-sized electrodes, while bipolar configurations have equal-sized electrodes. If you see a patient using a TENS unit with four electrodes, the unit has two channels and is not quadripolar.

Interferential Current Interferential current (IFC) is a therapeutic machine that has two interfering medium-frequency sinusoidal waves. The designation "medium-frequency" is an arbitrary classification that defines low frequency as frequencies less than 1000 Hz and medium frequency as those frequencies between 1001 and 10,000 Hz.[100] Most interferential currents are in the 3000 to 5000 Hz range.[100] One of the interfering currents produces a constant medium-frequency sinusoidal wave, while the other current is variable, so sometimes they create a higher frequency when combined and sometimes they create a lower frequency when they cancel each other out. Figure 9.3 is based on Denegar et al.,[101] and it illustrates how interference changes the effective frequency to what is known as a beat frequency that is delivered to the tissues. The **beat frequency** is essentially the net difference between the two interfering currents at any one time.

Because the IFC frequencies are in the medium range, the skin's impedance to the electrical flow is reduced, so the interferential current is more comfortable and can go deeper than conventional TENS units, which incorporate less comfortable low-frequency currents. The IFC beat

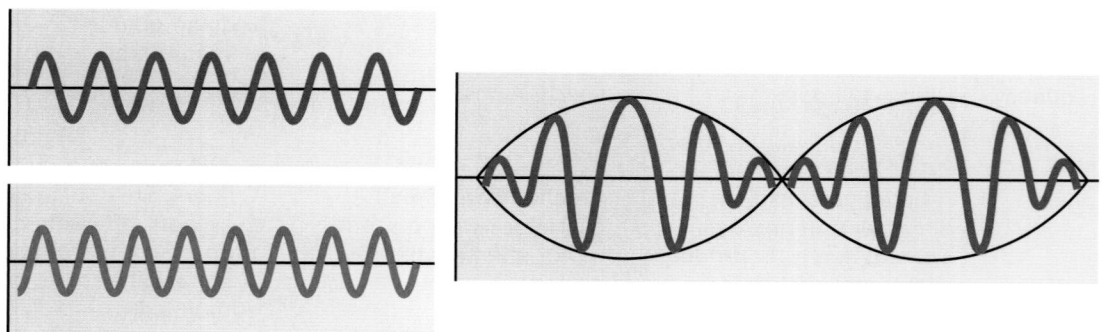

Figure 9.3 In interferential currents, the two medium-frequency sinusoidal waves of 5000 and 5100 Hz shown in this example are superimposed on each other to interfere with each other in order to sometimes produce a higher frequency to the tissues than either wave could produce alone. This is referred to as a beat frequency (bps) and is the difference between the two interfering frequencies : 5100 Hz -5000 Hz = 100 Hz or 100 bps.

Based on Denegar et al. (2016, p. 151).[101]

frequency can be altered to change the type of pain relief the IFC produces. Based on the information in table 9.11, when the IFC beat frequency is set at 60 to 100 bps, a conventional TENS effect will occur, but if it is set at 2 to 4 bps, an acupuncture-like TENS is produced.[101]

In addition to serving as a form of TENS for pain relief, IFC is also used for muscle contraction. The optimum stimulation to obtain a tetanic voluntary muscle contraction is 40 to 80 Hz.[102] Studies have demonstrated that IFC produces a more comfortable and better muscle contraction with a greater force production than does Russian stimulation.[103] Because IFC uses medium-frequency currents that have less skin resistance, it may be used to stimulate deeper muscle without being uncomfortable. Interferential current may be used to relieve muscle spasm by contracting the muscle to the point of fatigue.

Electrodes are used either in quadripolar or bipolar arrangement. The quadripolar application is used for pain relief while the bipolar may be used for either pain relief or muscle contraction.

High-Voltage Pulsed Current   High-voltage pulsed current (HVPC) is a monophasic current whose waveform has two rapidly occurring peaks and a relatively longer rest time to the next double peak as shown in figure 9.4. For this reason, it is described as a twin-peak, monophasic pulsed current. Its voltage, or electromotive force, ranges between 150 and 500 V. Another traditional arbitrary delineation, this time of volts, defines low-volt stimulators as those that deliver less than 150 V, while high-voltage stimulators deliver more than 150 V.

The pulse duration is the amount of time the two twin peaks occur. This is usually less than 200 ms.[104] Peak current amplitude is around 2 to 2.5 A, and frequency is usually 1 to 125 pulses per second (pps).[104] Although the voltage is usually 150 to 500 V, because each pulse is so short and there is a relatively longer time between each set of pulses, the current remains low. Because the current remains low, there is no ion movement to create biochemical changes in the tissue.

Because HVPC is monophasic, the clinician must select either negative or positive polarity for the patient's treatment. There is some evidence that wounds change their polarity as they go through the healing process.[105, 106] Although they discovered that either negative or positive HVPC heals a wound, Mehmandoust et al.[105] found that if the negative polarity was used to treat the wound for the first 3 d followed by a change to positive polarity for the rest of the treatment program, the formed tissue was stronger.

It has been recommended that when the treatment goal is to enhance granulation formation, negative polarity HVPC is used, and when it is desirable to improve a wound's anti-infection status or if a wound's healing process is slow, a positive polarity is used.[107]

In addition to healing promotion and pain relief, HVPC also assists in edema reduction and muscle spasm relaxation.[108, 109] It is thought that the edema reduction occurs through a combination of muscle pumping through muscle contraction and the effect HVPC has on reducing microvascular permeability.[100] Muscle spasm is forced to relax when HVPC produces muscle fatigue through electrically facilitated repetitive contractions.[109]

High-voltage pulsed current treatment often uses monopolar electrodes with a small active electrode and a larger dispersive electrode. Sometimes more than one active electrode is used. The active electrodes are placed over the treatment area, and the dispersive electrode is placed away from the treated area. The active electrodes are smaller, so the current concentrates over the treated area.

Neuromuscular Electrical Stimulation (NMES)

Neuromuscular electrical stimulation is known as NMES. (Although it won't be presented here, another type of electrical stimulation in the same family as NMES is functional electrical stimulation [FES]. This electric modality is used to enhance functional abilities of neurologically impaired patients.) One type of NMES, Russian stimulation, falls within the category of muscle-strengthening electrical modalities; it uses a sinusoidal-wave alternating current of 2500 Hz with burst modulations.[110] On the other hand, most NMES stimulators use a balanced, asymmetrical biphasic pulsed current.[110] The current is balanced because even though the waveform is asymmetrical, the total charge in the positive and negative portions of one pulse is equal.

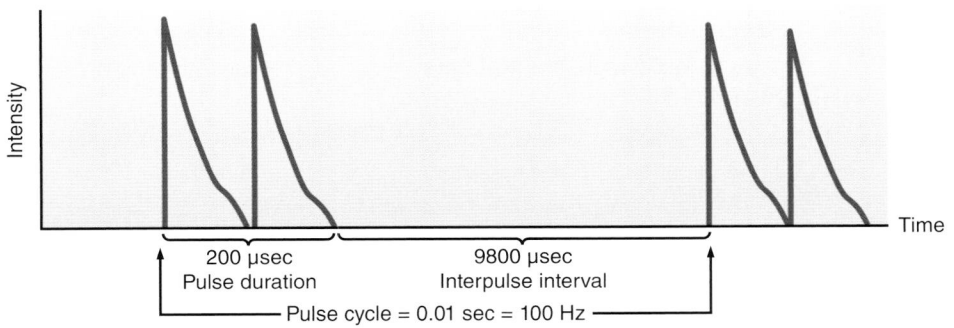

Figure 9.4   HVPC waveform example.

As the name may imply, NMES produces a muscle contraction. However, NMES stimulates the nerve to facilitate a muscle contraction, not the muscle fiber. An electrical stimulation obtains a reaction from the larger nerve fibers more quickly than from the smaller nerve fibers. These larger nerve fibers innervate the faster muscle fibers, the Type II fibers; since the nerve fibers are larger, their resistance is less, so their impulses are sent more quickly. Since the Type II muscle fibers are used for fast-action activities and fatigue quickly, electrical stimulation to their nerves (and subsequently the muscle fibers) causes rapid fatigue of the muscle. Unlike normal activity, Type II muscle fiber's nerves are stimulated simultaneously, further adding to a more rapid muscle fatigue. Table 9.12 has a short list of comparisons of muscle activation when it occurs during normal movement and when it is produced by electrical stimulation.

This modality is most often used to strengthen muscle, aid in neuromotor reeducation, prevent disuse atrophy, and relax muscle spasm. Since each of these functions involves setting parameters that produce a muscle contraction, regardless of the desired treatment goal, the parameters will be similar for each of these purposes. In clinical situations where an injured patient is being treated, an alternating current with a balanced, asymmetrical biphasic pulsed waveform will be selected rather than Russian stimulation with its burst-modulating alternating current because it produces a better muscle response.[114, 115] The pulse frequency should be above that which produces a muscle tetany; most often, the pulse frequency is set at 50 pps.[101] Increasing the pulse frequency above that increases the muscles' rate of fatigue.[101] The pulse duration ranges from 200 to 800 ms. The normal range of pulse duration is 300 to 400 ms.[110] The intensity is set to a level that produces a muscle contraction and is still comfortable for the patient.

Electrode placement for NMES usually involves a bipolar arrangement. The electrodes are placed over the proximal and distal ends of the treated muscle or muscle group. Larger electrodes are more comfortable and will disperse the current over a larger area, so greater current intensity is required when the larger electrodes are used. The farther apart the electrodes are placed, the deeper the current will penetrate, so a greater muscle contraction is achieved.

Indications, Precautions, and Contraindications

With few exceptions, the precautions and contraindications for these electrical modalities are similar. Since some of these modalities relieve pain while others create a muscle contraction, their indications will be different, but their warnings for use are essentially the same. As seen in table 9.13, many of the precautions and contraindications for electrical stimulation are similar to those for other modalities. In some specific patient cases those items listed as precautions will actually be contraindicated, while in other cases they may be permissible, but caution should be combined with careful observation for any potentially harmful result.

Some of these precautions may appear obvious, while others may have more subtle explanations. For example, in the presence of skin diseases, the need for precautions in the use of any electrical modality may be obvious. The need may be less obvious in the presence of obesity. The reason in this case is that, depending on its thickness, the patient's fat tissue may create too much resistance for results to be beneficial.

CLINICAL TIPS

Most of the precautions and contraindications for the different electrical modalities are similar if not the same. Since each mode delivers an electrical current to the tissues, their negative effects on specific body segments or conditions will be the same.

TABLE 9.12 Muscle Activation: Normal vs. Electrically Facilitated Responses

Activity	Normal muscle response	Electrically facilitated response
Muscle fiber recruitment	Type I, slow-twitch, endurance fibers recruited first; Type II, fast-twitch, power fibers recruited during forceful activity	Type II, fast-twitch fibers recruited first; Type I, slow-twitch fibers recruited with increased intensity of stimulation
Muscle fiber firing	Asynchronously	Synchronously
Rate of fatigue	Slow because of firing sequence	Rapid because of firing sequence
Muscle changes with facilitation	Isometric exercise: increase strength	NMES better strength increase than with isometric only*

*Based on Parker et al. (2003)[111]; Walls et al. (2010)[112]; Laughman et al. (1983)[113]

TABLE 9.13 Indications, Precautions, and Contraindications of Electrical Stimulation

Indications, precautions, and contraindications	ELECTRICAL STIMULATION			
	NMES	HVPC	IFC	TENS
BENEFICIAL EFFECTS				
Reduce pain		●	●	●
Relieve spasm		●	●	●
Prevent or reduce edema formation	●	●	●	
Increase blood flow	●	●		
Neuromotor performance	●	●	●	
Reduce acute inflammation	●	●	●	●
Reduce chronic inflammation	●	●	●	●
Promote open wound healing		●		
CONDITIONS AFFECTING TREATMENT				
Deep vein thrombosis	●	●	●	●
Cold sensitivity	●	●	●	●
Raynaud's disease or urticaria	●	●	●	●
Impaired circulation or peripheral vascular disease	●	◐	◐	◐
Impaired sensation	◐	◐	◐	◐
Malignancy or radiation therapy	●	●	●	●
Pregnancy	●	●	●	●
Skin diseases	◐	◐	◐	◐
Hypertension	●	●	●	●
Electronic implants	●	●	●	●
Metal implants	●	●	●	●
Obesity	◐	◐	◐	●
BODY SEGMENTS AFFECTING TREATMENT				
Open epiphysis	◐	◐	◐	◐
Regenerating nerves	◐	◐	●	●
Reproductive organs	●	●	●	●
Eyes	●	●	●	●
Carotid sinus; anterior neck	●	●	●	●
Chest, heart	●	●	●	●
Head	●	●	●	●

● Indicated. In the presence of specific conditions it is safe to apply the modality, or when specific effects are desired, the modality may be effectively applied.

◐ Precaution. This is a relative contraindication. In some instances the modality will be contraindicated, and in others it may be applied with caution.

● Contraindicated. These are absolute conditions or locations where the modality should not be applied.

Summary

Therapeutic modalities are a part of the total rehabilitation program. They are used primarily in the first half of the program. There are a variety of modalities from which to choose, each with its own specific indications, precautions, and contraindications for use. The three categories of modalities presented in this review chapter included superficial and deep thermal modalities and electrical stimulation. Within each of these categories are specific modalities with their own advantages and disadvantages. A brief overview of superficial heat and cold modalities, thermal and nonthermal ultrasound, and therapeutic electrical currents, including TENS, IFC, HVPC, and NMES, was presented. These modalities are some of the more commonly used modalities used in rehabilitation programs to optimize treatment outcomes.

LEARNING AIDS ━━━━ ━━━━━━━ ━━━━━ ━━━━━━ ━━━ ━

Key Concepts and Review

1. Explain why superficial heat is contraindicated during the inflammation phase of healing.

During the first 72 h after injury, there is a risk of bleeding because only the presence of a weak fibrin plug stems the bleeding. Heat modalities cause vasodilation and increase blood flow; these effects would increase the risk of renewed bleeding at the injury site.

2. Identify the main differences between superficial heat and cryotherapy.

Cryotherapy reduces blood flow; causes vasoconstriction; reduces capillary permeability, cell metabolism, chemical activity, oxygen uptake, tissue elasticity, inflammation, and edema formation; and increases tissue viscosity. Superficial heat, on the other hand, has the opposite effect in each of these areas.

3. Discuss the differences between treatment effects of ultrasound at 1 MHz and 3 MHz.

Heating is deeper with 1 MHz ultrasound than it is with 3 MHz ultrasound, but heating of the tissue with 3 MHz occurs more quickly and is maintained by the affected tissues for a longer time. Heating depth of 1 MHz is up to 5 cm (2 in.); heating depth of 3 MHz is less than 2.5 cm (1 in.).

4. Identify contraindications for ultrasound.

Contraindications of ultrasound include refraining from using it over areas of deep vein thrombosis, skin diseases, electronic implants such as cardiac pacemakers, open epiphysis, reproductive organs, the eyes, the carotid sinus, chest, heart, head, or areas of malignancy. It should not be used if the patient is receiving radiation treatments or is pregnant. Thermal ultrasound should not be used over areas of acute inflammation or recent injury.

5. Outline TENS treatment options that may be used to relieve pain.

Specific TENS parameters are dependent upon the type of pain being treated and which nerve fibers are to be impacted. Acute pain is treated with conventional TENS (low amplitude, high pulse frequency, and short pulse duration) to affect the A-beta nerve fibers. Acupuncture-like TENS (high intensity, high amplitude, low pulse frequency, with medium pulse duration) is used for either trigger points or subacute pain to facilitate A-delta nerve fibers so opiates are released through pain control mechanisms in higher nerve centers. Intense TENS is used for more chronic pain conditions and targets the C-fibers to create a noxious stimulation with some muscle contraction. Intense TENS uses a high amplitude intensity with variable pulse frequency and longer pulse duration.

6. List another type of electrical stimulation that may be used to relieve pain in addition to TENS, and explain how it is different than TENS.

In addition to TENS, interferential current (IFC) is often used to relieve pain. Rather than using biphasic, monophasic, or pulsatile waveforms, IFC uses two asynchronous interfering sinusoidal currents to reduce pain. It can affect deeper tissue than TENS can affect.

7. Present examples of electrical stimulation that may be used in the first half of a rehabilitation program and what the reason might be for using them.

Since an injury usually exhibits pain, swelling, and muscle spasm, electrical stimulation (ES) modalities such as HVPS, IFC, and TENS could be used to relieve pain and reduce muscle spasm. Edema would also be affected if IFC or HVPS was used. Since HVPS and IFC can manage all three injury problems, either one of these would be best to use immediately after the injury. As the injury heals, the muscles may remain weak. One option to strengthen the muscles in the early phases of rehabilitation is to use either HVPS or NMES to facilitate muscle contractions isometrically while the injury is still limited in its ability to function. If an open wound persists after an injury, the HVPS may be used to encourage the healing of the wound.

Critical Thinking Questions

1. For the scenario at the beginning of this chapter, what modality would you use to enhance the joint mobilizations that you are going to use to improve Stephen's right shoulder mobility? Justify your selection of this modality. What other modality options do you have if that modality is not available? Identify the specific parameters you would use to treat Stephen, and explain why you would make these selections.

2. A volleyball player who underwent an anterior cruciate ligament reconstruction is having excessive pain after the surgery. You decide to treat her with TENS to relieve her pain. Which kind of TENS would you use, and what would be the parameters you would set on the unit? How long would you have her continue with the TENS unit? After the pain subsides, you notice that she cannot fully extend her knee when she performs her straight-leg raises (SLRs). What modality could you use to encourage full knee extension during her SLRs? Justify your selection and explain why you selected this modality over others.

3. An intercollegiate gymnast suffered a grade II ankle sprain on a dismount off the rings during a competition last weekend. He did not come to you until 4 d after it happened because he thought it would get better, but it is now severely swollen and painful to the point where he needs crutches to walk across campus. What do you want to manage first? Why? List in order of importance the problems you will treat, and explain why you put your list in this order. Identify a modality that would best help you to achieve the goals you have set for the next 3 weeks of his rehabilitation program.

Lab Activities

1. One of the school's wrestlers injured his back in a match and underwent a partial discectomy 4 d ago. He was discharged from the hospital yesterday and is coming into the clinic today to begin his rehabilitation program. You realize that he will be the first patient that your clinic has seen for a surgical back repair; there are no protocols in place for this rehabilitation situation, so you decide to create one before he begins his rehabilitation program. Write a protocol for your department about the treatment and rehabilitation of a postoperative partial disc extraction. You need only include the protocol through the early proliferation healing phase.

2. A new patient has come into your facility for your examination and treatment. He is a 38-year-old stockbroker who works on the stock exchange floor, but on the weekends he enjoys playing basketball with his friends. He has noticed increasing pain occurring more often and more intensely over the past month in his neck and upper shoulders region. He has more pain at the end of the workday but not as much over the weekend when he is more active. During the week, he spends most of his days either looking up at the ticker tape running across the wall near the ceiling or bent over a computer. He has a forward head, round shoulder posture, and you notice that his scapulae are protracted and anteriorly rotated. He has several trigger points in his cervical and shoulder muscles. His pain is likely caused by the two extreme positions he assumes at work. Since he has been working at this job for over 15 years, you know that the problems he now has are the result of cumulative stress. Your first concern is to get his complaints of pain under control and to start him on changing his posture and body mechanics to reduce his body's repetitive stress. How are you going to achieve these goals? What modalities will you use to help you to achieve them? What parameters will you set for each of the modalities? How will you determine when you no longer will need to use these modalities?

10

Aquatic Rehabilitation Exercise

Objectives

After completing this chapter, you should be able to do the following:

1. Identify and discuss the physical properties of water that affect the ability to exercise in water.
2. Define and explain the difference between assistive and resistive aquatic equipment, and give examples of each.
3. List precautions and contraindications for aquatic exercise.
4. Identify three advantages of aquatic therapeutic exercise.
5. List an aquatic exercise for each body segment and identify its purpose.

Before Bobby Gall became a rehabilitation specialist, he had been a swimming instructor at the local beaches during the summer. He was well aware of the physical properties of water and of ways it can be used either to assist or resist a body in water. In his current job as aquatic rehabilitation clinician at the city's largest sports medicine facility, he feels his position is a perfect fit for him because it combines his sports medicine knowledge with his love for the water.

Bobby's patients have various kinds of injuries and are at different levels in their rehabilitation programs. Bobby enjoys this situation because it allows him to use various pieces of exercise equipment while taking advantage of water's properties. For example, with Pam Herslie, a patient who is non–weight bearing on her right knee's tibial plateau fracture, he uses the water to eliminate weight bearing to help her perform lower-extremity activities. With Olivia, who is resolving her hip adductor weakness, he uses water as resistance to provide strength activities. Olivia exercises in shallow water so that she encounters greater weight-bearing forces, but Bobby has Pam exercise in the deeper end for non-weight-bearing activities. Other patients of Bobby's use water dumbbells for resistance activities of the upper extremity and trunk, maximizing the water's drag and viscosity effects. Bobby appreciates the variety of exercises and his ability to use aquatic exercises throughout a rehabilitation program. He has created progressive and challenging aquatic programs not only for Pam and Olivia but also for all of his rehabilitation patients.

In matters of style, swim with the current; in matters of principle, stand like a rock.

Thomas Jefferson, 1762-1826, third U.S. president and author of the Declaration of Independence

Thinking outside the box can be challenging, but it can also be fun. When we create rehabilitation programs for our patients, creativity is important. Many rehabilitation clinicians have a swimming pool available to them but do not use it. Often the best exercises we can create for patients are aquatic exercises.

This chapter provides information that you may apply to what you have learned regarding exercise from previous chapters. General concepts and principles of aquatic exercise are introduced first. Examples of exercises for the trunk, lower extremities, and upper extremities are then presented.

Water-based treatment has existed for a long time. The ancient Greeks and Romans used water therapeutically. The development of whirlpools and Hubbard tanks stimulated the therapeutic use of water in the early 1900s. Recently there has been a resurgence of interest in aquatic therapy, emphasizing its use in exercise rather than its more traditional effects. This chapter addresses the use of water as a therapeutic exercise component in rehabilitation rather than its use as a thermal modality.

Aquatic rehabilitation is the application of rehabilitative exercise in water. Exercise in water is advantageous when the patient cannot perform land-based exercises; it allows the patient to begin exercises sooner than would otherwise be possible. It also offers a way to exercise on an injured lower extremity during the time the patient is non–weight bearing. An aquatic rehabilitation (aquatic therex) program can offer the patient a total exercise regimen that includes activities for cardiovascular conditioning, flexibility, strength, and muscle endurance. It can be instituted early in a rehabilitation program and can continue past the time when the patient can perform land-based exercises.

Physical Properties and Principles of Water

Before you can apply aquatic exercises, you must understand how water affects the body's ability to move and exercise. Although some of water's properties can be determined by formulas, we will not focus on the precise mathematical applications here. It is important only to appreciate that these formulas can help us to understand the impact of water properties on exercise.

Specific Gravity

Specific gravity is also called **relative density**. It refers to the density of an object relative to the density of water.[1, 2] It is, then, a ratio of an object's weight to the weight of an equal volume of water. The specific gravity of water is 1. If an object has a specific gravity greater than 1, it will sink in water since its relative weight per volume is more than that of water. If an object has a specific gravity of less than 1, it will float in water. If the object's specific gravity is 1, it will float just below the water's surface.

Specific gravity for the human body varies from one person to another and from one body segment to another.[2] The person's specific gravity depends on the body's composition of lean and fat mass and the distribution of body fat. The specific gravity of fat is 0.8, bone is 1.5 to 2.0, and lean muscle is 1.0.[3] The average range of specific gravity for the human body is 0.95 to 0.97.[4] Since the specific gravity of the average human body is less than 1, people will usually float. Women usually have more body fat than men, so women float better than men. A lean, muscular person may have a specific gravity of 1.10; an obese person may have a specific gravity of 0.93.[5] These wide variations in individual specific gravities lead to a wide range of abilities to float. Patients who are more muscular and have less fat mass may have a difficult time floating, so they may need flotation devices during aquatic exercises.

Buoyancy

Archimedes' principle of buoyancy states that a body partially or fully immersed in a fluid will experience an upward thrust of that fluid that is equal to the weight of the fluid the body displaces.[6] Buoyancy and specific gravity are closely related in that a body with a specific gravity of less than 1 will float because the weight of the water it displaces is more than the weight of the full body. For example, if a person has a specific gravity of 0.95, 95% of the body is submerged and 5% of the body floats above the water's surface. The amount of water displaced is 95% of the body weight. Specific-gravity values, in essence, indicate the amount of the body that floats and the amount that is submerged; the weight of the body or part of the body submerged is equal to the weight of the water it displaces.

Center of Buoyancy

Center of buoyancy is the center of gravity of the displaced fluid and the point at which the buoyant force acts on the body. In water, two opposing forces act on the body. Buoyancy is the upward force, and gravity is the down-

ward force. Each has a center point of balance. When a floating body is in equilibrium, the center of buoyancy and the center of gravity are in vertical alignment with each other (figure 10.1). In this position, the body is balanced. If the center of buoyancy and the center of gravity are not in vertical alignment with each other, the body is out of equilibrium and will tend to roll or turn. For example, if you place a kickboard between your knees, the center of buoyancy will cause your lower extremities to move upward to float.

Hydrodynamics

Hydrodynamics is the branch of physics that explores the motion of solid objects in fluids and the forces imparted on those objects by the fluid. The fluid's resistance to movement, the size and shape of the object moving, and the speed of the object all govern movement through water. Some of the factors that affect a body's movement through fluid are interrelated and are important for the clinician to understand when he or she makes decisions about the aquatic exercises to include in a patient's rehabilitation program.

Viscosity

Viscosity is the resistance to movement within a fluid caused by the friction of the fluid's molecules. Properties that influence viscosity include *cohesion* (the attraction of water molecules to adjacent water molecules), *adhesion* (the attraction of water molecules to the person's body), and *surface tension* (the attraction of water molecules on the surface to each other).[7] Movement within the water is resisted by the adhesion of water molecules to the person

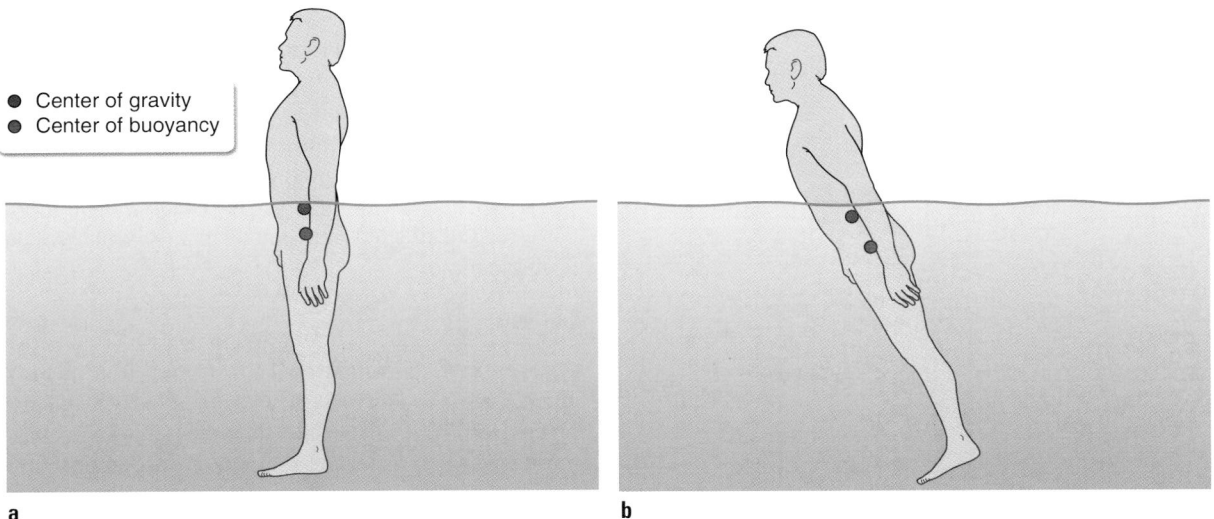

Figure 10.1 When the center of buoyancy and the center of gravity are not in vertical alignment, a person must actively work to keep from rolling in the water. *(a)* The body is in equilibrium; the centers of gravity and buoyancy are aligned vertically. *(b)* The body is not in equilibrium; the centers of gravity and buoyancy are not aligned vertically.

in the water and the cohesion of water molecules to each other. Surface tension provides resistance when a body or body segment tries to break the water's surface.

Drag

Drag is the water's resistance to a body that is moving through it. The three types of drag are form drag, wave drag, and frictional drag.[7]

Form Drag   **Form drag** is the resistance that an object encounters in a fluid. The amount of form drag is determined by the object's size and shape.[8] A larger object has more drag than a smaller object. A broad object has more drag than a streamlined object. Form drag is directly related to turbulence.[9] The greater the form drag, the greater the turbulence. Turbulence produces a low-pressure area behind the object that tends to pull the object backward, like what is seen behind a speedboat moving on a lake (figure 10.2).

A streamlined object moving through water produces a laminar flow—a smooth movement of water that causes a minimal amount of resistance. There is less form drag because there is less turbulence. The water molecules all travel at the same speed past the moving body. Friction of the fluid is minimal because the water molecules separate easily, moving smoothly behind the object.

On the other hand, a broad object produces a turbulent flow as it moves through the water. The object has more form drag because of the greater turbulence created behind it. The layers of the water move irregularly as they run into the object and rush to move past and behind it. This causes a circular movement of the water layers as they rejoin behind the object. This circular motion of water layers pulling against the moving object is called an **eddy**. In essence, the turbulence creates a backward pull on the forward-moving object, adding to the effort the object must make to move

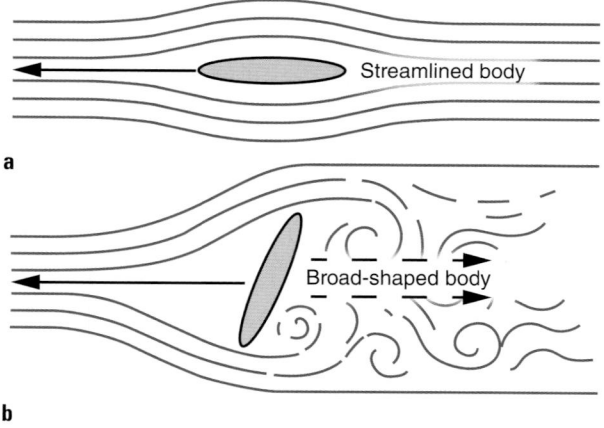

a

b

Figure 10.2   Form drag: *(a)* laminar flow (which produces minimal form drag) and *(b)* turbulent flow. Form drag is caused by turbulence behind an object moving through a fluid.

through the water. Because of the disturbance caused by the eddy, a wake, or trail, is left in the water (seen as either bubbles behind the body or white water, depending on the amount of turbulence created).

Form drag can be used in an aquatic therex program as a means of altering resistance to exercises. A change in the position of the body or body segment can increase or decrease form drag. For example, moving the arm horizontally in the water with the palm down causes less form drag than with the hand in a vertical position. Shortening or lengthening the body's extremity decreases or increases the form drag, respectively, since a longer lever arm pushes more water than a shorter one. Adding equipment such as hand paddles increases the surface area of the hand, and adding long paddles increases the lever-arm length; both provide additional form drag to increase the resistance of an exercise.

Wave Drag   **Wave drag** is the water's resistance because of turbulence caused primarily by the speed of the object in the water.[10] The greater the speed of the object, the greater the wave drag. Wave drag is reduced if movement remains underwater because less wake is produced.[11] The amount of water wake is an indication of wave drag. Swimming pools often have a splash gutter around the periphery to reduce wave drag for swimmers.

Exercises performed in calm water produce less resistance than those performed in turbulent water. The person can create wave drag during an exercise by changing positions often and rapidly. Increasing the speed of an exercise also increases the wave drag, thereby increasing the exercise's resistance. For example, walking in water provides the body with 5 to 6 times the resistance that walking in air does. Running in water, however, increases the resistance to more than 40 times that of air.[12]

Frictional Drag   **Frictional drag** is the result of water's surface tension. This is not a factor in rehabilitation, but it becomes an important element for competitive swimmers. Frictional drag can add crucial milliseconds to a race time; swimmers reduce frictional drag by shaving body hair before competition.[13] Recently, custom-made bodysuits constructed from unique new fibers have reduced frictional drag.[14]

Hydrostatic Pressure

Pascal's law states that pressure from a fluid is exerted equally on all surfaces of an immersed object at any given depth (figure 10.3).[15] The more deeply the object is immersed, the greater the pressure it encounters. Atmospheric pressure at the surface is 14.7 psi (pounds per square inch). For every foot of submersion, water pressure increases by 0.43 psi.[5] Hydrostatic pressure can positively affect edema both by reducing postinjury edema and by allowing exercise without the risk of increasing it.

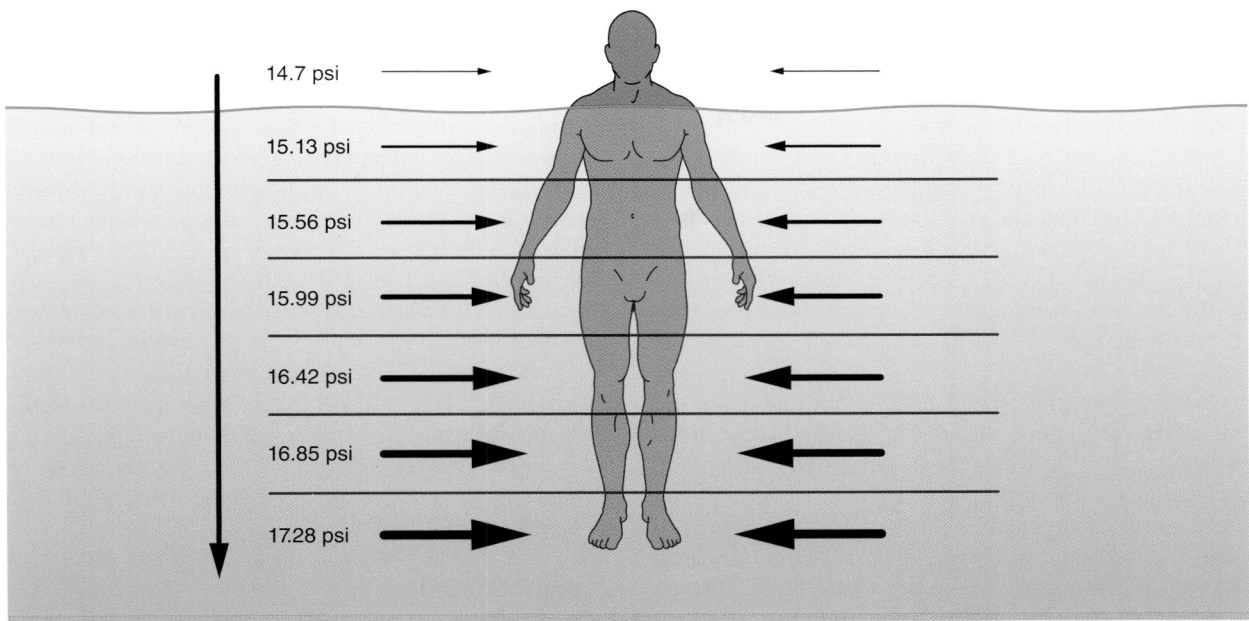

Figure 10.3 Pascal's law.

Weight Bearing in Water

Since buoyancy and gravity are opposing forces acting on a body in water, the more deeply the body submerges in water, the less weight is borne by the lower extremities (figure 10.4). Because a male's center of gravity is higher than a female's, the specific percentage of body weight borne at different depths varies slightly from female to male. For example, with the body immersed to the xiphoid process, females bear 28% of their weight, whereas males bear 35% of their weight.[16] Note that individual percentages will vary depending on body structure and weight distribution. In most cases, the percentage differences between

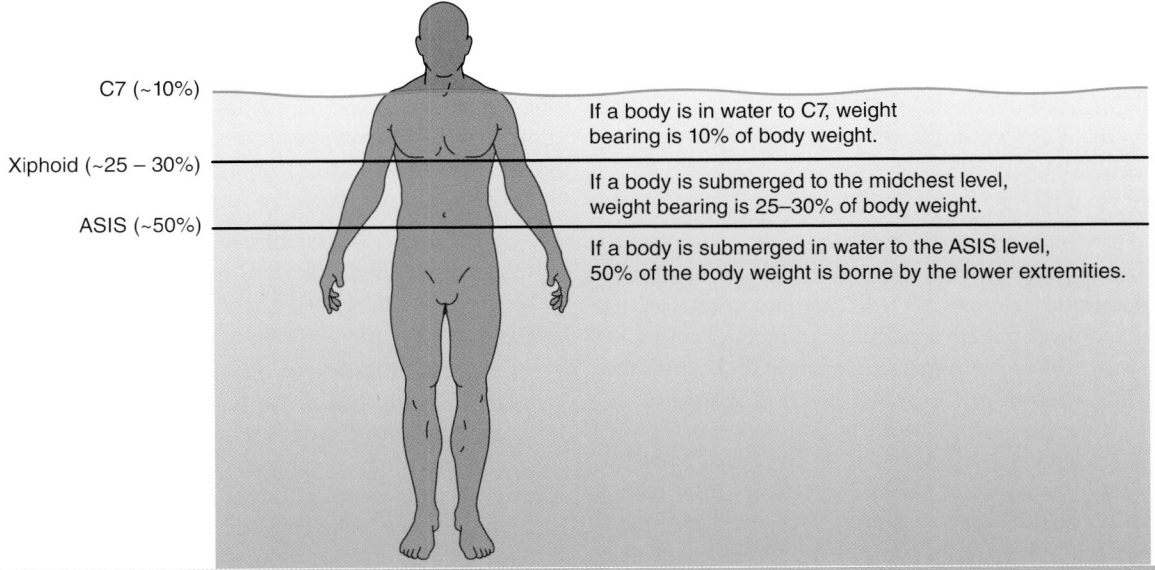

Figure 10.4 Weight bearing in water at different depths.

men and women are not enough to require a distinction between the sexes when it comes to determining the most appropriate water depth for exercises. Figure 10.4 may be used as a general rule for males and females.

These percentages provide useful information, especially in the early stages of rehabilitation. For example, an injured basketball player who is partial weight bearing to 50% on the left lower extremity can perform left leg exercises in water that is at anterior superior iliac spine (ASIS) level. As the patient is permitted to bear more weight on the limb, he or she can perform the exercises in shallower water.

Changing walking speed in the water changes the weight-bearing forces in the water.[17] Generally, the faster a person walks in the water, the higher the weight-bearing percentages. For example, if you walk at a slow pace, you can be in water that is at a level below the waist for you to be 50% weight bearing. If you walk at a fast rate, however, 50% weight bearing occurs in water above the axilla level.

Indications, Advantages, Precautions, and Contraindications

Although aquatic exercise has advantages over other forms of exercise, it is not for everyone. Before deciding to use an aquatic rehabilitation program, the clinician must be aware of the indications, as well as the limitations and dangers, of this type of system.

Indications

As mentioned, an aquatic rehabilitation program is indicated when the patient has many of the typical signs and symptoms associated with musculoskeletal injuries. These include pain, edema, muscle spasm, loss of motion, weakness, limited endurance, and restricted weight-bearing status.[18] Aquatic activities can also serve as a method of maintaining cardiovascular conditioning or normal status of the uninvolved extremities.[19]

Advantages

The indications point to several advantages to using aquatic exercises. Aquatic exercise can be especially beneficial when weight bearing is restricted. Patients who are limited in dry-land activities may perform a range of activities in the water while obtaining secondary effects from the water. The warmth of the water causes a relaxation of muscles.[19] The buoyancy reduces joint compressive forces to allow movement and positioning with reduced pain.[20, 21] The warmth of the water also reduces pain sensation by bombarding the sensory system with temperature input and decreasing the painful noxious input that travels the same pathways.

The reduction of joint compressive forces and the relaxation of muscles permit better movement of the injured area. Buoyancy equipment can further help to reduce stress on muscles in the affected area and permit greater ease of movement. The reduction of gravitational forces on the body allows for activity in water when weight bearing on land is not permissible. The minimal weight bearing required to walk in water makes it possible for muscles to function properly in the gait sequence. This encourages the maintenance of muscle tone and proper muscle recruitment and recruitment sequencing, and it prepares the patient for ambulation on land. Weight bearing can be progressive if the patient walks in water of decreasing depths: the shallower the water, the greater the weight bearing. The patient's ability to begin exercises sooner also helps to prevent deconditioning, a detriment that can delay the patient's return to full participation.

Precautions

As with any exercise, the rehabilitation clinician must be aware of precautions and must take special care to administer the aquatic rehabilitation program with these precautions in mind. When in doubt about the patient's ability to perform an aquatic program, the clinician must consult the physician in advance.

- *Fear of the Water.* A patient's fear of water often calls for encouragement and patience. It is advisable to use a vest, even in shallow water, for reassurance. The patient should begin in shallower water if the injury permits. You may have to give the patient some assistance and hands-on physical support until he or she becomes more comfortable in the water. No patient who has an excessive fear of the water should be forced to perform an aquatic rehabilitation program.

- *Medications.* Some medications that affect heart rate, blood pressure, respiration, or cardiorespiratory function may affect the patient's ability to exercise in the water. The clinician should check with the patient's physician or pharmacist before permitting the patient to go into the water.

- *Ear Infections.* If the patient has a tendency to develop chronic ear infections, he or she should apply proper protective ear devices before entering the water. Exercises should be designed so the patient's head is kept above the water to reduce the risk of infection.

- *Specific Conditions.* Patients with certain systemic or compromising diseases such as diabetes, cardiovascular disease, or seizure disorders should be carefully monitored while in the water. If the person is sensitive to the pool chemicals, it is essential to observe for and take steps to prevent unwanted side effects.

No patient should ever be in the pool alone, even if he or she is a good swimmer. Someone should always accompany patients during aquatic exercise.

Contraindications

Under certain conditions or in certain situations, patients should not be allowed in the pool for aquatic rehabilitation. These conditions or situations are absolute contraindications that, if ignored, could lead to serious consequences.

- *Illness.* A patient who has a contagious infection and is at risk of transmitting the infection to others should not be allowed in the water. A severe cold or the flu warrants keeping the patient out of the water until he or she has recovered. Any urinary tract infection should be resolved before the patient is allowed in the water. If the patient has a temperature of 100 °F, aquatic exercise must be postponed. Not only is a fever a problem in that it indicates an illness; it may rise further because of the temperature of the water and the exercise.
- *Open Wounds.* Open wounds should be healed before a patient is allowed in the pool. After surgery, the healing time is usually about 7 d. However, if any portion of the surgical scar is open, the patient should remain out of the water.
- *Other Medical Conditions.* Some conditions are not usually found in the young population but need to be mentioned as a point of information. Conditions that are absolute contraindications for a person's participation in an aquatic program include tracheostomy, severe kidney disease, presence of a nasogastric tube, fecal incontinence, radiation treatments within the past 3 months, and a history of uncontrolled seizures.

CLINICAL TIPS

Precautions and contraindications relate to the use of medications, various medical conditions, and illness. The clinician should be aware of anything that may warrant caution with the patient in the water or even contraindication of the patient entering the water. If unsure, the clinician should contact the patient's physician before beginning aquatic rehabilitation with the patient.

Aquatic Rehabilitation Principles and Guidelines

As with rehabilitation on land, aquatic rehabilitation follows a progression. It begins with range-of-motion and flexibility exercises, progresses to strength and muscle endurance exercises, and then advances to coordination and agility activities before the patient performs functional and performance-specific activities. A treatment session begins with a warm-up and ends with a cool-down.

The length of the warm-up depends on the temperature of the water. Therapeutic pools used exclusively for rehabilitation are often set at 92 to 98 °F (33-37 °C). Swimming pools are usually set at a lower temperature, 80 to 85 °F (27-30 °C).[22] The cooler the pool temperature, the longer the warm-up should be.

A cool-down is particularly important if the treatment session included cardiovascular activities. Cool-down activities can include activities such as walking, easily treading water, or sculling in deep or shallow water. It is important to remind the patient to rehydrate after exercises in the pool. Because of the warm water temperature, the patient will perspire while exercising and will not realize it.

Principles Related to Water Properties

The clinician determines the essential exercises of the aquatic rehabilitation session on the basis of specific findings and gears the session toward correcting the deficiencies observed. The same progression principles are used for aquatic exercises as for dry-land exercises. Because of the properties of water discussed earlier, other factors enter into the selection of exercises. These factors include hydrostatic pressure, drag and turbulence, and buoyancy.

Hydrostatic pressure can affect the edema of a segment. It is better to exercise a swollen extremity in deep water than in shallower water because of the greater hydrostatic pressure at greater depths.

A longer lever arm increases form drag. The straighter the limb is kept during movement, the greater the water resistance. It is best to start with a shorter lever arm and progress to longer ones as strength improves. You can make additional changes in lever arm length by changing the position of the resistive equipment. The farther away from the body's core the resistive object is positioned, the greater the resistance force it offers to the body.

The properties of water can be used to create resistance for a body segment. Increasing the speed of the activity in water causes increased resistance to movement. Moving objects toward the surface of the water and increasing resistive surface area by using specific equipment or floats can increase water resistance to help build strength. Exercising in various water depths also changes the weight bearing and resistance.

Buoyancy can make an exercise easier or more difficult, depending on the relative positions of the center of buoyancy and the center of gravity. Buoyancy becomes a greater factor for the body in deeper water.

Aquatic Exercise Progression

Although we have noted that an aquatic rehabilitation program can serve to maintain cardiovascular conditioning and the status of the uninvolved extremities, we will not consider such exercises in detail. The emphasis here is on the injured segment. Keep in mind that cardiovascular activities are usually performed in deep water unless in-water treadmills are available. Deep-water cardiovascular exercises include activities such as running, treading water, and swimming. If it is desirable to exercise the uninjured extremities, the more advanced exercises presented later in this chapter may be used.

In recent years, a variety of new equipment has appeared in the aquatic exercise market. Aquatic equipment can be divided into safety equipment and exercise equipment.

Early-Phase Exercises

The early portion of an aquatic rehabilitation program includes gait-training activities in appropriate-depth water, range-of-motion exercises, and perhaps early strengthening activities, if these are indicated and tolerated. Gait training emphasizes the correct manner of ambulation, proper posture, and good balance. The rehabilitation clinician should rely on knowledge of proper posture and proper gait timing and sequencing, as discussed in chapters 6 and 7, to assist and instruct the patient in correct posture and gait techniques. The goals in this phase are to achieve normal gait in water and to restore normal range of motion.

It is beneficial to use buoyancy equipment in range-of-motion exercises. Buoyancy equipment allows the extremity to move to the water's surface where range-of-motion gains are easiest to achieve. Figure 10.5 provides examples of different buoyant equipment for the extremities and trunk. The kickboard shown in figure 10.5b may also be used as a buoyancy mechanism for the trunk or lower extremities as well as the upper extremities.

At the surface, drag is at a minimum, so movement requires less effort. Resistance exercises in the beginning are low level and are provided without resistive devices. Use of the body segment's own drag in the water is sufficient in the early stage of strengthening activities. The speed of movement is kept slow at first so that the water offers less resistance. Koury[22] recommends limiting initial bouts of resistance exercises to one or two sets of 10 to 15 repetitions, but the specific numbers of sets and repetitions are individually determined and are based on the patient's level of fitness, tolerance, and ability and the program goals. Increasing the repetitions or increasing the sets makes the exercise progressive. The method selected to provide progression is determined by the patient's tolerance, normal activity demands, rate of healing, and fitness level. Figure 10.6 demonstrates examples of upper- and lower-extremity resistance equipment that may be used in more advanced aquatic exercises.

Middle-Phase Exercises

As the patient progresses in both healing and ability, program short-term goals are revised to reflect the patient's progress, and the program's focus moves from flexibility and mobility to muscle strength and endurance. Restoration of muscle strength and endurance—the goal of the middle phase—receives more emphasis during this time.

Viscosity-producing drag and buoyancy-permitting motion are now used to provide resistance to increase strength. Speed of motion and lever arm length are other variables that alter resistance. Deeper water offers additional resistance because it increases pressure on the extremity and increases stability demands.

Progression with resistive equipment includes starting with short objects and progressing to longer objects. Using lower-profile objects is less difficult than exercising with higher-profile objects. The more drag an object provides, the greater the resistance. The more turbulence the object produces, the greater the resistance. The farther from the extremity's axis of motion the object is placed, the greater the resistance it offers. Each of these ways of increasing resistance creates an additional level of difficulty.

As was done in the early-phase exercises, you can increase the intensity of an exercise by increasing the repetitions or sets. This change will help improve endurance more than strength, but there will also be strength gains at a lower rate. This principle is discussed in chapter 13.

Advanced-Phase Exercises

The later stages of the aquatic therex program present a progression toward achieving the goal of restoring the ABCs of proprioception—agility, balance, and coordination. This goal prepares the patient to withstand the stresses that will be applied during land-based activities.

Gait-training activities advance to include walking at a faster pace or running, side-stepping, cariocas, and retrograde walking. Hopping, jumping, squatting, and other sudden changes in direction are also appropriate in this phase. Coordination exercises with eyes open and eyes closed are included as well.

CLINICAL TIPS

The rehabilitation clinician moves the patient through a sequence of water-based exercises in accordance with the principles of progression for other forms of rehabilitative exercises. Goals are set for each phase; once the goals are achieved and the patient achieves sufficient healing to move to the next level, new goals with increases in resistance and exercise demands are placed on the patient, just as with a land-based rehabilitation progression.

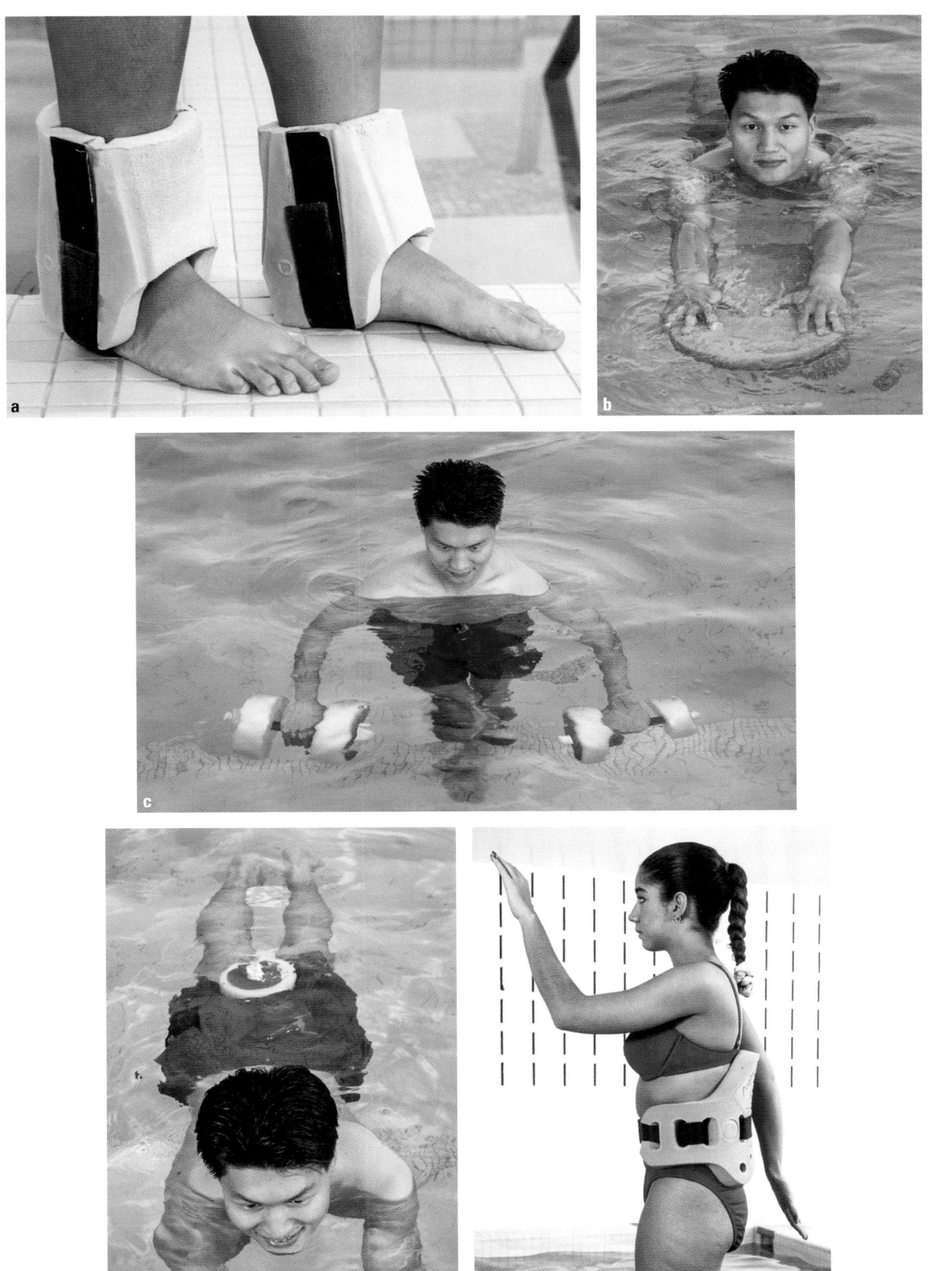

Figure 10.5 Examples of buoyant equipment. *(a)* For lower extremity, *(b, c)* for upper extremity, and *(d, e)* for trunk.

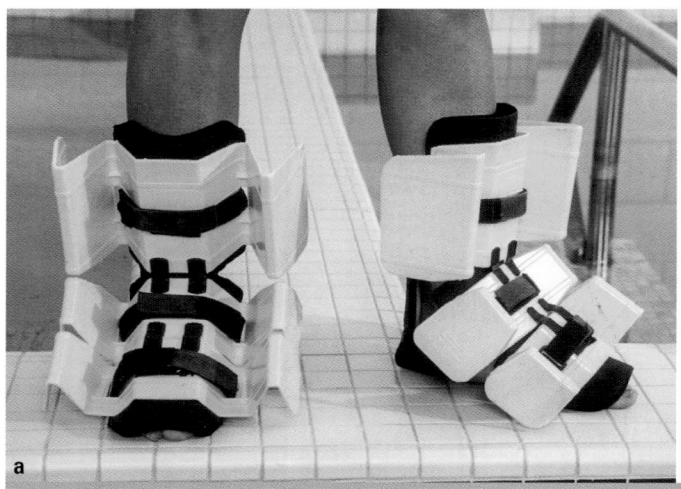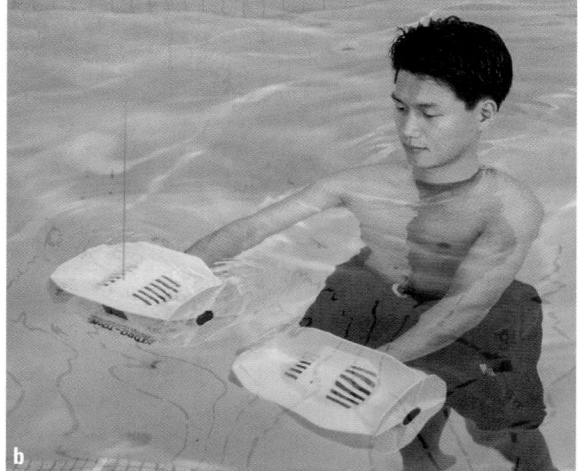

Figure 10.6   Resistive exercises for the extremities. *(a)* Boots for the lower extremities and *(b)* bells for the upper extremities.

Aquatic strength activities continue to increase in intensity if the rehabilitation clinician uses more aggressively resistive equipment, increases the exercise speed, requires more than one activity simultaneously, increases repetitions and sets, or changes the shape or size of the resistive equipment.

Land-based rehabilitation exercises may have started during this phase or during the middle phase. Whether or not the aquatic rehabilitation program continues depends on the patient's interest in the program, the clinician's preference, rehabilitation goals, time constraints, and equipment and pool availability.

End-Phase Exercises

If a patient continues in the pool for rehabilitation, this is the final stage of water-based exercises. Because of normal advancement to land-based rehabilitation exercises, aquatic exercises now either constitute only a fraction of the total time in the rehabilitation program or are discontinued entirely; however, some patients may prefer to continue in the water because of the satisfaction they receive from their workouts. The goal in this rehabilitation phase is to prepare the patient for the specific demands of his or her normal activity.

Exercises during this phase mimic the skill demands of the patient's sport; they include aggressive coordination, agility, and speed activities, and they reinforce the performance of specific skills while using proper posture. High-demand aquatic activities may include plyometrics, such as box jumping drills and bench stepping in the water. Performance-specific activities can include the use of equipment such as a golf club, tennis racket, or baseball bat in the water.

Progression Guidelines

Progression requires close observation and accurate patient feedback. You should observe the patient's rehabilitation program response and performance quality. Patients who perform the required exercises correctly and swiftly and who meet the exercise goals advance to the next level of difficulty. Throughout the aquatic program you must also periodically and routinely examine a patient's range of motion, strength, and balance and record improvements or changes.

The patient must communicate to the clinician any increases in pain or swelling or other symptoms after a treatment session. If there is no aggravation of the injury, the patient continues to progress in the program, working to achieve the goals set for each exercise. It is essential to advance the patient at a rate that will provide for a continued overload but not so quickly that she suffers a reinjury or fails to adapt to the stresses. For example, you may set a goal of performing a specific exercise for three sets of 15 repetitions; once the patient has achieved that goal for 2 consecutive treatment days, then the goal for that exercise increases or advances to a more difficult or challenging exercise.

Deep-Water Exercise

Even patients who cannot swim can exercise in deep water. Because of its advantages, deep-water exercise warrants special attention. We will look briefly at the benefits of this type of exercise.

The most obvious benefit of deep-water exercise is that it involves no weight bearing and no impact forces. This is particularly important if the patient wants to exercise but either cannot tolerate impact forces or is non–weight bearing. For example, running in deep water may be appropriate for a basketball player with patellar tendinopathy who cannot run on land without pain. Deep-water running can help keep the person's cardiovascular fitness level and strength intact during the rehabilitation process. A runner with a stress fracture is another example of a patient who can benefit from deep-water running.

Since gravity is opposed by buoyancy in deep water, the forces of gravity on a submersed body are minimal. If weights are applied to the ankles, a slight traction force is produced between the force of gravity and the counterbalance force of buoyancy in the joints. This can be important for a patient who has low-back pain secondary to either facet irritation or intervertebral disc compression.

Deep-water exercises are essentially concentric activities. Trauma to acutely injured tendons, muscles, or bones is reduced by avoiding eccentric activity, yet good strengthening can be provided with deep-water exercises.

Aquatic Rehabilitation Exercises

The following sections present a variety of aquatic exercises for the spine, lower extremities, and upper extremities. First, though, a few special points relevant to water-based exercise deserve mention. The first point concerns refraction in water and its effect on observation. **Refraction** occurs when light rays move from the air through water and bend because of the difference in density between air and water. This bending of the light rays makes the bottom of the pool appear closer to the surface than it actually is.

Some Recommendations for Optimal Benefits

During deep-water exercises, the body should remain in good alignment to minimize stresses and to use muscles effectively. The head is out of the water and in proper alignment with the rest of the body. The clinician should correct the patient with forward positioning of the neck or upward positioning of the chin to prevent an excessive cervical lordosis. The lumbar and thoracic spine is in correct alignment as discussed in chapter 6 in relation to proper standing posture (figure 10.7). Buoyancy vests or belts help the patient maintain a good postural alignment in deep water. If the spine is not in a neutral position, the center of gravity and the center of buoyancy will not be in vertical alignment. It is difficult to maintain a vertical position in deep water when the spine is not in good alignment.

To keep the spine in good alignment, the patient should lift the chest and maintain some tension in the abdominals and gluteals. This preserves good spinal alignment in the water just as it does on land.

Arm activity during deep-water exercises should occur from the shoulders, not the elbows. When running in water, the arms, as in land running, are used in a pumping action, with the activity initiating at the shoulders.

As in ground running, hip flexion and extension coincide with knee flexion and extension in water running. The ankle goes into plantar flexion during hip extension and into dorsiflexion as the hip moves into flexion.

Throughout the deep-water running activity, the spine remains in neutral with a slight forward inclination of the body (figure 10.8). The movement through the water is produced by the extremities, not the trunk. It is necessary for the trunk muscles—the abdominals and the back extensors—to act as stabilizers of the trunk as the body is propelled through the water by all four limbs.

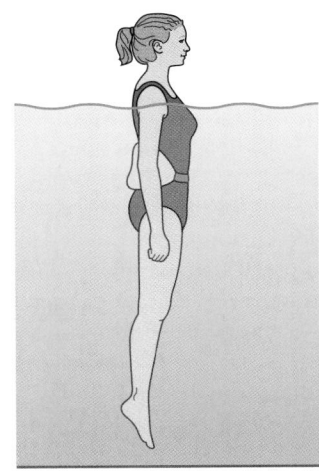

Figure 10.7 Correct vertical alignment in deep water.

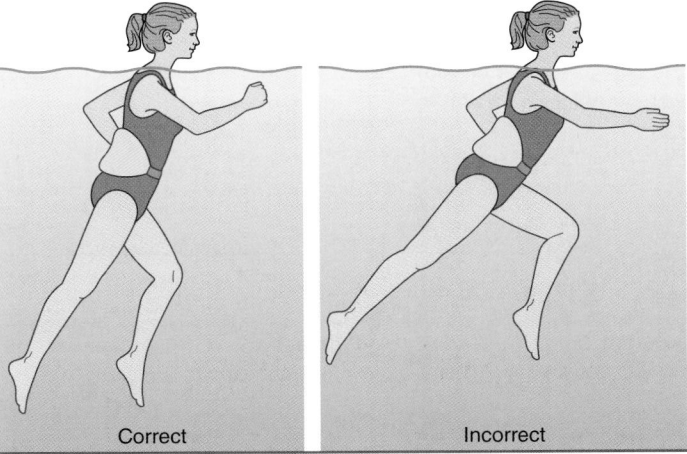

Correct   Incorrect

Figure 10.8 Position for deep-water running.

It also makes the submerged portion of the patient's body appear distorted (figure 10.9). The submerged body segments appear to be flexed at a different angle than the body segments that are not in the water. This can make it difficult for someone standing at poolside to accurately judge the position of the body or body segment. At times it may be necessary for the clinician to get into the water with the patient to make sure the positioning is correct, especially if the patient has difficulty with proprioception and cannot align him- or herself correctly without tactile guidance.

A note about deep-water safety: The patient should wear a vest or ski belt while performing deep-water exercises. The use of fins can make deep-water exercises more difficult, so the goals of the exercise are determined before the decision to use them is made.

A note about exercises in shallow water: A patient exercising with the feet on the bottom of the pool should wear aquatic shoes. These shoes may enhance balance,[23] provide friction resistance, and protect the patient's feet from abrasions.

The exercises described here are intended only as suggestions and are presented in a progressive series. The exercises are far from all-inclusive. Indeed, the range of possible exercises is limited only by the patient's abilities and your imagination and knowledge. If you know the goals of the rehabilitation program, understand the limitations of the injury, know the patient's abilities, and have an appreciation of the water's physical properties, you can incorporate a broad selection of appropriate exercises into an aquatic rehabilitation program.

A final point is that you should determine the depth of the water for the exercise according to the patient's confidence in the water and weight-bearing status and the goals for the treatment session.

Suggestions for exercises along with their purposes are presented in the following sections. For many of the strength exercises, however, descriptions do not specify which muscles the activity is designed to strengthen. Using your knowledge of kinematics and aquatic principles, try to identify the muscles for which each exercise is intended. As a hint, remember that most aquatic exercises are performed using concentric muscle activity.

Exercises for the Spine

The patient should maintain a neutral spine throughout all activities. This keeps the vertebrae in good alignment, places minimal stress on the spine, and uses the spine and trunk most efficiently, effectively, and correctly. If the patient cannot maintain proper spinal alignment during an exercise, the intensity, complexity, or demand level should be decreased and the patient should concentrate on a lower-level exercise until he or she has mastered spinal alignment at that level. If the patient has difficulty identifying correct spinal alignment with even the basic exercises, it may be necessary for the clinician to get into the pool and use tactile stimulation to help the patient find and maintain proper muscle recruitment and alignment.

You will see that many of the exercises described here are similar to land exercises. When patients perform them in warm water, the activity is often easier and more comfortable.

Spine Exercises in Shallow Water

The following sections describe only a few of many exercises that could be used for the spine. They begin with the cervical spine and move to the pelvis and advance from easiest to most difficult.

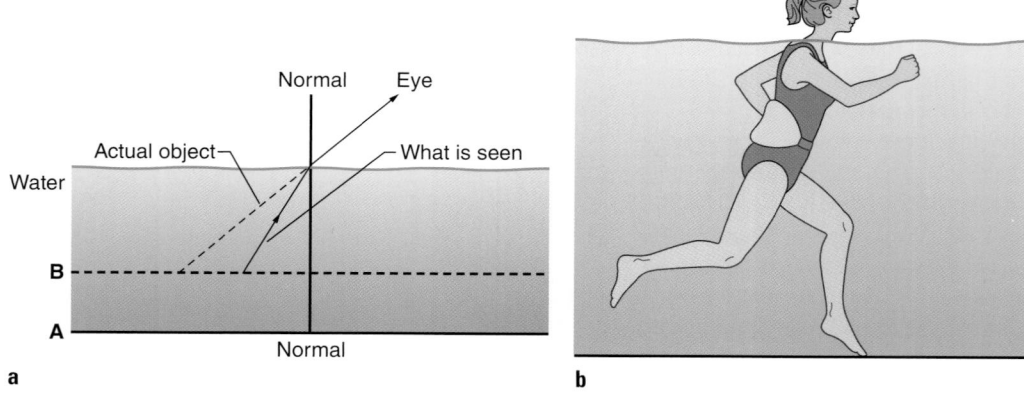

Figure 10.9   (a) Refraction of light causes rays reflected from the true bottom of the pool (A) to appear at a false bottom (B). (b) Refraction can create illusions in the alignment of body segments.

Neck Stretches

Position: To stretch the lateral neck, the patient holds the right arm down and across the front of the body.

Action: The patient side-bends the neck to the left, as seen in figure 10.10*a*. Reverse the neck and arm positions to stretch the left lateral neck. Figure 10.10*b* shows an alternative stretch in which the left hand is over the head. In this position, the patient provides a gentle stretch with the left arm while keeping the opposite arm behind the back. Substitutions for these exercises should be corrected.

Substitution: The most common substitutions are flexing the neck forward, rotating it to the stretch side, and flexing the trunk rather than the neck. In the neck flexion stretch in figure 10.10*c*, the patient places both hands on the back of the head and performs a gentle pull of the head forward and downward with the hands as the chin is tucked toward the chest. Instruct the patient to use only the weight of the arms and not add additional force in the stretch. The levator scapulae stretch (10.10*d*) is similar to that seen in figure 10.10*b* except that the neck is rotated slightly to face toward the axilla. Substitutions to watch for include rotating the neck too far, side-bending the trunk, and flexing the trunk.

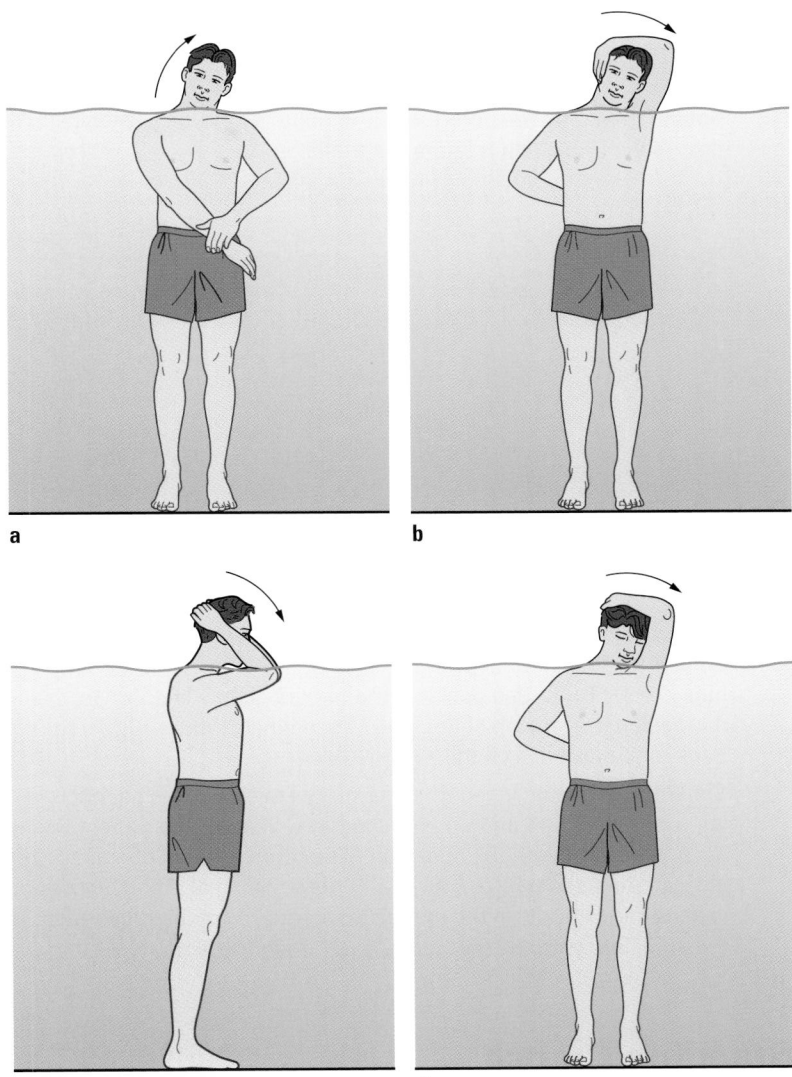

Figure 10.10

Spine Extension–Flexion

Position: Standing with hands on the pool wall and feet shoulder-width apart, the patient keeps the elbows straight throughout the exercise.

Action: The hips are pressed forward toward the wall, then backward. During the move forward, the chest is lifted upward (figure 10.11*a*); when moving backward, the patient tries to make the spine rounded (figure 10.11*b*).

Substitution: A common substitution is to rock on the feet rather than stretching the spine, or using the hands on the wall to push and pull the body forward and backward.

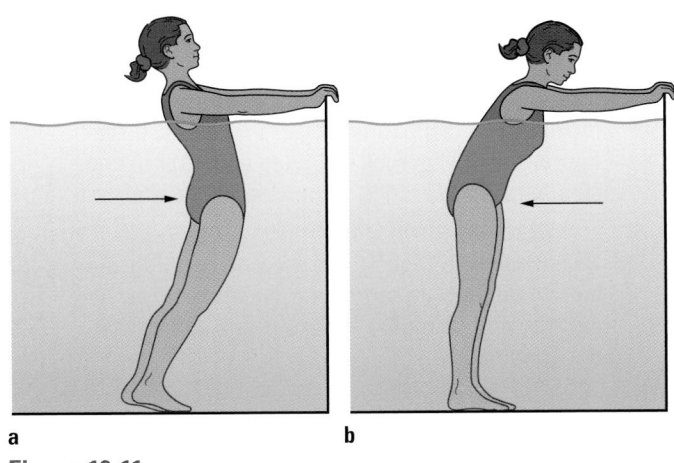

Figure 10.11

Lateral Stretch

Position: The patient stands with the feet shoulder-width apart.

Action: The patient raises one arm overhead and reaches upward and across the body (figure 10.12), feeling a stretch on the arm-elevated lateral trunk side.

Substitution: Substitutions include leaning to the side from the hips, extending or flexing the trunk, and rotating the trunk.

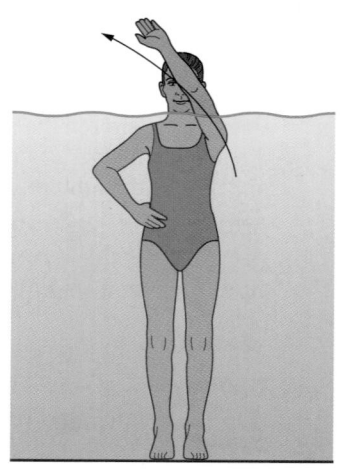

Figure 10.12

Pelvic Roll

Position: With the back against the pool wall, the patient supports himself or herself by holding onto the edge of the pool.

Action: With the lumbar spine kept flat against the pool wall and the abdominals tensed (pulling the navel to the spine), the legs are lifted until the knees and hips are at 90°. In this position, the patient slowly lifts the pelvis off the wall by increasing the tension of the lower abdominals (figure 10.13). The pelvis is rolled back to the wall before the legs are lowered.

Substitution: If pain is reported during this exercise, the patient is likely substituting with hip flexors and arching the back. Instruct the patient to keep the lower back in contact with the pool wall. If the correct position cannot be maintained, instruct the patient to alternately lift only one leg at a time until enough strength is acquired to perform the exercise properly. Another substitution is pushing off the pool floor with the feet rather than lifting the legs.

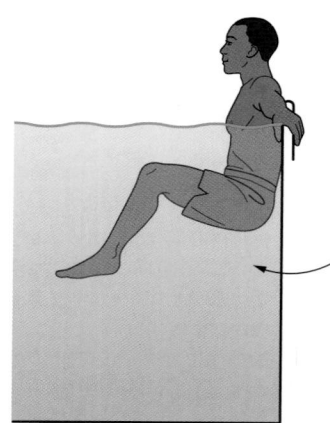

Figure 10.13

Standing Crunch

Position: The patient stands with a flotation device or a ball against the chest.

Action: The abdominals are contracted to flex the spine, and the position is held for 5 to 10 s (figure 10.14a). A pelvic tilt should be maintained throughout the exercise. This exercise can be modified to include rotational crunches as seen in figure 10.14b. The trunk is rotated about 10° to one side before the crunch is performed. The motion is repeated to the opposite side.

Substitution: Substitutions include pushing the ball down with the arms, not maintaining pelvic neutral, and using the hips to rotate rather than the abdominals.

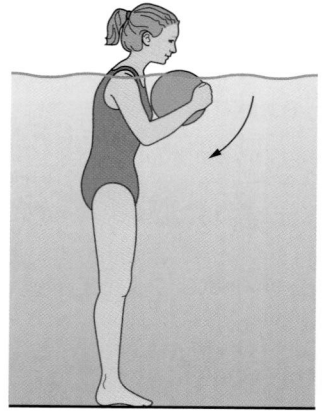 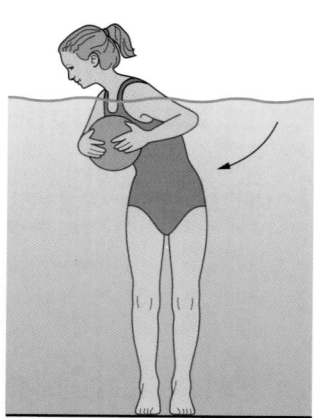

a   b

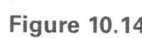

Figure 10.14

Trunk Rotation

Position: In a neutral standing position with the abdominals tightened, the patient grasps a kickboard and holds it in a horizontal position on top of the water throughout the exercise.

Action: Slowly and in a controlled manner, the patient rotates the trunk to one side and then to the other, maintaining tension in the abdominals throughout the movement (figure 10.15). The motion should not cause any pain. If pain is present, the motion should be restricted to a pain-free range. The exercise can be advanced by placing the kickboard under the water or holding the kickboard vertically in the water throughout the exercise. Holding the kickboard away from the body rather than next to it also increases resistance.

Substitution: Substitutions include rotating with the hips and knees rather than the abdominal muscles and pushing the board with the arms rather than keeping the board and arms in the same position throughout the range of motion.

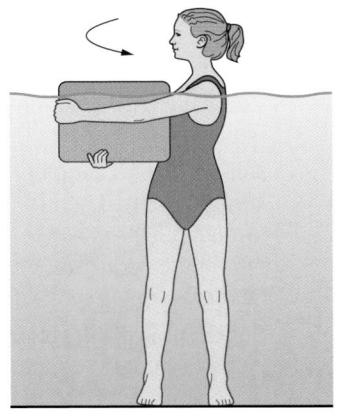

Figure 10.15

Wall Push-Off

Position: The wall push-off strengthens the thoracic spine. Standing away from and facing the pool wall, the patient keeps the spine straight and does not bend at the hips or the back during the exercise. The feet are kept in the same position throughout the exercise.

Action: The patient begins the exercise with the hands on the pool wall and the arms straight. He or she then leans forward by dorsiflexing the ankles and bends the arms until the chest comes close to the pool wall (figure 10.16) and finally pushes away from the wall until the arms are straight.

Substitutions: Substitutions include not keeping the spine straight and leading with the hips.

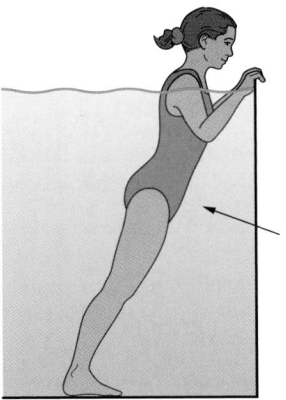

Figure 10.16

Pull-Down

Position: The feet are shoulder-width apart, the knees are slightly flexed to relieve low-back stress, and the spine is in neutral.

Action: The patient moves arm bells from in front of the body downward toward the sides (figure 10.17). The elbows maintain a partially flexed position, and the spine is in neutral throughout the motion. As strength improves, the elbows maintain an extended position throughout the exercise.

Substitution: A common substitution is trunk flexion to move the dumbbells.

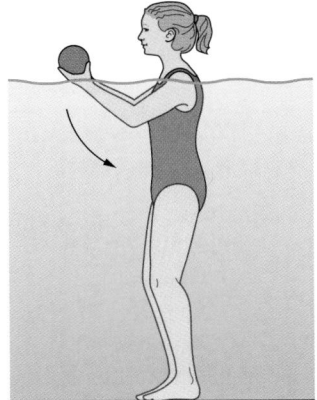

Figure 10.17

Spine Exercises in Deep Water

The patient must have good trunk control in order to perform the deep-water spine exercises. Someone who has difficulty with the exercise should perform it in waist-high or chest-high water first.

Double-Leg Lift

Position: With flotation devices in the hands or under the arms, the patient maintains a neutral spine throughout the exercise.

Action: The patient lifts the legs to a 90° hip flexion position with the knees extended (figure 10.18). The abdominals must remain contracted throughout the exercise. If a neutral spine position cannot be maintained during this exercise, the patient either begins with a single-leg lift or flexes the knees so the hips and knees are at 90° at the top of the motion.

Substitution: If the patient substitutes by arching the back, neutral spine is lost. Another substitution is flexing the knees to shorten the lower extremity's lever arm length.

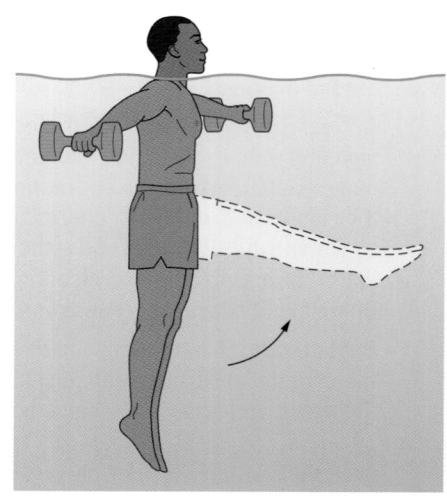

Figure 10.18

Trunk Rotation

Position: Using a flotation tube, the patient maintains a vertical position in the water.

Action: The hips and knees are flexed, and the oblique muscles are used to rotate the hips first in one direction (figure 10.19a) and then to the opposite side (figure 10.19b). The exercise is more demanding if the knees are fully extended.

Substitution: Substitutions include initiating the exercise with the hips or the shoulders rather than the abdominal obliques.

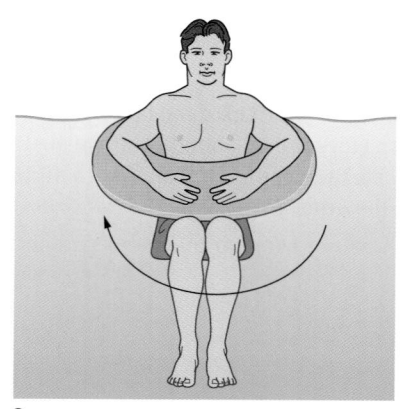 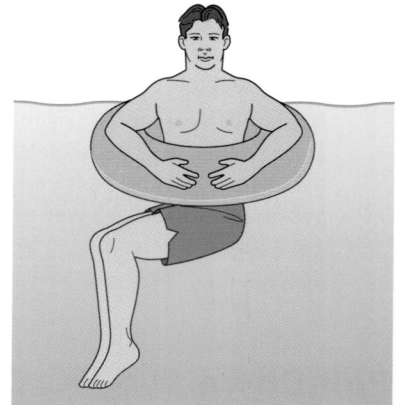

a   b

Figure 10.19

Lateral Flexion

Position: Using a flotation tube or other flotation device, the patient flexes the hips and knees to 90°.

Action: The patient maintains this position while lifting both hips laterally toward the left ribs, returning to the start position, and then lifting both hips laterally toward the right ribs (figure 10.20a). You can make this exercise more difficult by having the patient supine in the water with a flotation device at the waist and a small flotation tube or bells at the feet (figure 10.20b).

Substitution: A common substitution

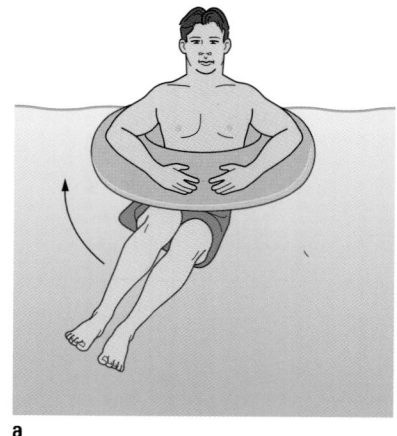 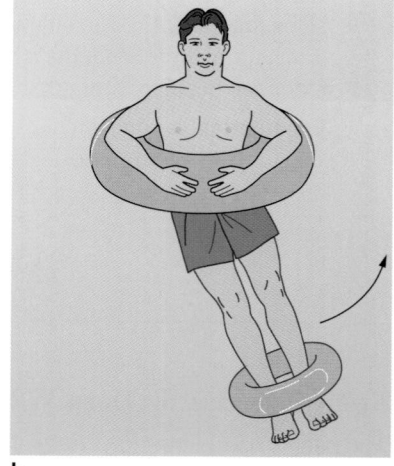

a   b

Figure 10.20

is arching the back and moving the legs in an arc around to the other side rather than moving back to the start position before lifting to the opposite side.

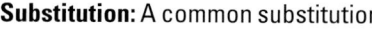

Exercises for the Lower Extremities

Exercises in this section begin with the simpler exercises in shallow water and advance to deep-water exercises. The patient may progress to some deep-water activities while still needing to continue with some shallow-water activities. A patient moves from shallow- to deep-water exercises when the short-term goals of each exercise are achieved and the patient is comfortable moving to deep water.

Ambulation and Balance Activities in Shallow Water

The following are examples of shallow-water exercises. You can increase difficulty by increasing the depth of the water in which the patient performs the activity. The patient should maintain body control throughout each exercise.

Forward Walking

Position: The patient may find it more comfortable to wear water shoes when exercising in shallow water. This exercise is useful as a gait-training exercise.

Action: Encourage the patient to maintain a correct gait pattern, as outlined in chapter 7, while in the water. Look for correct trunk stability. If necessary, the patient may use buoy lines or may walk along the side of the pool, holding on for balance in the beginning.

Substitution: Substitutions include any gait deviations that may be expected during land walking. The patient's specific substitution may relate to the injury. For example, if the knee is injured, the patient may not be willing to flex it enough during the swing phase and may opt instead to rise up on the contralateral toes to clear the involved extremity's foot during its swing phase.

Backward Walking

Position: This is another shallow-water activity. This exercise works particularly on the extensor muscles of the trunk and lower extremities. It is also good for balance and coordination.

Action: Emphasize normal stride backward with a good toe-to-heel pattern, normal and equal stride length, and proper weight shifting. The patient should maintain proper trunk alignment.

Substitution: The most common substitution is a forward trunk lean.

Toe Walking

Position and Action: The patient walks on the toes. This exercise is good for strength and proprioception.

Substitution: Substitutions to watch for include not rising up as high as possible on the toes and letting the heel touch the floor during the contralateral extremity's swing.

Heel Walking

Position and Action: The patient walks on the heels. This is a strengthening exercise for the dorsiflexors and is a proprioceptive exercise as well.

Substitution: Substitutions include hip flexion, forward trunk lean, not maintaining a high toe lift, and allowing the toes to touch the floor after midstance.

Single-Leg Balance

Position: The patient stands on the involved leg.

Action: The patient lifts the contralateral leg forward in a non-weight-bearing position and holds that position for 30 s (figure 10.21*a*). To advance this exercise, you can have the patient stand on the involved leg while moving the uninvolved leg forward and backward (figure 10.21*b*) or sideways (figure 10.21*c*). This exercise focuses on improving static balance. The trunk should remain stable and erect throughout the exercise, with tension maintained in abdominal and gluteal muscles.

>continued

Single-Leg Balance >*continued*

Substitution: Substitutions include using the trunk to move the extremity, flexing the weight-bearing or non-weight-bearing knee, and leaning the trunk.

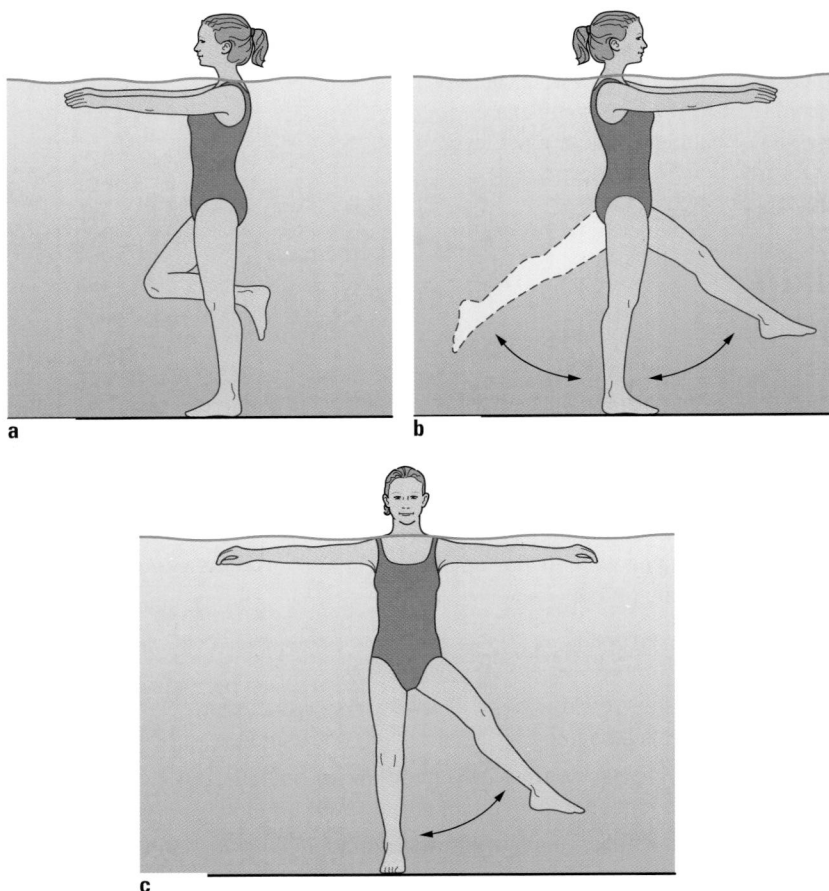

Figure 10.21

Lunge

Position: The patient begins by standing on both feet, shoulder width apart, with weight equally distributed.

Action: The patient performs a forward lunge by taking a large step forward and then bringing the back leg up to meet the front leg. This activity is good for increasing strength and range of motion of the hip and knee. Good upright trunk alignment is necessary throughout the exercise. The patient can also do backward lunges and side lunges to increase hip extension and hip abduction, respectively; these exercises are good for balance and strength as well.

Substitution: Substitutions include trunk lean, not using proper weight transfer, and not flexing the knee sufficiently.

Grapevine

Position: The grapevine is also referred to as a carioca or braid step. The patient stands with feet together.

Action: The patient first steps to the side with the first leg, then back (crossing behind the first leg) with the second leg, out to the side again with the first leg, then in front (crossing in front of the first leg) with the second leg. This exercise is good for improving proprioception, coordination, and balance.

Substitution: A substitution is rotating the trunk rather than facing the same direction while moving in the water.

Running

Position and Action: Similar to walking in the water, water running should imitate the technique of land running as much as possible. The patient should use the arms to keep an upright posture and should avoid the tendency to lean forward. Running forward, running backward, and cutting can all be performed in shallow water as a prelude to land running.

Substitution: The primary substitution is using the trunk rather than the legs to obtain sufficient speed and motion. The patient must wear water shoes when running in shallow water.

Hip Exercises in Shallow Water

Good trunk stability is important during all of the following hip exercises. You instruct the patient to maintain vertical trunk alignment and maintain tension in the abdominals throughout this activity. If the patient cannot demonstrate good trunk alignment, it may be necessary to work on the previously presented trunk activities in addition to the lower-extremity exercises presented here.

Hip Extension

Position: This activity stretches the hip flexors and strengthens the hip extensors. The patient stands in a backward–forward straddle position with the involved leg behind. The spine is kept in neutral throughout the exercise. Keeping the abdominals tense will help ensure correct spinal alignment.

Action: The involved knee remains extended, and the hip is pushed forward while the heel stays on the floor (figure 10.22). The gluteals are tightened during the exercise.

Substitution: Substitutions include arching the back, lifting the heel off the floor, and flexing the knee.

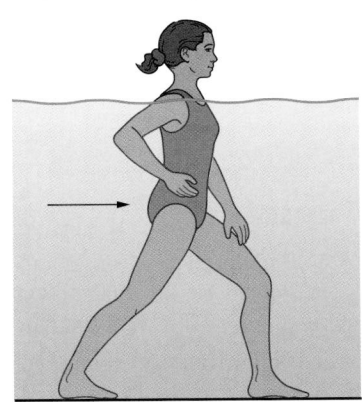

Figure 10.22

Hip Adductor Stretch

Position: This exercise stretches the hip adductors. The patient stands in a side-straddle position.

Action: The uninvolved knee is flexed as the weight is shifted to that side without leaning to that side. The involved knee extends, and the trunk is kept in an upright position (figure 10.23).

Substitution: Substitutions include lateral trunk bending or rotation, hip flexion on the involved side, and hip lateral rotation.

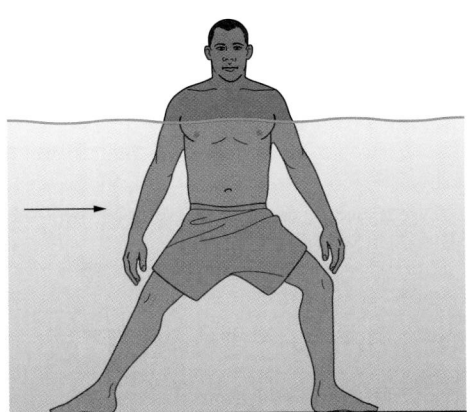

Figure 10.23

Hip Medial–Lateral Rotation

Position: These exercises can be used to stretch one group as they strengthen the opposing muscle group. The patient may need to hold onto the pool wall or rail. The knee and hip of the involved extremity are flexed, with the sole of the foot on the shin of the opposite leg.

>continued

Hip Medial–Lateral Rotation >continued

Action: The knee of the involved leg rotates outward as far as possible to stretch the medial rotators (figure 10.24a). To stretch the lateral rotators, the knee moves inward toward the opposite leg (figure 10.24b). The trunk should remain in neutral throughout the exercise, and the pelvis and back should not rotate.

Substitution: Substitutions include rotating the pelvis or trunk and rotating the entire body on the standing extremity.

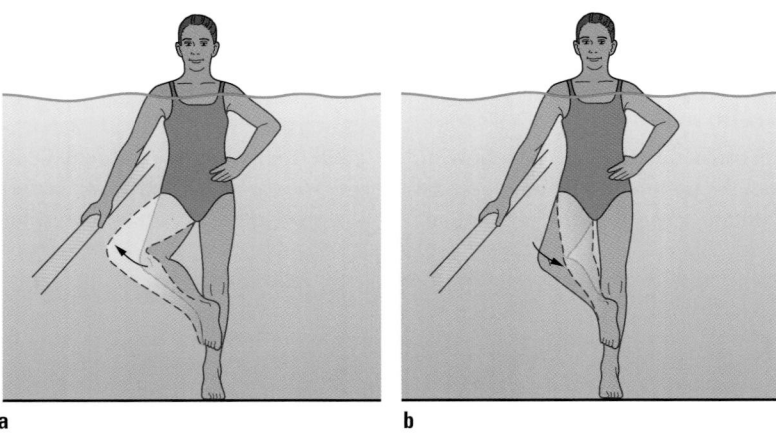

a   b

Figure 10.24

Figure-8

Position: This alternative to the rotation exercise just described offers resistance more than it increases range of motion. While grasping the pool side, the patient moves the exercising leg to a position of hip abduction with lateral rotation. The knee remains extended throughout the exercise.

Action: Using the water as the resistive force, the patient draws figure-8s in the water with the entire limb, initiating the movement from the hip, not the knee or ankle, while keeping the knee extended. Progressions from this exercise can include proprioceptive neuromuscular facilitation patterns in the water and breaststroke kicking.

Substitution: The common substitutions for this exercise include rotating the pelvis, flexing the knee, moving the trunk, and rotating from the knee or ankle.

Knee Exercises in Shallow Water

The first two knee exercises that follow are flexibility exercises; the others are strength exercises. The initial strength exercises should use only the limb as the source of resistance. As the patient's strength and control improve, attach drag equipment to the limb or have the patient perform the exercise faster as long as he or she maintains control of the limb.

Quadriceps Stretch

Position and Action: This stretch is similar to the land exercise in which the patient grasps the ankle of the involved leg behind the buttock, which is positioned with the knee flexed and the foot behind the body, and tries to pull the foot toward the buttock. The knee remains pointing directly downward, and the trunk remains in a neutral position.

Substitution: Substitutions include flexing the hip, flexing the trunk, and placing the foot on the side of the hip rather than behind it.

Hamstring Stretch

Position: The patient places the involved foot on the pool wall or on a step.

Action: The knee begins slightly flexed, but as the stretch is applied the knee is positioned fully extended (figure 10.25). Good trunk alignment is maintained throughout the exercise with trunk forward lean coming from the hip, not the back.

Substitution: Substitutions include posterior rotation of the pelvis and extending the hip.

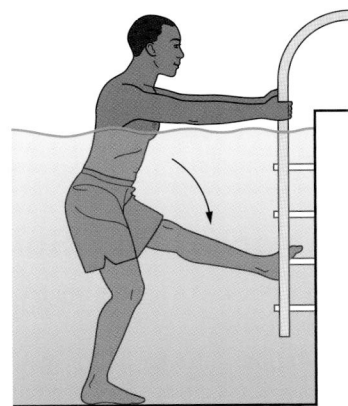

Figure 10.25

Single-Leg Bicycle

Position and Action: The patient flexes and extends the involved hip and knee in a cycling pattern while holding onto the side of the pool (figure 10.26). The trunk remains in neutral and does not move. This exercise is more difficult if the patient performs it without holding onto the side of the pool.

Substitution: Substitutions include using the trunk to move the lower extremity and using the arms for force transfer rather than using lower-extremity strength. Also, hip abduction or rotation may be observed; any substitution should be corrected so the hip, knee, and ankle maintain vertical alignment.

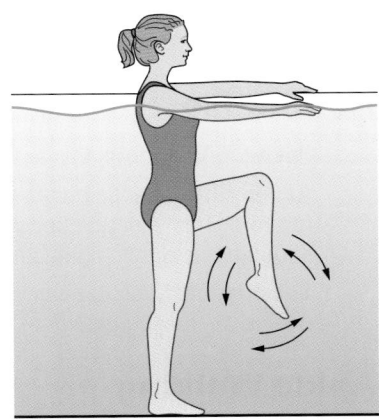

Figure 10.26

Squat

Position and Action: With the feet shoulder-width apart, the patient slowly bends the knees until the thighs are almost parallel with the pool floor. The spine should remain in a neutral position throughout the exercise, and the knee does not move forward of the foot. This exercise is more difficult if the patient performs it without holding onto the side of the pool or performs it only on the involved leg. In a further progression, the patient performs a squat jump so that he or she lifts off the pool floor.

Substitution: Hip flexion, hip hiking, hip abduction, and weight transfer to the uninvolved extremity are all substitutions to watch for and correct in this exercise.

Step-Up

Position: The involved leg is placed on the top of a box, stair, or platform.

Action: The patient steps onto the box by lifting the body upward, using the knee and hip muscles (figure 10.27). The trunk remains in a neutral position throughout. This exercise can be performed with the patient standing in front of, behind, or at the side of the box for forward step-ups, reverse step-ups, or lateral step-ups, respectively.

Substitution: Substitutions are trunk lean and hip hike, both common in this exercise.

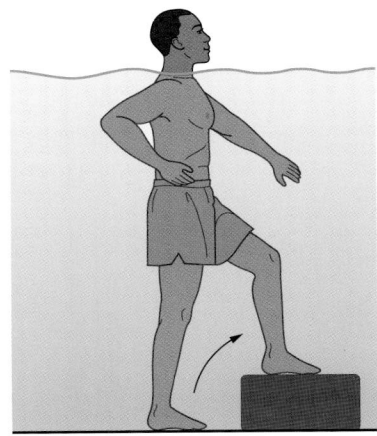

Figure 10.27

Ankle Exercises in Shallow Water

The ankle exercises outlined here are similar to those often performed on land, but the water is an ideal place to begin these exercises when weight bearing on the extremity is limited. In these situations, the patient begins in deeper water and progresses to shallower water as more weight bearing is permitted.

Gastrocnemius–Soleus Stretch

Position: The patient stands facing the pool wall and places the involved leg behind him or her and the uninvolved leg in front.

Action: The heel of the involved leg stays in contact with the pool floor, the knee remains extended, and the body weight is moved forward onto the hands and front lower extremity. This exercise stretches the gastrocnemius. To stretch the soleus, the lower extremity is brought forward slightly, the involved knee is bent, and the heel is kept on the pool floor as the weight is moved forward.

Substitution: Substitutions include flexing the hips, raising the heel off the pool floor, flexing the knee, outwardly rotating the foot, and laterally rotating the entire extremity.

Heel Raise

Position: To perform this activity, the patient initially may need to hold onto the side of the pool for stability.

Action: The patient slowly rises up onto the toes while the knees remain straight. The body should not lean or move forward. This exercise becomes more difficult if the patient does not hold onto the side of the pool. It is also more difficult if he or she stands only on the involved limb or moves to shallower water.

Substitution: Substitutions include rocking the body forward rather than moving the body directly upward with the heel raise, flexing the knee, and transferring weight to the uninvolved extremity.

Ankle Walking

Position and Action: The patient walks the length or width of the pool, first on the toes, then on the heels, then on the lateral sides of the feet, and finally on the medial sides of the feet. Progressions include increasing the stride length, increasing the speed, moving to shallower water, and using resistive equipment.

Substitution: Substitutions include knee valgus or varus positioning, hip rotation, and body lean.

Hopping

Position: The patient stands with feet shoulder-width apart with hips and knees flexed.

Action: The patient jumps forward, using the arms to assist while holding the spine in neutral (figure 10.28). The knees flex to absorb the impact-landing forces. Progression of this exercise includes advancing from double-leg to one-leg hops, moving to shallower water, increasing the repetitions or sets, and increasing the speed.

Substitution: Substitutions include flexing the trunk to lose spinal neutral and not landing vertically.

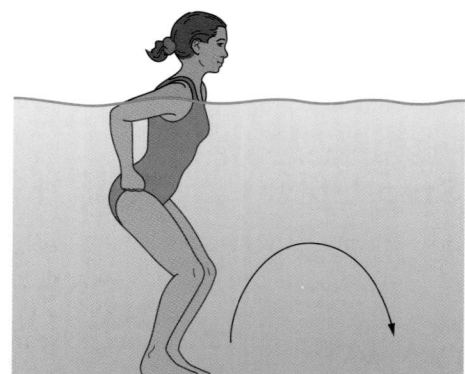

Figure 10.28

Ambulation Activities in Deep Water

The following activities are appropriate when weight bearing is restricted. Cycling and running in deep water can also serve as both cardiovascular activities and lower-extremity exercises. The most common substitution for any exercise in this group is using the trunk or arms rather than the lower extremities for power and motion.

Stride Walking

Stride walking is the use of exaggerated strides that are initiated from the hips. The spine should remain in neutral during the exercise.

Cycling

Cycling is performed with the patient in a vertical position. The patient mimics a bicycle motion with exaggerated hip and knee movement. The motion can be either forward or backward.

Running

Running in deep water, as with walking activities, is a good exercise for patients who must remain non–weight bearing. Running in deep water can include jogging or sprinting. The running form used is as close to land running as possible. The trunk should remain in neutral throughout the running phase.

Cross-Country Skiing

The patient performs a reciprocal motion of the arms and legs, similar to the cross-country skiing action, while maintaining a neutral spine position as seen in figure 10.29.

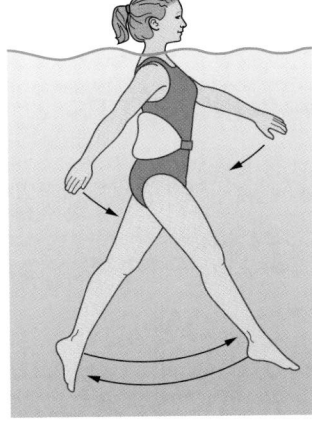

Figure 10.29

Hip Exercises in Deep Water

Deep-water exercises are more difficult than shallow-water exercises because, in addition to staying afloat, the patient must maintain an upright posture and a stable trunk during the exercise. Instructions to keep abdominal muscles tense and keep the chest elevated can be useful cues. The use of a flotation belt can help the patient in the early phases of deep-water exercise. Substitutions in these exercises will be most notable in trunk movement; trunk movement is indicative of poor core control, which becomes readily apparent when the body is not stabilized by contact with the floor of the pool. If the patient cannot maintain trunk stability in any of these exercises, he or she either may not be concentrating on performance or does not have the core or hip strength needed for the exercise. If the latter is the reason, instruct the patient to perform the exercise in shallower water, concentrating on core and hip stability, before advancing to deep water.

Jumping Jack

The elbows and knees are kept straight, and the spine is in neutral (figure 10.30). The arms begin in an abducted position. As the hips are abducted, the arms are adducted, and vice versa.

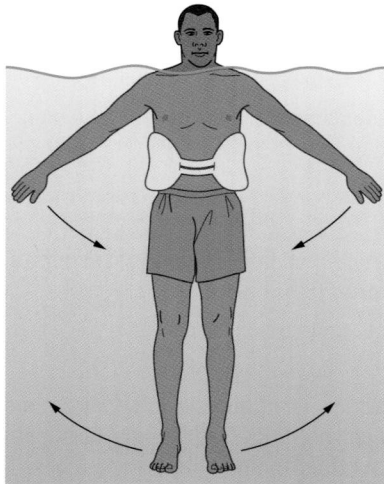

Figure 10.30

CLINICAL TIPS

Substitutions observed in deep-water exercises will be most notable as excessive trunk motion during extremity movement. Undesirable trunk motion is indicative of trunk, spine, and hip weakness, which becomes apparent when the body is not stabilized by contact with the floor of the pool. If the patient cannot maintain trunk stability during deep-water exercises because of deficient core control, begin exercises in shallow water, emphasizing core and hip stability exercises before advancing to deep water.

Double-Knee Lift

The patient lifts both legs together, bringing the knees toward the chest while the spine remains in neutral (figure 10.31).

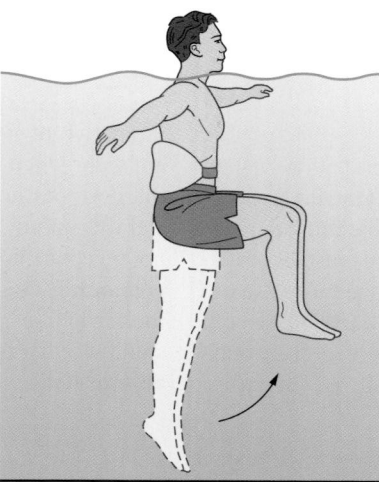

Figure 10.31

Flexion With Lateral Rotation

The patient is in a vertical position with the spine in neutral (figure 10.32). The legs move together simultaneously into hip flexion and lateral rotation and then they return to the starting position.

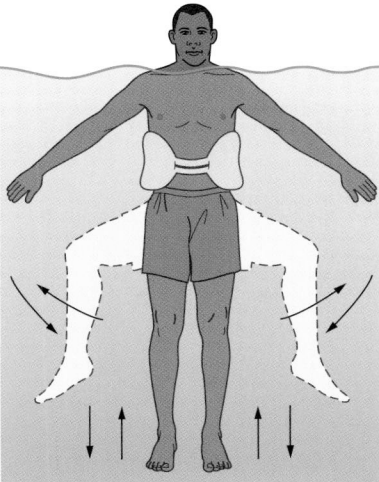

Figure 10.32

Hip Abduction

In a vertical position, the patient keeps the knees extended and the spine in neutral. The hips are both abducted simultaneously and then returned to the starting position (figure 10.33a). This exercise is more difficult if the patient performs abduction with the hips in 90° flexion, as seen in figure 10.33b.

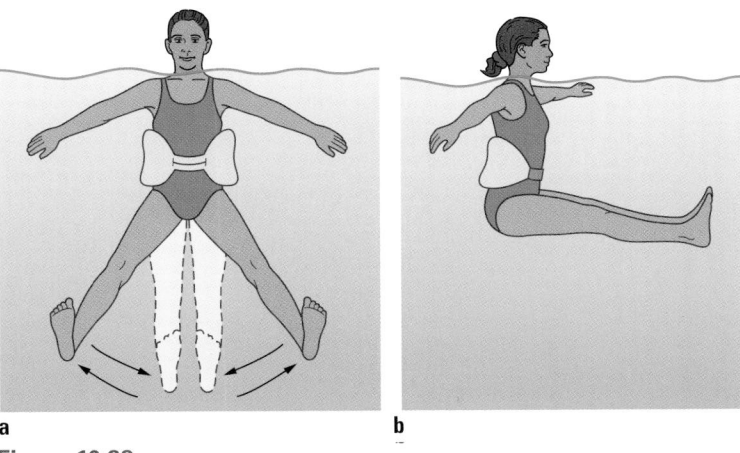

a   b
Figure 10.33

Flutter Kicking

Flutter kicking prone or supine, with two legs or with one, is useful for the hip. A substitution for this exercise is initiating the movement from the hip rather than the knee.

Knee Exercises in Deep Water

The knee exercises suggested here become more difficult if the patient performs them with both legs simultaneously or with resistance attached to the feet. Trunk and hip control is maintained throughout the exercises.

Double-Knee Bend

In a vertical position with the spine in neutral, the patient simultaneously flexes both knees while keeping them pointing directly downward (figure 10.34). The substitution for this exercise is flexing the hips.

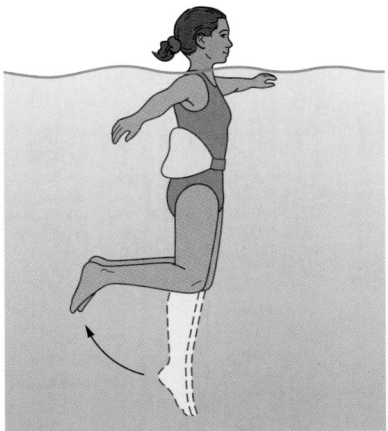

Figure 10.34

Seated Knee Extension

With the hips flexed to 90° and the thighs together, the patient extends the involved knee to full extension (figure 10.35). A vertical trunk position is maintained throughout the exercise. To make this exercise more difficult, have the patient extend both knees simultaneously. The common substitution is extending the hips. The trunk may also flex if the patient does not have good trunk control.

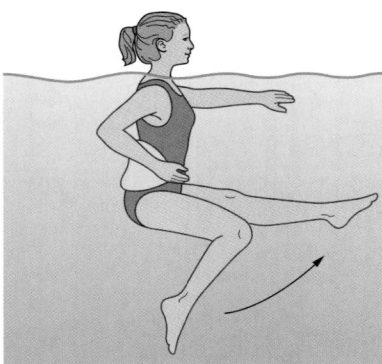

Figure 10.35

Exercises for the Upper Extremities

As with the lower-extremity exercises, the following exercises for the upper extremities do not constitute a complete list but are merely some suggested activities for use in rehabilitation. Although weight bearing is not the issue for the upper extremity as it is for the lower extremity, aquatic exercises can offer another way of rehabilitating the extremity. A mixture of activities can help to maintain the patient's interest in the rehabilitation program, and the variety can be enjoyable for the clinician as well.

Shoulder Exercises in Shallow Water

Our presentation of upper-extremity exercises starts with the shoulder and progresses through the upper extremity, beginning with stretches and advancing to strength exercises.

Pectoralis Stretch

Position: The patient stands in water above shoulder level with the arms elevated to shoulder level, elbows extended.

Action: The patient horizontally abducts the shoulders, squeezing the shoulder blades together. The palms should be facing upward.

Substitution: A common substitution is shoulder shrugging.

Capsule Stretch

Position and Action: With the involved arm at shoulder level, the patient grasps the elbow of the involved arm with the uninvolved hand and pulls the involved arm across the chest to stretch the posterior capsule (figure 10.36a). To stretch the anterior capsule, the patient clasps the hands behind the back and tries to lift the hands upward (figure 10.36b). Figure 10.36c demonstrates the inferior capsule stretch with the patient's hands overhead.

Substitution: Arching the back and flexing the trunk are substitutions in this exercise.

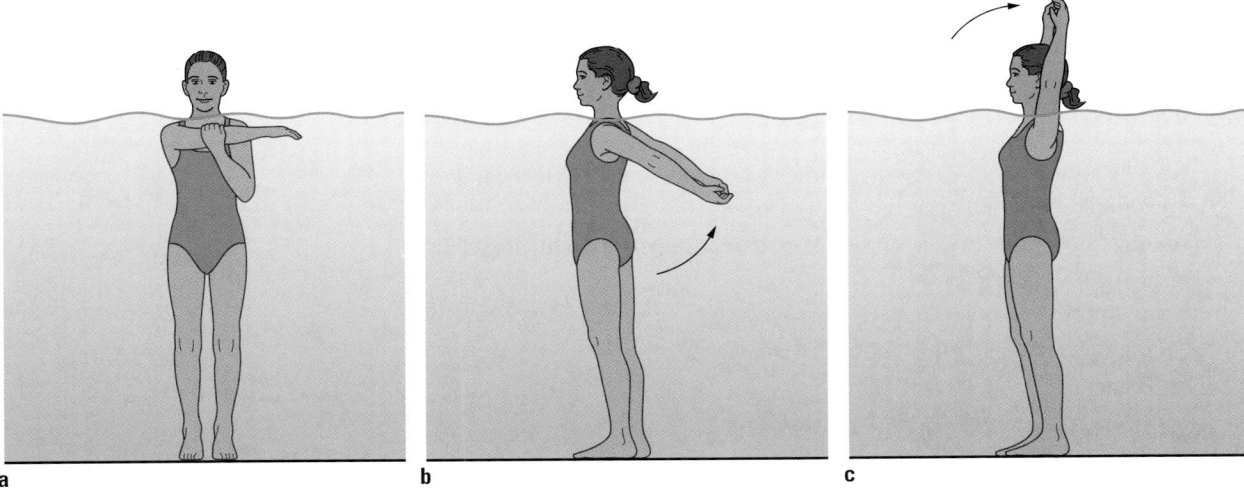

a   b   c

Figure 10.36

Lateral Rotator Stretch

Position: The patient places the involved hand on the low back.

Action: Keeping a neutral spine and erect posture, the patient flexes the elbow and reaches upward as high as possible on the back with the hand (figure 10.37a). In an alternative stretch, the patient grasps a bar or stair rung behind the back and tries to bend the knees (figure 10.37b).

Substitution: Forward trunk flexion and wrist extension are substitutions in this exercise.

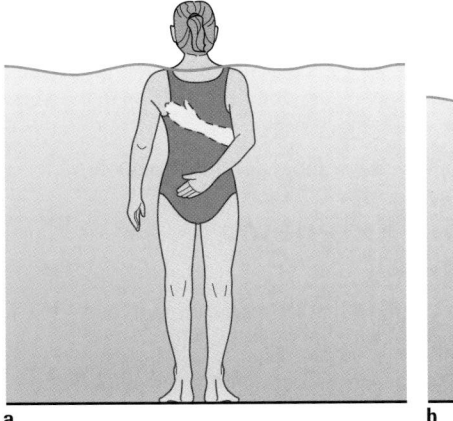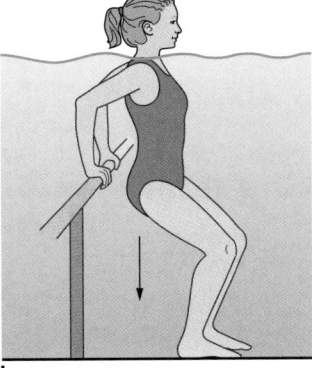

a   b

Figure 10.37

Medial Rotator Stretch

Position: The patient stands with the involved side near the pool wall. The elbow is at the side and flexed to 90° with the palm on the wall.

Action: The patient rotates the trunk away from the wall while keeping the hand in contact with the wall surface and the elbow at his or her side (figure 10.38). This exercise stretches the medial rotators.

Substitution: Substitutions include extending the elbow, rotating the pelvis rather than the trunk, and stepping away from the wall.

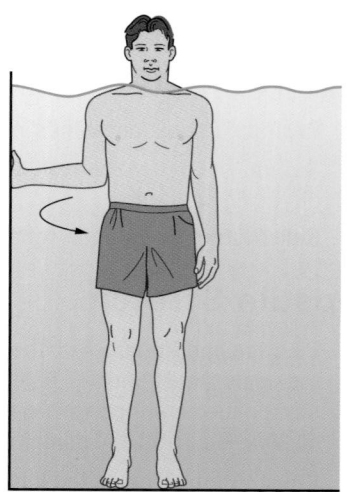

Figure 10.38

Shoulder Press-Down

Position: This is a shoulder-strengthening exercise. Using dumbbells or another flotation device, the patient allows the arms to elevate under the water as the elbows flex until the upper arms are at shoulder level and in an abducted position.

Action: The patient then pushes the dumbbells downward until the elbows are extended (figure 10.39).

Substitution: Using the trunk to push down by flexing the trunk forward is a common substitution.

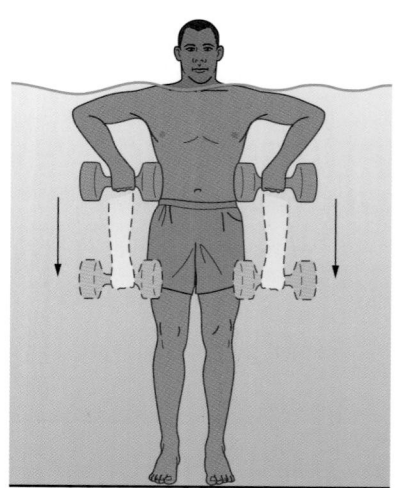

Figure 10.39

Shoulder Abduction–Adduction

Position and Action: Using resistive devices and keeping the elbows extended, the patient abducts the shoulders until the hands are at shoulder level and then returns to the starting position. The trunk remains in a neutral position throughout the activity.

Substitution: Trunk flexion is the most common substitution.

Shoulder Flexion–Extension

Position and Action: This exercise is similar to the preceding one, but the shoulder moves from flexion with the arm at shoulder level to hyperextension with the hand moving past the hips (figure 10.40).

Substitution: Trunk flexion is the most common substitution.

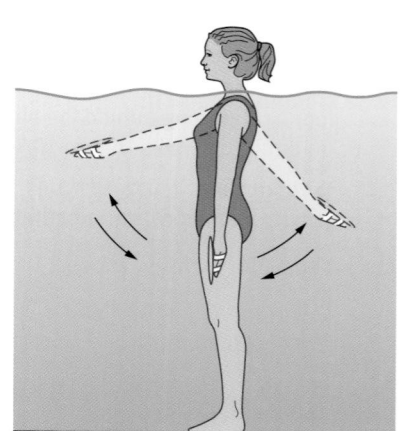

Figure 10.40

Horizontal Abduction–Adduction

Position: The patient keeps the arms at shoulder level and the elbows straight. The spine is kept in neutral.

Action: With resistive devices in the hands, the patient moves the shoulders through horizontal abduction and horizontal adduction.

Substitution: Arching and flexing the back during horizontal abduction and horizontal adduction, respectively, are the substitution patterns for these movements.

Medial Rotation–Lateral Rotation

Position and Action: With the elbow at the side, the spine in neutral, and a resistive device held in the hand, the patient moves the shoulder into lateral rotation and then medial rotation. If resistance in only one direction is desired, on the return to the starting position the hand is rotated so that the hand's profile in the water is reduced.

Substitution: Substitutions include shoulder abduction during lateral rotation or adduction during medial rotation.

Elbow and Forearm Exercises in Shallow Water

Stretching exercises are often more comfortable when performed in water. Elbow stretches can be particularly uncomfortable, and the elbow may be stretched more effectively with less discomfort in the pool than on land. Strength exercises can also be useful when performed in the pool. Consider the following activities.

Elbow Extensor Stretch

Position and Action: To increase elbow flexion range of motion, the patient actively flexes the elbow as far as possible and then applies additional force by using the contralateral hand to push the hand toward the humerus (figure 10.41).

Substitution: A common substitution is shoulder flexion.

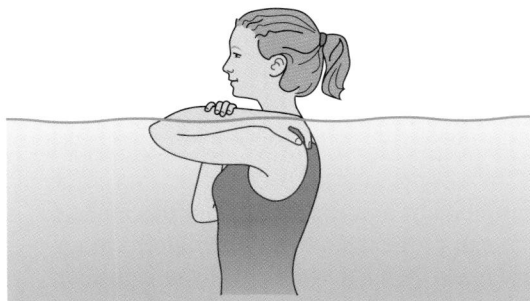

Figure 10.41

Elbow Curl

Position and Action: Using a resistive device to strengthen the elbow flexors, the patient flexes the elbow as the shoulder is abducted and as the hand is moved toward the water's surface. The shoulder and trunk are kept in a stable position throughout the exercise.

Substitution: Trunk extension is a common substitution.

Supination–Pronation

Position: With the elbow kept at the side at 90° of flexion, the patient grasps a resistive device in the hand, keeping the device underwater.

Action: The forearm is slowly moved from a palm-up position through a full range of motion to a palm-down position and then to the starting position.

Substitution: The trunk and shoulder are not kept in stable positions throughout the exercise.

Elbow Extension

Position and Action: With the elbow held at the side and a resistive device in the hand, the patient moves the elbow from a fully flexed to a fully extended position, keeping the device underwater throughout the motion. The hand remains in a palm-down position.

Substitution: Substitutions include trunk flexion and shoulder extension.

Upper-Extremity Exercises in Deep Water

Because so many of the deep-water exercises for one upper-extremity joint simultaneously engage the other upper-extremity joints, we consider all the deep-water upper-extremity exercises together.

Bent-Arm Pull

Position: With the body kept in a vertical position, the patient keeps the arms and forearms at approximately shoulder level.

Action: As one shoulder moves into hyperextension with the elbow flexed, the contralateral shoulder moves to 90° flexion, with its elbow moving from flexion to full extension (figure 10.42). The upper extremities then reverse their positions.

Substitution: A substitution is trunk rotation.

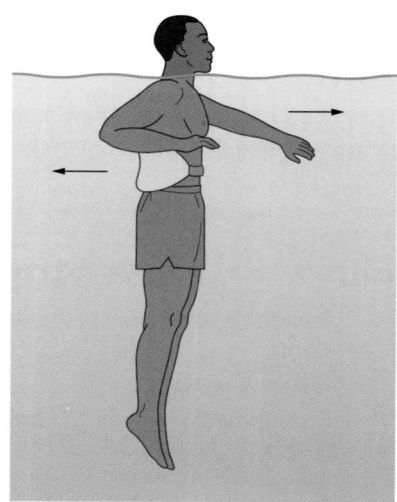

Figure 10.42

Straight-Arm Pull

Position and Action: With the body in a vertical position, the elbows extended, and the trunk stable and erect, the patient alternately swings the shoulders forward into flexion and then backward into hyperextension (figure 10.43). As the shoulder flexes, the hand faces upward; as the shoulder extends, the hand faces downward.

Substitution: Substitutions include flexing the elbow, using the trunk rather than the shoulder to provide the motion with trunk flexion during shoulder extension and trunk extension during shoulder flexion, and abducting the shoulder.

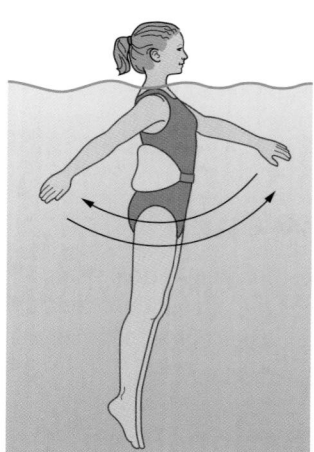

Figure 10.43

Arm Circles

Position: In a vertical position, the patient places the arms at shoulder level, keeping them submerged.

Action: With the elbows in extension, the arms move in circles clockwise and counterclockwise (figure 10.44). Changing the size of the circles, changing the speed of movement, or attaching resistive devices to the hands can alter the resistance. The motion is best performed with the shoulders in the scapular plane.

Substitution: Flexing the elbows is the most common substitution.

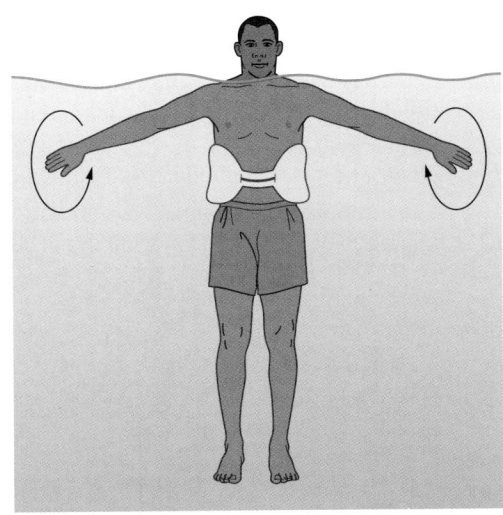

Figure 10.44

Breaststroke

Position: With the body in a vertical position, the patient keeps the arms at shoulder level but underwater.

Action: Shoulders begin in horizontal adduction and move through a full range of motion to end in horizontal abduction.

Substitution: Substitutions include moving the trunk into flexion, dropping the arms downward, and not moving the shoulders through an entire range of motion.

Shoulder Press

Position and Action: With the body in a vertical position, the patient pushes both upper extremities horizontally forward at shoulder level from the chest as in a bench press (figure 10.45). To increase the resistance of this exercise, you can add resistive devices, increase speed, or increase the number of repetitions.

Substitution: Losing pelvic neutral is a substitution, especially when resistance is added.

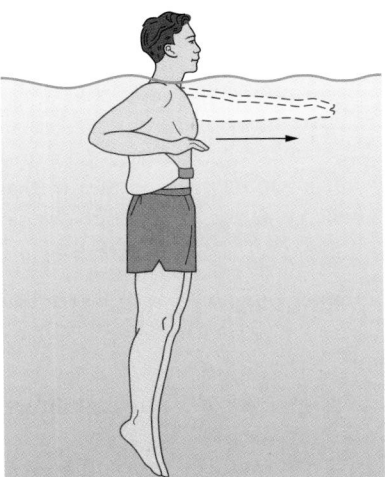

Figure 10.45

Elbow Press

Position and Action: With the body in a vertical position, the patient flexes and extends one elbow and shoulder, alternating the motion with the contralateral extremity. The forearm remains in pronation to offer resistance by the hand during the movement (figure 10.46). The movement occurs in an up-and-down motion in front of the body.

Substitution: Substitutions include not moving the extremities through a full range of motion and moving the arms to the sides of the body.

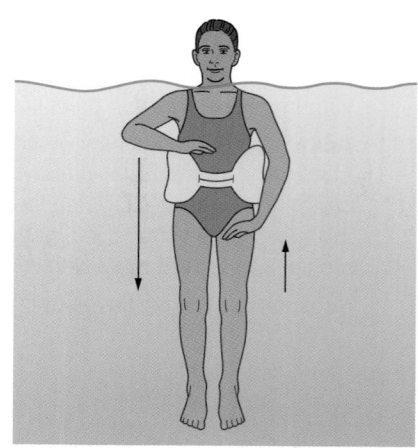

Figure 10.46

Wave

Position: In a vertical position, the patient places the upper extremities at shoulder level in abduction.

Action: With the elbows in extension, the wrists are alternately flexed and extended through their full range of motion.

Substitutions: Substitutions include flexing the elbows, dropping the arms toward the sides, and not moving the wrists through the full motion.

CLINICAL TIPS

Many water-based rehabilitation exercises are similar to dry-land exercises. As with dry-land exercise, most aquatic exercises for the spine and lower and upper extremities can be made more demanding through a progression of modifications. Throughout each exercise, the patient's spine must remain in neutral with proper engagement of core muscles; techniques for engaging the core are presented in chapter 17.

Summary

Specific gravity is the density of an object relative to that of water. The specific gravity of water is 1, so anything with specific gravity greater than 1 will sink and anything with specific gravity less than 1 will float. The specific gravity of the average body is 0.95 to 0.97. Moving the body in water causes resistance in the water; this is drag. There are three types of drag, but with each of them, the more drag a body has, the more resistance the water creates. Drag can be used as a resistive force just as buoyancy can be used as an assistive force for the body in water. Water exercises may be used early in a rehabilitation program if the body segment cannot bear weight or if it is too weak to withstand dry-land resistive forces. The deeper in the water a patient's body is located, the less weight is borne by the lower extremities. Devices are available to assist with flotation in water, while other devices are available to provide additional drag or resistance. As with any rehabilitation program element, there are advantages, disadvantages, and contraindications for aquatic exercise; the clinician must be aware of these before including aquatic exercise in a rehabilitation program.

LEARNING AIDS

Key Concepts and Review

1. Identify and discuss the physical properties of water that affect the ability to exercise in water.
The physical properties of water, including specific gravity, buoyancy, center of buoyancy, and hydrodynamics, influence the way a patient can exercise in water. Water has a specific gravity of 1. If a body's specific gravity is less than 1, the body will float, but if the specific gravity is more than 1, the body will sink. Buoyancy occurs when the specific gravity is less than 1. If a body is to remain upright while floating, the center of buoyancy must be in vertical alignment with its center of gravity; if it is not, it is difficult for the patient to maintain an upright position. Drag is the resistance to movement in

water; the greater the drag, the more resistance there is. Drag can be influenced by changing the speed of movement, turbulence, surface area being moved, and water depth.

2. Define and explain the difference between assistive and resistive aquatic equipment, and give examples of each.

Assistive devices in the water support the body to aid in buoyancy; examples are the kickboard and the flotation belt. Resistive equipment in the water increases the drag and makes it more difficult for a body to move; examples are paddles and boots.

3. List precautions and contraindications for aquatic exercise.

The most common precaution relates to the patient's fear. Other precautions include medications that can compromise the patient's situation, ear infections, and certain medical conditions. A patient who has uncontrolled seizures, for example, may be endangered in a pool and must be closely observed. Contraindications include illness, open wounds, and medical conditions that may be dangerous for either the patient or others in the pool; in these cases, the patient must not be allowed in the pool.

4. Identify three advantages of aquatic therapeutic exercise.

Aquatic exercises can begin early in the rehabilitation program. Patients with non-weight-bearing conditions can begin water exercises before land exercises. Aquatic rehabilitation can relax muscle spasm and pain, and it adds variety to a patient's rehabilitation program.

5. List an aquatic exercise for each body segment and identify its purpose.

An example of a trunk exercise is the lateral stretch in shallow water, used to improve flexibility. An example of a lower-extremity exercise is step-ups in shallow water, which increase the strength of the knee muscles, especially the quadriceps. An upper-extremity exercise is the shoulder press-down with water dumbbells, used to strengthen the shoulder depressors.

Critical Thinking Questions

1. Why is it that some of the patients you place in the pool have no trouble floating, while others must work to keep their heads above water? What principle causes this phenomenon?

2. If the patient you are rehabilitating is non–weight bearing on an injured ankle but wants to perform cardiovascular activities in the pool, what program will you design for him? What water depth should he be in for resistive exercises?

3. The softball player whose shoulder you have been rehabilitating fears going into the water. You would like to have her in the pool, since water activity would improve her shoulder motion and rotator cuff strength. What would you do to encourage her to get into the pool and to alleviate her fears? What would be your initial exercises with her, and at what water depth would you place her?

4. You are using the pool to rehabilitate a gymnast with a hip strain until she can perform land exercises without pain. Her motion is good, but her strength is limited in all hip motions, especially abduction. List three resistive exercises that you will include in her pool program, and provide a two-step progression for each one.

5. Identify a simple core stabilization exercise that you would use for a patient with a recent back injury, and include a four-step progression for the exercise. What would your criteria be for advancement from one level to the next?

Lab Activities

1. While standing in waist-deep water, move your hand through the water, maintaining the hand underwater, in the following ways:

   A. With the fingers together and the hand parallel to the surface but under the water

   B. With the fingers together and the hand perpendicular to the surface but under the water

   C. With the fingers apart and the hand perpendicular to the surface but under the water

   D. With the hand grasping a paddle and perpendicular to the surface but under the water

   Rate the movements in activity 1 from easiest to most difficult to perform. Which one was easiest and which one was most difficult, and why?

2. Walk across the pool in waist-high water. Walk across the pool in chest-high water. Walk across the pool in neck-deep water. Walk at the same speed at each depth. Which depth was the most difficult to walk in? Why? At which depth did you feel the most body weight applied through your feet? Why?

3. Now run across the pool at the same depths as in activity 2. Which depth was the most difficult? Why?

4. While maintaining pelvic neutral in chest-deep water, perform a single knee-to-chest exercise, alternating legs. Now repeat the activity in deep water. Which was the more difficult exercise and why?

5. While maintaining pelvic neutral in chest-deep water, perform a shoulder flexion–extension exercise, alternating arms. Now repeat the activity in deep water. Which was the more difficult exercise and why? What do you have to do at each depth that you do not have to do at the other depth? What do the results of this activity and activity 4 teach you about rehabilitation exercises in the pool?

6. Create an aquatic program for a lower-extremity injury suffered by a basketball forward. Start the program with the patient NWB and progress to partial and then full-weight-bearing activities. Don't forget to design exercises to include pelvic stabilization during lower-extremity exercises and functional and sport-specific activities in the final phase.

7. Create an aquatic program for an upper-extremity injury in a softball pitcher. Don't forget to design exercises to include pelvic stabilization during lower-extremity exercises and functional and sport-specific activities for this windmill pitcher in the final phase.

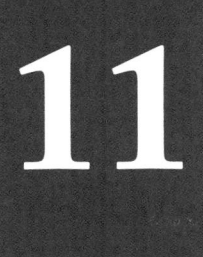

Manual Therapy

Objectives

After completing this chapter, you should be able to do the following:

1. Discuss the three techniques of Swedish massage strokes and their indications, precautions, and contraindications.
2. Explain the progression of myofascial restriction after an injury.
3. Discuss the techniques for myofascial release.
4. Explain the leading hypotheses for the mechanism of myofascial trigger points.
5. Discuss the spray-and-stretch trigger point release theory.
6. Explain the concave-on-convex and convex-on-concave rules.
7. Define joint mobilization, manipulation, and grades of movement.
8. Discuss the direction of glide and traction in relation to the treatment plane.
9. Explain the theoretical basis for proprioceptive neuromuscular facilitation.
10. Discuss how PNF can be used to improve flexibility and strength.

Neil Dean, athletic trainer for a Division III college, had never seen scar tissue adhesions like the ones he encountered in his most recent rehabilitation case. Over 6 months ago, one of the softball players, Pam, had suffered a severe cleat laceration along her entire forearm when an opposing player sliding into home plate ran the sole of her shoe into Pam's forearm. The forearm required more than 30 stitches. Although Pam hadn't suffered any immediate loss of motion from the scar, she was now losing some elbow and wrist motion because the scar tissue was pulling on both joints. When Neil palpated the forearm, he could feel a lot of hard, unyielding scar tissue adhesions below the skin. He knew he had to soften the scar tissue and mobilize the tissue below the skin if Pam were to have normal elbow and wrist motion. He also knew he would have to show Pam some soft-tissue techniques that she could perform on her own throughout the day to reinforce his efforts in the athletic training clinic.

Beyond all doubt, the use of the human hand, as a method of reducing human suffering, is the oldest remedy known to man.

James Mennell, *Manual Therapy*

Manual therapy is the application of skilled hands-on techniques to treat and improve the status of neuromusculoskeletal conditions. Any manual therapy is a combination of art and skill. The quality of the clinician's manual therapy techniques is directly related to the amount of time dedicated to learning and practicing them. True mastery of manual therapy, like mastery of musical or athletic performance, requires practicing many hours, analyzing your results, and adjusting your application as you learn and master your manual therapy skills. Anything worth learning is worth learning well. If you want to be a master clinician, then daily practice is required.

Although subjective reports of manual therapy's effectiveness abound in the literature, it is very difficult to objectively measure the effectiveness of manual therapy. We can use manual therapy for several orthopedic and sport-related injuries and the secondary problems that occur as a result of those injuries. A variety of structures, including joints and soft tissues, can be affected by applying manual therapy. The application, direction, duration, and amplitude of a force in this type of therapy is very difficult to quantify and can vary from one health care provider to another. Clinicians approach applications differently, and patient conditions vary. Therefore, most of the reported benefits are based on anecdotes rather than quantitative research.

The most familiar manual therapy techniques are joint mobilization and massage. Other manual therapies that are less familiar, but perhaps recognizable, are techniques such as soft-tissue mobilization, trigger point release, myofascial release, muscle energy, strain–counterstrain, and instrument-assisted soft-tissue mobilization. Even exercises such as proprioceptive neuromuscular facilitation, manual resistance, stretching, and stabilization may be considered manual therapy techniques. Manual therapy techniques are sometimes classified under the umbrella term of *alternative*

medicine, complementary and alternative medicine (CAM), or *alternative therapy.*

Manual therapy techniques address soft tissue and more specifically the collagen of soft tissue. Even joint mobilization affects joint motion by affecting changes in the soft tissue (capsule and ligaments) that surrounds the joint, not the bone ends that form the joint. When applying manual therapy techniques, you may be affecting not only the target tissue but other local tissues as well. For example, a deep massage technique targeting deeper muscle tissue will also affect the skin, subcutaneous tissue, superficial muscle, and myofascial structures overlying those deep muscles.

Most manual therapy techniques are aimed at altering pain and function by affecting the body neurologically and mechanically.[1-3] Manual therapy techniques approach these goals primarily by neurological stimulation and by mechanically altering fascia.[1] Mechanical manual therapy techniques stimulate the skin's neural A-beta receptors, creating a response within the nervous system. Higher and lower neural stimulation in manual therapy application reduces pain.[4, 5]

Figure 11.1 is a model of the neural and mechanical changes in soft tissue that manual therapy can bring about. Manual therapies are used to alter connective tissue through plastic deformation to break down adhesions and improve flexibility.[6] These changes result in improved mobility, relaxation of muscle spasm, and increased function, which produce pain relief.[2]

Manual therapy can be divided into two main categories: direct techniques and indirect techniques. **Direct techniques** are maneuvers that load or bind tissue and structures.[7] These techniques direct the treatment force at the point where tissue mobility is limited. Techniques such as stretching, joint mobilization, trigger point release, muscle energy technique, and Rolfing fall into this category. The goal of these techniques is to move the point of restriction closer to the normal range of motion.

Indirect techniques are the opposite of direct techniques. These techniques apply treatment forces to move the tissue away from the direction of limitation, thereby

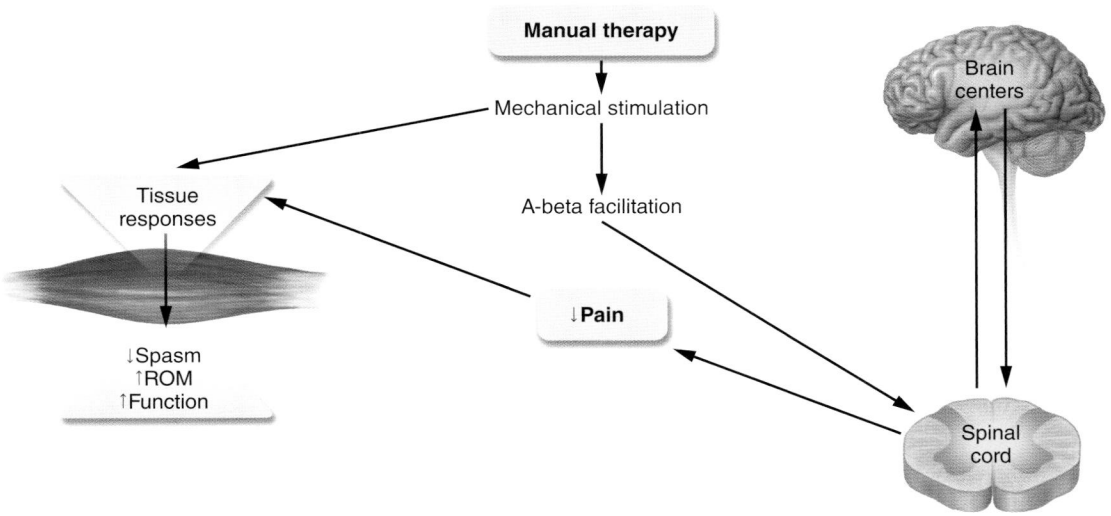

Figure 11.1 Effects of manual therapy. Mechanical effects result in neurological and soft-tissue responses that reduce pain, improve mobility, and aid in restoring function.

Based on theory of Bialosky et al. (2009).[2]

shortening or relaxing the tissue. Some techniques refer to this point of limitation as the barrier. Strain–counterstrain, or positional release therapy, is an example of this technique. The purpose of this technique is to relax tissue or help it to "let go" and allow more motion.[4] The underlying theory is that by shortening the restricted tissue, that tissue can relax and unwind so that normal motion can then occur, much like you would put slack on a knotted rope to allow

you to untie the knot. Once the knot is untied, the rope can extend to its normal length.

The sidebar Examples of Direct and Indirect Manual Therapy Techniques is a brief list of examples of direct and indirect manual therapy techniques that give you an idea of how manual therapy can be applied. Many of these techniques are covered in this chapter.

Examples of Direct and Indirect Manual Therapy Techniques

Direct Manual Therapy Techniques (apply treatment at the point of restriction)

Stretching exercises

Joint mobilization

Manipulation

Mulligan technique (NAGS, SNAGS, MWMs)

Myofascial release

Trigger point release

Muscle energy

Rolfing

Proprioceptive neuromuscular facilitation (PNF)

Neural mobilization

Cupping

Instrument-assisted soft-tissue mobilization (IASTM)

Indirect Manual Therapy Techniques (apply treatment away from the point of restriction)

Strain–counterstrain (positional release therapy [PRT])

Integrative manual therapy

Although there are many types of manual therapy, all have several principles in common. For whatever manual therapy technique you use, keep these principles in mind:

- Obtain verbal consent before touching the patient.
- Before you apply the technique, explain what will be done and what sensations to expect.
- Place the patient in a comfortable position.
- Place yourself in a comfortable position.
- Always use good body mechanics.
- Your fingernails should be clean and trimmed. As a general rule, the nail should not extend beyond the end of the fingertip.
- Obtain feedback from the patient throughout the treatment so you can apply the technique properly with appropriate pressure.
- Warn the patient in advance about any potential discomfort, and ask her to tell you when she wants less pressure or discomfort during the treatment.
- Assess the patient's condition before, during, and at the conclusion of the treatment.
- The appropriate manual therapy technique must be correctly applied for a successful result.
- Always respect precautions and contraindications.

For any manual therapy technique, having the skill to apply and deliver it is only half of the job. The other half is to know not only what to do but also why it should be done and to understand the outcome before it is achieved.

> ### CLINICAL TIPS
>
> Clinicians must not only have knowledge of manual therapy techniques, they must also have the skill to administer them. Skill is acquired only through practice. As with any skill, the amount of practice and repetition you perform will determine how skillful you become.

Critical Analysis

At the foundation of any manual therapy technique is the clinician's ability to think critically and analyze the patient's condition to determine the appropriate course of action. This involves understanding the injury and the healing process, identifying the structures and problems involved, analyzing the problems and the factors that cause them, deciding on a plan of action, and critically appraising the results of the treatment to determine its effectiveness.

Critical analysis and examination with continual reassessment are keys to effective manual therapy. This means that the clinician must assess the results of each treatment to determine whether the treatment is having the desired effect. Assessment may be as simple as palpating the treated region to determine changes in mobility or asking the patient what he or she feels after the treatment compared to before. Goniometric measurement, assessing quality of movement, and strength assessment are effective and easy-to-use tools for evaluating treatment. If gains are not made, then the clinician must reassess and either modify the technique or identify other techniques that will achieve the desired goals.

There is no cookbook method for applying manual therapy. You must be able to use your skills of observation, palpation, analysis, and applying therapeutic techniques. As with other aspects of rehabilitation, analysis and deductive reasoning are vital to a successful treatment outcome. The rehabilitation clinician is essentially a detective in search of answers to problems.

Whatever manual therapy techniques you choose, your selection is based on individual findings, not on rote protocol or cookbook decisions. Always approach an injury with an open mind and maintain flexibility in your choice of treatment options. Each patient must be assessed to determine the best individual course of treatment. A successful treatment program depends on your examination and assessment skills as much as your treatment skills.

Massage

Massage is the systematic and scientific manipulation of soft tissue for remedial or restorative purposes.[6] Massage affects various systems of the body through its influence on reflex and mechanical processes. Many types of massage are used in achieving a variety of goals. Some of these variations are presented in Examples of Popular Massage Techniques. Since Swedish massage is the classic therapeutic massage technique,[8, 9] it is the one described here. This section is an introduction to massage.

Effects of Massage

Controversy exists among investigators who have researched the effects of massage. There is some dispute between those whose research has found beneficial effects and those whose research has not. Although it has long been thought that massage provides beneficial effects, it has only been within the past 20 to 30 years that investigations have sought to confirm or disprove those beliefs. Effects identified through these investigations may be divided into four primary categories:[10]

1. Mechanical Benefits. Mechanical benefits include improvements in the tissues' ability to move because of reduced adhesions,[11] changes in the range of motion of joints,[12] increased mobility of muscle tissue,[13] and reduc-

Examples of Popular Massage Techniques

Swedish—Classic therapeutic technique that uses flowing and kneading strokes to affect tissue.

Deep tissue—Deep-pressure or cross-friction strokes are used to treat tight or restricted tissues, especially connective tissue.

Shiatsu—A Japanese technique in which the clinician uses finger and thumb pressure applied to acupuncture points to relieve pain and stress.

Reflexology—Reflexology also makes use of acupuncture points but focuses on the feet and hands, which contain acupuncture points associated with body organs. Treatment is intended to improve organ health, and thereby, overall health.

Thai—An active technique that includes stretching of body segments and pulling digits such as fingers and toes to recenter the body's energy.

Hot stone—Stones heated to a little over 38 °C (100 °F) are positioned on specific body locations to relax muscles and improve circulation to recenter the body's energy. Sometimes used with Swedish massage or other massage techniques.

Sport—Often used either before or after competition in what is known in nonmedical circles as a rubdown. It is used on healthy tissue to relax muscles.

---

tion in tissue stiffness.[14] Mechanical effects improve blood and lymph flow, promote the mobilization of fluid,[15, 16] and stretch and break down adhesions to ultimately help reduce edema and improve tissue mobility.[17]

2. Neurological Effects. Improved neurological effects result in a combination of pain reduction and muscle spasm relaxation.[18] There is evidence that massage reduces neuromuscular excitability so that muscles with injury-related spasm can relax.[19] Additionally, research indicates that pain subsides because massage facilitates the release of beta-endorphins, thereby affecting the gate-control mechanisms of pain.[20]

3. Physiological Effects. Several physiological effects result from massage application. Blood flow to the area increases along with an increase in localized skin temperature.[21] Even muscle temperatures improved up to 2.5 cm (1 in.) deep after massage, indicating an increase in muscular blood flow.[22] Other physiological effects include increased parasympathetic activity; this is evident from physical changes after massage such as a reduction in heart rate and blood pressure.[23] Massage also has been shown to reduce the production of cortisol, a stress hormone, in the body.[24]

4. Psychological Effects. One of the psychological effects of massage is relaxation.[25] Another psychological benefit of massage is reduced anxiety.[26]

Swedish Massage Strokes

Although many massage terms are French words, the techniques presented here are the Swedish massage techniques. The reason for the seemingly odd pairing of the French terminology with the Swedish techniques is that this form of massage was first introduced by Peter Ling of Sweden, who traveled widely in Europe where French was the primary language of diplomatic circles at that time. Table 11.1 provides a review of the various Swedish massage applications with accompanying figures.

Contraindications

Massage is contraindicated when the technique may aggravate the condition or cause additional harm to the patient. Contraindications include infection, malignancies, skin diseases, blood clots, and any irritations or lesions that may spread with direct contact.[27] Deep-tissue massage is also contraindicated when the patient is on anticoagulants (blood thinners).[27]

Precautions

When you apply massage to the patient, both the patient's skin and your hands should be clean. Your hands should be warm and your nails trimmed to prevent lacerations or abrasions. Rings, watches, and wrist jewelry should be removed for the same reason. A lubricant is used to reduce friction when applying effleurage. Less lubricant is used with pétrissage, and even less is used with friction massage. Too much lubricant with friction massage is counterproductive, and too much lubricant with pétrissage makes it difficult to lift or grasp the tissue.

Application

Massage is a direct soft-tissue technique. Before beginning the massage, position the patient comfortably with the body segment to be massaged properly exposed. If the massage is to reduce edema, elevate the part to enhance lymphatic flow. Obtain verbal consent to touch the patient. Explain the procedure and tell the patient to inform you if he or she feels pain with the massage.

When using effleurage or pétrissage, the pressure of the massage strokes should be toward the heart, and the hands should not lose contact with the skin. On the return stroke,

TABLE 11.1   Swedish Massage Strokes

Stroke		Technique	Application	Purpose
Effleurage		Hands glide over skin with hands flat, fingers together.	Start and end of massage. Stroking motion begins distally and moves proximally toward the heart. Pressure is uniform in each stroke, with subsequent strokes either deeper or lighter. Elevating the segment during treatment aids edema reduction.	Relax muscle, reduce pain, relieve edema, relax the patient.
Pétrissage		Fingers are kept together but flex at MCP joints to lift and knead tissue.	Skin and underlying tissue are kneaded and lifted to improve tissue mobility, relax muscle, and promote circulation. When using two hands, one moves clockwise and the other counterclockwise, passing by each other to lift tissue. Applied during the midmassage treatment session.	Mobilize deeper tissue to improve muscle circulation and relaxation.
Friction		Finger or thumb pads or elbow moves in small areas.	Small cross-fiber or circular motions are used to mobilize specific tissue.	Break adhesions or soften scar tissue to improve area mobility.
Tapotement		Percussion of tissue or tapping of tissue in a rhythmic manner, usually with the hands or fingers.	Hands are cupped, with motion occurring from relaxed wrists to tap on a surface, or if fingers are used, the fingers of one hand alternate with those of the other hand to create a gentle slapping of the surface.	Release lymph or fluid and mucous blockage or stimulate afferent nerves.

continue lightly touching the body part. Keep your hand in good contact with the part and your fingers together, not spread apart. The rhythm of the stroke should be even and slow to promote relaxation. Maintain a comfortable position during the treatment and use proper body mechanics.

When using friction massage, warn the patient that some discomfort may be felt but that it will not be long-lasting. The thumb or finger pads are used on a small, localized area. The massage is applied in a cross-fiber pattern perpendicular to the tissue's fiber arrangement. A firm, consistent pressure and rhythm are also important. A small area at a time is massaged until the discomfort of the massage subsides and you can palpate an increase in tissue mobility.

Myofascial Release

Myofascial release is a close relative to massage. Myofascial release involves manual contact with the patient and uses the sense of touch in evaluating the problem and the effectiveness of the treatment, just as massage does. Massage and myofascial release also both include the use of pressure and tissue stretch to produce soft-tissue results.

As with massage, there are many methods of myofascial release, but they all are essentially variations of the same principle: the use of manual contact for evaluation and treatment of soft-tissue restriction and pain with the goal of relieving those symptoms to improve motion and function. There are different names for these techniques, including myofascial release, myofascial stretching, strain–counterstrain, Rolfing, and soft-tissue mobilization. As with other manual therapy applications, empirical research results on the efficacy of myofascial release remain elusive. Case studies, clinical observations, and anecdotal reports of those who have recorded treatment results are currently the best barometer by which to judge the effectiveness of myofascial release. Ultimately, treatment effectiveness must be assessed by the results of your own applications on the patients you treat. In this section, some of the more commonly used generic myofascial techniques are introduced.

Before we describe the various myofascial release techniques, we discuss their theoretical basis. The myofascial release systems cannot be appreciated without understanding this.

Fascia

Fascia is a continuous sheet of connective tissue that surrounds and integrates tissues and structures throughout the body.[28] Fascia varies in density and thickness and is interconnected with the structures it surrounds.[29] (See figure 11.2a and 11.2b.) It can affect the relationship among the structures it encompasses (their physical orientation to each other, their chemical relationship, or their physiological relationship, such as what tissues are served by which blood vessels or nerves).[29] Fascia is vital for tissue form, lubrication, nutrition, stability, integrity, function, force transmission, perception of movement, and support.[29, 30]

Fascia throughout the body is divided into three layers. (See figure 11.2c and 11.2d.) The superficial layer is attached to the undersurface of the skin and varies in thickness, depending on the body segment, body surface, and sex; it tends to be thicker in the lower extremities than in the upper extremities, thicker on the posterior than on the anterior body surface, and thicker in females than in males.[30] Within this superficial layer lie capillaries, lymph vessels, nerves, and fat.[29, 31] Because this layer is a loosely knit structure made of fibroelastic and loose connective tissue, it permits the skin to move in many directions over the underlying structures.[29, 32] It is also an area where edema accumulates after injury or surgery.[32]

Deep fascia is dense connective tissue that surrounds and separates deeper structures, such as muscle, tendon, joints, ligaments, and bone.[29] Deep fascia is thicker than superficial fascia, about 1 mm thick on average. Deeper structures such as muscle are also more easily separated from their fascia than structures adjacent to superficial fascia.[32] Because of its stiffer, firmer structure, deep fascia is less able to accommodate edema, which can cause problems, such as compartment syndromes in the lower limb.[32] Deep fascia not only surrounds muscle structures but also merges with retinacula, which surround joints and maintains tendon positioning during motion.[32] Retinacula and their deep fascial connections provide joint stability and assist in proprioception.[33-36]

The final fascial layer is subserous fascia, which surrounds internal organs. Its loose areolar connective tissue contains channels where fluid helps to provide the organs with lubrication.[29] Myofascial release techniques do not treat fascia surrounding visceral organs.

Fascia contains collagen, elastin, cellular components, and ground substance.[35] (See figure 11.2e.) The elastin within fascia allows the structure to return to its original shape when applied stresses are released. Fascia also responds with plastic deformation when prolonged forces are applied.[35] Creep and hysteresis are properties of fascia and are affected by myofascial release techniques.[37, 38]

Although fascia has high tensile strength and can tolerate multidirectional compression, stretch, and shear forces, an injury can profoundly affect it. Depending on the load, duration, and type of stress applied to the fascia, its normal biomechanics can be altered to cause either a temporary or a permanent deformation. Injury to fascia causes a change in the biochemical structure of the ground substance; scar tissue that forms after injury can interfere with normal fascia functions.[39] When fascia either restricts normal motion or does not provide skin, subcutaneous, muscle, and other tissue with normal support, lubrication, and its other functions, fascial dysfunctions can result in loss of

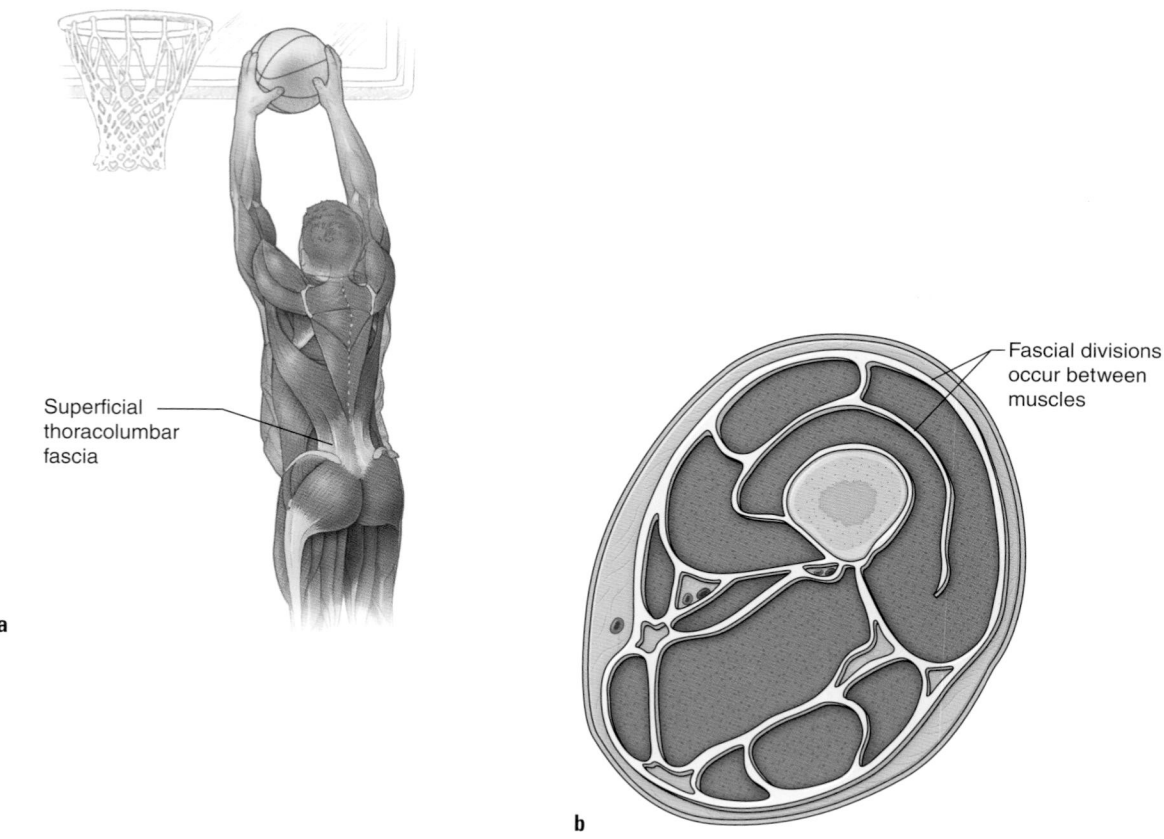

Superficial thoracolumbar fascia

a

Fascial divisions occur between muscles

b

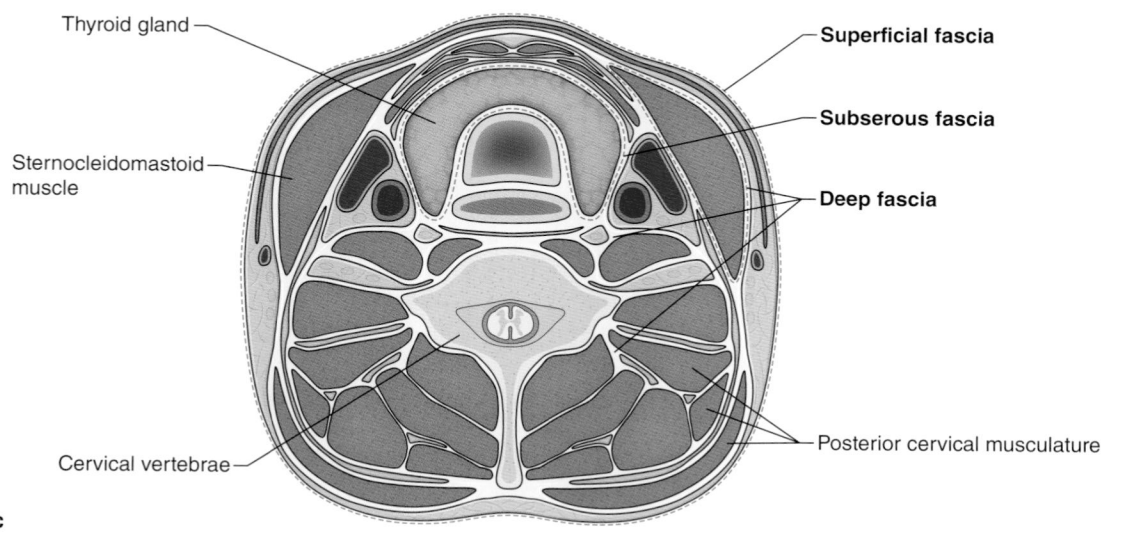

Thyroid gland

Sternocleidomastoid muscle

Cervical vertebrae

c

Superficial fascia

Subserous fascia

Deep fascia

Posterior cervical musculature

Figure 11.2 Components of the fascial system. Notice how fascia is an integral part of each of the structures in the area. *(a)* The superficial thoracolumbar fascia. *(b)* The deep enveloping fascial containers. *(c)* Notice how fascia provides form. *(d)* Note the relationship between fascia and the blood and lymph vessels. *(e)* Fascia contains collagen, elastin, cellular components, and ground substance.

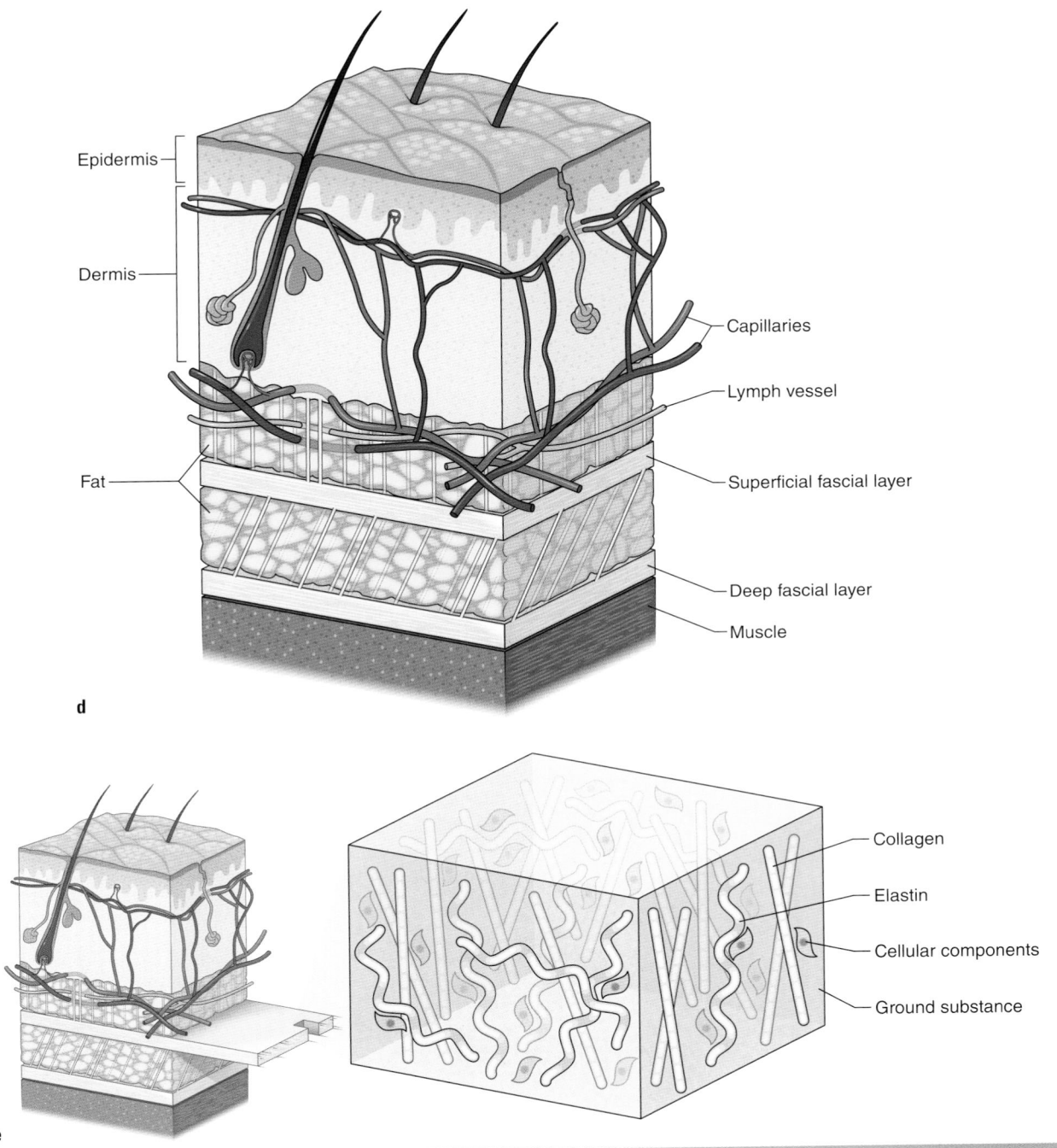

Epidermis

Dermis

Fat

Capillaries

Lymph vessel

Superficial fascial layer

Deep fascial layer

Muscle

d

Collagen

Elastin

Cellular components

Ground substance

e

Figure 11.2 >*continued*

functional capacity, extended disability, and prolonged symptoms after injury.[40-42]

Myofascia maintains an intimate relationship with the muscles it surrounds. Each muscle and its fascia provide the combined contractile and noncontractile properties of muscle.[43] As part of muscle's noncontractile tissue, myofascia assists in increasing muscle strength during eccentric contractions; therefore, damage to fascia affects its muscle's functional capacity.[43] Myofascia is important

to muscle for many reasons, perhaps especially for the vital assistance it provides to permit normal muscle function.

Nonacute Biomechanical Forces

Injury impairs myofascia's function, eventually leading to pain, loss of motion, and reduced function and performance.[4, 44] Muscle dysfunction causes additional changes in the myofascia.

In pathology that occurs over time—for example, the swimmer who has developed poor posture—muscle imbalances occur. As noted in figure 11.3, the process may start with a minor trauma or injury. It causes a change in the muscle that results in an imbalance of muscle strength between an agonist group and its antagonist group.[45, 46] Muscle imbalances lead to changes in neuromuscular response and coordination, which lead to further imbalances, until the structure reaches a point where the imbalance and resulting increased tissue stress cause symptoms that impair performance and require treatment.[46]

The patient can inadvertently start this pathological cycle through the activities he or she repeatedly performs.[47] If the swimmer with poor posture concentrates on pectoralis strengthening without also working on antagonist strength, or uses only strokes that emphasize anterior and not posterior muscles, eventually muscle imbalances occur. Awareness of muscle imbalance is important in treating patients with loss of motion. Muscle imbalances are discussed more thoroughly in chapter 13.

Other gradually changing factors can produce fascial changes that with time will ultimately affect performance or cause pain: leg length differences; inadequate rehabilitation from previous injuries; worn, poorly constructed, or ill-fitting shoes or protective equipment; prolonged activities that overstress supportive structures; and poor ergonomics.[48, 49] Over time, imbalances of strength, flexibility, and fascial mobility create imbalanced systems that render the patient susceptible to injury. When muscle changes, its surrounding fascia also changes to maintain its relationship with muscle. These changes also change normal recruitment patterns.[50]

Myofascial techniques release restricted areas, but exercises for flexibility and strength reset neurological programming. In other words, myofascial techniques work to make the fascia more mobile, and exercises work to help the patient regain normal muscle function. Together they produce positive changes in the affected tissues.[51]

Acute Biomechanical Forces

The muscle system is part of the fascial continuum, so when it is affected by pathology or acute injury, its function is compromised.[29] Once altered, the fascial tissue loses its sliding ability, which then places pressure on the mechanoreceptors, causing pain and loss of functional capacity.[29, 44] Acute injury may necessitate immobilization. When connective tissue is immobilized, the scar tissue matrix that ensues can send out tendrils that attach to and restrict neurovascular and lymph vessels and reduce local metabolism, increase cross-link formation, and restrict mobility.[52]

In addition to the scarring that occurs with acute injury, spasm can influence the fascial system by producing prolonged tightness in one area that causes another area to compensate with prolonged looseness, initiating a cycle of imbalance and fascial pathology.[53] It is important to evaluate for fascial restrictions in both acute and nonacute injuries.

Terminology

The term *myofascial release* is often used for the techniques described here, but it is actually a misnomer. Myofascial release implies the treatment of myofascia. Although myofascia can certainly be the target of treatment, it is not always the targeted tissue or the only tissue treated. For example, myofascial release techniques can be used after edema and immobilization to treat the fascia associated

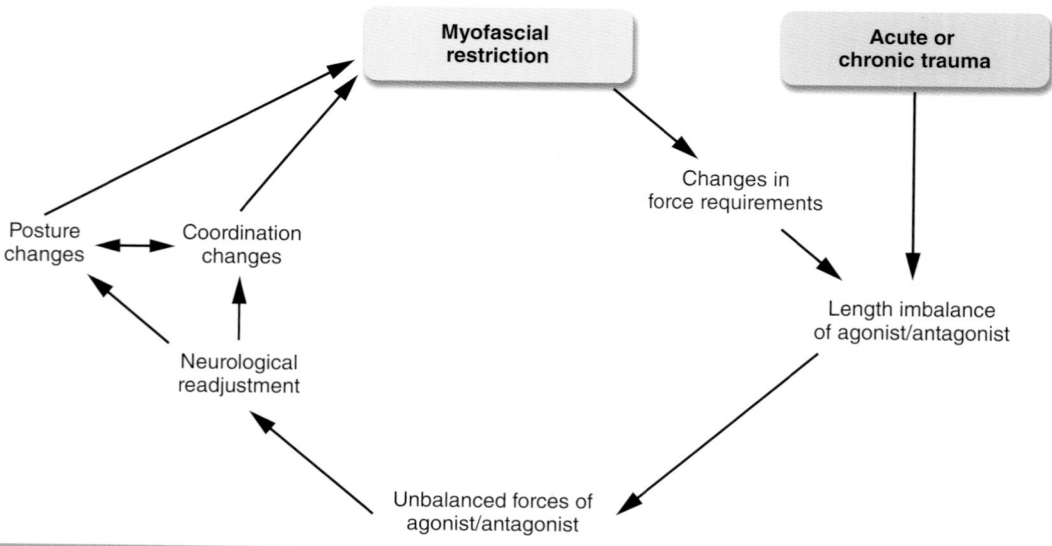

Figure 11.3 Pathology of myofascial restriction: Myofascial restriction can occur either within a short time from acute injury and scar-tissue formation or gradually from minor but progressive changes secondary to repeated low-level stress.[32] As a muscle changes, its fascia also changes to maintain its intimate relationship with the muscle.

with skin, subcutaneous tissue, and other superficial structures with limited mobility, not the muscle's fascia. Even when the target tissue is myofascia, other structures may be affected by treatment because of secondary restrictions in the area.

Palpation

Palpation is fundamental in myofascial release. Not only is it required for an examination of the area, but palpation is performed throughout the treatment. The soft tissue's extensibility, movement, end-feel, and response to treatment are palpated during and after the treatment. Adjustments are made as the area is palpated and examined during the treatment.

Normal tissue has no tenderness when palpated. Normal tissue also has a springy end-feel that can be palpated when pressure is released. Tissue mobility varies according to the body part and tissue type, but end-feel springiness is consistent. In myofascially restricted tissue, pain occurs with palpation, and restriction with a loss of springiness is palpated by the clinician. When the treatment is effective, the clinician feels tissues release during the treatment. This release is the treatment goal and is necessary to restore tissue mobility and balance.[4, 44] The release that is palpated has been described as the tissue giving way, letting go, relaxing, or melting like ice when a hot knife goes through it.

Superficial to Deep Structures

When examining and treating with myofascial release techniques, you should move from superficial structures to deeper structures to avoid a mistake in identifying the structure or tissue that is restricted. Techniques should be applied with the least amount of force that is appropriate for achieving the established goals. More force is often indicated when scar tissue adhesions and reduced mobility are present, but the additional force should be applied only after you examine and assess the area and determine the patient's tolerance.

Autonomic Effects

Neuroreflex changes can sometimes result from the use of myofascial techniques.[54] Fascial restriction can cause autonomic changes, so it is not surprising that when restriction is released, the autonomic system can be affected.[35] If pain and fascial restriction cause changes in skin color, moisture, temperature, and sensation, then their release will also cause changes in those signs and symptoms.

Afferent sensations are transmitted to the dorsal horn of the spinal cord. The dorsal horn is a processing center that receives and redirects information. It can send an impulse directly out the spinal cord as a reflex efferent response, or it can send the information to the subcortical or cortical level of the brain, where it is interpreted and a response is formulated and returned down the spinal cord.

The patient may experience an autonomic response when the myofascial treatment is particularly effective.[55] The patient's sympathetic system is stimulated, producing symptoms such as increased pulse rate, sweating, and blood pressure changes. Less intense responses include sensations of burning, tingling, stinging, or heat in the area being treated.[56] Although these sympathetic responses are unusual, you should be aware that they may occur, and you should be prepared to respond appropriately.

Treatment Techniques

There are many ways to apply myofascial techniques; table 11.2 illustrates several of them. Figures 11.4 and 11.5 demonstrate methods of applying myofascial release techniques.

TABLE 11.2 General Myofascial Techniques

Stroke		Technique	Application	Purpose
J-stroke		Finger or thumb pad is used to move skin against underlying tissue.	Finger or thumb pad is used to apply downward pressure to pull skin over underlying tissue, using a J-stroke in one small area at a time.	Relieve restricted fascial and scar tissue adhesions in small, localized areas.
Oscillation		Fingers are most often used in a cupped position to roll back and forth over muscle.	One or both hands working in the same direction move in a rhythmic, oscillating manner. The movement is relaxing for the patient and comfortable.	Relax muscle spasm.

> continued

TABLE 11.2 > *continued*

Stroke		Technique	Application	Purpose
Wringing		Both hands are used simultaneously to release tissue restriction.	Hands move in opposite directions to each other, applying a deep-tissue force to move underlying structures against each other.	Release multidirectional deep-tissue restrictions.
Stripping		Deep-tissue release.	One hand anchors the tissue while the other hand, elbow, or forearm is used to apply a downward and pulling force to stretch tissue below the skin.	Release adhesions of scar tissue or adherent fascia.
Arm or leg pull		Traction of extremity is applied throughout the extremity through a full range of hip or shoulder abduction motion.	Clinician grasps wrist or ankle then leans body weight away from limb to provide traction. Clinician walks the limb into abduction while passively rotating the limb until resistance is perceived. Resistance releases with continued traction; then abduction continues through the motion.	Used with conditions of generalized tightness within the extremity.

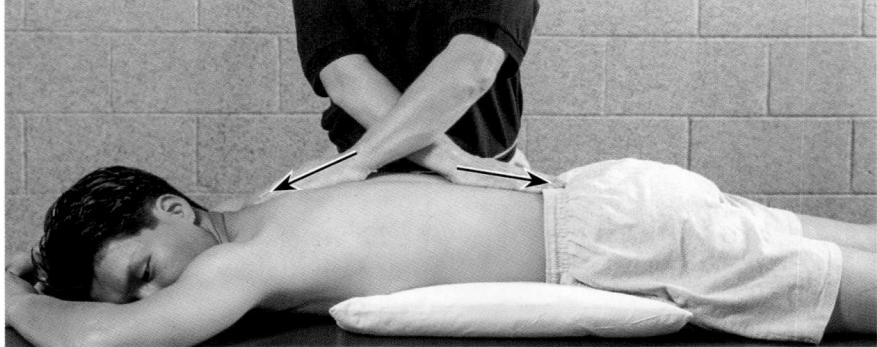

Figure 11.4   In longitudinal myofascial release, fascial tissue between the hands is stretched.

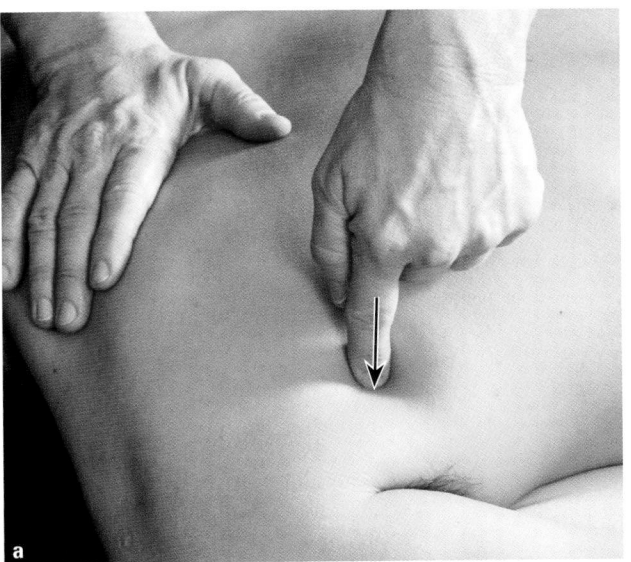
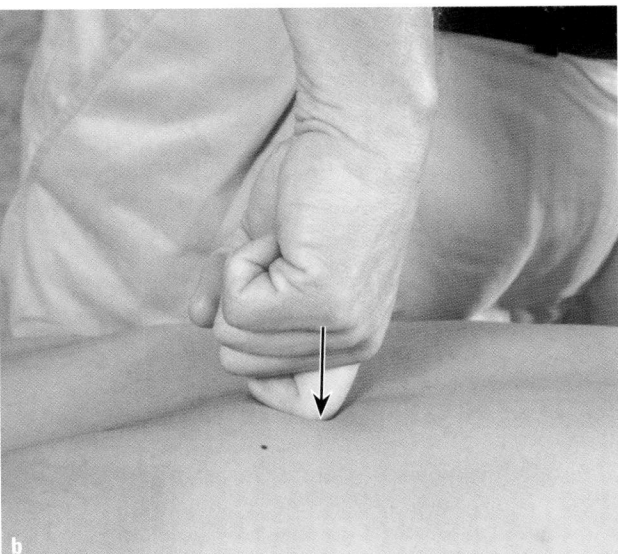
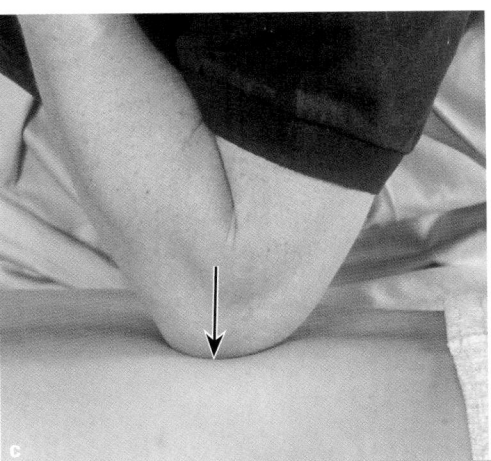

Figure 11.5 Alternative myofascial release applications using stripping or oscillation techniques: *(a)* finger pad, *(b)* knuckle, *(c)* elbow.

Contraindications

Myofascial release technique contraindications include malignancy, aneurysm, hypermobile joints, recent fractures, hemorrhages, sutures, osteoporosis, local infections, and acute inflammations.[56] As always, respect contraindications, and avoid treatment in the presence of these conditions.

Precautions

As with any treatment, you should be aware of precautions with this application. Myofascial release is used cautiously on new scars. The new tissue is fragile because of its reduced tensile strength. It also may have increased sensitivity and limited tolerance to pressure.

Use care on patients with complex regional pain syndrome (CRPS) or reflex sympathetic dystrophy (RSD). Patients with this condition may experience exacerbated pain; myofascial release treatments should avoid pain.

Also avoid bruising. This is a particular concern when techniques tend to be more aggressive. Bruising results in additional scar tissue formation.

Application

Like massage, myofascial release is a direct soft-tissue technique. Before beginning the technique, obtain verbal consent to touch the patient. Position the patient comfortably with the body segment to be treated properly exposed. Explain the procedure and warn the patient before treatment that sensations of pain, tingling, burning, and warmth may occur and are normal with this technique. Also instruct the patient to tell you of any sensations experienced during the treatment.

As mentioned, palpation is fundamental in myofascial release. Determine the depth and breadth of the myofascial restriction. If the restriction is in a small, localized area, use J-strokes or oscillation techniques. For myofascial restrictions over a larger area, use wringing, stripping, or arm or leg pull techniques. The depth of your technique will correlate with the depth of the myofascial restriction palpated.

Myofascial Trigger Points

Myriad terms are used interchangeably with myofascial trigger point. Some of the more commonly used terms are myalgia, fibrositis, muscular rheumatism, fibroplastic syndrome, myositis, and myofasciitis. The clinical definition of a trigger point is a hyperirritable point in a skeletal muscle that is palpable as a nodule within a tight band of the muscle and produces referred pain when compression is applied to it.[57] Trigger points are a common cause of muscle pain.[58]

A study of shoulder girdle muscles in normal subjects without shoulder pain revealed that 98% of those subjects had latent trigger points in various shoulder girdle muscles,[59] and a later study demonstrated active trigger points in all subjects with shoulder pain.[60] Both active and passive trigger points have been identified in patients with chronic tension headache; of interest is the fact that 30% of the control group without headaches within this study were also found to have trigger points.[61] Another study found that trigger points in scapular upward rotators had enough impact on those muscles to change their activation patterns during shoulder elevation activities.[62] Myofascial pain and trigger points not only affect muscle activation, but they also affect function and performance and complicate recovery from injury if they are not recognized and addressed.[62]

Two of the most recognized names in the study of myofascial trigger points are Janet Travell and David Simons. They devoted their professional lives to understanding and treating trigger points. Most of the information presented here is the result of their findings. For additional information on trigger points, see Travell,[63] Simons,[64] and Travell and Simons.[65-67] Of course, several other investigators are working toward a better understanding of trigger points; Travell and Simons are pioneers in this effort.

Definition of Trigger Point

Travell and Simons define a **trigger point** as a hyperirritable point in a skeletal muscle that is palpable as a nodule within a tight band of the muscle and produces referred pain when compression is applied to it.[57]

As the definition indicates, a myofascial trigger point involves a taut band of muscle tissue and its surrounding fascia; hence the name. A central focal point of local tenderness can be palpated as a nodule within the taut band.[68, 69] Compression of this point often refers pain to other areas or causes an autonomic response.

Travell and Simons[65, 66] identify two types of trigger points: active and latent. An **active trigger point** is one that is always tender and produces referred pain whether the muscle is active or inactive.[70] The muscle also displays weakness and reduced motion. When an active trigger point is palpated with a rolling pressure crosswise against the muscle fibers, the muscle fibers are stimulated to produce a localized twitch response. This palpation technique is called a snapping palpation and is performed using firm, constant pressure and moving the fingertips across the muscle fibers as if plucking a guitar string. The local twitch response is an involuntary contraction of the muscle fibers in response to the snapping palpation.[65] Sometimes this response is incorrectly called a *jump sign*. A **jump sign** is also a reflex response but is a reaction of wincing or withdrawal.

A **latent trigger point** is painful only when it is palpated.[65] Like active trigger points, it has a taut band that demonstrates a twitch response when manually examined.[71] Normal muscles do not have these areas of tenderness or pathology.

Trigger Point Characteristics

Trigger point tenderness is often described as a dull ache or a sharp, stabbing pain[43] and can be merely uncomfortable or very intense; the severity of complaints is directly proportional to the irritability of the trigger point. Pressure on the trigger point elicits a referred pain pattern that is unique for each muscle.

Trigger point referral patterns do not follow neurological referral patterns; this is an important distinction. The sensation of trigger point referral pain is also different from neurologically referred pain. Trigger point pain is often a deep ache. Occasionally, a trigger point pain is a sharp or stabbing pain, and only on rare occasions is it described as burning.[65] Referred sensation from peripheral nerve entrapment or nerve root irritation, on the other hand, is evidenced by prickling, tingling, or numbness.

Myofascial trigger point pain becomes amplified by muscle activity (especially strenuous activity), passive stretch of the muscle, direct pressure of the trigger point, prolonged stationary periods followed by moving (such as getting up in the morning or standing after prolonged sitting), repeated or sustained muscle activity, and cold.[58, 70] Conversely, myofascial trigger points are relieved with short periods of rest; heat accompanied by slow and sustained stretches; short-term, low-level activity; and specific treatment techniques that are discussed later in this chapter.

Trigger Point Hypotheses

Trigger points can be activated by various factors, including injury, overload, fatigue, and cold.[72] Acute injuries can also activate trigger points. Overload of the muscles from a prolonged stationary posture, prolonged muscle immobilization in a shortened position, and nerve compressions are the most common causes of gradual trigger point onset;[73] prolonged poor posture creates muscle overload and overwork fatigue within those muscles.[74]

Although we do not yet know the physiological pathology involved in the development of trigger points, several hypotheses have been presented by various authors to advance our understanding.[69, 75] Of these hypotheses, we will address the three most prevalent postulates that have been put forth by investigations. Each hypothesis has supporters and detractors, and none of them has been accepted by a consensus. These hypotheses center on histopathology, neuroelectropathology, and a combination of these two.

Travell and Simons[65] provide support for the histopathological hypothesis. Their hypothesis about the causes and creation of trigger points has been disputed but not disproved.[65, 73, 76] Their hypothesis involves the contractile activity of a muscle. During contraction of a normal muscle fiber, calcium that is stored in the fiber's sarcoplasmic retic-

ulum is rapidly released when the contraction begins and then reabsorbed in the presence of ATP when the contraction ends. This process is triggered by a brief nerve impulse called an action potential. A contraction is the result of the shortening of the sarcomere when its cross-bridges pull the actin and myosin filaments over each other (figure 11.6).

If an injured muscle fiber's sarcoplasmic reticulum is damaged, its calcium is released without an action potential, stimulating the sarcomere to produce a sustained contraction. This sustained calcium release that causes sarcomere contraction creates an energy crisis because of the resulting ischemia. Ischemia occurs because the muscle fibers' sustained contraction limits capillary blood flow in the region, causing oxygen deficiency within the muscle cells so they cannot provide enough ATP to relax the contraction. Without sufficient ATP, the sarcomere's filaments cannot disconnect from each other; therefore, they remain fixed in their contracted position. The energy crisis that occurs as a result of this cycle is demonstrated in figure 11.7, which is based on the hypothesis put forth by Simons and colleagues.[57] In partial support of this histopathological theory, there has been some evidence to suggest that a metabolic pathology of local tissue exists in trigger points.[58, 77] These findings did not support ischemia

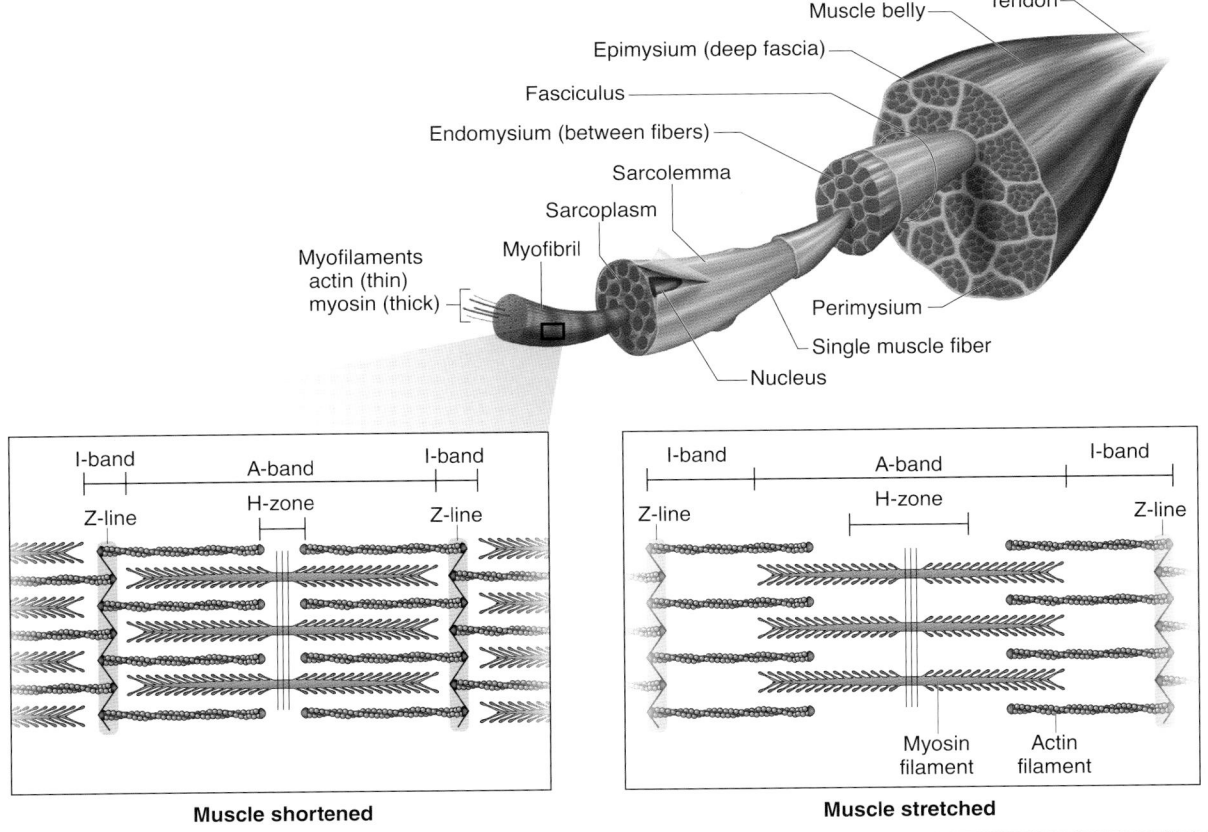

Figure 11.6 Normal skeletal muscle structure and a sarcomere in shortened and lengthened conditions.

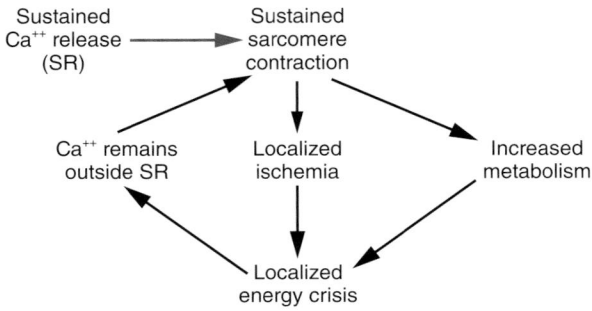

Figure 11.7 Histopathological hypothesis of myofascial trigger points. An energy crisis occurs when continuous calcium release produces sustained contraction of the sarcomere. Ischemia prevents ATP from entering, and the sustained contraction of the sarcomere increases ATP, but as long as calcium is present and ATP is deficient, sarcomere contraction continues.

as the basis for pain, but they did agree with the presence of some metabolic issue affecting trigger points.

Investigators who dispute Travell and Simons' hypothesis of ischemia have presented a theory based on neurological pathologies as the cause of trigger points and their associated sensory, motor, and autonomic changes.[78, 79] Supporters of this hypothesis believe that it explains the referral of pain to distant sites, and they believe treatment should focus on nerve roots rather than on muscle.

We know that smaller Type I muscle fibers are recruited first during submaximal activity and are deactivated last.[80, 81] Related to this concept is the Cinderella hypothesis, which refers to the fact that these Type I fibers are recruited first, remain activated for a prolonged time, and are afforded short recovery times; hence, these fibers are susceptible to pain and damage.[82] Studies have demonstrated that low-level activation after as little as 30 min causes trigger point pain in muscles.[83] Previous studies have shown spontaneous electrical activity in trigger point muscle fibers but not in adjacent or surrounding normal muscle fibers.[84, 85] It is believed that repetitive low-level muscle stress provides just enough stimulation that acetylcholine leaks from the motor nerve terminal to trigger a depolarization of the synaptic membrane.[83, 86] This opens the sodium channels to produce sustained activation of very localized muscle fibers.[68, 87] Figure 11.8 provides a model of this mechanism.

The third hypothesis regarding the cause of trigger points is the integrated hypothesis, which was developed by Simons[84] and has been further expanded upon by Gerwin.[68, 69] The integrated hypothesis assimilates certain aspects of the other two theories. Of the three hypotheses, this is the most widely accepted model for understanding the pathophysiology of trigger points.[88] This hypothesis indicates that a dysfunctional motor end plate provides sustained contraction of isolated muscle fibers, as was presented in the neuroelectrical hypothesis.[57] Sustained

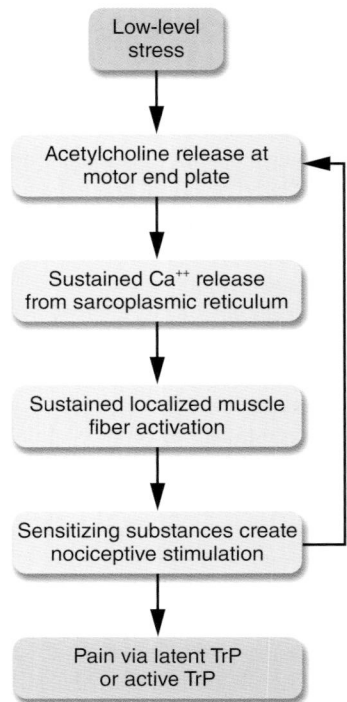

Figure 11.8 Neuroelectrical pathology hypothesis of myofascial trigger points. Low-level stress provides enough stimulation to cause leakage of acetylcholine across the motor end plate. This process then facilitates calcium release, which promotes the sustained contraction of localized muscle fibers.

muscle fiber contraction creates a combination of localized ischemia and increased metabolic needs, which together create a sustained energy crisis.[57] Lacking sufficient energy (ATP) to return calcium to the sarcoplasmic reticulum and reverse the polarized membrane potential, the muscle cells remain locked in contraction.[81] It is thought that ischemia and the ensuing local **hypoxia** trigger the release of chemical neural sensitizers that lead local nociceptors to produce pain.[76]

Gerwin and colleagues[68] expanded this hypothesis with new information about local effects of this hypoxia and ischemia: The area becomes acidic secondary to the ischemia, further adding to the continued presence of acetylcholine and the stimulation of nociceptors. The continued acetylcholine release triggers calcium release for ongoing sarcomere contraction without an action potential. A lower pH and inflammatory chemicals present in the area contribute to pain by stimulating nociceptors.[89-91] Input into the central nervous system from these nociceptors in the muscle may produce functional changes in the central nervous system, creating referred pain.[81] Figure 11.9 illustrates the integrated hypothesis and how the two previous theories combine to create the integrated theory of myofascial trigger point pain.

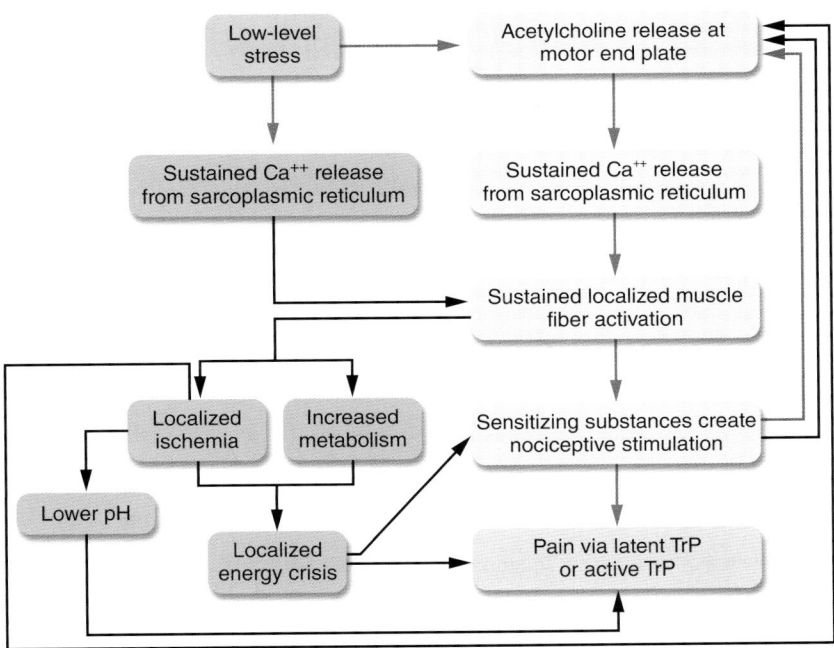

Figure 11.9 Integrated hypothesis of myofascial trigger points. An increased metabolic need and ischemia due to reduced blood flow from sustained muscle fiber contraction create a localized energy crisis that combines with a dysfunctional motor end plate's leaking of acetylcholine to produce a myofascial trigger point. Lowered pH levels and continued ischemia cause chemicals to be released, sensitizing nociceptors, which connect to the central nervous system, referring pain and stimulation to other nerve centers.

Pain changes muscle activation both in sequential timing compared to other muscles[92] and in strength output. Therefore, as a result of trigger points, significant changes occur: Pain increases and muscle function, strength, and mobility are reduced.[93] If muscle function remains altered, especially after injury, there is risk of secondary changes occurring to surrounding myofascia that result in scar tissue and fascial adhesions, loss of flexibility and range of motion, decreased mobility, and impaired function.[94]

In spite of other hypotheses, the integrated hypothesis theory of trigger point pathology remains pertinent and most popular. It gains further support when combined with the convergence projection theory.[76, 95] This theory indicates that a noxious stimulation in one area is interpreted by the central nervous system as coming from a different source of pain. So what may start as a local reaction can refer pain to other regions.[76, 95]

When trigger points occur because of either acute injury or repetitive demands placed on the muscle, irritating or noxious chemicals are released.[57, 66] The release of nerve-sensitizing substances such as histamine, serotonin, kinins, and prostaglandins (mentioned in chapter 2) may be the cause of continued, localized, runaway metabolic activity. Travell and Simons[57, 66] propose that these substances, which are released after an injury, increase the metabolic demands and sensitize afferent nerve endings to make them hyperirritable to produce referred pain, autonomic and motor neuron responses, and trigger points. Studies have demonstrated that there is, in fact, an increase in these noxious chemicals at the site of trigger points.[81, 96, 97]

Trigger Point Examination

As part of the total treatment plan, the causes of the patient's pain must be accurately assessed to rule out trigger points as a possible factor. Observation and examination of the patient's posture, range of motion, weakness patterns, pain areas, and history are all required in assessing the patient's injury and determining rehabilitation needs. It is sometimes easier to identify patterns if the patient indicates the areas of pain on a human figure drawing.

A compression test over the muscle can detect taut bands, nodules, and local and referred pain.[57] A local twitch response confirms the presence of a trigger point.[57] A taut band is palpated by passively stretching the muscle until the taut fibers are pulled to the point of discomfort without pain while the muscle remains relaxed. The taut band feels like a short cord within the muscle. Begin at the band's distal attachment and palpate with either the pad of the thumb or two or three fingers along the taut band toward the fibers' proximal attachment to locate the trigger point within the band. It is an area of increased tenderness and feels like a hard ball within the taut band.[57]

A local twitch response is elicited along the taut band with a snapping palpation of the band. A snapping palpation

We currently have only hypotheses to explain trigger points. A *hypothesis* is an idea that provides an explanation of some phenomenon but is untested. A *theory* uses scientific inquiry and experimentation to test a hypothesis; investigative findings encourage the scientific community to prove, disprove, or modify the hypothesis until an acceptable theory emerges. Explanations of trigger points are still in the hypothesis stage. Although several investigators have published research results to advance various hypotheses, no results have yet provided enough evidence to move to an acceptable theory.

Of these investigations, the hypothesis that has achieved the most attention, in terms of both agreement and detraction, has been the modified integrated hypothesis. Supporters back up the hypothesis that ischemia and hypoxia—reduced local blood flow within the trigger point with a resistance to outflow from the vicinity—create and sustain the trigger point and its symptoms with effects occurring from both the mechanical and the neural and histological pathways. On the other hand, several noted investigators have also presented evidence to declare this hypothesis to be extremely erroneous.[75, 98, 99] This volley of responses from noted researchers on the topic provides an informative and educational perspective on the progress that has occurred in recent years on topics related to myofascial trigger points. Although we have a long way to go before we have all the answers, evidence appears to be leaning toward the modified integrated hypothesis that was initially put forth by Simons[84] and expanded upon by Gerwin and colleagues[68, 69] as the most sound approach for now. The evidence on which they base their conclusions includes some key research findings:

1. *Muscle overload or repetitive loading.* This damages muscle fibers; this type of injury, which leads to capillary constriction, is consistent with trigger point development.[100]

2. *Ischemia.* Hypoperfusion occurs in myofascial pain.[101] Ischemia leading to tissue hypoxia is seen in trigger points.[102] It is thought that persistent muscle contraction creates ischemia, which facilitates the release of inflammatory mediators to trigger nociceptors.[68]

3. *Local lowered pH causes pain.* Trigger points have significantly reduced pH levels.[89] Reductions in local pH levels result in the activation of nociceptors, creating muscle pain.[103]

4. *Spontaneous electrical activity.* Electromyographic (EMG) studies have found spontaneous electrical activity (SEA) in trigger points;[85] investigators now believe that this EMG activity is likely the result of a dysfunctional motor end plate.[104] This end plate noise is thought to be the result of an excessive release of acetylcholine, a substance that also causes taut bands to form in muscles.[105] Taut bands contain trigger points.[106]

5. *Changes in chemistry with ischemia.* Ischemia promotes low ATP and higher calcium concentrations.[100] In these situations, higher acetylcholine levels are present, creating continual motor end plate discharge.[107]

6. *Segmentally contracted sarcomeres.* In vivo segmentally contracted sarcomeres and smeared Z-lines have been reported in tissue taken from either the myofascial trigger point region or the taut band region of skeletal muscle.[69]

In summary, when localized muscle fibers are stressed beyond their tolerance levels, the fibers are injured. With injury comes a sequence of events that include capillary constriction, ischemia, and lower pH levels, which lead to pain, increased acetylcholine levels, elevated calcium levels, and continued sarcomere contraction. These findings from a variety of investigators have been the source of conclusions that have led to the development of the modified integrated hypothesis. This hypothesis is not yet at the level of what can be considered theory, but it is the best evidence we have for now.

---

is produced by first placing the muscle in a relaxed, neutral position and then strumming the fibers with pressure perpendicular to the fiber alignment, much like strumming a guitar. In a positive response, the taut band twitches.[57] The more closely the pressure is applied to the trigger point of the taut band, the more vigorous is the response. This technique works most effectively on superficial muscles.

Trigger Point Treatment

Travell and Simons[57, 66] and Cyriax[108] advocate the use of trigger point injection as an effective method of treatment, but this invasive treatment is not appropriate for rehabilita-tion clinicians. If an active trigger point does not respond to the treatment techniques presented here, refer the patient to a physician who can inject the site.

Treatment goals for myofascial trigger points include relieving pain, resolving factors that cause trigger points, and restoring mobility, strength, and optimal function. As muscles regain appropriate balance and restore their normal firing patterns, normal function returns along with relief of pain. Since dealing with pain is the first priority in myofascial trigger point treatment programs, the techniques used to accomplish this are presented here. Corrections of muscle imbalances and muscle recruitment patterns are specifically discussed in part IV; therefore, keep in mind that while only specific treatments for myofascial trigger points are discussed here, the rehabilitation to resolve trigger points must also include stretching and strengthening muscles and correcting muscle performance.

Travell and Simons' trigger point treatments are direct techniques. Four primary methods (spray-and-stretch, pressure release, stripping, and modalities) are discussed briefly here. For additional information, refer to the Travell and Simons texts,[57, 66] the source of the techniques described next.

Spray-and-Stretch

An aerosol counterirritant coolant is commonly used in a technique known as spray-and-stretch to treat myofascial trigger points. The aerosol container provides a very narrow stream that instantly feels cold when applied to the skin, triggering an afferent sensory response to the central nervous system.[57] Travell and Simons[57] indicated that this technique followed by a stretch was the most effective noninvasive method of treating trigger point pain.

Before application, the patient should be instructed to relax. Applying just enough pressure on the trigger point area to produce the referred pain may help the patient understand why your treatment is not being applied directly to the painful area but to the source of pain. The patient is placed in a comfortable position with the skin exposed and the body part supported to permit full relaxation. Before treatment, the part is moved through its full range of motion so you and the patient can evaluate changes made by the treatment. With the muscle anchored at one end, the vapocoolant spray is applied in a sweeping motion in parallel strokes in only one direction over the length of the muscle and its referred pain pattern. As the vapocoolant is applied at a distance of about 30 cm (12 in.) from the skin in a rhythmic, unhurried fashion at the rate of about 10 cm/s (4 in./s), a slow, continual, passive stretch is applied progressively to the muscle.[57]

For optimal results, a single area of the skin should receive no more than three strokes of cold; no cold stream should be repeated over the same area before rewarming (figure 11.10). Correctly spraying the coolant in this manner causes the stimulation of afferent beta receptors to facilitate the gate control pain mechanism in the spinal cord.[57] On the other hand, repetitive strokes applied incorrectly to the same area create a cold modality treatment that does not produce the desired beta receptor response. The stretch force should be light enough that it does not elicit a stretch reflex from the muscle but strong enough to be effective. As the muscle releases, you must be able to detect the relaxation before you place the muscle in a new stretch position that takes up the slack and provides the same level of tension on the muscle as was present before the muscle responded to the treatment.

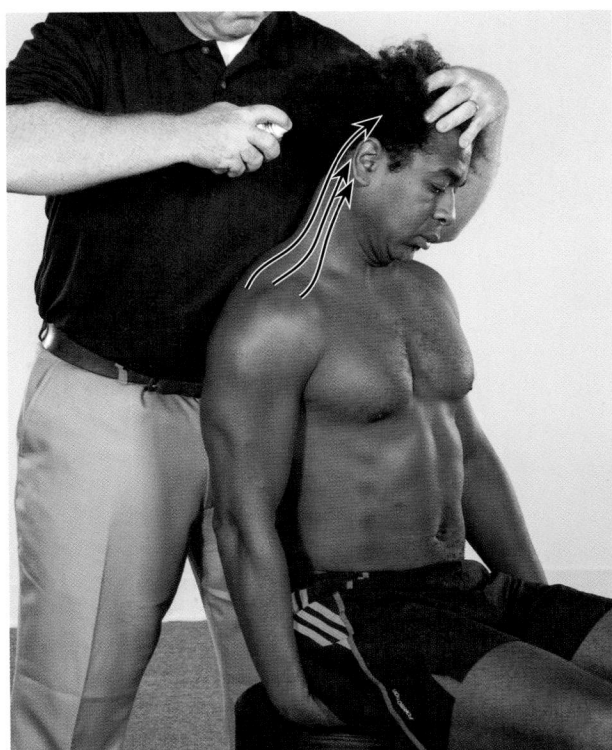

Figure 11.10 In the spray-and-stretch technique, a narrow vapocoolant stream is applied in sweeps that include the muscle's length, its trigger points, and its referred pain areas. It is applied in a rhythmic fashion while a gentle stretch is applied to the muscle. Do not repeat spray applications over the same skin.

Once the treatment is completed, releasing the stretch force occurs smoothly and gradually, not quickly. A hot pack can be immediately applied to further relax the muscle before another application. The patient can also help during the stretch by contracting the antagonist, but you must monitor the contraction, making sure it is submaximal and not too aggressive, since you do not want a co-contraction of the agonist and antagonist. The spray-and-stretch technique can be repeated for several cycles after the skin has been rewarmed, depending on the results of treatment, the patient's response, and the desired goals. Once the spray-and-stretch treatment is completed, the patient actively stretches the treated muscle to enhance treatment results.[109]

It is believed that this technique is effective because of two mechanisms, although they have not been confirmed through research. The gate control theory of pain presented by Melzack[110] and the modified gate control theory advanced by Castel[111] postulate that sudden cold and touch sensations stimulate A-beta fibers to inhibit pain receptor transmission (figure 11.11). The second factor is mechanical: If a muscle is stretched, its sarcomere elongates and releases the actin and myosin elements enough to terminate the sustained muscle fiber contraction.[74]

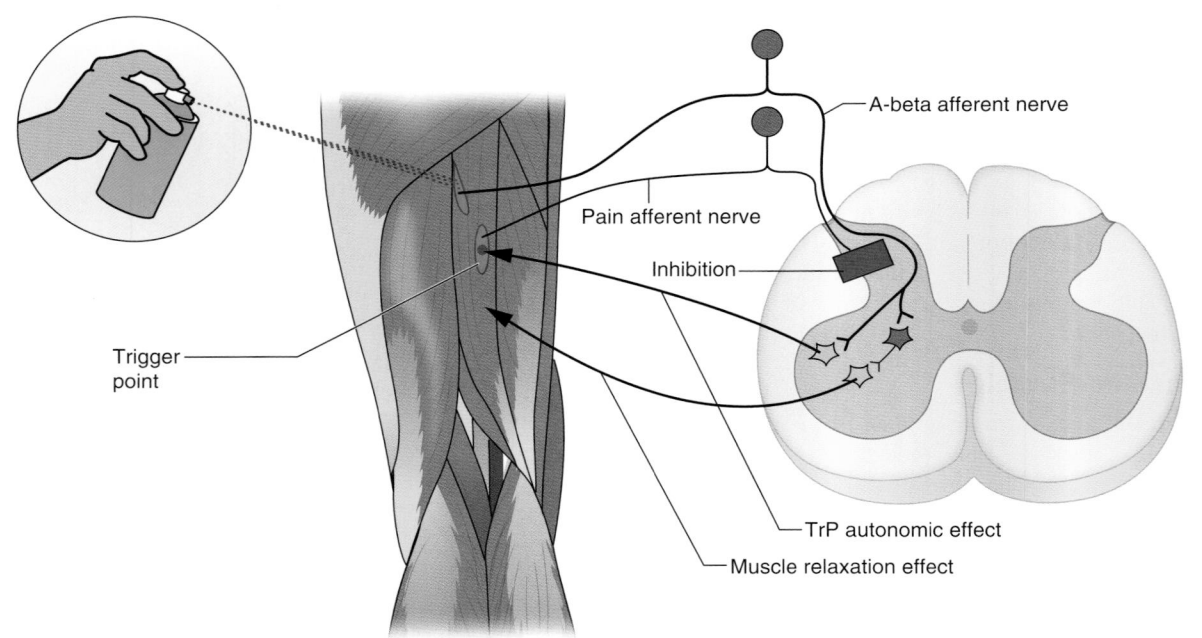

Figure 11.11 Effect of trigger point release on neural pathways: The sudden cold and touch afferent stimulation facilitate a presynaptic inhibition to "close the gate" to pain transmission. The cooling sensation moves along the faster beta fiber to reduce pain and reduce spasm via the autonomic reflex system.

Pressure Release

Another myofascial trigger point release technique is pressure release of the nodule within the fibrous band. In this technique, the muscle is passively placed into a mildly lengthened position with pressure applied slowly and progressively over the trigger point into the tissue's resistance to the point of discomfort without pain. The pressure and stretch are maintained until the clinician feels the tension in the muscle release.[57] The patient will report reduced discomfort when the muscle releases and may indicate that it feels as if the clinician relaxed the pressure, although the pressure has remained consistent throughout the treatment. Once the muscle fibers "let go," either pressure is increased or a stretch is applied to the new barrier, to the patient's initial level of discomfort. This process is repeated until the patient reports no pain with increased pressure or stretch. At that time the stretch and pressure are slowly released. The patient then actively stretches the muscle, helping the muscle to develop a "memory" for the new length. Hanten and colleagues[112] found that this technique of pressure release followed by stretching provided the best and most effective decrease in trigger point pain levels. Kashyap and colleagues[113] found that pressure release not only decreased trigger point pain levels but also improved range of motion.

Stripping or Other Myofascial Applications

A third technique of myofascial trigger point relief is stripping. In this technique, a deep-tissue stroking is applied with the finger pads. A firm pressure is used along the length of the taut band.[57] The pressure increases progressively with each successive pass along the muscle's trigger point. A milking movement from the distal to the proximal end of the muscle goes over the trigger point at the rate of about 2.5 cm (1 in.) every 3 s. As the effects of the technique become apparent, the taut band relaxes, the trigger point nodule softens, and the area ceases to be tender and no longer refers pain. As with the other myofascial trigger point treatments, active stretching exercises are used once the clinician completes the hands-on application.

The pressure of the stripping technique is thought to cause a reflexive **hyperemia** that returns the site to a normal condition.[57] Improving local blood flow restores normal chemical levels to relax taut muscle fibers, relieve pain, and allow electrophysiological return to pre–trigger point levels.[57]

Modality Application

Various modalities have demonstrated beneficial effects when applied to myofascial trigger points. Therapeutic ultrasound—1 MHz at 1.5 W/cm² for 7 min—applied over trigger points resulted in significant improvements in pain intensity and range of motion.[114] Other modalities that have demonstrated success are hot packs and cold packs,[115] electrical stimulation,[114] massage,[116] injections and acupuncture,[117] and dry needling.[118] Regardless of the modality used, clinicians should include active stretching exercises after applying the modality.[119, 120] The proprioceptive neuromuscular facilitation (PNF) techniques of contract–relax and reciprocal inhibition are also effective when combined with soft-tissue mobilization in relaxing myofascial trigger points.[121, 122] Proprioceptive neuromuscular facilitation is presented in detail later in this chapter.

Precautions

Before trigger point treatment is administered, an accurate history should be taken and the patient's condition assessed to determine whether this type of therapy is indicated. Trigger point therapy is not effective on scar tissue adhesions.

The patient should relax for optimal treatment results. Inform the patient what sensations to expect and what you will do before you begin the application; this will help the patient to relax during the treatment. The stretch applied should be passive, without any contraction of the agonist. If the patient can isolate the antagonist, and if you can monitor the patient's response, contraction of the antagonist may improve treatment results as long as the stretched muscle remains relaxed. Spray-and-stretch is not as effective if it is applied too quickly or repetitively over the same area. The stretch should be applied slowly and should span the area but should not cause painful spasm or prevent the patient from relaxing.

The cause of the myofascial trigger point must be corrected for the treatment to succeed, particularly if the cause is poor posture or chronic stress of the muscle. In these cases, the cause is corrected with flexibility and strengthening exercises and patient education.

Prolonged direct pressure over nerves and blood vessels should be avoided. Pressure release techniques should not be used if the patient complains of tingling or numbness.

Trigger Point Applications

This section describes the most commonly found myofascial trigger points. Signs and symptoms, pain-referral patterns, and the treatment applications of spray-and-stretch and pressure release are also included.

In each of the myofascial trigger point images, the black or white X identifies the location of the trigger point; the darkest concentration of color represents the region of most intense referred pain, and the speckled areas show where there are less frequent or less intense pain-referral patterns.

Once the muscle with the specific pain pattern is identified, the clinician palpates the muscle to confirm the presence of trigger points. All trigger points within the muscle should be assessed since it is common for more than one to be present and tender. The clinician treats the most severe trigger points first and then reassesses the remaining trigger points before treating them since they may become positively affected by treatment provided to the more severely affected trigger points.[57] Since the most effective trigger point treatment techniques are pressure release and spray-and-stretch, those are the techniques presented.

Cervical, Thoracic, and Lumbar Spine Myofascial Trigger Points

Each spinal segment has its myofascial trigger points. The cervical spine muscles are presented first, followed by the thoracic and lumbar spine. The thoracic and lumbar spine myofascial trigger points are presented together since they may send referred pain throughout both regions and also occur along muscles that extend through both regions.

Trigger Point Releases for the Cervical Spine

The upper trapezius, levator scapulae, sternocleidomastoid, and scalenes are the cervical muscles that are most often affected by myofascial trigger points. These muscles are presented here.

Upper Trapezius

Referral Pattern: Posterior neck, mastoid process, temple, and posterior region of head, occiput, and angle of jaw (figure 11.12*a*).

Location of Trigger Point: Junction of the angle between the neck and shoulder.

Patient Position for Palpation: Supine.

Muscle Position for Palpation: Slight slack in the muscle with the patient's head tilted slightly toward the shoulder on the side of pain.

Pressure Release Treatment: Either grasp the muscle at the juncture between the neck and shoulder portion of the muscle (figure 11.12*b*) or apply a caudally directed pressure over the trigger point after applying the stretch into some cervical flexion and lateral flexion to the opposite side.

Spray-and-Stretch Treatment: Apply a mild stretch by laterally flexing the head to the opposite side and flexing the neck. The direction of the spray coolant strokes are swept upward from the acromion process toward the base of the skull (figure 11.12*c*).

> continued

Upper Trapezius *> continued*

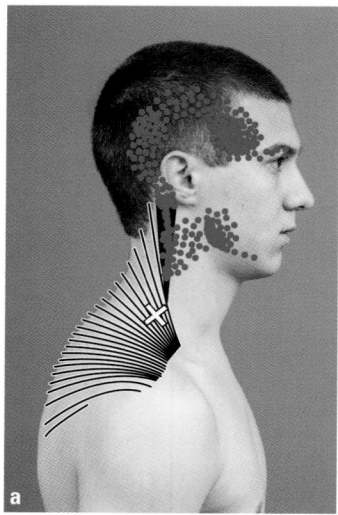
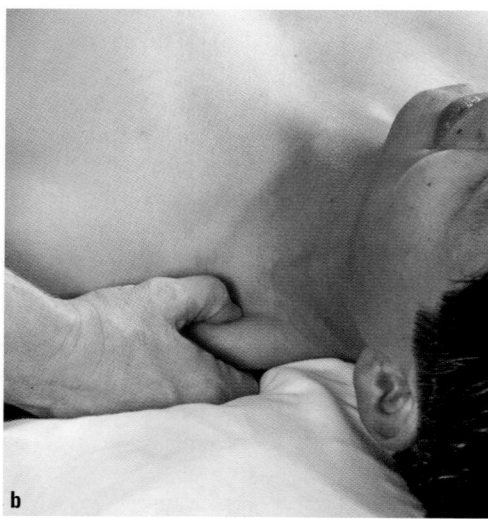
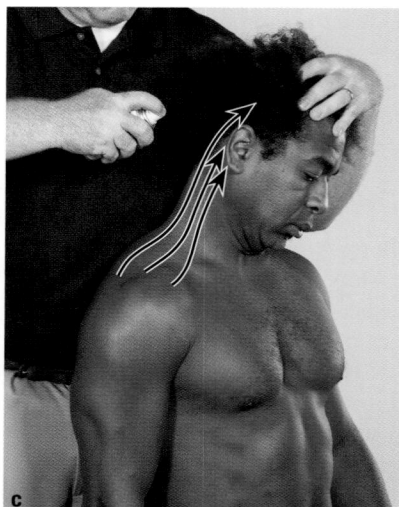

Figure 11.12

Levator Scapulae

Referral Pattern: The site of most intense referred pain from the levator scapulae occurs at the angle between the posterior neck and the shoulder with occasional referral along the vertebral border of the scapula or to the posterior shoulder (figure 11.13*a*).

Location of Trigger Point: Either at the distal insertion of the levator scapulae on the vertebral angle of the scapula or at the angle of the posterior neck.

Patient Position for Palpation: Supine or side-lying for pressure release. Sitting for spray-and-stretch.

Muscle Position for Palpation: Muscle is slightly relaxed, with clinician or a pillow supporting the patient's head.

Pressure Release Treatment: Finger is on the trigger point as in figure 11.13*b*. Place the neck into slight flexion and rotation to the opposite side, then place firm pressure on the myofascial trigger point nodule. Stabilize the patient's shoulder with your opposite hand as shown.

Spray-and-Stretch Treatment: The same-side arm is anchored, and the head is tilted forward and to the opposite side. A steady stretch is applied while the spray coolant strokes are swept from the base of the skull downward along the path of the muscle (figure 11.13*c*).

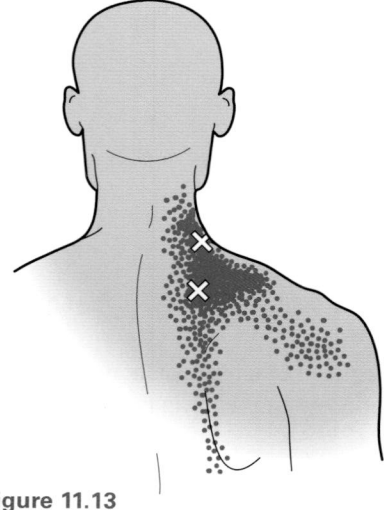
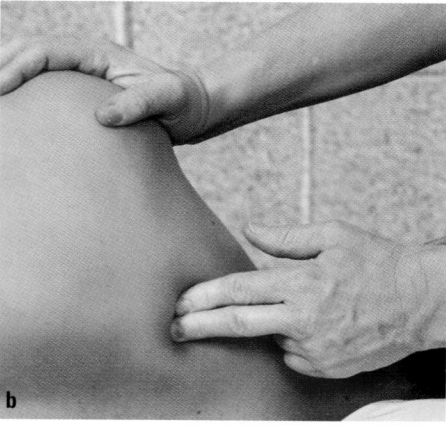
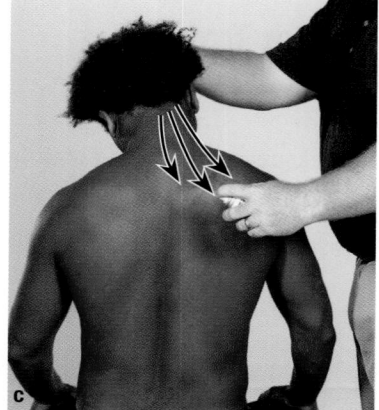

Figure 11.13

Sternocleidomastoid

Referral Pattern: Both the sternal and clavicular heads can refer pain into the face and head. The most common referral areas are in and behind the ear, around the eye, the forehead, cheek, teeth, tongue, pharynx, and the upper aspect of the sternum.

Location of Trigger Point: There are multiple trigger points for this muscle, as seen in figure 11.14a.

Patient Position for Palpation: Supine.

Muscle Position for Palpation: Head is tilted to the same side.

Pressure Release Treatment: A pincer grasp on the muscle at the trigger point or a vertical pressure can be applied to the muscle (figure 11.14b). Once you have positioned your hand, gently stretch the neck into extension and ipsilateral rotation, and apply pressure until the patient reports some discomfort.

Spray-and-Stretch Treatment: Spray-and-stretch is applied with the patient sitting, the same-side arm anchored, and the neck positioned in extension and rotation to the opposite side if the clavicular head is being treated (figure 11.14c). If the sternal head of the muscle is being treated, the neck is rotated to the same side and extended. The spray coolant strokes are swept from the clavicle upward toward the head.

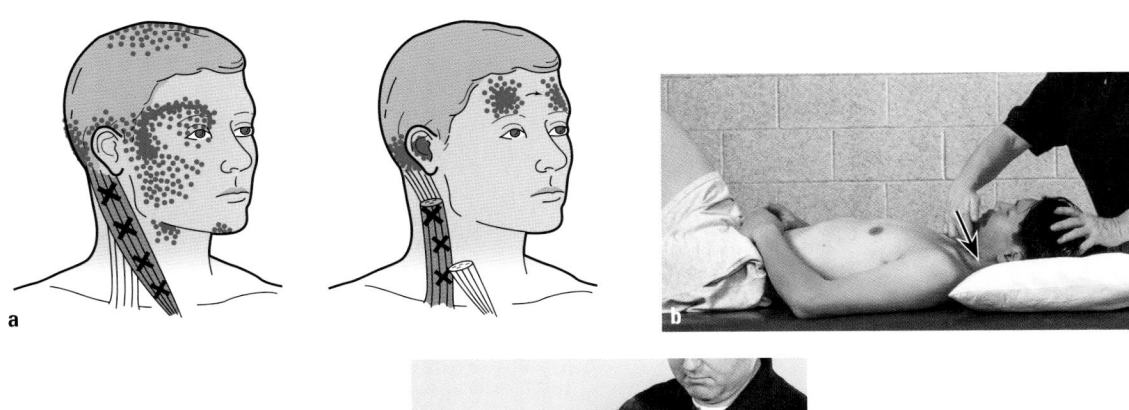

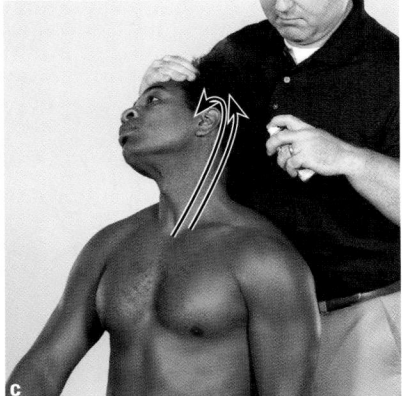

Figure 11.14

Scalenes

Referral Pattern: We consider the scalene muscles—anterior, medius, and posterior—together. Trigger points of these muscles are seen in people with a forward-head posture. The pain-referral patterns for the scalenes include pain along the anterior chest, lateral shoulder and arm, vertebral border of the scapula, radial forearm and hand, posterior thumb and index finger and metacarpal, and interscapular areas (figure 11.15a and b).

Location of Trigger Point: Locate the posterior sternocleidomastoid, cephalad to the clavicle. The scalenes lie just lateral to the sternocleidomastoid. Identify the external jugular vein as it crosses over the anterior scalene; the anterior scalene's myofascial trigger point is just caudal to the external jugular vein. The scalenus medius is deep; it is found just lateral to the anterior scalene and just above the clavicle. The subclavian artery lies between the

> continued

Scalenes *> continued*

medius and anterior scalenes and can be palpated as it passes over the first rib behind the clavicle. The cervical transverse processes can be palpated when pressure is applied to the scalenus medius.

Patient Position for Palpation: Supine for pressure release (figure 11.15c). Sitting for spray-and-stretch.

Muscle Position for Palpation: Have a pillow under the head for comfort, and slightly relax the scalenes by tilting the head to the same side.

Pressure Release Treatment: Gently stretch the specific scalene being treated by laterally flexing the head to the contralateral side. Use finger pad to press directly on trigger point. Referral may be reported into the shoulder or arm.

Spray-and-Stretch Treatment: Applied with the patient sitting and the arm anchored (figure 11.15d). The neck is positioned in extension with the head rotated away from the side being treated. The vapocoolant strokes are swept from the cephalad insertion of the muscles downward and along the shoulder and arm.

Notations: Take care to avoid applying pressure over the blood vessels in this area. These muscles are frequent sites of myofascial trigger points in people with forward-head postures.

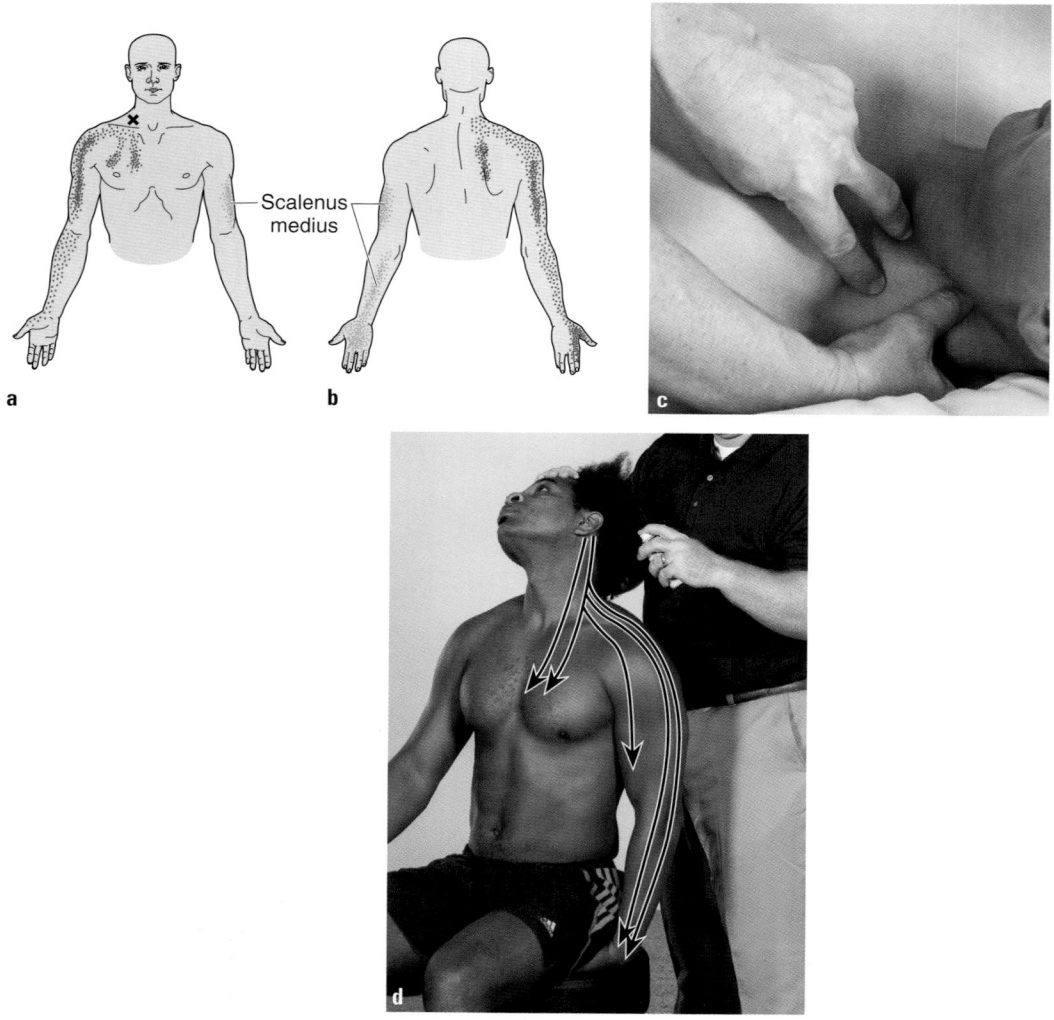

Scalenus medius

Figure 11.15

Trigger Point Releases for the Lumbar Spine

Muscles in the thoracic and lumbar regions that can refer pain into the thoracic, lumbar, and sacral areas include the thoracic and lumbar paraspinals and the quadratus lumborum. The only muscle presented here is the quadratus lumborum.

Quadratus Lumborum

Referral Pattern: Typical quadratus lumborum pain can be either a deep ache or a sharp pain. The superficial fibers can refer pain along the iliac crest or greater trochanter, or the pain can wrap around to the outer groin. The deep fibers refer down to the sacroiliac joint or lower buttock (figure 11.16*a*).

Location of Trigger Point: The superficial trigger points are located laterally, just cephalad to the iliac crest or distal of the 12th rib. The deep trigger points are located just lateral to the paraspinal muscles.

Patient Position for Palpation: Side-lying on the uninvolved side.

Muscle Position for Palpation: The top arm is placed over the head to elevate the lower ribs, and the top hip and knee are flexed with the knee on the table to lower the ilium (figure 11.16*b*). If the area is too tight or painful for the patient to lie in this position, the top leg should be placed on the bottom leg or on a supportive pillow to reduce the stretch of the muscle.

Pressure Release Treatment: Apply pressure over the myofascial trigger points that reproduce the patient's referred pain while the muscle is on a gentle stretch.

Spray-and-Stretch Treatment: Spray-and-stretch treatment is applied with the patient in a position similar to that for trigger point release, but with the top leg forward of the bottom leg and distal thigh and positioned off the table to allow a stretch (figure 11.16*c*). The spray coolant strokes are swept in a cephalad-to-caudal motion.

Notations: This muscle's referral pattern often gives the false sign of a disc syndrome and is neglected as a source of low-back pain. The pain, which can be intense, can accompany deep inhalation or can make walking painful.

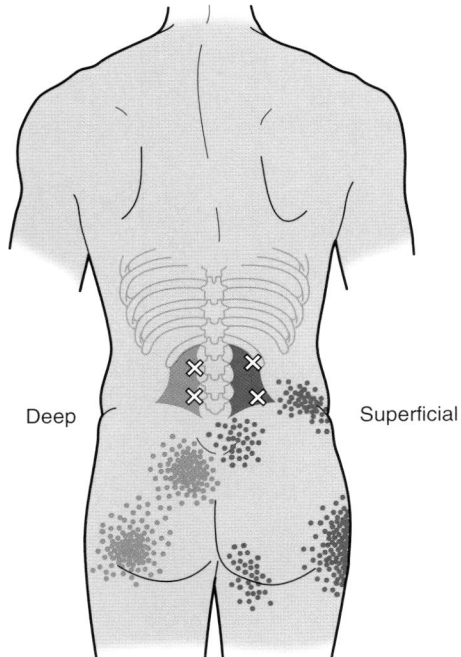

Deep   Superficial

a

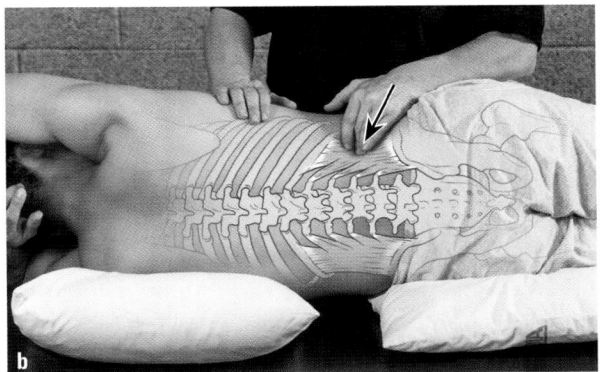

b

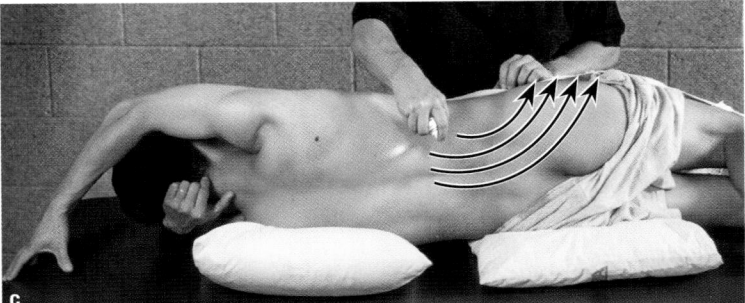

c

Figure 11.16

Upper-Extremity Myofascial Trigger Points

Although myofascial trigger points can be found through-out the upper extremity, we see them more often in the shoulder girdle region than in more distal aspects of the extremity. Since trigger points of other upper-extremity segments occur infrequently, only the frequently occurring rotator cuff muscles are presented in this upper-extremity section. For other upper-extremity trigger points, please refer to the Travell and Simons text.[66]

Trigger Point Releases for the Rotator Cuff

When shoulder injuries occur, the rotator cuff is a frequent site of myofascial trigger points. A patient complaining of pain over the deltoid insertion region is likely suffering from a myofascial trigger point within the rotator cuff. Common rotator cuff trigger points are found in the infraspinatus and subscapularis muscles, although the supraspinatus and, less often, the teres minor also are subject to trigger points.

Supraspinatus

Referral Pattern: Can refer pain into the arm. The referred pain pattern is a deep ache that occurs around the lateral shoulder in the middle deltoid area down to the deltoid insertion (figure 11.17*a* and *b*).

Location of Trigger Point: The two sites that are most common for this muscle are at the juncture of the middle third and lateral third of the muscle and at the junction of the middle third and medial third of the muscle. Of these, the more tender site is the more medial trigger point located just above the scapular spine, about 2 to 3 cm (0.8-1.2 in.) lateral to the vertebral border.

Patient Position for Palpation: Seated or side-lying on the uninvolved side.

Muscle Position for Palpation: Relaxed with the arm at the side.

Pressure Release Treatment: Some pressure is applied over the trigger point site just above the scapular spine, 2 to 3 cm (0.8-1.2 in.) lateral to the vertebral border as the shoulder is placed into medial rotation until some discomfort is felt (figure 11.17*c*).

Spray-and-Stretch Treatment: Spray coolant is swept from the proximal supraspinatus insertion, across the muscle and acromion, over the deltoid, and down the arm to the elbow (figure 11.17*d*).

Notations: The clinician applies the stretch by adducting the arm and raising the patient's hand behind the back upward toward the opposite scapula.

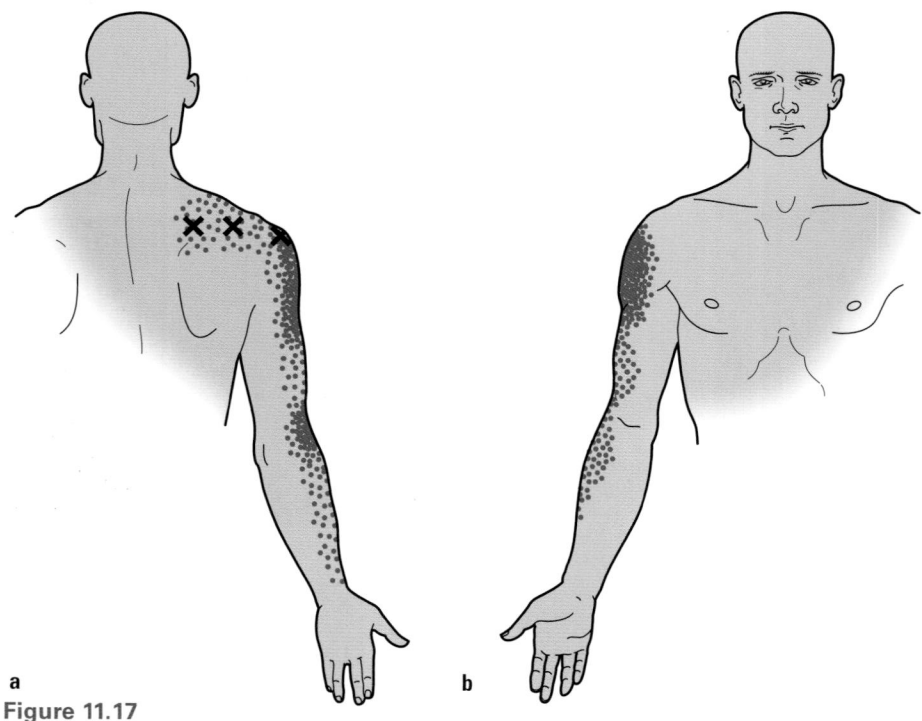

a   b

Figure 11.17

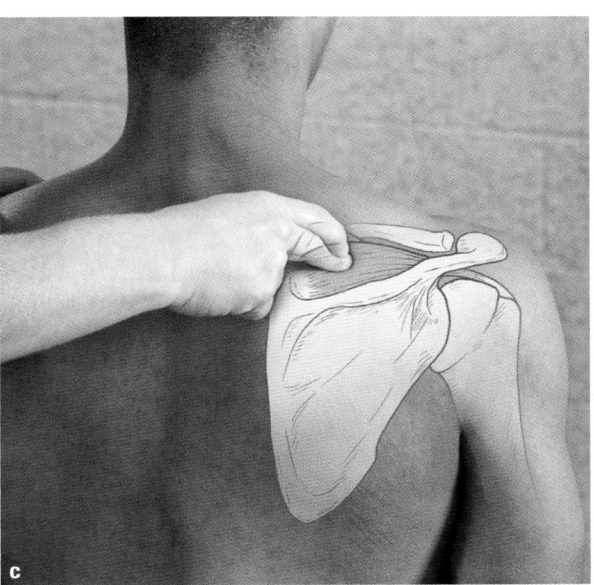
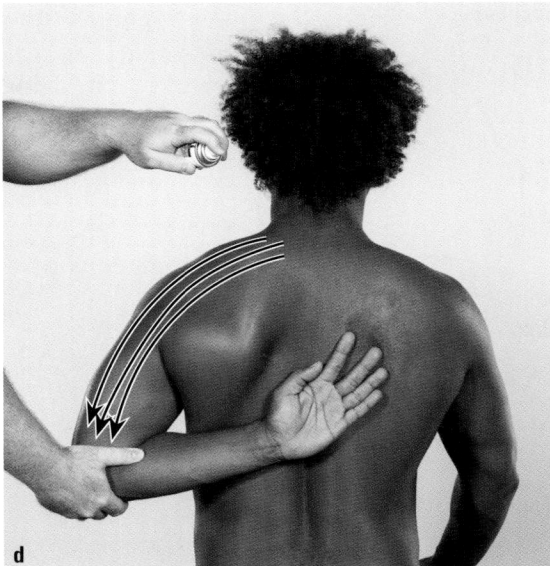

Figure 11.17 >*continued*

Subscapularis

Referral Pattern: The subscapularis refers pain to the posterior wrist and to the inferior aspect of the posterior shoulder region where the humerus meets the trunk. It can also occasionally refer pain into the scapula, down the posterior arm to the elbow, and circumferentially around the wrist (figure 11.18*a* and *b*).

Location of Trigger Point: Lateral anterior region of the scapula.

Patient Position for Palpation: Supine.

Muscle Position for Palpation: The arm is abducted comfortably away from the body to about 60° to 90°. The clinician stands between the patient's arm and side, facing the patient and supporting the patient's arm while applying traction to slide the scapula laterally, away from the ribs.

Pressure Release Treatment: The finger pads of the clinician's treatment hand are moved past the teres major and latissimus dorsi to palpate the anterior surface of the scapula. The best approach is to move the finger pads from the superior–lateral aspect of the axilla next to the ribs at a downward and medially directed angle as the scapula is passively protracted. Continue to move the fingers in this direction until the palpation hand feels the firm surface of the anterolateral scapula. Pressure in a cephalic direction toward the spine is applied to the subscapularis once the trigger point has been located, and the shoulder is moved into lateral rotation to stretch the subscapularis. Only enough pressure to cause initial discomfort is applied; once the patient reports no discomfort, the pressure and lateral rotation increase until the patient once again reports discomfort, at which time the position and pressure are held until the trigger point releases. The process is repeated until no discomfort with a stretch and pressure is reported (figure 11.18*c*).

Spray-and-Stretch Treatment: Spray-and-stretch is applied with the patient supine and the arm in partial abduction and lateral rotation. Spray coolant sweeps start at the lateral trunk and move over the axilla and along the posterior arm. As the sweeps are repeated, the arm is moved into more abduction and lateral rotation until it is positioned overhead in full abduction and lateral rotation (figure 11.18*d* and *e*).

Notations: This is a very tender trigger point on most people, but it is especially tender on pathological shoulders.

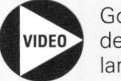
Go to HK*Propel* and watch video 11.1, which demonstrates finding and treating subscapularis trigger points.

> *continued*

Subscapularis > *continued*

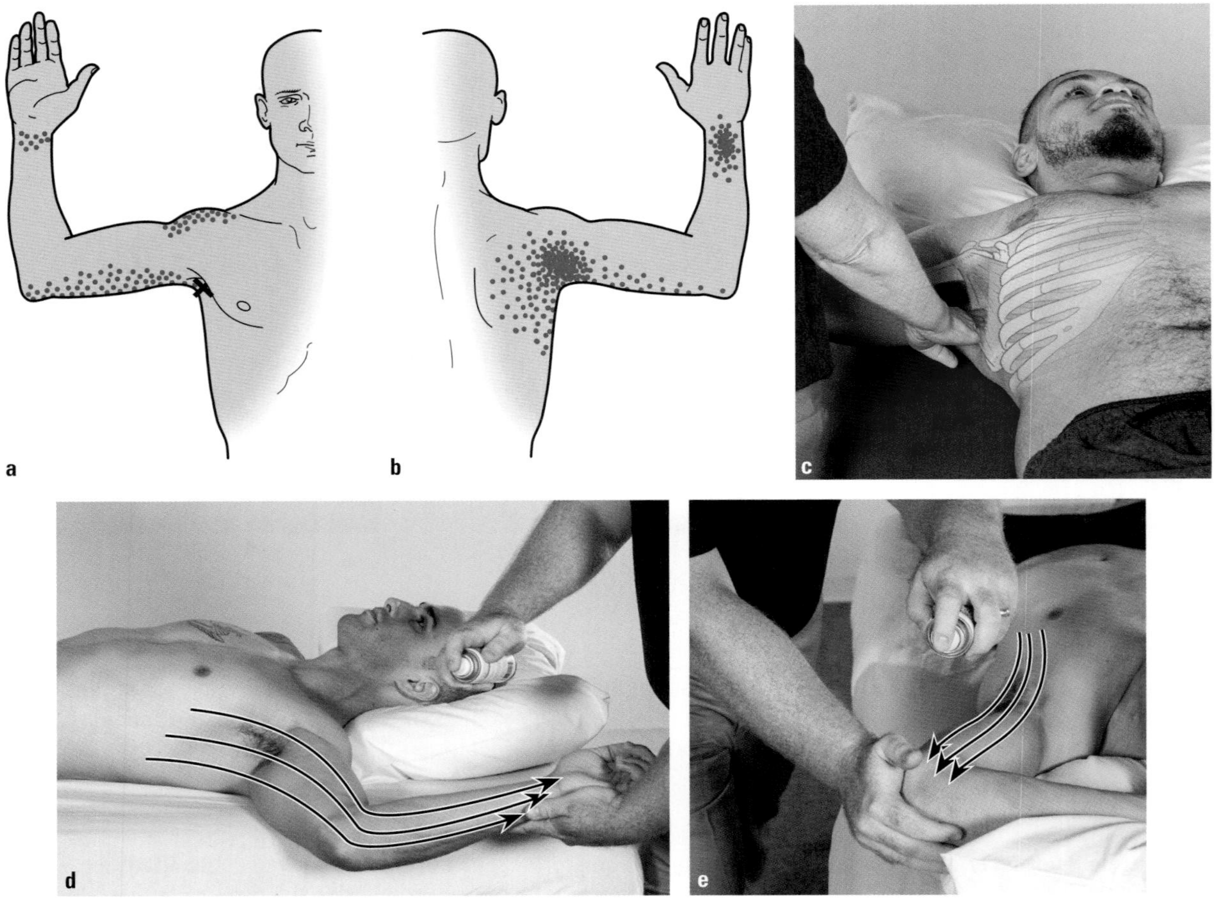

Figure 11.18

Infraspinatus

Referral Pattern: Most often refers to the anterior shoulder, anterior arm, wrist, and radial fingers (figure 11.19*a* and *b*). On occasion, vertebral border scapular pain or pain at the base of the skull can also occur. Pain can be felt deep in the anterior shoulder as well.

Location of Trigger Point: The superior aspect of the muscle inferior to the scapular spine and along the vertebral border.

Patient Position for Palpation: Side-lying on opposite side.

Muscle Position for Palpation: Arm is relaxed at the patient's side.

Pressure Release Treatment: Once the trigger point is located, pressure by the finger pads is applied over the central trigger point located along the tender band within the muscle while the muscle is stretched into medial rotation to the point of discomfort without pain (figure 11.19*c*).

Spray-and-Stretch Treatment: Spray coolant sweeps are applied from the vertebral border upward to the shoulder and then either up to the head or down the upper extremity (figure 11.19*d*).

Notations: Progressively stretch the muscle by moving the arm either behind the back with the shoulder in medial rotation or horizontally in front and across the body with medial rotation.

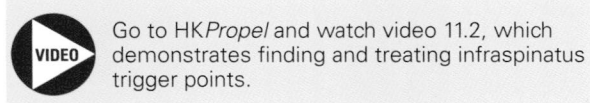

Go to HK*Propel* and watch video 11.2, which demonstrates finding and treating infraspinatus trigger points.

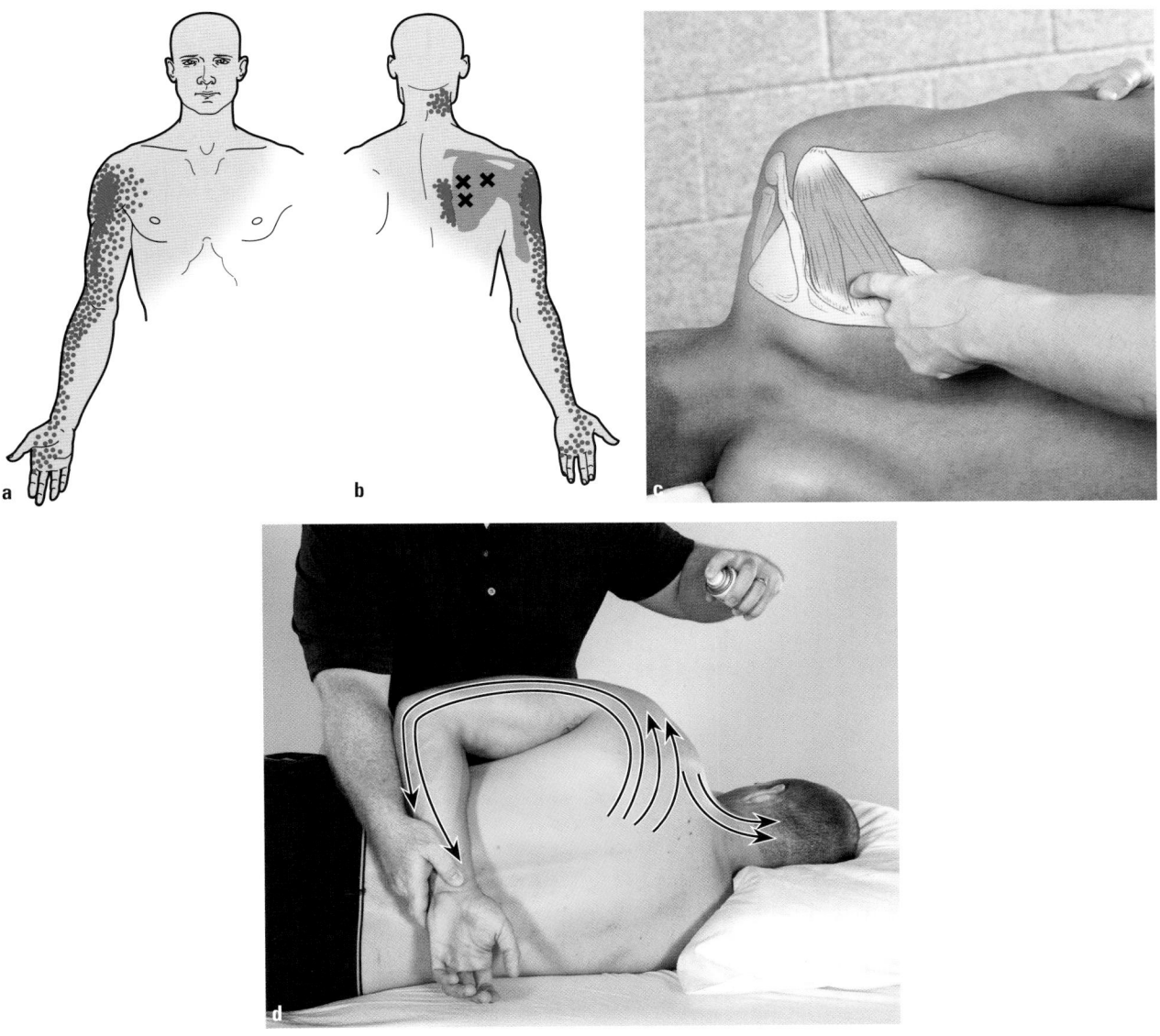

Figure 11.19

Lower-Extremity Myofascial Trigger Points

Although any lower-extremity muscle may develop a myofascial trigger point, only a few of the more frequently seen ones will be noted here. Foot myofascial trigger points are presented first, and the hip trigger points are presented last.

Trigger Point Releases for the Foot and Ankle Muscles

Myofascial trigger points of the intrinsic and extrinsic foot and ankle muscles focus on only a couple of muscles. One intrinsic muscle and three extrinsic muscles are presented here.

Abductor Hallucis

Referral Pattern: From the heel along the medial edge of the foot near the medial arch (figure 11.20a).

Location of Trigger Point: In the muscle belly distal and anterior to the navicular tubercle.

> continued

Abductor Hallucis > *continued*

Patient Position for Palpation: Supine.

Muscle Position for Palpation: Relaxed in a comfortable position.

Pressure Release Treatment: Direct pressure over the trigger point in the muscle belly (figure 11.20*b*) while stretching the toe into adduction and extension.

Spray-and-Stretch Treatment: With the ankle in neutral, the great toe is adducted toward the others and extended while the spray coolant strokes move from the plantar heel toward the toes (figure 11.20*c*).

Notations: The abductor hallucis brevis refers to the medial heel with some radiation into the medial arch.

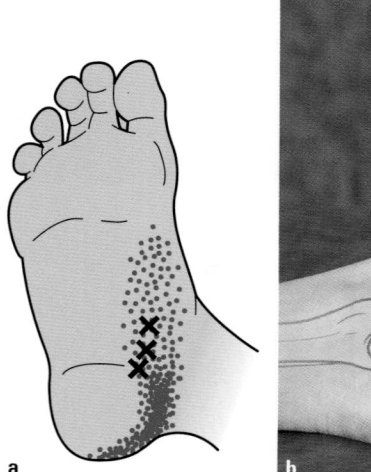
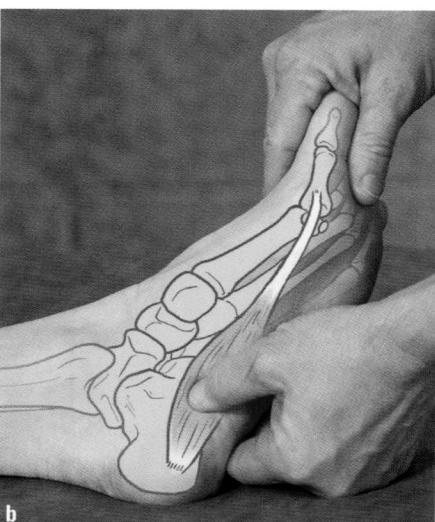
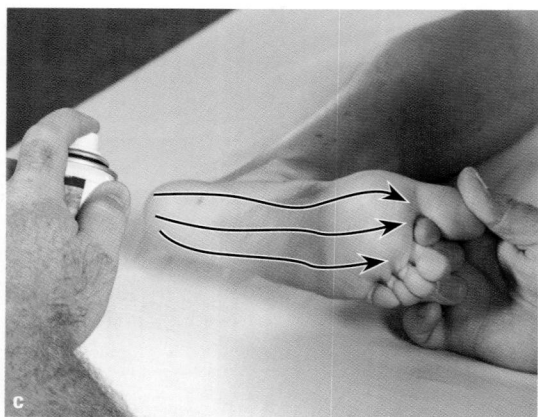

a b c

Figure 11.20

Gastrocnemius

Referral Pattern: There are four trigger points with different referral patterns. They can refer pain to the medial arch with spillover into the medial calf (figure 11.21*a1*), close to the lateral border of the mid-portion of the lateral gastrocnemius head (figure 11.21*a2*), close to the medial border of the medial gastrocnemius head (figure 11.21*a3*), and slightly distal to the posterior knee on the lateral head of the gastrocnemius (figure 11.21*a4*).

Location of Trigger Point: Trigger point causing medial arch pain is in the proximal medial belly distal to the knee (TP$_1$). The trigger point for the lateral calf is in the mid-belly of the lateral calf at the fullest portion of the calf (TP$_2$). The trigger point causing central posterior knee pain is located at the joint line of the knee toward the lateral edge of the medial belly (TP$_3$). The trigger point for lateral posterior knee pain is located in the lateral calf belly distal to the knee joint (TP$_4$).

Patient Position for Palpation: Prone.

Muscle Position for Palpation: Relaxed in a comfortable position with a pillow under the leg.

Pressure Release Treatment: Either a flat thumb pressure or a pincer grasp can be used (figure 11.21*b*). If the muscle is taut, a flat pressure is easier and more comfortable to administer. Trigger point release is best performed with the ankle in slight plantar flexion to place the muscle on slack; once the trigger point is located, apply stretch, moving the ankle into dorsiflexion until the patient reports discomfort. A pincer grasp of the lateral head is easily used with the thumb on the lateral border and the fingers at the midline groove between the two gastrocnemius heads. Flat pressure should be used in the popliteal area.

Spray-and-Stretch Treatment: With the patient in prone and the foot over the edge of the table. While the rehabilitation clinician uses his or her hand or knee to dorsiflex the ankle with pressure over the ball of the patient's foot, he or she applies the spray coolant strokes from above the knee in a distal direction toward the plantar foot (figure 11.21*c*).

Notations: Nocturnal cramps are often associated with these trigger points.

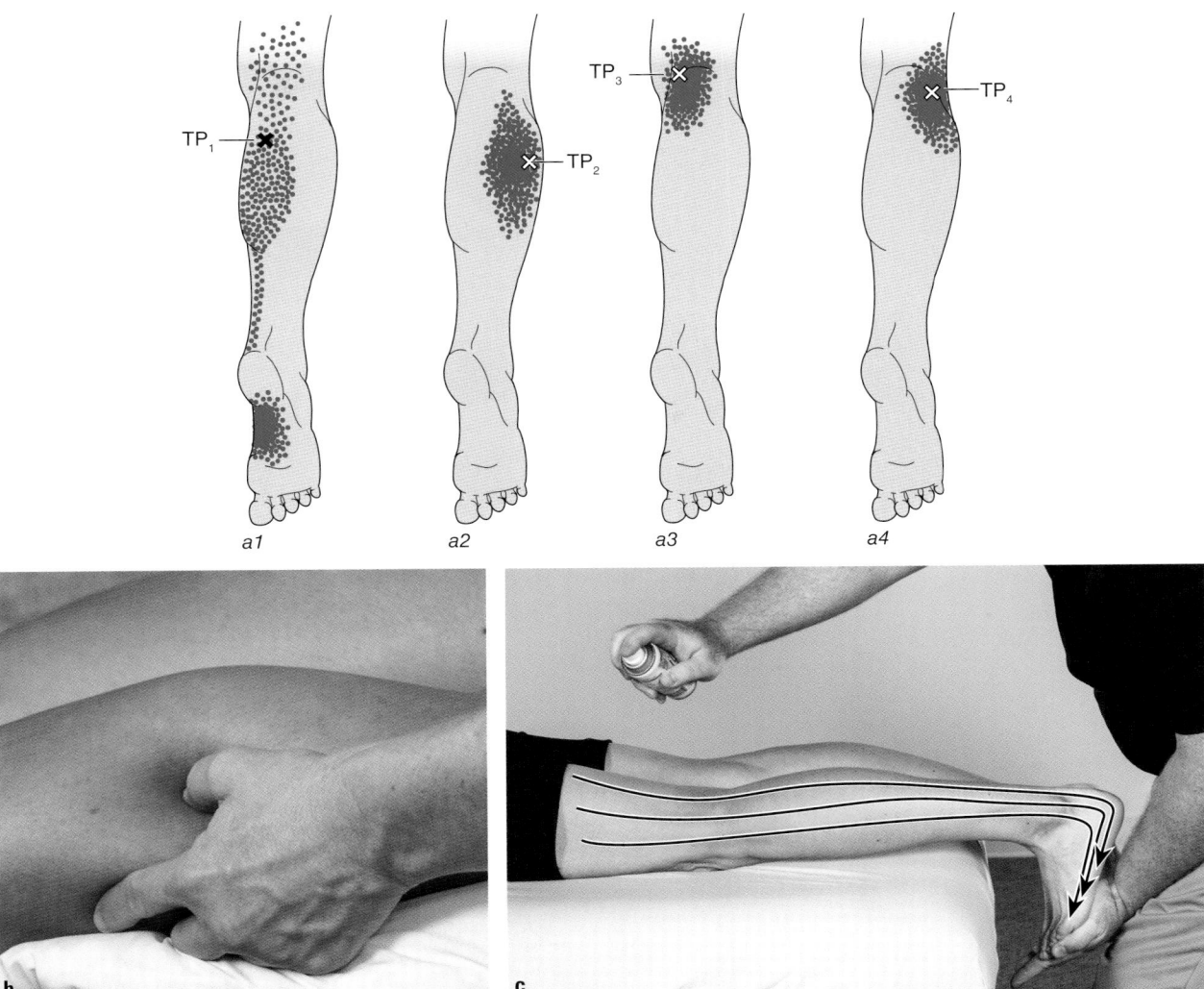

Figure 11.21

Soleus

Referral Pattern: The most common site of pain referral from the soleus is into the posterior and plantar heel area and into the distal Achilles. Unlike the gastrocnemius, the soleus does not cause nocturnal cramps in the calf. The soleus occasionally refers pain into the upper calf and rarely into the ipsilateral sacroiliac joint (figure 11.22a).

Location of Trigger Point: The trigger point for pain referral into the heel lies about 2.5 cm (1 in.) distal to the end of the gastrocnemius and just medial to the midline (TP$_1$). The trigger point for diffuse pain into the calf is located at the lateral proximal edge of the muscle belly (TP$_2$). The trigger point for pain into the ipsilateral sacroiliac is at the lateral distal edge of the muscle belly (TP$_3$), lateral and proximal to TP$_1$. Sometimes it refers to the heel, mimicking TP$_1$.

Patient Position for Palpation: Prone or kneeling.

Muscle Position for Palpation: Relaxed in a comfortable position with a pillow under the leg.

Pressure Release Treatment: Trigger point release uses either a pincer or flat-pressure application. The patient can be either in prone with the knee flexed to keep the gastrocnemius slack (figure 11.22b) or in a kneeling position. The distal trigger points are located just distal to the medial and lateral gastrocnemius muscle belly bulges. Direct pressure to the patient's tolerance is applied after the muscle is placed on stretch into dorsiflexion and maintained until the trigger point relaxes and the pain subsides; this treatment procedure is repeated until there is no discomfort.

> continued

Soleus *> continued*

Spray-and-Stretch Treatment: Performed with the knee in flexion. The patient can be kneeling or prone (figure 11.22c). As the ankle is passively dorsiflexed, the coolant spray is swept from proximal to distal across the posterior extremity and into the plantar foot.

Notations: Heel pain during weight bearing and nocturnal deep heel pain may be primary complaints, and dorsiflexion is limited.

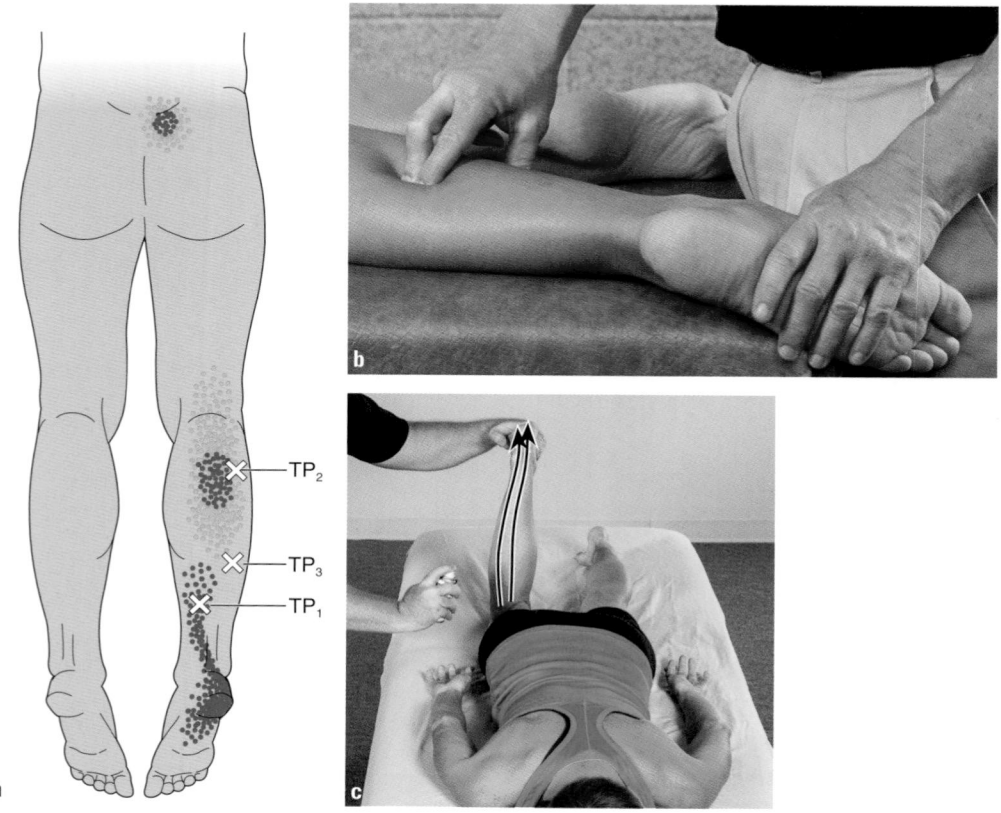

Figure 11.22

Tibialis Posterior

Referral Pattern: Pain can refer into the Achilles tendon with spillover into the midcalf proximally and the heel, instep, and plantar foot and toes distally (figure 11.23a).

Location of Trigger Point: Between the soleus and the medial border of the posterior tibia.

Patient Position for Palpation: Prone.

Muscle Position for Palpation: Relaxed in a comfortable position with a pillow under the leg.

Pressure Release Treatment: Because the tibialis posterior is the deepest muscle of the extremity, it is not possible to make direct contact with it with deep pressure. The ankle is moved into dorsiflexion with eversion, then deep pressure applied to more superficial muscles is used to apply indirect pressure on the tibialis posterior (figure 11.23b).

Spray-and-Stretch Treatment: Applied with the patient prone and the foot over the edge of the table. The ankle is stretched into dorsiflexion and eversion as the coolant spray sweeps begin at the posterior knee and traverse distally into the plantar foot (figure 11.23c).

Notations: Because the tibialis posterior works harder to stabilize the foot when ambulating on uneven surfaces, active trigger points in this muscle make it painful for the patient to walk or run on these surfaces.

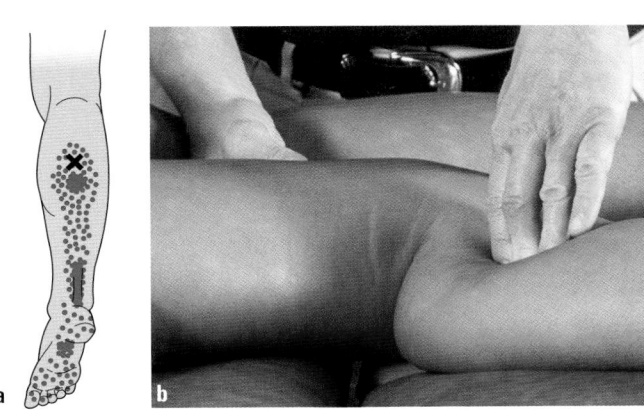
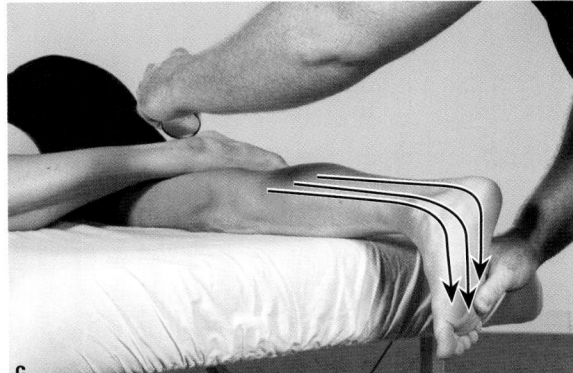

Figure 11.23

Trigger Point Releases for the Knee Muscles

Although the quadriceps is often the muscle most affected by knee injuries, the hamstrings are the muscle group with more myofascial trigger points. In addition to the hamstrings, trigger points of the popliteus are presented.

Hamstrings

Referral Pattern: In the gluteal fold and posterior knee with overflow along the muscle and into the distal medial calf (figure 11.24*a*).

Location of Trigger Point: Trigger points for both the medial and lateral hamstrings are located about 8 to 12 cm (3-4.5 in.) proximal to the knee.

Patient Position for Palpation: Patient is supine for medial hamstrings and prone or side-lying for lateral hamstrings.

Muscle Position for Palpation: For either the medial or lateral hamstring trigger point palpation, the knee is flexed. When treating the medial hamstrings, the hip is also abducted.

Pressure Release Treatment: Apply a mild stretch to the hamstrings first with hip flexion, then either a pincer grasp or a flat pressure can be used for the medial hamstrings, but the lateral hamstrings are best approached with a flat pressure (figure 11.24*b*). Extend the knee to intensify the stretch.

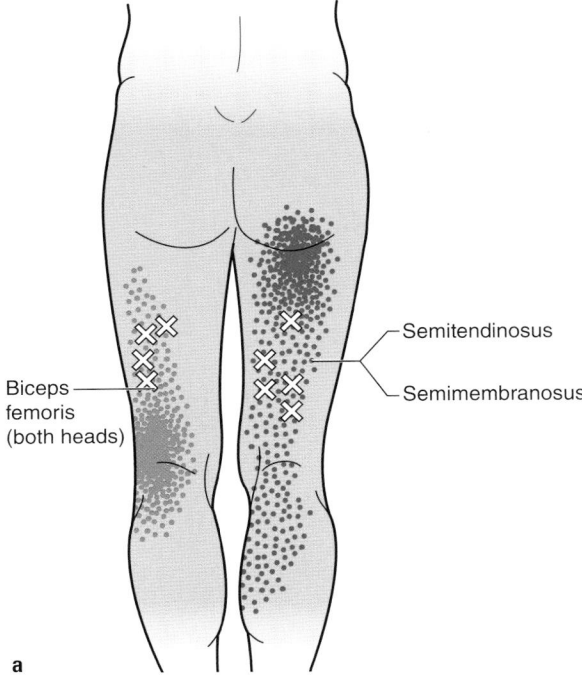
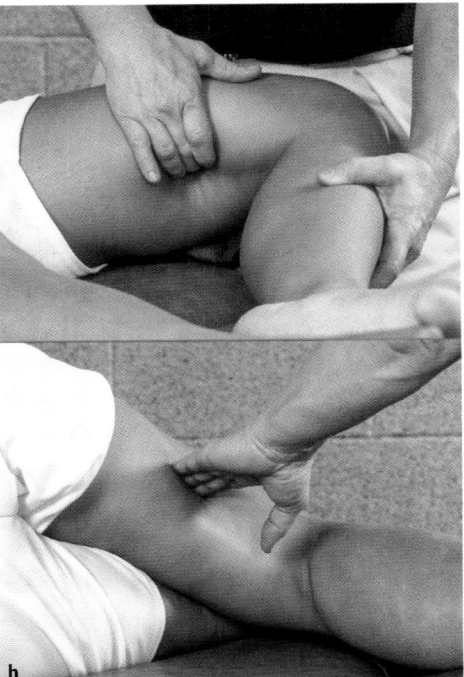

Figure 11.24

> continued

Hamstrings *> continued*

Spray-and-Stretch Treatment: Spray-and-stretch of the hamstrings is performed with the patient supine and the opposite extremity in extension. The involved extremity is supported at the ankle by the rehabilitation clinician. The initial distal-to-proximal coolant spray sweeps are performed with the extremity abducted to passively lengthen the adductor magnus. Once the extremity is abducted as far as possible (the thigh should be almost parallel with the tabletop), the coolant sweeps move in a proximal-to-distal direction while the hip is moved into flexion and adduction; the knee is maintained in extension throughout the motion (figure 11.24c). Once the extremity reaches a vertical position, the clinician stops the movement and dorsiflexes the ankle and extends the coolant application to the calf. Passive adduction is then resumed to the end of adduction motion while in full hip flexion.

Notations: Pain in the semimembranosus and semitendinosus is often described as a sharp pain, whereas referred pain from the biceps femoris is more often a deep ache.

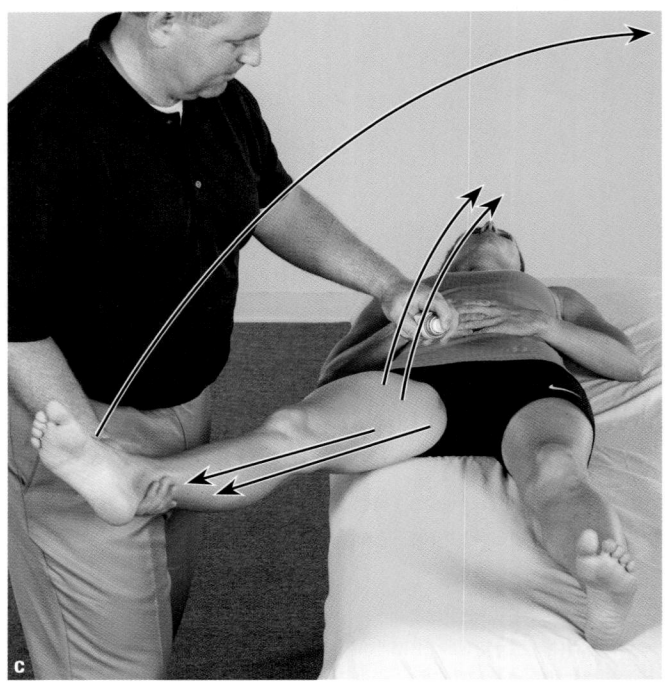

Figure 11.24 *> continued*

Popliteus

Referral Pattern: Posterior knee pain (figure 11.25a) occurs during activities such as running, walking down stairs and hills, and squatting. The patient may complain of knee pain when fully extending the knee.

Location of Trigger Point: At the muscle's tibial insertion. Locate the muscle's medial aspect between the semitendinosus tendon and the medial gastrocnemius head. Since the popliteus is covered by the soleus, passively moving the soleus laterally will expose the popliteus.

Patient Position for Palpation: Prone.

Muscle Position for Palpation: The knee is partially flexed, the limb laterally rotated slightly, and the ankle in moderate plantar flexion so the calf muscles are relaxed.

Pressure Release Treatment: Stretch the popliteus by placing the knee into extension and lateral tibial rotation. A flat pressure is applied in a downward and anterior direction medially (figure 11.25b).

Spray-and-Stretch Treatment: Spray-and-stretch is performed with the patient prone. Coolant sweeps begin distally and move along the muscle's path in a proximal direction as the limb is laterally rotated and the knee extended but not locked (figure 11.25c).

Notations: Posterior knee pain is rarely caused only by this muscle's trigger point. It is usually accompanied by pain associated with trigger points from the gastrocnemius, biceps femoris, or both.

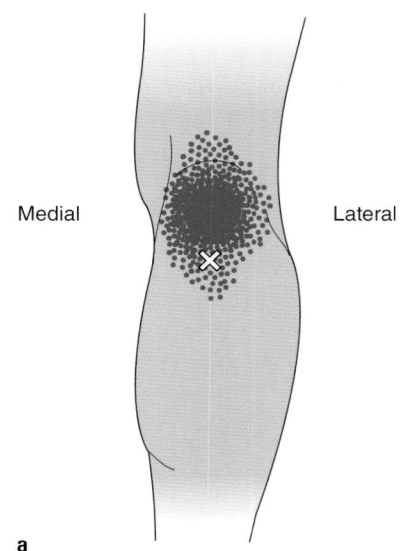

Medial

Lateral

a

Figure 11.25

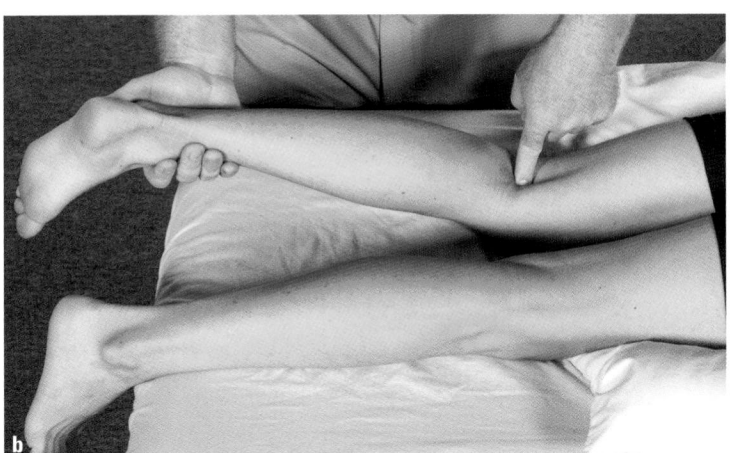
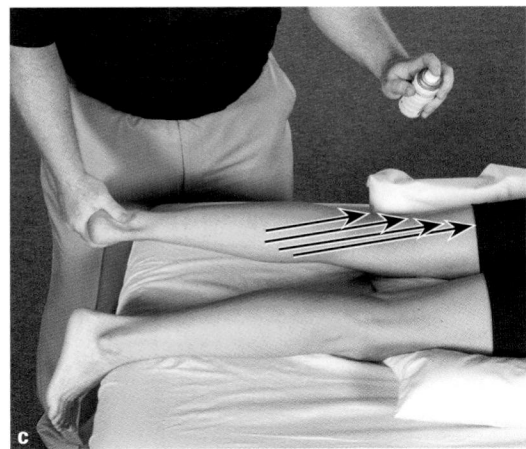

Figure 11.25 *> continued*

Trigger Point Releases for the Hip Muscles

Hip myofascial trigger points can occur with either hip pathology or back pathology. Occasionally hip referral patterns can be confused with sacroiliac-based problems or sciatica. Careful notation of the patient's report of type of pain experienced and aggravating factors can often allow the clinician to focus on the appropriate source of pain complaints. Of the muscles in the hip, myofascial trigger points in the gluteus medius and gluteus minimus are most commonly observed.

Gluteus Medius

Referral Pattern: Pain is along the posterior iliac crest, down the sacrum, and into the lateral posterior gluteal area (figure 11.26a).

Location of Trigger Point: The trigger points are along and immediately inferior to the iliac crest.

Patient Position for Palpation: Side-lying with the affected hip on top.

Muscle Position for Palpation: The hip is flexed and supported with a pillow between the knees and under the bottom hip for comfort.

Pressure Release Treatment: Thumb or finger-pad pressure on the trigger points against the ilium is used along the iliac crest at the tender sites with the muscle on slight stretch into adduction until their relaxation is palpated (figure 11.26b).

Spray-and-Stretch Treatment: Spray-and-stretch is applied with the patient side-lying. The hip is adducted and extended behind the uninvolved extremity for stretch to the anterior fibers and adducted and flexed in an anterior position relative to the uninvolved extremity for stretch to the posterior fibers. Parallel coolant spray sweeps are made from the iliac crest, over the lateral thigh to the knee (figure 11.26c; ● = greater trochanter).

Notations: Pain from the gluteus medius is aggravated by walking, lying supine, side-lying on the affected side, or sitting in a slouched position. Patients with Morton's toe are more susceptible to trigger points here.[66] Ambulating with the hip medially rotated, unilateral standing, falling on the hip, playing prolonged tennis matches, walking on soft sand, and doing aerobics are all activities that can contribute to activation of these trigger points.[66]

 Go to HK*Propel* and watch video 11.3, which demonstrates finding and treating gluteus medius trigger points.

> continued

Gluteus Medius *> continued*

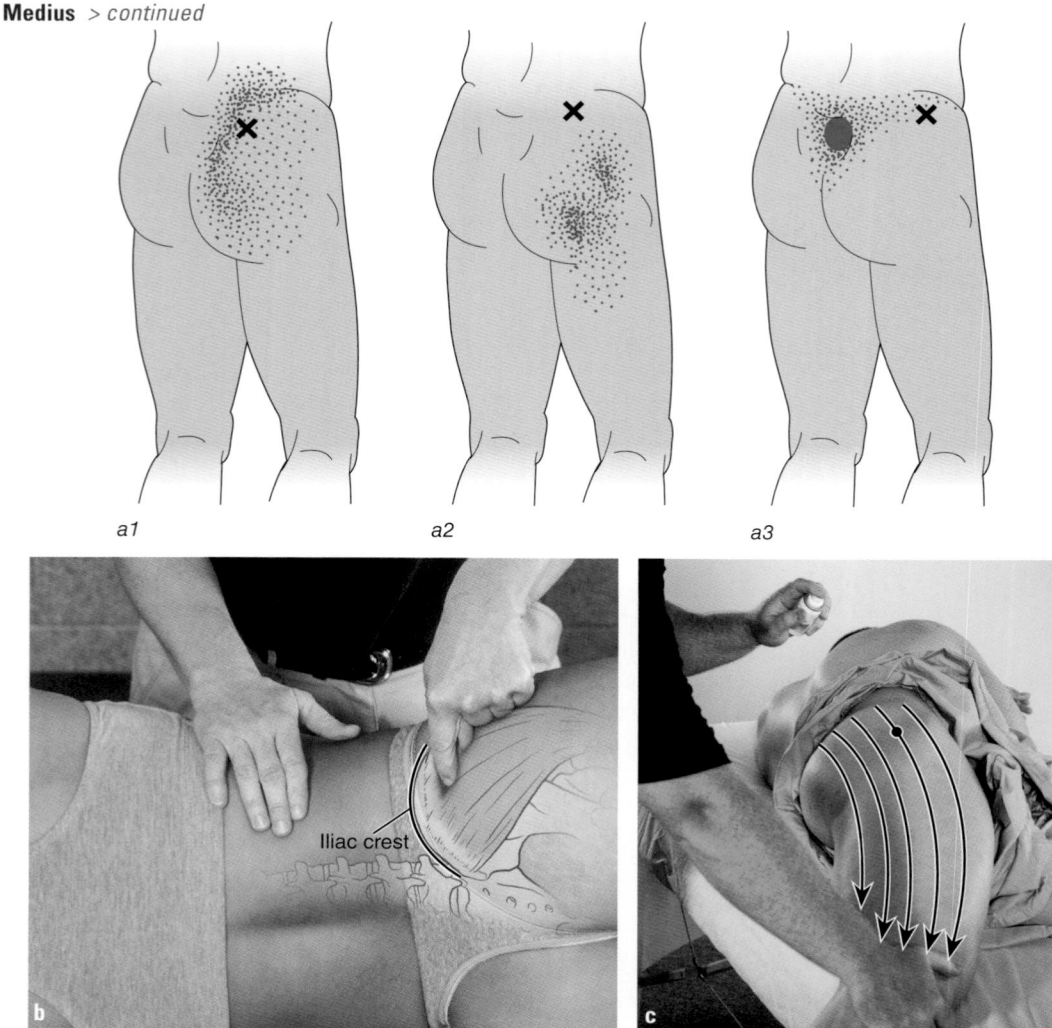

a1　　　　　a2　　　　　a3

Iliac crest

Figure 11.26

Gluteus Minimus

Referral Pattern: Pain-referral pattern is (1) over the lower lateral buttock, down the lateral thigh, and into the lateral leg to the ankle for anterior trigger points or (2) over the lower posterior buttock and posterior thigh and into the proximal posterior calf for posterior trigger points (figure 11.27*a*).

Location of Trigger Point: Several trigger points are located in the gluteus minimus, anteriorly and posteriorly. Anterior trigger points lie deep to the posterior border of the tensor fasciae latae muscle and can be located by offering resistance to find the tensor fasciae latae; just posterior to this muscle's border and inferior to the iliac crest is the anterior gluteus minimus. The trigger point found most often is located in the posterior gluteus minimus muscle cephalic to the greater trochanter about midway between the muscle's proximal and distal insertions. Other posterior trigger points are located just above the middle and lateral piriformis.

Patient Position for Palpation: Supine for anterior trigger points (figure 11.27*b*; ● = greater trochanter; ■ = ASIS); side-lying with the affected leg on top for posterior trigger point treatment.

Muscle Position for Palpation: The gluteus medius and maximus should be relaxed; supportive pillows between the lower extremities should be used for optimal effectiveness.

Pressure Release Treatment: A flat palpation is used for all trigger points. The gluteus medius and maximus should be relaxed; supportive pillows should be used for optimal effectiveness. The anterior fibers are treated just distal to the ASIS and lateral and deep to the tensor fasciae latae. To locate the tensor fasciae latae, the clinician palpates

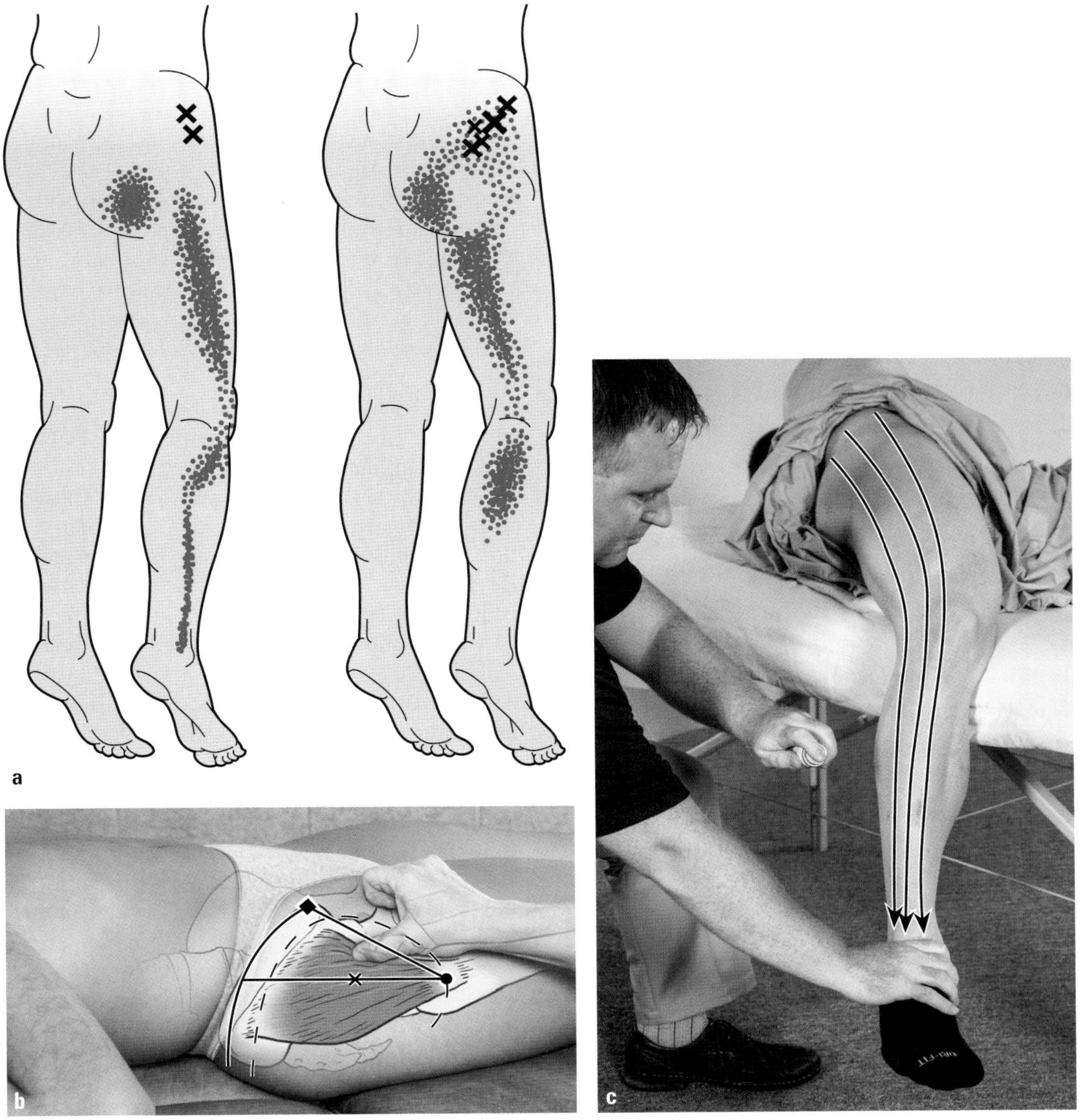

Figure 11.27

for the muscle and simultaneously provides light resistance to hip medial rotation. The posterior trigger points are treated with the hip slightly flexed and adducted.

Spray-and-Stretch Treatment: Spray-and-stretch is applied with the patient in side-lying with the buttock close to the table's edge (figure 11.27 c). With the hip in adduction and supported by the rehabilitation clinician, coolant spray is applied in sweeping strokes from the iliac crest down the lateral thigh to the lateral lower leg and ankle for the anterior trigger points and along the posterior hip, thigh, and calf for the posterior trigger points. The stretch force is applied with the hip in extension and adduction for the anterior fibers and in 30° flexion and medial rotation for the posterior fibers.

Notations: Pain from the gluteus minimus occurs with getting out of a chair and with walking.[66]

 Go to HK*Propel* and watch video 11.4, which demonstrates finding and treating gluteus minimus trigger points.

Muscle Energy

Like many manual therapy techniques, muscle energy techniques (MET) have their origin in osteopathic medicine. Fred Mitchell, DO, originally developed MET that others have since modified.

Definition of Muscle Energy

According to Greenman,[123] "muscle energy is a manual technique that involves the voluntary contraction of a muscle in a precisely controlled direction, at varying levels of intensity, against a distinct counterforce" applied by the clinician. Muscle energy technique uses the muscle's own energy to relax and lengthen muscles through autogenic or reciprocal inhibition.[124, 125] If a submaximal muscle contraction is followed by stretching that same muscle, it is autogenic inhibition MET; if a submaximal muscle contraction is followed by stretching of that muscle's antagonist, it is reciprocal inhibition MET.[125] Muscle energy technique differs from proprioceptive neuromuscular facilitation (PNF) techniques in that the isometric contraction is performed at lower forces compared to PNF.

Muscle Energy Theory

Muscle energy theory is based on the premise that joint malalignments occur when the body becomes unbalanced.[123] Malalignment may be the result of a muscle spasm, a weakened muscle overpowered by a stronger muscle, or restricted joint mobility. The muscle contraction used to correct a malalignment is usually a gentle submaximal isometric contraction. The patient controls the magnitude of contraction, and the clinician positions the patient and provides the resistance to change the treated joint's alignment.

In malalignments, movement is restricted by what Mitchell identifies as a barrier.[126] A **barrier** is not the end of the existing range of motion but a resistance that is felt when a part is moved through its passive range of motion. For example, you can passively move the lower limb of a patient with a tight hamstring in a straight-leg raise. Although the hip may be able to go through its full motion, you will feel a resistance because of tightness in the hamstring at some point before reaching the end of the motion. Where in the motion this resistance is felt depends on how tight the hamstring is.

Briefly reviewing principles of muscle physiology can help you understand how METs work. When the patient contracts a muscle against an external resistance, the contracting muscle causes a neurological response in other muscles.[127] Specifically, the contracting muscle causes relaxation of the antagonist and contraction of synergists through the responses of Golgi tendon organs (GTOs) and muscle spindles via spinal cord and higher center reflexes. The contraction of the agonist reciprocally inhibits its antagonist, allowing the antagonist muscle to relax and lengthen. This relaxation is thought to occur because the isometric contraction creates a latency period when the muscle is relaxed and cannot contract.[128] This relaxation period stimulates the GTO so the muscle's tone decreases, allowing the muscle to stretch to its new length.[129] Repeated contractions combined with passive stretches then provide additional gains in motion and improved muscle balance. For example, if the hamstring is found to be overactive and tight, passively take the hamstrings to the barrier point in a straight-leg raise stretch and then provide a counterforce against a submaximal isometric rectus femoris contraction. Through reciprocal inhibition, the hamstrings will relax, and you will be able to stretch the muscle to a new length.

On the other hand, when a muscle sustains a contraction through autogenic inhibition, tension in the muscle activates the GTO, which responds by inhibiting the contraction. If we use the same example as above, passively take the hamstrings to the barrier point and then provide a counterforce against a submaximal isometric hamstring contraction. Through autogenic inhibition, the hamstrings will relax, allowing you to stretch the muscle to its new length.

It is believed that these submaximal muscle contractions and changes in muscle length also affect the surrounding fascia and connective tissue.[123] Since muscle energy is an active technique, requiring the active participation of the patient, muscle physiology is affected, and it may sometimes result in postexercise soreness secondary to metabolic waste buildup and a change in the muscle's fascial length.[123] You should warn the patient that muscle soreness may occur, and in order to minimize that result you should avoid overpowering the patient or overdoing the activity. Remember, the isometric contraction used is of minimal force. Contraindications to MET include recent or nonunion fractures, significant joint disease, or recent surgery.[130]

Components of Muscle Energy Technique

Muscle energy techniques require several factors to be successful: an accurate determination of the cause and best treatment of the malalignment, a specific joint position, a precise active muscle contraction performed by the patient, an appropriate counterforce produced by the rehabilitation clinician, and an applied stretch force that results in increased motion without pain.[123]

Before you can determine the appropriate MET to apply, you must determine through an examination the presence of a malalignment and the cause of the malalignment. Once you determine that muscle energy can help to correct the patient's deficiency, you must determine the most effective position and technique to use. The injured segment is then positioned at the end of the barrier, and the patient is instructed in the amount, duration, and direction of the isometric force. While the patient actively contracts the muscle, you apply the appropriate resistive counterforce with the correct direction, duration, and magnitude.

Isometric contractions are used for muscle energy techniques. The isometric output is only about 57 g (2 oz) of force.[123] The isometric contraction is not strong, but it should be sustained for 5 to 10 s, and the muscle's length should not change while contracting.[123]

> ## CLINICAL TIPS
>
> Muscle energy techniques are used to treat joint malalignment. These techniques involve the precise and controlled voluntary contraction of a muscle against a counterforce provided by the rehabilitation clinician, followed by relaxation and then a passive stretch until a new barrier to motion is reached.

After the isometric contraction, it is important for you to allow the muscle to fully relax before you stretch the segment to a new barrier position. This allows the muscle to enter its refractory period (time of relaxation) after its contraction, and it enables you to achieve optimal stretch results. There are different schools of thought about the duration of the stretch; some advocate maintaining the stretch for 30 to 60 s[124] while others recommend the stretch be held for only a few seconds before moving to the next barrier.[123] One study compared the results of MET using these two timing variables and found no significant differences between stretching for the longer time and the shorter time.[131] The technique is repeated three to five times for the best results.[123, 124] The greatest changes occur after three repetitions;[124] clinical observations indicate that there is little additional benefit to using more than five repetitions.[123]

Application

An example is included here to demonstrate how MET may be used to relieve pain. In this example, isometric contractions are used in a MET applied to a soccer player who collided with another player and suffered a direct blow to the left anterior ilium. The contusion is resolved, but she continues to complain of groin pain that goes down her left leg. The physician has ruled out a disc injury and reports to you that the problem may be coming from her pelvis. You prepare to evaluate and treat the patient's injury:

1. *Assessment of the Problem.* Your examination reveals that the left ilium has rotated inward on its vertical axis (inflare). Other tests for lumbar dysfunction have ruled out injury to the low back. You determine that MET would be an appropriate treatment.

2. *Specific Joint Position.* With the patient lying supine, the left lower extremity is placed in a figure-4 position with the left knee flexed, the hip abducted, flexed, and rotated so the outside of the ankle is placed on the distal right thigh. Stabilize the patient's pelvis by placing your right hand on the right anterior superior iliac spine and the left hand on the patient's medial left knee. Then apply enough pressure on the knee to move the left hip to its end position of lateral rotation, the barrier point.

3. *Precise Active Contraction by the Patient.* Ask the patient to submaximally contract isometrically in an attempt to move the thigh into medial rotation, pulling the knee toward the right shoulder as you provide resistance to prevent the motion from occurring. The isometric contraction is held for 5 to 10 s.

4. *Appropriate Counterforce.* The amount of resistance applied by the patient is not great: 57 g (2 oz) of resistance. Since the contraction is isometric, you must instruct the patient to match your force and not overpower the resistance you provide (figure 11.28).

5. *Stretch Force.* Instruct the patient to relax while you support the extremity at its end position, wait to feel the muscles fully relax, and then apply a stretch into lateral rotation and abduction by pushing the left knee toward the table to the new barrier. The process is repeated three to five times. After the final repetition, passively return the leg into hip and knee extension. Reexamine for sacroiliac alignment and pain level. In this example, autogenic inhibition MET has been used.

Most muscle energy techniques must be accompanied by exercise to effectively treat the problem. You must understand the mechanics of the change that occurs with MET to correctly use the accompanying active stretches.

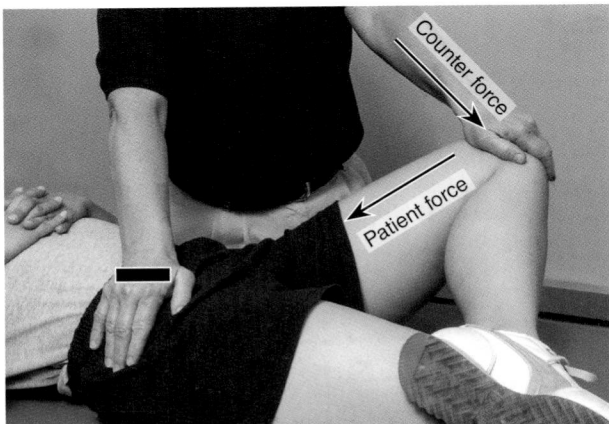

Figure 11.28 Muscle energy technique to correct left ilium inflare. Patient is isometrically moving the left hip into medial rotation while the clinician is providing a counterforce.

For example, you could instruct the soccer player with the iliac dysfunction to perform a stretch on her own that is similar to the position used in the treatment. The patient must also progress to strengthening exercises that support the stretching exercises, such as hip lateral rotation and hip abductor strengthening exercises.

Except for the general concepts introduced here, muscle energy is not used in this text except as it applies to the spine and sacroiliac joint. Therefore, muscle energy is addressed again in chapter 17. Specific techniques, including examination, assessment, and application of MET, are introduced as part of the spine and sacroiliac treatment regimen.

Proprioceptive Neuromuscular Facilitation

Proprioceptive neuromuscular facilitation (PNF) is both a manual technique and an exercise technique used to make gains in either motion or strength. Although the technique was originally designed for use in the rehabilitation of neurologic pathologies, over the years it has expanded into the orthopedic arena. Sherrington, a neurophysiologist, provided the basic concepts that were used and expanded upon by Herman Kabat, MD, during the late 1940s and early 1950s to develop PNF exercise techniques.[132] Since PNF was added to orthopedic treatment procedures, it has proven useful in restoring flexibility, strength, and coordination to injured muscles and joints.[128, 133-136]

Facilitation and Principles of Application

Proprioceptive neuromuscular facilitation incorporates impulses from the afferent receptors of skin, muscle, tendon, visual, and auditory neurons to facilitate a response from motor neurons, which produce desired actions.[137] How these receptors are stimulated to produce the actions is summarized in table 11.3.

Knott and Voss[132] and Voss, Ionta, and Myers[137] have presented several principles for maximizing the facilitation of these receptors:

1. *The clinician's hand placement is important for providing appropriate facilitation of the deep-touch and pressure receptors.* The hands are placed on the surface side toward which the extremity is to move to stimulate those muscles.[138] For example, if the patient's hip is moving into extension with the knee flexing and the ankle plantar flexing, the hamstrings and plantar foot should be the points where the clinician places his or her hands. To see the significance of this, you can perform a simple test. With a person lying supine, place one hand on the hamstrings and one hand on the quadriceps. Ask the person to maximally resist you in a straight-leg raise, and judge the amount of resistance the person provides. Now place your hands only on the quadriceps and have the person repeat the movement. You should have greater resistance when both of your hands are on the quadriceps surface and less resistance with one hand on the hamstrings and one on the quadriceps. With tactile input to both surfaces, the afferent stimulation is mixed, producing both facilitation and inhibition of the anterior muscles. When both hands are on the correct surface, optimal facilitation occurs.

Manual contact using appropriately applied pressure also helps guide the patient's extremity in the correct direction. The contact is firm and reassuring, not painful or hesitant.

2. *Verbal cues are given in a moderate tone if the patient is providing a maximal output.* If additional force is desired, a stronger, sharper verbal command is given.[139] Verbal cueing and guidance from the clinician during the activity stimulate the patient's auditory receptors to send messages to increase or decrease muscle activity.[137] The wording should be one- or two-word phrases, simple and meaningful. "Push!" or "pull!" "hold" or "relax," and "rotate" or "across" are all simple commands that give

TABLE 11.3 Applications for Optimal Recruitment During Proprioceptive Neuromuscular Facilitation

Application	Afferent facilitation	Resulting effect
Hand placement	Tactile stimulation	Gate control theory: pain reduction by increased beta afferent facilitation
Visual observation of action	Visual stimulation	Optimized correct motion sequence
Brief verbal cues	Auditory stimulation	Increased muscle response
Practicing the motion passively	Proprioceptive stimulation	Optimized normal motion sequence
Joint compression and distraction	Increases proprioceptive input	Increased muscle response
Quick stretch at start of motion	Facilitates GTOs and muscle spindles	Increased muscle response

the patient clear instructions. The commands are timed correctly with the activity.

Verbal input is used often in athletic events. It's used when cheering a team or player during competition. To get a patient to perform an exercise at a maximal output, verbal cues encourage him or her to do the most work possible. Verbal cues in PNF provide the same stimulus. They are also needed to help the patient to correctly perform the desired activity. Cueing with brief, well-timed words and phrases facilitates an improved muscle response.

3. *The technique should not be painful.* Pain will produce a reflex withdrawal and cause an inhibition rather than a facilitation of activity.[140]

4. *Proper instruction in the PNF pattern before the start of exercise is important if the muscles are to receive optimal facilitation.* The patient should receive simple instructions that include the sequencing of activities, the diagonal pattern, and appropriate speed of activity.[141] If the patient understands the exercise and knows what is expected beforehand, he or she will be better able to perform the activity and elicit an accurate response from the muscle. Being able to see the movement before performing the exercise provides additional valuable feedback.[142]

Taking the patient's limb passively through the activity before performing the exercise gives the patient visual and proprioceptive feedback about the desired direction and pattern of movement. If you do not do this before the exercise, you will find not only that the patient is confused about what to do but also that the output of the muscle is significantly less. The more confidence the patient has about being able to perform the pattern correctly, the stronger the motion will be.

5. *Providing traction to separate the joint surfaces and approximation to compress the joint surfaces stimulates the joint's proprioceptive nerve endings to ultimately improve muscle response.*[143] As a rule, traction occurs with pulling motions and approximation occurs with pushing motions. If a joint is very irritable, traction or approximation may aggravate it; the clinician must use caution and good judgment before applying joint compression or distraction.

6. *A quick stretch applied immediately before the beginning of the movement pattern uses the stretch reflex to help the muscle to produce a stronger initial response.*[144] A quick stretch stimulates the muscle spindles and Golgi tendon organs.[144] This causes increased response from the muscle. A stretch may be contraindicated with some injuries. Once again, caution and good judgment are needed before a quick stretch is applied.

7. *Rotation is an important component of the diagonal motion.* It begins distally and progresses toward the proximal muscle groups as the patient continues through the motion. Rotation begins the pattern, and by mid-ROM the rotation movement should be finished.[132]

8. *The motions are performed precisely and through a smooth range of motion.*[132] The movement is not jerky. Isometric contractions should build until maximal output from the patient's muscle is achieved. No motion is produced during an isometric activity, and the rehabilitation clinician does not break the isometric hold. Smooth and controlled movement during isotonic motion is comfortable, so optimal participation of the desired muscles results. Jerky or erratic movement creates inefficiency of motion and is not as effective as smooth, full motion.

9. *The clinician must use good body mechanics.* The application of manual resistance in PNF techniques requires the rehabilitation clinician to use his or her own body efficiently and safely and to conserve energy. Proper body mechanics makes this possible.

Patterns of Movement

The premise underlying PNF is that central nervous system stimulation produces mass movement patterns, not straight-plane movements.[145] Natural motion does not occur in straight planes but in mass movement patterns that incorporate a diagonal motion in combination with a spiral movement.[145] In other words, all major parts of the body move in functional patterns that have three component motions. These diagonal patterns include the motions of flexion and extension. Because the patterns are diagonal, they also include motions either toward and across the midline (adduction) or away from and across the midline (abduction). Rotation is the third motion involved in PNF patterns. Figure 11.29 demonstrates these components. Although PNF can be used for the trunk as well as the extremities, discussion of PNF here is limited to the upper and lower extremities, since these are the areas primarily treated with PNF in orthopedic and sport-related rehabilitation.

The movement patterns are referred to as D1 (diagonal 1) and D2 (diagonal 2). Since flexion and extension are the great motions, they are the anchor terms used in referring to these D1 and D2 patterns. D1 and D2 flexion patterns start in the extended position and move into flexion through

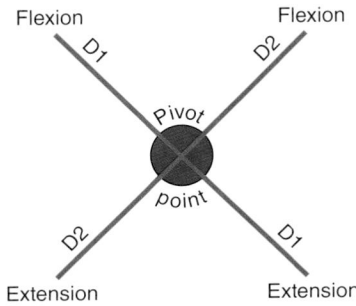

Figure 11.29 PNF patterns: Neural facilitation of motion causes movement to occur in diagonal planes of component motions, not straight-plane motions.

their diagonal patterns. D1 and D2 extension patterns start at end-flexion positions and move through the range of motion to their end-extension positions. Therefore, D1 and D2 flexion and extension patterns are named for the primary direction into which the limb is moving.

How the triplanar motions are combined into their movement patterns is easier to remember if you realize that in the upper extremity, lateral rotation always goes with flexion, and in the lower extremity, lateral rotation always goes with adduction. For example, when the shoulder starts in extension and moves to the end of its flexion motion, it always starts with medial rotation and ends with lateral rotation whether the third accompanying movement is adduction or abduction (figure 11.30a and b). Likewise, when the extremity moves into extension, the shoulder starts in flexion with lateral rotation and moves into extension with medial rotation, and the varying motion is abduction in the D1 pattern or adduction in the D2 pattern.

Because lateral rotation and adduction move together in the lower extremity, the varying motions are flexion and extension. Therefore, when the hip moves into flexion and adduction in the D1 pattern, the rotational movement is

lateral. When it moves into flexion in the D2 pattern, abduction and medial rotation are the accompanying motions (figure 11.30c and d). In the D1 extension pattern, the hip moves into extension with medial rotation and abduction. In the D2 extension pattern, the hip moves into extension with lateral rotation and adduction.

These are natural patterns that you see every day in sport and daily activities. For example, when you throw a ball overhand, the shoulder starts in abduction, flexion, and lateral rotation (D2 flexion position). When the ball is thrown, the follow-through ends with the shoulder in extension, adduction, and medial rotation (D2 extension position). Kicking a soccer ball also demonstrates the PNF pattern: As the ball is kicked, the limb moves from extension, abduction, and medial rotation (D1 extension position) to the follow-through position of flexion, adduction, and lateral rotation (D1 flexion position). When you sit in a relaxed position with your feet up and hands behind your head, the shoulder is in flexion, abduction, and lateral rotation (D2 flexion), and your lower extremities are extended in front of you, crossed, in adduction and lateral rotation (D2 extension).

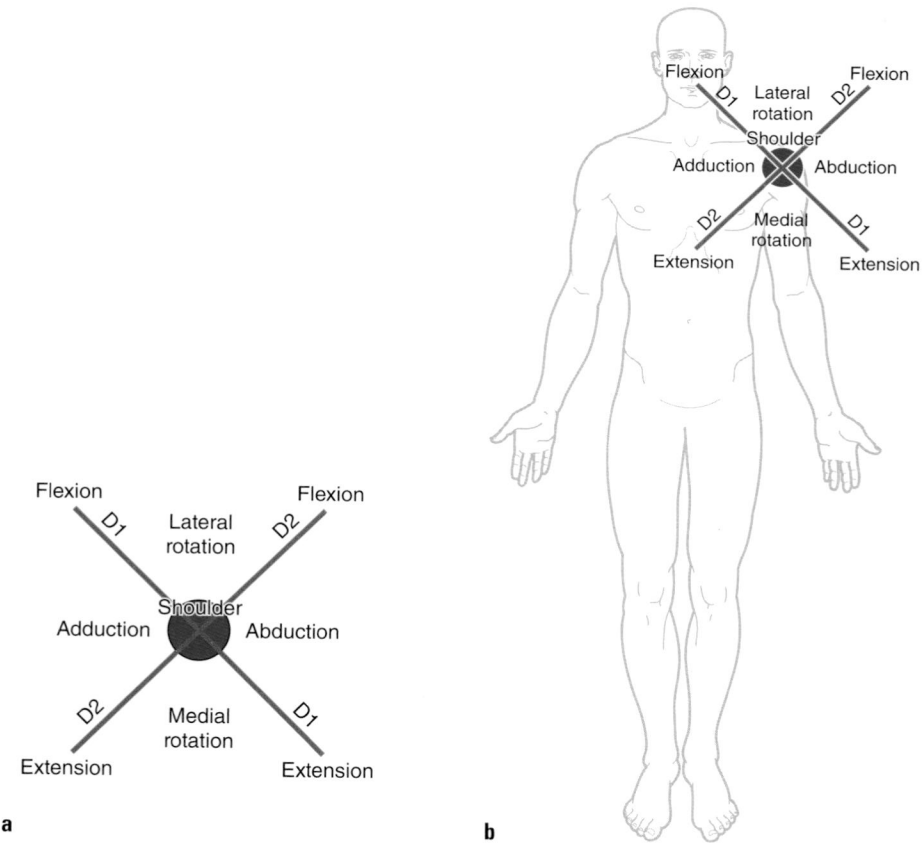

a

b

Figure 11.30 *(a)* Lateral rotation is associated with flexion, while medial rotation is associated with extension in the upper extremities. *(b)* Shoulder PNF patterns D1 and D2. *(c)* In the lower extremities, adduction and lateral rotation occur together, and abduction and medial rotation occur together. *(d)* Hip PNF patterns D1 and D2.

Chapter 11 • Manual Therapy   **323**

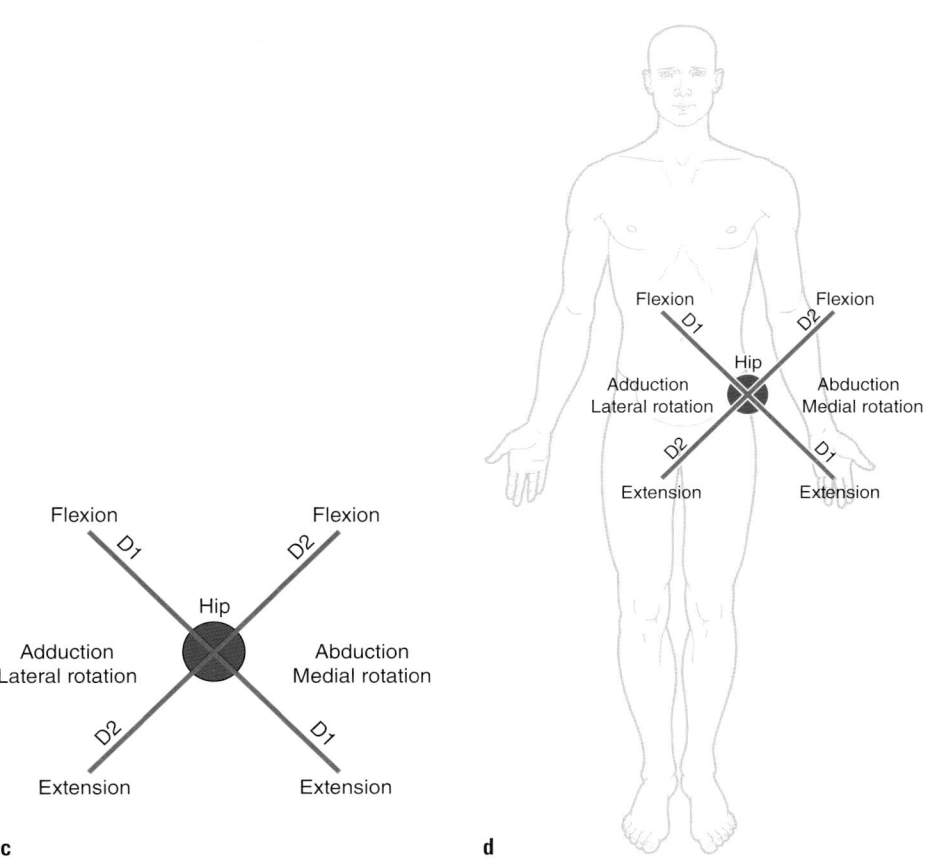

Figure 11.30 >*continued*

If you remember these natural positions, the patterns of movement for the segment of the extremity beyond the shoulder and hip should make sense. Figures 11.31 and 11.32 illustrate the positions of the other joints in D1 and D2 patterns.

In each pattern, the joints go from one extreme pattern position to the other by the time the full range of motion is completed. For example, if the patient begins in D1 extension with the shoulder extended, abducted, and medially rotated, the elbow extended, the forearm pronated, the wrist ulnarly extended, and the fingers and thumb extended, the end position will be the D1 flexion position—in shoulder flexion, adduction, and lateral rotation; elbow flexion; forearm supination; radial flexion of the wrist; and flexion and adduction of the fingers and thumb. Note that the elbow and the knee can be moved from flexion to extension or extension to flexion with any of the patterns. The position of the elbow or knee at the end of the pattern is the opposite of the joint's position at the beginning of the movement.

Remember that motion begins at the proximal joint and progresses distally. Rotation starts at the beginning of movement and is completed by the time the extremity is halfway through its full range of motion. For example, when performing a PNF D2 extension pattern on an upper

extremity, by the time the shoulder is halfway through extension and adduction, shoulder rotation is completed.

Essentially, all that has been written about PNF in recent years has been based on the works of Knott and Voss.[132] The patterns of movement, techniques, and principles most commonly used today center on the information these authors provided to the health care community. For the best results, they advocate the use of the principles presented here.

Terminology

Proprioceptive neuromuscular facilitation techniques can be confusing if you do not understand the terminology. The most common problem is confusing the agonist and the antagonist for a movement. The terms are used relative to the motion that occurs. The *agonistic muscle pattern* occurs when the muscle is contracting toward its shortened state. The *antagonistic muscle pattern* occurs when the muscle is approaching its lengthened state. The antagonistic pattern of motion is diagonally opposite to the agonistic pattern.

For example, if the lower extremity moves into hip flexion, flexion is the agonistic pattern, so the agonists are the hip flexors and quadriceps, and the antagonists are the

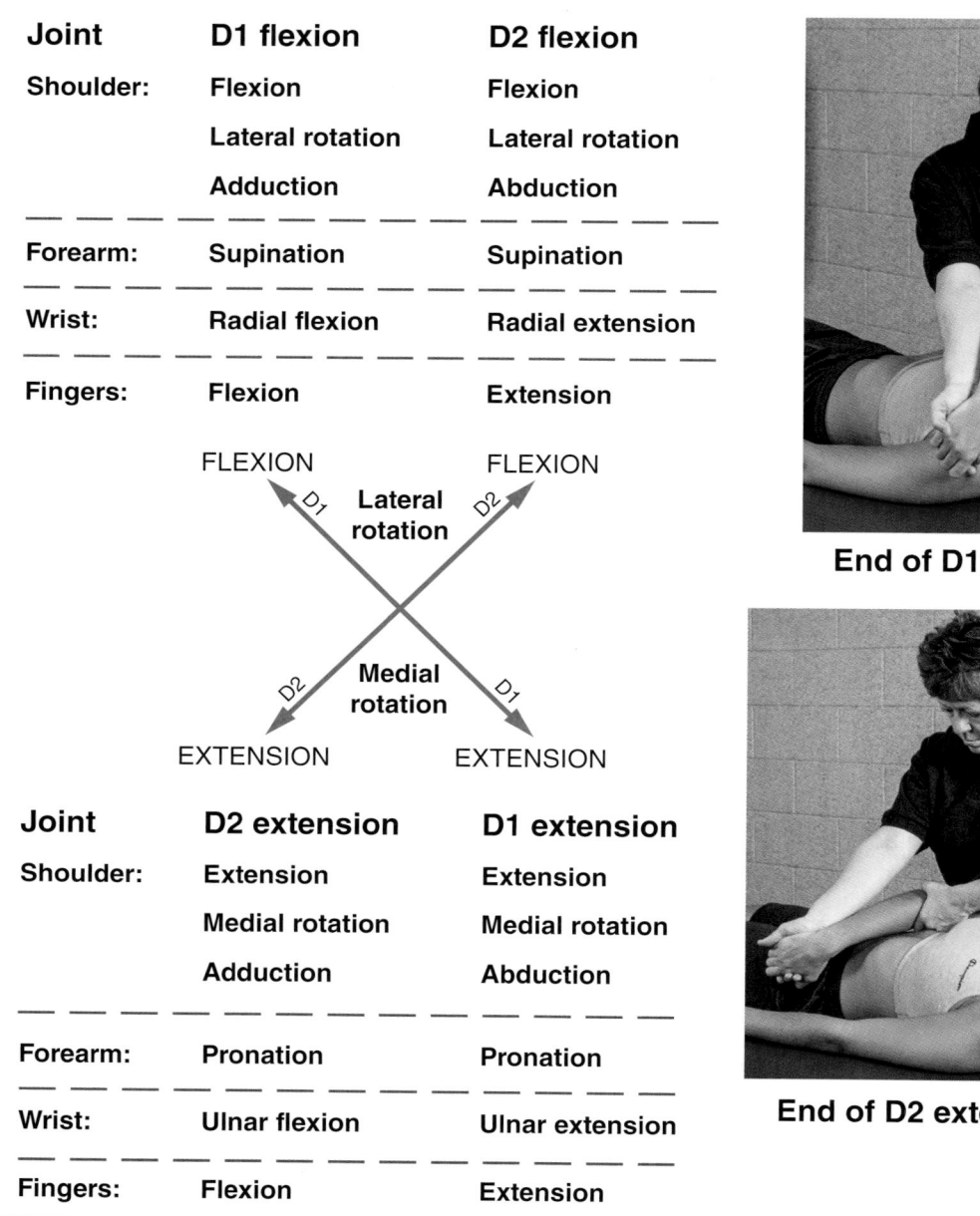

Joint	D1 flexion	D2 flexion
Shoulder:	Flexion	Flexion
	Lateral rotation	Lateral rotation
	Adduction	Abduction
Forearm:	Supination	Supination
Wrist:	Radial flexion	Radial extension
Fingers:	Flexion	Extension

FLEXION   FLEXION

D1   Lateral rotation   D2

Medial rotation

D2   D1

EXTENSION   EXTENSION

Joint	D2 extension	D1 extension
Shoulder:	Extension	Extension
	Medial rotation	Medial rotation
	Adduction	Abduction
Forearm:	Pronation	Pronation
Wrist:	Ulnar flexion	Ulnar extension
Fingers:	Flexion	Extension

End of D1 flexion pattern

End of D2 extension pattern

Figure 11.31 Upper-extremity PNF patterns.

gluteus maximus and hamstrings. Therefore, if a stretch using a hold–relax technique is used to increase hamstring flexibility, the terminology used properly would be this: "The limb is moved to the end range of the agonist (hip flexion, knee extension) pattern, then a maximal isometric contraction of the antagonist (hamstrings) occurs, followed by complete relaxation of the antagonist (hamstrings). The extremity is then moved to the new end range in the agonist (hip flexion, knee extension) pattern." Because the limb is moving to shorten the quadriceps, hip flexion is the agonist pattern, and the hamstrings are the antagonist muscles.

Stretching Techniques

As previously mentioned, PNF can be used to make gains in either flexibility or strength. Whether a PNF technique is used to gain mobility or strength, the principles and movement patterns presented previously hold true. The specific PNF stretching techniques include *hold–relax, contract–relax,* and *slow reversal–hold–relax* (figure 11.33). Regardless of the specific technique used, bouts are repeated until no apparent flexibility or muscle length gains are observed. All three of these PNF stretch techniques are

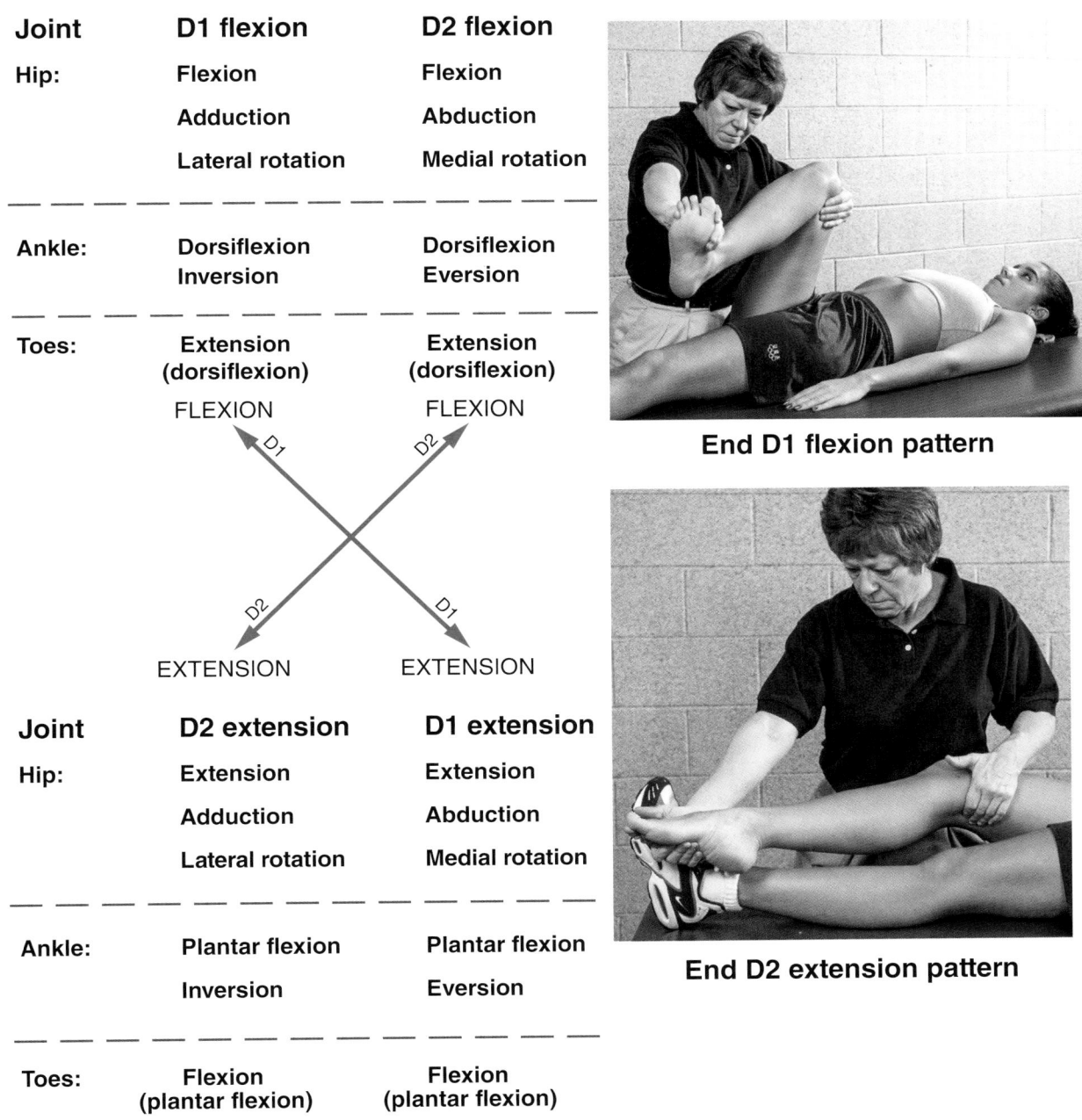

Joint	D1 flexion	D2 flexion
Hip:	Flexion	Flexion
	Adduction	Abduction
	Lateral rotation	Medial rotation
Ankle:	Dorsiflexion	Dorsiflexion
	Inversion	Eversion
Toes:	Extension (dorsiflexion)	Extension (dorsiflexion)

FLEXION ... FLEXION

D1 ... D2

D2 ... D1

EXTENSION ... EXTENSION

End D1 flexion pattern

Joint	D2 extension	D1 extension
Hip:	Extension	Extension
	Adduction	Abduction
	Lateral rotation	Medial rotation
Ankle:	Plantar flexion	Plantar flexion
	Inversion	Eversion
Toes:	Flexion (plantar flexion)	Flexion (plantar flexion)

End D2 extension pattern

Figure 11.32 Lower-extremity PNF patterns.

useful when the primary factor that restricts full motion is insufficient length of the antagonist, because of either muscle spasm or muscle inflexibility. The sidebar PNF Techniques for Gaining Flexibility summarizes the three PNF techniques for improving flexibility.

How motion gains are made using PNF remains a point of discussion among investigators. It has been thought that greater motion occurs with both the hold–relax and the contract–relax techniques through the activity of the GTOs, causing relaxation of the muscle to provide increased motion gains, but this may not be the case; there is enough evidence to indicate that other theories may provide additional rationales for these gains, but there is no conclusive evidence for any of these theories.[128, 144] These theories include four physiologically based mechanisms: (1) Autogenic inhibition occurs when GTOs send an inhibitory stimulus because the muscle either contracts or is stretched;[128] (2) reciprocal inhibition, as mentioned earlier,

PNF Techniques for Gaining Flexibility

Isometric contractions are maximally held 6 to 10 s; relaxation occurs for 2 to 3 s; all concentric contractions are smooth and against resistance.[132, 137]

- **Hold–Relax.** An extremity is brought to end motion in agonist pattern, isometric contraction of restricted muscle (antagonist), relax, passive motion to new end range in agonist pattern (to stretch restricted muscle).
- **Contract–Relax.** Extremity is brought to end motion of agonist, isotonic contraction of antagonist (restricted muscle), relax, passive movement to end range in agonist pattern (to stretch restricted muscle).
- **Slow Reversal–Hold–Relax.** Limb starts in the shortened position of the agonist (opposing muscle). The antagonist (restricted muscle) contracts concentrically to move to its shortened position (bringing restricted muscle to its end shortened range), isometric contraction of restricted muscle, relax, stretch by unopposed concentric contraction of agonist (opposing) muscle.

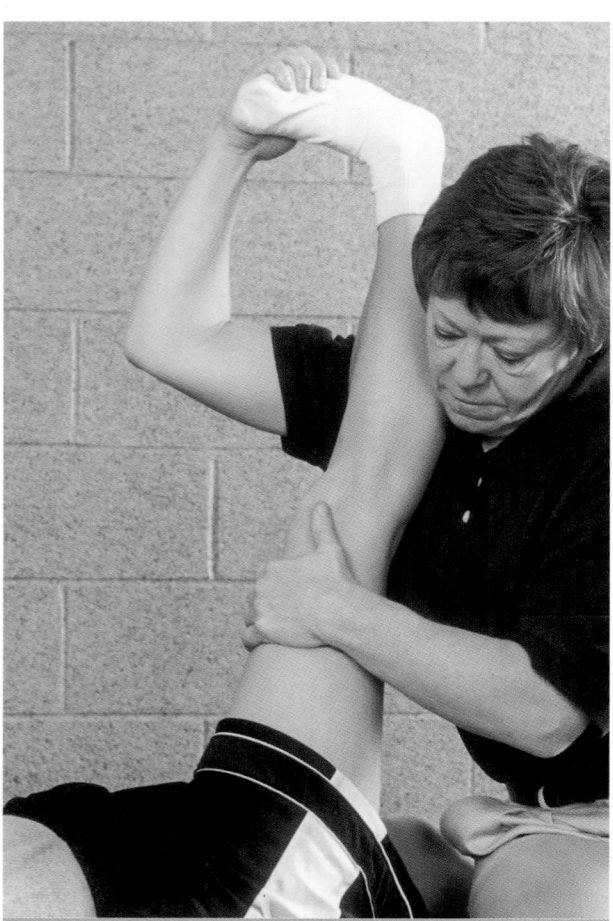

Figure 11.33 PNF stretching uses techniques of hold–relax, contract–relax, and slow reversal–hold–relax.

occurs when a muscle's opposing muscle contracts;[146] (3) stress relaxation occurs when a musculotendinous unit is under constant stretch, so its viscoelastic properties succumb to creep;[128] and (4) the gate control theory of pain triggers when noxious and non-noxious stimuli compete for the same afferent nerve connection, but repeated noxious stretch stimuli allow adaptation to the stress, so pain reception decreases over time.[128, 146] It may be that PNF improves flexibility through more than one of these mechanisms.

Although true PNF techniques incorporate three planes of motion, many clinicians using PNF stretching techniques with orthopedic patients fail to incorporate all three planes. Some clinicians limit movement to only the flexion–extension plane of motion.[147] Clinicians may, for example, use the hold–relax stretching technique but apply it only to hamstrings. This is not truly PNF but a grossly modified version of it.

Hold–Relax

The *hold–relax* technique uses an isometric contraction of the tight muscle to relax it before it is moved to its new stretch position.[148] In other words, an extremity is passively moved through an agonist pattern to its end position; at that point, an isometric contraction of the antagonist (restricted) muscle is held, then the muscle relaxes before the limb is passively moved to the new end position in the agonist pattern. Using a specific example, if the hamstrings are being stretched, the limb is passively moved through the flexion pattern to the end-motion position. In this position, the hamstrings contract isometrically for about 6 to 10 s, after which they relax completely. Once they are relaxed within about 2 to 3 s, the limb is passively moved into its greater flexion range until the new end-motion position is reached. This process is repeated until additional gains in motion do not occur.

This technique is used to relax muscle spasm and increase motion. For example, if a biceps brachii is in spasm and limits elbow extension, the hold–relax technique can be used to facilitate biceps relaxation. To begin the technique, the shoulder, elbow, and forearm are passively moved to their end range in shoulder and elbow extension and forearm pronation, and then the biceps performs an isometric contraction with a simultaneous maximum effort by the biceps against shoulder and elbow flexion and forearm supination resistance for about 6 to 10 s. The patient then relaxes the biceps, and the elbow, shoulder, and forearm are passively moved into greater end-motion positions. This process is repeated four or five times or until the desired results are achieved.

Contract–Relax

The *contract–relax* technique is another option for patients who have limited range of motion. In this technique, the limb is passively moved through its agonist pattern to its end-range position. The antagonist (restricted) muscles then perform a maximal isotonic contraction, moving the limb against resistance throughout the range of motion to the start of the agonist pattern. Once the antagonist muscles relax, the limb is passively moved to the end range of the agonist pattern. Bouts are once again repeated until additional motion does not occur. If we continue with the hamstrings as the specific example, the patient's lower extremity is passively moved through a flexion pattern (either D1 or D2) with knee extension and hip flexion in a hip flexion agonist pattern. At the end of the agonist motion, the clinician provides maximum isotonic resistance against the antagonist muscles (hamstrings and hip extensors) as the limb moves through the D1 or D2 extension pattern. When the patient relaxes the muscles, the clinician moves the limb passively into the agonist muscle pattern to stretch the antagonist (hamstrings). Again, this process is repeated four or five times or until the desired results are achieved.

Slow Reversal–Hold–Relax

In the *slow reversal–hold–relax* technique, the limb is positioned at the end-motion position of the agonist. The (restricted) antagonist then provides a concentric contraction to move the limb against resistance to the antagonist's end position. At this end-range position, the antagonist isometrically contracts maximally for 6 to 10 s. This maximal contraction is followed by a 2 to 3 s relaxation, and then the agonist muscles concentrically contract to actively move the limb to the start position (agonist's end position). As with the other techniques, this one is also repeated. Continuing to use the hamstrings as our example, the patient's limb is passively moved to the end of either the D1 or D2 flexion pattern. The patient then contracts the hamstrings concentrically to move through either the D1 or D2 extension pattern; once at the end of this motion, the patient performs a maximal isometric contraction of the hamstrings for 6 to 10 s. The clinician then tells the patient to relax completely, and once this occurs, the patient actively moves the limb through the D1 or D2 flexion pattern to its new end position by contracting the quadriceps and hip flexors.

Various investigations have compared the types of short-term passive, active, and combination stretching procedures. Many investigators conclude that PNF stretches are more effective than other active or short-term passive stretches.[135, 146, 149-152] Others conclude that the three stretching techniques are essentially no different from one another in providing flexibility gains.[153-156]

Strengthening Techniques

As previously mentioned, PNF can be used for muscle strengthening as well as for improving flexibility. Although the goal may change, patterns of motion and basic facilitation techniques of PNF remain the same; how those patterns and applications are applied is the only thing that changes. The D1 and D2 flexion and extension patterns are the same for both stretching and strengthening. Performing the D1 and D2 patterns throughout the full range of motion in all three planes of movement, with the motion initiated at the proximal joint and rotation ending halfway through the pattern, is also the same for both stretching and strengthening. Of course, the basic facilitation methods presented in table 11.3 are also important to remember for strengthening techniques. There are four primary PNF strengthening techniques for both the lower and the upper extremities: *repeated contractions*, *rhythmic stabilization*, *slow reversal*, and *slow reversal–hold*.

CLINICAL TIPS

PNF terminology can be confusing. If you keep in mind the example of strengthening the quadriceps, it may be easier to remember. Using this example, since the extremity moves into a straight-leg raise, this is the agonistic muscle pattern, so the quadriceps and hip flexors move to their shortest position (straight-leg raise); in this position, the hamstrings are the antagonistic muscles. If the PNF pattern moves the extremity in the antagonistic pattern, the extremity moves into hip extension and knee flexion.

Repeated contractions is a technique where the clinician provides a quick stretch at a weak point in the muscle pattern followed by a resistive isotonic contraction of the agonist. The quick stretch stimulates the muscle spindle of the agonist, facilitating a stronger contraction.157 Repeated contractions are used to facilitate a specific muscle group that is weak or fatigued within the D1 and D2 patterns. Repeated contractions can be used at multiple points within the diagonal pattern. Points to remember when using this technique include the following:

1. The quick stretch of the agonist may occur at any position within the range of motion.
2. There is no pause between the quick stretch and subsequent isotonic contraction of the agonist.
3. This technique can be repeated multiple times within the pattern.

4. Include all three planes of motion when providing isotonic resistance.

Rhythmic stabilization uses isometric activity of the agonists and antagonists. The rehabilitation clinician offers resistance that does not break the isometric activity of the antagonist and then immediately offers resistance to the isometric activity of the agonist. This produces a co-contraction to improve stabilization. The technique is repeated several times without movement of the extremity, with no pause between the contractions. It can be repeated at several points within the range of motion. Isometric contractions are first performed in an antagonistic pattern and then in an agonistic pattern to facilitate a reversal of antagonists, thereby promoting improved muscle response.[158] Rhythmic stabilization is most often used early in a rehabilitation program when the muscles are very weak, motion is limited, or muscular effort is restricted. Points to remember with this technique include the following:

1. There is no pause between contractions of the agonist and antagonist.

2. The isometric contraction does not have to be maximal.

3. The contraction occurs first in the antagonist pattern, then in the agonist pattern.

4. Include all three planes of motion when providing resistance in both agonist and antagonist patterns.

5. The isometric resistance may occur at any position within the extremity's range of motion.

Slow reversal is a technique whereby the clinician provides resistance starting at the end of an agonist position.

Using either a D1 or a D2 pattern, resistance is provided as the extremity moves through the antagonist pattern. This motion is immediately followed by resistance through the agonist pattern of motion to return to the start position. Facilitation of the agonist is increased with a maximal resistance against its antagonist first.[132] For example, if the hamstrings (agonist) are the weak muscle group, the clinician applies resistance to the lower extremity D2 pattern going into hip flexion–abduction–medial rotation (antagonistic pattern). At the completion of the antagonistic movement pattern, the rehabilitation clinician reverses hand positions on the patient's lower extremity to provide resistance to D2 going into hip extension–adduction–lateral rotation moving into an agonistic pattern. In this case, the knee is extended with hip flexion and flexed with hip extension. Points to remember when using this technique include the following:

1. Begin at the end range of the agonist pattern in either D1 or D2 and resist throughout the antagonist pattern first.

2. Immediately follow this pattern by providing resistance throughout the agonist pattern to the position where the first resistance movement started.

3. All three planes of motion occur as the extremity moves through the pattern's range of motion.

4. Motion begins proximally, and rotation is completed by the time the extremity reaches mid-flexion or mid-extension positions in its range of motion.

The *slow reversal–hold* technique is the same as the *slow reversal* except that an isometric hold is performed

PNF Techniques for Gaining Strength

- *Repeated Contractions.* At any weak or fatigued point within the D1 or D2 pattern, a quick stretch is applied to the agonist immediately followed by isotonic contraction of the agonist in the continued diagonal pattern. There is no pause between the quick stretch and the isotonic contraction of the agonist. The technique can be repeated throughout the diagonal pattern.

- *Rhythmic Stabilization.* An extremity is positioned within a D1 or D2 pattern of motion. Antagonist muscle contracts isometrically against clinician-provided resistance and is instantly reversed with isometric contraction of the agonist to cause a co-contraction of agonist and antagonist. There is no pause between antagonist and agonist isometric contractions.

- *Slow Reversal.* Starting at the end position of an agonist pattern in either D1 or D2, the extremity moves via concentric contraction of antagonists through the ROM against resistance provided by the clinician. Once the motion is completed, the extremity is resisted concentrically as it immediately moves through the agonist pattern.

- *Slow Reversal–Hold.* As in the slow reversal, the extremity starts at the end position of an agonist pattern in either D1 or D2 and is resisted by the clinician as it moves concentrically into the antagonist pattern to the end of motion. A 6 to 10 s isometric contraction is provided at the end motion before the agonist muscles are resisted concentrically as the extremity returns to the starting position. An isometric hold can also be provided at any weak point within the pattern.

at the end of the motion or at any weak point within the pattern. All other elements of the techniques are the same. Using the isometric hold may facilitate additional strength output.[159] Since these two techniques are essentially the same with the exception of the addition of the isometric in the slow reversal–hold technique, the points to remember are the same. The isometric should be held for 6 to 10 s. The sidebar PNF Techniques for Gaining Strength provides a quick reference for the four PNF strengthening techniques.

Other Manual Therapies

There are many other manual therapy techniques. Three of them are briefly discussed here. The purpose here is to introduce you to manual therapies you may have heard of, not to provide you with enough information to use them adequately after reading this section. If this introductory material piques your interest, we encourage you to seek out resources and formal instruction on the techniques.

Strain–Counterstrain

Lawrence Jones, an osteopath, originated strain–counterstrain (S–CS) during the 1960s after several years of clinical application and development of techniques.[160] Strain–counterstrain was first called spontaneous release by positioning[161] and later positional release. It is an indirect soft-tissue treatment technique because the dysfunctional segment is placed in a position of ease rather than at the point of restricted movement.[162]

Theory

The goal of Dr. Jones' strain–counterstrain treatments was to relieve what he called tender points. **Tender points** are small areas of tenderness about the size of a dime or smaller that are located in subcutaneous, muscle, tendon, ligament, or fascial tissue.[163, 164] Like trigger points in Travell and Simons' descriptions,[57] they are areas of local tenderness, but unlike trigger points, they do not evoke the same referred pain, do not have a taut band, and do not produce autonomic reactions.[164] Some clinicians feel that tender points, trigger points, and acupuncture points are all similar and occur because of trauma or dysfunction.[165, 166] Each of the therapies that address these differently labeled points aims to reduce tissue tenderness and thereby improve the patient's condition.[165]

Dr. Jones theorized that myofascial tender points are created by either acute injury or body dysfunctions that occur over time and result in incorrect neural output from muscle spindles, causing pain at the tender point sites. Neuromuscular changes occur because somatic dysfunction results from either acute or chronic injuries; when a muscle is injured, its antagonist shortens or *counterstrains*.[167] When the muscle is then suddenly stretched, the muscle spindles react by further shortening the already shortened muscle. Jones hypothesized that the proprioceptors that have already reconfigured their set points because of previous muscle shortening interpret the stretch of the shortened muscle as an overstretch. These reactions produce an ongoing somatic dysfunction;[163] shortening of the muscle results in restricted joint motion, pain, and body segment dysfunction.

Treatment Principles

The patient must be assessed before a S–CS treatment application. The patient's history can reveal problems that may have caused the somatic dysfunction. Factors such as prolonged sitting in poor posture, an acute injury, or a leg length difference may be the source of dysfunction. The clinician identifies this source of somatic dysfunction and locates the tender points associated with the problem. These tender points are used to diagnose the areas of strain. They are identified as fibrotic soft tissue that is palpable and tender to pressure that would not ordinarily cause pain or discomfort.[163]

Once the tender point is located, some pressure is applied to it to monitor tenderness, and the joint is passively placed in a comfortable, shortened position where tenderness to pressure over the tender point is relieved. This position is known as a **position of comfort** and is often fine-tuned by the clinician until the patient has no

Strain–Counterstrain Treatment Steps

1. *Locate tender point.* Identify the location for treatment.
2. *Place in a position of comfort.* With light pressure on the tender point, the joint is passively positioned in flexion or extension and fine-tuned using rotation or abduction–adduction to further reduce pain until no pain is present.
3. *Position is held 90 s.* The clinician monitors the tender point while passively maintaining the position of comfort, allowing the tender point to fully relax.
4. *Joint is returned to neutral position.* Motion occurs passively and slowly to maintain relaxation of the muscle.
5. *Reassess tender point.* Decreased tenderness and evidence of the tender point should be apparent if treatment has been successful.

pain or discomfort. For example, if the clinician positions a joint in flexion, it may be necessary to abduct or rotate it slightly to further relieve the patient's pain or discomfort. Moving the pressure over the tender point slightly may also change the patient's pain. As the clinician continues to monitor the tender point, sometimes the clinician may feel the tender point pulsating; it is thought that this may be blood flow returning to the area as tissue is restored to its nonpathological status.[168]

When the segment is in a position of comfort, the affected muscle spindles relax. After the position has been passively held for about 90 s and the clinician feels the tender point relax, the joint is slowly and passively returned to a neutral position from the position of comfort. This prevents the muscle spindle reflex from recurring, so pain is relieved.[169] The tender point is then reassessed to determine whether the treatment has been successful; the tender point should be significantly less tender to palpation, and there should be a noticeable decrease in its size.[168] These treatment steps are presented in the sidebar Strain–Counterstrain Treatment Steps. Usually related to these tender points is the presence of other tender points.

Some of them may be in the local area and others may be remote from it.[163] Most tender areas are located in tissues that undergo mechanical stress, most notably those that have significant postural demands.[165] The clinician must find these tender areas and treat each of them for all pain to be relieved. Dr. Jones spent several years mapping more than 200 tender points throughout the body and identifying the positions required for easing them.[168]

The **mobile point** is the position into which the patient is passively placed and is the point of maximum tissue relaxation;[167] this is a position from which any change produces an increased tissue tension that a clinician can palpate.[162] As mentioned, fine-tuning the position of either the mobile point or the tender point pressure is sometimes required for an effective treatment. Other treatment regimens can also improve efficacy. These include identifying and treating the most sensitive tender points first; treating more proximal tender points before more distal ones; and when tender points are in rows, treating the middle ones before the peripheral ones.[169] Posterior muscles are usually treated in extension, while anterior muscles are most often treated with the joint in flexion. Tender points

Strain–Counterstrain Treatment Considerations

- *Fine-tune treatment.* This can occur either by slightly adjusting the location of the digit applying pressure over the tender point or by making minor changes in the position of comfort, including rotation or abduction–adduction adjustments to further decrease tender point pain.

- *Treat more sensitive tender points before less sensitive tender points.* This may reduce the tenderness in other tender points.

- *Treat more proximal tender points before more distal ones.* More proximal tender points may have a direct effect on more distal ones.

- *When tender points are in rows, treat the middle ones first.* More distal tender points from the center of a line of tender points may have developed secondarily to the central ones, so they may lessen or resolve when central tender points are treated first.

- *Treat posterior tender points in extension and anterior tender points in flexion.* Tender point treatment is an indirect technique, so the treatment occurs with the muscles in shortened positions.

- *Midline and near-midline tender points are treated with flexion or extension.* Those are the motions that are most restricted when tender points occur near the midline.

- *More lateral tender points are treated with lateral flexion and rotation.* Those motions are more often affected by tender points away from the midline, and they will affect the lateral tender points more than straight flexion or extension motions.

- *Extremity tender points are sometimes found on opposite sides of pain.* There could be several reasons for this, including referral from the somatic dysfunctional area, misinformation provided by a facilitated neural segment, or incorrect proprioceptive information.

- *Move the treated segment slowly and passively to its neutral position.* This prevents restimulation of inappropriate neural firing.

- *Inform patient that soreness may occur for 24 to 48 h after treatment.* New adjustments and resetting muscle length may produce some discomfort.

that are located near the midline are most often treated in either more flexion or extension, depending on whether the tender points are in anterior (flexion) or posterior (extension) muscles. Those tender points located away from the midline usually respond better with more side bending or rotation positioning. Tender points in extremities are sometimes located on the opposite side from where the pain occurs. Patients should be informed that they may feel some soreness after a treatment, but this discomfort should subside rather quickly. These considerations in strain–counterstrain treatment are listed in the sidebar Strain–Counterstrain Treatment Considerations.

As with any treatment, there are contraindications to the use of strain–counterstrain techniques. These contraindications include acute inflammations, open wounds, healing fractures, sutures in place, and recent hematoma.[167, 168] Before any application of manual therapy, explain to the patient what you intend to do and what sensations the patient should expect. It is also important to receive feedback from patients during the treatment about pain and intensity levels and how they change with changes in applications or joint positions; communication is key to a successful treatment whenever manual therapy techniques are used.

There are published research investigations of strain–counterstrain techniques and applications. Unfortunately, most of them are case studies that deal with pain reduction or range-of-motion gains in isolated subjects.[170] Although evidence is weak at this point, there seems to be enough to indicate that these techniques can produce immediate relief of pain.[171] As with other manual therapies, empirical research is difficult to find with strain–counterstrain.

It is important to note that, as with many manual therapies, strain–counterstrain is not a technique in which proficiency comes quickly. Dr. Jones did not believe a person became proficient with strain–counterstrain techniques until he or she had practiced 8 h a day for 2 years.[169]

Rolfing

Ida P. Rolf, an American with a PhD in biochemistry, lived during the first half of the 20th century (1896-1979) when women with doctorates in the sciences were rare. She developed an interest in homeopathic and alternative medicine while on a leave of absence from her work, studying mathematics and atomic physics in Switzerland. Her interest and work evolved into what she referred to as structural integration. By the mid-1900s, her treatment techniques became known worldwide. She eventually opened a school in Boulder, Colorado, the Rolf Institute; there are now five institutes around the world teaching what is now known as Rolfing. The technique intertwines Dr. Rolf's observations, knowledge, and exposure with a range of topics beyond biochemistry, including osteopathic manipulation and yoga control of body motion.

Theory

Dr. Rolf based her techniques on the realization that fascia surrounds all tissue and body structures, so it also influences those tissues and structures when it is modified. She observed that the body centers on a vertical line of pull created by gravity. It was her theory that the body is most efficient and healthy when it can function in an aligned and balanced arrangement. With gravity's continual pull, stresses and injuries occur to pull the body out of its normal alignment; imbalance occurs and causes the body to become painful, malaligned, and inefficient. Dr. Rolf's philosophy and techniques focus on improving the body's posture so that all functions, including breathing, flexibility, strength, and coordination, are optimally efficient.

Gravity and the body have a constant relationship. The body is in a constant battle with gravity, and unless the body is optimally conditioned, gravity wins. Factors such as fatigue, injury, age, and body configuration predispose the body to develop imbalances and lose its war with gravity. Dr. Rolf was a strong believer in the link between form and function. If the body is to perform its normal functions, it must have an appropriate form in which to do it.[172] The goals of Rolfing are to place the body's large anatomical segments (the head, neck, shoulders, trunk, pelvis, and legs) in line with each other relative to gravity and to integrate each of those segments with each other in both structure and function.[173] Dr. Rolf believed that integrating these segments would also improve mental, emotional, and spiritual health.[173]

She based her treatments on the notion that they needed to occur in a specific series and that once the body's structure changed, changes in other areas such as metabolism, emotion, psychology, and function would follow.[172]

Treatment Principles

The treatment techniques of **Rolfing structural integration** include 10 sessions, each one focusing on a central theme, goals, and sequence of structural interventions.[172] The 10 sessions are divided into three categories, *sleeve sessions, core sessions*, and *integrating sessions*.[174]

The goals of the treatments are to balance and realign the body in all planes. If these goals are accomplished, pain is resolved, imbalance is no longer an issue, and the body performs most efficiently. As outlined by Bernau-Eigen[173] and James and colleagues,[175] goals for each session are different and progressive; they are outlined in table 11.4.

Treatments include not only manual therapy to release fascia but also instruction in becoming aware of the proper alignment of body segments.[176]

TABLE 11.4   Rolfing Treatment Sessions and Goals

Session	Focus	Goals
Session 1	Breathing	Release the fascial layer below the skin's surface.
Session 2	Posture	Free up and reorganize fascial planes in the feet and legs.
Session 3	Spinal elongation	Reorganize the lateral alignment, using this session as a transition between superficial and deep fascial layer treatments.
Session 4	Leg stability	Release the deep fascia closest to the spine and balance the pelvis and back structures.
Session 5	Balance of the trunk over the legs	Release the deep fascia closest to the spine and balance the pelvis and back structures.
Session 6	Pelvis and lower extremity stability with improved trunk mobility	Release the deep fascia closest to the spine and balance the pelvis and back structures.
Session 7	Balance in rhythm of head movements	Balance head and neck.
Session 8	Lower-body integration	Integrative session where superficial, middle, and deep fascial layers are worked with and integrated.
Session 9	Upper-body integration	Integrative session where superficial, middle, and deep fascial layers are worked with and integrated.
Session 10	Specific correction of static and dynamic activities throughout the person	Integrative session where superficial, middle, and deep fascial layers are worked with and integrated.

Based on Bernau-Eigen (1998); James (2009). [173, 175]

- **Sleeve Sessions.** The first three of the 10 sessions are the sleeve and include, in order of sequence, sessions on respiration, balance through the legs and feet, and sagittal balance. The first session deals with breathing and muscles involved in respiration. Elements of concentration include the superficial fascial layers of the arms, diaphragm, and ribs. During the second session, treatment deals with left-to-right standing balance, concentrating on weight distribution and balance of muscle activity in the feet and legs. In other words, the patient is made aware of frontal plane balance and is guided to correct imbalances. The last of the sleeve sessions focuses on the relative position of the head, shoulder girdle, and hips in a standing position. In this session, the positions of the body's segments from a sagittal view are investigated to make the patient more aware of what is proper alignment.

- **Core Sessions.** The second group of sessions, 4 through 7, are the core sessions, and they include the base of the core (midline of the legs), abdomen (psoas for pelvic balance), and sacrum (weight transfer from head to feet) and the relationship of the head to the rest of the body (primarily the occiput–atlas relationship, then to the rest of the body).[172] The fourth session starts at the feet, focusing on the medial arches of the foot and extending awareness of position and balance up the legs and to the lower pelvis. Session 5 focuses the patient's attention on the trunk, with particular attention paid to the deeper abdominal muscles and the spinal curves. Once trunk awareness and correction of position occur, the session 6 focus is directed back to the legs, pelvis, and lumbar spine and how these are not only connected but corrected in their alignment. The final session in this group, session 7, focuses on the head and neck, providing guidance in their proper alignment with the rest of the body.

- **Integrating Sessions.** The last three sessions are the integrating sessions and include two sessions on balance between the upper and lower girdles and a final session on balance throughout the whole system. What the patient has learned in earlier sessions serves as the basis for these last three sessions. During the eighth and ninth sessions, the patient's activity-specific demands determine how the previous sessions' gains are applied. The tenth session pulls together all of the information from the previous sessions, allowing the patient to proceed in the confidence that his or her body is now in balance and can perform optimally.

The focus of the sessions alternates between the upper and lower body.[174] The even-numbered sessions focus on pathologies of the pelvis and lower extremities, while the odd-numbered sessions focus on the trunk, neck, head, and upper extremities until the last session, which focuses on the entire body.[174]

Dr. Rolf thought that since gravity tends to shorten fascia, Rolfing techniques should lengthen fascia. Once an evaluation is completed to identify the shortened segments, part of the Rolfing technique involves the application of firm strokes with gentle pressure to affect fascial restrictions. This procedure is sometimes described as mildly uncomfortable.[177] Although not everyone responds within 10 treatment sessions, Dr. Rolf intended for patients to complete the course of treatment within a few months of starting it.[174] Treatment sessions are usually delivered once per week, but they are sometimes delivered as often as twice a week or as infrequently as once every 3 weeks.[174]

Some people may need additional techniques for a successful outcome. Other Rolfing strategies include active stretches and instruction in proper realignment of body segments by enhancing awareness of bad movement patterns and imbalances. Results vary between patients, but common outcomes include a sense of increased height; improved general well-being; greater strength, flexibility, and coordination; increased energy levels; and enhanced confidence.

Instrument-Assisted Soft-Tissue Mobilization

Instrument-assisted soft-tissue mobilization (IASTM) involves the use of specially designed instruments to manipulate soft tissue.[178-180] The technique has become more popular in recent decades and is considered an evolution of the traditional Chinese medicine, gua sha (pronounced "gwa shaw").[181] Gua sha is a 2000-year-old[181] technique that uses tools made from hard material to scrape the skin to reduce pain and stretch both underlying muscle and soft tissue to reduce soft-tissue pathology.[182] Instrument-assisted soft-tissue mobilization involves repeated mechanical stimulation of soft tissues, at various depths, patterns, and intensities, to facilitate tissue healing, improve range of motion, inhibit pain, and improve patient-reported function.[183, 184]

Theory

After injury, the inflammation and proliferation phases of tissue healing can result in fibrosis and formation of scar tissue in the injured soft tissue.[179] Scar tissue limits perfusion to the injured soft tissue, which restricts the supply of oxygen and nutrients to the area and interferes with the formation of collagen and the regeneration of tissues.[179, 185] In theory, instrument-assisted soft-tissue mobilization stimulates the remodeling of connective tissue through increased fibroblast proliferation and increased collagen synthesis, thereby breaking down scar tissue, adhesions, and fascial restrictions.[53, 178, 184, 186] The mechanical stimulation of IASTM also increases blood flow and nutrient supply to the injured tissue, thereby facilitating tissue healing.[53, 186-188]

Instrument-assisted soft-tissue mobilization is also hypothesized to improve range of motion by improving the extensibility of soft tissues.[189] When mechanical stress is exerted on the musculoskeletal fascia, the proprioceptive input sent to the central nervous system is modulated, resulting in a change of the tension in the tissue-related motor units.[190] It is thought that joint motion improves by decreasing muscle stiffness and altering stretch tolerance by the mechanical stimulation provided by IASTM.[183] Furthermore, the friction from the instrument is thought to decrease the tissue's viscosity, making it softer and more pliable, thereby allowing for improved mobility.[191]

In addition to the mechanical effects of IASTM, the technique is theorized to produce effects by means of a nociceptive mechanism. By varying the depth of the technique, the A-alpha and A-beta nerve fibers are stimulated. These nerve fibers inhibit the transmission of nociceptive stimuli, or pain, via the gate control theory of pain control. A superficial IASTM stroke will stimulate mechanoreceptors theorized to decrease musculoskeletal pain.[192-194]

Adhesions, scar tissue, restricted range of motion, and pain can independently or in combination impair function. As mentioned, IASTM is believed to facilitate tissue healing, improve soft-tissue mobility and range of motion, and decrease pain. Based on these effects, it could be inferred that function would then improve. Improved patient-reported function after IASTM treatments have been demonstrated by several studies.[195-197] When IASTM was combined with a rehabilitation program including flexibility, neuromuscular reeducation, and strengthening exercises, patient-reported function improved.[198-200]

A systematic review by Cheatham and colleagues[178] in 2016 concluded that the literature measuring the effects of IASTM is still emerging. Research findings challenge the efficacy of IASTM, but there is some evidence that supports its ability to increase range of motion.[178] A systematic review by Seffrin and colleagues[184] in 2019 indicated that current literature provides support for the use of IASTM for improving range of motion in noninjured people and for relieving pain and patient-reported function in both noninjured and injured people. Of interest, they did not find a profound difference in treatment effects between different IASTM tools.[184]

Treatment Principles

Many variations have appeared since IASTM became popular in Western cultures. Modern-day IASTM tools vary in material (e.g., stainless steel, plastic, jade, buffalo horn) and design[184] as shown in figure 11.34. These tools scrape along the skin to create petechial hemorrhages on the skin, relieve pain, or move deeper structures below the skin to improve soft-tissue mobility. Modifications of these tools' use include providing soft-tissue mobilization without scraping the skin to effect a mechanoreceptor response to decrease pain.

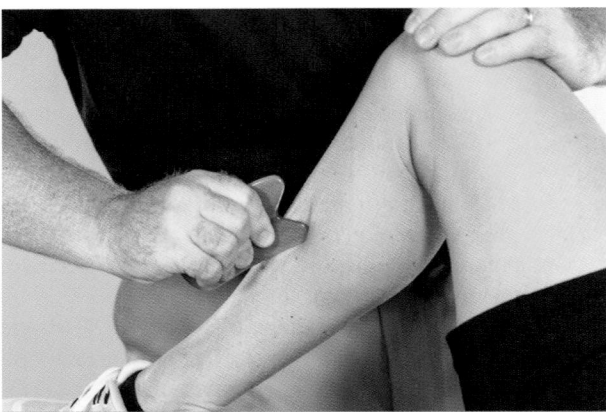

Figure 11.34 Gua sha tools used to mobilize soft tissue along posteromedial calf.

Graston is a form of IASTM whose tools are based on those used with the gua sha technique. These stainless-steel tools come in six shapes for different body segments. Before using these tools, clinicians must attend workshops to be instructed in their use. As with most other IASTM equipment, Graston tools mobilize soft tissue. Thus far, there has been no known investigation to demonstrate that the Graston technique surpasses other IASTM applications in achieving this goal.[201]

In addition to tools for specific techniques, several other tools are available for general application in soft-tissue mobilization. There are too many to describe each of them, but figure 11.35 provides a few examples. Some of them work to specifically treat myofascial trigger points, and others are more useful in improving soft-tissue mobility and inhibiting pain.

With the exception of the Graston tools, most manual therapy tools are relatively inexpensive. Probably most important, using these tools reduces the stress on the clinician's hands that occurs with the application of manual techniques. Recall that Seffrin and colleagues[184] did not find a profound difference in treatment effect between different IASTM tools. Clean the devices after each use to avoid spreading contamination from one patient to the next.

There are several proposed application protocols with IASTM, including Graston technique,[202] RockBlades,[203] Fascial Abrasion Institute,[204] and ASTYM,[205] to name a few. All of these companies and techniques fit under the umbrella of IASTM. Differences in protocol and technique include fiber direction with strokes, angle of tool, depth, rate, duration of application, and frequency of treatments. Parameters are dependent on the specific goal of the treatment.

As with other manual therapy techniques, there are contraindications for the use of IASTM. Contraindications

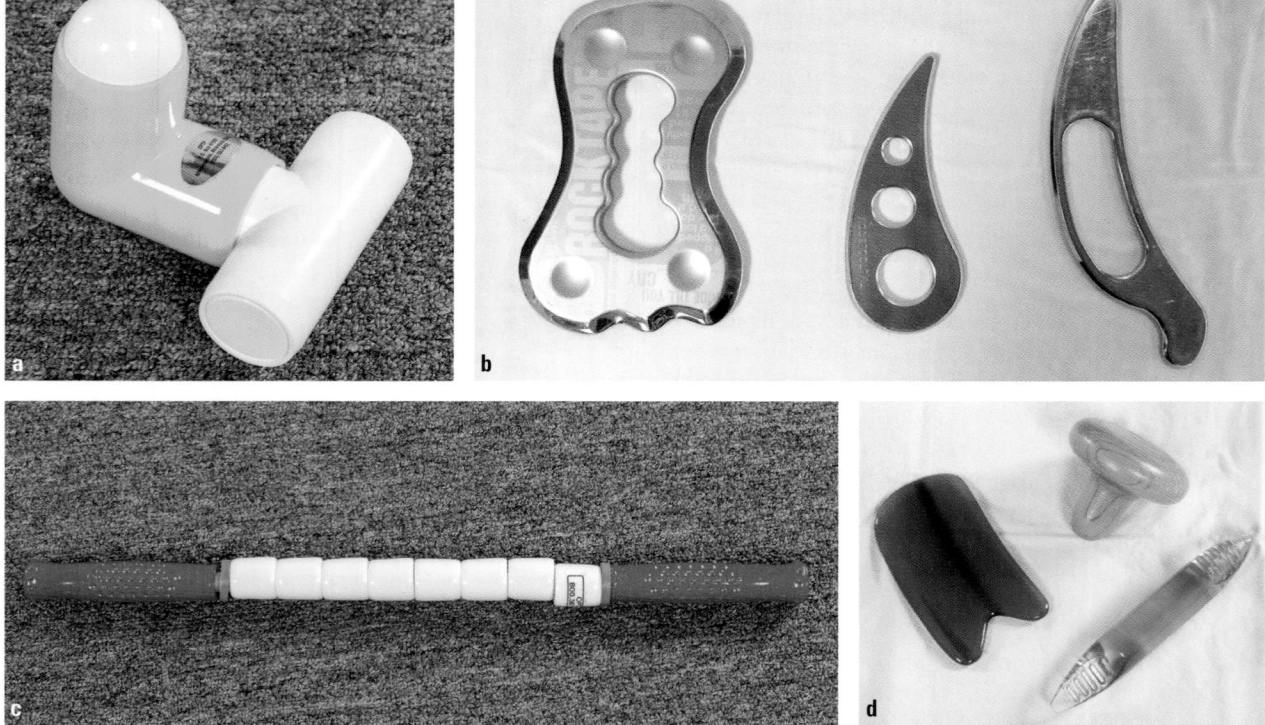

Figure 11.35 Various soft-tissue mobilization tools. *(a)* Knead tool; *(b)* RockBlade Mallet tool and TML tools; *(c)* roller stick; *(d)* gua sha tool, wooden knob, and ceramic polymer tool.

include open wounds, unhealed sutures, thrombophlebitis, skin infections, hematomas, myositis ossificans, unstable fractures, uncontrolled hypertension, and anticoagulant use.[179] Precautions for IASTM include cancer, kidney dysfunction, lymphedema, varicose veins, rheumatoid arthritis, osteoporosis, and steroid use.[179] Side effects may include bruising and soreness.

Joint Mobilization and Manipulation

Joint **mobilization** is one of the most commonly used manual therapy techniques in the treatment of restricted joint motion.[206] **Manipulation** and mobilization are not new concepts. Hippocrates (460-355 BC) used these techniques in his medical practice, and he recorded various methods of manipulating bones and joints. This section will focus on joint mobilization and briefly discuss joint manipulation.

Through the years, a variety of approaches to mobilization and manipulation have been developed. More recent schools of thought have been influenced by the teachings of manual clinicians such as Geoffrey Maitland,[207] Freddy Kaltenborn,[208] James Cyriax,[108] James Mennell,[209] and Stanley Paris.[210] The sidebar Manual Therapy Schools of Thought identifies the main distinctions of each of these manual clinicians' approaches.

Definition of Joint Mobilization and Manipulation

Joint mobilization is on a continuum with manipulation. They both involve passive movement of a joint, but mobilization is under the patient's control since it is performed at a slower speed and a voluntary muscle contraction will stop the movement. Manipulation is performed by the clinician at such a speed that the patient cannot stop the passive joint motion that the clinician produces. **Joint mobilization** is defined as "a manual therapy technique comprising a continuum of skilled passive movements that are applied at varying (low) speeds and amplitudes to joints with the intent to restore optimal motion, function, and/or to reduce pain."[211] **Joint manipulation** is defined as "a passive, high-velocity, low-amplitude thrust applied to a joint complex within its anatomical limit with the intent to restore optimal motion, function, and/or to reduce pain."[211] This section will focus on joint mobilization.

Joint Motion

The two types of joint motion are physiological and accessory. **Physiological joint motion** is movement that the patient can do voluntarily, such as flexion and abduction. **Accessory joint motion** is necessary for normal joint motion to occur, but cannot be voluntarily performed or controlled.

The two types of accessory joint motion are joint play and component motion. Both component motion and joint play are necessary for full motion. **Component motion** is not capsular but accompanies physiological motion. The rotation of the clavicle during shoulder flexion is an example of a component motion. **Joint play** occurs within the joint and is determined by the joint capsule's laxity. If you grasp and passively twist a finger, you can feel the joint play of the metacarpophalangeal joint. Joint play is necessary for full motion to occur, but a person cannot actively control joint play. For example, you can passively rotate your third metacarpophalangeal joint, but you cannot rotate it

---

Manual Therapy Schools of Thought

- *James Cyriax.*[108] Uses selective tension techniques to identify faulty structures in the examination. Emphasizes the need for soft-tissue massage and often uses injection of muscle trigger points. Believes the disc is the primary source of low-back pain and uses nonspecific spinal techniques designed to move the disc to relieve nerve root pressure.

- *Freddy Kaltenborn.*[208] His arthrokinematics techniques incorporate the influence of muscle function and soft-tissue changes in the manifestation of the patient's loss of function. The techniques are eclectic and very specific.

- *Geoffrey Maitland.*[207] Uses primarily passive accessory movements to restore function after an extensive assessment based on information from the patient's subjective examination (history) and the evaluator's objective assessment. The movements are oscillations, the techniques are specific, and the goal is to relieve what he terms "reproducible signs."

- *James Mennell.*[209] Believes that joint play is key to normal joint function. Emphasizes the importance of the small accessory movements as necessary for full joint motion to occur. Techniques are more specific for the extremities than for the spine.

- *Stanley Paris.*[210] Incorporates both chiropractic and osteopathic orientations in his eclectic approach to normalization of arthrokinematics, especially joint play and component motions. As a general rule, the patient's pain is not used to guide treatment.

actively; however, if you did not have that passive rotation, full active flexion–extension and abduction–adduction motion of the joint would not be possible.

Arthrokinematics

Arthrokinematics refers to the motions between the bones that form a joint. Five types of arthrokinematic motion occur within joints: roll, slide, spin, compression, and distraction. These motions permit greater motion of a joint and can occur only with appropriate joint play. This concept is vital to understanding how joint mobilization and manipulation work and how they can be applied.

Most joint surfaces are concave, convex, or both. Joints that have one concave and one convex surface are called *ovoid* (figure 11.36a). Joints that have a surface that is concave in one direction and convex in another with the opposing surface convex and concave in complementary directions are called *sellar* or *saddle joints* because of their similarity to a saddle (figure 11.36b). The shape of the joint determines its arthrokinematic motions.

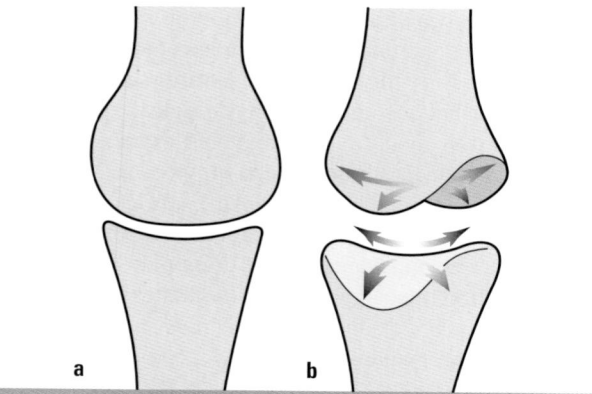

Figure 11.36 Joint surfaces of *(a)* ovoid and *(b)* sellar joints.

Roll

Roll occurs between joint surfaces when a new point of one surface meets a new point of the opposing surface, similar to when a bowling ball rolls down the lane; each point on the ball encounters a new point on the wood surface (figure 11.37). Rolling is accompanied by sliding or spinning in a normal joint. Roll of the concave end occurs in the direction of the bone's movement. For example, if a knee moves into flexion, the roll of the tibial plateau of

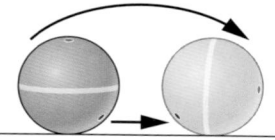

Figure 11.37 In a roll, different points on one surface come in contact with different points on the second surface.

the joint will be in the same direction as the shaft of the tibia, or posterior.

Slide

Slide occurs between joint surfaces when one point of one surface contacts new points on the opposing surface (figure 11.38), like a skier going down a hill. Like rolling, sliding does not usually occur by itself in normal joints. When a passive mobilization technique is applied to produce a slide in a joint, the technique is referred to as a *glide*. The more congruent a joint is, the better it responds to gliding mobilization techniques to gain mobility. Glide (slide) and roll occur together, sometimes moving in the same direction, and sometimes moving in opposite directions, depending on the joint's configuration and on which joint surface is moving. Joint mobilization forces are most often applied in the direction of the joint's slide.

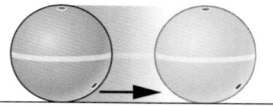

Figure 11.38 In a slide, one point on one surface comes in contact with different points on the second surface.

Spin

Spin occurs in a joint when one bone rotates around a stationary axis (figure 11.39). Like roll and slide, spin does not occur by itself during normal joint motion.

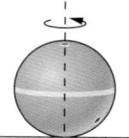

Figure 11.39 In a spin, a segment rotates about a stationary mechanical axis.

CLINICAL TIPS

The more congruent a joint is, the better it responds to gliding mobilization techniques to gain mobility. Joint mobilization forces are most often applied in the direction of the joint's slide.

Compression

Compression is a decrease in the space between two joint surfaces (figure 11.40). Compression adds stability to a joint. Compression also normally occurs in a joint when a muscle crossing that joint contracts, pulling the bone ends together. During roll, some compression occurs on the side in the direction of the motion.

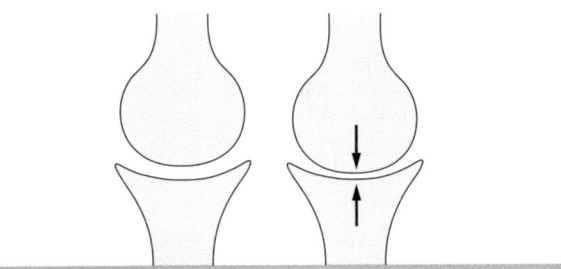

Figure 11.40   Compression.

Distraction

Distraction of a joint occurs when the two surfaces are pulled apart (figure 11.41). A gentle distraction can relieve pain in a tender joint. Distraction is often used in combination with joint accessory mobilization techniques to further stretch the capsule. Distraction can also make mobilization techniques more comfortable.

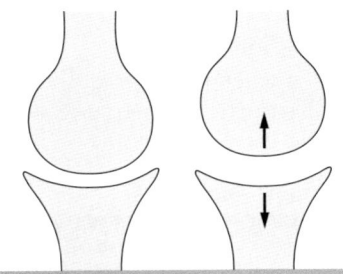

Figure 11.41   Distraction.

> **CLINICAL TIPS**
>
> If a joint rolls, it will also have a specific amount of slide as it moves through its range of motion. Full motion occurs only if the quantity of both the roll and the slide are normal.

Concave and Convex Rules

Knowing the shape of the joint being treated and keeping in mind the concave and convex rules (figure 11.42) are basic to the application of correct mobilization techniques. Using these rules, one joint surface is mobile, and the other is stable. The concave-on-convex rule states that the convex surface is stable and the concave joint surface slides in the same direction as the bone movement (figure 11.42a). The convex-on-concave rule states that the concave surface is stable and the convex joint surface slides in the opposite direction of the bone movement (figure 11.42b). For example, if the thigh is stabilized to prevent the femur from moving at the knee, the tibia's concave joint surface slides posteriorly when the tibia moves posteriorly from extension to flexion (concave surface moves on convex

surface). In contrast, if the glenoid is stabilized at the shoulder, the convex humeral head surface slides inferiorly as the humerus is moved superiorly into abduction.

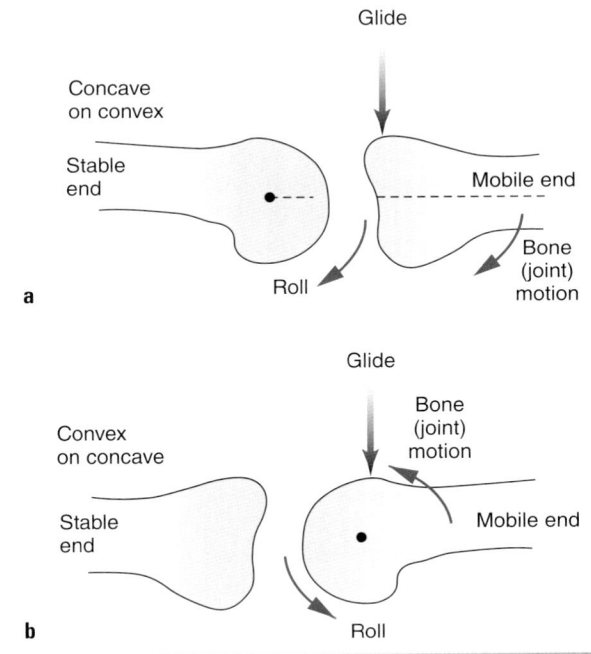

Figure 11.42   Rules for concave and convex joint surfaces. *(a)* Concave-on-convex rule: Joint mobilization glide force is applied in the direction of bone motion. *(b)* Convex-on-concave rule: Joint mobilization glide force is applied in the opposite direction of bone motion.

 Go to HK*Propel* and watch video 11.5*a*, which demonstrates concave-on-convex joint motion, and video 11.5*b*, which demonstrates convex-on-concave joint motion.

Keeping in mind that a mobilization force is applied in the direction of the joint's slide, if you want to increase knee flexion, your mobilization force on the tibia is in an anterior-to-posterior (AP) direction. If you want to increase knee extension, you apply a posterior-to-anterior (PA)

> **CLINICAL TIPS**
>
> To remember in which direction to apply the glide force, think of a joint as being like either a knee or a shoulder: either concave-on-convex or convex-on-concave, respectively. If you visualize the joint ends as being either one of these, then you know that if it is like a knee, you apply the glide force in the same direction that the bone moves, and if it is like a shoulder, you apply the glide force in the direction opposite to the bone's movement.

mobilization force on the tibia. On the other hand, when mobilizing a convex surface such as the talus of the ankle mortise, if you want to increase dorsiflexion, you apply an AP force on the talus, and to increase plantar flexion you apply a PA force on the talus. Table 11.5 provides guides for mobilizing most of the major joints of the body.

Capsular Patterns of Motion

All joints have normal ranges of motion, but various problems can prevent normal motion. When loss of normal motion results from restriction in the joint capsule, specific characteristic changes occur in the joint's pattern of motion and are referred to as **capsular patterns**. The sidebar Capsular Patterns of Motion Seen When Motion Loss Occurs Secondary to Capsular Pathology describes the capsular pattern for most joints. When you examine a joint's range of motion, knowing both the joint's normal degrees of motion and the typical pattern of capsular restriction is crucial. When restricted motion and a capsular pattern are present, full joint motion is attained, and capsular tightness is resolved using joint mobilization techniques. A capsular pattern indicates that a significant loss of motion is caused by capsular restriction and must be treated by

joint mobilization to effectively improve range of motion. A noncapsular pattern of restricted range of motion indicates that structures other than the capsule are preventing normal motion; however, a joint's capsular mobility should always be examined to eliminate any capsular restriction as a cause of lost motion.

Effects of Joint Mobilization

Of the manual therapies, joint mobilization has had the greatest amount of scientific evidence to support its efficacy.[212] Joint mobilization studies performed on the spine,[213-216] lower extremities,[217-222] and upper extremities[223-226] demonstrate the beneficial effects of joint mobilization. Additionally, many clinicians anecdotally report consistent positive results from their treatments. Although the reason for these benefits is yet to be verified, it is presumed that beneficial chemical, physiological, or mechanical changes are produced by joint mobilization techniques.

Neurophysiological Effects

Although there is no empirical evidence to demonstrate how joint mobilization techniques relieve pain, there are

TABLE 11.5 Examples of Concave-on-Convex and Convex-on-Concave Joints

Joint	Stable segment	Moving segment	Rule for joint mobilization
Glenohumeral	Glenoid fossa	Humeral head	Convex on concave: Humeral head slides opposite to humerus motion.
Forearm: proximal joint	Ulna	Radial head	Convex on concave: Round radial head slides opposite to forearm motion.
Forearm: distal joint	Head of ulna	Ulnar notch of radius	Concave on convex: Concave ulnar notch slides in the same direction as forearm motion.
Wrist	Distal radius and ulna	Proximal carpal row	Convex on concave: Convex proximal carpal row slides opposite to wrist motion.
Metacarpophalangeal and interphalangeal joints	Convex metacarpal	Concave proximal phalanx	Concave on convex: Concave phalanx slides in same direction as finger motion.
Hip	Acetabulum	Femoral head	Convex on concave: Femoral head slides opposite to femoral shaft motion.
Knee	Femur	Tibia	Concave on convex: Slide of tibia is in same direction as tibial motion.
Talocrural	Tibia-fibula mortise	Talar dome	Convex on concave: Talus slides opposite to foot motion.
Metatarsophalangeal and interphalangeal joints	Convex metatarsal	Concave proximal phalanx	Concave on convex: Concave phalanx slides in same direction as toe motion.

Capsular Patterns of Motion Seen When Motion Loss Occurs Secondary to Capsular Pathology

Glenohumeral	Lateral rotation is more limited than abduction. Abduction is more limited than medial rotation.
Elbow	Flexion is more limited than extension.
Forearm	Supination and pronation are equally limited at the proximal radioulnar joint. Pronation and supination are equally limited at the distal radioulnar joint.
Wrist	Flexion and extension are equally limited. Radial and ulnar deviation are equally limited.
Finger	Abduction is more limited than adduction of the thumb CMC. Flexion is more limited than extension of the MCPs and IPs. Abduction is more limited than extension in the MCPs.
Hip	Medial rotation and abduction are grossly limited. Flexion is more limited than extension. Generally, there is no limitation of lateral rotation.
Knee	Flexion is more limited than extension.
Ankle Talocrural Subtalar	Plantar flexion is more limited than dorsiflexion. Inversion is more limited than eversion.
Midtarsal joints	Limited in dorsiflexion, plantar flexion, adduction, and medial rotation. No limits of abduction and lateral rotation.
Foot and toes 1st MTP 2nd–5th MTP IP joint	Extension is more limited than flexion. Dorsiflexion is more limited than plantar flexion. Variable. Fixation in dorsiflexion with plantar flexed IP joints.
Lumbar spine	If a left facet is limited: Forward bending (FB) produces a deviation to the left. Side bending right (SBR) is limited. Side bending left (SBL) is unrestricted. Rotation left (RL) is limited. Rotation right (RR) is unrestricted.
Cervical spine	If a left facet is limited: FB produces some deviation to the left. SBR is restricted. SBL is comparatively unrestricted. RL is comparatively unrestricted. RR is most limited.

CMC = carpometacarpal; MCP = metacarpophalangeal; IP = interphalangeal; MTP = metatarsophalangeal.

several theories that outline how the techniques modulate pain.[215, 220, 227] One theory is that joint mobilization facilitates the gate control mechanism.[228-230] Small-amplitude joint mobilization oscillations stimulate the mechanoreceptors that inhibit the transmission of nociceptive stimulation from the spinal cord and brain stem. Small-amplitude and mild joint mobilization oscillations also affect muscle spasm and muscle guarding.[231] Inhibition of nociceptive stimulation results in relaxation, resulting in secondary pain reduction.[232] Another theory based on a mechanism-based approach to pain management theorizes that joint mobilization techniques activate descending inhibitory pathways using serotonin, noradrenaline, adenosine, and cannabinoid receptors in the spinal cord to produce analgesia.[233] Joint mobilization is also postulated to reduce glial cell activation in the spinal cord, thereby modulating pain.

Nutritional Effects

We know that synovial fluid provides nutrition for joints.[234] We also know that joint motion is important for synovial fluid movement, which provides adequate nutrition for the entire joint surface.[235] Distraction or small gliding movements can cause synovial fluid movement within the joint.[236, 237] Since the avascular articular cartilage within a joint depends on synovial fluid movement for its nutritional needs and nutrient–waste exchange, joint mobilization can help provide this nutrient exchange to prevent the deleterious effects of joint swelling and immobilization.[235]

Mechanical Effects

More aggressive mobilization techniques can improve the mobility of hypomobile joints.[238] Immobilized joints that have lost their normal mobility develop collagenous adhesions and thickened connective tissue.[38] Mobilization techniques that stretch collagen structures into their plastic range of deformation increase the tissue's mobility and improve the joint's motion.[207] Mobilization not only stretches capsular tissues but also loosens or breaks down adhesions to improve mobility.[208] There is also some evidence to indicate that a reduction in motion restrictions may be a secondary effect of joint mobilization's inhibitory effects on joint afferent receptors.[239]

Cavitation

Occasionally, mobilization or joint movement produces a cracking sound. The sound is called **cavitation**.[240] It is thought that when tension is produced in a synovial joint, increased pressure within the joint causes a vaporization of gas within the synovial fluid.[241] When the gas is liberated as the gas bubble forms then collapses, the joint space expands. The collapse of the gas bubble causes the noise.[242, 243] It takes about a half hour for the gas to be reabsorbed into the synovium; until then, the joint cannot be cracked again.[240] Initial reports indicated that the gas formed was nitrogen, but it is now believed to be carbon dioxide.[241, 244]

After this cracking, joint mobility often increases. This is believed to occur because of the expansion of the joint capsule from the increased pressure and the reflex relaxation of surrounding muscles through stimulation of inhibitory mechanoreceptors.[210] This increased joint mobility can be advantageous or disadvantageous. It is advantageous for hypomobile joints. For hypermobile joints, a reduction of muscle tone along with an increase in joint laxity can lead to increased joint stress and pain; the muscles reflexively tighten and cause additional discomfort. Although "cracking" one's back or neck may

offer temporary relief, Paris and Patla[210] believe that such joint cracking may increase the risk of spinal disc injury. When cracking occurs repeatedly in the spine, the joints become unstable.[245] Conversely, when joint cavitation occurs repeatedly in the extremities, as when cracking the knuckles, the joint capsule eventually becomes thickened and increases the joint's stiffness.[210]

Application of Joint Mobilization

Before you apply joint mobilization, you must identify the forces and excursions that can and should occur as well as what is considered normal for the person and the joint. These issues are discussed in the following sections.

Grades of Movement

According to Maitland,[207] movements used in joint mobilization are divided into four grades, I, II, III, and IV. Manipulation is grade V. The grading is based on the amplitude of the movement and where within the available range of motion the force is applied. Grades I and IV are small-amplitude movements performed at the beginning and end of the joint's available range, respectively. Grades II and III are large-amplitude movements. Grade II movement does not reach the limits of the range, whereas grade III movement is performed up to the limit of the available range. These grades overlap somewhat, as seen in figure 11.43. Grade V is the manipulation grade and is a small-amplitude, high-velocity thrust beyond the end range of a joint's restriction; this grade is not included in this section.

The amount of motion within each grade is relative to the specific joint and to the available motion in that joint. For example, a normal glenohumeral joint has larger grade I, II, III, and IV movements than a severely restricted glenohumeral joint and certainly more motion than a normal L4-5 joint.

Grades I and II are used to relieve joint pain. Oscillations in these grades stimulate joint mechanoreceptors to inhibit nociceptive feedback into the joints.[207] These grades often are also used before and after treatment with grades III and IV—beforehand to relax the joint and afterward to relieve discomfort that the more aggressive grades may have caused.

Grades III and IV are used to gain joint motion. These grades stretch the capsule and connective-tissue structures that limit joint mobility.[207] They may be uncomfortable, but they are not painful.

Oscillatory motions are often used with the various grades of movement. However, sustained joint-play motions can also be used. The sustained techniques involve only three grades: I, II, and III. Their grade definitions are slightly different from those of oscillatory motions: Grade II goes to the end point of resistance, and grade III is essentially a stretch of the joint, going toward a normal joint's limit (figure 11.44). The techniques discussed here use the oscillatory motions, since they are the most common.

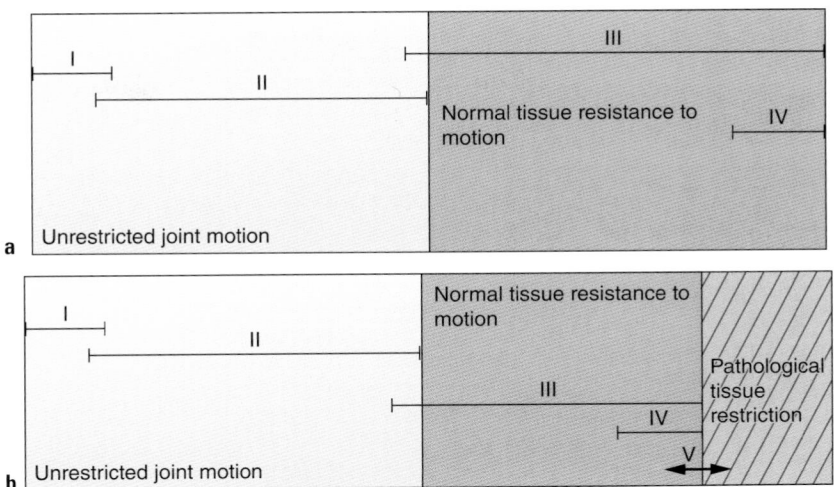

Figure 11.43 Grades of movement in a normal and a restricted joint. Grades I and II do not reach the limits of movement. Grades III and IV do reach the limits of movement. Grade V reaches the limit of movement and extends beyond the end range of a joint's restriction. Grades I and IV are small amplitude, while grades II and III are large amplitude. *(a)* Joint mobilization grades applied to a normal joint. *(b)* Joint mobilization grades applied to a restricted joint.

Adapted from Maitland (1991).[207]

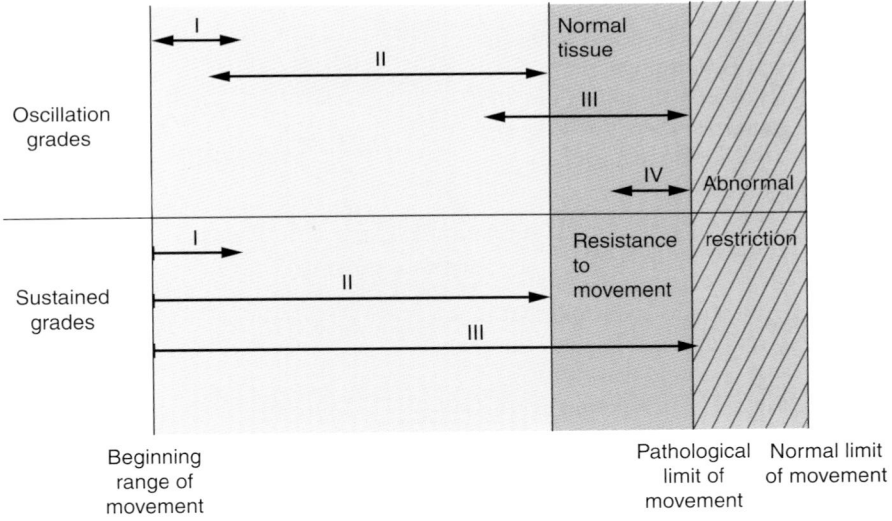

Figure 11.44 Sustained versus oscillation mobilization.

Movement Diagram

A movement diagram is a visual aid that can sometimes be helpful in determining which mobilization grade to use in a treatment. It is particularly helpful for visual learners who can apply the movement diagram to each joint's movement to understand where resistance to motion and pain within the motion occur. Such visualization can help in identifying the most appropriate grades of joint mobilization to use in treatment, especially for early users. Either physiological or accessory movements can be diagrammed. A movement diagram is shown in figure 11.45. **AN** is the normal range

of motion of a joint; **A** is the beginning of motion, and **N** is the normal limit of a motion. **L** is the abnormal limit of motion. **H** indicates a joint's hypermobile range. **AB** is intensity; the **A** end of the **AB** line is 0 intensity, and as you move up the line, the intensity increases until you reach the maximum intensity at **B**.

To complete the diagram, you mark on the movement diagram where throughout the range of motion the patient first reports pain. Figure 11.46 provides examples of different patients' movement diagrams. If you look at the examples in figure 11.46, you can get an idea of how to use

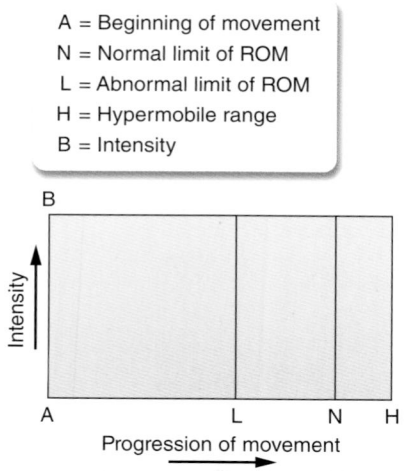

A = Beginning of movement
N = Normal limit of ROM
L = Abnormal limit of ROM
H = Hypermobile range
B = Intensity

Figure 11.45   Movement diagram. Any joint's movement can be configured to this diagram.

the diagram. Notice that **P** represents pain. A mark for P_1 indicates where in the range of motion the pain starts, and the intensity of the P_1 pain is demonstrated by where along the **AB** line the P_1 mark is placed. The **P** line is drawn according to the patient's description of changes in the pain as the joint capsule is moved through its motion. P_2 is the intensity of pain at the end of capsular motion. R_1 indicates where you first feel resistance during passive movement of the joint's capsule, and R_2 is the intensity of the resistance at the end of its motion. The path of **R** is drawn in correlation with the **AB** line to reflect how the resistance intensity changes as you continue to move the joint to the end of its motion. If the patient has pain at rest before your assessment begins, the **P** curve begins at **A** and is placed at a height on the vertical scale (**AB**) that corresponds to the intensity of pain reported by the patient.

Think of the **AB** line as a 10-point scale, dividing the line into 10 segments. If the pain is mild, the mark is placed on the lower third (1-3/10) of the **AB** line; if pain is moderate (4-6/10), the mark is placed within the mid–one-third section of the vertical line (figure 11.46b). If the patient reports the start of pain at 50% of possible motion, P_1 is placed at the midpoint of the **AL** line (figure 11.46a). If the pain occurs gradually but progressively over the length of the motion, a gradually sloping upward line is drawn, but if pain begins suddenly and quickly intensifies, a steep line is used.

To determine where **R** is drawn, you passively move the joint through its available accessory range and indicate on the graph where the start of the restriction can be palpated. If the restriction begins

(a) Pain occurs at 50% of the motion and intensifies quickly.

(b) Pain occurs at a moderate intensity at rest but changes little throughout the motion.

(c) Resistance is felt about $2/3$ through available motion and is moderate by the end of the motion.

(d) Resistance occurs early in the motion and steadily increases throughout the motion.

(e) Resistance is more significant than pain. Resistance occurs early and steadily increases, whereas pain is minor and occurs toward the end of the motion.

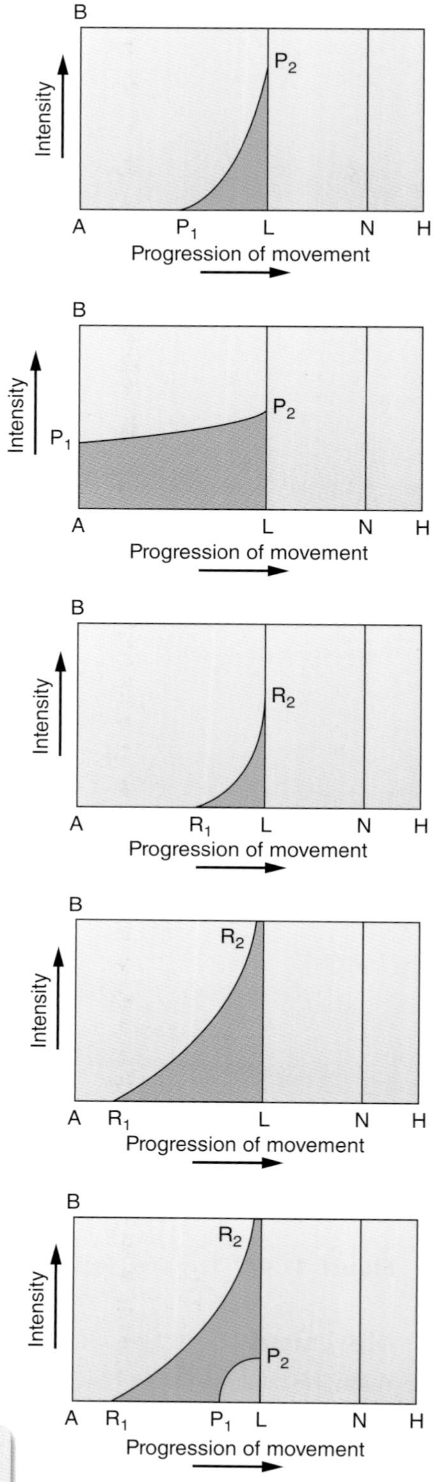

A = Beginning of movement
B = Intensity (0-10)
H = Hypermobile range
L = Abnormal limit of ROM
N = Normal limit of ROM

Figure 11.46   Examples of various combinations of pain and resistance levels and qualities drawn on movement diagrams.

abruptly and provides a rapidly progressive restriction of motion, a steep, rapidly climbing line is drawn. If restriction is more gradual, a line with a gentler slope is drawn (figure 11.46c and d).

Once you complete a movement diagram, you can easily assess the treatment needs and determine whether to attend to the patient's pain or to joint restriction first (figure 11.46e). If the pain is not significant, you may choose to treat the restriction first; if pain appears more intense, increases more quickly than resistance, or dominates resistance on the movement diagram, pain should be addressed before restriction is treated.

Until you understand joint mobilization techniques and mobilization grades and develop the skill to palpate and evaluate pain and resistance, it is a good idea to draw a movement diagram on paper or in your head. It will help you determine what you need to treat first and what grades of mobilization are most appropriate.

Normal Joint Mobility

Learning to distinguish between normal and abnormal joint mobility requires practice and familiarity with each patient. Because joint mobilization is a manual therapy, you must develop your sense of touch so you can detect what is normal for a joint. This is done only through practice on normal subjects. Once you can identify normal mobility, abnormal mobility is easier to recognize. Also, mobility that is normal for one joint may not be normal for another; for example, the mobility of a glenohumeral joint is not normal for a wrist joint.

Normal mobility also varies for different populations and depends on factors such as age, disease, occupation, sport, and position in a sport. For example, a 40-year-old man will not have the same normal lumbar spine mobility as his 15-year-old son. Age plays a role in what is considered normal joint mobility, so what is considered normal for the father may be abnormal for the son.

Athletes from different sports also demonstrate various degrees of normal joint mobility. For this reason, it is important to compare the joint being treated with the contralateral side in determining normal mobility for that person. For example, a baseball pitcher may have a hypermobile anterior glenohumeral joint when compared with a football lineman, but his mobility is normal for a pitcher. A ballet dancer may have a hypermobile hip compared with a shot-putter, but this is normal for dancers. You must consider the specific needs and demands of a sport or activity and even of a position within the sport when determining a person's normal joint mobility.

Close-Packed and Loose-Packed Positions

The relative position of the joint surfaces must be considered before applying joint mobilization techniques.

In a **close-packed position**, the joint surfaces are most congruent with each other (table 11.6). The convex surface of one bone is at its maximum congruence with the opposing concave surface of the other bone. The ligaments and capsule are taut, and the joint surfaces cannot be easily separated with traction. Joints are not usually mobilized in a close-packed position, but this position can be used to stabilize an adjacent joint before applying mobilization forces to another joint. For example, if you want to mobilize a proximal interphalangeal joint, the metacarpophalangeal joint can be positioned in full flexion, its close-packed position, to stabilize the proximal segment.

A **loose-packed position** is any position that is not close packed. The articular surfaces are not completely congruent, and some portions of the capsule are lax. Both examinations and early mobilization techniques are performed with a joint in its maximum loose-packed position. This position is a joint's **resting position**. See table 11.6 for a list of resting and close-packed positions for the joints. As a general rule, extremes of joint motion are close-packed positions, and midrange positions are resting positions.

A joint's resting position is the position in which the joint has its greatest laxity and is at its "maximal looseness."[208] Each joint has its unique resting position, as seen in table 11.6. When a joint has normal mobility within its resting position, it has maximal mobility, which allows it to function throughout its normal range of motion. If a joint does not have normal mobility but exhibits a capsular pattern of movement, it is restricted in its normal capsular motion, resulting in not only a unique pattern of mobility but also pathology in its function. Normal function must be restored by addressing the source of dysfunction, returning the capsule to its normal mobility.

Although each joint has a resting position, there is evidence to indicate that not all shoulders have the same resting position.[246] When treating your patient, it becomes necessary to identify that patient's joint-specific resting position. Using table 11.6 as a guide, then, you position the joint in the stated resting position. From there, you must use trial and error to identify the correct resting position for your patient's joint. By providing some distraction with the joint in the recommended resting position, you change the position slightly in one plane at a time until you identify the position in which you palpate the greatest amount of translational or rotational movement; you then maintain that plane's position and find the resting position for another plane until you have found the greatest amount of motion for that joint in all of its available planes of movement. This is that joint's resting position for that patient. As you gain experience, the time it takes to acquire the resting position shortens significantly until it takes you less than 2 s to find the resting position of even more complex triplanar joints, such as the shoulder and hip.

TABLE 11.6   Resting and Close-Packed Joint Positions

Joints	Resting	Close packed
Fingers and thumb		
Metacarpophalangeal	1: Mid-flexion/ext and mid-abduction/add 2–5: 20° flexion	1: Full opposition 2–5: Full flexion
Interphalangeal	20° flexion	Full extension
Wrist	0°	Full flexion or full extension
Forearm		
Proximal radioulnar	70° elbow flexion with 35° supination	Full pronation or full supination
Distal radioulnar	10° supination	Full pronation or full supination
Elbow		
Humeroulnar	70° elbow flexion with 10° supination	Full extension, forearm supination
Humeroradial	Full elbow extension with full supination	90° flexion, 5° supination
Shoulder girdle		
Glenohumeral	55° flexion with 20°–30° horizontal abduction	Full abduction with full lateral rotation
Sternoclavicular	Relaxed arm at side	Full shoulder elevation
Acromioclavicular	Relaxed arm at side	90° shoulder abduction
Hip	30° flexion, 30° abduction with slight lateral rotation	Full extension, medial rotation, and abduction
Knee		
Tibiofemoral	20°–30° flexion	Full knee extension with tibial lateral rotation
Patellofemoral	Full knee extension	Knee flexion
Tibiofibular	10° plantar flexion	Full dorsiflexion
Ankle and midfoot		
Talocrural	10° plantar flexion	Full dorsiflexion
Subtalar and midtarsal	Midrange of inversion and eversion	Full inversion
Forefoot and toes		
Metatarsophalangeal 1	20° dorsiflexion	Full dorsiflexion
Metatarsophalangeal 2–5	20° plantar flexion	Full dorsiflexion
Interphalangeal	20° plantar flexion	Full dorsiflexion

 Go to HK*Propel* and watch video 11.6, which demonstrates finding resting positions.

Indications

There are two main indications for the use of joint mobilization techniques. The first is joint pain. Grade I and II oscillations relieve pain.[207] The other indication is a hypomobile joint, which is determined by a capsular pattern of joint motion and less mobility than the contralateral joint. Grades III and IV improve joint mobility.[207]

Precautions and Contraindications

Absolute contraindications to joint mobilization grades III and IV include hypermobile joints, malignancy, tuberculosis, osteomyelitis, osteoporosis, recent fracture, ligamentous rupture, and herniated discs with nerve compression.[207] Joint effusion is a contraindication, since the capsule is already swollen from the extra fluid in the joint. Grade I and II mobilizations may be used to relieve pain, but grade III and IV techniques are avoided for these conditions. The rehabilitation clinician's skill and the patient's situation determine relative contraindications. Relative contraindications are also precautions and include oste-

Rules for Application of Joint Mobilization Treatments

As with other manual therapy techniques, you should understand the following rules and use them as guidelines for all joint mobilization treatments:

1. The patient should be relaxed.
2. Obtain patient consent before using joint mobilization techniques.
3. Before application, explain to the patient the purpose of the treatment and what sensations to expect.
4. Joint physiological and accessory mobility are assessed before and after the treatment. It may be necessary to check accessory mobility at various points within the physiological range.
5. Compare the joint to be treated with the contralateral joint to determine what is normal for the patient.
6. Determine treatment goals before treatment.
7. Grades I and II are used to relieve pain. Grades III and IV are used to increase mobility.
8. Stop the treatment if it is too painful for the patient.
9. Initial mobilization is performed in a resting position.
10. One segment, usually the proximal joint segment, is stabilized, while the other is mobilized.
11. Your hands should be as close to the joint as possible.
12. The larger the surface area of hand contact you have, the more comfortable the technique will be for the patient. When you use the entire hand, the fingers should be together, and as much of the finger and palm surface as possible should contact the patient's extremity.
13. Always use good body mechanics, and use gravity to assist the mobilization technique whenever possible.
14. The direction of the mobilization force is either parallel or perpendicular to the treatment plane. The treatment plane lies on the concave articulating surface, perpendicular to a line from the center of the convex articulating surface (figure 11.47). Traction and compression are applied perpendicular to the treatment plane, and glides or slides are applied parallel to it. The treatment plane can change with a change in a joint's position. Carefully determine the joint's treatment plane before application.
15. Always apply the concave-on-convex and convex-on-concave rules when determining in which direction to apply the mobilization force.
16. Emphasize one plane of motion at a time, although more than one plane may be treated in a session.
17. The patient's response determines the selection of oscillating or sustained techniques. Oscillation is used more often than sustained techniques for pain relief. Gains in range of motion can be achieved by either oscillation or sustained techniques. Sustained techniques are commonly used at the hip where the weight of the limb is difficult to support while providing oscillating techniques.
18. The patient's comfort and tolerance determine the duration of treatment. Oscillation techniques should be applied smoothly and regularly at the rate of two to three oscillations per second and should be repeated for 1 to 2 min for pain and 20 to 60 s for tightness. Sustained techniques are applied for only about 10 s in painful joints and repeated several times between bouts of rest. For tightness, sustained techniques are held for 10 to 30 s, depending on the patient's tolerance, and repeated three to five times.
19. Begin and end mobilization treatments for increasing range of motion with grade I or II distraction oscillations to facilitate relaxation at the start of treatment and relieve pain after treatment.
20. Progression is determined by the patient's response to the treatment. You must assess the patient's response to treatment in terms of pain, changes in joint mobility and range of motion, and the patient's psychological reaction to determine whether you should change the mobilization techniques. Progression can involve increasing the length of the treatment, increasing the grade if treating a hypomobile joint, or changing the joint to a less loosely packed position.
21. Mobilization techniques to improve motion should be accompanied by therapeutic exercise to reinforce the gains made with the manual treatment. Flexibility exercises after joint mobilization help to reinforce the gains made with mobilization.

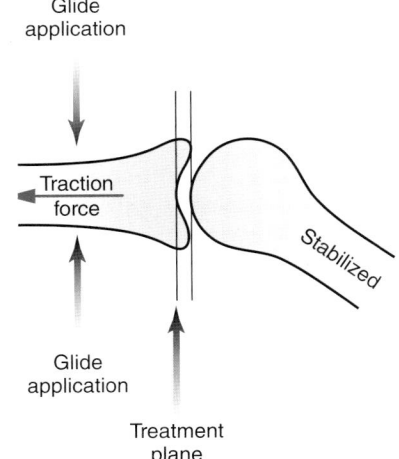

Figure 11.47 Direction of force application. The application is either perpendicular (traction or compression) or parallel (glides) to the treatment plane.

oarthritis, pregnancy, flu, total joint replacement, severe scoliosis, poor general health, and a patient's inability to relax.[207] Precautions should also be taken when treating hypermobile joints using the pain-relieving grades. If you doubt whether to use joint mobilization, err on the side of caution and refrain from its use.

Since joint mobilization plays such a crucial role in regaining mobility within a rehabilitation program, specific mobilization techniques are presented in part IV, Rehabilitation of Body Segments. Only the most commonly used maneuvers are presented.

NAGS, SNAGS, and MWMs

Although these techniques are not what many people consider to be joint mobilization in the purest sense, Brian Mulligan, a New Zealand manual therapist, developed a variation on traditional joint mobilization techniques that is presented in the next section. Mulligan theorized that injuries caused changes in a joint's normal position and resulted in loss of physiological motion.[247] Many of his techniques are performed with the patient standing or sitting. As with most other manual therapies, empirical results are lacking, although case studies with successful results are in the literature.[247] Several randomized controlled trials have compared the Mulligan concept with other interventions and report decreased pain and improved movement with Mulligan techniques.[248-251] Mulligan's applications primarily involve three techniques: NAGS, SNAGS, and MWMs. Each of these techniques has the same goals: abolish pain, increase range of motion, and produce immediate results.[252] During assessment, the rehabilitation clinician will identify a "comparable sign" as described by Maitland.[207] The technique of NAGS, SNAGS, or MWMs is then used to decrease pain and improve range of motion. NAGS and SNAGS focus on the spine and specifically treat the facet joints. MWMs is the only technique that is used for extremity joints in addition to spinal joints. Mulligan says that his treatment techniques must be painless during their application, so if they do produce pain, they should be abandoned as a means of treatment.[253]

NAGS

Natural apophyseal glides (NAGS) are passive oscillations applied between the middle and end range of available motion to relieve pain and increase motion, and they are used primarily in the cervical and upper thoracic region of the spine.[253] This technique is used for cervical spine levels 2 through 7 and thoracic spine levels 1 through 7. With the patient sitting, the patient's head is held and positioned by the clinician's chest and abdomen and one upper extremity with slight traction applied while a finger of the opposite hand is used to apply rhythmic glides to the specific restricted facet. After no more than six mobilization bouts, movement and pain are reassessed.[253] Several sets of treatment may be required to observe a change.[253] It is important that the patient have no pain with this technique. NAGS are useful for grossly restricted spinal movement and in highly irritable conditions.

SNAGS

Sustained natural apophyseal glides (SNAGS) are used to treat the cervical, thoracic, and lumbar spine. It is also used to treat ribs and the sacroiliac joints.[247] SNAGS are used both to relieve pain and to improve mobility. For this technique, the facet is moved to its end-range position and held. This technique adds active motion during the treatment. As with NAGS, the patient is usually weight bearing, either sitting or standing; if the patient's pain occurs in standing, then the patient stands for treatment, but if pain is present in standing and sitting, treatment starts with the patient seated, then later progresses to the patient standing once treatment goals are achieved in the sitting position.

Once the clinician identifies the spinal level involved and the direction of restricted movement, the hands are positioned at the site, and the patient moves to the position just before the point in the motion where pain occurs. Once in that position, the clinician applies the gliding force along the affected facet. At that point, the patient performs the symptomatic movement and moves the facet to the end position of the joint; if the technique is applied correctly, the patient should be able to move painlessly to the end of motion.[253] At the first treatment session, no more than three bouts should be applied. SNAGS are most effective when symptoms are provoked by a movement but are not present when the patient is at rest. Effects are usually experienced at the first treatment session.[254] SNAGS are not used for multilevel spine pain or with a highly irritable symptomatology.

MWMs

Mobilizations with movement (MWMs), as with Mulligan's other techniques, are intended to relieve pain and increase joint motion. This application uses a combination of a sustained passive accessory glide mobilization and simultaneous active and pain-free physiologic motion.[252] The mobilization is sustained without restricting the patient's active movement.[255] While sustaining the accessory glide, the patient performs 3 sets of 10 repetitions into the restricted motion.[255] If patient mobility and pain have not improved, the clinician reassesses and adjusts the treatment plane or direction of mobilization.

Mulligan advocates using MWMs to treat pain and motion restrictions of the extremities since, when successful, MWMs restore motion in both directions of a plane of movement (e.g., flexion and extension in the sagittal plane).[253] This differs from more traditional joint mobilization, which increases joint motion in only one direction (flexion or extension in the sagittal plane).[253]

Mobilizations with movement usually can be done in only one direction.[253] MWMs are always performed into resistance but without pain. Using MWMs to correct positional faults in the extremities is different than when MWMs are used in spinal treatments; applications to the facets in the spine occur in the direction of active motion, but in the extremities mobilizations are applied in a direction that is different from the joint's glide.[253]

An example from Mulligan's text on the subject,[253] improving dorsiflexion–plantar flexion after an ankle sprain, is appropriate since ankle sprains are common injuries. It is based on the idea that small changes occur in physiological motion after injury. Mulligan's theory indicates that when the anterior talofibular ligament is sprained, the fibula creates a positional fault since it is forced inferiorly and anteriorly because the sprained ligament pulled on it when it experienced the force that caused the injury. Therefore, to correct this positional fault, the clinician's thenar eminence grasps the fibula proximal to the malleolus and passively glides it superiorly and posteriorly in an oblique direction. As the clinician holds the fibula in this position, the patient actively dorsiflexes and plantar flexes the ankle. Both motions, the fibular passive positioning and the active ankle motion, should be pain free. As seen in figure 11.48, Mulligan advocates applying a tape strip over the distal fibula (proximal to the malleolus) pulling in an oblique direction laterally around to the posterior and medial leg.[253]

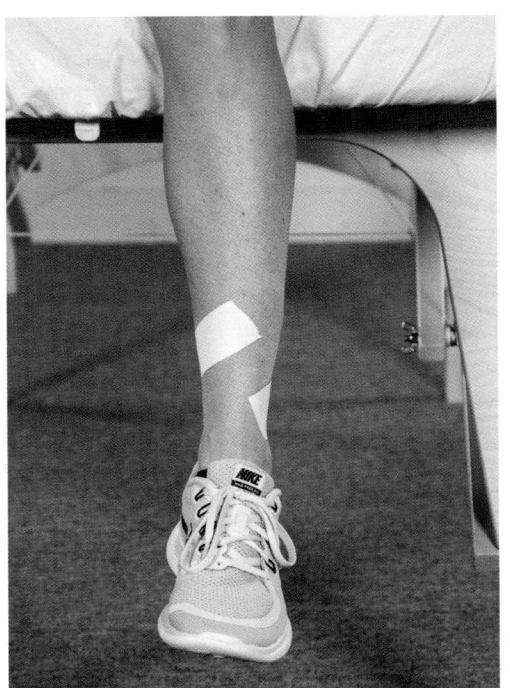

Figure 11.48 Taping to support fibular repositioning after treatment with MWMs to gain dorsiflexion and plantar flexion motion after a lateral ankle sprain.

Joint Manipulation

As described earlier in this section, manipulation is on a continuum with mobilization and is defined as "a passive, high-velocity, low-amplitude thrust technique applied to a joint complex within its anatomical limit with the intent to restore optimal motion, function, and/or to reduce pain."[211] Following the Maitland system,[207] a manipulation is a grade V joint movement.

In manipulation verbiage, the restriction of normal joint mobility is referred to clinically as *hypomobility*, *fixation*, *loss of end-play*, or *barrier*, and the patient problem is referred to as *somatic dysfunction* or *joint dysfunction*.[256] It is important to understand that a manipulation is performed within the normal physiologic capacity of the joint but not performed through the anatomical limit of the joint (figure 11.49).

There have been many studies, especially regarding the spine, that support the efficacy of joint manipulation.[257-260] The reported effects of manipulations include decreasing stiffness,[261] decreasing pain,[262] and improving passive range of motion.[263] From a mechanism-based approach to pain management, pain reduction through manipulation is thought to occur through a number of mechanisms, including activation of the peripheral neurochemical analgesic systems (cannabinoid and adenosine); activation of descending inhibitory pathways using serotonin, noradrenaline, adenosine, and cannabinoid receptors in the spinal cord, producing analgesia; reduction in central nervous system excitability; restoration of joint and connective tissue mobility, thereby removing possible mechanical irritants which stimulate nociceptors; and an increase in the expression and release of mediators that reduce inflammation.[233] Restoration of joint and connective tissue mobility has been described as a mechanical phenomenon that occurs by stretching collagen structures into their plastic range of deformation to increase the tissue's mobility and improve joint motion.[207]

Systematic reviews suggest that spinal manipulation is likely to reduce pain and improve function for patients with chronic low back pain, and overall patient outcomes are shown to be better than those of sham treatments.[264, 265] Spinal manipulation has also been associated with improved muscle function in the lumbar multifidus[266] and deep neck flexors.[267] These findings suggest that when used as part of a multimodal approach, spinal manipulation may provide a window of opportunity to maximize the effectiveness of spinal stabilization programs when used appropriately.

A clinical prediction rule was developed by Flynn et al.[268] for classifying patients with low-back pain who are likely to respond to spinal manipulation. This clinical prediction rule and the supine thrust "Chicago Roll" spinal manipulation technique used in the study were later validated by

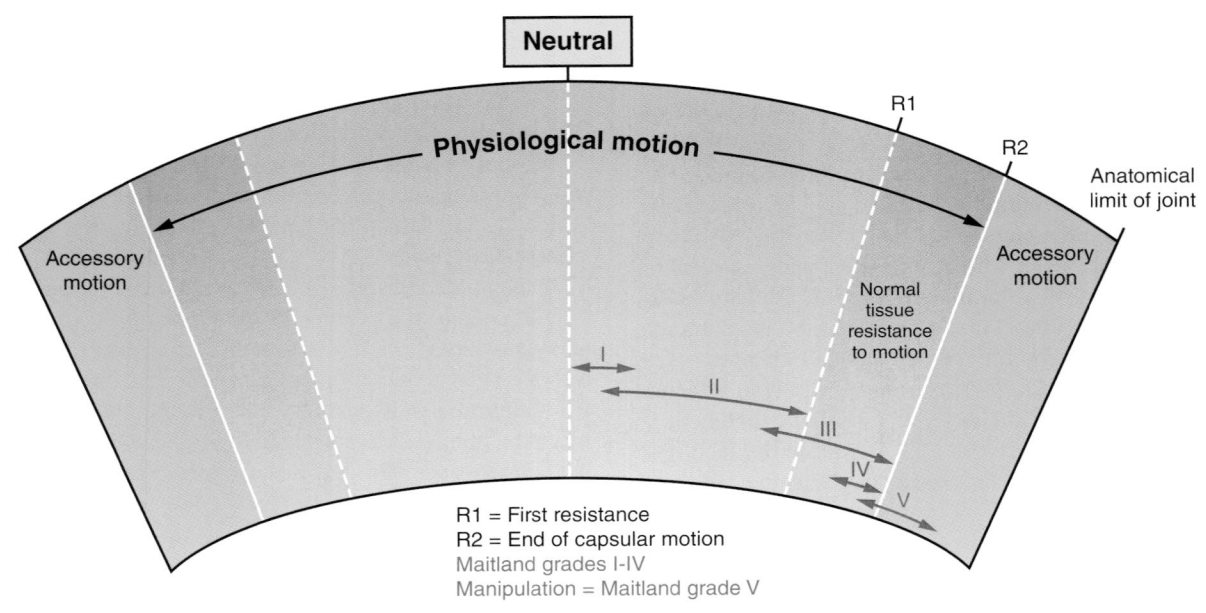

Figure 11.49   Physiologic motion, accessory motion, and anatomical limit of joint motion with Maitland grades of movement, including grade V joint manipulation.

Childs and colleagues.[269] The clinical prediction rule was once again tested by Cleland and colleagues,[270] who found that not only was the supine thrust technique effective in decreasing pain and disability but so was a side-lying thrust manipulation. These findings indicate that the low-back pain clinical prediction rule is generalizable to additional thrust manipulation techniques. In fact, manipulation has not been found to be segment specific or joint specific in the lumbar spine.[271] Investigation of research has led to two clinical treatment guideline recommendations for use of spinal manipulation in the lumbar spine, both of which are based on strong evidence: (1) the recommendation to use thrust manipulation for acute low-back pain to reduce pain and disability and (2) the recommendation to include thrust or nonthrust joint mobilization for subacute and chronic low-back pain and related leg pain.[272] Evidence is not yet strong enough to support a clinical prediction rule regarding thoracic spine manipulation, because there are mixed results in the literature regarding its benefits.[273-280]

Contraindications for joint manipulation include bone pathology, ligamentous laxity, fractures, dislocations, rheumatoid arthritis, aneurysm, joint infections, bleeding disorders, cord compression, cauda equina compression, and nerve root compression with progressive neurologic deficit.[281, 282] Precautions include spondylolisthesis, advanced degenerative joint disease with spondylosis, nerve root compression, disc herniation or prolapse, pregnancy,

anticoagulant therapy, arterial calcification, benign bone tumors, osteopenia, adverse reaction to previous manual therapy, and psychological dependence on high-velocity low-amplitude thrust (HVLAT) manipulation.[281, 282] There are possible adverse effects of spinal manipulation, including trauma to the spinal cord and pneumothorax,[281] acute vertigo,[283] vascular accidents,[284] rib and vertebral fractures, and cauda equina syndrome.[284] Research indicates the risk of adverse effects is low,[285-288] and it is primarily associated with treating the cervical spine.

Before performing a joint manipulation, you must identify the appropriate dysfunction, exclude any contraindications, consider any precautions, and obtain patient consent for the treatment. The performance of a joint manipulation consists of four phases: the orientation phase, preload phase, thrust phase, and resolution phase.[289] In the orientation phase, the patient is positioned into the appropriate treatment position. It is also important for the rehabilitation clinician to be in good postural positioning to perform the technique. The joint is taken to the end of the restriction in the preload phase. In this phase, you should produce pre-thrust tissue tension. In the thrust phase, a HVLAT is performed. The joint is then relaxed in the resolution phase. High-velocity low-amplitude thrust treatments should be pain-free. As with any manual therapy technique, you should then reassess for treatment effectiveness.

CLINICAL TIPS

The performance of a joint manipulation consists of four phases.

1. *Orientation phase:* The patient and clinician are situated in the proper position for the joint manipulation technique, and the joint is taken to the restrictive barrier.
2. *Preload phase:* The clinician produces prethrust tissue tension.
3. *Thrust phase:* HVLAT is performed.
4. *Resolution phase:* The joint is relaxed.

HVLAT Manipulation Techniques

It is imperative to have a complete understanding of joint anatomy and mechanics, indications, contraindications, and the possible adverse effects associated with the use of joint manipulation before considering it as a treatment technique. Patients can be injured if the techniques are not executed correctly. It takes time and a lot of practice to acquire the skills of mobility testing and HVLAT technique application. You must also obey the laws of your state regarding the use of HVLAT techniques. This section includes a review of a few examples of HVLAT techniques. To make the descriptions easier to understand, the clinician is referred to as "she," and the patient is referred to as "he."

Supine Thrust "Chicago Roll" Manipulation
The example is for treating the left sacroiliac (SI) joint and the right lower lumbar joints.

- **Orientation Phase:** The patient is supine with his hands clasped behind his head. The rehabilitation clinician stands on the right side. The clinician moves the patient's shoulders to side-bend them away. The clinician then crosses the patient's left ankle over the right and moves the lower extremities to side-bend them away. The patient is now in left side-bending (figure 11.50*a*). The clinician then places her cephalad arm through the left elbow triangle so the dorsum of her hand is resting on the patient's sternum. She rotates the patient's trunk toward her. She then places the heel of her caudad hand over the patient's left ASIS. If the patient does not have the mobility to rotate far enough to allow placement of the cephalad arm, the clinician may place her hand on the patient's left scapula or posterior shoulder region to provide the trunk rotation (figure 11.50*b*).

- **Preload Phase:** The clinician rotates the patient's trunk to the right further until she feels the left ASIS come into her hand. She then applies compression through the ASIS toward the table to produce prethrust tissue tension to the barrier.

- **Thrust Phase:** The clinician applies a HVLAT manipulation, directing the left ASIS posterior and inferior toward the table.

- **Resolution Phase:** The clinician brings the patient back to a neutral resting position.

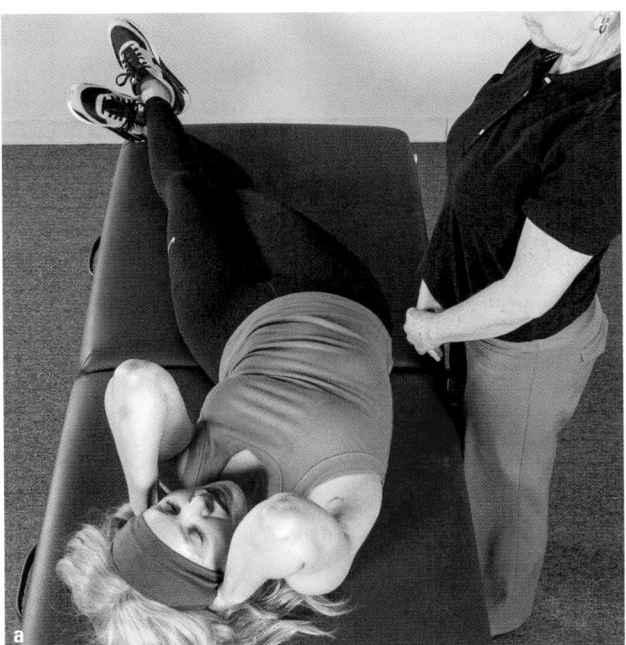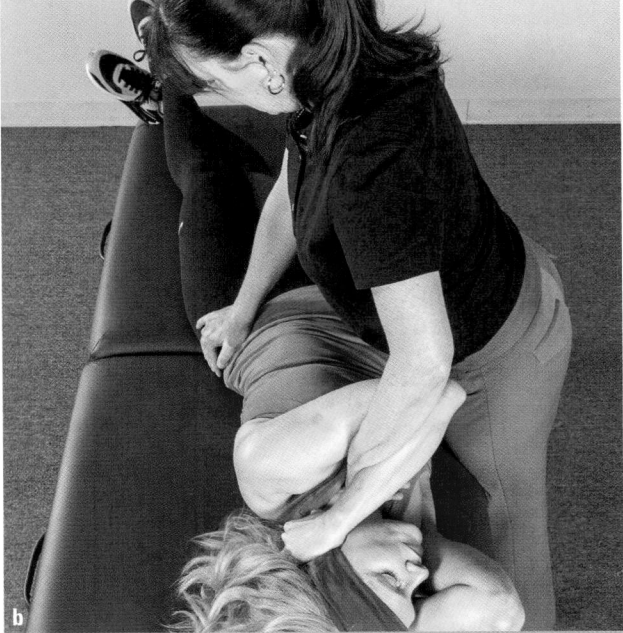

Figure 11.50 Supine thrust "Chicago Roll" manipulation.

Go to HK*Propel* and watch video 11.7, which demonstrates supine thrust "Chicago Roll" manipulation.

Mid-Thoracic Anterior to Posterior Thrust Manipulation   This technique is used to treat T4 through T10.

- **Orientation Phase:** The patient is side-lying with his hands interlaced behind his neck and elbows placed in front of his chest. The rehabilitation clinician faces the patient and places her caudad hand in a pistol position, with the scaphoid tubercle on one transverse process of the vertebra and the middle phalanx of the middle finger on the opposite transverse process (figure 11.51*a*). The cephalad hand supports the patient's head. With the cephalad hand, the clinician flexes the patient's trunk to the barrier, then backs off slightly from that point. While maintaining this position, the clinician rolls the patient supine until the dorsum of her caudad hand meets the table (figure 11.51*b*). A pillow can be placed between the clinician and patient for comfort.

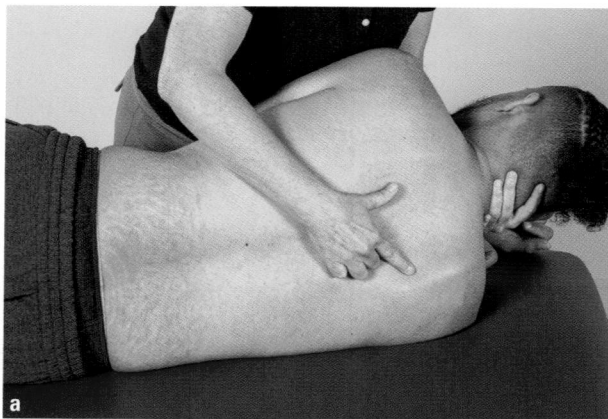

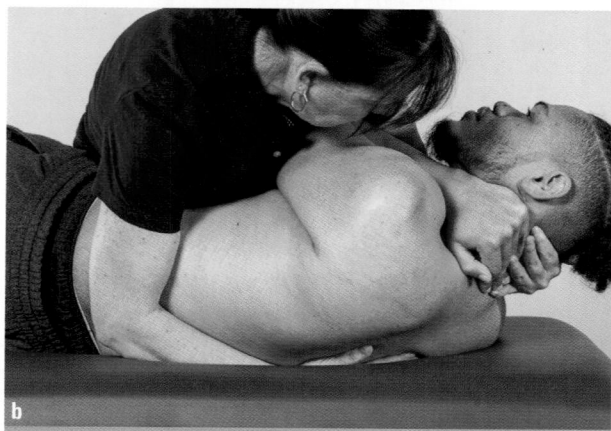

Figure 11.51   *(a)* Pistol position for thoracic spine placement. *(b)* Mid-thoracic anterior thrust manipulation.

- **Preload Phase:** The clinician fine-tunes to the barrier with trunk flexion and produces gentle prethrust tissue tension by gently leaning into the patient's forearms.
- **Thrust Phase:** The clinician applies a HVLAT manipulation in the anterior-to-posterior and cephalad direction through her trunk.
- **Resolution Phase:** The clinician brings the patient back to a neutral resting position.

Cuboid Whip Manipulation   Cuboid syndrome is a cause of lateral midfoot pain and is theorized to arise from injury and disruption of the calcaneocuboid joint.[290, 291] Cuboid syndrome has been associated with inversion ankle sprains and appears to be more prevalent in ballet dancers.[292, 293] The primary movement of the calcaneocuboid joint is medial and lateral rotation around an anterior–posterior axis.[290] Cuboid syndrome is theorized to result from forceful eversion of the cuboid while the calcaneus is inverted, thereby disrupting the congruency of the calcaneocuboid joint.[294]

If an examination determines that the patient has cuboid syndrome and has no contraindications for the treatment, the cuboid whip manipulation is recommended.[290, 293-295]

- **Orientation Phase:** The patient is positioned in prone with the limb relaxed and in 70° to 90° of knee flexion (figure 11.52). The rehabilitation clinician cups the dorsum of the patient's foot, placing the thumbs on the plantomedial aspect of the cuboid with the ankle in neutral.
- **Pre-load Phase:** The cuboid is passively moved to the end of restriction using slight pressure through

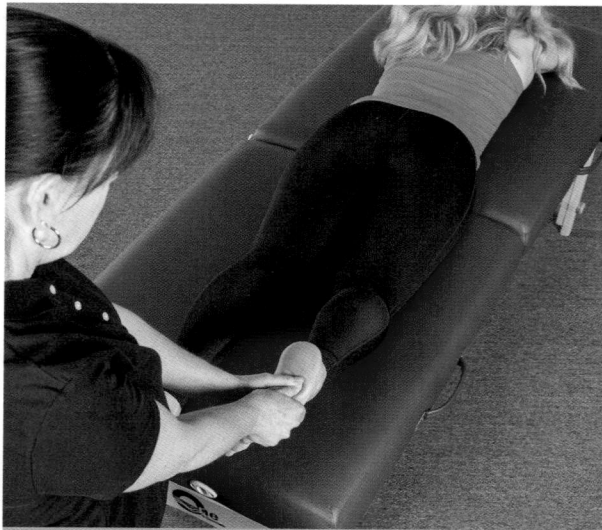

Figure 11.52   Cuboid whip manipulation.

the clinician's thumbs in an inversion-plantar flexion direction to preload tissue tension to the barrier.

- **Thrust Phase:** The clinician applies a HVLAT manipulation to the cuboid by abruptly whipping the foot into inversion and plantar flexion.
- **Resolution Phase:** The joint is relaxed. It is common to hear a pop or to feel a shift during the thrust.[294]

Dorsal Lunate Manipulation An example of a commonly used manipulation technique for the upper extremity is in the case of a perilunate dislocation. The lunate can be displaced volarly with a fall on an outstretched hand (FOOSH) injury.[296] Additionally, in carpal tunnel syndrome, the lunate may be displaced volarly, thereby narrowing the carpal tunnel and increasing pressure on the median nerve.[297] If the clinician's examination reveals that the patient's lunate is displaced volarly and the patient has no fracture or contraindications to manipulation, a lunate manipulation may be performed.

- **Orientation Phase:** The patient is either supine or seated. The rehabilitation clinician supinates the patient's forearm. The clinician grasps the patient's hand in hers and places her thumbs on the volar surface of the lunate with the patient's wrist in neutral. See figure 11.53.
- **Preload Phase:** Using slight pressure through the clinician's thumbs in a dorsal direction, the lunate is taken to the end of restriction to preload tissue tension to the barrier.
- **Thrust Phase:** The clinician abruptly whips the lunate in a dorsal direction by delivering a HVLAT manipulation to the lunate.
- **Resolution Phase:** The joint is then relaxed.

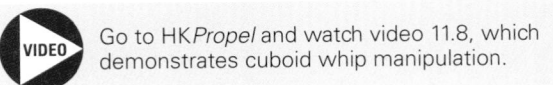
Go to HK*Propel* and watch video 11.8, which demonstrates cuboid whip manipulation.

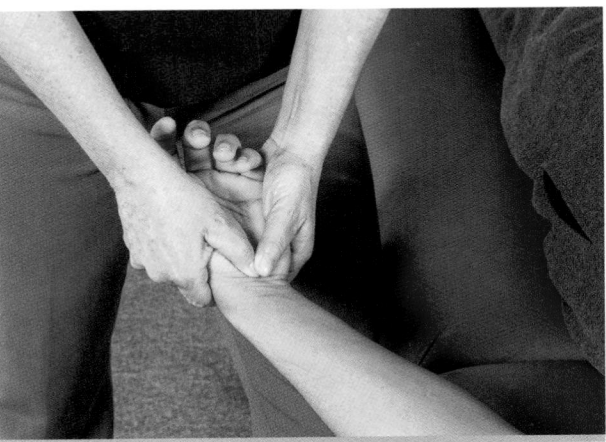
Figure 11.53 Dorsal lunate manipulation.

Summary

A clinician who uses the hands to affect tissue is performing manual therapy. Many kinds of manual therapy affect different tissues and structures. Only a few manual therapy techniques are presented in this chapter: massage, general myofascial release techniques, trigger point treatments, joint mobilization and manipulation, and PNF. Other manual therapy techniques are briefly introduced. Although the empirical evidence for the effectiveness of manual therapy remains sparse, evidence is growing. Each of these techniques has precautions, indications, and contraindications that clinicians must respect. Each technique also has a specific method of application that the clinician must both understand and practice in order to become proficient at using it to help patients. Before the application of manual therapy techniques, it is necessary to obtain verbal consent from the patient, or from a parent if you are working with a minor. Manual therapy techniques are not performed in isolation; instead they are performed with other manual therapy techniques and nonmanual therapy interventions as part of an integrated approach to patient care.

LEARNING AIDS ▬▬ ▬▬▬▬▬▬ ▬▬▬ ▬ ▬ ▬

Key Concepts and Review

1. Discuss the three techniques of massage and their indications, precautions, and contraindications.

The massage techniques used most commonly in rehabilitation include effleurage, or stroking; pétrissage, or kneading; and friction massage. They relieve pain, relax muscles, reduce swelling, and mobilize adherent scar tissue. Tapotement is a type of massage used in cases where fluids need to be dislodged. Massage should be avoided in the presence of infection, malignancies, skin diseases, blood clots, and any irritations or lesions that may spread with direct contact. Precautions include having clean hands and body surface to be treated, obtaining patient (or parent) consent and explaining the procedure before application, removing jewelry that may interfere with the application, using warm hands and massage media, and draping the body part appropriately.

2. Explain the progression of myofascial restriction after an injury.

Myofascial restriction occurs after an injury when secondary effects such as excessive or prolonged edema, scar tissue formation, and adhesions occur between the newly formed tissue and adjacent structures. Immobilization after an injury can also lead to myofascial restriction and loss of tissue mobility.

3. Discuss the techniques for myofascial release.

The primary techniques for myofascial release are J-stroke, oscillation, wringing, stripping, and arm or leg pull. J-stroke and oscillation are used on smaller areas of restriction, whereas wringing, stripping, and arm or leg pull are used on larger areas or more general restrictions.

4. Explain the leading hypotheses for the mechanism of myofascial trigger points.

Three hypotheses explain myofascial trigger points and focus on histopathology, neuroelectropathology, and a combination of these two. The histopathological hypothesis indicates that during contraction of a normal muscle fiber, calcium that is stored in the fiber's sarcoplasmic reticulum is rapidly released when the contraction begins and then reabsorbed in the presence of ATP when the contraction terminates. This process is triggered by a brief nerve impulse called an action potential. A contraction is the result of the shortening of the sarcomere when its cross-bridges pull the actin and myosin filaments over each other. If an injured muscle fiber's sarcoplasmic reticulum is damaged, its calcium is released, stimulating the sarcomere to produce a sustained contraction. This sustained calcium release and sarcomere contraction create an energy crisis because of the ischemia that results. Ischemia occurs because the muscle fibers' sustained contraction limits capillary blood flow in the region, causing oxygen deficiency within the muscle cells so they cannot provide enough ATP to relax the contraction. Without sufficient ATP, the sarcomere's filaments cannot release from each other, and therefore they remain fixed in their contracted position.

The second hypothesis is based on neuroelectrical pathology. It uses concepts of the Cinderella hypothesis, which refers to the fact that Type I fibers are normally recruited first, remain activated for a prolonged time, and are afforded short recovery times; hence, these fibers are susceptible to pain and damage. Studies have demonstrated that low-level activation after as little as 30 min causes trigger point pain in muscles. Previous studies have shown spontaneous electrical activity in trigger point muscle fibers but not in adjacent or surrounding normal muscle fibers. It is believed that repetitive, low-level muscle stress provides just enough stimulation that acetylcholine leaks out of the motor nerve terminal to trigger a depolarization of the synaptic membrane. This facilitation opens the sodium channels to produce sustained activation of very localized muscle fibers.

The third hypothesis is the integrated theory, which is a combination of the other two hypotheses. This hypothesis indicates that a dysfunctional motor end plate provides sustained contraction of isolated muscle fibers, as is presented in the neuroelectrical theory. Sustained muscle fiber contraction creates a combination of localized ischemia and increased metabolic needs, which together create a sustained energy crisis. Lacking sufficient energy to return calcium to the sarcoplasmic reticulum and reverse the polarized membrane potential with an inability to reduce acetylcholine quantities, the muscle cells remain locked in contraction. It is thought that ischemia and the ensuing local hypoxia trigger the release of chemical neural sensitizers that facilitate local nociceptors to produce pain. Input into the central nervous system from these nociceptors within the muscle may result in functional changes in the central nervous system, creating referred pain.

5. Discuss the spray-and-stretch trigger point release theory.

According to the gate control theory of pain, the sudden, brief application of cold inhibits the pain–spasm cycle and provides muscle relaxation and pain relief, especially when accompanied by a stretch.

6. Explain the concave-on-convex and convex-on-concave rules.

Joint mobilization techniques are based on these rules. The concave-on-convex rule states that concave joint surfaces slide in the same direction as the bone movement, and the convex-on-concave rule states that convex joint surfaces slide in the direction opposite to the bone's movement.

7. Define joint mobilization, manipulation, and grades of movement.

Joint mobilization is the passive movement of a joint with a force applied at a speed that enables the patient to stop the movement at any time. Movements in joint mobilization are divided into four grades. Grade I is small-amplitude movement in the beginning range of motion, grade II is large-amplitude movement in the middle of the nonrestricted range of motion, grade III is large-amplitude movement to the restricted range of motion, and grade IV is small-amplitude movement to the restricted range of motion. Manipulation is a grade V technique involving a high-velocity, low-amplitude thrust performed at the limit of the range of joint motion. The speed of the technique is such that a patient cannot stop the movement.

8. Discuss the direction of glide and traction in relation to the treatment plane.

Glide movements during mobilization should be parallel to the treatment plane, and traction is perpendicular to the treatment plane.

9. Explain the theoretical basis for proprioceptive neuromuscular facilitation.

Proprioceptive neuromuscular facilitation incorporates the inhibitory and excitatory impulses from the afferent receptors of skin, muscle, tendon, visual, and auditory neurons that facilitate a response from the motor neurons, resulting in a desired action.

10. Discuss how PNF can be used to improve flexibility and strength.

Improvement in either flexibility or strength is accomplished using PNF because this technique uses optimal relaxation during stretching exercises and optimal muscle recruitment during strengthening exercises to achieve the desired changes. It does this through increased neural recruitment by afferent stimulation of the central nervous system. To achieve increased flexibility, the CNS is stimulated to optimize muscle relaxation to produce motion gains. During strengthening activities, increased CNS stimulation results in greater stimulation of its muscle fibers with reduced facilitation of its GTOs to allow for greater muscle output.

Critical Thinking Questions

1. What problem would you suspect if, during a myofascial release treatment, a patient began to sweat and become pale? What steps would you take to relieve the symptoms? Why might this occur?

2. A patient you are treating for a shoulder injury has range-of-motion measurements of 120° flexion, 90° abduction, and 40° lateral rotation. How would you improve this patient's range of motion? Why? If the patient's motion were 100° flexion, 125° abduction, and 70° lateral rotation, would your selection change? Why?

3. A patient who had surgery on his ankle 3 months ago has severe joint and soft-tissue restriction of all motions. There is more loss of plantar flexion than of dorsiflexion, and the soft tissue around the ankle feels very stiff. What techniques would you use to improve motion, and why? Which techniques would you emphasize the most, and why?

4. A patient complains of scapular area pain with some arm movements and has headaches. What are the possible causes of the patient's complaints? What treatments would you initiate, and why would you select those techniques? Would you give the patient any home program? If so, what would it include?

5. If you were Neil Dean, the athletic trainer in the scenario at the beginning of this chapter, what techniques would you use to relieve the soft-tissue adhesions of Pam's forearm? What home activities would you give her to increase soft-tissue mobility on her own?

Lab Activities

1. Apply grades I, II, III, and IV joint mobilization techniques to the tibiofemoral joint in anterior–posterior glides on your lab partner. Feel what the relative amounts of force and motion are for each grade. Now apply the same grades to your lab partner's number 2 MCP joint. What are the relative amounts of force and motion for this joint? How do they compare with those of the knee joint? Where in the mobility of the joint do you feel the resistance begin?

2. Apply mobilization grades I, II, III, and IV to your lab partner's glenohumeral joint. Feel for where the resistance begins. Does it become greater as you move the humerus through the glenoid fossa, or does it stay at a relatively consistent level of resistance throughout the mobilization? Draw it out on a movement diagram. How does the amount of mobility for each of the grades compare with those you found in the knee and MCP joints?

3. Locate a trigger point in your partner's scalenes and apply a trigger point release technique. How much pressure should you apply? How much stretch should you apply while you apply the pressure release? What will be your guidelines in determining the amount of pressure used? Can you feel the trigger point relax as you continue to hold the pressure on it?

4. A patient with rotator cuff repair has had the left arm in a sling for the past 3 weeks. He comes to you today, 3 weeks after the surgery, because his physician wants him to begin rehabilitation today. How can you determine if the patient will need manual therapy? How can you determine what type of manual therapy he will need? What kinds of problems would you expect him to have at this stage? What would today's treatment include? What would you avoid doing with him today? How will you know if your techniques are beneficial? Justify each of your answers.

12

Range of Motion and Flexibility Rehabilitation

Objectives

After completing this chapter, you should be able to do the following:

1. Define the differences between range of motion and flexibility.
2. List and discuss the deleterious effects of prolonged immobilization.
3. Discuss the mechanical properties of plasticity, elasticity, and viscoelasticity of connective tissue.
4. Explain the physiological properties of creep and stress–strain and how they affect stretching techniques.
5. Discuss the neuromuscular influences of the muscle spindle and GTO on stretching muscle.
6. Discuss the differences between PROM, AAROM, and AROM in rehabilitation.
7. Discuss the dynamic, static, and pre-contraction methods for stretching.
8. Identify two mechanical assistive devices used to increase range of motion.
9. List contraindications, indications, and precautions of stretching.
10. Discuss the selection of a stretching exercise program.

II

As a senior athletic training student, Darwin is on his first day at his new sports medicine clinical rotation. His first patient today is a new patient: Mr. O'Bay, a 55-year-old golfer with a shoulder injury. Darwin knows from his experiences at his last clinical site that he will measure the shoulder, elbow, wrist, and hand ranges of motion in all their planes of movement. He also knows that Mr. O'Bay had a rotator cuff repair, but he does not know when the surgery was performed, what specific repair was used, or the physician's postoperative restrictions on shoulder motion. He anticipates, though, that there will be some limitations and precautions. Although there should be no limitations on Mr. O'Bay's elbow, wrist, and hand motions, if the shoulder is immobilized in a sling, there may be some loss of motion in the elbow that must be evaluated and addressed.

What wound did ever heal but by degrees.

William Shakespeare, 1564-1616,
English playwright, poet, and actor

As you well know and as William Shakespeare indicates, it takes time for a wound to heal. In this chapter we will delve into the ideas and techniques designed to regain and maintain flexibility, including the proper times to integrate these interventions within a rehabilitation program. We will briefly review the physiological principles that affect tissue length changes, discuss the deleterious effects of prolonged immobilization, define the differences between range of motion and flexibility, identify normal range-of-motion values throughout the body, and discuss the various methods and progressions for achieving full motion.

By the end of this chapter, the consequences of establishing or not establishing normal motion and of delaying this part of the rehabilitation process should be clear. You will also know the techniques and skills needed for restoring range of motion, and you will learn about precautions and the progression of flexibility in rehabilitation.

Defining Flexibility and Range of Motion

IIIIIIIIIIIIIIIIIIIIIIIIIIIIIIIIIIIIIIIIIIIIIIIIIIIIIIIIIIIIIIIIIIIIIIIIIIIIIIIIIII

Range of motion and flexibility are closely related. Although the terms are often used interchangeably, their definitions are different.

Flexibility refers to a musculotendinous unit's ability to elongate when a stretching force is applied. The extent of a structure's flexibility is related to its stiffness, suppleness, or pliability. Prolonged loss of flexibility can reduce range of motion.

Range of motion is the amount of mobility of a joint and is determined by the soft-tissue and bony structures in the area. The status of soft tissues—including muscles, tendons, ligaments, capsule, skin, subcutaneous tissues, nerves, and blood vessels—affects a joint's range of motion. If a patient has impaired flexibility, range of motion is also limited.

Clinically, range-of-motion measurements quantify both range of motion and flexibility, as well as neuromuscular control to some extent. The control of muscle activity that produces active range of motion is centrally mediated. You will learn more about muscle activity in chapter 13. Although there is a technical distinction between range of motion and flexibility, clinical interpretations make differences less clear. For this reason, many clinicians use the terms *range of motion* and *flexibility* interchangeably.

CLINICAL TIPS

Although flexibility is a musculotendinous unit's ability to elongate and range of motion is a joint's mobility, loss of a muscle's flexibility may affect a joint's ability to move through its full motion. Likewise, if a joint is restricted in its mobility, a muscle may not be able to move throughout its full length. There are specific ways to delineate whether reduced motion is the result of joint or muscle changes in some body segments; these methods are presented in the specific body segment chapters in part IV.

Connective-Tissue Composition

IIIIIIIIIIIIIIIIIIIIIIIIIIIIIIIIIIIIIIIIIIIIIIIIIIIIIIIIIIIIIIIIIIIIIIIIIIIIIIIIIII

Mobility of the musculoskeletal system is determined by the composition of connective tissue and the orientation of the various soft-tissue structures. Connective tissue is mainly composed of two types of structures: cells and extracellular matrix. The cells of most interest in connective tissue are fibroblasts, the cells that create the connective tissue components collagen, elastin, reticulin, and ground substance. These components make up the extracellular matrix. The quantities of each of these substances vary according to the specific structure and determine the characteristics of the structure. For example, there is more collagen in ligament and more elastin in skin.

Collagen provides tissue with strength and stiffness. Although there are several different types of collagen in the body, Types I, II, and III are the ones of primary concern in the musculoskeletal system. Recall from chapter 2 that the collagen fibers bind themselves together; the more binding between the fibers, the greater the tensile strength and stability of the structure. Type I collagen fibers are five times as strong as elastin fibers.

Elastin fibers provide a structure with extensibility. Elastin fibers can withstand elongation stress and return to normal length. Tissues that have more elastin have more flexibility.

Reticulin fibers are essentially Type III collagen fibers. They are weaker than Type I. They are particularly important during repair after injury.

Ground substance is a structureless, organic gel-like material that reduces friction between the collagen and elastin fibers, maintains spacing between the fibers to prevent excessive cross-linking, and transports nutrients to the fibers.

There are three kinds of connective tissue in the body, and they are classified according to their density and arrangement. The fiber arrangement of **areolar (loose irregular) connective tissue** is irregular and loose, with relatively long distances between the cross-links. Loose connective tissue's open network is composed primarily of thin collagen and elastic fibers interlaced in several different directions. This arrangement provides the structure with tensile strength as well as pliability. Fascia of skin and fascia surrounding muscles and nerves are examples of areolar connective tissue. Loose irregular connective tissue lies between structures in areas where motion occurs, such as joint capsular fascia, intermuscular layers, and subcutaneous tissue. Areolar connective tissue permits movement in all directions.

A tendon is an example of a structure containing more highly organized connective tissue, with regular parallel collagen fibers and more cross-links. This arrangement allows **dense regular connective tissues** to resist high-tensile loads and still provide some flexibility. Ligaments are similar to tendons in their structure except that their fiber arrangement is not quite as regular, but they are still within this category of dense regular connective tissue. Ligament collagen fiber arrangements are primarily parallel, but there are also spiral and oblique arrangements.

On a continuum between the structural extremes in the arrangement, orientation, and quantity of fibers and cross-links in skin and tendons are structures such as ligaments, capsules, and fascia. Even within these tissue categories, fiber arrangements vary. For example, ligaments that must resist higher forces have more organized fiber arrangements with greater quantities of cross-links than other ligaments that undergo less stress.

The third type of connective tissue, **dense irregular connective tissue**, is similar to dense regular connective tissue, but its arrangement is not parallel. Dense irregular connective tissue is multidimensional in its fiber pattern.

Such an arrangement allows the tissue to provide resistance to forces in multiple directions. Such tissue provides for tensile strength but has little extensibility to deform. Examples of this connective tissue are found in joint capsules, aponeurosis expansions of tendons, and bone periosteum.

Therefore, connective tissue can influence all structures of interest to the rehabilitation clinician. It provides structure and strength to healthy tissue, and as part of scar tissue formation, it can be either detrimental or beneficial during healing. Since it lies within and between structures, connective tissue also affects the motion and function of structures when a body segment is immobilized, as we will see in the following section.

Effects of Immobilization on Connective Tissue

Connective tissue is continually replaced and reorganized as a normal body function. During this ongoing reorganization process, connective tissue tends to shorten.[1] Fortunately, normal daily activities overcome this tendency so that functional motion is preserved. However, if motion is restricted, either voluntarily or passively, rapid changes occur in the structure and function of connective tissue. After an injury, it is sometimes necessary to immobilize the area in order to protect it and permit the healing process to occur unimpeded. Immobilization, however, can also be detrimental. Depending on how long an area is immobilized, the changes that occur in connective tissue can be either reversible or permanent. Restricted range of motion can contribute to functional deficits and decreased quality of life; it is also associated with an increased risk of developing osteoarthritis.[2, 3] Although it does not take long for changes to occur, the longer a part is immobilized, the more difficult it becomes to restore the part to normal.

CLINICAL TIPS

Connective tissue supports the body and provides it with its framework. It is composed of many kinds of cells and fibrous and ground substances that form in various combinations, depending on the specific connective-tissue type. The primary fibers include collagen, reticulin, and elastin; collagen gives strength to tissue, while elastin provides resilience to withstand stresses. The proportions of these fibers vary between different types of connective tissue, and these variations account for the fact that connective tissues differ in the types, orientations, and linking of their fibers, which affect their ability to withstand stress.

To understand the problems involved in restoring normal range of motion and other lost parameters to an affected area, you must first understand the changes that occur with immobilization. Immobilization affects all tissue, from bone to skin.

General Changes in Soft Tissue

Soft-tissue changes are seen after even 1 week of immobilization and are increased by edema, trauma, and impaired circulation.[4] Immobilization causes a loss of ground substance, which in turn results in less separation and more cross-link formations between collagen fibers.[5, 6] The fiber meshwork contracts, and the tissue becomes dense, hard, and less supple.[5] Even if an uninjured joint is immobilized for 4 weeks, the dense connective tissue that forms prevents normal motion.[7]

After an injury, the newly formed fibrin and collagen fibers arrange themselves in a haphazard way when the injury is immobilized.[8] An increase in the formation of cross-links impairs motion. Although cross-links are necessary for collagen strength, too many cross-links can restrict the normal movement of collagen tissue (figure 12.1). After 2 weeks of immobilization, an injured joint has reduced motion because of these connective tissue changes.[9] Remember that as scar tissue forms, the natural process of wound contraction will augment the injured area's loss of motion.

When edema is present during immobilization of the segment, fibrosis increases,[10] probably because of the increased tissue fluid protein and metabolites the swelling

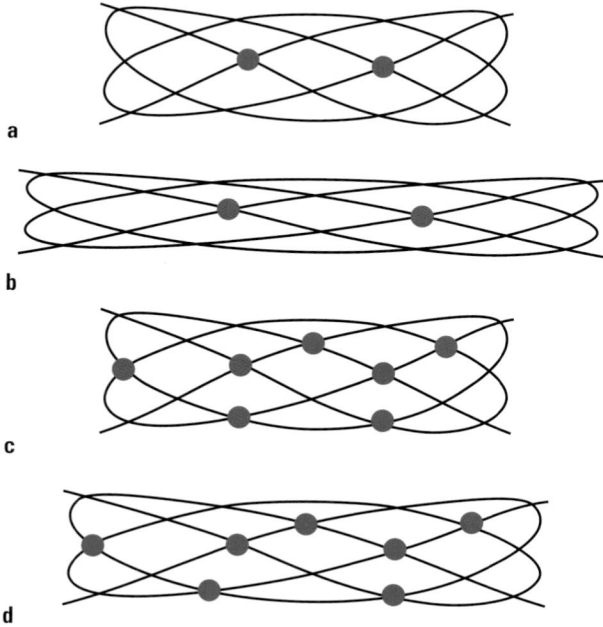

Figure 12.1 Schematic of collagen cross-links and how they reduce tissue mobility. Parts *(a)* and *(b)* are normal cross-links; *(c)* and *(d)* are excessive cross-links. Parts *(a)* and *(c)* are at resting length; *(b)* and *(d)* are stretched. An excessive number of cross-links prevents tissue from achieving full extensibility.

contains, along with deficient local metabolism caused by the immobilization. In essence, when an area has edema, the edema contains substances that cause the fluid to coagulate and become more solid. It is similar to setting gelatin, which starts out as a water mixture that becomes more solid when immobilized in a container. The result in the human body is that the tissue that is surrounded by the fluid becomes less mobile because it is bound to the coagulating fluid, leading to fibrosis. Fibrosis further increases when circulation is impaired, either because of age or local conditions. When edema remains in an area for a long time, it acts like a glue to bind down local tissue structures, reducing tissue mobility.

Even when an area is immobilized, connective tissue continues its normal process of remodeling and reorganizing.[11] Without movement, collagen creates a dense, hard meshwork of sheets or bands with a loss of normal suppleness as it re-forms. Collagen fibers then develop between the connective tissue's reticular fibers and between structures, "gluing down" the area. The result is restricted motion where otherwise normal areolar connective tissue would have permitted one tissue type to freely move over another. Muscle tissue becomes restricted by its own fascia, tendons lose their ability to move against adjacent tissues, and ligaments adhere to joint capsules.

Immobilization produces structural weakness as well as a loss of tissue mobility.[12] Weakness occurs because of a decrease in collagen mass. This is believed to occur because of the reduction in normal stresses on the immobilized part. On the other hand, Klein and colleagues[13] demonstrated that if motion is allowed in a non-weight-bearing extremity, the integrity of the ligaments is not lost. Additionally, bone density declines in immobilized, non-weight-bearing limbs.[13] Therefore, when possible, activity should begin early in rehabilitation for extremities with weight-bearing restrictions until weight bearing and a full rehabilitation exercise program are allowed.

Effects on Muscle Tissue

Changes in muscle tissue after immobilization and disuse include reductions in muscle fiber size, reductions in the number of myofibrils in the muscle, and reduced oxidative capacity.[12, 14, 15] As these changes occur, there is an increase in the amount of fibrous and fatty tissue in the muscle and a reduction in the intramuscular capillary density.[12] These changes, which cause the muscle to become smaller and weaker, occur after 2 weeks of immobilization.[16] The longer a muscle is immobilized and inactive, the greater the number of muscle fibers that degenerate, and the greater the amount of fibrous and fatty tissue that infiltrates the muscle.[15] As the muscle becomes weaker and loses its motion during the time it is immobilized, the normal neural feedback system of movement is also impaired. The combination of these factors, along with changes in the ligaments, impairs proprioception and neuromuscular control.[16-18]

Histological changes observed in immobilized muscle include decreased levels of adenosine triphosphate (ATP), adenosine diphosphate (ADP), creatine phosphate (CP), creatine, and glycogen.[12] When the immobilized muscle contracts, more than the normal level of lactic acid is produced.[12] These changes, along with a reduction in mitochondrial production and size, cause a reduction in the oxidative capacity of the muscle, which causes the muscle to fatigue more quickly and easily.

Several clinical observations can be made about immobilized muscle. The most obvious change is that the muscle is smaller. It also cannot produce as strong a contraction and cannot sustain activity for as long a time as it could before immobilization. The muscle is also slower to respond to a stimulus when it contracts, and it becomes fatigued more quickly.

Many of these changes occur within the first few days of immobilization. A decrease in muscle size (atrophy) and mitochondrial production occur within the first 5 to 7 d of immobilization.[14, 19] The rate of atrophy, however, varies from one muscle to another. For example, when the lower limb suffers disuse, the quadriceps becomes weaker and smaller more readily than the hamstrings.

Effects on Articular Cartilage

Articular cartilage also suffers changes from immobilization. These changes depend on the position of immobilization, the duration of immobilization, and whether or not the joint bears weight during immobilization. With immobilization, the mechanical properties decay: The cartilage becomes thinner, the proteoglycan concentration decreases, and the matrix organization declines.[20] The articular cartilage of joint surfaces that are not in contact with each other also changes. In addition, necrosis of articular cartilage occurs when there is constant pressure between the joint surfaces during immobilization.[21] Immobilization also increases the amount of fibrofatty tissue that ultimately becomes scar tissue within the joint.[5]

Buckwalter[20] indicated that joints suffer irreparable damage with continued or prolonged immobilization. He found that these changes include contracture of the joint because dense, fibrous tissue forms around the joint and in muscles that cross the joint; reduction of the articular cartilage lining of the joint surfaces; and replacement of the normal joint cavity with fibrofatty tissue.[20] The time required before the process becomes irreversible has not yet been established in humans. In rats, it occurs after 4 weeks of immobilization.[7] More recent findings indicated that even 1 week of immobilization with contact between the joint segments produced irreversible changes in articular cartilage in rats.[22] In rabbits, reversible changes occurred with 2 weeks of immobilization, but irreversible

changes were seen when knee joints were immobilized for 6 weeks.[23] Studies performed on animals also demonstrate that the longer an extremity is immobilized, the longer it takes to establish pre-immobilization parameters. For example, rabbits that had knees immobilized for 2 weeks took 2 months to restore motion, and only 64% of the rabbits with knees immobilized for 6 weeks regained partial or full motion after 4 months of remobilization.[23] Presumably, humans follow similar paths of degradation and restoration during episodes of immobilization and remobilization, with longer recovery times required for longer periods of immobilization. This recovery delay was presented in chapter 2.

Effects on Periarticular Connective Tissue

Periarticular connective tissue is soft tissue that surrounds a joint, including structures such as ligaments, joint capsules, fascia, tendons, and synovial membranes. As with muscle and articular cartilage, all these structures are adversely affected by immobilization, and their connective tissue becomes thick and fibrotic. As has been discussed, the ground substance, a viscous gel that contains glycosaminoglycans (GAGs) and water, separates the collagen fibers, lubricates the area, and keeps the fibers gliding freely. During immobilization, the GAG and water content in the ground substance is reduced, causing a diminution of extracellular matrix.[5] The combination of changes in ground substance, increased collagen cross-links, and continued normal collagen processing diminishes tissue mobility and strength.[5] The clinical impact of these changes is a loss of motion and weakened structures in the affected joint.

Time of Immobilization and Tissue Healing Timeline

With all these dramatic changes from immobilization, it makes sense to minimize the duration of immobilization. Immobilization is important and necessary after some injuries and surgeries. It is in the best interest of the patient, however, to base the time of immobilization on the course of injury and healing timeline that was discussed in chapter 2.

Recall that collagen formation is well underway 7 d after an injury. The injury has gone from inflammation to proliferation and is entering the start of the remodeling phase. By day 21, the remodeling phase is in full swing, and a permanent structure is emerging. Although there are exceptions, gentle range-of-motion activities may usually start by day 7 and certainly should be instituted by the third week after injury or surgery.

From a biological standpoint, the initiation of range-of-motion activities depends on the severity of the injury, the tissue and body part involved, and the surgical repair technique used. From a practical standpoint, it is also determined by the patient's ability and status, the philosophy of the physician, the physician's confidence in his or her own surgical repair, and the abilities of the rehabilitation clinician.

Effects of Remobilization on Connective Tissue

In the late 20th century, orthopedic injuries were commonly immobilized for several weeks after surgical repair. Since that time, our discoveries about the deleterious long-term effects of this practice, along with findings about the benefits of early remobilization, have led to the elimination of prolonged immobilization in postinjury and postoperative care. Just as there are many disadvantages to prolonged immobilization, there are many advantages to early remobilization.

Collagen in all tissue is affected by remobilization. Immobilization causes collagen to be misaligned during its development;[9] this causes a reduction in tensile strength. Remobilization effectively improves its strength.[24] In addition to this important understanding of remobilization, specific tissues have additional specific responses to being moved after immobilization. However, the longer a body segment is immobilized, the less its structures will be able to return to their former levels, both chemically and physically.[7, 25, 26] Long-term changes have been found when immobilization occurs for 1 week,[22] and more permanent results occur with 4 weeks of immobilization.[25] The following few paragraphs summarize the advantageous effects of mobilization.

Effects on Muscle Fibers

Muscle fibers recover from immobilization if its duration has not been excessive. Initially, the recovery is rapid, but as it continues, the rate of improvement slows before full recovery occurs.[27] Injured muscle responds best to a short period of immobilization followed by active motion.[28] Movement causes a more rapid absorption of hematoma, an increase in tensile strength, and improved myofiber regeneration and arrangement for an effective overall recovery.[29] With immobilization, adhesions of muscle to fascia reduce the muscle's flexibility and affect joint range of motion.[30] Techniques for treating these restrictions are discussed in chapter 11.

Effects on Articular Cartilage

Articular cartilage will suffer less degeneration if both joint motion and weight bearing are allowed on a limited basis.[31] Controlled weight bearing or loading of articular cartilage may even encourage the repair of damaged cartilage.[32]

Research findings consistently indicate that a joint, after injury, responds best to a rehabilitation program that provides controlled loading and movement, which stimulate proteoglycan and chondrocyte production.[33]

Effects on Periarticular Connective Tissue

Timely remobilization of periarticular connective tissue prevents abnormal cross-link formation and helps to maintain the fluid content of the extracellular matrix so that proper fiber distance can be maintained.[34] Fatty tissue buildup around the joint limits mobility and must be broken by techniques such as stretching and joint mobilization.[35, 36] Stretching techniques are discussed later in this chapter, and joint mobilization is discussed in chapter 11.

CLINICAL TIPS

Although immobilization is sometimes necessary for tissue to heal properly, clinicians must understand the deleterious effects that long-term immobilization has on human tissues. The longer a segment is immobilized, the longer it takes for the segment to achieve optimal rehabilitation results. Restricted range of motion can contribute to functional deficits and decreased quality of life.

Connective Tissue Mechanical Properties and Behavior in Range of Motion

Even when an extremity is not immobilized, injury or surgery causes scar tissue formation. As scar tissue forms, it can lead to adhesions of adjacent tissue and increased fibrosis. When loss of motion occurs, it is because connective tissue extensibility diminishes.[37, 38] Connective tissue is in joint capsules, ligaments, tendons, and fascia. Although muscles are not composed primarily of connective tissue as these other structures are, muscles are surrounded by an extensive fascial network that affects their flexibility and response to stretch.[39] Therefore, flexibility of all tissues that rehabilitation clinicians deal with is influenced by connective tissue.

To determine the most effective ways to increase the range of motion of injured parts, it is important to review the physiology of connective tissue. Stretching exercises can affect the noncontractile element of all connective tissue. Because collagen gives tensile strength, resilience, and form to a structure, it is also the main cause of restricted range of motion; therefore, it should be the primary target of stretching exercises.

Remember that body parts respond to forces in three dimensions. When stress is applied, a structure's response depends on the direction, duration, and magnitude of the force and the specific elements affected.

Mechanical Properties of Connective Tissue

To effectively apply stretch forces to connective tissue, you must first understand its mechanical properties. Connective tissue is elastic, viscoelastic, and plastic and possesses all three qualities simultaneously. When connective tissue is stretched, all three qualities may be affected. If we separate the properties and look at them individually, it might be easier to understand how collagen functions and what we can do to influence it. Plasticity allows the connective tissue's length to change, while elasticity allows some restoration of normal length following an applied stress. As previously mentioned, the effectiveness of the stretch depends on the amount of collagen and elastin in the gross structure. The effectiveness of the stretch also depends on the amount of force applied, the duration of the stretch, the temperature of the tissue, and the physical properties of collagen.

Elasticity

Elasticity is the ability of a structure to return to its normal length after the application of an elongation force or load (stress). This restoration of length occurs because of the structure's stored potential energy. Elastic material is commonly symbolized by a spring in engineering models (figure 12.2a). A rubber band easily demonstrates elasticity. If you give a rubber band a brief pull, then release the force, the rubber band returns to its normal length.

Viscosity and Viscoelasticity

Viscoelasticity is a property of substances that are both elastic and viscous. **Viscosity** is the resistance to an outside force that causes a fluid-like, permanent deformation. Resistance occurs from a cohesion of molecules that provides a shearing force to resist a change in structural shape. No potential energy is stored in a viscous object, so there is no energy to permit its return to normal length; the energy is released as heat before it can be stored. An example of a viscous substance is tar. A hydraulic cylinder represents viscosity, as in figure 12.2b. **Viscoelasticity**, then, is the ability of a structure to use its elastic properties to resist a change of shape when an outside force is applied but an inability to completely return to its former state after changing shape because of its viscous properties. A combination of a spring and a hydraulic cylinder represents viscoelasticity (figure 12.2c). We see viscoelasticity demonstrated when we stretch the hamstrings. After a stretch, there is an increase in hamstring length; if we examine the hamstring a little later, some of the length that was originally gained is maintained because of the viscous component, but some is lost because of the elastic component.

Plasticity

Plasticity is the ability of a substance to undergo a permanent change in size or shape after a deforming force is applied. Viscosity and plasticity create similar effects in human tissue. An example of plasticity is pulling a ball of putty; the putty changes in length and does not return to its former condition when you release your force. Plasticity is represented by a block, as seen in figure 12.2d. If the force applied to the block is greater than the structure can withstand, the structure will lengthen; if the applied

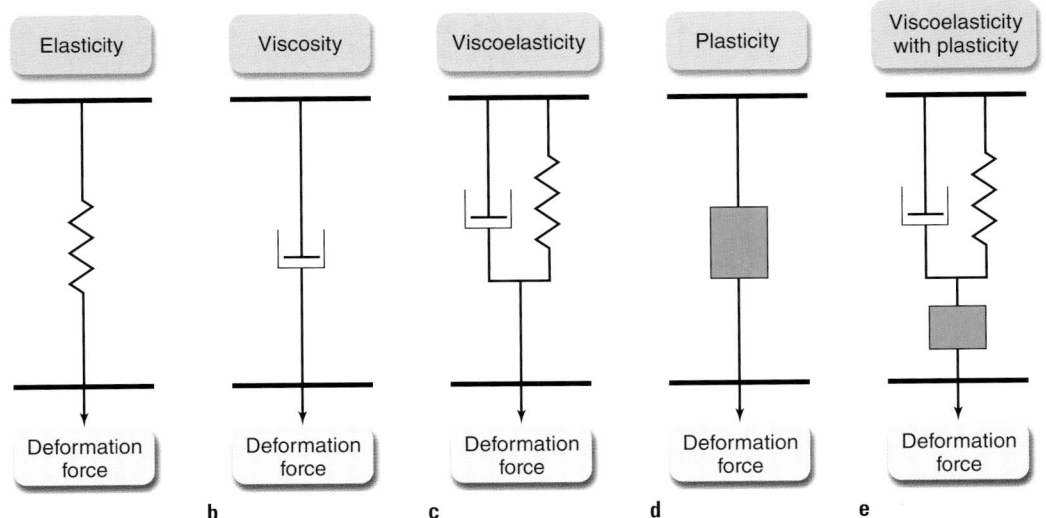

Figure 12.2 Models of tissue resistance against forces of deformation: *(a)* elasticity, *(b)* viscosity, *(c)* viscoelasticity, *(d)* plasticity, and *(e)* viscoelasticity with plastic components.

force is less than the structure's resistance to change, no lengthening will take place. We see this phenomenon with the plasticity of collagen: A change in length occurs when the applied force is greater than the force that attaches the collagen fibers to one another.

Figure 12.2e diagrams the combination of plastic and viscoelastic elements working against a resistance force, but it fails to identify how tissues with these characteristics resist deformation forces applied to them. Since biological tissue has both plastic and viscoelastic elements, figure 12.3 is a more practical representation of the body's tissue response to a load. When a load is applied to the structure in this model (figure 12.3b), the tissue responds with its viscous and elastic elements first, followed by plastic deformation when the viscoelastic components are used up. When the load is released (figure 12.3c), there is some change in the structure's length because of the plastic deformation, but there is also some return toward normal length because of the elastic elements of tissue. It is important to understand that before plastic elements can be affected by a stretch, the elastic and viscous elements must reach their end points first.

Physical Properties of Connective Tissue

The physical behaviors of connective tissue in response to stretching exercises include force relaxation and creep. They are both time-dependent responses that rely on the duration of the outside force and the rate at which it is

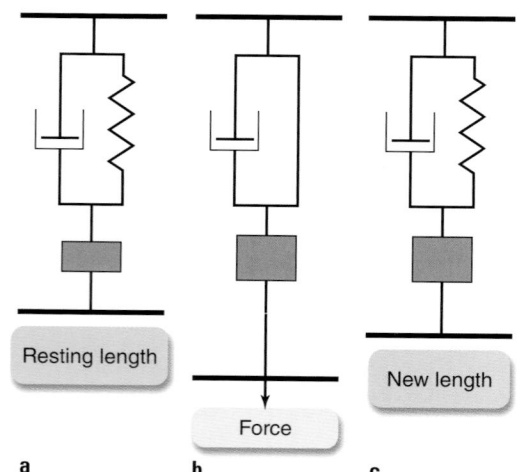

Figure 12.3 An illustration of the integration of plastic and viscoelastic qualities of tissue resistance working against a force to increase the tissue's length. *(a)* Tissue without a force resisting its length. *(b)* Tissue unable to withstand a force with plastic tissue changes occurring after viscous and elastic elements have reached their end limits. *(c)* Plastic changes remain after the stretch is released and viscoelastic qualities are returned, resulting in new tissue length.

applied. **Force relaxation**, or **force deformation**, is the amount of force that is applied to maintain a change of length or other deformation of tissue. It results in a relaxation of the tissue. If the force is applied too quickly and viscoelastic and plastic changes result that are faster or greater than the tissue can tolerate, an injury can occur. Also, there is more viscoelastic resistance to rapid change than to slowly applied forces; for example, removing a stick from a bucket of tar quickly is more difficult, with the tar providing greater resistance to change, than if the stick is removed with a slowly applied upward force. Likewise, collagen resists rapidly applied deformation forces. Thus it is easier to affect changes in tissue length with slowly applied elongation forces.

Creep

Creep is the elongation of tissue when a load, usually low level, is applied for an extended time to cause plastic deformation.[40] The result is a permanent change in the tissue's length. Creep is time dependent, so a load that is applied for a longer time is more effective in causing a change in tissue length than a load that is applied and released quickly. Increasing the tissue's temperature increases the rate of creep.[41] In functional terms, applying heat to a muscle before and during a stretch improves range of motion and permits a better stretch.[41, 42]

Recall that if a load is applied in the elastic range, the structure gradually returns to normal length once the load is released.[43] This force level does not cause a permanent change in tissue length.[44] The load applied must reach the end of the viscous and elastic ranges and affect the plastic range of deformation of the tissue to result in permanent change in tissue length.[45]

A structure's length can also be affected by structural fatigue. Fatigue occurs when a structure is loaded repeatedly below the failure point until the cumulative stress results in failure;[46] the greater the load, the fewer the repetitions needed for failure to occur. The point at which structural fatigue causes tissue failure is referred to as **fatigue failure** or the **endurance limit**. When structural fatigue occurs in bones, it is called a stress fracture; when it occurs in tendons, it is called tendinopathy.

Stress–Strain

The load required to change the length of connective tissue is directly related to the tissue's strength, and the tissue's strength is directly related to its ability to resist a load. This relationship is defined by **Hooke's law**, which states that the strain (deformation) of an object is directly related to the object's ability to resist the stress (load), and it is illustrated by the stress–strain curve.[47] **Stress** is a force that changes the form or shape of a body. Connective tissue is subject to three types of stress: tension stress (stretching force), compression stress (from muscle contractions and weight bearing on joints), and shear force (force applied parallel to the cross section of the tissue).

Strain is the amount of deformation a structure undergoes when a stress is applied. All structures have a stress–strain curve that represents their own specific ability to resist deforming forces. Although various body tissues' stress–strain curves may differ in timing and magnitude, they share the same general characteristics. The specific reactions of a tissue to a load are illustrated in figure 12.4.

The initial portion of the stress–strain curve is the toe region. In connective tissue, the collagen fibers have a wavy crimp arrangement at rest. The toe region accounts for 1.5% to 5%[48] of the total collagen fiber lengthening that is possible. As a force is applied, the fibers stretch into the elastic range. As the slack in the collagen is taken up when a stretch force is applied, it loses its wavy appearance. At a macroscopic level, resistance is felt when the tissue reaches the end of its elastic limit. In the elastic range, a collagen fiber elongates 2% to 5% beyond its resting length.[49] The tissue's full normal range of motion is in the elastic range. If the force is released in this range, the tissue will return to its prestretch length.

At the yield strength point, the stress loads the tissue beyond its elastic range and into its plastic range. Tissue loaded into this range undergoes permanent elongation. This is the result of a few of the collagen fibers failing to withstand the stress, creating a disruption of some cross-links. Collagen fibers fail through a number of mechanisms, including a failure of the force-relaxation response when a load is applied too quickly for the collagen's viscoelastic and plastic adaptations to occur. Fibers also tear if the creep response causes too much deformation too quickly. This deformation can occur either in one episode or from accumulated stress from a number of lesser loads. This failure of isolated collagen fibers occurs unpredictably and results in an increase in range of motion.[50]

Two factors beyond the plastic range should be mentioned. **Ultimate strength** is the greatest load that a tissue can tolerate. After this point, the fiber length changes without the application of any additional load. The point of ultimate strength is not usually a goal in stretching. There may be a necking region prior to failure of the tissue, where the tissue's resistance to the strength force noticeably decreases so that less stress is needed to cause a change in the tissue's length. When this occurs, tissue failure or rupture is often imminent if the application of stress continues.

Fatigue failure is the point at which the tissue cannot tolerate continued stress, and so it ruptures. In collagen, this occurs when the fiber is stretched to 6% to 10% beyond its resting length.[49, 51]

The general shape of the stress–strain curve appears in figure 12.4, but the specific shape of the curve varies from one structure to another. The initial portion in the toe region of the curve is curvilinear, but as the stress–strain curve moves from the elastic to the plastic region, the curve becomes more linear.[52] Several factors, known and unknown, influence a tissue's specific curve; some of these factors include an individual's sex, height, and body mass index (BMI).[48]

Some additional factors influence the failure point of an entire body structure rather than just its connective tissue content. Tissue width is one of these factors. A structure's larger cross-sectional size indicates more fibers, so more stress is required to produce failure of the structure. The tissue's slack length is another factor. Longer tissues can withstand greater forces because they have more slack. For example, if two pieces of rope have the same number of fibers but one is twice as long as the other, the longer rope can tolerate more deformation before breaking. The microstructure of the tissue and the orientation of the structure to the forces applied also influence the ability of the ligament or tendon to withstand deforming loads.[53]

Stiffness of tissue is its resistance to deformation when stress is applied to it.[54] The more stiffness tissue has, the greater its ability to maintain its original shape. At the other end of the spectrum, tissue with **compliance** is easily deformed.[55] Compliant tissue stretches with low-level forces, while tissues with stiffness can resist deformation with high-level forces.

Hysteresis

Repetitive stretching with submaximal loads can also be effective in increasing range of motion. Heat energy, a by-product of stress, is released when stress is applied to tissue. As local tissue is heated with repetitive stretches, the tissue is more easily stretched. When tissue cannot

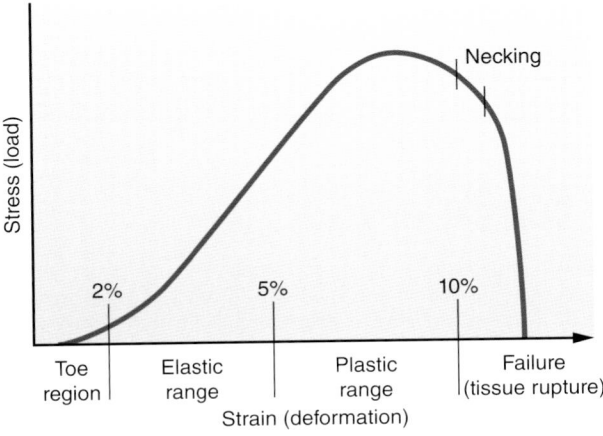

Figure 12.4 Generic stress–strain curve. Although different tissues have different specific configurations, all tissues abide by the stress–strain curve concept. Some tissues may have a larger toe region and others may have a more abrupt stress–strain ratio, but all tissues have a stress–strain curve that contains toe, elastic, plastic, and failure regions.

keep pace with the forces, with each successive load application, it elongates more. This response is **hysteresis**. When a stress force is released, the tissue returns to its normal length at a different rate from the rate at which it was stretched, as seen in figure 12.5.

As the tissue changes length and is heated with repeated stretches, higher-level loads are tolerated in subsequent repetitions, as seen in figure 12.6. In other words, the tissue's failure load increases, so a greater force can be applied to produce additional tissue deformation (lengthening).[56] This principle is used when a **proprioceptive neuromuscular facilitation (PNF)** stretch is applied, released, and then reapplied to a patient's hamstrings; in the second stretch, the patient's hamstring is stretched farther and the patient can tolerate a slightly greater stretch force.

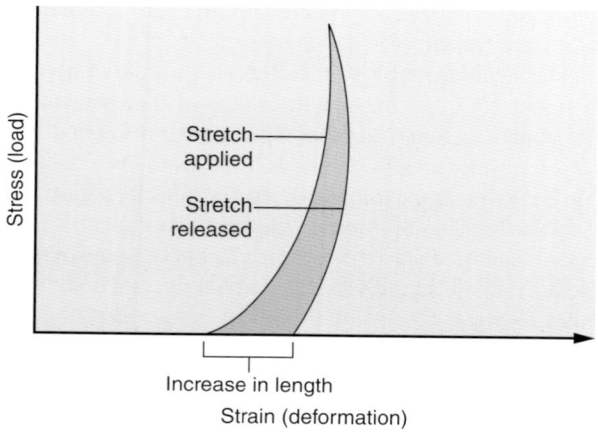

Figure 12.5 Hysteresis. Heat released by stress application causes tissue to have more pliability, allowing for an increase in tissue length.

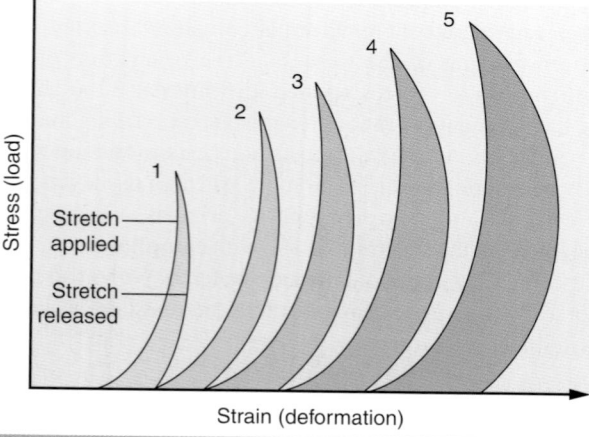

Figure 12.6 Deformation with hysteresis in repetitive stretching. As tissue is stretched repetitively, the overall length of a structure increases, and the tissue can tolerate increasing applications of stress.

Rehabilitation and Using the Physical Properties of Connective Tissue

So, now that we understand all of the physical properties of connective tissue, why is it important to us in rehabilitation? There are two good reasons why this information is important. Before we discuss these reasons, recall that tissue healing occurs over four phases. During the inflammation phase, there is no collagen formation, but during the proliferation phase it starts to appear. In the inflammation phase, injured tissue is at its weakest, relying only on the fibrin plug for tensile strength. As collagen forms, tensile strength increases. Finally, in the remodeling phase, we see a conversion of Type III collagen to the stronger Type I collagen and a completion of the maturation process.

Here are the important rehabilitation points relative to the physical properties of connective tissue we have just identified. First, tissue does not have the strength to withstand significant stresses during the inflammation phase. If we apply stresses during this time, we may further damage tissue. Second, once healing moves into the proliferation phase, we may begin mild mobilization of tissue since it is during this time that Type III collagen is being laid down in a disorganized fashion, improving healing tissue strength; Type III collagen is pliable enough to be influenced by motion. As collagen converts from Type III to Type I and tissue maturation progresses over time, it becomes less influenced by our attempts to increase mobility. This resistance to change occurs as the collagen becomes more resilient to applied stresses and as the adhesions that have formed between the newer fibers and the surrounding tissues become more permanent. Given this healing progression, the best time to influence collagen arrangement is during proliferation and in early remodeling. Figure 12.7 demonstrates the relationship between healing, the degree of risk to tissue when a force is applied to it, and the ability to influence and change collagen arrangement throughout the healing process.

CLINICAL TIPS

A tissue's mechanical properties, such as plasticity, elasticity, and viscoelasticity, affect its response to force and thus to stretching. A stretch exercise must move tissue beyond its elastic range and into its plastic range to have long-term effects on tissue mobility or flexibility.

Neuromuscular Influences on Range of Motion

In addition to the physical and mechanical properties of connective tissue, neurological factors influence the

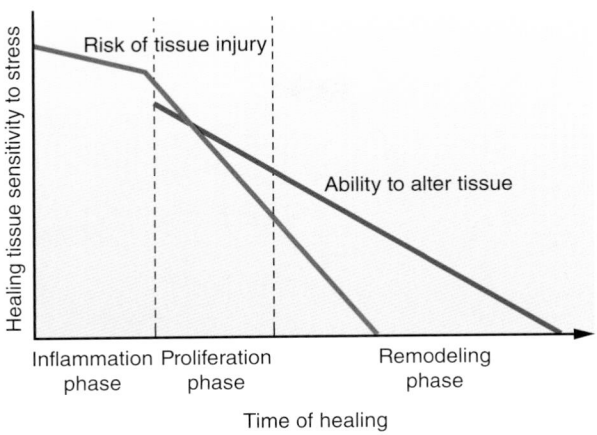

Figure 12.7 Relationship between hazards of tissue mobilization and time to influence collagen change after injury occurs. The further into the remodeling phase healing tissue advances, the less effective stretching activities will be in changing scar tissue length or mobility.

effectiveness of stretching techniques in increasing range of motion. Neurological components that affect a muscle's ability to respond to a stretch force include the muscle spindle and the Golgi tendon organ (GTO). The muscle spindle is much more complex than the GTO.

Muscle Spindle

There is a variation in the ratio of muscle spindles to muscle fibers between individual muscles. The more precise the movement required of a muscle, the lower the ratio of muscle fibers to muscle spindles.[57] A typical muscle fiber is an **extrafusal fiber**. Muscle spindles vary in length and diameter, but all lie between and are parallel to the extrafusal muscle fibers. The muscle fibers that contain the muscle spindles are the **intrafusal muscle fibers**.

Entering the intrafusal muscle fiber are three efferent nerve fibers: alpha, beta, and gamma nerves, as noted in figure 12.8. Exiting the intrafusal fibers are the Ia, Ib, and II afferent, or sensory, fibers. The muscle spindle is composed of these nerve fibers, the intrafusal muscle fibers, and the sac that surrounds these structures. There are two types of intrafusal fibers, and each has a different function within a muscle spindle. One type, the **nuclear bag fiber**, has an enlarged center region with two or three nuclei stacked beside each other.[58] The shorter, thinner fibers are **nuclear chain fibers**, and their nuclei are in single file in the center region.[58] Although both are sensitive to stretch, the nuclear bag fiber has more elasticity and is, therefore, sensitive to the velocity of the stretch.

An afferent Ia nerve fiber wraps around the center region of the intrafusal fibers. This nerve ending is sometimes called a *primary ending* or an *annulospiral ending*. The secondary or II afferent nerve endings are at the ends of the

intrafusal muscle fibers, primarily on nuclear chain fibers, and are sometimes called *flower-spray endings* because of their appearance. Because of the structure of Ia nerve fibers, they respond much more quickly to stimulation than the II nerves. The Ia nerve fibers are sensitive to a quick stretch, while both Ia and II nerve fibers respond to a static stretch.[59-61]

Because the intrafusal fiber attaches to the connective tissue surrounding extrafusal muscle fibers, the intrafusal muscle fiber is sensitive to changes in the muscle's length. Both afferent nerve fibers in the muscle spindle transmit signals to the spinal cord about changes in the muscle's length and the velocity and duration of a stretch. An efferent response sent to both the intrafusal and extrafusal muscle fibers causes the muscle to react to the stimulation. Gamma efferent fibers transmit to the intrafusal muscle fibers, and alpha efferent fibers transmit to the extrafusal muscle fibers; stimulation of the extrafusal fibers produces the muscle's contraction. Once the muscle contracts and shortens, stress and stimulation of the muscle spindles cease.

In addition to stimulating the muscle in which they lie, a muscle's group I nerve fibers send branches to synergistic muscles and antagonistic muscles. The result is simultaneous stimulation of synergistic muscles and inhibition of antagonistic muscles.[62] Group II nerve fibers also transmit to the synergistic and antagonistic muscles, but they use another neuron link to complete the transmission. The impact of stimulating synergistic muscles is made more apparent in chapter 11 during the discussion of proprioceptive neuromuscular facilitation (PNF).

Golgi Tendon Organs

Like the muscle spindle, the **Golgi tendon organ (GTO)** also functions as a protective mechanism. Golgi tendon organs are not as sensitive to stretch as muscle spindles, but they are very sensitive to contraction and tension in a muscle.

Golgi tendon organs, located at the distal and proximal muscle–tendon junctions, are long, delicate, tubular capsules that contain a cluster of Ib nerve fibers. These nerve fibers originate on the tendon's fascicles. The protection performed by the GTO is known as **autogenic inhibition**.[63] When the GTO is stimulated, its activity causes simultaneous inhibition of the alpha motor neuron of its own muscle and internuncial activation (between afferent and efferent neurons) of the antagonistic muscle.

The result of the combined reactions of the muscle spindle and the GTO is evident in functional activities. If a muscle stretches quickly, the muscle spindle produces a **monosynaptic response**, which is a rapid reflex motor response resulting from a direct neural connection between a sensory (afferent) and motor (efferent) nerve in the spinal cord without an intermediary neuron. A monosynaptic response is the most rapid response because only two

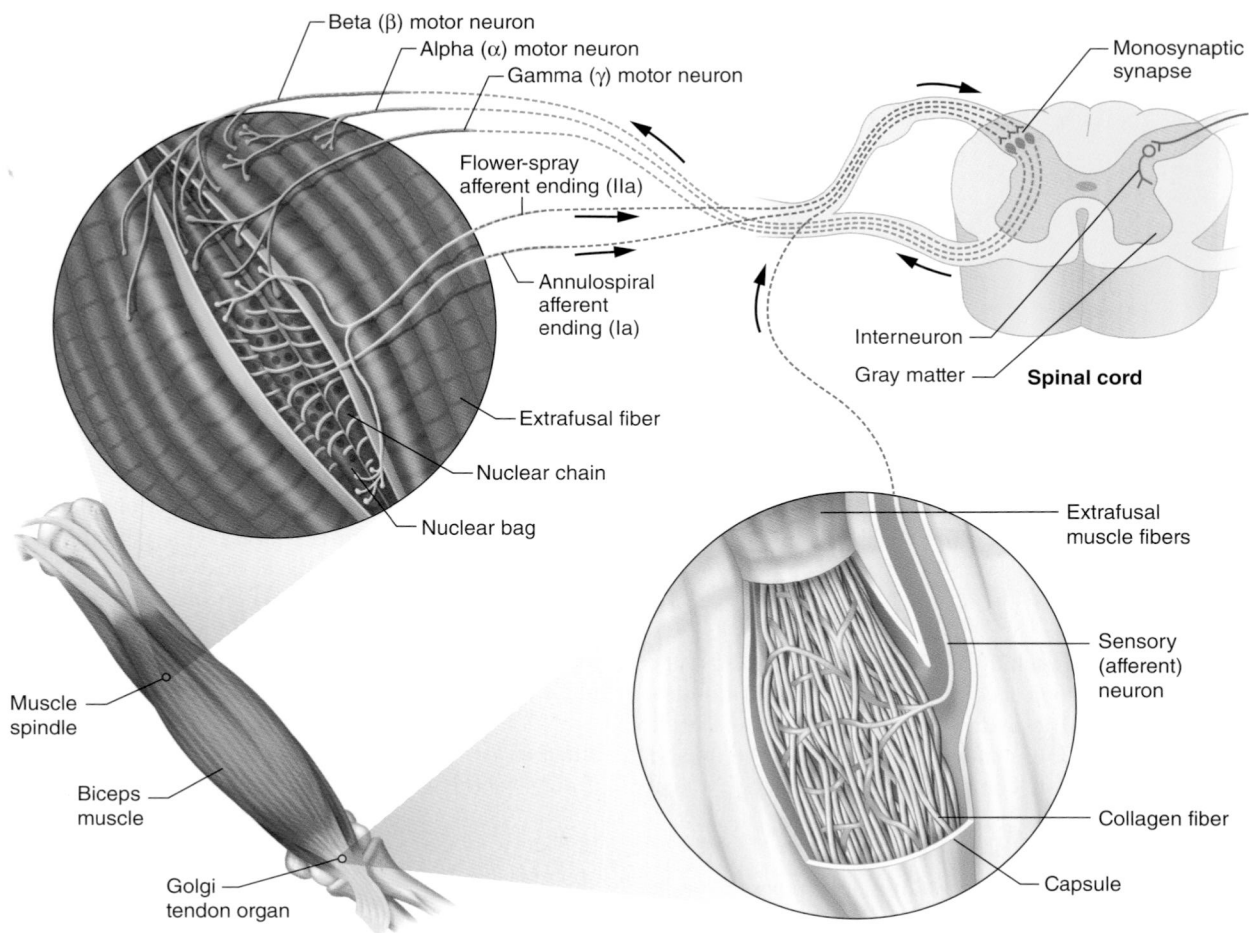

Figure 12.8 Muscle spindles within the muscle and Golgi tendon organs within the musculotendinous junction are neural receptors that are sensitive to changes in muscle length and tension.

nerves are involved. If a stretch force is applied too quickly, the muscle being stretched reflexively responds secondarily to stimulation of the muscle spindle. This reflex potentially occurs with ballistic stretching and is discussed later in this chapter. On the other hand, if a stretch occurs more slowly, the GTO inhibits muscular contraction. This application may actually provide better relaxation of the muscle to improve the effectiveness of the stretch.

Determining Normal Range of Motion

Before you can determine whether a joint has deficient range of motion (ROM), you must first know what normal motion is. Table 12.1 illustrates the dispute among authors about what is considered normal, although all are within close range of one another. Differences are likely due to the specific populations the investigators measured to collect

their data. Measurement results are affected by the age and sex of subjects and the positions in which measurements are taken. Regardless of whose data are used, they provide rehabilitation clinicians with a guideline for expectations of normal ROM.

Each patient's normal range of motion for an injured joint is determined by examining the uninjured contralateral joint. It is also based on the demands of the individual's activities. For example, normal ranges of motion for shoulder lateral rotation are different for a baseball pitcher and a football lineman.

It is important for you to become familiar with normal ranges of motion. Without this knowledge, it is difficult to determine when a problem exists.

Limited range of motion is often multifactorial, and so the treatment plan must be comprehensive. If problem areas are not identified, proper rehabilitation programs cannot be designed, nor can the program succeed.

TABLE 12.1 Various Authors' Judgments of Normal Ranges of Motion (in degrees)

Joint motion	Hoppenfeld[64]	Daniels and Worthingham[65]	AAOS[66]	Kendall et al.[67]	Kapandji[68, 69]	Esch and Lepley[70]	Gerhardt and Russe[71]
Shoulder							
Flexion	180	—	180	180	180	170	170
Extension	45	50	60	45	50	60	50
Abduction	180	—	180	180	180	170	170
Lateral rotation	45	90	90	90	80	90	90
Medial rotation	55	90	70	70	95	80	80
Horizontal abduction	—	—	—	—	—	—	30
Horizontal adduction	—	—	135	—	—	—	135
Elbow							
Flexion	135+	145–160	150	145	145–160	150	150
Forearm							
Supination	90	90	80	90	80	90	90
Pronation	90	90	80	90	85	90	80
Wrist							
Extension	70	70	70	70	85	70	50
Flexion	80	90	80	80	85	90	60
Radial deviation	20	—	20	20	15	20	20
Ulnar deviation	30	—	30	35	45	30	30
Thumb, carpometacarpal							
Abduction	70	50	70	80	50	—	—
Flexion	—	—	15	45	—	—	—
Extension	—	—	20	0	—	—	—
Opposition	Tip of thumb to tip of 5th finger (all authors agree)						
Thumb, metacarpophalangeal							
Flexion	50	70	50	60	80	—	—
Thumb, interphalangeal							
Flexion	90	90	80	80	80	—	—
Digits 2–5, metacarpophalangeal							
Flexion	90	90	90	90	—	—	—
Extension	45	30	45	—	—	—	—
Digits 2–5, proximal interphalangeal							
Flexion	100	120	—	—	—	—	—
Digits 2–5, distal interphalangeal							
Flexion	90	80	—	—	—	—	—
Subtalar joint							
Inversion	—	—	35	35	52	30	40
Eversion	—	—	20	20	30	15	20
Ankle, talocrural							
Dorsiflexion	20	—	20	20	20–30	10	20
Plantar flexion	50	45	50	45	50	65	45

>continued

TABLE 12.1 >*continued*

Joint motion	Hoppenfeld[64]	Daniels and Worthingham[65]	AAOS[66]	Kendall et al.[67]	Kapandji[68, 69]	Esch and Lepley[70]	Gerhardt and Russe[71]
Knee							
Flexion	135	135	135	140	135	135	130
Hip							
Flexion	120	115–125	120	125	120	130	125
Extension	30	15	30	10	30	45	15
Abduction	45–50	45	45	45	45	45	45
Adduction	20–30	—	30	10	30	15	15
Medial rotation	35	45	45	45	45	33	45
Lateral rotation	45	45	45	45	60	36	45

CLINICAL TIPS

Normal range-of-motion requirements are different for each joint, each patient, and each sport and position. The clinician must know not only the normal ranges of motion for each joint but also the expectations for joint motion within specific activities and sports. What is considered normal motion for a joint may actually be deficient motion if the patient does not have enough motion to perform a desired activity.

Range-of-Motion Activities

Range-of-motion activities are a basic intervention for initiating movement in the rehabilitation program. We have already discussed how important appropriately timed movement is to healing tissue. Range-of-motion activities are used to maintain or improve soft-tissue or joint mobility in an effort to minimize loss of tissue flexibility and contracture formation.[34] Range-of-motion activities also nourish articular cartilage through synovial fluid movement.[72] This section will not discuss ROM activities to improve impaired mobility. The principles of soft-tissue and joint mobilization are discussed in chapter 11, and stretching is addressed in the next section of this chapter.

Types of Range-of-Motion Activities

There are four types of ROM activities: passive range of motion (PROM), active-assistive range of motion (AAROM), active range of motion (AROM), and resistive range of motion (RROM). The specific technique used depends on many factors, including phase of tissue healing, patient pain level, postoperative status, integrity of tissue repair, patient general health, and physician preference.

Passive Range of Motion

Passive range of motion is the amount of motion achieved without the assistance of the patient. The movement is produced by an external force such as another person, gravity, or a device. No voluntary muscle contraction occurs. See figure 12.9. Passive range-of-motion activities are indicated when tissue is acutely injured or in the inflammatory phase of tissue healing; when patients cannot move the part themselves—for example, when they are in pain, paralyzed, or on complete bed rest; or when they are not supposed to

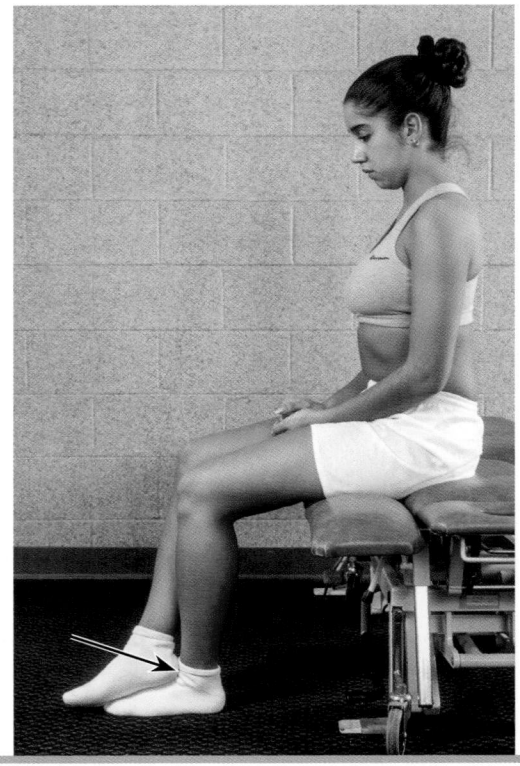

Figure 12.9 PROM for left knee flexion. The uninvolved right extremity pushes the involved left knee into passive flexion.

move actively, as may be the case if they have had a recent tissue repair or reconstruction. Denard and Ladermann[73] found that immediate PROM after total shoulder arthroplasty provided a more rapid return to function than a delayed ROM protocol.[73] The general goals of PROM are to minimize adhesions, maintain connective tissue mobility, maintain muscle elasticity, assist with circulatory and vascular mechanics, promote synovial fluid movement, and decrease or inhibit pain. Passive range-of-motion activities do not improve muscle strength or function.

Continuous passive motion (CPM) refers to PROM performed by a machine. After major surgery, the physician may prescribe the use of a CPM machine for the involved segment. See figure 12.10. A CPM machine does not harm the surgical site, but it provides immediate postoperative motion, reduces pain, and lessens edema that can otherwise limit postoperative motion.[74] A study by Liao and colleagues[75] concluded that when CPM is used, early application with initial high flexion settings accompanied by rapid progress improved knee function.[75] The use of CPM machines is not as prevalent today as it was when they were first introduced; surgeons have discovered that early active motion within safe bounds can also produce similar beneficial results.

Specifically designed splints provide passive prolonged stretching of restricted tissue. Splints that apply a very low-level, continuous stretch force for several hours are beneficial with very mature or restricted scar tissue.[76] They commonly use a three-point lever-and-spring system to provide a low-level, continuous load. These devices stretch connective tissue surrounding joints, but they do not change muscle length. The magnitude of the load and the angle at which the stretch is applied are adjusted to meet the patient's needs. A splint is worn for several hours at a time, most often overnight, to cause effective plastic deformation of connective tissue.[77] It is common for the

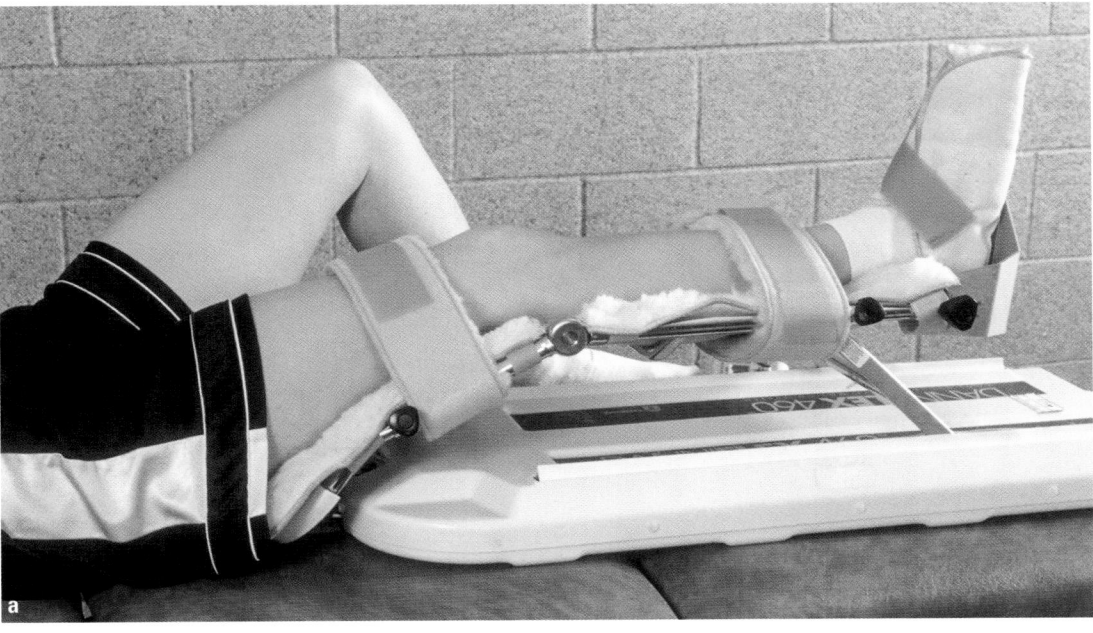
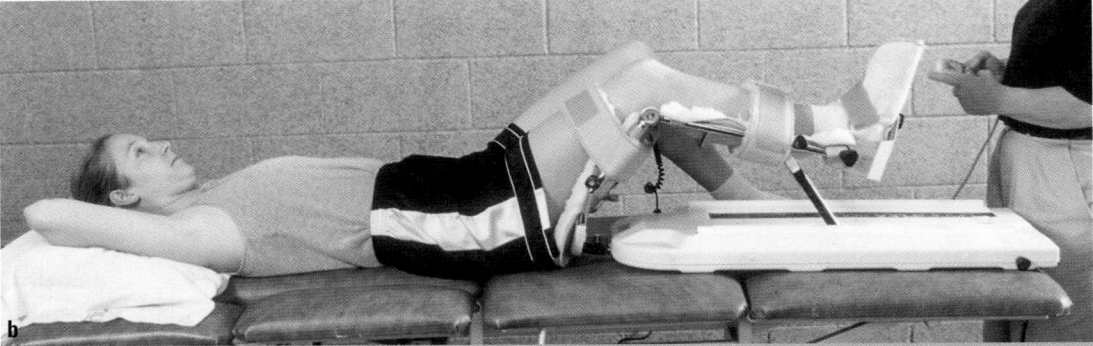

Figure 12.10 Continuous passive motion machine: Range-of-motion limits for *(a)* extension and *(b)* flexion can be set at desired levels as needed.

patient to take a few days to become accustomed to wearing the splint for long periods; several days of gradually increasing time are often required before the patient adjusts to tolerating the splint enough to wear it throughout the night or for an entire day.

Active-Assistive Range of Motion

Active-assistive range of motion is ROM that is performed with a combination of voluntary muscle activity and passive assistance from an outside force. AAROM activities are indicated when the prime movers are weak and unable to move the segment through the desired ROM or when a surgical repair is not yet healed enough to allow AROM. See figure 12.11. The general goals of AAROM are similar to those of PROM with the addition of providing a stimulus for neuromuscular control. Active-assistive range of motion is the steppingstone between PROM and AROM.

Active Range of Motion

Active range of motion is the amount of unrestricted movement produced at a joint by the patient without assistance. With AROM, the movement is solely produced by active contraction of muscles that cross a joint. Active range-of-motion activities are indicated when the muscle is strong enough to move the segment through the desired range or when a surgical repair is sufficiently healed and can withstand the forces of active movement. The general goals of AROM are to maintain elasticity and contractility of muscle, improve neuromuscular control, and develop coordination and motor skills for functional activities. As we have already discussed, restricted ROM can contribute to functional deficits and can affect quality of life. It is important to progress to AROM activities as soon as the tissue can safely tolerate the stress of active movement.

Resistive Range of Motion

Resistive range of motion is motion that occurs with resistance applied to the movement. Resistive range of motion is also referred to as strengthening exercises or progressive resistive exercises and is covered in chapter 13.

Stretching Techniques

When an injury results in deficient range of motion, several techniques may be applied to restore mobility, depending on your preference and skill, the type of tissue restriction involved, the extent of the injury, and the duration of the loss of motion. In the previous section we discussed ROM interventions, and in chapter 11 we discussed joint mobilization and various techniques of soft-tissue mobilization to improve mobility. In this section we will present another common method of increasing range of motion: stretching exercises.

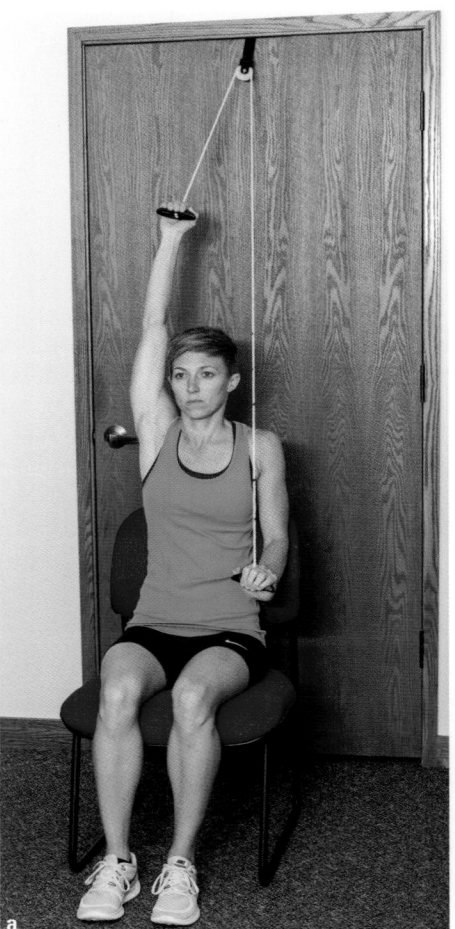
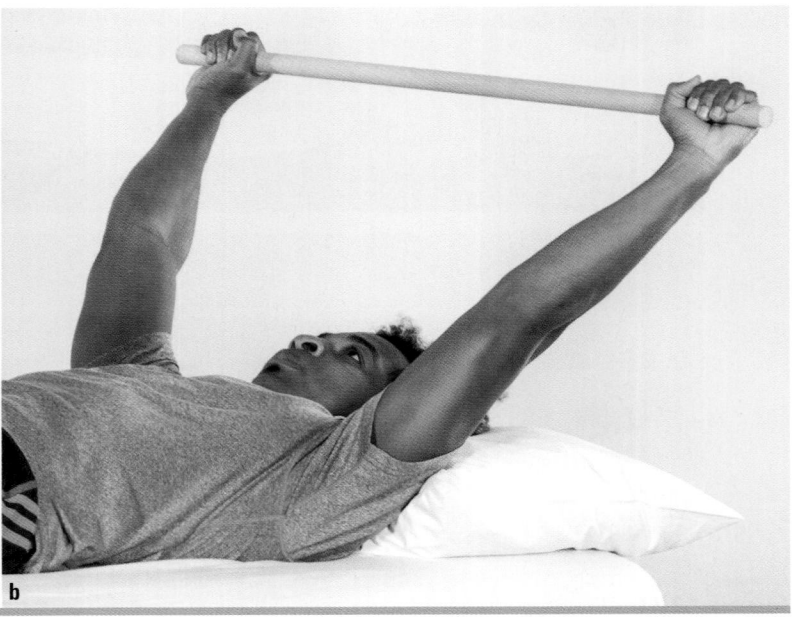

Figure 12.11 AAROM for shoulder flexion. *(a)* A pulley or *(b)* a wand can be used to allow the uninvolved side to assist the involved side into shoulder flexion.

Researchers have investigated various methods and techniques in search of the best and most effective way to improve flexibility and gain range of motion. Studies performed on normal populations have led to disputes over whether there is any benefit to pre- and postexercise stretching.[78-84] There is also unresolved disagreement among investigators about which kind of stretching technique (static,[85, 86] dynamic,[84, 87, 88] or proprioceptive neuromuscular facilitation[89, 90]) produces the most effective results. Comparison studies have shown no significant differences between static and PNF stretching[90-92] or between static and dynamic stretching.[93-95] When all three techniques are compared, all three show increased gains in flexibility without significant differences in their results.[90, 96, 97]

Unfortunately, research on the benefits of flexibility exercises in rehabilitation has been scarce. Most of the research has involved assessing the effects of stretching techniques on the healthy gastrocnemius medialis[86, 90, 98] or on hamstrings that are tight or have been injured in the past but not on recent strains, which are of more concern to rehabilitation clinicians.[99-101] Most research studies of stretching have been performed using healthy, uninjured people or animals. Some investigations are not sound, objective, or reproducible. We still need answers about the best and most effective stretching techniques to apply to damaged and healing tissue.[102-104]

There have been a few studies that have indicated benefits with a gentle loaded stretch.[101, 105, 106] A study by Apostolopoulos and colleagues[107] found that stretches between 30% and 60% of maximum range of motion did not cause tissue inflammation, whereas a stretch of 90% of maximum range of motion (with pain) caused inflammation. As you know, with injured tissue one of our goals is to limit inflammation; a gentle loaded stretch has been supported by research. Given the limited amount of research on stretching techniques for damaged and healing tissue, as rehabilitation clinicians we must rely on our knowledge of injury, healing, and connective tissue physiology and pathophysiology more than on research evidence to determine the best way to stretch an injured area.

The other factor we rely on to learn the benefits of flexibility exercises in rehabilitation is anecdotal information from experienced clinicians; these professionals have consistently stated that positive results occur when flexibility exercises are used after injury. Therefore, although research data are lacking, we can conclude with sufficient confidence that stretching does improve the status of injured body segments. The main techniques of stretching include dynamic stretching, static stretching, PNF stretching, and ballistic stretching. Ballistic stretching is a rapid reciprocating or bouncing movement that pushes tissues beyond their normal range of motion, and it is not used in rehabilitation because of the risk of injury.[108] That is not to say, however, that ballistic stretching is not beneficial; there is evidence that ballistic stretching can yield positive results when used in the conditioning of healthy people.[109, 110] Since this text deals with rehabilitation, not conditioning of healthy people, ballistic stretching is not discussed here.

Evidence for Effects of Stretching in Rehabilitation

The literature is filled with investigations on the various types of stretching and their effects on the body. Unfortunately, little agreement exists on the following main factors: (1) how mobility is gained, (2) what physiological changes are produced with stretching, (3) how long stretching effects last, and (4) the duration and repetition of stretching that produces optimal rehabilitation results after injury.

For a long time, clinicians have assumed that motion increases after stretching exercises because muscle–tendon units or joint structures are stretched into their plastic range; however, this may not be the case. It has been demonstrated that if a person performs stretching exercises, gains in flexibility occur because tissue lengthens with the application of stretch forces.[84, 117, 118] Some investigators have found that stretching improves flexibility by reducing muscle stiffness and tonic reflex activity, thereby allowing the muscle to lengthen.[94, 97, 119] Other investigators have concluded from their research that increased flexibility is the result of an increased tolerance to stretch forces rather than an actual physical change in tissue.[89, 99, 120, 121] Needless to say, studies of flexibility gains from stretching

Evidence in Rehabilitation

Evidence for the use of stretching in rehabilitation has been sparse. Research on injured tissue and stretching is lacking in the literature. Some studies that compared stretch load and range of motion provided results that can cross over to rehabilitation. Studies that included stretch to discomfort,[111-113] stretch to pain,[114, 115] maximum stretch with no pain,[116] and gentle stretch to the point of first tension[101] present conflicting results as to whether stretching is beneficial. A study by Apostolopoulos and colleagues[107] found that stretches between 30% and 60% of maximum range of motion did not cause tissue inflammation, whereas a stretch of 90% of maximum range of motion (with pain) caused inflammation. Wyon and colleagues[106] also found that a gentle stretch produced the greatest gains in increasing active and passive range of motion compared to strength training and moderate-intensity and high-intensity stretches.

have produced varied results; it may be that the different muscles, techniques, and durations used in different studies create different outcomes.[122] Regardless of these variations, the important point for clinicians is that studies consistently indicate that all modes of stretching are acutely effective at improving range of motion.[86, 90, 123-127]

The literature about stretching effects on other muscle–tendon parameters is also confusing because some studies reveal detrimental effects to strength and power output and muscle activation after stretching activities,[128-130] while other investigators have shown either no change or improvement in these parameters.[95, 131-134] Reviews of the current literature on this topic identify an important reason why studies may find that stretching has negative effects on muscle activation and performance: The duration of stretch used in most of these studies is much greater than that normally used in routine stretching programs.[83, 135, 136] Keep in mind that the duration of stretches, frequency of stretches, and duration of studies vary widely among the investigations; with so many variables, it is not surprising that little or no consensus has been reached on recommended methods, durations, and frequency of stretching techniques. Future research on these matters will require stretch routines to be more similar to normal protocols if clinicians are to glean useful information from the results.

How long do the effects of stretching endure? This is an important question for clinicians and their patients as well as healthy people who want to improve flexibility. Investigations published in this area demonstrate that after 5 to 30 min, the gains made were significantly reduced.[83, 101, 137-142] One study reported significant gains persisting for about 3 min once the stretch was relaxed.[143] Additional studies had varying results, with significant longer-term results lasting up to about 6 to 30 min.[83, 144, 145] The most important thing to take from these studies is that although large gains in flexibility were lost within a rather short time, the end measures still showed more motion than was recorded before stretching exercises were performed. In other words, all subjects who stretched realized improved flexibility, albeit less than they immediately experienced after the stretch. It is presumed, then, that with routine, repetitive stretching, a person's flexibility improves. For this reason, the clinician should consider instructing the patient to perform stretching exercises several times throughout the day for optimal mobility gains, especially in the early days of the rehabilitation program.

When we try to identify how long and how often to stretch, we again are confronted with a wide variety of investigative results. Most studies have looked at 15 s, 30 s, and 60 s stretches.[83, 96, 98, 146-150] Some investigators have found that stretching for one 30 s stretch provides the best results,[96, 148, 151] while others have demonstrated effective changes with three 15 s stretches.[152, 153] Several studies have shown that it is not the length of the stretch as much as the total time that produces the best results.[154-156] Thomas

and colleagues[157] concluded that stretching at least 5 d per week for at least 5 min per week is beneficial to promote range-of-motion improvements in healthy individuals. Since they tested healthy individuals and not injured tissue, you must take this into consideration when making decisions on how to instruct a patient to stretch.

Based on research, the American College of Sports Medicine (ACSM) and the Physical Activity Guidelines for Americans from the U.S. Department of Health and Human Services (HHS) recommend that healthy people perform stretching exercises for 10 to 30 s up to the point of tightness or discomfort for two to four repetitions at least 2 to 3 d per week. Keep in mind that these recommendations are for healthy people; clinicians will use their own best judgment based on a combination of the research, patient needs, and the clinician's professional experience to determine the most effective results for their patients.

When it comes to providing useful information about how stretching or flexibility affects recovery after injury, published studies can be inaccurate or misleading if not interpreted correctly. For example, studies that have looked at stretching or flexibility exercises after an injury include comparisons of stretching along with other types or groups of exercises, modalities, or manual therapy techniques; they do not isolate the effects of stretching exercises on injured segments.[158-161] Marom and colleagues[162] conducted a lab study where they applied nondamaging stretch intensities directly to fibroblast and myoblast monolayers that had been induced with cellular microdamage. Their findings indicate that a nondamaging stretch of 3% to 6% of resting length accelerates the migration of fibroblasts and myoblasts during wound gap closure.[162] This is encouraging for tissue healing; however, findings cannot be extrapolated directly to rehabilitation because it is not known how the extracellular matrix and surrounding structures transmit loads with injured tissue. Furthermore, a stretch load of 3% to 6% would be difficult to accurately determine and execute in the clinic.

Some investigations have demonstrated that applying flexibility exercises as part of a warm-up before activity or competition actually reduces muscle strength or performance.[81, 132, 136, 163] However, a systematic review by Behm and colleagues[97] indicated static stretching and PNF stretching more than 10 min before activity had trivial effects on muscle performance unless extreme stretching protocols were used. Additionally, there is some evidence that higher-frequency dynamic stretching provided improved performance.[97] An important point is that these studies all pertain to power activities performed with normal body segments by uninjured people. They say nothing about how flexibility exercises affect a muscle's ability to perform therapeutic exercise during a rehabilitation program, nor can they be applied to such a case. This is a topic sorely lacking attention in the investigative world.

By now you should realize that most of the research on stretching parameters has occurred on normal subjects. The effects of stretching on injured tissue have not been established.[164] Most of the studies on injured tissue have investigated either "tight" hamstrings that were not injured but qualified for the studies by having less than normal flexibility[96, 99] or previously injured hamstrings that were fully healed at the time of the investigation.[101] It is difficult to draw conclusions about the influence of stretching in rehabilitation because high-quality studies are lacking in this area.[165] This lack of research on the effects of stretching injured tissue makes it difficult to identify the best program to use in regaining lost motion after an injury. Until investigations on this topic can provide clinicians with reliable information, it is important to understand the different types of stretching and how they may affect uninjured tissue; this information along with anecdotal information from experienced clinicians is currently our best evidence from which to determine the best-practice approaches to stretching recent injuries.

Dynamic Stretching

Dynamic stretching includes active flexibility exercises performed by the patient without outside assistance from either another person or equipment. **Dynamic stretching** is a rhythmic, controlled, and smooth motion from a neutral position to an extreme end of movement and then either back to the start position or to the other extreme end of movement within a plane of motion[84] (figure 12.12). Research on dynamic stretching demonstrates that this type of stretch is most beneficial for someone performing power-based activities or activities that require speed of motion.[83, 84, 88, 163, 166] Various investigators have identified different parameters for dynamic stretching, including 30 s bouts for five sets[87] or three sets[131] to two sets of 15 s bouts[132] and four sets of 12 to 15 s bouts.[129] Dynamic stretch duration does not appear to influence muscular performance as long as fatigue is not a factor.[84] Dynamic stretches are not usually used in early rehabilitation programs because they require strength and proprioception, factors that are lacking during the first half of rehabilitation. Such stretches, however, may be considered during the advanced phase of rehabilitation as the patient moves into the functional and performance-specific exercises before returning to normal activities.

Static Stretching

Static stretching includes a variety of methods, including short-term and long-term stretches. **Static stretching** involves placing a muscle or muscle group at the end of its motion and holding the position for a specific amount of time, then relaxing the stretch and repeating it. This technique may be performed by the individual (figure 12.13a) or with the use of equipment or another person (figure 12.13b). A typical example of a short-term passive stretch is when the clinician moves the patient's injured part through its range of motion and applies an over-pressure stretch at the end of the motion.

Based on the results of the studies cited previously, along with our clinical observations and experience over the years, we feel the best application of a static stretch is one that is performed for either 15 s for four repetitions or

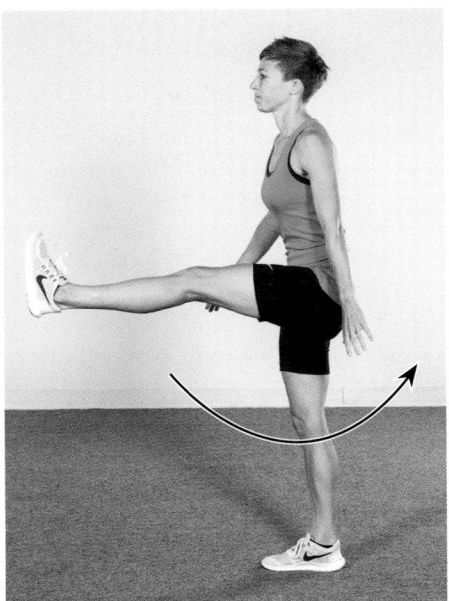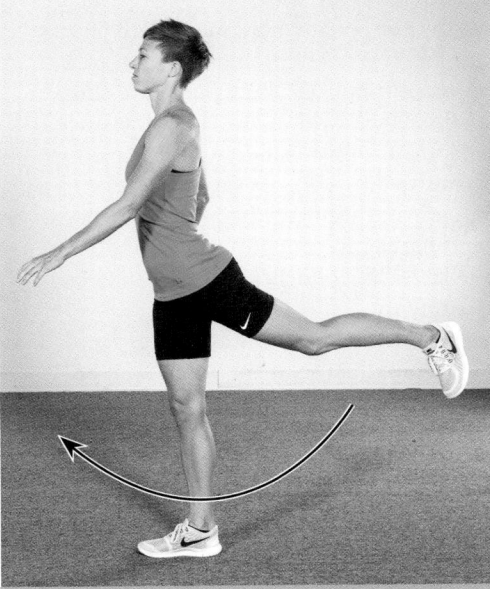

Figure 12.12 Dynamic stretches are performed by the person using a smooth, controlled, and rhythmic motion to gain flexibility. This is most commonly used by healthy athletes in events that require power or speed.[84, 164]

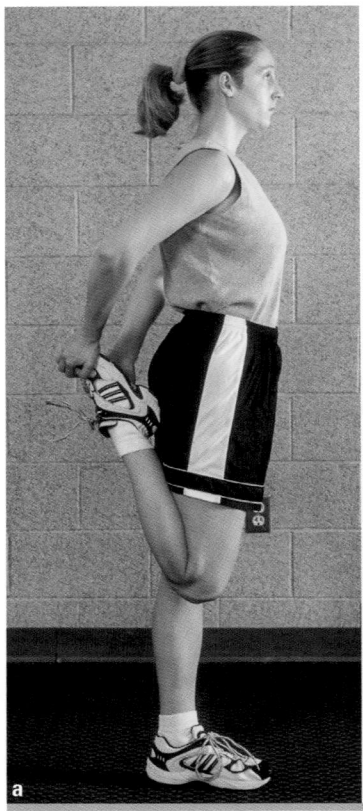
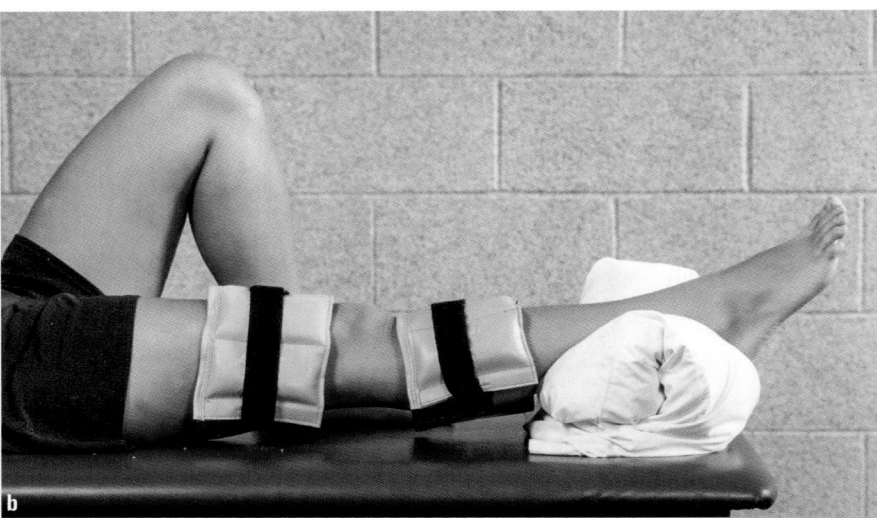

Figure 12.13   The muscle or muscle group being stretched is held at its end position for a specific amount of time. *(a)* The individual performs the stretch actively to the quadriceps. *(b)* The stretch here is provided by gravity and further assisted by weights on the leg.

30 s for one to two repetitions; either program is repeated at least three times a day. Which program we select depends on the patient; we use the shorter-term stretches and more repetitions with those who are older, have less balance, have a low pain tolerance, or are more inclined to be less compliant in their home exercise program, and we select the one- or two-repetition 30 s stretches for younger patients with good balance, with higher pain tolerances, and who are compliant with rehabilitation instructions given to them. Consistency is key. It takes 3 weeks of a static stretching routine to see decreased muscle stiffness occur.[167] If patients are participating in sport activities or strengthening exercises, the stretches should also be performed after their activity.

During a static stretch, the part is moved to the end of its motion.[168] The proximal segment of the joint being stretched is stabilized to prevent its movement while a firm but not excessive pressure is applied to the joint's distal segment. A steady pressure is applied until the soft tissue's slack is taken up and the muscle is taut. To apply the stretch, the joint is then moved slightly beyond this point. The patient should feel a stretch or tension, but not pain. A systematic review by Apostolopoulos and colleagues[165] found that stretching into moderate discomfort yields the

best results.[165] If a two-joint muscle is stretched, one joint is positioned in the muscle's lengthened position, then the second joint, until maximum muscle length is achieved. The stretch is repeated one to four times, depending on the patient and the duration of the stretch.

Reciprocal Inhibition

Because of the phenomenon of antagonist inhibition, if the person contracts the opposing muscle, relaxation of the stretched muscle occurs.[169] This relaxation of the antagonist results in a more effective stretch of the agonist. For example, a better stretch occurs when the patient actively contracts the quadriceps as the hamstrings are stretched.

It is believed that a strong relationship between muscles and their antagonists affects muscle flexibility. When a muscle becomes tighter, its antagonist becomes weaker. It is believed that an agonist muscle is shortened over time when its antagonist remains weak, creating an imbalance between the two and resulting in a loss of motion.[170] On the other hand, if the antagonist is facilitated, the agonist becomes inhibited, which allows a restoration of normal flexibility.

You can perform this quick experiment on yourself to see the impact of agonist inhibition on increasing muscle flexibility. Do not perform this activity if you have a lumbar disc injury or lower extremity radicular symptoms. In a standing position, first evaluate your hamstring flexibility by placing your foot on a surface such as a chair seat or tabletop. Keeping both knees straight and the standing foot facing forward, reach with your opposite hand for the foot on the elevated surface. Lean forward from your hips (hinge) until you feel a stretch in the hamstrings. Now tighten the quadriceps of the stretch leg and see how much farther you can move your hand toward your toes.

The effects of this reciprocal inhibition demonstrate the need to accompany any stretching technique with strengthening exercises to maintain newly acquired muscle length. Strengthening exercises also help restore balance between agonist and antagonist muscle groups.

Prolonged Static Stretch

The most effective stretches involve the steady application of force over a length of time. Low-intensity, long-duration stretching is the most effective way to acutely decrease passive torque.[171] This prolonged passive stretch produces better results in more mature connective tissue, primarily because of the length of time it is applied. Although research has yet to define how long a prolonged stretch should be applied, Kottke, Pauley, and Ptak[1] suggested 20 min in clinical applications, Ono and colleagues[172] suggested 30 min, and Starring and colleagues[173] found benefits with 15 min stretches. Although reduced-load prolonged stretching seems to be the most effective of all stretching techniques, it also appears to be the least investigated.

A prolonged static stretch must be applied with a reduced load. Two articles by Warren, Lehmann, and Koblanski[41, 174] reported that the amount of time required for a prolonged stretch to change connective tissue length is inversely proportional to the amount of force used; however, they investigated healthy tissue. As with short-term stretches, research is lacking on prolonged-stretching effectiveness on healing tissue. One study investigated normal subjects with a prolonged stretch of 3 min but used full body weight as the force; the investigators found significant immediate linear increases in motion because of the great amount of force applied over a 3 min period, but no lasting effects from the stretch.[175] Most of the time, however, prolonged stretches applied to healing tissue are not that intense, so to counterbalance the reduced force application, stretch time is increased. A prolonged stretch is effective in increasing motion, probably because of a number of factors, including its impact on the tissue's stress–strain curves and the creep phenomenon, adaptation to stretch tolerance, and changes in tissue length, all of which have been discussed earlier in this chapter.

For prolonged stretches, the segment must be stabilized to permit the load to stretch the correct tissue. This stabilization can be provided either by the weight of the body or segment or by a mechanical device such as a weight or strap. The stretch is applied slowly and steadily to the point of tightness. The segment is then secured in this position and held for the desired amount of time. If a two-joint or multijoint muscle is stretched, the other joint or joints the muscle crosses should be placed in a position that elongates the muscle. For example, if the hamstrings are stretched with the knee in extension, the patient should sit to elongate the hamstrings at the proximal end where they cross the hip joint.

The patient commonly does not feel much, if anything, when the stretch is first applied. Within a few minutes, however, the patient feels the stretch's effect. The minimum prolonged stretch duration is usually 15 to 20 min; if the patient cannot tolerate the stress, the force should be reduced to allow the patient to stretch for the desired time. Sometimes even with a lighter force it is necessary to gradually increase the stretch time to give the patient time to adapt. For example, the patient may tolerate only 5 min to start, but the clinician gradually increases the time as the patient adapts until sufficient time, 20 to 30 min, is achieved.

The part placed in a prolonged stretch can feel very stiff at first when the stretch load is removed. The patient should be cautioned about this before releasing the stretch. The stretch force should be released slowly. As the stretch is released, the patient is advised to simultaneously contract the stretched muscle to reduce the discomfort. Gentle, active range-of-motion activities following the stretch release help relieve the stiffness.

Pre-Contraction Stretching: Proprioceptive Neuromuscular Facilitation

The unique combination of active and passive stretching is sometimes referred to as pre-contraction stretching. **Pre-contraction stretching** uses active contraction of either the muscle being stretched or its antagonist before the stretch force is applied.[176] Proprioceptive neuromuscular facilitation is the most common example of this stretching technique.[176] Although PNF is also used as a strengthening technique, it is useful for gaining mobility. A more extensive discussion of PNF principles is presented in chapter 11 along with the other manual therapy techniques.

Indications and Precautions for Stretching Techniques

Before applying a stretch to increase range of motion, you must first know when stretching is indicated, when you should not use stretching, and precautions for its use.

Indications

As part of the patient examination performed before treatment, the clinician determines deficiencies in range of motion, identifies the structures causing the loss of motion, and assesses the status of the tissue. Is the loss a result of recent scar tissue formation, adherent and mature scar tissue, spasm, edema, postural deformities, or weakness of opposing muscles? If ligaments, capsules, muscles, fascia, skin, or other soft tissues are shortened because of scar tissue adhesions, stretching exercises and fascial mobilization techniques are indicated. These techniques are also indicated in the presence of contractures and structural deformities from injury or posture changes over time. If weak muscles are overpowered by opposing overactive structures, flexibility of the restricted structures must accompany strengthening of the weak muscles for the rehabilitation program to be optimally effective. If muscle spasm or edema contributes to reduced motion, the rehabilitation program must include modalities and activities to address these problems first. Fascial mobilization techniques are used in the presence of restricted scar tissue and postinjury soft-tissue adhesions; these techniques are presented in chapter 11.

Contraindications

Although stretching is usually safe, it is contraindicated when certain conditions are present. These conditions include recent fractures when immobilization is necessary for healing and movement is detrimental to it, a bony block that restricts motion, infection in a joint, acute inflammation in a joint, extreme or sharp pain with motion, and when shortening of soft tissue actually contributes to an area's stability.

Precautions

Precautions are taken to ensure the most effective application of the stretch and to prevent harm from a stretch. Before applying any treatment, in addition to obtaining patient consent, you should always explain to the patient what you will do and what sensations and results to expect. A patient who is apprehensive and unable to relax will not respond effectively to stretching interventions.

The force applied in a stretch should cause sensations of tension, perhaps unpleasant, in the segment stretched, but there should be no pain, nor should there be any residual pain after release of the stretch. This is true for both active and passive stretching. It is important that the patient understand that during active stretches, the sensation of a stretch is necessary, but it should be without pain. Residual pain beyond a brief transitory tenderness, especially when accompanied by new edema within a 24 h post-treatment period, is an indication that the stretch has been too aggressive. In this case, the stretch force should be reduced in the next treatment to continue to improve mobility but without these undesirable post-stretch symptoms.

The release of a stretch force is as important as its application. Both the application and the release should be performed slowly. A quick application or release of a stretch, especially release of a prolonged stretch, can be very uncomfortable. Begin applying the stretch slowly, and do not apply more force until you know the patient can tolerate it. Some tenderness and stiffness are normal after release of a stretch, especially a prolonged stretch. As mentioned earlier, these symptoms can be relieved by contracting the stretched muscle as the stretch is released and after the stretch with gentle, active range-of-motion exercises.

If a stretch is painful, gentle traction applied to the joint during the stretch may relieve the pain. If this does not relieve the pain, reduce the stretch load. A stretch should not be painful.

A stretch force affects all soft tissue in the area where the force is applied. Knowing exactly which tissues are affected has thus far eluded researchers. Just like tissues affected by scar tissue, the structures affected by a stretch may include joint capsule, ligaments, surrounding tendons, muscles, fascia, nerves, skin, and subcutaneous tissue.

Vigorous stretching of areas that recently have been immobilized for a while should be performed with extreme caution and even avoided in the early stretching stages. Recall that immobilization reduces the tensile strength of many connective tissue structures, including tendons and ligaments, so caution must be used.

Stabilization of the area is necessary to properly apply the stretch force in the correct direction and to the correct structures. During both active and passive stretches, the part is positioned so the stretch force affects only the targeted structures. For example, if a patient is stretching the left hamstrings in a standing position with the left foot on a chair or bench, the left foot should be facing the ceiling, not rotated; in the rotated position, the hip adductors, not the hamstrings, are stretched.

When stretching a muscle that traverses two or more joints, the other joints must be positioned so that the muscle is elongated throughout its entire length. In other words, every joint a muscle crosses is placed so that the muscle is stretched at that joint for an appropriate elongation of the muscle to occur. For example, to stretch the quadriceps, place the hip in extension with the knee in flexion so the rectus femoris portion of the quadriceps is fully lengthened.

In active and passive stretches, the muscle stretched should be relaxed for optimal results. If a muscle tenses, it will resist the stretch and make the stretch ineffective. For this reason, careful positioning and understanding of positional biomechanics is important. For example, standing bent over from the waist to touch the floor with the fingertips is an ineffective position for stretching the hamstrings because the hamstrings must tense to maintain this position and cannot relax. Likewise, if a passive stretch is too forceful and causes a reflex or voluntary muscle contraction, the stretch will be both ineffective and painful to the patient.

Once full range of motion is achieved after an injury, maintenance flexibility exercises are used. Connective tissue will continue to contract as scar tissue continues to heal, so loss of motion will also continue. This is why a patient can achieve full range of motion in one rehabilitation session and return for treatment the next day with less than full range of motion. Until the healing process is complete, it is important to maintain full range of motion once it is achieved.

Exercise Progression

Two common questions about therapeutic flexibility exercises are "When is the best time to use ROM and stretching exercises?" and "Which stretching exercises should I use?" The information presented in this chapter and in chapter 2 provides the answers.

If motion is permitted immediately after an injury, active range-of-motion exercises may be all that is needed to regain full ROM. Active motion performed by the patient is the first choice because it does not require outside assistance, so the patient can perform it often and independently throughout the day when it is convenient. Frequent flexibility exercise sessions throughout the day, especially during the proliferation and into the early remodeling phases of healing, can be an effective way to increase flexibility.

Following an acute injury or major surgery, passive range of motion (PROM) or, in some cases, a continuous passive motion machine (CPM) will allow for mobility exercises without stressing the healing tissue. Recall that in the inflammation phase of tissue healing the tissue cannot withstand loading; however, it is important to maintain connective tissue mobility and muscle elasticity and to minimize adhesions. In the case of tendon repairs, such as a rotator cuff repair, the physician may have specific PROM guidelines for you to follow.

Other techniques may be needed after immobilization. To some extent, the method of regaining mobility depends on the length of immobilization, the tissues affected by the immobilization, the patient's motivation, and the rehabilitation clinician's facilities and availability. Recall that collagen appears in a wound as early as 3 to 5 d after an injury. By the seventh day, collagen may abound, and the forming scar tissue begins to contract. This contraction continues into the final phase of healing and requires stretching exercises to maintain range of motion even after full motion has been achieved.

If scar tissue is relatively new and still easily pliable, active and short-term passive stretches are effective for increasing motion. PNF stretching techniques can also be used with success, assuming the patient has the muscle control for these types of exercises. When scar tissue is more mature and well into the remodeling phase, however,

prolonged-stretching techniques should be the main part of the stretching program. Short-term and active stretches performed throughout the day help to reinforce the effects of the prolonged stretches.

In difficult situations where scar tissue is more than 3 to 4 months old and range of motion is still deficient, prolonged-stretch machines or devices are more beneficial to achieve maximal range of motion. With proximal interphalangeal (PIP) joint flexion contractures, superior results were achieved by wearing a PIP orthosis device, which provided a low-load prolonged stretch, for a minimum of 6 h per day.[177]

Special Considerations With Stretching

As with the application of any therapeutic intervention, the application of stretching techniques requires common sense and consideration of the specific structure to be stretched.

Spine

The most important consideration in stretching the spine is to avoid any stretch that causes pain or a change in sensation down an extremity. Stretching structures that affect trunk or neck mobility without increasing disc pressure is ideal.

Upper Extremity

When stretching the glenohumeral joint, the scapula must be stabilized. If it is not, the stretching force is distributed into the scapular muscles, and gains in motion may not be actual gains in the intended area.

When stretching the elbow, remember that several muscles acting at the elbow also cross the shoulder, so the shoulder should be positioned and stabilized before stretching the elbow. Because the elbow flexors and extensors work in either forearm supination or forearm pronation, stretches for those muscles should be performed with an awareness of whether these positions affect the stretch's effectiveness. One possible side effect of vigorous elbow stretching is myositis ossificans, especially in youth. For this reason, elbow stretches should be performed with caution. Active stretches and reciprocal inhibition techniques may help prevent this problem.

CLINICAL TIPS

The anatomy of the structure to be stretched determines the most appropriate stretch application. The clinician must be familiar with the anatomy and biomechanics of the musculoskeletal system.

When stretching the wrist, the distal force is applied over the metacarpals, not the fingers. The patient's fingers should remain relaxed during the stretch since the extrinsic finger flexors and extensors cross the wrist and can affect the stretch if they are not relaxed. Stretching any of the digits begins distally and moves proximally, including each joint a finger tendon crosses one at a time.

Lower Extremity

The ankle and foot contain many joints and soft-tissue structures. When stretching these areas, the location where the joint's tendons cross and the appropriate application of force must be considered.

The position of the hip affects knee stretches. Since both the knee flexors and extensors cross the hip joint, the effectiveness of the stretch is determined by the position of the hip during the stretch.

When stretching the hip, the pelvis must be stabilized. If the pelvis is not stabilized, just as with the scapula during shoulder stretching, movement occurs in this segment, and an increase in hip range of motion is sacrificed to the pelvis.

Caution must be used when stretching hip rotators with the knee in flexion and the force applied at the tibia. This position offers the clinician a tremendous lever arm advantage and reduces the force required to cause hip joint subluxation, especially in patients who have under-gone prolonged immobilization, recent fracture, or recent dislocation.

Summary

Many factors influence a person's range of motion and flexibility, both normally and after injury. One of the major issues after injury is scar tissue formation and adhesions of that scar tissue to adjacent and surrounding tissues. If this is not managed properly, long-term loss of motion may result in long-term effects on a person's function and ability to perform. Other factors influencing mobility include tissue viscosity, elasticity, plasticity, and neural input. The clinician must be aware of how to influence these factors to obtain optimal rehabilitation results. There are several types of range-of-motion and stretching techniques to increase flexibility and mobility. Each has its advantages and indications, so the clinician must be aware of which techniques are most appropriate for each patient. In rehabilitation, the most effective stretches are static stretches that are held for 15 to 30 s and repeated one to four times three times a day. In the advanced stages of rehabilitation and in performance, dynamic stretching is the most effective technique. When an injured site has severe or well-healed scar tissue adhesions, low-load prolonged stretches of at least 15 to 20 min will be more effective than any other type of stretch to change tissue mobility.

LEARNING AIDS

Key Concepts and Review

1. Define the differences between range of motion and flexibility.
Range of motion is the amount of mobility of a joint, and flexibility is the musculotendinous unit's ability to elongate with the application of a stretching force. The terms are closely related and are often used interchangeably.

2. List the deleterious effects of prolonged immobilization.
Immobilization affects different tissue types differently, but some generic changes are seen in all tissues. These include a loss of ground substance, which in turn results in less separation and more cross-links between collagen fibers. The fiber meshwork contracts, so the tissue becomes dense, hard, and less supple. The more severe effects occur with more prolonged immobilization. If a normal joint is immobilized for 4 weeks, the dense connective tissue that forms prevents normal motion.

3. Discuss the mechanical properties of plasticity, elasticity, and viscoelasticity of connective tissue.
Connective tissue's plastic quality allows its length to change when a force is applied, while its elasticity allows some return toward normal length. Viscoelasticity is a combination of elastic and viscous properties that allows either a change in length or a return to former length after stretching, depending on the speed, duration, and magnitude of the stretch force applied.

4. Explain the physiological properties of creep and stress–strain and how they affect stretching techniques.
Creep permits a gradual change in tissue length with the prolonged application of a low-level stretch force. The stress–strain curve describes a tissue's ability to withstand stresses and the subsequent strains they produce on the tissue. If a stretch force is applied beyond a tissue's elastic limits, deformation occurs.

5. Discuss the neuromuscular influences of the muscle spindle and GTO on stretching muscle.
The muscle spindle and GTO are neuromuscular protective mechanisms that try to reduce the stress–strain

forces on the musculotendinous unit. The muscle spindle is more sensitive to stretch, and the GTO is more sensitive to muscle shortening.

6. Discuss the differences between PROM, AAROM, and AROM in rehabilitation

Passive range of motion (PROM) is the amount of motion achieved without the assistance of the patient. The movement is produced by an external force, and there is no voluntary action from the patient. Active-assistive range of motion (AAROM) is performed with a combination of voluntary activity of the muscles and passive assistance from an outside force. Active range of motion (AROM) is the amount of unrestricted movement produced at a joint by the patient without assistance.

7. Discuss the dynamic, static, and pre-contraction methods for stretching.

Dynamic stretching is a type of flexibility exercise that the person performs without the assistance of others. It is a rhythmic, controlled, and smooth motion from a neutral position to an extreme end of motion and then back to the start position within a plane of motion. It is used more by healthy individuals or in the advanced phase of rehabilitation. Static stretching involves placing a muscle or muscle group at the end of its motion and holding the position for a specific amount of time, then relaxing the stretch and repeating it. This technique may be performed by the individual or with the use of equipment or another person. This technique is most often preferred in rehabilitation. Pre-contraction stretching involves contraction of either the muscle being stretched or its antagonist before the stretch force is applied. Proprioceptive neuromuscular facilitation is the most common technique in this category that is used in rehabilitation. Ballistic stretching is also in this category, but it is not used in rehabilitation because it creates too high a risk of injury.

8. Identify two mechanical assistive devices used to increase range of motion.

CPMs and splints are commonly used as external devices to gain additional motion. CPMs are sometimes used after surgery to counteract the deleterious effects of immobilization. Splints can be used to apply prolonged stretch to joints restricted by mature or very restricted scar tissue.

9. List contraindications, indications, and precautions of stretching.

Indications for stretching include a shortening of ligaments, capsules, muscles, fascia, skin, and other soft tissue by scar tissue or adhesions. Some precautions include explaining to the patient the technique and expected sensations before application, applying and releasing the force slowly and steadily, and avoiding pain. Contraindications include recent fractures, inflammations, infections, and extreme pain.

10. Discuss the selection of a stretching exercise program.

The type of flexibility exercise applied depends on a number of considerations, including the age of the scar tissue, the stage of healing, available equipment, the patient's motivation and pain tolerance, and the tissue involved. If the scar is in the early remodeling phase of repair, active exercises may be sufficient. If the scar tissue is more mature, a more prolonged stretch that affects the plastic range of the tissue is indicated.

Critical Thinking Questions

1. How would you stretch the quadriceps muscle if you did not want to fully lengthen the rectus femoris? In what position is the rectus femoris included in the quadriceps stretch? Try these two positions with a partner. Does the knee motion change in the different positions? If so, what does that tell you?

2. Over the course of a week, stretch a partner's hamstrings using a different technique each day: a passive technique with a 15 to 30 s hold, a contract-relax-stretch PNF maneuver, a ballistic stretch, and a prolonged stretch for 15 min. Measure the hamstring length each day before you begin the stretch exercise and again immediately after the stretch is released. Record each day's findings and which stretch technique is used each day. Which technique gives you the greatest change in hamstring length? Why does this occur? Do any of the physical properties of creep, stress–strain, or hysteresis influence the changes?

3. Explain why active range of motion is not usually as great as passive range of motion. Can you think of exceptions to this generalization and explain why they occur?

4. If a patient had a condition in which the GTOs did not respond to stimuli, what would be the result? Could this be harmful during normal activity?

5. What is the most effective stretch for a patient who has a tight Achilles tendon? Why would you select that stretch?

Lab Activities

1. Perform PROM and AAROM and instruct your lab partner in AROM on the following joints.

    A. Ankle

    B. Knee

    C. Hip

    D. Shoulder

    E. Elbow

    F. Wrist

2. Perform dynamic, static, and pre-contraction stretches on the upper extremity and lower extremity.

3. Outline the progression of mobility intervention to normalize motion for a rotator cuff repair patient. Start with the inactive phase of rehabilitation and progress through the advanced phase of rehabilitation.

13

Muscle Strength and Endurance

Objectives

After completing this chapter, you should be able to do the following:

1. Explain why slow-twitch fibers are used for endurance activities and fast-twitch fibers are used more in explosive power activities.

2. Provide an example of strengthening exercises for the coracobrachialis and the biceps muscles, and explain why they must have different considerations.

3. Identify Lombard's paradox, and explain why it is useful in an activity such as getting up from a chair.

4. Explain why a muscle's length–tension relationship changes throughout its range of motion.

5. Identify the various types of dynamic activity.

6. Discuss the differences between open and closed kinetic chain activity.

7. Explain what position a muscle working against gravity must be in to provide the maximum resistance against the patient.

8. Explain why a muscle can provide more force during an eccentric contraction than during a concentric contraction, and explain how to use this concept with a patient who has less than grade 3 strength.

9. Describe the two main approaches clinicians use to determine how long a patient may rest between strength exercise sets.

10. Identify and justify three OKC and three CKC activities that could be used by L.C. from the chapter opening scenario to advance Leanne's rehabilitation program and add more resistance.

||||||||||||||||||||||||||||||||||||||||||||||||||||||||||||||||||||||||||||||||||||||||||||||||||||||||||||||||||||||||||||||||||||||||||||||||||||||||||||||||||||||||||||||||||||||||

Now that L.C. has achieved good range of motion in Leanne's knee, he is ready to begin a more advanced strengthening program. Early in the season, Leanne injured her right knee during her intercollegiate team's gymnastics practice. She underwent rehabilitation but continued to have difficulties with the knee throughout the season. Three weeks ago she underwent an arthroscopy for a medial meniscal repair.

L.C. wants Leanne to progress in her rehabilitation program with effective, efficient, and appropriate strengthening exercises, but he's having difficulty deciding what equipment to use. Fortunately, his facility has a nice variety of rehabilitation equipment. Now that Leanne can bear full weight on the extremity, he wants to do a combination of open and closed kinetic chain activities. Until now, L.C. has used manual resistance and free-weight resistance to provide strengthening activities, but at this point in Leanne's program, more resistive exercises are indicated.

The block of granite, which was an obstacle in the path of the weak, becomes a stepping stone in the path of the strong.

Thomas Carlyle, 1795-1881,
Scottish historian, essayist, and philosopher

As you might guess from the quote by Mr. Carlyle, this chapter is about muscle strength and endurance. As you read this chapter, you will discover that although much is known about muscle strength, much is yet to be learned. We have come a long way in the past few years in advancing our knowledge; this has led to changes in how we manage strength within rehabilitation programs. This text does not come close to presenting the body of knowledge available, but we discuss the importance of having muscle strength, the methods of achieving it, and the ways in which clinicians can maximize the development of muscular strength and endurance in rehabilitation programs.

As you read this chapter, keep in mind that many of the concepts presented are not black and white but shades of gray. There is not necessarily a single answer for even simple questions such as *What is the best number of repetitions for increasing muscle endurance?* The "best" answer for each patient will emerge through your ability to combine the knowledge you obtain from this text, your coursework, and your own observation skills and common sense.

One can never have too much knowledge. Knowledge leads to understanding, understanding leads to appreciation, appreciation leads to insight, and insight leads to wisdom in application. The greater your understanding of the whys and hows, the more effective will be your application of the knowledge you have.

This chapter briefly reviews neurophysiology, muscle anatomy, and how the muscular and neurological systems work together to create movement. We spend a little more time on those concepts that directly affect muscle strength and endurance. The progressions provided in this chapter will give you additional skills to design and build your own rehabilitation program for any patient, regardless of obstacles or complications associated with the patient's injury.

Neurological Structure and Function

||||||||||||||||||||||||||||||||||||||||||||||||||||||||||||||||||||||||||||||||||||||||||||||||||||||||||||||

Before we get to the muscular system, we need to review how the neurological system "talks" with the muscular system so muscles function properly. Most of the information presented here about the neurological elements is a review of your basic anatomy and physiology course content. As we delve into the more complex aspects of muscle activity, some information may be review and some may be new; all of it, however, is relevant to understanding how muscles work.

Neurological Structure Relevant to Muscle Function

There are many sensory receptors that provide input to the central nervous system to influence the neuromuscular system. Figure 13.1 indicates that the central nervous system receives sensory input from muscles, joints, and skin. The sensory receptors on the skin—including free nerve endings that perceive pain and temperature, Meissner's corpuscles that receive light touch sensation, and Pacinian corpuscles that perceive pressure sensation—transmit afferent impulses to the central nervous system. Table 13.1 lists the somatosensory receptors. As you may recall, these impulses are interpreted at various levels within the central nervous system, including the spinal cord, brain stem, cerebellum, and cerebral cortex. Once received and interpreted, a response is transmitted down the spinal cord through appropriate spinal pathways to the anterior horn, along efferent nerves to the motor structures that respond to the impulses they receive.

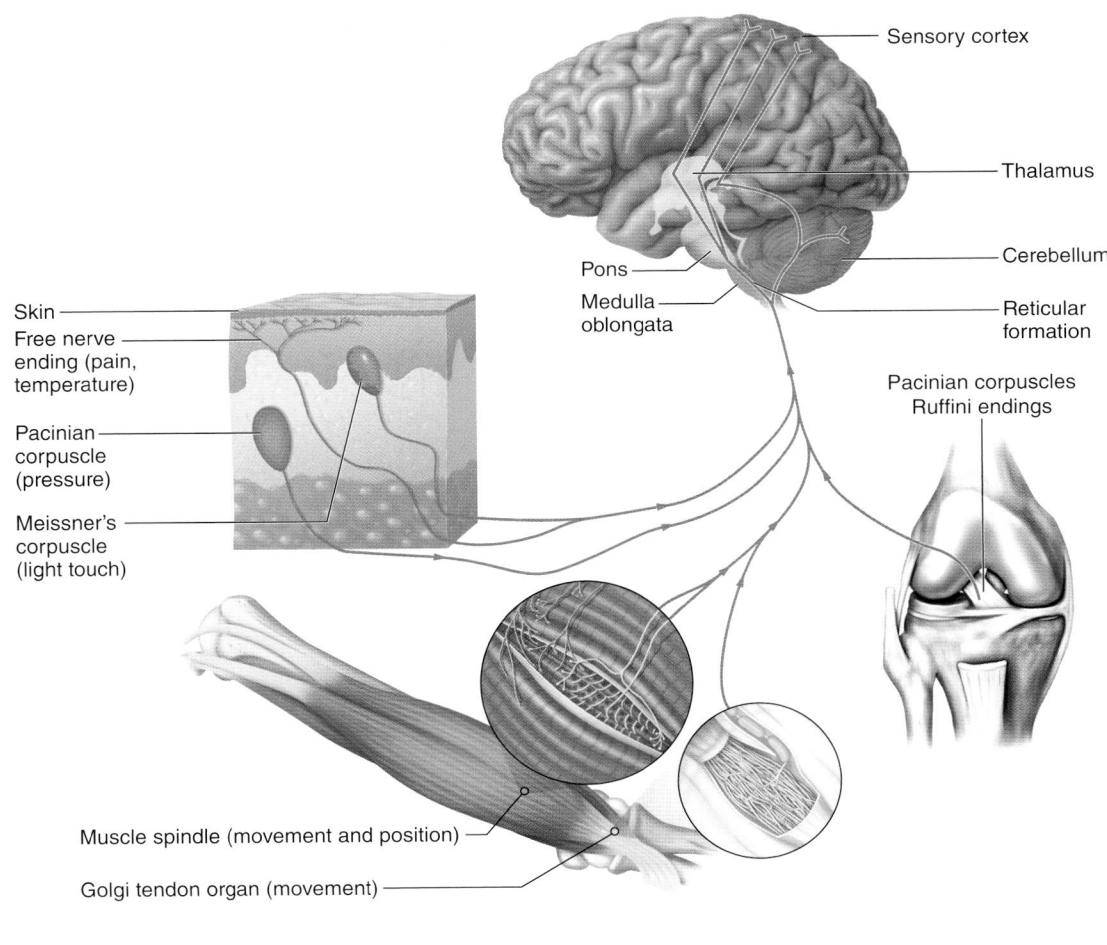

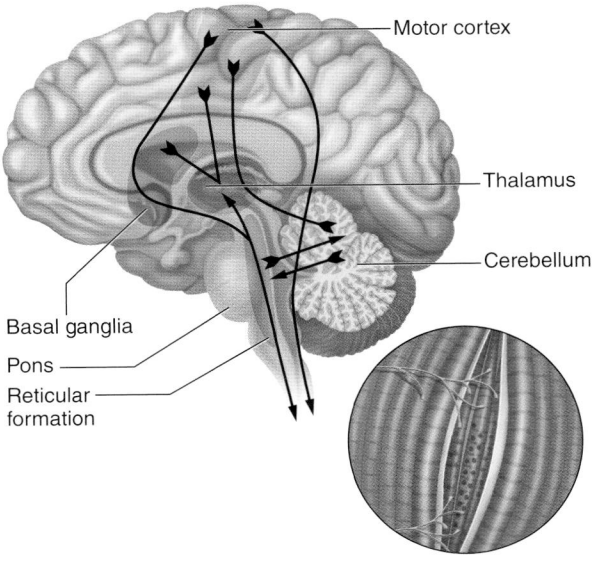

Figure 13.1   Neural pathways: *(a)* sensory (afferent); *(b)* motor (efferent).

TABLE 13.1   Somatosensory Receptors of the Skin

Receptor name	Group name	Conducting nerve fiber	Sensations	Locations
Free nerve endings	Nociceptor; thermoreceptor; mechanoreceptor	A delta fiber, C fiber, or A beta fiber	Pain, itch; temperature; touch, pressure, stretch	Epidermis; dermis; base of hair follicles
Meissner's corpuscle	Mechanoreceptor	A beta fiber	Light and discriminative touch, vibration, pressure and shear	Epidermis; dermis
Merkel's disc	Mechanoreceptor	A beta fiber	Light and discriminative touch	Epidermis; base of hair follicles
Pacinian corpuscle	Mechanoreceptor	A beta fiber	Deep pressure, high-frequency vibration	Lower dermis
Ruffini endings	Mechanoreceptor; thermoreceptor	A beta fiber, C fiber	Sustained pressure; low-frequency vibration; temperature: warm receptor	Dermis
Krause end bulbs	Thermoreceptor	A delta fiber	Temperature: cold receptor	Dermis

Neurological Function Relevant to Muscle Function

When an impulse is strong enough to produce an action potential, the motor neuron fires, and all of the muscle fibers that it supplies respond; this response is in accordance with the **all-or-none principle**. Throughout the entire muscle, a few or many motor units are facilitated to fire at one time. As a rule, the more motor units recruited, the stronger the muscle's contraction response. The efferent stimulation of an electrical impulse, an action potential, moves along the motor neuron to the neuromuscular junction. At this junction, the action potential causes the release of acetylcholine, which stimulates the sarcolemma to release its calcium ions, beginning the muscle activity just described. When this occurs just once, the result is a muscle twitch.

This muscle twitch may not involve the entire muscle or cause a full muscle contraction, but it does include enough muscle fibers that it may make the segment move. We know that one motor unit innervates several muscle fibers. These fibers are spaced throughout the muscle and are not necessarily adjacent to one another.[1] Because the lengths of the nerve's motor end plates vary according to the distance between the motor point and the muscle fiber that the nerve stimulates, the impulse does not reach all of the muscle fibers at the same time.[2] This causes an asynchronous firing of the muscle fibers. Although it may sound counterintuitive, this asynchronous firing of a single motor unit produces a smooth muscle contraction. Therefore, whether the muscle response is a twitch or a larger, more forceful contraction, the muscle's motion occurs throughout its length.

The wall, or membrane, of a nerve or muscle cell has a **resting membrane potential**, also referred to as *resting potential*. There are positive and negative ions in the intracellular and extracellular fluids of the nerve and muscle cells. The extracellular fluid contains many sodium (positive) and chloride (negative) ions. Inside the cell are many potassium (K^+) ions, protein molecules (A^-), and some chloride (Cl^-) ions (figure 13.2a). This distribution of ions produces a cell's resting potential. If microelectrodes are placed on the inside and the outside of a cell, they will

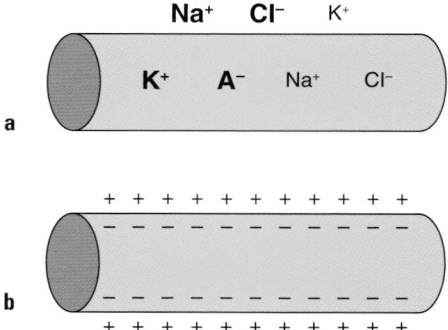

Figure 13.2 *(a)* Resting membrane potential. Notice the imbalance of negative and positive charges between the cell's interior and exterior. *(b)* Arrangement of charges on the membrane of an axon. Because potassium tends to want to leak out of the cell, the sodium–potassium pump works to maintain a balance of a negative charge inside the cell and a positive charge outside the cell.

show that an axon's intracellular fluid carries a charge of 70 to 90 mV. Figure 13.2*b* illustrates the interior negative charge and exterior positive charge of the cell membrane. There is a natural tendency to try to attain ion equilibrium. The task of keeping the ion concentration balance in check—because the potassium tends to "want" to leak out of the cell and sodium to leak into it—is the responsibility of the sodium–potassium pump. This constant activity level produces an average net resting membrane potential of approximately –85 mV.

Muscle Structure and Function

Now let's move from nerve to muscle cells and take a microscopic perspective to see how muscle fibers and the entire muscle react when nerves stimulate them.

Microstructure

You already know the structure of muscles and their surrounding fascial tissue. Figure 13.3 serves as a visual review, illustrating muscle's macro- and microstructures.

A **motor unit** is composed of the nerve, or motor neuron, and the muscle fibers that it innervates (figure 13.4). The number of motor units in any healthy muscle depends on the size and function of that muscle. For example, in small muscles that primarily perform finely tuned activities, such as the intrinsic muscles of the hand, the ratio of muscle fibers to neurons is small; larger muscles that are used primarily for gross motor activities, such as the gastrocnemius, have a much higher ratio of muscle fibers to neurons.[3] The neurons innervating larger muscles are themselves larger with larger cell bodies and thicker axons.[4, 5] The sidebar Muscle Fibers in a Motor Unit in Different Skeletal Muscles provides some examples of the average numbers of muscle fibers in the motor units of various muscles. Note that the eye muscles have fewer than 10 muscle cells innervated by one neuron, while postural muscles that play a role in standing have a ratio of 1000 muscle cells to one neuron.[6]

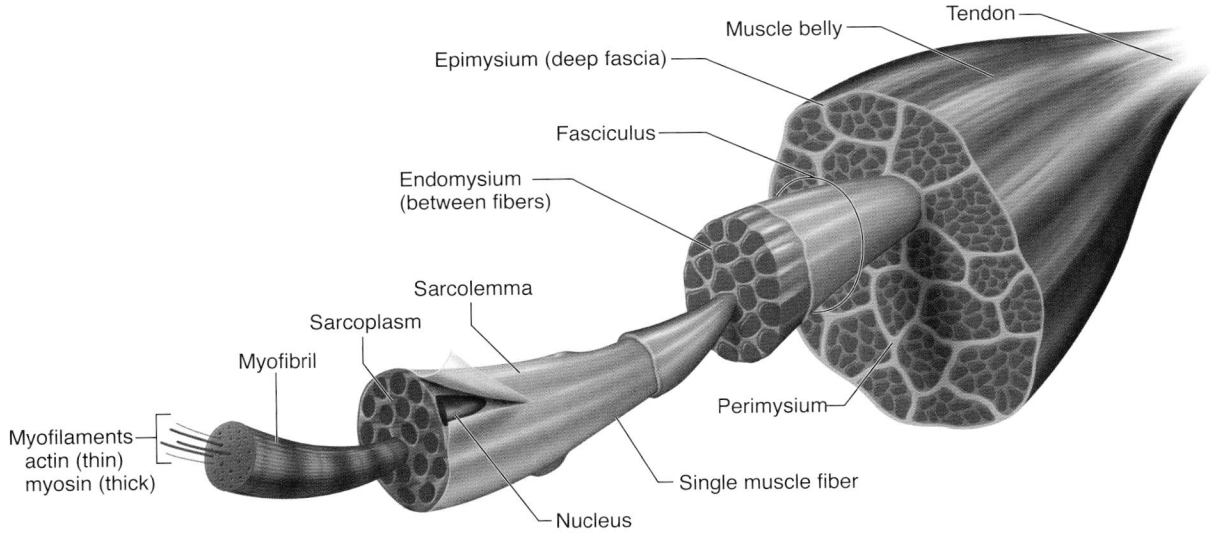

Figure 13.3 Muscle structure.

Muscle Fibers in a Motor Unit in Different Skeletal Muscles

The number of muscle fibers in a motor unit varies greatly depending on the size and function of each muscle. Examples of muscles that have a relatively high number of muscle fibers per motor unit include the following:

- Medial gastrocnemius, approximately 1600 to 1900 fibers per unit
- Biceps brachii, 750 fibers per unit
- Opponens pollicis, 595 fibers per unit
- Tibialis anterior, approximately 560 to 660 fibers per unit
- Brachioradialis, more than 410 fibers per unit[9]

By contrast, the platysma muscle of the neck has only about 25 muscle fibers per motor unit, and the tensor tympani muscle of the middle ear has only about eight muscle fibers per motor unit.[9]

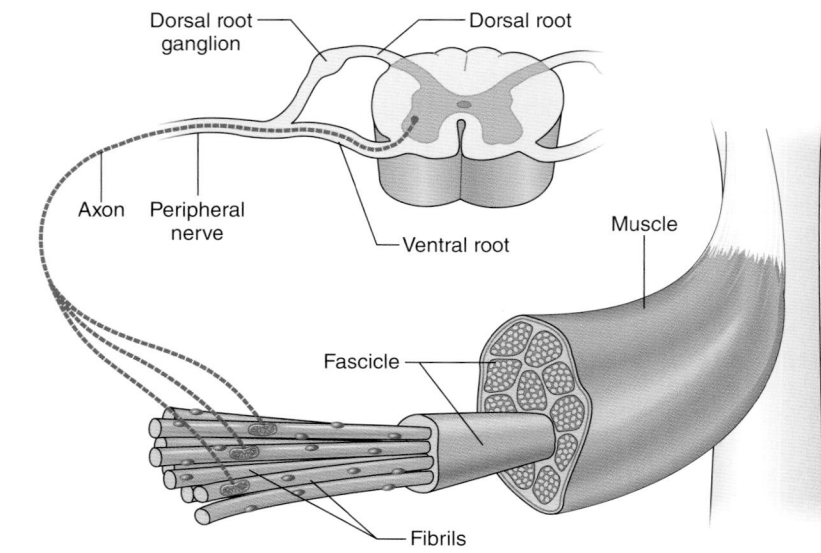

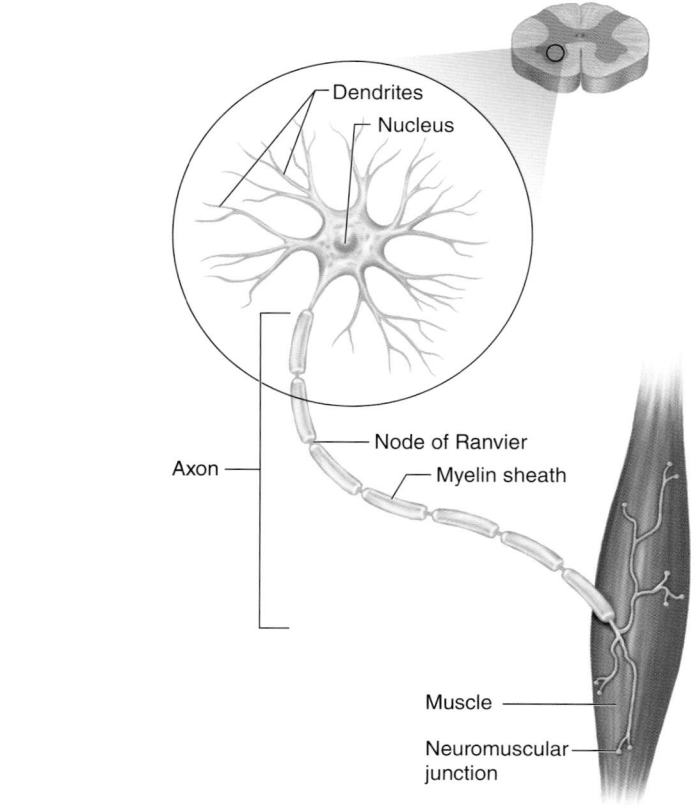

Figure 13.4 Motor unit: *(a)* Schematic drawing of the components of a motor unit—the anterior horn cell, its axon and terminating branches, and the muscle fibers it innervates. *(b)* One neuron from the spinal cord with its axon extending into the muscle. The number of muscle fibers a single motor unit innervates can range from a few to several thousand.[7, 8]

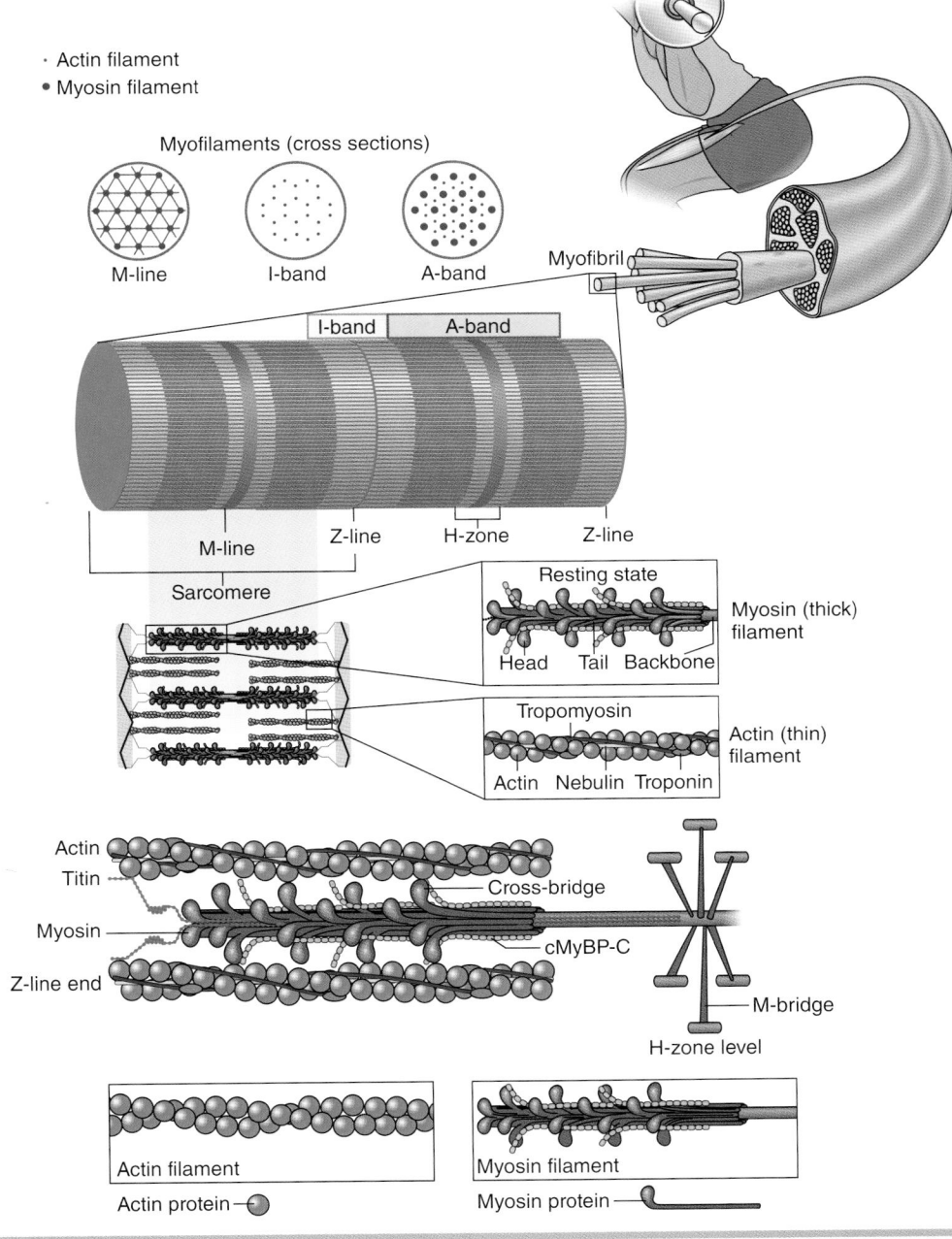

- Actin filament
- Myosin filament

Myofilaments (cross sections)

M-line   I-band   A-band

Myofibril

I-band   A-band

M-line   Z-line   H-zone   Z-line

Sarcomere

Resting state

Myosin (thick) filament

Head   Tail   Backbone

Tropomyosin

Actin (thin) filament

Actin   Nebulin   Troponin

Actin
Titin
Myosin
Z-line end

Cross-bridge
cMyBP-C

M-bridge

H-zone level

Actin filament
Actin protein

Myosin filament
Myosin protein

Figure 13.5 Actin proteins are like round balls connected together to form a long-chain filament, while myosin proteins are oblong with heads on them that face away from the center of the filament they form. Note the hexagonal arrangement of thin filaments around thick filaments and the triangular arrangement of thick filaments.

At muscle's most basic functional level, we find sarcomeres. Figures 13.5 and 13.6 depict the actin and myosin elements of sarcomeres and the arrangements these filaments have within the basic sarcomere structure.

Figure 13.6 shows how actin and myosin are arranged parallel to each other between protein structures labeled with various names: Z-discs, Z-lines, or Z-bands. Actin filaments are anchored on either end of the sarcomere to the Z-lines. The myosin filaments are in the larger filaments.[10] Large protein molecules, called nebulin, extend along the length of the actin filaments along with two other protein structures, tropomyosin and troponin.[11] The myosin fila-

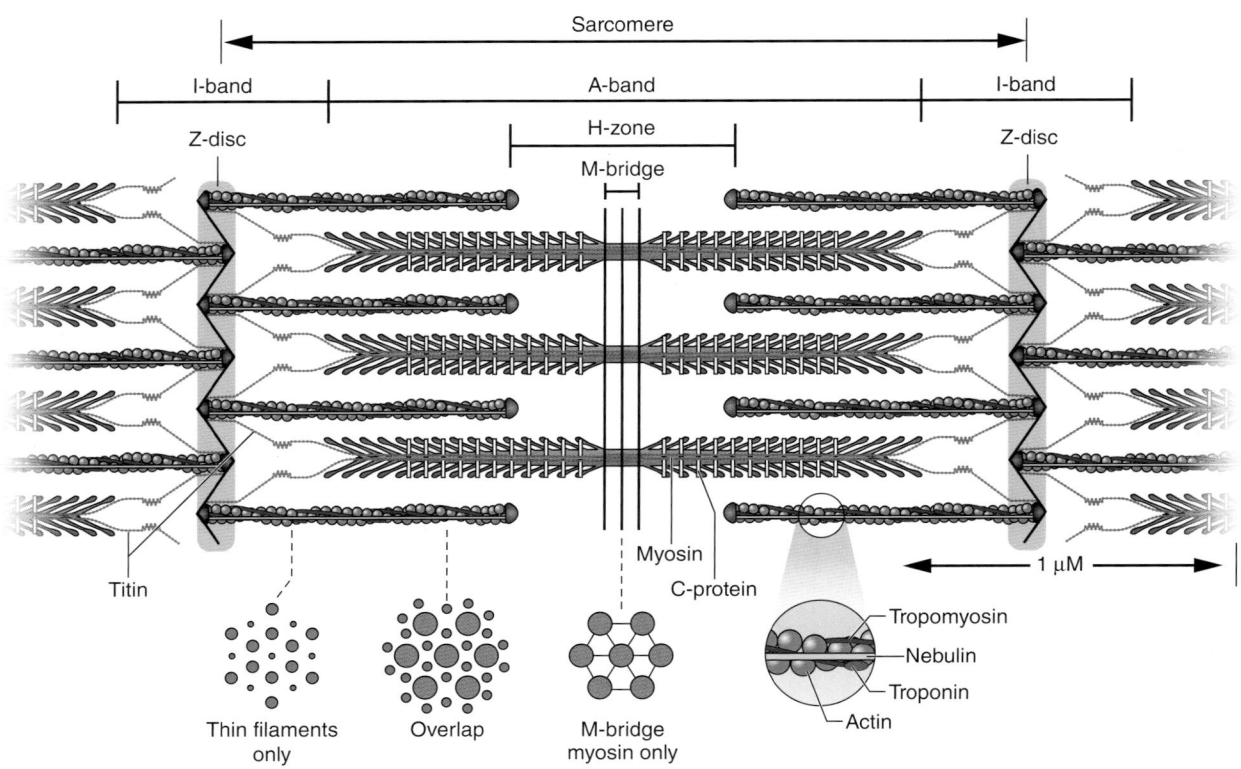

Figure 13.6   Elements of a sarcomere.

ments are in the equatorial center of the sarcomere. They are anchored with each other at the M-bridge (M-line) in the center of the H-band. They are tethered to the Z-bands by six parallel strands of titin, which are giant elastic protein strands that not only keep myosin filaments centered within each sarcomere but also provide passive elasticity to a muscle.[12-14] The titin strands from each end of the sarcomere meet and overlap with each other at the M-bridge in the middle of the larger myosin filament.[10] The Z-bands contain a number of proteins that signal various molecules throughout the muscle to provide normal muscle function.[15]

Sarcomere Function

Muscle function involves a complex interaction between the neurological and muscular systems. The systems work interdependently to provide smooth muscle activity. Energy and chemical interactions are required for these unique intersystem functions. How all of these elements work together is briefly reviewed here.

Recall that when a motor unit is stimulated by an excitatory impulse called an **action potential**, the myosin heads flex and create cross-bridges with actin filaments to pull the actin filaments toward the center of the sarcomere, so the Z-discs move toward the sarcomere's equatorial center, shortening the sarcomere. The theory that describes this process is the *sliding filament theory*. The sarcomere's

length changes because the actin and myosin filaments slide over each other, not because the filaments change length; only the relative sizes of the areas of the sarcomere that contain myosin (I-bands) or actin (H-bands) change, as demonstrated in figure 13.7.

CLINICAL TIPS

The sarcomere's structure can be summarized as follows:

- The sarcomere is from Z-line to Z-line.
- The A-band is dark and contains both actin and myosin filaments.
- The H-band is the center section of the A-band that does not contain actin filaments.
- The M-line (M-bridge) lies within the center of the H-band.
- The I-band is lighter and contains only actin filaments, and it is transversely bisected by a Z-disc (also referred to as a Z-band or Z-line).
- The M-line is the equatorial center of the sarcomere within the H-band and contains myosin but not actin filaments. The M-line anchors the myosin filaments.
- The Z-disc serves as the border of the sarcomere and is the site where actin filaments on either side of the Z-disc are anchored.

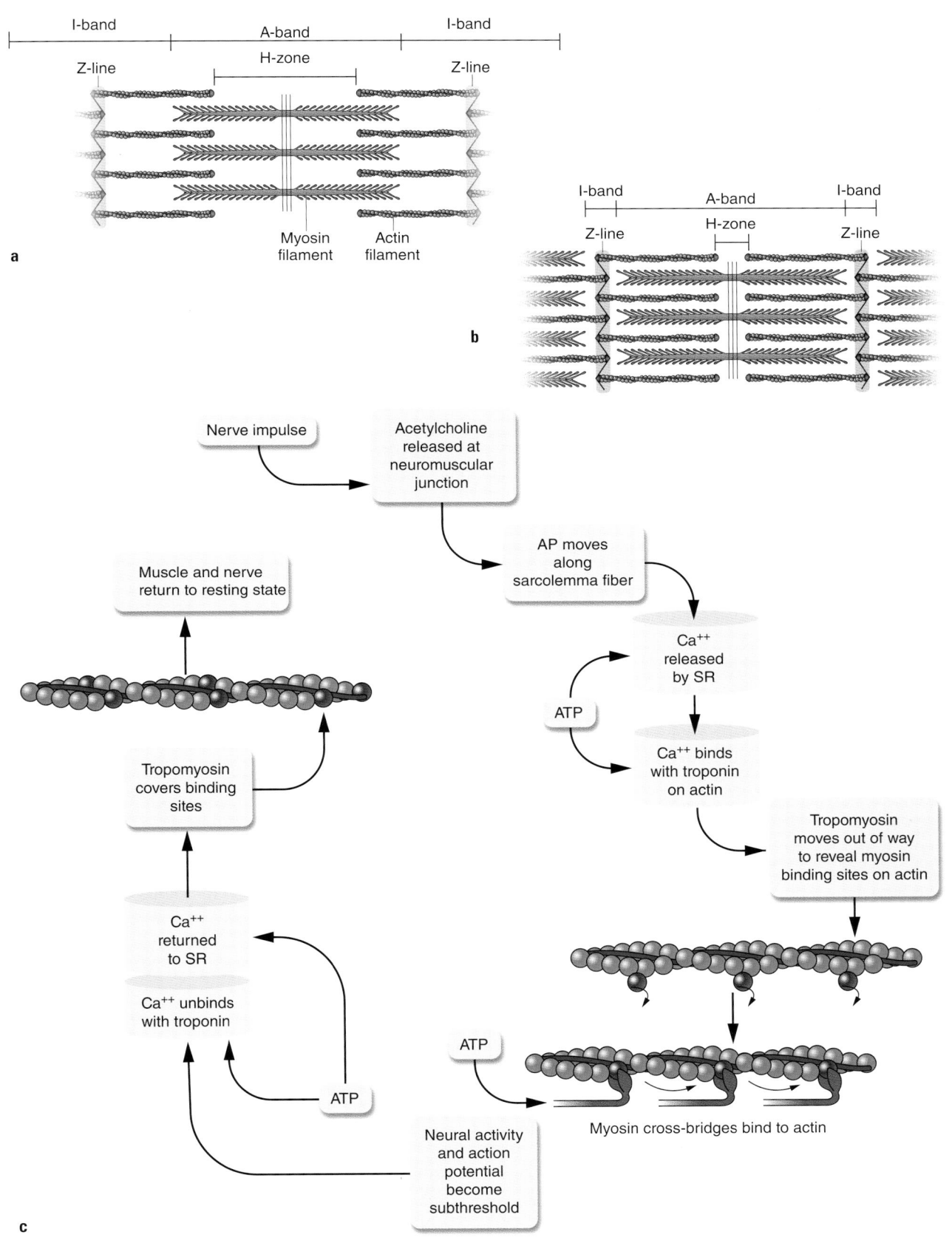

Figure 13.7   Changes in sarcomere length: *(a)* on stretch; *(b)* shortened; *(c)* sequence of muscle fiber contraction.

The biochemical process that causes this sarcomere shortening is rather complex and occurs instantaneously. There are two tubular systems vital to the activity of the sarcomere. The **sarcoplasmic reticulum** is an internal tubule system that is arranged parallel to the sarcomere and surrounds it in a fishnet mesh arrangement that terminates near the Z-discs. The transverse tubule (T-tubule) system extends into the inner aspects of the fiber to encircle the myofibrils and runs perpendicular to the sarcoplasmic reticulum. The T-tubules terminate near the Z-bands between two sarcoplasmic reticulum tubules in a triad arrangement, as seen in figure 13.8.

Sarcomere Energy System

Myosin heads contain an enzyme, myosin **ATPase**, which is a catalyst that hydrolyzes (breaks down) the **adenosine triphosphate (ATP)** into **adenosine diphosphate (ADP)** and phosphate for energy production.[16] This energy activates the myosin head. As long as calcium ions are present and ATP hydrolysis occurs to permit the cross-bridges to recock, the process continues and muscle activity is sustained. This series of attaching and releasing occurs at an asynchronous rate throughout a muscle's fibers, with some attaching while others are releasing during muscle activity.

ATP plays different roles twice within the sarcomere contraction process. It is hydrolyzed (broken down via an aqueous chemical reaction) into ADP and phosphate, and it re-forms to break the connection between actin and myosin. When it is hydrolyzed, energy is produced that provides for the power stroke for the movement of actin over myosin. When it is re-formed after the power stroke, it breaks the connection between the two myofibril filaments so the process either stops or is allowed to restart to maintain a muscle contraction. If ATP is not present but calcium is, sustained muscle contraction occurs, such as that seen in **rigor mortis** after death.

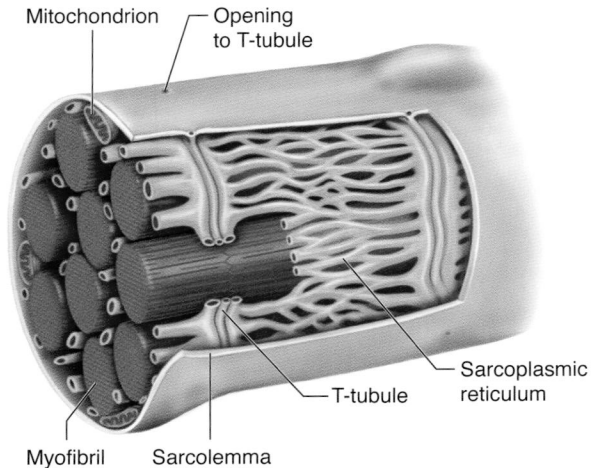

Mitochondrion — Opening to T-tubule

Myofibril   Sarcolemma

T-tubule

Sarcoplasmic reticulum

Figure 13.8 Tubule system.

Muscles of the Body

Having reviewed the microfunction of muscle, we can appreciate how those microscopic elements ultimately create muscle activity. As we look at the muscle as a whole, that which occurs at the microscopic level is simply magnified to create functional body movement.

Muscles of the body have four main functions: movement, posture, joint stability, and heat production.[17] Among the most obvious is motion production. Muscles provide actions, make us mobile, and allow us independence. If we look beyond skeletal muscle, we see that cardiac muscle pumps blood throughout our bodies, and smooth muscle moves substances needed for survival through our organ systems.

If we focus only on skeletal muscle, we see other functions as well. For example, skeletal muscles enable us to maintain our posture. As we move, muscles continually adjust to meet the demands that gravity and other forces place on our bodies so that we can remain upright. Since gravity is a constant force, muscles must change their activity as we change positions.

There are physiological characteristics that are unique to skeletal muscle and are vital for normal body function. It is important for clinicians to know what these characteristics are so that, when an injury occurs, they can design rehabilitation programs that will restore muscle health and function. These important characteristics that enable skeletal muscle to function normally are listed in table 13.2.

Types of Muscle Fibers and Muscles

When muscles contract, they normally shorten at both ends, so functional motion must include the stabilization of one muscle end while the other end performs the desired activity. Therefore, other muscles must stabilize the nonmoving end of the body segment. Stabilization of the nonmoving end requires greater activity and more muscle recruitment to accomplish higher-demand activities. For example, if you flex your elbow to bring a cup of water to your mouth, some muscles are recruited at the wrist and shoulder to stabilize those joints while the elbow moves. However, if you flex your elbow with a 9 kg (20 lb) dumbbell in your hand, not only do all of those muscles work harder, but more muscles are recruited to provide the added stability needed to move the heavier weight.

Muscles can be classified in a number of different ways: according to their shape, size, function, or fiber arrangement. Along with different muscle types, we have different muscle fibers. These are briefly reviewed in this section.

TABLE 13.2 **Unique Physiological Characteristics of Skeletal Muscle and the Role They Play in Normal Muscle Function**

Characteristic	Significance
Excitability	Motor unit response requires a threshold stimulation that is followed by a delayed (latent) response, and then in sequential order there is an electrical (neural) response, a metabolic (energy) response, and a mechanical (contraction) response.
Contractility	Series elastic components of the muscle respond to electrical and metabolic activity to contract.
Viscosity	The faster the rate of contraction, the greater the viscosity: More force is required to move a resistance at faster speeds than the same resistance at slower speeds.
Extensibility	Muscle can be stretched without changing its structure: Daily motion causes muscle heat to allow connective tissue to stretch, but immobility causes stiffness and loss of extensibility.
Elasticity	Elastic elements of muscle allow it to be stretched and return to normal length, but stretched plastic elements of muscle will produce a new muscle length.
Stiffness	Stiffness is resistance to change in shape or length. A slow stretch is more effective at increasing muscle length than a rapid stretch. Muscle tone is passive tension; weaker muscles have less tone than stronger muscles.
Contracture	Failure of a muscle to relax. Fatigue results in contracture; it is better to stretch after exercise than before exercise to return the muscle to its resting length.
Fatigue	Muscle fatigue causes inadequate neural propagation, insufficient energy supplies, impaired excitation-coupling (Ca^{++} release), or hydrogen accumulation that impairs energy systems and muscle contraction. Muscle fatigue reduces strength, force, and power.
Tetany	Normal muscle function that results in voluntary muscle contraction.

Fast- and Slow-Twitch Fibers

It should be mentioned that muscle fiber classifications have been updated to reflect more recent identifications of additional fibers. Fibers I, IIA, and IIB were identified as the original fibers. However, more recently 7 human muscle fiber types have been recognized; from slowest to fastest they have been named I, IC, IIC, IIAC, IIA, IIAB, and IIB.[18] Each of these fiber types are still discussed in terms of their speed. For convenience sake, some researchers place all 7 fiber types within the original 3 classifications since they fall within those original categories.[18] In an effort to keep things simple, these 3 categories will be discussed.

Skeletal muscle contains **fast-twitch** and **slow-twitch fibers**. The ratio of these fiber types is genetically determined and varies not only from one person to another for the same muscle but also within the person from muscle to muscle. In other words, one sprinter may have more fast-twitch fibers in the quadriceps than another sprinter does, and she may have more fast-twitch fibers in her quadriceps than in her hamstrings. It is generally agreed that muscle fiber types can convert from one type to another;[18-20] however, the process by which this transition occurs remains unknown.[21] The general consensus is that this conversion occurs within each division of fibers, and less often between the main divisions of fiber types; for example, one version of a Type II muscle fiber may convert

to another Type II during anaerobic training.[22] It should be noted, however, that it has recently been demonstrated that a shift from Type II to Type I is possible with specific training regimens.[23] Additional research is needed in this area.

An antigravity muscle, such as the soleus, tends to have more slow-twitch fibers than a muscle that is used more for locomotion and for fast or powerful movements, such as the quadriceps.[23, 24] No muscle has all fast-twitch or all slow-twitch fibers; a combination of these fibers is in all muscles, but those with more fast-twitch are used for power and explosive activities, while those with predominantly slow-twitch fibers are used for endurance or antigravity activities.

The two fiber types have different appearances, metabolic capacities, and contraction characteristics. Their names are based on their relative speed of activity. Figures 13.9 and 13.10 display the visual differences and the differing contraction rates, respectively, between fast- and slow-twitch fibers, and table 13.3 lists the differences between the three fiber types.

From a rehabilitation perspective, it is important to remember that the ratio of fast- and slow-twitch fibers varies from one person to another. Other factors being equal, if you rehabilitate two patients with knee injuries, the patient with more fast-twitch fibers in the quadriceps will produce a stronger output than the patient with fewer

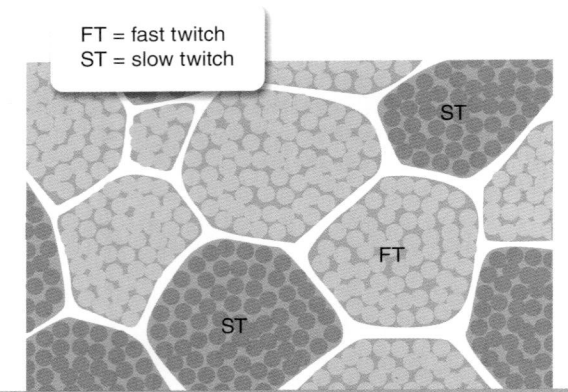

Figure 13.9 Fast- and slow-twitch fibers in a cross-section of a muscle. Slow-twitch fibers are stained darker because they are rich in mitochondria and myoglobin for their primary role, sustained muscle activity.

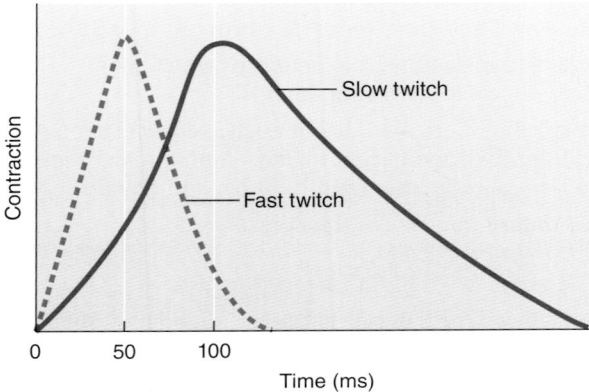

Figure 13.10 Contraction–relaxation curves for fast-twitch and slow-twitch skeletal muscle fibers.

fast-twitch fibers in the muscle and will demonstrate more speed during power activities. This is one reason that it is fruitless to expect two patients to perform equally, even if they are the same size and have similar injuries.

CLINICAL TIPS

Because of their characteristics differences, slow- and fast-twitch fibers have different functions. The slow-twitch fibers have a slower-acting myosin ATPase, and the fast-twitch fibers have a faster-acting myosin ATPase, so ATP is converted more quickly to produce energy faster for fast-twitch fibers than for slow-twitch fibers. The extensive sarcoplasmic reticulum of the fast-twitch fibers provides a more efficient delivery of calcium ions to permit a quicker fiber response to stimulation. However, because slow-twitch fibers have more mitochondria, more myoglobin, and more glycogen stores, they are better equipped for prolonged or sustained activity.

Although the differences between the two fast-twitch fibers are not yet fully understood, the Type IIA fibers are recruited more often during muscle activity than the other Type II fibers. Since Type IIB fibers require a stronger stimulus to fire, they are not recruited in low- or medium-intensity activities but are used in high-intensity activities, such as the 100 m swim. Type IIB fibers are the fastest; Type IIA fibers are a transitional type between Type I and Type IIB fibers because Type IIA fibers have qualities of both.

While both Type IIA and Type IIB fibers are fast-twitch, the Type IIA fibers are more important for moderate-resistance activities and for activities that require a combination of anaerobic and aerobic energy systems, such as the 400 m run. Type IIB fibers are more important for explosive resistance activities and for activities that use the purely anaerobic energy system. One reason that fast-twitch fibers can produce stronger forces than slow-twitch fibers is that their motor units contain more muscle fibers. The greater number of responding muscle fibers produces a greater force.

Muscle Types

Skeletal muscles may be categorized in different ways. For example, some discussions refer to muscle groups as slow-twitch or fast-twitch, depending on the predominance of the muscle's fiber types. Muscles may also be referred to as either prime movers or assistant movers, based on which muscles are primarily responsible for a specific movement and which ones merely assist in performing the motion. Skeletal muscles may also be described as either movers or stabilizers, depending on their function for a specific body motion or segmental activity. A muscle can also be recognized as an agonist, or prime mover, for a specific motion while its opposing muscle, which produces a motion in the opposite direction, is the antagonist.

Skeletal muscles may also be identified as either one-joint, two-joint, or multi-joint muscles; this definition is based on the number of joints the muscle and its tendon cross from its proximal to its distal insertion. Skeletal muscle that crosses more than two joints (multi-joint or polyarticular) in the body are exceptional and include some of the spinal muscles and the extrinsic muscles of the fingers and toes. Two-joint muscles are technically polyarticular muscles; there are several of these muscles in the upper and lower extremities. These two-joint muscles are more commonly referred to as biarticular or two-joint muscles rather than multi-joint muscles. Studies have found that monoarticular and biarticular muscles act differently during both isometric and isotonic motions.[25]

Monoarticular Muscles

Monoarticular, or single-joint, muscles cross only one joint, so their function occurs primarily at that joint.[26] Monoar-

TABLE 13.3   Differences Between Types of Muscle Fibers

Characteristics	Type I	Type IIA	Type IIB
Speed	Slowest	Fast	Fastest
Axon size	Smaller	Large	Larger
Fiber size	Smaller	Moderate	Larger
Color	Red	White	White
Conduction velocity	Slow: 100 ms	Fast: 50 ms	Faster: 25 ms
Fatigue resistance	Greatest	Moderate	Least
Recruitment threshold	Lower	Moderate	Higher
Firing rates	Lower minimum and maximum	Moderate minimum and maximum	Higher minimum and maximum
Capillary density	Higher	Moderate	Lower
Mitochondria	Greater number	Moderate number	Smaller number
Fuel consumption efficiency	Higher	Moderate	Lower
Myosin ATPase	Slow acting	Intermediate acting	Fast acting
Oxidative capacity	Higher	High	Lower
Glycogen stores	Lower	High	Higher
Energy system used	Oxidative system	ATP-PC system	Glycolytic system
Force produced	Lower	High	Highest
Activity	Endurance, aerobic	High-intensity activity, less than 2 min	Max-intensity bursts, no more than 30 s

ticular muscles provide force during movement.[27, 28] They produce force mainly through concentric contractions during functional activities.[29]

The amount of force a monoarticular muscle produces is related to its length; a muscle's ability to generate tension is based on the length of its fibers.[30] Also, because of limitations of the sarcomeres, a muscle's ability to shorten is limited to about 70% of its resting length.[31-36] This physiological factor is a distinct disadvantage for monoarticular muscles; once they reach their length at maximum contraction, they cannot produce any additional force. If the body had to rely only on monoarticular muscles, motions we currently perform with ease would become very inefficient, and they would require a lot more energy to perform.[37-39] Without a combination of monoarticular and biarticular muscles, our systems would require a lot more muscles and a lot more energy. This is not to say that monoarticular muscles are unimportant in functional activities; only that they work synergistically with biarticular muscles to allow us to complete our movements effectively.[40]

There are more monoarticular muscles than biarticular muscles in the body. Tables 13.4 and 13.5 list the monoarticular and biarticular muscles in the extremities.

Biarticular Muscles

While monoarticular muscles provide the force during functional activities, muscles that cross two joints—biar-

ticular, or two-joint muscles—provide the direction, control, and stabilization of functional movement.[41] Monoarticular muscles usually perform either isometrically or concentrically during functional activities, while biarticular muscles work more often eccentrically than concentrically.[28, 42, 43] Unlike the monoarticular muscles that shorten during functional activities, biarticular muscles usually shorten at one joint while lengthening at another joint, so their length–tension relationship remains essentially unchanged.[44] Positive work is produced at the shortening end of the muscle and negative work occurs at its lengthening end, so energy demands are reduced, making the muscle's activity energy efficient.[44] Since these interactions of positive and negative work within the muscle counterbalance each other to reduce energy needs for an activity, using biarticular muscles in this manner requires significantly less energy than if monoarticular muscles were used to perform the same activities.[37, 38]

 Go to HK*Propel* and watch video 13.1, which demonstrates multi-joint muscles: Positioning for strength.

As part of their system of efficient movement, biarticular muscles also abide by Lombard's paradox. Normally, skeletal muscles contract and relax according to the concept

TABLE 13.4   Monoarticular Muscles of the Lower and Upper Extremities

Joint	Muscle	Action
Hip	Gluteus maximus	Hip extension, lateral rotation
Hip	Gluteus medius	Hip abduction, medial rotation
Hip	Gluteus minimus	Hip abduction, medial rotation
Hip	Gemellus superior	Hip lateral rotation
Hip	Gemellus inferior	Hip lateral rotation
Hip	Obturator internus	Hip lateral rotation
Hip	Obturator externus	Hip lateral rotation
Hip	Quadratus femoris	Hip lateral rotation
Hip	Piriformis	Hip lateral rotation
Hip	Adductor brevis	Hip adduction
Hip	Adductor longus	Hip adduction, medial rotation
Hip	Adductor magnus	Hip adduction, medial rotation
Hip	Gracilis	Hip adduction, medial rotation
Hip	Pectineus	Hip adduction, flexion
Hip	Psoas	Hip flexion
Hip	Iliacus	Hip flexion
Knee	Vastus medialis	Knee extension
Knee	Vastus lateralis	Knee extension
Knee	Vastus intermedius	Knee extension
Knee	Popliteus	Femoral lateral rotation in CKC
Ankle	Soleus	Ankle plantar flexion
Shoulder	Posterior deltoid	Shoulder horizontal abduction
Shoulder	Middle deltoid	Shoulder abduction
Shoulder	Anterior deltoid	Shoulder horizontal adduction
Shoulder	Supraspinatus	Shoulder abduction
Shoulder	Infraspinatus	Shoulder lateral rotation
Shoulder	Teres minor	Shoulder extension
Shoulder	Subscapularis	Shoulder medial rotation
Shoulder	Teres major	Shoulder extension
Shoulder	Coracobrachialis	Shoulder flexion
Elbow	Brachialis	Elbow flexion
Elbow	Triceps, medial and lateral heads	Elbow extension
Forearm	Supinator	Forearm supination
Forearm	Pronator	Forearm pronation
Forearm	Pronator quadratus	Forearm pronation

of reciprocal inhibition: when a muscle contracts, its opposing muscle relaxes.[45] However, when we perform functional activities such as getting up from a chair or jumping or running, opposing biarticular muscles of the lower extremities contract together to create those activities. Lombard's paradox says that antagonistic muscles, rather than acting according to the laws of reciprocal innervation, co-contract to produce an efficient system of movement.[46]

To understand how Lombard's paradox creates efficiency in biarticular muscle activity, we must first recall that when a muscle contracts, it produces force throughout its entirety, resulting in movement at both ends of the

TABLE 13.5   Biarticular Muscles of the Lower and Upper Extremities

Extremity	Muscle	Actions
Lower extremity	Sartorius	Hip flexor; knee flexor
Lower extremity	Rectus femoris	Knee extensor; hip flexor
Lower extremity	Biceps femoris, long head	Hip extensor; knee flexor
Lower extremity	Semimembranosus	Hip extensor; knee flexor
Lower extremity	Semitendinosus	Hip extensor; knee flexor
Lower extremity	Gastrocnemius	Ankle plantar flexor; knee flexor
Upper extremity	Biceps brachii	Shoulder flexor; elbow flexor; forearm supinator
Upper extremity	Triceps brachii, long head	Shoulder extensor; elbow extensor

muscle as the fibers shorten toward the center.[47] When we move from sitting to standing, the hip and knee extend together: The hamstrings and rectus femoris both contract at both joints in spite of the fact that they are antagonistic muscles at both of these joints. So, if both of these antagonistic muscles are contracting, how can motion occur at either joint? The reason has to do with their moment arms. At the hip, the hamstring muscles have a longer moment arm, so they have a mechanical advantage over the rectus femoris to create hip extension. At the knee, the moment arm of the rectus femoris is longer than that of the hamstrings, so extension is the resultant force at that joint. In other words, these two muscles create a net resultant moment at each of these two joints; the net moment at the hip produces extension because of the greater moment arm of the hamstrings at the hip, and at the knee it is extension because of the greater moment arm of the rectus femoris at that joint. Additionally, as the hip extends, it allows the rectus femoris to lengthen at the hip, adding potential force at the knee (related to its length–tension relationship); likewise, as the knee extends, the hamstrings gain tension from their length–tension relationship to provide additional extension force at the hip. Figure 13.11 provides a visual representation of Lombard's paradox at the hip and knee. Lombard's paradox applies to other activities besides rising from a chair; in the lower extremities, these include stair climbing, jumping, hopping, running, and squatting.

When rehabilitating body segments with biarticular muscles, the clinician must consider the impact of this anatomical arrangement from both an exercise perspective and a functional perspective. For example, if a patient is undergoing rehabilitation of a knee after anterior cruciate ligament reconstruction (ACL-R), exercise positioning becomes important when either stretching or strengthening biarticular muscles. If the clinician is to improve quadriceps flexibility, a stretch exercise must include a position that places the rectus femoris in a stretch position at both the hip and knee joints. Flexing the knee with the patient sitting is not beneficial in providing an effective stretch for the rectus femoris since it is being stretched at the knee

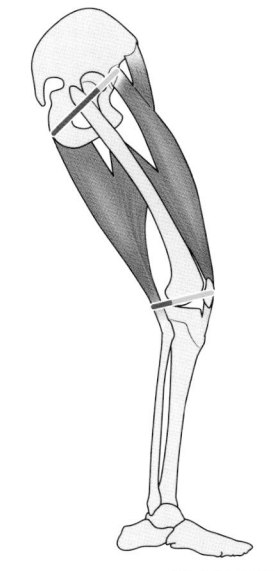

Figure 13.11 Lombard's paradox explains how opposing muscles both contract to produce efficient motion during functional activities. The red line is the moment arm of the hamstrings, and the yellow line is the moment arm of the rectus femoris.

but shortened at the hip; no stretch occurs. An accurate rectus femoris stretch must be performed with the hip in extension and the knee in flexion.

Strength exercises are also needed to produce optimal results for a biarticular muscle. For example, for the ACL-R patient to strengthen the hamstring muscles, in what position should the strength exercises be performed? It depends on the clinician's goals. Research has demonstrated that biarticular muscles are optimally activated when they contract from both attachment sites.[48] Therefore, if it is the clinician's goal to obtain as much output from the hamstrings as possible, then the patient should be positioned in hip extension and knee flexion.

From a functional perspective, the clinician must assess the rectus femoris and hamstrings' ability to work together as opposing forces to create movement. Coordination and timing of the activity may require reeducation to produce optimal performance and reduce the risk of re-injury.[49] It is appropriate to use functional activities such as a sit-to-stand exercise in the early rehabilitation program and then advance to more complex biarticular activities such as stair climbing, jumping, hopping, and running as the patient progresses.

Muscle Strength and Power, Endurance, and Recovery Related to Rehabilitation

Before we discuss how to improve muscle function in a rehabilitation program, we must identify the components involved. These components are important, for they play important roles in returning the patient to optimal function.

Muscle Strength and Power

Strength is the maximum force that a muscle or muscle group can exert. Several factors determine one's ability to produce strength; some can be changed with exercise and some cannot. Age and heredity determine sex, body structure, muscle size, height, and limb lengths. People with a slight build will not be as strong as those with a larger frame, women are generally weaker than men, and older patients are usually weaker than younger patients. Strength can change, however, with exercise,[50] and regular exercise can also alter muscle fiber types[23, 51, 52] and improve muscle recruitment by improving the efficiency of the neural response system.[53, 54] All of these factors play important roles in strength and in the ability to make strength gains.[55-57] Lifestyle certainly influences muscle strength; if a patient performs only the activities of daily living, that person's strength will be less than that of someone of the same age, sex, size, and build who exercises on a regular basis. The patient who does not exercise will have fewer Type II muscle fibers and more Type I muscle fibers, and the patient will have less muscle tone than someone who participates in sports; sudden movements and quick responses will also be slower than those of a more active person.[58, 59]

Before we can discuss the elements of strength, we have to identify how we determine someone's strength. There are various ways. A commonly used clinical method for examining a patient's strength uses the clinician's manual resistance in either an isometric or an isotonic contraction.[60] The results can be used to establish the resistance level at which to start the patient's rehabilitation exercises. This method is not foolproof, and occasionally it requires some adjustment in weight, even by the most experienced clinicians, but it provides a starting point for early rehabilitation strengthening.

The amount of force a muscle produces depends upon various factors. Some of these factors may be manipulated, and others are inherent in the person. We will limit this discussion to those elements that may be influenced by the clinician in a rehabilitation program.

Joint Angle

Joint movement is the result of a muscle's pull on the joint. The amount of force causing rotation of the joint (movement) and the amount of force directed at compression or distraction of the joint (stability or instability, respectively) are determined by the angle of the joint and the vector forces produced. Since movement around a joint is rotational, the force produced is **torque**. Remember that torque is determined by the amount of applied force and the length of the moment arm: $T = F \times d$ (torque = force $\times$ distance). As the joint moves through its range of motion, the moment-arm length changes, causing a change in the muscle's torque. For example, when a patient performs a biceps curl, as the elbow moves from 90° flexion to 125° flexion, the moment arms of the resistance and the biceps shorten. Since the moment arm of the resistance (weight) undergoes a greater change than the moment arm of the biceps, the weight gets easier to lift by the time the patient reaches the end of elbow flexion, as seen in figure 13.12. Based on the torque formula and from a purely mechanical standpoint, the greatest torque production occurs when the muscle's moment arm is at its greatest length; this length occurs when the muscle's line of pull is perpendicular to the joint. Although moment-arm length often has a direct impact on a muscle's ability to provide force,[61] there are other influences that make torque production analysis more complicated than this concept alone.[62]

How does this concept apply to rehabilitation? You must keep it in mind whenever you have a patient perform a weight-resistive exercise. It will affect how you position the patient in relation to where the maximal resistance will occur within the muscle's motion. For example, for the elbow, you must decide where in the motion you want the patient's elbow flexors to experience their greatest resistance: at the beginning, middle, or end of elbow flexion. If you choose to provide the greatest resistance at the beginning of the exercise, the patient will perform the exercise in supine, and you will access the maximum length of the sarcomeres, but if you want the muscle to work against maximal resistance with an optimal moment arm for the biceps, you will place the elbow at 90°. On the other hand, if your goal is to work the muscle against it greatest resistance at the end of elbow flexion, then the patient will perform the exercise in a prone position when both sarcomere length and moment-arm length are short and at their lowest force levels. Since the biceps is a biarticular muscle, you must also be aware of the shoulder's position during resistive exercises.

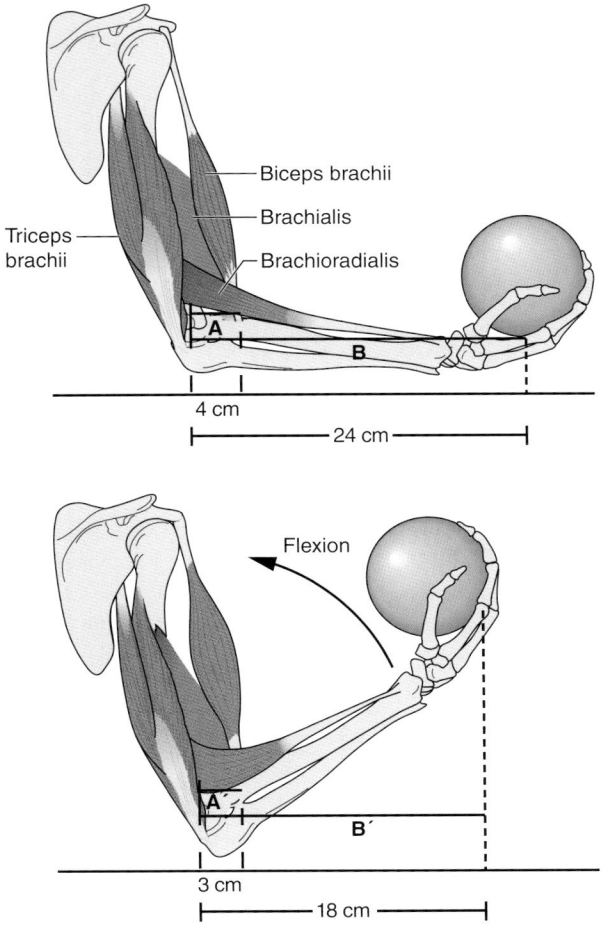

Figure 13.12 Change in biceps moment-arm length (A to A′) and change in resistance lever-arm length (B to B′) with different joint angles.

Another way torque around a joint is affected is by the length of the muscle or resistance moment arm. You can optimize the muscle's moment-arm length by positioning the muscle so its moment arm is perpendicular to the resistance force. You can also change the length of the resistance moment arm by shortening it to reduce the force against which the muscle must work. For example, a patient lifting the lower extremity in a straight-leg lift will reduce the amount of force exerted against the hip flexor muscles by bending the knee to shorten the resistance moment arm; the patient will find it easier to lift the limb when the knee is flexed than when it is fully extended.

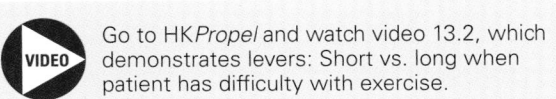

Go to HK*Propel* and watch video 13.2, which demonstrates levers: Short vs. long when patient has difficulty with exercise.

Length–Tension Relationship

One of the factors that determines a muscle's force production is the muscle's length.[63] However, distinctions should be made between a sarcomere's length and a whole muscle's length; although a whole muscle responds according to its sarcomere contraction, its length is affected by additional factors that do not affect sarcomeres. It makes more sense to look at a sarcomere's length first.

A sarcomere's ability to produce force and the shape of its length–tension curve are defined by the number of cross-bridges between the actin and myosin strands.[64] Gordon and colleagues[63] provided the first sarcomere force–length curve that demonstrated the change in isometric force of a single muscle fiber as the relative position of the actin and myosin strands overlapped. The optimal number of cross-bridge connections occurs at the resting length.[65] When the sarcomere is either stretched or shortened from that resting length, fewer cross-bridges are present, so its strength decreases. Figure 13.13*a* shows this relationship.

As with the sarcomere, the force produced by a muscle changes with its length (figure 13.13*b*); however, some important differences add to a change in the muscle's length–tension configuration. When a muscle contracts, several sarcomeres are engaged throughout its entire length. A whole muscle has different fiber types and different sarcomere lengths, so the entire muscle will demonstrate a smoother curve than one sarcomere, and the optimal length region will be larger.[66]

In addition to this length difference, other factors contribute to a whole muscle's force production. One of these factors involves both active and passive elements. The active component is the motor unit; the passive component includes its tendons and the connective tissue surrounding the whole muscle, its fascicles, and its fibers. A muscle's ability to actively produce force lessens as the length of the muscle diminishes.[63] When shortening, a muscle uses only its active component; however, when muscle tension occurs as a muscle lengthens, the muscle's passive components also play a role in creating that tension. Since tension occurs in tendons and fascia as a muscle lengthens, this tension is added to the tension that is created by the cross-bridges, so more force is produced by a muscle as it elongates. This concept has a direct effect on the application of eccentric exercises; these activities will be presented later in this chapter.

In addition to using passive muscle components to increase whole-muscle force production, we can use these passive components for their elastic qualities. When a muscle either passively or actively lengthens rapidly before it shortens, its passive components, the surrounding connective tissue structures, become taut and produce an additional resistive force because of their elasticity and the release of kinetic energy from that elasticity.[67] The optimal

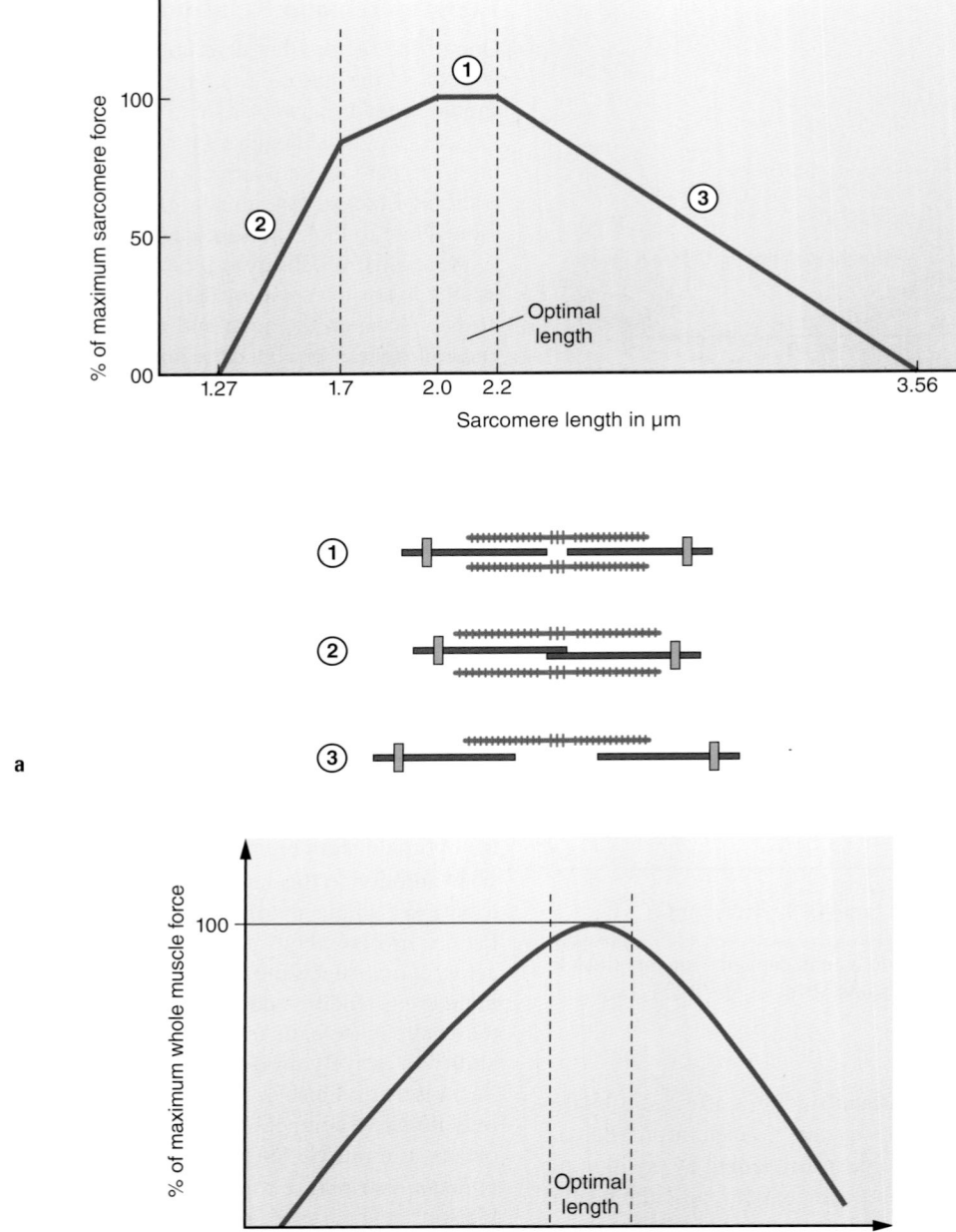

Figure 13.13 *(a)* Sarcomere length is related to the relative positions of actin and myosin fibers, while sarcomere strength is related to the number of cross-bridge connections. *(b)* Like the sarcomere, the whole muscle produces its greatest force when it is at its optimal length, and it weakens as it becomes either shorter or longer than its optimal length.

length of a muscle for producing force—because of the release of elastic energy from the passive elements and the position of actin–myosin cross-bridges in the active elements—is slightly beyond its resting length[68] (figure 13.14). However, if we stretch the muscle beyond that point, separation between the actin and myosin occurs and reduces the number of cross-bridges available. The result

is less force rather than more,[69] so care must be taken to apply a stretch but not an overstretch to create this force reduction.

Given the effects of this elastic release of kinetic energy on a muscle's length–tension relationship, there are several concepts that are important to rehabilitation. When we want to achieve a maximum muscle force, it is helpful to produce

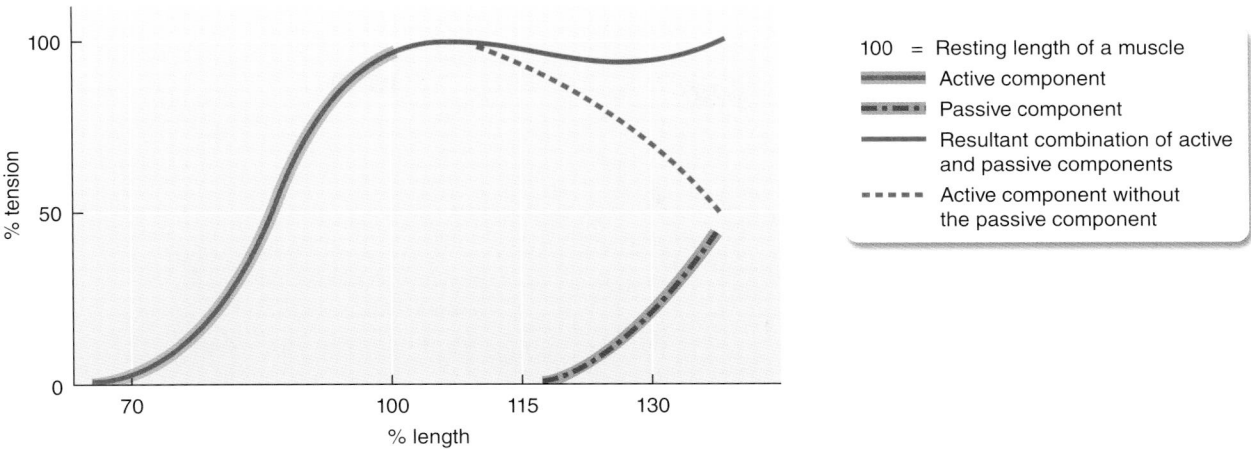

Figure 13.14 Length–tension relationship of a whole muscle: Because of the active and passive muscle tissue elements, a muscle produces its greatest strength slightly beyond its resting length.

a quick stretch of the muscle to use this elastic energy component. We apply this concept to exercises throughout a rehabilitation program. For example, in early strengthening exercises, the clinician may apply a quick manual stretch to the patient's muscle immediately before the patient moves into a concentric motion to increase the muscle's concentric force. Later in the rehabilitation program, the patient may incorporate a quick stretch immediately before executing a resistive or power exercise to facilitate optimal output and to improve performance during a functional activity. This technique is normally used in functional activities such as jumping and throwing.

Another factor in rehabilitation related to length–tension has to do with positioning the muscle for a resistive exercise. The length–tension relationship tells us that as the muscle shortens from its resting length, it becomes weaker. Based on the length–tension graph in figure 13.14, we know that a muscle's strength declines in a progressive yet smooth manner as the muscle shortens. The clinician, therefore, positions the muscle accordingly given the goal of the exercise. For example, if the muscle's strength suddenly decreases or fails at a point in the range of motion instead of declining steadily, the clinician may want to concentrate exercises at that point to restore a normal strength decline. Imagine that a patient with a quadriceps strain has excessive weakness in the midrange of knee extension to the point that when she tries to do a unilateral squat, the leg collapses. To resolve this problem, the clinician may decide to use exercises that work the quadriceps only in the range of 75° to 100° so the patient can restore the strength that is appropriate for that part of the muscle's range of motion.

Another way to use the concept of greater force occurring during an eccentric contraction is during the early phase of strengthening in a rehabilitation program. For example, a patient has a post-surgical condition and cannot lift the extremity; let's say you are working with a steel-worker who recently had an ACL-R. He cannot perform a straight-leg lift because of muscle weakness. Since he does not have the strength to perform a concentric movement, start him with an eccentric activity: While he is supine, passively lift the leg into a straight-leg raise position, and then tell him to slowly lower the leg to the treatment table while you release your support of the limb. Keep your hands close to the extremity in case he needs some help to perform the activity. The first time may be difficult for him, so he may need some assistance, but as the neuromotor elements and passive tissue tension "kick in," the exercise will become something he can do.

If we examine figure 13.14 and look only at the active component, we realize that not only does the muscle weaken as it gets shorter, but it also weakens as it extends beyond its optimal length. This important concept has a direct impact on patients who are treated for postural abnormalities such as those that were mentioned in chapter 6. As a poor habitual posture creates pathologically long and short muscles, those muscles become weak because they move from their optimal resting length. Investigations of Grossman and colleagues[70] demonstrate that when a muscle's resting length either increases or decreases, changes occur in the muscle's ability to create force. Additional studies have also demonstrated that sarcomeres in series are added when a muscle undergoes an adaptation by anatomically lengthening and are removed when the muscle's resting length adapts to a shortened anatomical position.[71] Figure 13.15 summarizes the findings of Grossman and colleagues[70] to provide a visual image of the strength changes that occur with postural changes.

It is no wonder then that the patient who has developed an anatomical postural change experiences weakness and fatigue in both the lengthened and shortened muscles. The

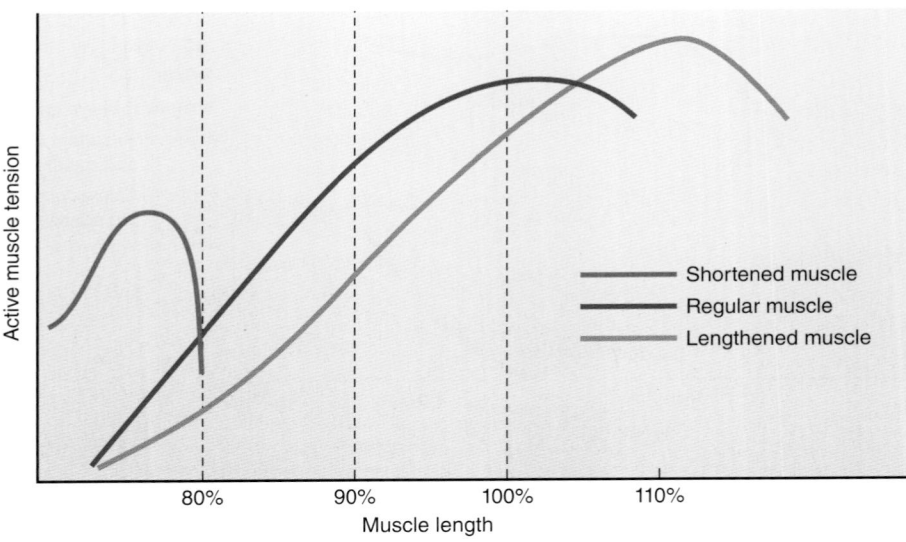

Figure 13.15 Based on the findings of Grossman and colleagues,[70] muscles change with changes in resting lengths. A muscle adapts to applications of continuous low-level stress by changing length and strength, removing sarcomeres on the shortened side and adding sarcomeres on the lengthened side. Both changes weaken the muscle. Although a lengthened muscle has greater tension in its lengthened position, notice how much weaker it is than a muscle with normal length throughout most of its range of motion. Likewise, the tension of a muscle that has undergone anatomically adaptive shortening falls far short of that of the normal-length muscle.

Based on the findings of Grossman et al. (1982).[70]

rehabilitation clinician must be aware of these anatomical and physiological changes so they may be appropriately addressed in the patient's rehabilitation program.

Force–Velocity Relationship

Just as the length–tension relationship affects the muscle's ability to create force, the force–velocity relationship affects the muscle's ability to produce power.[69] In essence, the force–velocity relationship is the definition of power since velocity includes the element of time. **Power** is strength applied over a distance for a specific amount of time. Power is a factor in most athletic events because it involves the body's ability to produce speed with strength. The volleyball player who can leg-press 180 kg (400 lb) in half the time it takes a basketball player to press the same weight has twice the power of the basketball player. Power is represented mathematically by this formula:

$$P = F \times d / T$$

where P = power, F = force, d = distance, and T = time.

Work is force × distance. In other words, power is work performed over a specific amount of time. Power increases when the same amount of work is performed in less time or when more work is performed in the same amount of time. In essence, power is directly related to the strength a muscle produces or the distance it can move; it is inversely proportional to the time it takes to perform the task.

Based on the power formula, when a muscle shortens, the force produced is inversely proportional to the veloc-

ity of shortening. It is assumed that this occurs because there is insufficient time for actin and myosin to attach to each other, so there are fewer cross-bridge connections available during a higher-velocity shortening.[72, 73] For example, patients who lift 22.5 kg (50 lb) quickly will find that same weight easier to lift when they lift it more slowly. Figure 13.16 shows the graphic representation of how a muscle's force production changes as its speed of contraction increases.

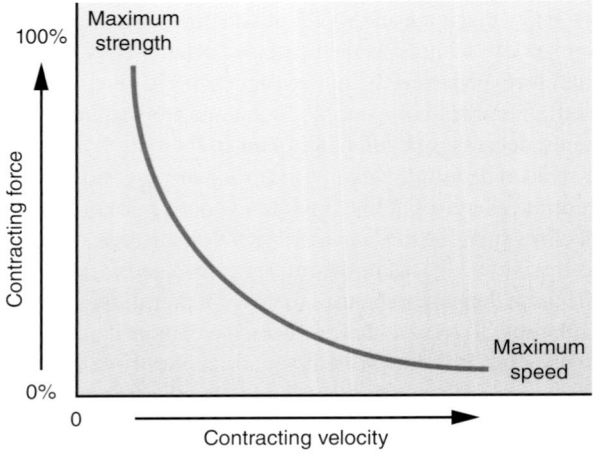

Figure 13.16 Force–velocity curve as it relates to concentric muscle contractions. The faster a muscle shortens concentrically, the less strength it can produce.

On the other hand, as a muscle lengthens, the force it produces is directly proportional to the velocity of movement; therefore, a muscle can oppose more resistance during a lengthening activity than during a muscle-shortening activity. One study showed that force production using a muscle-lengthening activity is 120% to 160% more than with a muscle-shortening activity.[74, 75] Other investigators believe that this figure is close to 130%.[74] This concept will be dealt with in more detail later in this chapter when types of muscle activity are presented.

Speed is a factor in power-based activities; such activities also depend on additional factors such as coordination, accuracy of movement, and performance timing.[76-80] Because of their importance, these elements are incorporated into a rehabilitation program once strength improves because, to some extent, they depend on the patient's strength.

When it is time to include power exercises in the patient's rehabilitation program, remember that the strength the patient can demonstrate during slow, controlled exercises will not be available for faster, more functional motions. High-velocity activity can only be produced at a fraction of the patient's maximum ability to produce force. The exercises included and the level of resistance forces provided in power exercises are determined based on the patient's age, sex, skill level, size, and goals.

Muscle Endurance and Recovery

Muscle endurance and the ability of a muscle to recover from fatigue after an exercise or activity are important concepts that must be considered in any rehabilitation program. To some extent, a muscle's endurance and ability to recover are related, and both may be improved with rehabilitation. Muscle endurance determines how long it takes a muscle to reach fatigue, and muscle recovery determines how long that muscle needs before it can resume performance activities at a pre-fatigue level.

Muscle Endurance

Muscle endurance is the ability of a muscle or a muscle group to perform repeated contractions against a less-than-maximal load. A muscle's endurance, or ability to prolong activity, depends on the status of the energy systems available and the quantity of forces resisted. With advanced conditioning levels, circulatory and local metabolic exchanges improve. The more work the muscle must do against resisted forces, the more quickly muscle fatigue will occur. Muscle endurance is related to the muscle's strength, and it is affected by the amount of resistance it must work against. For example, if a person's 1RM on a bench press is 136 kg (300 lb), that person will be able to lift 68 kg (150 lb) for more repetitions before fatiguing than if he lifts 113 kg (250 lb). Therefore, if a gain in endurance is the desired goal, it would be appropriate to use a lower weight that allows more repetitions before fatigue occurs.

There is also an intimate relationship between muscle endurance and muscle strength that must be borne in mind when designing a patient's rehabilitation program. Gains in muscle strength and muscle endurance lie on a continuum of exercise repetitions and intensity.[81] High-intensity, low-repetition exercises, at one end of this continuum, emphasize primarily strength gains. Low-intensity, high-repetition exercises, at the other end of the continuum, produce primarily muscle endurance gains.

Before we can begin a discussion of endurance exercise repetitions, we must first return to the topic of muscle strength improvement in rehabilitation and how it is attained. Although strength gains have been found to occur with high-intensity exercises, the recommended numbers of repetitions and sets vary among investigators.[22, 82-89] Reasons for this variability may include the specific programs and populations chosen for each study.[50] The American College of Sports Medicine (ACSM) has made recommendations based on the initial conditioning level of a healthy person.[50] Unfortunately, there are currently no general strength recommendations or guidelines for patients in orthopedic or sports injury rehabilitation programs.

Until these guidelines for injuries are identified, we can develop a reasonable rehabilitation strength program if we use investigations of normal populations as a guide. We know that high resistance and low repetitions more directly improve strength, while low resistance and high repetitions develop muscle endurance. Exercises to achieve either strength or endurance have a recommended range of repetitions based on various studies of normal groups. The number of repetitions recommended for strength gains ranges from 3 to 5 repetitions in one source[22] to 3 to 9 repetitions in another[90] to 8 to 12 repetitions in yet others.[89, 91] For lower-intensity exercises aimed at building muscle endurance, the recommended number of repetitions ranges from 10 to 15[86, 92] to 10 to 25.[50, 89, 92]

In addition to exercise repetitions, exercise intensity must be determined in a program design; this intensity is the amount of resistance the muscle works against. Healthy muscle can resist a 1RM without injury risk, so studies on normal subjects have determined that moderate-intensity resistance—70% to 90% of the 1RM—can be used to provide gains in both strength and muscle endurance.[50] Researchers have found that strength gains in untrained individuals occur when an exercise provides resistance levels of about 60% of the muscle's maximum (1RM).[93, 94] The ACSM[50] has provided guidelines for strength gains that depend on a person's conditioning level: For individuals at a low level or intermediate conditioning level, it is recommended that they use a resistance level that is 70% to 85% of 1RM and perform 8 to 12 repetitions for 1 to 3 sets. Those at a high conditioning level use a resistance at 70% to 100% of their 1RM and perform 1 to 12 repetitions for 3 to 6 sets.

Rehabilitation programs usually cannot use high-intensity exercises even though strength gains are needed, especially in the early stages of rehabilitation.[95] The patient's pain or weakness during early rehabilitation usually limits the resistance that can be tolerated, or postoperative precautions restrict the use of high-resistance weights.[96] In such cases, it helps to remember that the patient can still achieve strength gains using low-resistance, high-repetition exercises. For example, if a gymnast develops a patellar tendinopathy and cannot tolerate much resistance during a leg press exercise, the weight is adjusted to a lower resistance and the patient performs more repetitions, providing quadriceps strength gains without overstressing the joint. Later in the program, as quadriceps strength improves and pain declines, the patient can use higher-resistance and lower-repetition exercises.

The number of repetitions a patient performs depends on several factors, including the patient's pain tolerance, the phase of the healing process, and the demands on the patient after return to normal activities. For example, a football defensive lineman requires strength and power, and so his rehabilitation program is primarily strength based; a soccer player's program involves endurance exercises; and a basketball player—whose sport demands both strength and endurance—will have a program that emphasizes both strength and endurance exercises. If a patient begins a rehabilitation program one week after surgery, the resistance exercises are mild so as not to cause undue stress on newly forming tissue; in such a case, regardless of the patient's sport demands, the strength program begins with low-resistance, high-repetition exercises so new tissue is not overstressed.

High-resistance, low-repetition exercises produce **hypertrophy** of the fast-twitch, Type II muscle fibers.[97] Moderate-resistance, higher-repetition exercises produce a more general increase in hypertrophy by affecting the size of both Type I and Type II fibers.[98]

As a rehabilitation clinician, you must be knowledgeable about various kinds of injuries and the performance requirements of various activities, and you must use good judgment to determine what level of resistance exercises to incorporate into a patient's therapeutic exercise program. Appropriate rehabilitation programs are designed to meet the demands to which the patient will eventually return.

If we use the research just presented, we can adapt the findings to provide general recommendations for strengthening rehabilitation patients: If your primary emphasis is strength, perform no more than 10 repetitions, but if your goal is primarily endurance increases, repetitions from 15 to 25 are advised. One to three sets is recommended for either strength or muscle endurance gains. Studies have demonstrated that performing more than one set of an exercise results in long-term strength improvement, with evidence indicating that three sets is optimal.[99, 100] The closer the exercise resistance is to the patient's maximum resistance (10RM for patients), the fewer the repetitions performed; the further from the patient's maximum resistance the exercise resistance is, the more the repetitions performed. The relationship between muscle strength and muscle endurance, relative to the repetitions used to make gains in each of the parameters, is visually demonstrated in figure 13.17.

Muscle Recovery

Working a muscle optimally and to fatigue requires a recovery period between exercise sets. Several studies have addressed the relationship between fatigue and recovery of muscles in isometric, isotonic, and isokinetic activities. Since fatigue may be caused by inadequacies of one or more of three systems—neural,[101] energy,[102] or sarcoplasmic reticulum[103]—the rate of a muscle's recovery depends upon the source of fatigue.[104] It also depends on the muscle's fatigue capacity.[105] We know that of the three sources of fatigue, calcium deficiencies (from the sarcoplasmic reticulum) that cause M-wave reduction[106] recover first, within about 4 min. Energy sources recover next, in about 20 min, elevated hydrogen levels—which decrease muscle's pH and interfere with energy production and muscle contraction—return to normal in about 35 min, and neural elements recover most slowly, within an hour.[107] Many investigations have been performed on muscle fatigue and recovery and have produced a wide range of results;[2, 101, 107-117] the varying results are likely due to a combination of variables, such as different definitions of fatigue, different types of exercises used, varying durations of exercise, different muscles used in the study, different populations studied, and different parameters measured.

We know that recovery from isotonic exercise occurs more slowly than recovery from isometric exercise, but the recovery curves have similarities.[118] As seen in figure 13.18,

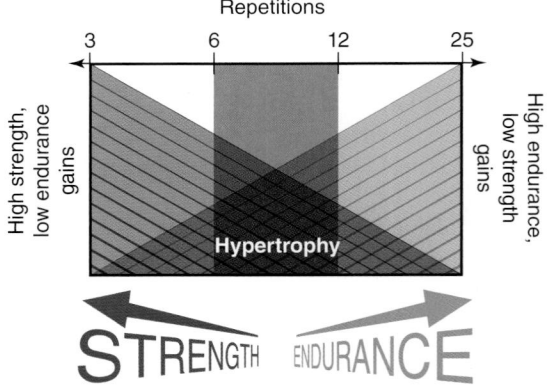

Figure 13.17   Relationship between muscle strength and endurance. Greater strength gains are achieved with fewer repetitions and higher resistance, whereas greater endurance gains are achieved with more repetitions and lower resistance. Hypertrophy occurs with 6 to 12 repetitions for 3 to 6 sets.[98]

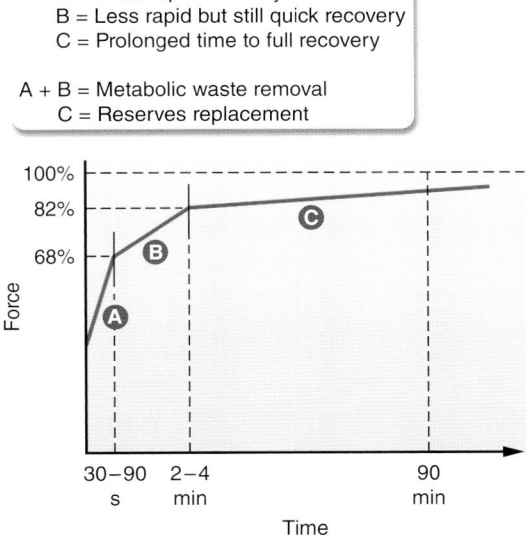

A = Initial rapid recovery
B = Less rapid but still quick recovery
C = Prolonged time to full recovery

A + B = Metabolic waste removal
C = Reserves replacement

Figure 13.18 Based on Stull and Clarke,[118] muscle recovery after an exercise bout to fatigue occurs most quickly within the first minute.

based on research of Stull and Clarke,[118] the recovery rate is rapid within the first 30 to 90 s. The rate of recovery then declines slightly over the next couple of minutes before making a final rate change to a very gradual return to full recovery that takes place over a longer period. The exact time of recovery depends on the study design and the type of exercise investigated, but all researchers have found a similar curve for the recovery pattern. When the activity is isokinetic, it takes approximately 4 min for a muscle to recover to 90% to 95% of its initial torque levels after an exercise bout to fatigue.[119] Recovery from isometric and isotonic exercises to fatigue occurs most rapidly in the first minute—58% and 72%, respectively.[118] After the first minute, the recovery from isometric activity occurs at about a 35% faster rate than from isotonic activity.[120] In all of these types of exercise recovery, there is an initial burst of recovery within 30 to 90 s. This recovery burst is followed by a slightly slower but still rapid recovery.[110] In the final phase of recovery, it takes more than 40 min for the muscle to return to pre-fatigue strength levels.[121] On the basis of his findings in a classic study, Lind[110] extrapolated the probability that it would take more than 90 min for a muscle to fully recover.

Given these results, we can make a generalized summary of appropriate rest periods between sets for a patient who is in the strength phase of a rehabilitation program. As a rule, rest periods may last 30 to 60 s between sets. Another option is to follow a 1:1 ratio between the time it takes to perform a strength exercise and the rest time between sets. Later in the strength program, the patient may need more or less rest, depending on the intensity of the exercise and the patient's goals.

Since it is not practical to wait 90 min for nearly full muscle recovery, and the remaining recovery after the initial recovery phase is minimal, we can use this research information from normal subjects as a basis for determining rest intervals for rehabilitation patients. If our goal is to either develop an increase in muscle size or gain muscle endurance, shorter recovery times should be used;[122] a 30 s rest between sets is sufficient. If the primary goal is strength gains, then a 1 to 3 min rest between sets may be more beneficial.[122] Finally, a longer rest period of 3 to 5 min may be used when developing power in a muscle.[122]

CLINICAL TIPS

The required rest between sets varies based on the rehabilitation goal:

- Muscle endurance: 30 s
- Muscle hypertrophy: 30 s
- Muscle strength: 1 to 3 min
- Muscle power: 3 to 5 min

These fatigue recovery findings are essential considerations in a patient's rehabilitation program. For example, if you are treating a hockey player with a quadriceps strain and she performs a leg press to fatigue, you should allow a 1/2 to 1 min recovery before the next exercise set. If you are using an isokinetic machine to rehabilitate the quadriceps, the recovery time should be 2 to 4 min. With the use of isometric exercises, the rest between sets should be about 1 min.

Muscle Recruitment

Muscle use and activation are complicated procedures that are both immediate and systematic. The body has a very organized system by which muscle fibers and entire muscles are engaged to produce the smooth motions, explosive actions, and precision with which we can create our desired activities. An understanding of muscle recruitment is pertinent to creating a rehabilitation program, so a brief review is presented here.

Muscle Fiber Recruitment

Activities of daily living (ADLs) and other low-intensity activities require little muscle involvement. The CNS recruits smaller motor units to perform these activities. Smaller motor units are composed of slow-twitch muscle fibers, and they are recruited before larger motor units.[123, 124] They are recruited earlier because they produce less force, but they are also better than larger motor units at resisting fatigue.[123] This means that common low-level activities such as standing or sitting can be performed for long durations because the muscle fibers performing them are fatigue resistant. When greater force or power is required, larger motor units are added to the smaller ones to produce the desired outcome.[123]

During fast and power-producing activities, the Type II motor units are recruited first.[9, 123] This recruitment of fast-twitch motor units over lower-threshold slow-twitch motor units enables one to produce optimal power and strength for explosive activities and rapid changes in direction.[98] When you need to jump quickly or run fast, your body bypasses the slow-twitch muscle fibers to enable a more rapid response by those muscle fibers that can meet the need. Such a neural-driven mechanism allows for an efficient and effective motor system, whether the goal is to challenge a world-record high jump or save a child from drowning.

Whole-Muscle Recruitment

Similar to muscle fiber selection, whole-muscle recruitment also depends on the specific activity that is to be performed. One of the first deciding factors in which muscles are recruited is the strength that is required for the intended task. Muscle strength is determined by several factors, including the muscle's cross-sectional size, the geometric distribution of the muscle fibers, the neural innervation ratio (muscle fibers within a motor unit), the number of motor units, and the types of muscle fibers.[9] When muscles are used during daily activities, usually not all fibers are involved. However, when a muscle's motor units are activated, the muscle as a whole moves or creates force in response to that activation, regardless of how many motor units respond. How many motor units are activated determines the force of the muscle's contraction.[125]

Whether a few or many motor units are firing, there is organization in muscle recruitment that is systematic but varies according to the changes in environmental demands or restrictions.[38] Studies have found that monoarticular and biarticular muscles act differently during both isometric and isotonic motions.[25] Biarticular muscles are responsible for controlling the direction of joint movement during a motor activity, while the monoarticular muscles are activated to contribute force, or torque, to produce the motion.[126] This may make inherent sense when we think about the fact that when a biarticular muscle contracts, it will move both of its joints, so the degrees of motion are much greater for a biarticular muscle than for a monoarticular muscle. It is assumed that if a monoarticular muscle activates to move a joint, the biarticular muscle also activates to both stabilize and control joint motion to achieve the desired activity.[48, 127] Another important feature of monoarticular muscles is that they are recruited before biarticular muscles during low-level activities.[29]

In terms of the sequence of muscle recruitment, stabilizing muscles activate early in a joint's movement system.[128] This makes intuitive sense too. Like a tennis player, who must stop running toward the ball to hit it so that his swing can move from a stable base, joints must also move from a stable base to achieve the desired motion. Therefore, smaller muscles close to a joint are activated immediately before motion to stabilize the segment. For example, immediately before you lift a box from the floor, the core muscles engage to stabilize your trunk. It is often found that in persons with pain, these stabilizing muscles are weaker and are not recruited correctly.[129-131] Another example is the shoulder muscles activating to stabilize the shoulder when the elbow moves so that shoulder motion does not interfere with the desired elbow activity.

Keeping these concepts in mind, the patient's rehabilitation program should include recruitment reeducation activities that restore proper muscle activation sequencing. We know that when an injury occurs, whether a stabilizing muscle is injured or not, its function is going to be affected for the simple reason that all function of the injured site is affected.[132] The longer a recovery takes, the greater the loss will be in a muscle's ability to perform at preinjury levels.[133]

Types of Muscle Activity

Although some authors refer to the types of muscle activity as muscle contraction, that is not entirely accurate. Contraction implies a shortening of the muscle, but as you will see, a muscle does not always shorten when it acts. Therefore "muscle contraction" is referred to here as *muscle activity, muscle tension,* or *movement.* There are two types of muscle activity, static and dynamic. **Static activity** is **isometric**. **Dynamic activity** is divided into **isotonic** and **isokinetic**. Isotonic activity is further divided into **concentric** and **eccentric** movements. Since the clinician must have intimate knowledge of these types of strength exercises, they are presented here in terms of both their identification and how they are used in rehabilitation.

Static Activity

Static, or isometric, activity is produced when muscle tension is created without a change in the muscle's length. Static activity is not only used in rehabilitation but is also part of ADLs and sports. Trunk muscles act statically to provide a stable base for upper- and lower-extremity movements. Shoulder muscles act statically as shoulder stabilizers when a person moves the elbow and hand.

The advantage of isometric exercise is that this type of activity can strengthen a muscle without imposing undue stress on injured or surgically repaired structures. For example, in situations such as a recent fracture or a surgical repair in which movement is restricted or limited, isometrics are used early in the rehabilitation program until motion is permitted. Isometrics are also used when the muscle is too weak to provide sufficient resistance against gravity or other external forces. The disadvantage of isometrics is that strength gains are isolated to no more than 20° to 30° within the angle at which the isometric is performed (10° to 15° on either side of the isometric position).[134-136] It is important to caution the patient to avoid a **Valsalva maneuver** during isometric exercises. Valsalva occurs when the patient holds his or her breath, causing an increase in intrathoracic pressure. This can impede venous return to the right atrium, leading to an increase in peripheral venous pressure (increasing blood pressure) and reducing cardiac output because of lowered cardiac volume. Patients who hold their breath during exercise should be reminded to breathe in order to avoid this risk.

During a maximal isometric exercise, tension within the muscle decreases rapidly.[137, 138] At 5 s, the tension is 75% of the tension exerted at the start of the isometric activity. By 10 s, the strength drops to 50% of the original tension (figure 13.19). Because of this fatigue factor, no one can produce a sustained maximal contraction. An example of this is when you help to carry a stretcher with an injured person on it. As the upper-extremity muscles holding the stretcher begin to fatigue, the muscles start to burn, and the transport team has to stop because someone will need a rest if it takes more than a short time to carry the patient. At the other end of the spectrum, however, a muscle can provide submaximal isometric tension for prolonged periods and repetitive events.[139, 140] For example, postural muscles often work at submaximal levels for extended periods without fatiguing.

This fatigue factor is important to remember when a patient performs isometric exercises in a rehabilitation program. Maximal isometric activity need not be performed for more than 5 to 10 s at a time; 6 s is the recommended duration for one maximal isometric exercise.[141] Since patients often count faster than the actual time, telling the patient to hold the contraction for 10 s may really result in a 6 s hold! The number of repetitions and the frequency of exercise throughout the day depend on the condition of the muscle, the ability of the body part to move, and the phase of the healing process.

If a patient performs isometric exercise during a time when motion is restricted, strength gains will be limited to a few degrees on either side of the position in which the exercise is performed. Therefore, if the injured part can be moved to different positions, it would be advantageous to have the patient perform the isometric exercise in different positions throughout the range of motion to obtain strength gains in more than one small part of that ROM.

Strength gains are achievable if the muscle's effort is 66% to 100% of its maximum output.[141] Efforts at 35% to 66% of maximal isometric output produce some gains in strength, but the increase is slow. Most daily activities, apart from sport activities, produce periodic tensions of 20% to 35% of maximum; this level of output maintains strength. A muscle that is immobilized or inactive may experience a loss of strength ranging from 8% a week[142] to 5% a day.[143]

It takes about one week of therapeutic exercise to increase a muscle's strength by 5%[142] to 12%.[143] These numbers may vary from one study to another because of the different protocols and subjects researchers used, but all the data make a similar point: The rate of strength lost is much more rapid than the rate of strength regained. In essence, it may take up to a week to recover the strength lost in one day of inactivity. This highlights how important it is to keep a muscle active if such activity causes no deleterious effects. If an injured part must be immobilized, isometric exercises can become very important in retarding atrophy and weakness.

CLINICAL TIPS

The rate at which muscle strength is lost during times of inactivity or immobilization is much higher than the rate at which that loss of strength can be recovered. It may take up to a week to recover the strength lost in a day of inactivity.

Dynamic Activity

The term *dynamic* in relation to activity implies a change in the position of a muscle. Dynamic strength activity is further defined by the specific types of activity that occur.

Isotonic Activity

Isotonic activity is dynamic in that it involves a change in the muscle's length. If the muscle shortens as it produces force, the activity is called *concentric*. If the muscle lengthens as it works, the activity is called *eccentric*. Although you can isolate muscle activity to produce either concentric or eccentric motion, most sport and daily activities involve the use of both concentric and eccentric actions. For example, lifting a weight during an elbow curl is a concentric

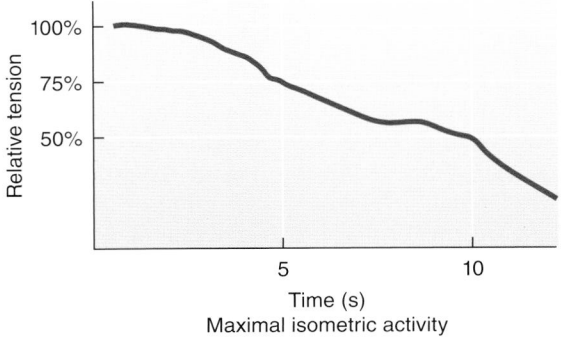

Figure 13.19 Based on Sesboüé and Guincestre,[137] maximal isometric force production falls rapidly from 100% to 50% in about 6 s.

Based on Sesboüé and Guincestre (2006).[137]

action, and lowering the weight is an eccentric action. Likewise, jumping for a basketball rebound is a concentric action that is preceded and followed by an eccentric action.

Because of a muscle's passive components, an eccentric action can produce anywhere from 20% to 40% more force than a concentric action.[144] Wilmore and Costill[145] have averaged out that range and indicate that eccentric activity produces 30% more force than concentric activity. For example, if an 18 kg (40 lb) weight can be lifted in an elbow curl exercise concentrically, the same muscle can lift 23.5 kg (52 lb) eccentrically when the arm is lowered. It is believed that the muscle's noncontractile elements provide the additional forces during eccentric activity that permit increased muscle loading.

There are several other differences between concentric and eccentric activity. Although it takes more energy to perform a concentric action, there is evidence to indicate that greater strength gains occur with eccentric exercises.[146, 147] It has been demonstrated, however, that a combination of concentric and eccentric exercise is important in optimizing strength gains.[74] As the speed of a concentric activity increases, the muscle's ability to produce force decreases. The opposite is true for eccentric exercises: As speed increases with eccentric exercise, the force increases initially, then eventually levels off or decreases as progressively increased speeds of motion are performed. The differences in speed and force production of concentric and eccentric activity are demonstrated in figure 13.20.

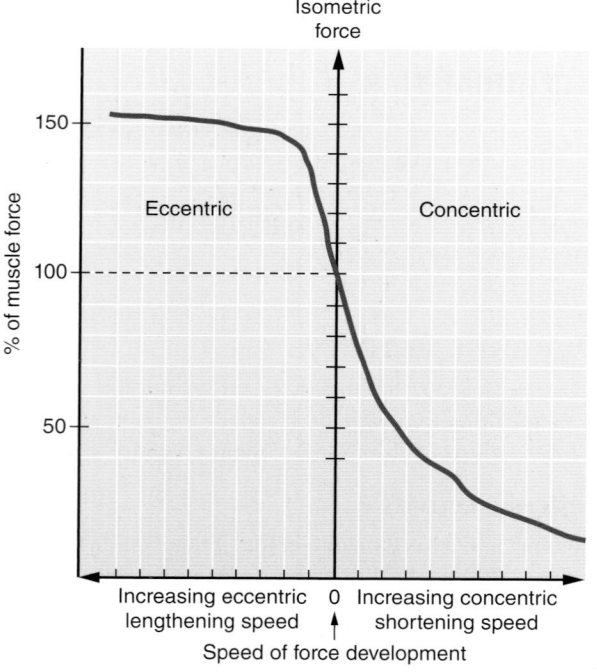

Figure 13.20 Concentric–eccentric force-velocity curve. The faster a muscle works concentrically, the less strength it produces; but when it works eccentrically, greater forces can be produced until a maximum is achieved.

There is also a greater likelihood of delayed-onset muscle soreness (DOMS) with eccentric exercise. More recent investigations indicate that this is the result of a combination of damage occurring to muscle membranes and a secondary inflammatory reaction within the muscle.[74]

The term *isotonic* means "having the same tension." It is, in fact, inaccurate because the amount of tension produced by a muscle varies throughout the range of motion. The amount of tension produced depends on moment arms and the physiological principles previously discussed. When selecting the amount of resistance for an isotonic exercise, the clinician must realize that the greatest amount of tension a patient can create during an isotonic activity is actually the force that the muscle or muscle group can produce at its weakest position in the motion. For example, if a patient can lift 18 kg (40 lb) in an elbow curl, that weight is the maximum the elbow flexors can exert at their weakest point in elbow flexion. If the patient performs the exercise while standing, the weakest point occurs when gravity is at its greatest, with the elbow at 90° flexion. The elbow flexors can lift more than 18 kg at the beginning of the motion and at the end of the motion as gravity's moment-arm length shortens. They can also lift more in the beginning of the motion, where the muscles are at their greatest physiological length, than they can at the end of the motion when they are at a physiological disadvantage. Because the elbow flexors can lift no more than 18 kg at 90°, that is the maximum weight the patient lifts through the full range of motion. Similarly in this example, because the weight feels lighter in the beginning and at the end of the motion where gravity's moment arm is shorter, the patient lifts the weight more quickly during those parts of the motion. As the weight becomes more difficult to move around the 90° point, the patient's movement slows.

Isokinetic Activity

Isokinetic activity is a dynamic activity in that it involves motion. It differs from isotonic activity, however, in that the velocity remains at a specific speed. Isokinetic means "having the same motion" and refers to the unchanging speed of movement that occurs during these activities. Whereas the speed of motion remains constant, the amount of resistance provided to the muscle varies as the muscle goes through its range. Returning to the example of the elbow curl, if the exercise is isokinetic, the patient's elbow moves through its motion at a uniform speed, but maintaining that uniform speed requires varying the amount of resistance. In that part of the motion where an isotonic exercise would be easy, the resistance in an isokinetic exercise would be greater, and where the isotonic exercise would normally be more difficult, the resistance offered isokinetically would be less in order to accommodate the varying strength of the muscle as it goes through a constant motion. For isokinetic exercises to be performed properly, the patient produces a maximal muscle contraction throughout the exercise. Isokinetics is sometimes called **accommodating resistance** exercise because of the change in resistance given throughout a range of motion. Today's equipment makes it possible to perform isokinetic activities both eccentrically and concentrically. Although isokinetics was very popular during the 1970s and 1980s, closed kinetic chain activities are the current trend.

Open and Closed Kinetic Chain Activity

A kinetic chain is a series of rigid arms linked by movable joints. This is a mechanical description of the body. **Open kinetic chain (OKC)** and **closed kinetic chain (CKC)** activity within the body are identified in terms of the distal segment of the extremity, the hand or foot. The kinetic chain is open when the distal segment moves freely in space. Kicking and throwing a ball are open kinetic chain activities. A kinetic chain is closed when the distal segment is weight bearing and the body moves over the hand or foot. Landing during running and performing a handstand are closed kinetic chain activities. Generally, open kinetic chain athletic activities produce high-velocity motions such as throwing a ball or swinging the distal leg while running. Closed kinetic chain activities occur more often in lower-extremity functional activities; they place lesser shear forces on the joints,[148] so they are generally safer to use earlier in a rehabilitation program.[149, 150]

Both OKC and CKC activities involve a relationship between one joint and the others within the chain. This is important to remember in rehabilitation because if you ignore the other joints within the chain, success will be elusive. The function of a single joint is not exclusive: The function of one joint determines the function of the other joints within the kinetic chain. Abnormal stresses applied to an injured joint are transmitted to and absorbed by other structures within the kinetic chain and can cause additional problems if those stresses are not tolerated by those other areas. For example, if a baseball pitcher has weak shoulder muscles and cannot keep the arm elevated correctly during the pitch, he may develop elbow pain from the additional stress transmitted by abnormal forces to the elbow from the shoulder.

Lower-extremity activities in ADLs and sport use a combination of open- and closed-chain movements, but many lower-extremity rehabilitation exercises focus on closed kinetic chain activities. Closed kinetic chain exercises may be used to improve strength, power, stability, balance, coordination, and agility and are capable of generating large forces but relatively low velocities of movement. Lower extremity open and closed kinetic chain activities are functional in that they occur in normal activities from walking and standing to running and jumping.

In a CKC system, no link within the chain can move independently; movement of one segment affects all others. For this reason, the inadequacies of a weak link in the chain can be compensated for by the other links, but at the cost of additional stresses on those links.

Open kinetic chain activities are also part of daily activities and sport. Examples of OKC activities include kicking, throwing, and lifting lower-body weights in a seated position, as in performing knee extensions. The running and walking cycles both include an OKC segment. In an OKC, any link in the chain is free to move independently of the other links. Generally, the forces generated by an OKC are small, but the velocities are large. When a body segment functions in an OKC, it is non–weight bearing. The contrast between OKC and CKC activities are listed in table 13.6.

TABLE 13.6 Comparisons Between Open Kinetic Chain and Closed Kinetic Chain Activities

Feature	Open kinetic chain	Closed kinetic chain
Movement	Usually isolated to one joint	Involves multiple joints
Planes of motion	Uniplanar	Triplanar
Muscle involvement	Usually one muscle or muscle group	Multiple muscles including co-contraction for stability
Rehab involvement	Isolates weak muscle for strength gains of specific muscles	Utilizes muscles functionally as groups
Force effects	Low force, high velocity	High force, low velocity
Chain position	Non–weight bearing	Weight bearing
Anchored segment	Proximal segment	Distal segment
Advantage	Isolates muscle or joint for strength and ROM gains	Promotes neuromotor control, co-contraction, proprioception
Forces increased	Acceleration forces	Joint compression forces
Forces reduced	Resistance forces	Joint shear forces
Performance activities	Rapid motions	Forceful motions

Open and closed kinetic chain activities are produced in both upper and lower extremities (figure 13.21). But different stresses are applied to the body by the two types of activities. The differences in stresses occur because the motion is different. In OKC activity, the stabilized proximal segment provides the foundation upon which the distal segment moves; in other words, activation of proximal extremity muscles provides a secure base for movement.[151] For example, shoulder muscles activate isometrically to stabilize the proximal upper extremity before the fingers and wrist muscles move the hand. In CKC activity, there is compression of the joints, and stabilization occurs because of the coactivation of opposing muscle groups. In a squat, the quadriceps works eccentrically while the hamstrings activate to counteract knee flexion. The result is stabilization of the knee through the simultaneous activity of opposing muscle groups.

In an OKC activity, the hand or foot moves, while in a CKC activity the hand or foot is anchored, or not moving. It is usually easier to identify OKC versus CKC activity in the lower extremity. When the person stands on the lower extremity, the limb is in a CKC activity; if that limb then kicks a ball, it performs an OKC activity. The upper extremity does not always present as clear a picture. For example, if a person performs a military (overhead) press, she uses her arms in an OKC activity because the hands are moving; however, if she performs a chin-up on a stationary bar, she is performing a CKC activity because the hand is anchored to the unmoving bar.

If we continue our focus on the knee, only the hamstrings work in OKC knee flexion. In OKC knee extension, the quadriceps performs the motion while the hamstrings remain quiet. During OKC knee extension, quadriceps moment changes as the knee moves from flexion to extension. The moment is the product of the amount of force (weight of the leg) and its moment-arm length (the perpendicular distance from the joint to the distal end of the limb). In other words, as the knee moves into extension, the work required by the quadriceps to lift the weight of the leg segment increases because the moment arm of the resistive force (gravity) increases. This change not only requires more quadriceps strength as the knee moves

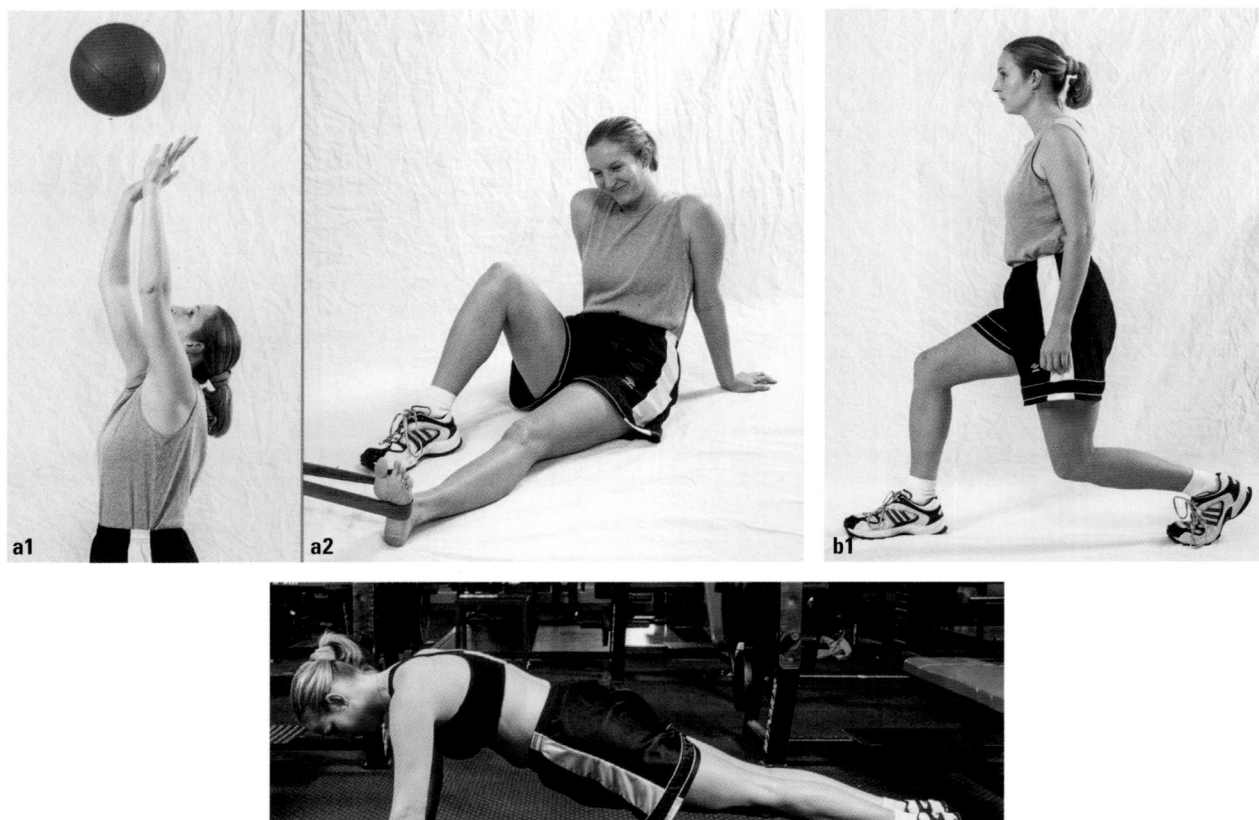

Figure 13.21 *(a)* Open and *(b)* closed kinetic chain activities for the upper *(a1, b2)* and lower *(a2, b1)* extremities.

toward terminal extension, but in an OKC, the knee joint suffers a high shear force with an active contraction of the quadriceps as the muscle moves the knee from flexion to extension, especially during the last 30°.[152] The quadriceps tendon creates this shear force by causing an anterior translation of the tibia as it pulls the knee into extension. In a CKC, the shear force is counteracted by a co-contraction of the hamstring with the quadriceps.[153] Co-contraction produces less stress on the knee during terminal extension and increased stability of the joint through the simultaneous contraction of the hamstrings and quadriceps during a closed kinetic chain exercise.

Although CKC exercises and the co-contraction they promote may provide more joint stability,[154] in situations when the patient cannot bear weight it may be necessary to use open kinetic chain exercises. The advantage of OKC activities in these situations is that strengthening activities are not delayed until weight bearing occurs. Another advantage of open kinetic chain exercises is that specific weaker muscles can be targeted. This point highlights one precaution for the use of CKC exercises: Because more than one muscle group is active during CKC exercises, the substitution of stronger muscles rather than the correct use of weaker muscles is always a possibility, and this incorrect performance must be corrected when observed. A rehabilitation program should include a combination of open and closed kinetic chain exercises for optimal results.[155-157]

CLINICAL TIPS

Muscles have various gradations of activity; from the least active to the most active, these are passive range of motion (PROM), active-assistive range of motion (AAROM), active range of motion (AROM), and resistive range of motion (RROM).

Strength Program Design

As you have already learned, there are many parts of a rehabilitation program. Since this chapter deals specifically with strength, its content will only deal with those issues that pertain to muscle strength and muscle endurance. Within a muscle strength and endurance portion of a rehabilitation program, variables that should be considered include (1) goals and a plan for muscle strength and endurance gains, (2) identification of the most appropriate types of exercises to use to achieve those goals, (3) the required overload for strength gains, and (4) a progression of exercises that produces the desired results. Each of these factors is presented in this section.

As with any element of a rehabilitation program, for the muscle strength and endurance part, the clinician should have a sound rationale for each exercise. The program should meet the needs of each patient as determined by the patient's examination results, the deficiencies found, and the demands of the activities to which the patient intends to return. The strength portion of a rehabilitation program may emphasize strength or muscle endurance or a combination of the two.

Create a Plan

Before the clinician can decide what the patient needs to do, a plan must be developed. That plan is based on the problems that are found during the patient's examination. Each part of the plan is designed to resolve one of the problems.

With an appropriate rehabilitation program, those problems will diminish until they are resolved entirely. As the program has its effect, the problems will change, and the plan must address those changes. For example, during the early phase of rehabilitation, a patient with a surgically repaired dislocating shoulder may start with isometric exercises in the early strength segment; however, as the program progresses, isotonic exercises will replace those isometric exercises. And later in the rehabilitation program, strength exercises will progress to even more challenging forms.

At each level of rehabilitation, plans change, goals change, and problems change. These changes require the clinician to perform periodic examinations to keep the rehabilitation goals and treatment program current to best meet the patient's needs.

Identify Exercises

Although each program is tailored to each patient's needs, there is a general strength progression followed in all rehabilitation programs. At the most basic level, a program may start with isometric exercises. These exercises are used with patients whose strength is minimal (grade 1/5 or 2/5) or who are limited in their motion because of injury precautions, limited ability, or postoperative restrictions. Once the patient can move beyond isometric exercises, isotonic exercises are used to replace those isometric exercises. It may be that not all muscles can start isotonic exercises at the same time, and some may start with light weights and high repetitions while others may start with heavier weights and lower repetitions. It may be that some isotonic exercises include only eccentric exercises, while others will include both eccentric and concentric motions. These factors are determined by the patient's goals, strength, and specific injury.

Isotonic exercises start in straight-plane motions so the weak muscles can be specifically targeted. The idea is to isolate the weak muscles and prevent stronger muscles from performing the work so the desired strength increases occur. Allowing stronger muscles to overpower the weak muscles promotes erroneous firing patterns, resulting in muscle imbalances and pathological movements.[158] Once these weak muscles gain strength, multiplanar exercises are used to encourage proper sequential muscle activation for normal activities.

There is an exception to the use of straight-plane strength exercises before multiplanar exercises. That exception occurs when the exercises are designed to focus primarily on motor development. Motor control retraining exercises focus more on muscle sequencing and firing patterns than on strength.[159] These exercises use repetitive motion patterns without resistance to develop proper control of motion.[160] Proprioceptive neuromuscular facilitation (PNF) is also used to correct muscle firing patterns.[55] Once the muscles achieve their proper firing patterns, strength exercises are used to restore muscles to proper strength levels. This technique is used mainly in body segments where muscle firing patterns are dysfunctional after an injury.[161]

As strength gains occur in the weak muscles, multiplanar activities are added to the strength program. Since normal motion is multiplanar, usually involving all three planes of motion, strength exercises should be designed to mimic these motions. As muscle firing sequences and multiplanar motions occur correctly, normal function returns.

Multiplanar activities are usually added in the early days of the third rehabilitation phase and are followed by functional exercises. Functional exercises are a prelude to the final rehabilitation phase when the program advances to performance-specific exercises. These functional exercises may include something as simple as stair climbing or tossing a medicine ball or something as complex as plyometric exercises. From these exercises, the patient usually advances quickly to the performance-specific exercises that include normal activities.

The rate of this strength progression rests on several factors. These factors include the severity of the injury, the type of injury, the involved body segment, the patient's age, specific healing factors, the patient's long-term goals, and the physician. The rehabilitation clinician must be aware of each of these factors and progress a patient from one type of strength exercise to the next only when it is appropriate to do so.

CLINICAL TIPS

Progressing from the easiest exercises to the most difficult, a strength exercise progression includes the following: isometric exercises; concentric or eccentric exercises and other isotonic exercises that start with single-plane movements; diagonal-plane movements when the muscle can correctly fire sequentially; functional exercises; and finally, performance-specific exercises.

Provide a Progressive Overload

Most research on strengthening and strengthening programs has been performed on healthy subjects;[162] therefore, once again we must use investigative results based on normal subjects as a guide for strength development in rehabilitation programs.

Providing a progressive overload of exercises in rehabilitation is fundamental to muscle strengthening. To continue to produce strength gains, the load must progressively increase. This concept is sometimes referred to as the **overload principle**. An overload for muscles occurs when they are stressed beyond their normal capacity.[163] An overload becomes progressive when changes in strength occur. Strength occurs through the manipulation of two factors: intensity and volume.[163] Intensity refers to the amount of resistance, and volume refers to the number of repetitions; as we have already discussed, these two factors are related to each other on the strength-continuum scale, and changing either the amount of resistance or the number of repetitions will alter muscle strength.

The intensity is the resistance, weight, or force against which the muscle works to improve its strength. In healthy individuals, the amount of resistance used in an exercise is usually determined using the 1RM system; however, a one-repetition maximum is often an inappropriate and unreasonable base to determine the amount of resistance a patient can tolerate without harming the injured area. Because of this injury risk with using 1RM, the clinician will usually use one of two options instead: (1) identify the patient's 10RM[123] and begin a resistance exercise at that weight, or (2) estimate, based on manual muscle testing (MMT),[164] an appropriate beginning weight and then make adjustments according to the patient's ability to perform against that weight. For example, if the clinician performs an MMT and determines that the patient's elbow flexors are a grade 4, she may decide to have the patient use 4.5 kg (10 lb) in an elbow curl, but if the patient can perform 15 repetitions when the goal is 8 repetitions, then the clinician will adjust the weight, increasing the resistance to meet the desired exercise goal.

Table 13.7 lists the recommendations for the optimal numbers of repetitions to achieve gains in muscle strength, endurance, and power. You will notice that as repetitions decrease, the amount of resistance a muscle can tolerate increases. Estimates of the amount of resistance to use in either strength or endurance exercises are provided by the American College of Sports Medicine Position Stand on resistance training.[50] Although these recommendations are based on normal subjects, clinicians may use them as a guide for their patients, making adjustments for the condition and situation of each patient. Also note that the resistive force recommendations cover a wide range, with the lower end of each range more applicable to novice,

TABLE 13.7 Repetition and Intensity Recommendations for Improving Muscle Strength, Endurance, and Power

Goal	Repetition range	Intensity range[b]
Strength	3-5[a,b,c] 8-12[d]	Higher resistance = 60%-100% of max
Endurance	10-25[b] 20-28[c] 25-35[d]	Light to moderate resistance = 30%-60% of max
Power	1-2[e] 3-5[b]	Upper body resistance = 0%-60% of max Lower body resistance = 30%-60% of max

Note: Estimates provided are based on research performed on normal subjects, using a 1RM.

[a]Weiss et al., 1999;[82] [b]Ratamess et al., 2009;[50] [c]Campos et al., 2002;[22] [d]Schoenfeld et al., 2015;[165] [e]Baechle et al., 2008.[90]

younger, untrained, or weaker persons and the higher end more suitable for advanced individuals.[50]

As the patient continues to work against a resistance force, that level of resistance will eventually not be an overload because the muscle's strength adapts to the resistance. Therefore, as the patient's strength improves, the exercise difficulty must also increase. For example, if a biceps muscle lifts 8 kg (18 lb) repeatedly from one exercise session to the next without changes to the exercise, its strength will be maintained at that level but will not increase.[166] A new goal is set to continue making strength or endurance gains: Either the intensity or the volume must increase. Which one is manipulated will depend on the goals for the patient. If muscle endurance is to improve, then additional repetitions may be added to the exercise; however, if additional muscle strength is the goal, then additional resistance will be used to provide a new overload for the muscle.

When a muscle cannot actively exercise or the patient is restricted from moving the injured area, **cross-training** can produce strength gains.[55, 167] Cross-training occurs when the contralateral part is exercised, resulting in strength gains on the opposite extremity. This form of training, sometimes also referred to as *cross-education,* has been around since the 1800s and has been used with varying degrees of success. The results depend primarily on the amount of resistance provided to the exercising extremity: The greater the effort of the extremity, the better the results. This type of exercise is a useful technique that you can apply in rehabilitation programs when the patient's injured area is restricted, perhaps because it is in a cast or splint, and there are limited possibilities to exercise the part.

Use Specific Exercises

A rehabilitation program incorporates specific exercises to achieve the most important long-term goal, the patient's return to his or her normal performance level. This concept is based on the **SAID principle**: **S**pecific **A**daptations to **I**mposed **D**emands.[168] This principle means that the muscle will adapt and perform according to the demands placed on it. As we have mentioned, if a patient lifts low weights for high repetitions, the muscle will gain endurance. If a patient wants to gain strength, resistance should be closer to his or her maximum resistance with low repetitions.

The SAID principle also means that exercises should mimic stresses placed on a muscle during functional activities to produce appropriate strength gains. If a patient's sport calls for a specific activity, such as holding a pike position on the parallel bars in gymnastics, then the strength exercises for that patient should include isometric hip flexor and abdominal exercises. If the patient's job is to lift and move boxes throughout the day, then the rehabilitation program should include repetitive lifting activities.

In the early stages of a rehabilitation program, rapid gains in strength are commonly seen in a debilitated or deconditioned muscle. This occurs without a change in the muscle's size during the first 3 to 5 weeks of exercises.[57] Many believe that these initial strength gains are primarily the result of neural adaptations within the neuromuscular system.[55, 98, 169]

We know that reflex inhibition of the muscle occurs with injury or inactivity.[170, 171] Immediate weakness is present after surgery as well.[172] These sudden declines in strength are attributable to decreased neural activity. Because neural adaptations occur quickly after injury, it is postulated that they are also readily affected by attempts to restore the injured part.[173]

Strength is influenced by both muscle fiber and neural control.[24, 174] The initial rapid gains in strength are attributed to improved neuromuscular recruitment, efficiency, coordination, and motor unit reeducation.[55, 112] Many researchers believe that improved neural activation results in an increased activation of synergists with a better coordination and co-contraction of the synergists, an inhibition of the antagonists, and improved activation ability and sensitivity to facilitation of the prime movers.[175] A learning factor also affects the neural element of muscle activity.[55]

The rate of strength gains in normal, healthy muscle depends on a number of factors, including age and sex of the patient.[166] In rehabilitation, evidence to date on this topic appears to be anecdotal only; clinical observation has indicated that the rate of strength gains in rehabilitation decreases as a rehabilitation program advances in time and duration (figure 13.22).[176] Once the neural components are restored, the gains are primarily made through muscle fiber hypertrophy.[55] The greatest strength gains occur in the early stages of a therapeutic exercise segment of a

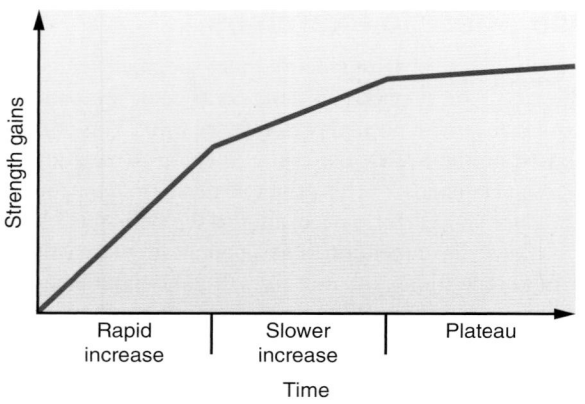

Figure 13.22 Rate of strength gains in a rehabilitation program.

rehabilitation program, which suggests that neural changes are more significant than muscle size changes, especially in rehabilitation.[55] Primary hypertrophic changes occur more commonly in patients who have lifted weights over a longer period of time or who use drugs to enhance hypertrophy.[177]

In the early stages of a rehabilitation program, especially in cases of prolonged muscle inactivity, the initial exercise efforts should emphasize facilitation of the neural elements of the atrophied muscle. In addition to active exercise, electrical stimulation to assist in the facilitation of these neural pathways and in the facilitation of proper muscle response may expedite recovery.

If a severe injury or surgery requires a long rehabilitation program, you will likely see a recovery sequence that begins with a rapid increase followed by a slower increase and then a plateau. This sequence of changes may occur in one cycle, or it may recur in more than one cycle before the rehabilitation program is completed. The pattern is individually determined and is not predictable. If the patient reaches a plateau early in the program before achieving final goals, you should explain that this is common and that gains will come if the patient persists in the program. These plateau times can be difficult for the patient, since it may seem that no amount of effort produces gains. Patience and perseverance are essential to staying motivated during this time. Sometimes the psychological lift of having a day off from the rehabilitation program can have a rejuvenating effect.

Programs of Goal Progressions

This final section has a lot of overlap with one of the topics just presented: progressive overload. Setting program goals for muscle strength and endurance is similar to setting goals for other deficits or problems. Each deficient muscle or muscle group is identified, precise strength levels are determined, goals are set according to those current strength deficits, and finally, a plan of treatment to restore those deficient strength levels is made. The strength exercise plan includes a progression of exercises that ultimately reach the final goal of optimum strength restoration. This system may be most easily demonstrated with an example.

Let's use the example of a volleyball player with a biceps strain. When it is time to start his strength program, the muscle's strength is determined to be 3+/5; he can tolerate only slight resistance in an antigravity position. The clinician decides to start with low-resistance, high-repeti-

---

Evidence in Rehabilitation

A 2015 study presented an interesting, supportive discussion of augmentation of traditional strength training methods after injury or surgery.[178] These authors noted that several investigations had identified persistent weakness in the quadriceps after injury, despite rehabilitation efforts to restore knee function. They pointed out that if this deficiency endured, it could lead to either additional injury or osteoarthritis. They argued convincingly that the quadriceps weakness persisted because of the presence of neuromuscular deficits. Pietrosimone and colleagues[178] referred to this deficit as *arthrogenic muscle inhibition* and described it as a reflexive neurogenic inhibition that likely served as an acute protective response to the injury that never resolved. As weakness persisted, they indicated that changes in the higher cortical levels also occurred, further advancing quadriceps inhibition.

Pietrosimone and colleagues[178] offered an addendum to traditional rehabilitation to treat this dysfunctional inhibitory condition. They advocated addressing the neurophysiological impairment before the start of a traditional program, with the goals of resolving the pathology and restoring normal neuromuscular pathways. Once this underlying problem was addressed, traditional rehabilitation would prove to be beneficial in fully restoring quadriceps strength. Modalities they advocated to pursue these goals included a selection of manual therapy, neuromuscular nerve stimulation, biofeedback, and other applications that would diminish the neuromuscular inhibition.[178]

Although they advocated treatment of arthrogenic muscle inhibition for quadriceps rehabilitation, they noted that traditional therapeutic exercises, including strength exercises, are required for a successful outcome.[178] If these investigators are correct, it makes sense that if you have a patient who has difficulty making strength gains, using these techniques to "reboot" the neuromuscular system may be beneficial.

tion exercises as a way to start building strength without overstressing the muscle. She has him perform one set of antigravity biceps curls for 15 repetitions. He completes the exercise without any problems. The clinician decides to set a goal of 3 sets of 15 repetitions before he advances to a more difficult resistance exercise. He can perform the second set without any trouble, but the last couple of repetitions are more difficult. He begins the third set but can only complete 12 repetitions before he fails to move the elbow through a full range of flexion motion. The clinician will have him repeat this exercise, 3 sets of 15 repetitions, at the following treatment sessions until he can complete 3 sets of 15 repetitions through a full range of motion for 2 consecutive treatment sessions. Once that goal is achieved, the clinician changes the goal because the biceps has adapted to this level of resistance and needs another exercise to continue the overload progression. Since he is so weak, the clinician has the patient stay with the same number of repetitions but adds 1.5 kg (3.3 lb) of resistance to the exercise. He will continue with that weight until he can lift it for 3 sets of 15 at one treatment session; she will then progress him to another level of strength, adding more resistance to further improve his strength. As he gains strength, she may change more than just the resistance. What she changes may be determined by a number of variables, including the available resources, patient interests, specific goals, and equipment availability.

In summary, patients are advanced in their rehabilitation programs based on when they achieve the goals for each exercise. Strength exercise goals are centered on repetitions, sets, and resistance. These goals are set for each exercise, and when patients achieve that specific goal for that specific exercise, the goals change to the next level of exercise. That next level may be an increase in weight, repetitions, or number of sets, based on the needs of the patient and the final long-term goals. This goal-based increase in weights, repetitions, or number of sets provides a progressive overload. A progressive overload can be applied using various progression methods. Several programs, advocated by a number of professionals over the years, have been used rather widely in rehabilitation. Some traditional examples are provided here.

DeLorme and Watkins Exercise Progression

DeLorme and Watkins[179] provided a system that still serves as a basis of progressive strengthening in rehabilitation circles today.[180] These researchers used 10RM as a maximum strength determination. They advocated the use of 3 bouts, or sets, of exercise, 10 repetitions each: The first set is performed at 50% of maximum, the second set at 75% of maximum, and the final set at 100% of the 10RM (table 13.8).

TABLE 13.8   DeLorme and Watkins Strength Progression

Set	Repetitions	Weight
1st	10	50% of 10RM
2nd	10	75% of 10RM
3rd	10	100% of 10RM

Oxford Technique Exercise Progression

Zinovieff, a physician who worked at England's United Oxford Hospitals, published a revision of the DeLorme program that he named the Oxford Technique.[181] Zinovieff found that with the DeLorme system, his patients were too fatigued to complete the final set of 10RM exercises. He suggested reversing the system, starting with the 10RM on the first set of 10 repetitions and progressively reducing to 75% and then 50% on each successive set of 10 repetitions (table 13.9).

TABLE 13.9   Oxford Technique of Strength Progression

Set	Repetitions	Weight
1st	10	100% of 10RM
2nd	10	75% of 10RM
3rd	10	50% of 10RM

DAPRE Exercise Progression

A number of authors have advanced a variety of other resistive exercise progressions. One familiar system is the DAPRE (Daily Adjusted Progressive Resistive Exercise) technique.[182] This is a complex system of daily exercise (6 d per week) progression that meets the patient's ability to tolerate increased resistance. Table 13.10 illustrates the establishment of an RM and number of repetitions along with the determination of the next session's exercise weight.

The essential element of DAPRE is that in the third and fourth sets of exercise, the patient performs as many repetitions as possible. The number of repetitions the patient can

CLINICAL TIPS

Several commonly used progressive overload systems are available. A clinician may vary his or her system from patient to patient or develop a system that works best for the individual clinician. Whatever system a clinician uses, however, should be based on sound research and good anecdotal findings.

TABLE 13.10   DAPRE System of Strength Progression

TECHNIQUE		
Set	**Repetitions**	**Weight**
1st	10	50% of working weight
2nd	6	75% of working weight
3rd	As many as possible	100% of working weight
4th	As many as possible	Adjusted from third set*

ADJUSTMENT GUIDELINES		
Number of repetitions performed during prior set	**Fourth-set weight adjustment based on third set**	**Next-day weight adjustment based on fourth set**
0-2	Wt; redo set	Wt; redo set
3-4	By 0-5 lb	Keep the same
5-7	Keep the same	By 5-10 lb
8-12	By 5-10 lb	By 5-15 lb
13 or more	By 10-15 lb	By 10-20 lb

*See "Adjustment guidelines."

The number of repetitions performed on the third set determines the weight used on the fourth set. The next treatment day's starting weight is determined by the number of repetitions performed on the fourth set of the previous treatment.

Based on Knight (1985).[182]

perform on the third set determines the amount of weight added for the fourth set of the day as well as for the start of the next treatment session.[182]

Based on Knight's design,[182] the intent of the program is to have the patient perform as many repetitions during the set as possible. The goal is 5 to 7 repetitions. If the patient does 8 to 12 repetitions, the weight change is minimal, but if the patient performs 15 to 20 repetitions, the weight change is significantly larger. This program continues until the strength of the injured part is within 10% of the strength of its non-injured counterpart. Once this goal is achieved, the emphasis shifts to other deficiencies such as muscle endurance or coordination, and the DAPRE program is continued twice a week to maintain strength.

Most rehabilitation clinicians develop an exercise routine that seems to work best for them in achieving progression of a patient's strength. In the early stages of strengthening a person whose strength and muscle endurance are both deficient, low resistance with higher repetitions is recommended. It has been demonstrated that high repetitions with low resistance and high resistance with low repetitions both provide increases in strength.[22, 83, 86] Since this is the case, it is safer for the injured segment to receive reduced stress with lower resistance in the earlier stages of strengthening when the injury is not yet fully healed.

The program that the rehabilitation clinician chooses depends on individual preferences, his or her judgment about which program would benefit the patient most, and available time. The programs we have considered have been shown to be beneficial for making strength gains. As a patient achieves a set goal of weight, repetitions, or number of sets, some rehabilitation clinicians increase the patient to the next goal at the time of the next treatment session, while others may want the patient to be able to reach the same goal for two or three sessions before advancing to the next goal. In part, the decision about how many times to perform a specific goal before advancing to a new goal may be based on the patient's age, physical conditioning level, long-term goals, and athletic performance level.

For example, a clinician treating a 60-year-old recreational runner may decide that the patient should be able to perform a strength exercise goal for three consecutive treatments before advancing to the next goal level, while another patient the clinician is treating, a 20-year-old Olympic sprinter, will advance to the next treatment session after achieving his goal for only one treatment session. As you gain experience with many patients who have varied rehabilitation exercise needs, you will find a system that works best for you. Until then, we recommend that you keep an open mind, try different programs, and investigate the systems presented here as well as others to see what produces the best results for you. Whether you use an existing program or design one yourself, the key element for success is that it must be progressive and based on objective goals; it must continue to stress the patient's muscles for continued improvement toward the rehabilitation goals. Experienced professionals adjust rehabilitation programs and exercise goals according to what produces the best results for each patient.

Summary

Intimate cooperation and coordination between the muscular and neural systems provide the body with a very complex physiochemical mechanism that creates movement. This mechanism enables muscles to exert strength and build endurance. How clinicians restore and develop these two abilities is determined in part by how the injured muscles are rehabilitated. Clinicians must be aware of the anatomy and biomechanics of each muscle and remember that monoarticular muscles function differently than multiarticular muscles. Since most of the research on muscle strength, endurance, and power is based on normal muscle, clinicians must adapt these findings to choose exercises and progressions for each patient, consistent with the patients' needs and the best practices of the profession. Clinicians must choose numbers of sets and repetitions of muscle activity and resistance levels appropriate for each patient, and recovery applications that will best produce muscle strength or endurance. The clinician must also understand how changes in body positions may affect resistance and

the body's ability to withstand that resistance. Muscles perform at different levels and in different ways to provide movement, assist movement, or stabilize movements. The clinician must know how a muscle functions and how to rehabilitate it to work at its best.

LEARNING AIDS

Key Concepts and Review

1. Explain why slow-twitch fibers are used for endurance activities and fast-twitch fibers are used more in explosive power activities.

The slow-twitch fibers have a slower-acting myosin ATPase, and the fast-twitch fibers have a faster-acting myosin ATPase, so ATP is converted more quickly to produce energy for fast-twitch fibers than for slow-twitch fibers. The extensive sarcoplasmic reticulum of the fast-twitch fibers provides for a more efficient delivery of calcium ions to permit a quicker fiber response to stimulation. However, because slow-twitch fibers have more mitochondria, more myoglobin, and more glycogen stores, they are better equipped for prolonged or sustained activity.

2. Provide an example of strengthening exercises for the coracobrachialis and the biceps muscles, and explain why they must have different considerations.

The coracobrachialis is a monoarticular muscle, while the biceps is a biarticular muscle, so the biceps position during the exercise must be considered from both the shoulder and elbow insertion points of the muscle. Monoarticular muscles are generally used for concentric activity, while biarticular muscles are used for both concentric and eccentric activity. A biarticular muscle often concentrically works at one end and eccentrically works at the other to create an energy-efficient system of movement.

3. Identify Lombard's paradox, and explain why it is useful in an activity such as getting up from a chair.

Lombard's paradox says that antagonistic muscles, rather than acting according to the laws of reciprocal innervation, co-contract to produce an efficient system of movement. When we move from sitting to standing, the hip and knee extend together: The hamstrings and rectus femoris both activate at both joints in spite of the fact that they are antagonistic muscles at these joints. Even though these opposing muscles act simultaneously during this activity, they can create motion because of the length of their moment arms and because of how their biarticular forces are used for efficient movement. At the hip, the hamstring muscles have a longer moment arm, so they have a mechanical advantage over the rectus femoris to create hip extension. At the knee, the rectus femoris moment arm is longer than that of the hamstrings, so extension is the resultant force at that joint. In other words, these two muscles create a net resultant moment at each of these two joints; the net moment at the hip produces extension because of the greater moment arm of the hamstrings at the hip, and at the knee it is also extension because of the greater moment arm of the rectus femoris at that joint. As the hip extends, it allows the rectus femoris to lengthen at the hip, adding additional force capability at the knee (related to its length–tension relationship); likewise, as the knee extends, the hamstrings gain tension from their length–tension relationship to provide additional extension force at the hip.

4. Explain why a muscle's length–tension relationship changes throughout its range of motion.

The optimal number of cross-bridge connections are available at the resting length.[65] When the sarcomere is either stretched or shortened from that resting length, fewer cross-bridges are present, so its strength decreases.

5. Identify the various types of dynamic activity.

Dynamic activity includes muscle tension with movement. Dynamic activity is divided into isotonic and isokinetic activity. Isotonic activity is further divided into concentric and eccentric activity.

6. Discuss the differences between open and closed kinetic chain activity.

Open kinetic chain activity occurs when the distal aspect of the limb is not fixed and joints in the chain can move independently of each other; closed kinetic chain activity occurs when the distal aspect is fixed or anchored so movement of one joint affects the motion of the others in the chain.

7. Explain what position a muscle working against gravity must be in to provide the maximum resistance against the patient.

Whenever gravity's resistance arm is perpendicular to the limb, limb segment, or body, it produces its greatest moment.

8. Explain why a muscle can provide more force during an eccentric contraction than during a concentric contraction, and explain how to use this concept with a patient who has less than grade 3 strength.

When shortening, a muscle uses only its active component; however, when muscle tension occurs as a muscle lengthens, the muscle's passive components also play a role in creating that tension. If a patient cannot lift a limb or body segment against gravity, begin with an eccentric movement to facilitate neuromotor and passive components to lower the segment against gravity.

9. Describe the two main approaches clinicians use to determine how long a patient may rest between strength exercise sets.

One option is that rest periods may last 30 to 60 s between sets. As another option, a 1:1 ratio between the time it takes to perform a strength exercise and the rest time between sets may be used. Later in the strength program, the patient may need more or less rest, depending on the intensity of the exercise and the patient's goals.

10. Identify and justify three OKC and three CKC activities that could be used by L.C. from the chapter opening scenario to advance Leanne's rehabilitation program and add more resistance.

Since free weights have already been used, she could advance to OKC exercises such as the NK table for knee flexion and knee extension, active knee extension with combined hip flexion with full quad activation to mimic gymnastic movements, Theraband resistance for knee extension and knee flexion, knee extensions on knee extension machine, and hamstring curls on knee flexion machine. Closed kinetic chain exercises for the knee can include standing squats to a pain free depth, leg press machine, standing terminal knee extension against Theraband resistance, partial lunges in a pain-free range of movement, wall squats with isometric holds throughout the available pain free range of motion, and Swiss ball hamstring curls in hip extension.

Critical Thinking Questions

1. If you provide manual resistance to a patient's shoulder flexors, will the position in which the patient has been placed make any difference? Why or why not?

2. What steps could you take to improve performance if a patient could not lift his lower extremity in side-lying without assistance because of weakness? How would your selection improve the patient's performance? How would it enable the patient to perform a straight-leg raise independently?

3. Explain four techniques that you could use to change the resistance without changing the amount of weight in a shoulder flexion exercise.

4. Explain the characteristic differences between fast-twitch and slow-twitch muscle fibers.

5. For a patient who has weakness in the quads, describe three progressive open kinetic chain and three progressive closed kinetic chain exercises you could use to strengthen the quads. What, if anything, would determine whether you started with the open or closed kinetic chain exercises?

6. If a patient could not bear weight on the lower extremity, not because of medical restriction but because of apprehension, what progression of activities would you select so that the patient could progress to weight bearing? What obstacles would you have to overcome for the patient to gain confidence that the leg would support him or her?

7. In which position can a patient lift a heavier dumbbell in elbow flexion, in a seated or in a supine position? Where in the motion is the weight most difficult for the patient to lift? Why? Is it a good idea to have the patient perform an elbow curl in both positions? Why? What other elbow-curl exercise would be an adequate substitute for a dumbbell exercise?

8. List six progressive exercises you would give Leanne in the chapter's opening scenario just prior to her beginning performance-specific activities. What is your justification for each exercise, and what are your criteria for progression?

Lab Activities

1. Have your lab partner lift 2 to 4 kg (5-9 lb) in shoulder flexion in a standing position, supine position, and prone position. Where in the range of motion for each exercise did the patient encounter the most difficulty? Why? Of what relevance is this to you in setting up a patient on a strengthening program?

2. Have your lab partner perform a lateral step-up. Identify all the possible ways she could substitute and not use the muscles correctly for this exercise. For each error, indicate what you would suggest to patients so they would perform the activity correctly.

3. Perform a forward step-up exercise and then return to the start position. What muscles are used going up the step? What muscles are used going down backward and forward; are they the same or different muscles? What type of muscle contraction is used to go up and to go down?

4. With your forearm on a table and grasping a bar with a weight at its end, move your forearm all the way from full pronation to full supination and back to the start position. Explain which muscle and what type of muscle contraction is occurring throughout the range of motion in both directions. How would this information influence a rehabilitation program for the elbow or wrist?

5. Ask your lab partner to lie prone and to isometrically contract the hamstrings at $0°$, $45°$, $90°$, and $120°$ of knee flexion while you provide maximal resistance against your partner at each position. Compare the force produced at each of these angles. Describe the differences. Consider the length–tension curve and the moment arm of the hamstrings. How does this information affect how you might start a patient on an early strength program?

6. Perform the following activities. Identify the primary muscle(s) performing the activity and what part of the motion is concentric and what part is eccentric:

   A. Getting up from a chair

   B. Sitting down in a chair

   C. Doing a modified push-up

   D. Doing an abdominal curl

   E. Doing an elbow curl

   F. Doing a French curl

   G. Walking up stairs

   H. Walking down stairs

   I. Performing a vertical jump

   What does this show you about activity or performance? How is this relevant to establishing a strengthening program for a patient?

7. Identify how you could have a patient perform a quadriceps strengthening exercise using the following methods:

   A. Manual resistance

   B. Body-weight resistance

   C. Rubber band or tubing

   D. Free weight

   E. Machine weight

   F. Isokinetics

8. A shot putter suffered a rotator cuff strain and has been undergoing a rehabilitation program. This is his first day of strength exercises. How will you determine what exercises and how many repetitions he should start with today? Provide a justification for each exercise. What is the determining factor in the number of repetitions he will perform for all of his strength exercises? Indicate a progression of strength exercises for the rotator cuff for this patient. How will this patient's program differ from that of a baseball pitcher who has also suffered a rotator cuff strain and is at the same stage in his rehabilitation program? Why?

14

Neuromotor Control and Proprioception

Objectives

After completing this chapter, you should be able to do the following:

1. List the locations of afferent receptors involved in proprioception.
2. Identify the CNS sites that relay proprioceptive information to the motor system.
3. Discuss the elements of proprioception.
4. Identify the systems that control balance.
5. Describe the neural processes involved in developing coordination.
6. Describe a progression of proprioceptive exercises for the lower or upper quarter.

Proprioception has been a topic of interest for rehabilitation clinician Amanda Lizbett ever since one of her college professors, Dr. C. Michaels, explained the importance of proprioception during a rehabilitation course. Since taking that course, she has been intrigued by any topic related to the neurophysiology of proprioception. She understands the interrelationship between balance, coordination, and agility, and she is fascinated by how so many body systems must all work together to generate both simple and complex motions, from standing and walking to highly skilled sport activities.

Carter, the school's star decathlete, is recovering from a hip injury, and Amanda started him on simple proprioceptive activities early in his rehabilitation program. Now he is ready to begin more intensive agility and sport-specific activities. Therefore, Amanda has designed an agility program that will challenge Carter's neuromechanical system and progress him to a full return to his sport.

In order to change, people need to become aware of their sensations and the way their bodies interact with the world around them.

Bessel van der Kolk, MD, 1943, psychiatrist, author, researcher, and educator

The human brain is an incredible supercomputer. Our collective understanding of how the brain works is growing steadily, but we have only just scratched the surface when it comes to knowing what the brain does for us every moment of every day. In the preceding quote, Dr. van der Kolk describes the need to know how our bodies feel and interact with our surroundings. He is referring to how vital this is in his field of mental health. But if this awareness is necessary for our mental health, imagine how vital it is for our physical performance. If the body is to perform at peak efficiency, our neuromechanical system needs to be fully functional. This system includes balance, body position, coordination, motor control, and agility. Correct execution of all of these functions requires our brains to be acutely aware of how our bodies interact with our surroundings and how our surroundings interact with us.

The elements of the neuromechanical system form a complex performance unit that is based on strength and flexibility. If a muscle is too weak to move a body part, the brain knows that the muscle cannot control the movement of that part. If limited flexibility prevents a muscle from engaging in the full motion that is needed to perform an activity, or if the muscle cannot work long enough to complete an activity accurately, the brain detects these deficiencies and cultivates compensatory strategies. Once these substitution strategies become engrained, they make the rehabilitation process longer and more challenging.

It is certainly necessary for people to have good flexibility, muscle endurance, and strength to perform well, but proprioception is crucial if one is to execute any skill with accuracy, consistency, and precision. Proprioception is fundamental to correct performance, and correct performance requires agility, balance, and coordination (figure 14.1). Proprioceptors play a vital neurosensory role in the

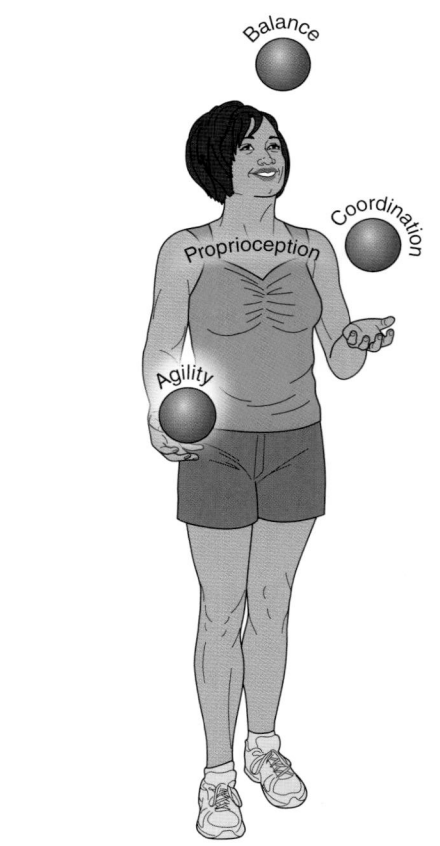

Figure 14.1 Components of proprioception.

patient's execution of motor skills, and they are a key factor in the ability to perform tasks with dexterity, mastery, and proficiency. To optimize proprioception in any activity, we must first understand what proprioceptors are and how they affect execution and skill. We review them here so that you will better understand the important role neuromotor factors play in the outcome of a rehabilitation program.

Proprioception has been defined in various ways by different investigators.[1] It begins within the general category of somatic receptors. Somatic receptors are sensory receptors (other than the specialized sensory receptors in the eyes, ears, nose, and mouth) that provide afferent information to the **central nervous system (CNS)**. Although there are various ways to classify sensory receptors, perhaps the easiest way to do it for this chapter is to identify three groups based on the information they provide: (1) **Exteroceptors** provide information on the external environment, (2) **interoceptors** (or *interoreceptors*) provide information about the body's internal environment, and (3) proprioceptors provide information on the position of the body or a body part in space.[2] **Proprioception** is the body's ability to transmit position sense, interpret the information, and respond consciously or subconsciously to stimulation through appropriate execution of posture and movement,[1] whereas **kinesthesia**, a term commonly used when discussing proprioception, is the sensation of limb movement and positions.[3] In other words, proprioception is the sensory information the body receives about motion and position, which the body interprets and responds to appropriately, and kinesthesia is an awareness of motion and position. Kinesthesia is operating when we sense that a limb is moved passively, and proprioception is responsible for the afferent stimulation that actively moves and positions the limb. Many people use these terms interchangeably.

For the past 400 years, people have investigated how the body processes information so we can know where a joint is and where it is moving without looking at it.[4] Much has been discovered over the last 100 years.[3] Since joint-position sense and motion awareness both involve joints, the prevalent view during the 20th century was that joint receptors are responsible for joint position and motion awareness.[3] This notion was expanded to include input received from skin, muscles, and tendons when it was discovered that these structures contained mechanoreceptors that facilitated proprioceptive responses. These mechanoreceptors include those listed in table 14.1. **Mechanoreceptors** are specialized afferent nerve endings that respond to mechanical stimulation such as pressure, tension, and vibration.

Proprioception is what enables us to know what position our fingers are in without looking at them. It is what maintains our balance when we stand. It is what enables us to write smoothly. It is what enables us to jump, run, and throw. It is what permits us to adjust our delivery when we miss the goal on a jump, move from asphalt to a gravel surface, or correct our overshooting of the target with our next throw. Although we must first have the flexibility and muscle strength, power, and endurance to be able to perform these activities, proprioception gives us the agility to change our direction of movement quickly and efficiently, the balance to maintain our stability, and the coordination to produce the activity correctly and consistently. Proprioceptors, therefore, are important to performance, whether it is the activities of daily living, working tasks, or complex athletic activities. Proprioceptors feed information into higher neural centers where that information is processed, interpreted, and assimilated to provide musculoskeletal output known as balance, coordination, and agility; the better the proprioceptive system works, the better we can perform.

TABLE 14.1 Mechanoreceptors

Receptor	Location	Function	Responds to
Pacinian corpuscles	Deep in the dermis, joint capsule, and ligaments	Mediate pressure and vibration sensations	Strong pressure, vibration
Meissner's corpuscles	Skin just below the epidermis, especially fingers, lips, and external genitalia (hairless skin)	Light touch and vibration	Low-threshold response to low vibrations, light touch
Ruffini endings	Joint capsule (flexion side), ligaments, and deep skin layers	Contribute to position and motion	Extension with joint rotation, skin stretch, and sustained pressures
Merkel nerve endings	Skin and mucosa	Provide touch information	Tissue displacement, pressure, and texture
Muscle spindles	Interspersed within muscle contractile fibers	Detect stretch and muscle movement	Muscle stretch
Golgi tendon organs	Musculotendinous junctions	Detect muscle tension	Muscle stretch and contraction
Golgi-Mazzoni corpuscles	Joint capsules	Detect pressure	Joint compression

Neurophysiology of Proprioception

As we now realize, although muscle spindles[5] and skin receptors[6] are the primary proprioceptors, receptors located in tendons, ligaments, and joints also serve in additional supporting roles.[7] These other receptors have unique abilities to respond to different stimuli (figure 14.2). Now that we have reviewed how proprioception works, let us take a closer look at the neural elements involved in proprioception.

Cutaneous Receptors

Most researchers believe that cutaneous **afferent receptors** do not play a major role in proprioception.[8] Evidence

suggests that they provide cues about skin stretching and fingertip touching, but they do not have a major impact on joint proprioception in healthy people. Investigations have shown that when a segment is injured, it loses normal proprioception.[9] Other investigations have shown that injured body segments with cutaneous input from bracing or splinting improve their proprioception.[10] The neural processes responsible for these proprioceptive changes are not clear, but it is more likely that they are caused by central nervous system interpretation and response than by proprioceptive receptor dysfunction.[9]

Muscle and Tendon Receptors

Neuromuscular principles that affect rehabilitation involve more than just muscles shortening and lengthening. Several

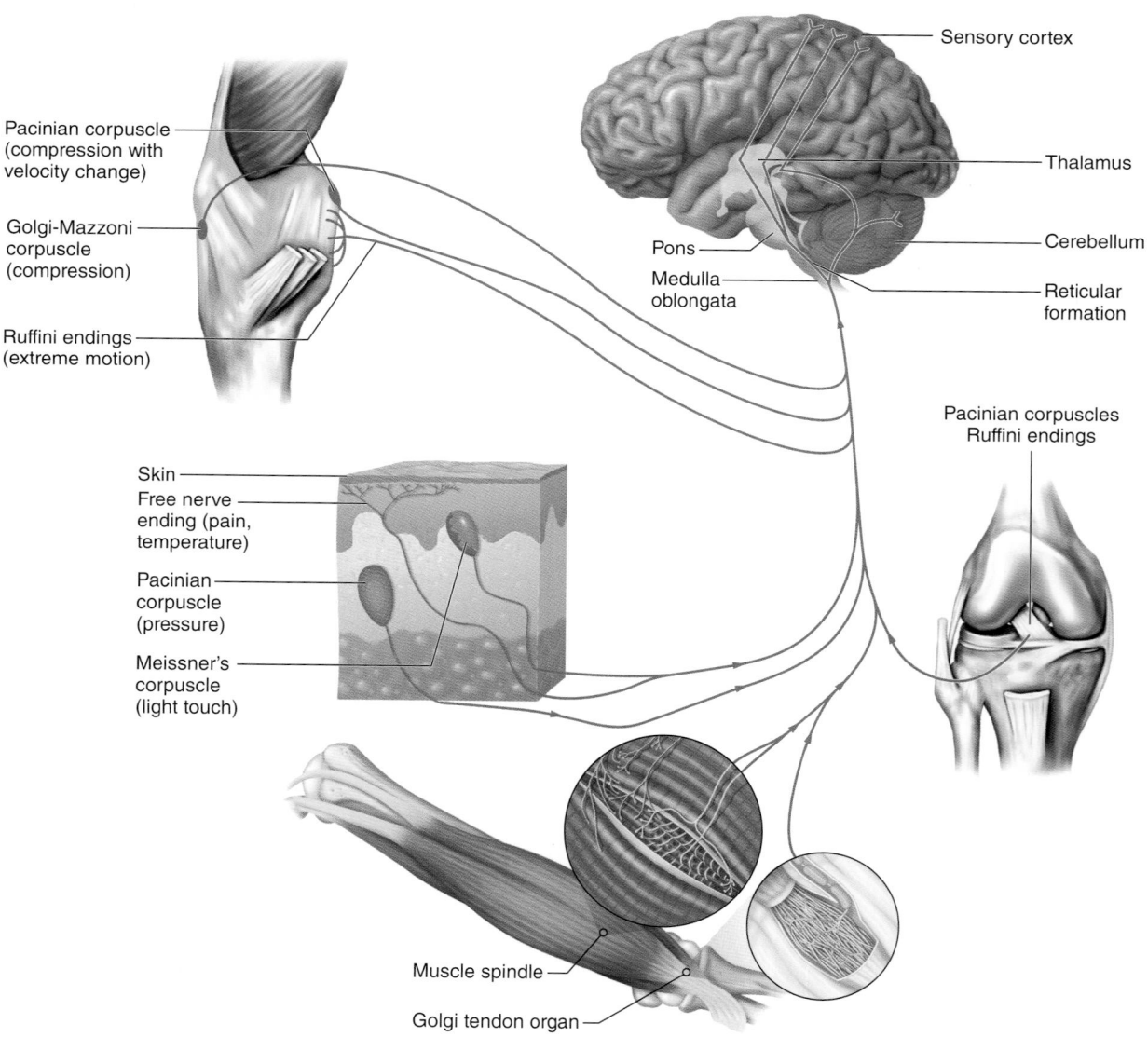

Figure 14.2   Proprioceptive afferent receptors are located throughout the body in skin, joints, ligaments, muscles, and tendons.

factors influence neuromuscular performance; one example is the stretch–shortening principle. The stretch–shortening principle is based on our knowledge about the two components of the neuromuscular system, the mechanical components and the neurological components. These components have important roles in the performance of functional and proprioceptive tasks such as plyometric activities. Plyometric activities are discussed in chapter 15.

Mechanical Components

The mechanical components can be divided into contractile elements and noncontractile elements. The contractile elements move on and with each other during active movement. While the noncontractile elements are passive in nature and function, the assistance they provide the contractile elements improves performance.

Contractile Components

The **contractile components (CC)** are the myofibrils, which contain the sarcomeres, the contractile elements of the muscle. Muscle is the only structure in the body that actively shortens or lengthens to cause motion. The contractile elements of the muscular system control the noncontractile elements.

Studies have demonstrated that when an active muscle lengthens, two things happen: The speed with which the cross-bridges detach increases, and the number of cross-bridges between actin and myosin increases.[11, 12] The end result is greater strength with a quicker release of connections between the two fibers. These activities are important if the muscle is to move quickly during a rapid lengthening while maintaining good strength and control.

Noncontractile Elements

The noncontractile elements, or components, include the muscle's tendons and the connective tissue surrounding the muscle and its fibers. The noncontractile elements are named according to their arrangement and are identified as a **series elastic component (SEC)** and a **parallel elastic component (PEC)**. The tendons, sheath, and sarcolemma are the primary structures that make up the SEC, and the muscle's connective tissue composes the PEC.[13]

Interaction of the Series Elastic Component, Parallel Elastic Component, and Contractile Component

When a muscle actively shortens, the component responsible for the muscle's ability to move the extremity or resist a force is the CC. As the muscle continues to shorten, a stretch is applied to its SEC.

When a muscle actively lengthens, as in an eccentric activity, the components responsible for producing the force are the CC, SEC, and PEC.[14] The SEC and PEC offer resistance to the movement as the muscle elongates. The

CC controls the speed and quality of the movement. When a muscle elongates, the contribution of the passive component force makes it unnecessary for the active component to produce the equivalent force as was the case during the shortening activity. For example, if a force of 4.5 kg (10 lb) is needed to lift a weight during a shortening activity, the active component, the muscle itself, must produce all 4.5 kg of force in order for the weight to be lifted. If the same weight is moved during a lengthening activity, only 3 kg (7 lb) of force needs to be produced by the active component because 1.3 kg (3 lb) is produced by the passive components, the SEC and PEC. In other words, the muscle itself works less to produce the same force during the lengthening activity because its noncontractile elements provide some of the force.

Since less work is required from active components during eccentric exercise, less energy is used during eccentric exercises. Although the exact differences in eccentric and concentric forces vary depending on the muscle groups investigated, this example demonstrates that less active force is required of the muscle during eccentric activity than during concentric activity. Stated another way, if equally active muscle output is generated in concentric and eccentric activity, a greater total force will be produced during eccentric activity.

At faster speeds of eccentric activity, a muscle can produce greater forces than at lower speeds, but the opposite is true for concentric activity.[13] The importance of this principle will become apparent in chapter 15 during the discussion of specific plyometrics.

Neurological Components

The proprioceptors that play important roles in stretch–shortening muscle activities are the **muscle spindles** and **Golgi tendon organs (GTOs)**. The muscle spindle is stimulated by sudden changes in the muscle's length, such as during an eccentric movement. Eccentric movement produces a stretch, or **myotatic reflex**, to facilitate a muscle shortening.[15] The **stretch reflex** is the most basic sensorimotor response system because it does not involve an internuncial neuron but instead goes directly from the afferent sensory nerve (muscle spindle) to the spinal cord, where it makes contact with the efferent motor neuron to permit a rapid response by the muscle. Because no additional nerves are involved in the relay process, the stretch reflex is one of the fastest reflexes in the body.[16] It is also called a **monosynaptic response** because there is only one neural connection.[17]

Normally, the GTOs play an inhibitory role in muscle activity.[18] As the muscle shortens, GTOs are stimulated to send impulses to the spinal cord that relay, via an internuncial neuron, messages to limit the force produced by a muscle. Because of this internuncial neuron, this reflex is slightly slower than the muscle spindle reflex.

The **muscle spindles** and **Golgi tendon organs** are the primary afferent receptors of muscles and tendons.[19, 20] Current thought now identifies the muscle spindle as the most important proprioceptor, with the skin's mechanoreceptors a distant second in providing position and motion information.[3, 21-23] Although the evidence is not as strong, it is suspected that Golgi tendon organs also play a contributing role in providing proprioception.[3] There is some evidence to indicate that Golgi tendon organs provide some input to proprioception, but it is difficult to separate Golgi tendon organ activation from the muscle.[20] They are complicated structures that produce complex neuromuscular responses not only from the muscles and tendons where they are located, but also from the associated **antagonistic** and **synergistic** muscles, which are stimulated to assist with the desired movement. The GTO detects tension within a muscle and so responds to both contraction and stretch, and its stimulation results in muscle relaxation.[18] The muscle spindle, on the other hand, responds to the stretch of a muscle. Its activation leads to a contraction of the muscle. A muscle's GTOs and muscle spindles can determine joint position because of their sensitivity to the length of the joint's muscles. This capability also enables them to help stabilize the limb.[17]

Joint Receptors

Most afferent receptors of a joint lie within the connective tissue of a joint's capsule and surrounding ligaments; their main purpose is to influence proprioception in end-range positions. As seen in table 14.2, they are divided into fiber type groups II, III, and IV and include both proprioceptor and **nociceptor** receptors. As you can see from table 14.2, the small-diameter nerves conduct more slowly than the large-diameter nerves because they are not myelinated and because their size creates more resistance to conduction than the larger-diameter fibers (consider the difficulty of moving a gallon of water through a drinking straw versus

a garden hose). These nociceptors do not play a role in proprioception, but they can evoke a flexion response to cause a joint to unload and thereby protect it.[24, 25]

In the last several years, investigators have realized that joint receptors are not the primary facilitators of motion and position perception.[26, 27] This is obvious in light of the fact that proprioception is not lost after joint replacement surgery.[19, 28] Since joint receptors activate when joints move into their end ranges, they are not believed to play a significant role in kinesthesia and proprioception but are used more as motion-limit detectors.[20] However, there is one exception: The finger joints use joint receptors in midrange movements.[29]

Other Receptors

Ligaments also contain receptors. Although receptors have been identified in knee and shoulder ligaments, the most thoroughly investigated ligament receptors are those in the knee's anterior cruciate ligament. These receptors are generally not active in the middle ranges of movement but are stimulated when the ligament is stressed in its lengthened state. When stimulated by ligament tension, they produce an inhibitory response of the **agonistic** muscles.[30]

As important as it is to realize that many different afferent receptors in many structures are affected by joint movement, it is also important to understand that they do not work independently.[31] What may be the most profound recent discovery about proprioception involves the upper neural centers and how information is received. There is now evidence to demonstrate the neural system's complexity in response to facilitation: (1) The CNS is instrumental in not only grouping but also interpreting afferent input to create movement and position information, and (2) input into the upper centers is not from individual afferent receptors but from groups, or populations, of receptors.[20] In other words, the brain responds to information provided by several muscle-spindle afferent nerves from groups

TABLE 14.2   Joint and Ligament Afferent Receptors

Receptor	Fiber	Conduction speed	Types	Stimulated by
Group II	Large diameter, thick myelination	High-speed conduction	A-alpha and A-beta = Ruffini endings, Pacinian corpuscles, Golgi-Mazzoni corpuscles	Proprioception (touch): pressure, vibration, skin stretch, joint compression
Group III	Small diameter, thin myelination	Slow conduction	A-delta fibers	Pain: mechanical and thermal. Pain is acute, sharp, bright, prickling.
Group IV	Small diameter, no myelination	Slower conduction	C fibers	Pain: mechanical, thermal, chemical. Pain is burning, slow, aching, long-lasting.

of muscles during movement—not just signals from one muscle or from single afferent nerves—and responses are generated by a complicated mix of peripheral receptor and central nervous system signals.[21, 23, 32-36] In essence, local afferent nerves throughout the body work together to produce a complete picture of joint position and motion for the CNS. Such input allows the CNS to process and interpret the input to produce an accurate response.

To make this easier to understand, think about what it would be like to try to correct a baseball pitcher's delivery if you watched only the pitcher's hand. You could not accurately identify the required changes unless you had the complete picture of the pitcher's performance by watching the entire delivery and analyzing all of the joint movements and positions. Similarly, the CNS cannot determine the position of an extremity unless it receives input from all sensory, motor, and joint receptors. Therefore, it makes sense that proprioception is not produced by one or two afferent receptors but by several of them sending information to the neural system, which then processes all of the information to produce an appropriate response.

Central Nervous System Proprioceptor Sites

Once the afferent nerves have sent their message to the CNS, the body's motor response is determined by the location within the CNS that interprets the stimuli and initiates the efferent reaction. Several areas within the central nervous system activate in response to proprioceptive stimuli; in essence, many cortical and subcortical sensorimotor levels are activated and become involved in integrative processing of stimulation for movement tasks.[37] Although a number of areas within the brain can be activated by proprioceptive input, the three primary areas are the **spinal cord**, **brain stem**, and **cerebral cortex**.

Spinal Cord

When an impulse goes from a dorsal root afferent nerve either to an internuncial connecting nerve or directly to an efferent nerve in the spinal cord and then immediately out the ventral root to the muscle, it is called a **spinal reflex**. This is an efferent response in its simplest form. The reflexes that do not use an **internuncial neuron** produce a more rapid response than those that use an internuncial nerve. This is because of the additional time it takes to transmit from one nerve to another. The fewer the connections between neurons, the more rapid the reflex response. These rapid proprioceptive reflexes are often used to protect an area through muscle splinting or rapid withdrawal motion. For example, a joint that is under excessive stress is protected by the sudden activation of the muscle's flexion-reflex response to suddenly reduce the

load on a joint. Reflexes provide joint stability, especially when there is a sudden change of direction or position. The joint proprioceptors, muscle spindles, and GTOs all work together to produce a reflex response that provides the joint with stabilization to prevent injury during activities.[38]

Brain Stem

The brain stem is the primary proprioceptive correlation center. The proprioceptors relay information via interneurons in the spinal cord that maintain desired body and segment position or posture and either connect to or are part of the ascending pathways to the brain stem (figure 14.3). The brain stem also receives input from other areas such as the eye's visual afferent centers and the ear's vestibular afferent centers to help maintain balance. The brain stem then sends excitatory or inhibitory efferent stimulation to produce an appropriate response. We will consider the importance of these sensory systems in the Balance section. Think of the brain stem as a central switchboard through which incoming and outgoing information is continually sent to and from higher brain centers.

Cerebral Cortex

Sensory pathways travel to the cortex of the **cerebrum** (figure 14.3). This is the highest level of the brain and the location of consciousness—the center of volitional control of movement. It is here that correct movement is learned and consciously controlled and corrected before it becomes an automatic response. To understand this process, think about how you learned to type on your computer. When you were first learning, you were very conscious of what your fingers were doing and where they were on the keyboard. Now, after several years of typing, you do not have to think about what you are doing because the activity has become automatic. You make fewer mistakes and perform the activity faster than you did as a beginning typist. This occurs with any activity that is practiced repeatedly; conscious performance becomes automatic performance, and cognitive awareness of the activity is not required.

CLINICAL TIPS

After the afferent nerves send their input to the CNS, the body's motor response depends on an integrated response from higher central nervous system centers. These CNS centers lie within the spinal cord, brain stem, and cerebral cortex.

Proprioception requires a wide range of functions from simple to complex. Complexity, however, is relative since even the simplest function involves complex neuromuscular connections. The elements of agility, balance, and

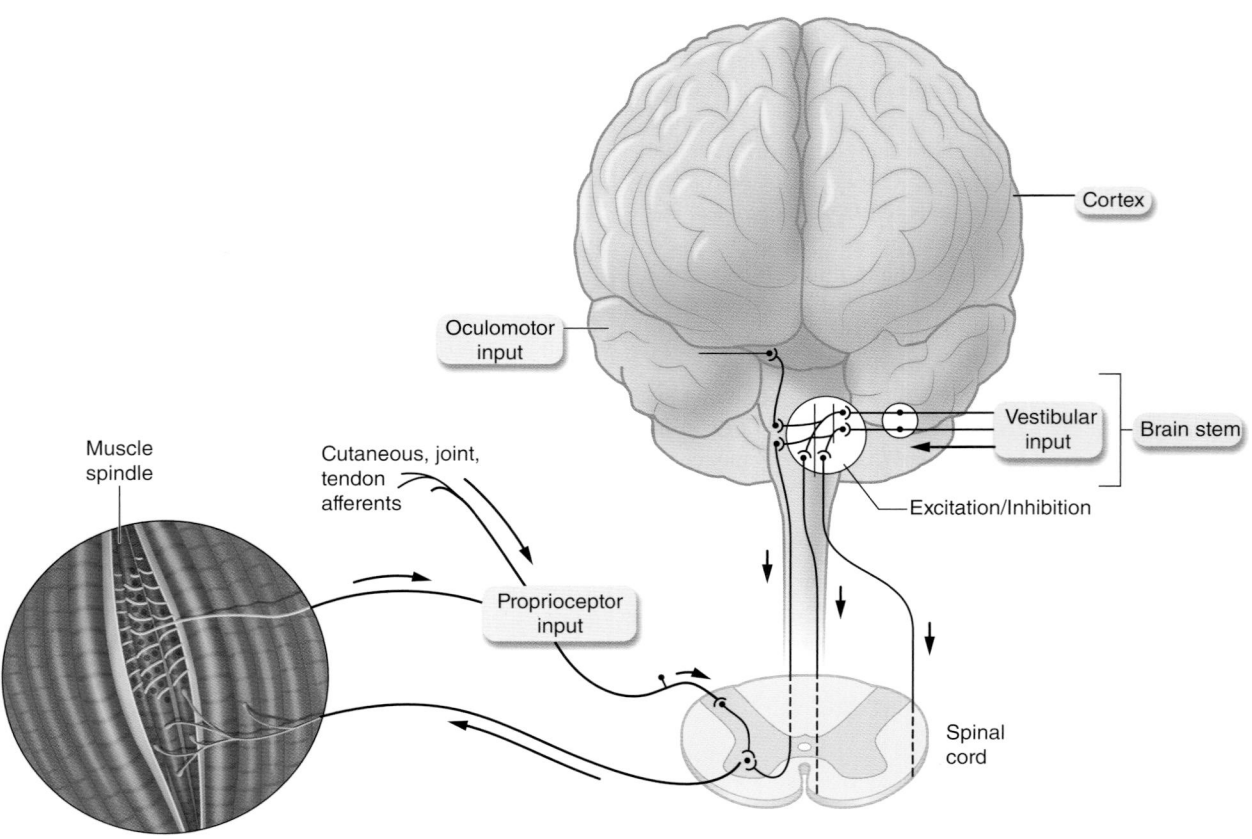

Figure 14.3   Balance pathways include oculomotor, vestibular, and proprioceptor pathways. These three neural pathways for balance result in inhibitory or excitatory stimulation to affect the body's motor response.

coordination are all interrelated because they are influenced and controlled by the body's proprioceptors. These functions are discussed here in order of their complexity, beginning with the simplest and progressing to the more highly challenging functions.

Balance

Balance is fundamental to most activities, including such simple ones as standing still. Correct performance of nearly every activity requires balance. A person who lacks good balance risks injury. If balance is not restored after an injury, the risk of reinjury increases significantly.[39]

Balance is the body's ability to maintain equilibrium by controlling its center of mass over its base of support. Balance is important in both static and dynamic activities. Standing and sitting are static balance activities. Walking, running, jumping, hopping, and dancing are examples of dynamic balance activities.

Balance is influenced by strength and the CNS.[40, 41] It is because strength influences balance that strength is emphasized before proprioception in a rehabilitation program. As we have mentioned, the subcortical brain receives sensory input from the vestibular system, the visual system, and the proprioceptors. The combination of input from the ears, eyes, and proprioceptors enables us to maintain balance and posture.[42-44] If you have ever had an ear infection, you may remember the difficulty you had in keeping your balance. You may also have experienced vestibular upset with some unsteadiness after getting off a fast amusement-park ride. An example of a balance test that eliminates vestibular input is repetitively turning your head from left to right while standing on one leg. A simple test to highlight the importance of visual input for balance is to stand on one foot with your eyes open and then close your eyes. You will quickly discover that without visual input, it is more difficult to maintain balance. So, too, when proprioceptors are damaged after surgery or injury, balance is impaired since one of the three balance input systems is damaged.

Other factors can influence balance, such as cognitive awareness of balance and previous injuries. For example, a patient's ability to focus on balance is basic to the cognitive portion of the proprioceptive system, and a patient's ability to perform skills on different playing surfaces is directly related to the proprioceptive system. It stands to reason, then, that to further develop balance, providing

CLINICAL TIPS

Sustained joint position contributes to proprioception. Chapter 6 discusses position and posture, as well as the impact that posture has on the body. Similarly, the positions of bones, joints, and muscles influence balance, proprioception, and gait, which was discussed in chapter 7.

For example, if a patient demonstrates a resting posture in which the left pelvis is more anteriorly tipped than the right and the left shoulder is higher than the right shoulder, several proprioceptive elements become engaged. Because this posture places the body's center of mass more to the right side, the left hamstring is lengthened by the pelvis's position. This lengthened state excites its muscle spindles.[45] However, because this is a maintained posture, the information the muscle spindles send to the CNS is continuous but diminished. The brain stem and cortex adapt to this low-level, unfluctuating information, so the body perceives this new length of the hamstring as "normal." This is an example of neuromechanical adaptations that occur due to a maintained posture.[45]

the patient with distracting activities during balance or placing the patient on different surfaces will further engage proprioceptors. In static standing, the ankle appears to be the proprioceptive component that is critical to achieving good balance[41, 46] and postural control.[47] Therefore, ankle injuries or a history of ankle injury without rehabilitation to restore balance may increase a patient's susceptibility to reinjury, regardless of how long ago the ankle injury occurred or what current lower-extremity injury is being treated. This relationship between previous injuries and current balance underlines the importance of obtaining a thorough history before beginning a rehabilitation program.

Vestibular System

The **vestibular system** within the inner ear is responsible for sending messages to the CNS about static position and motion. The vestibular system includes three semicircular canals, one in each of the three major planes; these detect changes in position and help the body to maintain an upright posture. The inner ear also has two sacs. One sac, the **saccule**, regulates equilibrium; the other, the **utricle**, senses forward–backward head motion. Both sacs respond to gravity and are sensitive to head and body motions. The inner ear provides a vestibular-ocular reflex. This allows the eyes to remain steady when the body is in motion.

Oculomotor System

Vision provides feedback about the position of the body in space. This feedback system is the **oculomotor system**.

As we have already noted, with your eyes closed it is more difficult to maintain good balance than with your eyes open. If you dive underwater with your eyes closed or are in water in which vision is poor, you can become disoriented and unaware whether you are upright in relation to the water's surface and bottom. If you sit in an environment that contains a lot of activity, the oculomotor and vestibular systems work together to determine whether you or the environment is moving. Sometimes the oculomotor system does not interpret the feedback correctly, and you have a sense of moving when, in fact, you are staying still and it is the environment that is moving. This may occur when your car is stopped at a light but the car next to you is moving forward—you may have a sense that you are moving backward.

Patients who must perform activities that require rapid changes of position, such as figure skaters, gymnasts, or dancers, must learn to disregard the visual input so they do not get dizzy. The vestibular system provides rapid feedback about the change in position that occurs in these activities, but the athlete uses the technique of visual fixation—focusing on one object and disregarding other moving objects—to prevent dizziness and loss of balance.

CLINICAL TIPS

Balance involves three systems—the vestibular system, the oculomotor system, and the proprioceptive system. The rehabilitation clinician can perform simple tests to evaluate the patient's reliance on each system for his or her balance by eliminating one at a time. Results of these tests are used to clinically identify deficiencies in proprioception. Many of these tests may be used as exercises to improve balance.

Proprioceptive System

The proprioceptive system is sometimes referred to as the **somatosensory system**. We have already discussed the importance of a good proprioceptive system for balance. We have also mentioned that when injuries occur, the resulting impairments to the system can increase the risk of reinjury.[48]

Balance must be restored using exercises as part of the rehabilitation program. These include exercises that begin at a basic level and progress to more complex, functional, and specific activities as the patient's balance improves. These exercises and functional activities are discussed in later chapters, but you may quickly realize that tests to assess balance often also serve as early balance exercises and activities in a rehabilitative program.

Balance Exercises

Both laboratory research and clinical tests are available to measure balance. Although the clinical tests usually are less complicated and require little or no equipment to administer, they have proven to be reliable tools for assessing balance deficiencies, and they are easily converted to treatment techniques. Since we are interested in using these tests as rehabilitation exercises, we will look at some of the more common clinical static and dynamic balance tests used as exercises. The difficulty of these exercises changes as the patient's ability improves, proceeding from static to dynamic. The simplest are static exercises, and these are used before dynamic exercises. Although static balance ability does not usually translate to dynamic balance ability,[53] static balance exercises are a good starting point from which the clinician can advance a patient's balance exercise program.

Perhaps the simplest static balance exercise is the **Romberg test**. In this exercise, the patient stands with feet together and eyes closed. The normal result is for there to be no loss of balance. Most adults should be able to perform this stance without difficulty for 30 s.[54] A slightly more difficult static exercise is the stork stand, or single-leg stance, in which the patient stands only on the injured leg with arms at the sides. The exercise goal is to maintain this position for 30 s without touching the other foot to the floor or using the arms for balance.[55] Normal balancing ability in this position for persons 60 years old and older is 20 s.[56] Individuals in the 45- to 55-year range also begin to demonstrate a reduced ability in balance activities,[57, 58] so for an older patient the clinician may set a goal for this exercise of less than 30 s. Once the patient can achieve this goal, the exercise advances to a single-leg stance with the eyes closed; eyes closed eliminates oculomotor feedback and forces the patient to rely more heavily on the other two balance systems.

Elimination of the vestibular system occurs when the person performs a single-leg stance while rotating the head from one side to the other. The patient should be able to perform each of these balance activities for 30 s (less for older patients) without losing balance before advancing to more difficult exercises. Additional ways to advance this exercise include placing the patient on progressively less stable surfaces and starting with a single-leg stance with eyes open, then eyes closed, then eyes open with head rotation. In the most challenging static exercise for the proprioceptive system, the patient has eyes closed during head rotation while maintaining balance in a single-limb stance.

More difficult balance exercises are dynamic exercises. Some clinicians refer to these balance maneuvers as functional activities, but this is not entirely accurate since they do not always reproduce the activities of daily living or sport performance. They are, however, a progression from static exercises because the patient must maintain balance while in motion.[53] As with the static balance exercises, some dynamic exercises are based on tests that assess a patient's balance. Because these dynamic balance exercises include motion, they may also be considered a form of coordination exercise. Of these dynamic-test-as-exercise applications, perhaps the most commonly used is the Star Excursion Balance Test (SEBT).[59] Since it is also used as a rehabilitative exercise in this text, it may be referred to as the Star Excursion Balance Exercise (SEBE).

The SEBE is performed on a grid marked off on the floor (figure 14.4). It has eight lines extending out from a center point at 45° angles from their adjacent lines, similar to spokes on a wheel, or a star, hence its name.[53] The lines are labeled according to the stance leg: anterior, anteromedial, medial, posteromedial, posterior, posterolateral, lateral, and anterolateral. While standing on the injured limb, the patient extends the non-weight-bearing lower extremity out along each spoke as far as possible without bearing weight on the limb while maintaining good balance and not moving the stance foot or the arms. The patient reaches as far as possible on each spoke without losing balance.

Of the eight spokes, the anteromedial, medial, and posteromedial reaches were found in one study to be the most important reaches of the test for predicting deficiencies.[60]

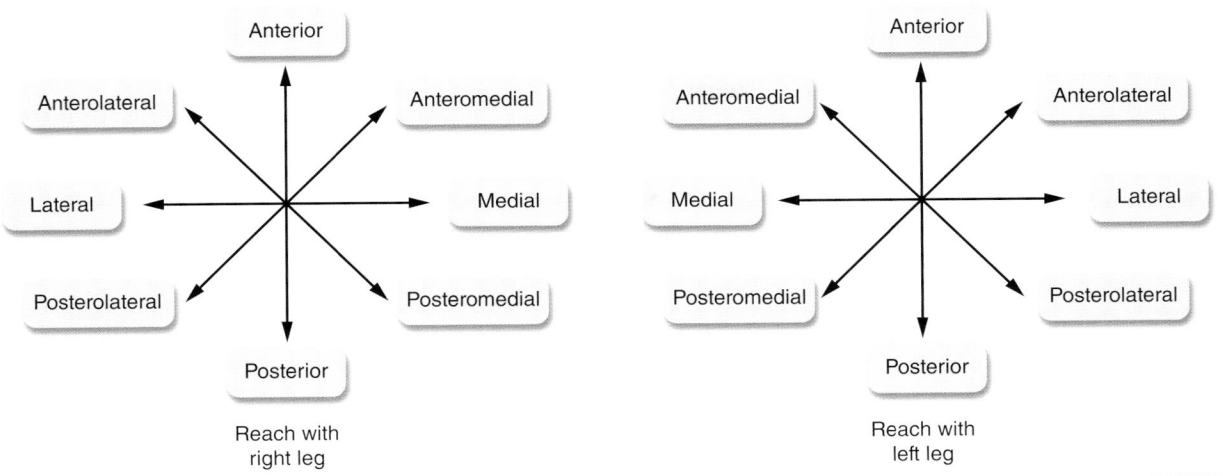

Figure 14.4 SEBE (Star Excursion Balance Exercise) diagram. The weight-bearing limb is the injured limb.

Therefore, if there are time restrictions, the patient may use only these three spokes rather than all eight. A balance exercise that uses only the anterior, posteromedial, and posterolateral spokes is called the Y-balance.[61, 62] However, when patients use the Y-balance test rather than the SEBT, they have different anterior reach results, so results between the two systems should not be compared.[62] Either method, however, is reliable.[60, 63]

An upper-extremity dynamic balance exercise based on a test called the upper-quarter Y-balance test (UQYBT)

is a takeoff on the SEBT.[64] For simplicity's sake, we will call this exercise the arm balance exercise (ABE). In this exercise, the patient is in a regular push-up position with the feet no more than 12 in. apart. The patient reaches with the uninvolved arm as far as possible in medial, posterolateral, and superolateral directions while maintaining balance on the involved upper extremity (figure 14.5).[64] The line labels are referenced according to movements relative to the weight-bearing extremity. The patient reaches as far as possible without losing balance on the weight-bearing arm.

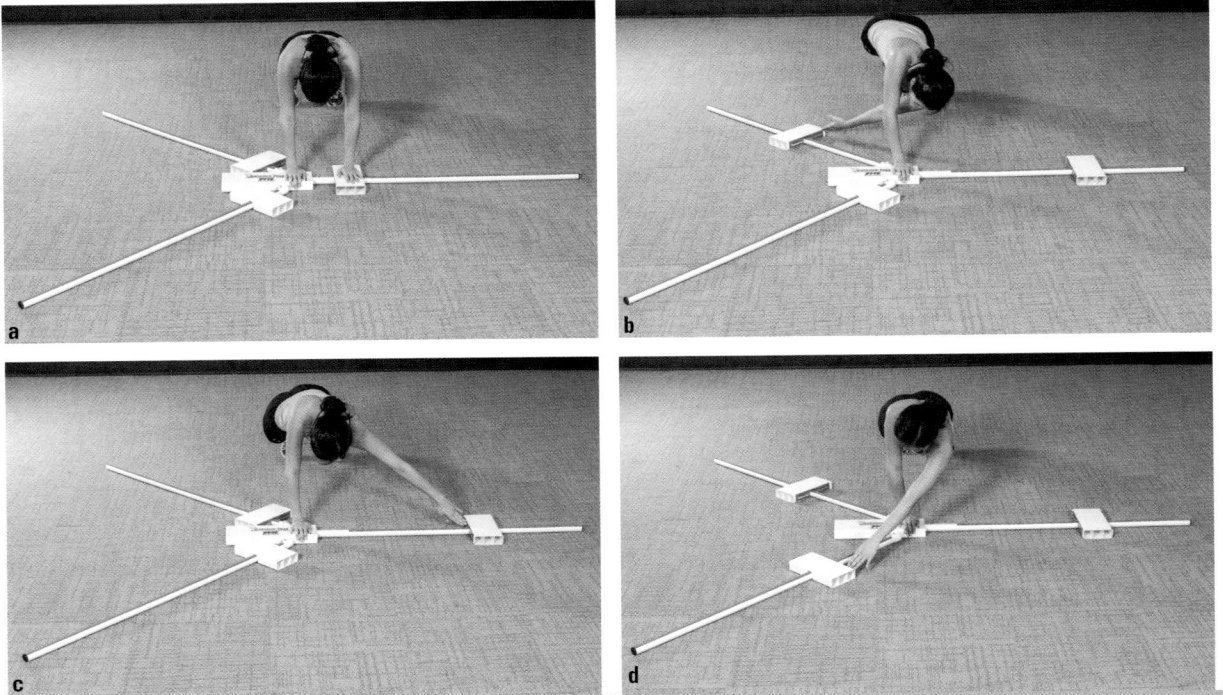

Figure 14.5 ABE (arm balance exercise) demonstrated for right upper extremity.

Coordination

Coordination is another proprioceptive function that is fundamental to dynamic activities. **Coordination** is the complex process by which a smooth pattern of activity is produced through a combination of muscles acting together with appropriate intensity and timing. Several muscles are involved in a coordinated activity. As in balance, these muscles produce movement by the actions of a complex neurological network of sensory receptors, internuncial neurons, ascending and descending corticospinal pathways, and efferent nerves. Some muscles are stimulated to provide an activity, while others are inhibited to permit the activity, and still others are facilitated to provide synergistic or stabilizing responses to permit the desired motion to occur. Each muscle must provide an accurate response in both timing and intensity for the activity to be coordinated. If a muscle is too weak to provide the appropriate response, the activity will be uncoordinated and undesirable. For example, if a volleyball player does not have enough strength in the scapular rotators, the arm cannot be positioned correctly to hit and place the ball accurately. A soccer player who has weak hip abductors on the standing leg has neither the stability needed to stiffen the body nor the base needed for the opposite leg to kick the ball well.

If muscles are weak, they must work harder than they should to achieve a specific output. This causes an irradiation of stimulation, called **overflow**, to other muscle groups.[65] We see this in a simple activity such as opening a jar. If the cover comes off with little effort, minimal activity of the hand and arm is required. However, if the cover is stuck and more effort is needed, the arm muscles increase tension, the grip gets tighter, the jaw muscles clench, and the entire body tenses as we try to open the jar. Likewise, when a muscle lacks the strength to provide appropriate motion, it tries as hard as it can to perform the activity and in so doing stimulates otherwise inactive muscles to assist, causing incoordination.[66] This results in undesired and inefficient movements; the body's preference is for efficient, desirable movement.[67] For this reason, the patient must achieve adequate strength gains before you include advanced coordination activities in a rehabilitation program.[68]

Components of Coordination

There are specific requirements for coordinated movement. Let's briefly look at them so that the logical progression of therapeutic exercises for improved coordination will be clear.

Activity Perception

Probably the most basic element of coordination is the awareness of **volitional** muscle activity. An awareness of joint position and movement is fundamental to the ability to perform activity. Proprioception is essential to this awareness.[69] Vision is also important, for it provides feedback about performance results: Have the muscles created the desired outcome? Vision is important to the development of accurate motions, especially when one is learning a new activity and motor patterns are being established.[70]

Feedback and Feedforward

The body's motor system relies on a combination of two systems for performance, feedback and feedforward.[71] In the feedback system, an action occurs and, with input from the muscular, visual, auditory, and several other afferent systems, the neurological system interprets the result of that action and makes adjustments as needed to correct the action. We use this system when we perform new activities and learn to perfect them. For example, when we throw a ball, our body makes calculations about the accuracy of the throw: Was it far enough? Did it land where we wanted it to land? Was it too high, too low, too short, too far? On the next throw, adjustments are made based on the body's calculations to make the throw more accurate.

The body also uses a feedforward process in its response to the environment. In this system, actions are based on information from previous knowledge and activity that enable the body to perform with accuracy and predictability.[72] The process is based not on error correction but on previous experience, so the body can anticipate the expected performance and produce it as it was produced before. If you have ever gone down stairs thinking you have reached the final step only to find that you have one more to go and are suddenly "missing" the final step and losing your balance, you have experienced your feedforward system in action.

Many of the activities we learn begin with the feedback process, then convert to the feedforward process as we become more accurate with them. Standing, walking, running, riding a bike, and throwing a ball are all examples of activities that have been learned through the feedback process and then converted to the feedforward system once they become automatic and no longer require our conscious correction. The body can also adapt quickly to sudden changes, realigning feedforward messages when changes in feedback information provide new or temporary information.[73, 74] For example, a skilled field-goal kicker who must kick a football with a 20 mph wind coming from his left knows the adjustments he must make to kick the ball so that it lands between the goalposts.

The feedback process involved in learning coordinated movement is similar to programming a computer. An activity is performed, the CNS evaluates the quality of the performance, the body sends information to the CNS to make adjustments to correct the undesired movements, and the activity is repeated with the adjustments made. The proprioceptors are among the most important elements in this feedback process.[72] The sensory afferents send information to the spinal cord for reflex adjustments or to the brain stem and cerebrum, where input from the activity is received and either acted upon or sent to the **cerebellum**, where muscle position and length adjustments are made during the next performance (figure 14.6). Cognitive-response information is relayed from the cerebellum to the brain stem, where it is integrated with other response feedback the brain stem has received from other upper neural centers and sent down the spinal cord for adjusting performance.

Repetition

As the activity becomes more accurate with repetition and adjustments, the performance becomes more consistent. To visualize this, we could use an analogy from cross-country skiing. The more that the tracks on a trail are used, the deeper they get and the easier it becomes to stay within them. Deviation from the tracks becomes less likely the more the trail is used.

Repetition is a requirement for the development of accuracy and coordination.[75] As the activity is repeated, the required effort decreases, and there is less chance of overflow to the wrong muscles. Eventually, an activity engram is developed that can be repeated precisely and accurately.[76] An **engram** is an effect or performance that is impressed upon the CNS through repetition. Coordination develops based on the number of times an engram is practiced.[75] Thousands of repetitions are required to achieve proficiency.[75] Once learning occurs, the coordinated activity becomes automatic, and it moves from the cognitive centers of the brain to the secondary motor areas.[77]

Inhibition

In the development of coordination, it is important to inhibit undesired muscle activity. **Inhibition** cannot be trained directly.[78] It must be facilitated by precise, slow, and controlled activity until the engram is developed and the patient can increase speed of execution without producing unwanted muscle responses.[78] In the early developmental stages of coordination, the activity should not be so difficult that the patient's performance causes an overflow of unwanted muscle responses. Given that early coordination requires cognitive awareness and conscious correction, it is best that the patient not be distracted with too many activities. Such distractions will lead to imprecise patterns of movement because the patient will not be able to concentrate adequately on any one activity. For example, the first time you drove a car, you may have turned off the radio so you could concentrate on your driving.

Inhibition is part of the computer-like adjustment process that eventually results in coordinated activity. When we apply this concept to a new rehabilitation activity or skill, we should start the patient with basic activity to eliminate the overflow to other pathways until a coordinated pattern is established. As the desired motion becomes an engram, the activity is modified to be more difficult because the ability to inhibit undesired activity will have improved.

> ### CLINICAL TIPS
>
> The components of coordination include perception of activity, feedback, performance adjustment, and repetition. The development of coordination involves repetition for improved performance and progression of activities from simple to more complex as performance improves.

Development of Coordination

The progression of coordination starts with simple activities and moves to ones that are more complex. Increasing the speed of the activity, increasing the force, or increasing the complexity are all ways to advance the difficulty of coordination exercises. All coordination activities require repetition if they are to be learned and executed accurately. This means that any coordination exercise in a rehabilitation program should include many repetitions. This is especially important as the program progresses to functional and performance-specific exercises.

Accuracy of performance is vital to the development of coordination. The rehabilitation clinician must be sensitive to this when the patient is performing the exercises. Once the patient begins to fatigue and coordination becomes less accurate, the activity should be stopped. Continued execution of uncoordinated motions will include undesired movement in the engram. Remember this when you are scheduling coordination exercises in a treatment session. The coordination activities should come early in the session when fatigue is less of a factor than it will be toward the session's end.

Agility

Agility is the ability to control the direction of the body or a body segment during rapid movement. Athletic agility

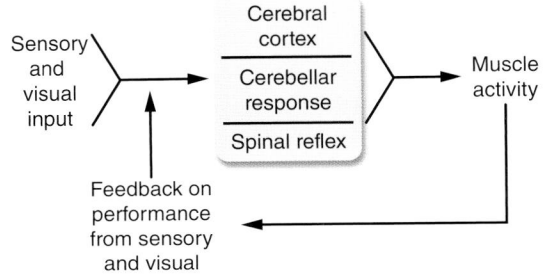

Figure 14.6 Feedback system for coordination.

requires a number of qualities: flexibility, strength, power, speed, balance, and coordination. It involves rapid change of direction and sudden stopping and starting.

Most sports require agility in the lower extremities. A football receiver must be able to cut suddenly to the left or right to evade a defensive player, and a soccer forward must zigzag down the field to move the ball around an opponent. Upper-extremity agility is required when a piano player moves the fingers rapidly across the keyboard and when a soccer goalie uses the hands to suddenly block a shot.

Agility is a highly advanced skill that requires a base of coordination, flexibility, strength, and power. Balance has been shown to directly affect one's agility and performance.[79] Adequate flexibility provides a base for speed and power. Since power is needed for agility, and power is force times distance divided by time ($F \times D/T$), one can increase power by increasing the distance through which the body part moves. Therefore, normal flexibility produces greater power than restricted flexibility. Power is important because the greater the power, the more quickly an athlete can move.

Strength is also a component of agility. A patient with good strength can control the inertia that forceful movement creates. If a 90 kg (200 lb) patient cannot control his or her weight during movement, that movement will be ineffective. Strength is a controlling factor in a patient's maneuverability.

As with coordination activities, rehabilitation for agility should begin with simple exercises and progress to more complex activities as skill level improves. The ultimate goal of agility exercises is for patients to perform all the agility activities their sport or normal activities may require. The early stages of agility exercises involve the execution of simple activities in simple drills. These activities are usually components of an athletic skill or specific job requirement, and they are performed at slower-than-normal speeds. As the patient achieves goals and new goals are established, the activity becomes more complex, and the speed approaches normal rates.

CLINICAL TIPS

Agility is an advanced skill that is built on flexibility, strength, power, balance, and coordination. Each of these elements must be achieved before agility can be included in a rehabilitation program.

Agility activities in a rehabilitation program resemble the patient's sport or work activities. It is your responsibility as a rehabilitation clinician to understand the demands of the patient's sport position or occupation so you can provide appropriate agility exercises. For example, agility activities for a basketball player should include both functional exercises (such as lateral-line sprints, figure-eight cone running, sudden-stop activities, and running backward) and performance-specific activities (such as dribbling on a fast break, layups, and one-on-one drills). Agility exercises for an assembly-line worker may include performance-specific exercises such as rapid eye–hand coordination activities to pull an object off the assembly belt, package it, and send it to be boxed before the next object appears. Performance goals for the exercise progressions of these activities are determined by the speed of the activity, the ability to suddenly change direction, the competence to use the injured and noninjured extremities equally in all directions, and smoothness and accuracy of execution.

Rehabilitation Exercises for Proprioception

Agility, balance, and coordination all reside under the umbrella of proprioception exercises. Agility, balance, and coordination naturally follow flexibility and strength within a rehabilitation program. Coordination and agility are often intimately related, and they can be difficult to separate except in very basic exercises. With the more advanced agility exercises, there is a similar relationship between agility and functional activities; they are often difficult to separate from one another. There is an important general progression of proprioception exercises, whether you are working with upper- or lower-quarter injuries. Proprioception exercises should be a routine part of a rehabilitation program.

General Concepts

Some concepts related to exercise for proprioception have already been introduced but are important enough to be repeated. Balance is achieved first, followed by coordination, and finally agility. The order is important because agility depends on coordination and coordination depends on balance. Balance exercises start with static activities and progress to dynamic activities as balance improves.

All exercises for proprioception progress from simple to complex. Simple exercises include activities in which the patient has only one or two items that require skill or concentration. Simple exercises also include only enough muscle activity to produce the desired result without overflow to unwanted muscles. Simple exercises are performed slowly and deliberately in controlled situations and environments. Distractions should be avoided when high-level concentration is needed.

Progression from simple to complex occurs only after the patient has mastered the simple exercise by achieving the goals established for the exercise. You can make the activity more complex by having the patient perform the simple activity at a faster pace or by requiring a more powerful output with control. Progression from simple to more complex can also include exercises that require the patient to perform more than one task simultaneously. A task becomes more complex when one of the feedback mechanisms is restricted, as when the patient performs the simple activity with eyes closed. Progression to exercises that mimic sport or work activities occurs as soon as the patient's abilities allow.

The patient must perform the activity accurately. To encourage this, the difficult proprioceptive activities occur early in the rehabilitation treatment session rather than later when the patient is more fatigued and coordination is more difficult.

Lower-Quarter Progression

Although specific exercises are addressed in part IV with rehabilitation programs for specific areas of the body, a brief description of proprioceptive programs is presented here.

Static balance activities begin with the single-leg stance with eyes open, using all three balance feedback systems. The patient stands on the foot of the involved leg with arms at the sides. The goal is to stork stand for 30 s, holding the arms at the sides without touching the elevated foot to the floor or to the stance leg. Patients who have difficulty with the single-leg stance can begin with a stance in a tandem position, with the toe of one foot touching the heel of the foot in front of it (figure 14.7a); this is more difficult with the injured leg in the back position. Without using the arms to balance, the patient stands in this position for 30 s with eyes open. After accomplishing either the single-leg stance (figure 14.7b) or the tandem position with eyes open for 30 s, the patient performs it with the eyes closed for 30 s to eliminate the visual input, and then with eyes open while rotating the head left to right for 30 s to eliminate the vestibular input. Balance activities progress from a single-leg stance on the floor to a single-leg stance on an unstable surface such as a mini-trampoline, foam rubber pad, or one-half foam roller, eyes open, eyes closed, eyes open with left-to-right head rotation (figure 14.7c), and eyes closed with left-to-right head rotation.

You can also increase difficulty in a single-leg stance by having the patient perform a distracting activity such as playing catch with a teammate or a trampoline rebounder. This can become even more challenging if the ball is

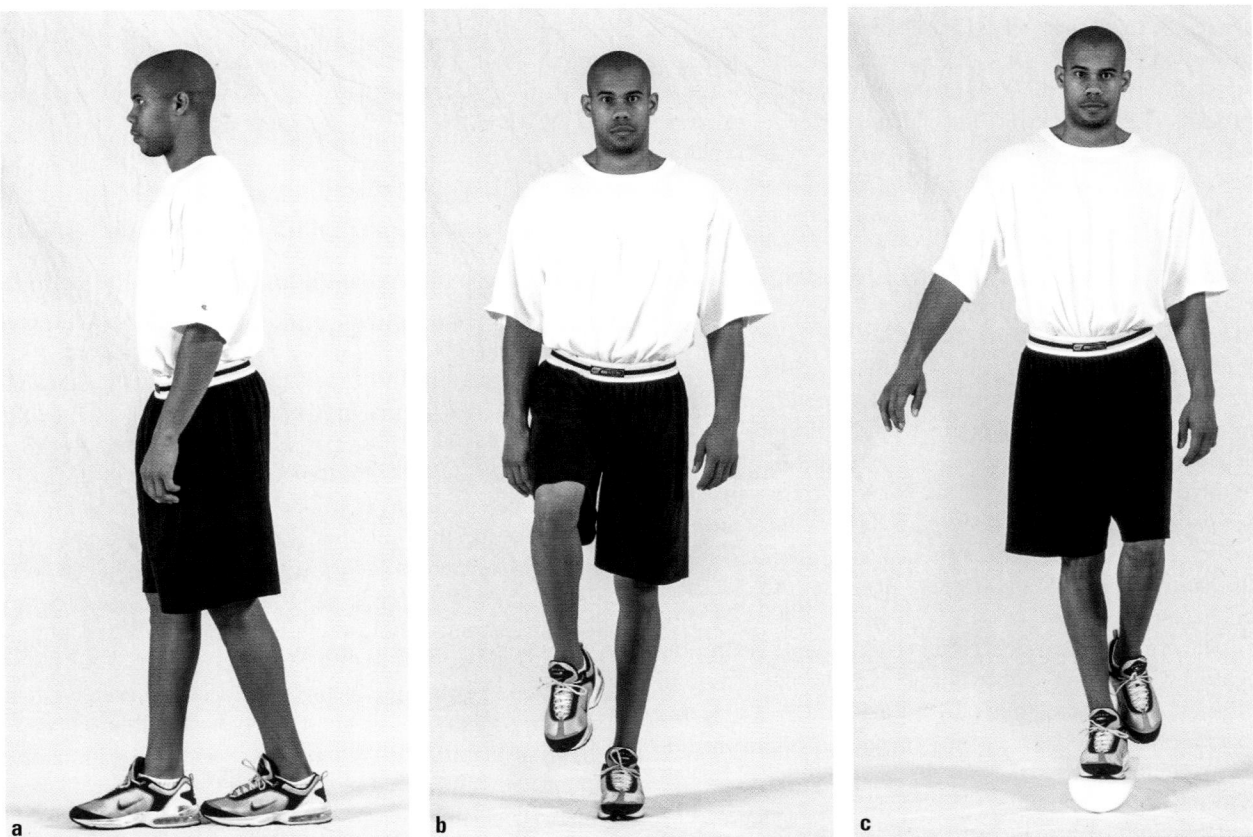

Figure 14.7   Static balance progression: *(a)* tandem stance balance, *(b)* stork stand balance, *(c)* stork stand on one-half foam roller.

weighted or if the patient stands on an unstable surface. If the patient normally participates in a ball-related sport, it is useful to use that ball to play catch to provide the patient with an emotional connection to his or her sport during the rehabilitation process.

The patient can also perform static balance activities in a sport-specific position. For example, a gymnast can perform the single-leg stance on a balance beam or with the hip in lateral rotation. A tennis player can perform static balance activities on the balls of the feet while in hip and knee flexion. A wrestler can perform static balance activities on the unstable surface of a wrestling mat.

After having mastered static balance, the patient progresses to dynamic balance. These activities include sport demands such as running, lateral movements, and backward movements. Lateral movements might include lateral shuffles or leaps to a target for accuracy, later advancing to dynamic activities for speed such as jumping, cutting, twisting, and pivoting. They begin as low-level activities, performed at a slow speed with balance and control, and progress to faster speeds. Some activities, such as jumping, can begin with the use of both legs but then progress to unilateral activities as the patient gains skill, confidence, and accuracy in execution. It may be necessary to remind the patient to maintain core control during these activities, especially in the early days of their execution. Plyometrics, discussed in chapter 15, can be incorporated into the later stages of proprioceptive exercises within the rehabilitation program. Plyometrics is a specialized system of exercises used only in the final stages of a program when the patient has appropriate strength, flexibility, and control.

In the final stages of these dynamic movements, exercises advance to mimic specific performance requirements. These exercises represent the true agility activities required of the patient in his or her normal activities. You must know the required activities and understand the stresses applied in the patient's sport or job to be able to design this part of the rehabilitation program. If the patient is returning to a job, then the tasks required during normal working activities are used as the performance-specific exercises in the final rehabilitation phase. These exercises fine-tune the patient's agility and restore his or her confidence in a successful return to work without fear of reinjury or performance deficits. Many of these exercises are discussed in chapter 15.

The use of braces, sleeves, and tape to enhance proprioception with ankle and knee injuries is still a matter of some dispute. As was previously mentioned, there is evidence that proprioception input from skin and subcutaneous sensory receptors helps in the perception of motion.[3, 23, 80] There is also evidence that proprioceptive function may improve with bracing.[81-83] One investigator found that the benefit of joint support (orthotics or bracing) is inversely proportional to the proprioceptive ability of the joint,[84] so injured people

who demonstrate balance deficiencies may benefit from using a brace or orthotic until proprioception is restored. It seems that the investigators who found no benefit to using braces performed their investigations on normal people[85] or on those whose injuries and rehabilitation occurred more than 2 years earlier.[86] Since it has been demonstrated that people with proprioceptively deficient knees rely on their cutaneous proprioceptors more than uninjured people do,[87] it may be that tape or other types of support are effective because they facilitate these cutaneous receptors to act as position-sense monitors. Most studies on proprioception and kinesthesia have been able to demonstrate an improved awareness about joint position or joint sense, but no evidence thus far demonstrates that joint stability is enhanced during functional activities with the use of such devices.[88] Complicating the decision to use braces or sleeves even more, one study offered evidence that healthy people did improve their proprioceptive performance with the use of prophylactic bracing.[81]

Although we have learned that cutaneous receptors are the "second-string" receptors the body uses for proprioceptive information,[3] there is conflicting evidence about the benefits of braces and sleeves;[89] therefore, you must decide whether to use them on an individual basis. If the patient feels more confident and performs better when wearing a brace or splint, the device may provide enough psychological benefit to warrant its use.

Upper-Quarter Progression

Although most lower-extremity sport activities are arguably closed-chain activities, upper-extremity activities are both open and closed chain. The patient's performance requirements in relation to open- or closed-chain activities will determine the extent of the proprioceptive exercises used in the rehabilitation program. A well-rounded program includes both open and closed kinetic chain activities, but end-program emphasis is determined by the demands of the patient's normal activities. For example, a baseball pitcher's demands are open kinetic chain, so most proprioceptive exercises for a pitcher should be of this type. A gymnast performs both open and closed kinetic chain activities and thus should do a combination of open and closed kinetic chain proprioceptive exercises, but a cyclist performs closed kinetic chain activities, so the program for this patient should include primarily closed kinetic chain exercises.

Initial open kinetic chain proprioceptive exercises can include proprioceptive neuromuscular facilitation (PNF) rhythmic stabilization techniques. Rhythmic stabilization can progress to closed kinetic chain exercises. In a closed kinetic chain, the exercise can progress from co-contraction without movement, to movement on a stable surface, to movement on an unstable surface. For example, the patient can either be on a Swiss ball and move his or her body with the hands anchored on the floor, or be positioned with hands moving the ball and the body supported on a table (figure 14.8). This activity can start with bilateral support and then advance to using only the involved arm. As with lower-quarter exercises, upper-quarter cues should include patient reminders to maintain core stability and proper neck and back alignment throughout the exercise progression.

1. Patient lies prone on a Swiss ball with feet off the floor. Patient begins with both hands on the floor and then raises the uninvolved arm to balance for 30 s (figure 14.8*a*).

2. Patient lies prone on a table with lower extremities on the table, and hands move the Swiss ball. The Swiss ball is rolled outward, and the position is held for 30 s (figure 14.8*b*).

3. Progressions for both exercises can include the patient's moving the ball using only the involved arm to propel the ball forward and backward and from side to side. Patient reminders to maintain an engaged core and proper spinal alignment may be required for any of these exercises.

4. Further progression can include resistance to movement—for example, on a Fitter or with manual or band resistance (figure 14.9).

Active and passive repositioning can be useful for early proprioceptive gains.[90] Passive repositioning involves the rehabilitation clinician moving the patient's uninvolved upper extremity into a position while the patient's eyes are closed; while keeping the eyes closed, the patient then moves the injured upper extremity into the same position.[90] When a mistake occurs, the patient visually compares to correct the position and repeats the exercise.

In active repositioning, the rehabilitation clinician passively moves the injured arm into a position and then

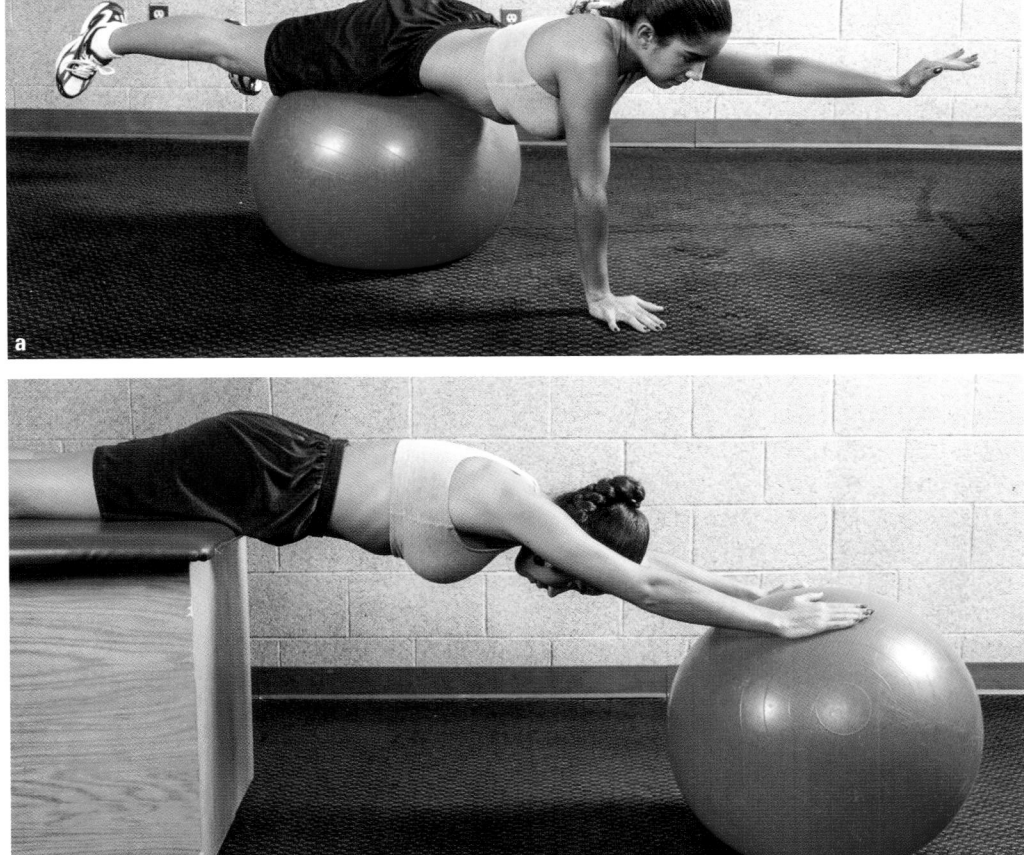

Figure 14.8 Proprioception exercises for the upper quarter on the Swiss ball: *(a)* Patient is supported by a Swiss ball only. *(b)* Patient is supported by a table while moving a Swiss ball.

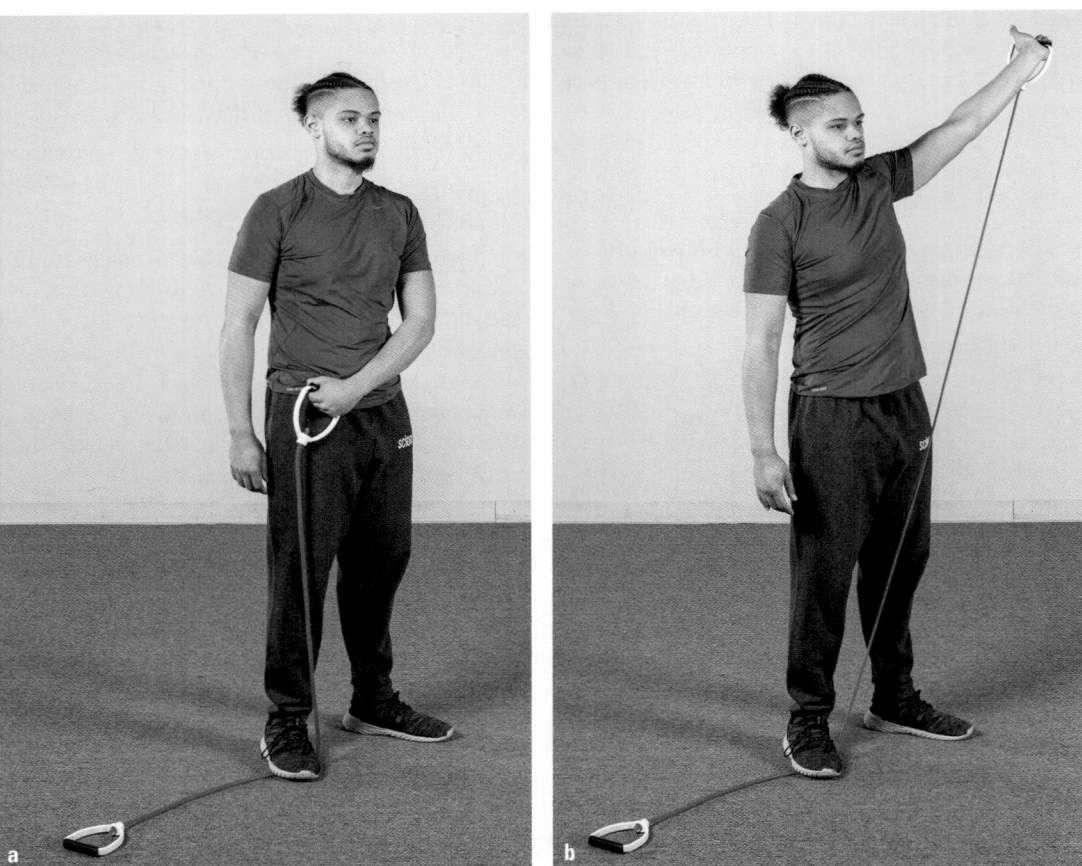

Figure 14.9 Resisted proprioceptive exercise: *(a)* start by securing the resistance tube with the contralateral foot, and *(b)* move the upper extremity in an overhead and diagonal direction.

returns it to the starting position. While keeping the eyes closed, the patient then reproduces the position of the arm in which it was placed by the clinician.[90]

Both of these activities can be performed in straight-plane, diagonal, and functional positions. The best response is achieved in functional positions near the end of the joint's range of motion.[91]

Functional exercises can be easily incorporated into an upper-quarter program. Proprioceptive neuromuscular facilitation (PNF) exercises using manual resistance, machines, and tubing provide for strength and propriocep-

tive gains. Proprioceptive exercises increase in difficulty as the patient achieves goals that are set for each exercise. Refer to chapter 11 for information, theory, and application of PNF exercises. PNF activities are beneficial at this point of the rehabilitation process because they require multiple muscles to work efficiently together to influence multiple joints to achieve a common rehabilitation outcome.

Summary

Proprioception is the body's perception of where it is in space in relation to its environment. Receptors in muscles, tendons, ligaments, capsules, and skin send information into the central nervous system, where it is processed before impulses trigger a response. Proprioceptors are important for balance, balance is important for coordination, and coordination is important for agility. Proprioception provides the information that the neurological system needs to assign meaning, intent, and accuracy to musculoskeletal position and activity. When a body segment is injured, the proprioceptors for that segment are also injured. Therefore, the rehabilitation program must include progressive exercises that develop the proprioceptors and restore them to their optimal function.

CLINICAL TIPS

Rehabilitation exercises to improve balance, coordination, and agility follow exercises for flexibility and strength gains. Exercises begin with static balance, then progress to dynamic balance, then coordination activities, then agility drills before moving on first to plyometrics, then to functional activities, and finally to performance-specific activities. Exercises for the lower and upper extremities within each of these exercise groups progress from simple to complex and emphasize accuracy through repetition.

LEARNING AIDS

Key Concepts and Review

1. List the locations of afferent receptors involved in proprioception.

Afferent receptors are found in skin, muscles, tendons, and joints.

2. Identify the CNS sites that relay proprioceptive information to the motor system.

The afferent receptors transmit information to one of three CNS sites: the spinal cord, the brain stem, or the cerebral cortex. The most rapid reflexes involve quick transmission and response from the spinal cord. The slowest responses are sent from the cerebral cortex, where conscious execution of the response is initiated.

3. Discuss the elements of proprioception.

The elements of proprioception are balance, coordination, and agility. Balance is fundamental to coordination, which in turn is fundamental to agility. A patient must have good balance, coordination, and agility to fully meet the demands of his or her sport or job. Specific exercises are used to restore these functions. These exercises can be initiated early in a rehabilitation program with simple activities and progressed to more complex activities as the patient advances. Agility requires good coordination; coordination requires good balance; and balance requires functioning afferent input from three sources, one of which is proprioceptors.

4. Identify the systems that control balance.

Balance is influenced by three systems: the vestibular, oculomotor, and proprioceptive systems. These all are influenced by posture and deliver input to the CNS to provide both static and dynamic balance.

5. Describe the neural processes involved in developing coordination.

Coordination includes the process of perceiving an activity, getting feedback from the CNS about the result of the activity, and correcting the activity through a series of repetitions and changes until the activity is performed correctly and without the need for cerebral cortex input.

6. Describe a progression of proprioceptive exercises for the lower or upper quarter.

Rehabilitation exercise for proprioception progresses from easy to difficult, from static to dynamic, from slow to fast, and from simple to complex. As a rehabilitation clinician, you must understand the complexity and requirements of the patient's sport or work to be able to include appropriate proprioceptive exercises that will eventually enable the patient to return to full participation.

Critical Thinking Questions

1. If a patient stands on one leg with eyes shut, which balance system is eliminated? How can the other two balance systems be eliminated or challenged in a stork-stand activity?

2. Would you expect a patient with an ankle sprain to have difficulty balancing on one leg? Why? List three progressive exercises that you could use to improve this patient's balance. What would be your criteria for advancement from one exercise to the next?

3. Coordination exercises are more effectively performed in a treatment session before the patient becomes fatigued. Why is this? When during the day's program would new coordination exercises make any difference in performance? Why?

4. Identify three criteria that should be met before a patient advances from balance to coordination activities and from coordination to agility activities. You should be able to explain to the patient why you are setting these criteria.

5. List three agility exercises you would provide Carter on his first day of agility training in the chapter's opening scenario. Provide two progressions for each exercise and your criteria for each progression.

Lab Activities

1. Use a five-exercise progression, beginning with the easiest and progressing to the most difficult, to challenge your lab partner's lower-quarter proprioception. The first exercise should be a static balance activity; subsequent activities should progress to the final exercise in agility. Grade your lab

partner's ability to perform each exercise level as you would in a patient's note. Indicate with each exercise what makes the exercise more challenging than the previous one. How will you determine when the patient is ready to proceed to the next level? What goals will you set?

2. With your lab partner seated on the table's end, instruct your partner to keep his or her eyes closed and move the leg into 45° of knee flexion. Measure the knee with a goniometer and record the position. Repeat this activity three times. Now instruct your partner to move the opposite leg to 45°, hold the position for 5 s, and then relax the limb. With the eyes still closed, have your partner extend the knee to 45° again. Measure the knee with a goniometer and record the position. Repeat this activity three times.

3. Have your lab partner stand on one leg, the arms at the sides, and the non-weight-bearing thigh hanging comfortably but not actively adducted to the weight-bearing extremity. Have your partner stand for 30 s with eyes open. An error occurs if the arms come away from the sides, the non-weight-bearing extremity moves away from the body or the ankle wraps around the weight-bearing limb, the trunk moves out from alignment with the hips, or the non-weight-bearing foot touches the ground. Count the errors. Repeat the exercise with the eyes closed. What is the difference between the two activities? Why? Identify two other ways the stork-stand exercise can be made more challenging for a patient. How would you determine when the patient could advance from one exercise to the next?

4. You and your partner should each perform the UQYBT exercise. You should normalize your scores by dividing your scores by your own arm lengths (from the C7 spinous process to the tip of the longest finger when the shoulder is abducted to 90°)[64] before you and your partner compare your results. Explain any differences that exist between the two of you.

15

Functional and Performance-Specific Development

Objectives

After completing this chapter, you should be able to do the following:

1. List three considerations for plyometric program execution.
2. Outline a progression of four plyometric exercises for either a lower- or an upper-extremity program.
3. Explain the difference between functional exercise and performance-specific exercise.
4. Identify the contributions of functional and performance-specific exercise to a rehabilitation program.
5. Discuss the differences between basic and advanced functional activities.
6. Discuss considerations for implementing a plyometric program.
7. List factors that can be varied in a progression of functional and performance-specific activities.
8. Identify precautions for functional and performance-specific exercises.
9. Outline a sample progression from functional through performance-specific exercises, including plyometric exercises, for either the lower or the upper extremity.

Dawn Misty works with the university's tennis team. At the end of last season, Christian Carl, the star singles player, underwent a shoulder superior labrum from anterior to posterior (SLAP) and capsular repair. He has progressed well through his rehabilitation program and is now ready to begin functional activities. Dawn knows that the functional activities will quickly progress to performance-specific activities before Christian returns to his regular tennis routine. It has been several weeks since Christian has swung a tennis racket, and he has a lot of apprehension about whether he will be able to return to competition. Dawn is confident that he will do well once he has completed the performance-specific phase of his rehabilitation program.

For the past few weeks Dawn has had Christian get accustomed to holding a tennis racket by having him bounce a ball on the ground and in the air with his elbow near his side. Now it is time for Christian to begin ground strokes. Dawn has outlined the progression of the program she has designed for Christian, informing him that the program will move at his pace and will allow him and his shoulder to become accustomed to one level before advancing to the next level. Christian has confidence in Dawn's ability and judgment because she has done an excellent job of bringing him this far along in his rehabilitation program. He knows that if she feels he can do an activity, he probably can do it.

All progress takes place outside the comfort zone.

Michael John Bobak, 1977, contemporary artist

This chapter addresses an important but often neglected aspect of rehabilitation: functional and performance-specific activities that lead to normal performance. Too often the patient's program focuses on restoring flexibility, strength, power, and endurance, while the functional and performance-specific demands are not addressed. As Mr. Bobak indicates in his quote, progress is rarely comfortable. As a patient is introduced to more challenging activities, the expectation is that the patient will find this stage of recovery difficult and uncomfortable—not necessarily painful, but mentally and physically challenging as the patient approaches the resumption of preinjury activities. Therefore, during the later stages of the rehabilitation program, rehabilitation clinicians should prepare their patients to withstand the specific stresses of their normal activities and help them to regain the required skills. Patients must also have confidence that they will be able to return to full and regular participation.

Most healthy people want to perform at their best, even if not at exceptional levels. That preinjury attitude must be regained if a patient is to return to full participation. To restore that attitude, the rehabilitation clinician must include functional and performance-specific exercises in the final stage of the rehabilitation program.

The rehabilitation clinician must understand and appreciate not only the patient's sport or occupation but also his or her responsibilities or activities. Offensive and defensive football players encounter different stresses and demands, just as the defensive line and defensive back positions have different requirements. A volleyball setter and a volleyball hitter have different needs; a warehouse manager and a warehouse worker have different performance expecta-

tions. The clinician should know what the patient's sport or job performance requirements are and should also know how to incorporate those performance requirements into the rehabilitation program.

Once the basic parameters of flexibility, strength, endurance, and proprioception have been restored, specific exercises mimicking necessary skills are added to the program. This will restore the patient's confidence in his or her performance capabilities and will also provide an avenue for renewing the skills that were lost after the injury.

Definitions, Goals, and Foundations

Before we can discuss particular functional and performance-specific programs and exercises, we must understand what functional exercises and evaluations are, as well as the rationale and objectives for each, and the goals we set for them. Once you realize how a rehabilitation program progresses to its functional exercise portion and then to the performance-specific phase, it will be easier to develop exercises for each category in this final phase.

Final Phase Definitions

Functional exercises or activities are exercises that precede performance-specific exercises in a rehabilitation program. They commonly involve multiplanar activities, and they create stresses and demands greater than those of single-plane strength exercises. They may include precursor activities to performance-specific exercises such as walking before running or underhand tossing before throwing. They prepare the patient for the more advanced skills required for performance-specific activities. Sometimes functional activities use the same tools or equipment the patient may use for performance activities, but the equipment is not used in a performance manner. For example, a tennis player may use a racket to bounce a tennis ball into the air; although the ball and racket are used to play tennis, bouncing a ball with the racket in this way is not a part of the game. On the other hand, functional exercises may also include activities similar to performance activities but may use other equipment. As an example, a baseball pitcher may throw a sponge ball at a mirror to improve his windup before advancing to performance-specific exercises; the mirror and sponge ball are not baseball equipment, but a windup is part of a performance-specific activity.

Performance-specific exercises, or **activity-specific exercises**, are exercises that include drills or mimic tasks found within a specific sport or job. They differ from functional activities in that they are tasks specific to the person's sport or work performance. Performance-specific exercises also often incorporate equipment and tools used by that person during normal activities. For example, while an underhand toss with a medicine ball is a functional activity for a baseball outfielder, throwing a baseball overhand with 50% force for a shortened distance is a performance-specific, or activity-specific, exercise since that is the activity required of an outfielder, albeit with less force and distance than normal.

As part of the rehabilitation program for an employee, a work-conditioning or work-hardening program uses activity-specific tasks to prepare the injured worker to return to work safely with reduced risk of reinjury. Performance-specific exercises are included in the final phase of the rehabilitation program to mimic the stresses, demands, and skills of the sport or job to advance a patient toward a safe and prompt return to sport participation or normal activities. As with other types of rehabilitation exercises, the drills and activities are presented in a progressive manner as patients meet their exercise goals and develop their performance abilities with progressively more challenging and complex exercises.

In the rehabilitation of athletes, *sport-specific exercises* is the term often used instead of performance- or activity-specific exercises. Athletes in the final phase of their rehabilitation program go through a sport-specific phase; this is the performance-specific phase. When we rehabilitate an injured worker, activity-specific exercises include a range of activities from sitting at a desk properly to lifting and transferring heavy boxes; the activities included in a rehabilitation program are determined by the normal tasks involved in the person's job. Although "sport-specific" is not the right term to describe final-phase rehabilitation exercises for a person returning to work, the important thing is that the final phase of any rehabilitation program includes *specific tasks* that the person performs in his or her normal environment, be it in a sport, at a job, or in the home. Therefore, performance-specific exercises, activity-specific exercises, and sport-specific exercises are

all the same thing, but the exercises involved are individually determined and are based upon the performance needs of each patient.

Performance evaluation occurs throughout the therapeutic exercise program. **Performance evaluation** is an assessment of the patient's ability to perform and complete an exercise or skill safely and accurately before he or she is allowed to advance to the next level. The final performance evaluation occurs before the patient resumes full participation. In order to safely advance to each rehabilitation level, the patient must pass functional tests. The functional tests vary according to the patient's skill level and performance requirements. Examples of these tests are discussed later.

Performance evaluations should include return-to-play issues since that is the optimal goal of most sport-based rehabilitation programs. According to Creighton and colleagues,[1] the definition of **return to play (RTP)** is "the medical clearance of an athlete for full participation in sport without restriction (strength and conditioning, practice, and competition)." Although there are no commonly agreed-upon criteria for return to play for many injuries, most professionals agree that several criteria are required;[2, 3] measures for these include clinical examination of strength, range of motion, joint mobility, and more.[4, 5] Additional RTP assessment tools include testing and examination procedures such as functional testing, an objective clinical examination, and subjective information.[4, 6]

According to consensus statements provided by the American College of Sports Medicine,[7-9] there are several steps to determining a patient's return-to-play status. Performance evaluations and return-to-play decisions do not simply involve determining the patient's medical and psychological readiness and functional ability. Rehabilitation clinicians must also appreciate the demands of the patient's sport, know how to protect the patient with various orthotic or taping techniques, and understand how the patient's return to play may affect other athletes. What the rehabilitation clinician is essentially determining is the acceptable level of risk in returning a patient to normal participation.[1] This decision is based on several factors that include the healing status of the injury; individual factors that influence healing and performance such as age, sex, medical history, sport and position, and competitive level; signs, symptoms, and laboratory tests indicative of patient injury status; functional assessment of patient performance; and the patient's psychological readiness to return to play.[1] Performance evaluations and return-to-play decisions involve many factors.[10]

As part of the performance evaluation and return-to-play process, the final phase of the patient's rehabilitation program must include activities that will prepare the patient so that he or she is truly ready to perform optimally, not only during RTP testing but also during normal sport participation. Previous parts of the rehabilitation program have addressed some of the determinants of RTP such as strength, flexibility and mobility, proprioception, and neuromuscular control. The final portion of the program focuses on optimizing the patient's ability to perform the tasks, meet the demands, and develop the psychological readiness to return to play with minimal risk of reinjury.[11]

Final Phase Goals

To meet performance demands and satisfy RTP criteria, rehabilitation programs in this final phase have three goals. The first is to attain full functional levels of flexibility, strength, endurance, and coordination. The second is to achieve full functional ability so that normal speed, power, control, and agility are restored. The third goal is to restore the patient's skills and self-confidence to perform at least at a preinjury level. Performance-specific exercises target these final rehabilitation program goals.

The first and second goals are achieved through basic and advanced functional activities. These are discussed in the next section. The third goal is achieved after the patient advances through performance-specific exercises. Success builds self-confidence and failure damages self-confidence, so it is important that the clinician provide goals that are challenging yet achievable. Being both injured and unable to participate in normal activities often causes patients to doubt their abilities. Prolonged absence from normal activities also leads to a loss of some of the skills that were so natural before the injury. To reestablish a preinjury level of self-confidence, the clinician must incorporate a progression of performance-specific exercises that mimic the skills the patient needs for normal functions.[12] A final performance evaluation takes place before the patient returns to full participation; it is the patient's ability to participate in the normal activities that is the final test of a rehabilitation program.

CLINICAL TIPS

The three goals of the therapeutic exercise portion of a rehabilitation program are to (1) acquire full functional levels of flexibility, strength, endurance, and coordination; (2) acquire normal speed, power, control, and agility; and (3) acquire activity skills with the ability to perform at least at a preinjury level. The first two goals are achieved during the early and middle phases of the therapeutic exercise portion of the rehabilitation program. Functional and performance-specific exercises are added to the last phase of a program with the third goal in mind. Once the patient has accomplished all three of these goals and met RTP criteria, he or she can expect to return to full participation at optimal performance levels.

Foundations of Final Phase Rehabilitation

Functional exercises are a part of the total rehabilitation process, and they make a vital contribution to the patient's preparation and return to work or sports participation. These exercises must place unique combinations of stresses on the patient to produce unique results. The following sections deal with seven of these demands and the corresponding results.

Normal Motion

Normal activity requires normal motion. If normal motion is lacking, the patient places undue stress on areas that must compensate for the necessary motion, and these areas are then at risk for additional injury.[13] For example, if a tennis player does not have the normal shoulder flexion, rib cage rotation, scapular elevation, and shoulder lateral rotation needed to serve, he or she may develop a low-back injury by hyperextending the lumbar spine to hit the ball overhead.

The patient should be able to demonstrate normal motion; first passively, then actively. The patient is not expected to use all of the available range of motion all the time. However, normal motion is needed for the body to perform movements with appropriate variability to reduce stress on joints and soft tissue.[14, 15] When normal mobility is lacking, compensatory motions develop.[16]

Multifaceted Muscle Activity

Several types of strengthening activities are used throughout the resistive phase of a rehabilitation program. These activities include primarily single-plane exercises to isolate weaker muscles and improve their strength levels.[17] These exercises commonly include a mixture of isometric, concentric, and eccentric activities because most normal activities include combinations of these types of movements. Once muscles acquire basic, single-plane strength, the rehabilitation program advances to include activities in multiple planes of motion since they normally work with other muscles in such a manner. Functional movement is not only triplanar, but it also commonly involves rapid changes of performance requirements from one type of muscle activity to another. Even in the simple activity of running, the lower-extremity muscles undergo rapid changes of concentric and eccentric activity in their roles as accelerators, decelerators, and stabilizers during different parts of the running cycle.

Multiplanar Motion and Multiple Muscle Group Performance

Normal activities are not performed in single-plane movements, so multiplanar activities are added to an exercise program after weakened muscles have been strengthened.[18] Since functional activities involve the simultaneous use of all three planes of motion, they also recruit many muscle groups at one time to produce the desired activity.

Multiplanar motion is performed in a coordinated manner through the simultaneous facilitation and inhibition of many muscles. An activity like throwing a ball not only involves the shoulder, elbow, wrist, and hand muscles but also requires coordinated multiplanar motions from scapula, rib cage, pelvis, and lower-extremity muscle groups. Even normal walking requires synchronization of the muscles of the foot, ankle, knee, hip, pelvis, rib cage, scapulae, shoulder, elbow, forearm, and neck.

Stabilization and Acceleration Changes

Normal performance, including daily activities, requires that some muscles work to stabilize a part while other muscles work either to accelerate or decelerate a segment. Others are even required to change from stabilization to acceleration or deceleration tasks quickly during performance.[19] For example, in an overhand toss, the trunk must be stabilized so the scapula has a platform from which to allow the shoulder joint to move to propel the ball. Even during a deceptively uncomplicated activity such as walking, the hip and leg muscles stabilize and limit lateral movement during part of the gait cycle and then convert to accelerators during other parts of gait as the body moves forward.

Proprioceptive Stimulation

Proprioception is the awareness of body movement and position. Proprioception is vital to performance. Proprioceptive skills, basic and advanced, must be finely tuned and prepared to meet the demands of the activity to which the patient will return. Functional exercise performance requires proprioception and neuromuscular training; improvement of the patient's functional performance correlates directly with his or her proprioceptive development.[20, 21]

Agility and Power Development

Agility and power are essential requirements for most sports.[22] Agility is needed for the basketball player to dribble the ball downcourt, for the volleyball player to dive and pass the ball to the setter, and for the hurdler to time each jump correctly. Power enables the sprinter to reach the finish line first, the defensive end to sack the quarterback, and the crew team to sprint to the finish. Agility and power are required in a gymnast's floor exercise, an ice skater's triple Lutz, and a water polo player's scoring a goal. Agility and power must improve as the patient increases his or her ability to perform functional activities. Progressive functional exercises provide a graduated increase in stress and, therefore, advance the patient's ability to perform at a level

of agility and power sufficient for optimal performance at sport-specific activities.

Agility and power performance require complex neuromotor skills. This is where plyometrics comes into play in many sport-based rehabilitation programs. Plyometric exercises are not only a precursor to performance-specific exercises but also serve as a transition from the strengthening phase to the final performance-specific phase of rehabilitation. Some plyometric exercises actually are specific sport activities.

CLINICAL TIPS

When instructing a patient in exercises that are the same activities required for normal performance of a sport or job, the clinician must remember these steps: (1) ensure proper posture during and after the task; (2) instruct the patient in the desired performance; (3) make sure that the patient understands the task to be performed; (4) have the patient perform the activity slowly, precisely, and without resistance; (5) add more complex tasks once basic tasks are performed correctly; (6) increase the activity's intensity as the patient's performance improves; and (7) perform the activity repeatedly to achieve the desired outcome.[23]

Confidence Development

As the patient successfully executes the performance-specific exercises that mimic the demands of the sport or job, confidence returns. By the time the patient is ready to resume full participation, he or she can perform with the level of skill that normal participation requires. This will provide the patient with the necessary self-confidence.[24]

Plyometric Exercises

Plyometrics is the use of a quick movement of eccentric activity followed by a burst of concentric activity to produce a powerful output from a muscle. It is a brief, explosive activity with maximum power production as its ultimate goal. You will recall from previous discussions that power is calculated as force times distance divided by time ($F \times d/T$). The quicker the time, the greater the power. For example, if a patient weighing 80 kg (176 lb) jumps 0.6 m (2 ft) in the air and takes 1 s to perform the activity, he produces 352 ft-lb per second of power (176 lb $\times$ 2 ft/1). If, however, he can jump the same distance in half the time, he will produce 704 ft-lb per second of power (176 lb $\times$ 2 ft/0.5).

The term *plyometrics* was coined in 1975 by an American track and field coach, Fred Wilt.[25] Its Greek origins are *plio* and *metric*, which mean "more" and "measure," respectively. Before Wilt coined the term, plyometrics was referred to as "jump training."[26] Although plyometric activities have been used since people first ran and jumped, plyometrics became popular in the late 1960s when people attributed the high-performance abilities of Eastern European Olympic athletes to the jump-training exercises used by their coaches.

Because of the muscle activation involved in plyometrics, it is sometimes referred to as stretch–shortening activity.[27] Although it has been used primarily in conditioning for healthy, uninjured people, more and more rehabilitation programs are also incorporating plyometrics.[28] Unfortunately, most of the published research has investigated uninjured persons,[29] not patients, so the effects and purported benefits of plyometrics for patients have been anecdotal, not scientific. Therefore, the references used in this chapter refer to uninjured individuals.

Many daily activities such as walking are essentially stretch–shortening activities. Plyometrics, however, is a more aggressive activity whose purpose is to improve a patient's output or performance through the use of several physiological and neuromuscular constructs.[30] As we will learn in this chapter, plyometrics is not for everyone, so the clinician must use discretion in the selection of patients whose rehabilitation program will include plyometrics.

Neuromechanical Components

At the foundation of functional and performance-specific development is the neuromuscular system's ability to perform as intended. This is known as neuromotor control. Remember from chapter 14 that **neuromotor control** is the proper activation and sequential recruitment of muscles to produce the correct response. Neuromotor control occurs because of a very complicated communication process between the musculoskeletal and nervous systems.[31] You may have noticed that some nervous system elements (i.e., proprioceptive parameters) are included in basic functional exercises and that agility is in the advanced functional exercises category. This is because proprioception is a transition neuromotor parameter that may be initiated early and may advance well into the rehabilitation program. Since the complexity of proprioceptive activities varies widely, balance is a basic functional goal that may be introduced early in a rehabilitation program. Agility, on the other hand, requires a great deal more neuromotor skill, so it is a more advanced function that enters later in the program.

Plyometrics uses specific mechanical and neural components of the neuromuscular system to create optimal performance results. The mechanical components are contractile and noncontractile elements; the neural components are the muscle spindles and the Golgi tendon organs (GTOs).

Many believe that during plyometric training, the GTO excitatory level is increased so that more stimulation is required before a response from the GTO occurs, and this elevated excitation requirement allows for an increased tolerance for additional stretch loads in the muscle.[32] As the stretch loads are better tolerated, there may be an ability to create a stronger stretch reflex, which results in additional power during the concentric phase of motion.[33]

The theory of the GTO's inhibitory role has been challenged more recently by evidence demonstrating that the GTO is stimulated during submaximal outputs and may actually store energy that is released during plyometric activity.[34] Therefore, the GTO may add to rather than detract from plyometric results. Obviously, this finding presents intriguing possibilities but requires additional investigation.

Working intimately together, the mechanical and neurological components produce the desired results of increased strength and power for athletic activity. The noncontractile, elastic elements of the mechanical component are important to force production in stretch–shortening exercises. A simplified example of the way noncontractile elements work is a rubber band model: If the rubber band is quickly stretched and then just as quickly released, it shortens rapidly. The greater the length to which it is stretched, the greater the force that is produced when the stretch is released. As the stretch increases, more stored (potential) elastic energy develops within the rubber band. If the stretch is released quickly, the stored elastic energy converts to kinetic energy, producing the rubber band's recoil. To test this concept, stretch a rubber band to about half of its fully elongated length, hold it at that length for 1 s, and then release one end. Notice the impact the rubber band makes on the other hand that is holding it. Now stretch the band to the same length as you did the first time, but this time do it quickly and release the stretched end the instant you reach the stretch point. Notice how much more of an impact the band makes on your hand.

Plyometric exercises provide an increased power output during concentric activity. This increased power, like that in the rubber band, has to do with the transfer of the elastic energy that is produced during eccentric activity immediately before concentric activity. In a muscle that moves eccentrically, the force produced by the noncontractile elements is elastic energy. As the muscle moves from eccentric to concentric activity, elastic energy is released, adding to the muscle's concentric force.[35]

It is believed that a muscle's increased output during plyometric exercise training may be the result of improved synchronization of muscle activity rather than an improvement in either strength or power.[36, 37] This finding indicates that a person's best performance is likely to occur when he or she can properly coordinate muscle firing activity. Although muscle synchronization is important, strength and power also have some influence—after all, they are required before synchronization can be optimized.[37]

Range of motion cannot be forgotten as a contributing factor to optimal plyometric performance. If a muscle can go through a greater range of motion, it can produce more optimal function.[38] For example, the patient who squats to only 30° of knee flexion does not jump as high as when he or she squats to 60° of knee flexion before takeoff. More force can be produced when more lengthening is permitted before concentric activity.

Another factor in improved performance with plyometric activity is improved neuromuscular coordination. As speed increases and the activity is performed more accurately, the manner in which muscle strength is used to execute the activity is improved.[39] Energy and movement are not wasted on ineffective, inefficient activity. Neuromuscular training involves the development of the engram as discussed in chapter 14.[40] Better coordination permits more power production directed to the desired motion since the activity can be performed more efficiently and in less time.

When speed and coordination of activity are improved, more power can be produced.[41] Studies have demonstrated that the use of an extremely brief interval between an initial eccentric contraction and a follow-up concentric contraction creates improved strength and power during the muscle's concentric phase.[36, 42, 43]

Plyometric Exercise Phases

Plyometric exercises are often divided into two or three phases. If divided into three phases they include the eccentric, amortization, and concentric phases.[28, 44] Since the middle phase is essentially a termination of the first phase and a transition to the third phase, some investigators identify only two phases, the prestretch or eccentric phase and the concentric or contraction phase.[28, 45] Since it is easier to examine plyometrics if we mention all three phases, and since the three-phase model is the one more commonly addressed in the research, we will use this model in our discussion. According to this model, the eccentric phase prepares the muscle, the amortization phase transitions the muscle, and the concentric phase is the outcome.

Eccentric Phase

The eccentric phase is also called the stretch phase, prestretch phase, or cocking phase, and it occurs when the muscle is prestretched as it actively lengthens.[46] The slack is taken out of the muscle, and its elastic components are put on stretch. This is the preparatory phase that "sets" the muscle as the person gets ready to perform the activity.[47] This phase uses muscle spindle facilitation, so the quality of the response is determined by the rate of the stretch. The muscle's response directly correlates with the quantity of the stimulation: the greater the stimulation, the greater the muscle's response.[48] The eccentric phase is an important phase of plyometric activity because it increases the

stimulation to provide for this increased muscle response; muscle output increases when a concentric contraction is preceded by a rapid stretch.[44, 49, 50]

The muscle spindle creates a more rapid muscle response when the stretch is rapidly applied, but if the stretch is applied slowly, the muscle accommodates to the facilitation and fails to produce the desired rapid response.[51] For this reason, the rate of the stretch is a more important factor than the amount of stretch. If a muscle lengthens quickly, it can produce more tension than if it is forced to elongate more slowly.[27] In addition, rapid elongation of a muscle adds stiffness to the muscle and provides elastic energy to assist on recoil of the muscle during the shortening phase.[50, 52] The best results occur when the eccentric phase is performed quickly and through a partial range of motion.[28, 36] If the range of motion through which the muscle moves is excessive, the time needed to move through that greater range causes a loss of elastic recoil energy, and if the motion is not performed quickly, then the energy is dissipated.[53] Based on research, it also appears that elastic energy is used in smaller amplitude motions with the elastic recoil primarily affecting the early phase of concentric activity.[35] Although there is disagreement on precisely how quickly the muscle must move through the stretch–shortening cycle, it is generally agreed that the faster it can perform the eccentric contraction, the better the utilization of the elastic energy produced.[54] Muscle stiffness improves the muscle's ability to store and use this energy.[55-57] Studies have demonstrated that with plyometric conditioning, muscle stiffness improves, and muscle stiffness has been shown to improve muscle response.[42, 56-58]

Amortization Phase

The eccentric phase is followed immediately by the amortization phase, which is simply defined as the amount of time it takes to change from eccentric to concentric motion.[44] Of all the phases, this is the one that varies most in descriptions of plyometrics. Some label this the transition phase or coupling phase.[28] The primary concern about the term *amortization* is that it is not an accurate description of what happens between the eccentric and concentric phases of plyometrics. This phase is extremely quick. For optimal results, the average duration of this phase during jumping should be 23 ms.[57] Contrary to this relatively "long" time, the ideal amortization phase is considered to be under 15 ms.[59] If too much time is spent in this transition phase moving from eccentrics to concentrics, the elastic energy produced during the eccentric phase is dissipated as heat and is wasted. A prolonged amortization phase also inhibits the stretch reflex.[42] Remember, the amortization phase is the transition phase. As clinicians, we are not concerned with the specific length of time of this transition phase, but we realize that the quicker the transition is from eccentric to concentric activity, the more forceful the movement will be.

Concentric Phase

The final phase, the concentric phase, is the result of the combined eccentric and amortization phases.[60] The concentric phase is the outcome phase. It is also referred to as the shortening phase, unloading phase, or propulsion phase. If the eccentric activity has been quick and the transition has occurred rapidly, the concentric phase will produce the desired powerful outcome, increased force, and improved speed of muscle shortening.[61]

If plyometric exercises are done correctly, the end result should be a higher jump,[62] a greater running economy,[55] or an improved explosive performance.[63] Over time, with practice and neurological facilitation, improved performance occurs because of a number of physiological effects produced by the plyometric exercises; in essence, an improved synchronous activity of motor units and an earlier recruitment of the motor units occur because these physiological modifications include an increased neural drive along with changes in muscle's elastic properties, improved synergistic coactivation, and inhibition of the body's neural protective mechanisms along with increased neuronal excitation.[64-69] In short, plyometrics bridges the gap between strength and explosive power by integrating the mechanical and neurological factors that influence these performance elements.[70]

Pre-Plyometric Considerations

Power production is important in most sports. For example, it is an important element in the execution of skills and performance in basketball, volleyball, gymnastics, track and field, baseball, softball, and skating. Since power is crucial for sport performance and plyometrics enhances neuromuscular efficiency, plyometric exercises should be considered for patients who are returning to power-essen-tial sports. Just as with functional and performance-specific exercises, before plyometrics can become part of a rehabilitation program, specific physical parameters must be met. For this reason, plyometric exercises are placed toward the end of the rehabilitation program before functional and performance-specific exercises.

Strength

Strength is basic to plyometric exercises.[30] The patient should have enough strength to adequately control his or her performance. As the difficulty of the plyometric exercise increases, the patient needs to have even more strength. One can minimize the potential for overuse injuries from plyometric activities with good pre-plyometric strength levels.

Greater strength provides for better output during the plyometric exercise. Recall that if $F \times d/T = P$, then the greater the force, the greater the power. Since force is a measure of strength, power is directly related to strength. In addition, the greater the muscle cross section because of hypertrophy, the more elastic elements there will be to provide additional eccentric strength. Minimum recommended strength levels for plyometric exercises vary, and they depend on the severity of the plyometric exercise. For more rigorous lower-extremity plyometric exercises, the recommendation for healthy people is that they be able to perform a squat with 60% of body weight for five repetitions within 5 s.[25] Unfortunately for patients, there are no established minimum strength requirements for performing plyometrics in a rehabilitation program. Since plyometric exercises are used in the latter phase of rehabilitation when tissue strength is approaching optimal levels, the clinician's assessment of the patient's abilities should be combined with recommendations for healthy individuals, the clini-

Evidence in Rehabilitation

Although most research investigations into plyometric exercise use lower-extremity activity, a recent study looked at the effects of a plyometric program on the upper extremity. Swanik and colleagues[71] used two 8-week programs, one with weight training only and one with combined weight training and plyometrics, to assess changes in upper-extremity kinematics. At the end of the 8-week programs, the authors found that although both programs decreased the time required to perform all three phases of a plyometric ball toss and increased scapular upward rotation, only the program that included both plyometrics and strength training improved shoulder medial rotation range of motion.[71] The authors speculated that decreases in amortization phase time may have occurred at least in part because of changes in muscle spindle and GTO sensitivity: Decrease in GTO inhibition may improve muscle spindle facilitation. If muscle spindle sensitivity increases, the muscle may perceive length changes more readily to enable a more forceful contraction in the concentric phase of plyometric movement. They speculated that with greater motion occurring over less time, power production increases.

The authors hypothesize that since the primary problems leading to shoulder injury include prolonged abduction and lateral rotation positioning, limited upward scapular mobility, and limited glenohumeral medial rotation, using plyometric exercises that reduce these factors may prove to be beneficial in injury prevention. Given their findings and conclusions, adding plyometric exercises to the latter portion of a rehabilitation program may further ensure the patient's safe return to normal sport participation.

cian's experience, and common sense in decisions about whether and how to use plyometrics. A logical approach is to start with lower-impact and low-stress plyometrics, then progress as the patient responds appropriately.

Flexibility

Flexibility is another pre-plyometric exercise requirement.[37] As mentioned earlier, greater flexibility permits a greater lengthening of the muscle. A muscle that lacks good flexibility cannot generate the forces or create the control for optimal plyometric results. The muscle is also at risk for injury because the reduced flexibility leads to a diminished level of force absorption, needed especially for impact and deceleration stresses.[72] For example, the patient who can flex her knee to only 60° will be unable to absorb the forces imposed on her when she jumps from a 40 cm (16 in.) box. However, the patient who can fully flex her knees and hips can absorb the impact stresses much more effectively to prevent the forces from being transmitted up the extremity.

Patients must be individually assessed for the flexibility they need for plyometrics. Clinicians must evaluate patients for their actual flexibility and determine the minimum amount of flexibility needed to safely perform each plyometric exercise.

Proprioception

Another pre-plyometric consideration is proprioception as discussed in chapter 14. The patient must have agility, balance, and coordination to control the rapid and forceful movements of plyometric activities.[37] The amount of control required depends on the complexity and severity of the plyometric activity. For example, a plyometric activity such as jumping rope is not as complex or as intense as the plyometric activity of bounding with vertical jumps. Although both activities require agility, balance, and coordination, the patient's abilities are more challenged with the bounding and vertical jump activities. For this reason, it makes sense not to include even simple plyometric exercises in a rehabilitation program until the patient can perform some of the basic dynamic proprioceptive activities discussed in chapter 14.

Because flexibility, strength, and proprioceptive elements are prerequisites to plyometric exercises, the sequential progression of a rehabilitation program is important. As noted in chapter 1, each treatment component builds on the previous one and, in turn, serves as a foundation for the next one. Likewise, there are progressions within each plyometric parameter. Plyometrics is no different from any other type of rehabilitation exercise we have already discussed; it must progress from the simple to the more difficult.

Plyometric Program Design

A plyometric exercise program is designed to improve the patient's overall coordination, efficiency, speed, and power output in preparation for sport participation. Just as a patient with a 4-/5 grade on muscle strength cannot be expected to lift the same weights as when he has a 5/5 grade, a patient should not be expected to perform high-level plyometric exercises on the first attempt. A graduated progression is crucial to avoiding injury and providing a successful outcome. The progression is from general exercises to more sport-specific activities, from simple to complex, and from low-stress to high-stress activities. When designing a plyometric program, a number of variables may be changed to provide a progression: intensity, volume, recovery, and frequency. Only one variable, however, is changed at a time.

Intensity

Intensity is the degree, extent, or magnitude of effort applied during an exercise or activity. In strengthening, it is the amount of weight used; in flexibility, it is the force applied to the stretch; in proprioception, it is the complexity of the agility, balance, or coordination activity. In plyometrics, it is the stress of the activity.[73] You can change stress in plyometrics by using weights during the activity, increasing the height of the vertical jump, increasing the distance of the horizontal jump or the throw, increasing the weight of the medicine ball, or increasing the speed of the activity. You can also increase stress by changing the complexity of the exercise. For example, hopping with one leg is more intense than hopping with two legs, and hopping side to side is more challenging than hopping in place.

Volume

Volume is the total quantity of work performed during one session. Volume in lower-extremity plyometric exercises is measured in total number of foot contacts for jumping activities and in distance for bounding activities during the session.[73] Volume in the upper extremity and in medicine ball exercises is measured in the total number of repetitions and sets. Selection of the volume of plyometrics depends on the intensity and goals of the session.

Although no guidelines have been established for rehabilitation programs, normal athletic lower-extremity conditioning guidelines for beginners at low intensity levels are 60 to 100 foot contacts.[25] The rehabilitation clinician must know the patient's ability and the stresses that the activity will place on the healing tissue. This knowledge, combined with observations of the patient's performance quality, will determine the appropriate volume and intensity of plyometric exercise to include in the rehabilitation session.

Recovery

Recovery is the amount of rest time between sets or exercise groupings. The amount of rest time determines whether the plyometric exercises will be more effective in improving power or improving muscular endurance. The shorter the rest period between exercise sets, the more the emphasis is on endurance; longer rest times will provide for more improvement in power.[74] As a general guideline, rest periods of 45 to 60 s between sets or exercise groupings promote power increases.[25] This translates to a work-to-rest ratio of 1:5 to 1:10.[25] For example, if an exercise set takes 5 s to perform, the recovery could be 25 to 50 s. If the exercise set takes 10 s to perform, the recovery could be 50 to 100 s. Again, these recommendations are based on findings with healthy, uninjured subjects and may have to be adjusted in rehabilitation.

If muscle endurance is a goal with plyometric exercise, the recovery time between exercise sets is less; the general guideline is about 30 s.[74] This amount of rest time does not allow for an optimal recovery of the muscle, so muscle endurance improves.

Plyometric exercises can also be used to develop aerobic conditioning through the use of a circuit program in which the patient performs various exercise groupings for 12 to 20 min with less than a 2 s rest between the exercises.[25] A circuit program can develop aerobic, power, and muscle endurance levels.

Frequency

Another variable is the frequency with which plyometric activities are used in a rehabilitation program. Frequency depends on the exercise intensity and the patient's tolerance and ability to recover. The time needed for recovery from plyometric exercises is determined, at least in part, by the severity and type of the exercises. Recovery times range from 24 h for light plyometrics to 72 h for aggressive plyometrics.[75] As a general rule of thumb, you should allow at least 48 h between plyometric exercise sessions, but if the exercise session has been particularly intense, a longer recovery time may be necessary. After plyometric exercise, muscles undergo an inflammatory response and require time to sufficiently recover before they can respond appropriately to another bout of plyometrics.[75] Your judgment, common sense, and knowledge of stresses and the patient's abilities are essential to determining frequency for a patient's program.

Plyometric Program Considerations

Because plyometric activities are generally more intense than other types of exercises, you must consider several special issues when using them in a patient's rehabilitation exercise program. Even if the patient has satisfied the pre-plyometric requirements and has the necessary flexibility, strength, and proprioceptive abilities, other criteria for safe participation must also be met. Plyometric exercises must also be performed on an appropriate surface, and progression and goals must be determined appropriately.

Age

Although most children use plyometric activities every day—activities such as running, jumping, hopping, and skipping—one must use plyometrics carefully with children and youth ages 8 to 13. Plyometric activities for prepubescent and early-pubescent patients should remain at low volume and low intensity.[76] For example, jumping with both feet and without the use of boxes or weights is low-intensity jumping. Prepubescent muscles and bones are weaker than adult structures, so they do not tolerate the same physical stresses as adults.[77] Because of variations in physical maturity between individuals, it may be a safe rule of thumb to prohibit patients under age 16 from participating in moderate- to high-intensity plyometrics.

Studies have demonstrated the benefit of plyometric exercises for young athletes.[78, 79] Advocates for plyometrics indicate that it may improve bone strength and reduce the risk of injury when incorporated into a preparticipation exercise program.[80] Evidence demonstrates that plyometric programs improve the neural adaptations of young athletes, thus improving their coordination in performance.[81] Using plyometric activities as part of the terminal phase of rehabilitation for young performers during a time of their natural age-related neural development may complement their motor skill and strength development.[82] Strength and general health benefits have also been seen with the addition of plyometric exercises for youth athletes.[83]

Body Weight

The design of a plyometric program must take into account the patient's weight. Patients weighing 100 kg (220 lb) or more cannot perform the same plyometric exercises that lighter patients engage in.[73] The stresses imposed on tendons and joints may be too great for safe participation by these patients in higher-intensity plyometric activities. For example, a 113 kg (250 lb) patient may be able to perform single-leg hops for only half the distance that a 68 kg (150 lb) patient can. The intensity of plyometric exercises for heavier patients should be selected cautiously.

Competitive Level

Patients involved in competitive sports are more appropriate candidates for moderate- and high-level plyometric exercises than are those in recreational activities. The competitive patient has more advanced performance goals than the recreational patient and typically has more intense sport participation requirements. Although rehabilitation programs for all patients may include some level of plyometric exercises, only the competitive patients require higher-intensity plyometric activities.

Surface

The best surfaces for plyometric lower-extremity activities are those that have some "give" to them. Although plyometrics may be performed indoors or outdoors, the surface should be one that yields to absorb some of the impact stress of the plyometric activity. Ideal surfaces include spring-loaded floors, mats, and grass. Harder surfaces such as asphalt, concrete, and carpet or rubber over concrete should be avoided. Although the surface should be able to absorb some of the impact forces produced during the activity, it should not be so yielding that it reduces the tissue's elastic recoil, the crucial element of plyometric activity. If the surface prevents sufficient amortization or slows the person's transition or concentric phase, it is probably too soft. This is an important consideration for all plyometric activities, but especially for the higher-stress activities.

Footwear

Shoes that offer good support, have a solid heel counter, and provide some cushion for shock absorption are the best shoes to wear for plyometrics. A shoe can offer too much absorption and thus be too spongy, causing instability instead of stability in landing. Additionally, if the shoe is too big and the patient's foot slides in the shoe, force production will be diminished. In either case, the person may report a sense of instability or find that he or she cannot perform the exercise properly, or you may be able to observe instability at the foot landing or takeoff during the exercises. Shoes should be in good condition, not be excessively worn, be tied properly, and fit well.

Proper Technique

Technique is probably the most important special consideration. Proper foot position is an essential factor in jumping activities. The patient should land on the midfoot and then roll forward to push off from the balls of the feet.[77] The patient should not land on the balls of the feet or the heel, since these landing techniques increase the impact forces and thereby increase stress applied at the foot, ankle, and knee. Midfoot landing also allows a shorter amortization time so that a more powerful concentric motion can occur.

The trunk should remain upright so that summation of forces from the back, abdominals, and arms can be used. The arms can contribute 10% of the force of the plyometric jump, so both the timing of activities and posture are important factors.[77]

The quality of the execution is important. As a rehabilitation clinician, you must carefully observe the patient's quality of performance. As the patient fatigues, performance quality will decline. This can result in two problems: risk of injury and development of an improper engram. It is important to know the proper exercise technique and to observe the patient's performance closely so that you can discontinue the exercise when performance begins to deteriorate.

Progression

A gradual progression from simple to difficult, from few to more, and from general to specific is vital to avoid injury in plyometric activities. The patient's body must be given time to adapt to new stress levels in order to avoid overstress injuries. As we have seen, there are a variety of ways to implement progression into a program.[28] The rehabilitation clinician must monitor the injury and note undesirable responses to activity and activity progressions. The stresses of plyometrics may cause an inflammatory response,[75] and rehabilitation clinicians should have alternate plans if unwanted responses occur.

Goals

The program's goals are individually dictated by the patient and by the demands of the patient's sport. The specific exercises within the program are determined by each patient's sport-specific requirements. For example, a long jumper will have a different plyometric jumping program than a basketball player, and a volleyball player will have a different jumping program than a wrestler. You must understand the stresses, skills, and demands of the patient's sport so that you can incorporate appropriate plyometric exercises into the rehabilitation program at the proper time.

You assess the patient's plyometric performance throughout the rehabilitation sessions. Any time you introduce a plyometric activity, you take initial measurements of the patient's performance. For example, in a standing jump, you measure the jump height the first time the patient tries the jump. As the patient progresses through the program, more intensive plyometric activities are introduced. Each time the patient performs a new activity, you record initial performance values for the new activity and establish new goals. Additional measurements are taken either at specific intervals, such as every week, or when the patient is ready to advance to a more difficult activity. These recordings help the clinician to maintain objective measures of improvement. They also provide additional motivation and goals for the patient.

Plyometric Precautions and Contraindications

As you know, there are precautions for any rehabilitation exercise. Because plyometric activities can be vigorous, you must consider additional precautions before deciding to incorporate them into a rehabilitation program:

- *Time.* Because plyometric activities place such high stresses on the body, they should not be performed for extended periods of time. They also should be performed in the early part of the rehabilitation session before the patient becomes fatigued and begins to lose strength, flexibility, and coordination. The time to perform the plyometric activities is after the warm-up but before other exercises and activities are begun.

- *Postexercise delayed onset muscle soreness (DOMS).* Because plyometric activities are more strenuous than other exercises, patients may experience postexercise soreness. Delayed onset soreness is common, especially when plyometric exercises are first introduced into the program or when the intensity changes.

You must also know about several explicit contraindications to plyometric activity:

- *Acute inflammation.* Plyometric exercises must be avoided with acute inflammatory conditions. The intensity of these exercises can increase the inflammation.

- *Postoperative conditions.* Persons with immediate postoperative conditions should not engage in plyometric exercise. The tissues cannot tolerate the stress of such exercises and are highly vulnerable to injury.

- *Instability.* Gross joint instability, until strength is sufficient to control the joint, is a contraindication. Strength is a prerequisite to any plyometric exercise. Strength provides the control needed for the safe and effective performance of plyometric exercise.

CLINICAL TIPS

As with any rehabilitation element, the clinician must be keenly aware of the precautions and contraindications associated with plyometrics. Precautions about the use of plyometrics relate to the time the patient spends on these activities and to vulnerability to postexercise soreness. There are also a few frank contraindications to the use of plyometrics in a rehabilitation program.

Equipment for Plyometric Activities

Equipment for plyometric activities need not be elaborate or expensive. In fact, most plyometric exercises require little or no equipment. In the following sections, we review some of the most commonly used items.

Cones

Plastic barriers or traffic cones are used as jump obstacles or for sprint activities. Their plasticity makes them safe for patients to land on if they should lose their balance or accidentally hit one of them during an activity. These cones come in various sizes from 20 to 60 cm (8 to 24 in.) (figure 15.1).

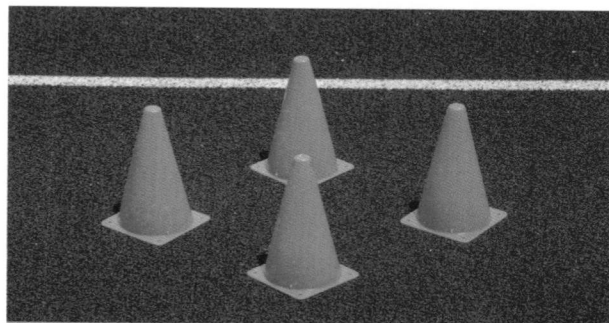

Figure 15.1 Plyometric cones.

Boxes

Commercially made boxes come in a variety of heights, ranging from 15 to 106 cm (6 to 42 in.), and various designs. Regardless of its composition or design, the box's top should have a nonslip surface. The lower boxes are used for less intense activities and the higher ones for more intense activities (figure 15.2). Higher boxes are generally not used with younger patients.

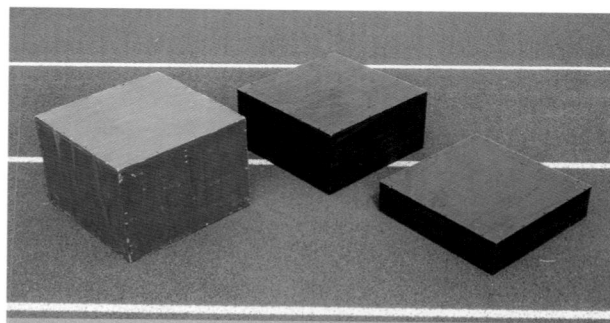

Figure 15.2 Plyometric boxes.

Hurdles

Track hurdles are used for more advanced plyometric exercises. Some are adjustable within ranges of 15 to 100 cm (6 to 40 in.). A low hurdle can be easily constructed from two cones and a dowel (figure 15.3). Rehabilitation equipment catalogs also have lower hurdles that may be used.

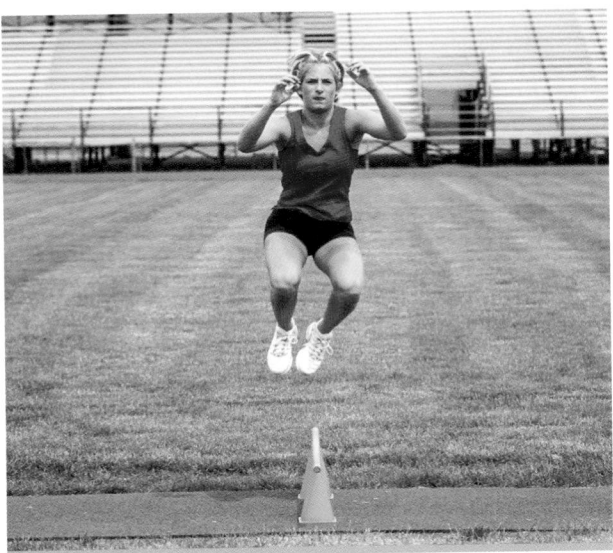

Figure 15.3 Plyometric hurdle constructed from cones and a dowel.

Medicine Balls

Medicine balls are useful in plyometric activities for the upper extremities and trunk, and they also provide additional resistance for lower-extremity plyometrics. They come in a variety of sizes, weights, and surface compositions. The leather-covered balls are limited to indoor use because moisture shortens the life of the cover. Balls should be of a manageable size and should have a surface that permits the patient to maintain an adequate grasp. If one-hand activities are required for the exercise, the ball should have a diameter that will accommodate the patient's hand size (figure 15.4).

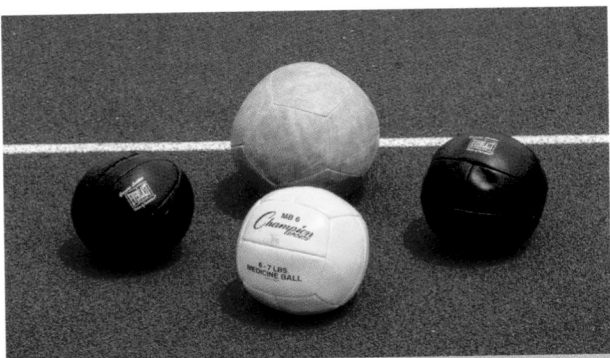

Figure 15.4 Medicine balls.

Other Equipment

A variety of other equipment can be used for plyometric activities. Jump ropes, stairs, and barriers are examples of items that are usually readily available. Their specific use depends on the goals of the exercise and the imagination of the rehabilitation clinician.

Lower-Extremity Plyometrics

Once the patient has the necessary strength, flexibility, and coordination, and the tissues have healed enough to tolerate the stresses of such activity without further damage or inflammation, plyometric exercises may become a part of the rehabilitation program.

Exercise Progression

A lower-extremity plyometric exercise progression involves six types of exercises: jumps-in-place, standing jumps, multiple jumps and hops, bounding, box drills, and depth jumps.[25] The exercises described next are based on Chu and Myer's[25] textbook on plyometrics.

Jumps-in-Place

Jumps-in-place are repeated jumps that begin and end in the same place. They can range in intensity from low to high. The low-intensity jumps are good early activities for developing a brief amortization phase. The specific goal, to develop a short amortization phase with a rapid rebound, often serves to develop the patient's jump technique. Jump-in-place exercises should relate to the patient's sport. For example, a two-foot ankle hop is suitable for a basketball player, and a hip-twist ankle hop is well suited to a skier. As the patient progresses, he or she can perform more difficult jumps-in-place or can advance to another type of jump exercise.

Two-Foot Ankle Hop   Have the patient jump in place using only the ankles. The patient should jump as high as possible. The knees will bend, but only slightly (figure 15.5). This exercise is particularly good for patients who play basketball.

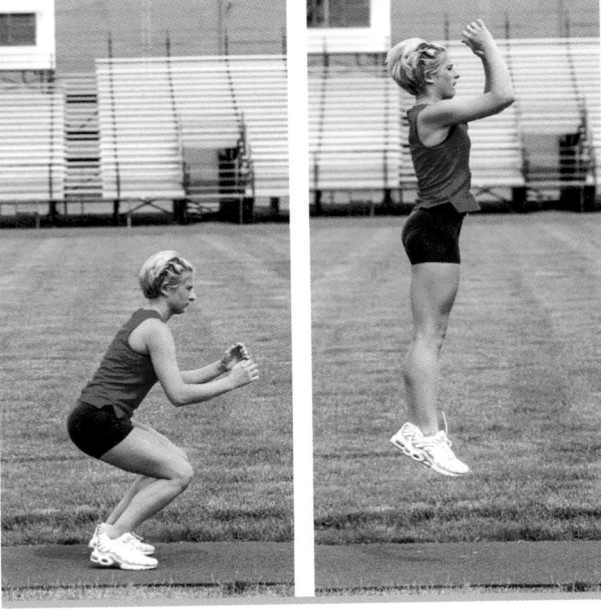

Figure 15.5 Two-foot ankle hop.

Hip-Twist Ankle Hop   With the feet together, the patient jumps and twists 90° to the left, returns to the start position, and then repeats the activity to the right. The patient should twist from the hips, not the knees (figure 15.6). This exercise is particularly good for patients who ski.

Standing Jumps

Standing jumps are single jumps that emphasize a maximal effort with motion occurring either vertically or horizontally. Recovery after each attempt is necessary for a maximal effort each time. A progression of this type of jump could consist, for example, of beginning with a standing long jump, progressing to a jump over a cone, and advancing to a standing long jump with a sprint. Standing jumps can be performed in a forward direction or laterally and can involve the use of barriers. Patients can combine standing jumps with multiple jumps, running, or sprinting in different directions.

Standing Long Jump   The patient's feet are shoulder-width apart. Have him or her explode from a semisquat position to jump as far forward as possible. The patient should use the arms to assist (figure 15.7). This exercise is particularly good for patients who swim or participate in track.

Standing Jump Over Barrier   Have the patient, with feet shoulder-width apart, jump upward and over a cone, landing on both feet simultaneously. The patient should keep the hips over the knees and feet (figure 15.8). You can add cones from 0.9 to 1.8 m (3-6 ft) apart for multiple jumps. This exercise is particularly good for patients who are figure skaters or basketball players.

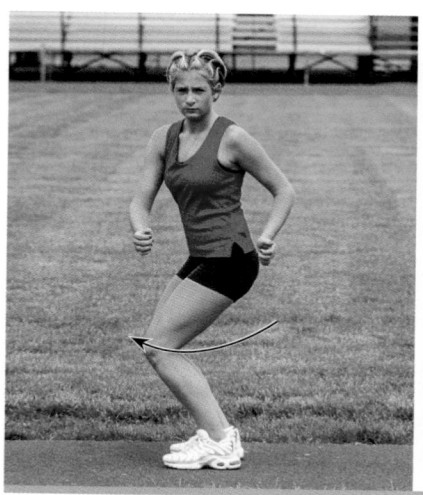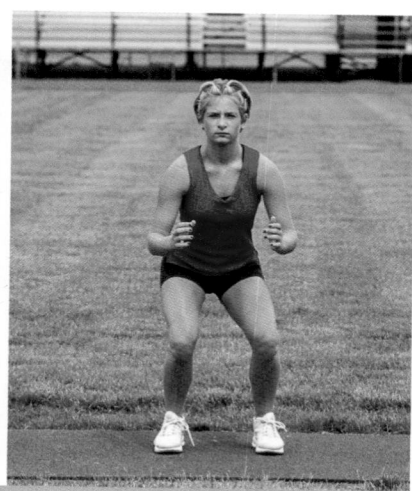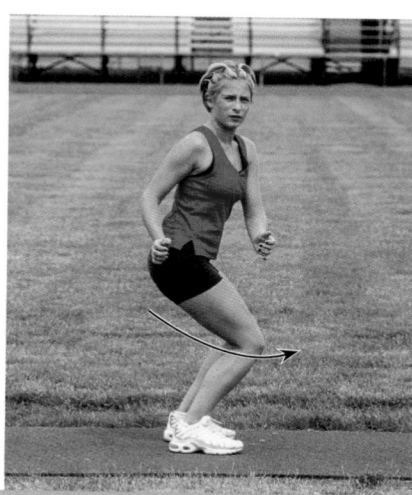

Figure 15.6   Hip-twist ankle hop.

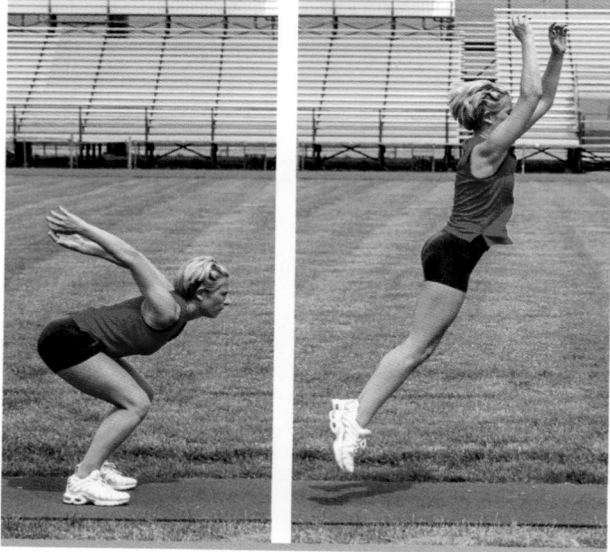

Figure 15.7   Standing long jump.

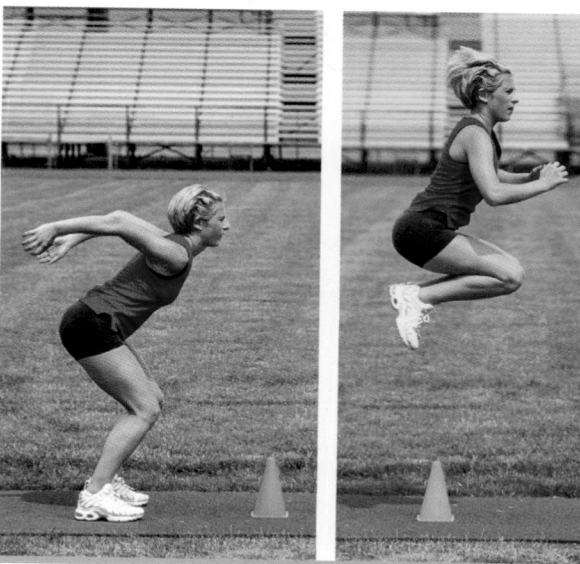

Figure 15.8   Standing jump over a barrier.

Standing Long Jump With Sprint   Using the arms to assist, the patient jumps as far forward as possible. Immediately after landing, he or she sprints forward as fast as possible for 10 m (figure 15.9). Add sprints to left and right for additional activities. This exercise is particularly good for patients who play hockey, participate in track, or play football.

Multiple Jumps and Hops

Multiple hops and jumps combine the skills of jumps-in-place and standing jumps. The patient tries to jump as high as possible and repeats the jumps without resting. The total distance in each set of exercises is usually kept under 30 m.[25] The jumps can be performed with one or two legs, in a straight line or in multiple directions, with or without barriers. Forward hops over a cone is an example of a simple multiple-hop exercise. The single-leg hop and a series of stadium-step hops are examples of more difficult multiple hops.

Single-Leg Hops   The patient jumps from the left leg, propelling as far upward and forward as possible, using arm movement to assist, and then lands on the same leg. The patient uses the forward movement of the right non-weight-bearing leg to propel forward for the next jump, landing on the right leg. Remind the patient to keep hips and knees directly over the landing foot (figure 15.10).

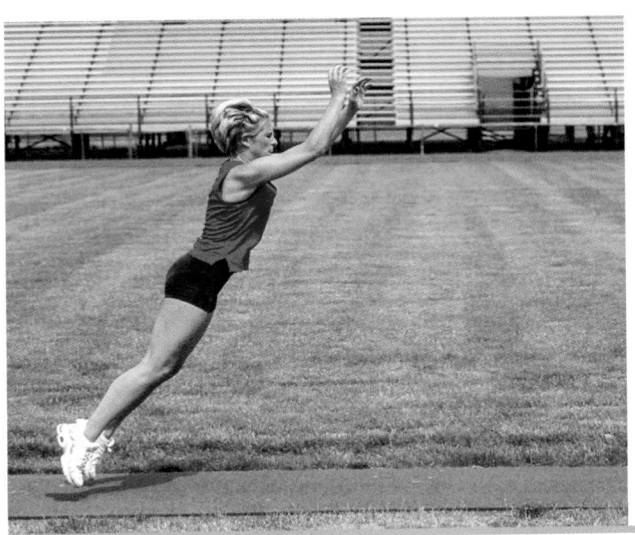
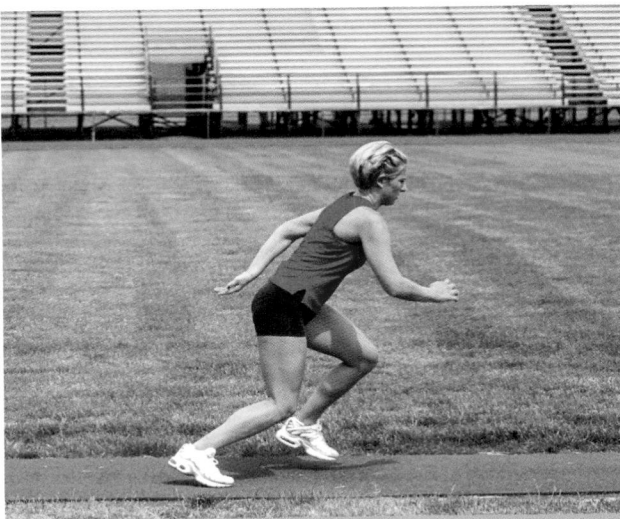

Figure 15.9   Standing long jump with sprint.

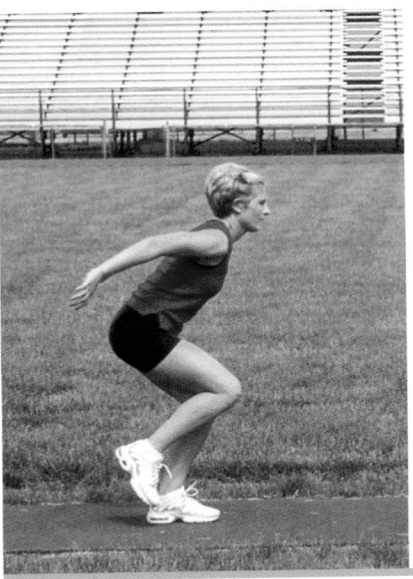
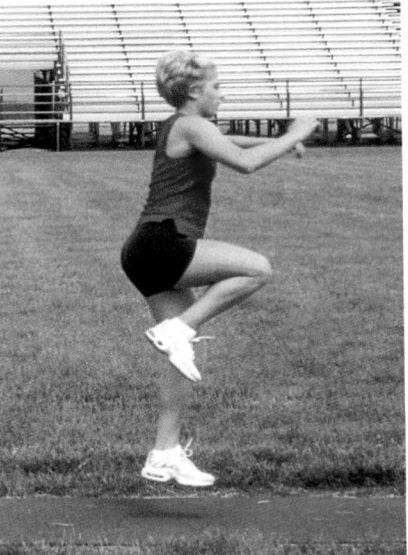
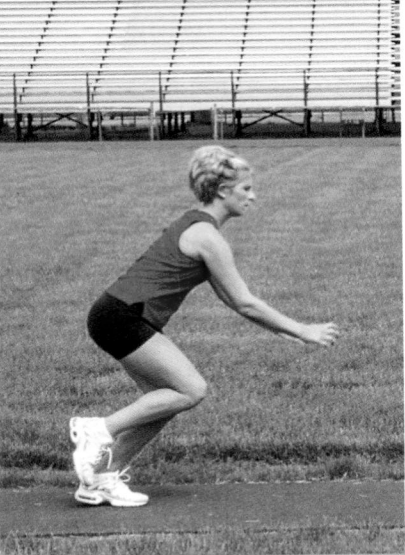

Figure 15.10   Single-leg hops.

Stadium Hops   The patient jumps onto one step at a time using both legs. The movement is rapid, light, and continuous up the stairs, without stops or hesitation. The patient progresses to taking two steps at a time or using one leg or alternating legs (figure 15.11). This exercise and the single-leg hops previously described are particularly good for patients who wrestle or play hockey.

Bounding

Bounding exercises are an exaggeration of the running stride. They are used to improve stride length and speed. These exercises are most commonly used for patients in track and field events. Distances usually exceed 30 m.[25] A simple bounding exercise is skipping; an advanced bound-ing exercise is single-leg bounding. Skipping and bounding are explosive activities with the patient exploding quickly from landing and jumping upward and forward.

Skipping   The patient lifts the right leg with the knee bent to 90° while also lifting the left arm with the elbow bent to 90°. Then the patient alternates with the opposite extremities (figure 15.12).

Single-Leg Bounding   While on the right leg, the patient moves forward and upward as far as possible by using the momentum of the left leg and both arms to propel forward, landing on the right leg. The patient continues the forward and upward movement, this time landing on the left leg (figure 15.13).

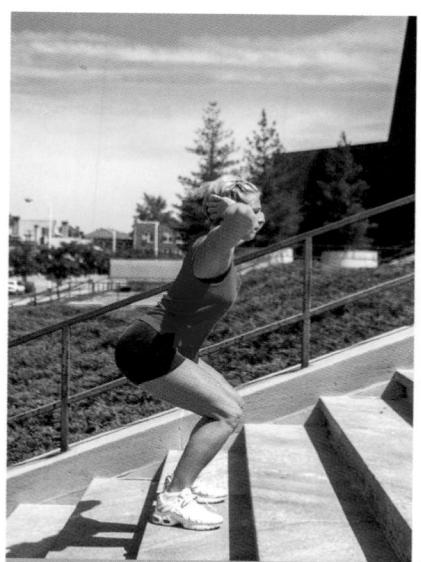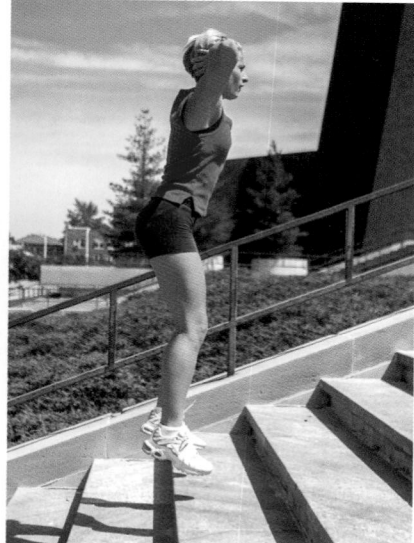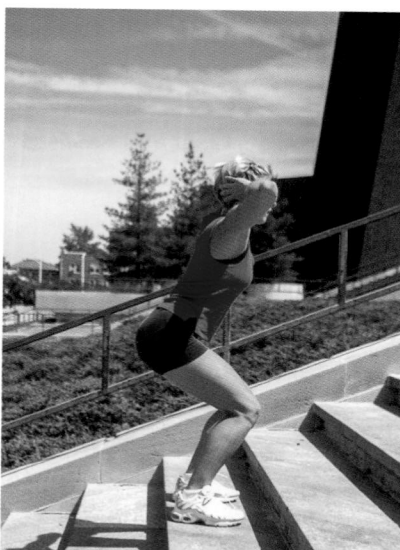

Figure 15.11   Stadium hops.

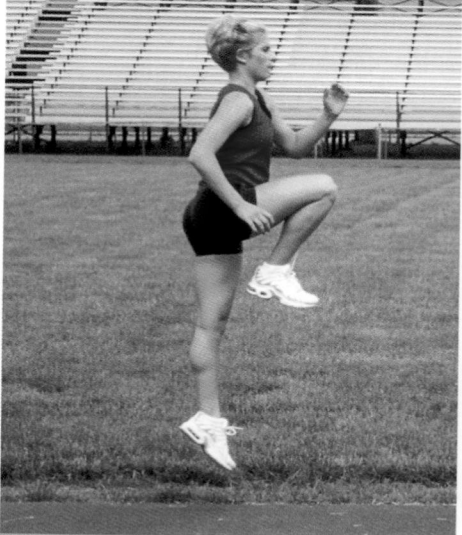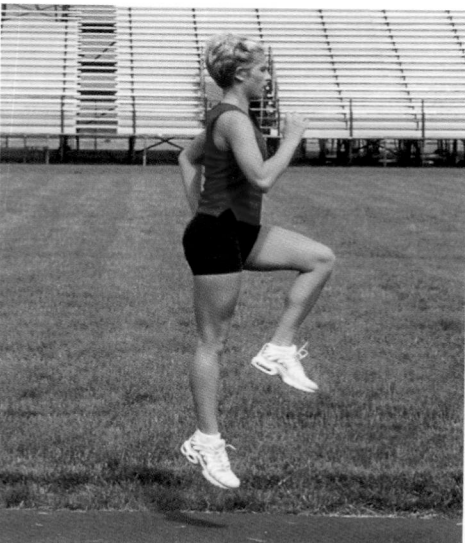

Figure 15.12   Skipping.

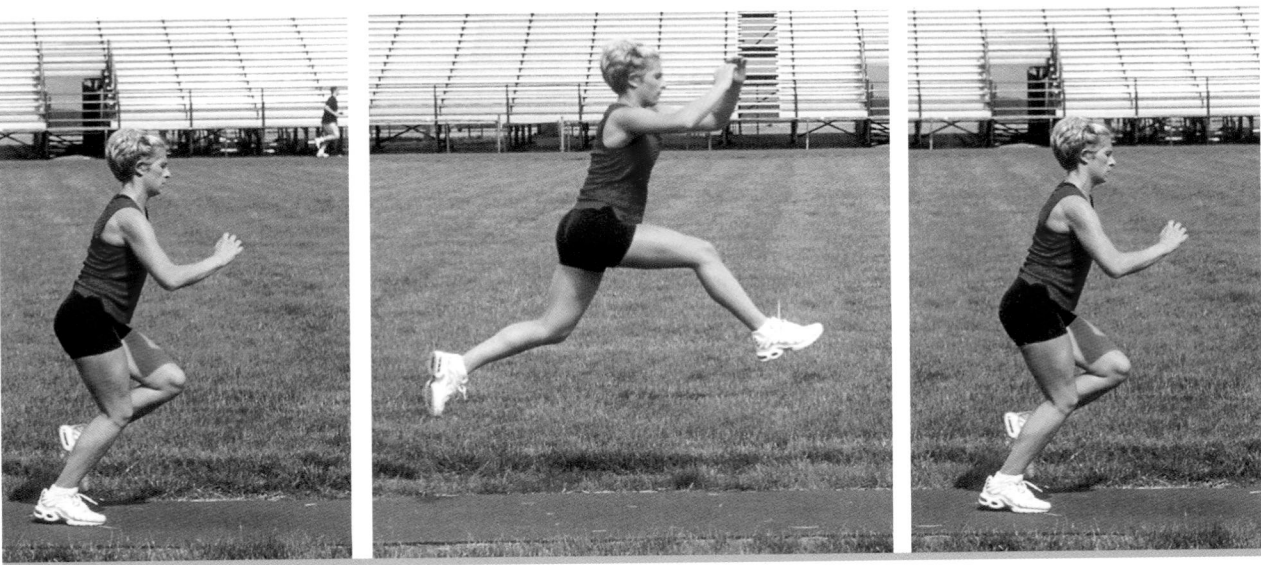

Figure 15.13 Single-leg bounding.

Box Jumps

Box drills involve the more advanced skills required for multiple jumps and hops because the jumps and hops are performed onto and off boxes of varying heights. These exercises can be low or high intensity, depending on the box height. Both exercises use vertical and horizontal jumps.

Front Box Jump Begin with a box about 30 cm (12 in.) high. Jump onto the box with both feet (figure 15.14). Step down and repeat. The difficulty can be increased by increasing the box height or by using one leg, alternating left and right.

Pyramiding Box Hops Place up to five boxes of progressively increasing height about 0.6 to 0.9 m (2-3 ft) apart in a line. Jump onto the first box, onto the floor on the opposite side, and then onto the next box, repeating to the end of the row. Use the arms to assist in the motion (figure 15.15).

Depth Jumps

Depth jumps are the most aggressive plyometric exercises. They are box jumps of greater intensity in that patients are challenged by the combination of their own weight and

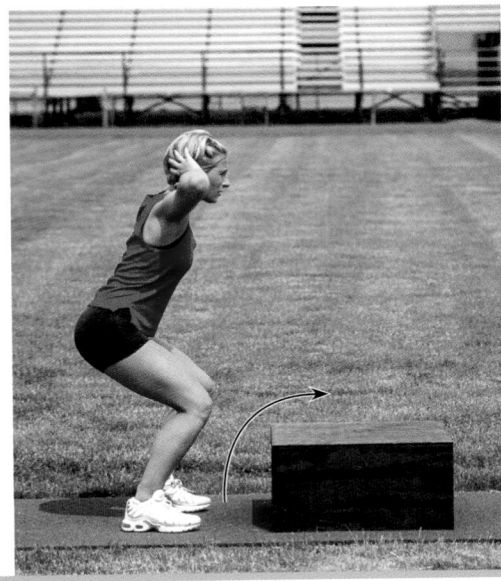 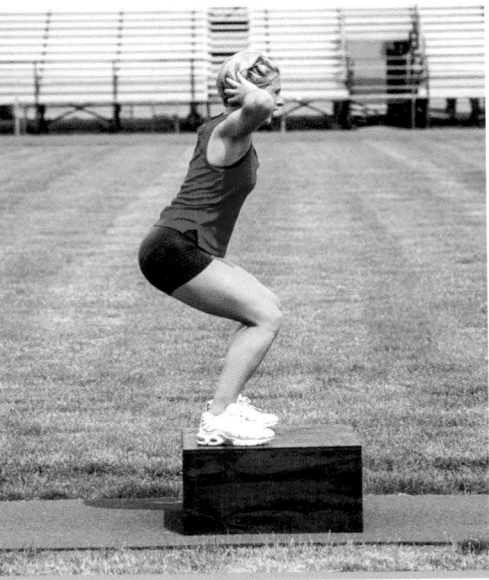

Figure 15.14 Front box jump.

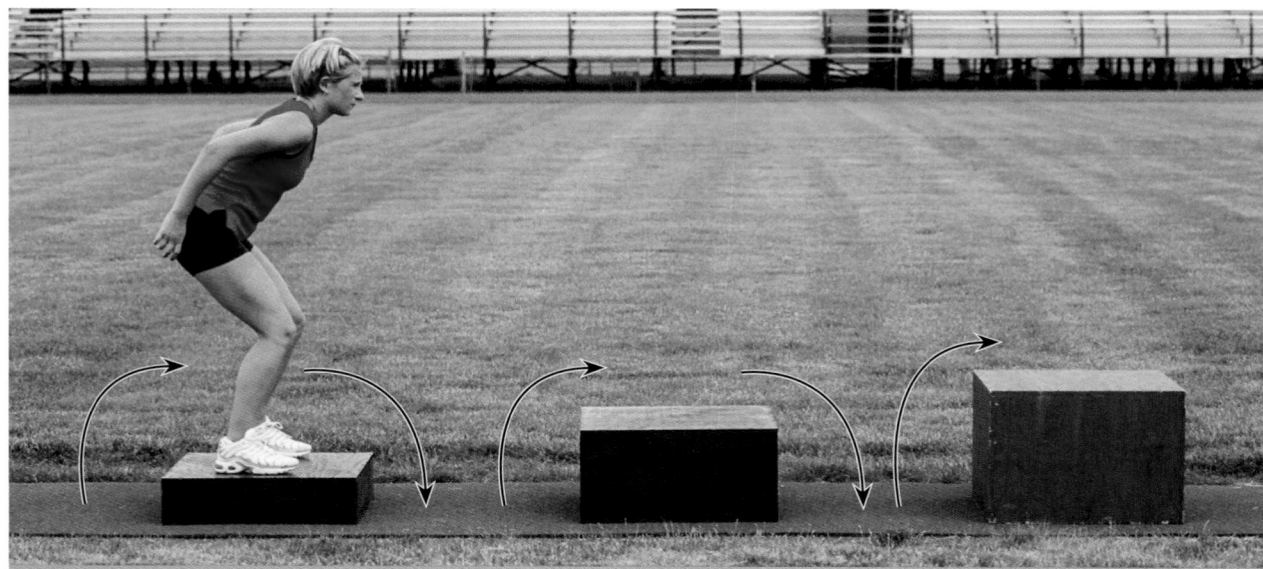

Figure 15.15 Pyramiding box hops.

the acceleration of gravity. The motion in depth jumps includes stepping—not jumping—off a box, dropping to the ground, and then immediately rebounding upward. These are intensive exercises that the patient must perform with caution. Jumping off the box is avoided in these exercises because a jump will increase the distance to the floor and will significantly increase the stresses applied to the patient's joints.

You must select a box height for depth jumps carefully. A box of excessive height increases the risk of injury and requires the muscles to absorb greater impact forces from the higher drop. Also, the time required to absorb the force makes the amortization time too long to be effective. Select the maximum box height carefully. If the patient takes too much time during the transition phase to move from eccentric to concentric, the box is too high. Although boxes up to 4 ft high are available, these are rarely used in plyometric rehabilitation programs.

Chu and Myer[25] recommend determining a box height for depth jumps using the following procedure. The person performs a standard jump-and-reach test, and the target point the person achieves is marked. The person then performs a depth jump from a 45 cm (18 in.) box and tries to reach for the same point attained on the test. If the mark is attained, the box height increases by 15 cm (6 in.) increments until the person cannot achieve the target. The first box at which the person cannot achieve the target point is the depth-jump box height. If the person cannot reach the target point from the 45 cm box, either the box should be lowered or the person should not perform the activity until he or she gains strength.

An example of progression using depth jumps starts with a simple depth jump in which the patient steps down from a box and jumps vertically, using both feet. The patient subsequently advances to a much more difficult depth jump—a single-leg depth jump in which the patient lands on one foot and jumps as high as possible from the one leg. A more challenging progression can include using a higher box or using more than one box and jumping onto the second box from the ground.

Double-Leg Depth Jump
The patient steps off a 30 cm (12 in.) box, landing on the floor with both feet. As rapidly as possible, the patient then jumps upward as high as possible, using the arms to reach upward (figure 15.16).

Single-Leg Depth Jump
The patient steps off a 30 cm box, landing on the left leg only. The patient then springs upward as high as possible from the left leg. The exercise is then repeated with the right leg (figure 15.17).

CLINICAL TIPS

Lower-extremity plyometric exercises use various types of jumps, as well as bounding and box drills, in various combinations to provide a progression of intensities. The clinician determines which plyometric exercises to use based on a number of factors, such as the patient's age and competitive level, body size and type, and demands of the patient's sport and the position played within that sport.

Exercise Selection

Although the various types of plyometric exercises provide a progression of difficulty from low to high intensity, you must analyze each exercise to determine its relative

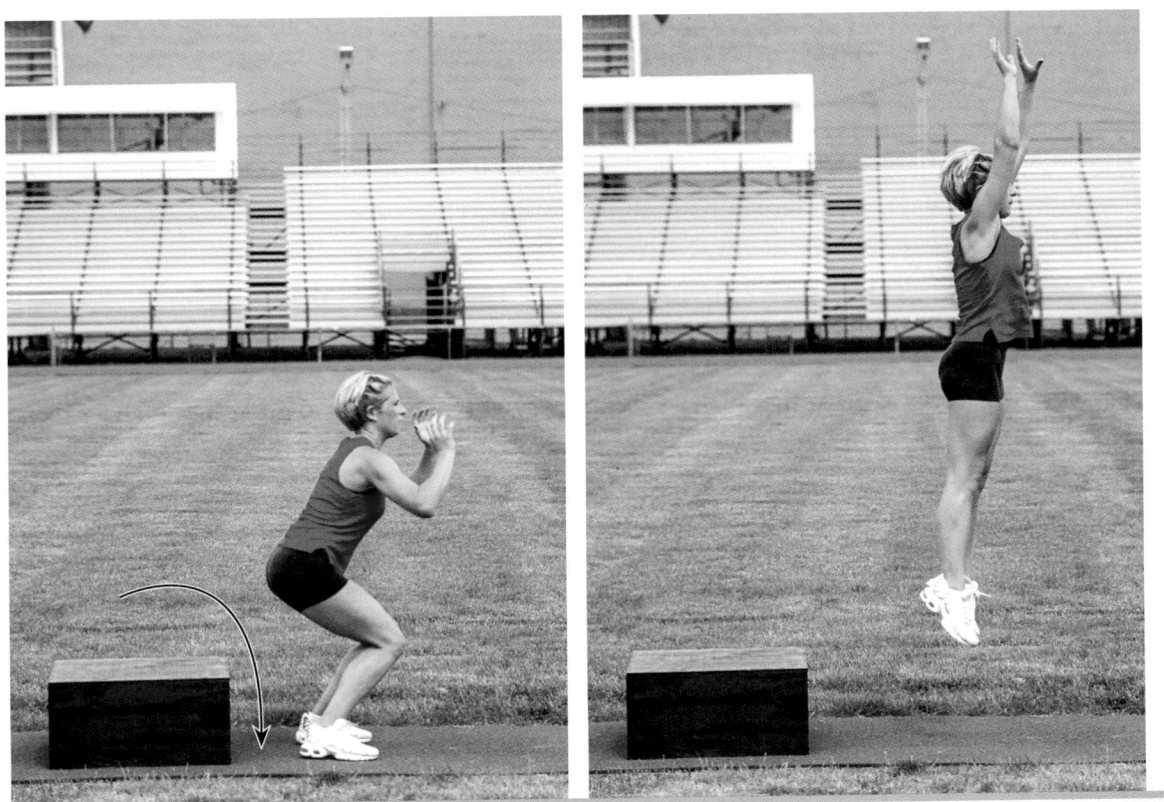

Figure 15.16   Double-leg depth jump.

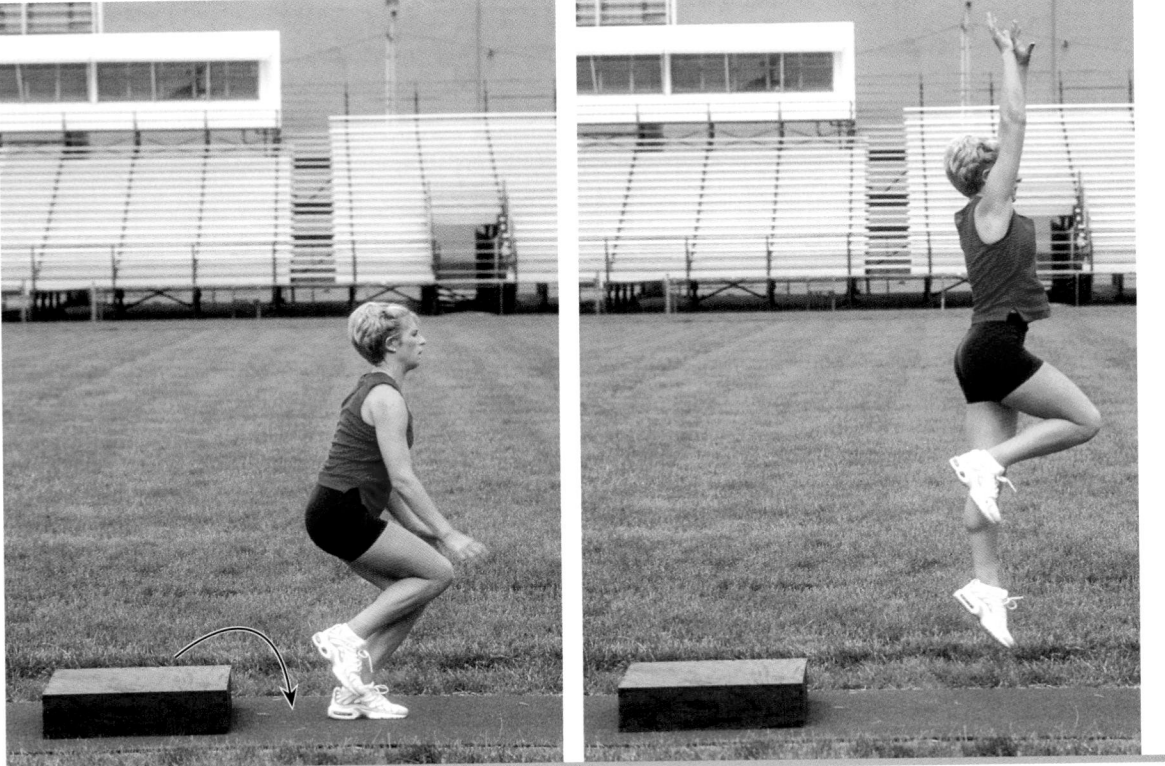

Figure 15.17   Single-leg depth jump.

intensity. For example, a high-level standing jump may be more intense than a moderate-level box jump.

The selection of exercises for a patient's rehabilitation program depends on the demands of the patient's sport and the level of participation of that patient. For example, you may give one patient plyometric exercises that include varying intensities of multiple jumps and hops; another patient may be more appropriately stressed with box jumps and depth jumps. Two patients in the same sport, one at a recreational level and the other at an intercollegiate competitive level, have different requirements because of the different competitive demands. This issue is a prime consideration in exercise selection.

Figure 15.18 provides an example of a plyometric progression for a college-level competitive volleyball athlete who is nearing the functional phase of the rehabilitation program. The lower-extremity example is based on the recommendations in Chu and Myer.[25] This program is meant only to provide you with ideas and concepts of sequencing plyometric activities.

Specific exercises are determined by the patient's activity demands. As much as possible, running, jumping, and plyometric exercises should mimic the activities that the patient will be performing once he or she returns to full participation.

Upper-Extremity and Trunk Plyometrics

We will consider upper-extremity and trunk exercises together because many of the upper-extremity exercises with medicine balls strongly influence the trunk muscles and vice versa. The exercises that are specific to either the upper extremity or the trunk are indicated. Because the trunk plays a vital role in stabilization during upper-extremity activities, the strength of the muscle groups in the trunk is important to the strength of the upper extremity. The trunk muscles also perform trunk movement during most upper-extremity activities.

Plyometrics for the upper extremity and trunk have essentially the same considerations as those for the lower extremity. The exercises should be specific to the sport demands, should provide a progression of difficulty to present a challenge and promote the desired gains, and should be performed with controlled speed of movement.

LOWER-EXTREMITY PLYOMETRIC PROGRESSION EXAMPLE FOR VOLLEYBALL

Plyometric activity	First level	Second level	Third level
Tuck jump with thighs parallel	10 jumps	10 jumps	10 jumps
Alternate bounding	Use double arm action, 25 yards	Single arm action, 25 yards	Single arm action, 25 yards
Jump over barrier	Forward, both legs together, 15 repetitions	Forward-backward, both legs, 20 jumps	Forward-backward, single leg, 20 jumps
Lateral jumping over barrier	Both legs together, 6" height, 15 times	Single leg, 6" height, 15 times	Single leg jump onto box, 15 times
Zig-zag hopping	Both legs together, 10 yards	One leg, 10 yards	One leg, forward and backward, 10 yards
Lunge jump	Alternating forward leg, landing on both feet, 10 times each leg forward	Alternating forward leg, landing on one foot, 10 times	One leg for 15 times and then the other leg for 15 times
Box depth jump	Double leg forward, 10 repetitions	Single leg forward, 10 repetitions	Single leg forward and backward 10 repetitions

Figure 15.18 Sample of a lower-extremity plyometric program for a college-level competitive athlete.
Based on Chu and Myer (2013).[25]

You can provide progression by changing the intensity. This may be accomplished by changing the weights of the medicine balls, the speed of the activity, and the distance the medicine balls are passed. Passing medicine balls includes tossing and throwing. Tossing is defined as passing a ball a short distance with the arm below 90° of shoulder flexion; throwing is defined as passing the ball a long distance with the arm above 90° of flexion.[25] Passing exercises can be performed with either a partner or a Rebounder—a trampoline inclined so that it returns the ball to the patient (figure 15.19).

Figure 15.20 provides examples of medicine ball plyometric exercises for the upper extremities and trunk. The chest-pass photo shows the patient executing a chest pass from a distance of about 3 m (10 ft), using the forward

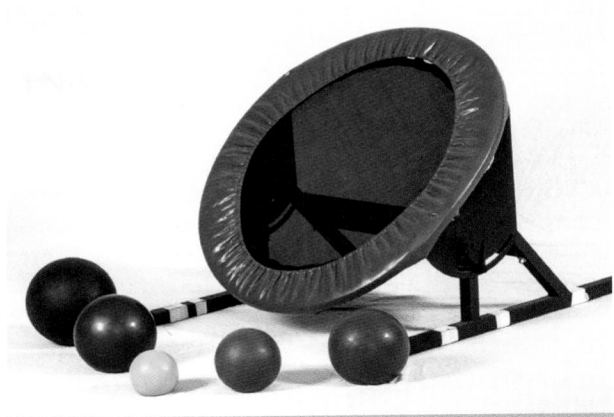

Figure 15.19 Rebounder and medicine balls.

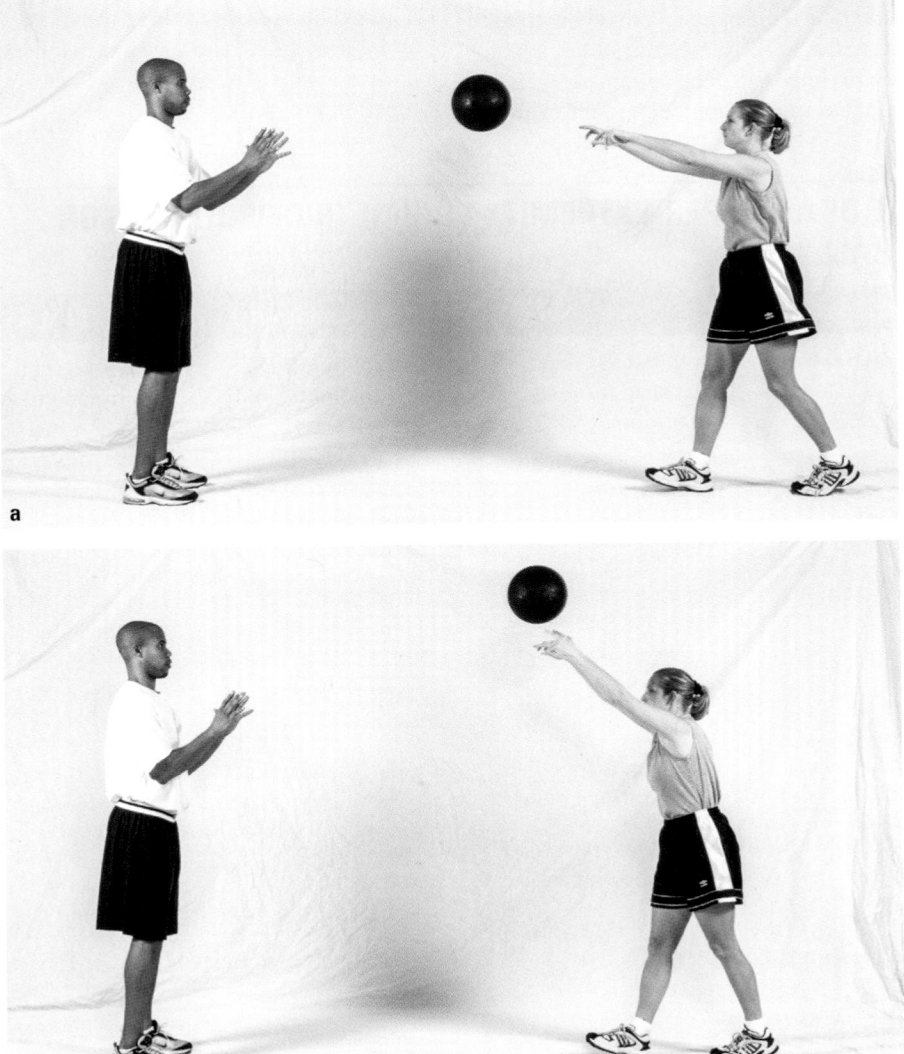

Figure 15.20 Upper-extremity and trunk plyometrics: *(a)* chest pass; *(b)* overhead throw. Note the erect position of the trunk, allowing force from the lower extremities to be transmitted through the trunk to the upper extremities.

movement of the legs to coincide with the snap of the ball. Follow-through should continue until the arms are fully extended in front of the body and the backs of the hands face each other. In the overhead throw, once again the patient uses leg movement to coincide with arm motion so that the ball is released from behind the head. The patient moves body weight from the back to the front leg as the ball is released. Follow-through is with the arms straight, upward, and forward as shown in figure 15.20. During both of these activities, the trunk muscles are kept taut and the back is held straight to allow force from the legs to be transmitted through the trunk to the arms.

As with lower-extremity plyometrics, upper-extremity and trunk plyometrics should be specific to the patient's needs. They should provide specific challenges that will permit the patient to make gains in the muscles most challenged by the patient's sport. The SAID principle is as important in plyometric exercises as it is in other strength exercises. As a review, the SAID principle is an acronym for Specific Adaptations to Imposed Demands and refers to the body's ability to adapt to stresses applied through exercise.

Figure 15.21 is an example of an upper-extremity progressive plyometric program for a basketball player. As with the lower-extremity program shown in figure 15.18, it only serves as an example and should not be taken verbatim from this text.

Rehabilitation Progression From Plyometrics to Functional to Activity-Specific Exercises

As is often the case for athletes undergoing rehabilitation for an injury, there is an overlap of plyometric and functional activities—while some of the patient's program incorporates plyometric exercises, other aspects of the same treatment session may also include functional exercises. As the patient nears the end of the plyometric section of rehabilitation, this overlap becomes even more apparent.

Figures 15.22 and 15.23 provide examples of how to progress a patient through a lower-extremity return to function program.

EXAMPLE OF AN UPPER-EXTREMITY PLYOMETRIC PROGRAM FOR BASKETBALL

Plyometric activity	First level	Second level	Third level
Medicine ball throws to wall	Both hands, standing overhead throws, 10 repetitions with 2 kg	Standing rotational throwing both hands, 10 repetitions L side towards the wall, 10 repetitions R side towards the wall, 2 kg	Half kneeling rotational throwing both hands, 10 repetitions L side towards the wall, 10 repetitions R side towards the wall, 2 kg
BOSU ball push-up	Push up with both hands on BOSU, 10 repetitions	L hand on BOSU, then push up to move over BOSU to place R hand on BOSU, 10 repetitions	L hand on BOSU, then push up to move over BOSU to place R hand on BOSU, 15 repetitions
Medicine ball wall dribbles	Both hands together, 12 repetitions, 2 kg	L hand, then R hand, 12 repetitions, 2 kg	L hand, then R hand, 12 repetitions, 3 kg
Medicine ball sit-up throws	Both hands, overhead throws, 10 repetitions with 2 kg	L hand, then R hand overhead, 10 repetitions, 2 kg	L hand, then R hand overhead, 10 repetitions, 3 kg
Plyometric push-ups	On knees, 10 repetitions	On feet, 10 repetitions	On feet, 15 repetitions
Medicine ball chest pass	Both hands, 10 repetitions, 2 kg	Both hands, 10 repetitions, 3 kg	L hand, then R hand, 10 repetitions, 3 kg

Figure 15.21   Example of an upper-extremity plyometric program for a basketball player.

BALANCE AND AGILITY PROGRESSION PROGRAM

1. Beginning level

A. Double-weight support for balance: static

 1. Stand with eyes closed, feet together, 30 s

 2. Stand in tandem-stance position, 30 s each

 - Eyes open
 - Eyes closed
 - Eyes open, head rotating left to right
 - Eyes closed, head rotating left to right

B. Single-weight support for balance: static

 1. Stork stand with eyes open, 30 s

 2. Stork stand with eyes closed, 30 s

 3. Stork stand with eyes open and head rotating left to right, 30 s

 4. Stork stand with eyes closed and head rotating left to right, 30 s

 5. Stork stand with eyes open while on unstable surface, 30 s each

 - Trampoline
 - 1/2 foam roller

 6. Stork stand with eyes closed while on unstable surface, 30 s each

 - Trampoline
 - 1/2 foam roller

 7. Stork stand with eyes open and rotating head left to right while on unstable surface, 30 s each

 - Trampoline
 - 1/2 foam roller

 8. Stork stand with complex activity

 - Stork stand on ground while playing catch
   - Sport ball
   - Medicine ball
 - Stork stand on uneven surface while playing catch
   - Sport ball
   - Medicine ball

2. Intermediate level: dynamic activities

A. Two-leg support: balance board, wobble board

B. One-leg support: trampoline jumping

C. One-leg support: hopping

D. Treadmill retrowalking

E. BAPS board

F. Fitter

G. Step-up exercises

3. Advanced level

A. Running activities (start at reduced speeds and distances, and progressively advance to normal speeds and distances)

B. Jumping activities (bilateral support)

 1. Lateral jumping

> continued

Figure 15.22 Example of a balance and agility progression program.

    2. Forward–backward jumping

    3. Command jumping

  C. Hopping activities (unilateral support)

    1. Lateral hopping

    2. Forward–backward hopping

    3. Command hopping

  D. Cariocas

  E. Plyometric box jumping

4. Preinjury level

  A. Sport-specific running, jumping, cutting activities at full speed

  B. Normal sport-specific drills

  C. Resumption of sport participation

  D. Mimic work activities (start at low reps, advance to more reps or more time)

Note: Jumping and hopping activities may start as exercises performed in place, but then can progress to line, target, and zigzag jumping and hopping exercises.

Figure 15.22 *>continued*

LOWER-EXTREMITY FUNCTIONAL AND PERFORMANCE EXERCISE PROGRESSION

1. Non-weight-bearing exercises

  A. Proprioceptive neuromuscular facilitation

  B. Joint reposition sense activities

2. Partial-weight-bearing exercises

  A. Aquatic exercises

  B. BAPS board

  C. Stationary bike

3. Full-weight-bearing exercises

  A. Lunges
- Partial depth
- Full depth (90°)

  B. Running
- Running on level surface 50% maximum speed, 1/4 normal distance
- Running on level surface 75% maximum speed, 1/4 normal distance
- Running on level surface 100% maximum speed, 1/4 normal distance
- Running on level surface 100% maximum speed, 1/2 normal distance
- Running on level surface 100% maximum speed, full normal distance
- Running on incline surface 75% maximum speed, 1/2 normal distance
- Running on incline surface 75% maximum speed, 3/4 normal distance
- Running on incline surface 75% maximum speed, full normal distance
- Running on incline surface 100% maximum speed, full normal distance

  C. Sprinting
- Sprinting on level surface 50% maximum speed, 1/4 normal distance
- Sprinting on level surface 75% maximum speed, 1/4 normal distance

Figure 15.23 Example of a lower-extremity functional and performance exercise progression.

- Sprinting on level surface 100% maximum speed, 1/4 normal distance
- Sprinting on level surface 100% maximum speed, 1/2 normal distance
- Sprinting on level surface 100% maximum speed, 3/4 normal distance
- Sprinting on level surface 100% maximum speed, normal distance

D. Jumping and hopping
- Jumping rope, both feet
- Jumping rope, one foot
- Jumping lines, both feet forward, backward
- Jumping lines, one foot forward, backward
- Jumping lines, both feet zigzag forward, backward
- Jumping lines, one foot, zigzag forward, backward
- Box jumps, 6-in. boxes, two feet, forward
- Box jumps, 6-in. boxes, two feet, sideways
- Box jumps, 6-in. boxes, one foot, forward
- Box jumps, 6-in. boxes, one foot, sideways
- Box jumps of increasing heights with sequences above repeated

E. Agility
- Cariocas, 50% speed, both to left and to right
- Cariocas, 75% speed, both to left and to right
- Cariocas, 100% speed, both to left and to right
- Circle-8s with same sequence as cariocas, starting with large circles and reducing the size to tight circles
- Zigzag sprints with same sequence as cariocas
- Command drills with sudden changes in direction of any agility exercise on command

Note: Any of these exercises can be made more difficult by increasing distance or number of sets, or using weights with the exercise.

Figure 15.23 *>continued*

Activity-specific exercises are introduced in the last segment of the rehabilitation program. These exercises are dictated by the patient's activity demands.

Functional-Level Exercise Basics

In a good rehabilitation program, functional exercise and functional evaluation occur from the very beginning of rehabilitation and transition to performance-specific exercises as the patient progresses in the program. Before a patient advances to functional activities, the rehabilitation clinician must confirm that the patient has met the requirements of flexibility, strength, endurance, and other parameters to perform functional activities. For example, before a football lineman can push a football sled, he or she must have enough strength in the subscapularis, infraspinatus, latissimus dorsi, and serratus anterior to resist the sled's weight. Before a volleyball player can perform box jumps, there must be a functional degree of mobility in the thorax and strength in the quadriceps. A gymnast must be able to stork stand on the ground before advancing to a one-legged jump.

Functional exercises require multiplanar abilities. Basic functional exercises such as a single-leg stance may occur early in a patient's rehabilitation program, provided the

patient can bear full weight, has appropriate mobility, and has enough strength to balance and recover from loss of balance in any plane. The rehabilitation clinician must be aware of the stresses these exercises place on the body and must know the patient's limits and abilities.

As the rehabilitation program progresses with improvements in each of the required parameters, more complex functional activities are added. These exercises may include lower-extremity activities such as side shuffles, cariocas, hops, backward running, or exercising on a slide board. More complex upper-extremity functional exercises include juggling, PNF movement with rubber tubing, throwing or dribbling a ball against a wall, or playing "rock, paper, scissors." Exercise selection to a great extent is determined by the patient's sport or work requirements.

The primary difference between functional exercises and exercises for gains in range of motion or strength is that functional exercises are multiplanar, while exercises intended to make specific gains in isolated muscles or muscle groups are not usually multiplanar. The primary difference between functional exercises and performance-specific activities is that while both are multiplanar, the performance-specific activities are drills that are used in a specific sport or work environment, and they involve skills required for that sport or job demand. Some sports and jobs have overlapping performance-specific and functional activities.

Functional and Performance-Specific Exercises

Progression from complex functional to more specific skill activities requires the clinician to break down the skills required in a sport or job to provide the patient with exercises that offer a fundamental skill review first. Once the fundamental skills are mastered, the next step is combining these basic skills into more complex performance activities. In addition to flexibility, strength, muscle endurance, and neuromotor control, these advanced performance activities require agility, speed, power, and control. Depending on the requirements of the advanced performance skill, some basic skill exercises can be started earlier in the program while the patient is still working to achieve proficiency in other areas. For example, the patient can start basic coordination exercises such as bouncing a basketball before he or she has achieved full range of motion or full strength.

Functional exercises and activity-specific exercises are combined in this section because they often overlap within a program, and the division between functional activities and activity-specific exercises is sometimes difficult to define. Experienced clinicians can discern which of these activities can be incorporated early and which ones must wait until more healing occurs or until the patient develops other skills.

Progression of Functional and Performance-Specific Exercises

Each of these factors must be considered for both functional and activity-specific exercises. The complexity of each factor may vary depending on the specific exercise and the complexity of the desired outcome for each patient.

Force and Intensity

Any activity or performance skill requires delivery of a force with a specific intensity. Forces and their intensities vary in type and quantity depending on the activity and the outcome desired.[84] The intent of any functional or performance exercise is to provide an overload in accordance with the SAID principle described in chapter 13. Just as with strengthening, the skill's force or intensity starts light and increases as the patient can tolerate increased loads. For example, in an upper-extremity functional exercise such as a basketball chest pass, the patient may begin without any equipment and concentrate on the technique. As the skill is reacquired, a light medicine ball such as a 0.9 kg (2 lb) ball may be used, then increasing to 1.8 kg (4 lb) and so on until the patient becomes proficient with the desired medicine ball weight.

Speed

Speed is the rate at which an exercise or activity is performed. In the beginning, the speed is slower so that the patient can master the correct execution. As skill improves, the exercise speed increases. For example, an injured track athlete may begin running at half normal speed for a specific distance but then increase the speed as his or her ability to handle increased stresses improves. In an upper-extremity exercise such as throwing, the patient may begin throwing at one-quarter to one-half normal speed and increase the throwing speed as technique improves.

Specific speeds for initial functional exercises during this phase of rehabilitation are individually established and are determined by a variety of factors. Examples of these factors include the length of time the patient has been out of full participation, the severity of the injury, the person's competitive level, preinjury distances for distance-related activities, motivation level, and goals for return to participation. As a rule of thumb, initial functional or activity-specific exercise speed may be one-quarter to one-half the normal or preinjury speeds and progress from there to three-quarter speed and then to full speed. This is a very general rule, however, and you must always consider the patient's condition and abilities, as well as the demands of the exercise.

Distance

Distances for functional activities range from short to long. The greater the distance, the greater the activity's stress level. In lower-extremity activities, increasing distance may include increasing the patient's running distance or jumping distance. In the upper extremity, it may include throwing or hitting a ball farther or swimming farther.

As in determining functional exercise or specific performance speeds, one establishes distances in initial exercises individually and according to the factors already discussed. A general guideline, though not a fixed rule, is to start with no more than one-quarter to one-half the preinjury distance. Initial distance, however, may be significantly less for a patient such as a marathoner who has been out of competition for 4 months and had a preinjury running distance of 16 km (10 mi) per workout, or for an outfielder who must throw a ball 55 m (180 ft). The rehabilitation clinician uses his or her best judgment and knowledge of healing and performance demands to determine the most appropriate distances for initial functional exercises. It is better to underestimate than to overestimate the patient's ability to withstand stresses. You can avoid aggravation of an injury when you underestimate, but you can provoke it when you overestimate.

Complexity

An exercise's complexity refers to how advanced the activity is and how challenging it can be to perform. Functional and performance-specific exercises both progress from simple to complex. Each progressive level places more demands on the patient's ability and skill. For example, in the lower extremity, a jumping progression may begin with a simple standing jump activity and progress to multiple jumps-in-place, to a forward or backward jump, and to multiple forward or backward jumps. Upper-extremity functional exercises may begin with a simple activity such as bouncing a tennis ball into the air from the racket. From this early functional activity, the patient progresses to a performance-specific activity such as a forehand stroke, to a backhand stroke, to a combination of backhand and forehand strokes against a wall, and to a combination of backhand and forehand strokes with another player across a net.

You can also increase complexity by having the patient perform a simple functional exercise and then progress to a number of simple activities at one time or combine them with a performance activity. For example, a single-leg stance with eyes open becomes more complex when you have the patient catch a ground ball while stork standing. The progression continues if you have the patient catch the ground ball while single-leg standing on an unstable surface.

The rehabilitation clinician determines on an individual basis how complex the initial functional exercise should be, how quickly the complexity should increase, and when progression should occur to performance-specific exercises. You must consider the factors already outlined and make your best judgment. Remember, the patient should master the basic exercise and perform it correctly before progressing to more complex activities; you do not want the patient to establish poor movement patterns.[85]

Support

Support refers to the number of extremities that are bearing weight during the activity. In simple standing, support is bilateral; in a stork stand, support is unilateral. Unilateral stance is more difficult than bilateral stance. Jumping on one leg is a progression from performing the same activity on two legs. Throwing a ball with one hand overhead is more difficult than throwing a ball with two hands overhead; performing a push-up with one hand is more difficult than performing it with two hands.

Type of Exercise

The type of exercise determines whether the activity is basic or advanced. Once the exercise mimics a specific performance skill or is a component of a performance skill, it is a performance-specific exercise. The progression of performance-specific exercises follows the same principles as for other types of exercises. For example, a common functional exercise progression for an injured cross-country athlete may include walking on toes on a treadmill, carioca on a treadmill, and then a combination of walking

and jogging for time or distance on a treadmill. When goals for these activities are achieved and the patient's performance of the skill is correct, performance-specific exercises include running a mile outdoors at half speed, increasing distance or intensity until the patient has attained near-normal levels, and then increasing to three-quarter speed with the patient maintaining the previously achieved intensity and distance. Once normal speed and distance on level ground are achieved, hill work may proceed.

Early performance-specific activities are light so that the patient can concentrate on execution. Instruction in the correct performance of a skill is required at each stage of the progression, but especially in the beginning when it has been a while since the patient has been able to perform the skill. Once performance is accurate and appropriate, activity goals become more challenging. From accurate performance, goals advance to include parameters such as speed, intensity, distance, or other competition requirements, all while maintaining performance accuracy.

Throughout the progression of functional and performance-specific activities, the exercises should be difficult enough to challenge the patient without causing failure. The judgment and evaluative skills of the rehabilitation clinician are crucial in these decisions. As patients near the end of the therapeutic exercise regimen and approach their return to full participation, they must have full confidence in their abilities and in the restoration of the injured part. The progression from functional exercises through the final stages of performance-specific exercises must be carefully planned to create a natural sequence that will promote this confidence.

Some exercises in a treatment session may be at different demand levels than others. For example, one exercise may be at half speed while another exercise is at three-quarter force. The session may include a simple exercise and another that is much more complex. Selection of each exercise level is based on the person's ability to execute each skill.

CLINICAL TIPS

The rehabilitation clinician must understand the skill and performance demands of the patient's sport or work in order to develop a functional-to-performance program. A carefully planned program includes early inclusion of basic functional activities with modifications as the patient's skills improve. Advancement to performance-based, or performance-specific, exercises begins with low-level skills and increases in complexity as the patient masters the appropriate skills. Changes in force and intensity, speed, distance, complexity, support, and type of exercise are used to provide a logical progression of difficulty as the patient masters each level of performance until normal performance with full confidence is achieved.

Precautions for Functional and Performance-Specific Activities

Performance-specific exercises are more complex, more challenging, and more rigorous than functional exercises. This is generally so because they include more complex and simultaneous movements, and more accuracy and skill are required for correct execution. Because of the increased demands such activities impose, there are also precautions that one must respect in assigning these advanced therapeutic exercises to a patient.

At each session, you present the patient with specific goals for that session. The exercises for that session are designed to achieve those goals. Do not move to more complex skills until those goals are achieved. If skill patterns are performed incorrectly, you must correct the performance to avoid making incorrect engrams.[85] Movements and activities you design for the rehabilitation session should mimic the movement requirements of the patient's sport or work.

Patients should warm up before performing the performance-specific program you have outlined for the day. You should give them feedback about their performance, correcting for any errors in technique, throughout their treatment sessions. At the end of each session, give the patient your general assessment of his or her performance for the day, and explain what you expect to include in the next treatment. If you want the patient to work on a technique or maneuver before your next session, be specific in your instructions about the intensity, frequency, duration, and expected outcomes of the home program.

Explain the Exercise to the Patient

Before patients perform an exercise, they should understand how to perform it, what its goals are, and what positions or movements to avoid. For example, the clinician demonstrates or explains a single-leg stance on a trampoline by telling the patient that the eyes should remain open, the arms should be kept at the sides, and the position should be maintained for 30 s. During execution, cues are provided to correct the patient's performance. The cues should be constructive and should include specific suggestions about how to improve the execution.[86] For example, simply telling patients "Don't move!" is not helpful because they may not know how to stop moving; instead, the instruction "Unlock your knee" or "Stand with your weight equally distributed between the ball of your foot and heel" may be a more useful hint for performing a single-leg stance without moving. Having the patient perform the exercise on the uninvolved extremity first often proves to be very helpful because it provides internal feedback about correct performance.[87] This is especially helpful if the clinician tells the patient to note how the muscles feel when standing on the uninvolved leg and then tells him or her to achieve the same feeling when standing on the injured leg.

Avoid Pain and Swelling

Residual pain and swelling within 24 h after a treatment session should be avoided. Any increase in pain or swelling indicates that the exercise is too aggressive for the injured area. With pain, strength is reduced, and other detrimental effects result.[88] If this occurs, the clinician returns the patient to the previous level of exercise until the injured part can tolerate additional stress.

Whenever the program advances, the clinician should watch for pain and edema and tell the patient to report any symptoms that occur post-treatment.

Understand Tissue Integrity

The rehabilitation clinician must be aware of the healing sequence and the time needed for tissue to complete the healing process. He or she must consider the tissue's structural integrity and understand the amount of stress involved in each functional exercise before including any functional activity in the rehabilitation program. Tissue healing and tensile strength were presented in chapter 2.

Know the Patient's Confidence Level

Patients must have confidence in their ability to execute functional and performance-based exercises, and they must be confident that the injured part will tolerate the stress of the activity. If the patient is not prepared mentally or emotionally to handle a particular functional or performance-specific exercise, you must start with one that is less stressful and less complex that the person feels able to perform.[89] When patients lack full confidence for fear of reinjuring the segment, what is often needed is a slower progression of performance-specific exercises with longer times at one level before advancing to the next level. This gives the patient more time to develop confidence in the injured segment through repetition of activities. In such cases, the clinician should point out the quality of the patient's performance, demonstrating that the injured segment can perform the required activities.

Be Aware of Progression Tolerance

As mentioned, performance-specific exercises are introduced at lower-than-normal speed, intensity, and difficulty.

CLINICAL TIPS

Since performance-specific activities increasingly challenge the patient's skills, consider several important precautions in this part of the rehabilitation program. The patient must understand the exercise, and the rehabilitation clinician must be aware of the patient's healing process and of his or her confidence and tolerance levels. Proper execution of each skill must occur before the patient advances to the next skill.

Increases in these parameters occur one at a time until the exercise is equivalent to normal performance. The body must be allowed to adapt to increased stress levels before each goal is changed. This will ensure that the patient's confidence will grow and that tissue overload will not be excessive, thereby preventing additional injury.

Performance Evaluation of Functional and Performance-Specific Activities

Evaluation and assessment are vital parts of the rehabilitation process all the way to the end of this final rehabilitation phase. As with earlier phases of the rehabilitation program, the clinician continues to use examination, evaluation, and assessment skills throughout this final phase to determine the patient's progression to return to play or work. Throughout this final phase, the rehabilitation clinician evaluates the patient's ability to perform both functional and performance-specific exercises. Advances in the program occur only after the patient performs to expected levels and achieves established goals. With the stork stand, for example, the patient does not progress until he or she can stork stand with eyes open for 30 s. Only after the patient passes that goal does the next phase of balance proceed. Then the patient may stork stand on an uneven surface or on the ground with eyes closed or with head rotations. The specific exercise goal in the next sequence depends on the demands of the patient's normal activities.

CLINICAL TIPS

Step-by-step evaluation determines when the patient should advance to the next stage in the functional and performance-specific exercise program. The final evaluation, whose purpose is to determine whether the patient is ready to return to normal and full participation, is highly individualized.

The final evaluation occurs before the patient returns to full participation. The patient's performance in the evaluation determines his or her readiness to return to normal and full participation. Final examination includes highly specific performance drills and tests. These tests should be as objective as possible and should mimic the person's required performance as much as possible, whether it is for work or for sport. For a gymnast, the examination may include performance of dismounts, tumbling skills, or apparatus skills. For a basketball player, the examination includes performance of dribbling, shooting, cutting, or passing drills. For a warehouse worker, the examination includes performance of lifting specific weighted objects and moving them within a specified distance using proper body mechanics and safety techniques. Because specific activities vary greatly from job to job, sport to sport, and

between positions within a sport or worksite, you must be familiar with the patient's needs. You may need to obtain the supervisor or coach's help, or acquire a job description from the employer, in designing performance exercises and tests for some skills. It is the goal of the final examination, however, to demonstrate to the patient, the medical team, and the supervisor or coach that the person is able and ready to withstand the stresses of full participation.

The tests for determining readiness to return to full participation must fulfill certain criteria, some of which have been previously mentioned. One criterion is that the examination tool should be as objective as possible.[2] The tests should be repeatable so that they can be used both in initial examination and in final examination to measure changes and assess whether or not the patient has achieved the appropriate goals.[90] The tests should provide useful information to the patient and medical team about the progress and status of the patient's performance. They should also be able to show whether the exercise program is providing the advancement of parameters needed for return to participation.

In the final examination, your observation and assessment of the patient's performance are critical. All activities should be performed without hesitation, and the use of each extremity should be appropriate, without favoring of the injured segment. The patient should move quickly, stabilize appropriately, and demonstrate self-confidence with all maneuvers. Based on the patient's performance, you should be unable to identify which extremity has been injured.

Examples of Functional Performance-Specific Progression

This chapter has included information on the final steps in a rehabilitation program. We know that this is the time when the patient starts preparing to return to his or her sport or work. The most difficult parts of the rehabilitation process have been completed, and now the focus moves from the general need for mobility and strength to the more specific needs that enable the patient to return to cross-country truck driving or home construction or softball pitching or pole vaulting.

In these last steps of the program, the clinician continues to advance the patient by creating activity and exercise progressions that move the patient from low-level activities to normal sport or work activities. Part of that work or sport performance involves relearning the skill. The patient must advance from conscious to subconscious, or automatic, performance. This process involves practice and repetition. It also involves a gradual increase in complexity of the activity as the patient improves at each skill level (figure 15.24).

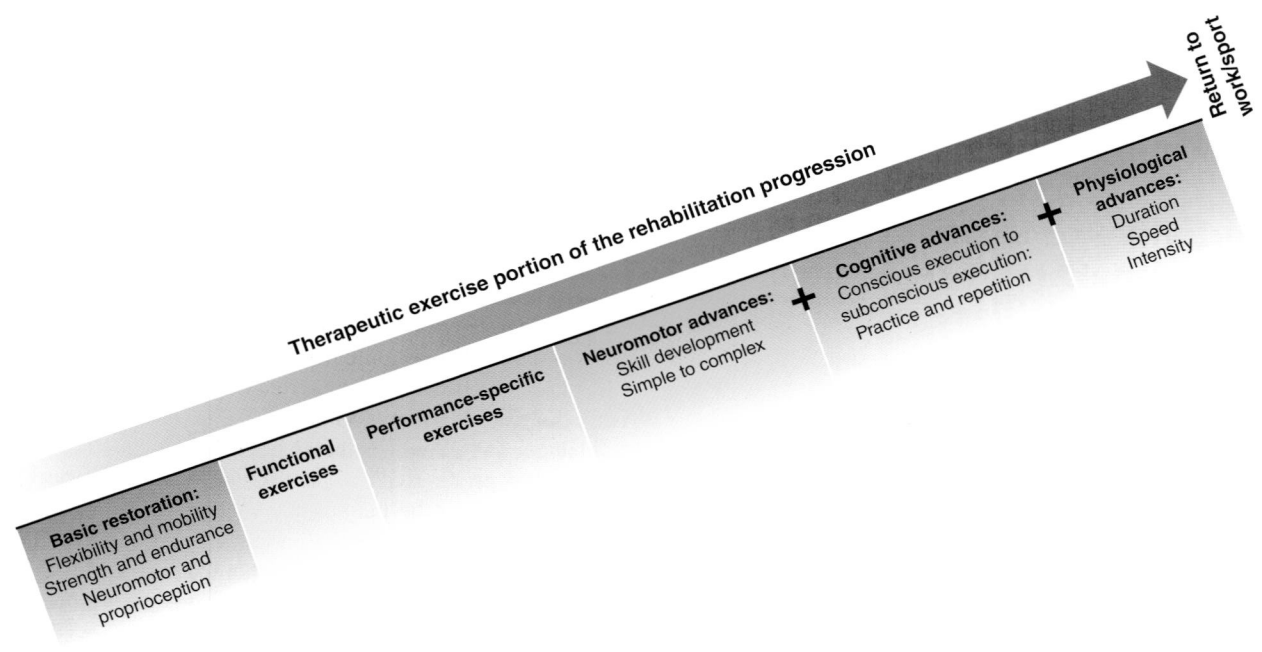

Figure 15.24   The exercise portion of a rehabilitation program is represented as a progression of exercises from the early days of rehabilitation to the final days just before the patient is discharged from your care. The activities in the final phase are designed to meet the specific demands the patient will face when returning to work or sport.

This neuromotor education promotes a physiological change in the body's ability to meet the increasing demands of the skill activity. These changes are accomplished by changing the duration, speed, repetitions, and intensity of the activity.

All of these aspects are included in the clinician's design of the activity-specific phase of the patient's rehabilitation program. Keep these topics in mind as you go through the examples in this section. Envision a patient that you have witnessed in the clinic and how you might design this phase of that patient's program.

Functional Capacity Evaluation

There are many ways to determine an injured worker's progression in this phase of rehabilitation. Just as there are specific activities for examining an athlete's function and performance, there are different ways to examine how well a worker performs before allowing that person to return to the workforce. In addition to the activities and tests already mentioned, there are commercially available programs that may be used to determine if a patient is ready to return to his or her job.

These programs have been developed to enable companies to manage injured workers and return them to work safely. The programs are based on functional capacity evaluations (FCEs). A variety of FCE programs or systems are available from a number of vendors.[91, 92] Each

of these vendors requires clinicians to attend an instructional program before they are allowed to use their FCE system. There are no information or training standards for certifying those who perform FCEs, but the vendors often issue a certificate to clinicians who have completed their training programs.

OccuPro is an example of a company that provides FCEs that have demonstrated good reliability in upper-extremity testing.[93] Another example is WorkWell Systems; their system has also demonstrated good reliability.[94] These systems all use a variety of tests; the patient's performance for each test is graded and sometimes timed. The tests may vary from one system to another, but there are also tests that these systems have in common. Examples of the overlapping tests include assessment of activities such as grip strength testing, standing, lifting, sitting, carrying, and squatting.

Lower-Extremity Example

This section presents functional and performance-specific exercises for the lower extremity and then describes testing that could be included as part of the assessment before the patient is allowed to return to unrestricted activity.

Functional Exercises

Any functional exercise should be preceded by a simple warm-up activity. Simple functional exercises for the lower extremity can begin relatively early with a non-weight-bearing exercise such as proprioceptive neuromuscular facilitation. Partial-weight-bearing use of the BAPS board can also begin early in the therapeutic exercise program. As patients become weight bearing, they can start to do the single-leg stance, first with eyes open, then with eyes closed, and then with head rotation. This activity can progress from the floor to a BAPS board (figure 15.25), trampoline, half foam roller, or balance board (figure 15.26) and then to combining the balance activity with another activity such as ball catching. Single-leg stance activities will then progress to dynamic movement activities such as lunges, single-leg squats (figure 15.27), and backward step-ups and step-downs (figure 15.28). Treadmill activities such as cariocas, backward walking, and sideways walking are also functional activities.

Performance-Specific Exercises

Walking, walking combined with jogging, and jogging without walking intervals are included in performance-specific exercises. From jogging, the patient progresses to running. Running activities begin with a forward jog on a flat surface, then progress to increased speed and distance, and then move on to lateral runs and cuts and sudden changes in direction. In figure 15.29*a*, the patient pushes forward from the left foot to the right foot and then moves laterally to the left foot before retracing the steps to the starting position, moving from one position to the next as quickly as possible. Figure 15.29*b* shows

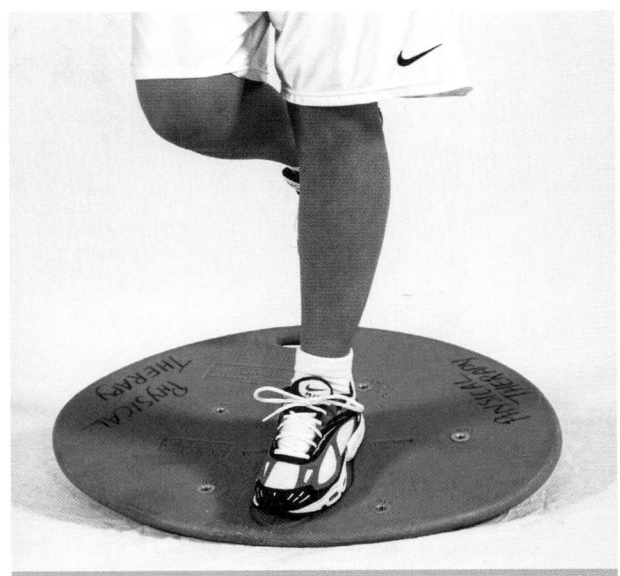

Figure 15.25   BAPS board.

W-sprints that require the patient to sprint forward to the first marked spot or cone, then backpedal to the second marker, and then sprint forward to the next, repeating the series as illustrated to complete the exercise. These could be used for football defensive backs. Figure 15.29*c* shows a figure-8 run, which uses markers or cones around which the patient runs in a figure-8 pattern. These could be used

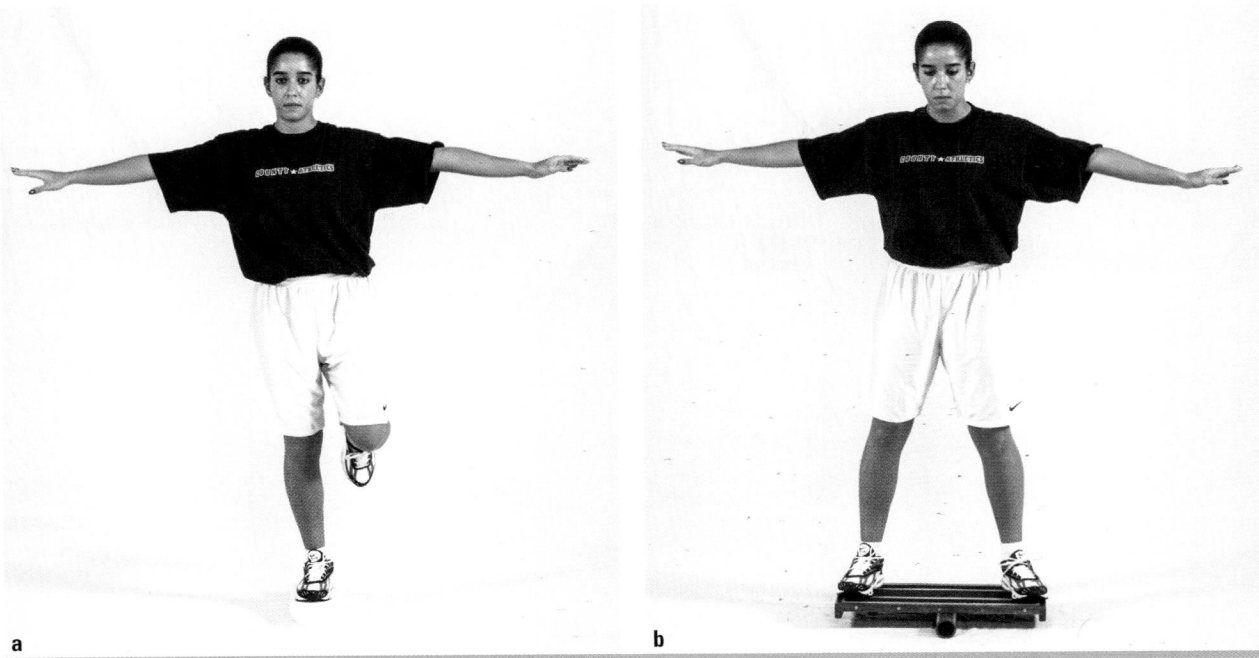

a   b

Figure 15.26   Balance activities: *(a)* stork stand on half foam roller and *(b)* balance board. It is best to leave the arms at the sides, rather than extend them, while holding the positions.

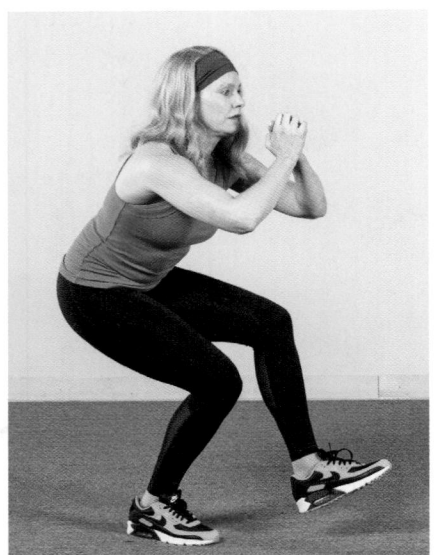

Figure 15.27 Single-leg squat.

for a soccer player. The exercise in figure 15.29d is similar to the W-sprint except that the patient runs straight ahead, pivots on the right outside leg to cut sharply to the left, runs straight ahead for a designated distance, and pivots on the left outside leg to cut sharply to the right until the end of the course. This exercise could be used for lacrosse players. Each of these exercises can become more difficult if you require either a faster pace or smaller distances between the sudden motion changes.

Upper-Extremity Example

As in the discussion of the exercise program for the lower extremity, this section describes functional exercises and activity-specific exercises for the upper extremity.

Functional Exercises

Like lower-extremity functional work, upper-extremity functional exercises may begin early in the program with proprioceptive neuromuscular facilitation (figure 15.30). Partial-weight-bearing activities on a Swiss ball can sometimes be used early in the program as well. Closed kinetic chain activities such as weight-bearing exercises, first on a stable surface and then on an unstable surface, can be used once full weight bearing is permissible.

A patient in a push-up position with hands on a BAPS board or wobble board is an example of a closed kinetic chain activity on an unstable surface. Both hands are on the board while the patient moves the board. An example using the BOSU ball has the flat portion of the ball facing up with the patient's hands on the sides of the platform in a push-up position. A tennis ball is placed on the top of the BOSU ball, and the patient has to move the tennis ball into the indented center of the BOSU ball. In another push-up position example, the patient can start with both hands on the floor, lift one hand off the floor while maintaining trunk stability, and then switch arms. In another example with the patient in a push-up position, the patient moves the Fitter platform from side to side.

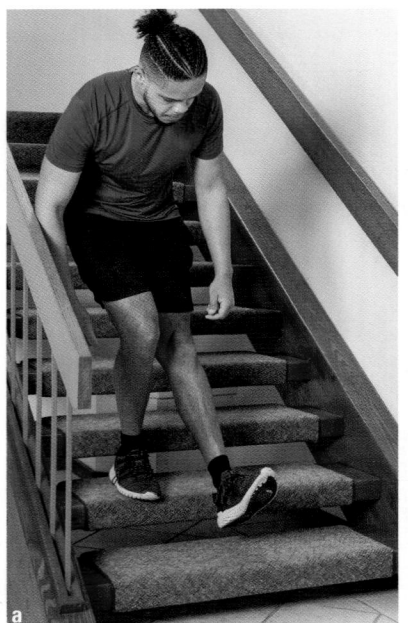
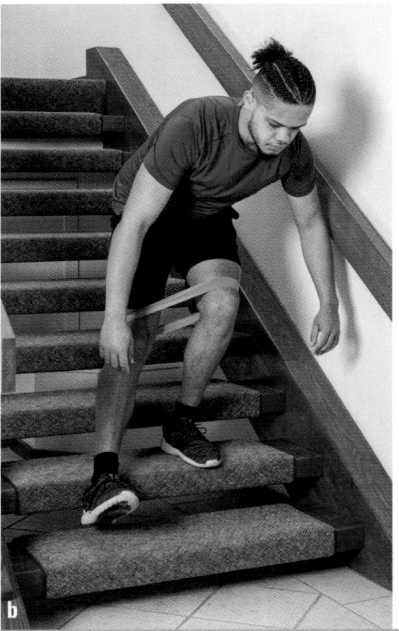

Figure 15.28 Backward step-ups for gluteus, hamstring, and quad strength without use of paraspinals. Can be performed (a) without a resistance band, or (b) with a resistance band around the knees for additional strength for the gluteus complex.

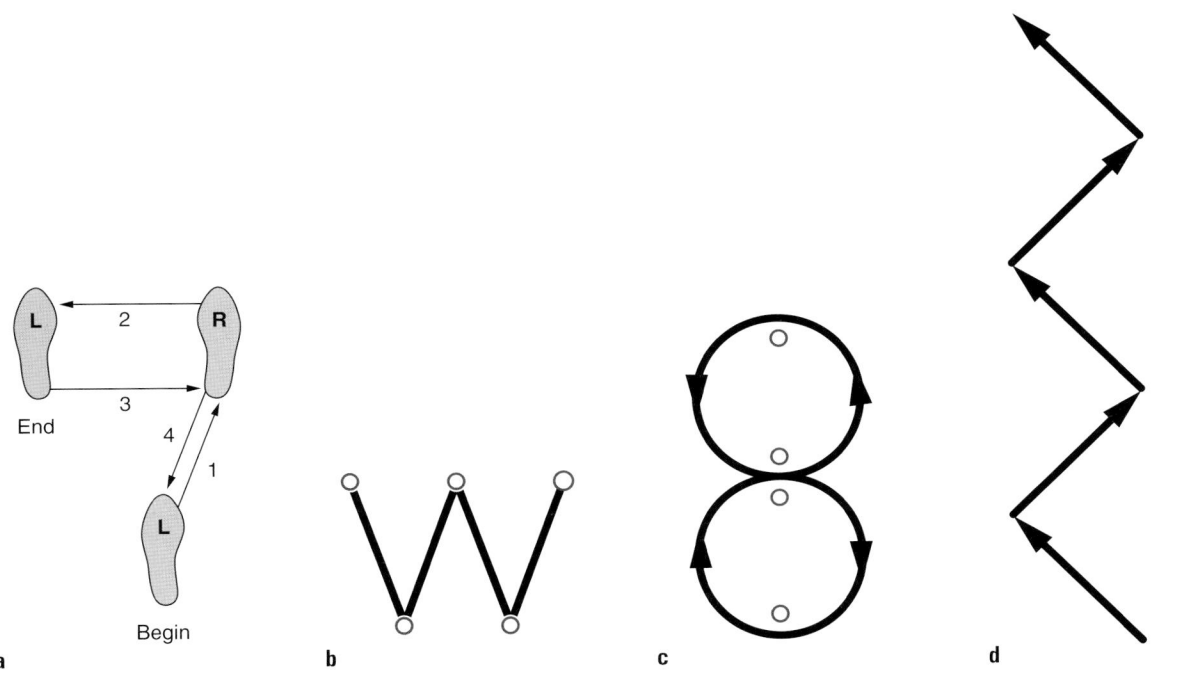

Figure 15.29   Agility drills: *(a)* 90° lunge, *(b)* W-sprint course, *(c)* figure-8 course, *(d)* Z-course (zigzag).

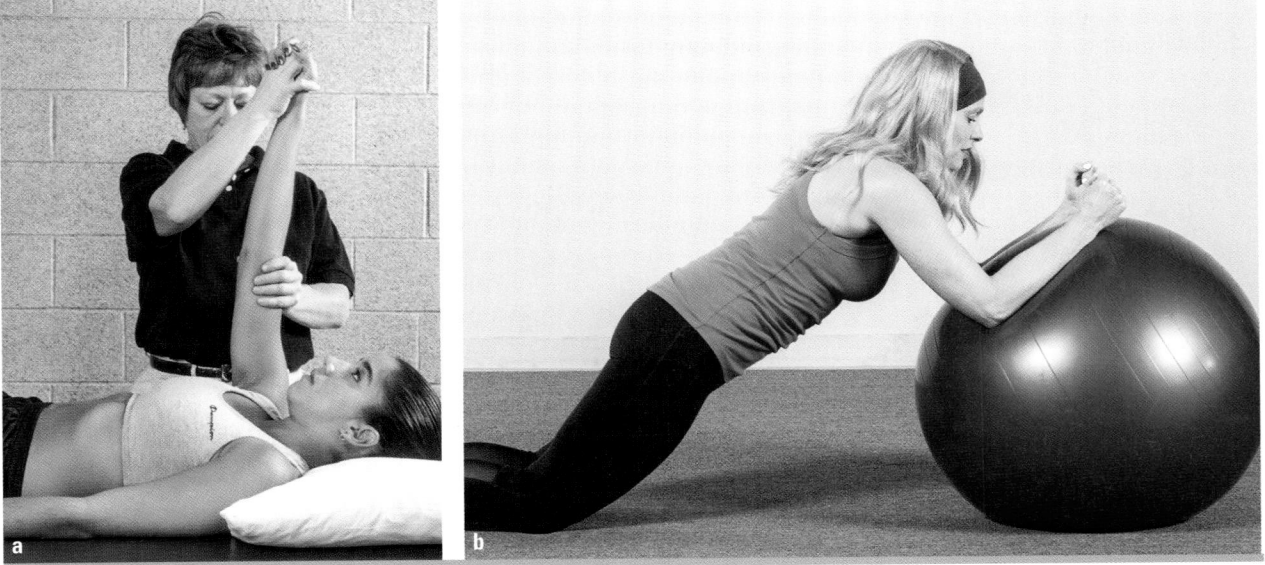

Figure 15.30   Functional exercise progression for the upper extremity: *(a)* open kinetic chain, and *(b)* closed kinetic chain.

All of these push-up position exercises can progress from a modified push-up position on hands and knees to a full push-up position on hands and toes. The patient should have adequate scapular muscle strength, rotator cuff strength, and large shoulder muscle and other upper-extremity strength, along with proper range of motion, before beginning more complex functional exercises.

Complex functional exercises for the upper extremity may include a variety of shoulder, elbow, or wrist and hand activities, depending on the performance demands to which the patient will return and his or her functional deficiencies. Examples of these types of activities include PNF-pattern movements using rubber tubing, throwing a foam ball at a mirror to watch for follow-through motion, bouncing a ball between the legs and around the back, lying prone on a roller stool and using the arms to propel the stool, or juggling. As with lower-extremity functional exercises, the upper-extremity exercises involve multiple joints and planes of movement and require the patient to perform complex activities in preparation for advancement to performance-specific exercises.

Performance-Specific Exercises

Having achieved proper stabilization, strength, range of motion, and control, the patient progresses to such exercises as those required for competitive shot putting, javelin throwing, golf, tennis, or swimming. A progression of throwing begins with shortened distances for reduced speed and distance. As previously mentioned, early per-

formance-specific sessions emphasize correct technique and advance to increased performance demands only after the skill is retrieved. These parameters include progressive increases in distances, numbers of throws, and severity of throws. See figure 15.31 for an example of a throwing progression program.

A golf progression may begin with the putter and short irons for putting and chipping activities with a partial swing and then progress to longer irons, fuller swings, and finally to the woods with a full swing. For each club, the swing begins as a partial swing and increases to a full swing as the patient gains progressive control of the club. Repetitions also increase as the patient's endurance improves. See figure 15.32 for an example of a golf progression program.

SPORT-SPECIFIC BASEBALL OR SOFTBALL PITCHING AND THROWING PROGRESSION PROGRAM

1. Beginning level

A. 0-45 ft distance
50% normal speed
30 throws, 2 sets

B. 40-45 ft distance
50% normal speed
30 throws, 4 sets

C. 40-45 ft distance
75% normal speed
30 throws, 3 sets

D. 40-45 ft distance
75% normal speed
30 throws, 5 sets

E. 60 ft distance
75% normal speed
30 throws, 3-4 sets

F. 60 ft distance
75% normal speed
30 throws, 5 sets

2. Intermediate level

A. 60 ft distance
100% normal speed
30 throws, 3-4 sets

B. 100 ft distance
75% normal speed
30 throws, 3-4 sets

C. 100 ft distance
75% normal speed
30 throws, 5 sets

D. 100 ft distance
100% normal speed
30 throws, 3-4 sets

E. 100 ft distance
100% normal speed
30 throws, 5 sets

F. 150 ft distance
75% normal speed
30 throws, 3-4 sets

G. 150 ft distance
75% normal speed
30 throws, 5 sets

H. 150 ft distance
100% normal speed
30 throws, 5 sets

3. Advanced level

A. 180 ft distance
75% normal speed
30 throws, 3 sets

B. 180 ft distance
75% normal speed
30 throws, 5 sets

C. 180 ft distance
100% normal speed
30 throws, 3 sets

D. 180 ft distance
100% normal speed
30 throws, 5 sets

Figure 15.31 Example of a baseball or softball pitching and throwing progression program.

4. Precompetition level

A. Pitch off mound
100% normal speed
30 pitches, 3-4 sets

B. Pitch off mound
100% normal speed
30 pitches, 5 sets

Note: All throwing sessions begin with a warm-up and end with a cool-down. Warm-up and cool-down throws are performed as light, arcing tosses. A rest of 3 to 5 min between sets is allowed. If the patient experiences pain with a progression to the next level, he or she should return to the previous level for another session. If the patient is not a pitcher, throwing progression follows the same routine as listed, but the distances vary according to the sport (e.g., discus, javelin, football) and are determined by the distances and weights used within the sport.

Figure 15.31 >continued

SPORT-SPECIFIC GOLF PROGRESSION PROGRAM

1. Beginning level

A. Putts and chips
20 putts, varying distances
10 chips

B. Putts and chips
20 putts, varying distances
20 chips

C. Putts and chips
20 putts, 3 sets
20 chips, 2 sets

D. Putts and chips
20 putts, 3 sets
20 chips, 3 sets

2. Intermediate level

A. Short irons, no more than three clubs
Partial swing, 1 × 20 each

B. Short irons, no more than three clubs
Partial swing, 2 × 20 each

C. Short irons, no more than three clubs
Partial swing, 3 × 20 each

D. Short irons, no more than two clubs
Full swing, 1 × 20 each

E. Short irons, no more than two clubs
Full swing, 2 × 20 each

F. Short irons, no more than two clubs
Full swing, 3 × 20 each

G. Long irons, no more than three clubs
Partial swing, 1 × 20 each

H. Long irons, no more than three clubs
Partial swing, 2 × 20 each

I. Long irons, no more than three clubs
Full swing, 2 × 20 each

J. Long irons
Full swing, 3 × 25 each

K. All irons
Full swing, 1 × 20 each

3. Advanced level

A. Woods
Partial swing, 2 × 20 each

B. Woods
Full swing, 2 × 20 each

C. Woods and irons
Full swing, 1 × 20–25 each

4. Preparticipation level

A. Par-three course

B. Nine-hole course

C. Return to regular play

Note: All sessions begin with a warm-up and end with a cool-down. A rest of 3 to 5 min between sets is allowed. If the patient experiences pain with an increase to the next level, he or she should return to the previous level for another session.

Figure 15.32 Example of a golf progression program.

We have already briefly looked at a progression of tennis exercises. A simple stabilization exercise such as bouncing the ball on the floor with the racket can begin once the scapular stabilizers and rotator cuff can maintain proper control. This activity advances to bouncing the ball in the air with the racket. More advanced exercises progress from a forehand to a backhand to overhead and serve strokes. See figure 15.33 for a general outline of a progression.

A swimmer's progression may begin with the use of a stroke for a short distance or with alternating strokes for short distances and performing the stroke for no more than half normal speed. Distances and speed increase as

---

SPORT-SPECIFIC TENNIS PROGRESSION PROGRAM

1. Ball bounce

Bounce the tennis ball on the racket into the air. Start by grasping the racket on the neck and advance to the handle.

A. 50 bounces with a palm-down grip
B. 50 bounces with a palm-up grip
C. 50 bounces alternating between palm down and palm up

2. Forehand strokes

Forehand strokes only against a backboard or wall

A. 50% power: 5 × 10
B. 75% power: 3 × 20
C. 100% power: 3 × 40

3. Backhand strokes

Backhand strokes only against a backboard or wall

A. 50% power: 5 × 10
B. 75% power: 3 × 20
C. 100% power: 3 × 40

4. Alternate strokes

Alternate between backhand and forehand strokes against a wall or backboard

A. 75% power: 5 × 15
B. 100% power: 3 × 30
C. 100% power: 4 × 40

5. Overhead serve

Overhead serve against a wall or backboard

A. 50% power: 5 × 10
B. 75% power: 3 × 20
C. 100% power: 3 × 40

6. Game

A. Play one set of tennis
B. Play two sets of tennis
C. Play three sets of tennis
D. Play full match of tennis

Note: All sessions begin with a warm-up and end with a cool-down. The patient should try to hit a specific target or targets on the backboard or wall. If the patient experiences pain with advancement to the next level, he or she should return to the previous level for the next 2 to 3 sessions before returning to the higher level.

Figure 15.33 Example of a tennis progression program.

tolerated. See if you can develop your own example of a swimmer's progression program using these guidelines.

Preparing a warehouse worker to return to work includes knowing the patient's job description or job demands and understanding the daily activity and stresses his or her body undergoes during the workday. It may be necessary for the clinician to visit the patient's workplace to fully understand the return-to-work needs. Once the tasks are identified, they are broken down into specific elements, just as with the sports activities presented in this section. For example, if the worker's schedule includes walking throughout the warehouse for 80% of the shift, then early skill activities may include walking for a specific distance. If the patient must lift containers that can weigh up to 60 lb, then early functional activities include instruction in proper lifting, and later performance exercises begin a progressive lifting program up to or greater than the patient's job requirements.

Other work tasks may include lifting objects from the floor to a waist-high shelf, chest-high shelf, or overhead. If the patient is required to climb ladders, crawl in small spaces, or sit at a computer, these activities become part of the rehabilitation program. Each required task or skill is identified and included in the patient's performance-specific program, starting with easy exercises until the patient performs the task properly, and then adding time or resistance until normal activities are performed without difficulty. As described earlier in this chapter, several companies have assessment tools that may help the clinician to determine when the injured worker can return to work.

Depending on the patient's employer, it may be possible to have the patient perform some tasks in the workplace as a partial workday. When such an arrangement is not possible, the clinician must provide substitute activities in the clinic, and if work endurance is an important issue, the clinician may require the patient to attend extended sessions.

We want to emphasize that the progressive functional and performance-specific exercise programs presented here are only examples. Specific programs vary depending on the patient's needs, abilities, level of competition, length of time away from the activity, and degree of injury. The programs described in this chapter offer only general guidelines and demonstrate how to progress and change the parameters of functional and performance-specific exercise programs. Your creativity as a clinician is an important tool during this phase of rehabilitation.

Final Step Before Full Return to Participation

When the performance-specific phase of rehabilitation ends, the only step remaining is to ensure that patients are fully ready to return to their required activities. This is done by performing final tests. These tests are important

and should not be neglected. They confirm the clinician's determinations and provide patients with the final piece of evidence they may need to feel safe performing any activity. The true test of rehabilitation program success comes when patients return to their previous level of performance.

For that to happen, a patient must meet four specific criteria:

1. The acute signs and symptoms of the injury are resolved, and no pain or edema is present.
2. The patient demonstrates full range of motion; normal strength, muscle endurance, and cardiovascular endurance; and appropriate proprioception, agility, and coordination in relation to the required performance skills.
3. The patient performs all activities at least as well as he or she could before the injury. You should be unable to identify the area that was injured if the patient is performing the activities appropriately.
4. The patient has the confidence to perform without any hesitation or doubt or any modification of performance or mechanics.

If these criteria are met and the patient can pass all tests, the clinician and patient have achieved the goals established at the start of the rehabilitation program.

Test Selection

Several performance-based lower-extremity tests can be used.[95-98] The tests chosen should reflect the patient's required activities as accurately as possible and should be as objective as possible. To measure gains in performance, you should use the same test to evaluate performance when the patient begins the functional exercise phase and when he or she prepares to return to full activity.

Lower-Extremity Tests

Lower-extremity tests can be classified as running tests for time and distance, jumping tests for height and distance, and agility tests.[97, 99] The running tests can be either sprints or timed long-distance runs, depending on participation and performance demands.

Jumping tests can include a standing vertical jump, a step-and-jump, a repeated jump for distance, and a single jump for distance. A volleyball player's jump test is more functional if it is either a standing or a step-and-jump test, whereas a long jumper's test is more functional if it is a run-and-jump-for-distance test.

Agility tests use cariocas, zigzag runs, figure-8 runs, shuttle runs, and box runs, to name a few.[100] Whatever activities are selected, the distances, angles, and sizes of the turns and circles should be the same on the pretest as on the posttest for accurate comparisons. Goals should also be predetermined. The goals may be defined either with reference to established norms or by the athlete's preinjury performance ability.

Lower-extremity testing for the industrial patient returning to work includes repetitive squatting, squat-lifting objects similar in weight and size to those at their work, climbing ladders, and using stairs.[93] The tests used depend upon the demands of the person's normal responsibilities.

Upper-Extremity Performance: Final Testing

It is more difficult to examine the upper extremity and obtain objective and measurable criteria than it is for the lower extremity. This is because of the greater variability of upper-extremity activities. If a speed gun is available, it is fairly simple to measure the speed of a patient's throw. However, if you do not have a speed gun or the patient's activity does not involve throwing, measuring the skill objectively is more difficult. There are a number of generic upper-extremity performance assessment tests that can be used to determine a patient's readiness to return to sport participation.[101-104] There is also a limited number of tools that measure such specific performance abilities as overhead activities[105] and softball throws.[106]

Final goals are individually determined and are based on the patient's preinjury performance. The injured industrial technology worker may need to be able to input computer data for a specific amount of time. A retail store stocker may need to demonstrate an ability to lift 40 lb overhead. For a golfer, it may be his or her score on 18 holes of golf. For the swimmer, it may be the ability to perform an event in the same amount of time as in preinjury performances. For the tennis player, measuring a serve with a speed gun is simple, but evaluating other types of performance may be more difficult. Establishing goals such as hitting a specific target across the net on a given number of consecutive forehand and backhand shots, and using that number for pretest and posttest performance guidelines, may be a way of establishing an objective measure. When establishing any goal in this manner, you should consult with the supervisor or coach to arrive at realistic and achievable goals.

Summary

Plyometric exercises serve as a bridge between strengthening exercises and functional and performance-specific exercises. Before initiating a plyometric program, the clinician must consider several factors, including program design, contraindications, and necessary equipment. Functional exercises are those that precede performance-specific activities in a rehabilitation program. They commonly involve multiplanar activities and produce greater stresses and demands than single-plane strength exercises, and they involve more muscle groups. They may include precursor activities to performance-specific exercises, such as walking before running or underhand tossing before throwing. They prepare patients for the more advanced skill demands they will experience in their specific activities. Performance-specific exercises include drills used for a specific sport or specific job tasks. Functional activities prepare the patient for performance-specific activities. The clinician must understand the physical requirements of both functional and performance-specific tasks and be able to relate them to the demands patients will face when they return to normal activities. Whether the patient is a basketball player or a steel mill worker, a soccer player or a computer analyst, a tennis player or a plumber, the clinician must understand the elements and skills that each patient must perform so they can be appropriately integrated into the rehabilitation program. The final step in the program is an assessment of the patient's ability to perform activities to which he or she will return. If the patient passes these tests, the rehabilitation program is complete and the goals are satisfied.

LEARNING AIDS

Key Concepts and Review

1. List three considerations for plyometric program execution.

When designing a plyometric program, one must consider the patient's physical condition and the sport's demands. Specifically, the patient should have adequate flexibility, strength, and proprioception before beginning a plyometric program. Special considerations also include factors such as the patient's age, weight, level of competition, footwear, the surface, proper technique, progression, and goals.

2. Outline a progression of four plyometric exercises for either a lower- or an upper-extremity program.

A lower-extremity plyometric exercise progression for a basketball player might begin with a two-foot ankle hop and progress to a single-foot ankle hop, side-to-side hops, standing jump-and-reach, long jump with lateral sprint, and box depth jumps.

3. Explain the difference between functional exercise and performance-specific exercise.

Functional exercises are used in a rehabilitation program from its early stages to its final stages. Functional exercises are activities that precede performance-specific exercises in a rehabilitation program.

They commonly involve multiplanar activities and produce stresses and demands on performance muscle groups that are greater than those required for strength exercises in order to prepare the patient for more advanced skill activities. In later rehabilitation stages, performance-specific exercises prepare the patient to return to normal activities by mimicking the stresses and skills required during those activities. Final testing uses activities or drills that are specific to the patient's sport or work demands and activities that mimic the maneuvers and movements that will be required when the patient returns to full participation. This testing assesses whether the patient is ready to resume normal activities.

4. Identify the contributions of functional and performance-specific exercise to a rehabilitation program.

Both types of exercise are used to ready the patient physically for the stresses and demands of his or her activity and to prepare the patient mentally. Successful execution of functional and performance-specific activities will result in the patient's discovery that the injured segment can withstand normal stresses.

5. Discuss the differences between basic and advanced functional activities.

Basic exercises begin early in the rehabilitation program to assist in achieving flexibility, strength, endurance, and proprioception. Advanced exercises, however, include more complex functional performance exercises that prepare the patient for performance-specific exercises.

6. Discuss considerations for implementing a plyometric program.

Several factors should be considered when implementing a plyometric program including age, body weight, competitive level, surface, footwear, proper technique, progression, and goals.

7. List factors that can be varied in a progression of functional and performance-specific activities.

Functional exercises proceed from slow to fast, simple to complex, low force to high force, short distance to long distance, and bilateral support to unilateral support. A progression of functional exercises features a steady change to allow for advancement according to the SAID principle. Functional exercises include some characteristics unique to functional exercises and some characteristics common to most exercises.

8. Identify precautions for functional and performance-specific exercises.

Precautions include some that were discussed in previous chapters, such as explaining the exercise to the patient, avoiding pain and swelling, considering tissue integrity when designing exercises, knowing the patient's confidence level, and being aware of the patient's progression tolerance.

9. Outline a sample progression from functional through performance-specific exercises, including plyometric exercises, for either the lower or the upper extremity.

The progression and selection of exercises depend on the patient's specific task demands, especially as he or she nears the final stages of the program. A lower-extremity program may include a progression that begins with non-weight-bearing use of the BAPS board that can start early in the therapeutic exercise program. As the patient becomes full weight bearing, stork standing can be introduced, first with eyes open, then with eyes closed, and finally with eyes open and head rotation left to right. A progression of this activity can go from using the floor to using either a trampoline or a half foam roller or a balance board and then to combining the activity with another activity such as ball catching. Stork-standing activities can then progress to dynamic movement activities such as lunges, single-leg squats, forward and backward step-ups and step-downs, walking, and jogging. Running activities begin with a forward jog on a flat surface, proceed to increased speed and distances, and then move on to lateral runs and cuts and sudden changes in direction.

Critical Thinking Questions

1. On the basis of the scenario at the beginning of this chapter, what would you do to improve Christian's confidence in his tennis abilities? What activities would you have him do on the first day of his functional program? List three levels of progression, and give your criteria for advancement. When would you have him start overhead activities and serves?

2. When would you decide that Christian could return to full participation? What would your criteria be for this, and why have you set these criteria?

3. A volleyball player who injured his knee and has completed the rehabilitation program up to the performance-specific exercise level is very anxious to return to full sport participation. You estimate that it will be another week before he has completed the performance-specific exercise portion of the program. What will your first day's activities include, and how will you establish a progression

of activities? What are your criteria for each level of progression? What specific activities must he be able to perform before he may resume full volleyball participation?

4. A cross-country competitor is now ready for performance-specific exercises. She has been running short distances for no more than 2 min without difficulty. What distance, speed, and terrain progression will you give her over the course of the next 2 weeks? Write up a 2-week progression of functional activities that will move her to full sport participation.

5. A patient with an ankle sprain is now ready for plyometric exercises. What are the criteria that she has to meet before these exercises can be included in the rehabilitation program? How will you measure these criteria to be sure she is ready?

Lab Activities

1. Have your lab partner perform each of the following jumps as well as possible for one repetition, measure the height achieved with each jump, and record the results. Instruct your partner to begin each jump from the standing position. Allow a few practice jumps before doing the test jumps.

    A. Jump 1: Quickly bend the knees to approximately 60° and jump.

    B. Jump 2: Slowly bend the knees to approximately 60°, hold for 3 s, and jump.

    C. Jump 3: Quickly bend the knees to approximately 120° and jump.

    D. Jump 4: Quickly bend the knees to approximately 120°, hold for 3 s, and jump.

    E. Jump 5: Step off a step stool or box, then immediately jump up.

    F. Jump 6: Jump up onto a box, then immediately jump off and jump upward.

    Which jump produced the greatest height? What is the physiological reason for your results? In what important way do these results relate to a plyometric rehabilitation program?

2. Design a functional upper-extremity program of five exercises for your patient who is a computer programmer. Identify the goals for each activity, have her perform the activity, and score the performance. Explain your scoring criteria, and report your lab partner's score. Identify how you would know when to progress from one exercise to the next exercise (What goals have you set for each exercise?).

3. Design a performance-specific upper-extremity program for your lab partner who is a baseball outfielder. Identify the goals for each activity, have him or her perform the activity, and score the performance. Explain your scoring criteria, and report his or her score. Identify how you would know when to progress from one exercise to the next exercise. How does this program differ from the one you set up for the computer programmer? Why?

4. Design a functional lower-extremity program for your partner who is a volleyball player. Identify the goals for each activity, have her perform the activity, and score the performance. Explain your scoring criteria, and report your partner's score. Identify how you would know when to progress from one exercise to the next exercise.

5. Design a sport-specific lower-extremity program for your lab partner who is a 4 × 400 m relay runner. Identify the goals for each activity, have him perform the activity, and score the performance. Explain your scoring criteria, and report his score. Identify how you would know when to progress from one exercise to the next exercise. How does this program differ from the one you set up for the volleyball athlete? Why?

6. You are in the final phase of a rehabilitation program for a basketball forward who is recovering from a lateral ankle sprain. Design a progressive functional and performance-specific exercise program in preparation for return to play. Have your partner perform each exercise you include in the program to see if you have provided a progression of the exercises, moving from the easiest to the most difficult. Assuming no delays or backward steps in ability to perform the exercises, outline how you would progress her in the program and what criteria you would use to determine when to progress.

Creating the Rehabilitation Program

Objectives

After completing this chapter, you should be able to do the following:

1. Identify the qualities a rehabilitation clinician should have in order to provide patients with a successful rehabilitation program.

2. Explain why examination and assessment are important parts of a rehabilitation program.

3. Identify the four phases of a rehabilitation program, and briefly describe what is included in each phase.

4. Discuss the types of interventions that are usually included in each of the rehabilitation exercise phases.

|||||||||||||||||||||||||||||||||||||||||||||||||||||||||||||||||||||||||||||||||||||||||||||||||||||||||||||||||||||||||||||||||||||||||||||||||||||||||||||||||

Linda and David are working together on their capstone project before they graduate in May. They are creating a case study of a patient they each had an opportunity to work with on their most recent student clinical rotations. Although their clinical rotations ended before the patient completed the rehabilitation program, Linda followed the patient during the first part of her rehabilitation and David followed her through her middle phase, and so they are confident that they will be able to create an extensive and thorough program that the patient would have followed had they had the opportunity to see the patient through her final phase to return her to pitching softball. Their confidence comes from the experiences they have had throughout their final student year as well as the knowledge they have acquired about what a complete rehabilitation program should include.

A goal without a plan is just a wish.

Larry Elder, 1952-,
lawyer, author, media personality

Now that we have looked at the elements of therapeutic interventions and investigated their impact on rehabilitation, this chapter reassembles these elements, putting them into a workable template for a rehabilitation program. Therefore, we will put together the concepts, theories, and techniques that have been presented in parts I, II, and III of this book into a model that may be used and modified for the topics presented in the remaining chapters in part IV. As Mr. Elder indicates, you need to develop a plan to approach a problem and achieve your goal; this chapter creates the skeleton upon which you will develop a rehabilitation program, create a plan, and provide any patient you treat with the optimal goal of efficient and effective return to function. This chapter also includes information that you should have when designing a therapeutic exercise program but which was not discussed in earlier chapters. You should read this chapter before proceeding to part IV; this chapter presents the framework upon which all rehabilitation programs are designed.

By now it should be clear that rehabilitation clinicians wear many hats throughout a patient's rehabilitation program. As we saw in chapter 1, the clinician is a combination of detective, problem solver, innovator, and educator who follows the laws of physics, physiology, and kinesiology through acquired knowledge, skill, logic, and common sense to achieve the ultimate goal of returning patients to full function as efficiently and safely as possible. The detective work involves examining the injury's status, determining its underlying causes, and continually reassessing the patient's response to the interventions provided.

As a problem solver, the rehabilitation clinician must be able to adjust treatment programs, manual therapy techniques, exercises, and progression sequences when a patient does not respond as expected. As an innovator, the clinician tries to develop rehabilitation plans that achieve treatment goals while remaining interesting and stimulat-

ing for every patient in order to encourage compliance. If the selection of equipment is limited, innovation becomes even more important because it requires the clinician to be a "MacGyver," devising imaginative alternatives to make the program interesting and challenging with minimal resources.

Throughout a rehabilitation program, the clinician is an educator. The patient is educated about the dos and don'ts after an injury—what activities are important to perform and what activities should be avoided to protect the injury and to promote an uneventful yet progressive healing process. The patient is also educated with regard to the injury, the rehabilitation process, the rationale for specific interventions, and the importance of compliance with home exercises.

The rehabilitation clinician's knowledge, understanding, observation skills, examination skills, application skills, and ability to employ common sense and logic all contribute to the success of the rehabilitation process. Rehabilitation involves applying all of these skills and talents at the proper time to provide a balanced program for the patient—one that provides appropriate stresses with the necessary degree of protection to advance the patient efficiently and effectively toward the goal of safe return to function as quickly as possible.

Along with all of these caveats associated with putting a rehabilitation program together, the final one is that the rehabilitation clinician should make the program fun for both the patient and the clinician.

CLINICAL TIPS

The rehabilitation clinician is a combination of detective, problem solver, innovator, and educator who follows laws of physics, physiology, and kinesiology through acquired knowledge, skill, logic, and common sense to achieve the ultimate goal of returning a patient to full function as efficiently and safely as possible.

Rehabilitation Program Contents

The specific elements and the complexity of a rehabilitation program are determined by a variety of factors. These include the magnitude of the injury, the type of injury, the body segment involved, the patient's health, age, and activity level, the patient's response to the injury (physical, emotional, and psychological), and the patient's goals. All must be considered in the injury examination and rehabilitation program design.

CLINICAL TIPS

Factors that determine specific elements in a rehabilitation program, and which must be factored into the patient's examination and program design, include the magnitude of the injury, the type of injury, the body segment involved, the patient's health, age, and activity level, the patient's response to the injury (physical, emotional, and psychological), and the patient's goals.

Examination

Before providing treatment in a rehabilitation program, the rehabilitation clinician examines the injury to determine where in the healing process the injury is and how irritable it is. If the injury is very irritable, regardless of the healing stage, the treatment must begin gently and must consist primarily of modalities to calm the area. If the patient had reconstructive surgery 3 d ago, the initial treatments are not aggressive. If, on the other hand, the injury is not very irritable and is well along in the healing process, the clinician can be more aggressive in the first treatment. Whatever the initial treatment includes, the clinician must carefully observe the patient's and the injury site's responses, both during the treatment session and before the start of the next session. The course of the current treatment is always determined by the injury's response to the previous session.

Likewise, treatments are assessed for their effectiveness within a session. This requires the clinician to examine and assess a patient or a specific tissue both before and after treatment. How else can you know if a treatment has produced any benefit? The clinician's mantra should be *Assess, Assess, Assess!*

Maintenance of Conditioning Level

Periodically throughout this book, we have emphasized the importance of maintaining cardiovascular health and the conditioning levels of noninjured body segments. Although this is a vital aspect of a total rehabilitation program, it is not specifically presented in part IV; however, you should always include exercises to address these needs in a rehabilitation program. The exercises discussed in this part of the book include only those that are relevant to the injured segment and its injury.

Interventions

As discussed in chapter 5, your interventions with the patient include both procedural interventions and patient education and instructions. Patient education is one of your most powerful interventions. Educating patients about the clinical diagnosis, the prognosis, and the plan of care will help them to understand the rehabilitation process. Patient instructions about postural awareness, edema reduction principles, body mechanics, and proper execution of therapeutic exercises provide them with the tools they need to improve their function and well-being as they progress through their rehabilitation programs.

Procedural interventions include modalities, manual therapy, and therapeutic exercises to decrease pain, edema, and muscle spasms and to improve range of motion, flexibility, strength and endurance, neuromotor control and proprioception, and patient function. Which interventions you use will depend on the phase of tissue healing and the patient's specific problems and goals.

Modalities

Modalities were introduced in chapter 1 and were discussed more extensively in chapters 3 and 9. Modalities are used to modulate pain, reduce edema and muscle spasm, and promote tissue healing.[1, 2] They also serve as preliminary adjuncts to the total rehabilitation program; they should not be the primary means of treatment throughout the entire program. Once pain modulation and healing are under way, manual therapy and therapeutic exercises become the primary emphasis in the rehabilitation process.[3] However, electrical stimulation modalities may be used beyond the first rehabilitation phase to facilitate muscle activity, especially if the muscle is too weak to provide the desired response to therapeutic exercise.[4, 5]

An injury does not have to become entirely pain free before therapeutic exercises begin, and in fact most of the time it is not desirable to delay exercises until the patient is completely pain free. Pain and swelling are monitored throughout the rehabilitation process, especially in the first half of the program when the newly forming tissue is more susceptible to overstress from exercise than it is later. Both pain[6-8] and edema[9-11] act as neural inhibitors, reducing the patient's rehabilitation progress and his or her ability to perform therapeutic exercises and functional tasks. Modalities are used to modulate these symptoms.

Manual Therapy

In chapter 11, several manual therapy techniques were discussed. Most manual therapy techniques are aimed at relieving pain and improving mobility.[12-14] The manual therapy techniques most clinicians are familiar with include soft-tissue mobilization techniques and joint mobilization. The techniques you use will depend on the patient's specific problems and your treatment goals.

Soft-Tissue Mobilization

You may want to refer to chapter 11 to review specific soft-tissue mobilization techniques. You must examine the patient's injury to decide whether soft-tissue treatment may be appropriate. Keep in mind that this treatment is often necessary after injury. An extensive selection of soft-tissue techniques is available. However, the specific technique used depends on the clinician's familiarity, experience, knowledge, and skill level. Soft-tissue techniques can also be combined with manual stretching techniques, depending on the treatment goals.

Joint Mobilization

As presented in chapter 11, joint mobilization is a complex technique entailing either accessory movements or physiological movements. When using joint mobilization, you should remember that the movement is produced not by your hands but by your body; this gives you a better perception of the movement and produces a more comfortable sensation for the patient. The hands are the vehicles through which your body produces the joint motion.

Joint mobilization is not used in all conditions. It is used to treat pain or when capsular patterns of movement indicate that motion loss is attributable to capsular restriction.[15] Positive results from mobilization should usually occur within 4 to 5 d.[16] Recall from chapter 11 that joint mobilization is appropriate to treat pain using grade I and

II movements or to treat restricted joint mobility using grade III or IV movements. Joint mobilization movements can be oscillatory or sustained. Please refer to chapter 11 to review these techniques as needed.

Most of the joint mobilization techniques presented in part IV are based on a combination of Kaltenborn's[15] and Maitland's[17] works. The techniques applied in this text are not the only possible ones; scholars and clinicians have developed a number of variations.

Therapeutic Exercise

Many therapeutic exercise techniques are available to clinicians. For example, range-of-motion exercises, flexibility exercises, strengthening exercises, endurance exercises, neuromotor control activities, proprioception exercises, and functional training may be items and techniques you select for your patient's program. The exercises and techniques you use will depend on the examination findings, the phase of tissue healing, and the treatment goals.

Progression

You should have a reason for every intervention you use in a rehabilitation program. Programs may be similar from one patient to another, but they should never be the same because no two people are the same, and they will not respond to an injury—or a rehabilitation program—in exactly the same way.

Rehabilitation progression is based on several factors, including severity of injury, phase of tissue healing, patient age and general health, response to interventions, and activity, occupation, or sport demands of the patient.

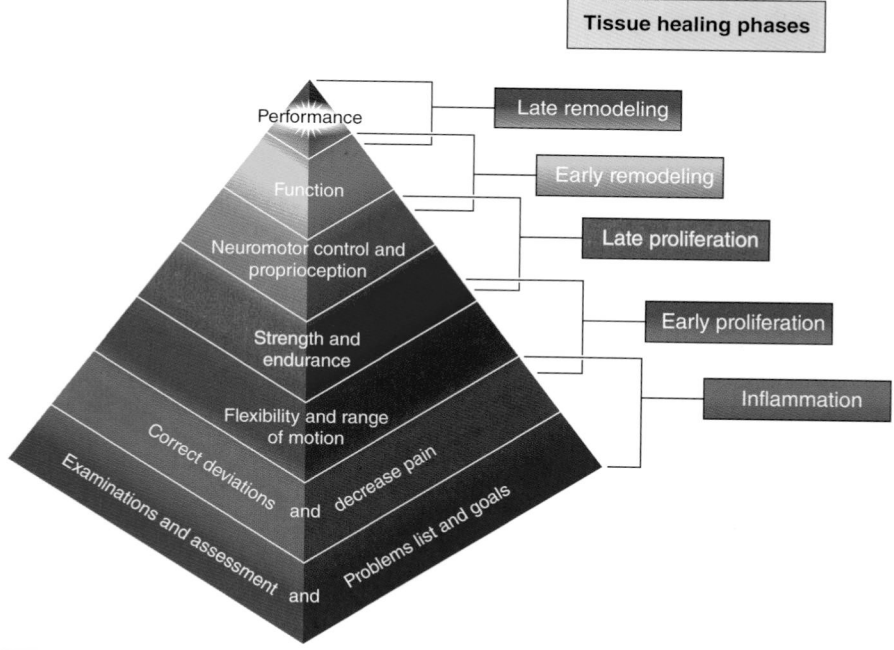

Figure 16.1 Pyramid demonstrating the components and progression of a rehabilitation program with respect to tissue healing phases.

Evidence in Rehabilitation

Barton and colleagues[19] performed an intensive study to identify best-practice guidelines in the management of patellofemoral pain. They combined systematic reviews of high-quality level 1 investigations with interviews of international specialists who had extensive clinical experience and research knowledge in the management of patellofemoral pain. They concluded that best-practice patellofemoral pain management included a multimodal rehabilitation approach. These interventions included modalities for pain control, patient education, manual therapy techniques, gait training, and a variety of exercises for flexibility, strength, and improved function.[19]

These practices are beneficial for more than just patellofemoral joint pain. As we have mentioned throughout this text, they are important to include in any rehabilitation program. Some elements are needed more than others in specific cases, but they are all available to clinicians to provide effective rehabilitation for their patients.

Progression also follows a hierarchy of function, which is outlined in the rehabilitation program pyramid presented in chapter 1. See figure 16.1 to see how these components correlate with the phases of tissue healing.

Evidenced-based practice (EBP) also guides the progression of a rehabilitation program. Program decisions are made based on information obtained through research and investigation, the clinician's experience and skill set, and the patient's needs and goals.

Remember the familiar advice of Hippocrates: Do no harm.[18] If you are unsure about whether to advance a patient's program, do not do so until you are sure it is appropriate. If you have any doubt about whether an exercise or technique may cause edema or increased pain later, consider lessening the intensity. As you learn more about each patient's ability to tolerate the stresses of the interventions, and as your judgment of rehabilitation progressions improves with experience, you will more accurately gauge the appropriate stress levels for each patient.

Phases of Rehabilitation

The rehabilitation program can be divided into four phases or stages: (1) inactive, (2) active, (3) resistive, and (4) advanced. These phases correlate with the tissue healing progression from the time immediately after an injury up to the point where heavy stresses may be safely applied near the end of the healing process. Each rehabilitation phase overlaps with the phase on either side of it. The progression of each phase of rehabilitation is determined by the tissue healing progression, and it also follows the hierarchy of function outlined in the rehabilitation program pyramid. See figure 16.2 to see how the phases of rehabilitation coincide with the phases of tissue healing and the

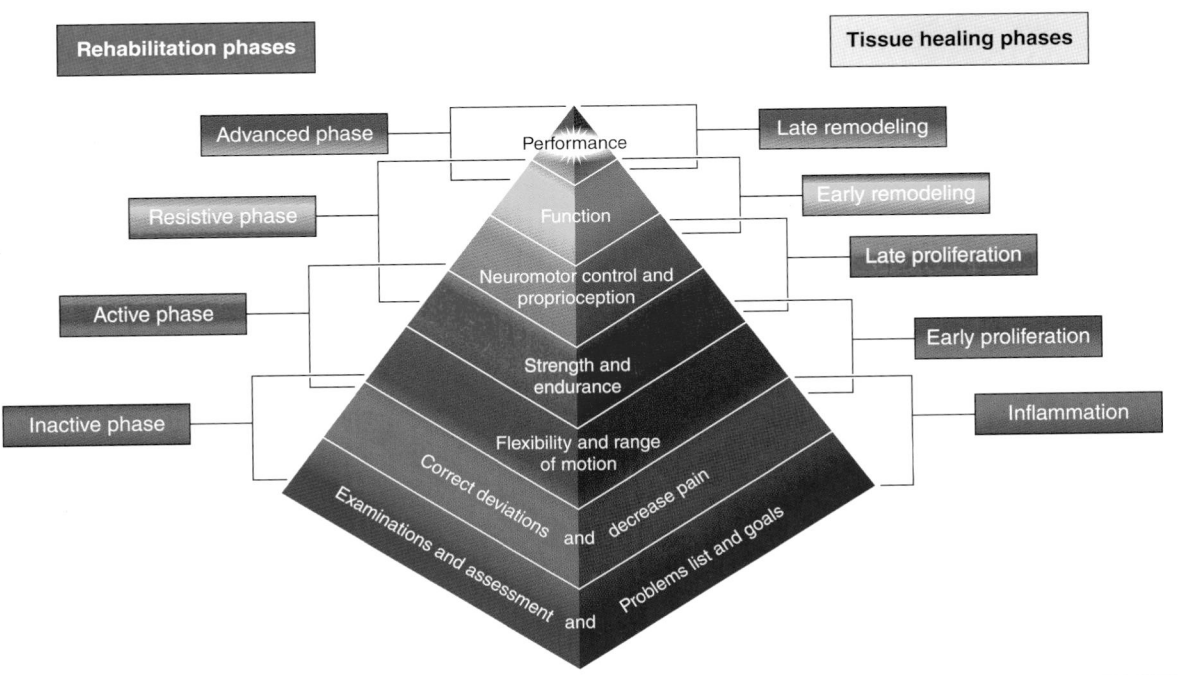

Figure 16.2 Phases of rehabilitation coincide with the phases of tissue healing in a rehabilitation program.

pyramid that displays the components and progression of a rehabilitation program.

The phases of rehabilitation can also be associated with specific therapeutic interventions. In the early phases of rehabilitation, modalities are used to control pain, muscle spasm, and edema associated with the initial injury and the early phases of healing. In the later phases of rehabilitation, manual therapy and therapeutic exercises are added as the tissue can better tolerate stress, and the treatment goals shift to improving function. See figure 16.3.

Phase I: Inactive Phase

The early part of the rehabilitation program is especially important since it addresses the injury's initial problems: pain, muscle spasm, and edema. The rehabilitation clinician may not be involved during the first phase of tissue healing, hemostasis, but the first phase of rehabilitation begins during the inflammation phase. The injured region is weak and vulnerable; therefore, this is a time of relative inactivity for the injured segment. Treatment focuses on relieving the immediate problems that the injury creates for the specific structures and their surrounding tissues. If these problems are controlled and healing is encouraged in an optimal environment, advancement to the remaining phases can occur as expected. The clinician attends to these symptoms while also being careful to avoid causing additional damage. Refer to figure 16.3 to see that this rehabilitation phase corresponds with the first phase of tissue healing.

The general goals of this phase are to *relieve* pain, edema, and muscle spasm. An additional goal is to maintain proper conditioning in the unaffected body segments and the cardiovascular system. Since the injured tissue is in the inflammation phase, caution must be part of the treatment protocol. Remember that for the first several days after an injury, the only substance holding the injury site together and preventing additional bleeding is the weak and fragile fibrin clot. Aggravating the injury site is contraindicated.

Therapeutic modalities are effective tools for achieving the goals of the inactive phase.[1] Later in this phase, when inflammation is waning, manual therapy techniques that focus on reducing pain, spasm, and swelling are appropriate. Motion and exercise of the injured segment are usually not performed during this phase so that the fragile healing tissue will not be damaged. Depending on the injury's severity, location, and onset, the patient's age and health, and other factors, early range-of-motion activities may begin at the end of this phase.

Patient education and instructions are particularly important during the inactive phase. Instructions about such topics as edema reduction, sling and splint positioning, proper use of ambulatory aids, body mechanics, and ergonomics all encourage patients to participate in the healing process and promote their own well-being.

Phase II: Active Phase

Phase II begins once the injured segment is past the inflammation phase and is in the early proliferation phase. Tissue strength is increasing through collagen fiber development, and structures are becoming resilient enough to tolerate some stress. Therefore, mild activity of the injured segment may be permitted. Pain, edema, and muscle spasm are no longer the major focus but are minor issues that are still resolving. Appropriate therapeutic modalities may

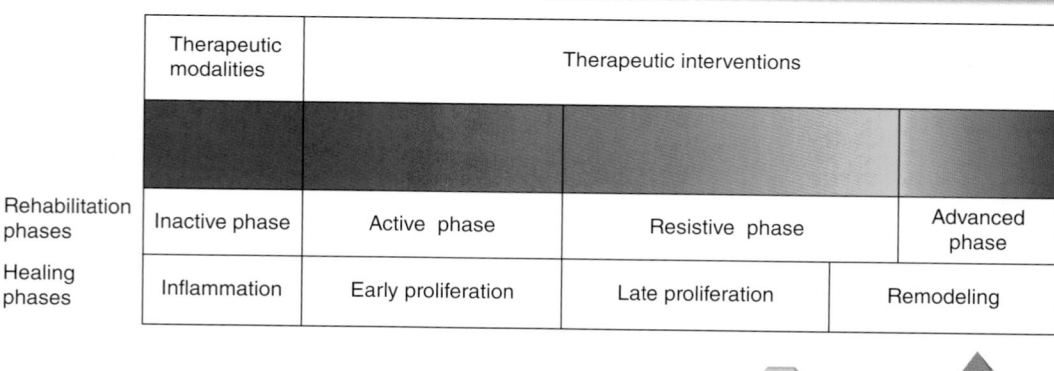
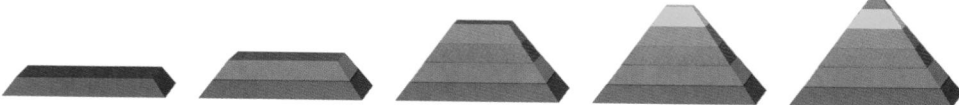

Figure 16.3 Phases of rehabilitation.

continue to be used during this phase to further alleviate any lingering symptoms of the injury and to mitigate any soreness or edema that may develop from beginning the active phase of rehabilitation. During phase II, the secondary effects of inflammation are resolved and eliminated as pertinent problems. Phase II of rehabilitation extends into the beginning of late proliferation of tissue healing.

General goals during this rehabilitation phase are to resolve any remaining inflammation signs and symptoms, improve mobility, normalize gait and posture, and begin to improve strength, endurance, proprioception, and neuromotor control. Treatment in this phase includes range-of-motion exercises and may include mobility techniques such as joint and soft-tissue mobilization. In the case of lower-extremity injuries, gait activities begin in this phase of rehabilitation. Although concepts of posture and postural awareness were presented during phase I of rehabilitation, phase II is when exercises to improve and correct posture are begun.

If any exercises were started during late inflammation, they were likely range-of-motion exercises. In the active phase, as tissue stability increases, early strength and simple static proprioception exercises may begin, but this decision is based on a number of factors such as the severity of the injury, the tissue that is injured, the location of the injury, and the patient's age and general health. The closer to the inflammation phase the injury is, the more cautious the clinician must be with the amount of stress applied to newly developing tissue. In some cases, exercises may not be permitted until 3 to 4 weeks after injury;[20-22] when exercises are delayed for longer periods than this, the risk of serious and permanent changes in the injured site's mobility becomes significant.[23, 24]

Range of motion and flexibility are important factors to restore during the active phase and are the primary exercises in this phase. Along with joint and soft-tissue mobilization techniques, passive, active, and assistive exercises can be used to improve motion, but the type of tissue and the location of the injury will dictate if the motion exercises are active or passive. For example, active exercises are generally used before passive motion exercises in the hand,[25] but passive motion activities are initiated before active exercises after musculotendinous injuries of other segments such as the knee or shoulder.[26, 27]

Normal gait is necessary for normal function. Just as the clinician assesses and corrects the patient's improper execution of exercises to achieve desired goals, he or she must also assess and correct improper gait to restore normal ambulation.

Likewise, postural alignment must be assessed and corrected in this rehabilitation phase. In good postural alignment, the body is balanced so that stress applied to the body segments is minimal. In some cases, poor posture may have been the cause of the injury, so unless posture is corrected, the patient's injury will recur. For example, poor posture is a contributor to glenohumeral impingement.[28]

Early nonresistive strengthening exercises are included in phase II; the tissue involved, type of injury, patient issues, and physician preference are some factors that determine when nonresistive strength exercises begin. If strengthening is initiated in rehabilitation phase II, it will occur in the mid- to late portion of this phase; early strengthening exercises will likely include isometrics and easy concentric, concentric–eccentric, or eccentric exercises that use no more than the weight of the body segment. Isometric exercises are often performed at either multiple angles, midrange, or in an anatomic position, depending on mobility and the physician's motion restrictions. As the neuromuscular system is facilitated with nonresistive exercises, simple static balance activities are added at the end of phase II. These types of exercises may be included at the end of this phase because the injured tissue is becoming more resilient and better able to tolerate initial neuromuscular control and proprioception activities.

Phase III: Resistive Phase

By the time the patient progresses to the rehabilitation program's resistive phase, range of motion is nearly or completely restored. Edema and pain are no longer problems. Tissue healing has progressed to the end of proliferation and during this phase will move into early remodeling. Muscle strength, endurance, and proprioception have improved somewhat but remain deficient. This phase is called the resistive phase because our primary focus is on using resistance exercises to completely restore any deficiencies in strength, muscle endurance, and neuromotor function. Tensile strength of the injured tissue is much greater than in earlier phases. Throughout this phase, therapeutic exercises become progressive in their intensity, complexity, and rigor as the injured segment becomes stronger and more resilient.

Phase III begins in the late proliferation phase and progresses into the early remodeling phase of tissue healing. Precisely when this phase begins depends on the specific injury, the physician's preference for progression, and the patient's response to the program. Usually, however, resistance begins during later proliferation. The resistive phase is often delayed when rehabilitation involves structures with delayed healing or tenuous tissue. General goals during phase III include maintaining the parameters that have been restored and restoring the patient's strength, muscle endurance, neuromotor control, and agility to normal levels.

If range of motion and flexibility have not been restored, you can be more aggressive with your mobilization and stretching techniques in late phase III to seek normal mobility. Depending on the structures involved, you may use deeper soft-tissue techniques, more aggressive stretching techniques, and grade IV joint mobilization techniques to restore full mobility.

Strength exercises are initially performed in a straight plane. They progress to diagonal functional patterns when the patient has enough strength to control the extremity correctly through a functional motion. It is common for strength exercises to begin with high repetitions and low resistance.[29] This approach reduces stress on joints and tissues that may not yet be strong or stable enough to tolerate the shear or overload forces produced by heavy resistance. With lower resistance and higher repetitions, the primary gains are in muscular endurance, with secondary gains in muscle strength. Exercises later in this phase include more aggressive resistance training and muscle endurance exercises as the tissue's healing and maturation progress.

Proprioception and neuromotor control exercises progress as healing continues through this phase. The exercises advance from basic static exercises to more complex static activities and then to more challenging dynamic balance and agility exercises. The exercises throughout this phase prepare the patient for the stresses of functional and performance-specific activities in the next phase.

Phase IV: Advanced Phase

Once the goals of phase III are achieved, the patient moves into the final phase of rehabilitation, the advanced phase. It is called the *advanced phase* because exercises during this phase mimic the stresses that the patient will encounter when he or she returns to normal activities. By the time the patient reaches this final phase, mobility, flexibility, strength and muscle endurance, proprioception, and neuromotor control are all at normal or near-normal levels; the patient is now ready for more advanced, aggressive activities that further stress the injured area in preparation for a return to his or her normal activities.

Patients often lack confidence in their ability to return to previous activities; fear of reinjury is common.[30] During this phase, one of the clinician's goals is to instill confidence in the patient by having the patient perform skilled activities that demonstrate restored competence and complete healing of the injured segment.

At this point, the only real physical deficit lies in the patient's functional and performance abilities, so the general goals in this phase are to restore these abilities as well as to renew the patient's confidence in his or her ability to perform all the functional activities of an occupation or sport. Flexibility and strength activities are now at maintenance levels, and the major emphasis is on finely tuning the patient for a smooth transition to normal function in whatever environment the patient will return to.

Functional and performance-specific exercises are a vital part of the final phase of rehabilitation. Functional activities should evolve to a progression of performance-specific exercises. Functional activities begin with reduced stress, speed, force, and distance and increase in each of these parameters as the patient's body adjusts to the stresses. As the patient improves, the focus moves from functional activities to performance-specific exercises. If the patient is a volleyball athlete, exercises in this phase begin with volleyball drills at a slow, controlled speed and progress into game play activities. If the patient is a construction worker, exercises in this phase may begin with tasks such as wearing a tool belt and progress to exercises that mimic all of the activities the patient will encounter on the job. The patient who demonstrates normal confidence and performance in these activities has achieved the final goals of the rehabilitation program and may be discharged.

Progression of Rehabilitation Phases

The interventions for each phase lie on a continuum (figure 16.4). On the continuum are all the previously presented parameters, as well as interventions corresponding to the phases. The diagram outlines the progression of a rehabilitation program—including range of motion, strength, endurance, proprioception, neuromotor control, functional and performance-specific exercises—through the active, resistive, and advanced phases. (No exercise occurs during the inactive phase as the injured segment begins to heal.) All exercises in a rehabilitation program flow from one level to the next and are based on the tissue healing phases.

Figure 16.4 may give you a mental image that helps you to advance a patient in a rehabilitation program. A good rehabilitation program progresses in a challenging yet safe manner. A good progression matches the patient's healing rate and challenges the patient without causing negative effects such as increased pain, swelling, or a reduced ability to function.

Each time you see a patient, you evaluate the patient's status both before and during treatment. You must not only determine how the patient reacted to the previous treatment but also ensure that healing is occurring as expected. As the patient's injury moves through the phases of tissue healing, the patient also progresses through the corresponding phases of rehabilitation.

If, in your evaluation, you find signs and symptoms of new tissue inflammation between treatment sessions, you must determine why this is occurring. As long as the injured segment remains in the inflammatory phase, the patient cannot advance to the next rehabilitation phase. If the patient has an inflammatory reaction to a part of the treatment program, you must identify what caused it and then treat the inflammation before the patient can advance further. Once you have identified what caused the reaction, you make adjustments to the next treatment so that the patient can advance without another setback. Perhaps you overestimated the injured site's ability to tolerate an

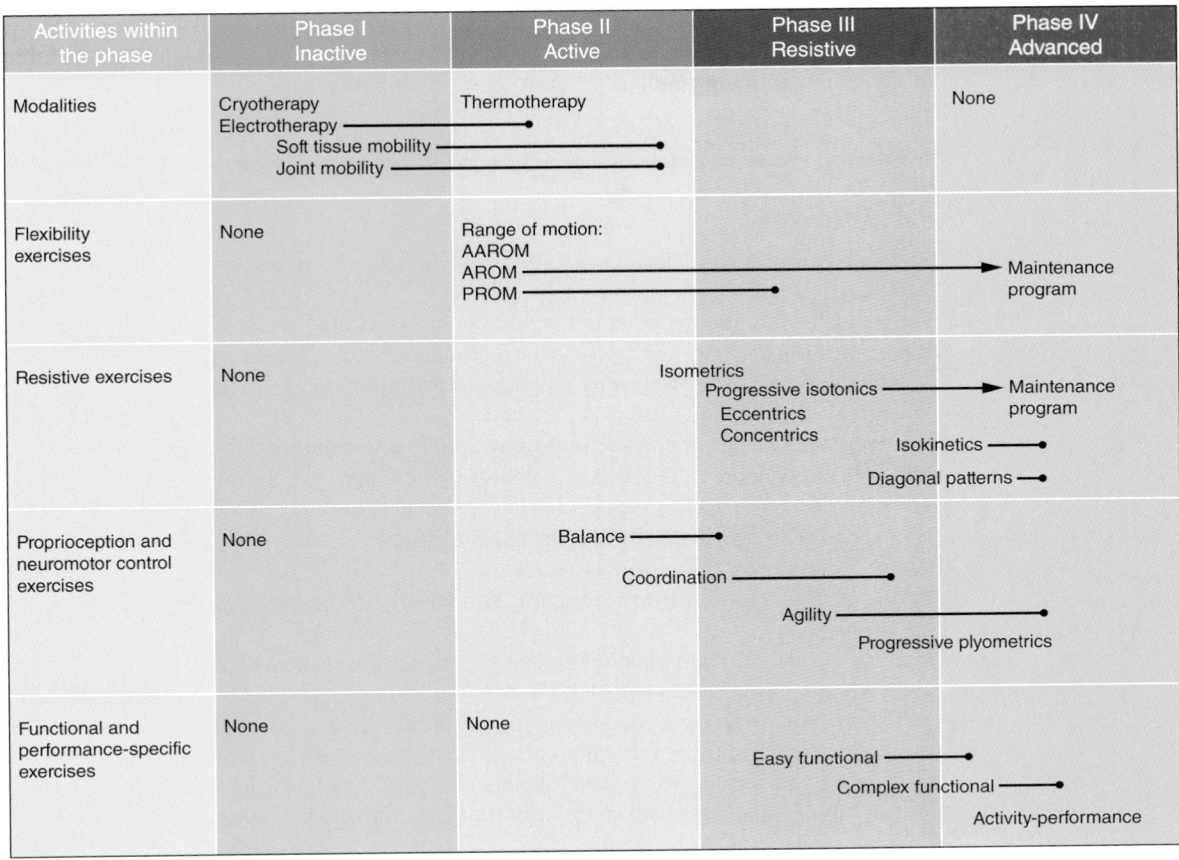

Activities within the phase	Phase I Inactive	Phase II Active	Phase III Resistive	Phase IV Advanced
Modalities	Cryotherapy Electrotherapy ——————	Thermotherapy • Soft tissue mobility ————————• Joint mobility ————————•		None
Flexibility exercises	None	Range of motion: AAROM AROM ———————————————→ PROM ——————————————•		Maintenance program
Resistive exercises	None		Isometrics Progressive isotonics ————————→ Eccentrics Concentrics Isokinetics ————• Diagonal patterns —•	Maintenance program
Proprioception and neuromotor control exercises	None	Balance ————• Coordination ————————• Agility ————————• Progressive plyometrics •		
Functional and performance-specific exercises	None	None	Easy functional ————• Complex functional ————• Activity-performance	

Figure 16.4 Rehabilitation program continuum. The progression of interventions after the inactive phase is based on a tissue's ability to withstand stresses as it moves through healing.

exercise's new stress level; now that you have a better idea of what the injury can tolerate, you can provide more appropriate exercises.

Individualization of a Rehabilitation Program

You must design a rehabilitation program specific for each person.[31] Two patients with grade II ankle sprains will not necessarily progress at the same rate, so you cannot expect them to follow the same timeline. These patients may even need different exercises. The injury and the body's response to it, the patient's abilities and goals, and the way the patient responds to both the program and the clinician all determine the interventions selected, the rate of progression, and the final outcome of the rehabilitation program.

The clinician should continually assess the patient's performance; examine outcomes before, during, and after each session to see whether the treatment has had the desired effect; and be ready to alter treatments if undesirable effects occur. It is essential to obtain information from the patient about post-treatment responses in order to accurately assess the effects of the treatment program. If increased pain, swelling, and other deleterious effects occur after treatment, the program has been too stressful. *Progression without regression* should be the rehabilitation clinician's creed. In other words, the program should challenge the patient enough to improve all parameters without overstressing the injury.

Summary

This chapter provided you with an overall perspective on the important elements and progressions of a rehabilitation program. A template was provided that includes the four phases of a rehabilitation program. Rehabilitation phases coincide with the tissue healing phases. The initial rehabilitation phase focuses on relieving deleterious effects of inflammation, while the three remaining phases include a variety of interventions designed to create a progressive path for the patient's optimal recovery. Each of the rehabilitation phases contains specific types of interventions that are in accord with tissue strength and maturation changes that occur throughout the healing process. Although each patient responds differently to rehabilitation, all patients follow a similar path through the rehabilitation process to achieve an optimal outcome. This chapter provided an outline that may be used to design any rehabilitation program for any injury.

LEARNING AIDS

Key Concepts and Review

1. Identify the qualities a rehabilitation clinician should have in order to provide patients with a successful rehabilitation program.

The rehabilitation clinician is a combination of detective, problem solver, innovator, and educator who follows laws of physics, physiology, and kinesiology through acquired knowledge, skill, logic, and common sense to achieve the final goal of returning a patient to full function as efficiently and safely as possible.

2. Explain why examination and assessment are important parts of a rehabilitation program.

Before providing treatment, the rehabilitation clinician examines the injury to determine where in the healing process the injury is and how irritable it is. Likewise, the rehabilitation clinician must examine and assess a patient's or specific tissue's status before, during, and after treatment; there is no other way to determine if the treatment produces the desired outcomes.

3. Identify the four phases of a rehabilitation program, and briefly describe what is included in each phase.

The four phases in a rehabilitation program include the inactive phase (phase I), where modalities and gentle manual therapy techniques are used to reduce inflammation and encourage healing. Later in the phase, gentle manual therapy techniques can be used to decrease pain and edema. The active phase (phase II) is when manual therapy and range-of-motion and flexibility activities are used to restore mobility, nonresistive exercises are used to begin development of strength and neuromotor control, and static balance exercises are used to improve proprioception. In the resistive phase (phase III), strength and endurance exercises, as well as more challenging static and dynamic proprioception exercises, are used to restore strength, endurance, and proprioception. In the advanced phase (phase IV), the final phase of rehabilitation, functional and performance-based activities are used to restore confidence and return the patient to full and optimal function.

4. Discuss the types of interventions that are usually included in each of the rehabilitation exercise phases.

In the active phase, joint mobilization, soft-tissue mobilization, and active, active-assistive, and passive exercises are used to improve mobility. Nonresistive exercises are used to improve neuromuscular control. Beginning static balance activities are used to improve proprioception. In the resistive phase, a progression of resistive strengthening exercises is included along with more challenging exercises to improve proprioception. Multiplanar diagonal activities and functional exercises are initiated. The advanced phase includes more advanced functional exercises, and finally, performance-specific exercises to improve confidence and restore the patient's prior level of function.

Critical Thinking Questions

1. If you were discussing the opening scenario with Linda and David, what do you think they should have included in the progression of their patient's rehabilitation program? What should they use to determine when their patient should progress through the different rehabilitation phases?

2. You are rehabilitating two patients; one is recovering from a severe ankle sprain, and the other had an anterior cruciate ligament reconstruction. Identify how their rehabilitation programs would be the same and how they would differ.

3. Outline a rehabilitation program for a 17-year-old patient who suffered a second-degree ankle sprain. Create a timeline for his recovery, and itemize the types of activities you would include in each phase of his rehabilitation program. He is using crutches because it is too painful to walk without them, but the physician has told you that he can advance to full weight bearing as tolerated. There is moderate swelling and reduced soft-tissue mobility; joint range of motion is limited and demonstrates a capsular pattern in sagittal and frontal plane motions. Strength is difficult to assess

because of his pain, but given the severity of his injury and his time on crutches, you assume that he has weakness in all ankle and foot muscle groups. He wants to return to playing and competing with his high school's soccer team as soon as possible.

4. As you move any patient through a rehabilitation progression, identify how you would determine when the patient can move from phase I to phase II, from phase II to phase III, and from phase III to phase IV.

Lab Activities

1. Present to your lab partner a case-study scenario that he or she will use to outline a rehabilitation program. Your lab partner should make up a different case-study scenario to give to you. After each of you works on creating the rehabilitation program for the case study you have been given, compare the two programs. How are they the same? How are they different?

2. Create a list of at least four different injuries and the rehabilitation programs you have participated in or observed during your clinical experiences. List with them the severity of the injury and the activities involved in the rehabilitation programs. Can you see how the severity of the injury relates to the speed with which the patient advances in the rehabilitation process? What other factors did you notice that affect the progression and duration of the rehabilitation program?

3. Outline a rehabilitation program for the following conditions:

    A. Mild ankle sprain in a high school football lineman

    B. Elbow dislocation in a college wrestler

    C. Moderate lumbar strain of a 70-year-old man who is a type 2 diabetic

    D. Moderate rotator cuff strain of a flight attendant

    Include within each phase the likely elements (e.g., modalities, manual therapy, active stretching, isometrics, etc.) that you would use to advance the patient through the rehabilitation program. Identify what factors would have to be considered as the patient progresses in the program.

4. Work with your lab partner to create a list of differences between rehabilitation programs for two people with a moderate wrist sprain: a 19-year-old golfer and a 69-year-old golfer, each of whom wants to return to golfing.

PART IV

Rehabilitation of Body Segments

The quality of a person's life is in direct proportion to their commitment to excellence, regardless of their chosen field of endeavor.

Vince Lombardi, 1913-1970, NFL football coach

Parts I, II, and III established the groundwork for this final part of the book. Having acquired the information from the earlier parts, you are now prepared to fully understand, appreciate, and apply the information presented in part IV. Part IV is where you will put all the information and knowledge you have gained in the other parts into comprehensive rehabilitation programs. Each chapter in part IV is dedicated to a specific body segment; each contains information specific to that body segment and rehabilitation techniques that may be used. Each chapter presents the more commonly seen injuries that require rehabilitation.

Case studies are presented throughout each chapter. No answers are given for the questions that follow each case study because the studies are meant to stimulate discussion between students and their instructors. There is no single right answer for every question because the answer is driven by the particulars of the case and is to some extent flexible, as dictated by the rehabilitation clinician's preferences and the equipment available.

The rehabilitation programs presented are not divided by sport or activity, for an ankle sprain is an ankle sprain, regardless of whether it occurs in basketball, volleyball, or at work, and regardless of whether the patient is a teenager, college student, or retired person. The only point where a rehabilitation program for an injury will deviate substantially from one person to another is in the final stages of rehabilitation, when patients begin functional and performance exercises that will enable them to return to their regular activities.

Although timelines of normal progression are provided, part IV is not a cookbook for the rehabilitation of injuries. A cookbook is not needed, nor is it practical since every patient is unique and responds differently to injury and postinjury treatment. Part IV provides suggestions for exercises and treatment techniques, but for application, you will depend on the knowledge you have gained throughout this text to use those suggestions in an effective program you design for each patient.

Part IV begins with chapter 17, which provides sacroiliac and spine information. The axial skeleton is presented first because many upper- and lower-extremity problems are related to the core, the spine, and the sacroiliac and pelvic regions. The sacroiliac and spine are also important considerations in the rehabilitation of upper and lower extremities because core strength is vital for stability and performance in both upper and lower segments. Thus, the sacroiliac and spine are presented before the extremity chapters.

Chapters 18, 19, and 20 move to the lower-extremity segments; the final chapters (21 to 23) include rehabilitation programs for the upper extremities. The lower-extremity chapters are chapter 18 on the hip, chapter 19 on the knee and thigh, and chapter 20 on the foot, ankle, and leg. The upper-extremity chapters are chapter 21 on the shoulder and arm, chapter 22 on the elbow and forearm, and chapter 23 on the hand and wrist.

It would be nearly impossible to list all the exercises that could be included in a rehabilitation program for these segments. Exercises outlined in these chapters include the more commonly used activities as well as some that are unique. As always, the clinician's knowledge of injury healing, awareness of the patient's abilities, the facilities and equipment available, and the clinician's own imagination are the only limiting factors. A rehabilitation program can be fun and challenging both for the patient and for the rehabilitation clinician. The clinician can provide imaginative, stimulating exercises for the patient so both enjoy the process. As you read these next few chapters, see whether you can think of exercises in addition to those presented that would challenge and stimulate a patient in a rehabilitation program.

Spine and SI Joint

Objectives

After completing this chapter, you should be able to do the following:

1. Describe the closed sacroiliac ring and the lumbopelvic–hip complex, how they are related, and how they are important for functioning of the extremities.

2. Define the terms used in discussing sacroiliac stability, *form closure* and *force closure*.

3. Identify the third element in lumbopelvic–hip stability, and explain how it works with the other two.

4. Explain what the core muscles are and why they are important to function.

5. Identify three sacroiliac pathologies and their muscle energy release techniques.

6. Discuss the progression, or series of steps, involved in the rehabilitation of core muscles.

7. Identify three progressive spinal stability exercises.

8. Describe three flexibility exercises for the cervical spine and lumbar spine.

9. List precautions for a rehabilitation program for disc lesions.

10. Discuss the differences between rehabilitation programs for a lumbar strain and for a facet injury.

Will Floid has been a clinician in the city's largest sports medicine clinic for the past 2 years, ever since he graduated from Gilbert College, where he received his degree in athletic training. One of Will's fellow clinicians is Pam. She has been working with Bob for the last few weeks since Bob hurt his back while snowboarding. Pam has been helping Bob to improve his core strength as well as the strength of his larger trunk muscles and hip stabilizers.

Today Will has on his schedule a patient he will see for the first time, Violet Jann, a gymnast on the city's high school team. Will knows that Violet has pain in the low-back region, but he doesn't know where her pain originates. He knows that her pain could be related to the spine, the sacroiliac joints, or even the hip, so he goes through his mental list of ways to rule out each of these segments to come up with the real cause of Violet's pain. He has successfully treated back patients before, so he feels prepared to see this new patient. Even so, Will decides to ask Pam for advice on how to advance a core strengthening program since Pam has been progressing Bob through his rehabilitation program for the last few weeks. Will and Pam know that even though Violet's symptoms may be due to her sacroiliac joint and Bob's symptoms are from his lumbar spine facet sprain, core strength is important for both.

Life doesn't make any sense without interdependence.

Erik H. Erikson, 1902-1994,
German-American developmental
psychologist, author, educator

This chapter introduces the fun part of rehabilitation, applying the science that we have been learning and letting our imaginations create rehabilitation programs. We will begin to blend the science of rehabilitation with the art of imagination. We can now apply our scientific knowledge in an artful manner to provide patients with complete, stimulating, and challenging rehabilitation programs that will offer them a safe and speedy return to full participation and normal activity.

Clinicians are often more comfortable working with patients who have injured their extremities than patients with injuries to the less familiar spine and sacroiliac regions. As a result, they may devote less time and attention to these regions, and they may not enjoy working with patients who suffer injuries to the sacroilium or spine. This chapter will help you to understand that injuries to these segments, like injuries to the extremities, are approachable and treatable. You will develop an understanding of the relationship that several different regions of the body have with each other. The cervical spine, thoracic spine, rib cage, lumbar spine, sacrum, and pelvis are linked together and work together to provide a reliable platform from which the arms and legs can derive power and movement. Erikson's statement is timely and relevant, not only in reference to the human condition, but also with regard to the axial region of the body. Our body's efficient functioning depends on the neuromotor relationship between the pelvis, sacrum, rib cage, and spine. Because our arms and legs attach to that region, one can argue that their functions also rely upon the interdependence of the axial parts of the body.

The spine is composed of several different segments. Any segment can have injuries that do not affect the others. Any segment can also be injured in a way that affects or is affected by other regions. Between the regions of the spine, there are both similarities and unique features. For example, only in the thoracic region is each vertebra joined to a rib. The cervical spine includes the first spinal segment, the atlas, and the nerve bundle of the brachial plexus. The lumbar region contains the lumbar plexus nerve bundle, the largest vertebral bodies, and connections to the sacrum. Among the similarities that exist throughout the spine, vertebrae in the three regions all have spinous processes and transverse processes, and they are all separated by discs.

The sacro-pelvis unit is prone to unique injuries, and it also has unique examination procedures and techniques. This structure also has a unique anatomical configuration in that it forms a complete, closed system in which malalignment at one segment alters alignment at another segment within the unit. The rehabilitation clinician must appreciate each of these concepts to fully understand how the sacroilium and pelvis influence the rest of the spine as well as the upper and lower extremities.

This region of the body is complex. So is the shoulder. So is the ankle. There are many segments of the body that we as health care providers still have much to learn about, yet we do not hesitate to deal with injuries to these other segments. One of the goals of this chapter is to help you to appreciate the simplicity of this region and to lessen any fears you may have of treating this central segment of the body.

Many texts are devoted to spine and pelvis anatomy and function, so this chapter by no means deals with all there is to know about the spine and pelvis. The aim is to present information to enable you to rehabilitate spine, sacral, and pelvic injures that you will encounter as a rehabilitation clinician. Catastrophic injuries that include spinal cord injury resulting in paralysis are treated with rehabilitation exercises but not necessarily with the goal of returning the patient to sport participation or previous work tasks, so they will not be addressed here.

Special Rehabilitation Considerations

While the appendicular region of the body includes the extremities, the axial region includes the main axis of the body: the head, neck, thorax, and pelvis. The upper section of the axial region is often divided into the head, neck, and chest, while the lower section includes the trunk, lumbar, and pelvic areas.

When dealing with injuries and rehabilitation of the axial portion of the body, the clinician must realize that pain referral patterns can make clinical diagnosis difficult. Some facts to keep in mind include these:[1-3]

- The cervical spine can refer into the thoracic spine.
- The neck can refer into the shoulder and upper extremity.
- The shoulder can refer into the neck.
- The lumbar spine can refer into the sacroiliac or hip.
- The sacroiliac can refer into the lumbar spine.
- The hip can refer into the lumbar spine.
- Pain down the lower extremity does not necessarily indicate sciatica.

Additionally, the clinician should realize that back injuries can sometimes involve more than one problem. For example, a patient with pain shooting down the lower extremity may not only have back and leg pain but a facet injury as well. Poor posture often complicates a patient's

injury,[4] so the clinician should routinely perform a posture assessment as part of the examination. Improper use of body mechanics, such as chronically picking up a book bag from the floor incorrectly or sleeping in the wrong position, can continue to aggravate a patient's injury.

Since the lower portion of the spine has more injuries than the upper portion,[5] this chapter will contain more information about the lower spine and pelvis than about the upper spine. The cervical and thoracic spine sections will not be overlooked, however. Many of the topics discussed in this chapter, such as core recruitment and pelvic stability, influence the upper spine because of its muscle attachment sites. The cervical spine is also influenced by posture[6] and rib rotation during respiration,[7] both of which have been discussed in previous chapters and will be addressed in this chapter as well.

In the lower portion of the axial skeleton, the sacroilium and the pelvis create a sacroiliac ring, which is a closed ring connecting the left and right hemipelvises together. Each hemipelvis, consisting of an ilium, pubis, and ischium, is connected anteriorly at the pubic symphysis joint and posteriorly by the sacrum and its two sacroiliac joints. The pelvis is a platform to which three large levers are attached and upon which they act; these levers are the spine and the two lower extremities.[8] Because of the direct attachment of these segments to the pelvis, they can influence the pelvis, and likewise the pelvis can influence the function of these three segments. The pelvis, lumbar vertebrae, and hip joints together are often referred to as the lumbopelvic–hip complex.[9] Here are two examples of how these segments are related to one another: (1) An anteriorly tilted pelvis places the hips in more flexion, while a posteriorly tilted pelvis produces more hip extension, and (2) a lordotic lumbar spine causes the pelvis to tilt anteriorly (figure 17.1).

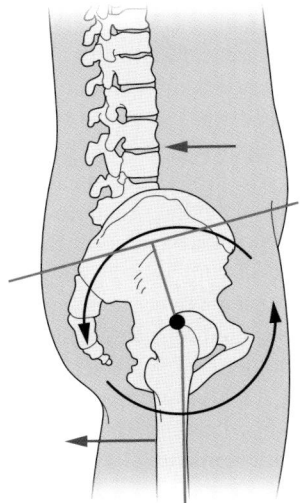 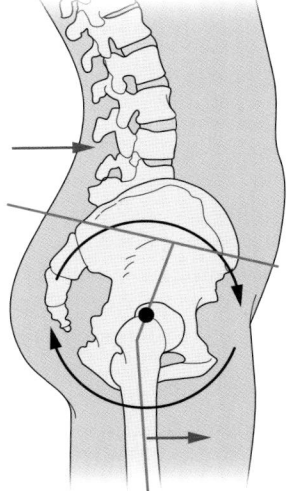

Figure 17.1 Movement relationships between the pelvis and hips and between the pelvis and spine. Notice with the tilting of the pelvis that the hip position changes, and the relationship between the pelvis and lumbar spine also changes.

Given the anatomical relationship between the lumbar spine and the sacrum, it should not be surprising that the lumbar spine, sacrum, and pelvis also have a functional relationship. Treatment of the spine has evolved over time. Treatment formerly consisted of bed rest for extended periods, but thankfully, medical professionals have realized how detrimental immobility is to the lumbar spine and sacroiliac region. Current treatments include minimal rest and progression into activity much more quickly than in the past.[10]

Although the sacroiliac joints are the largest joints in the spine complex, motion within these joints is known to be small;[11] how small is a matter of dispute. Various investigations have produced different results.[12] For example, in the sagittal plane, the plane with the most motion, studies report from 3° to 17° of motion, with linear motion between the posterior superior iliac spines and the sacrum ranging from 4 mm to 8 mm.[13] Although the amount of mobility measured within the sacroiliac joints may be small and variable, there is now general agreement that this region is responsible for back and pelvic pain.[14, 15]

It has also recently become generally accepted that stabilization of this region is important for relieving pain and transmitting force up and down the kinetic chain between the extremities and trunk.[16, 17] Investigations have shown that the converse is also true: dysfunction in the sacroiliac joints promotes back and pelvic pain.[16] It is therefore important to have good mechanical relationships within the spine, sacroiliac joints, and pelvis for people to be pain free and to function well in their daily and sport activities. Before we can discuss stabilization, questions must be answered.

One of the first questions is, what is lumbopelvic–hip stabilization? Several different terms have been created to define it. You may have heard of some of these: core stabilization or stability, lumbar stabilization or stability, pelvic stabilization or stability, trunk stabilization or stability, spinal stabilization or stability. It can get confusing with so many terms being used to define the same concept.

Stabilization

Having recognized that these terms are essentially synonymous, we ask what it is that provides this stabilization. The pelvis provides stability in three ways: through its form closure, force closure, and neuromotor control.[18, 19] **Form closure** refers to the stability of the pelvic ring provided by the joint's shape and structure, while **force closure** refers to the stability provided by the dynamic forces acting on the pelvis.[18] **Neuromotor control** is the proper activation and sequential recruitment of muscles to produce the correct response.[20] All three of these elements must be functioning properly and working together to create optimal lumbopelvic–hip stabilization.[21, 22]

Form closure is the result of both the joint's shape and the ligaments that support it.[23] The sacroiliac joints have

a unique joint configuration with articular surfaces that change with age. While the articular surfaces of these joints are relatively smooth in younger people, by the time a person reaches the middle years of adulthood, these surfaces become ridged and grooved, more so in males than in females.[24] There are also a number of ligaments that provide added stability to this very congruent joint.[25] It is important to realize that these ligaments undergo frequent stress because of the forces transferred up and down the kinetic chain through the pelvis during functional activities.[26]

Force closure adds to the stability of the sacroiliac joints through the activation of muscles that are aligned to act as a corset, providing active protection of the joints and secondary reinforcement to the ligaments.[25] Such an arrangement allows for the transfer of forces up and down the system from the trunk to the legs and from the legs to the trunk.[25] Various muscles around the hips, pelvis, and trunk work to varying degrees to provide this active stability during movement. The muscles that can provide the greatest impact are those that are arranged in a transverse fashion relative to the sacroiliac joints; these include the transverse abdominis and pelvic floor muscles.[25] It is not surprising, then, to realize that these two muscle groups are very important in providing force closure and pelvic stabilization, especially during functional activities.

Neuromotor control is important to the normal function of any body segment.[20] Injury and pain often create disruption of normal neuromotor control.[8, 27] It is when this disruption of neuromotor control occurs that muscles function inappropriately, further adding to dysfunction and pathology.[28] In other words, patients with sacroiliac pain have poor recruitment of these muscles compared to those without pain.[28] It is therefore important to promote correct muscle activation and timing to provide optimal stabilization during movement of the lumbopelvic–hip complex.

Neuromotor control occurs through a combination of feedforward and feedback systems.[20] A feedforward system is used when a stress or load is anticipated and muscles are "set" in advance to create the stability needed to manage the anticipated load. Feedback systems are used to make the adjustments needed to stabilize the body or a body segment when the load changes or is different than expected. Although spinal and core stability involve both systems, the feedforward system is typically used to stabilize the spine during upper- and lower-extremity activities. For example, the transverse abdominis normally fires before the shoulder muscles when the body prepares to throw an object,[29] but this timing is lacking in persons with a history of low-back pain.[30] Therefore, neuromotor control is an important element in the triad it creates with form closure and force closure; when all are working properly, the three together create stability and promote core health.

An important question yet to be answered is, how should clinicians restore this optimal stabilization? The answer is easier than you may think. If any ligaments providing form closure are injured, they are treated like any other sprain with modalities and manual treatments to relieve pain and spasm and to minimize other immediate secondary effects of injury. Once these structures are injured, they will heal, but they will not be able to support the joints as they previously did, so the clinician must focus on the force closure structures to compensate for this. The clinician's goals are not only to strengthen the stabilizing muscles but also to help them to fire appropriately.[31, 32] Because this is so important, neuromotor control of the core muscles will be a recurring theme of this chapter.

CLINICAL TIPS

Lumbopelvic–hip stabilization relies on the interaction of three important elements: (1) form closure of the sacroiliac joints' unique structural congruency; (2) force closure created by the local and global muscles of the core, and (3) neuromotor control provided by sensory input and feedback to and from the central nervous system. All three systems create an environment in which stability, refined movement, and power transmission occur.

Importance of the Core in Axial Function

Although many terms can be used for **lumbopelvic stabilization**, we will use the term *core stability*, which should make it less confusing as we go through the chapter. Since there are nearly as many definitions as there are terms to describe lumbopelvic stabilization, we will use this definition: the ability to maintain and control proper sacroiliac positioning to provide trunk stability with correct movement over the pelvis and lower extremities, allowing optimal function and performance of the extremities.[33] A word picture that may be helpful is a boat tied to a dock. The boat is moving, but it isn't free to float away and move in any direction. There is a constraint to its movement in the relationship the boat has to the dock.

The foundation for any successful movement is stability.[34] The body is designed to provide stability during functional movement through its "core" muscles; the shoulder joint is stabilized by scapular muscles,[35] and the hip is stabilized by gluteal muscles.[36] The spine is also stabilized by its core.[37] Because the core is so important to spinal stability, we will spend time examining its mechanics, pathology, and rehabilitation.

The Core

We know that the spine by itself cannot support any significant load; by itself, it collapses with no more than 5 lb (about 2 kg) applied to it.[38] Therefore, it receives a signif-

icant amount of support and stability from its surrounding muscles. As previously mentioned, trunk stability is often discussed in relation to what is known as the core. Some people think of the core as a box or cylinder of muscles in which the top consists of the diaphragm, the bottom is the pelvic floor, the front and sides are the abdominal muscles, and the back is the paraspinals and gluteals (figure 17.2).[39] So when we speak of the core, we are referring to the muscles of the pelvis and trunk and their ability to provide stability and control for functional movement.[33] Basic biomechanical principles tell us that if there is to be a power transfer, it has to occur through stable structures. Because the pelvis and trunk are the means by which power is transferred between the upper and lower extremities,[40] these elements that make up the core must be strong and stable since they are important to performance; therefore, they need to be included in either conditioning or rehabilitation programs.[41]

Stability within the lumbopelvic–hip region is essential to the performance of difficult tasks, such as athletic feats or lifting or moving heavy objects at work. Neuromotor control is important not only when you must produce a great deal of muscular force, but also when you perform less rigorous activities such as walking and breathing.[42-44]

Since there is a relationship between poor posture and back pain,[45] it stands to reason that posture plays a vital role in both recovery from and prevention of injuries.[46] As discussed in chapter 6, if an injured patient has poor posture and nothing is done to correct it, the poor posture will continue to affect the injury and make recovery more

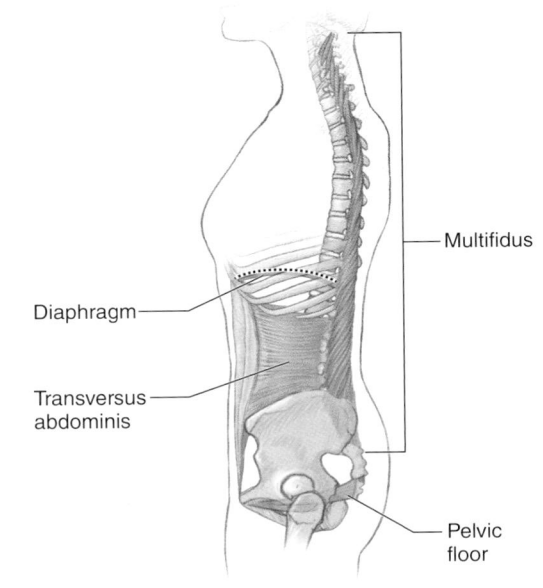

Figure 17.2 Core muscles form a box or cylinder at the innermost level of the trunk.

difficult.[47] Instruction in techniques to maintain proper posture and to use proper body mechanics should be a part of the rehabilitation program and will be discussed later in this chapter.

The art and science of treating lumbopelvic–hip injuries include the science behind the physiology and biomechanics of spinal, sacral, and pelvifemoral exercises and the art of knowing how and when to use them to create individualized rehabilitation programs. This chapter provides a partial list of exercises commonly used to treat injuries to this region.

Interest in the core developed in the latter half of the 20th century after Kennedy[48] suggested that the abdominal muscles brace the spine by increasing intra-abdominal pressure to stabilize the trunk during movement. Since then, we have understood the importance of intra-abdominal pressure in spine support and stability.[49] When intra-abdominal pressure is created, it converts the trunk into a solid cylinder to withstand compressive and shear loads placed on it.[50] Both the diaphragm and pelvic floor muscles increase intra-abdominal pressure when activated.[44, 51] The pelvic floor and multifidus muscles are coactivated when the transverse abdominis contracts.[52, 53] Since the diaphragm activates during upper-extremity activities, it is presumed that the diaphragm has the dual responsibility of providing not only respiration but also postural stability.[54] So for this intra-abdominal pressure to be produced during difficult activities that require core stability, there must be a coordinated and synchronous effort of the abdominal muscles, pelvic floor, and diaphragm.[50]

Stiffness is a factor in the prevention and treatment of injuries,[27] including low-back pain. Stiffness is the result of a combination of active and passive elements.[55] The passive elements are the ligaments, capsules, and fascia that surround the lumbar spine and trunk region. The active elements are the muscles. The region's superficial and deep muscles play a role in providing stiffness for the spine. A strong muscle is stiffer than a weak one.[56] If a sacroiliac ligament is injured, then the muscles in the area must compensate for the ligament's loss of normal stiffness; therefore, strong muscles are important to the rehabilitation of pelvis and back injuries.

Investigators, authors, and clinicians have identified the core muscles in different ways.[57] Some identify the core as including both active and inactive elements,[58] while others include muscles from the cervical region and diaphragm[59] to the thigh muscles.[33, 60] In defining the core muscles, Bergmark[61] distinguished between the trunk movers and the trunk stabilizers, referring to the trunk stabilizers as *local muscles* and the trunk movers as *global muscles*. He identified the **local muscles** as those muscles close to the center of the body that provide stability because their moment-arm lengths are too short to provide significant movement.[61] He identified the **global muscles** as those that

provide gross trunk motions because they are sufficiently distanced from the center of motion and have longer moment arms that cover many more spinal segments.[61] It was not long after Bergmark's ideas were presented that Panjabi and his group provided a rationale through their development of a biomechanical model in which both the local and global muscles are needed for spinal stability.[38] It may seem irrelevant, then, to distinguish between local and global muscles. However, their functions are different, so we need to understand these differences before we can design a rehabilitation program that includes core stability.

The global, or superficial, muscles include the rectus abdominis ventrally, the external oblique muscles ventrally and laterally, and the quadratus lumborum and erector spinae muscles dorsally.[62] The erector spinae is composed of large paraspinal muscles that span several vertebral levels; these muscles include the longissimus and iliocostalis. The local, or core muscles, sometimes known as the stabilizers, include the transverse abdominis, pelvic floor muscles, diaphragm, multifidus, and internal oblique muscles.[32, 61-63] Although this distinction between the superficial and deep muscle groups continues to exist, it is important to remember that both groups provide stability during functional movement.[64]

Not only are these superficial and deep trunk muscles and their neuromotor functions important for force transmission and overall stability during activities, but a deficiency in core stability places other body segments at risk of injury.[9, 31, 65] Core instability has been linked to knee injuries, including anterior cruciate ligament injuries[66] and patellofemoral pain syndrome.[67] Other lower-extremity injuries related to instability and imbalances include ankle sprains.[67, 68]

When discussing methods of providing core stability, we therefore have to consider more than the trunk muscles (figure 17.3). Hip muscles must also be included since not only do they provide hip motion but, because of their attachment to the pelvis, they also influence pelvis and trunk motion.[67, 69] Weakness or restricted motion in these muscles can lead to low-back pain and injury.[70] Hip muscles attached to the pelvis and hip or thigh directly influence the stability of the pelvis and sacroiliac joints; these muscles include the quadratus lumborum, hip extensors, hip abductors, and hip rotators. There is evidence that patients with low-back pain have deficiencies in hip abductors and rotators.[67] Evidence also indicates that people with low-back pain demonstrate poor muscle endurance and have delayed activation of hip extensor and hip abductor muscles.[71] There is also evidence that poor core stability affects upper-extremity injuries.[72] On the other hand, there is also evidence to demonstrate that having good core stability helps prevent musculoskeletal injuries.[65] Therefore, these muscles should also be included in a core rehabilitation exercise program.

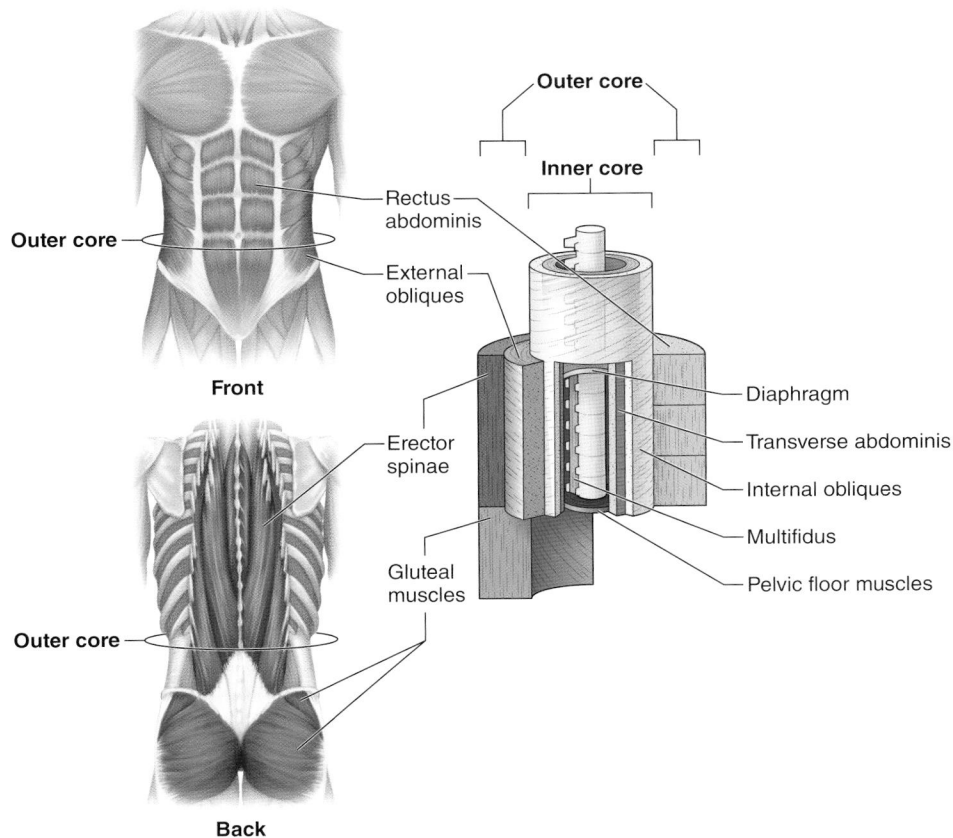

Figure 17.3 Stabilization also requires activation of the larger outer core muscles. These muscles include the external obliques, rectus abdominis, erector spinae, and gluteal muscles.

Pelvic Neutral

We know now that a stable pelvis serves as a platform from which the extremities can perform their activities.[33] A stable pelvis should be basic to performance. Investigations on uninjured athletes have demonstrated that performance improved when core stability exercises were used.[73] Therefore, core stability exercises should be a part of a rehabilitation program. Before you can incorporate *pelvic neutral* in rehabilitation programs, you must first know what pelvic neutral is, why it is important, and how to teach it to patients.

As we have discussed, core stability relies primarily on the strength and control of transverse abdominis, multifidus, diaphragm, and internal oblique muscles and secondarily on the large trunk movers, hip rotators, and the gluteal muscle group. The quadratus lumborum and latissimus dorsi also play a role in stability through their attachment to the thoracolumbar fascia.[74-76] Clinicians should design programs that improve the endurance and strength of all these core muscles before functional and performance-specific activities are begun.

Before exercises for these muscles begin, however, the patient must be taught to find the pelvic position that places the least amount of stress on its joints and supporting structures and allows for optimal lumbopelvic–hip complex function (to allow stability and force transmission) to occur. This position is referred to as pelvic neutral. **Pelvic neutral** is a postural position where the least amount of stress is placed on the lumbopelvic–hip complex. In this position, the head, arms, and trunk are balanced on the pelvis; minimal joint stress occurs, and minimal muscle activity is needed to hold the position. Sometimes the position is called *lumbar neutral,* or *neutral spine,* which is not necessarily accurate because pelvic neutrality doesn't guarantee spinal neutrality.

Pelvic neutral can be difficult to find for someone who is not accustomed to being in this position, especially those with low-back pain. Patients can often achieve pelvic neutral in the sitting position, especially during initial instructions when the concept is unfamiliar. With the patient sitting with the hips and knees at 90°, the patient places his or her index and middle fingers on the left and right anterior superior iliac spines (ASIS). The patient then rocks the pelvis as far as possible posteriorly and notes the end position, then rocks the pelvis as far as possible anteriorly, noting the end position. Now the patient rocks between these extremes, moving through a progressively smaller range of motion until arriving at the mid-position of the range. This is the patient's pelvic neutral; this position is the center of pelvic motion where the spine should be balanced over the pelvis. In this position, the shoulders, trunk, and head should sit directly above the ischial tuberosities (figure 17.4). Each person's pelvic neutral is unique; it depends on the person's available range of motion and ability to move the pelvis. In each case, however, people will have their head, trunk, and shoulders in better alignment when they are in pelvic neutral.

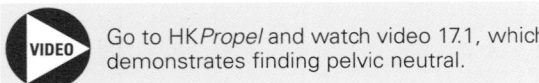

Go to HK*Propel* and watch video 17.1, which demonstrates finding pelvic neutral.

Once the patient can find and hold pelvic neutral, emphasize the need to maintain this position during all activities. Maintaining this position can be difficult, especially at first when the patient might be accustomed to a very different posture and the muscles might lack the strength and endurance to maintain it. However, as the patient's strength and endurance improve, and with frequent reminders, the patient will become better able to hold this position and feel comfortable in it.

Maintaining pelvic neutral requires some tension and endurance in the core muscles. The exercises presented on the next few pages can be used in the early exercise phase when the patient has difficulty maintaining pelvic

neutral during arm and leg motions. The purpose of these exercises is to have the patient learn how to perform simple arm and leg movements while maintaining pelvic neutral. You should pay careful attention to the patient's performance in order to make corrections and to encourage correct performance.

Special Sacral, Ilial, and Pelvic Considerations

Earlier in this chapter we saw that the sacroiliac joints provide for a load transfer between the spine and the lower extremities. The SI joints are also closely related to functions of the upper and lower extremities through the interconnections of the muscles and fascia of the body.[8] From our knowledge of how the body works, we know that if there is dysfunction or weakness in one segment, other segments pick up the slack so that we can continue to perform normal activities. For example, it has been shown that people with reduced cervical disc height and associated segmental motion loss also increased their mobility at cervical segments on either side of the reduced segment.[77] The position of the sacroiliac joints also influences the other spinal segments up the chain.[78] Even cervical posture will change when SI joint positioning changes.[79]

Since forces move up and down the kinetic chain through the sacroiliac joints, these joints may experience more stress, and thus face an increased risk of pathologies, because of dysfunction in the extremities.[80] Before we investigate these pathologies, we need to recall some biomechanical aspects of the sacroiliac joints.

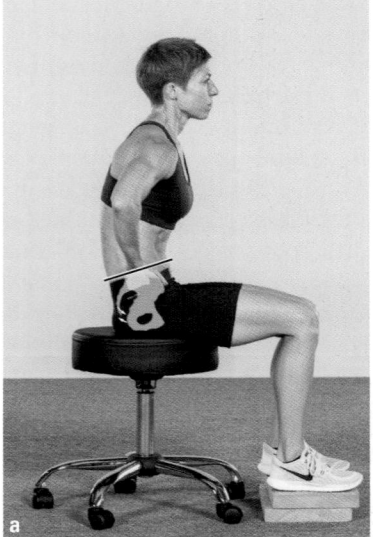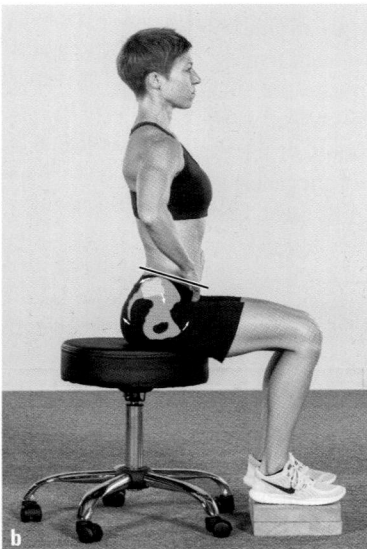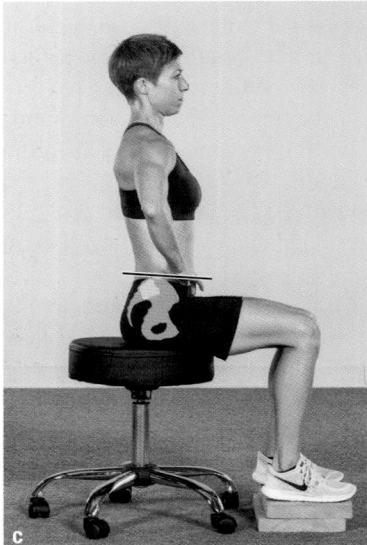

Figure 17.4   Finding pelvic neutral. Instruct the patient to move to *(a)* the extreme end of posterior pelvic tilt and *(b)* the extreme end of anterior pelvic tilt. *(c)* Then, the patient slowly moves between the extremes, gradually reducing the amount of motion until the pelvis is centered in the middle between the extremes of motion. This is pelvic neutral for this patient.

Sacral and Ilia Mechanics

The sacrum rotates anteriorly and posteriorly in the sagittal plane. Although the motions are limited, they are complex. Sacroiliac motion actually occurs as triplanar movement.[81] These motions are given unique names to reflect the fact that the sacroiliac motions are triplanar; the terms were initially coined and defined by Weisl[82] in the mid-1950s. He indicated that **nutation** occurs when the proximal sacrum (sacral base) moves into an anterior tilt relative to the ilium; **counternutation** is a posterior tilt of the proximal sacrum (sacral base) relative to the ilium.[82] Since either the sacrum or the ilium may move, these motions are relative to the position of these two structures; it does not mean that the sacrum is always the moving structure. For example, figure 17.5a shows nutation as either the sacrum moving anteriorly or the ilium moving posteriorly, and figure 17.5b illustrates counternutation with the sacrum moving posteriorly or the ilium moving anteriorly.

Because the sacrum is part of the spine and attached to the spine, sacral motion occurs during lumbar motions.[83] When a person is standing, the sacrum is in a nutated position.[23] When the lumbar spine moves into flexion as a person reaches for the toes while standing (figure 17.6a), the sacrum remains in nutation for the first 60° of trunk flexion. The relative positions of the pelvis and the sacrum do not change until ligaments and muscles tighten to affect their relationship; from that point to the end of the trunk

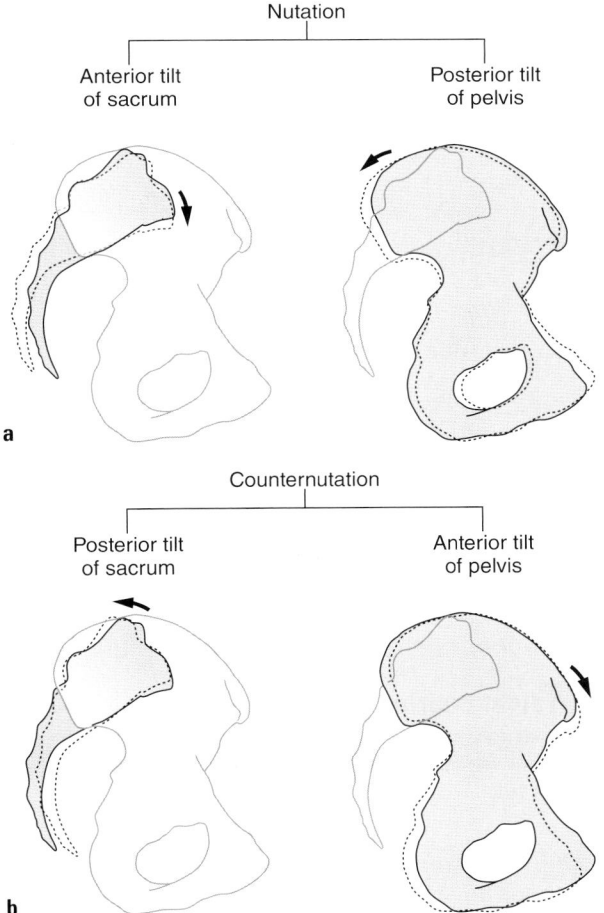

Figure 17.5 *(a)* Nutation occurs with either an anterior tilt of the sacrum or a posterior tilt of the pelvis. Notice that the pubic bone moves forward or the iliac moves posteriorly. *(b)* Counternutation occurs with either a posterior tilt of the sacrum or an anterior tilt of the pelvis. Notice that the ischial tuberosity moves posteriorly or the ilium moves anteriorly.

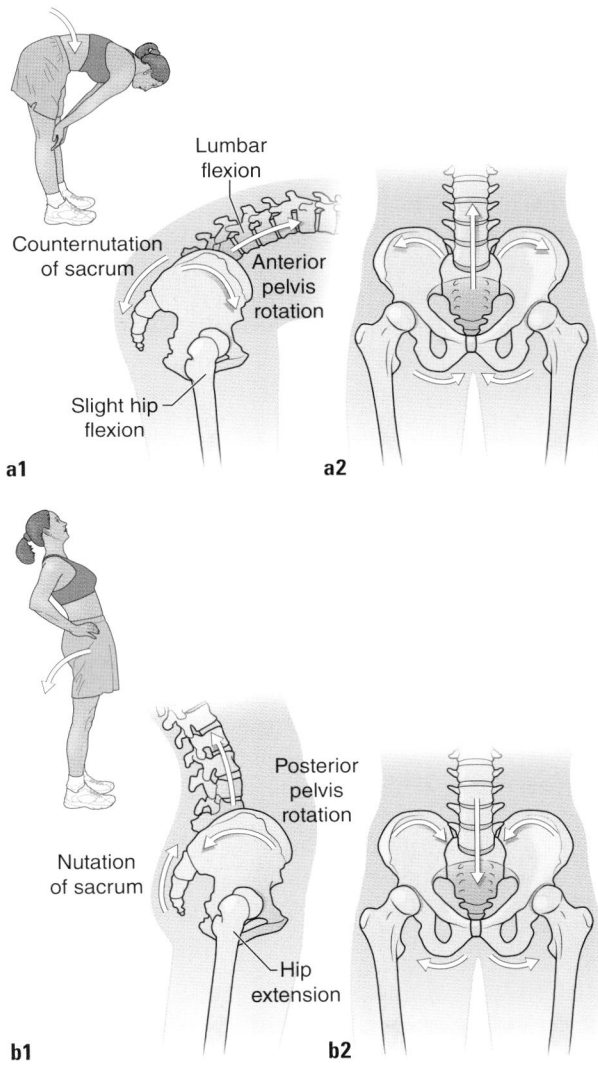

Figure 17.6 Lumbar motions with sacral motions. *(a1)* During standing lumbar flexion, the pelvis rotates anteriorly and the sacrum's end-motion is counternutation relative to the iliac crests, *(a2)* causing the ischial tuberosities to move closer together and the iliac crests to move apart. *(b1)* During standing lumbar extension, the pelvis has a slight posterior rotation while the sacrum moves into nutation relative to the iliac crests, *(b2)* causing the ischial tuberosities to move apart and the iliac crests to move closer together. Notice that during anterior pelvic rotation the hip flexes, and during posterior pelvic rotation the hip moves into extension.

flexion motion, the sacrum moves into counternutation.[84, 85] Sacral counternutation also causes the ischial tuberosities to move closer together and the iliac crests to move apart. When the lumbar spine moves into extension, there is some posterior pelvic rotation, and the sacral base rotates forward into nutation, causing the ischial tuberosities to move apart and the iliac crests to move closer together (figure 17.6b). The significance of these motions will become clearer when we discuss the examination and assessment of pelvic dysfunction later in this chapter.

During nutation and counternutation, a number of coupled motions occur. **Coupled motions** occur when a motion in one plane cannot be produced without an associated motion in another plane. Coupled motions must occur for a joint to have its full range of motion. This is the case for both nutation and counternutation. For example, during nutation of the SI joints, as the sacral base rotates forward and downward, the iliac crests move closer together, and the ischial tuberosities move farther apart.[86] The accompanying movements of counternutation include the iliac crests moving farther apart while the ischial tuberosities move closer together.[86] Recall that the pelvic ring is a closed system, so the motion of one segment directly affects another. When the sacral base rotates forward, it moves the ilia toward each other during nutation and the ischia away from each other; the opposite occurs with counternutation.

Since the sacrum is part of both the spine and the pelvic ring, as trunk and spine motions occur, the innominate bones (ilium, ischium, and pubis) of the pelvic ring also move. These innominate bones are collectively referred to as the pelvis. Therefore, during trunk flexion, the pelvis moves into an anterior tilt, and during trunk extension, the pelvis tilts posteriorly. Keep in mind that in weight bearing, sacral nutation produces the same osteokinematic motion as posterior rotation of the pelvis, and counternutation produces the same osteokinematic motion as anterior rotation of the pelvis.[85]

Since the innominate bones of the pelvis make up the socket portion of the hip joint, hip motion and position affect the pelvis and sacroiliac joints, and likewise, they are affected by the pelvis and SI joints. However, the relationship between these structures is different when the person stands or moves. For example, the hips are extended when a person stands with a posteriorly tilted pelvis, and when the pelvis is in an anterior tilt, the hips are flexed, as seen in figure 17.1. On the other hand, figure 17.6 shows that when a person bends to touch the toes, anterior pelvic tilt occurs with hip flexion, and the reverse is true when the person again stands erect. Although these variations in motions are different, the relative alignment between the pelvis and hip joints is the same. Table 17.1 is based on the information from Lee[85] and shows coupled motions that occur with lumbar movements when standing.

Functional movements such as walking or running often include each hemipelvis moving in opposite directions. As demonstrated in table 17.2, when one hip moves into flexion while the other maintains an extended position, the pelvis on the flexed-hip side tilts anteriorly in the sagittal plane, so the ilium flares out in the frontal plane while the extended-leg pelvis tilts posteriorly and the ilium moves inward. During actions such as walking, stair climbing, and sport activities, when one hip moves opposite the other, the sacrum rotates on a diagonal axis that runs from one sacroiliac joint to the opposite inferior lateral angle (figure 17.7). These diagonal axes will become apparent when we discuss torsion pathologies of the sacroiliac joints.

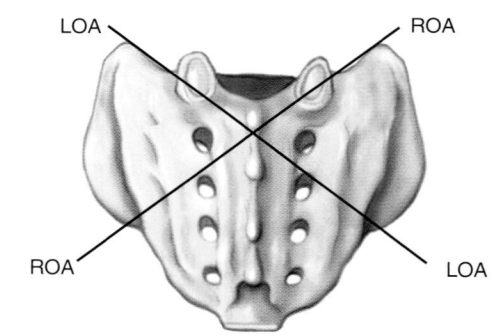

Figure 17.7 Diagonal axis of the sacroiliac joints. LOA = left oblique axis; ROA = right oblique axis.

TABLE 17.1 Lumbosacropelvic and Hip Motions During Weight Bearing

Lumbar motion	Sacral motion	Pelvis motion	Hip motion
Forward bending	Nutation, then counternutation	Anterior tilt	Flexion
Extending	Nutation	Posterior tilt	Extension
Sidebending to the left	Left sidebends to L; right sidebends to R	Left rotates anteriorly; right rotates posteriorly	Left adducts; right abducts
Rotating to the left	Nutation on left side	Left rotates posteriorly; right rotates anteriorly	Left laterally rotates; right medially rotates

Note: Lumbar sidebending and rotation motions to the right have reversed motions from those stated for left sidebending and rotation. Based on Lee (2004).[85]

TABLE 17.2   Pelvifemoral Motions During Gait

Gait phase	SAGITTAL PLANE				FRONTAL PLANE		Transverse plane	Diagonal plane
	Right femur	Left femur	Right pelvis	Left pelvis	Right ilium	Left ilium	Entire pelvis	Sacrum
Right heel strike	Extending	Flexing	Posteriorly tilting	Anteriorly tilting	Inwardly flaring	Outwardly flaring	Rotating right	Rotating right
Right toe-off	Extension, moving toward flexion	Flexion, moving toward extension	Moving toward anterior tilt	Moving toward posterior tilt	Moving toward outward flare	Moving toward inward flare	Rotating toward the left	Rotating toward the left
Right swing phase	Flexing	Extending	Anteriorly tilting	Posteriorly tilting	Outwardly flaring	Inwardly flaring	Rotating left	Rotating left

Diagonal sacral rotations occur on these diagonal axes during ambulation because the sacrum is wedged between the two hemipelvic segments, which move in opposite directions to each other. As seen in table 17.2, when a person moves the right limb forward, the right sacrum rolls posteriorly around a medial–lateral axis at heel strike and anteriorly on the left sacrum as the left limb moves through as toe-off. Posterior sacral rotation (counternutation) is the open-pack position of the SI joint that occurs during the end of the swing phase of gait; this mobile position allows for the absorption of force during initial contact with the ground. Nutation, on the other hand, is the close-pack position of the SI joint[87] that occurs toward the end of the weight-bearing phase; having the sacrum in an anteriorly rotated (close-pack), rigid position provides additional leverage for propulsion immediately before the foot leaves the ground.[88] This sagittal plane rotation of the sacrum also helps produce a rotation around a diagonal axis.[17]

Because the pelvis is a closed ring, when one of the innominate bones moves, the other bones of the pelvis also move; therefore, the pubic bones correspond to iliac motion during walking. You may remember from anatomy that the sacrum has an inferior lateral angle (ILA) lateral to its inferior apex. The right and left ILAs are located just lateral to and on either side of the cornua (figure 17.8). The left and right sacrotuberous ligaments connect their ipsilateral ischial tuberosities to the inferior sacrum. Each ligament lies at about a 45° angle superior to and medial from the ligament's distal insertion on its respective ischial tuberosity to its proximal insertion on the inferior–lateral sacrum. You will need to identify each of these structures during an SI examination.

Maintaining Pelvic Neutral Through Core Recruitment

Once a patient locates pelvic neutral and has a sense for where it is and how to achieve it, the patient must activate core muscles and strengthen them to maintain that position

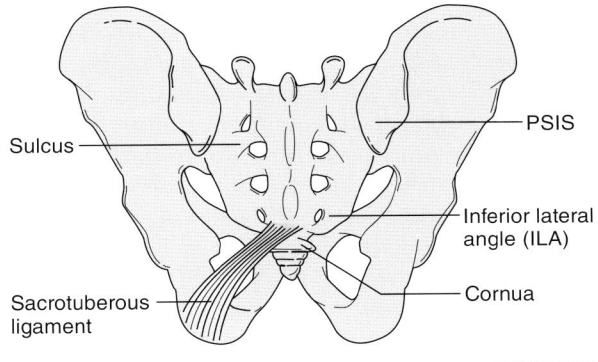

Figure 17.8   Sacroilium.

and stabilize the lumbopelvic–hip complex. This process begins with facilitation of the local muscles: diaphragm, pelvic floor, transverse abdominis, and multifidus. It has been demonstrated that there is a synergistic relationship between the transverse abdominis, internal oblique, and pelvic floor muscles.[89, 90] Contracting either the pelvic floor muscles or the abdominal stabilizing muscles will cause an accompanying contraction of the other.[89-91] If your examination reveals deficiencies in the secondary global muscles, exercises for these muscles are also included.

CLINICAL TIPS

The primary muscles involved in core stability are those that are closest to the center of the body; these include the pelvic floor muscles, diaphragm, transverse abdominis, internal obliques, and multifidus. While most of these muscles provide stability rather than substantial motion, the internal oblique muscles provide both stability and trunk motion. The secondary muscles for core stability provide motion as well as some stability; these include the hip muscles and the larger global muscles of the trunk.

504   Rehabilitation of Musculoskeletal Injuries

Local Core

The local core muscles are essential for stabilizing the trunk so that we can perform functional activities with our extremities, so recruitment of these muscles deserves attention. These muscles and the methods of recruiting them for core stability are described next.

Diaphragm Recruitment   For the diaphragm to be recruited for inhalation, the rib cage must move into an exhaled position first.[92] An example of a diaphragm recruitment exercise is performed in the hook-lying position as shown in figure 17.9. Use a balloon to provide resisted exhalation to better recruit the abdominal obliques for a complete exhalation.[93] The patient positions himself or herself in a slight posterior pelvic tilt to lift the hips off the table using the hamstrings and abdominals. Then the patient takes a balloon and exhales into it, trying to squeeze all the air out of the lungs and into the balloon. The patient pauses 3 to 5 s, maintaining the exhaled position without letting the obliques relax and without deliberately flexing the abdominal muscles. Without allowing air to escape from the balloon and without pinching the neck of the balloon, he or she keeps the obliques engaged, places the tongue at the roof of the mouth, and inhales slowly through the nose. The patient lowers the tongue and exhales into the balloon again, then pauses as before. The patient performs three exhalations; after the fourth inhalation, the patient relaxes and lets the air out of the balloon.

Go to HK*Propel* and watch video 17.2, which demonstrates balloon blowing to recruit the diaphragm.

Another exercise to facilitate diaphragm neuromotor control is performed with the patient standing and facing a desk or table with both hands on the tabletop. During the first exhalation, the patient rounds the thorax by slightly pushing into the table to protract the scapulae. The patient performs a slight posterior pelvic tilt by bending the knees slightly and allowing his or her knees to move slightly forward while keeping the heels on the floor. The patient pauses for 3 to 5 s at the end of the exhalation with the ribs positioned in inward rotation. The patient then maintains this position and pressure through his or her hands on the table, while inhaling slowly through the nose. The patient expands the posterior rib cage while filling the lungs without shrugging. This exercise is performed 3 times, then the patient relaxes after the fourth inhalation. This exercise promotes diaphragm activity by maintaining inward rotation of the rib cage during inhalation. This position has been demonstrated to improve diaphragm recruitment during inhalation.[94]

These two respiration exercises can be performed in any position. As patients develop proper diaphragm control, they move to more functional positions that are used during daily activities.

Abdominal Hollowing and Abdominal Bracing

Two exercises that help patients facilitate the transverse abdominis, internal oblique muscles, and pelvic floor muscles are abdominal hollowing and abdominal bracing.[91] **Abdominal hollowing** is when the abdomen is drawn in to facilitate the action of the transverse abdominis and multifidus muscles, and **abdominal bracing** occurs when more of the abdominal and back muscles are activated to co-contract.[95] There is disagreement about which is the

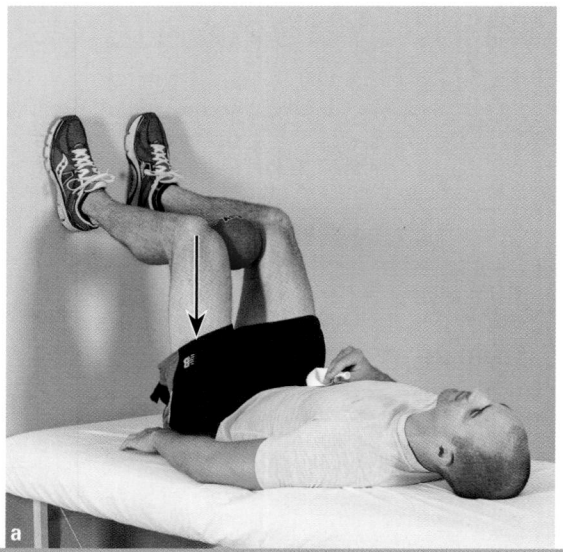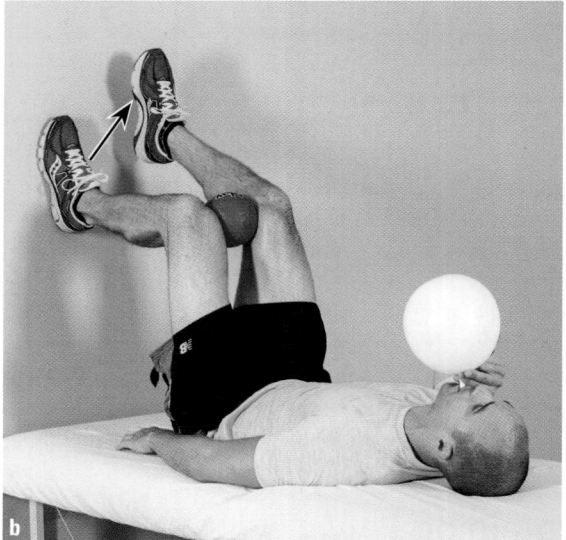

Figure 17.9   Diaphragm recruitment exercise from Boyle and colleagues, 2010.[93] *(a)* Before the start of the exercise, the patient positions his back flat on the table with the hamstrings performing a slight posterior pelvic tilt. With the feet at the same level on the wall, the left knee is shifted down and medially. *(b)* The exercise is performed in the start position with the right foot off the wall.

better exercise since abdominal hollowing recruits the transverse abdominis and multifidus muscles but does not facilitate the rectus abdominis and external oblique.[96] Abdominal bracing, however, facilitates the transverse abdominis as well as the internal and external obliques.[62] Although both activation methods are used during core exercises, it is generally agreed that abdominal bracing provides for better recruitment of core muscles than abdominal hollowing and provides more pelvic and spinal stability.[95, 97, 98] Because both local and global muscles are needed for optimal core control, exercises for both groups should be used in a rehabilitation program.[99]

Although studies have reported no difference in muscle recruitment whether patients are in a supine hook-lying, prone, sitting, or standing position,[100] you may find that they more readily grasp the concept and recruit the correct muscles when they begin in a supine hook-lying position with the hips and knees flexed and the feet on the floor. The patient first positions the spine in a neutral position (pelvic neutral). The clinician then instructs the patient to maintain this neutral position and to hollow the abdomen by pulling the navel in and up toward the spine (figure 17.10*a*).[101] It is important that the patient not suck in the belly but instead tense the muscle to draw in the abdomen. It is also important that the patient perform the activity slowly and breathe normally during the exercise. The position is held for 5 s to start and is then repeated. As the patient improves control, the duration of the hold may be increased up to 30 s or more.

 Go to HK*Propel* and watch video 17.3, which demonstrates abdominal hollowing and abdominal bracing.

If the patient has difficulty with this exercise, the use of a blood pressure cuff or specifically designed lumbar biofeedback pressure cuff may be helpful to serve as a biofeedback mechanism.[102, 103] With the patient in a supine hook-lying position, the pressure cuff is placed comfortably beneath the patient's low back. The cuff is inflated to 40 mmHg. The patient moves into a pelvic neutral position and is instructed to "Pull your navel up and in toward your spine." The clinician can monitor whether the patient has successfully performed the activity by monitoring the blood pressure cuff gauge. If the pressure jumps significantly, then the patient has lost pelvic neutral and moved into a posterior pelvic tilt; if the pressure decreases significantly, the patient has moved into an anterior pelvic tilt. Allow the patient to see the blood pressure gauge as a visual feedback mechanism. Palpation of the abdominals may also help the patient with correct muscle recruitment. Once the patient can pull the navel to the spine without more than a 5 to 10 mmHg change in the blood pressure gauge

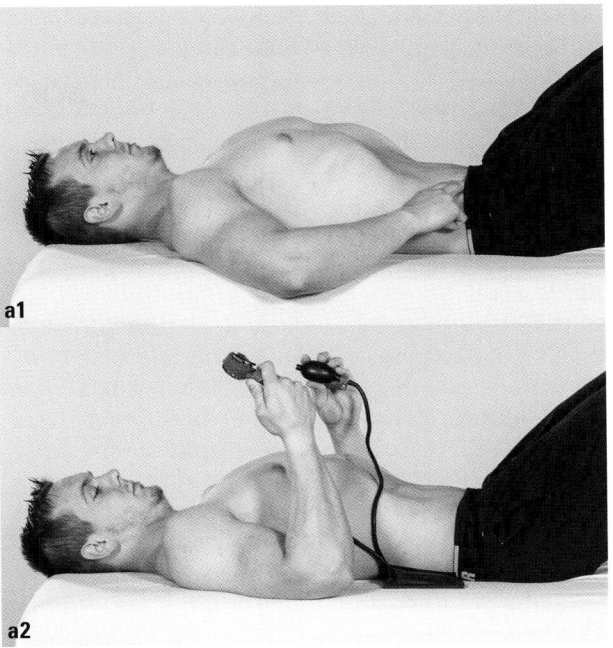

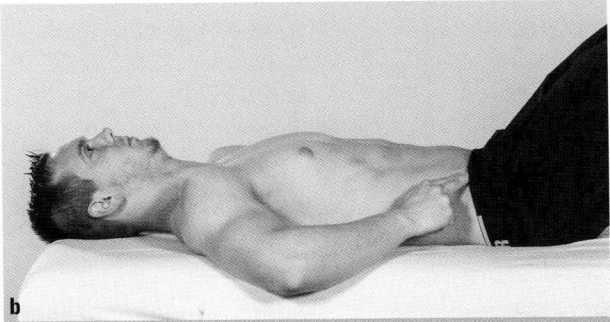

Figure 17.10 Abdominal hollowing *(a1)* without a blood pressure cuff and *(a2)* with a blood pressure cuff; *(b)* abdominal bracing.

reading, correct recruitment of the transverse abdominis has occurred.[96, 104, 105]

Another technique used to facilitate transverse abdominis activity and provide the patient with tactile feedback is to have the patient place finger pads about 2 cm (1 in.) medial and superior to the anterior superior iliac spine.[106] The patient should feel these oblique abdominal muscles pull in, not push out, when the abdominal hollowing exercise is performed correctly. In each of these exercises, the goals are correct execution and gains in strength and control along with the development of muscle endurance. If the patient cannot recruit the transverse abdominis correctly (pushes the abdomen out rather than pulling it in) after being given verbal instruction and tactile cues, have the patient practice independently for several minutes until he or she can draw in the abdomen. It may take a while for patients to recruit the transverse abdominis, especially if they have never correctly recruited core muscles before.[39]

How much activation of these muscles is needed to provide stability? A maximal contraction is not needed for most functional activities. It has been found that the amount of force these core muscles must exert during functional activities is far less than maximal when the person maintains a neutral position.[107] Therefore, maintaining a pelvic neutral position and a sustained submaximal contraction are essential for optimal function and performance.[108]

Once patients can create a consistent contraction of these local core muscles, demonstrating a good hollowing performance, they advance to controlling the amount of contraction. It is usually easy to identify a maximal contraction, so have the patient contract the transverse abdominis as much as possible, then tell the patient to relax to 50% of that contraction and hold it. From there, instruct him or her to relax to 50% of that submaximal contraction (50% of the 50%). This is approximately the amount of force needed to maintain core stability during functional activities (25% of maximal contraction).[97] Of course, with activities that require extreme effort, the contraction intensity also increases, but 25% is an average recommendation for daily functional activities.[97, 109] The patient should be encouraged to maintain this 25% core tension throughout the day, allowing it to become an automatic and natural condition.

Abdominal bracing is an activation of all the abdominal muscles to create stiffness of the trunk. It is thought that with increased muscle activity, a secondary extensor muscle activation occurs.[95] This anterior, lateral, and posterior muscle tension provides stiffness without restricting the muscle's ability to provide motion.[95]

Patient instructions should first include moving the pelvis into a neutral position. The next instruction should be to tense all of the abdominal and back muscles without drawing in or flaring out the muscles (figure 17.10*b*).[110] This protects the spine against external forces and provides more stability than abdominal hollowing.[111] It also encourages activation of the diaphragm, an important stabilizer. The patient should breathe normally during this activity and activate the anterior and posterior muscles simultaneously. The clinician should see no changes in the position of the pelvis, spine, or abdominal wall, and the clinician should palpate around the abdominal wall to check for enough muscular tension to resist a light inward press of the fingers on the abdominal wall.[112]

Multifidus Recruitment   Research demonstrates that the multifidus is activated when the transverse abdominis is activated.[52, 113] In people with back pain, however, the multifidus is often atrophied and is not recruited in the normal feedforward system.[114] Investigations show that people with low-back pain experience pain relief once they can recruit core muscles, which include the multifi-

dus.[115] Although the multifidus is small and located next to the spinal column, it may be palpated if the patient can relax the erector spinae muscles.

Although the multifidus contracts when the transverse abdominis activates in normal persons, this may not be the case for people with a history of back pain. Therefore, it is best to start with exercises that isolate the muscle in these people. Specific verbal and tactile cues during muscle-isolating exercises can help. With the patient sitting in pelvic neutral, instruct the patient to place the finger pads of both hands on top of the lumbar spinous processes and slide the fingers laterally off the spinous processes into the paraspinal gutter between the spinous processes and the bulk of the erector spinae (figure 17.11).[104] Then tell the patient to push the muscle under her fingers against her fingers without pushing out the larger muscle located immediately lateral to the finger pads.

For patients who cannot manage this task, have them lie prone with hands in the lumbar region as described and then extend the trunk to feel the erector spinae muscles activate. Tell the patient that this larger muscle should not be activated when recruiting only the multifidus. If the patient is performing the multifidus isometric isolation exercise correctly, a slight increased resistance or slight bulging of the muscles against the fingers will be felt.[104] Tension in the muscle should occur without changing the position of the pelvis. Once she can perform the activity, instruct the patient to hold the isometric for about 10 s, then relax and repeat. Muscle reeducation, strength, and control along with development of muscle endurance are goals for this exercise.

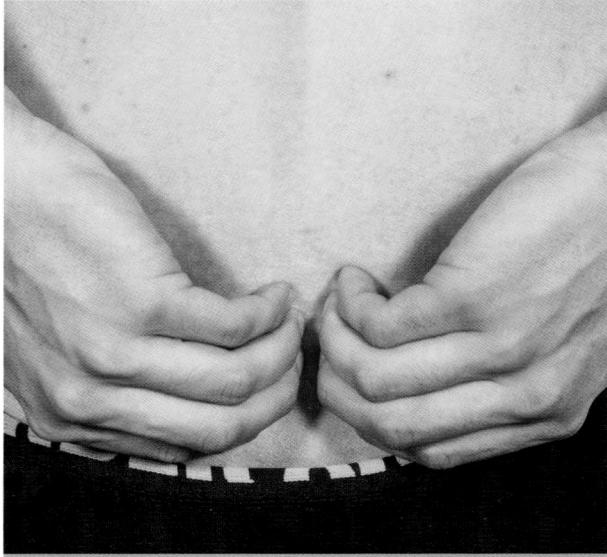

Figure 17.11   Recruitment of the multifidus may be difficult for a patient with a history of low-back pain. Instructions to palpate the muscle during activation will provide tactile feedback to help the patient to recruit the correct muscle.

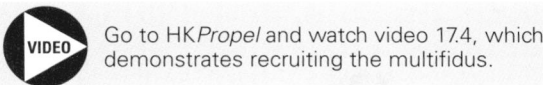

Go to HK*Propel* and watch video 17.4, which demonstrates recruiting the multifidus.

Global Core

As we have discussed, global core muscles include the trunk muscles that are farthest from the trunk's center and are considered the "movers" of the trunk and spine. These muscles include the rectus abdominis, external obliques, erector spinae group, and quadratus lumborum muscles.[61] Often these muscles lack normal strength after an injury; if deficiencies are found on examination, the clinician must include specific exercises to isolate and strengthen any weakened global muscle, just as he or she would for any extremity injury.

Since these muscles usually have had some level of activity, and, unlike the local core muscles, have not been dormant, special considerations on how to "awaken" these muscles are not needed. Specific exercises to strengthen these global core muscles are provided later in this chapter. Note, however, that in patients with low-back pain or dysfunctional local core muscles, the global core muscles may be recruited improperly during functional activities, and they may need retraining or reeducation during the rehabilitation program.[116]

Combining Local and Global Core Muscles

Once the patient can activate the transverse abdominis and multifidus muscles individually, the clinician instructs the patient to activate both at once. Since it has been demonstrated that the local muscles are often not recruited, especially in patients with a history of low-back pain,[117] the patient must first learn to enlist these muscles before engaging other muscles for functional activities.[118, 119] The next step is to perform abdominal bracing activities, recruiting both local and global abdominals and posterior muscles. The final step in the progression is to maintain pelvic neutral and recruitment of core stabilization muscles while executing functional and performance-specific activities.

Basic to all functional and performance-specific activities is the concept of how we use the body to perform those activities. How we use the body is known as *body mechanics*. Before we continue our discussion of the spine, we must address the importance of proper body mechanics.

Body Mechanics

Body mechanics refers to the way the body is positioned and used during activity. Incorrect body mechanics increases the stresses that are placed on certain body segments; correct body mechanics makes the most effective use of the body's forces and lever systems. An awareness of good body mechanics is important to the rehabilitation clinician from both a personal and a treatment perspective.

From a personal perspective, the use of proper body mechanics improves your efficiency during application of your own daily activities, treatments, manual therapy, and exercises. It conserves your energy and makes the most effective use of your body. From a treatment perspective, a knowledge of correct body mechanics helps you to provide patients with the proper exercises. The right exercises will enhance the patient's performance and will include corrective techniques to prepare the patient for a safe return to normal activities.

Basic Principles

A few basic concepts are important to remember regardless of the activity that is being performed. The first principle is that the spine should retain its normal curves (figure 17.12). Neutral spinal position has slight lumbar lordosis, thoracic kyphosis, and cervical lordosis. In this position, each vertebra is in correct alignment with the adjacent vertebrae, as discussed in chapter 6. In this position the stress on the pelvis and spine is minimal, and the vertebrae are balanced.

A neutral spine permits forces from the lower extremities to be properly transmitted to the trunk and upper extremities. It is easier to understand this if you think of the legs, trunk, and arms as three sections connected in series. When the sections are all rigid and stiff, forces transfer

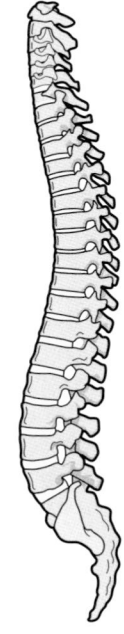

Figure 17.12 Neutral spinal alignment. Minimal stress occurs on the spine when the spine is properly aligned with normal spinal curves being retained.

easily from one section to another, but if the middle section, the spine, is a spring rather than a rigid structure, it is more difficult to transfer forces from one section to another. When the middle segment is not rigid, the forces produced in the lower segment are absorbed by the "spring," and the arms must develop their own forces—a far more difficult and strenuous method of delivering forces needed for many athletic activities.

For this reason, it is important for patients to perform difficult tasks in proper spinal alignment, especially those that require significant force transmission. For example, a football lineman squats with the core engaged and the spine in good, straight alignment to use the driving force from the legs. The warehouse worker does the same thing during a squat to transfer the lifting force from the legs to the arms. The rehabilitation clinician must also maintain a straight back so the power of the legs, not the arms, is the primary source of manual resistance forces created for challenging rehabilitation exercises.

If the back is not "straight" or "stiff" and rigid, less force is transferred from the lower extremities to the trunk and upper extremities. To illustrate the significance of this, have a friend bend over from the waist so that his or her back relaxes its normal spinal curvature, and then push on your friend's shoulders to move the person off balance. Now have your friend bend at the hips but keep the core engaged and the spine straight as you again push his or her body off balance. You will find that with proper body mechanics and the power the legs provide, there is increased stability and resistance to outside forces. This example demonstrates that when the body must produce forces sufficient to resist external loads, spinal stiffness and rigidity are necessary and are achieved by engaging the core and establishing a "straight" spine.

Lowering the body's center of mass increases the body's stability. This stability is important for resisting outside forces. For example, if you push your friend while he or she is standing fully upright, it will be easier for you to move your friend than if he or she squats to lower the body's center of gravity. This is one reason linemen in football and rugby are in a squat position.

Broadening the base of support is another method of providing increased stability. If your friend stands with feet together, it is much easier to push him or her off balance than if the feet are apart. A broader base of support produces a larger area for the center of gravity to move within before balance is lost. When you move an object, standing with a broad base of support increases your stability.

Another principle of good body mechanics is to stand in the direction of force application. This enables you to transfer force from the legs. For example, when you throw a ball forward, your feet are in a backward–forward split stance. This permits a transfer of forces from the back leg to the front leg as you throw the ball. To appreciate this concept, throw a ball with your feet in a side-by-side stance and then with your feet in a backward–forward split stance. You will find that the ball goes farther with the split stance. If you need to transfer an object or exert a force from one side of the body to the other, the best stance is a side-by-side stance with the feet in line with the shoulders. For example, if you are resisting a patient's straight-leg raise with the patient supine on the table, your stance should be side by side as you face the table. This way, as the patient raises his or her leg, your weight can transfer from the leg you have positioned near the patient's foot (lower) to the one you have positioned near the patient's hip (upper). You will be able to use a body-weight shift from your lower-positioned leg to your upper-positioned leg as the patient's leg moves through its motion.

Abdominal strength is important for force transfer from the lower to the upper extremities. Strong, core stability from both local and global muscles provides the support needed to keep the spine aligned and to transfer forces from the legs to the arms. When arm and leg movement are assisted by trunk stability and spinal stiffness, they produce the desired activity with the desired force. You can see this if you have someone resist your shoulder flexion-to-extension movement. You should feel your abdominals tighten as you extend the arm against the resistance. You should also feel the abdominals tighten when you perform hip flexion against resistance. For these reasons, an injured person's rehabilitation program should include abdominal strengthening exercises for trunk stability.

Body Mechanics During Daily Activities

Correct body mechanics is important when performing daily activities because it conserves energy, makes for efficient and effective use of the body, and reduces stress on the back and other segments. Knowledge of these techniques enables you to instruct patients on ways to minimize stress on an injury.

Patients routinely lift and carry objects such as book bags, backpacks, boxes, athletic gear, and gym bags. The way an object is lifted depends on its size and weight. It is important to test the weight of the object before lifting it. If an object is heavy, the proper way to lift it is to approach it head on. This means facing the object, standing as close to the object as possible, and standing so that when your back is properly aligned and you flex at the hips and knees, your arms fall directly over the object. As you flex your knees to lift the object, the knees should never be higher than the hips. Bending the knees more than 90° imposes a great deal of stress on the knee's meniscus. Additional lowering of the trunk occurs by pushing the hips backward, bending the knees to no further than 90°, and keeping the chest and head up and the core engaged. With the abdominals tightened, you lift the object by straightening the lower extremities as you move to a standing position (figure 17.13). The object is kept close to the body to reduce its force (force equals weight × distance). The farther away from the body the object is, the more force is needed to lift it.

While carrying objects in only one hand, it is best to shift the object periodically from one side to the other, especially when carrying an object for more than a short time. The load is minimized when the object is kept close to the body and no higher than waist level.

To push or pull an object, you place your legs in the direction of movement (side-by-side if the object is being moved left to right; backward–forward if the object is to be moved toward or away from you) as demonstrated in figure 17.14. You then move the object by transferring your weight from one leg to the other. If the object is to be moved from the right side of the body to the left, you place your legs in a side-by-side stance, grasp the object, and move your body weight from the right to the left leg. If the object is to be moved from a position in front of you to one farther away, you begin in a backward–forward stance, grasp the object, and shift your body weight from the back leg to the front leg to move the object. The legs, not the arms, provide the force to move the object. Your arms are only there to grasp the object and transmit the force from your legs to the object.

The easiest way to push or pull heavy objects is to keep your back extended, lower your center of mass, and use a wide forward–backward stance. Keeping your center of mass low will help you to use lower-extremity forces to move the object (as seen in figure 17.14). Pushing is

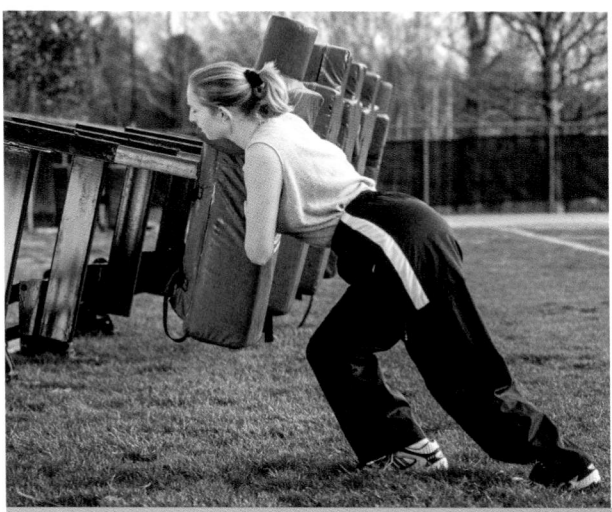

Figure 17.14 Proper pushing technique. The spine remains flat and extended with the core engaged to provide force transfer from the legs through the trunk to the upper extremities.

easier than pulling because you can make better use of your body's weight.

Rising from a chair uses the same principles as bending. As figure 17.15 shows, the back is in proper alignment, the bend occurs at the hips and knees, and the spine is kept in alignment by keeping the chest up.

The proper technique for transferring the body to the floor is to go down first on one knee and then the other

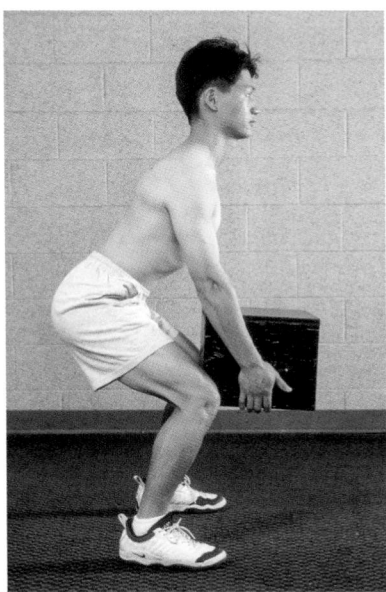

Figure 17.13 Proper lifting technique. The back remains unchanged throughout the activity; the legs are used by flexing the hips, knees, and ankles to move or lift an object.

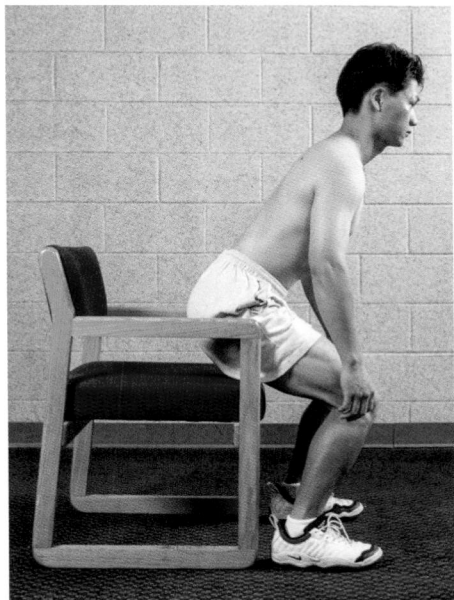

Figure 17.15 Proper sit-to-stand position. The spine remains properly aligned while the hips and knees flex to move the center of mass from sitting to standing. The center of mass must remain over the feet throughout the activity.

before placing the hands on the floor in a quadruped position. From there, walk the hands out to get into a prone position, and then roll into either a side-lying or a supine position. Use this technique in reverse to return to a standing position.

 Go to HK*Propel* and watch video 17.5, which demonstrates proper body mechanics for sit to stand.

Athletic Events

Athletic activities, unlike daily activities, demand optimal transmission of forces from the lower extremities to the upper extremities. Isometric abdominal strength with core and trunk stability is important for transmitting these forces. Maintenance of correct spinal alignment is important for force production and transmission.

It is beyond the scope of this text to describe proper body mechanics for the execution of all activities. However, based on the information presented here about body mechanics, the rehabilitation clinician should have a concept of the proper posture and position for the execution of many activities. For example, a canoeist must have correct spinal alignment to transmit forces from the legs to the arms to move the canoe quickly and forcefully (figure 17.16); likewise, a gymnast must engage her core as she goes into a kip on the uneven bars. A weightlifter's back must be extended as he lifts the weight overhead (figure

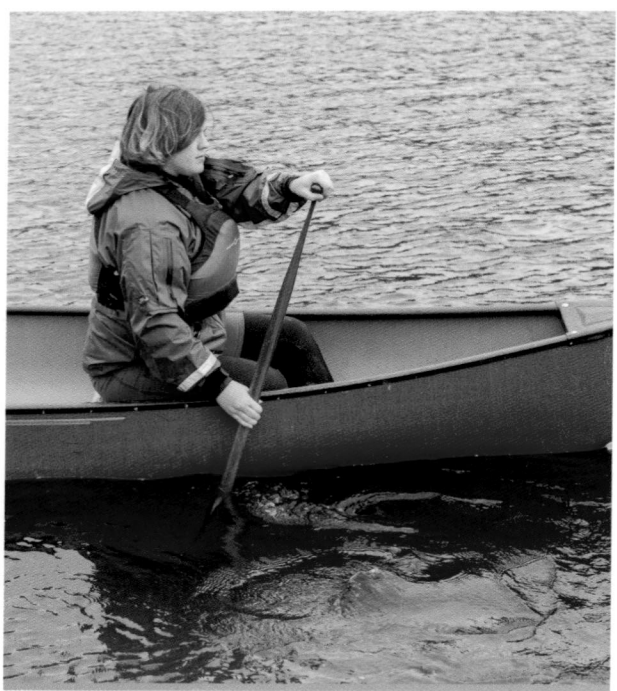
Figure 17.16 Canoeist with proper technique.

17.17), and a shot-putter must transfer lower-extremity forces to the upper extremity by keeping the back straight to propel the shot for maximum distance. In all of these examples, the desired force production requires a stiff, flat, rigid spine for proper transfer of energy. And all of these tasks require forces well beyond those needed to perform normal daily activities. As a result, the body mechanics is different for these tasks than for normal, nonchallenging daily activities.

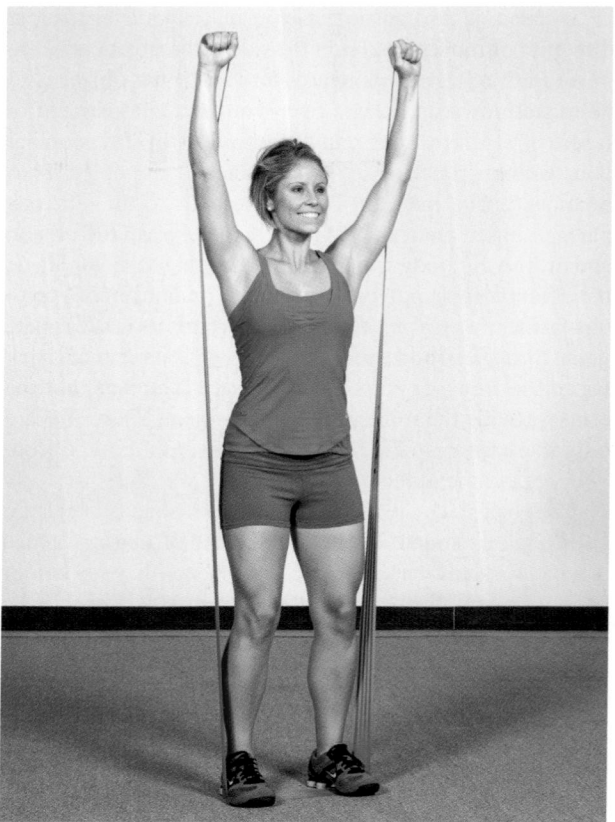
Figure 17.17 Weightlifter using proper mechanics.

The Rehabilitation Clinician's Daily Activities

Just as the patient must learn to use the body efficiently and effectively, the rehabilitation clinician must use his or her body correctly to be effective, competent, and proficient in the application of rehabilitation techniques. That is, rehabilitation clinicians must use good body mechanics.

Your body weight should be equally distributed over both feet. Your feet should be positioned in correct alignment in accordance with the direction of the forces you are applying, and the force you use should be produced by the legs rather than the arms. Remember to keep your core engaged and your trunk stable so that your powerful leg muscles, not your arm muscles, provide the force. Transferring body mass from one lower extremity to the other as you move or resist the patient's extremities through a range of motion reduces the demands on your body. Keeping the upper extremities relaxed but in proper alignment makes it easier for you to achieve the transfer of forces from the lower to the upper extremities. Figure 17.18 demonstrates the use of proper body mechanics when working with patients.

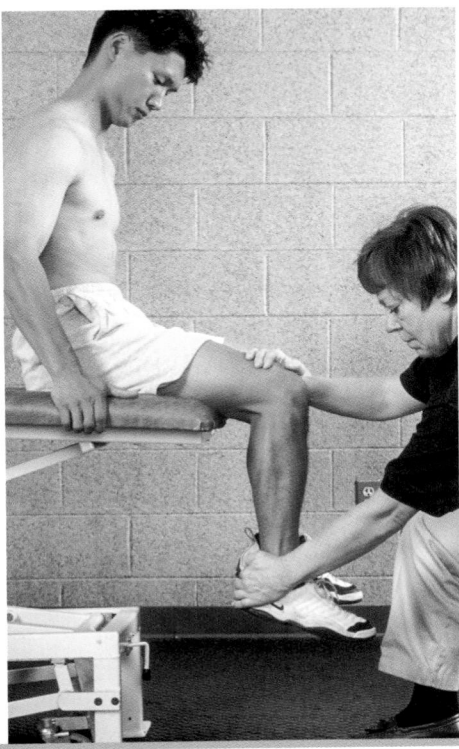

Figure 17.18 Rehabilitation clinician demonstrating proper body mechanics while offering manual resistance to knee flexion.

 Go to HK*Propel* and watch video 17.6, which demonstrates proper body mechanics for a clinician while providing manual resistance.

CLINICAL TIPS

Proper body mechanics is fundamental to proper posture, regardless of an activity's level of difficulty. Important principles include maintaining normal spinal curves while performing daily activities, and using correct body mechanics for proper force transfer while lowering the center of mass, and keeping the base of support broad during difficult tasks. Patients must perform daily and athletic activities using correct body mechanics, and rehabilitation clinicians must pay attention to their own use of proper body mechanics as well.

Examination of the Spine and Sacroilium

Identifying the proper treatment for injuries to the spine and sacroilium requires observational skills and a knowledge of normal spine and SI function. Before the clinician can construct an appropriate rehabilitation program, the patient and his or her injuries, position, and movement dysfunction must be assessed.

As with other manual techniques, the reliability and validity of the sacroiliac and vertebral tests are not strong.[120-122] Special tests involve both a patient's subjective report of pain and a clinician's subjective assessment of test results, so it is not surprising that research outcomes are neither consistent nor concrete. There is often a gold standard for diagnosing various injuries, but these gold standards are usually beyond the realm of practicality for clinicians. For example, the gold standard for diagnosing SI dysfunction is anesthetic blocks using either computed tomography (CT) or fluoroscopic-assisted injection.[123] However, it has been found that when a group of clinical test results are compiled in what is known as a cluster of tests during an examination, the collective data become more useful;[124] the specificity and sensitivity of cluster test results have been shown to be within acceptable margins, ranging from 60% to 91%.[15, 125]

Special Tests for the Sacroilium

Selecting the appropriate tests to assess sacroiliac joint dysfunction is challenging for a variety of reasons, including the complexity of the joint mechanics and the clinician's experience level.[124] Thus it is best to use several tests to strengthen your clinical decision making. Two studies compared the sensitivity and specificity of six tests and concluded that testing produced the best statistical strength when the patient demonstrated three or more positive tests.[15, 126] Table 17.3 provides a list of commonly used sacroiliac pain provocation tests with their sensitivity and specificity ratings.

Special Tests for the Spine

There are a number of special tests that may be used for the spine. As with any body segment, these special tests are designed to either confirm or exclude a particular diagnosis from the clinician's list of potential diagnoses. Some of the more commonly used special tests for the spine are listed in table 17.4. As with the SI tests, the more positive tests a patient displays, the more confidence you can have that your clinical diagnosis is accurate.[138]

Many of these tests have low sensitivity and higher specificity. These ratings indicate that such tests are good at ruling out people who do not have the problem for which the test examines, but they don't do a very good

TABLE 17.3 Common Sacroiliac Tests With Their Sensitivity and Specificity Ratings

Test	Other names	Sensitivity	Specificity	Notes
Thigh thrust	Oostagard test; 4-P test; sacrotuberous stress test; POSH test	80%[128] 36%[129]	100%[128] 50%[129]	Performed only if hip joint is normal
Mennell's	—	54-70%[130]	100%[130]	
Resisted hip abduction	—	87%[128]	100%[128]	Performed in side-lying, full extension, and 50° abduction
Sacral thrust	Sacral clearing test	63%[131]	75%[131]	
FABER	Patrick's test	34%[132] 69%[129] 72%[133]	92%[132] 16%[129] 67%[133]	Also a special test for the hip
Seated flexion	Piedallus sign	9%[134]	93%[134]	Others have identified low sensitivity and specificity.[130, 135, 136]
Pubic stress	—	81%[130]	99%[130]	
Prone knee bend	Nachlas test	44%[137]	83%[137]	
Gaenslen's	—	71%[128] 31%[132] 71%[129] 62%[133] 52%[124]	26%[128] 94%[132] 26%[129] 33%[133] 74%[124]	

Note: The more positive test results you obtain from your examination, the more confidence you will have in your diagnosis.[127, 128, 133]

TABLE 17.4 Commonly Used Special Tests for the Spine

Test	Sensitivity	Specificity
Spurling (cervical compression test)	30%[139]	93%[139]
Cervical distraction	40-43%[140]	100%[140]
Rib fracture compression	Unknown	Unknown
Forward bend scoliosis (Adam's test)	92%[141]	60%[141]
Valsalva maneuver	70%[142]	91%[142]
Crossed straight leg (well straight-leg test)	29%[143]	88%[143]
Straight-leg raising (Lasègue test)	91%[143]	26%[143]
Posteroanterior mobility	82%[144]	81%[144]
Prone instability	72%[144]	58%[144]
Slump	84%[145]	83%[145]
Slump knee bend (femoral slump)	100%[145]	83%[145]
Passive lumbar extension	84%[146]	91%[146]

Note: Results provided by references are rounded off to the nearest whole number. If a test has high sensitivity, it will likely produce a positive result when the condition is present. If a test has high specificity, it will likely produce a negative result when the patient does not have the condition.

job of telling the clinician when the patient does have the problem. For this reason, clinicians are apt to use several tests to confirm a diagnosis. This is a common practice. Using several tests to determine a diagnosis improves the accuracy of that diagnosis.[147]

Hicks and colleagues[148] found that when one test was used to assess patients with low-back pain, the sensitivity was 94% and the specificity was 28%, but if at least three tests were used, the sensitivity went down to 56% but the specificity went up to 86%. Many special tests used in orthopedics and sports medicine do not have excellent records for diagnostic accuracy, and several other tests have not been tested for their accuracy. These are additional reasons why clinicians should use a cluster of tests to improve the accuracy of their diagnoses. The greater the number of positive test results, the more confident the clinician can be that the diagnosis is accurate.[149]

Rehabilitation Interventions

Since the axial skeleton and its related soft tissues provide stability during body motion, these are obviously important structures for functional activities. We often simply refer to this body mass as the *trunk* or *core*. Trunk stability improves with co-contraction of anterior and posterior trunk muscles.[61] Unfortunately, because of the locations,

Evidence in Rehabilitation

The Ober test, as introduced by Dr. Frank Ober in the mid-1930s, was a test he used to determine if his patients needed spinal surgery.[150] His test is commonly used to assess femur abductor tightness or ITB tightness. However, recent research indicates that the Ober test may not actually be testing abductor or ITB tightness.

Research has demonstrated that the position of the acetabulum determines the amount of coverage of the acetabulum on the femur,[151] the position of the femur,[152] and the movement of the femur.[153] Based on these findings, some researchers have theorized that the Ober test is less a test of the femur and more a test of the acetabular position. Willett and colleagues[154] transected the ITB and the hip capsule to determine which structures had a stronger influence on the cause of a positive Ober test. These researchers determined that even with a transected ITB, the Ober test remained positive, while transection of the hip capsule generated a negative Ober test. The implication is that the position of the pelvis may influence the position of the femur, generating hip capsule torsion, which is the source of a positive Ober test. Tenney and colleagues,[155] Kage and Naidu,[156] Shori and Joshi,[157] and Basu and colleagues[158] determined that exercises using muscles to perform a posterior pelvic tilt (i.e., hamstrings, abdominals, and ischiocondylar adductor) were more effective in producing a negative Ober test than ITB stretching. Further research is needed to determine the cause of a positive Ober test and the clinical implications of the test results.

positions, and fiber alignment of the muscles surrounding the trunk, there is no single exercise that works all of these muscles. It has been shown, however, that the transverse abdominis and multifidus are the only muscles that are normally activated in all trunk motions.[63] Based on what we know of the spine and the importance of stabilization, several issues must be addressed in a rehabilitation program for any patient presenting with sacroiliac or spine pain, regardless of the patient's injury. Patients with neck, back, and sacroiliac pain commonly present with similar deficiencies, including the following:

1. *Reduced proprioception.*[159] Deficiencies in proprioception, balance, and coordination during activity result in inadequate or unsafe performance.
2. *Reduced muscle endurance.*[160] Although strength is a significant factor, especially in the athletic and blue-collar worker population, muscle endurance is perhaps a more important factor because it is required for good posture and for performing the activities of daily living. Muscle endurance may be more deficient than strength, and it must be restored to ensure the safe performance of functional activities. The internal obliques, external obliques, and transverse abdominis must work together during basic functional tasks such as walking.[43]
3. *Lack of muscle coactivation.*[161] If the trunk muscles do not co-contract during difficult activities, spinal stiffness and stability are insufficient, resulting in an increased injury risk.
4. *Delayed core muscle recruitment.*[162] If stabilizing muscles fail to fire when they should, stability is lost, and more stress is placed on other supporting structures such as muscles, joints, and ligaments. Additionally, not only is injury risk increased, performance decreases.

5. *Incorrect diaphragm use.*[163] The diaphragm has a necessary role in spinal stability as well as in respiration.[164] As a stabilizing muscle, the diaphragm changes its function during activity, but when pain interferes with its function, its ability to support and stabilize is lost.[44]
6. *Hip muscle strength imbalances.*[71] Since the hips provide a base for the lumbar spine, if hip strength is deficient, especially the extensors and abductors, their weakness will directly affect the spine.
7. *Reduced stability.*[16] All of these factors contribute to create trunk instability. This instability not only increases a person's injury risk but also prevents optimal performance by limiting force transfer through the trunk and reducing efficiency.

Given these problems, one of the goals for treating a patient with axial pain is to resolve them. A rehabilitation program for a patient with these symptoms and problems should include the following:

1. Flexibility and mobility activities for the spine, pelvis, and hips
2. Proprioception and balance activities
3. Muscle endurance, reeducation, retraining for coactivation and recruitment during daily activities
4. Muscle strength exercises
5. Instruction in core recruitment to enhance spinal stability during difficult tasks
6. Exercises for cervical and upper thoracic muscles for head position and posture endurance
7. Exercises for the larger trunk muscles, the trunk movers, in all planes of motion along with coactivation activities

8. Hip muscle strengthening exercises
9. Progression to functional, work-specific, and performance-specific activities that simultaneously incorporate spinal stabilization

Flexibility Activities

Flexibility activities for the spine and pelvis include both manual techniques and exercises. Manual techniques are used when there are either soft-tissue or joint restrictions that impede normal mobility or range of motion. These techniques are usually incorporated to varying degrees into the first two phases of rehabilitation, the inactive and active phases, and they continue until the goals for their inclusion in the program are achieved.

Vertebral Artery Insufficiency

Before any manual technique for the spine is used on a patient, it is important to first test for vertebral artery insufficiency. Although such a problem is rare, injury to the cervical spine or poor posture may create vertebral artery compromise or insufficiency.[165, 166] Unknowingly treating patients with such a condition can create serious complications such as brain stem ischemia. Since the vertebral artery supplies blood to the medulla oblongata, the part of the brain that controls cardiac and respiratory functions, circulatory compromise can affect these functions.[167] Therefore, it is very important to check for vertebral artery insufficiency before beginning treatment to the cervical spine.

The ability to detect vertebral artery insufficiency with certainty is disputed.[165] However, since no definitive tests have yet come to light, clinicians rely on the existing tests before they administer manual therapy. These clinical screening tests try to temporarily occlude a vertebral artery on one side or the other to identify a patient who is at potential risk of vertebral artery injury during a cervical treatment.[168]

To identify patients with potential vertebral artery insufficiency, static and dynamic tests are performed before cervical treatment. These tests are particularly important if the patient reports any symptoms of vertebral artery involvement: dizziness, light-headedness, nausea, blurry vision, tinnitus, headaches, or facial sensory deficiencies.[169, 170] If any of these tests produces any of these symptoms, it is an indication that the vertebral artery is being occluded.

The two active tests should be performed before the passive tests.[171] The patient may be sitting or standing with the clinician positioned behind the patient. In the first active test, the clinician stabilizes the patient's shoulders and has the patient rotate the head and neck maximally to the left and to the right, holding each end position for about 10 to 30 s. In the second test, the clinician holds the patient's head stable while the patient rotates the body to

the left and to the right,[172, 173] holding each position for about 10 to 30 s. If the patient reports symptoms in the first test but not the second test, the problem is related to the vestibular system. Symptoms produced with the second test may indicate vertebral artery compromise.[172] A positive test should be reported to the physician, and the patient should avoid positions in cervical rotation until further examination is provided.

The five static tests are passive and can be performed with the patient sitting, standing, or supine, although supine is the best position for achieving the greatest motion; sitting offers the additional benefit of gravitational pull on the artery. The patient is more likely to relax in supine with the clinician's hands supporting the head off the end of the table. The clinician places the patient's head and neck into each of the following positions and holds each position for 10[171] to 30 s:[174, 175] (1) maximally rotates the patient's head and neck to the left, (2) maximally rotates the head and neck to the right, (3) maximally extends the patient's neck with exaggerated lordosis in the mid-cervical region, (4) maximally rotates and extends the head and neck to the left, and (5) maximally rotates and extends the head and neck to the right. While each position is held at its end range, the clinician observes the patient's eyes for either changes in pupil size or nystagmus and asks the patient to report any symptoms. Although there is some dispute over which of these tests is most likely to reveal a positive result when the condition is present,[176, 177] it is probably better to perform these tests than to risk unknowingly treating a patient with vertebral artery insufficiency.[165, 178]

 Go to HK*Propel* and watch video 17.7, which demonstrates vertebral artery insufficiency.

Soft-Tissue Mobilization

Because there are so many types of soft-tissue mobilization techniques, only a couple of techniques are identified in this chapter. Keep in mind, however, that other soft-tissue mobilization techniques may be more appropriate than those presented here, depending on the individual and the specific injury. The techniques listed in table 17.5 are the specific Travell and Simons[179] trigger point release applications for the spine that are found in chapter 11. If the rehabilitation clinician observes pain-referral patterns identified with these muscles, he or she should use some of these techniques.

Figure 17.19 shows a soft-tissue mobilization technique that you can instruct the patient in and that does not require assistance to perform. It uses either one or two old tennis balls that have lost their compression. If two balls are used, they can be either taped together or placed together in a sock. One tennis ball may be used if the area is small. The patient lies on the tennis balls, which are placed under a

TABLE 17.5 Spinal Muscles With Commonly Found Trigger Points

Spine segment	Muscle with trigger points
Cervical	Upper trapezius
	Levator scapulae
	Sternocleidomastoid
	Scalenes
Thoracic and lumbar	Paraspinals
	Quadratus lumborum

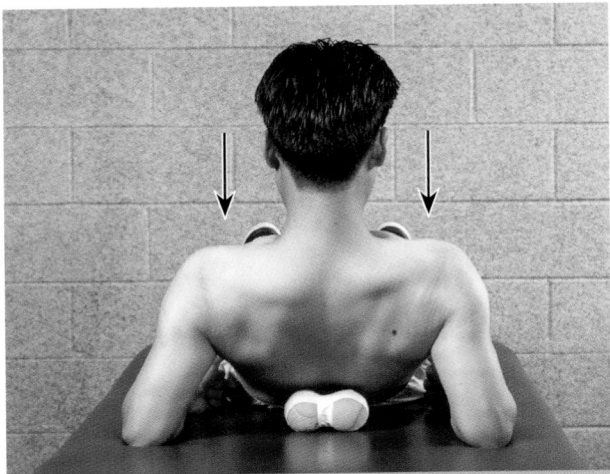

Figure 17.19 Tennis ball release. The patient lies down and relaxes so his body weight pushes the tennis balls into a trigger point or area of fascial restriction.

tender, restricted soft-tissue area. The patient lies on the tennis balls until the tenderness is gone and he or she feels only the pressure of the tennis balls. The patient then rolls over the balls to move them to another location of restriction and discomfort, and the technique is repeated. If tissue is normal, the tennis balls will not create pain. This technique can be performed in the thoracic and lumbar areas; it can also be used in other soft-tissue restricted areas of the body such as the hip and thigh.

Joint Mobilization

Obviously, the degree of movement in spinal joint accessory motion is very different from that in extremity joints. In learning how to determine normal movement, you will have to evaluate many vertebral movements on many patients of varying ages and with various conditions. Normal accessory movement in the lumbar spine is different from that in the cervical spine, and joint accessory movement in a 19-year-old patient is different from that in a 50-year-old. You must recognize and consider these normal variations when assessing and treating a patient with joint mobilization.

Joint mobilization is used to reduce pain or improve mobility. Since it is common to find a hypermobile vertebral joint adjacent to or near a hypomobile joint,[172] each spinal level should be assessed before joint mobilization is applied. The hypermobile joint should not be mobilized, but the restricted joint should be treated to improve its motion.

There are some basic principles to know before we discuss specific application techniques. When the cervical spine and head are in normal alignment, the lower cervical and lower lumbar spines are curved somewhat anteriorly. Because the best position for joint mobilization is an open-packed position, these areas of the spine should be placed in slight flexion to place the joints into a mid-position before mobilization is performed. Rotating the head to the nonpainful side opens the vertebral foramen of C2 to C7 on the painful side.[180] You can also open these foramina by laterally tilting the patient's head away from the painful side. Mobilization techniques differ for the upper and lower cervical spine.

The clinician's body weight supplies the force needed for joint mobilization, not the fingers, thumbs, or hands. Using body weight to supply force rather than the hands provides several benefits: it frees the fingers and hands to focus on joint movement, allowing more sensitive palpation; it is more comfortable for the patient; it imposes less stress on the clinician's fingers, thumbs, and hands; and it conserves the clinician's energy.

Initial mobilization techniques should be gentle. There should be no increase in patient symptoms because of the treatment. Examination before, during, and after the application is necessary for you to decide the appropriate treatment grade. The primary factors indicating the need for lighter mobilization grades are muscle spasm and pain: gentle grade I and II mobilization are used. Refer to chapter 11 for joint mobilization grades, indications, precautions, and contraindications.

Although there are several mobilization techniques for the spine, only a few for each area of the spine are presented here. The primary techniques described include central posterior–anterior (PA) and unilateral PA mobilizations. The symbols used to record these techniques

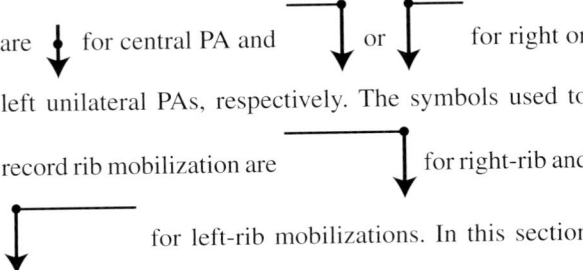

we will consider additional techniques for some specific sites. We recommend that once you begin practice as a qualified health care provider, you participate in continuing education courses to develop an understanding and

Evidence in Rehabilitation

In 2015, Shank Ganesh and colleagues[181] published an article on the effects of joint mobilization applied to the facet joints of the lumbar spine. They wanted to see if changes that occurred as a result of applying joint mobilization to the spine remained for longer than just immediately post-treatment. The authors applied a grade III PA oscillation for 30 s at each level from T12 to L1 through L5 to S1 unilateral facet joints. They measured each subject's straight-leg raise motion before and after treatment, comparing the results to a control group. Twenty-four hours later, the measures were repeated. They found the immediate-change effects remained over the 24 h time frame. This study is important in that it demonstrates that there may be more than immediate beneficial effects from joint mobilizations. It will be interesting to see what other benefits may occur with joint mobilization when there are changes in other factors, such as the amplitude of force applied or the duration of treatment.

appreciation of more complex maneuvers. You should also keep in mind as you go through the techniques presented here that there are a number of variations and styles of joint mobilization applications; the ones presented here are only examples.

Cervical Spine The most commonly used cervical spine joint mobilization techniques are outlined in the following sections. Descriptions of these techniques will primarily emphasize hand placement. The specific grade applied is determined by the patient's condition and the treatment goals, but remember that grades I and II are used for pain relief and grades III and IV are used to improve range of motion. Regardless of the grade applied, hand placement is the same unless otherwise indicated. Refer to chapter 11 for a review of joint mobilization.

Joint Mobilization of the Cervical Spine

Spinal mobilization techniques are divided into three sections: cervical, thoracic, and lumbar spine segments. As you apply joint mobilization techniques, you must know how to position the patient in order for the treatment force to occur parallel to the plane of the joint. As you learn these joint planes and how to position the client, it is sometimes useful to have a spine model nearby to visually identify each vertebral level's position before joint mobilization techniques are applied.

Longitudinal (Distraction) Movement

Resting Position: Normal alignment of the head with the body.

Mobilization Technique: Distraction.

Indications: Relaxing technique used to gain patient's confidence.

Patient Position: Supine.

Rehabilitation Clinician and Hand Positions: The rehabilitation clinician stands or sits by the head of the table, facing the patient. The patient's head is grasped and supported with one of the rehabilitation clinician's hands behind the head; the thumb and fingers are at the occiput. The other hand is placed under the chin (figure 17.20).

Mobilization Application: While maintaining the position of the upper extremities, the rehabilitation clinician leans back to produce a gentle longitudinal pull of the neck.

Notations: The hand on the chin is for positioning only; no force is directed into the chin. This is often the technique used to initiate a mobilization treatment session.

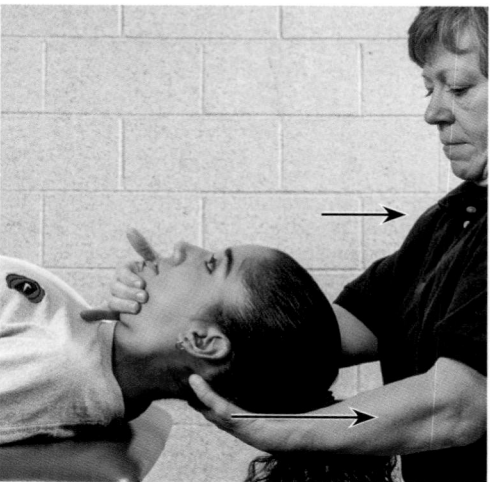

Figure 17.20

Central PA Mobilizations

Resting Position: The cervical spine is in good alignment to allow the rehabilitation clinician to identify the level being treated. Usually this is a position of proper alignment relative to the entire spine or slight cervical flexion to expose a specific joint. Instructing the prone patient to slightly tuck the chin tends to flatten the cervical spine to provide good alignment for joint mobilization.

Mobilization Technique: Anterior glide.

Indications: Midline pain, unilateral pain, or spasm; decreased mobility.

Patient Position: The patient lies prone with his or her hands under the forehead and the chin slightly tucked. If a mobilization table or specifically designed prone pillow is available, either of these may be more comfortable for the patient; in either of these cases, the patient's hands are not under the forehead, but the arms are placed more comfortably at the sides.

Rehabilitation Clinician and Hand Positions: The rehabilitation clinician stands at the head and places the thumbs on the spinous process with the fingers relaxed, along the sides of the neck (figure 17.21). C1 and C3 are usually too difficult to palpate, but C2, C4, C5, C6, and C7 can usually be readily identified.

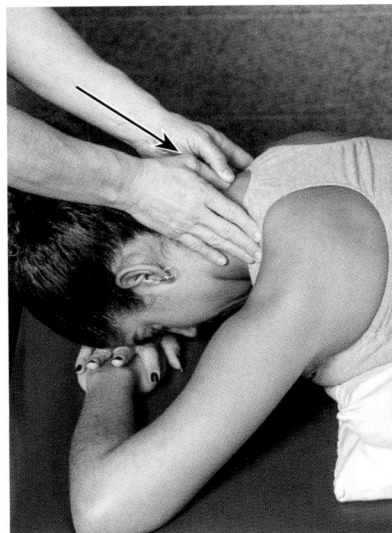

Figure 17.21

Mobilization Application: The rehabilitation clinician applies PA pressure with the thumbs through movement of his or her trunk over the hands. The mobilization force is directed at a 45° angle because of the cervical facets' orientation. This angle usually coincides with the line of the patient's mandible.

Notations: The mobilization grades should be gentle at first; depending on the treatment goals, grades I and II are used to relieve pain while grades III and IV improve joint mobility.

Unilateral PA Mobilizations

Resting Position: The cervical spine is in good alignment to allow the rehabilitation clinician to identify the level to be treated. Usually this is a position of proper alignment relative to the entire spine or slightly flexed to expose the specific joint.

Mobilization Technique: Anterior glide on the articular pillar to either the left or the right of the spinous process; usually the painful side.

Indications: For lower cervical spine and for unilateral neck pain; decreased mobility.

Patient Position: The patient lies prone with his or her hands under the forehead and the chin slightly tucked.

Rehabilitation Clinician and Hand Positions: The rehabilitation clinician stands on the side that is to be treated. The thumbs are placed on the articular pillar and with the downward force angled about 30° medially (figure 17.22).

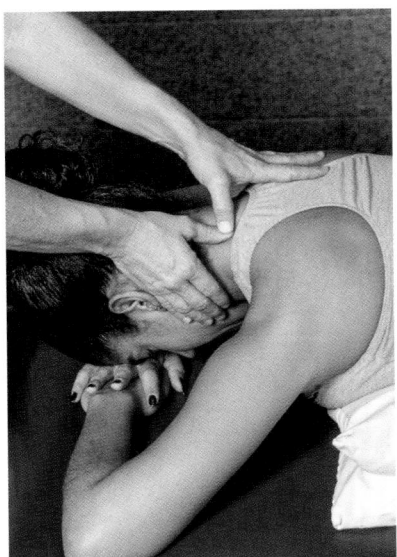

Figure 17.22

Mobilization Application: The pressure is applied by the thumbs in a PA direction with a constant medially directed pressure to maintain position on the articular pillar. In this example, the right thumb is the palpating thumb, while the left thumb delivers the mobilizing force. Notice that the vertical thumb position and 45° angle of the arm allow the clinician to change force angles to be able to apply the mobilization force parallel to the plane of the joint.

Notations: The head may nod slightly, but there should be no rotation motion if the pressure is applied correctly.

Thoracic Spine Look at the bony arrangement on a skeleton to see how the position and relative alignment of the spinous processes change from the cervical to the lumbar spine. The angle of the joint mobilization force must change as these angles change to produce a force in the plane of the joint. This is a crucial point to keep in mind as you perform mobilization techniques along the spine. Joint mobilizations for the thoracic spine are presented here. If you apply the mobilization force in the correct alignment, the patient will not feel uncomfortable, and you will feel the greatest amount of motion at that angle. Therefore, if the patient reports pain or discomfort with your mobilization, apply the force at a slightly different angle; if the angle is correct, the patient's pain during your application goes away.

Joint Mobilization of the Thoracic Spine

As you perform joint mobilization on the thoracic spine, remember that the spinous process is located one full level below the level of its vertebra. Since thoracic vertebrae attach to their corresponding ribs, costovertebral mobilizations are also performed within this spinal segment.

Central PA Mobilizations

Resting Position: The thoracic spine should be relatively parallel to the floor with the patient prone on the treatment table. A pillow is placed under the patient between the pelvis and mid-thoracic spine to achieve this parallel position.

Mobilization Technique: Anterior glide.

Indications: Central or unilateral symptoms.

Patient Position: The patient lies prone with his or her hands under the forehead and the chin slightly tucked.

Rehabilitation Clinician and Hand Positions: The thumbs are placed directly over the spinous process (figure 17.23a), with the fingertips spread across the back to act as stabilizers for the thumbs. The thoracic segment being treated determines where the rehabilitation clinician stands. He or she stands at the head (figure 17.23b) if the upper segments are treated and at the side (figure 17.23c) if the middle and lower segments are treated.

Mobilization Application: The pressure is applied so the thumbs create a line perpendicular to the back's surface; therefore, the thumb positions will change slightly as the hands move along the thoracic spine. The force is transmitted from the clinician's trunk through the arms to the thumbs. Both thumbs may deliver the mobilization force, or the lower thumb palpates while the upper thumb delivers the force. The fingers remain relaxed so the clinician can use them to perceive joint motion.

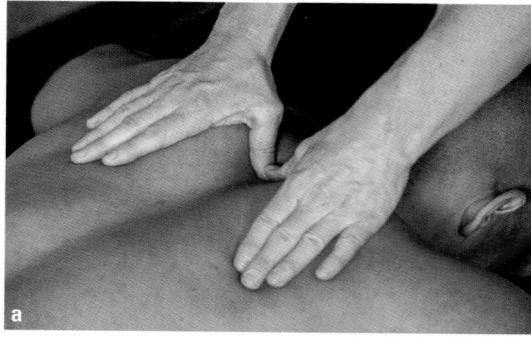

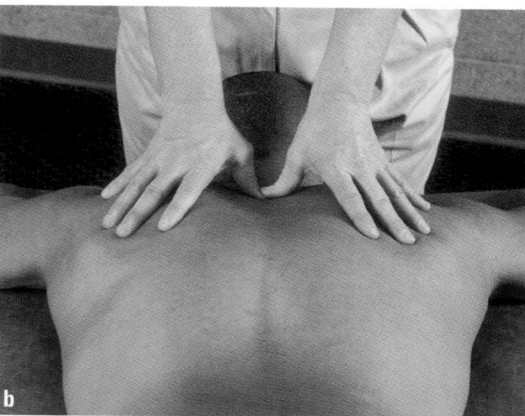

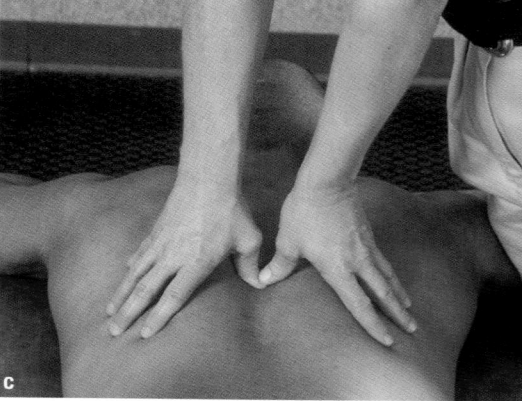

Figure 17.23

Unilateral PAs

Resting Position: As in the previous technique, the thoracic spine should be relatively parallel to the floor with the patient prone on the treatment table.

Mobilization Technique: Anterior glide on either the right or the left side of the spinous process.

Indications: Used for unilateral symptoms.

Patient Position: The patient lies prone with the head turned to the side being treated. The arms hang over the side of the table.

Rehabilitation Clinician and Hand Positions: The rehabilitation clinician stands on the side being treated and places his or her hands on the patient's back, with the thumb pads on the transverse process of the painful side and the fingers buttressed over the back (figure 17.24). The transverse process is located by placing one finger on the spinous process

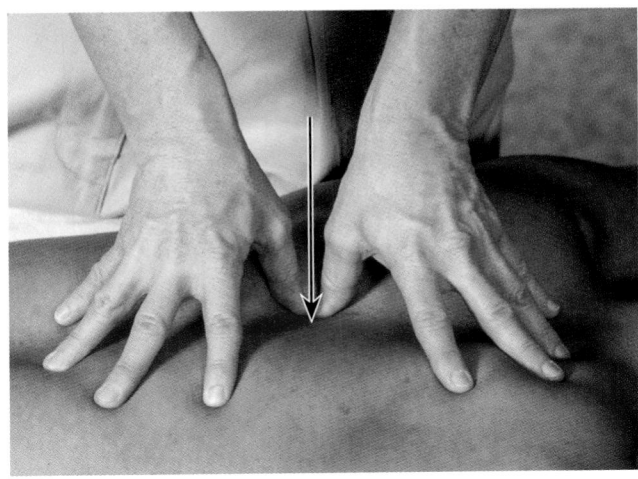

Figure 17.24

of the vertebra immediately above the vertebra to be treated and another finger immediately lateral to that point and in touch with the first finger; this is the transverse process. Remember that thoracic spinous processes extend one level below their vertebrae, so if you want to treat the T7 transverse process, go lateral to the T6 spinous process. The rehabilitation clinician's shoulders and arms are directly over his or her hands.

Mobilization Application: The force is directed perpendicular to the surface.

Notations: Rehabilitation clinician's hand motion occurs as a result of trunk and leg movement, not thumb movement. The side of treatment is usually the painful side.

Unilateral Costovertebral PAs

Resting Position: As with previous thoracic mobilizations, the thoracic spine should be relatively parallel to the floor with the patient prone on the treatment table.

Mobilization Technique: Anterior glide over the costovertebral joint.

Indications: Painful and restricted rib joints.

Patient Position: The patient lies prone with the head turned to the side being treated. The arms hang over the side of the table.

Rehabilitation Clinician and Hand Positions: The costovertebral joint is located by placing two fingers adjacent and lateral to the spinous process; the lateral edge of the lateral digit is over the joint. The ulnar border of the rehabilitation clinician's hand is placed over the costovertebral joint in alignment

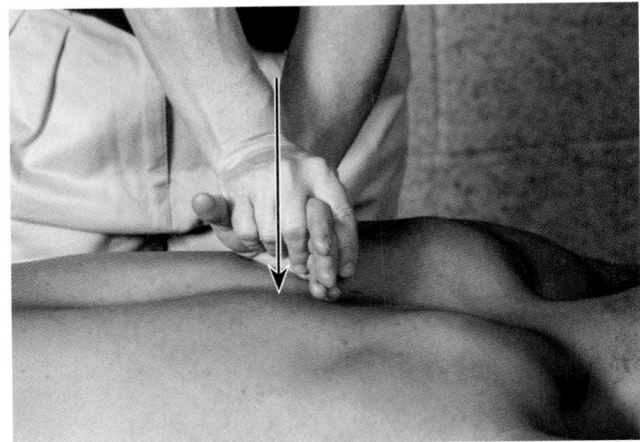

Figure 17.25

with the patient's rib. The other hand is placed on top of the second metacarpal and digit (figure 17.25). Be sure the placement of the ulnar border is approximately two finger widths from the spinous process.

Mobilization Application: The pressure is applied perpendicular to the surface from the trunk through the shoulders and into the hands.

Notations: The two-finger-width positioning for the treatment application is based on the patient's finger width, not the rehabilitation clinician's.

Lumbar Spine Like the cervical and thoracic areas, the lumbar spine is treated with central and unilateral PA movements. In addition, rotation mobilizations can be performed as a gross technique affecting the lumbar spine as a whole rather than treating individual vertebral levels. The following sections describe the various mobilizations for the lumbar spine.

Joint Mobilization of the Lumbar Spine

As features of the largest vertebrae, the lumbar spine's spinous processes are usually easily located. Even though these vertebrae are relatively large, it can be difficult to palpate the transverse processes because of the muscle and fascia mass overlying them.

Central PA Mobilizations

Resting Position: The lumbar spine should be relatively parallel to the floor with the patient prone on the treatment table. A pillow may be needed under the patient's abdomen from the pelvis to the mid-thoracic region to maintain a level lumbar spine.

Mobilization Technique: Anterior glide.

Indications: For hypomobility and central or unilateral pain and derangements.

Patient Position: The patient lies prone.

Rehabilitation Clinician and Hand Positions: The rehabilitation clinician stands to the side of the patient at the lumbar spine level. The ulnar side of one hand, with the other hand reinforcing the treatment hand, may be used to apply the treatment force (figure 17.26). The rehabilitation clinician's shoulders are directly over his or her hands.

Mobilization Application: Pressure is applied directly downward through the shoulders from the trunk.

Notations: Maintain elbow extension while applying the treatment force.

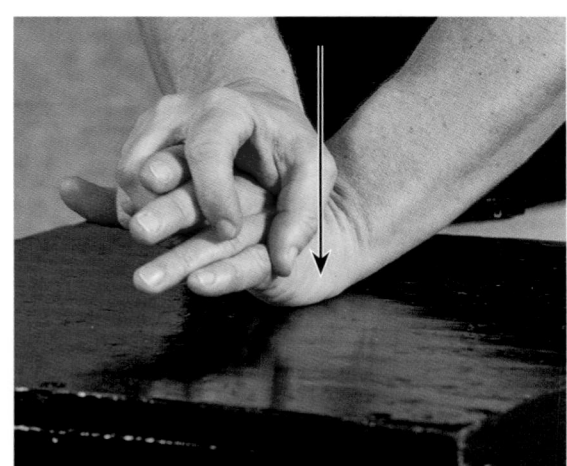
Figure 17.26

Unilateral PAs

Resting Position: The lumbar spine should be relatively parallel to the floor with the patient prone on the treatment table. A pillow may be needed under the patient's abdomen to maintain a level lumbar spine.

Mobilization Technique: Anterior glide on either the right or the left side of the spinous process.

Indications: For unilateral symptoms.

Patient Position: The patient lies prone with the head turned to the side being treated.

Rehabilitation Clinician and Hand Positions: The rehabilitation clinician stands on the side to be treated and places the thumbs immediately lateral to the spinous process, at the level being treated, with the fingers spread across the back to provide stability and support to the thumbs (figure 17.27).

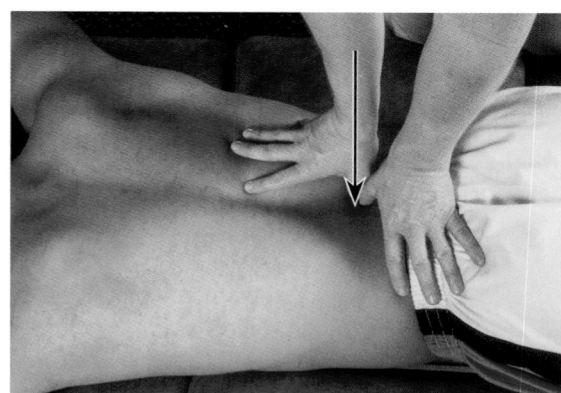
Figure 17.27

Mobilization Application: The pressure is applied directly downward through the shoulders.

Notations: The rehabilitation clinician's shoulders are placed directly over his or her hands with the fingers relaxed.

Rotation

Resting Position: Patient position for all grades is side-lying, but specific position depends upon the grade. The lumbar vertebrae are positioned in mid-range flexion–extension by the amount of hip flexion.

Mobilization Technique: Gross movement rotational glide.

Indications: Unilateral restriction of movement or unilateral back or leg pain.

Patient Position: The patient lies on the unaffected side with a pillow under the head. The top shoulder is near the table's side, and the elbow is flexed with the forearm resting on the side. The lower-extremity position depends on the grade of pressure being applied. For grades I and II, the hips and knees are flexed, with the top leg slightly more flexed than the bottom limb. In grade III, the top shoulder is extended slightly more posteriorly, and the trunk is slightly rotated so that the chest faces the ceiling and the torso is in a three-quarter position. The bottom leg is more extended than in grades I and II; the top leg is flexed forward of the bottom limb with its medial femoral condyle on the table or just off the edge, and the ankle is hooked around the bottom leg. Grade IV position has the top knee more extended and the distal tibia off the table (figure 17.28c).

Rehabilitation Clinician and Hand Positions: The rehabilitation clinician places his or her mobilizing hand on the pelvis. For grade III, the rehabilitation clinician places the stabilizing hand on the patient's shoulder and the mobilizing hand on the pelvis with the fingers pointing forward. If the desired lumbar motion is more into extension, then the hand is placed over the iliac crest with the clinician standing near the shoulder (figure 17.28b), but if the desired lumbar motion is flexion, the hand is placed over the greater trochanter with the rehabilitation clinician standing near the pelvis. For grade IV, the rehabilitation clinician may need to kneel on the table behind the patient or lower the table so the force can be directed more easily from the rehabilitation clinician's shoulders to the hand on the pelvis. The rehabilitation clinician's knee behind the patient's back can also assist in stabilization.

Mobilization Application: For grades I and II, the rehabilitation clinician should produce a gentle rocking motion of the pelvis (figure 17.28a). The rocking motion is produced with movement caused by the hand on the patient's pelvis, not the hand on the shoulder.

Notations: Motion for each grade should be a rotatory motion of the pelvis, not posterior-to-anterior or inferior-to-superior.

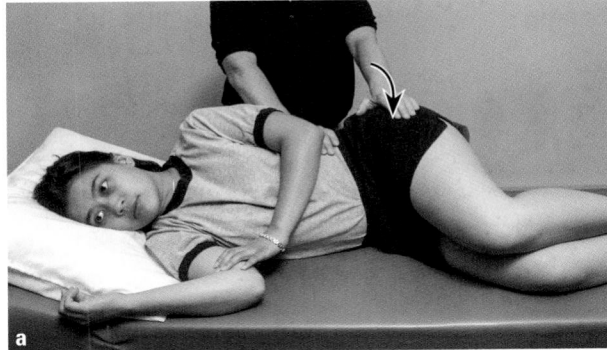
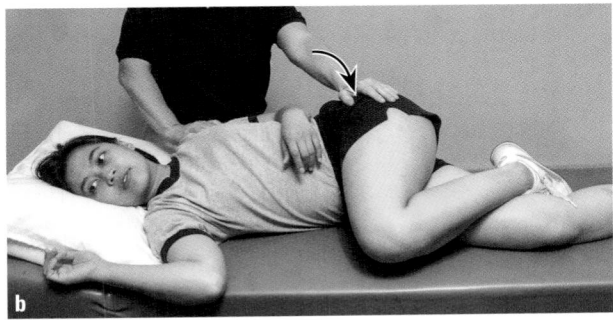
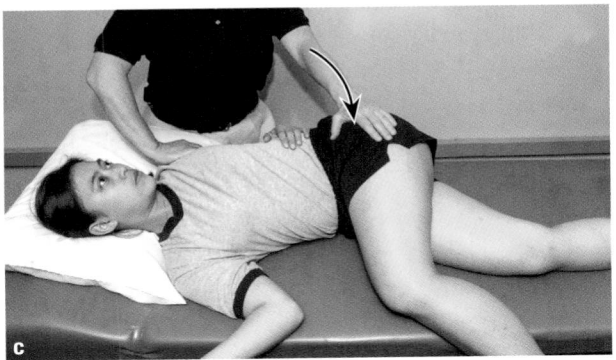

Figure 17.28

Flexibility Exercises

Because the lower cervical spine is related to the upper thoracic spine and the lumbar spine is related to the lower thoracic spine, sacrum, and hips, some of the flexibility exercises for cervical and lumbar regions of the spine overlap into these respective areas. Unless otherwise indicated, the stretch is performed, as presented in chapter 12, throughout the day with 1 to 4 repetitions at each session;

the shorter the hold, the more repetitions performed. If a 30 s hold is used, 1 to 2 repetitions is sufficient, but if a 15 s hold is used, the exercise is repeated 4 times.

The description of each flexibility exercise in the following sections includes the correct manner of execution and common errors or substitutions that should be avoided.

These substitutions occur when patients try to produce as much motion as possible without increasing their symptoms. You should watch for these patterns carefully and correct them as they occur to prevent patients from stretching ineffectively.

Flexibility Exercises for the Cervical, Thoracic, and Lumbar Spine

Exercises listed here are active exercises with overpressure. If the patient experiences pain with overpressure, then the exercise is performed to the motion's end range where there is no pain. As motion improves, additional stretching tension may be tolerated without pain. The exercises presented here begin with cervical stretches and progress down the spine to the lumbar and hip regions. Since the flexibility of hip muscles directly affects the spinal column, stretches for them are included here.

Axial Extension

Body Segment: Cervical.

Stage in Rehab: Active or resistive.

Purpose: This exercise helps the patient restore normal cervical alignment and correct posture.

Positioning: The patient lies supine on a firm surface, such as a tabletop or the floor. A pillow is not used.

Execution: The patient places the fingertips of one hand on the cervical spinous processes and the other hand under the chin (figure 17.29a). The neck is then pushed into the fingertips as the patient tucks the chin, pushing it back with the front hand.

Possible Substitutions: Tilting or rotating the head rather than moving it straight posteriorly.

Notations: As the patient finds this activity easier to perform, he or she can do it while sitting. The patient places the index finger and thumb of one hand on the chin and the fingertips of the other hand along the upper cervical spine. With the chin tucked, the patient pushes the chin back with the chin hand and feels with the other hand as the cervical spine is pushed into that hand (figure 17.29b).

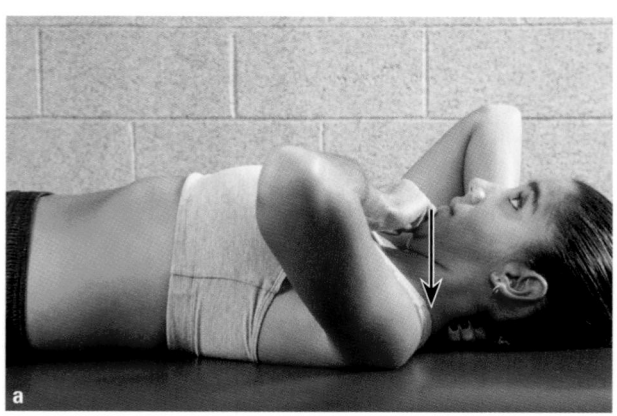
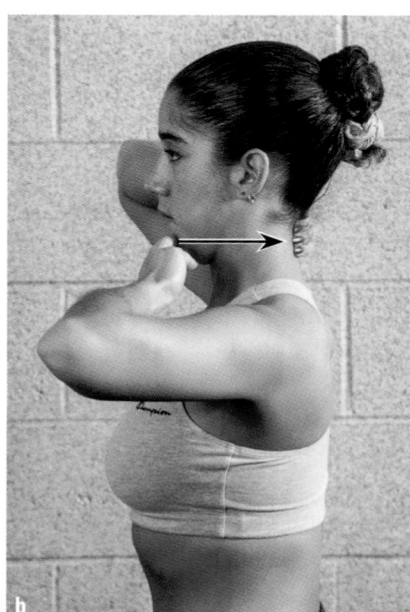

Figure 17.29

Cervical Retraction

Body Segment: Cervical.

Stage in Rehab: Starts in active and continues throughout.

Purpose: This exercise is used to stretch the posterior cervical muscles and improve posture.

Positioning: Sitting, standing, or supine.

Execution: The chin is tucked, and the head is pulled back while the chin stays at the same level (figure 17.30). The head does not tilt up or down during this activity.

Possible Substitutions: Tilting the head upward and moving the cervical spine into lordosis.

Notations: Also called the turtle exercise because of the motion involved.

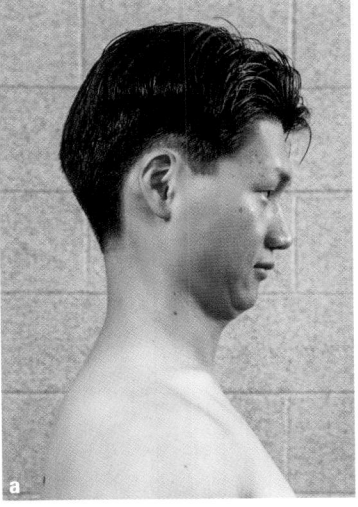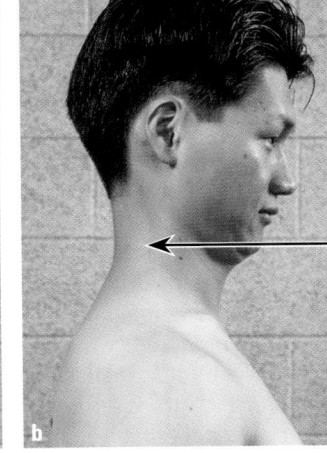

Figure 17.30

Cervical Flexion

Body Segment: Cervical.

Stage in Rehab: Starts in active phase and continues throughout.

Purpose: Stretch the posterior muscles.

Positioning: Sitting.

Execution: With the chin tucked, the patient bends the head forward, trying to touch the chin to the chest.

Possible Substitutions: The common substitution for this exercise is not to curl the neck but to use the lower cervical spine as a fulcrum while the upper cervical spine stays straight. If this occurs, instruct the patient to unwind the neck, beginning with the upper spine and rolling downward. Remind the patient not to pull with the arms since this will produce unnecessary force on the posterior neck.

Notations: The patient should feel a stretch in the posterior cervical muscles. Slight overpressure can provide additional stretch: The patient places his or her hands on the crown of the head and relaxes the shoulders. The weight of the arms will provide sufficient stretch, so instruct the patient not to pull the head but to let the arms relax and the elbows hang down (figure 17.31).

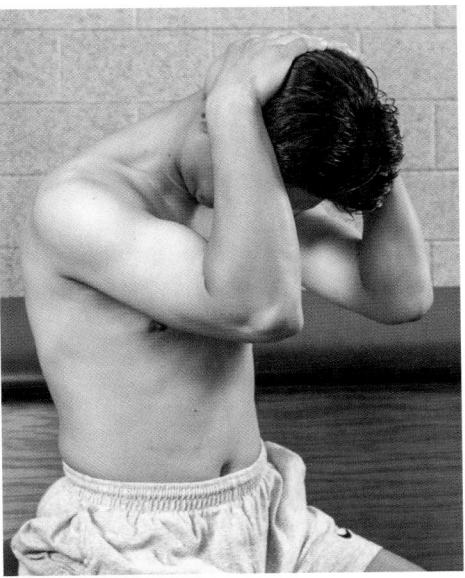

Figure 17.31

Upper Trapezius Stretch

Body Segment: Cervical.

Stage in Rehab: Starts in active and continues through the later stages.

Purpose: Isolate the upper trapezius muscle.

Positioning: Sitting; sometimes it may be necessary to start the patient in a supine position so that cervical rotation and forward flexing are minimized.

Execution: The patient grasps the wrist or forearm of the side to be stretched with the opposite hand and pulls it across the body. The head is tilted away from the shoulder (figure 17.32*a*). Leaning the head to the opposite side increases the stretch.

>continued

Upper Trapezius Stretch >*continued*

Possible Substitutions: Common substitutions for this exercise are allowing the shoulder to shrug upward, rotating the neck, or bending the head forward, rather than directly sideways. If these substitutions occur, correct the patient by instructing him or her to stabilize the shoulder by sitting on the hand, and to keep the nose in a forward position.

Notations: An alternative stretch uses a stretch strap that is draped over the treated shoulder. The toes of the opposite foot are used to anchor the strap to the floor (figure 17.32b). The patient aligns the strap from the anchoring toes to under the elevated heel and takes up the slack using the hands in front of the body to pull on the strap. A towel or other pad is placed on the shoulder, under the strap, for comfort. The heel is then moved to the floor so the strap becomes taut, applying pressure on the upper trapezius. While in this position, the neck is laterally stretched away from the strap until the patient feels a stretch on the side of the neck.

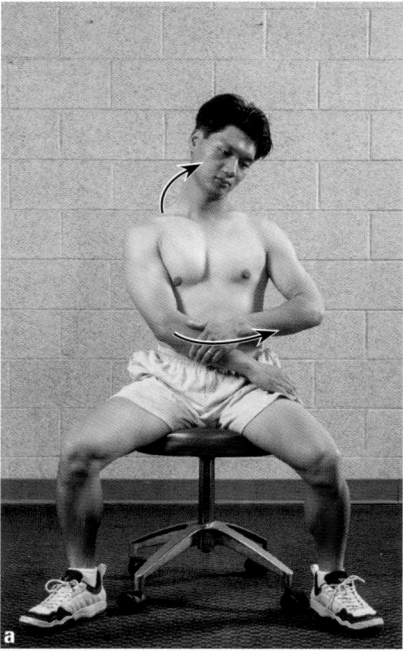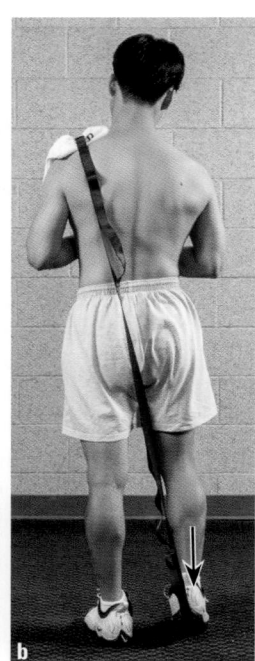

Figure 17.32

Scalene Stretch

Body Segment: Cervical.

Stage in Rehab: Starts in active phase and continues through the later phases.

Purpose: Isolate the scalenes in three different positions.

Positioning: Because the scalenes have three different parts, there are three positions for stretching them. These stretches can be performed in sitting or supine positions.

Execution: The arm on the side being stretched is anchored under the hip in all positions, and the opposite hand is placed over and across the top of the head and above the ear on the stretch side. For the posterior scalene, the face is turned to the opposite axilla (figure 17.33a). For the medius, the patient faces forward while the head is tilted

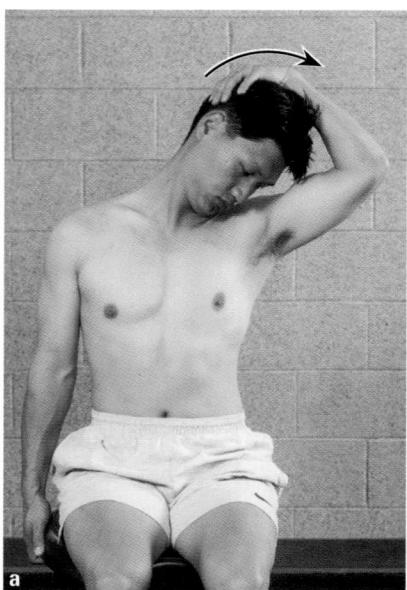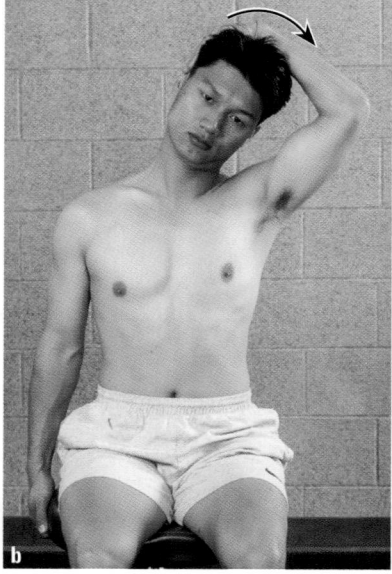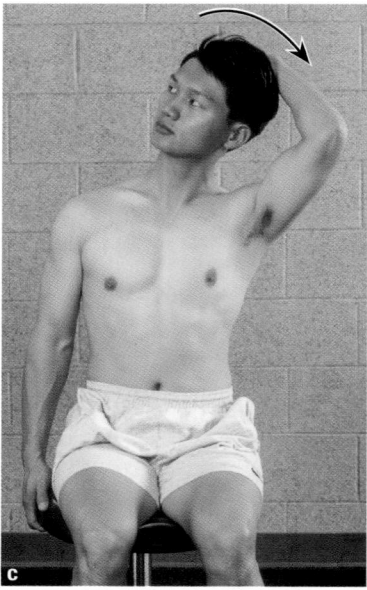

Figure 17.33

laterally (figure 17.33*b*). To stretch the anterior scalene, the face is turned to the ipsilateral side and the patient looks to the ceiling (figure 17.33*c*). The hand over and across the top of the head applies a gentle force that produces a stretch sensation without discomfort or pain.

Possible Substitutions: The common substitutions for this exercise are to move the shoulders or to lean sideways during the stretch. If either substitution occurs, have the patient perform the exercises in supine, and make the patient aware of the substitution.

Spinal Twist

Body Segment: Thoracolumbar.

Stage in Rehab: Begins in the active phase and continues throughout the later stages.

Purpose: Stretch the middle and low back.

Positioning: Sitting on the ground or in a chair.

Execution: On the ground, the patient crosses one leg over the opposite outstretched leg so that the crossing foot is placed lateral to the outstretched knee. The elbow on the outstretched-leg side is placed on the outside of the flexed knee, and the opposite arm is placed behind the body with the elbow straight. The patient then twists the body around toward the straight arm, pushing the elbow on the knee to provide the stretch.

   If performing this exercise in a chair, the patient uses a straight-backed chair without arms. The feet are firmly planted on the floor, and the trunk is rotated toward the back of the chair. With one hand placed on the chair back, the other hand is placed on the lateral knee as shown in figure 17.34. The patient uses the hands to provide the stretch.

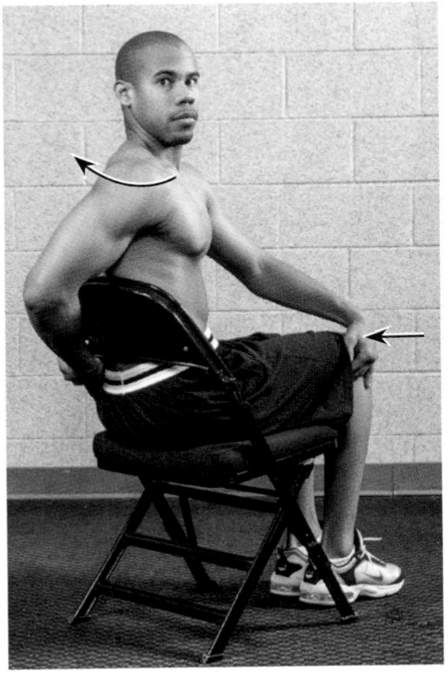

Possible Substitutions: A common substitution for this exercise is to allow the hips to rotate with the stretch. Instruct the patient to apply a hand on the outside of the thigh or knee to hold the hips in place during the chair-twist stretch. To correct the substitution when the stretch is performed on the floor, the patient should use the hand on the knee to apply a stabilizing force.

Figure 17.34

Notations: The thighs should not move during the stretch.

Quadratus Lumborum Stretch

Body Segment: Thoracolumbar.

Stage in Rehab: Starts in the active phase and continues through all phases.

Purpose: Stretch the quadratus lumborum and latissimus dorsi.

Positioning: The patient sits on the floor. One thigh is parallel to the wall with the knee flexed so that the sole of the foot of that leg is placed on the inner thigh of the opposite leg, which is extended out to the side and almost perpendicular to the wall (figure 17.35). The side being stretched is adjacent to the wall.

Execution: The arm farther from the wall is anterior and medial to its ipsilateral leg, and the hand nearest the wall is placed on the wall to push the trunk laterally, away from the wall. The hips remain on the floor, and the pelvis doesn't tip anteriorly or posteriorly.

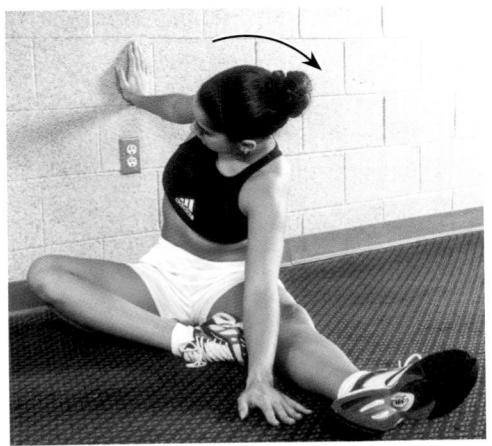

Figure 17.35

Possible Substitutions: A common substitution for this stretch is to move into lumbar extension or lumbar flexion, or to rotate the trunk. Instruct the patient to lean sideways only as far as sagittal movement of the spine permits.

Notations: In an alternative position that offers more stretch, the patient places the wall arm over the head with the shoulder in lateral rotation and full abduction and leans toward the opposite side toward the extended knee.

Prolonged Side-Bending

Body Segment: Thoracolumbar.

Stage in Rehab: Starts in the active phase and continues throughout the later phases.

Purpose: Stretch the lateral trunk area. This activity can also be used to open a closed facet.

Positioning: The patient is side-lying with the tight region on the top and a rolled towel or pillow supporting the portion of the trunk that is directly under the tight region.

Execution: The top arm is placed overhead, and the top leg is in extension (figure 17.36). Increasing or decreasing the size of the rolled towel or pillow can alter the degree of stretch. This position is held for anywhere from 5 to 15 min, depending on the patient's tolerance.

Possible Substitutions: Trunk flexion and rotation are common substitutions with this exercise. The patient must remain in a straight-aligned position of the trunk relative to the pelvis to attain optimal results.

Notations: Depending on the position and where the rolled towel or pillow is placed, this exercise can be used to stretch out the middle or lower thoracic area or the lumbar area. This stretch may require the use of more than one towel or pillow, depending on the patient's tolerance and the amount of restriction present. The patient may not feel a stretch initially, but as the stretch position continues, the patient will report a stretch sensation.

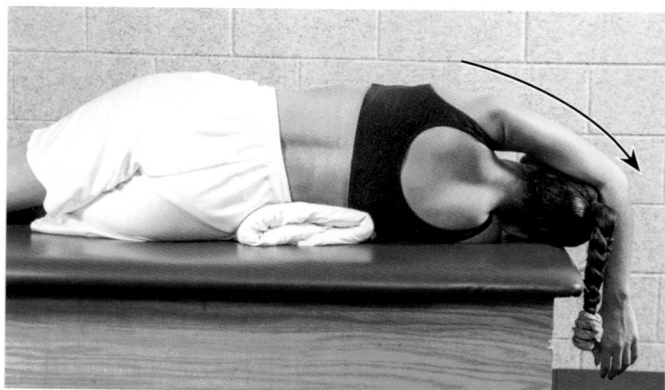

Figure 17.36

Bent-Over Stretch

Body Segment: Thoracolumbar.

Stage in Rehab: Starts in the active phase and continues throughout.

Purpose: Stretch the lumbar and thoracic spine.

Positioning: The patient sits in a chair with the feet flat on the floor and shoulder-width apart.

Execution: Starting from the neck, the patient slowly flexes forward and continues to roll the spine into a C as the body flexes forward during exhalation. The patient can wrap the hands around the ankles from inside the legs to outside the ankles and pull to give an additional stretch. When returning to the starting position, the patient places the hands on the knees and pushes with the arms to move upright rather than using the trunk muscles.

Possible Substitutions: Bending from the hips is the most common substitution. Instruct the patient to roll and feel each segment moving as he or she curls to the end position.

Notations: Because poor rib inward rotation restricts the mobility of the thoracic spine, thoracic motion may be limited. Abnormally limited motion in the thoracic ribs or spine can reduce shoulder motion and inhalation. An important cue is to instruct the patient to exhale as he or she is flexing during this activity.

Lumbar Rock

Body Segment: Lumbar.

Stage in Rehab: Starts in the active phase and continues throughout the later phases.

Purpose: Stretch the low back and hips.

Positioning: The patient is on the hands and knees with elbows straight, hands shoulder-width apart, knees under the hips, and hands under the shoulders.

Execution: The back is arched during exhalation, and the hips are pushed back toward the ankles as the shoulders go down toward the floor while maintaining thoracolumbar flexion and rib cage inward rotation (figure 17.37*a* and *b*). Without moving the hands or knees, the patient then moves forward to the starting position and continues forward until he or she is in a press-up position (figure 17.37*c*).

Possible Substitutions: A common substitution is to move the hands rather than keeping them stationary. If you observe this, remind the patient to maintain hand positions.

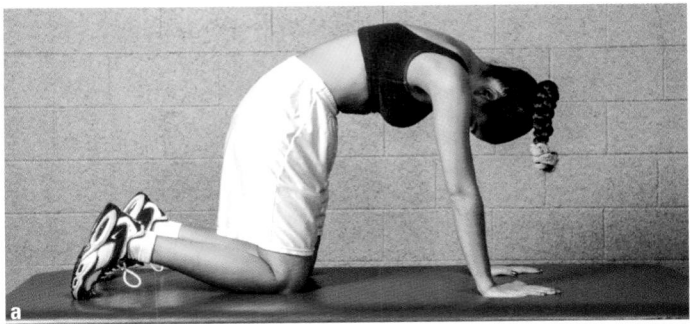
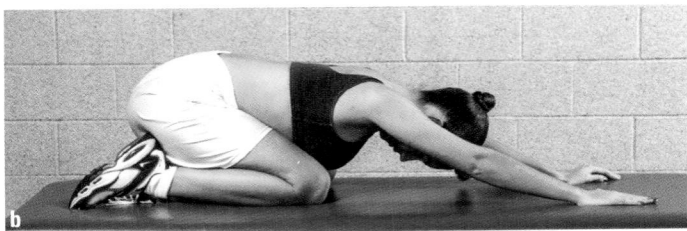
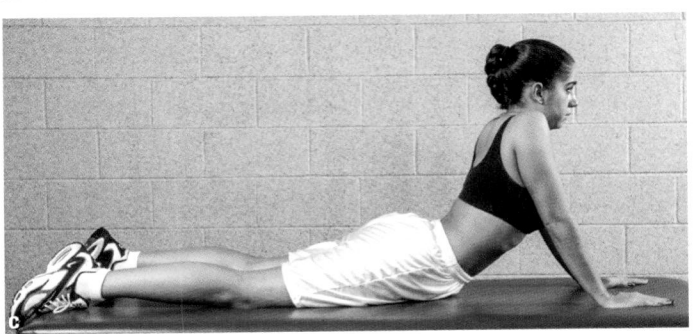

Figure 17.37

Knees to Chest

Body Segment: Lumbar.

Stage in Rehab: Starts in the active phase and continues throughout the later phases.

Purpose: Stretch the low back and hips.

Positioning: Supine with knees and hips flexed and feet on the floor.

Execution: For a single knee-to-chest exercise, the patient first tightens the abdominal muscles to stabilize the pelvis, then lifts one knee to the chest. The knee is passively held to the chest by the arms.

In the more aggressive double knees-to-chest stretch, the patient stabilizes the pelvis by tightening the abdominal muscles, then raises one knee to the chest. While keeping the knee up, the patient raises the other knee to the chest and pulls both knees to the chest with the arms. To lower the legs, the reverse occurs, with the patient lowering one leg at a time.

Possible Substitutions: The most common substitution is moving the back into lumbar extension as the knee moves toward or away from the chest. To prevent this, remind the patient to exhale to engage the abdominal muscles before lifting and lowering each leg.

Notations: In the double knees-to-chest stretch, one leg at a time is raised and lowered to prevent the back from arching.

Lateral Trunk Stretch

Body Segment: Lumbar.

Stage in Rehab: Starts in active phase and continues throughout the later phases.

Purpose: Stretch the lateral lumbar spine.

Positioning: The patient lies supine with the hips and knees flexed, feet flat on the floor, and arms away from the sides.

Execution: One knee is crossed over the other, and the top leg pulls the bottom leg toward the top-leg side while both shoulders remain in contact with the floor (figure 17.38).

Possible Substitutions: A common substitution is to allow the ipsilateral shoulder to come off the floor so less stretch is applied. Remind the patient of the importance of shoulder stabilization if you observe this error.

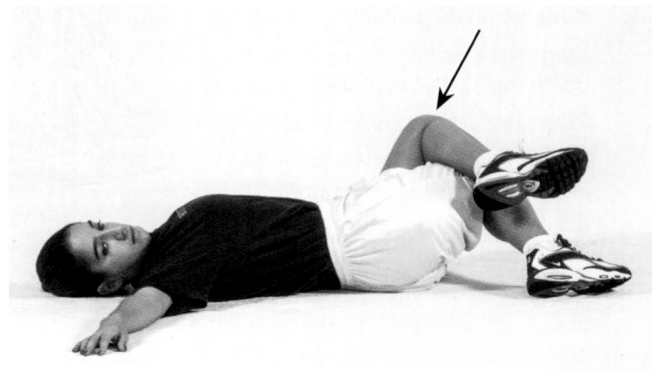

Figure 17.38

Notations: For a more localized stretch to the lumbar spine, the hip is flexed to approximately 90°.

Thomas Hip Flexor Stretch

Body Segment: Hip.

Stage in Rehab: Starts in the active phase and continues throughout the later phases.

Purpose: Stretch the iliopsoas muscle to reduce lumbar spine stress.

Positioning: The patient sits on a table so that the hips are halfway off the table. The patient rolls back to lie supine with both knees to the chest.

Execution: One thigh is grasped behind the knee, and the leg being stretched is lowered off the end of the table. The thigh of the leg being stretched (the lowered leg) should be kept in alignment with the body's midline, without hip rotation or abduction and with knee flexion to 90° (figure 17.39).

Possible Substitutions: Lateral rotation and abduction of the stretched hip are common substitutions. If the patient does not have enough flexion of the nonstretched hip, the back may arch off the table. Remind the patient to firmly pull the nonstretched leg to the chest.

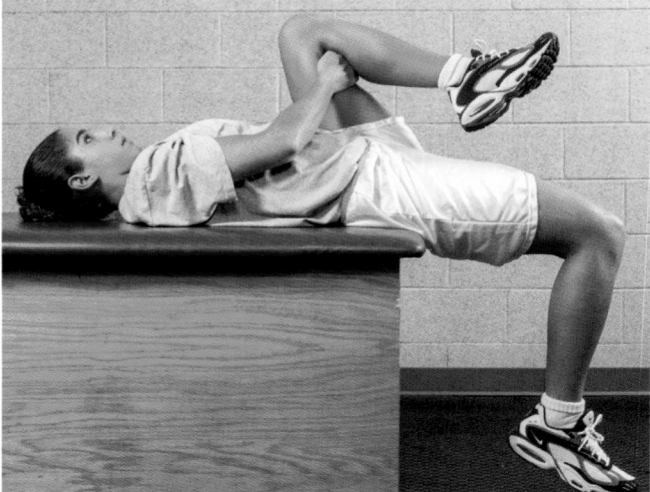

Figure 17.39

Notations: With normal flexibility in this stretch position, the thigh rests comfortably on the table with the back in full contact with the table. This stretch may also be used as a prolonged stretch using straps to secure both the flexed and the stretched hips in place so the patient does not have to work to hold the stretch. If this stretch is used as a prolonged stretch, it is not started until the resistive phase of rehabilitation. A patient may tolerate a 5 min stretch at first, then gradually progress to tolerating longer-duration stretches.

Straight-Leg Raise

Body Segment: Hip.

Stage in Rehab: Starts in the active phase and continues throughout the later phases.

Purpose: Stretch the hamstrings.

Positioning: Supine.

Execution: The patient places the hands behind the thigh of one lower extremity while the other lower extremity remains extended. The patient then extends the knee of the limb that the hands are supporting until he or she feels a stretch in the posterior thigh or behind the knee (figure 17.40).

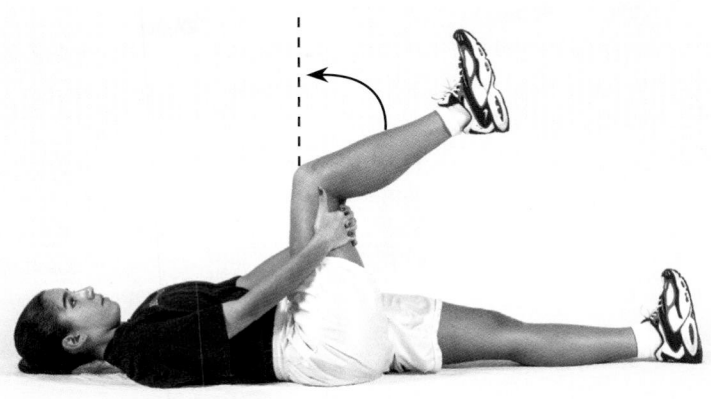

Figure 17.40

Possible Substitutions: The common substitution for this exercise is to flex the opposite hip to relieve the stretch. Remind the patient to keep both knees fully extended throughout the exercise.

Notations: Hamstring tightness can contribute to low-back inflexibility. Although a variety of methods are available to stretch the hamstrings, this exercise places minimal stress on the spine.

Piriformis Stretch

Body Segment: Hip.

Stage in Rehab: Starts in the active phase and continues throughout the later phases.

Purpose: Stretch the lateral rotators, especially the piriformis.

Positioning: The patient lies supine with the knees flexed and feet flat on the floor.

Execution: The knee of the involved leg is crossed on top of the other, and both knees are brought to the chest. The patient grasps the lower knee and uses it to pull both knees toward the chest (figure 17.41a).

Possible Substitutions: A common substitution is to provide less rotation of the stretched hip. The knees should be adequately crossed to aim the knee of the stretched leg toward the opposite shoulder when the knees are brought to the chest.

Notations: The piriformis is a common source of low-back pain. In an alternative piriformis stretch, the patient is on hands

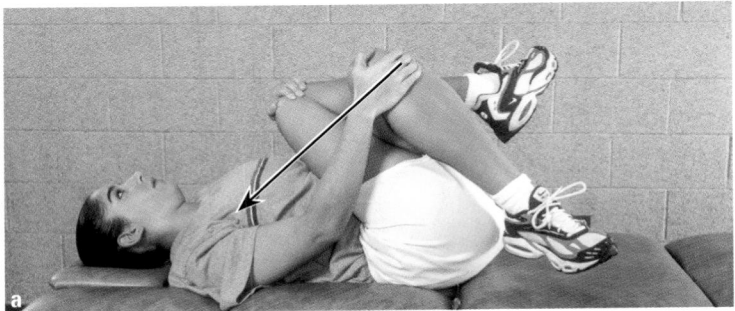

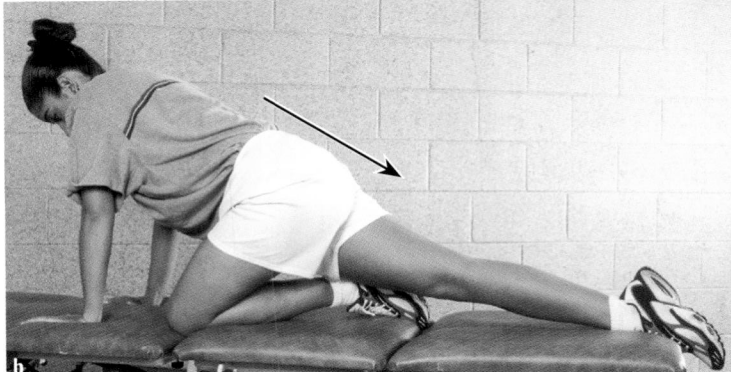

Figure 17.41

and knees with the involved leg and foot crossed in front of the uninvolved knee and behind the involved hip as shown in figure 17.41b. The patient pushes the hips backward, keeping the uninvolved knee extended and the knee of the involved leg flexed and rotated. A common substitution when this exercise is performed is shifting body weight toward the uninvolved side rather than keeping the weight equally distributed over both hips. Instruct the patient not to rotate the hips or pelvis but to move straight back if you observe this substitution.

Iliotibial Band (ITB) Stretch

Body Segment: Hip and thigh.

Stage in Rehab: Starts in the active phase and continues throughout the later phases.

Purpose: Stretch the tight lateral muscles and soft tissue.

Positioning: Supine with the knees extended.

Execution: The extremity to be stretched is flexed and crossed over the other so that the foot of the top leg lies lateral to the opposite knee. The hand on the nonstretched side grasps the crossed-over knee and pulls it toward the floor (figure 17.42).

Possible Substitutions: The common substitution for this exercise is to lift the ipsilateral shoulder off the floor. Placing the arm on the floor at 90° of abduction may help prevent the shoulder lift. Teach the patient the proper stabilization of the trunk for this exercise.

Notations: Tightness in the ITB can affect the low back.

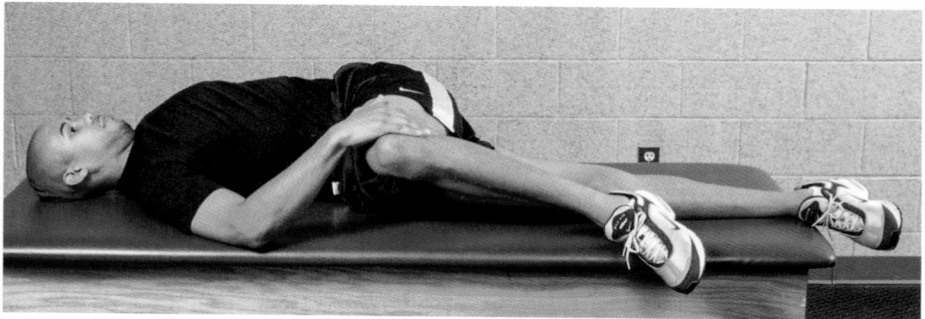

Figure 17.42

Lateral Shift

Body Segment: Lumbar.

Stage in Rehab: Active phase.

Purpose: Correct a lateral shift and realign the spine.

Positioning: The patient stands sideways next to the wall, with the side that has the lumbar lateral shift farthest from the wall.

Execution: Keeping the shoulders level by flexing the elbow and keeping the arm adjacent to the lateral trunk and in contact with the wall, the patient shifts the pelvis sideways to the wall (figure 17.43a).

Possible Substitutions: The common substitution for this exercise is a tilting of the shoulders away from the wall or a leaning of the hips into the wall, or both. If this occurs, either have the patient perform the exercise in front of a mirror or place your hands above the shoulders, but not touching them, and instruct the patient to perform the exercise without letting the shoulder touch your hands.

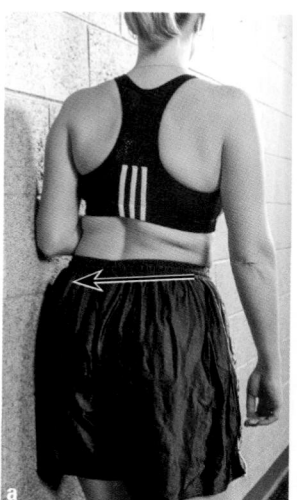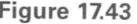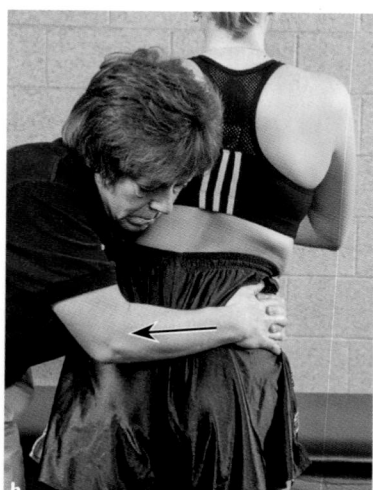

Figure 17.43

Notations: When performing the stretch passively, the rehabilitation clinician stands next to the patient on the side opposite the lumbar shift. The rehabilitation clinician then encircles the patient's waist and clasps his or her hands together on the opposite hip (figure 17.43b). The rehabilitation clinician stabilizes the patient's trunk by leaning a shoulder into the patient's ribs while pulling the pelvis toward him- or herself. If a lateral shift is present, this is one of the first exercises to be used.

Standing Extension

Body Segment: Lumbar.

Stage in Rehab: Starts in the active phase and continues into later phases.

Purpose: Increase trunk extension and relieve tension in the lumbar spine after prolonged sitting or a prolonged forward-bending position.

Positioning: The patient stands and places both hands in the small of the back.

Execution: The patient then leans backward from the waist, leading with the shoulders and keeping the knees and hips extended.

Possible Substitutions: A common substitution is moving the hips posteriorly and flexing the knees to lean backward from the knees. If this occurs, have the patient perform the exercise with his or her back against a kitchen countertop or other firm structure at waist level to stop the hips from moving posteriorly.

Stability and Strength Exercises

As with injuries to other body segments, the rehabilitation clinician first reduces pain, muscle spasm, and edema and then applies techniques and exercises to improve mobility and flexibility. The next level in a rehabilitation program involves strength and muscle endurance. When dealing with spine, core, trunk, and pelvic injuries, stabilization exercises must be included as part of the strengthening portion of the rehabilitation program.

Stability Exercises

To some extent, core stabilization has already been presented. We have presented information on the importance and function of a strong core, how to recruit core muscles, and the muscles included in local and global core muscle groups. This section provides an abbreviated list with explanations of some exercises that strengthen core muscles.

Core muscle strengthening exercises at the most basic level involve two groups of exercises called *dead bug* and *bird dog* exercises. The dead bug exercises involve moving the arms or legs from a supine position, while the bird dog exercises are performed on hands and knees and involve similar extremity movements while recruiting the core muscles to provide stability.[182] These supine (dead bug) and quadruped (bird dog) exercises are outlined here from easiest to more difficult. Table 17.6 provides a progressive list of these exercises. The next progression from these exercises moves the patient to standing exercises, using rubber band and tubing resistance for either upper- or lower-extremity activities. The goal of these exercises is to recruit core muscles during simple extremity motions while performing alternating extremity movements; they serve as precursor activities for performing more difficult and complex stabilization activities.

Not all patients with back injuries need to perform dead bug or bird dog exercises, and some may be able to progress rapidly through them. Any difficulty the patient has with any of these exercises indicates that core sta-

TABLE 17.6   Progression of Dead Bug and Bird Dog Exercises for Early Core Stabilization Exercises

Type of exercise	Name of exercise
Dead bug in supine	1. Stabilization with arm movement
	2. Stabilization with leg movement
	3. Stabilization with ipsilateral arm and leg movement
	4. Stabilization with contralateral arm and leg movement
Bird dog in quadruped	1. Arm raise in quadruped
	2. Leg raise in quadruped
	3. Arm and leg raise in quadruped
	4. Arm and leg raise with resistance in quadruped

bility is inadequate; in these cases, the patient continues the exercise until it is performed correctly; after that the exercise is discontinued or the patient progresses to the next level of exercise.

When to insert these exercises into the patient's rehabilitation program will depend on the patient's status. Some patients may be able to begin them even during the inactive phase, provided their signs and symptoms are relatively minor. However, if a more severe injury limits the patient's ability to perform them, then it is best to wait until the person can do so without pain. Since the dead bug exercises are less intense than the bird dog exercises, they are usually started earlier in the program. None of these exercises should produce pain; if they do, the clinician should be sure the patient is performing them correctly, or wait to add them until the patient can do them without pain.

Dead Bug Exercise Progression   The *dead bug* exercises, or *bug* exercises, are so named presumably because of the position in which they are performed. Remember before each exercise to remind the patient to recruit the core muscles during performance.

The rehabilitation clinician should correct the patient if lumbar extension or an anterior pelvic tilt occurs during any exercise. This includes telling the patient what is being done incorrectly and giving specific instructions on how to correct the performance. If the patient cannot maintain stability or proper breathing techniques during any exercise, even with your verbal and tactile cueing, the patient should return to exercises at the previous level of difficulty.

These exercises may appear to be easy, but if you try them, you quickly realize that when they are performed correctly, they are not as simple as they may seem. They can be made even more difficult by having the patient lie either on a foam roller that is positioned longitudinally from sacrum to cervical spine during the exercises or on a Swiss ball; unstable surfaces make the exercise more difficult to perform correctly.[183]

Each exercise is performed with proper core recruitment before its execution. The patient begins with the supine dead bug exercises and then advances to the bird dog exercises in the quadruped position. Any of these dead bug exercises can be made more difficult by having the patient perform arm and leg motions in a diagonal pattern rather than in straight-plane motions. This change requires additional action from the oblique muscles.

Supine Stabilization With Arm Movement

Exercise Type: Dead bug.

Stage in Rehab: Active and early resistive.

Positioning: Supine with knees and hips flexed, feet flat on the table.

Execution: One arm is raised overhead and then the other, in an alternating fashion (figure 17.44). The trunk is stabilized, with no movement occurring in the spine or pelvis while the arms are moving.

Cues and Notations: Patients are cued to perceive their body weight rolling toward the opposite direction without the legs or pelvis rolling as well. The patient must breathe normally while performing the movement.

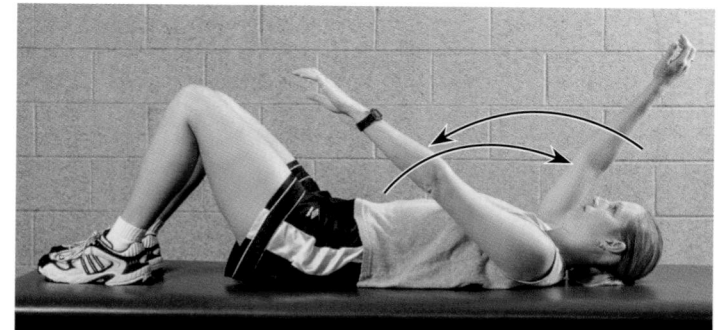

Figure 17.44

Supine Stabilization With Leg Movement

Exercise Type: Dead bug.

Stage in Rehab: Active and early resistive.

Purpose: Instruct trunk mechanics similar to that of the gait cycle with diaphragm breathing.

Positioning: Supine hook-lying position.

Execution: While in a neutral spine position, the patient raises one knee up toward the chest and then extends the leg from the knee without moving the hips as the abdominal muscles are contracted more tightly to maintain pelvic neutral (figure 17.45).

Cues and Notations: The hips should not rise up or rotate, and the back should not arch. The motion should be smooth. The patient returns the leg to the starting position and repeats the movement with the opposite leg.

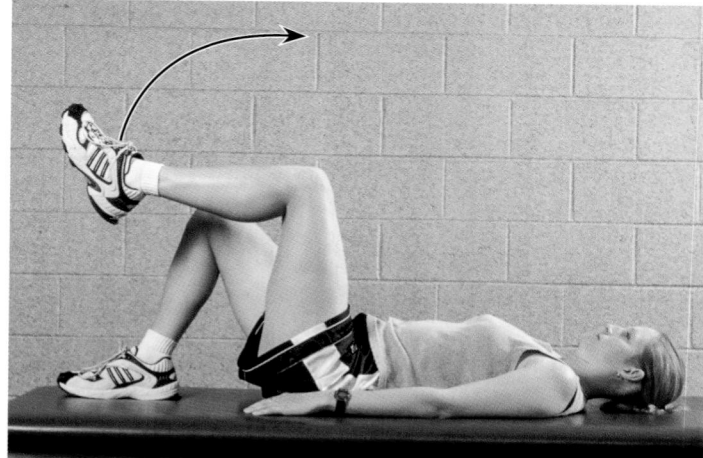

Figure 17.45

Supine Stabilization With Arm and Leg Movement

Exercise Type: Dead bug.

Stage in Rehab: Active and early resistive.

Purpose: Strengthen the abdominal muscles and stabilize the spine during arm and leg movement similar to that of the gait cycle.

Positioning: Supine hook-lying position.

Execution: One arm and the opposite leg are raised simultaneously and then lowered while pelvic neutral is maintained (figure 17.46). The movement is repeated with the contralateral arm and leg.

Cues and Notations: The movement should be smooth, and very little trunk motion should occur. The pelvis is maintained in neutral throughout the exercise. The back should not roll from one side to the other and should not arch off the floor.

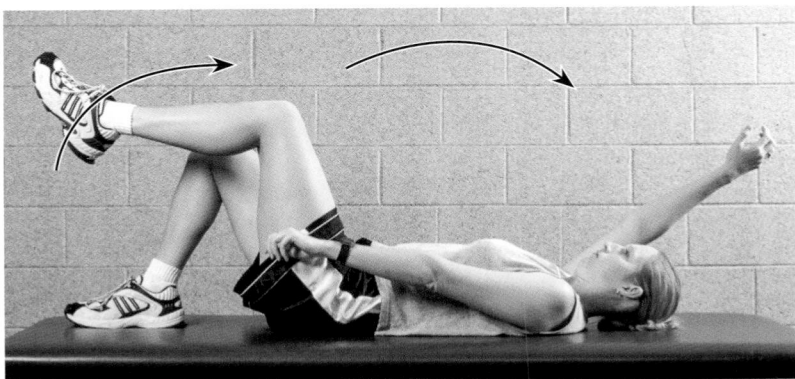

Figure 17.46

Supine Stabilization With Arm and Unsupported Leg+ Movement

Exercise Type: Dead bug.

Stage in Rehab: Active and early resistive.

Purpose: This is a more severe exercise for strengthening the abdominal muscles and maintaining core engagement during independent arm and leg movement.

Positioning: Supine hook-lying position.

Execution: The neck and shoulders should remain relaxed throughout the exercise. The abdominal muscles remain tightened as the patient lifts the arms and legs off the floor. The patient gradually extends one leg while flexing the arm on the same side, then reverses the position with the extremities on the opposite side (figure 17.47).

Cues and Notations: The back should not lift off the floor, and the hips should not roll. This exercise facilitates muscle activity as during the gait cycle.

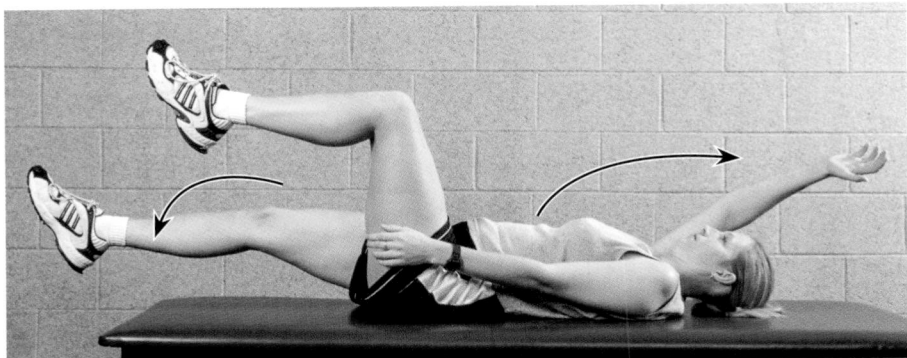

Figure 17.47

Bird Dog Exercise Progression   As with the dead bug exercises, not all patients will need instruction in these exercises. The rehabilitation clinician's examination and assessment of the patient will determine the patient's needs. The patient should maintain an engaged core throughout each of these exercises. When they are performed correctly, the patient's pelvis remains stable and does not rock or roll from side to side during an exercise. A long stick or dowel (1 to 1.3 m; 3 to 4 ft) may be placed across the patient's low back to provide tactile and visual feedback on pelvic position and movement during the exercise. If the patient sees the stick drop on one side during the exercise, he or she knows that the hips have rotated and that core control has not been maintained.

Quadruped Arm Raise

Exercise Type: Bird dog.

Stage in Rehab: Active and early resistive.

Purpose: Spinal stabilization.

Positioning: Quadruped position in a position of exhalation.

Execution: One arm is raised with the instruction to reach forward without allowing the body to move forward, and then repeat on the opposite side (figure 17.48).

Cues and Notations: The hips and pelvis remain stable throughout the exercise. The patient should shift the center of mass toward the ipsilateral knee of the elevated arm without elevating the pelvis on that side.

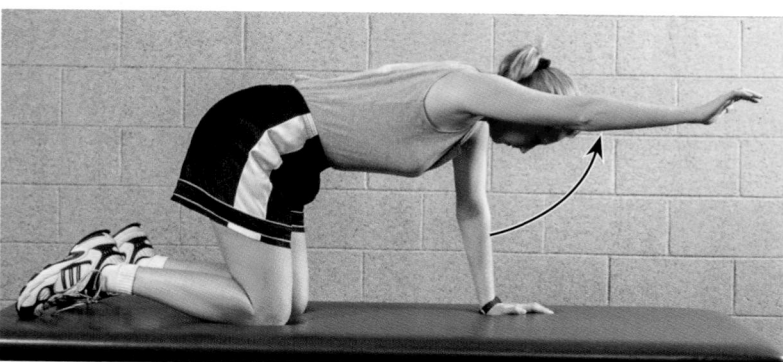

Figure 17.48

Quadruped Leg Raise

Exercise Type: Bird dog.

Stage in Rehab: Active and early resistive.

Purpose: Enhance pelvic stabilization.

Positioning: The patient is in a quadruped position.

Execution: The patient extends one leg, extending the hip and knee by tightening the buttocks and hamstrings. No twisting of the pelvis, trunk, or back should occur throughout the motion.

Cues and Notations: The extremity's motion should be smooth and steady. Cue the patient to lift the leg without lumbar extension. The actual height of the lifted leg is not relevant because it will vary from patient to patient. They may shift to the weight-bearing leg that is on the table.

Quadruped Arm and Leg Raise

Exercise Type: Bird dog.

Stage in Rehab: Active and early resistive.

Purpose: Enhance stabilization and strengthen spine extensors.

Positioning: Quadruped position.

Execution: The patient lifts and reaches forward with one arm and lifts the opposite leg without lumbar extension, and then repeats the motion with the other arm and leg (figure 17.49).

Cues and Notations: Shifting of the center of mass to the right and left is to be expected, but the pelvis should not drop or elevate on one side or the other. Tactile cues may be needed to help the patient with proper execution.

 Go to HK*Propel* and watch video 17.8, which demonstrates the bird dog exercise with corrections for maintaining proper core engagement.

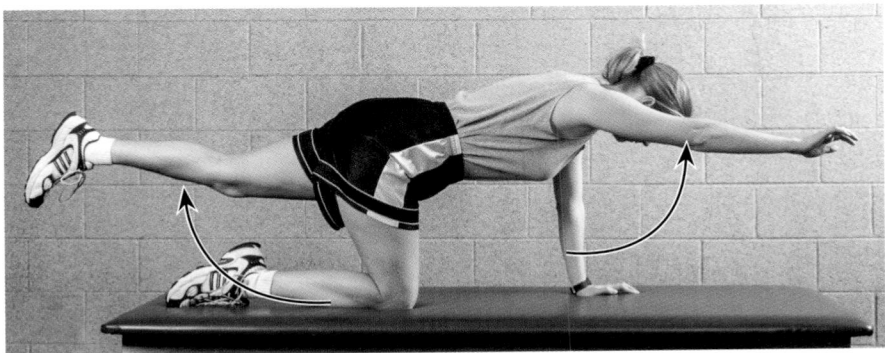

Figure 17.49

Quadruped Arm and Leg Raise With Manual Resistance

Exercise Type: Bird dog.

Stage in Rehab: Active and early resistive.

Purpose: Enhance stabilization and strengthen spine extensors and abdominal muscles.

Positioning: Quadruped position with the lumbar spine in neutral. The patient lifts the arm on the side of the back that is painful and also lifts the opposite leg.

Execution: The rehabilitation clinician grasps the hand in a handshake position. The rehabilitation clinician and patient then play "tug of war." The rehabilitation clinician provides a push-pull resistance to the patient while moving from left to right so the angle of the force in the tug of war varies (figure 17.50). Since the patient must maintain core stability throughout the exercise, this exercise allows for a good transition from single-plane to multiplanar activities while engaging the core.

Cues and Notations: The patient should maintain core control throughout the activity.

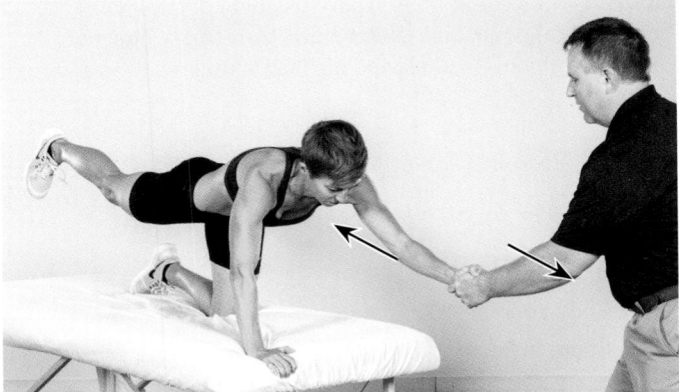

Figure 17.50

Trunk Stability Exercises   Once the patient has mastered these movements, core stabilization exercises progress to more dynamic activities to advance toward functional movements while the core is engaged. Resistive activities that include diagonal lower- and upper-extremity exercises with a resistance band are added during this time. The clinician watches the patient's performance to ensure that the patient can maintain core stability while moving the extremities. As the exercise becomes more physically demanding, the core and trunk move less so that the body has a solid platform to distribute forces without insult to the spine or SI joints. The patient may need to perform exercises in front of a mirror for visual feedback if your verbal and tactile cues fail to correct the patient's form during these activities. The resistance does not need to be severe; a light resistance, especially early in this phase, allows the patient to perform the exercise correctly and to maintain proper control but still create a progression.

Strength Exercises

Goals for these exercises are to increase muscle strength and muscle endurance. Exercises listed in this section begin with the mildest and proceed to more challenging exercises, first for the neck and then for the lower back. Exercises you can use for strengthening, in addition to the suggestions presented in this section, include activities such as aquatic, Swiss ball, and foam-roller exercises.

Strengthening exercises from other chapters that should be included for low-back pain (LBP) patients involve muscles from both the shoulder and hip that are attached to the back.[184, 185] The latissimus dorsi, rhomboids, trapezius, quadratus lumborum, hamstrings, gluteus maximus, gluteus medius, and hip lateral rotators should

all be strengthened as part of a total lumbar stabilization program.

Cervical Exercises   Two distinct advantages of isometric exercises are that they can begin early in the rehabilitation program and that the patient can perform them independently throughout the day. Depending on the severity of the patient's injury, healing process, and presenting signs and symptoms, isometric exercises may be started as early as the late inactive or early active rehabilitation phase. If isometrics are started earlier than the resistive rehabilitation phase, they should be performed at submaximal intensities.

Isometric exercises may produce some strength gains without unduly stressing the joints since no motion occurs during the exercises. Each isometric exercise is maximally held for a count of 6 s, the muscles relax, and then the exercise is repeated. Typically, isometric exercises are performed for 5 to 10 repetitions for one or two sets.[186]

After isometric exercises, more aggressive exercises for strengthening the cervical muscles are begun. These are labeled "resistive cervical exercises." They are performed with manual resistance or with various types of equipment such as resistance bands, pulleys, or machines. It is important to be careful using machine resistance; if performed incorrectly, it can place too much stress on the cervical spine and increase the risk of injury. Proper cervical alignment must be maintained throughout the exercises with movement occurring at each segment—the lower cervical spine should not be used as a fulcrum. If the patient reports pain with any exercise, the clinician must watch the patient perform the exercise to make sure that he or she is doing it correctly before the exercise is changed or removed from the program.

Strength Exercises for the Cervical Muscles

Isometrics

Body Segment: Cervical.

Stage in Rehab: Active phase.

Purpose: Early strengthening in all planes.

Positioning: The patient is sitting or supine with the neck in a midrange and properly aligned position.

Execution:

1. Forward flexion: The patient places the palms of the hands on the forehead and tries to touch the chin to the chest while providing resistance to the motion with the hands on the forehead (figure 17.51*a*).

2. Extension: The patient places both hands behind the back of his or her head while trying to tilt the head backward, resisting the motion with the hands (figure 17.51*b*).

3. Lateral flexion: The patient places one hand just above the ear, resisting the motion of bringing the ear to the shoulder on the same side (figure 17.51*c*). Repeat the exercise to the opposite side.

4. Rotation: The patient places one hand on the side of the face and resists the movement of rotating to look over the same-side shoulder (figure 17.51*d*). Repeat the exercise to the opposite side.

Possible Substitutions: A common substitution for each of these exercises is to perform them out of proper cervical alignment.

Cues and Notations: Each exercise should be performed with the head and neck in correct postural alignment. Patients who have difficulty identifying correct postural alignment should perform the exercises in front of a mirror until they can maintain correct alignment during the exercises.

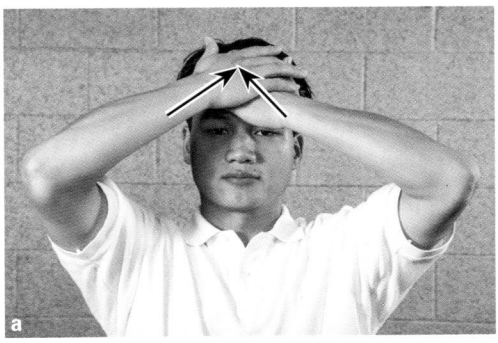
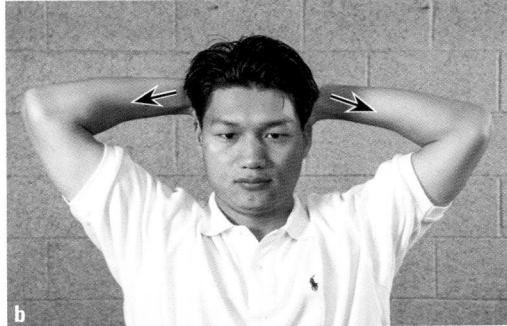
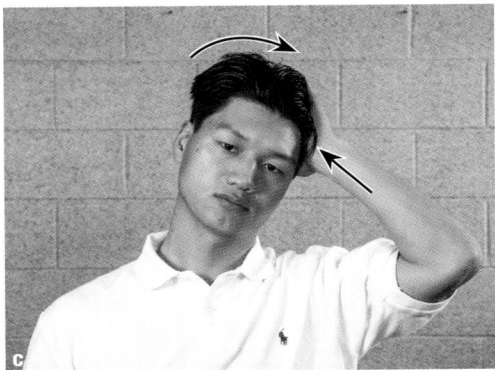
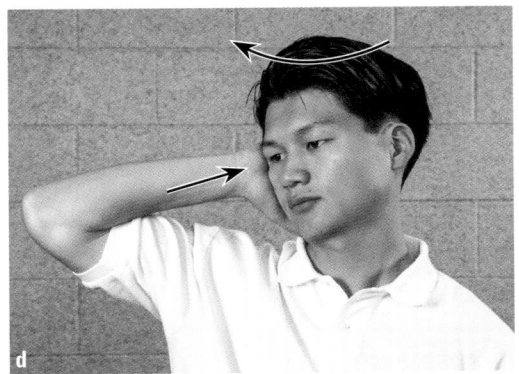

Figure 17.51

Prone Neck Retraction

Body Segment: Cervical.

Stage in Rehab: Active phase.

Purpose: Strengthen the posterior cervical muscles and encourage correct cervical alignment.

Positioning: Prone with the head off the end of the table.

Execution: Keeping the chin tucked, the patient lifts the posterior head toward the ceiling (figure 17.52). The scapulae can also be squeezed together. At the top of the movement, the position is held for 5 to 10 s.

Possible Substitutions: The neck moves into hyperextension and is tilted up toward the ceiling.

Cues and Notations: Instructing the patient to keep the chin tucked and describing the activity as "like opening and closing a drawer" may give the patient a visual image that will help.

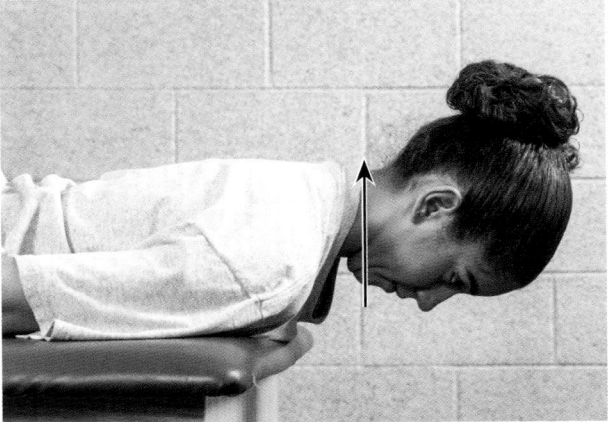

Figure 17.52

Side-Lying Head Lifts

Body Segment: Cervical.

Stage in Rehab: Active phase.

Purpose: Strengthen the lateral neck muscles.

Positioning: Side-lying with the head hanging down toward the table or off the end of the table.

Execution: Keeping the chin tucked in good alignment, the patient lifts the head toward the top shoulder, going through a full arc of cervical motion.

Possible Substitutions: The neck moves into a forward-head position, hyperextends rather than maintaining proper alignment, or does not move in an arc.

Cues and Notations: Give verbal cues for correct alignment and movement.

Upper-Back Exercises   Because many of the shoulder muscles are located in the upper-back region, many upper-back exercises are also shoulder exercises.

Strength Exercises for the Upper Back

Prone Fly

Body Segment: Upper back.

Stage in Rehab: Active phase.

Purpose: Strengthen the rhomboids, middle trapezius, and cervical and upper thoracic spine extensors.

Positioning: Prone on a bench with the arms hanging down to the floor. The patient can also lie prone at the end of a treatment table with the shoulders and head off the end of the table.

Execution: The patient lifts dumbbells toward the ceiling while squeezing the scapulae together (figure 17.53).

Possible Substitutions: People often perform this exercise incorrectly by raising the arms but not squeezing the scapulae together.

Cues and Notations: The patient should be instructed to go through the full scapular retraction motion, squeezing the shoulder blades together. If it is too difficult for the patient to perform the exercise with elbows near extension, flexed elbows may allow for improved scapulae retraction.

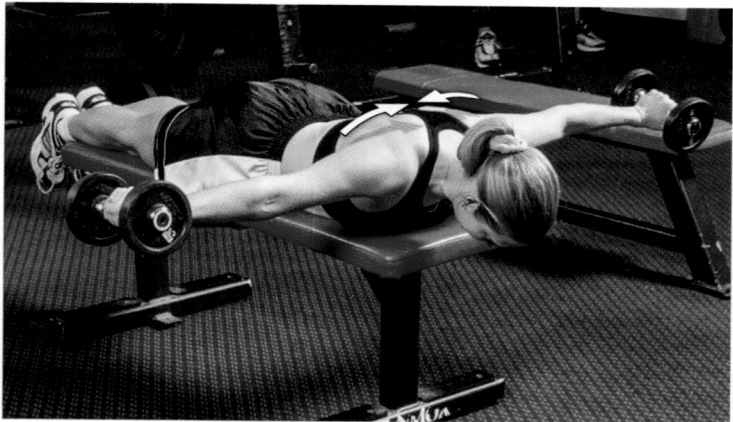

Figure 17.53

Upright Row

Body Segment: Upper back.

Stage in Rehab: Resistive phase.

Purpose: Strengthen the upper back, trapezius, and deltoids.

Positioning: The patient uses pulleys, weights, or resistance bands with hands close together while standing erect.

Execution: Standing with the abdominal muscles tightened to maintain a pelvic neutral position and the feet shoulder-width apart, the patient lifts the device upward toward the chin, keeping the elbows higher than the wrists (figure 17.54).

Possible Substitutions: Keeping the elbows down rather than up provides less resistance for the deltoids and rotator cuff.

Cues and Notations: Instruct the patient to keep the elbows up and wrists straight.

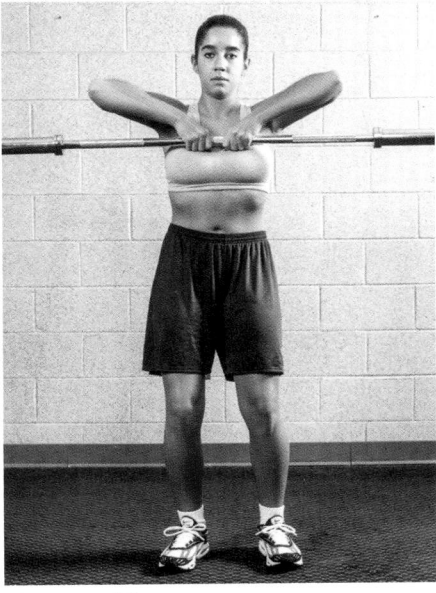

Figure 17.54

Upright Press

This exercise is also called a military press.

Body Segment: Upper back and neck.

Stage in Rehab: Resistive phase.

Purpose: Strengthen the deltoids, trapezius, and trunk stabilizers.

Positioning: Seated or standing with weights grasped in hands, elbows flexed, and weights positioned at shoulder level.

Execution: The abdominal muscles are tightened to maintain trunk stability and to prevent the back from arching as the patient lifts the weight straight up and overhead toward the ceiling (figure 17.55).

Possible Substitutions: Arching the back and shrugging the shoulders are common substitutions.

Cues and Notations: Provide verbal cues to correct for these errors: Instruct the patient to maintain pelvic neutral or abdominal bracing and "pull the shoulder blades into your back pocket."

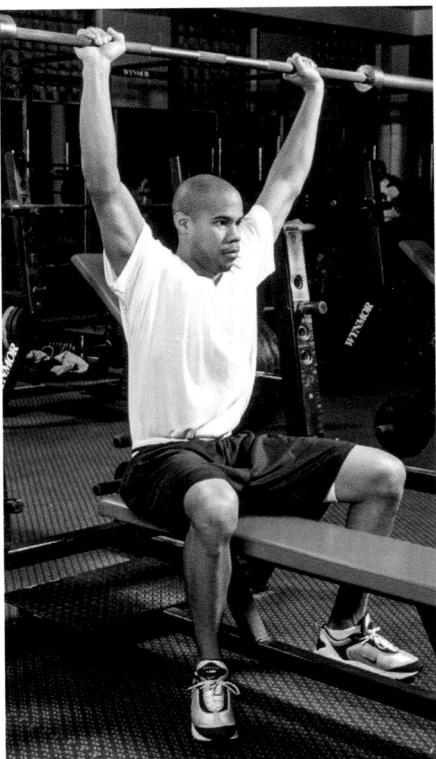

Figure 17.55

Bouhler Exercises

Body Segment: Middle and lower back.

Stage in Rehab: Active phase.

Purpose: Strengthen the middle back muscles and lower trapezius.

Positioning: The patient stands with the back to the wall and heels about 2.5 cm (1 in.) from the wall with hands at the sides. Shoulders are abducted to move the hands overhead with elbows next to the ears and elbows extended. The abdominals are tightened to maintain pelvic neutral and prevent the back from arching as the arms move overhead.

Execution:

1. The patient pushes the thumbs to the wall, holds the position for 5 s, relaxes, and then repeats (figure 17.56a).
2. The patient positions the thumbs facing each other and repeats the movement with the backs of the hands to the wall (figure 17.56b).
3. The arms are positioned at a 45° angle from the horizontal and then pushed backward to the wall, with the elbows straight and the scapulae retracted together (figure 17.56c).

Possible Substitutions: Common errors include arching the back and standing too far from the wall. Good lumbar stability with an engaged core helps ensure correct execution.

Cues and Notations: In each position, the patient must tighten the abdominal muscles to stabilize the trunk and prevent the back from arching. A progression of these exercises is to position the patient in prone to perform the exercises (figure 17.56d) or to add weights while the patient is in prone.

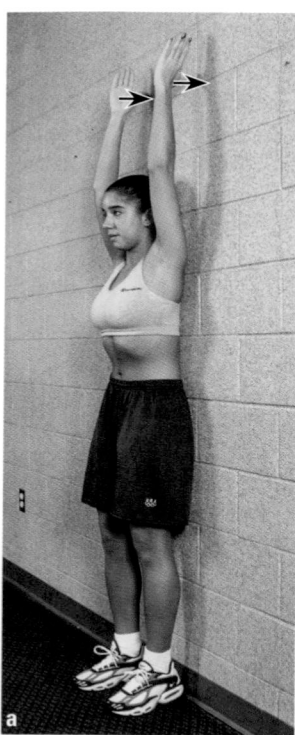 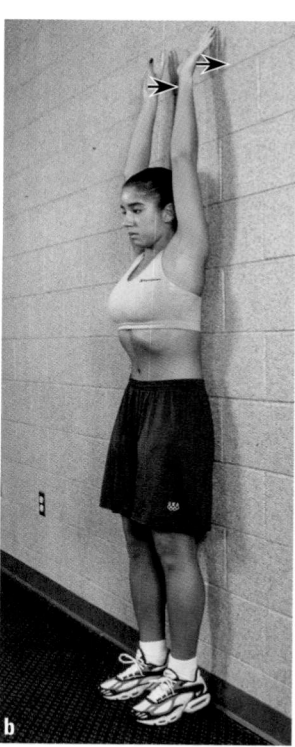 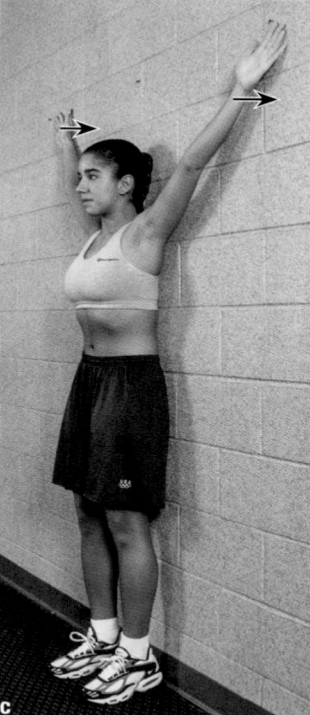

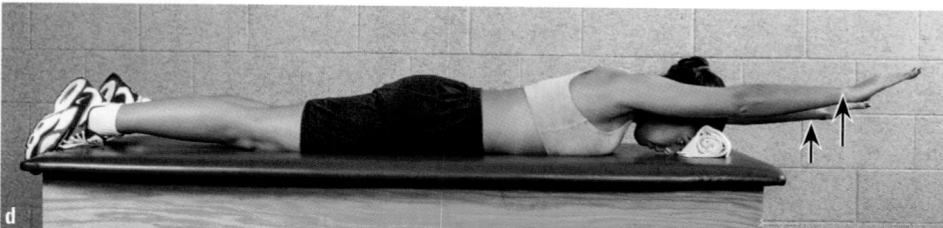

Figure 17.56

Low Back, Abdominal, and Pelvic Exercises   In many ways, we have already presented exercises for the low back, abdominal, and pelvic regions. However, most of those exercises have involved the core; specifically, the local core. The exercises presented here deal more with the global core muscles. The artful application of these exercises means you must be able to judge the degree of difficulty of each of these exercises and incorporate them at an appropriate time in the strengthening program. Since most of the exercises listed in this section deal with the global core, they are useful for pelvic or lumbosacral stabilization.

One of the exercises in this section is the abdominal curl, or full sit-up. However, it is listed here with a caveat: It is not recommended for abdominal strengthening because of the high loads the activity places on the spine.[187] Therefore, a patient who has LBP caused by disc dysfunction may experience harm with this exercise. Additionally, the exercise does not recruit abdominal muscles as effectively as the crunch exercise does.[187]

Strength Exercises for the Lower Back, Abdomen, and Pelvis

Posterior Pelvic Tilt

Body Segment: Lumbar.

Stage in Rehab: Active phase.

Purpose: Strengthen the gluteals and abdominal muscles and encourage a posterior pelvic tilt position.

Positioning: Supine with hips extended or in a supine hook-lying position. Arms relaxed at the sides.

Execution: The patient activates the inner core muscles, pushes the back to the floor during an exhale, and activates the hamstrings and gluteal muscles to roll the pelvis posteriorly (figure 17.57).

Possible Substitutions: Common errors include using the rectus abdominis rather than the local core, hamstrings, and gluteal muscles to move the pelvis, arching the back rather than performing a pelvic tilt, and pushing the abdomen outward.

Cues and Notations: This exercise is not recommended in standing or lifting since it puts pressure on the posterior discs.[188] Exceptions include hyperextension conditions such as spondylosis or facet injuries.

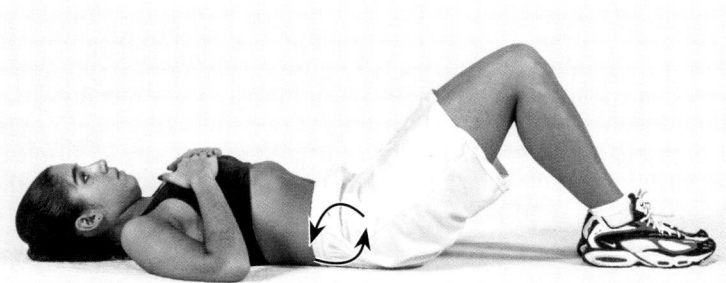

Figure 17.57

Abdominal Curl

Body Segment: Lumbar.

Stage in Rehab: Resistive phase.

Purpose: Strengthen the rectus abdominis and obliques.

Positioning: Legs are extended with the patient supine. This exercise may start with the patient's arms at the sides and then advance to the arms across the chest and then hands on the shoulders. As the patient advances, the hands are placed behind the head.

Execution: The chin is tucked to the chest, and the neck and upper trunk are slowly curled toward a sitting position. The end position is not a full sitting position (figure 17.58). The abdominal muscles should be tensed so the umbilicus

>continued

Abdominal Curl >*continued*

moves inward toward the spine. The spine should curl throughout the movement. Holding the top of the position for several seconds or holding weights in the hands makes the exercise more difficult. The feet are not anchored in this exercise because that would permit the hip flexors to perform the exercise instead of the abdominal muscles.

Possible Substitutions: The back should not arch, and movement should occur as a curling up starting from the neck and proceeding to the low back. The patient should not pull on the neck; if this occurs, instruct the patient to relax the head into the hands.

Cues and Notations: This exercise is not advocated and should be used with caution since the lumbar discs may experience increased pressures.

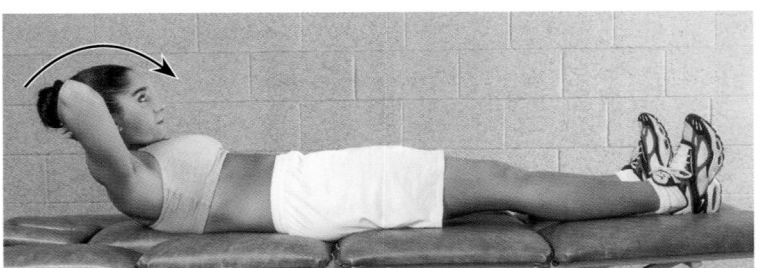

Figure 17.58

Abdominal Crunch

Body Segment: Lumbar and lower thoracic.

Stage in Rehab: Resistive phase.

Purpose: Strengthen the rectus abdominis and obliques.

Positioning: The patient lies supine with the knees flexed, feet flat on the floor, and hands behind the head.

Execution: The abdominal muscles are tightened by pulling the navel to the spine, and the head and shoulders are lifted upward toward the ceiling. There is no curling movement (figure 17.59). The position is held for 1 to 5 s at the top of the motion. If hands are behind the head, they do not pull on the neck; the head should rest into the hands.

Possible Substitutions: The patient is performing the exercise incorrectly if the trunk moves toward the knees rather than toward the ceiling. Elbows should remain in the frontal plane with the scapulae retracted as the patient lifts the upper trunk. If the patient complains of LBP, it is likely that either the muscles are too weak to perform the exercise correctly or the patient is not maintaining enough tension in the abdominal muscles during the motion and is hyperextending the lumbar spine. If the patient persists in pulling on the neck with the hands behind the head, reposition the hands on top of the head instead.

Cues and Notations: If this exercise is too difficult for the patient with the hands behind the head, the arms can be placed by the sides or across the chest rather than on or behind the head. The exercise becomes more difficult if the patient has the legs flexed but in an unsupported position with the feet off the floor.

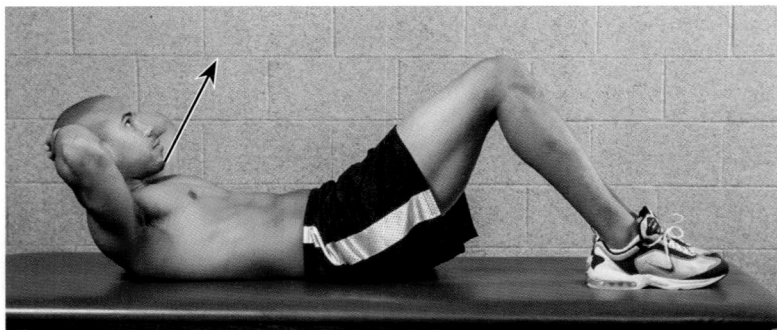

Figure 17.59

Oblique Abdominal Curl

Body Segment: Lumbar.

Stage in Rehab: Resistive phase.

Purpose: Strengthen the internal and external obliques.

Positioning: The patient is supine with the hips and knees flexed and feet on the floor.

Execution: The patient rotates the hips to one side so that he or she is lying on the back while on one hip and the other hip is facing the ceiling. With hands on shoulders, or in the more difficult position, on top of or behind the head, the patient curls toward the top hip, trying to lift the head and shoulders upward and forward as much as possible (figure 17.60). The feet are not anchored.

Possible Substitutions: A common error is starting the rotation at the end of the motion rather than beginning the rotation at the onset of movement and continuing throughout the range of motion.

Cues and Notations: An alternative method is for the patient to lie supine in a hook-lying position with the hips and knees flexed and the feet on the floor. The patient places the left foot onto the right knee and the right hand behind the head. In this position, the patient brings the right elbow toward the left knee while performing a crunch. Difficulties with this method are that hip rotation can be easily substituted for trunk rotation, trunk rotation can begin too early or too late in the motion before the patient lifts the shoulders upward, or the rotation can be performed with momentum rather than muscle contraction.

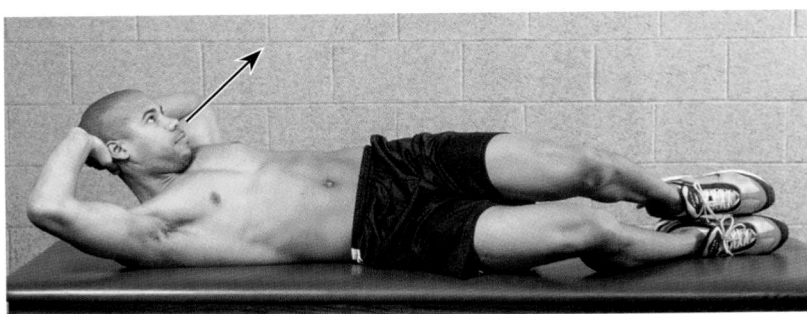

Figure 17.60

Supine Leg Exercises

Body Segment: Lumbar.

Stage in Rehab: Resistive phase.

Purpose: Strengthen the lower rectus abdominis and facilitate core engagement.

Positioning: The patient lies supine in a hook-lying position. Hands are at the sides or resting across the abdomen.

Execution: The core remains engaged throughout this exercise.

1. Both legs begin with the hips and knees flexed to 90°. The patient slowly lowers the foot of one flexed leg to the table and then returns the extremity to the start position while maintaining pelvic neutral. The activity is repeated with the other limb.
2. One hip is flexed to 90° with the knee extended and foot pointing toward the ceiling. The leg is slowly lowered to the floor (figure 17.61*a*).
3. The patient alternately moves one hip into extension from the start position of 90° flexion while bringing the other lower extremity toward the start position so that both limbs are moving simultaneously but in opposite motions without either foot touching the table (figure 17.61*b*).
4. In this next progression, the patient starts with both knees in extension and both hips flexed so the feet are elevated toward the ceiling. The patient slowly lowers both limbs to the floor without letting the low back arch (figure 17.61*c*).
5. A V-sit-up is performed while the pelvis maintains its neutral position (figure 17.61*d*).

>continued

Supine Leg Exercises >*continued*

Possible Substitutions: Core control is lost during the exercise so the pelvis rolls from one side to the other or the back flexes or hyperextends.

Cues and Notations: Remind the patient to maintain a neutral position and keep the abdominal muscles tense. If the patient can advance to the next-level exercise but cannot perform the next exercise correctly, flex the knees to shorten the lever-arm length of the lower-extremity resistance arm so that he or she performs the exercise without losing core control.

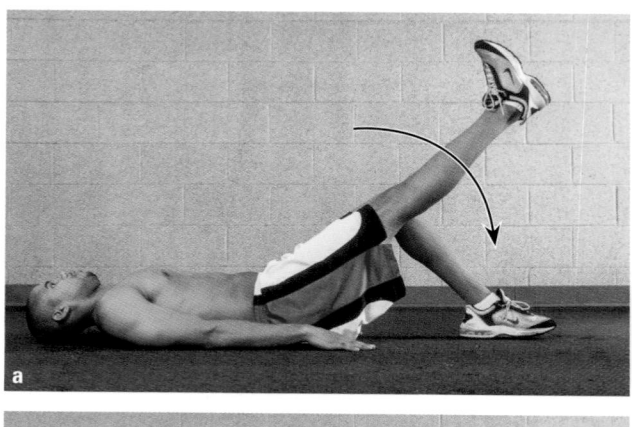 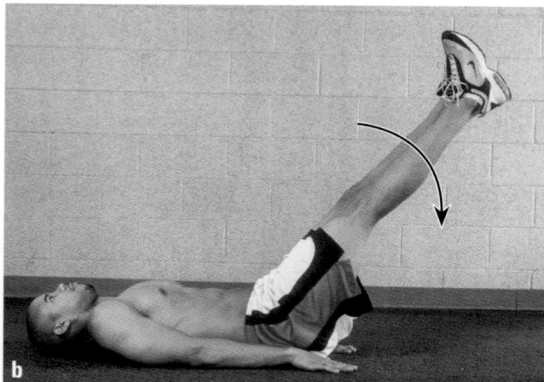
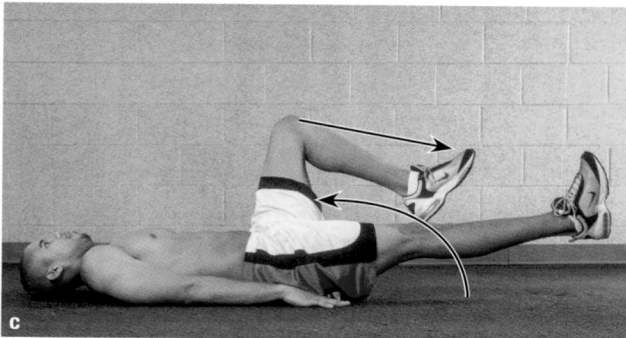 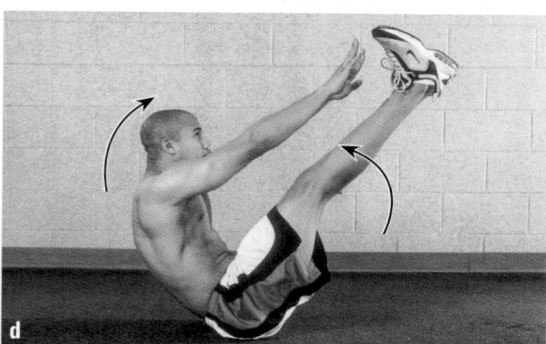

Figure 17.61

Bridging

Body Segment: Lumbar.

Stage in Rehab: Resistive phase.

Purpose: Strengthen the trunk extensors and emphasize stabilization.

Positioning: The patient is in a supine hook-lying position.

Execution:

1. The patient lifts the hips off the floor until the thighs form a straight line with the trunk (figure 17.62*a*). The position is held for 5 to 30 s.

2. The next progression of this exercise is to perform the bridge and then lift each leg to march in place without performing lumbar extension. The patient must use the abdominal muscles and buttocks while performing this exercise to maintain a straight line from the trunk to the supporting thigh.

3. A more advanced version of this exercise has the patient in the same bridging position, keeping abdominal, buttock, and lower-back muscles in good tension to maintain the position. The patient first brings one knee into full extension without moving the hips, then lowers it, and then performs the motion with the other leg (figure 17.62*b*).

Possible Substitutions: The hips should not drop or roll toward the unsupported side.

Cues and Notations: A stick placed across the hips and parallel to the floor will alert the patient if the pelvis position changes. If the stick either falls off or dips on one side, stability is lost.

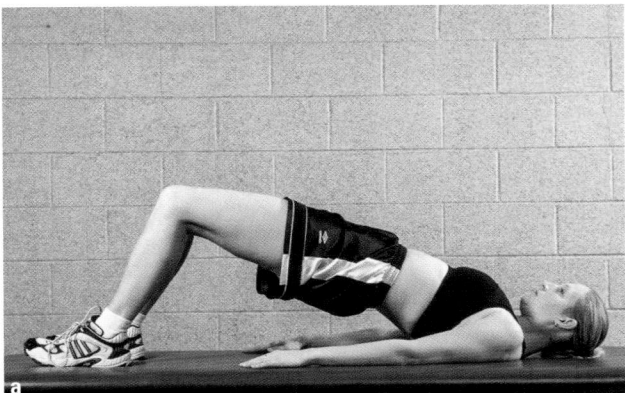 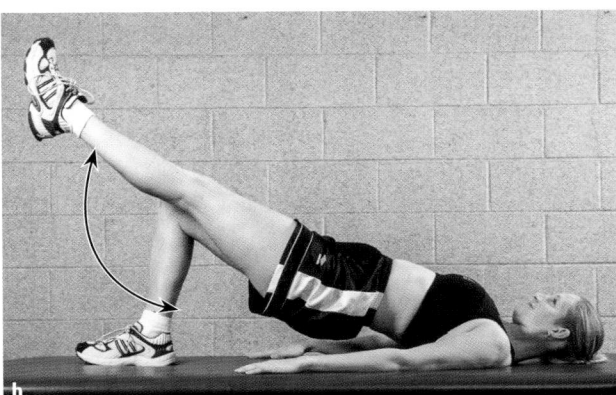

Figure 17.62

Prone Plank

Body Segment: Lumbar.

Stage in Rehab: Resistive and into advanced phase.

Purpose: Strengthen the abdominals.

Positioning: The patient is prone with the hips and knees in extension and the elbow positioned under the shoulder. Weight is borne on the toes and elbows.

Execution: Without performing lumbar extension, the patient lifts the body so it forms a straight line from the shoulders to the feet (figure 17.63). The position is held for 5 to 30 s.

Possible Substitutions: The trunk sagging into extension and flexing the hips are common substitutions.

Cues and Notations: The patient may need verbal or manual cues to properly align the trunk with the lower extremities if the patient has poor body awareness. If the exercise is too difficult, reduce the time of the hold. The exercise can move from the elbows to the hands, although patients may report discomfort at the wrists with prolonged positioning.

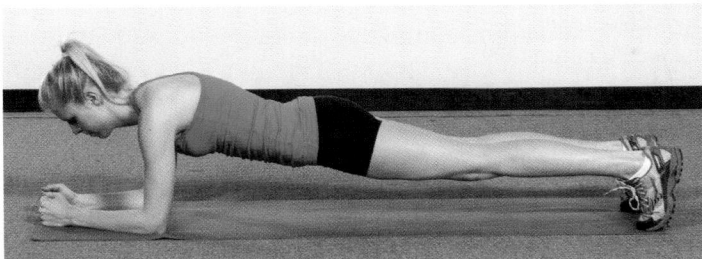

Figure 17.63

Side Plank (Side Bridge)

Body Segment: Lumbar.

Stage in Rehab: Resistive and into advanced phase.

Purpose: Strengthen the obliques and quadratus lumborum.

Positioning: The patient is side-lying with the hips and knees in extension and the elbow positioned under the shoulder. Weight is borne on the bottom lateral foot and elbow.

Execution: Without lumbar extension, the patient lifts the hips so that the body forms

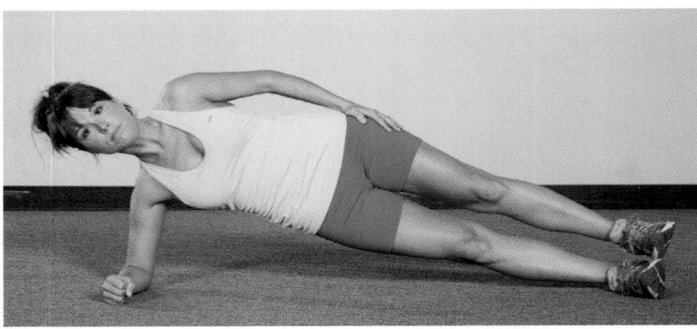

Figure 17.64

one line from the shoulders to the feet (figure 17.64). The position is held for 5 to 20 s.

Possible Substitutions: Trunk flexion or lateral rotation is often a substitution pattern. The lateral trunk may sag rather than maintaining a straight line with the lower extremities.

Cues and Notations: Tell the patient that the lower extremities may feel as though they are behind the trunk when they are actually in good alignment. If the exercise is too difficult, reduce the time of the hold, begin with a hip-hike exercise in standing position, or have the patient perform the exercise with the weight on the side of the knee rather than the feet.

Side-Lying Sit-Up

Body Segment: Lumbar.

Stage in Rehab: Later resistive phase and into the advanced phase.

Purpose: Strengthen the quadratus lumborum and obliques.

Positioning: The patient is side-lying with the feet anchored and the legs extended and in line with the trunk.

Execution: Hands are placed across the chest or in the more difficult position behind the head. The patient curls sideways toward the top hip as far as possible, trying to curl rather than lift from the hips (figure 17.65).

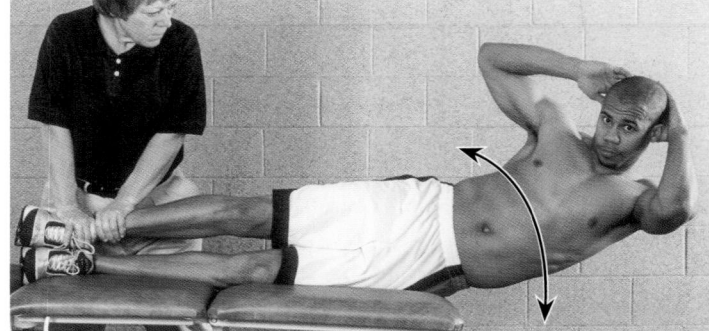

Figure 17.65

Possible Substitutions: Moving into trunk flexion during the exercise is the most common substitution.

Cues and Notations: Remind the patient to exhale to avoid lumbar extension throughout the exercise and to hold a good alignment between the trunk and legs. Instruct the patient to maintain tension in the gluteal muscles to prevent trunk flexion. If the patient pulls himself up with the hands behind the head, reposition the hands on top of the head.

Lateral Trunk Rotation

Body Segment: Lumbar.

Stage in Rehab: Later resistive phase and into the advanced phase.

Purpose: Strengthen the obliques and quadratus lumborum.

Positioning: The patient lies supine in a hook-lying position.

Execution: A resistance band or a pulley system is secured around the knees and anchored to a stable object near the patient's side, as shown in figure 17.66. The feet are either on a bench or flat on the floor. The patient begins with the knees and hips rotated toward the pulley or band anchor, then rotates the knees away from the anchor or pulley by initiating the movement with the abdominals and back muscles. The patient should avoid lumbar extension throughout the activity.

Possible Substitutions: Initiating the movement from the knees rather than the trunk is the most common substitution. Arching the back indicates overuse of back muscles and lack of use of abdominals.

Cues and Notations: Use tactile feedback with your hands on the patient's back and abdomen to facilitate the correct recruitment pattern.

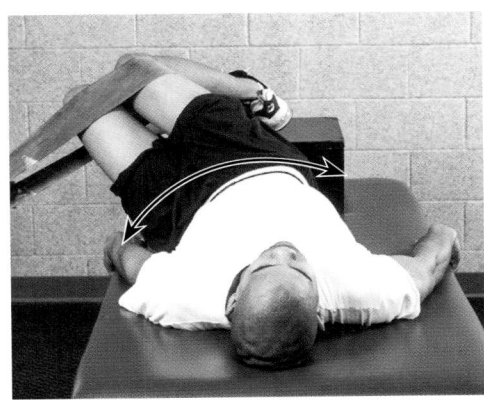

Figure 17.66

Lunges

Body Segment: Lumbar.

Stage in Rehab: Later resistive phase and into the advanced phase.

Purpose: Strengthen the abdominal, thigh, and gluteal muscles. This exercise also facilitates correct trunk stability during lower-extremity activities.

Positioning: The patient is standing in an exhaled position without lumbar extension.

Execution: Keeping the abdominal muscles tightened, the patient moves to a lunge position, lowering the body smoothly, and then returning to a standing position (figure 17.67).

Possible Substitutions: Moving into lumbar extension; flexing, tilting, or rotating the trunk; and moving the hips and shoulders out of the frontal plane.

Cues and Notations: Use verbal cues to remind the patient to avoid back extension, to avoid holding his or her breath, and to keep the pelvis in the same plane as the shoulders. If this is difficult to perform, have the patient take smaller lunge steps until control is achieved.

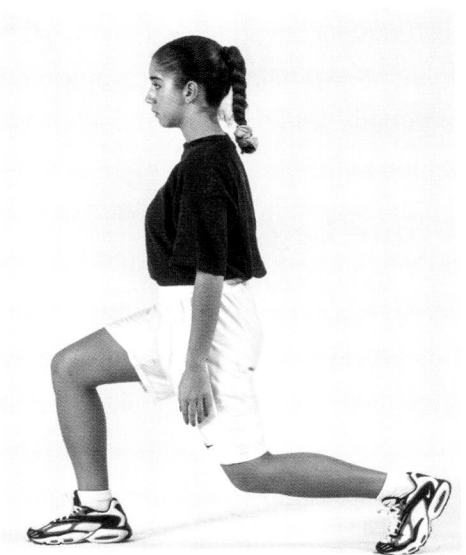

Figure 17.67

Prone Trunk Extension

Body Segment: Lumbar.

Stage in Rehab: Later resistive phase and into the advanced phase.

Purpose: Strengthen the lower-back extensors, gluteals, and hamstrings.

Positioning: The patient lies prone over the end of a table, a Swiss ball, or a Roman chair so that the hips are at the edge of the object and are flexed to 30°. Either another person (figure 17.68a) or the equipment (figure 17.68b) anchors the feet. A chair set below the patient may prevent the patient from flexing too far forward. The dot on the photo indicates the point from which movement occurs.

Execution: With the hands at the sides or in the small of the back, the patient contracts the gluteal muscles to lift the trunk to align with the lower extremities. Advancing the hands from their position behind the back to across the chest and then overhead progressively increases resistance and exercise difficulty. Since this is an advanced exercise, patients should not perform it until there is good strength in the abdominal muscles and trunk extensors; they should be able to first perform side sit-ups and trunk rotations in standing with a medicine ball without difficulty or pain.

Possible Substitutions: The most common substitutions include arching the back rather than using the hip muscles to lift the trunk and bending from the back rather than at the hips.

>continued

Prone Trunk Extension >*continued*

Cues and Notations: Reposition the patient if he or she cannot flex at the hips. Instructing the patient to keep the chest elevated, to tighten the buttocks rather than lifting with the back muscles, and to bend from the hips will remind the patient to maintain a proper back position. The rehabilitation clinician provides verbal cueing and tactile correction if the back arches.

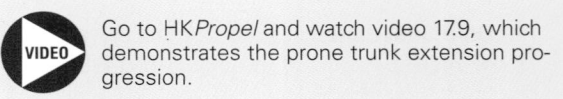

Go to HK*Propel* and watch video 17.9, which demonstrates the prone trunk extension progression.

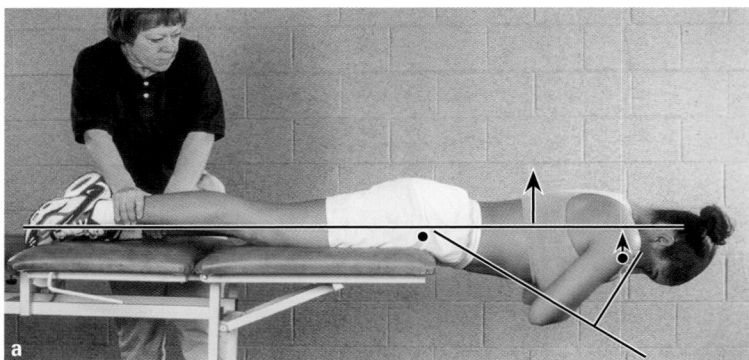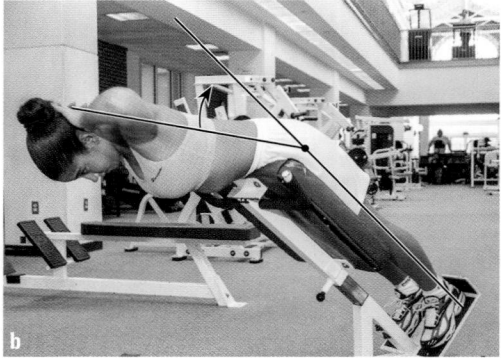

Figure 17.68

Prone Leg Lift

Body Segment: Lumbar.

Stage in Rehab: Later resistive phase and into the advanced phase.

Purpose: Strengthen the trunk extensors, abdominal muscles, and gluteal muscles.

Positioning: The patient is in the reverse position of that for the prone trunk lift. This time the trunk and pelvis are supported on the table or Roman chair, and the legs are off the table or apparatus.

Execution: The patient squeezes the buttocks to lift the legs until they are parallel to the floor. The pelvis must remain in neutral to avoid lumbar extension, and it is supported on the apparatus so flexion occurs at the hips, not the spine (figure 17.69; the dot indicates the point from which movement occurs).

Possible Substitutions: Movement is initiated from the back, not the gluteals, and the patient swings the legs upward using momentum so the back hyperextends.

Cues and Notations: Instruct the patient to squeeze the buttocks to lift the legs and to control the speed of the lift. Motion should occur from the hip joints and not the lumbar spine. If this is difficult, instruct the patient to flex the knees slightly to shorten the lever-arm resistance of the lower extremities.

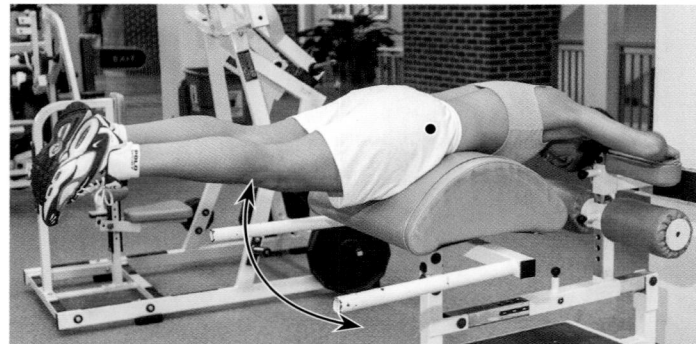

Figure 17.69

Lat Pull-Down

Body Segment: Lumbar.

Stage in Rehab: Resistive phase.

Purpose: Strengthen the latissimus dorsi.

Positioning: The exercise uses an overhead pulley bar, with the patient's hands positioned shoulder-width or slightly farther apart and the elbows extended.

Execution: The abdominal muscles remain taut throughout the exercise, and the core remains engaged to avoid lumbar extension. The hips and knees are slightly flexed to relieve stress on the back. The patient brings the bar downward toward the thighs while keeping the elbows in near-extension (figure 17.70).

Possible Substitutions: Common errors include flexing the elbows too much, shrugging the shoulders, or flexing the trunk.

Cues and Notations: The latissimus dorsi plays an important role in providing stabilization to the thoracolumbar spine because the muscle originates from the lower thoracic spinous processes, lumbar fascia, and iliac crest and has interdigitations with the external oblique muscles.

 Go to HK*Propel* and watch video 17.10, which demonstrates the lat pull-down for back strengthening.

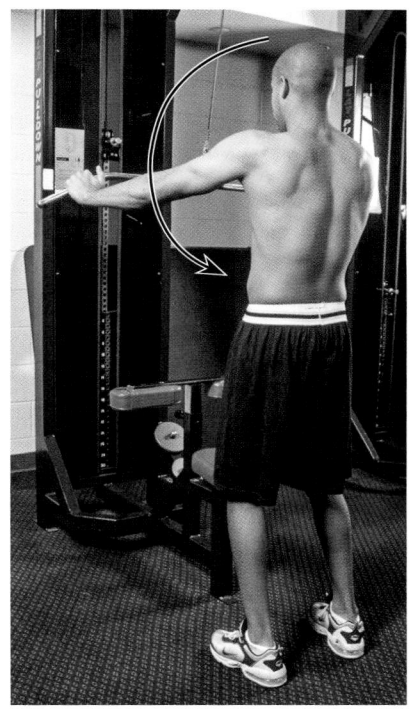

Figure 17.70

This is clearly not an exhaustive list of strength exercises for the spine. These exercises, however, provide rehabilitation clinicians with a starting list that may be used throughout the strengthening phases of a rehabilitation program. They may also spur rehabilitation clinicians to think of or develop other exercises for their patients to meet their specific needs.

Proprioception and Balance Exercises

Proprioception and balance activities occur early in a spine and sacroiliac rehabilitation program. Proprioception and core strengthening exercises begin as part of neuromotor control. Since balance is, at least in part, related to strength,[85] it is not surprising that one way to achieve improved joint and body position and posture sense is to improve core strength.

These balance and stability activities are presented as the dead bug and bird dog exercises seen earlier in this chapter. Once the patient progresses from these exercises, additional balance activities focus on more dynamic movements. Many of these activities and exercises are presented in chapter 14. These more advanced exercises may start with static exercises such as balancing with eyes closed while standing on the floor, then advancing to standing on unstable surfaces. Once static balance is achieved,

the patient progresses to dynamic balance activities. For example, the Star Excursion Balance Test is both a good test and a good exercise for back patients.[189]

Neuromotor Rehabilitation Techniques

As we have mentioned, the pelvis and spine serve to transfer force during functional body activities, so the stability of this region is fundamental to any performance. The more challenging the activity, the greater the demands for neuromotor readiness and stabilization forces.[190] During daily activities such as walking, the trunk relies on neuromotor control and coordination for efficient movement of the body's mass from one lower extremity to the other. When an injury occurs, normal neuromotor control is hampered, so muscles fail to perform their tasks.[191]

Investigations have shown us that patients with axial pain often have lost their ability to use core muscles correctly, and this places them at increased risk of injury.[192] When muscles are not recruited as they should be, stress increases on other joints and muscles, reducing dynamic stability and creating inefficient movement.[162, 193-195] The cause of a patient's axial pain may very well be the result of a deficient core.[196] Therefore, for patients with spine injuries, it is important for rehabilitation clinicians to devote time early in rehabilitation to reeducating and developing core muscles to provide the stability needed for both healthy performance and reduced injury risk.[65, 67, 197]

Early performance-specific activities while working on neuromotor control may include simple daily movements such as getting out of bed, walking, transferring to sitting or standing, and stooping while engaging the core muscles. More advanced activities may include jogging or lifting weighted objects from the floor while using trunk stabilizers. Sport-specific activities will include a progression of activities; for example, when throwing, the patient may begin with a step-and-toss activity, then advance to short overhead throws, then short overhead pitches, and finally normal throws or pitches, with each progressive activity performed with proper engagement of trunk-stabilizing muscles.

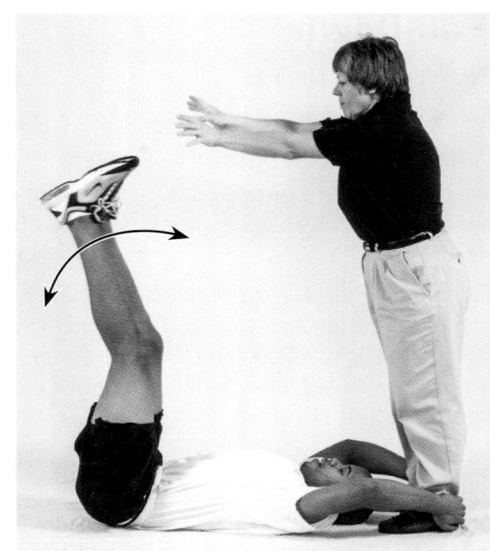

Figure 17.71   Resisted leg lifts.

CLINICAL TIPS

Progression of core activation, stabilization, and use includes these steps: (1) improve neuromotor control of the trunk muscles; (2) perform trunk stabilization activities, such as abdominal hollowing exercises for spinal stability; (3) perform activation exercises for the multifidus; (4) perform abdominal bracing to activate local and global muscles; (5) engage core muscles while performing simple daily activities; and (6) engage abdominal bracing and trunk stability during performance-specific activities.

Agility and Coordination Exercises

Once patients have achieved their goals for strengthening and neuromotor control, they are ready for trunk rotation activities and plyometric exercises that involve higher forces, quicker movements, and functional multiplanar motions. Pelvic stability should always be maintained throughout the execution of these exercises. Since many agility and coordination exercises are available, and the exercises chosen for a rehabilitation program are based on individual patient needs, only a few suggestions are included here.

Resisted Leg Lifts

This exercise is performed with the patient supine on the floor and the rehabilitation clinician standing at the patient's head. The patient's knees are extended, and the hips are flexed to approximately 90°. The patient lifts the legs overhead as the clinician pushes the patient's lower extremities to move the hips into extension (figure 17.71). This exercise is performed quickly but with control. The patient must keep his or her back flat on the floor; the back must not arch throughout the exercise.

Medicine-Ball Exercises

Medicine-ball exercises are easy to create and include in a trunk rehabilitation program. Figure 17.72 depicts two

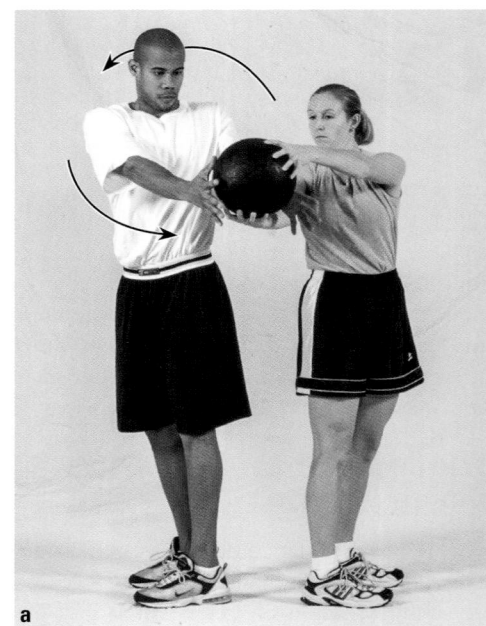

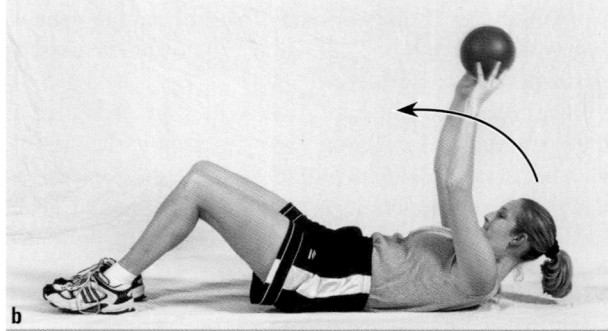

Figure 17.72   Medicine-ball exercises. *(a)* Trunk rotations. *(b)* Medicine-ball toss can be performed in a straight plane or rotationally to facilitate oblique activity.

medicine-ball exercises. Medicine-ball exercises include activities such as ball passing low or high, trunk rotations, and abdominal curls with ball catching. Other examples include ball bouncing while in a horizontal prone position on a Roman chair and abdominal crunches in a supine position on a Roman chair while holding a small medicine ball in either hand with the shoulder in abduction. If you know the muscle's function, your imagination can provide you with any number of exercises to achieve the patient's strength goals.

Alternative Rehabilitation Applications

In earlier times, back programs involved bed rest as the initial course of treatment. Two clinicians were among the first to institute exercise as a means of treating back pain. These early pioneers in the rehabilitation of back pain patients included Williams and McKenzie. Although their programs are no longer followed as dutifully as they were when they were first presented to the health care community, they are of value because some of the exercises and specific aspects of their theories remain beneficial and continue in use today.

Williams' Flexion Exercises

For many years, Williams' flexion exercises were the accepted back-exercise regimen. Paul Williams was an orthopedic surgeon who believed that lordosis was the cause of low-back pain. Williams' flexion exercises are a series of six exercises that emphasize flexion and include activities to reduce lumbar lordosis.[198] These are the six exercises (figure 17.73):[198]

- Exercise 1: Sit-up in a flexed-knee position to strengthen the abdominals

- Exercise 2: Pelvic tilt to strengthen the gluteal muscles
- Exercise 3: Single knee-to-chest and double knee-to-chest to stretch the erector spinae muscles
- Exercise 4: Seated reach to the toes with knees extended to stretch the erector spinae and hamstring muscles
- Exercise 5: In a quadruped position with one knee forward under the chest and the other hip and knee in extension to stretch the tensor fasciae latae and iliofemoral ligament
- Exercise 6: Starting in standing and moving to a full squat to strengthen the quadriceps muscles

According to Williams, these exercises should be performed 2 to 3 times a day with the number of repetitions of each being dependent upon the patient's physical ability and restrictions. In addition to these exercises, Williams advocated instructing the patient in proper posture and the maintenance of proper posture during functional activities. He believed that balance among the postural muscles was key to maintaining lumbar spine health.

It was Williams' contention that the success of a postural program depended to a great extent on the strength of the

CLINICAL TIPS

Williams' flexion exercises focus on placing the lumbar spine in a flexed position to reduce excessive lumbar lordotic stresses. Exercises are designed to (1) strengthen the abdominal, gluteal, and quadriceps muscles and (2) stretch the erector spinae, hamstring, and tensor fasciae latae muscles and the iliofemoral ligament.

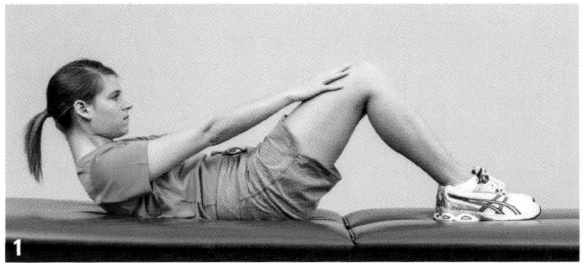
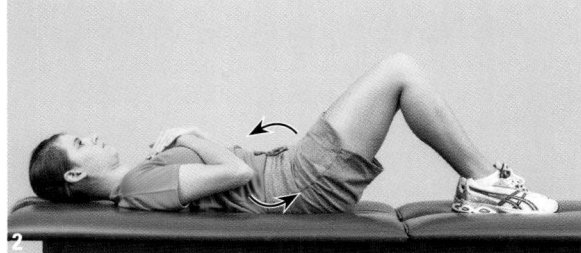
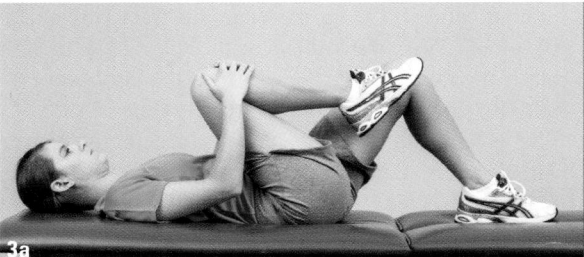
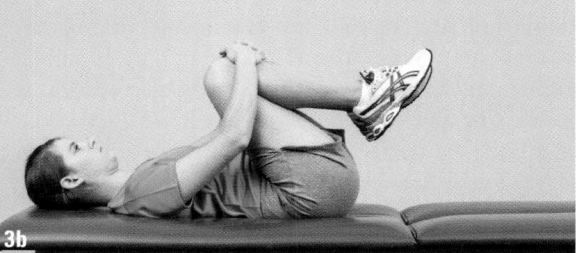

Figure 17.73 Williams' flexion exercises 1 through 6; see text for descriptions.

>continued

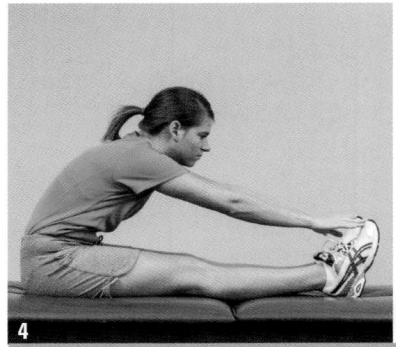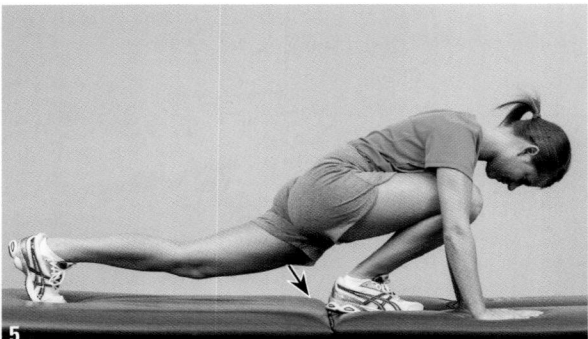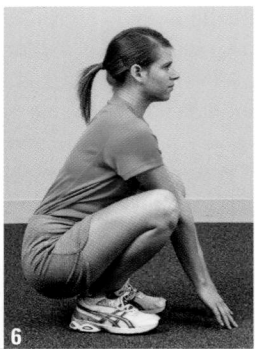

Figure 17.73 *>continued*

gluteus maximus and quadriceps muscles. He believed that if these muscles were strong, the person would rely less on trunk muscles for movement, thereby avoiding low-back stress; he believed that the spine should remain in a flexed position at all times, especially while exercising.[198]

McKenzie Back Program

Later, extension exercises became the exercises of choice because flexion exercises made many patients with disc injuries worse. Extension exercises, advanced by Robin McKenzie, a New Zealand physiotherapist, emphasize trunk extension aimed at relieving posterior pressure on discs.[199] His rationale was that the disc is the primary source of back pain. Disc problems occur because people spend a lot of time sitting and in other positions of flexion, not moving enough into extension to relieve disc pressures. He therefore primarily advocated extension exercises to relieve disc pressures. He also divided back problems into three progressive syndrome classifications: (1) postural syndromes, (2) dysfunctions, and (3) derangements.

According to McKenzie, *postural syndromes* are the first step in progressive chronic back pain. This condition is not severe, and it occurs during one's teen years and early 20s. The patient experiences back, neck, or interscapular pain, especially after prolonged sitting postures. The pain is intermittent in this stage, and the patient's examination is essentially negative.

Unfortunately, if no steps are taken to correct posture and habit, the condition may progress to the next syndrome, *dysfunction*. It is during this phase that early physical changes are noted. There is some loss of accessory joint movement, reduced range of motion, and diminished soft-tissue mobility. Neurological examinations during this phase, however, are negative. The patient may complain of stiffness and either intermittent or constant pain. It is imperative that posture and restrictions in soft-tissue and joint mobility be corrected to prevent the patient from advancing to the final phase.

McKenzie identified the third classification, *derangements*, as the most severe condition. By this time, the source of pain has changed from the inflammation of peripheral structures associated with postural syndromes to changes in the disc. Poor posture, over time, changes vertebral positions, leading to advanced stress that produces disc changes and degeneration. McKenzie further divided derangements into six progressive levels and one other pathology. The first six derangements deal with posterior disc pathology and the seventh involves anterior disc pathology.[199]

- *Derangement 1:* There is a mild disc bulge with either central or asymmetrical pain in the back. The pain results from irritation to the posterior annulus and the posterior longitudinal ligament caused by the bulging disc. Usually the pain subsides in a few days, but these patients need instruction in proper posture and body mechanics, and they need exercises to correct deficiencies.

- *Derangement 2:* The disc bulge is now moderate in size and may cause buttock pain. Examination reveals the patient to have a flat lumbar spine and some pain when changing positions or when in prolonged sitting. In addition to the exercises and posture activities for derangement 1, the patient may find relief when lying in a prone position.

- *Derangement 3:* The disc bulge is now more prominent, with pain occurring to the buttock or even the posterior thigh. Although no deformity is visible, the pain is more intense. At this time, the goal is to relieve the pain referred down the extremity and to "centralize" the pain, or move it more proximally until it is limited to the central spine. Repetitive exercises of trunk extension in a prone position are added to the previous exercises.

- *Derangement 4:* The pain is pronounced down one extremity to the knee, and the patient exhibits a shift of the lumbar spine. If the bulge occurs medial to the nerve root (figure 17.74*a*), the shift is to the same side as the pain, but if the derangement is lateral to the nerve root (figure 17.74*b*), the shift is toward the contralateral side of pain. This is the body's way to reduce stress on the nerve root. The first step in treating this derangement is to correct the lateral shift. Once the shift is reduced, extension exercises are used to centralize the pain, and then the patient follows the treatment program for derangement 1.

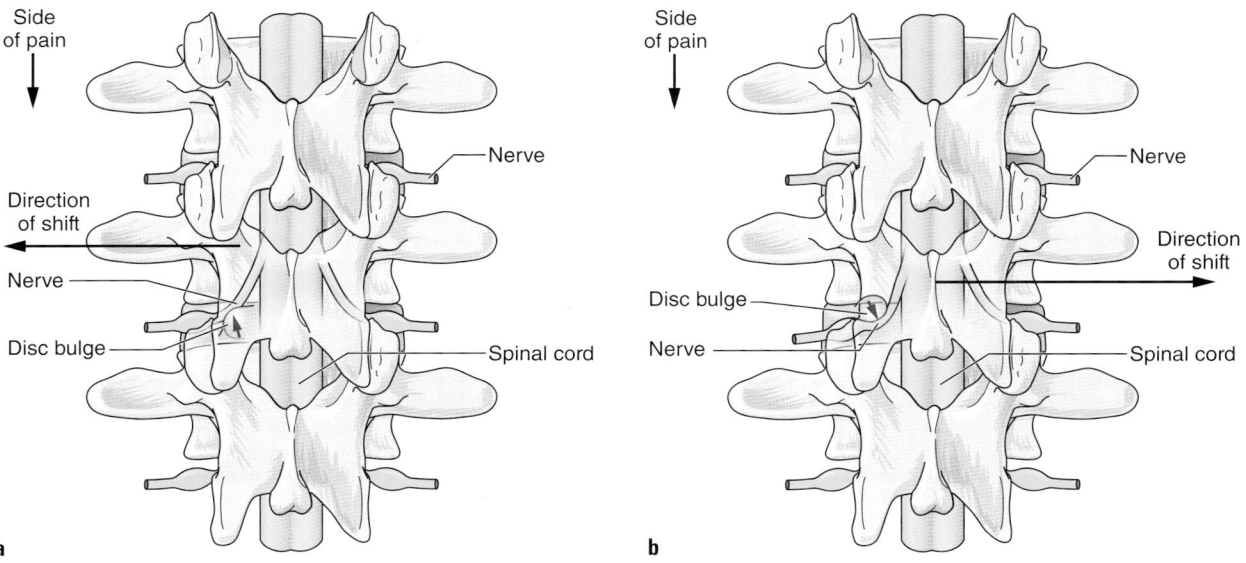

Figure 17.74 Disc bulge with pressure on nerve roots. *(a)* Bulge with pressure applied medial to nerve root. *(b)* Bulge with pressure applied lateral to nerve root.

• *Derangement 5:* Disc degeneration continues to where the patient experiences unilateral referred pain below the knee. No deformity is noted on examination, but the progressive bulge of the annulus fibrosis causes irritation of the nerve root and the dura mater. Although the patient's pain is more intense and fewer positions of comfort may be found, treatment goals are to centralize the pain through repeated extension exercises and to continue with other treatment aspects outlined for derangement 1. It is probably necessary to have the patient perform the extension exercises while side-lying or prone, not while standing.

• *Derangement 6:* In this derangement, the disc is herniated through the annulus fibrosis. The unilateral extremity pain is below the knee and may go into the foot. The patient reports feelings of paresthesia, weakness, and numbness. Treatment at this time includes reducing any shift that may be present, centralizing the pain, and having the patient avoid flexion for 2 to 3 months to allow the annulus fibrosis to scar over. Treatment also includes those procedures for derangement 1 as the patient tolerates them.

• *Derangement 7:* This derangement involves an anterior rather than a posterior bulge of the disc, and it causes a stretching of the anterior longitudinal ligament. This type of derangement is rare. Buttock and thigh pain may be seen with this condition, and the patient usually has a fixed lumbar lordosis. Treatment involves repeated flexion activities, first in supine and then in standing.

McKenzie's approach to treating back pain used a method he identified as *centralizing*, which progressively moves the pain from its more distal region in the extremities to a proximal and central location in the lumbar region.[199]

CLINICAL TIPS

McKenzie's progressive syndrome classifications include, from least to most problematic, postural syndromes, postural dysfunctions, and seven levels of postural derangements. The first six derangements are progressive levels of posterior disc pathology ranging from a mild disc bulge to a disc herniation, and the seventh derangement involves anterior disc pathology.

Since low-back pain is more tolerable than pain referred into the extremity, *centralizing* the pain is a key factor in his treatment of distal pain referred from the spine.[199] His idea included allowing the patient to control the pain and using simple exercises to treat the pain. To that end, McKenzie listed six exercises that are given to the patient in a sequential order[199] (figure 17.75):

• *Exercise 1:* Prone lying for 5 min. If the patient cannot lie prone, it may be necessary to place a pillow or two under the lumbopelvic area. As the patient's pain subsides, the pillows are removed one by one until the patient can lie prone without a pillow.

• *Exercise 2:* Once the patient can lie prone, the patient advances to lying prone on the elbows with the elbows under the shoulders for 5 min. The pelvis must be flat on the table. If the patient's ASISs are not on the table, have the patient place the elbows farther forward of the shoulders until the pelvis is flat on the table. As flexibility improves, the elbows are moved until they are directly under the shoulders.

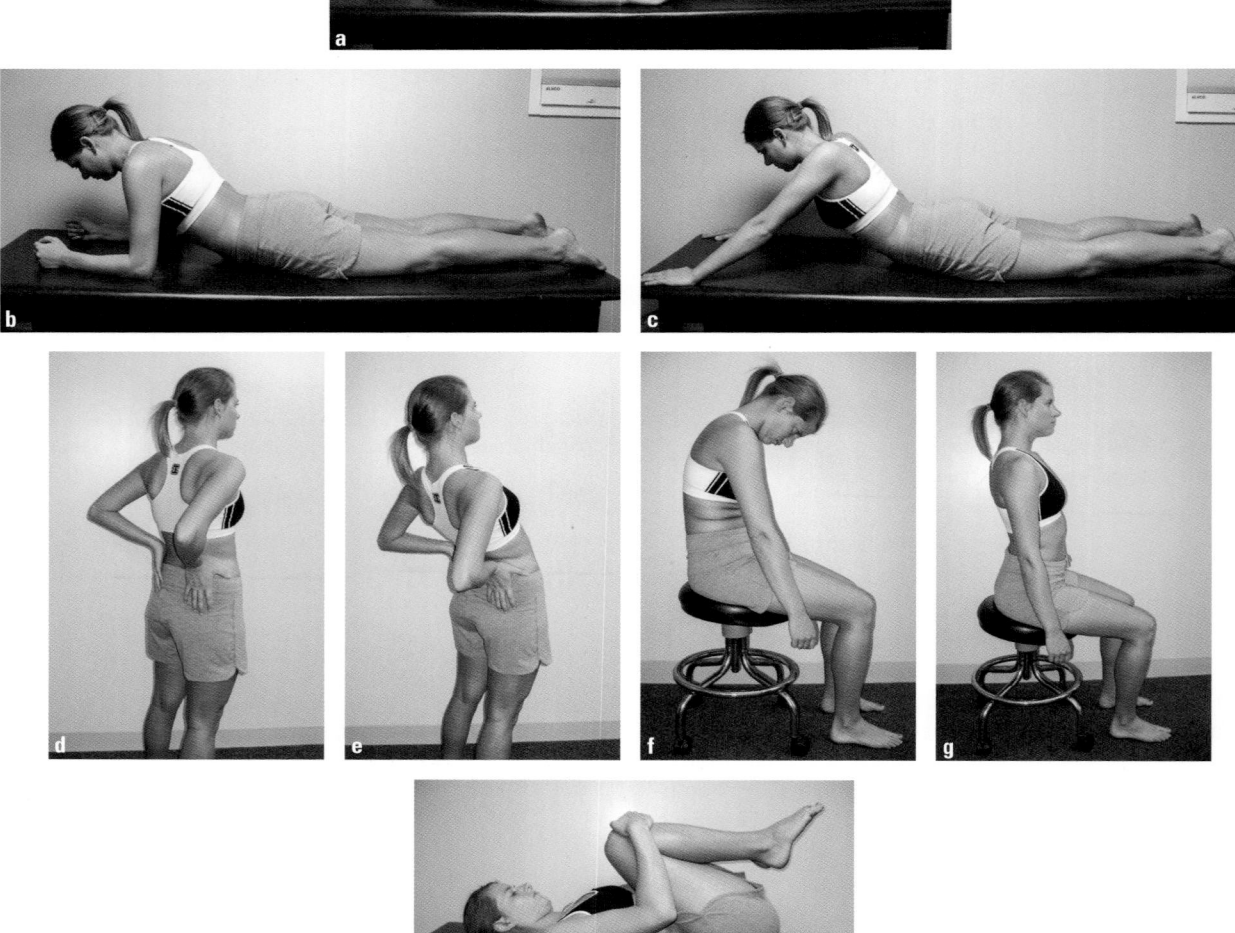

Figure 17.75   McKenzie exercises (see text for descriptions): *(a)* prone lying; *(b)* prone on elbows; *(c)* press-up; *(d)* standing extension, start position; *(e)* standing extension, end position; *(f)* cat-cow in sitting, start position; *(g)* cat-cow in sitting, end position; *(h)* both knees to chest.

© Peggy Houglum

- *Exercise 3:* Once the patient can lie prone with the elbows in the correct position, the exercise advances to prone press-ups. Once again, the ASISs should remain flat on the table as the elbows extend into a full press-up. The hands start near the shoulders to push the trunk upward, but if the pelvis cannot remain on the table, hand positions must be adjusted until flexibility gains are sufficient. This exercise is performed for 10 repetitions, 6 to 8 times a day. Each time the patient moves into the end of the push-up position, the patient remains in that position a few seconds to relax the spine and gluteal muscles before returning to the start position.

- *Exercise 4:* The next exercise is trunk extension in standing. The patient places both hands in the small of the back and extends the trunk backward from the waist, not the knees. This exercise is performed for 6 to 8 repetitions 6 to 8 times each day.

- *Exercise 5:* This is the seated "cat-cow" exercise. The patient begins in a slumped position with the lumbar spine curved posteriorly. Then the patient moves into an anterior pelvic tilt. Each position should be in the extreme end of possible motion. This exercise is repeated 15 to 20 times, 3 times a day.

• *Exercise 6:* The final McKenzie exercise is similar to a Williams flexion exercise. It is bringing both knees to the chest. It is repeated 10 times, 6 to 8 times a day. Each leg is moved to the chest and returned to the start position one at a time, with the first leg held to the chest while the other is brought up, then the first leg held in the start position while the second leg is brought down so the back does not arch during the motion.

McKenzie's overall concept of identifying a specific diagnosis and creating a rehabilitation program to manage these mechanical deficiencies has become what is known as Mechanical Diagnosis and Therapy (MDT).[200] Since his initial application of treatments for his lumbar derangements, an expansion of this approach has been developed and used successfully with other body segments.[200] This approach is used to help identify syndromes or pathologies that are mechanically based and have their own signs and symptoms, making them unique and distinguishable from other pathologies.[201, 202]

Putting the Components Together

Many rehabilitation clinicians today do not advocate the purist approach of either Williams' flexion exercises or McKenzie's extension exercises for spine patients. Instead, programs use a combination of activities and are individually customized for the problems and needs of the patient.[203] There are many individual differences among patients, types and degrees of injuries, and emotional and physical responses to both injury and treatment; for these reasons, there is no one way that successfully treats all axial system injuries or problems. It is important for the clinician to have an array of approaches to meet the problems and needs of each patient.

The patient's injury dictates the requirements for each program. However, it is important for spine rehabilitation programs to include cardiovascular exercises.[204, 205] Cardiovascular exercise has proven to be beneficial for spine patients and should be included in most cases.

In addition to cardiovascular activities, a rehabilitation program for the spine should routinely include spinal stability instruction, posture correction, and body mechanics instruction.[206] Muscle energy techniques and neuromotor activities focusing on proper muscle recruitment are also important. A complete rehabilitation program should also include flexibility exercises, strengthening exercises, and muscle endurance activities.[188, 207] Hip muscle tightness and weakness, especially in the hip rotators, is often correlated with low-back pain,[208-210] so the program should include flexibility activities for those hip muscles that have been assessed as having restricted motion.[211] The core and spine extensor muscles are key muscle groups that provide support and stability to the spine, so strength exercises for these groups should also be included. Recent evidence

indicates that patients with back pain have neuromuscular dysfunction causing the muscles either to fire in an incorrect pattern or to delay their firing.[32, 161, 193, 212, 213] Chronic low-back pain patients have deficient proprioception,[159, 214] but there is evidence to indicate that improvements occur with treatment.[160, 212, 215]

If one segment of the spinal column is hypomobile, it is common for an adjacent segment to be hypermobile.[216] One must carefully examine each vertebra's mobility before applying joint mobilization. Random joint mobilization applied to a segment in the absence of a pretreatment examination of its mobility may increase, not decrease, the patient's symptoms. Be sure you have assessed the area correctly before applying joint mobilization.

Before we look at specific injuries and their corresponding programs, let us use our battery of exercises and progressions to put together a generic outline of a spinal rehabilitation program. From this generic program, specific programs for specific injuries can be developed.

At first, modalities might be needed to modulate pain and control muscle spasm. Muscle energy techniques, soft-tissue mobilization, and joint mobilization, if appropriate, are also part of the program to resolve soft-tissue and joint restrictions. Neuromotor control involves motor relationships between the spine, pelvis, and sacrum through core recruitment and facilitation, and it is important to address this early in the rehabilitation program.

Flexibility exercises to correct range-of-motion deficiencies are usually incorporated in the active phase and continued throughout the program. Patients are instructed to perform these exercises throughout the day until they achieve normal motion; thereafter, they can be done just once a day and after vigorous activities to preserve the flexibility gains. Specific frequency recommendations will vary from patient to patient, depending on the pathology and other problems. Instruction in neuromotor control, core stabilization exercises, and body mechanics education must be part of the program before beginning strength exercises.

Once the patient demonstrates the ability to maintain an engaged core during simple exercises, he or she can progress to other activities such as pool exercises, trunk-strengthening exercises, and multiplanar activities. Resistive phase trunk-strengthening exercises such as abdominal crunches, oblique exercises, and bridging exercises strengthen global core muscles. As has been mentioned, the latissimus pull-down and other exercises that include shoulder muscles whose proximal insertion sites are located on the trunk are included among the strengthening exercises.

As the patient's trunk stability improves, he or she performs lower-extremity-strengthening exercises for the hip muscles, including hamstrings, since these muscles also affect the spine. Swiss ball exercises such as crunches, bridges, leg lifts, side sit-ups, and progressions of strengthening exercises for the abdomen and trunk can begin in the resistive phase of the program once the patient demonstrates pelvic stability with other resistive exercises. Recall that endurance and proprioception should be emphasized during this phase.

When the patient demonstrates core control and strength with Swiss ball and weight exercises in the resistive phase, more advanced strengthening exercises for the trunk begin in the advanced phase. These more difficult exercises include planks and side planks, trunk and hip extension exercises on the Roman chair, and abdominal crunches and standing trunk rotations using the medicine ball. Toward the latter half of the advanced phase, specific exercises needed for the patient's normal tasks are added to the program. For example, if the patient is to return to track and field as a hurdler, jumping and bounding exercises for quadriceps power gains are added.

The final aspect of the advanced phase includes the incorporation of drills that mimic performance-specific activities. The patient should be able to maintain core stability and spinal alignment throughout these activities. When the patient is pain free, has good strength and flexibility, and can perform functional activities without difficulty, a return to normal activities is the final step. Figure 17.76 presents the goals and treatment schedule for a generic rehabilitation program for the spine.

Because the spine is subject to a few unique injuries, there are additional special considerations for these injuries beyond the general rehabilitation program outlined in figure 17.76. Once these unique considerations are identified, rehabilitation programs are created to address them. As the patient progresses toward return to participation or return to work tasks, body mechanics specific to the spine and SI joints may also need to be addressed.

SI Joint and Spine

Stage I: Inactive phase	
0-2 weeks	**Inflammation phase: Inactive rehabilitation phase**
Goals	Relieve pain. Reduce edema. Relieve spasm. Demonstrate correct diaphragm inhalation. Maintain conditioning levels of unaffected body segments (MCL).
Treatment guidelines	Modalities such as electrical stimulation for pain, muscle spasm Muscle energy techniques Grade I and II joint mobilization for pain Soft-tissue mobilization Posture instruction Neuromotor control activities with diaphragm inhalation CV exercises and other extremity exercises for maintenance (ME) After first week: Begin active ROM
Precautions	Gentle motion after modalities and mobilizations to increase muscle relaxation; may be active or active-assistive No resistive exercises
Stage II: Active phase	
2-8 weeks	**Early proliferation phase: Active rehabilitation phase**
Goals	Achieve normal range of motion, flexibility, and tissue mobility. Progress activity level with diaphragm inhalation. Restore proprioception. Acquire muscle endurance for activities. Initiate trunk stability exercises. MCL. Eliminate pain, spasm, and edema.

Figure 17.76 A generic rehabilitation program for the spine.

Stage II: Active phase	
2-8 weeks	**Early proliferation phase: Active rehabilitation phase**
Treatment guidelines	AROM, PROM for motion gains Grade III and IV joint mobilization Soft-tissue mobilization to achieve normal tissue mobility Instruction in proper body mechanics during ADL Early proprioception exercises Home exercise program to reinforce treatment goals Early strength exercises ME
Precautions	Stay within pain limits of motion and exercise. Discomfort may be present during soft-tissue mobilization, but pain level should improve immediately after treatment. Watch for continued diaphragm inhalation during neuromotor control exercises and instruct trunk stability exercises without requiring rib cage and pelvic motion in preparation for required core activation during subsequent stages of rehabilitation.

Stage III: Resistive phase	
6-12 weeks	**Late proliferation phase: Resistive rehabilitation phase**
Goals	Maintain normal ROM. Use verbal and tactile cues to have patient maintain pelvic neutral throughout treatment session. Achieve normal strength and muscle endurance without lumbar extension. Maintain core stability during triplanar activities. MCL.
Treatment guidelines	Continued ROM exercises; convert to HEP Joint and soft-tissue mobilization PRN Diagonal exercises with UEs and LEs with core stability Aggressive strength and endurance exercises HEP for self-mobilization for soft-tissue maintenance ME
Precautions	Pain is the primary guideline. Patient must maintain core stability throughout all exercises; assist with verbal and tactile cues as needed. Correct patient for posture and body mechanics during more challenging tasks PRN.

Stage IV: Advanced phase	
12-18 weeks	**Remodeling phase: Advanced rehabilitation phase**
Goals	Perform functional (multiplanar) activities properly. Execute performance-specific exercises with core stability without lumbar extension. Return to normal participation without pain, and normal strength, mobility, and execution of activities.
Treatment guidelines	Functional exercises without compensation Performance-specific exercises without compensation
Precautions	Use verbal cues to correct for pelvic positioning.

CV = cardiovascular; ROM = range of motion; AROM = active range of motion; ME = maintenance exercise; MCL = maintain conditioning levels; PRN = as needed; HEP = home exercise program; UE = upper extremity; LE = lower extremity.

Figure 17.76   >continued

Special Rehabilitation Applications

In this section, a few common injuries to the spine, sacrum, and pelvis are explored with examples given for suggested evaluation tools and treatment considerations.

Posture and Lumbopelvic–Hip Dysfunction

Before we can discuss various spine injuries, we must first investigate factors that are often present regardless of the injury suffered. These factors have to do with posture. Recall from chapter 6 that proper posture encourages optimal function of everything from internal organs to muscles and bones. Improper posture, on the other hand, can reduce respiratory function, create additional physical stress, degrade support systems, and increase a person's risk of injury.[217] Unfortunately, people tend to start developing poor posture as youngsters. Children often mimic their parents in posture.[218] This is one way poor posture develops. Other ways include performing repetitive movements while in poor posture until it becomes "normal"[216] or maintaining a poor posture for prolonged periods so structural changes occur.[219] Regardless of the reason people develop poor posture, the end result is the same: increased soft-tissue and joint stresses and increased risk of injury.[220, 221]

Muscle balance is crucial to proper posture.[104] So is bone and ligament balance.[104] So is myofascial balance.[104] So is proprioceptive perception and input.[104] Muscle imbalance is often the first offender, leading to poor posture and additional stresses and injury.[217] Part of the problem is that we often overuse some muscles and underuse their opposing muscles. For example, when you sit at your computer for several hours to compose a paper, most of the muscles used include anterior flexor muscles: the scapular protractors, pectorals, and elbow flexors. Over time, muscles that are predominantly used tend to shorten.[219] At the same time, their opposing muscles tend to be stretched.[219] If a muscle is chronically stretched, it becomes weaker. Think of a rubber band that is kept at its fully stretched length for a long time; its ability to spring back to its original resting length diminishes. Therefore, in prolonged poor posture, the overused muscles become shortened and the underused muscles become lengthened and weaker with less tone.

Poor posture, then, creates muscle imbalances by changing muscle length and strength over time. As this posture is maintained, surrounding fascia changes in length to accommodate these changes, further compounding poor posture. As discussed in chapter 14, neural adjustments are made to adapt to these changes, so the improper posture is perceived by the body as "normal"; both proprioceptive and neuromotor firing sequences change as a result.[4] Without correction, poor posture becomes progressive, eventually resulting in bony changes along with more soft-tissue and neurological adaptations.[222]

Unfortunately, most people have poor postural habits.[104, 223] Therefore, rehabilitation clinicians play a crucial role in identifying and correcting postural deviations before they become significant, interfering with the patient's functions. Fortunately, it is not difficult to identify these postural deviations. A Czech physician who was a neurologist and physiatrist, Vladimir Janda,[224] has made this task relatively easy because of his investigations and identifications of postural deviation groupings. He grouped muscles into two classifications, those that are responsible for posture (which he called *tonic muscles*) and those that are responsible for movement (which he called *phasic muscles*).[186] Janda identified the tonic, or postural, muscles as the predominant system that experienced shortening,[225] presumably because of their continual low-level effort against gravity. Their opposing muscles, the phasic muscles, tend to lengthen and weaken.[225] Janda indicated that the tighter muscles activate before the lengthened muscles.[225] However, this may be primarily because the postural muscles have a larger number of Type I fibers, and these fibers are activated before Type II fibers because their recruitment threshold is lower.[226]

Based on his theory of muscle imbalance development, Janda identified two muscle imbalance systems, one for the upper body and one for the lower body.[225] They are both identified as crossed syndromes, primarily because of how they affect the body segments; he called the upper-body system the *upper crossed syndrome* and the lower-body system the *lower crossed syndrome*. These syndromes feature a cross-pattern arrangement with anterior muscles that are weak diagonally correlated with posterior muscles that are also weak, and anterior muscles that are tight diagonally correlated with posterior muscles that are also tight, so the alignment of weak and tight muscles forms a cross, or an X-shape, through the sagittal plane of the body. This arrangement also demonstrates a tight muscle on one side of the body aligned directly across from a weak muscle on the opposite side. Janda believed that although the severity of muscle imbalance may vary from one person to another, this pattern of tight and weak muscles is fairly consistent.[186] Each of these is presented next.

Upper Crossed Syndrome

Upper crossed syndrome is demonstrated in figure 17.77. This syndrome includes tightness of the suboccipital spinal muscles, upper trapezius, and levator scapulae posteriorly; this area of tightness crosses with tightness in the pectoralis major and pectoralis minor.[186] The anteriorly weak muscles include the deep cervical muscles that cross with the serratus anterior, rhomboids, and middle and lower trapezius posteriorly.[186] The typical posture of a person with upper crossed syndrome includes a forward head with a flat

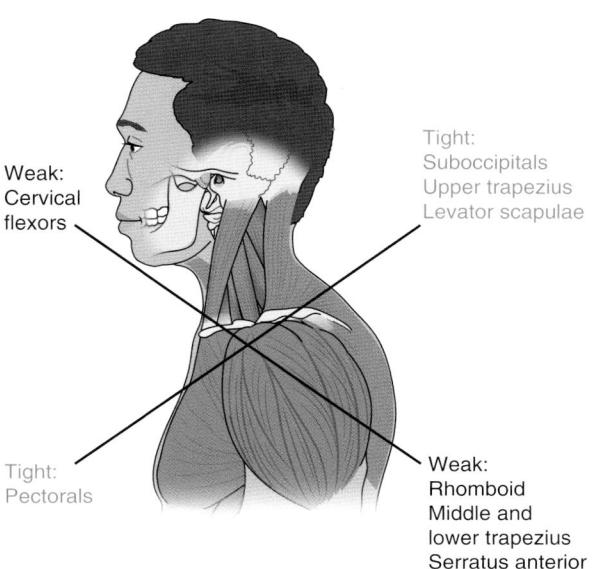

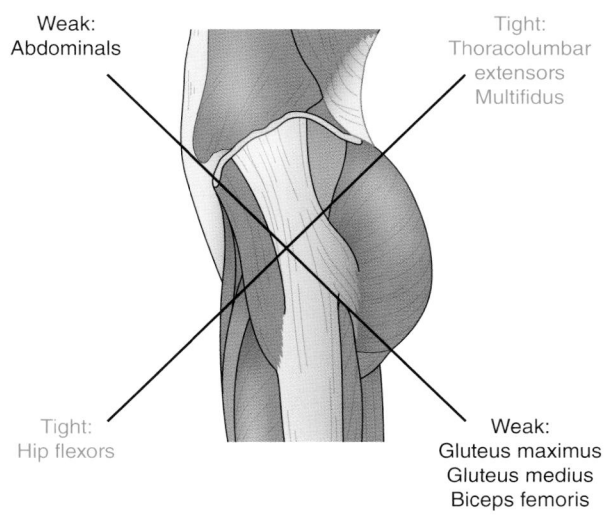

Figure 17.77 Upper crossed syndrome posture is recognized by the forward head, cervical lordosis with thoracic kyphosis, protracted scapulae, and abducted scapulae.

Figure 17.78 Lower crossed syndrome posture is identified by an exaggerated lumbar lordosis and anterior pelvic tilt.

lower cervical spine and upper cervical lordosis, thoracic kyphosis in the mid-thoracic region with extension above and below the kyphotic segment, protracted and winged scapulae, and medially rotated or abducted shoulders. This posture may range from mild to severe, depending on the severity of the person's pathology.

As you can see from the muscles affected by upper crossed syndrome, this pathology affects both the neck and the shoulders. Muscles are imbalanced, and this imbalance places excessive stress on them as well as on the joints, ligaments, and fascia.[224, 227] As these imbalances continue over time, osteoarthritic changes occur in joints.[228] Headaches, neck pain, thoracic outlet syndrome, and shoulder impingement result.[227, 229, 230]

Lower Crossed Syndrome

Lower crossed syndrome is illustrated in figure 17.78. This syndrome displays tightness anteriorly in the hip flexors (iliopsoas and rectus femoris), which is crossed with tightness in the posterior back extensor muscles (thoracolumbar erector spinae and multifidus); the weakened muscles include the abdominals (transverse abdominis) anteriorly, which are crossed with the posterior gluteal muscles (gluteus maximus, gluteus medius, and biceps femoris).[186, 230] This imbalance of muscles in the region results in an excessive anterior pelvic tilt that is identified as an exaggerated lumbar lordosis. Associated with this pelvic tilt and lordosis is hyperextension in the knees. Hip flexor tightness pulls the lumbar spine anteriorly to exaggerate the lumbar lordosis. Unfortunately, the weakened abdominal and gluteal muscles lack sufficient strength to counteract

this pull from the hypertonic muscles. The anterior pelvic tilt moves the hips into flexion, which results in the body's center of mass moving forward of the knees. This alignment of the body's line of gravity causes the knees to hyperextend, further lengthening (and weakening) the biceps femoris muscle posteriorly.

Therefore, lower crossed syndrome pathology affects the lower back as well as the lower extremities. It is not surprising that injuries commonly associated with this pathology include low-back pain, facet dysfunction, sacroiliac dysfunction, anterior knee pain, hamstring strains, and myofascial trigger points.[230, 231]

Upper and Lower Crossed Syndrome Rehabilitation

Unfortunately, people with upper or lower crossed syndrome posture often have both conditions (figure 17.79).[232] It is common for pathology in one body segment to affect adjacent segments. Like a spiral staircase, if one stair is positioned forward of the others, the adjacent stairs must compensate for that malposition by adjusting their positions or the structure will not stand. So, too, when tight muscles pull one vertebra in one direction, the spine must create a compensatory curve if the spinal column is to keep the body erect. This compensatory strategy can influence not only the spine, but also the entire kinetic chain.

Rehabilitation clinicians must be aware of these crossed syndromes and the impact they have not only on muscles, but also on fascia, neural facilitation, joints, and bones. Depending on the duration and severity of the pathological posture, any or all of these structures may be affected and may need to be addressed in treatment. Since poor posture results in multiple adaptations, treatment must be multifactorial.

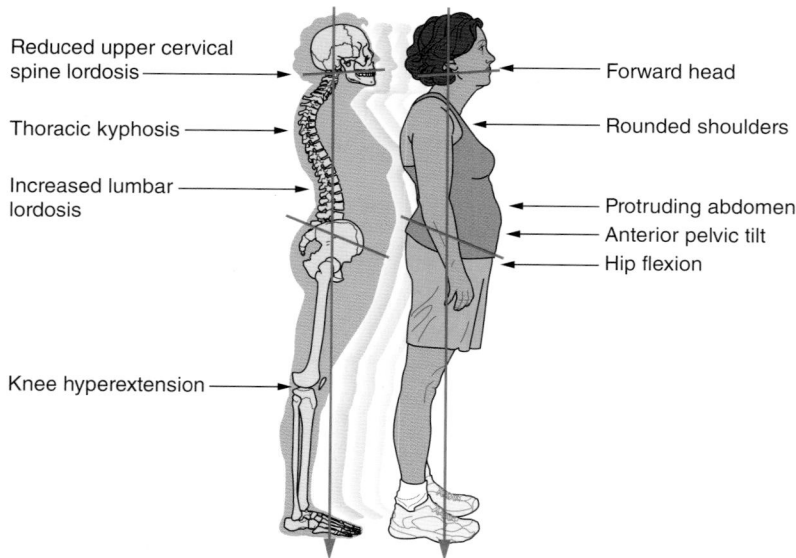

Reduced upper cervical spine lordosis

Thoracic kyphosis

Increased lumbar lordosis

Knee hyperextension

Forward head

Rounded shoulders

Protruding abdomen
Anterior pelvic tilt
Hip flexion

Figure 17.79   Upper and lower crossed syndromes often occur together. The posture that results from these syndromes includes forward head, rounded shoulders, reduced upper cervical spine lordosis, thoracic kyphosis, increased lumbar lordosis, protruding abdomen, anterior pelvic tilt, hip flexion, and knee hyperextension.

Elements of the rehabilitation program include patient education, postural changes, soft-tissue treatments, and correction of muscle imbalances with flexibility and strengthening exercises.[217] Posture education includes demonstrating to patients the difference between their current posture and correct posture with neuromotor control and inhalation from the diaphragm; it also includes discussing the hazards of continuing with incorrect posture. Clinical instruction to change posture often throughout the day, and to avoid any prolonged posture, helps to reduce muscle stress, especially for those who normally remain in prolonged positions to perform their daily tasks.

People with poor posture will have difficulty maintaining the proper posture, especially in the early phases of treatment. Until muscle imbalances are corrected, muscle endurance improves, and bad habits change, patients will only be able to hold the correct posture for short periods, after which they will slip back into their habitual posture. Proper posture can gradually become the new normal as muscles lengthen and strengthen and as patients keep remembering to correct their posture. This is challenging, though, because posture improves from the inside out through neuromotor control and reeducation. Rehabilitation clinicians must be persistent with reminders and rehabilitation programs and be supportive as patients make slow gains.

Several soft-tissue and joint techniques may be beneficial when tissues affected by these techniques develop secondary pathology resulting from poor posture. Myofascial release is often needed to help improve the flexibility and mobility of tight fascia that restricts muscles and joints.

Various techniques are appropriate for fascial restriction within the body segments. Since trigger points can develop as secondary results of poor posture, trigger point release techniques may also be appropriate if patients report trigger point pain patterns. Joint mobilization or muscle energy techniques may also be indicated if patients have had prolonged poor posture that creates joint mobility changes.

During your examination, you identified the muscles with restricted mobility and those that are weak. Before you restore strength to the weakened muscles, you must first correct the tightness—to address the strengthening first would limit the treatment's effectiveness.[231] Stretching exercises for each of the tight muscles are incorporated both in the clinic program and in the home exercise program. Clinic or home flexibility exercises may include the use of foam rollers, lacrosse balls, or Swiss balls in addition to exercises that may be performed throughout the day while in school or at work.

Once flexibility improves, strengthening the weak muscles you identified during your examination improves the patient's ability to maintain a proper posture. Since these muscles are primarily antigravity, or postural, muscles that must work continuously throughout the day, endurance exercises with high repetitions are the primary strengthening exercises used in the program. As patients begin to improve in both flexibility and strength, the rehabilitation clinician will observe positive changes in their posture.

Once the patient's muscle strength improves, the patient may continue to have difficulty maintaining appropriate posture throughout the day. During this time—when some strength gains have occurred, but strength levels are not yet normal—it may be appropriate to apply tape to the back or neck to provide tactile reminders when patients move out of good posture. This technique was presented in chapter 6. Tape should not be applied too soon in the program because muscles will not have enough endurance or strength to tolerate the posture requirements. The tape used is Cover-Roll Stretch Tape (BSN Medical Inc., Charlotte, NC) because it can stay on the skin for prolonged periods and is not affected by water. When the tape is used, the patient is instructed to remove it after 24 h or sooner if it causes burning, itching, or discomfort. It may be reapplied at the next treatment session as long as no skin irritation develops.

As patients progress through their rehabilitation and improve their posture, they often find that proper posture now feels normal. Once patients have achieved their rehabilitation goals, the rehabilitation clinician creates a maintenance program. Daily flexibility exercises for the formerly tight muscles, and a strength-maintenance program for the formerly weak muscles, is often enough to preserve good posture when performed 1 to 2 d a week.[233]

 Go to HK*Propel* and watch video 17.11, which demonstrates proprioceptive taping for posture.

Facet Injuries

Facet injuries can be frustrating to treat, especially if you do not consider the factors listed here. Facet injuries can also be difficult to identify. Rehabilitation clinicians must use their deductive skills to identify facet injuries.

Before we discuss facet injuries, we must first understand that in the spine, motion in one direction will facilitate motion in a different plane. This is because of the position of the facets. Although the precise motions that go together are a matter of some dispute,[234] they are called coupled motions. **Coupled motions** are those that occur in a joint together; one motion does not occur without the other. The coupled motions in the spine are lateral bending and rotation. There is disagreement over whether these coupled motions occur on opposite sides or on the same side.[234, 235] Researchers' inability to reach the same findings is based on such differences as the varied methods used in the studies, the original postures of the subjects studied, age factors, types of subjects investigated, and other considerations. In spite of the lack of consensus on normal coupling motions, many agree that with dysfunction, lumbar lateral flexion motion in the spine is coupled with rotation to the opposite side.[236-238]

You can determine your own coupling motions. In a standing position, flex your trunk laterally as far as you can go while keeping your feet flat on the floor. As you reach the end of your motion, notice how your trunk is positioned. Do you rotate to the side you flexed to or to the opposite side? You can also do this in the cervical spine. Standing in a proper cervical alignment, laterally flex your neck as far as possible and notice in which direction you rotate by the end of your lateral flexion. Many people agree that lumbar spine lateral flexion and rotation coupling occur in the opposite directions, but the same motions in the cervical spine couple in the same direction with each other.[239] If your cervical spine motions were to the same side when you performed the motion, now move into a slumped posture and repeat the exercise. You should notice that the coupling motions are now in opposite directions: Lateral flexion is to one side and rotation is to the other.

Fryette's Laws of Physiologic Spinal Motion

Coupled motions in the spine originate with concepts described by Harrison Fryette, an osteopathic physician, and are named after him. Although they are not actually laws of motion as much as they are observations and ideas, they are called "Fryette's laws of physiologic spinal motion," or more simply, "Fryette's laws of motion."[240] Fryette presented his ideas of coupled motions between facets both in a neutral position and out of a neutral position. He presented three laws that determine coupling motions of the spine.

Fryette's first law states that when the lumbar or thoracic spine is in neutral, side-bending occurs to the opposite side of that vertebral level's rotation. For example, in proper alignment, when the L3–4 spine laterally flexes to the right, it rotates to the left.[240] This law does not address the cervical spine because Fryette defined a neutral position as the position where the facet joint surfaces are not in contact with each other; adjacent cervical facet surfaces are always in contact with each other.[240]

Fryette's second law deals with coupled motions in pathological positions. Fryette indicated that when the spine is in either flexion or extension (out of a neutral position), the side-bending and rotation of the vertebrae will be toward the same side.[240] For example, if the lumbar spine is placed into a hyperlordotic position and the subject side-bends to the left, rotation to the left will also occur at the vertebral level. Since the facet joints are in contact when the vertebrae are out of their neutral position and the coupled motions occur to the same side, we may be able to conclude that since the cervical spine facet joints are also in contact with each other, they undergo the same coupling action: Rotation and side-bending occur to the same side.

Fryette's third law states that if motion in one plane occurs in the spine, motion in another direction is diminished.[240] The motions Fryette refers to are the three plantar motions of flexion-extension, rotation, and lateral flexion. His concept is easy to demonstrate on yourself with this exercise: Stand erect and rotate your spine to the left, noting the amount of rotation you have. Now stand and forward flex at the trunk and lumbar spine and while in that position, repeat the left rotation. You should find that you achieve less rotation in this position than when you are standing erect.

Facet Impingement and Positional Dysfunction

Fryette's laws help us to understand what occurs with facet-restricted motions. Facet restriction can occur from an impingement after a traumatic event where the facet surfaces on one side suffer an injury. A facet can be restricted in either flexion or extension, and this determines whether the restriction to motion is to the same side or to the side opposite the site of injury. The position the facet is in is called *positional dysfunction*. The motion the facet cannot perform is called a *motion restriction*. A positional dysfunction will always be opposite to the direction of its restricted motion. A facet joint in flexion is *open* since the two facet surfaces of the joint are apart; the upper facet surface cannot drop down into extension, so the two joint surfaces are "open." A facet joint in extension is *closed*; the upper facet surface cannot move upward and forward into flexion, so the two joint surfaces are "closed."

If a facet is restricted in its ability to open (flexing), the facet is stuck in extension and has motion restriction (it cannot move) in flexion; therefore, extension is the positional dysfunction and flexing is the restricted motion. Since rotation and side-bending are coupled with each other, they will also have motion restrictions in positional dysfunctions. In other words, if motion is restricted in rotation, side-bending is also restricted since these motions occur together. When there is a positional dysfunction of *(stuck in) extension*, rotation and side-bending are limited on the *side opposite to the problem facet*. In a positional dysfunction of *(stuck in) flexion*, side-bending and rotation are limited on the *same side as the problem facet*.

Since this concept can be confusing, let us look at an example of each condition. If a left facet has a positional

dysfunction of (stuck in) extension, rotation left, and side-bending left, the motion restriction will be flexion, right rotation, and right side-bending; the problem causing this situation is that the *left* facet will not open into flexion. The patient will be unable to move the spine into normal flexion, rotation to the right, and side-bending to the right, but movement into extension, left rotation, and left side-bending will not be impeded and will appear normal (figure 17.80).

On the other hand, if the positional dysfunction of *(stuck in) flexion* is present, restricted motion in side-bending and rotation will be *ipsilateral* to the problem facet. For example, if a patient has a positional dysfunction of (stuck in) flexion because the right facet will not close, the stuck position (positional dysfunction) will be flexion, rotation left, and side-bending left with motion restricted in extension, right rotation, and right side-bending; the patient will be unable to move the spine into normal extension, right rotation, and right side-bending, but movement into flexion, left rotation, and left side-bending will not be impeded and will appear normal (figure 17.81).

Table 17.7 includes a list of positional dysfunctions and motion restrictions most commonly seen. These dysfunctions are evaluated with the patient sitting on a table and the clinician sitting on a chair behind the patient so the clinician can position his or her eyes at the level of the patient's lumbar spine. The clinician palpates the transverse process of the spinal level below, at, and above the painful region. While palpating the left and right transverse processes with his or her thumbs, the clinician asks the patient to slowly perform lumbar flexion and extension by rolling the pelvis into an anterior and posterior pelvic tilt. The clinician compares the left and right transverse processes' prominence into his or her thumb in flexion and extension to determine the side of dysfunction. The clinician then repeats this process at adjacent levels to determine the level of the dysfunction.

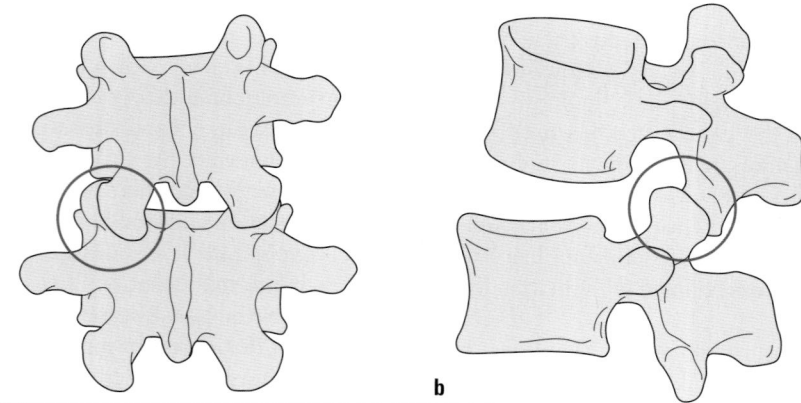

a   b

Figure 17.80   Left facet is stuck in extension: *(a)* posterior view; *(b)* side view. Positional dysfunction is extension, left rotation, and left side-bending. This vertebral level is restricted in its ability to move into flexion, right rotation, and right side-bending. This dysfunction is known as ERSL (extension, rotation, and side-bending left). The left facet will not open.

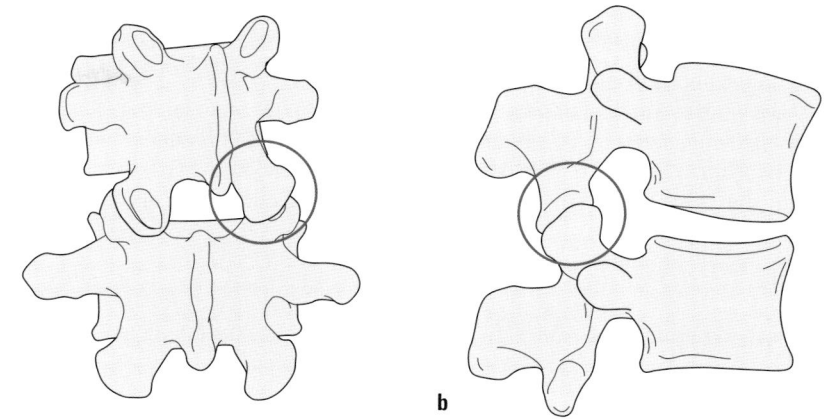

a   b

Figure 17.81 Right facet is stuck in flexion: *(a)* posterior view; *(b)* side view. Positional dysfunction, then, is flexion, left rotation, and left side-bending of the upper facet. This vertebral level is restricted in its ability to move into extension, right rotation, and right side-bending. This dysfunction is known as FRSL (flexion, rotation, and side-bending left). The right facet will not close.

TABLE 17.7 Facet Dysfunctions

Positional dysfunction (stuck in)	Motion restriction (cannot move into)	Problem
FRSL (Flexion, **R**ot L, and **SB L**)	Extension, Rot R, and SB R	**Right** facet will not close
FRSR (Flexion, **R**ot R, and **SB R**)	Extension, Rot L, and SB L	**Left** facet will not close
ERSR (Extension, **R**ot R, and **SB R**)	Flexion, Rot L, and SB L	**Right** facet will not open
ERSL (Extension, **R**ot L, and **SB L**)	Flexion, Rot R, and SB R	**Left** facet will not open

Note: Rot = rotation; SB = side-bending; L = left; R = right.

The source of the problem for these facet dysfunctions is also provided in table 17.7 to help you understand where the treatment will occur since the problem facet is the side where unilateral joint mobilizations are applied. Other signs and symptoms include radiating pain mimicking dermatomal distribution, tenderness of spinous processes, and reflex muscle spasm.

Facet Sprain

Sprains to the facet joint result in more trauma than impingement, so tissue injury is also greater. A more conservative treatment approach is needed. Additionally, soft tissue around the joint may also have been injured, and swelling and muscle spasm are common. A cervical collar may reduce pain. A forward-head position occurs because extension is painful. If motion loss occurs, a unilateral capsular pattern may develop. The capsular pattern for facets is limitation of rotation to the involved side and side-bending to the opposite side. For example, if a left cervical or lumbar facet has a capsular pattern, left rotation and right side-bending will be restricted, but right rotation and left side-bending will be free. Gentle ROM in pain-free movements and joint mobilization after modalities can relieve muscle spasm, pain, and edema. Later, grades III and IV joint mobilization are used to promote facet mobility.

Facet Treatment

Although a facet sprain is more painful than an impingement and must be treated with more caution, especially in the initial rehabilitation phases, their treatment courses follow similar procedures once the injury moves into stage II of rehabilitation. It may take a little more time with modalities and grade I and II joint mobilization to reduce pain with facet sprains. Once the initial acute pain is reduced for either condition, the clinician applies grade III and IV joint mobilizations to the painful facet, as the patient tolerates it.

As rehabilitation continues, flexibility exercises and strengthening are added to the rehabilitation program. Initially, neuromotor control exercises are prescribed. Extension activities may be painful, so they are approached as the patient tolerates them. Any postural pathology present should also be addressed in the program. Core strengthening may be necessary if deficiencies were noted during the patient's examination. As with any spinal rehabilitation program, cardiovascular activities should be routinely included in the program. If the patient fails to progress and pain persists, it may be necessary to refer the patient to a physician for injection into the facet joint to relieve the pain and subsequently allow the patient to complete the rehabilitation program.[241]

Case Study

Four days ago, a diver landed poorly in a dive during practice. She has had a stiff neck since that time. This morning she awoke and could not turn her head to the left. She presents to you with her head laterally flexed about 20° to the right, and she cannot look straight ahead. Her head is rotated to the right about 15°. It is painful for her to try to place her head in an upright and straight position, but she has no difficulty turning her head all the way to the right and looking over her right shoulder. Your palpation reveals tenderness over the C5 and C6 spinous processes, and there is some tightness in the muscles in the same area.

Questions for Analysis

1. What do you believe her problem is; what side of her cervical spine is the location of her problem?
2. Outline your treatment program, sequencing your treatment in a logical progression.

Sprains and Strains

Sprains and strains are among the most common back and neck injuries.[242, 243] If they are not appropriately examined and treated, sprains and strains become frustrating and aggravating injuries because they can linger and cause lasting disability.

The resulting pain and muscle spasm from acute sprains and strains must first be resolved in phase I with modalities and mild stretching exercises.[242] Sometimes these conditions respond to grade I and II joint mobilization,[242] but early response will depend on the severity of the pain and spasm and on the effectiveness of the modalities in relieving these problems.

Acute conditions require modalities in the initial treatment phase along with limited activity and stretching exercises. As spasm and pain are reduced, muscle energy techniques and soft-tissue mobilization are indicated if restriction is noted with palpation. Grade III and IV joint mobilization may be useful if the restriction is the result of joint hypomobility.

As with all spinal injuries, posture and body mechanics should be assessed and corrected as needed. Spasm will persist if the muscles are required to overwork in the presence of poor posture or body mechanics.

A progression of strengthening exercises should begin once the pain and spasm have diminished enough to allow active exercises. The muscles that need the most emphasis on strengthening are the local and global core muscles and the gluteal muscles. Figure 17.82 presents a rough timeline of events in a rehabilitation program for a lumbar sprain

Lumbar Sprain or Muscle Strain

Stage I: Inactive phase	
0-2 weeks	**Inflammation phase: Inactive rehabilitation phase**
Goals	Relieve pain. Reduce edema. Relieve spasm. Achieve diaphragm inhalation and neuromotor control. Maintain conditioning levels of unaffected body segments (MCL).
Treatment guidelines	Modalities such as ice and electrical stimulation (ES) for pain, muscle spasm Gentle PROM after ice and ES to relax muscles Muscle energy techniques Grade I and II joint mobilization in area of injury for pain Instruction in diaphragm inhalation and neuromotor exercises as tolerated CV exercises and other extremity exercises for maintenance (ME)
Precautions	Gentle motion and diaphragm inhalation after modalities and mobilizations to increase muscle relaxation; may be active or active-assistive No resistive exercises

Figure 17.82 Rehabilitation progression for lumbar sprain or muscle strain.

	Stage II: Active phase
2-6 weeks	**Early proliferation phase: Active rehabilitation phase**
Goals	Increase range of motion, flexibility, and tissue mobility. Maintain diaphragm inhalation in functional positions. Restore proprioception. Acquire muscle endurance for activities. Initiate trunk stability exercises. Early strength gains in core muscles with trunk stability. MCL. Eliminate pain, spasm, and edema.
Treatment guidelines	AROM of spine Grade III and IV joint mobilization Early neuromotor control exercises in supine and quadruped positions Learn body mechanics for daily activities (e.g., sitting, sit-to-stand, brushing teeth, shaving, picking up objects, etc.) with diaphragm respiration Early proprioception exercises Standing balance with neuromotor control Home exercise program to reinforce treatment goals Initiate core strength exercises with trunk stability Hip strength exercises ME
Precautions	Stay within pain limits of motion and exercise. Observe for continued diaphragm inhalation during neuromotor control exercises, and instruct patient in trunk stability exercises without requiring rib cage and pelvic motion in preparation for required core activation during subsequent stages of rehabilitation. May require postexercise modalities. Use flexibility exercises at end of treatment.
	Stage III: Resistive phase
6-12 weeks	**Late proliferation phase: Resistive rehabilitation phase**
Goals	Maintain normal ROM. Use verbal and tactile cues to have patient maintain core stability throughout the treatment session. Achieve normal strength and muscle endurance with core stability. Maintain core stability in triplanar activities. MCL.
Treatment guidelines	Continue with ROM exercises; convert to HEP Joint and soft-tissue mobilization PRN Diagonal exercises with core stability using pulleys or rubber bands for endurance and muscle control Add rotational exercises using body-weight resistance Add UE and LE exercises while with trunk and core stability ME
Precautions	Pain is the primary guideline. Patient must maintain neuromotor control or trunk stability throughout all exercises, depending upon the level of difficulty; assist with verbal and tactile cues as needed. Correct patient for posture and body mechanics PRN. Continue to include flexibility exercises at treatment conclusion.

>continued

Figure 17.82 >continued

Stage IV: Advanced phase	
12-16 weeks	**Remodeling phase: Advanced rehabilitation phase**
Goals	Perform functional activities properly. Perform performance-specific exercises without compensation. Return to normal participation without pain, and normal strength, mobility, and execution of activities without compensation.
Treatment guidelines	Functional exercises executed without compensation from lumbar spine Increased speed and agility of exercises Plyometric exercises without compensation from lumbar spine Performance-specific exercises executed without compensation from lumbar spine
Precautions	Use verbal cues to correct for pelvic positioning.

ES = electrical stimulation; PROM = passive range of motion; CV = cardiovascular; AROM = active range of motion; ROM = range of motion; UE = upper extremity; LE = lower extremity; MCL = maintain conditioning levels; ME = maintenance exercises; PRN = as needed; HEP = home exercise program.

Figure 17.82 >continued

injury. Keep in mind that each patient responds to a treatment protocol differently; therefore, patients may follow a similar progression of exercises and treatment, but no two persons may have the same timelines.

Spondylosis, Spondylolysis, and Spondylolisthesis

The following is a brief outline of considerations to keep in mind in a rehabilitation program for spondylosis, spondylolysis, and spondylolisthesis. Although these three conditions differ from one other, they all usually involve the lower lumbar spine that becomes irritated with extension movements. The two most important factors with patients who have any of these conditions are that the person should be taught to perform posterior pelvic tilt activities and she should avoid extension movements as much as possible. These patients must establish and maintain pelvic mobility and stability in more of a posterior-tilt position and strengthen the hamstrings, internal obliques, and transverse abdominis. In spondylolisthesis, the most severe of the three conditions, there is a forward displacement of the

Case Study

A javelin thrower injured his back last week in practice when he threw the javelin and felt a sudden pain in the right low-back area. He comes to you stating that he applied ice to the injury when it occurred. The pain is now better than it was last week, but he still has pain when he rotates his trunk to the left and to the right. He has pain when he gets up from a chair and when he gets out of bed in the morning. His pain is worse at the end of the day. His pain ranges from 3 to 6 on a 10-point scale. He has been taking it easy for a couple of days but still cannot practice because of the pain. His pain is located on the right side of his low-back area. He has no radiation of symptoms into the lower extremities, but he does get pain in the right buttock. When you examine him, you find that he cannot bend forward because of pain; side-bending to the left is too painful to perform, but side-bending to the right is okay. Trunk rotation is more painful to the left than to the right. His spine has a lateral shift to the right in the lumbar region. Palpation reveals muscle spasm with tenderness in the right paraspinals and quadratus lumborum muscles. Pressure over the right lumbar multifidus reproduces his buttock pain.

Questions for Analysis

1. What stage of the healing process is he in? How severe is the injury?
2. How irritable is his injury? What is the nature of the injury?
3. What do you include in your first treatment?
4. What is your treatment progression and what guidelines will you use to advance this patient from one level to the next?
5. What are some examples of specific exercises, including functional activities, you should use before the patient's return to full participation?

Case Study

A gymnast has seen an orthopedic physician because of persistent complaints of low-back pain that did not resolve after 2 weeks of modality treatments and reduced activity. The physician's diagnosis is a spondylolysis. The patient needs to work with you, completing a rehabilitation program before she can return to competition.

Questions for Analysis

1. What exercises would you have this patient avoid?
2. What progression of exercises and activities should her rehabilitation program include to return her to full participation?
3. What is a main concern for you about her pelvic neutral positioning, and how will you address it as you instruct her in her rehabilitation program?

---

vertebrae; since any extension movement is usually painful, it is extremely important for these patients to establish and maintain pelvic stability in a posteriorly tilted position.

A rehabilitation program for these patients involves the same exercises and progressions as for other back patients. The important difference, however, is that their pelvic position is different than what is commonly taught to back patients. An excellent set of exercises to initiate this stage of rehabilitation is the dead bug and bird dog exercises because the focus of those exercises is a posterior pelvic tilt. The least degree of posterior pelvic tilt that the person achieves without pain is the position he or she should maintain during rehabilitation exercises and activities such as standing still and walking.

Disc Lesions and Sciatica

Disc lesions can be unnerving conditions to deal with for both patient and rehabilitation clinician. You should be familiar with the factors identified here and consider them before establishing a plan of care.

A protruding or herniated disc can be a serious problem and often causes radiculopathy down one or both extremities, depending on the location of the protrusion. The mere presence of pain or symptoms down the leg does not mean that there is a disc herniation, but you should consider this a possibility until it has been ruled out. Other conditions such as facet injuries, muscle spasm, and myofascial pain can also refer pain down the lower extremity.

Patients diagnosed with disc lesions should avoid those positions and motions that aggravate or reproduce the patient's sciatica symptoms. These motions most commonly are forward flexing or flexing and twisting in the direction that further increases disc pressure.

Evaluation tools for disc lesions include a thorough history with subjective pain profile and complete objective examination. Included in the objective examination are special tests that help to eliminate all except the correct clinical diagnosis. Tables 17.3 and 17.4 identify many of these special tests, with which you should be familiar.

Patients who have disc lesions must learn to engage the core and perform motions with appropriate neuromotor control. These patients must also strengthen the abdominals, obliques, back extensors, and gluteal muscle groups, as was presented in the general spine program. They should also learn correct posture and body mechanics and eventually progress to performing all physical activities with appropriate core control and body mechanics.

Although not all authorities agree on its importance, some advocate the centralization of pain for disc lesions.[199] This means that if the treatment is appropriate, the patient will experience a gradual and progressive retreat of the sciatic pain from distally to proximally until the only pain remaining is localized to the back. It is the goal of treatment to ultimately relieve this central pain.

Typically, the use of extension exercises, flexibility and strengthening activities, and trunk stability training will accomplish this goal.[199] Exercises progress at the patient's own rate. Progression depends on the treatment results and the patient's feedback about the pain. If the pain recedes with treatment, the progression of exercises can continue; if the sciatic pain worsens, you must reevaluate the current exercises, first for how the patient performs them and second for appropriateness. It may be that the exercise has been introduced too soon for the patient to tolerate it. Use of the wrong exercises or failure to correct faulty execution may aggravate the disc lesion. It is vital that the clinician have a good understanding of the exercises and the stresses that each exercise produces.

Compression Fracture

A compression fracture in the spine exists when the vertebral body fractures, resulting in the height of the involved vertebral body becoming smaller than the ones above and below it. The cause of a vertebral fracture is primarily aging and osteoporosis,[244] but trauma can also cause a vertebral body fracture.[245]

The patient often has pain at the fracture site. If the fracture is due to trauma, it is usually the result of a high-velocity event, such as a motor vehicle accident. Treatment will require local soft tissue and pain management, as well as potential management for other regions of the body affected by the event.

If the fracture is due to osteoporosis, medical management or pharmacological management may be needed.[246] Rehabilitation is patient specific and requires individual modifications to meet each patient's needs. Fall prevention, strengthening the extensors of the trunk, cardiovascular fitness, and overall strength training to improve the patient's ability to perform activities of daily living should all be considered.[244, 246] Occasionally, if the patient's spine is unstable due to one or more fractures, surgical intervention is needed to stabilize the anterior aspect of the vertebral body.[245] Due to the location of the surgery and the individual nature of patient progression, communication between the rehabilitation clinician, surgeon, and patient is critical to ensuring a successful rehabilitation outcome.

Microdiscectomy

Occasionally, patients with a disc injury cannot succeed with conservative treatment and need surgery. A microdiscectomy is a common procedure in which a small incision is made in the center of the back at the site of the herniated disc. The muscles are moved out of the way, rather than cut, so postoperative recovery is less complicated. The surgeon bypasses the nerve root and cuts through the lamina to remove the part of the disc that is protruding and irritating the nerves.

Those patients who have undergone microdiscectomies follow a course of treatment similar to that for patients who have disc pathology without surgical correction. In a typical timeline, treatment begins about 1 week postoperatively and follows a logical progression. During the initial phase of rehabilitation, motion must be restricted to a pain-free range. The active phase of treatment includes pain modulation, flexibility exercises, neuromotor control with diaphragm inhalation, and instruction in proper posture and body mechanics. A cardiovascular program on a stationary bike, treadmill, elliptical, or other equipment is used in a progressive manner, using patient tolerance and heart rate as a guide. Also in the active phase, stretching exercises for the hamstrings, piriformis, and quadriceps are added.

In the early resistive phase, more flexibility, range-of-motion, and core exercises are added for trunk stability, and early strength exercises of progressive difficulty may begin if the patient tolerates them without pain. If post-surgical muscle tightness and soft-tissue restriction are present, they are treated with soft-tissue release and modalities. Disc patients must learn core recruitment techniques, use correct posture and body mechanics, and improve muscle endurance and strength of core, trunk, latissimus dorsi, and hip muscles to support the spine. As healing continues into remodeling, the advanced phase of the rehabilitation program begins. During this time, more intensive strength exercises and agility activities occur and evolve to the point where performance-specific routines are used to prepare the patient to return to normal activities.

Spinal Fusion

In more severe cases, a spinal fusion may be indicated. These surgeries are usually reserved for people with unstable spines, severe or multiple-level disc degeneration, or spondylolisthesis. Although some surgeons use local bone grafts for these fusions, a bone chip from the hip or pelvis is most commonly used to fuse two or more vertebral levels.[247] Hardware, such as metal plates, screws, and rods, may be used to hold the vertebrae together. After surgery, the patient's range of motion is restricted to allow the fusion to heal. In these cases the rehabilitation clinician must see to it that the patient does not disrupt the fusion site by excessively loading or rotating the spine.

During the inactive phase, modalities are used to modulate pain, swelling, and muscle spasm. Submaximal isometric activities may begin in this phase, depending on the physician's preference and the patient's status. In the active phase, the clinician instructs the patient in core recruitment and proper body mechanics. The patient also begins daily walking with appropriate core engagement and arm swing. Since the spine sits on the sacrum, limited pelvic shifting enables the body to learn to move safely without lumbar rotation. The dead bug exercise sequence is useful here; this sequence of exercises allows the body to relearn proper trunk movements, correct breathing, and walking without pain in the lumbar spine.

In the active phase, soft-tissue mobilization of the scar, proprioceptive exercises, and core stabilization exercises begin. Toward the end of this phase, advanced instructions in more advanced body mechanics are initiated. These advanced instructions may include techniques on lifting, lateral movements, and pushing and pulling activities. Cardiovascular activities on the treadmill, elliptical, or stationary bike and hip strengthening exercises with core stability also occur during this time. By the time the patient approaches the resistive phase, he or she may perform strengthening exercises for the body and trunk and begin easy agility exercises. As with other conditions, the progressive performance-specific program is begun in the advanced phase to permit the patient's return to normal activities.

As you can see, the programs for microdiscectomy and spinal fusion are similar. The primary difference is in the precautions for each of the conditions. This is because with the microdiscectomy there is removal of tissue but no tissue repair as there is with the fusion. Although both conditions have an inflammation phase after the surgical insult to the body, the fusion requires much more caution because the body must be given time to fuse the bones.

Case Study

A football defensive lineman injured his back in a game 4 weeks ago. He was referred to an orthopedic surgeon because of continued low-back and right lower-extremity pain. Magnetic resonance imaging revealed that he has a disc bulge of 3 mm at L4–5. The physician indicates that this patient is not a surgical candidate because the problem may be resolved with rehabilitation, corticosteroid injections, or Medrol dose pack. After his second injection, he reports significant relief from back and leg pain. He is now coming to you for a rehabilitation program.

His movements are not guarded when he enters the examination room. He does not appear to hesitate to walk or to get up from a chair. When he moves around the room, however, you notice that he has very poor body mechanics, bending from the back to sit down and bending and twisting sideways to retrieve his backpack. His examination reveals an SLR to 50° on the right and 55° on the left, and his medial hip rotation is 20° bilaterally. In a standing forward bend motion, he can touch his fingers to his knees; in a side bend he can touch 10 cm above his knee; and in backward bending he has normal motion. Forward bending produces some discomfort.

You notice that when he flexes forward, the motion starts in the upper thoracic spine, with the lumbar spine remaining hyperextended, while most of the motion comes from his hips. The neurological examination reveals no deficiencies in sensory, motor, or reflex innervation. The patient's gluteal muscles and abdominals each test at 4/5 strength. He cannot perform a side sit-up on the right side. The paraspinals, quadratus lumborum, and hip lateral rotators are all tender to palpation, especially on the right, and you can palpate restriction of soft-tissue mobility in those tender areas. There is some restriction of joint mobility to PA tests in the lower lumbar spine.

Questions for Analysis

1. What precautions would you observe in treating this patient?
2. What would your initial treatment program include for him today?
3. What techniques would you include in your first three treatment sessions?
4. What progression of exercises would you select for this patient, and what criteria would you use for progression from one level to the next in the program?

The rehabilitation process with the microdiscectomy may last from 6 to 10 weeks, but the fusion recovery may take 3 to 4 months, depending on the patient and the physician.

SI Joint Pain

Sacroiliac joint pain is usually due to a sprain or strain, depending on which structure is involved. However, while some treatments are similar to lumbar region sprains and strains, there are some differences.

When examining a patient with low-back pain, it is important to test the SI joint to determine if the patient's pain is coming from the lumbar spine or from the SI joints. If none of these tests elicit pain, the patient is probably experiencing pain from the lumbar spine rather than the SI joints. However, if three or more of these tests from tables 17.4 and 17.8 are positive, then the patient is experiencing pain of SI joint origin.[124] Before these tests are presented, we must realize some of the potential causes as well as signs and symptoms a patient with SI dysfunction or injury may present.

Etiology, Signs, and Symptoms

Susceptibility to SI pathology increases because of posture or activities that increase SI torque stresses. Patients who have excessive lumbar lordosis with an exaggerated forward pelvic tilt can place excessive stress on the SI joint

TABLE 17.8 Sensitivity and Specificity of Common Muscle Energy Tests for the SI Joint

Test	Sensitivity	Specificity
Standing forward-bend test	17%[1]	79%[1]
Seated forward-bend test	9%[a]	93%[a]
Kinetic (Gillet) test	8%[a]	93%[a]
	41%[b]	68%[b]
SI compression test	69%[b]	69%[b]
SI distraction test	60%[b]	81%[b]
Alignment test	Unknown	Unknown
Sphinx test	Unknown	Unknown
Iliac crest test	Unknown	Unknown
ASIS test	Unknown	Unknown
Pubic symphysis (spring) test	Unknown	Unknown

[a] Levangie.[134]

[b] Laslett et al.[124]

Data from Levangie (1999); Laslett et al. (2005). [134, 124]

and cause pain in the area.[248, 249] Patients are susceptible to sacroiliac and low-back pain if they have a leg length discrepancy, fall on the side or buttocks, misstep off a curb while running, run while twisting, or bend and twist the lumbar spine.[250-252] The patients most susceptible to SI injuries because of the stresses of their sports are soccer players, basketball players,[253] gymnasts, dancers, golfers, competitive rowers, rugby players, and track and field athletes.[123, 252, 254] Sacroiliac malalignments can occur with imbalances caused by injury or secondary spasm, weakness, loss of mobility, or repetitive activities requiring unilateral standing.[253] Some SI joint injuries result from classic types of injuries and stresses.

Before treatment is begun, the specific malalignment must be determined. A complete sacroiliac examination includes an investigation of posture, alignment, and lumbar range of motion. Landmarks most often accessed during a sacroiliac examination include the ASIS, posterior superior iliac spine (PSIS), sacral base, sacral sulci, sacral inferior lateral angles (ILAs), iliac crests, ischial tuberosities, sacrotuberous ligaments, and pubic symphysis.[255]

Therefore, malalignments of the SI joints can occur for a variety of reasons, and from a variety of forces applied to the region. For example, upslips, inflares or outflares, and pubic subluxations can occur when there is a sudden, sharp upward force applied from the foot up the leg as a person steps off a curb or stair and does not realize that there is another step. Falling on the buttock can lead to sacral flexion, pubic subluxations, and upslip injuries. Trunk rotation and bending activities can cause sacroiliac dysfunctions. Knowing the history will help to identify the problem. Table 17.9 shows common pathologies with their etiology along with commonly experienced signs and symptoms.

TABLE 17.9   Sacroiliac Dysfunctions, Common Causes, and Symptoms

Type of dysfunction	Dysfunction	Common causes	Signs and symptoms
Iliosacral	Pubic subluxation	Soccer; after pregnancy and delivery	Groin pain, buttock pain; patient may have only low-back pain.
	Iliac inflare	Direct blow; soccer	Groin pain; patient may or may not have leg pain.
	Iliac outflare	Falls; direct blow; soccer	Groin pain; patient may or may not have hip pain or leg pain.
	Anterior iliac subluxation (R upslip)	Past history of falling on buttock; sudden step off curb; hockey; basketball; motor vehicle accident (MVA)	Always on right (right upslip); pain often on opposite side; leg pain; low-back pain; coccygeal pain; nerve root pain.
	Posterior iliac subluxation (L upslip)	Same as for anterior iliac subluxation	Always on left (left upslip); often occurs with other spinal problems that haven't responded to treatment; often occurs with spinal flexion.
	Anterior iliac rotation	Usually occurs with other lesions	Long leg on side of lesion; should be the last to be treated.
Sacroilial	Sacral flexion	Occurs with bending and twisting activities or push–pull activities; MVA	Pain often on side opposite lesion; patient may report feeling as if back popped at the time of injury.
	Forward torsion: same letters (1st letter = sacral motion; 2nd letter = axis)	Bending with twisting motion; getting out of car quickly	Most common sacroiliac injury. Back or leg pain; buttock pain. Pain may be on side opposite lesion. Indicated as a right-on-right (R on R) or left-on-left (L on L) forward torsion.
	Backward torsion: opposite letters (1st letter = sacral motion; 2nd letter = axis)	Bending with twisting motion	Not as common as the forward torsions. Patient is flexed in trunk flexion 2° to pain and waddles like a duck; painful during movement into extension; may appear to have a disc lesion or may have pain in the buttock and lumbosacral region; indicated as a right-on-left (R on L) or a left-on-right (L on R) backward torsion.

Note: MVA = motor vehicle accident; L = left; R = right.

Sacroiliac and Iliosacral Lesions

Sacroiliac dysfunctions occur when either the sacrum cannot move on the ilium or the ilium is restricted in its movement on the sacrum. Based on these restrictions, dysfunctions are divided into two categories, sacroiliac and iliosacral.

The first half of the term indicates which part of the joint is restricted in its ability to move on the second half of the term; therefore, a *sacroiliac dysfunction* indicates that the sacrum is not moving on the ilium, while an *iliosacral dysfunction* is restriction of ilium movement on the sacrum. It is important to first determine which segment is restricted since treatment is designed to address either sacral or ilial restriction. The composite results of the motion tests provide the clinician with the information needed to determine a diagnosis and plan of treatment.

Treatment and assessment results of sacral-pelvic dysfunction are intimately linked with treatment selections identified only after the rehabilitation clinician has performed the pretreatment tests. Likewise, treatment results cannot be determined unless the rehabilitation clinician performs post-treatment tests. These tests are presented in the following section.

Special Tests of the SI Joint

There are specific factors to be examined when sacroiliac pathology is suspected. These factors determine either relative alignment or the quality and quantity of SI motion. A number of tests are used to examine and assess sacroiliac joint alignment.[124, 255] Only some of the most common ones are presented here.

These special tests may be divided into two categories based on their intent: identification of motion or identification of malalignment. The three tests that determine quality and quantity of motion are usually used before the alignment tests are performed.

Movement Tests and Kinetic Test   Three movement tests used to determine quality and quantity of motion are the standing forward-bend test (StFBT), the kinetic test (KT), and the seated forward-bend test (SitFBT). These tests identify differences in movement between the right and left sacroiliac sides. Some of these tests identify the presence of SI dysfunction and the side of the lesion. Some can also identify whether the problem is due to the ilium not moving on the sacrum (iliosacral dysfunction) or the sacrum not moving on the ilium (sacroiliac dysfunction).

- *Standing Forward-Bend Test.* The standing forward-bend test is sometimes called the *Piedallu's sign* and is performed with the rehabilitation clinician facing the patient's back and placing each thumb on the patient's PSIS and the hands on the iliac crests.[256] The rehabilitation clinician's eyes are at the same level as the patient's pelvis. Once the rehabilitation clinician properly positions his or her thumbs, the patient then bends forward (figure 17.83). If the SI joint is normal, the thumbs will move inferiorly as the patient bends forward; if there is a lesion, the thumb on the side of the lesion will either move upward or will not move as the other thumb moves inferiorly. This test only identifies the side of the lesion; it does not identify the kind of lesion.

- *Seated Forward-Bend Test.* The seated forward-bend test is performed with the rehabilitation clinician's hands as indicated in the standing forward-bend test. The patient is in a seated position with the knees apart and higher than the hips (figure 17.84). The

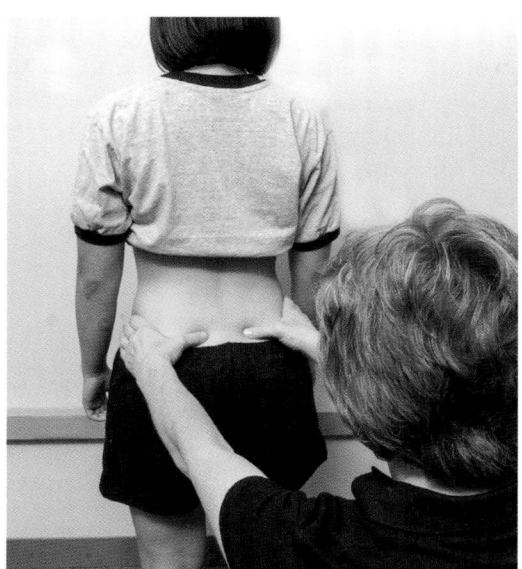
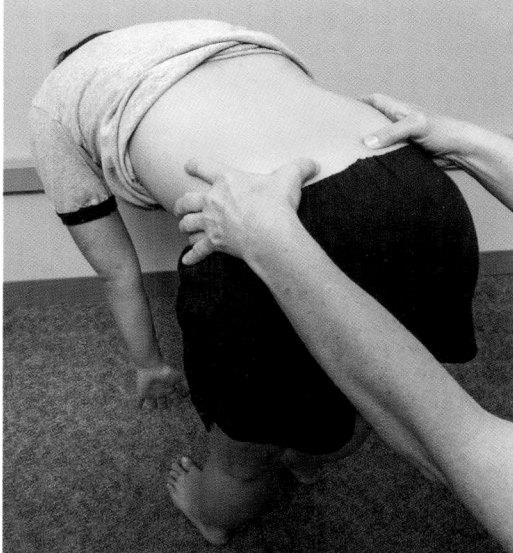

Figure 17.83   Standing forward-bend test.

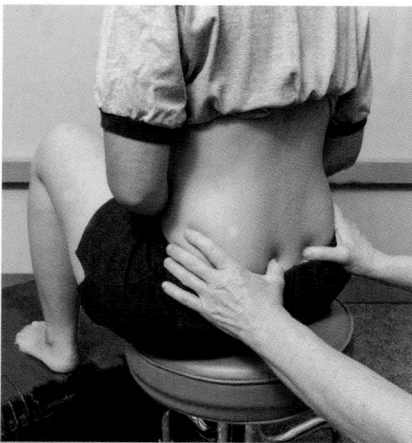
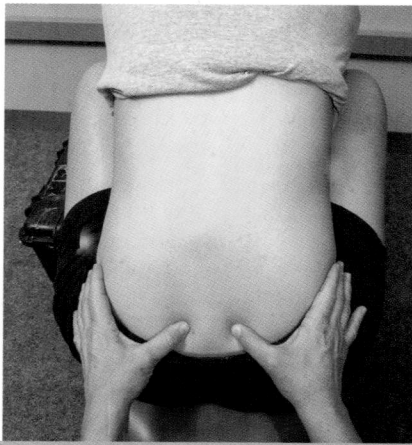

Figure 17.84 Seated forward-bend test

rehabilitation clinician's eyes are at the same level as the patient's pelvis. The patient bends forward; in normal movement, the thumbs should move inferiorly as they do in the standing forward-bend test. If a thumb either does not move or moves superiorly, the patient has a sacroiliac lesion on that side. With the ischial tuberosities anchored in sitting, movement of the sacrum occurs on the ilium; if movement does not occur, the sacrum on the side of restriction will not be able to move in its normal counternutation during lumbar flexion.

- *Kinetic Test.* In the kinetic test (also called the *Gillet test*, or *one-leg stork test*),[96] the patient stands with his or her back to the clinician. To evaluate the left, the rehabilitation clinician places one thumb on the left PSIS and the other thumb at the same level on the mid-superior sacrum (figure 17.85). The rehabilitation clinician's eyes are at the same level as the patient's pelvis. The patient then lifts the left knee

toward the chest; if the SI joint is normal, the left thumb moves inferiorly, but it stays at the same level if joint motion is restricted. This test checks for left iliosacral (ilium on sacrum) motion, so if the thumb does not move inferiorly, then the left ilium motion on the left sacrum is restricted.

With the thumbs and patient in the same start position, the patient then lifts the right knee toward the chest; if the SI is normal, the right thumb moves inferiorly, but motion is restricted if the thumb stays at the same level; this test checks for left sacroiliac (sacrum on ilium) motion. In this instance, if the right thumb does not move inferiorly, the left sacrum motion on the left ilium is restricted. The rehabilitation clinician then places the thumbs in a reverse position, with the right thumb on the right PSIS and the left thumb on the mid-superior sacrum at the same level as the right thumb, and repeats the two single-leg stance tests. Lifting the right leg

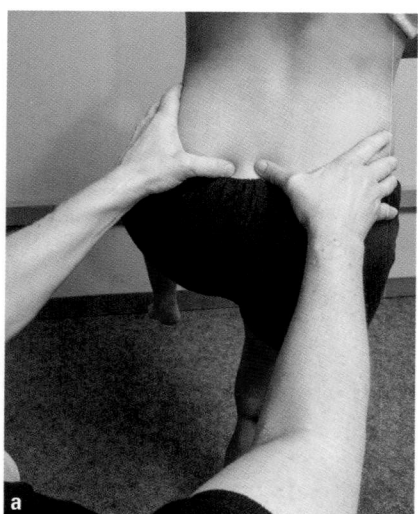
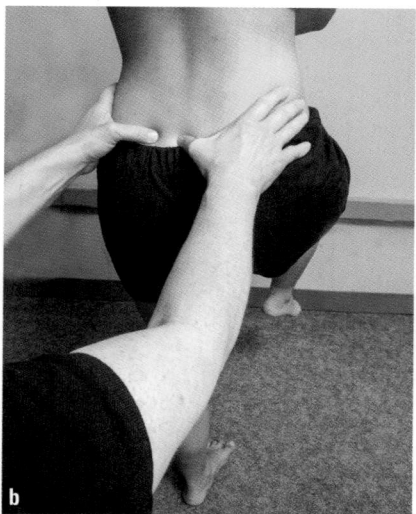

Figure 17.85 Kinetic test of the left sacroiliac joint. *(a)* Assess movement of the left ilium on the sacrum. *(b)* Assess movement of the sacrum on the left ilium.

and watching right thumb movement assesses right iliosacral motion (iliac motion on the sacrum), and lifting the left leg while watching left thumb movement assesses right sacroiliac motion (sacral motion on the ilium).

Alignment Tests The alignment tests are performed with the patient in supine and prone positions; the supine tests include examination of left and right iliac crest height, leg length (leg L), the distance of the ASIS to the umbilicus, the ASIS height (ASIS), and the height and springiness of the symphysis pubis (pube ht, pube spring). The prone tests include the sphinx test, and examination of positions of the sulcus (sulcus), inferior lateral angle (ILA), and sacrotuberous ligament (st lig). See table 17.10.

These tests are passive tests performed by the rehabilitation clinician. If the patient is supine, the rehabilitation clinician stands on the same side of the patient as the rehabilitation clinician's dominant eye. If the patient is prone, the rehabilitation clinician stands on the opposite side from the rehabilitation clinician's dominant eye. For example, if the rehabilitation clinician is right-eye dominant, he or she stands on the patient's right side when the patient is supine, and on the patient's left side when the patient is prone.

Alignment tests are used to identify malalignment and to reproduce the patient's complaint of pain. Pressure applied during the test will evoke the patient's pain when there is a positive sign. Malalignment is readily apparent and obvious; otherwise it is not present.

- *Sphinx Test.* The patient is positioned comfortably in a prone position while the rehabilitation clinician is standing to the side of the patient. The rehabilitation clinician palpates the right and left sacral sulcus, noting asymmetrical depth. The rehabilitation clinician slides his or her thumbs inferiorly along the border of the sacrum to the inferior lateral angle (ILA) of the sacrum on both sides. Again, the rehabilitation clinician takes note of asymmetrical height of the ILA, right compared to left. The patient is asked to prop up onto the elbows and rest in that position. The rehabilitation clinician again palpates the sacral sulcus and ILA on both sides, noting whether the landmarks have become symmetrical or remain asymmetrical. This test is used to determine the difference between a backward and a forward sacral torsion, which informs proper treatment (figure 17.86).

TABLE 17.10 Commonly Used Sacroiliac Tests

Purpose	Test	Positive results
Quality and quantity of motion	Standing forward-bend test (StFBT); also called Piedallus test	Identifies side of lesion.
	Seated forward-bend test (SitFBT)	Identifies side of sacroiliac lesion.
	Kinetic test (KT)	Identifies side of sacroiliac or iliosacral dysfunction.
Relative alignment in supine	Leg length (leg L)	Dysfunction present only if difference is easily noticed and significant.
	Left and right iliac crest height	Difference in height between the two should be notable if present.
	Distance of ASIS to umbilicus	Dysfunction indicated by obvious difference of 2.5 to 5 cm (1 to 2 in.).
	ASIS height (ASIS)	One will appear more superior if it is positive.
	Height of symphysis pubis (pube ht)	One side is higher than the other.
	Springiness of symphysis pubis (pube spring)	Pain occurs with spring test on one side.
Relative alignment in prone	Positions of left and right sulcus (sulcus)	One side will be deeper than the other.
	Positions of left and right inferior lateral angles (ILAs)	One side will be more posterior (relative to sacral alignment) than the other.
	Tension of left and right sacrotuberous ligaments (st lig)	One ligament will be looser than the other.

Note: FBT = forward-bend test; KT = kinetic test; leg L = leg length; pube = pubic bones; ASIS = anterior superior iliac spine; ILA = inferior lateral angle; L = left; R = right; St = standing; Sit = sitting; st lig = sacrotuberous ligament.

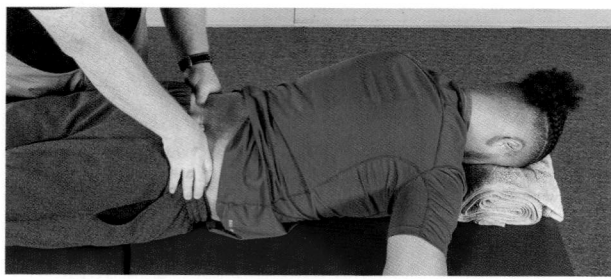

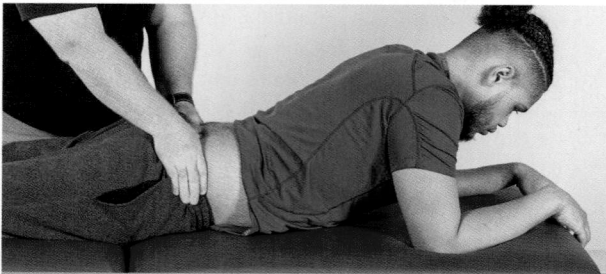

Figure 17.86 Sphinx test.

- *Leg Length Test.* Before performing the supine tests, the rehabilitation clinician places each thumb immediately under and in contact with the patient's medial malleoli. The patient performs a bridge and then lowers the hips to the examination table, and the rehabilitation clinician moves both hips and knees passively into extension. Leg length is assessed by comparing levels of medial malleoli; if leg length discrepancy is present secondary to SI dysfunction, the difference will be readily apparent (figure 17.87).

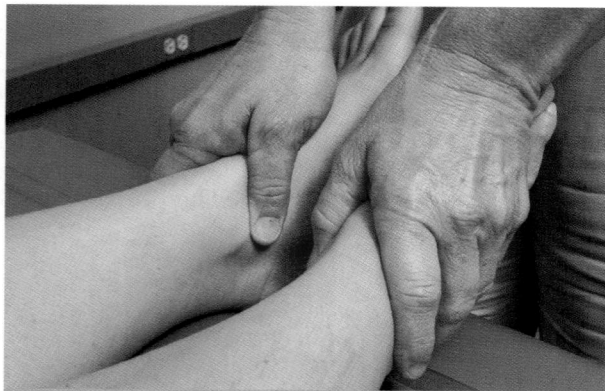

Figure 17.87 Leg length difference.

- *Iliac Crest and ASIS Tests.* With the patient supine, the rehabilitation clinician determines the heights of the iliac crests (figure 17.88) and ASIS (figure 17.89*a*). Placing the lateral index fingers with digits and wrists extended at the top of each iliac crest, the rehabilitation clinician looks directly down at the crests from a birds-eye view; obvious differences must exist to consider the result positive. When pal-

pating the ASIS, the rehabilitation clinician places a thumb on each ASIS and visualizes them from eye level. Each ASIS should be equal in height from the tabletop and with each other. If one ASIS is more posterior than the other, it will also appear more superior. The distance from each ASIS to the navel is determined by placing a thumb on each ASIS and rotating the hands to place the index finger at the navel (figure 17.89*b*); obvious differences between the distances will be approximately 2.5 to 5 cm (1 to 2 in.), if present.

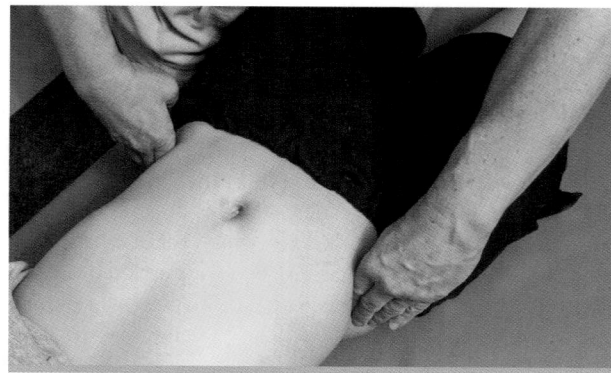

Figure 17.88 Iliac crest height test.

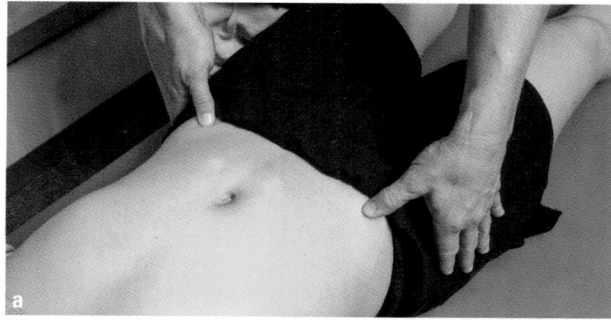

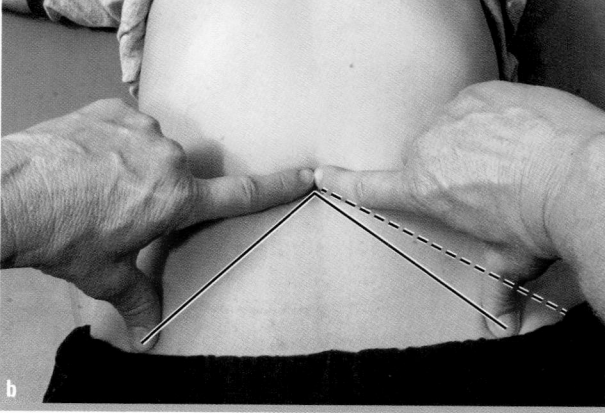

Figure 17.89 ASIS *(a)* height test and *(b)* to-navel tests. The solid line represents a normal result, while the dotted line indicates a positive result on the left. The differences between the left and the right are obvious when they exist.

- *Pubic Symphysis Tests*. The springiness of the pubic bones is tested by first locating the pubic symphysis; place the heel of one hand on the patient's abdomen with the fingers directed cranially and move the hand caudally until the heel of the hand contacts the superior portion of the symphysis pubis. Once the pubic bones are located, the rehabilitation clinician's hands are repositioned so the index fingers or thumbs are placed about 2 cm (<1 in.) laterally from the superior symphysis pubis joint to alight on the pubic tubercles. The rehabilitation clinician then presses down on the left, then the right pubic tubercle (figure 17.90); pain or restricted mobility of either pubic bone is a positive sign. Differences in height between the right and left pubic bones are assessed by placing a finger or thumb on each bone, observing the bones at eye level, and noting differences.

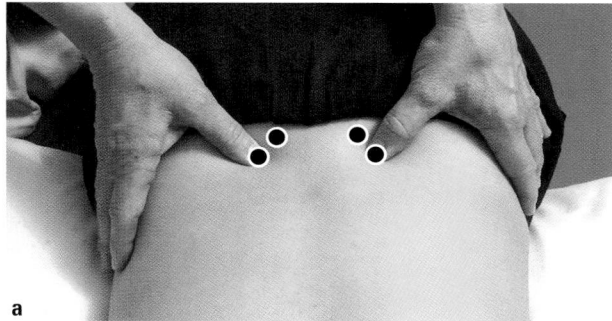

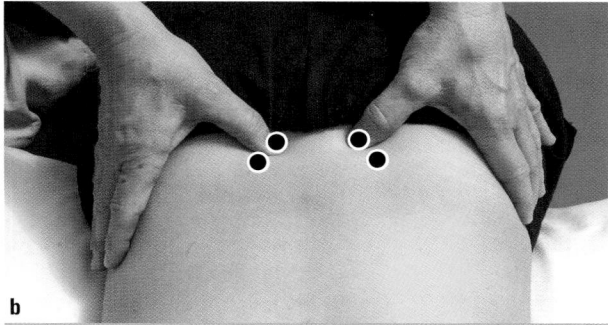

Figure 17.91 *(a)* PSIS examination and *(b)* location of right and left sulci.

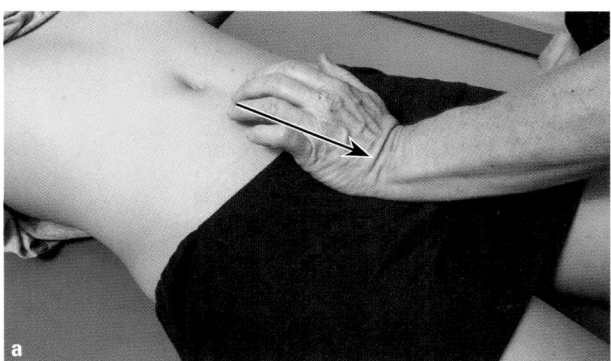

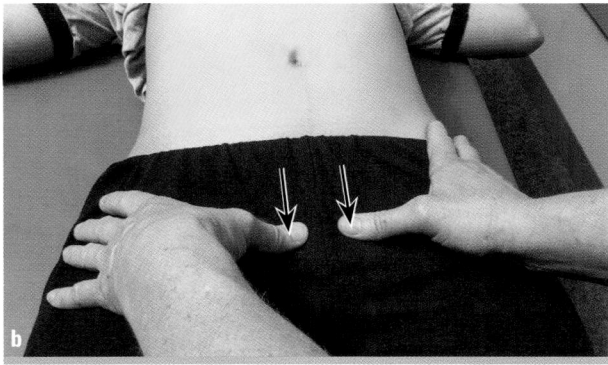

Figure 17.90 Pubic symphysis test: *(a)* locating symphysis pubis and *(b)* testing for springiness and height of each pubic tubercle separately.

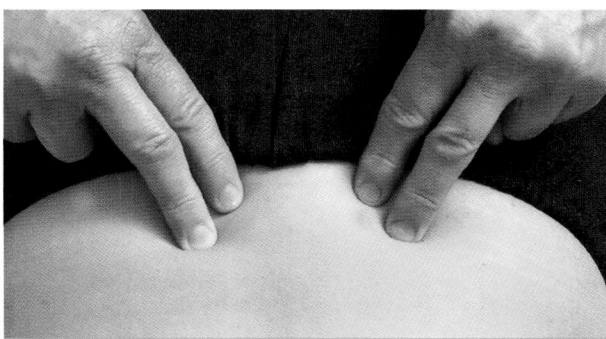

Figure 17.92 Sulcus and PSIS. The middle fingers indicate the location of the left and right PSISs, and the index fingers show the location of the left and right sulci, about 30° medial and inferior to their respective PSISs.

The right and left PSISs are examined in the prone position (figure 17.91a); they should be the same height. In the presence of dysfunction, one will appear either more superior or more inferior than the other. The left and right sulcus are also examined in the prone position (figure 17.91b). The left and right sulci are located at a point about 30° inferior and medial from the left and right PSISs, respectively (figure 17.92); the positions of the two should be the same relative to their respective PSISs and the

planes of motion, but if one is more posterior or anterior, it should be noted because this is abnormal (figure 17.91b). The height of the right and left inferior lateral angles (ILAs) are then examined (figure 17.93). To locate the ILAs, the cornua, the very end of the sacrum as it meets the coccyx, is palpated; the ILAs are about 1.5 to 2 cm (<1 in.) lateral to the cornua. The ILAs should be level with each other, but if one is more anterior or more posterior than the other, this malalignment should be noted.

There should be no pain with palpation or pressure on any of these landmarks; pain is an abnormal response. The sacrotuberous ligament lies between the ILA and the ipsilateral ischial tuberosity. Each left and right sacrotuberous ligament should be palpated in a crosswise manner to

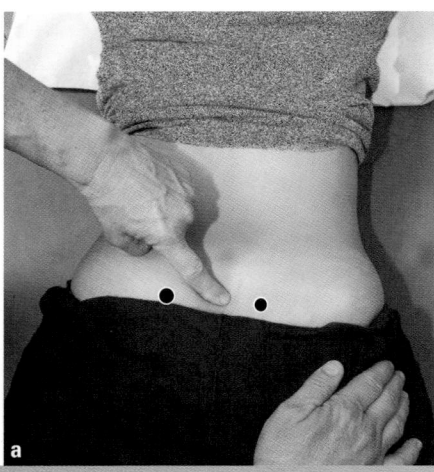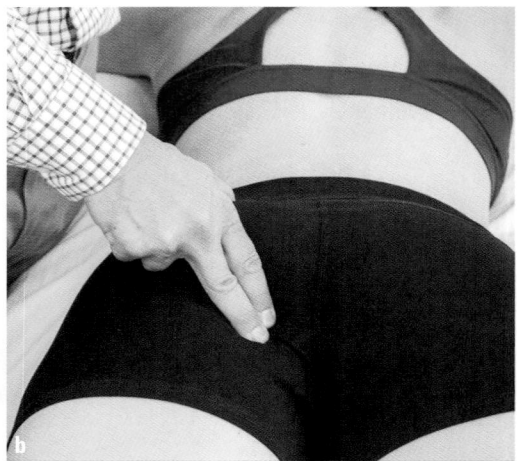

Figure 17.93   The rehabilitation clinician *(a)* locates the cornua and moves thumbs laterally to palpate the ILAs (black circles), and *(b)* palpates sacrotuberous ligaments (medial and superior to ischial tuberosities).

compare the tension in each ligament. The tension should be the same in each ligament, and the patient should have no complaints of pain with the palpation. If one ligament has more tension than the other, there may be malalignment in either the sacrum or the ilium on the tender side.

Additional Tests   Additional examinations include trunk range-of-motion tests for quality and quantity of motion and pain during any motion. If lateral flexion is limited and accompanied by signs of SI dysfunction, the spinal motion loss is probably of sacroiliac origin. If flexion–extension motion is limited, the problem may be iliosacral in origin.

Muscle Energy Techniques

Once the special tests are completed, the rehabilitation clinician gathers this information from the subjective (table 17.10) and objective (table 17.11) segments of the examination to identify the clinical diagnosis. Once the diagnosis is established, the rehabilitation clinician appropriately treats the patient. Immediately after the treatment is completed, the rehabilitation clinician reassesses the patient's sacroiliac alignment and pain level to determine the treatment outcome. If the proper diagnosis and treatment have been applied, the patient experiences significant pain relief, and retesting produces negative results at the first treatment. The treatment is usually supplemented with a home exercise to reinforce the treatment effects. After successful muscle energy technique treatment, the patient's rehabilitation program follows the generic program outlined earlier in this chapter.

Muscle energy techniques are a form of manual therapy that lend themselves well to the sacroiliac region. As was mentioned in chapter 11, muscle energy techniques treat either the spine or the extremities. Some muscle energy techniques for sacroiliac (SI) and iliosacral (IS) motions are presented here.

When muscle imbalances occur, malalignments result and restrict movement.[257] These issues were discussed previously. These restrictions, in muscle energy terminology, are *barriers* to movement. A **barrier** is not an end of movement but rather a resistance to movement. The objective of muscle energy is to relieve these barriers and restore balance.[257] Muscle energy allows the patient to control the muscle contraction, but the clinician must first place the patient's segment in the correct alignment and instruct the patient to produce a specific muscle contraction in a specific direction to promote optimal results.[258]

The clinician must avoid common errors that will interfere with optimal results. These errors include[257]

- not controlling the joint position or direction of movement,
- not applying a counterforce to the patient's force in the correct direction,
- not allowing enough time between the contractions to achieve complete muscle relaxation before moving the segment to a new barrier, and
- not providing enough instructions to enable the patient to perform the activity correctly.

Patients also make errors in their muscle energy performance. Some of the patient errors include[257]

- using too much force,
- not contracting in the correct joint or segment position,
- not holding the contraction long enough, and
- not completely relaxing after the contraction.

Muscle energy techniques involve some very precise applications. The rehabilitation clinician must remember and perform these correctly for optimal results. An isometric contraction is held for 3 to 10 s, and the amount of the

TABLE 17.11   Test Findings for Iliosacral and Sacroiliac Pathologies

Pathology	SitFBT	StFBT	KT	Leg length	Pube ht	Pube spring	ASIS	PSIS	Sulcus	ILA	st lig
ILIOSACRAL LESIONS											
R sup pubic subluxation	Neg	Pos R	Pos R	Short R	R sup	Pain R					
R iliac inflare	Neg	Pos R	Pos R		R ant	Pain R	↓ Dist R ASIS to umbilicus	R is lat			
R iliac outflare	Neg	Pos R	Pos R		R post	Pain R	↑ Dist R ASIS to umbilicus	R is med			
R upslip: ant iliac subluxation (always on R)	Neg	Pos R	Pos R	Short R	R sup	Pain R	R sup	R is sup	Varies	Shorter R	R is slack with high R isch tub tension in L st lig.
L upslip: post iliac subluxation (always on L)	Neg	Pos L	Pos L	Short L	L sup	Pain L	L sup	L is sup	Varies	Shorter L	Tension in R st lig L is slack.
R ant iliac rotation	Neg	Pos R	Pos R	Long R	R inf	Pain R	R inf				
SACROILIAC LESIONS											
L sacral flexion	Pos L	Pos L	Pos L	L long	Varies	Varies	Varies	Varies	L deep	L post	
Forward torsion L on L (same)	Pos R	Pos R	Pos R				L inf	L is sup	R deep	L post	Tension in L
Backward torsion L on R (opp)	Pos L	Pos L	Pos L				L inf	R is sup	R deep	L post	Tension in L

Note: FBT = forward-bend test; KT = kinetic test; pube = pubic bones; ASIS = anterior superior iliac spine; PSIS = posterior superior iliac spine; ILA = inferior lateral angle; L = left; R = right; Sit = sitting; St = standing; sup = superior; st lig = sacrotuberous ligament; isch tub = ischial tuberosity; inf = inferior; ant = anterior; post = posterior; opp = opposite; neg = negative; pos = positive.

contraction is only very light.[258] Typically, the patient tries to produce a maximal contraction, but the rehabilitation clinician must impress upon the patient the importance of applying only a light resistance force. Using the statement "use only 2 ounces of force" communicates that the rehabilitation clinician does not want strong resistance. The light

Evidence in Rehabilitation

We have pointed out more than once in this text that it is very difficult to get objective data from manual therapy techniques because some of the techniques are subjective, such as patient self-reports of pain or the clinician's palpation of a treated area. For this reason, most of the evidence about manual therapy treatment outcomes is in the form of case studies or case reports.[259, 260] One of the stronger objective studies of muscle energy techniques was performed by Wilson and colleagues.[261] It was a pilot study of low-back pain resolution that compared two approaches; both approaches used neuromuscular reeducation and strength exercises, but one also incorporated muscle energy techniques. Patients who received muscle energy techniques along with the neuromuscular reeducation and strength exercise did statistically better than those who did not receive the muscle energy treatment. Unfortunately, most studies lack the objective measures that offer the evidence needed beyond the case report level to provide clinicians with stronger guidance. More objective studies are needed in specific manual therapy topics like muscle energy techniques.

resistance is used to reset the feedback system between the intrafusal and extrafusal muscle fibers to a normal level of excitation; a forceful contraction only makes it more difficult to restore this balance.[258] Once the patient relaxes after the active contraction, the rehabilitation clinician pauses to ensure full relaxation of the muscle and then applies a stretch. As the segment is passively moved, the rehabilitation clinician pays attention to where the new barrier is felt; the segment is moved only to that point and not beyond. Once the new barrier is reached, the process is repeated 3 to 5 times. Because the muscles and joints are asked to move in a precise and controlled manner, neuromotor control is an element of muscle energy. Since muscle energy positioning is very specific to the dysfunction, specific exercises are presented in the Home Exercise section after each technique.

Most commonly encountered sacroiliac and iliosacral lesions and their appropriate treatments are described here. If a patient you are treating has more than one lesion, the sacroiliac lesions are usually treated first.[257]

Sacroiliac Lesions and Their Treatment Techniques

Here is why sacroiliac lesions are treated before iliosacral lesions: Iliosacral lesions usually affect the pelvis unilaterally, while sacroiliac lesions are usually torsional dysfunctions that affect the other hemipelvis. Sacroiliac lesions are usually the result of muscle imbalances, especially between the piriformis and psoas muscles.[257] This indicates that sacroiliac lesions have existed for a while before the patient reports pain. Therefore, treating sacroiliac lesions first is prudent not only in terms of affecting outcomes but also in being more efficient in the approach.

CLINICAL TIPS

The patient's muscle energy exertions should be very light so that the neuromotor feedback system between the muscle spindle fibers and the extrafusal muscle fibers will reset to lower, normal levels. Strong muscle contractions continue the greater feedback exchange, making it difficult for the joint to move to its normal length and for the muscles to fully relax.

Sacral Flexion

Characteristics: This treatment is for a sacroiliac lesion.

Mechanism: This injury can occur with a bending-and-twisting activity. Push–pull activities can also cause a sacral flexion injury. This injury occurs more commonly on the left than on the right, but it can occur on either side.

Features: The pain may sometimes be on the side opposite the injury. If the injury is on the left side, the left sulcus will appear deeper (more anterior) than the right, and the left ILA of the sacrum is palpated more posteriorly.

Treatment: The patient lies prone with the leg in 30° abduction and medially rotated. The patient's thigh is stabilized on the rehabilitation clinician's thigh, and the rehabilitation clinician's hand applies pressure to

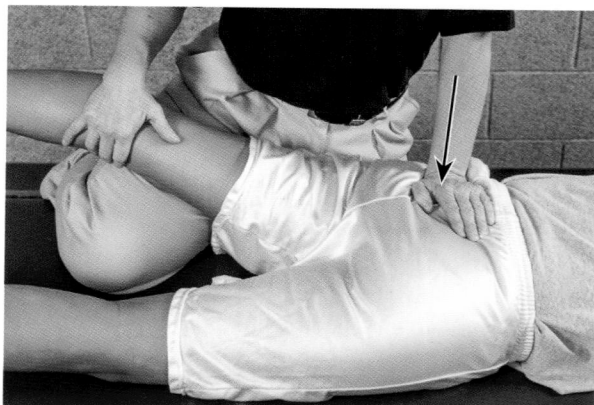

Figure 17.94

the left ILA (if the injury is on the left) (figure 17.94). The patient takes in a deep breath and holds it, then breathes slowly out while the clinician continues to exert constant pressure over the left ILA. The pressure is maintained as the patient breathes in again. This technique is performed 3 times. Sometimes a click can be palpated or heard on the maneuver.

Home Exercise: In the home exercise that accompanies this treatment, the patient lies with both knees to the chest. This facilitates sacral extension because the sacrum moves in the opposite direction of the lumbar spine—as the lumbar spine moves into flexion, the sacrum extends, and vice versa.

Sacral Torsion Sacral torsion is another sacroiliac lesion. There are two types of sacral torsion: forward and backward. These occur on the oblique axes of the sacrum. Each axis is labeled according to its location on the sacral base; the left axis is from the left sacral base to the right inferior lateral angle (ILA), and the right axis is from the right sacral base to the left ILA (see figure 17.7). Torsions are defined according to which axis they occur on and in which direction the sacral base opposite to the axis moves. For example, if it is a L on L torsion, the sacral axis is the left (second letter), and the right sacral base is rotated to the left (first letter), or forward. If it is a R on L torsion, the sacral base axis is the left, and the right sacral base is rotated to the right, or backward. When there is a R on R torsion, the left sacral base is rotated to the left (backward) on the right axis. As you can see, if the letters are the same (R on R or L on L), it is a forward torsion; if the letters are different (L on R or R on L), it is a backward torsion. Because a R on L and a R on R appear the same with a deep L sulcus and a posterior R ILA, we need to have a method to identify whether it is a forward or a backward torsion. Figure 17.95 illustrates the forward and backward sacral torsions.

The test used to determine whether the lesion is a forward or backward torsion is the sphinx test. With the patient lying prone on the treatment table, the rehabilitation clinician palpates the sacral sulci and ILA with both hands, noting which sacral sulcus is deep and which ILA is posterior. The patient then moves into a sphinx position with the elbows under the shoulders and the forearms and palms flat and forward on the treatment table. If the deep sulcus moves deeper so that the two sulci become even more asymmetrical, this is a positive sign, meaning it is a backward torsion, or the sacral base is stuck in a backward (posterior) position. If the sacral sulci become more symmetrical when the patient moves the spine into extension during the sphinx position, this is a negative result and indicates that it is a forward torsion, or the sacral base is stuck in a forward (anterior) position.

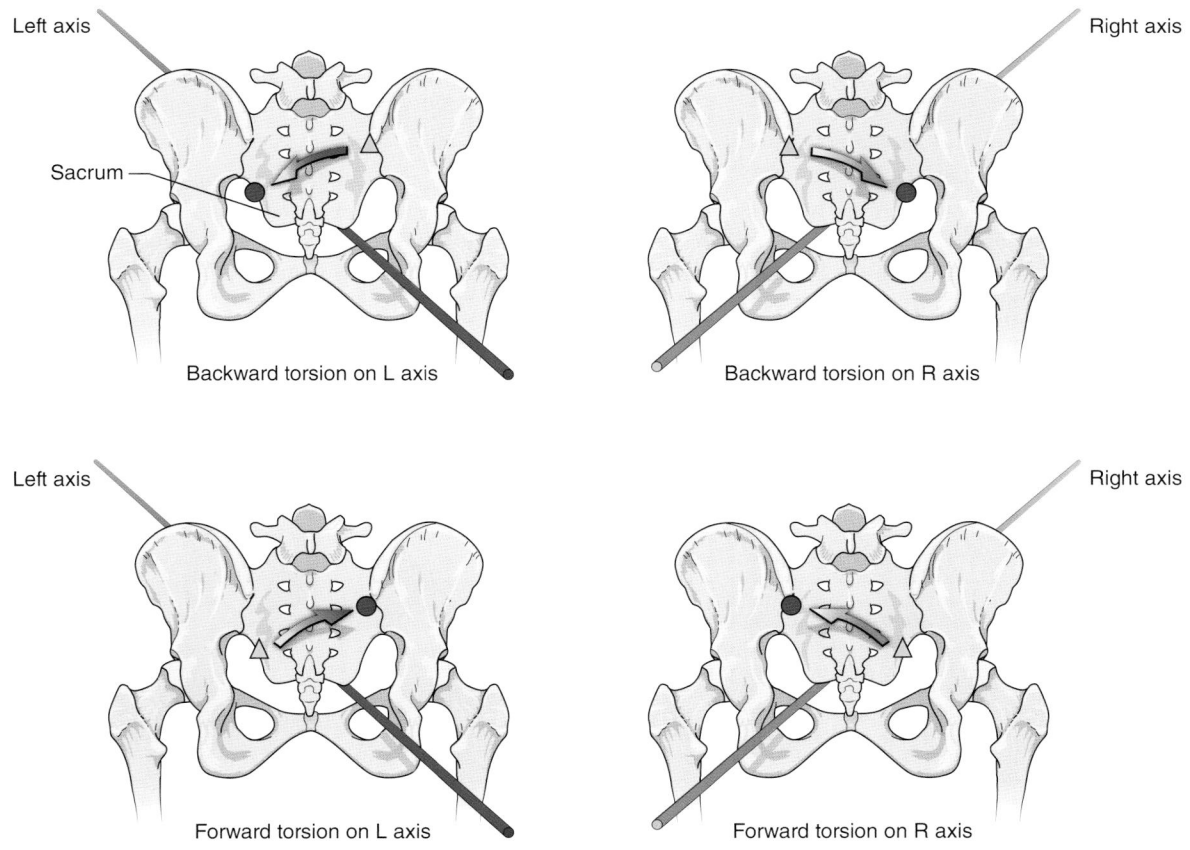

Figure 17.95 Sacral torsions may be either forward or backward torsions and may rotate around either the right or left oblique axis. A red circle indicates the structure is deep (anterior) compared to its contralateral structure. A yellow triangle indicates the structure is shallow (posterior) compared to its contralateral structure. In a backward torsion, the base of the sacrum moves backward, and in a forward torsion, the base of the sacrum moves forward.

Forward Torsion

Characteristics: The sacroiliac lesion of a forward torsion occurs primarily on the left and is more common than a backward torsion.

Mechanism: Simultaneous bending and twisting is the most common mechanism for this injury.

Features: The pain may be present in the back, buttock, or lower extremity, and it may occur on the opposite side. Because this is a torsion injury, one side of the sacrum is twisted on the other. For example, if the torsion is on the left, the left ILA is more posterior than the right ILA, but the right sulcus lies deeper than the left sulcus. The left piriformis is tight.

Treatment: The patient lies on the side of the injury, usually the left, with the knees and hips flexed to 90°. The patient then pushes up with his or her top hand to lift the trunk off the table and places the bottom arm behind the back. The patient then lies back down with the top arm hanging over the table toward the floor. The rehabilitation clinician places a hand in the L5–S1 joint space to monitor and maintain the spine in neutral

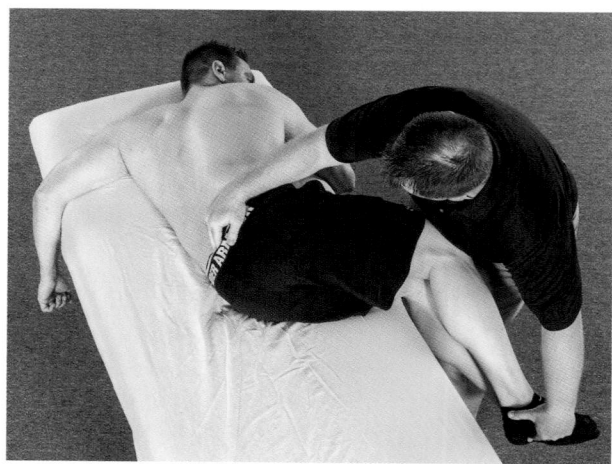

Figure 17.96

 Go to HK*Propel* and watch video 17.12, which demonstrates forward torsion muscle energy.

(figure 17.96). The patient's thighs are supported on the table to the knee, and the legs and feet are off the table. The rehabilitation clinician provides light resistance at the ankles as the patient produces an isometric lift of the feet toward the ceiling. The muscles relax, and the rehabilitation clinician lowers the patient's legs to the floor until a new barrier is felt by the hand at the L5–S1 joint space.

Home Exercise: The home exercise that helps correct a forward torsion is similar to the rehabilitation clinician's treatment. The patient assumes a side-lying position as described for the treatment: the bottom arm is behind the trunk and the top arm hangs to the floor while the knees and hips are flexed to 90° with the lower legs over the edge of the bed or table. The patient relaxes in this position for 5 to 10 min. This home exercise is performed 2 to 3 times daily until the area is stable.

Backward Torsion

Characteristics: This treatment is for a sacroiliac impairment that has very unique and classic signs.

Mechanism: Occurs with a combined bending and twisting motion, especially sudden motions.

Features: The patient cannot stand upright because extension is too painful. He or she cannot walk normally and may waddle like a duck with the lumbar spine in a forward-flexed position. Pain may be in the low back or buttock or may mimic nerve root pain.

Treatment: The patient stands facing a table and leans onto it with both ASISs on the edge of the table. The trunk is supported on top of the table. The rehabilitation clinician applies firm pressure on the sacrum, with the heel of the hand at the

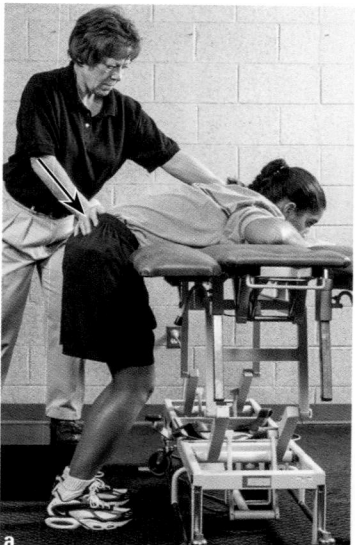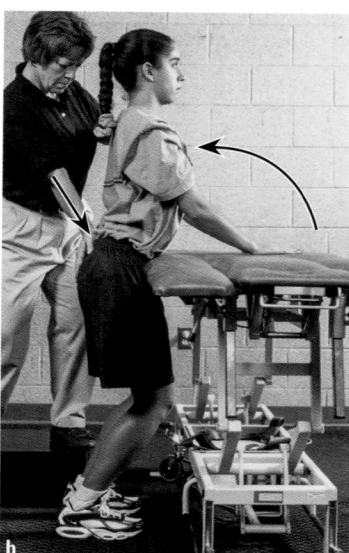

Figure 17.97 Backward torsion muscle energy treatment: *(a)* start position, *(b)* end position.

base and the fingers pointing toward the sacral apex (figure 17.97*a*). The pressure should be downward and firm throughout the motion. The patient then gradually walks the hands on the table, pushing with the arms against the table, and moves to a trunk-erect position (figure 17.97*b*). The movement may be uncomfortable, but the patient should be encouraged to continue to the end of the motion.

Home Exercise: The home exercises that the patient should do to promote correction of the backward torsion are press-ups or standing trunk extensions. If standing extensions are too painful, start with press-ups. If press-ups are too uncomfortable, the patient can begin by lying prone on a pillow (figure 17.98*a*), progressing to lying prone without a pillow (figure 17.98*b*), and then progressing to lying prone on elbows (figure 17.98*c*) before advancing to a press-up (figure 17.98*d*) and then to standing trunk extensions.

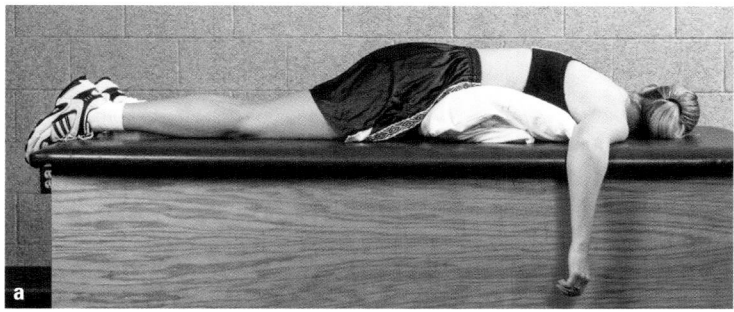

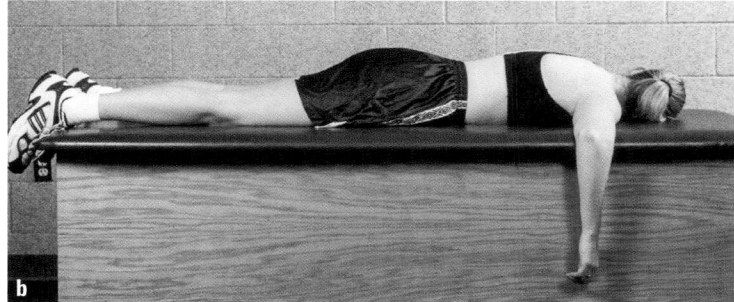

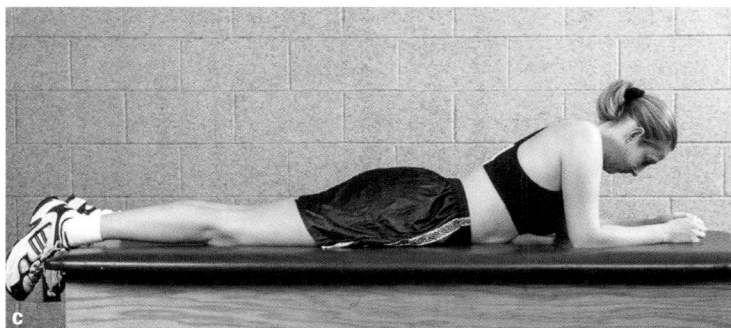

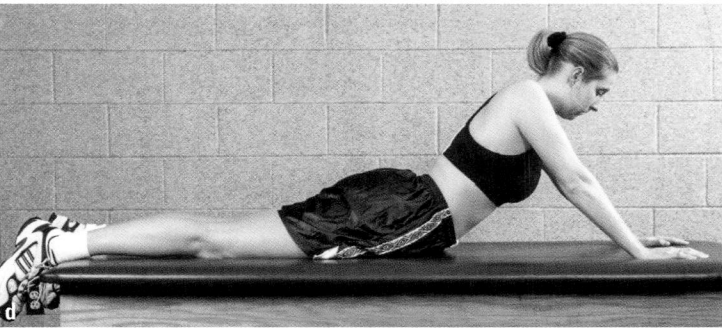

Figure 17.98

Iliosacral Lesions and Treatment Techniques Iliosacral dysfunctions are often the result of trauma.[257] For this reason, athletes are more commonly seen with these types of lesions than other populations. There is no need to memorize the signs and symptoms of the lesions described since they are listed here, but the rehabilitation clinician should be aware that an undiagnosed iliosacral lesion may be the source of persistent back pain, hip pain, or groin pain that does not respond to treatment.

Anterior Iliac Subluxation: Upslip

Characteristics: Iliosacral lesion—an upslip of the ilium whereby the ilium on the right is higher than the one on the left.

Mechanism: A fall on the buttock or stepping off a curb. It also occurs in sports such as basketball and hockey.

Features: Although the lesion always occurs on the right, the pain is sometimes on the left. Pain can also be located in the low back or coccyx or can mimic nerve root pain. The right leg appears shorter than the left leg, and the right iliac crest is higher. When palpated, the right sacrotuberous ligament feels slack compared to that on the left side.[256]

Treatment: The patient lies prone with the right leg in 30° of abduction and extension. The rehabilitation clinician grasps the tibia and fibula proximal to the ankle to maintain the leg position and takes up the slack of the leg. The patient takes in a deep breath and blows it out as the rehabilitation clinician takes up the slack of the leg again (figure 17.99). This is repeated 3 or 4 times. On the last repetition, the rehabilitation clinician has the patient cough twice and simultaneously provides a quick pull on the leg along the long axis of the leg.

Home Exercise: No exercise.

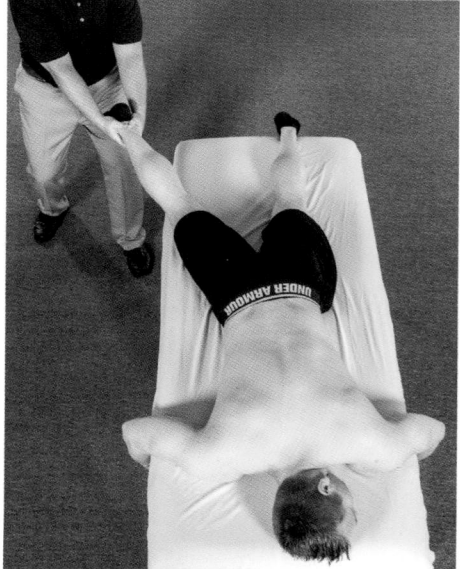

Figure 17.99

 Go to HK*Propel* and watch video 17.13, which demonstrates an anterior iliac subluxation (right upslip).

Posterior Iliac Subluxation: Upslip

Characteristics: This treatment is for an iliosacral lesion. This upslip always occurs on the left.

Mechanism: The left leg is the short leg this time, and the left sacrotuberous ligament is slack when palpated. The left iliac crest appears higher than the right.[256]

Features: The lesion commonly occurs with other spinal problems and should be investigated if the pain does not resolve with treatment.

Treatment: The patient is supine, and the left leg is held by the rehabilitation clinician, proximal to the ankle in 30° of abduction and flexion (figure 17.100). The slack is taken out of the leg, and the patient is instructed to take a deep breath in and then let it out as the rehabilitation clinician takes out additional slack. After the final repetition, the patient is asked to cough; simultaneously with the cough, the clinician provides a quick longitudinal pull on the leg.

Home Exercise: No exercise.

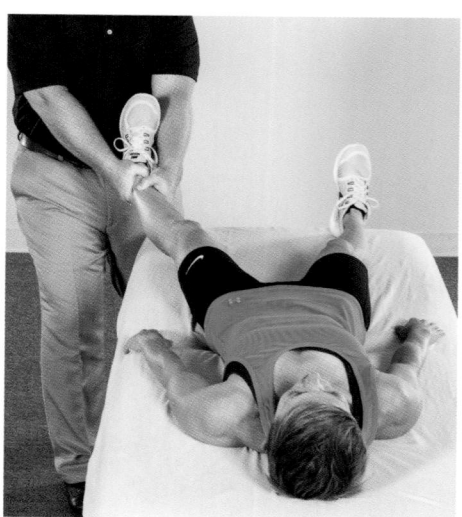

Figure 17.100

Anterior Iliac Rotation

Characteristics: The dysfunction is an iliosacral lesion that usually occurs with other lesions. It is also called an anterior innominate lesion. The patient complains of cervical or lumbar symptoms.

Mechanism: Usually occurs with other lesions.

Features: The iliac crest may be low on the same side as the injury, whereas the PSIS is high and the ASIS is low.

Treatment: The patient lies prone along the edge of the table with the leg of the involved side positioned over the side of the table and the foot on the floor. The rehabilitation clinician places his or her thumb in the sacral sulcus to monitor the SI joint. For control of

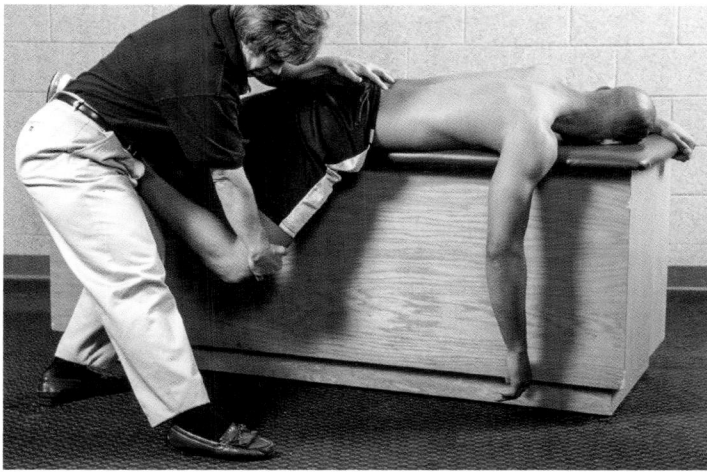

Figure 17.101

the leg, the foot is placed on the rehabilitation clinician's thigh and the knee is grasped (figure 17.101). The patient's 3 to 10 s isometric contraction toward extension is resisted. The patient is instructed to relax, and the leg is moved into flexion until its new barrier is felt in the sulcus. This exercise is repeated 3 to 5 times. If this is a secondary lesion, it is treated after the primary lesion.

Home Exercise: Pelvic tilt exercises and both knees-to-chest exercises.

Posterior Iliac Rotation

Characteristics: This iliosacral lesion is a posterior iliac rotation, or a posterior innominate lesion.

Mechanism: This lesion is seen after a fall or sudden hamstring contraction.

Features: The patient may use an antalgic gait and walk with reduced hip extension movement on the involved side. Patients with this injury usually complain of a lot of pain in the buttock or knee. The ilium is posteriorly rotated, and the ASIS, PSIS, and iliac crest can appear high. There may also be a short-leg appearance on the same side as the lesion.

Treatment: The patient lies in a prone position. The rehabilitation clinician places one hand on the ilium to monitor joint movement and the other on the anterior thigh proximal to the knee. Pelvic neutral is maintained while the hip is extended until the barrier is felt (figure 17.102). The barrier is detected when the monitor hand feels ilium movement as the hip is extended. The patient is then instructed to try to push the thigh to the table isometrically for 3 to 10 s. The patient then relaxes, and the thigh is passively moved into extension to the next barrier. The procedure is repeated 3 to 5 times.

Home Exercise: There are two home exercises for this iliosacral dysfunction. These exercises include press-ups and hip flexor stretches.

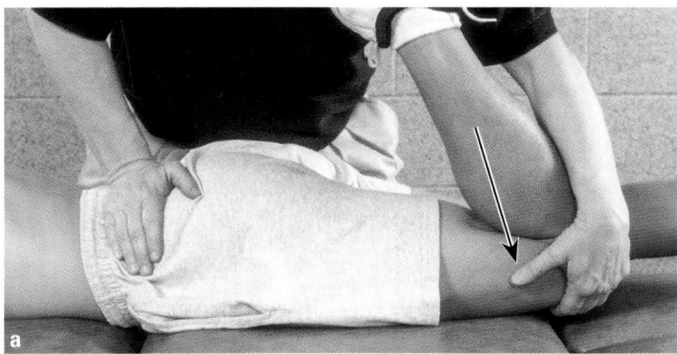
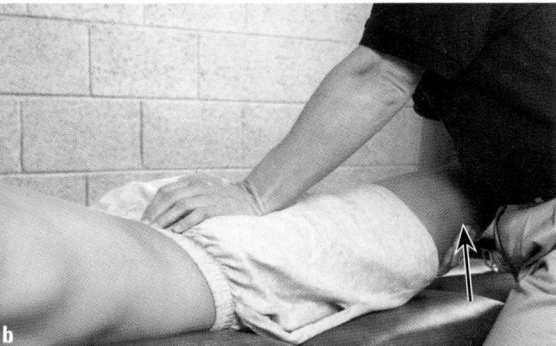

Figure 17.102

Pubic Subluxation

Characteristics: This is an iliosacral lesion. This lesion commonly occurs in combination with other SI lesions, especially upslips, or low-back injuries.

Mechanism: It is a pathology that occurs in soccer players. It occurs also during pregnancy or childbirth.

Features: The patient may complain of only low-back pain or may have groin or buttock pain. Pushing down on the left or right pubic bones (spring test) produces pain. If it is a superior lesion, the leg will appear shorter, but if it is an inferior lesion, the leg will appear longer.

Treatment: Treatment depends on whether the pubis is superior or inferior and involves a contract-relax-stretch technique. For a superior pubic subluxation, the patient lies supine with the leg on the involved side over the edge of the table. The rehabilitation clinician supports the hanging leg under the patient's thigh and stabilizes the ASIS on the opposite side (figure 17.103a). The patient performs isometric hip flexion for 5 to 10 s against the rehabilitation clinician. Once the leg muscles relax after the isometric contraction, the hip is passively moved into extension to its new barrier.

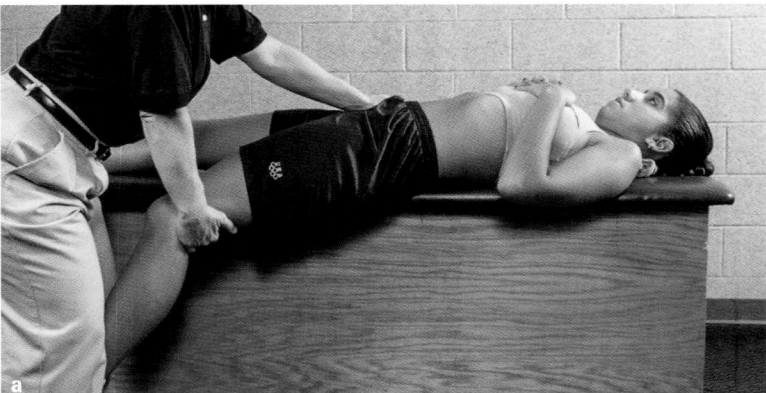

For an inferior pubic subluxation, the patient lies supine with the hip in flexion while the clinician places a hand under the ischial tuberosity to monitor its stability. The patient performs isometric hip extension against the clinician's hand on the proximal leg (figure 17.103b). A passive movement into hip flexion to the new barrier is performed after the patient relaxes the muscles.

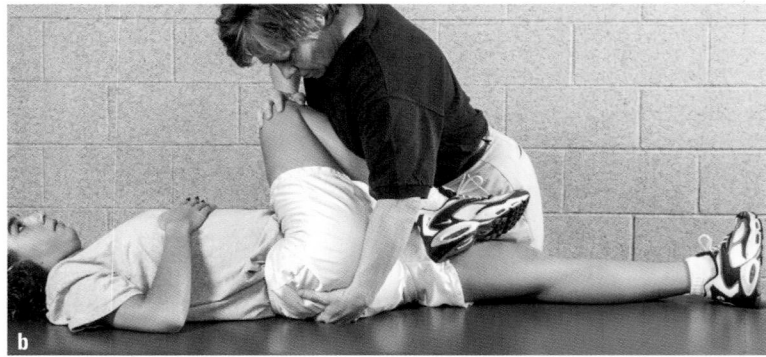

Occasionally, a treatment technique specific to superior subluxations or one specific to inferior pubic subluxations can be successful for either problem. The patient is supine with the hips and knees flexed and the feet on the table. The patient performs a series of isometric abduction exercises of both legs simultaneously as the rehabilitation clinician resists the movement (figure 17.103c). This is followed by a series of isometric adduction exercises with the rehabilitation clinician's forearm placed between the patient's knees during the isometric exercise (figure 17.103d). Sometimes a pop of the pubic bones may be heard.

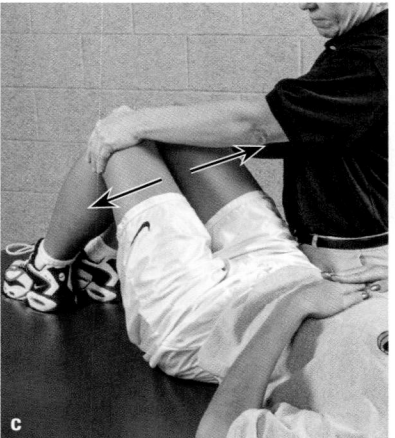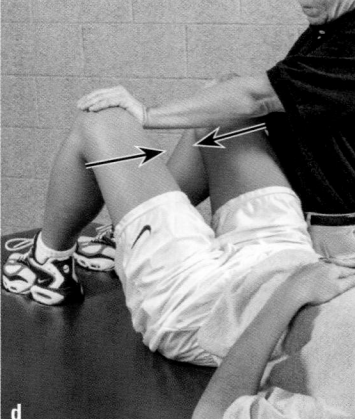

Home Exercise: Home exercises the patient should perform for superior pubic subluxation include a Thomas stretch. The inferior pubic subluxation home exercise is a single-knee-to-chest stretch.

Figure 17.103

Inflares and Outflares

Characteristics: Inflares and outflares are also referred to as innominate medial and lateral rotations, respectively.

Mechanism: Soccer players are commonly affected by inflares and outflares. Either falling on the iliac crest or receiving a direct blow are common mechanisms.

Features: These iliosacral conditions often produce groin pain. Leg and hip pain may or may not be present as well. They occur in soccer players and can result from a direct blow on the ilium. With an inflare, the distance from the ASIS to the umbilicus is shorter on the affected side. With an outflare, the distance is greater on the affected side than on the opposite side.

Treatment: The patient lies supine with the leg of the involved side flexed and across the opposite knee. The rehabilitation clinician's hand is either on the medial aspect of the knee or on the medial malleolus, with the forearm on the leg. The patient's lateral thigh rests against the rehabilitation clinician's hip (figure 17.104a). The rehabilitation clinician's other hand is used to stabilize the opposite ASIS. The patient performs an isometric hip adduction exercise for 5 to 10 s. When the muscle relaxes, the patient's leg is moved passively into hip abduction until the new barrier is felt with motion of the opposite ASIS. When the exercise series is complete, the patient's leg is passively moved into extension by the rehabilitation clinician.

An outflare is treated with the patient supine and the knee of the affected side brought across the trunk, toward the opposite shoulder. The rehabilitation clinician places his or her hand on the sulcus of the involved side. The hip is medially rotated passively. While maintained in this position, the patient performs a series of isometric exercises of simultaneous hip flexion, adduction, and medial rotation (figure 17.104b). Once the muscle relaxes after the isometric contraction, the rehabilitation clinician moves the extremity into greater hip flexion, adduction, and medial rotation until the barrier is felt when the sulcus moves beneath the rehabilitation clinician's fingers. Once the repetitions are completed, the extremity is returned passively to full extension.

Home Exercise: The home exercise position for an iliac inflare is supine with the leg flexed at the hip and knee and the leg positioned across the contralateral distal thigh. In this position, the knee is dropped out to the side to move the hip into abduction and lateral rotation. To perform the home exercise for an outflare, the patient moves the knee to the opposite shoulder and produces a series of hold–relax techniques, using the arms to position the lower extremity in the stretch.

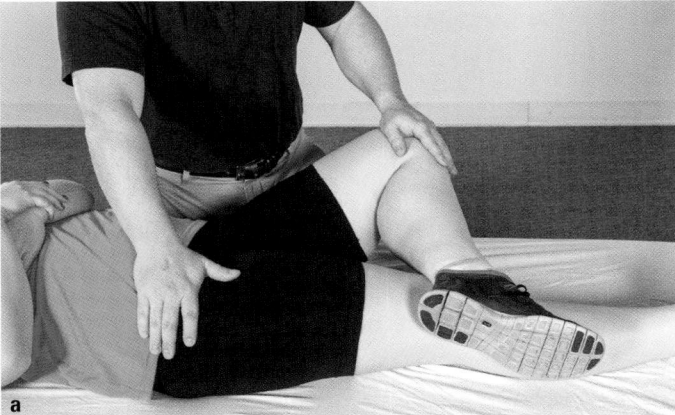

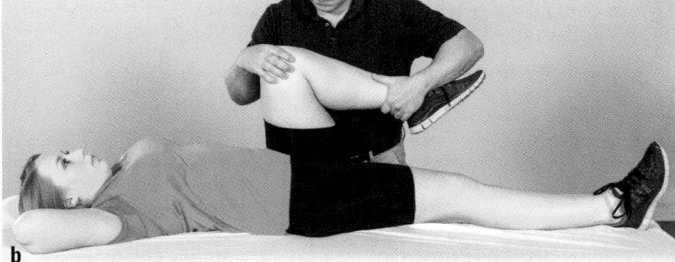

Figure 17.104

When the sacroiliac joint is treated, the low back and hip areas should also be addressed to eliminate other sites of injury or pain referral. Sacroiliac joint muscle energy techniques must be used in combination with lumbar and hip neuromotor control, flexibility, and strengthening exercises to provide an effective outcome. If the sacroiliac dysfunction was not caused by a traumatic injury, then as with any injury of gradual onset, the specific cause needs to be identified and corrected to prevent a recurrence.

If the SI joint is the source of pain, muscle energy techniques are usually very effective in relieving or reducing the pain. If the problem has not been long-standing, the patient usually experiences significant resolution within a few treatments. After muscle energy techniques, the general spine rehabilitation program is used to return the patient to optimal function. Core exercises, specific flexibility and strength exercises based on the patient's needs, functional training, and neuromotor activities are part of the rehabilitation program before performance-specific exercises are introduced.

Summary

This chapter focuses on the spine and sacroiliac joints and the treatment often used to approach injuries to this unique body segment. Before any manual techniques are applied to the cervical spine, tests should be performed for vertebral artery compromise. Rehabilitation clinicians now customize the exercises they select when they design rehabilitation programs for their patients. These programs include combinations of modalities, manual treatment, and exercises that restore patients to optimal functioning. Given the functional influence of the lumbopelvic–hip structures on the extremities, this chapter presents information about the muscles involved in neuromotor control, core stabilization, recruitment techniques for those muscles, and exercise progressions. Common sacroiliac dysfunctions with muscle energy examination and treatment techniques are presented as well. Some of the most commonly seen injuries include upper and lower crossed syndromes, sprains, strains, SI joint dysfunction, facet dysfunctions and injuries, and disc pathologies.

LEARNING AIDS

Key Concepts and Review

1. Describe the closed sacroiliac ring and the lumbopelvic–hip complex, how they are related, and how they are important for functioning of the extremities.

The sacroilium and the pelvis create a sacroiliac ring, which is a closed ring connecting the left and right hemipelvises together. Each hemipelvis, consisting of an ilium, pubis, and ischium, is connected anteriorly at the pubic symphysis joint and posteriorly by the sacrum and its two sacroiliac joints. The pelvis is a platform to which three large levers are attached and upon which they act; these levers are the spine and the two lower extremities. Because of the direct attachment of these segments to the pelvis, they can influence the pelvis; likewise, the pelvis can influence the function of these three segments.

2. Define the terms used in discussing sacroiliac stability, *form closure* and *force closure*.

Form closure is the result of both the sacroiliac joint's shape and the ligaments that support it. Force closure adds to the stability of the sacroiliac joints through the activation of muscles that are aligned to act as a corset, providing active protection of the joints and secondary reinforcement to the ligaments. Both are important in sacroiliac stability.

3. Identify the third element in lumbopelvic–hip stability, and explain how it works with the other two.

Neuromotor control, provided by sensory input and feedback to and from the central nervous system, is the third element in lumbopelvic–hip stability. Along with form closure and force closure, it creates an environment in which stability, refined movement, and power transmission occur.

4. Explain what the core muscles are and why they are important to function.

The core can be thought of as a box or cylinder of muscles in which the top consists of the diaphragm, the bottom is the pelvic floor, the front and sides are the transverse abdominis and internal obliques, and the back is the multifidus muscles. Outer muscles of the abdominal group anteriorly and the erector spinae and gluteal muscles posteriorly also provide support to this box or cylinder. The core provides stability and motion control of the trunk during the movement of the extremities. Since the pelvis and trunk are the means by which power is transferred between the upper and lower extremities, the core muscle groups should be included in both conditioning and rehabilitation programs.

5. Identify three sacroiliac pathologies and their muscle energy release techniques.

(1) Anterior iliac subluxation, or upslip: An anterior iliac subluxation is an iliosacral lesion that is always

on the right and often accompanies other spinal problems. A leg pull is performed with the patient in prone and the leg positioned in 30° abduction and extension. (2) Forward torsion: This is a sacroiliac lesion that occurs primarily on the left and occurs with twisting and bending motions. With the patient lying on the involved side, the legs are off the table, where resistance is provided to leg movement toward the ceiling. (3) Posterior iliac rotation: This iliosacral pathology occurs because of a fall or sudden hamstring contraction. With the patient prone, the hip is passively extended; the isometric force occurs in hip flexion.

6. Discuss the progression, or series of steps, involved in the rehabilitation of core muscles.

Progression of core activation, stabilization, and use includes these steps: (1) improve neuromotor control of the trunk muscles by focusing on using the diaphragm for respiration; (2) perform trunk stabilization activities, such as abdominal hollowing exercises, to recruit the diaphragm, transverse abdominis, and pelvic floor; (3) perform activation exercises for the multifidus; (4) perform abdominal bracing to activate local and global muscles; (5) progress neuromotor control with core activation while performing simple daily activities; and (6) engage abdominal bracing and trunk stability during performance-specific activities.

7. Identify three progressive spinal stability exercises.

Dead bug, bird dog, and abdominal strengthening exercises.

8. Describe three flexibility exercises for the cervical spine and lumbar spine.

- Cervical flexion: Bring the chin down to the chest, trying to move one cervical level at a time.
- Rotational stretch: While sitting in a chair, reach behind to grasp the back of the chair with the near hand, and use the opposite hand to keep the lower extremities stable.
- Both knees to chest: In a supine position, bring one leg to the chest, then the other leg; return to the starting position by reversing the procedure.

9. List precautions for a rehabilitation program for disc lesions.

Avoid positions that increase disc pressure and aggravate the sciatica; rule out other causes of sciatica; implement neuromotor control with diaphragm inhalation; strengthen abdominals, gluteals, and back extensors; exercises should progress at the patient's own pace; and the rehabilitation clinician should have a good understanding of the exercises and the stresses that are imposed by each exercise.

10. Discuss the differences between rehabilitation programs for a lumbar strain and for a facet injury.

Facet injury treatment includes gentle rotation and side-bending in a pain-free range of motion, as well as avoiding extension activities (pain will occur in rotation to one side and side-bending to the opposite side in the lumbar spine). Extension exercises do not have to be avoided in lumbar strains; rotation and side-bending are painful in the same direction and should occur in pain-free motions.

Critical Thinking Questions

1. Regarding the scenario presented at the beginning of this chapter, assume that Will examined Violet and diagnosed her with a right upslip after a poor dismount off the uneven bars during which she landed only on the right foot. What is another name for this dysfunction? What technique should he use to treat her?

2. What would be the signs and symptoms Will would have found when he examined Violet?

3. As you watch a junior high school baseball pitcher warming up, it occurs to you that he is not transferring the power from his leg to his arm but is using primarily shoulder muscles to provide force during his pitches. It is obvious to you that he needs to improve his technique, but before he can do so, he must first strengthen his core, then learn how to use it. Outline a progressive program you would design to accomplish these goals.

4. If you are treating a swimmer who competes in the 200 m breast stroke with spondylolysis, what exercises should be avoided? How can you improve her neuromotor control and strengthen her core muscles without aggravating her injury? Will your attempts to strengthen her abdominals irritate the spondylolysis? Why or why not?

5. A football lineman has been diagnosed with a forward torsion of his left SI. Identify his signs and symptoms and the likely cause of his dysfunction. What treatment and home exercise would you provide for him?

6. A gymnast reports to you that she has low-back pain, especially on the right. She noticed this the day after a particularly long practice on her balance beam dismounts. She notices some pain down the right leg but has no other symptoms besides the back pain. Your examination reveals that her lumbar range of motion is normal in extension, rotation to the right, and side-bending to the right, but she has pain and reduced motion when she tries to flex forward, side-bend to the left, or rotate her trunk to the left. Her muscles are in mild spasm on the right, and she finds it difficult to lie prone for very long. She is very tender to your PA joint assessments at L4 on the right side. What do you suspect is her injury? What will you do for her today? Outline the progressive program you will provide for her, including the home exercises and instructions you will provide throughout the program.

Lab Activities

1. Perform the supine diaphragm recruitment exercise presented early in this chapter. Could you detect hamstring activity? Could you detect left oblique activation without your deliberate contraction? Could you feel how difficult it was to slowly inhale after pausing for 3 to 5 s?

2. Have your partner perform a progression of dead bug stabilization exercises outlined in the chapter. Now perform the bird dog stabilization exercises. What short verbal cues did you give while instructing in these techniques? What strengthening exercises will you give your partner to improve neuromotor control? What will be the reps and sets you have him or her perform? Justify why you have selected these reps and sets.

3. Have your partner perform abdominal hollowing and abdominal bracing exercises in supine. Now have your partner perform them in a quadruped and then in a sitting position. During each exercise, correct your partner if he or she demonstrates lumbar hyperlordosis. In which of the three positions did your partner have the most difficult time avoiding lumbar hyperlordosis while performing the exercises? Was it more difficult to avoid lumbar hyperlordosis in the hollowing or in the bracing exercise?

4. Examine your partner's sacroiliac joints for proper alignment using all the examination techniques outlined earlier in the chapter. Be sure to locate each landmark appropriately.

5. Perform the following muscle energy techniques:
   A. Anterior iliac subluxation
   B. Sacral flexion
   C. Forward torsion
   D. Anterior iliac rotation
   E. Pubic subluxation
   F. Inflare

   What will the malalignments be for each of these conditions? What home exercise will you provide for patients who present with these problems? How will you know if your treatment has been effective?

6. Have your lab partner lie prone; be sure to have him or her positioned comfortably and in a neutral position throughout the entire spine. Start at the upper cervical spine and palpate each spinous process through L5. Locate L4; first examine your partner's joint PA excursion at L4–5, and then apply grades I, II, III, and IV PA joint mobilizations to the joint. Determine the mobility of each joint throughout the spine. Where is there laxity and where is there restriction? Now examine another lab partner and repeat the process. How do they differ, or are they similar? Have each person on whom you performed a joint mobilization examination stand and bend forward while you observe the spine from a posterior view. Do the areas of restriction you found during the examination correlate with the range-of-motion restrictions you saw during active physiological motion? What does this indicate for you in terms of patient motion related to joint mobility?

7. Demonstrate one flexibility exercise and one strength exercise for each of the muscles or muscle groups in the following list:

A. Left scalenes

B. Right upper trapezius

C. Left sternocleidomastoid

D. Right quadratus lumborum

E. Left internal obliques

8. A 21-year-old male discus thrower began having left low-back pain after a long workout last week. He presents to you today with complaints of left low-back pain that goes into his left buttock. He does not remember an injury. Your examination reveals a deep sulcus and a posterior left ILA. He is tender to palpation of the left sulcus. What do you suspect is his problem? What will your treatment with him today include? What home exercise will you give him? What therapeutic exercises would you provide as part of his treatments? What other things would you include in his rehabilitation program? How would your assessment and treatment change if this patient instead presented with tenderness at his left L4 transverse process with restricted movement in flexion, right side-bending, and right rotation?

18

Hip

Objectives

After completing this chapter, you should be able to do the following:

1. Discuss how anteversion and retroversion change lower-extremity mechanics.

2. Explain the mechanical factors involved in a gait with hip abductor weakness, and explain how a cane or single crutch assists in normal gait.

3. Identify a joint mobilization technique for the hip, and explain its benefit.

4. Identify a flexibility exercise and a strengthening exercise for the hip.

5. Identify a proprioception exercise for the hip, and indicate its progression.

6. List precautions for a hip-dislocation rehabilitation program.

Eddie Jesness has worked with dancers for several years. He is responsible for the city ballet company's rehabilitation programs, and he is quite busy. Over the years, he has come to realize that the novice dancers' injuries tend to be acute, whereas the experienced dancers' injuries are more often chronic. Although he can resolve the acute injuries more quickly, Eddie sees the chronic injuries as a challenge—one that he can usually meet and resolve, much to his patients' delight.

Eddie's current patient, however, has been his greatest challenge yet. Margaret Duggs, the lead female dancer in the company, had been bothered with a groin strain for several months before she reported it. It occurred early in the season during rehearsal, and Margaret had dismissed it as minor and didn't believe it to be worth treating. But the problem did not go away, and now that the company is at the peak of its performance season, the injury becomes more aggravated with each performance. Still, Margaret refuses to take any time off to allow the injury to heal.

Before I injured my hip, I thought going to the gym was for wimps.

Bo Jackson, 1962-,
retired professional football and baseball player;
first player ever to be both an
NFL Pro Bowler and MLB All-Star

As we move through this chapter, it is important to understand the relationships the hip joint has with the body segments proximal and distal to it. In addition to its unique joint structure, the hip is the link between the trunk and the ground, underscoring its importance in closed kinetic chain function. If the normal position, length, strength, or function of any element of a body segment is lost or changed, the other elements of that segment are affected, and the relationship that segment has with its adjoining segments is also affected; the hip is no exception.

This chapter introduces basic considerations for hip-injury rehabilitation, focusing on topics relevant to treatment and rehabilitation program progression. Techniques for soft-tissue and joint mobilization and exercises for flexibility, strength, and proprioception are addressed. Specific injuries commonly seen in the hip are then discussed, along with program progressions for these injuries. Cases are presented in connection with some injury programs to help you conceptualize how a hip program is put together.

Special Rehabilitation Considerations

The hip is a stable joint with extensive range of motion in three planes. The socket is deep and reinforced with strong ligaments for stability. Strength and motion are important for the hip because it serves as a force transmitter for both lower- and upper-limb activities and provides motion and strength for propulsion in walking and running.[1]

Osseous Structures

The **acetabulum**, the hip socket, is in an inferior and anterolateral position. The femoral neck forms a 125° angle with the shaft of the femur, as shown in figure 18.1a.[2] An angle greater than 125°, called coxa valga (figure 18.1b), increases pressure into the joint, resulting in increased risk of osteoarthritis.[3] Coxa valga also increases the limb's functional length since the increased angle places the limb into adduction.[3] With an increased angle, the greater trochanter lies closer to the hip joint; this placement lengthens the gluteus medius but shortens its moment arm, thereby reducing its torque during single-limb stance.[3] A femoral neck angle less than 125°, called coxa vara (figure 18.1c), increases stress on the femoral neck, making it more susceptible to fractures.[3]

Because the femoral neck is rotated from the plane of the femur's long axis, the neck and the femur do not lie in the same plane. Normal alignment places the neck in a position that is rotated 15° anterior to the femur's frontal plane in the adult (figure 18.2). If the angle is greater than 15°, the femur is positioned in medial rotation; this condition is called **anteversion**. An anteverted hip has more range of motion medially and less range of motion laterally.[4] If the femoral neck's position is less than 15° to the femur's long axis, **retroversion** occurs to position the femur in lateral rotation. This condition occurs less often.[5] Anteversion and retroversion alter knee alignment and change the forces acting throughout the entire lower extremity. Anteversion leads to medial hip rotation, squinting patellae, or foot adduction, causing the person to ambulate with a toe-in gait.[6] Retroversion results in lateral hip rotation, frogeyed patellae, or foot abduction and causes the person to ambulate with a toe-out gait.[5] Anteversion and coxa valga each make the hip susceptible to dislocation.[7]

Anteversion is measured using different methods.[8] One measurement method commonly used is Craig's test; it is performed with the patient lying prone and the knee flexed to 90° (figure 18.3). The rehabilitation clinician moves the patient's thigh into medial rotation until palpation of the greater trochanter reveals that it is parallel to the tabletop.[9] A goniometer is then used to measure the difference between the tibial position and a line vertical to the tabletop. This value is the degree of anteversion.

120°-125°
> 135°
< 120°
a
b
c

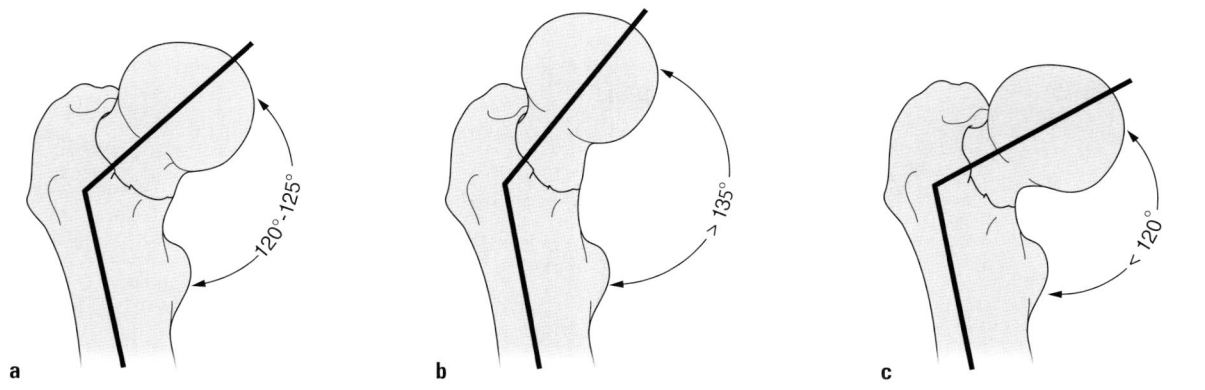

Figure 18.1 Femoral neck angles: *(a)* normal; *(b)* coxa valga—increased angle results in increased joint stress; *(c)* coxa vara—decreased angle results in increased femoral neck load.

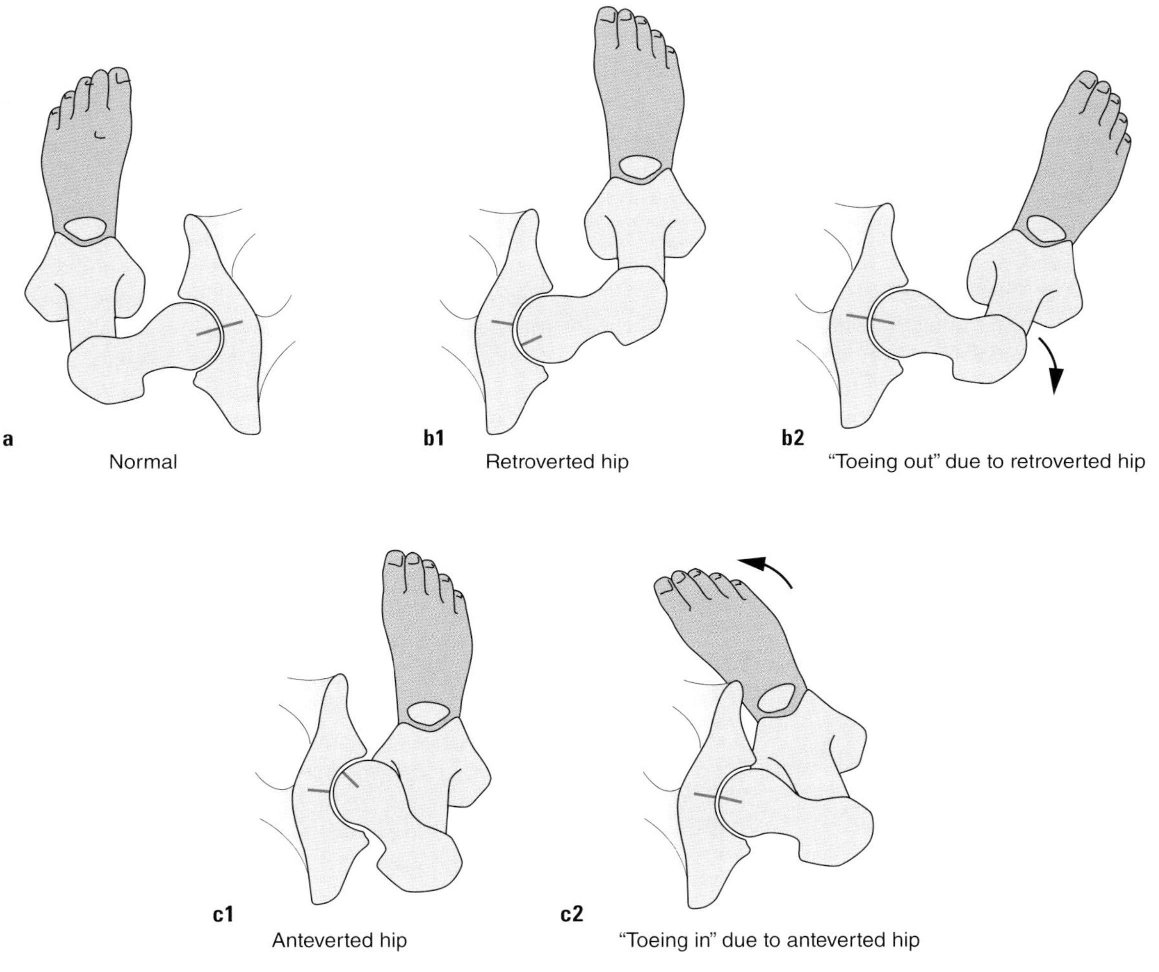

a
Normal
b1
Retroverted hip
b2
"Toeing out" due to retroverted hip
c1
Anteverted hip
c2
"Toeing in" due to anteverted hip

Figure 18.2 Femoral head–neck position relative to the femur's long axis: *(a)* normal, *(b1)* retroversion, *(b2)* retroversion with femoral head and acetabulum aligned, *(c1)* anteversion, *(c2)* anteversion with femoral head and acetabulum aligned. Notice the lower limb alignment changes with retroversion and anteversion.

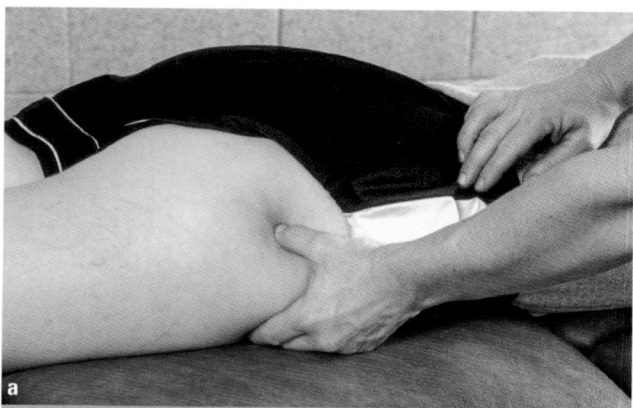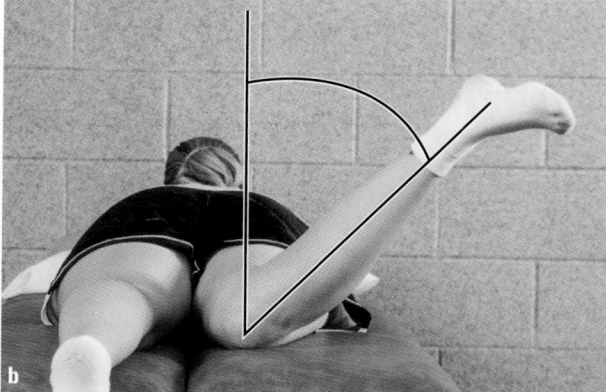

Figure 18.3 Craig's test for femoral anteversion: *(a)* Greater trochanter is positioned parallel to the tabletop, and *(b)* the angle between the tibia's position in 90° of knee flexion at this point and a vertical line is measured.

Neural Structures

Nerves entering the entire lower extremity must pass through the hip region. Nerve irritations can occur when soft tissues surrounding the hip impinge on a nerve.[10] The sciatic nerve passes beneath, occasionally through, the piriformis muscle and through the sciatic notch before it travels along the posterior thigh. Entrapment of the nerve in the piriformis region[11] or during a stretch of the hamstrings[10] can produce neural irritation distally.

A sensory branch of the femoral nerve, the lateral femoral cutaneous nerve, travels through the psoas major muscle and then passes under the inguinal ligament near the anterior superior iliac spine (ASIS). Compression of this nerve in the region of the inguinal ligament can cause aching and burning over the tensor fasciae latae in the anterolateral thigh, where the nerve provides sensory innervation.[12]

The obturator nerve enters the pelvis from upper lumbar nerve roots and provides sensory and motor innervation to the medial thigh. Entrapment of this nerve can cause medial thigh sensory changes and adductor weakness.[13]

Stabilization

As you should recall from chapter 17, there is a relationship between trunk stabilization and the hip muscles during functional activities.[14] Specifically, the hip extensors and abductors play a very important role in pelvic stability.[15] When you think about it, this makes sense. Since most athletic performances, some work activities, and efforts to reduce injuries depend on a stable trunk or pelvis, and the gluteal muscles attach to the pelvis, then hip stability is also important for these same purposes.[16-18] The hip muscles also provide a way for the power of the lower limbs to transfer up the chain to other body segments during upper-extremity activities such as pitching, golf, and tennis.[19-21] As is mentioned in chapter 21, assuming the patient performs with good sequential motion, the lower extremities and

trunk provide 51% to 55% of the total kinetic energy and force for overhead activities.[22] This means that if the hip muscles are weak, not only will less force be applied when needed, but there will be more stress on other segments in the chain to compensate for the weak hip muscles' inability to provide the needed forces. The hips must be the platform from which the pelvis functions, just as the pelvis is the platform from which the scapula functions, and the scapula is the platform from which the shoulder complex functions.[23] It is important, then, for the rehabilitation clinician to examine hip stability, especially the strength of the hip extensors and abductors, not only for hip-injury rehabilitation but also for treating any extremity joint, just as the rehabilitation clinician examines trunk stability for upper- and lower-extremity rehabilitation programs.[24-26]

Joint Mechanics

Pelvis movement has a direct influence on hip movement because the hip joint's socket is comprised of the pelvic bones. Pelvic motion alters hip positioning,[27] and hip abnormalities affect pelvic posture. An anterior pelvic tilt moves the anterior pelvis closer to the anterior femur, and a posterior pelvic tilt moves the posterior pelvis closer to the posterior femur. This change in the pelvis alters the hip so that an anterior pelvic tilt increases hip flexion and a posterior pelvic tilt increases hip extension. This is important to remember when examining a patient's posture; for example, a patient with an exaggerated lumbar lordosis is likely to have tightness in hip flexors as either a cause or a secondary result of the lordosis.

The body's center of mass shifts toward the supporting limb when a person moves from a two-limb to a one-limb stance. This weight transfer places frontal plane rotatory stress on the weight-bearing hip because gravity's pull on the non-weight-bearing limb drops the pelvis on that side. To minimize this pelvic drop and the rotatory forces accompanying it, the abductors on the weight-bearing leg work to keep the hips relatively level with each other.[28] The force required of the weight-bearing extremity's abductors is greater than the weight of the body because the abductors' moment-arm length is less than that of the body's center of mass (figure 18.4). If the abductors are not strong enough to counter the force of gravity that is pulling downward and laterally rotating the pelvis, the patient cannot achieve a normal gait. The patient either excessively drops the non-weight-bearing hip and downwardly rotates the pelvis to the non-weight-bearing side, or else the patient tilts the trunk to lean over the weak weight-bearing hip during stance on that limb to position the body's center of mass closer to the fulcrum, the hip joint.[29] If the center of mass moves far enough laterally to be positioned on top of or just lateral to this fulcrum, the abductors do not have to work nearly as much as they do in normal gait.

When a cane or one crutch is used on the side opposite the weakness, an upward force is transmitted through the appliance to counterbalance the downward gravitational force on the same side (figure 18.5). Because the moment arm from the cane to the fulcrum of motion (the weak hip) is longer than the moment arm of the body's center of mass, the amount of force that must be transmitted through the cane is relatively small. Therefore, patients who ambulate

with a cane or a single crutch in the hand contralateral to the lower-extremity injury need only apply light pressure on the handle to offset the gravitational pull and produce adequate compensation for the weak abductors.

Limb-length discrepancies can result from actual differences in length or from other unilateral differences such as genu valgus, coxa vara, rotated sacrum, or foot pronation, as well as from soft-tissue pathologies that create functional limb-length differences such as hip flexor tightness, abductor tightness, and muscle imbalances.[30-32] When one limb is shorter than the other, the pelvis rotates and drops on the shorter side, and the trunk bends away from the short limb when weight bearing on the short limb.[33, 34] The greater the discrepancy, the more notable are these compensations. If a less obvious limb-length discrepancy is suspected, shoe wear is the most observable indication that one exists. When a limb-length discrepancy exists, the rehabilitation clinician should assess all possible causes; correction or adaptation of the discrepancy may be needed to alleviate the patient's pain.

Limb-length differences can eventually lead to osteoarthritis of the hip in the longer limb.[35] This occurs because the longer limb is in a position of adducted angulation when weight bearing. This position produces increased joint incongruence, in which more weight is borne on the superior lateral aspect of the acetabulum. During

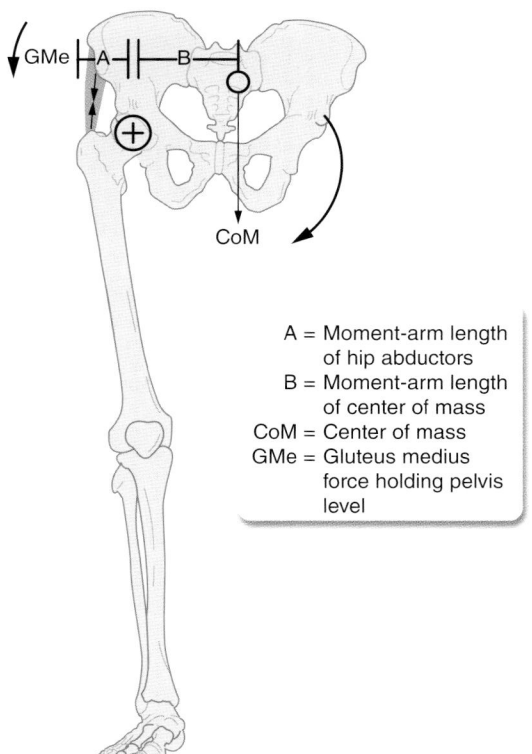

A = Moment-arm length of hip abductors
B = Moment-arm length of center of mass
CoM = Center of mass
GMe = Gluteus medius force holding pelvis level

Figure 18.4 Single-limb stance mechanics. The hip serves as the fulcrum from which the pelvis drops toward the nonsupporting side. Fortunately, the stance-limb hip abductors normally have enough strength to "pull" on the pelvis so it remains relatively level during single-limb stance.

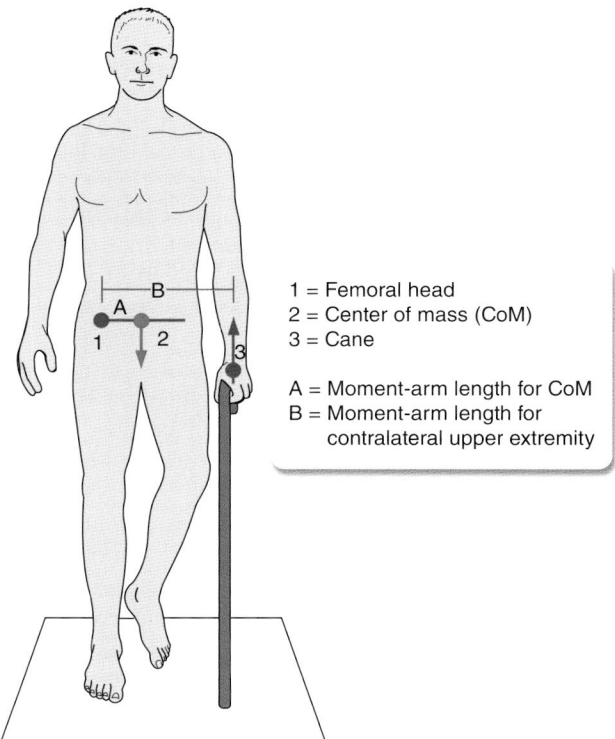

1 = Femoral head
2 = Center of mass (CoM)
3 = Cane

A = Moment-arm length for CoM
B = Moment-arm length for contralateral upper extremity

Figure 18.5 The force applied by the patient pushing down on the cane is minimal because the moment arm for it is much longer than the body's weight.

weight-bearing activities such as walking and running, the body's weight shifts to the shorter limb; consequently during this time, increased compressive forces act on the longer limb's hip joint abductors, thus increasing the demand on them to keep the pelvis level.

Stress-Reduction Concepts

One rule of thumb is that if a patient cannot ambulate normally, he or she must use assistive devices until normal ambulation is possible without them. An abnormal gait may result from pain, inadequate muscle control, or apprehension; if it continues, stresses will increase on the hip, back, or other lower-extremity segments, resulting in additional injury.[36] Once weight bearing is permitted, an assistive device is used only as much as needed to create a normal gait. As the problem causing the need for crutches or other assistive devices resolves, the patient is weaned off them. The clinician must correct the patient's gait throughout the process to ensure a normal gait as the patient transitions from walking with assistive devices to walking without them.

If the hip is painful, joint stress is reduced by shortening the stride length when walking or running. A smaller stride reduces the force and motion demands on the muscles, tendons, and ligaments. Applying a hip spica wrap for ambulation can also help to moderate stride length and reduce pain.

Rehabilitation Interventions

Reducing pain and managing inflammation are the primary initial goals for hip rehabilitation programs in phase I, the inactive phase; the various means of pain control include anti-inflammatory medication, reduced activity, and modalities. Some hip injuries are self-limiting in that pain determines the patient's degree of activity. In instances where neither the pain nor the injury is severe enough to restrict activity, the patient may wish to continue normal participation since continued activity will not make the condition worse; however, the recovery time may be longer because irritation continues to occur on a regular basis.

Rehabilitation beyond the inactive phase includes a progression of stretching or flexibility exercises, neuromotor control exercises, strength exercises, proprioception activities, and functional activities. When injuries result from predisposing factors rather than acute insult, those factors must be corrected to reduce the risk of recurrence. Phase II, the active phase, emphasizes flexibility with neuromotor control and proprioceptive activities. Since many hip muscles cross more than one joint, effective flexibility exercises require adequate stabilization of adjacent segments and the proper application of the stretch force.

In phase III, the resistive phase, strength and agility exercises are the main emphasis as the rehabilitation process moves toward preparing the patient for a return to normal activities. Because the hip is so closely aligned with the pelvis, rehabilitation must include pelvic and core stabilization exercises. Because the hip depends on the back, pelvis, knee, and ankle for its balance and quality of motion, exercises for deficiencies in these segments must also be a part of a hip's rehabilitation program. Many of these neuromotor control and coordination exercises for other body segments can be initiated in phase II. During this phase, strength exercises for the hip are restricted, but retraining and resistive exercises for these other segments will not place undue stress on the hip.

In phase IV, the advanced phase, the rehabilitation program concentrates on plyometrics and functional and performance-specific exercises in preparation for a return to normal activities. Patients can return to full sport or work participation when they are pain free, when muscle actions are normally balanced, and when their execution of performance-specific activity is normal.

CLINICAL TIPS

A rehabilitation program for the hip must be based on a knowledge of the hip's osseous, soft tissue, and neural structures, as well as an awareness of the normal expectations for joint mobility and joint mechanics. The rehabilitation clinician must also be familiar with methods of reducing stress in an injured hip.

Soft-Tissue Mobilization

Because of the neurological, myofascial, orthopedic, and organ systems that may refer pain into the hip region, it is prudent for the rehabilitation clinician to identify any differential diagnosis that could be contributing to hip or groin pain. If myofascia is the expected source of pain, treatment can proceed. If soft-tissue mobilization techniques do not produce some relief, you must reassess for other probable causes.

Soft-tissue mobilization techniques for the hip include deep-tissue massage, scar-tissue mobilization, cross-friction massage, and myofascial release, including trigger point techniques. The myofascial release techniques and pain-referral information were presented in chapter 11. Table 18.1 lists the muscles whose trigger points are common causes of pain.

CLINICAL TIPS

Soft-tissue pain referrals are common in the hip, especially among runners. The gluteus medius, gluteus minimus, and piriformis muscles are often the source of pain referrals secondary to trigger point development within them. Because of the frequency with which they occur, it would be useful for the clinician to remember their referral patterns and trigger point locations.

TABLE 18.1   Common Trigger Points of the Hip Region

Hip segment	Muscles with trigger points
Pelvic muscles	Gluteus medius
	Gluteus minimus
	Piriformis
Thigh muscles	Tensor fasciae latae
	Hamstrings

Joint Mobilization

The joint is configured as a convex femoral head on a concave acetabulum, so glide of the femur on the pelvis occurs in the direction opposite to movement during open-chain motion. The hip's capsular pattern has its most significant restriction of motion in medial rotation. Flexion and abduction are less limited, and extension is less limited than either flexion or abduction, while lateral rotation is unrestricted.[37, 38]

The hip joint's close-packed position is full extension, abduction, and medial rotation.[37] The resting position is 30° flexion and 30° abduction with slight lateral rotation.[37]

Whereas painful hip joints can benefit from grade I and II mobilization techniques, hip joints that display a capsular pattern of restricted movement can benefit from grade III and IV mobilization techniques. Because of the limb's weight, clinicians usually apply oscillating techniques with mobilization grades I and II and sustained applications with mobilization grades III and IV.[39]

Because the pelvis segment of the hip joint is firmly attached to the trunk, there is little need to stabilize the hip joint during joint mobilization. The weight of the pelvis acts as an anchor. Some mobilizations for the hip are included in the following sections.

Joint Mobilization of the Hip

Because the hip is a large joint with a distal segment that can sometimes be difficult to manage during joint mobilization, applications of joint mobilization at the hip often use sustained techniques rather than oscillations. Sustained mobilizations require less work from the clinician than oscillations.

Inferior Glide

This is also called a traction or distraction technique.

Joint: Hip.

Resting Position: 30° flexion and 30° abduction with slight lateral rotation.

Indications: To help regain joint play. In grades I and II, to relieve pain.

Patient Position: Supine.

Rehabilitation Clinician and Hand Positions: The rehabilitation clinician grasps the distal tibia and fibula of the affected limb and places the hip in a resting position.

Mobilization Application: The rehabilitation clinician leans backward, using his or her body weight to supply the traction force (figure 18.6a).

Notations: If the patient has a history of knee disorders, an alternative position for an inferior glide is to have the patient's leg over the rehabilitation clinician's shoulder. The rehabilitation clinician clasps his or her hands around the proximal thigh and applies the inferior glide (figure 18.6b).

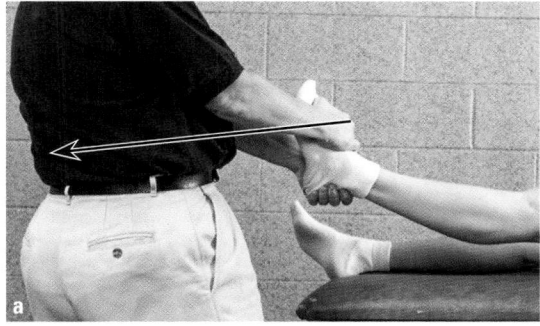

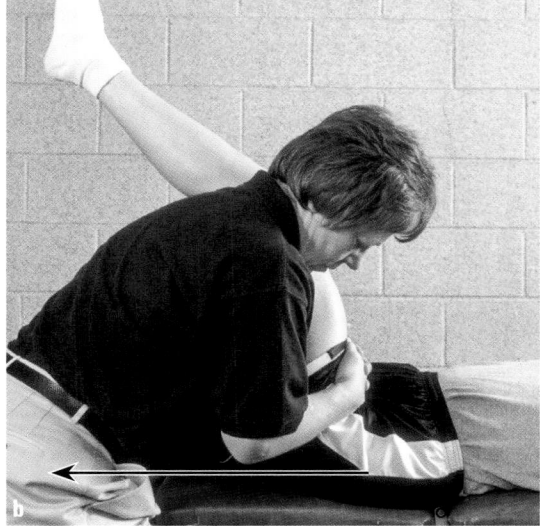

Figure 18.6

Lateral Glide

Joint: Hip.

Resting Position: 30° flexion and 30° abduction with slight lateral rotation.

Indications: To increase hip adduction.

Patient Position: Supine.

Rehabilitation Clinician and Hand Positions: The rehabilitation clinician stands at the patient's side by the thigh. A strap is secured around the patient's proximal thigh and the rehabilitation clinician's hips (figure 18.7a). The rehabilitation clinician places his or her cephalic hand on the lateral pelvis to stabilize it and the caudal hand on the distal thigh.

Mobilization Application: With the patient's thigh in slight flexion, the clinician transfers his or her weight from the front limb to the back limb, pushing his or her body against the strap to apply the traction force through the strap.

Notations: The patient's hip can be placed in various positions of flexion and rotation for application of superior or inferior distractions with the lateral glide (figure 18.7b and c).

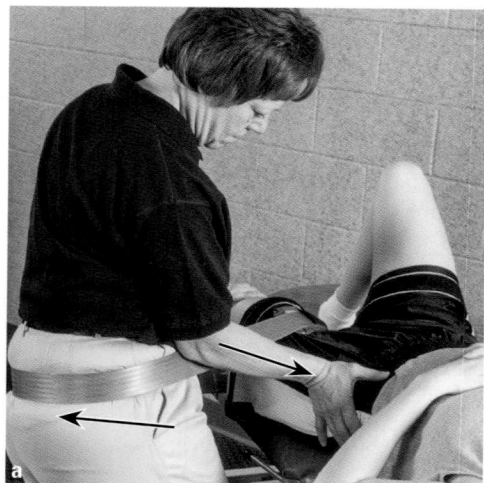
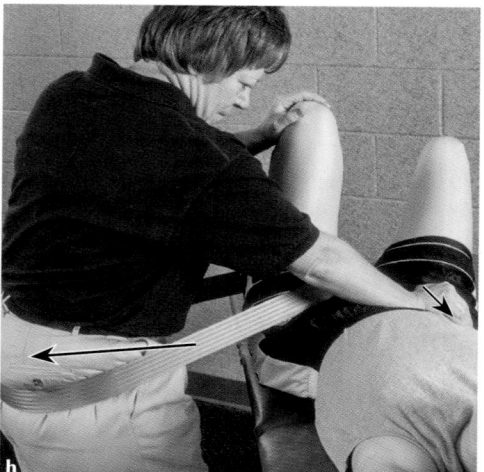
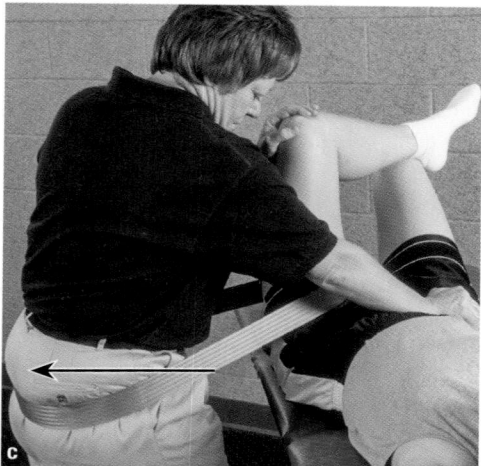

Figure 18.7

Posterior Glide

This test is also known as AP glide or dorsal glide.

Joint: Hip.

Resting Position: 30° flexion and 30° abduction with slight lateral rotation.

Indications: To increase hip flexion and medial rotation.

Patient Position: Supine with the hip and knee flexed.

Rehabilitation Clinician and Hand Positions: The degree of hip flexion depends on the technique used. When a belt is used, partial flexion of the joints is necessary, with the belt placed around the distal thigh and secured to the rehabilitation clinician's shoulder.

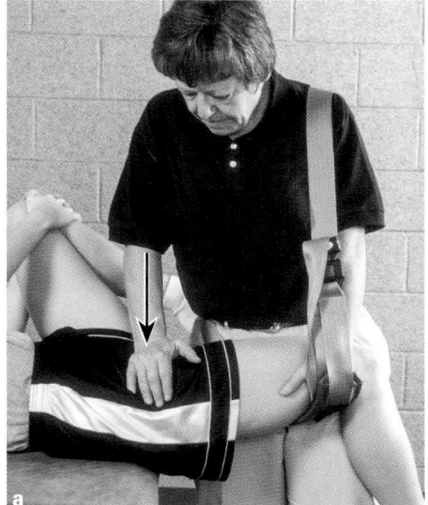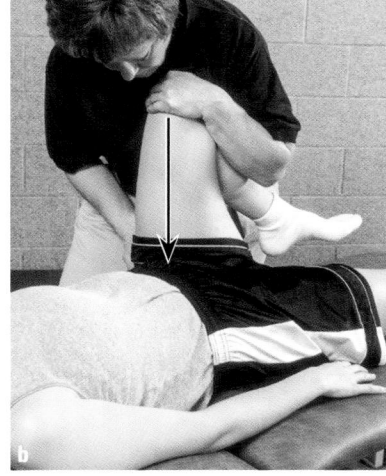

Figure 18.8

The rehabilitation clinician places the stabilizing hand under the belt and the mobilizing hand over the anterior proximal thigh just distal to the inguinal ligament.

Mobilization Application: With the elbow kept extended, the rehabilitation clinician applies a downward force on the proximal thigh, using his or her lower extremities, while the patient's thigh is kept stable with the belt (figure 18.8*a*).

Notations: An alternative position is with the hip in 90° flexion and about 10° adduction and the knee in full flexion. The rehabilitation clinician applies the posterior glide force through the long axis of the femur by leaning his or her body weight into the femur (figure 18.8*b*). Care must be taken not to apply the mobilizing force through the patella.

Medial Glide

Joint: Hip.

Resting Position: 30° flexion and 30° abduction with slight lateral rotation.

Indications: To increase hip abduction.

Patient Position: The patient is side-lying on the unaffected hip while the clinician supports the distal thigh and knee and positions the thigh in slight abduction and flexion (figure 18.9).

Rehabilitation Clinician and Hand Positions: The mobilizing hand is placed on the proximal thigh between the greater trochanter and pelvis.

Mobilization Application: The mobilizing force is applied downward, parallel to the joint's plane.

Notations: If the patient is large compared to the clinician, the assistance of another clinician may be needed to support the patient's limb. This technique may also be performed with the patient in supine.

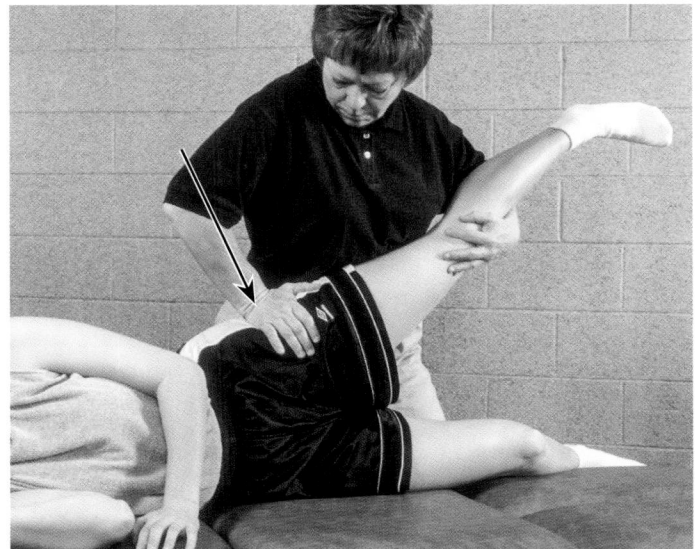

Figure 18.9

Anterior Glide

This test is also known as PA glide or a ventral glide.

Joint: Hip.

Resting Position: 30° flexion and 30° abduction with slight lateral rotation.

Indications: To increase hip extension and lateral rotation.

Patient Position: Prone with the knee flexed.

Rehabilitation Clinician and Hand Positions: The rehabilitation clinician supports the distal thigh using the stabilizing hand or a strap.

Mobilization Application: The mobilizing hand applies a downward force through an extended elbow; body weight exerts the force (figure 18.10a). The hip can be placed in various rotation positions for additional techniques.

Notations: In an alternative position, the patient is prone, with the hips on the edge of the table and the noninvolved lower extremity supporting the body weight with the lower-extremity foot on the floor. The rehabilitation clinician can either support the patient's distal thigh in one hand or can have a stabilizing strap over the shoulder and wrapped around the distal thigh (figure 18.10b).

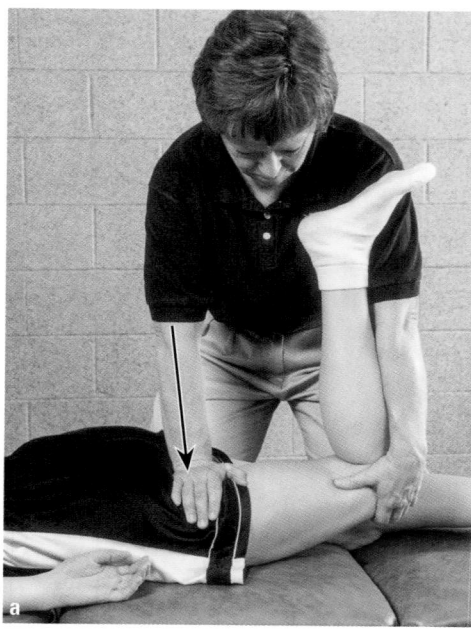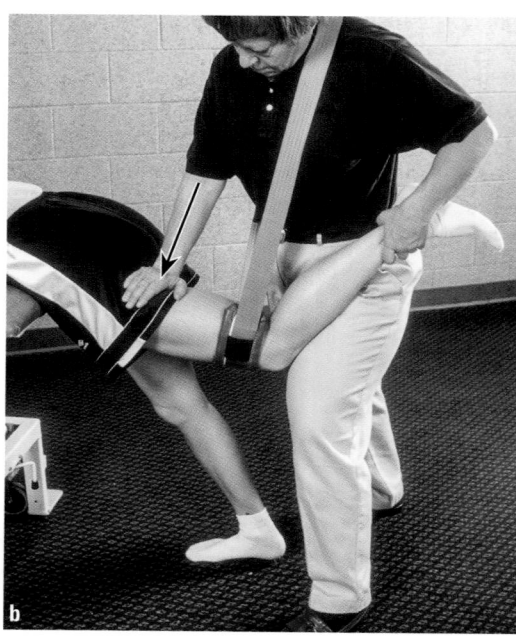

Figure 18.10

CLINICAL TIPS

The rehabilitation clinician uses joint mobilization of the hip to improve joint play and general hip mobility, as well as specific hip motions. Patients can also apply self-mobilization techniques as part of their home exercise programs.

Self-Mobilization

The patient can perform self-distraction using a stretch strap. The patient is supine with the strap anchored around the foot and the anterior hip; the knee and hip are placed in flexed positions, about 90° each (figure 18.11). A pad is placed on the anterior thigh for comfort. Keeping the opposite hip flexed with hands supporting the thigh, the patient pushes the involved foot against the strap, trying to extend the hip and knee.

In an alternative position, the patient places a weight cuff around the ankle and stands with the foot off a step, allowing gravity to create a distraction force on the hip. The position is maintained for several minutes as tolerated.

Flexibility Exercises

Several muscles cross the hip joint, acting not only on the hip but also on the knee, back, and pelvis. For effective stretching at the hip, these segments must be positioned appropriately. It is important to position the patient so the

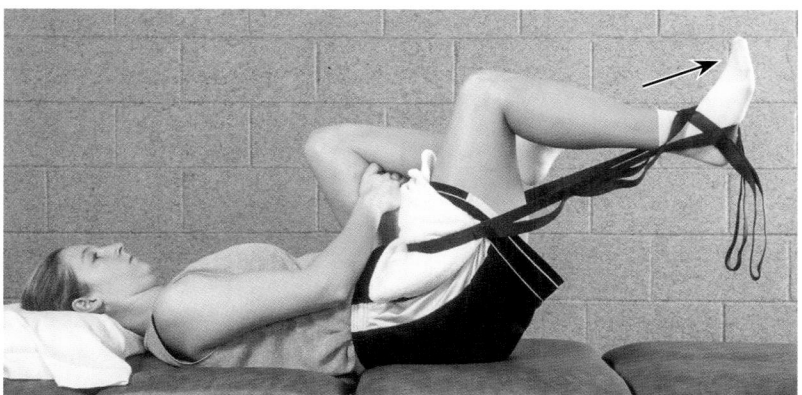

Figure 18.11   Joint mobilization: Self-mobilization distraction can be used to relieve pain and to improve general hip joint mobility.

muscle is not working during the stretch exercise, so for each flexibility exercise, note which muscles are used to maintain the body's position. There is usually a variety of stretches that may be used for any one muscle. The following sections present hip flexibility exercises using more than one position.

As with other body segments, active stretches are held for 15 to 20 s and are repeated about four times each, or they are held for 30 s for 1 to 2 repetitions. They should

be repeated at least 3 to 4 times throughout the day. As with any stretch, active contraction of opposing muscles can improve the results by enhancing the relaxation of the stretched muscle. Enough force should be applied to move the muscle to a point at which the patient perceives a stretch without pain. Prolonged stretches are most effective in altering tissue length in mature scar tissue and connective tissue.

Flexibility Exercises for the Hip

Since the hip is adjacent to the lumbar spine and pelvis proximally and to the knee distally, these segments must be properly stabilized during stretching exercises for optimal and accurate execution. Some hip muscles cross these joints as well, so knowing how to position the lumbosacral region and knee is important in achieving the desired stretch.

Lower Lumbar Rotation

Body Segment: Lateral hip muscles.

Stage in Rehab: Active phase.

Purpose: Increase flexibility of lower lumbar muscles.

Positioning: The patient flexes the involved hip and knee and rotates the thigh across the body, keeping the ipsilateral shoulder on the ground.

Execution: The weight of the leg provides the stretch, but additional force on the stretch can be supplied by the contralateral hand pushing on the thigh (figure 18.12).

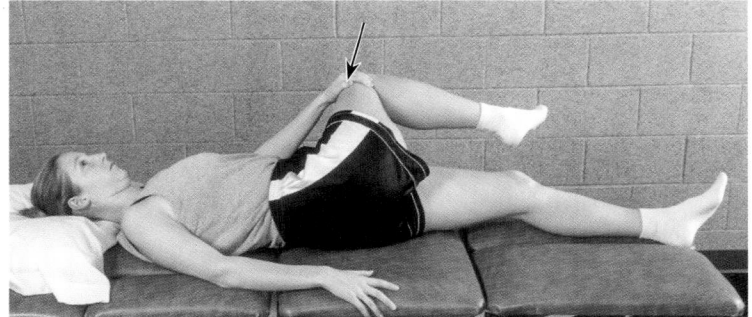

Figure 18.12

Possible Substitutions: Rotating the body with movement of the thigh. The ipsilateral shoulder must be kept on the ground. If necessary, the arm can be placed outward, away from the side, to prevent the shoulder from rising up.

Notations: The stretch is felt in the lower back, buttock, and lateral hip. The more the hip is flexed, the lower on the hip the stretch occurs.

Tensor Fasciae Latae Stretch, Standing

Body Segment: Lateral hip muscles.

Stage in Rehab: Active phase.

Purpose: Increase flexibility of hip abductors.

Positioning: Standing with the affected side closest to a wall, about an arm's length from the wall.

Execution: The patient pushes the hips toward the wall, keeping both feet on the ground as the hand on the wall helps push the hip toward the wall (figure 18.13).

Possible Substitutions: Rotating the body or flexing the elbow.

Notations: The stretch should be felt on the lateral thigh.

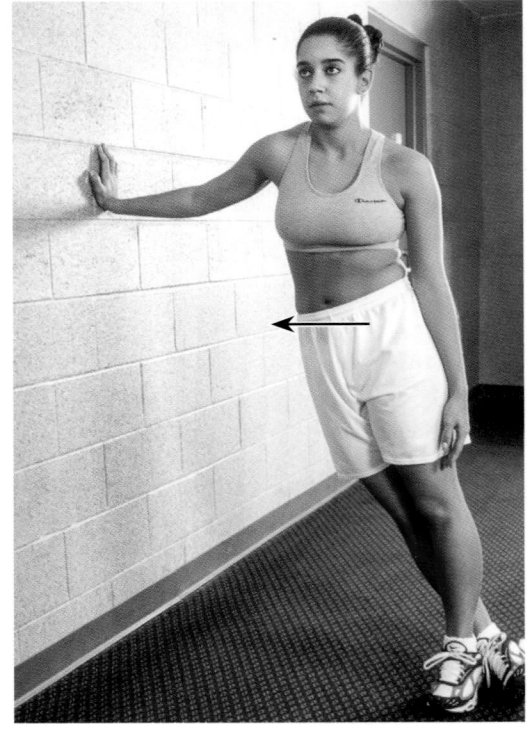

Figure 18.13

Tensor Fasciae Latae Stretch, Seated

Body Segment: Lateral hip muscles.

Stage in Rehab: Active phase.

Purpose: Increase flexibility of hip abductors.

Positioning: In long sitting, the patient has the uninvolved extremity's knee extended and the involved extremity flexed at the knee and hip; the foot of the involved extremity is flat on the ground lateral to the uninvolved knee.

Execution: The patient uses the hands to pull the involved knee across the body toward the opposite shoulder (figure 18.14).

Possible Substitutions: Rotating the trunk with the stretch or medially rotating the thigh.

Notations: Rotating the opposite thigh medially may stabilize the pelvis during the stretch.

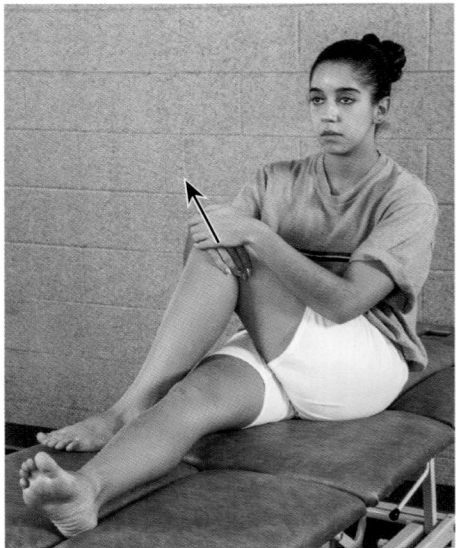

Figure 18.14

Tensor Fasciae Latae Stretch, Side-Lying

Body Segment: Lateral hip muscles.

Stage in Rehab: Active phase, resistive phase if used as a prolonged stretch.

Purpose: Increase flexibility of hip abductors.

Positioning: The patient lies on the uninvolved extremity with the top hip extended and the knee flexed.

Execution: The top extremity drops down behind the bottom extremity (figure 18.15).

Possible Substitutions: Rotating the trunk to place the top hip behind the bottom hip.

Notations: This position can be used as a prolonged stretch.

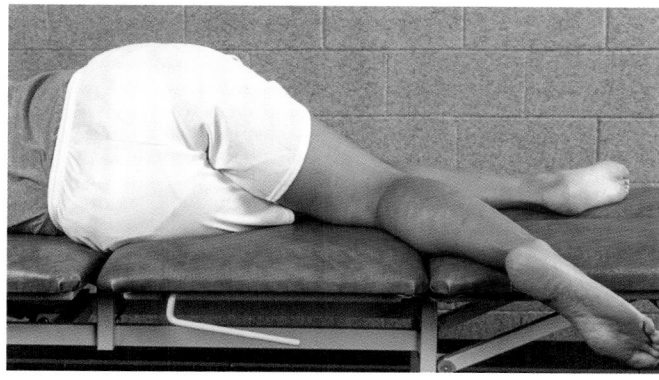

Figure 18.15

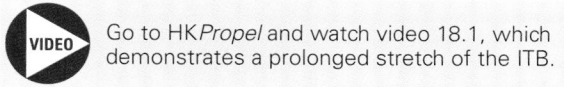

Go to HK*Propel* and watch video 18.1, which demonstrates a prolonged stretch of the ITB.

Standing Hip Flexor Stretch

Body Segment: Anterior hip muscles.

Stage in Rehab: Active phase.

Purpose: Increase flexibility of the hip flexors.

Positioning: The patient is standing and grasps the foot from behind.

Execution: The foot is grasped by the ipsilateral hand toward the buttocks while the knee remains pointing to the floor and the trunk remains upright (figure 18.16).

Possible Substitutions: Trunk flexion forward or moving the knee forward of the hip.

Notations: To include the rectus femoris in the stretch, the knee is flexed. If the knee is extended, the iliopsoas will be the only hip flexor muscle stretched.

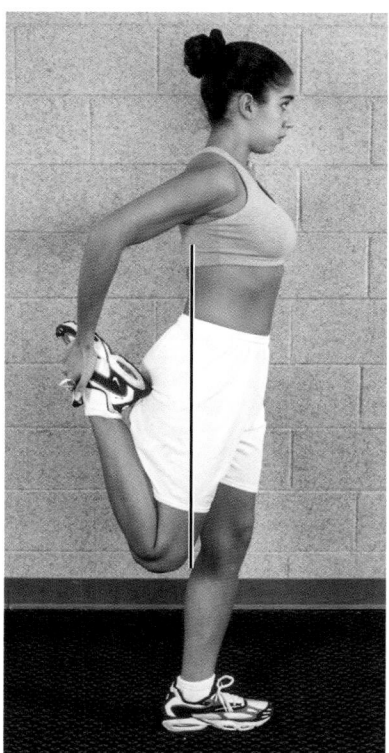

Figure 18.16

Kneeling Hip Flexor Stretch

Body Segment: Anterior hip muscles.

Stage in Rehab: Active phase.

Purpose: Increase flexibility of the hip flexors.

Positioning: The patient kneels on the involved extremity, and the opposite extremity bears weight on the foot in front of the kneeling limb.

Execution: The patient transfers weight from the back knee to the front foot (figure 18.17).

Possible Substitutions: Flexing the trunk forward.

Notations: The patient can apply additional stretch by trying to flex the kneeling knee, although this can be a difficult maneuver. A pad can be placed under the knee for comfort.

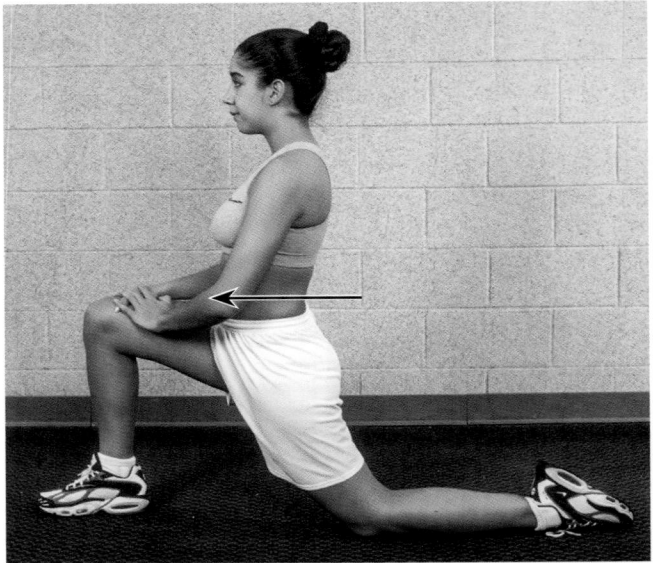

Figure 18.17

Prone Hip Flexor Stretch

Body Segment: Anterior hip muscles.

Stage in Rehab: Active phase, or resistive phase if used as a prolonged stretch.

Purpose: Increase flexibility of the hip flexors.

Positioning: The patient lies prone with the feet off the end of the table. A pillow may be placed under the stomach above the waist.

Execution: The patient flexes the involved extremity's knee until a stretch is felt in the anterior thigh or hip.

Possible Substitutions: Abducting the hip or rolling the trunk to face the stretching extremity. The lumbar spine may also hyperextend if the stretch is excessive.

Notations: Additional stretch is applied with greater pillow height or flexing the knee to lift the tibia off the table. This position can be used for a prolonged stretch (figure 18.18).

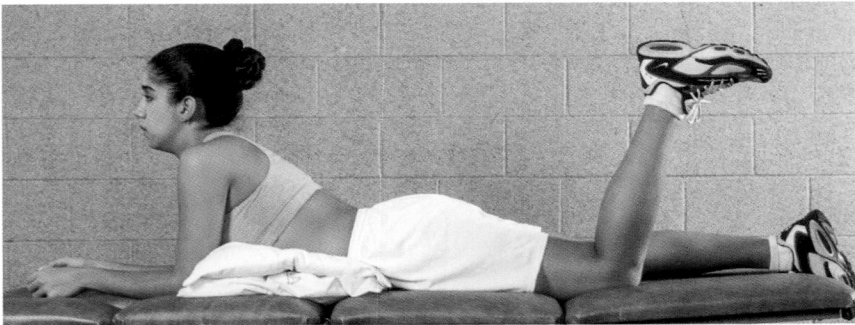

Figure 18.18

Thomas Hip Flexor Stretch

Body Segment: Anterior hip muscles.

Stage in Rehab: Active phase, or resistive phase if used as a prolonged stretch.

Purpose: Increase flexibility of hip flexors.

Positioning: The patient lies with the buttocks on the end of the table. The uninvolved extremity flexes at the hip and knee, and the extremity is brought toward the chest; this limb position is maintained by the patient's hands.

Execution: The involved extremity hangs over the edge of the table so that the mid- to upper thigh is at the edge (figure 18.19).

Possible Substitutions: Hip abduction and hip lateral rotation. Patient does not adequately secure the uninvolved lower limb, so the back arches.

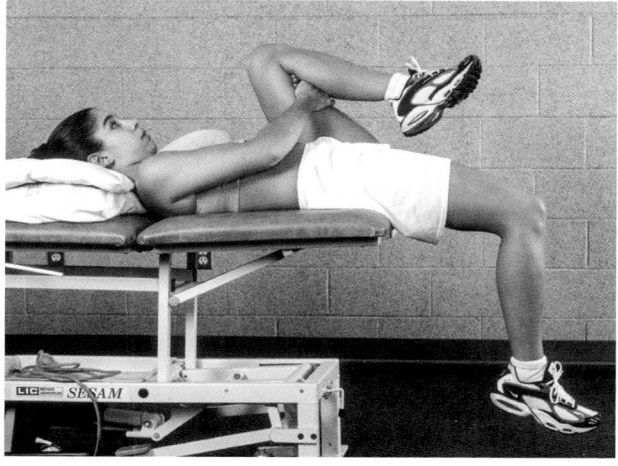

Figure 18.19

Notations: The alignment of the extremities can be positioned and maintained passively by the clinician or with use of stabilization straps. This position can be used as a prolonged stretch. If tolerated, weights can be applied to the ankle for additional stretch force during a prolonged stretch.

Adductor Stretch in Sitting

Body Segment: Medial hip muscles.

Stage in Rehab: Active phase.

Purpose: Increase flexibility of hip adductors.

Positioning: In sitting, the patient flexes and abducts the hips and knees to place the bottoms of the feet together. He or she pulls the feet toward the buttocks. In this position, the hands are on the ankles, and the forearms lie along the inner legs.

Execution: A stretch force is applied by the forearms on the tibias to lower the knees (figure 18.20).

Possible Substitutions: Flexing forward from the back. The back should be kept straight with the chest elevated, with forward flexion occurring from hip flexion.

Notations: The long adductors pass below the knee joint, so they are stretched when the knee is extended; the shorter adductors can be stretched with the knee flexed or extended.

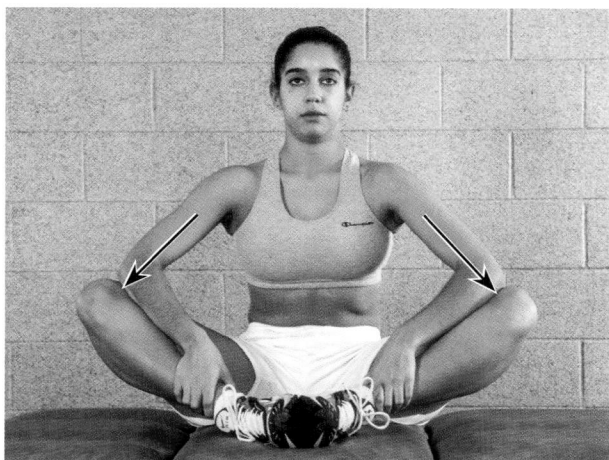

Figure 18.20

Adductor Stretch in Long Sitting

Body Segment: Medial hip muscles.

Stage in Rehab: Active phase.

Purpose: Increase flexibility of hip adductors.

Positioning: The patient is in long sitting with the hips abducted and the knees extended. With elbows extended, hands are on the floor between the lower extremities.

Execution: The patient flexes forward from the hips, keeping the back straight and chest elevated, while placing the weight on the hands to keep the groin muscles relaxed (figure 18.21).

Possible Substitutions: Flexing from the back and lifting the pelvis off the floor.

Notations: Additional stretch is provided to the long adductors by rotating to the affected extremity and reaching for the toes.

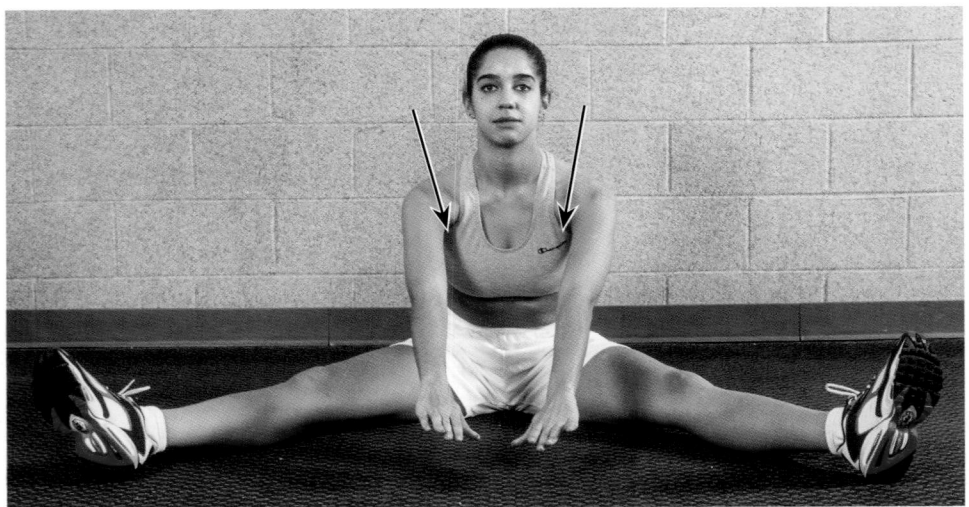

Figure 18.21

Adductor Stretch in Kneeling

Body Segment: Medial hip muscles.

Stage in Rehab: Active phase.

Purpose: Increase flexibility of hip adductors.

Positioning: The patient kneels on the uninvolved knee and places the involved extremity in abduction with the knee extended.

Execution: The uninvolved hip shifts laterally away from the involved extremity as the involved extremity is pushed downward (figure 18.22).

Possible Substitutions: Rotating the hip so the inside border of the involved foot rotates downward.

Notations: A pillow can be placed under the supporting knee for comfort, and the patient can use hand support if needed.

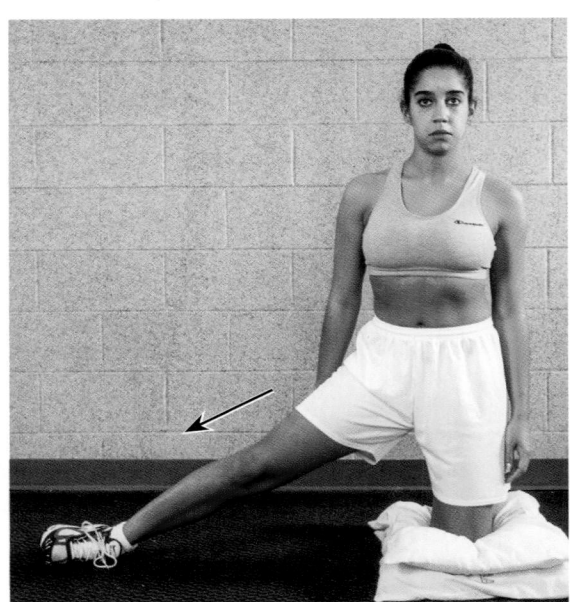

Figure 18.22

Adductor Stretch in Standing

Body Segment: Medial hip muscles.

Stage in Rehab: Active phase.

Purpose: Increase flexibility of hip adductors.

Positioning: The patient stands sideways to a supporting object that is about hip height or lower, depending upon the patient's limitations, and places the involved extremity's foot on top of the object (figure 18.23).

Execution: Keeping the medial border of the foot facing downward, the patient squats on the supporting extremity while pushing down on the involved lateral thigh.

Possible Substitutions: Rotation of the hip or pelvis.

Notations: A pad may be placed under the ankle for comfort.

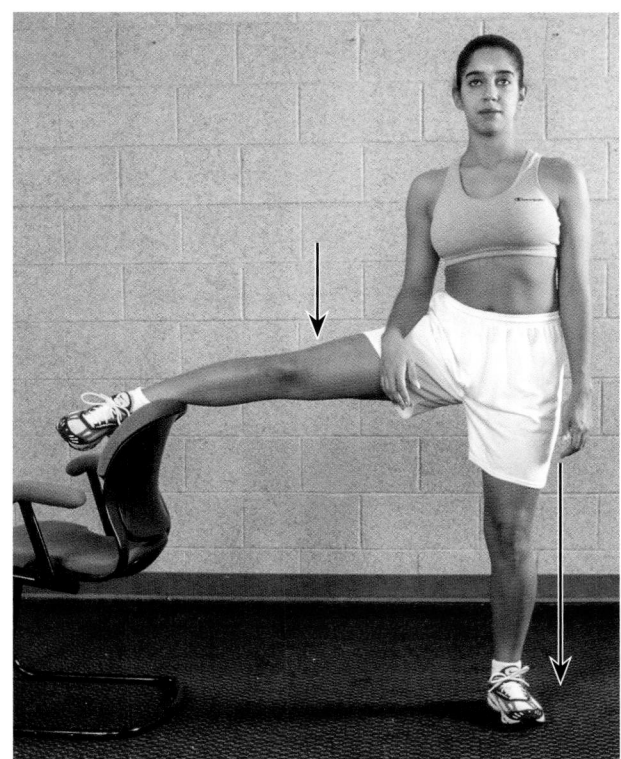

Figure 18.23

Hamstring Stretch in Standing

Body Segment: Posterior hip muscles.

Stage in Rehab: Active phase.

Purpose: Increase hamstring flexibility.

Positioning: In standing, the patient places the involved extremity on a supporting surface (figure 18.24). The height is determined by the tightness of the hamstrings: The tighter the hamstrings, the lower the surface height. The standing extremity should be positioned with the foot facing forward.

Execution: Keeping the back straight and the chest elevated, the patient leans forward from the hips toward the elevated foot and reaches forward with the opposite hand.

Possible Substitutions: The standing extremity should not laterally rotate; the body flexes forward from the hips, not the back, and the opposite hand reaches forward to keep the pelvis from rotating.

Notations: This exercise isolates the hamstrings and prevents the pelvis from rolling posteriorly.

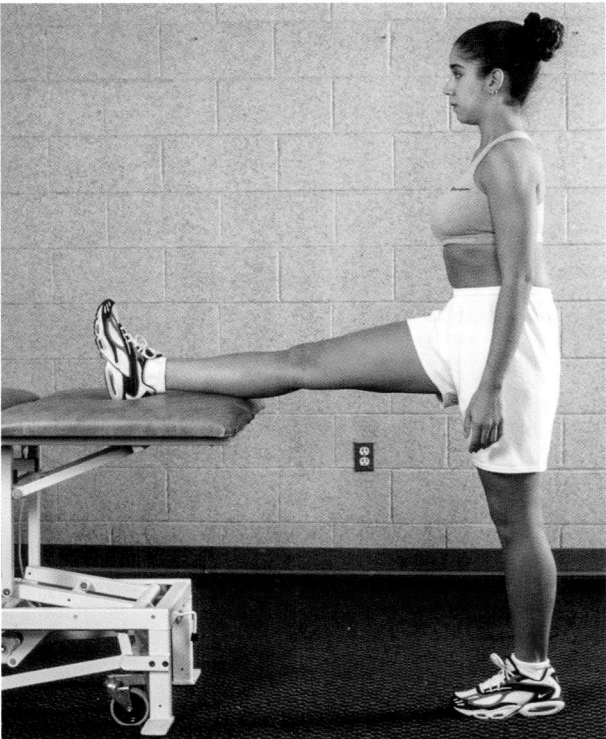

Figure 18.24

Hamstring Stretch in Supine

Body Segment: Posterior hip muscles.

Stage in Rehab: Active phase.

Purpose: Increase hamstring flexibility.

Positioning: The patient is supine with uninvolved hip and knee in extension.

Execution: The patient places his or her hands around the posterior thigh and pulls the knee toward the chest to 90° of hip flexion and then extends the knee (figure 18.25).

Possible Substitutions: Arching the back or posterior pelvic tilt.

Notations: The knee is extended until a stretch in the hamstrings is felt.

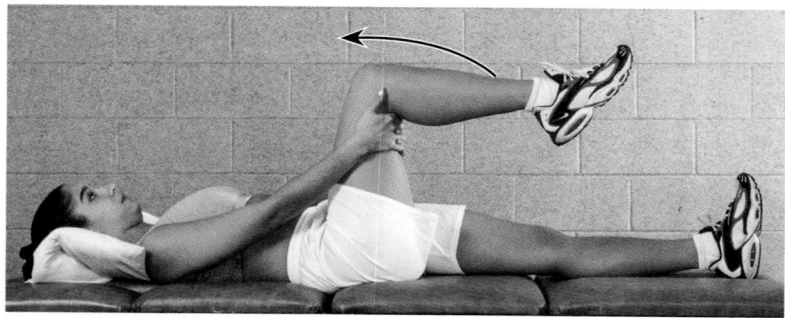

Figure 18.25

Gluteus Maximus Stretch in Supine

Body Segment: Posterior hip muscles.

Stage in Rehab: Active phase.

Purpose: Increase flexibility of hip extensors.

Positioning: As with the supine hamstring stretch, the patient is supine.

Execution: As the patient brings the involved extremity toward the chest, the knee remains flexed (figure 18.26).

Possible Substitutions: Posterior roll of the pelvis as indicated by the opposite extremity's rise off the table.

Notations: The patient hugs the knee toward the chest until a stretch in the gluteals is felt.

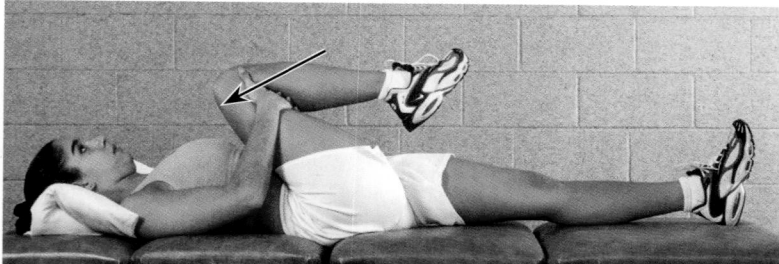

Figure 18.26

Piriformis Stretch in Supine

Body Segment: Posterior hip muscles.

Stage in Rehab: Active phase.

Purpose: Increase flexibility of lateral rotators.

Positioning: The patient is supine with knees flexed and crossed. The involved extremity is on top of the uninvolved extremity.

Execution: The knees are brought to the chest, and the patient pulls them toward the chest (figure 18.27).

Possible Substitutions: Rotating the pelvis.

Notations: The stretch should be felt in the posterior hip over the region of the piriformis.

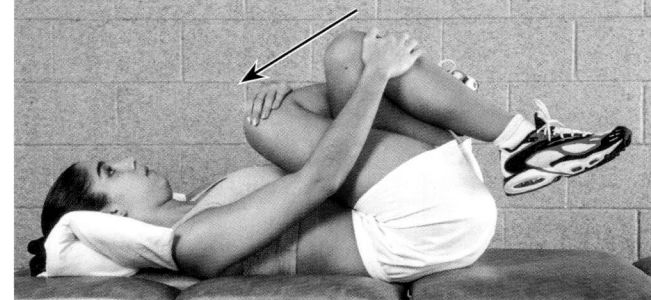

Figure 18.27

Piriformis Stretch in Quadruped

Body Segment: Posterior hip muscles.

Stage in Rehab: Active phase.

Purpose: Increase flexibility of lateral rotators.

Positioning: In a quadruped position, the patient crosses the involved extremity under the uninvolved extremity.

Execution: The patient leans the hips backward, keeping the uninvolved extremity's knee off the floor and pushing the limb and body toward the uninvolved foot (figure 18.28).

Possible Substitutions: Applying too much weight to the arms.

Notations: If there is a history of knee injury, this may be difficult for the patient to perform. This stretch permits the involved hip to adduct, flex, and medially rotate.

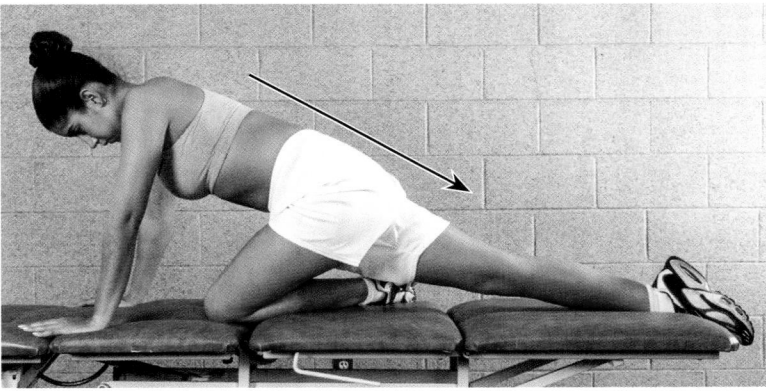

Figure 18.28

Piriformis Stretch in Standing

Body Segment: Posterior hip muscles.

Stage in Rehab: Active phase.

Purpose: Increase flexibility of lateral rotators.

Positioning: The patient stands and rests the involved extremity's knee flexed with the leg on a tabletop and the hip in lateral rotation and flexion.

Execution: The patient leans forward toward the tabletop from the hip, keeping the chest up and back straight.

Possible Substitutions: Rotating the body toward the stretch limb.

Notations: The patient's pelvis must remain square with the table.

Strength Exercises

As with other body segments, hip-strengthening exercises late in the active phase or early in the resistive phase may begin with isometrics that could be performed in various joint positions for optimal results. Isotonic exercises in the resistive phase include concentric and eccentric exercises; these exercises use gravity as resistance for the least difficult exercise and advance to various other forms of resistance, including manual resistance, weight cuffs, resistance bands, pulleys, and machines. Increased manual resistance and weight-cuff resistance are applied at the ankle. If less resistance is needed, the same amount of resistance can be placed more proximally on the extremity.

The exercises are performed in a smooth, controlled movement of the hip through a full range of motion. Substitutions using other muscles occur easily in the hip, so the patient must be carefully observed and corrected as needed by the rehabilitation clinician. Low-intensity, high-repetition resistance is replaced with higher loads and fewer repetitions as strength and control improve.

Because the trunk, knee, and ankle are so intimately connected to the hip, strength, motion control, and stabilization within each of these body segments are vital to hip stability and performance quality. Exercises to correct deficiencies that exist within any of these body segments must be part of a total hip rehabilitation program. Because exercises for these segments have been presented in previous chapters, they are not repeated here.

Isometric Exercises

The patient can perform isometrics independently against his or her hand or against a stationary object. To perform hip adduction in long or short sitting, the patient places either the hands or a rolled towel between the knees and tries to push the knees together (figure 18.29a).

Hip abduction isometrics are performed in sitting. The patient tries to move the thigh outward as he or she resists the motion at the lateral distal thigh (figure 18.29b).

Hip flexion is best performed while sitting in a chair. The patient places a hand on the distal thigh and resists attempts to lift the knee up. The patient should refrain from using the foot to push off the floor.

Hip extension is performed best in supine or standing. The patient squeezes the buttocks to set the gluteals.

All isometric exercises are performed using a buildup to maximal tension. The tension is held for 5 or 6 s and then gradually released to full relaxation before the exercise is repeated.[40] Isometrics are performed several times

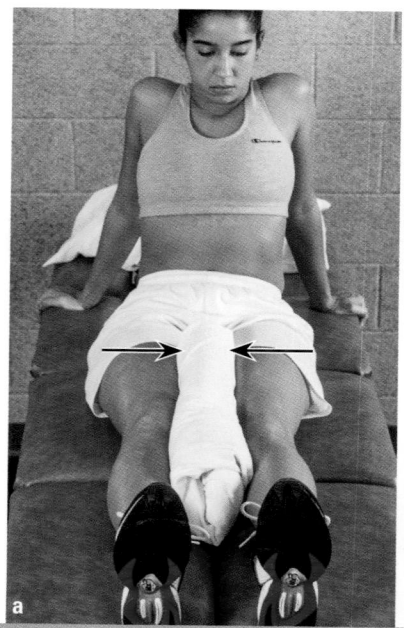
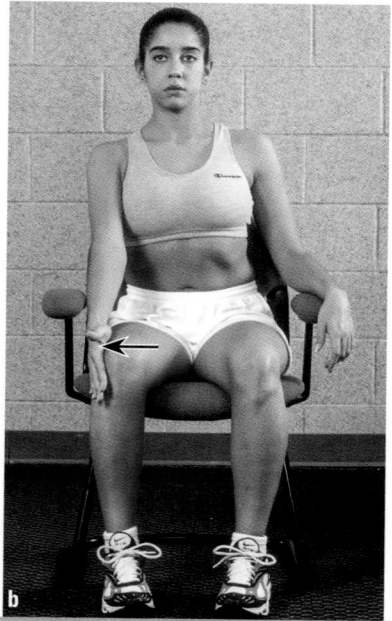

Figure 18.29 Isometric hip exercises create tension in the muscles without movement. They are often used during early rehabilitation when movement is restricted or when the muscle is very weak: *(a)* bilateral hip adduction, *(b)* right hip abduction.

throughout the day in sets of at least 10 repetitions. They may be used early in the rehabilitation program in either later phase I (inactive) or early phase II (active) when the muscle is very weak or when range of motion is limited either by immobilization or by restricted mobility. If isometrics are used in the inactive phase, they should occur with submaximal output.

Body-Weight Resistance Exercises

In a 68 kg (150 lb) patient, the lower extremity weighs about 11 kg (25 lb). This can be substantial resistance for a very weak hip muscle. Weight should not be added to the extremity until the patient can control movement against gravity through a full range of motion.

If the patient cannot lift the extremity against gravity, flexing the knee to perform the exercise shortens the resistance moment-arm length. If antigravity exercises are too difficult, the patient can perform the same activity in standing; gravity affects muscle activity less in this position, but the muscle strength is still needed to move the hip. Antigravity and other resistive strengthening exercises are presented in the following sections.

Strength Exercises for the Hip

In addition to their use after hip injuries, hip-strengthening exercises are often incorporated into core, spine, shoulder, and other lower-extremity rehabilitation programs. Here are a few examples of hip-strengthening exercises.

Hip Abduction Against Gravity

Body Segment: Hip abductors.

Stage in Rehab: Early resistive phase.

Purpose: Strengthen hip abductors.

Positioning: The patient lies on the uninvolved extremity with the bottom hip and knee flexed for stability.

Execution: The patient keeps the top knee and hip extended and lifts the extremity against gravity (figure 18.30).

Possible Substitutions: Lying more on the back, moving the hip into flexion, and rotating the hip outward.

Notations: The patient may feel as though the extremity is positioned behind the body rather than in line with the trunk; this is normal. If hip abductor weakness prevents the patient from lifting the lower extremity, begin this exercise with the patient standing.

Go to HK*Propel* and watch video 18.2, which demonstrates substitutions during side-lying hip abduction exercises.

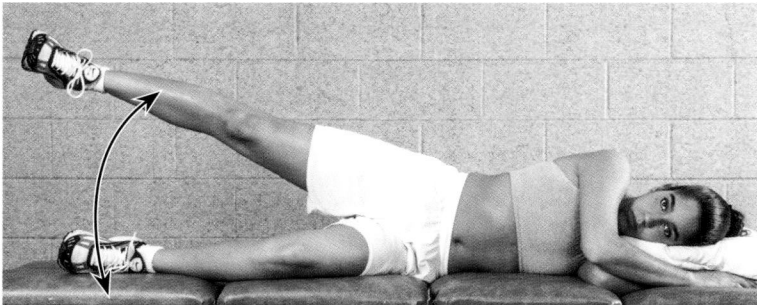

Figure 18.30

Hip Adduction Against Gravity

Body Segment: Hip adductors.

Stage in Rehab: Early resistive phase.

Purpose: Strengthen hip adductors.

Positioning: The patient lies on the involved side with the top extremity flexed at the hip and knee and its foot placed in front of the bottom knee.

Execution: Keeping the involved extremity's knee and hip extended, the patient lifts the extremity against gravity in the frontal plane (figure 18.31*a*).

Possible Substitutions: Rotating the hip, lying more on the back, and moving the hip into flexion rather than keeping it in the abduction plane.

Notations: If the patient lifts the fully extended top extremity into abduction and maintains that position while lifting the bottom extremity to meet the top extremity, the exercise is more difficult because greater trunk stabilization is required (figure 18.31*b*). An alternative position is with the top extremity placed on a supporting object such as the seat of a chair (figure 18.31*c*).

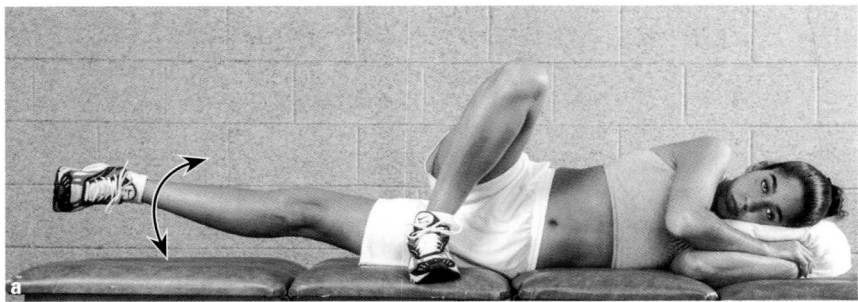

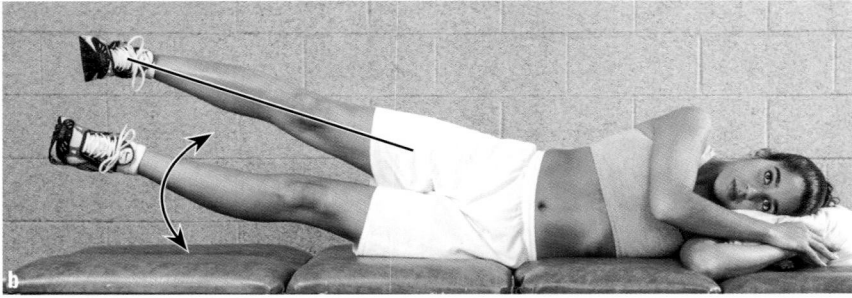

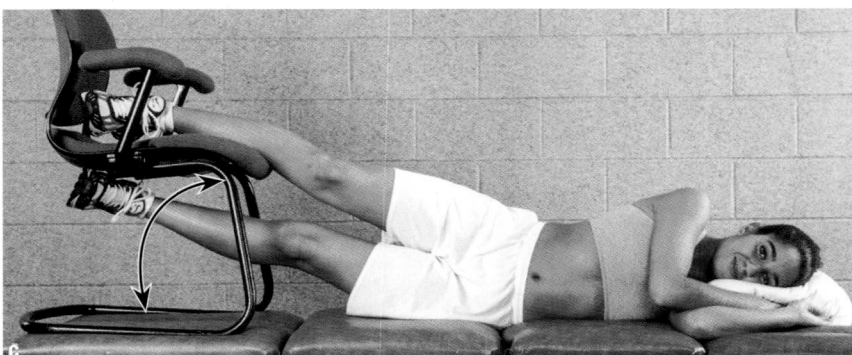

Figure 18.31

Hip Extension in Prone

Body Segment: Hip extensors.

Stage in Rehab: Early resistive phase.

Purpose: Strengthen gluteals and hamstrings.

Positioning: The patient is prone with the extremity either starting in extension on the table (figure 18.32*a*) or positioned in flexion with the extremity off the table and the toes on the ground (figure 18.32*b*). If the patient lies prone with the extremity over the edge of a table, the hip begins in flexion and must travel through a greater range of motion, providing resistance to the muscle through a greater range of motion.

Execution: The patient squeezes the gluteal muscles while lifting the extremity, keeping the knee extended to facilitate all hip extensor muscles. If the patient is to isolate the gluteals, the knee should be flexed, but remember that with a shorter moment-arm length when the knee is flexed, the resistance of the extremity is reduced.

Possible Substitutions: Hip rotation and trunk rotation.

Notations: Hip extension is limited to about 15°, so when the patient begins lying prone in a hip neutral position, the amount of motion the muscles produce is relatively small.

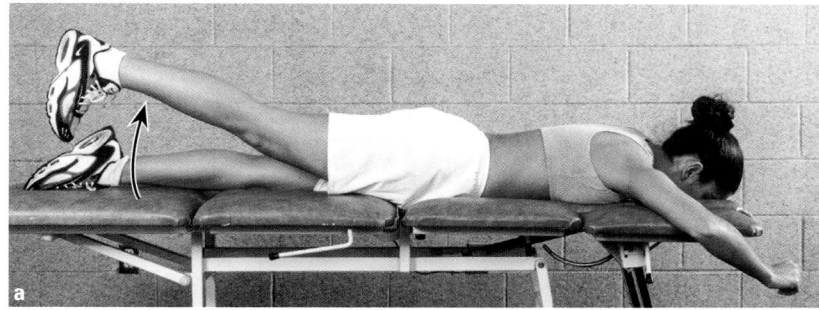

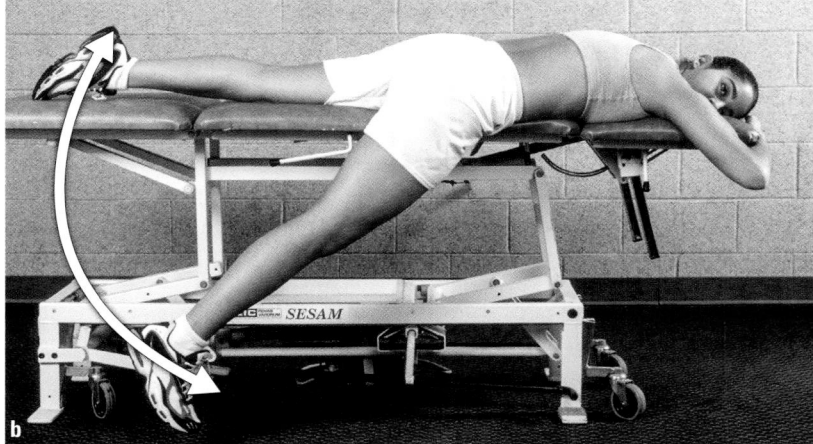

Figure 18.32

Bridge

Body Segment: Hip extensors.

Stage in Rehab: Early resistive phase.

Purpose: Strengthen gluteals, hamstrings, and spinal extensors.

Positioning: The patient is supine with hips and knees flexed and with the feet flat on the floor.

Execution: The patient tightens the gluteals. The hips are raised so that the thighs and trunk form a straight line. The patient then holds this position for several seconds.

Possible Substitutions: Dropping the hips, moving them into flexion, or performing an anterior pelvic tilt.

Notations: This exercise can be advanced to one-extremity support (figure 18.33).

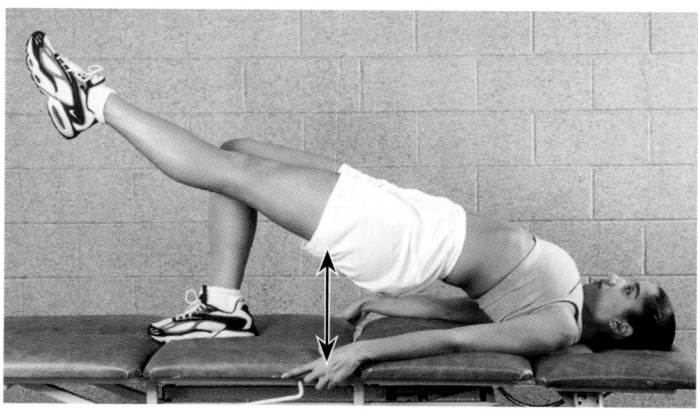

Figure 18.33

Figure-4 Lift

Body Segment: Hip extensors and lateral rotators.

Stage in Rehab: Early to middle resistive phase.

Purpose: Strengthen gluteals and lateral rotators.

Positioning: The patient lies prone; the involved extremity is flexed at the hip and knee, the hip is laterally rotated, and the ankle is under the uninvolved thigh. If the right knee is lifted, the face is turned to the left, and if the left knee is lifted, the face is turned to the right.

Execution: The patient lifts the flexed knee as high as possible (figure 18.34).

Possible Substitutions: Hip rotation or trunk rotation.

Notations: If the patient lacks enough flexibility for the position, he or she should place the involved extremity's ankle on top of the uninvolved extremity as proximal along the extremity as possible.

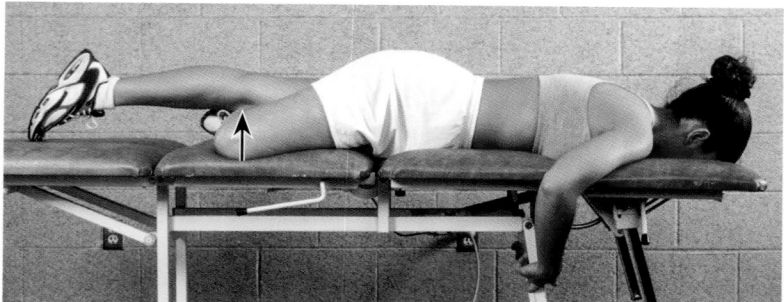

Figure 18.34

Straight-Limb Raise

Body Segment: Hip flexors.

Stage in Rehab: Early resistive phase.

Purpose: Strengthen iliopsoas and rectus femoris.

Positioning: The patient is supine or leaning back on the elbows in a semireclined position; the uninvolved extremity is flexed at the hip and knee with the foot flat on the floor.

Execution: The patient tightens the abdominal muscles and quadriceps and then lifts the limb about 0.5 m (about 18 in.) off the floor, keeping the knee extended.

Possible Substitutions: Arching the back (prevented with abdominal tensing), hip rotation, and hip abduction.

Notations: The patient may be asked to raise the limb as high as possible, but as the limb is raised more, the resistance becomes less because the angle of the force of gravity changes.

Evidence in Rehabilitation

Verrelst led a team of investigators who looked at the relationship between hip muscle strength and lower-extremity function.[41] Based on their findings, they concluded that the hip muscles play an important role in controlling the movements of the lower extremity. They found that people with weak hip abductors were at increased risk of exertional medial tibial pain. These investigators theorized that since the gluteus medius is the primary hip abductor that also produces lateral rotation of the hip, when the muscle is weak, it influences transverse plane movements of the lower extremity. They further theorized that since the gluteus medius has this influence in both frontal plane and transverse plane alignment, weakness in this muscle may be responsible for increasing the postural malalignments of femur adduction and medial femoral rotation. They speculated that such pathological alignment may further contribute to tibial stress fracture, chronic exertional compartment syndrome, and musculotendinous injuries.

The results of their investigations suggest that the rehabilitation clinician would be wise to examine hip abductor and lateral rotator strength when treating patients with other lower-extremity injuries. Weakness proximally changes the alignment of more distal elements, placing additional stresses on those distal segments.

Resistance-Band Exercises

Resistance bands or weighted pulleys can be used progressively once the patient can perform antigravity exercises through a full range of motion. In the descriptions of the exercises in the following sections, the involved extremity is the exercising extremity, so you should use upper-body support devices for balance as needed to achieve better execution. Reminding the patient to engage the core before performing the exercise will also provide stability.

Many resistance-band exercises can also be performed with the resistance attached to the uninvolved extremity so that the involved extremity must work to support and stabilize the body during activities for the uninvolved extremity. When exercises are used with this goal, upper-extremity support is limited or eliminated to elicit a greater effort from the weight-bearing hip. When the exercises are used for balance and proprioception, they can be executed as explained here or performed in the more challenging diagonal planes.

If the patient performs the exercise using a substitution pattern, correct the execution by providing verbal or tactile cueing (or both) or visual feedback with a mirror. If substitution continues with these corrections, the resistance may be too much for the patient to control properly; in this case, he or she should use the next-lightest resistance band. The motion should be full and should be controlled by the patient throughout the exercise.

Resistance-Band Hip Abduction

Body Segment: Hip abductors.

Stage in Rehab: Resistive phase.

Purpose: Strengthen hip abductors against resistance.

Positioning: With the band attached to a doorjamb, wall anchor, table leg, or around the ankle of the uninvolved leg, the patient places the band around the involved extremity's ankle. The patient stands sideways with the uninvolved side closest to the anchor site and takes the slack out of the band.

Execution: The patient tightens the quadriceps and gluteals and then abducts the extremity out to the side, keeping the pelvis level and the foot above but close to the floor to prevent hip hiking (figure 18.35). Cue the patient to engage the core to prevent substitutions. If the patient hikes the hip or laterally bends the upper trunk, have the patient perform the exercise in front of a mirror to watch for and correct these substitutions.

Possible Substitutions: Moving the hip into flexion, using a forward lean of the trunk, side-bending the upper trunk to the opposite side, and hiking the hip.

Notations: Once the patient performs this exercise correctly, it may be transferred to the home exercise program.

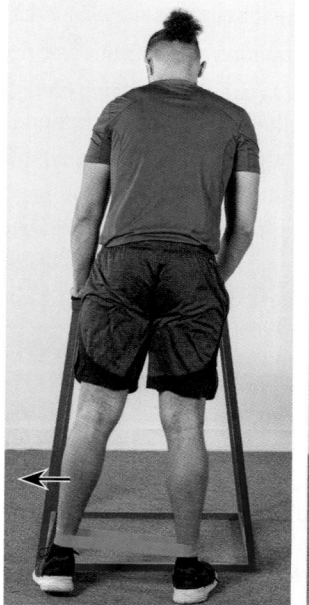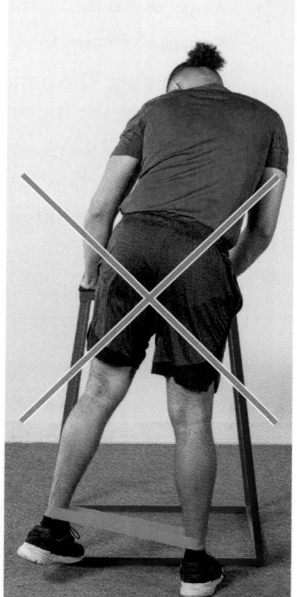

Figure 18.35

Walking Abduction

Body Segment: Hip abductors.

Stage in Rehab: Resistive phase.

Purpose: Strengthen hip abductors.

Positioning: A short-length circular band is wrapped around both ankles. The patient stands in a partial squat position with the back relaxed to maintain neutral spinal curves.

Execution: The patient takes a large step laterally and controls the opposite lower extremity as weight is transferred to the other limb. This motion occurs to the left and to the right limb (figure 18.36).

Possible Substitutions: Standing upright, flexing the back, taking small steps, moving body weight over the weight-bearing limb rather than keeping it between the two feet, flexing the trunk too far forward, and hiking the pelvis rather than abducting the hip.

Notations: If the patient is partial weight bearing or does not have the balance to walk during this exercise, he or she may perform it facing a wall with the hands on the wall for balance. In this position, the patient tightens the quadriceps and gluteals and extends the involved hip backward and outward to about a 45° angle.

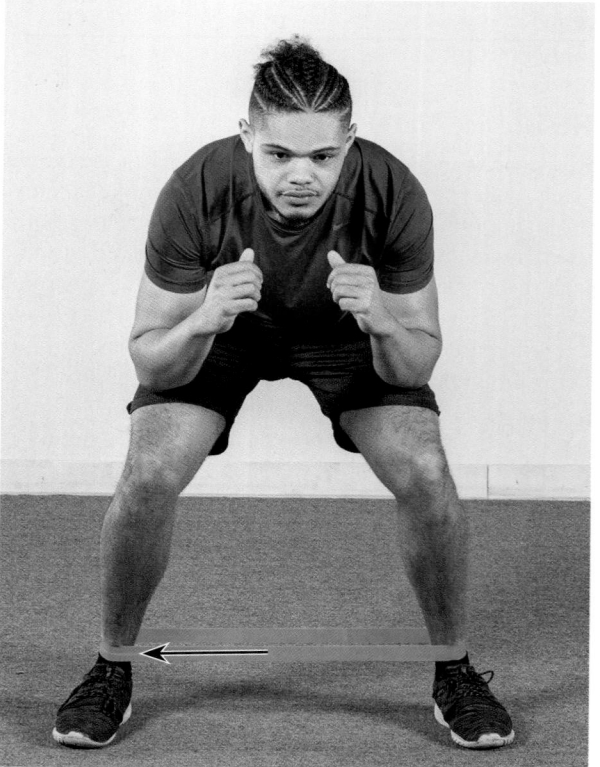

Figure 18.36

Standing Rotation

Body Segment: Hip abductors and lateral rotators.

Stage in Rehab: Resistive phase.

Purpose: Strengthen hip rotator abductors.

Positioning: The patient is standing sideways with the uninvolved side about 5 to 10 cm (2 to 4 in.) from the wall. The uninvolved extremity's knee is flexed to 90° and the lateral thigh, knee, and leg are pressed into the wall. The involved extremity is flexed slightly at the knee and should be in line with the ipsilateral shoulder and the second toe (figure 18.37).

Execution: The standing knee rotates laterally while the foot stays flat on the floor and the pelvis remains stable.

Possible Substitutions: Rotating the weight to the outside foot, rotating the pelvis away from the wall.

Notations: The motion is very small, so the patient must be cautioned that the foot should remain entirely on the floor and the pelvis should stay in contact with the wall.

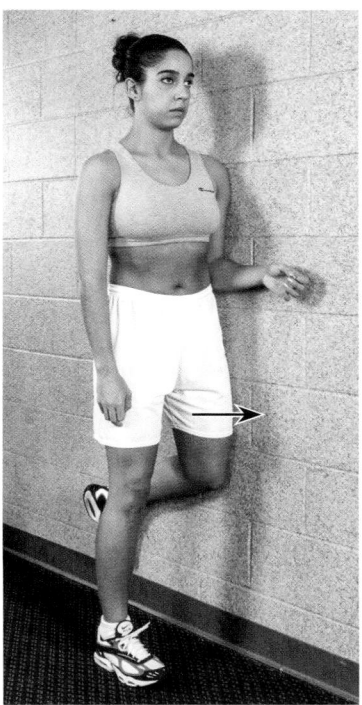

Figure 18.37

Hip Adduction With Resistance Band

Body Segment: Hip adductors.

Stage in Rehab: Resistive phase.

Purpose: Strengthen hip adductors.

Positioning: With the band anchored around a table leg, wall anchor, or doorjamb, the patient places the band around the involved extremity's ankle and stands sideways from the anchor site, with the involved side closest to the anchor site. The slack is taken out of the band.

Execution: The patient moves the extremity across and in front of the uninvolved extremity, keeping the knee extended without rotating the trunk or pelvis.

Possible Substitutions: Trunk rotation as the extremity moves across the body, flexing the hip too far forward, hip flexion, knee flexion, and trunk lean toward the band anchor site.

Notations: Once the patient performs this exercise correctly, it may be transferred to the home exercise program.

Hip Extension With Resistance Band

Body Segment: Hip extensors.

Stage in Rehab: Resistive phase.

Purpose: Strengthen gluteus maximus and hamstrings.

Positioning: With the band anchored around a table leg, wall anchor, or doorjamb, the patient places the band around the involved extremity's ankle and faces the anchor site with the slack out of the band.

Execution: The patient tightens the quadriceps and gluteals and extends the hip (figure 18.38).

Possible Substitutions: Backward trunk lean and knee flexion.

Notations: Once the patient performs this exercise correctly, it may be included in the home exercise program. These muscles are usually stronger than other hip muscles and will require a more resistive band. As discussed earlier in this chapter, hip extension is about 15°, so this motion is small.

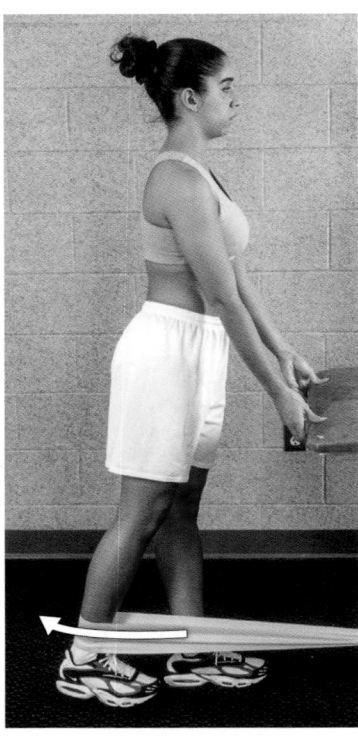

Figure 18.38

Hip Flexion Resistance with Resistance Band

Body Segment: Hip flexors.

Stage in Rehab: Resistive phase.

Purpose: Strengthen iliopsoas and rectus femoris.

Positioning: With the band anchored around a table leg, wall anchor, or doorjamb, the patient stands with the band around the involved ankle and his or her back to the anchor site, removing the slack from the band.

Execution: The patient tightens the quadriceps to keep the knee straight and then flexes the hip.

Possible Substitutions: Backward trunk lean and knee flexion during the exercise.

Notations: Once the patient performs this exercise correctly, it may be included in the home exercise program.

Medial Rotation Against Resistance Band

Body Segment: Hip medial rotators.

Stage in Rehab: Resistive phase.

Purpose: Strengthen hip medial rotators.

Positioning: The band is anchored between a closed door and the doorframe about 30 to 45 cm (12 to 18 in.) from the floor. With the uninvolved side closest to the band anchor, the patient lies prone on the floor with the band around the involved ankle. The involved extremity's knee is flexed to 90°, and the slack is taken out of the band.

Execution: The patient rotates the hip, moving the band away from the anchor site (figure 18.39).

Possible Substitutions: Pelvis rotation rather than hip rotation; extending or adducting the hip during the exercise.

Notations: This exercise may also be performed with the patient sitting in a chair.

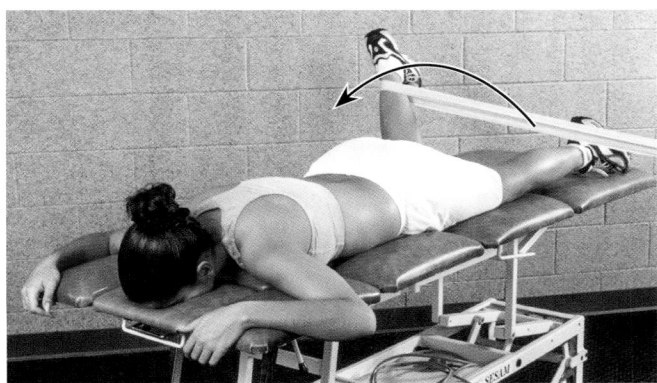

Figure 18.39

Hip Lateral Rotation Against Resistance Band

Body Segment: Hip lateral rotators.

Stage in Rehab: Resistive phase.

Purpose: Strengthen hip lateral rotators.

Positioning: With the band anchored as for hip medial rotation, the patient lies prone on the floor with the involved extremity closest to the anchor site and the band around the extremity's involved ankle. With the knee flexed to 90°, the patient takes the slack out of the band.

Execution: The patient pulls the involved extremity's foot toward the uninvolved extremity, keeping the knee at 90°.

Possible Substitutions: Rotating the pelvis, abducting the hip, or extending the knee.

Notations: This exercise may also be performed with the patient sitting in a chair.

Machine and Equipment Exercises

Many resistive exercises for the hip are the same as those used for the knee, as discussed in chapter 19. Some additional exercises are mentioned here, but chapter 19 includes other resistance exercises for both the hip and the knee. Some of these include step exercises, wall squats, mini-squats, the plié, lunges, sit-to-stand, and leg press machine exercises.

Reciprocal-Exercise Equipment   Reciprocal-exercise equipment can be useful for range-of-motion gains, strengthening, and coordination. These can be used early in strengthening work when the patient may not have antigravity strength but can tolerate resistance in an upright posture that does not require full antigravity strength. These exercises include activities on machines such as the step machine, ski machine, or stationary bike (figure 18.40).

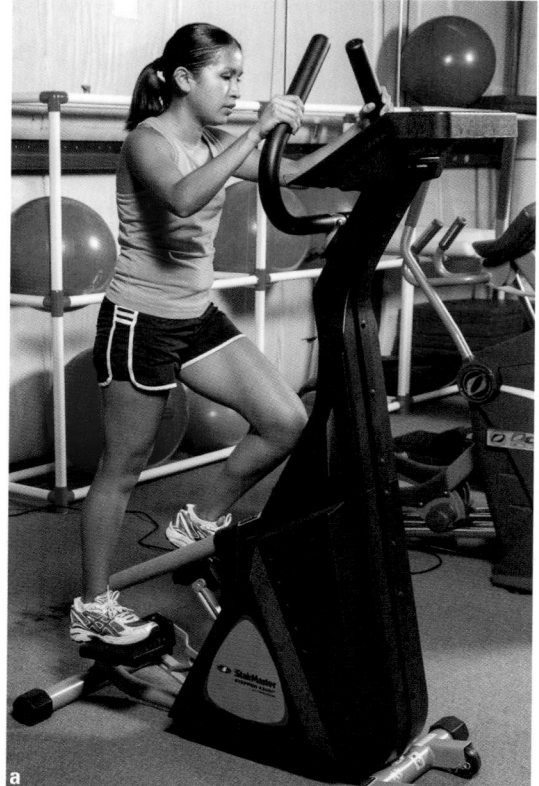

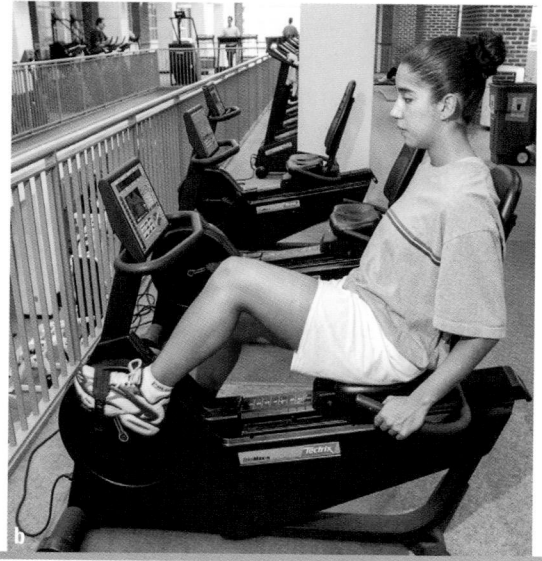

Figure 18.40 Reciprocal machines, such as the *(a)* step machine or *(b)* stationary bike, can be used to increase strength, ROM, and coordination.

Resistance Machines Machines are used primarily during phase III, the resistive phase, of the rehabilitation program. Machines have a number of resistance mechanisms, including weight pans, hydraulics, rubber, and asymmetrical cam systems. They all provide progressive resistance for a variety of exercises. Resistive increments

vary from one type of machine to another. The rehabilitation clinician should understand how to set up and use the facility's machines to deliver the desired results. You must instruct the patient in the proper use of these machines before they are used; you should not assume that a patient who has lifted weights before has always done it correctly. Instructions should include how to position the machine and the body for correct hip alignment, the need to choose weights that the patient can control throughout the motion, and how to perform the exercise without improper substitution.

Swiss Ball Exercises

Swiss ball exercises can involve activities such as bridging with leg curls, first with both legs and then with the involved extremity only. This exercise facilitates the hip extensors. Hip flexor exercises on the Swiss ball are performed with the patient prone with hands on the floor and anterior tibias on the ball. The patient pulls the knees toward the chest while maintaining balance on the ball (figure 18.41). Both of these exercises become more difficult when manual resistance is applied to the movement of the ball: The clinician's hands provide friction against ball motion during the exercise.

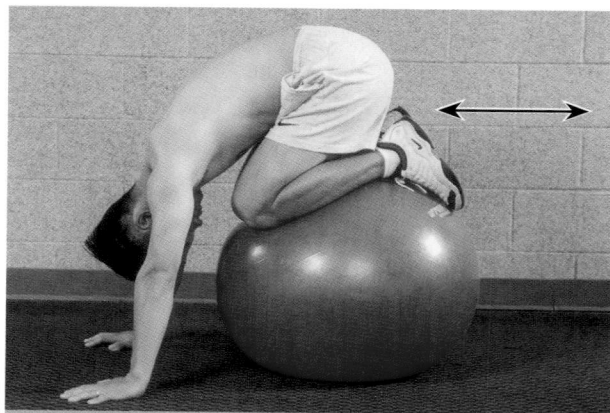

Figure 18.41 Swiss ball hip-flexion exercise: With legs on the ball, the knees and hips begin in an extended position. The patient pulls the knees toward the chest to end in the position shown.

Neuromotor Control and Proprioception Exercises

Neuromotor control requires proprioception as well as other components such as strength and balance. When these elements work together optimally, the result is neuromotor control. Neuromotor exercises are placed after strength activities in the rehabilitation program. Gains in neuromotor control and proprioception lead to advances in power and speed, so these activities occur in the rehabilitation program before plyometrics and agility activities.[42, 43]

Balance is a complicated motor activity that depends heavily on sensory information, and it is one of the key elements of neuromotor control. One of those sensory systems of balance is proprioception. Therefore, balance improves when proprioception improves. In fact, many exercises that improve the flow of proprioceptive information into the neuromotor system are balance activities.

Early Neuromotor and Proprioception Exercises

Proprioception exercises for balance begin early in the rehabilitation program, even before the patient can bear weight on the extremity. Joint proprioceptive activities performed early in the rehabilitation program can improve kinesthetic awareness.[44] When patients begin weight-bearing activities, those who do not bear weight properly may use the balance scale activities presented in chapters 19 and 20 for proper neuromotor development. Static balance activities are used before dynamic balance exercises. As with other lower-extremity injuries, progression during phase II (active phase) advances from weight-transfer activities and gait training to stork standing with eyes open and then eyes closed. Single-leg stance activities may be performed with head rotation to left and right and then combining those movements with eyes closed to further enhance proprioceptive and neuromotor reeducation.

Balance work begins with static activities and advances to distracting activities in which static balance is challenged while the patient performs other functions and dynamic activities. Examples of these activities include the resistance-band exercises performed with the uninvolved extremity while the patient balances on the involved extremity. This can be done on the ground or on a half foam roller, while stork standing on a trampoline or BAPS board and catching or bouncing a ball, or while using a balance board or other machine such as a Fitter or slide board.

As balance, proprioception, strength, and coordination improve, the patient progresses to the later resistive phase, advancing to agility exercises that demand higher levels of proprioceptive response and control. These include resistive weight-transfer activities, exercises using increased speed of movement, and finally, explosive exercises using jumping and plyometrics.

Advanced Neuromotor and Proprioceptive Exercises

Agility exercises are introduced in chapters 19 and 20. Some of these are rapid box exercises, such as rapid step-up and step-down activities, changes in direction from left to center to right box steps, and hopping over boxes.

Resistance bands can be used to increase the resistance of rapid direction-change exercises. With the band attached to the waist, the patient can be required to jump to different targets on the floor, change directions of movement, and

alternate patterns of jumps. Examples of these exercises are presented in chapter 20.

Plyometrics

Once neuromotor control is achieved, the patient can advance to the very final phases of the rehabilitation program. Not everyone's programs will include plyometrics, but those whose normal activities dictate an inclusion of plyometrics will benefit from their use.

Plyometric exercises maximize the use of the patient's agility, strength, power, and coordination. Plyometric activities are added to the rehabilitation program when the patient demonstrates good control in rapid agility exercises and has good strength and enough flexibility to perform the exercises safely.

Plyometric exercises such as drop-jump activities, lateral jumps, and cone jumps can be used for all lower-extremity injuries, including hip injuries. These activities are discussed in chapter 15.

Functional and Performance-Specific Exercises

A variety of functional exercises can be included in hip rehabilitation. Some suggestions for functional exercises include squats, step exercises, lunges, lateral lunges, cariocas, and stair running. Some basic exercises in this category may be started in the resistive phase of the program, while others that are more performance-specific are better added in phase IV, the advanced phase.

The main factor in determining which performance-specific exercises to use in a hip program is the patient's sport and position within the sport or the patient's work demands. If the sport includes primarily running activities, then those types of activities are included in the functional and performance-specific program. If the patient's activity includes rapid changes of direction, acceleration, and deceleration, then the performance-specific portion of the program includes those activities. If the patient's activity demands include squatting and lifting heavy objects up ladders, then those are added to the performance-specific program.

Speed, distance, repetitions, and difficulty of the exercises are all incorporated at a low level at first and then are increased progressively as the patient's tolerance for additional stresses improves. As the patient achieves each goal that is set, the rehabilitation program provides a continuous progression of activities that precisely mimic the demands of the patient's normal activity, as long as pain and other deleterious signs or symptoms are avoided.

As with other phases of the program, exercises in this phase build upon one another. Short-term goals in this phase ultimately end with the final goal of returning the patient to normal activities. Whatever the normal activity involves, the clinician breaks down its components to devise a progressive program of accomplishment. For example, if the patient is a triple jumper in track, the first goals during this phase may include jogging, then running, then sprinting. Each of these subsections has short-term goals. Perhaps the rehabilitation clinician sets a goal of the patient jogging 2 mi (3.2 km) in 20 min; once that is achieved, the running goal may be running the same distance in 18 min, and then the sprinting goal is sprinting 100 m in 12 s.

Once the patient is working to achieve sprinting goals, the rehabilitation clinician may include jumping drills that progress in their goals for distance, repetitions, and speed while also including sprinting drills in the same treatment session. These performance-specific goals may take anywhere from a few days to several weeks to accomplish; the rate at which goals in the advanced phase are achieved depends on the sport, the level and complexity of required skills, the patient's abilities, the injury, and the length of time the patient has been away from the sport or from work.

The patient may return to normal participation once he or she is pain free; has normal strength, flexibility, and agility; performs equally on the left and right lower extremities without hesitating or favoring the involved extremity; and uses both lower extremities normally.

Special Rehabilitation Applications

Although hip injuries do not occur as often as knee and ankle injuries, they can be just as disabling, and they need proper rehabilitation if the patient is to return to normal activities.[45] Younger patients whose bones have not matured sustain more growth plate injuries in the hip than ligamen-tous or musculotendinous injuries.[46, 47] Over the past few years, research advances and improved surgical techniques have provided the health care world with a new understanding of hip pathologies.[48] We are learning more about hip anatomy and biomechanics and the role they play in hip injuries. Musculotendinous and bone injuries have been the primary concerns,[49] but as we learn more, we realize that the acetabular labrum is also a frequent cause of hip pain in athletes.[50] We are finding that structural dysfunctions may be responsible for many of the labral hip injuries.[51]

Hip-pain complaints usually occur with injuries, but they also sometimes occur without a frank injury to the hip. Hip pain without a specific injury can sometimes be difficult to interpret because of the various possible sources. Pain in the hip joint itself commonly refers to the groin, the anterior or medial proximal thigh, or the knee.[52] Spinal-based pain can refer to the anterior hip, buttock, or thigh.[53] Sacral pain can refer to the buttock or the posterior or lateral thigh.[54] Internal organs and the abdomen can refer pain to the groin.[55] When a patient complains of pain in these areas without a specific history of injury, the clinician must eliminate these locations as sources of hip pain.

An examination occurs before a patient's rehabilitation program is designed. As part of that examination, special tests should reproduce the patient's pain so that the clinician can make a correct diagnosis. If tests for these possibly referring segments do not reproduce the patient's pain, but the pain is reproduced with special tests to the hip joint, the clinician can deduce that the pain is hip related. Please see table 18.2 for a list of tests specific for the hip joint.

Muscle-Imbalance Syndromes

Many of the soft-tissue injuries around the pelvis, hip, and thigh result from muscle imbalances.[62] These syn-

TABLE 18.2 Commonly Used Special Tests of the Hip Joint

Site or structure tested	Special test (other names)	Sensitivity	Specificity
ITB tightness (traditional view)	Ober's test	Unknown	Unknown
Femoroacetabular impingement	FADIR (FAIR test)	59%[56]	100%[56]
		88%[57]	83%[57]
Hip joint pathology	FABER (Patrick's test)	41%[56]	100%[56]
		57%[58]	71%[58]
Labral pathology	Scour test	62%[58]	75%[58]
Gluteus medius weakness	Trendelenburg test	72%[59]	76%[59]
Hip flexor tightness	Thomas test (iliacus test or iliopsoas test)	Unknown	Unknown
Rectus femoris tightness	Ely's test	56-59%[60]	64-85%[60]
Labral pathology	Anterior impingement test	75%[61]	43%[61]
Piriformis tightness	Piriformis test	88%[57]	83%[57]

dromes are characterized by tightness of a muscle group and weakness of its antagonist and compensatory muscle firing patterns in adjacent areas.[63] The resulting symptoms typically include pain and reduced function and can cause structural changes over time. Changes in myofascial tissue are also commonly seen. Unfortunately, these problems are often not addressed until an injury occurs as a result of these imbalances.

Hip Flexor Tightness

This problem is observed during postural assessments of patients with excessive lumbar lordosis. Hip flexors are tight and restricted, and the antagonists, the hip extensors, are weak and inhibited.[64] This imbalance is characterized by an exaggerated anterior pelvic tilt and increased lumbar lordosis in standing.[65] If this sounds familiar, refer to the presentation in chapter 17 on lower crossed syndrome. Lower lumbar spine dysfunctions, including disc degeneration, spondylosis, spondylolysis, or spondylolisthesis can develop.[66] Myofascial restriction is common in the lumbar paraspinals, quadratus lumborum, and latissimus dorsi.[67]

Objective examination findings demonstrate a positive Thomas test for hip tightness. In prone, assessment of muscle firing during hip extension in these patients reveals an asynchronous pattern. The most recent evidence indicates that normal firing sequence in prone hip extension is initiated by the medial hamstrings; next, the contralateral and then ipsilateral erector spinae fire, and the gluteus maximus fires last.[68] Excessive hamstring muscle firing is seen as a compensation for weak, inhibited hip extensor muscles.[69] This hamstring overuse is demonstrated during a supine one-legged bridge; the supporting limb quickly experiences a muscle cramp in the hamstrings when the gluteus maximus is inhibited or weak.[69]

Hip flexor restriction requires correction of shortened muscles, myofascial release of restricted soft tissue, correction of posture, strengthening of the weak muscles, and muscle reeducation to facilitate correct muscle firing patterns. When the antagonistic muscles are weak secondary to agonistic muscle tightening, lengthening the tight muscles often has a significant positive impact on strength changes in the antagonists.[63] Neuromotor control exercises, pelvic stabilization activities, and strengthening lower abdominals for pelvic support provide a base for posture correction. The use of electrical stimulation and instruction in muscle firing sequence patterns, beginning with slow sequences and progressing to more rapid firing sequences and finally to functional activities, can be helpful in muscle reeducation.

Patient who can perform some of their normal activities should be cautioned that their skills may be affected as the muscle firing patterns change. This can be frustrating for someone who has adapted sport-skill performance to compensate for these muscle imbalances.

Piriformis Syndrome

Buttock and leg pain are the most distinguishing symptoms of piriformis syndrome.[70] Pain can radiate distally into the thigh and leg, mimicking a lumbar nerve root syndrome. Running, standing, or prolonged sitting can aggravate the piriformis. Clinical examination reveals tightness of the piriformis that is often accompanied by weakness. When the patient is relaxed in supine, the involved extremity is more laterally rotated than the contralateral limb. Palpation reveals tenderness, tension, and soft-tissue (fascial) restriction in the piriformis muscle.[67] Activities that involve hip flexion, medial rotation, or adduction stretch the piriformis and produce pain.[45] Active trigger points are often the source of pain referral into the lower extremity.[67] Sciatic nerve irritation that occurs when a tight piriformis presses on the nerve can also refer pain into the lower extremity.[71] The 12% to 15% of the population whose sciatic nerves pass through the piriformis muscle[72] are more susceptible to this condition as the source of referred lower extremity pain from the piriformis.

Athletes in sports such as skiing, ice skating, gymnastics, and dance are more prone to piriformis syndrome.[45] Common causes of piriformis syndrome include sacroiliac dysfunction; limb-length discrepancies; running on canted surfaces, which creates a false limb-length difference; and muscle imbalances, including tightness of the piriformis, hamstrings, and lateral thigh muscles.[73, 74]

Rehabilitation includes correcting the underlying causes, myofascial release and trigger point release techniques, stretching exercises for the piriformis and other tight muscles, and strengthening exercises for the weak muscles, including hip abductors and medial rotators. If a limb-length difference is the cause, inserting a heel lift in the shorter leg's shoe will relieve pain symptoms, but resolution of muscle imbalances should not be ignored. Patients can usually continue their normal activities during treatment. Piriformis syndrome is a self-limiting condition in that pain is the limiting factor to the patient's ability to perform.

Acute Soft-Tissue Injuries

Injuries in this category include sprains and strains. Traumatic bursitis can also come under this heading, but bursitis will be discussed as it relates to repetitive stress, its more common etiology.

Case Study

A 25-year-old distance runner presents with complaints of right buttock and posterior thigh pain that has become progressively worse over the past 3 weeks. He has recently increased his distance from 6.4 to 9.7 km (4 to 6 miles). The pain occurs about 4.8 km (3 miles) into his run and remains. The patient reports that when he gets up from his desk after sitting for about 45 min, his right buttock is painful until he walks around for a few minutes. He had a back injury about 5 years ago that was treated successfully, so he has not had any back problems since then. Standing trunk motions do not elicit pain in any direction. When he lies supine on the treatment table, his right leg is laterally rotated about 20° more than his left. Placing the hip in 60° of flexion, adduction, and medial rotation elicits pain in the right buttock. Straight-leg raise is to 70° and negative for sciatic pain. Palpation of the right buttock reveals tenderness in the mid-buttock region to deep pressure. You can feel tightness in the piriformis. Resisted hip lateral rotation in this position is painful. Hip rotation is weak.

Questions for Analysis

1. What do you suspect is his problem?
2. What other tests should you perform to eliminate any other possible cause of the patient's problem?
3. What will be your first treatment for him today?
4. What instructions for home treatments will you give him before he leaves today?
5. What will your goals for the first week of treatment include?
6. What will you tell the patient when he asks you if he can continue running?

Groin Strain

Groin strains occur often in sports, with hockey and soccer players being most susceptible to them.[75] Any of the six adductor muscles may be involved.[76] The involved muscle is injured when it is either brought beyond its normal limits of motion or produces a rapid, forceful contraction.[77] Premorbid contributing factors include muscle tightness, weakness, or imbalances.[78] As with other muscle strains, the injury is usually at the site of the musculotendinous junction; this strain can be disabling in moderate or severe cases.

Since other injuries may mimic groin strains, differential diagnoses must be eliminated. Other possible conditions include osteitis pubis, stress fractures, avulsion fractures, and sports hernias.[79]

The patient has an antalgic gait favoring the injured limb, with an uneven stride cadence, shortened stride length, and reduced knee and hip motion. Muscle spasm, swelling, and tenderness to palpation of the injury site can also be present. Ecchymosis occurs in second- and third-degree strains.

The rehabilitation examination of the injured muscle includes resisted muscle activity tests to determine which motion produces the greatest pain response. Hip flexion with knee extension tests the iliopsoas; hip flexion with knee flexion tests the rectus femoris; hip flexion, lateral rotation, and abduction with resisted knee flexion test the sartorius; and resisted hip adduction tests the adductors.

Treatment in the inactive phase includes modalities to control pain and reduce spasm. Electrical stimulation to reduce muscle spasm, followed by assistive active range of motion and active range of motion exercises, are used to regain lost range of motion as soon as possible. If the patient displays an antalgic gait, a cane or crutches are needed until he or she demonstrates a normal gait. A hip spica wrap supports the muscle and reduces range of motion during ambulation to make walking more comfortable. Instructing the patient to ambulate with a shorter stride also reduces pain during gait. Aquatic exercises and reciprocal-motion machines can be helpful once the active phase starts after postinjury day 2 or 3. The patient begins with isometric exercises on day 2 or 3 and makes a gradual transition to the resistive phase with progressive resistive exercises when the limb can be moved in antigravity positions without pain. Eccentric exercises are included early in the resistive phase.

Once the patient can transfer weight from one extremity to the other correctly, stork standing and progressive proprioception and neuromotor exercises are used to develop balance; these exercises later advance to dynamic balance and agility exercises. Treadmill activities begin when the patient walks normally without crutches. The treadmill progression starts first with walking, then jogging, and finally running. The rate of progression on the treadmill depends on where in the healing process the patient is and if the patient is pain free during the activities. Agility activities on the treadmill are used when the patient demonstrates good muscle control and range of motion with closed kinetic chain exercises toward the end of the resistive phase; these treadmill agility activities may include cariocas, walking backwards, and side shuffles. Soft-tissue massage is helpful in reducing scar tissue adhesions and stimulating blood flow to encourage healing after day 5 to 10, depending on the injury's severity and the extent of tissue damage.

As with hamstring injuries, groin strains have a high reinjury rate.[80] Clinically, these injuries recur when scar tissue adhesions, which occur as part of the healing process, are not properly managed during rehabilitation. You must be confident that the injury is healed before you allow the patient to return to full sports participation because premature return to sport can result in reinjury.[79]

Resistance-band jumping, box drills, and lateral movements begin when good dynamic balance and muscle control are present in the early advanced phase. As with other rehabilitation programs, the patient advances from these activities to plyometrics, then functional exercises, and finally performance-specific exercises before returning to full activity.

Depending on the severity of the injury, the patient's program may span from less than a week to several weeks. Before returning to normal activities, the patient moves through a series of performance-specific tests to determine his or her readiness to return pain free and without deficiencies in performance.

Sprains

Hip ligaments are relatively strong. The joint is stable because of its deep socket and strong ligamentous support, and it does not succumb easily to outside forces.[2] Hip ligaments are not often injured, but they can incur sprains when a violent injury involving severe forces occurs. During these injury events, the hip is usually moved suddenly into a position of either combined extreme flexion, abduction, and lateral rotation or combined extreme flexion, adduction, and medial rotation. Passive seated hip rotation is often painful and limited after a hip ligament sprain.

When hip ligaments are injured, grade I and II joint mobilizations can relieve pain. Since the hip joint is relatively deep, very few modalities can reach it effectively. Aquatic exercises using small arcs of motion are beneficial early in the program, with progressions in the size of the arc as the joint improves. Flexibility and strength rehabilitation progress according to healing and patient response to treatment through the rehabilitation phases, as in other hip rehabilitation programs.

Femoroacetabular Conditions

Because of advances in recognition and arthroscopic procedures, additional sources of hip pain in the athletic population have been identified.[81] These pathological conditions are related to joint structure and mechanics and lead not only to pain but to more potentially serious effects. Just as important, there is a wider range of treatment options, especially with a timely diagnosis. We will focus on femoroacetabular impingement and acetabular labral tears.

Femoroacetabular Impingement

Femoroacetabular impingement (FAI) occurs when the acetabulum and femur contact each other prematurely during hip motion.[82] The normal anatomical configuration of the acetabulum with its labrum and the head–neck femoral component of the hip joint provide for extensive range of motion within the joint (figure 18.42*a*). In femoroacetabular impingement, the pathology's source may be either the femoral head or the acetabulum. A *pincer impingement* exists when the acetabulum covers more of the femoral head than it should. This is called over-coverage (figure 18.42*b*), and it causes the anterosuperior aspect of the acetabulum to pinch the labrum between the acetabular rim and the femoral head–neck region during hip flexion.[83]

Evidence in Rehabilitation

In the early 2000s, Ganz headed a group of colleagues who first began presenting information on femoroacetabular impingement and surgical treatment for it.[91] Since then, surgical repair of FAI now occurs throughout the world, but randomized controlled trials (RCTs) comparing this technique to other treatments are lacking.[92]

Additionally, nonsurgical treatment, including rehabilitation programs, injections, medications, and pain-relieving efforts, have found success in the treatment of FAI. Unfortunately, these systems have also lacked RCTs to authenticate their effectiveness.[93] Only very recently has there been an RCT study that looked at the effectiveness of FAI treatment programs, but the researchers compared a nonoperative to an operative method of treatment.[94] Clearly, more RCTs are needed to identify the most effective and appropriate treatment options for FAI patients.

To that end, a group of medical and health care professionals at multiple sites throughout Australia are in the middle of a long-term study to investigate and study the outcomes of operative and nonoperative FAI treatment protocols. Based on their research design that was presented in 2017, they intend to investigate a number of outcome measures, such as changes in joint integrity, muscle activation patterns, gait motions and moments, quality of life, and satisfaction outcomes. This is obviously a huge undertaking, but it is needed to help us further understand and ultimately achieve optimal management for FAI. Their results are likely to be anxiously awaited by health care professionals who are currently involved in the treatment of femoroacetabular impingement.

The other, more common, condition is the *cam impingement*.[84] Cam impingement occurs because the anterior–superior aspect of the femoral head–neck junction is aspherical (like a cam), with either a flattened or a convex contour, not its normal concave configuration (figure 18.42c);[85] this feature of the anterosuperior aspect of the femoral head makes premature contact with the acetabulum and labrum in motions that combine flexion and rotation in activities such as squatting.[86]

Often there is a combination of both of these anatomical variations with one condition predominant over the other (figure 18.42d).[82] Cam impingement is more often seen in young adult male athletes, while pincer impingement is more common in middle-aged and older females.[87] Femoroacetabular impingement has been shown to be a common cause of hip surgery in athletes in recent years.[88] Since the presence of femoroacetabular impingement has been identified as a major cause of articular damage and early osteophyte formation and osteoarthritis of the hip,[89] early recognition and intervention using corrective surgery seems to be the current preferred means of reducing the risk of these degenerative changes later in life.[85, 90]

A common history includes insidious onset of groin pain.[51] It may or may not have been preceded by an injury, and patients report intermittent pain at first but more frequent episodes with time. Patients with femoroacetabular impingement present with groin pain during extensive hip movements or when sitting in a low chair, putting on shoes and socks, or moving in and out of a car.[95] Reduced medial rotation of the hip and pain with passive combined flexion and medial rotation of the hip are additional positive findings.[95]

In the past several years, arthroscopic surgery rather than open surgery has become a popular method of correcting cam and pincer impingement pathologies.[88] One of the main advantages of arthroscopic procedures over the

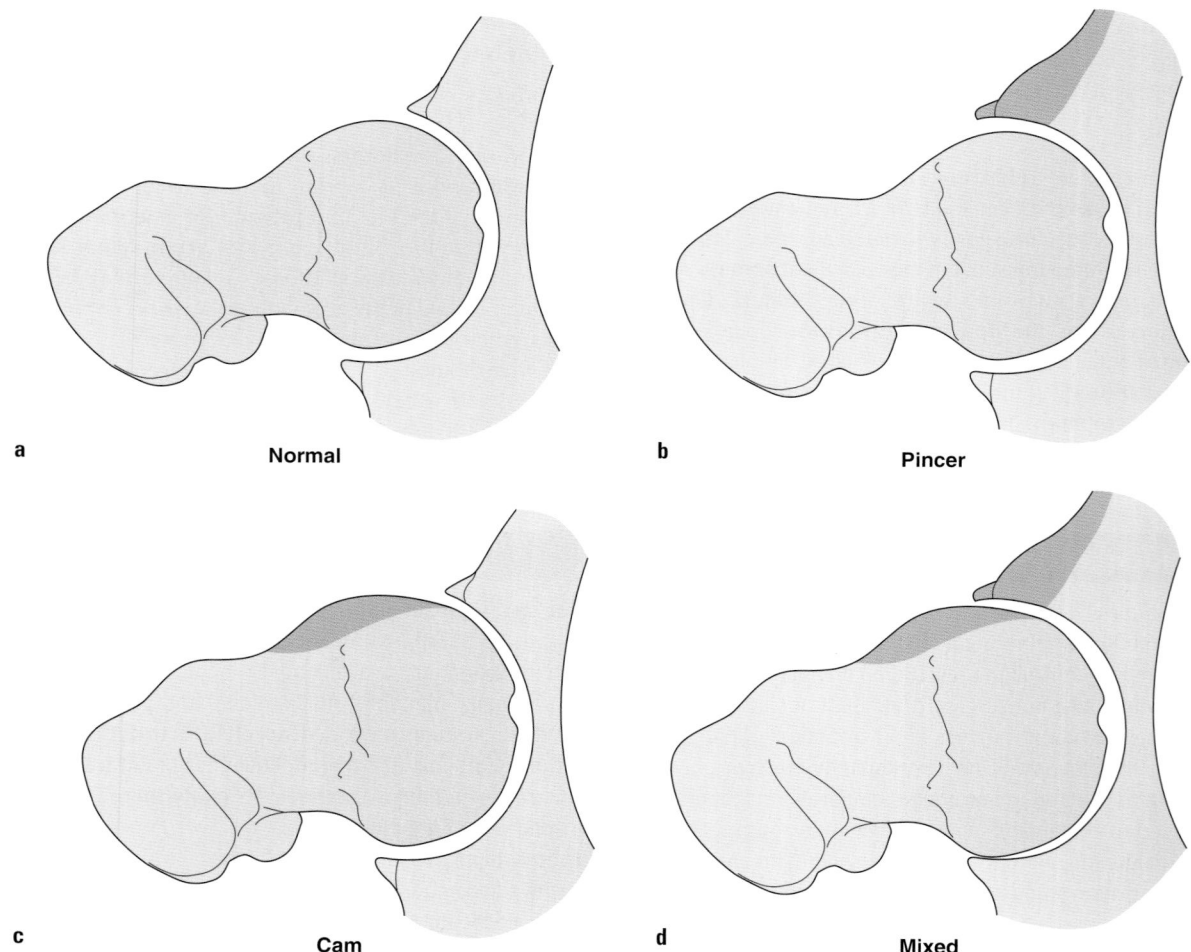

Figure 18.42 Configuration of the femoroacetabular joint. *(a)* Normal femur and acetabulum. *(b)* Pincer impingement between the femur and acetabulum occurs when the acetabulum covers more of the femoral head than it should. *(c)* Cam impingement occurs as a result of the femoral head being aspherical or the junction between the femoral head and neck being either flat or convex. *(d)* A combination of pincer and cam impingements is also seen.

open surgical approach is that the hip is not dislocated—a step often taken in the open surgical procedure[96]—so postoperative range-of-motion precautions required with surgical dislocation are not needed.[81] Goals of this arthroscopic surgery are to shave the bony elements that are causing the impingement while preserving the soft-tissue elements of the joint with special attention paid to the acetabular labrum.[97]

Postoperative rehabilitation for these arthroscopic procedures varies and depends on clinician and surgeon preferences, which are based on their experiences and the limited evidence currently available. The rehabilitation progression provided here is an amalgamation of available resources[81, 97-99] and personal professional experience with these postoperative patients. How rapidly a patient progresses through the rehabilitation program depends upon the extensiveness of the surgery, the tissues involved and the procedures performed, and the patient's response to both surgery and rehabilitation.

One of the main concerns after arthroscopic osteoplasty to correct FAI is avoiding excessive stress to the surgical site; excessive forces in this area pose a fracture risk.[100] This means that weight bearing and extreme motions in flexion, abduction, and lateral rotation are restricted for the first 3 to 6 weeks.[99, 100] Since bone remodeling takes 3 months, high-impact activities such as jumping and rotational activities are avoided during this time.[100]

The inactive phase of rehabilitation begins at postoperative day 1 with goals to protect the surgical site, relieve secondary effects of surgery (e.g., effusion, edema, pain, spasm) and prevent deconditioning of the unaffected body segments. If a continuous passive motion machine is used after surgery, it is used 2 to 6 h daily during the first 2 weeks.[99] A postoperative brace is sometimes used from 10 d to 4 weeks.[81] The purpose of the brace is to limit the hip's sagittal plane range of motion from either neutral or slight hyperextension to 80° to 90° of flexion. Weight bearing is initially limited to partial or toe-touch weight bearing.[81] Gait training may be needed if the patient cannot ambulate normally using crutches with these weight-bearing restrictions. Passive range of motion for the first 2 weeks is limited to hip rotation that is performed in 30° of hip flexion while supine, hip abduction to 15°, and passive hip medial and lateral rotation pain free in the prone position.[101] The patient is encouraged to lie prone at times throughout the day to prevent hip flexion contractures. A stationary bike without resistance can begin within the first postoperative week. Isometric exercises for all hip motions begin on day 2 with the hip in neutral.

Active range of motion begins in the active phase about 2 weeks after surgery. Once the surgical site is healed, aquatic exercises and gait training are added. Weight bearing progresses to full weight bearing by postoperative weeks 6 to 8. Gait training may be needed for the patient to ambulate normally with each progressive change in weight bearing. Early strengthening exercises before weight bearing begin during this phase. Open kinetic chain exercises such as clam abduction with resistive bands; quadriceps, hamstring, and gastrocnemius resistive exercises; and core exercises are important during this time.

When the patient is full weight bearing, the resistive phase begins with the use of greater resistive exercises; this is about week 8. Stretching for hip motion gains also begins, so the patient has full motion by about weeks 8 to 10. Bridging, planks, and other closed-chain exercises for the core are used in this phase. Balance exercise progressions begin once the patient is full weight bearing. Single-plane hip-strengthening exercises begin with high repetitions and low resistance and progress as tolerated.[97] Leg press, partial squats, heel raises, lunges, lateral lunges, and step-ups are also used in this phase. During open- and closed-chain exercises, sagittal plane hip range of motion during exercises remains restricted to no more than 90°. Particular emphasis is placed on strengthening hip extensors.[97] All exercises should be pain free.

The advanced rehabilitation phase occurs after 3 months and prepares the patient for normal activities. Multiplanar exercises are used in this phase, along with agility drills. Plyometric exercises may be used later in this phase. The final segment of this phase includes evolving from functional activities to performance-specific exercises. Once the patient successfully completes these exercises, the clinician does preparticipation testing to assess the patient's readiness to return to normal activities. The complete rehabilitation process may take up to 6 months.[97] Figure 18.43 illustrates this rehabilitation progression for postoperative femoroacetabular impingement.

Acetabular Labral Tears

Although acetabular labral lesions were once thought to be rare injuries, recent advances in diagnostic imaging have revealed the frequency of these incidents, especially in sports.[102, 103] The acetabular labrum is an integral structure that adds to the joint's functional stability.[104] Labral lesions lead to instability of the joint and early osteoarthritic changes.[105] The labrum is also important for proprioception and may help to distribute synovial fluid throughout the joint.[106] Labral lesions are often associated with femoroacetabular impingement.[89, 107] They are also the most common cause of mechanical symptoms such as painful clicking and locking or giving way in the hip.[108] When the anterior labrum is torn, pain increases with hip extension.[109]

The injury mechanisms for acetabular tears include repetitive pivoting, twisting, and cutting maneuvers in flexed hip positions.[103, 110] Either capsular laxity or FAI also occur because of these mechanisms.[111] Impingement occurs in the anterior and superior aspect of the hip as the femur moves closer to the acetabular rim,[112] so hip flexion

Femoroacetabular Impingement

	Stage I: Passive phase
0-3 weeks	**Inflammation phase: Passive rehabilitation phase**
Goals	Relieve pain. Reduce edema, effusion, ecchymosis. Relieve spasm. Protect surgical site. For first 2 weeks: Limit hip flexion to 30° with rotation, hip abduction limited to 15°. Prevent deconditioning of unaffected body segments.
Treatment guidelines	CPM machine first 2 weeks Electrical stimulation for pain, muscle spasm First 3-6 weeks: PWB; gait training PRN ROM exercises for knee and ankle muscle groups. Full hip rotation in prone Day 2: OKC exercises: quad set, hamstring set, hip isometrics, ankle strengthening Day 2: Stationary bike without resistance for hip ROM only Weeks 1-2: PROM in supine = abduction to 15°; supine hip rotation in 30° hip flexion; prone rotation pain free Week 2: AROM Week 2: Aquatic exercises and weight shifting, gait training in water Exercises for unaffected body segments HEP for pain, edema; prone lying during the day to maintain hip extension
Precautions	Encourage proper gait with PWB on crutches. Protect surgical repair. Encourage passive hip extension. All activities are pain free.
	Stage II: Active phase
3-6 weeks	**Early proliferation phase: Active rehabilitation phase**
Goals	No pain, edema, spasm. Weeks 2-4: Remove brace. Weeks 6-8: Full weight bearing without brace or crutches. After week 2: Full PROM of hip. Normal gait.
Treatment guidelines	Weeks 6-8: Gait training without crutches Week 3: Begin gentle active stretching exercises; start with hamstrings and progress as tolerated Stationary bike continues Balance activities when FWB Week 3: OKC exercises = clams, resistive-band exercises for quadriceps, hamstrings, gastrocnemius, core muscles HEP: Isometrics; AROM
Precautions	Avoid hip pain with exercises. Avoid extreme hip flexion and hip abduction. Do not use home exercises as treatment session exercises.

Figure 18.43   Example of rehabilitation progression for postoperative femoroacetabular impingement.

Stage III: Resistive phase

6-12 weeks	Late proliferation phase: Resistive rehabilitation phase
Goals	No pain, edema, spasm. Weeks 6-8: Full weight bearing. Weeks 8-10: Normal ROM. Increase strength of all deficient muscles and muscle groups. Normal gait.
Treatment guidelines	Weeks 6-8: Gait training without crutches Joint mobilizations, soft-tissue mobilizations PRN Increased balance, coordination activities Resistive exercises start with high repetitions, low resistance; remain pain free throughout all exercises Weeks 8-10: CKC exercises: bridging, planks, mini-squats, leg press, wall squats, heel raises, lunges, lateral lunges, step-ups HEP for strength gains; ROM
Precautions	Avoid hip pain with exercises. Use weight-scale exercises if weight transfer is incorrect. Resistive exercises: Limited to 90° of hip flexion. Place emphasis on hip extensor strengthening. Do not use home exercises during treatment sessions.

Stage IV: Advanced phase

12-32 weeks	Remodeling phase: Advanced rehabilitation phase
Goals	Maintain normal strength of all muscles. Maintain normal ROM of all joints. Normal sport and work performance.
Treatment guidelines	Plyometric exercises Functional exercise progression Performance-specific exercises and drills progression
Precautions	Correct performance PRN.

CPM = continuous passive motion; PWB = partial weight bearing; FWB = full weight bearing; ROM = range of motion; PROM = passive range of motion; AROM = active range of motion; PRN = as needed; HEP = home exercise program.

Figure 18.43 >continued

combined with rotation or twisting movements creates a simultaneous stress on the labrum during moments when it is pinched.

Surgical treatment of these labral tears is the treatment of choice.[88] Open surgical procedures are being replaced by more popular arthroscopic techniques for either debridement or repair of the labrum.[88] Because of the acetabular labrum's important role in hip joint stability, there is a growing emphasis on repairing the labrum rather than resecting the lesion.[113, 114]

If additional pathology exists, the surgeon will perform other procedures besides the arthroscopic acetabular labral repair. It is common to find FAI pathology that requires excision of bony pathology.[115] It is also common that

capsular laxity requires surgical repair during the labral procedure.[116] When additional procedures such as these are undertaken, additional postoperative precautions may be needed, especially during the early rehabilitation process. It is important to communicate with the surgeon to learn what procedure was performed and to learn the surgeon's protocol for precautions and progressions.

Postoperative rehabilitation after acetabular labral repair includes immediate protection of the surgical site. These efforts include weight-bearing restrictions and range-of-motion limits on rotation, flexion, and extension because these motions, based on the locations of most labral tears, typically add stress to the surgical site.[115] The duration of weight-bearing restrictions ranges from 2 to 6 weeks, depending on the size and location of the repair, and they start with partial or toe-touch weight bearing (about 20% of body weight).[108, 115] The surgeon must communicate the specific locations of the labral tears so the clinician avoids the motions that stress the surgical repair. During this initial phase, efforts to relieve the inflammatory effects of surgery also occur. Isometric exercises start a day or two after surgery. Early activation of core muscles along with the gluteals, deep hip rotators, hamstrings, and quadriceps begins as well.[115] A CPM machine is often used for the first 2 weeks after surgery to reduce pain and promote healing.[115] As with FAI surgery, a hip brace is worn for the first 2 weeks with hip flexion limited to motions within a 0° to 90° range.

Passive range-of-motion exercises in the inactive phase occur within the first week and include activities such as towel slides, piriformis stretch, and rocking forward and backward in a quadruped position while staying within the hip flexion limits allowed during this time.[117] With the patient prone, medial and lateral hip rotations can also be performed. All range-of-motion exercises should be pain free. Passive range-of-motion activities during this time help reduce the risk of capsular adhesions and encourage synovial motion to improve nutrition into the joint.[108] These passive motions include medial hip rotation and circumduction in supine and medial and lateral hip rotation in prone.[118]

Gentle joint mobilizations are also useful during this time to maintain mobility between the hip capsule and the acetabular labrum.[117] Along with hip motions, ankle pumps and knee flexion–extension motions should be used and are good exercises to include as part of the home exercise program. The patient should also be encouraged to lie prone throughout the day to prevent joint adhesions in flexion from occurring.

Isometric exercises begin on postoperative day 2 for the knee muscle groups and hip muscles.[118] Ankle resistive exercises can also start at this time, along with core activities. The patient begins using an upright stationary bike without resistance to encourage hip range of motion. The seat should be adjusted to allow no more than 90° of hip flexion.[119]

Within the second week after surgery, the patient can ambulate in the pool. Careful instruction on proper gait and weight transfer from right to left during pool ambulation will enhance the patient's ability to ambulate with crutches on land. After the third week, other exercises and jogging in the water can begin.

By the time the patient enters the active phase after the second week, pain, spasm, and edema should be resolved. The patient discards the brace after the second to fourth week. Around weeks 6 to 7, the patient achieves full knee extension without an extensor lag and can ambulate normally; at this point the crutches can be discarded. The patient may need instruction in proper ambulation if he or she cannot walk normally. Soft-tissue and joint mobilization continue in this phase to restore full mobility to the hip and its surrounding structures. Early neuromotor control activities can be initiated at this stage of healing. Active stretching exercises are added to the home exercise program once the patient demonstrates good exercise execution during treatment sessions. Side-lying hip abduction, extension, and adduction exercises in antigravity positions begin in week 3, along with jogging in the pool. Once the patient is full weight bearing, balance and other early neuromotor activities are added to the program. Resistive-band exercises for the knee and ankle and clam exercises for the hip also begin at week 3. Early resistance exercises for hip abduction and flexion occur during week 4 as long as they do not cause hip pain.

The resistive stage introduces more resistive exercises for the hip. During this phase, normal gait and full range of motion of the hip must occur if they haven't yet. More aggressive stretching exercises for hip flexors and adductors begin in weeks 6 to 8 but should cause no hip pain; the patient should feel the stretch in the muscles, not the joint. Single-limb balance activities give way to more difficult balance and coordination exercises. Closed kinetic chain exercises for the lower extremity include slide board activities, wall squats, heel raises, mini-squats, and leg presses. Open-chain exercises for the hip include resistive medial and lateral rotation in sitting. Resistance-band exercises for all hip motions, squats, lunges, side-walking with a resistance band, step-ups, and bridging can be used to increase hip strength. Resistive exercises begin with high repetitions and low resistance and progress as tolerated to increased resistance.[97] Strength exercises become more progressive as tolerated by the patient. Once the hip strength reaches 75%, jogging can begin, along with early agility exercises and triplanar activities. Agility exercises such as sport-cord resisted walking exercises, jogging on the treadmill, and low-level jumps on a padded surface are used in this phase. The home exercise program should include both strengthening and stretching exercises.

Once the final rehabilitation phase—the advanced phase—begins, the patient has no pain, full motion, and 85% of normal strength. By week 12 the patient is sprinting, performing functional rotational activities, and performing a variety of plyometric exercises. These plyometric exercises may begin with easy activities such as rope jumping and then progress to more functional plyometric exercises that are designed and based upon the skill requirements of the patient's normal activities. From these exercises, the patient progresses through a series of performance-specific exercises that mimic the skills and demands placed upon the patient during normal activities. This aspect of the rehabilitation program is designed by the rehabilitation clinician and includes performance-specific exercises the patient must perform once he or she returns to normal function. Once the patient passes the tests used in the final examination and assessment and all goals are achieved, the patient can safely return to normal activities. Figure 18.44 illustrates this program in a condensed version.

Acetabular Labrum Repair

Stage I: Passive phase	
0-2 weeks	**Inflammation phase: Passive rehabilitation phase**
Goals	Relieve pain.
	Reduce edema, effusion, ecchymosis.
	Relieve spasm.
	Protect surgical site.
	Early hip motion.
	After week 2: Full PROM of hip.
	Prevent deconditioning of unaffected body segments.
Treatment guidelines	CPM machine first 10-14 days
	Electrical stimulation for pain, muscle spasm
	First 2-6 weeks: PWB; gait training PRN
	First week: Easy PROM exercises for hip without pain: towel slides, piriformis stretch, quadruped rocking forward–backward, medial and lateral rotation with hip in neutral and within motion restrictions
	Manual PROM exercises for hip medial rotation and circumduction; medial and lateral rotation in prone; all motions pain free
	AROM exercises for knee and ankle muscle groups
	Full hip rotation in prone
	Day 2: OKC exercises: quad set, hamstring set, hip isometrics, ankle strengthening
	Day 2: Stationary bike without resistance for hip ROM only
	Day 2: Isometric exercises for hip abductors and extensors
	Week 2: Aquatic exercises and weight shifting, gait training in water
	Week 2: Distraction joint mobilizations
	Exercises for unaffected body segments
	HEP for pain, edema; prone lying during the day to maintain hip extension
Precautions	Encourage proper gait with PWB on crutches.
	Protect surgical repair.
	Limit hip flexion to 90° flexion, 0° extension, 25° abduction.
	Lie prone for several minutes throughout the day.
	All activities are pain free.
Stage II: Active phase	
2-6 weeks	**Early proliferation phase: Active rehabilitation phase**
Goals	No pain, edema, spasm.
	Weeks 2-4: No brace.
	Weeks 6-8: Full weight bearing without brace or crutches.
	Week 6: Full ROM.
	Normal gait.

Figure 18.44   Rehabilitation progression for postoperative acetabular labrum repair.   >continued

Stage II: Active phase	
2-6 weeks	**Early proliferation phase: Active rehabilitation phase**
Treatment guidelines	Weeks 6-7: Gait training without crutches when no extensor lag and normal gait Weight scale weight-shift exercises PRN Soft-tissue mobilization PRN Week 4: Joint mobilization for flexion, extension, medial, and lateral rotation Week 3: Begin gentle active stretching exercises; start with hamstrings and progress as tolerated Week 3: Full PROM Week 3: Antigravity exercises for hip abduction, adduction, and extension Weeks 3-4: Aquatic jogging Stationary bike continues without resistance Balance activities when FWB Week 3: OKC exercises = clams, resistance-band exercises for quadriceps, hamstrings, gastrocnemius, core muscles Week 4: Begin easy hip flexor and hip abductor resistance exercises HEP: isometrics; hip stretching
Precautions	Avoid hip pain with exercises. Do not use home exercises as treatment session exercises.

Stage III: Resistive phase	
6-12 weeks	**Late proliferation phase: Resistive rehabilitation phase**
Goals	No pain, edema, spasm. Weeks 6-8: Full weight bearing. Weeks 6-8: Normal ROM. Increase strength of all deficient muscles and muscle groups to 85%. Normal gait.
Treatment guidelines	Weeks 6-8: Gait training PRN Weeks 6-8: Emphasize stretching exercises for hip flexors and adductors Joint mobilizations, soft-tissue mobilizations PRN Increased balance, coordination activities Resistive exercises start with high repetitions, low resistance; remain pain free throughout all exercises Weeks 5-6: OKC and CKC exercises: planks; 3-way hip machine (no flexion); resisted medial and lateral rotation in sitting; wall squats; heel raises; lunges; lateral lunges; step-ups; slide board; and bridging, mini-squats, and leg press starting with two-limb and moving to one-limb resistance Week 6: Aquatic exercise; freestyle swimming Weeks 8-12: Jogging Weeks 10-12: Early agility activities Weeks 10-12: Triplanar exercises HEP for strength gains; ROM
Precautions	Avoid hip pain with exercises. Resistive exercises: Limited to 90° of hip flexion. Place emphasis on hip extensor strengthening. Do not use home exercises during treatment sessions.

Figure 18.44 >continued

Stage IV: Advanced phase	
12-32 weeks	**Remodeling phase: Advanced rehabilitation phase**
Goals	Normal strength of all muscles. Maintain normal ROM of all joints. Normal sport and work performance.
Treatment guidelines	Week 12: Functional rotational activities Weeks 12-16: Sprinting Plyometric exercises Functional exercise progression Performance-specific exercises and drills progression
Precautions	Correct performance PRN.

CPM = continuous passive motion; PWB = partial weight bearing; ROM = range of motion; PROM = passive range of motion; AROM = active range of motion; PRN = as needed; OKC = open kinetic chain; CKC = closed kinetic chain; HEP = home exercise program.

Figure 18.44 *>continued*

Total Hip Arthroplasty

A common surgical procedure for the hip is the total hip arthroplasty (THA), which is often referred to as a hip replacement, or total hip replacement (THR). The average age of a THA patient is 66,[120] although the procedure is performed on patients younger than 30 years old and as young as 11 years old with promising outcomes.[121] Many patients who have undergone THR return to sports activity.[122] Therefore, clinicians must understand the rehabilitation protocol to safely progress their patients toward the resumption of performance and work tasks.

For many reasons, a patient's hip joint may degenerate to the point that the best option to reduce pain and improve function is a THA. Degenerative joint disease (DJD), including primary osteoarthritis and secondary arthritis, is not only one of many reasons a patient may require a THA;[123] it is the primary reason total hip replacements are performed.[124] Research indicates another one of the causes of DJD is an FAI,[125] which was discussed earlier in this section. Osteoarthritis (OA) has several causes, including genetics, previous injury, age, and activity.[126] Independent of the reasons necessitating a patient's THA, it is the responsibility of the rehabilitation clinician to progress the patient through the physician's post-surgical protocol, observe precautions, and safely implement a rehabilitation program so the patient can return to optimal function.

Since 1962 when Sir Charnley of England surgically inserted the first human total hip joint replacement, many iterations of those first artificial joints have come and gone.[127] Likewise, changes in the surgical techniques have also evolved over the years.[128]

Since there are now a number of options available to surgeons, both in hardware and in surgical procedures, different surgeons may have different rehabilitation protocols they want clinicians to follow. Although physi-

cian preferences may vary in the details, there are many similarities between protocols. These days, patients will often be allowed weight bearing as tolerated (WBAT). Weight bearing is usually started postoperatively with either crutches or a walker and advances to ambulation without assistive devices as the patient progresses in the rehabilitation program. See chapter 7 for further discussion of how to properly use assistive devices.

Most THA rehabilitation protocols have an initial phase of soft-tissue management, wound care, and range of motion for the newly replaced hip. Around weeks 3 to 4, most protocols expand the exercises to include activities such as stationary bike, neuromotor control, and general strength for the muscles surrounding the hip. Weaning off the assistive device starts around 3 to 4 weeks after surgery, which is when the strengthening program is accelerated as the patient tolerates it. By the time the patient reaches the final phases of rehabilitation, normal gait, balance, strength, and mobility are restored. During the advanced phase, the patient then prepares for return to either sport, work, or normal functional activities. The rehabilitation protocol for a THA will have slight variations, particularly in the inactive and initial active phases, but the general progression will be similar to figure 18.45.

The primary concern in the inactive and early active phases of rehabilitation is to observe hip precautions. Hip precautions depend on the type of surgery performed.[129] For a posterior surgical approach for the THA, the patient must avoid hip flexion greater than 90°, avoid hip adduction past the midline, and avoid hip medial rotation beyond neutral. When the surgeon uses an anterior approach to perform the THA, the patient must avoid hip extension and lateral rotation beyond neutral and should not lie prone. If the surgeon selects a lateral THA approach, the patient must avoid moving the hip into extension beyond midline

Total Hip Replacement Rehabilitation Protocol

Stage I: Inactive phase	
0-1 week	**Inflammation phase: Inactive rehabilitation phase**
Goals	Relieve pain. Reduce edema, effusion, ecchymosis. Relieve spasm. Protect surgical site. Limit hip flexion motion to 90°. Prevent deconditioning of unaffected body segments.
Treatment guidelines	Modalities for pain and swelling relief Educate patient on hip precautions CPM machine first 2 weeks Electrical stimulation for pain, muscle spasm Weight bearing: As tolerated with assistive devices; gait training PRN ROM exercises for knee and ankle muscle groups AROM hip rotation in prone Day 2: OKC exercises: quad set, hamstring set, hip isometrics, ankle strengthening, AAROM in hip-knee flexion (heel slides) and in hip abduction as tolerated Week 1: Stationary bike without resistance for hip ROM only Week 2: AROM hip motions Week 2: Aquatic exercises and weight shifting, gait training in water Exercises for unaffected body segments HEP for pain, edema; prone lying during the day to maintain hip extension
Precautions	Encourage proper gait with WBAT on crutches or walker. Protect surgical repair. All activities should be pain free. For specific surgical approaches: (a) Posterior: Avoid hip flexion >90°; no medial rotation; no adduction past midline. (b) Anterior: Limit passive motions in extension, lateral rotation to midline; OK to move into extension or lateral rotation actively, but no passive motion. (c) Lateral: No extension with lateral rotation for 6 weeks.
Stage II: Active phase	
2-4 weeks	**Early proliferation phase: Active rehabilitation phase**
Goals	Continue to relieve pain, edema, spasm. Increase ROM while respecting precautions. Begin strength exercises. Weeks 2-4: Achieve full weight bearing. Achieve normal gait.
Treatment guidelines	Weeks 2-3: Gait training without crutches or walker, advancing to a cane Weeks 2-3: Soft-tissue mobilization PRN Week 3: Begin gentle active stretching exercises; start with hamstrings and progress as tolerated Stationary bike continues Balance activities when FWB Weeks 2-3: OKC exercises = clams, resistive-band exercises for quadriceps, hamstrings, gastrocnemius, core muscles; hamstring curls, heel raises, mini-squats, large arc quads, marching in place HEP: Hip isometrics; AROM

Figure 18.45   Total hip replacement rehabilitation protocol.

Stage II: Active phase	
2-4 weeks	**Early proliferation phase: Active rehabilitation phase**
Precautions	Avoid hip pain with exercises. Avoid extreme hip flexion, extension, and abduction. Do not use HEP exercises as clinic treatment session exercises.
Stage III: Resistive phase	
3-12 weeks	**Mid- and late proliferation phase: Resistive rehabilitation phase**
Goals	Reach a condition of no pain, edema, or spasm. Weeks 3-4: Achieve full weight bearing without assistive devices. Weeks 6-8: Achieve normal ROM. Increase strength of all deficient muscles and muscle groups. Improve balance and muscle firing through proprioceptive and neuromotor training. Achieve normal gait.
Treatment guidelines	Weeks 4-5: Easy walking program to begin as part of HEP Weeks 6-8: Gait training without crutches, walker, or cane PRN Joint mobilizations, soft-tissue mobilizations PRN Increased neuromotor and activities: Single-leg stance on hard, soft surfaces, eyes open, eyes closed, advancing to distracting activities during balance, dynamic balance activities Functional exercises: sit to stand, stairs, total body activities Resistive exercises start with high repetitions, low resistance; remain pain free throughout all exercises; body weight resistance exercises Weeks 6-10: CKC exercises: bridging, planks, mini-squats, leg press, wall squats, heel raises, lunges, lateral lunges, step-ups, resisted abduction, walking for distance Weeks 9-12: Multiplanar activities HEP for strength gains; ROM
Precautions	Avoid hip pain with exercises. Use weight-scale exercises if weight transfer is incorrect. Resistive exercises should be limited to 90° of hip flexion. Place emphasis on hip extensor strengthening. Do not use home exercises during treatment sessions.
Stage IV: Advanced phase	
12-32 weeks	**Remodeling phase: Advanced rehabilitation phase**
Goals	Maintain normal strength of all muscles. Maintain normal ROM of all joints. Achieve normal sport and work performance.
Treatment guidelines	Plyometric exercises Functional exercise progression: walking, elliptical, cycling, low-impact aerobics, Tai Chi, resisted weight machines Performance-specific exercises and drills progression
Precautions	Correct performance PRN.

ROM = range of motion; FWB = full weight bearing; WBAT = weight bearing as tolerated; LE = lower extremity; PRN = as needed; HEP = home exercise program; CKC = closed kinetic chain; AROM = active range of motion; OKC = open kinetic chain.

Figure 18.45 *>continued*

or lying prone and should avoid laterally rotating the hip. These hip precautions protect the surgical site from either disruption of the surgical scar or dislocation of the joint. The patient is usually instructed to adhere to these precautions for 4 to 6 weeks, but exactly how long they should be observed is debated.[130-133]

Other Conditions

The following are typically overuse injuries; they occur when repetitive stresses are applied so often that the body does not have time to recover. Among the conditions that fall into this category are bursitis, tendinopathy, and osteitis.

Bursitis

The most common bursitis in the hip is greater trochanteric bursitis, but other bursae surrounding the hip are also subject to irritation.[45] If the patient's symptoms persist in spite of treatment efforts, other diagnoses must be considered. Additional diagnoses that should be ruled out include lumbar disc injury, facet syndrome, fracture, nerve entrapment, inguinal hernia, abdominal visceral diseases, hip joint disease, and bone tumors. Additional diagnoses for males are testicular torsion and chronic prostatitis.

Two forms of bursitis in the hip region will be briefly described. Since any form of hip bursitis is essentially treated the same way, one program that is easily adapted for individual cases is presented after the two examples are described.

Greater Trochanteric Bursitis   The greater trochanteric bursa is susceptible to bursitis when the patient's running mechanics increase stress on the bursa; common causes include either a greater-than-normal adduction angle or running on a canted surface. Muscle imbalance between adductors and abductors, an increased Q-angle, limb-length discrepancy, and a wider pelvis are also precipitating causes for trochanteric bursitis.[134] Falling on the lateral hip can cause a traumatic bursitis. Pain in the lateral hip can radiate distally down the thigh or proximally into the lateral buttock. There is pain with lying on the involved side and crossing the legs, as well as when running or walking.

Iliopectineal Bursitis   Dancers and skaters are the athletes who most commonly experience iliopectineal bursitis, although it can occur in most sports. The iliopectineal bursa lies superficial to the anterior acetabulum and deep to the iliopsoas tendon. Sudden flexion–extension activities, especially resisted motions, can aggravate the bursa. The bursa lies adjacent to the femoral nerve and may irritate the nerve if the bursa becomes painful and swollen. Pain occurs with either stretch or contraction of the iliopsoas muscle. The pain is located at the bursa site in the inguinal area, but pain can also radiate into the hip, anterior thigh, or knee if the femoral nerve is also affected.[135]

Rehabilitation for patients diagnosed with hip bursitis commonly include ultrasound and thermal modalities.[136] Correction of underlying causes such as running mechanics and running surfaces is necessary and arguably the most

Case Study

A 16-year-old sprinter injured her left hip when she was practicing 3 d ago. She has continued pain in the proximal inner thigh with some discoloration along the middle aspect of the inner thigh. Pain prevents a normal gait. Your examination reveals hip abduction to 20°, limited by pain. The patient cannot adduct the hip against gravity. Hip flexion is 4/5 and painful but is not as tender as adduction. The inner thigh area feels tight and is tender to palpation from the middle thigh to the groin.

Questions for Analysis

1. What do you suspect is the patient's injury?
2. What other differential diagnosis tests will you do?
3. What will her treatment today include?
4. What instructions for home care will you give her today?
5. Outline the progression of the rehabilitation program you will provide for this patient. What modalities will you use on her, and why?
6. Once her scar tissue is mature, what manual technique will you use to reduce the risk of reinjury once she returns to sprinting?

The examination reveals tenderness to palpation over the greater trochanter, pain to direct pressure over the trochanter, pain with hip rotation, and tightness of the ITB as demonstrated with a positive Ober's test. Resisted abduction is tender because of the pressure placed on the bursa by the contracting muscles. Passive hip flexion with adduction and medial rotation press the bursa against the greater trochanter and cause irritation. The patient may stand with the involved extremity more abducted or may place more weight on the contralateral extremity to reduce pressure on the bursa.

important treatment step in reducing the risk of recurrence. Anti-inflammatory medications may be prescribed by a physician. Cross-friction massage reduces adhesions and pain.[137] Part of the home exercise program includes daily self-administered deep massage or myofascial treatment on a foam roller or other soft-tissue treatment device. Therapeutic exercises should include stretching exercises to increase the flexibility of tight muscles and strengthening to correct muscle imbalances. Since these injuries are nonacute, there is no inactive phase of rehabilitation, so exercises to correct deficiencies may begin soon after diagnosis. The one exception to this would be if the patient reports significant pain with activity.

Each step of the rehabilitation program follows the normal logical progression and stays within the patient's pain tolerance. Bursitis is self-limiting, and although activity modification may be helpful, total cessation of activity is left to the discretion of the rehabilitation clinician or the physician. Total activity restriction depends on factors such as the severity of the injury, the type of activity, the intensity of participation, and the required correction of mechanics.

Tendinopathy

The adductor longus, iliopsoas, and rectus femoris tendons are the most common sites of tendinopathy at the hip. Mechanisms of injury relate to overuse and can involve additional factors such as tightness, muscle imbalances, limb-length discrepancies, running on canted surfaces, increasing workloads too quickly, and incorrect mechanics. A gradual onset of pain in the groin (adductor longus) or inguinal area (rectus femoris or iliopsoas) is the primary complaint. The course of hip tendinopathy follows that of tendinopathy in other body segments, with a progression of pain into the patient's workout until daily activities such as walking and stair climbing are painful.

Examination reveals tenderness to palpation of the tendon. Crepitus may be felt. Stretching or resisted contraction can be painful. Flexibility is often reduced. Reduced stride length and diminished hip motion may be present in an antalgic gait.

Rehabilitation follows the same course as for other tendinopathies. First and foremost, the underlying causes must be corrected to minimize recurrence. Pain-relieving medications and modalities for pain control accompany therapeutic exercises. Stretching exercises and a graduated program of primarily eccentric strengthening exercises are used initially. Since there is no inactive phase preventing motion with this type of chronic injury, these exercises begin fairly soon after treatment begins. Other activities such as balance exercises, core exercises, and exercises for unaffected body segments should also be included in the program during this time. Cross-friction massage on the tendon is also used during early treatment to reduce adhesion formation and pain. Later, when the patient can

perform fast eccentric exercises without pain, other types of exercises are added. These additional exercises include concentric and concentric–eccentric exercises with progressive resistance.

If the patient continues to participate in normal activities during rehabilitation, that participation may need to be reduced during treatment, depending on the severity of the injury. As a rule of thumb, if the patient's pain does not respond to treatment or increases, the patient should be advised to reduce or sustain the normal workout load until the condition responds to the treatment program.

Snapping Hip Syndrome

Snapping hip, known by its medical name as **coxa sultans**, presents with an audible snapping or cracking sound. It can occur intra-articularly or extra-articularly and medially, laterally, or posteriorly in the hip region. It occurs more commonly in persons who perform repetitive hip flexion movements. In sports, these actions are seen most often in cyclists, runners, and dancers. It also is related to weakness of the hip flexors and hip adductors. It can be pathological or asymptomatic. It can be the result of various pathologies such as loose bodies, acetabular labral tears, synovitis, subluxation, or chondral injuries. It can also occur from a tendon or ligament snapping against a bone during movement.

On the lateral aspect, the ITB can be the source of snapping in the hip. The snapping occurs when a tight ITB moves across the trochanteric bursa during hip flexion–extension. The condition becomes more noticeable with medial rotation when the band is moved across the bursa. It can cause pain and irritation of the trochanteric bursa or the proximal ITB.

Another snapping malady found in dancers is the iliopsoas snap syndrome, which occurs when the hip is in about 45° of flexion and moving into extension. In this position, the iliopsoas snaps against the iliopectineal bursa and the anterior ridge of the acetabulum. Tightness of the iliopsoas or an anterior pelvic tilt can be the source of this syndrome, which can cause either bursitis or tendinopathy in the area if it persists.

A clicking sound that accompanies pivoting movements may result from a torn acetabular labrum. The pivoting motion of the femur catches the labrum when the hip is in extension. A torn acetabular labrum presents with a sharp pain into the groin or anterior thigh.

Patients with acetabular click syndrome should be referred to the physician for orthopedic examination and for diagnostic tests to rule out other diagnoses. Patients with either iliopsoas or ITB syndrome should learn proper stretching exercises to lengthen shortened structures, use stabilization techniques for proper pelvic and hip alignment, and strengthen muscles if imbalances exist. Special attention is paid to hip flexors and hip adductors since

Case Study

A 16-year-old male competitive figure skater has been diagnosed with right iliopectineal bursitis. His physician has referred him to you for treatment. The patient presents with tenderness in the inguinal area for the past 4 weeks. Over that time, the pain has increased to the point that it interferes with his practices. He cannot lift his partner during their practices without intense pain. He also experiences pain throughout the practice, especially when he pivots, jumps, or lands on the right limb. During the past week, he has noticed pain extending down the anterior thigh. Your examination reveals pain with resisted hip flexion and stretch into hip extension. The patient displays pain and weakness with resisted hip flexion. He has a moderate lumbar lordosis and weakness in the lumbar extensors, and his hip-extension firing-pattern test reveals increased scapular activity with gluteal firing occurring first in the sequence during hip extension.

Questions for Analysis

1. List your other differential diagnoses and the tests you will use to eliminate them.
2. What is your goal for treatment today, and what treatment will you give the patient today?
3. What home instructions will you discuss with him?
4. What will you tell the patient when he asks if he can continue his workouts?
5. Outline your program for the patient for the next 2 weeks. What functional activities will you include in his program before full return to competitive skating?

they are often inherently weak in patients with snapping hip syndrome. Deep-tissue massage can reduce adhesions, stimulate circulation, and reduce pain.

Rehabilitation for this condition includes finding the cause of the snapping hip syndrome and then applying heat modalities before stretching. It is also important to correct any muscle imbalances in strength or flexibility that may be present. Since the pathology does not require a time of inactivity, there is no inactive phase in the rehabilitation program, and the progression occurs according to patient tolerance. Foam roller and other soft-tissue mobilization techniques are used in addition to the corrective exercises. Sometimes a patient must refrain from activities, while at other times it may be enough to reduce the activity level.

In cases that are not resolved with medications, rest, and rehabilitation, surgery is used to correct the problem. In these cases, the tendon is usually released at the site of tightness or a Z-plasty is used to lengthen the tendon. After surgery, the patient begins a rehabilitation program within the first postoperative week. Initial treatments are geared to resolving postoperative responses such as effusion, ecchymosis, pain, and spasm. After the first week, however, flexibility exercises are started. By the end of weeks 2 to 3, resistive exercises to tolerance begin and progress as the patient tolerates. During this time, the clinician monitors the surgical site to ensure undeterred healing. During the next 3 to 8 weeks, the patient's strength and mobility improve along a steady progression. The clinician performs daily assessments to confirm that the program is providing optimal results. By week 8, the patient has full motion and near-normal strength levels without pain. At this time more vigorous resistive exercises, including multiplanar activities, agility exercises, and early-level plyometrics,

are added to the program. By the time the patient reaches the advanced phase, about 12 weeks postoperatively, functional activities give way to performance-specific exercises. Once the patient displays abilities equivalent to preoperative skills, he or she is returned to full and normal activities.

Fractures and Dislocation

Fractures fall into three main categories: traumatic, stress, and growth plate fractures. Traumatic fractures of the hip are rare in athletics and in the common workplace because of the great forces required; for this reason, the rehabilitation programs will not be presented in this text. Stress fractures, however, are more common. Growth plate fractures occur in younger athletes whose epiphyseal plates remain immature.

Stress Fractures

Bone continually undergoes remodeling according to stresses applied to it. Stress fractures occur in patients who suddenly increase their training intensity, thereby adding more stress than the bone's remodeling process can manage. Stress fractures are most often seen in distance runners and other athletes whose sport involves extensive running. The common sites of stress fractures are the pubic ramus, the femoral neck, and the subtrochanteric region of the femur. In patients with coxa vara, stress loads placed on the femoral neck may increase, predisposing these athletes to femoral neck stress fractures.

The patient reports a sharp, deep, localized pain that is aggravated by jumping and running. In the early stages, rest relieves the pain, but as the injury progresses, the pain continues during rest. Nocturnal pain may also be present.

Rehabilitation includes, most importantly, correction of the causative factors. There should be no weight bearing or partial weight bearing on crutches for up to 3 weeks. Exercises on reciprocal machines such as the stationary bike or upper-body ergometer, pain-free open kinetic chain exercises, and aquatic exercises, including deep-water running, can occur early in the program during restricted weight bearing. Hip, knee, ankle, and trunk exercises should be included in the program. As the patient progresses to full weight bearing with a normal gait and without pain, he or she performs progressive closed kinetic chain and proprioception exercises to make additional strength, balance, coordination, and agility gains.

Growth Plate Fractures

Slipped capital femoral epiphysis is a displacement of the femoral head from the femoral neck because of a weakness in the epiphyseal plate. This condition occurs in boys around age 13 to 16 and in girls around age 11 to 14. It is seen in youths who have predisposing factors such as a recent growth spurt, an imbalance of sex hormones and growth hormones, and an overweight or lanky build. The patient presents with an insidious, gradual onset of pain in the groin that can refer to the thigh and knee in chronic slips. Less often, the patient experiences an acute slipped capital femoral epiphysis that presents with a sudden onset of pain and disability after a traumatic event. Pain produces an antalgic gait.

Examination reveals restriction of hip medial rotation, abduction, and flexion, with the greatest restriction in medial rotation. During active hip flexion, the hip also moves into lateral rotation. In a relaxed position, the thigh is in greater lateral rotation than the contralateral limb. Hip abductors are weak.

Possible differential diagnoses with groin, anterior thigh, and knee pain must be investigated. Other possible diagnoses include fracture, tumor, hernias, strains, and contusions. An evaluation of the patient's history, hip motion, motion patterns, pain level, and strength helps the clinician to determine other possible sources of the patient's pain.

Treatment includes open reduction and internal fixation. After surgery, the patient is allowed partial weight bearing for 2 to 6 weeks. Gait training may be needed during partial weight bearing if the patient ambulates improperly. About 1 week after surgery, isometric exercises begin, along with open kinetic chain exercises as tolerated. Exercises also begin for the uninvolved body segments. After the surgical incision has healed while the patient is still partial weight bearing, aquatic exercises are used to achieve range-of-motion and strength gains. Once the surgically repaired site is healed, full weight bearing is permitted; at this time the patient continues to use the crutches until gait and hip control are normal. Stork standing and other proprioception exercises should progress as tolerated when unilateral weight-bearing activities are permissible. The rehabilitation progression follows that of other fractures once the patient is full weight bearing.

Dislocation

Because the hip socket is deep and the ligaments surrounding it are strong, the hip is rarely dislocated in sports: a large, violent force is required to disrupt the joint. One may see dislocations in high-energy sports with large external force applications such as downhill skiing, soccer, football, and rugby. Rarely are orthopedic injuries considered medical emergencies, but hip dislocations are emergencies because of the risk of arterial damage.

Case Study

A 17-year-old female soccer player reports that she has had progressive anterior hip pain for the past 4 weeks. The pain has increased to the point that it bothers her walking, climbing stairs, and standing. She ambulates with an antalgic gait, using a shortened stride length, and she maintains a flexed hip and a forward trunk lean throughout the gait cycle. Your examination reveals tenderness to resisted hip flexion that increases when resisted knee extension is applied simultaneously. Hip flexion is weak. Passive hip extension stretch with knee flexion in prone is more uncomfortable than hip extension with the knee extended. There is tenderness to palpation of the anterior inferior iliac spine, and pressure on this area reproduces the patient's pain.

Questions for Analysis

1. What do you suspect is the patient's problem?
2. What other differential diagnoses should you eliminate, and how would you accomplish this?
3. Explain what your treatment for her today will include.
4. What home instructions will you give the patient before she leaves today?
5. Outline the rehabilitation program you will place the patient on over the next 2 weeks. How will you decide when she is ready to resume full sport participation?

Rehabilitation of hip dislocations starts with up to 6 weeks of non-weight-bearing ambulation. During this time, isometric hip exercises and isotonic exercises for the knee and ankle are used to retard atrophy. Resistance-band exercises for the ankle and knee are performed several times a day. Manual resistance exercises can also be used. Activities that put the hip at risk for posterior re-dislocation include hip adduction, hip flexion, and trunk forward bending. For this reason, the patient must not cross the legs, sit in a chair with the hip at 90° or more to the trunk, or bend over from the waist for 12 to 16 weeks postinjury.

Once the patient is permitted partial weight bearing, active range-of-motion exercises such as heel slides can begin. All exercises should be pain free and should not include motion beyond active abilities. The patient uses crutches for about 6 to 8 weeks postinjury, until he or she can ambulate normally and demonstrate good hip control. Closed kinetic chain exercises begin when the patient begins weight bearing, but hip flexion beyond 90° is avoided for up to 12 to 16 weeks postinjury. Aquatic exercises may start around weeks 2 to 3.

Once the patient is full weight bearing, partial squats, step-up exercises, and heel raises are incorporated into the program. Swimming begins in about weeks 8 to 12 when the hip strength is sufficient to provide hip stability against the water's resistance; the breaststroke is avoided until week 16. The stationary bike can begin at weeks 6 to 8; treadmill walking begins during week 10 and is performed without an incline until week 12. Machine squats, leg press, and other resistance machines for the hip are appropriate after weeks 10 to 12. If the patient demonstrates good hip control, jogging may begin after weeks 14 to 16. The patient transitions to running, then to agility and participation-specific activities as he or she makes further gains in strength, control, and coordination, usually anywhere from week 20 to week 30.

Summary

Since lower-extremity stresses occur mainly during closed-chain activities, the hip's alignment, or misalignment, has an impact on other joints up and down the closed chain. A common problem is hip abductor weakness. This problem can occur as a primary factor that has been caused by an abductor injury or as a secondary factor caused by an injury to another segment. Regardless of the cause, the rehabilitation clinician must recognize the problem and correct it to reduce abnormal stresses on other elements of the closed chain. Injuries to the hip do not occur as often as to other joints, but they can be disabling, and they require accurate assessment and treatment for correction. Trigger point treatment, joint mobilization techniques, and progressive exercises from flexibility to functional activities were included in this chapter. Some of the more commonly seen injuries of the hip involve the acetabular joint and its labrum; both femoroacetabular impingement and acetabular labral tears are common among athletes who engage in activities of repetitive flexion with rotation and abduction. Sprains, avulsion fractures, and tendinopathies are also among the more common injuries found in the hip region. These injuries and other common pathologies of the hip were presented along with rehabilitation programs for them.

LEARNING AIDS

Key Concepts and Review

1. Discuss how anteversion and retroversion change lower-extremity mechanics.

Normal alignment places the neck in a line that is 15° anterior to the line of the femur in the adult. If the angle is greater than 15°, the hip is in anteversion. If it is less than 15°, the hip is in retroversion. Retroversion and anteversion change knee alignment and the forces that act throughout the entire lower extremity. Retroversion results in frog-eyed patellae, forefoot abduction, and a toe-out gait. Anteversion causes squinting patellae, forefoot adduction, and a toe-in gait. Anteversion makes the hip susceptible to dislocation.

2. Explain the mechanical factors involved in a gait with hip abductor weakness, and explain how a cane or single crutch assists in normal gait.

When the person stands on the involved extremity, the abductors are not strong enough to counter the force of gravity pulling the non-weight-bearing hip downward and laterally rotating the pelvis, so the person cannot achieve a normal gait. The patient either drops the non-weight-bearing hip and downwardly rotates the pelvis to that side or tilts the trunk to lurch over the weak hip during stance on the limb so that the body's center of mass is closer to the fulcrum, the weight-bearing hip joint. If the body's center of mass is moved far enough laterally to position it over the fulcrum, the abductors do not have to work, and the pelvis does not drop. If a cane is used on the side opposite the weakness, an upward force is transmitted through the cane to counterbalance the downward gravitational force on the same side. Because the moment arm from the cane to the fulcrum is longer than the center of mass's moment arm, the force that must be transmitted through the cane is relatively small.

3. Identify a joint mobilization technique for the hip, and explain its benefit.

Anterior glide increases hip extension and lateral rotation.

4. Identify a flexibility exercise and a strengthening exercise for the hip.

Thomas stretch is used to gain hip extension. A resistance-band exercise that resists hip extension is used to increase hip extensor strength.

5. Identify a proprioception exercise for the hip, and indicate its progression.

In a proprioceptive exercise progression for the hip, the patient stork-stands with eyes open, then with eyes closed, then with eyes open while rotating the head to the left and to the right, then stands on an unstable surface, then stands on an unstable surface while performing a distracting activity, and finally stands on the involved extremity while performing a resisted exercise with the uninvolved extremity.

6. List precautions for a hip-dislocation rehabilitation program.

Activities that put the hip at risk for re-dislocation include hip adduction, hip flexion, and trunk forward bending. Therefore, the patient should not cross the legs, sit in a chair with the hip at 90° or more to the trunk, or bend over from the waist for 12 to 16 weeks postinjury.

Critical Thinking Questions

1. If you were Eddie in the opening scenario, how would you manage Margaret's injury? Would you insist that she take time off from her performances? Would you rehabilitate the injury as if Margaret were not performing daily? Would you treat the injury to keep it from getting worse until the season is over and fully rehabilitate it then? Would you refuse to treat her unless she complied with your recommendations? Or would you use some other approach? Justify your decisions, and explain your treatment program.

2. If a patient complains of anterior hip pain, what possible differential diagnoses will you need to identify and rule out before beginning a rehabilitation program? (Hint: Do a mental review of all the structures from superficial to deep.) What differences would there be in the rehabilitation programs for those diagnoses?

3. If a gymnast sustained an anterior hip contusion on the uneven bars, what possible secondary problems would cause her to need rehabilitation? What would be your rehabilitation approach to these problems?

Lab Activities

1. Locate the trigger points on your lab partner for the following muscles. As you locate each one, indicate what the pain pattern would be if the trigger point were active.

   A. Piriformis

   B. Gluteus medius

   C. Gluteus minimus

   Where was your partner's most sensitive trigger point? Perform a treatment technique on it, and provide your partner with a home exercise for the tender trigger point.

2. Perform grade I, II, III, and IV joint mobilizations on your lab partner's hip joint for any motion. Examine the joint's total range of capsular mobility in a posterior glide. Where does the joint's resistance occur relative to the entire joint's mobility (draw the joint's movement diagram)? Is it the same for the other hip joint? How do your partner's joint excursion and point of resistance compare with those of two other people in your class? Of what relevance is this to your thoughts on hip joint mobilization?

3. Perform grade II and IV joint mobilization examinations on your lab partner's hip, and identify what motion restriction would be best treated with each mobilization:

   A. Anterior glide

   B. Posterior glide

   C. Distraction

Which one was the easiest to perform? Which one allowed you to feel the greatest motion within the joint? Given the size of the limb you treated, what accommodations did you have to make in order to manage the extremity during joint mobilization treatment?

4. Check your partner's sequential firing pattern during prone hip extension. Looking at when these muscles fire, what is the sequence? What is the normal sequence? Compare your partner's sequential firing pattern with that of the opposite limb. Are they the same? What would you do to correct the firing-sequence pattern if it were abnormal? Why should an abnormal firing-sequence pattern be corrected?

5. Examine your partner's hip ROM for flexion, extension, abduction, lateral rotation, and medial rotation. What are the ranges of motion for each movement? What is normal for each motion? Measure medial and lateral rotation of your partner's hip with your partner in seated and prone positions. Do you get differences between the two positions? Why?

6. Have your partner perform the tensor fasciae latae stretches in standing, sitting, and side-lying as demonstrated earlier in the chapter. Hold each stretch for 30 s. Observe and correct for substitutions. During which exercise did your partner feel the greatest stretch? What do you think is the reason for this?

7. Have your partner perform the hip flexor stretches demonstrated earlier in this chapter. Hold each stretch for 30 s. Observe and correct for substitutions. Which position created the greatest stretch for him or her? What do you think is the reason for this?

8. Instruct your partner in a piriformis stretch. Watch to ensure that the exercise is performed correctly, and give verbal cueing to correct for any errors. Reverse positions so that you are now the patient; have your partner instruct you in a different piriformis stretch, correcting with verbal cues any errors in your performance. What kinds of substitutions could each of you use in these exercises?

9. Have your partner perform each of the hip extension exercises in figures 18.32 and 18.33 for 10 repetitions. Which exercise was the most difficult? Why?

10. Using rubber tubing or bands that provide sufficient resistance, have your partner perform resisted hip extension and abduction, each for 10 repetitions. What are the possible substitutions for each exercise? What verbal cues should you use to correct these errors?

11. Have your partner perform two different exercises for proprioception. Which one was the easier one and which one was more difficult? How could you make them each more difficult?

12. Have your partner perform two plyometric exercises, and identify how you would determine when he or she has progressed in one to go to the next. What substitutions would you be looking for, and how would you correct them with verbal cues?

13. A cross-country runner strained his piriformis 3 weeks ago when he slipped on wet grass running up a hill. He has noticed that he is limping and does not have the stride length he usually has when he runs. He reports that he has pain with sitting, walking, and running. Why do you think he continues to have pain 3 weeks after the injury? What do you think will need to be resolved before he can resume racing without pain? Describe a progressive rehabilitation program, including all types of exercises you would incorporate into the program. What would be your guidelines for progression throughout the program?

14. Place a small screw or marble in your right shoe and walk with the object in your shoe. Now walk with a cane in your right hand, and then with the cane in your left hand. In which condition did you experience less discomfort while walking with a screw or marble in your shoe? Explain why you experienced less pain in one condition and more pain in the other.

19

Knee and Thigh

Objectives

After completing this chapter, you should be able to do the following:

1. Discuss the relationship and alignment between the patella and the femur.
2. Identify postinjury factors that influence strength output.
3. Define *quadriceps extensor lag* and *AMI* and explain their significance.
4. Outline a general progression of rehabilitation for a knee.
5. Identify three soft-tissue mobilization techniques for the knee.
6. Identify three joint mobilization techniques for the knee and the purpose of each.
7. Describe three flexibility exercises for the knee, and identify the structures they affect.
8. Describe three proprioception and balance exercises for the knee.
9. Identify three functional activities.
10. Identify three factors that influence PFPS.

||||||||||||||||||||||||||||||||||||||||||||||||||||||||||||||||||||||||||||||||||||||||||||||||||||||||||||||||||||||||||||||||||||||||||||||||||||||||||||||||

Three mornings a week, Steve Turnwell and his friends play a game of basketball at the university gym before going to work. It is their way of having fun and getting exercise at the same time. They have been following this routine since they were in their mid-30s, about 10 years ago. About 2 weeks ago, their routine was suddenly disrupted. Steve jumped to retrieve a rebound and landed in severe pain. He felt a searing pain in his knee. Several weeks later he underwent an anterior cruciate ligament reconstruction and was fitted with a knee immobilizer and placed on crutches.

Today he had his first rehabilitation appointment with Joan Runnae, a clinician who came highly recommended to Steve. After Joan completed an examination, she explained to Steve what she saw as primary problems and discussed how she thought they could best resolve those problems. Steve agreed with her and realized that this was not going to be an easy or short process, but he was willing to work with Joan to get back onto the basketball court. He liked Joan's approach and appreciated the way she could explain things in layman's terms better than the physician did, so he could understand what his injury was and what the surgeon did to repair it. He knew Joan would work him hard, but he also knew that if he wanted to play basketball again, he would have to work hard, and he was eager to start.

In addition to the commitment and consistency that would be required of Steve in his rehabilitation, Joan knew that the tissue's healing process had to be respected. Because it was less than a week since Steve's surgery, some stress to the newly formed tissue was important, but too much stress could be detrimental. While using caution with the knee, she could start Steve on more aggressive exercises for the hip and ankle without unduly stressing the repaired ligament. Joan sensed that Steve was the type of person who was eager and willing to work hard but would also understand precautions if he knew about them. As she does with all her patients, Joan would keep Steve well informed throughout his program about what he should and should not be doing and why.

I had a bad knee injury when I was about seventeen. I wasn't able to climb for about six months. It was kind of like a transformative time for me, because it was really hard for me not to be able to climb. It forced me to appreciate things without just climbing.

Chris Sharma, 1981-,
American rock climber, instructor, entrepreneur

Over the years, the approach to rehabilitation of knee injuries has evolved. The standard of care changes as we learn more and more about knee mechanics and healing. Research findings sometimes determine that current approaches are in error. Sometimes disappointment with previous treatment results spurs us to change our techniques to keep up with new discoveries. In recent years there has been a tremendous amount of research creating a wealth of knowledge on the knee. We still have much to learn, but investigators have given us new insights and information about knee biomechanics, improved surgical procedures, and updated rehabilitation techniques.

Mr. Sharma's insight into his perspective about his knee injury, and how that injury enabled him to turn something potentially negative into a positive, is not unique. However, his description of the experience gives us some insight into how valuable he found the rehabilitative process. Often that process can be lengthy and difficult, especially for the knee and thigh. In the opening scenario, Joan provided Steve with helpful explanation and perspective. This is the part of the rehabilitation process that can help many patients change their perspective from one of doom and gloom into a worthwhile, transformative learning experience. As medical knowledge evolves, techniques and concepts change and improve, so rehabilitation clinicians can offer their patients better explanations, communication, and programming, paving the way for better rehabilitation experiences.

Rehabilitation programs resolve many knee injuries in both athletic and nonathletic populations. This chapter deals with thigh and knee injuries and their rehabilitation. Thigh injuries could just as easily have been considered along with the hip in chapter 18. We will often refer you to other chapters because there is an intimate relationship between the thigh and knee and the thigh and hip. We have placed several thigh injuries in this chapter because of this intimate relationship; other thigh injuries that affect primarily the hip are discussed in chapter 18.

As with the other chapters in part IV, this one begins with general information that affects rehabilitation programs for knee and thigh injuries. This information is vital if the clinician is to design appropriate rehabilitation programs for injuries to the knee and thigh. This chapter presents specific rehabilitation techniques, including manual therapy and exercises for flexibility, strength, and coordination. Recommendations are also included for functional activities before the patient's return to full sport or normal activities. The final section of the chapter discusses rehabilitation programs for specific injuries commonly seen in the knee and thigh.

Controversy continues over the best surgical repair technique and the most appropriate postoperative and post-injury methods of rehabilitation for the knee. The evolution of surgical and rehabilitation procedures for knee injuries continues as new evidence comes to light. Some surgeons choose to remain conservative in their postoperative care, while others prefer a more accelerated approach to their surgical repairs. It is important for rehabilitation clinicians to work with physicians to provide successful outcomes for their patients. Both the physician's and the rehabilitation clinician's protocols for the rehabilitation of knee and thigh injuries should be based on current best-practice evidence, the severity of the injury, the structure injured, the specific repair technique used, and the tissue healing timeline. If there is to be an error, as with any rehabilitation program, it should be on the side of caution.

CLINICAL TIPS

Injuries to the knee and thigh that require particular therapeutic exercise approaches include ligament sprains, collateral ligament sprains, meniscus injuries, patellofemoral injuries, strains and contusions, and bone injuries. Although treatment guidelines for each of these injuries may exist, the clinician must always consider each patient's response and use that as the primary guideline in treatment progression.

Special Rehabilitation Considerations

The knee is one of the most often injured joints.[1-3] The forces applied to it during running, twisting, and lifting activities are complicated by the fact that there are two long lever arms on either end of the joint, making it susceptible to excessive stress. For as shallow a joint as the knee is, complete dislocation is surprisingly rare.[4] This may be so because of the strong static and dynamic structures that surround the joint. The ligaments and muscles of the knee give the joint strong support, so tremendous forces are needed to produce an injury. The more commonly seen knee injuries are discussed later in this chapter. This section deals with unique knee structures that support and protect the joint and are affected when injury occurs.

Knee Structure

At first glance, the knee appears to be a relatively simple joint, but it is actually quite complex. Within its anatomical structure are several elements that influence its function. When balance is deficient, the knee becomes susceptible to injury. To develop a therapeutic exercise program for any injury to the knee, clinicians must understand the knee's structures and how they work together.

Tibiofemoral Joint

The knee joint is actually two joints, the tibiofemoral joint and the patellofemoral joint. The tibiofemoral joint has a concave tibia platform comprising the distal aspect of the joint, with a convex femur proximally. This means that when you perform a mobilization technique to the joint, the concave tibia moves on the convex femur in the same direction as the physiological movement of the joint. In other words, a grade III or IV posterior glide of the tibia on the femur enhances flexion and an anterior glide enhances extension.

Capsule

The knee joint is the largest joint of the body; it is surrounded by a capsule that helps stabilize the joint by merging with the collateral ligaments.[5] The capsule also distributes the synovial fluid around the joint during movement and merges with many of the knee's bursae. If the joint capsule is restricted, a capsular pattern becomes apparent. The knee's capsular pattern is loss of flexion motion greater than loss of extension motion.[6] The joint is in a resting position when it is in about 20° to 25° of flexion and in a fully close-packed position in full extension with lateral tibial rotation.[7]

Ligaments

The collateral ligaments provide knee protection and stability against medial and lateral stresses.[8] The medial collateral ligament (MCL) attaches to the medial meniscus. This arrangement may be one reason the medial meniscus is often injured with MCL sprains. In addition to providing protection against valgus stresses, the MCL helps to restrict lateral rotation of the tibia on the femur. The lateral collateral ligament (LCL) does not attach to the lateral meniscus, and it is taut during medial rotation of the tibia on the femur and when the knee incurs varus stress. Because lateral forces on the knee produce valgus stresses more often than varus stresses, the MCL is the more frequently injured of these two ligaments.[9]

The anterior and posterior cruciate ligaments (ACL and PCL, respectively) are structures unique to the knee. Their position within the joint enables them to provide anterior–posterior stability as well as rotational stability.[10] Some fibers of each ligament are taut throughout the knee's range of motion.[11] Injury to either ligament can cause disabling knee instability.

The ACL and PCL are encased within a synovial membrane that provides the ligaments with their primary blood supply. If a partial tear of either ligament occurs, the synovial membrane may also become disrupted, compromising the ligament's vascular supply. If this happens, dehiscence, or erosion, of the ligament eventually results.

Within the past quarter century, the ACL has become the most researched structure of the entire musculoskeletal system.[12] This may be because of the frequency with which it is injured, especially in sports. The ACL protects the knee from anterior translation of the tibia on the femur. The PCL is not injured as often, but there is evidence that injury rates to the PCL have increased with the growth in sports participation.[13, 14] The PCL serves primarily to restrict knee hyperextension and posterior displacement of the tibia on the femur.[15]

All ligaments of the joint restrain rotational stresses at the knee. The cruciate ligaments twist and become taut during medial rotation of the tibia.[16] The collateral ligaments become taut to provide stability during lateral rotation of the tibia.[16] Rotation is a primary automatic motion of the knee in both weight bearing and non–weight bearing.[16] In weight bearing, the femur rotates on the tibia, and in non–weight bearing, the tibia rotates on the femur. Since all ligaments restrain rotation, injury mechanisms that produce excessive rotational forces can damage more than one ligament and subsequently can produce joint instability.

The knee's joint capsule and intra-articular structures, including the anterior and posterior cruciate ligaments, contain various neuroreceptors that provide the neural system with position information from the knee.[17, 18] We know that the ACL contains afferent mechanoreceptors that affect the knee's stability.[19] The joint capsule has mechanoreceptors (Ruffini nerve endings) that are sensitive to pressure and deformation.[20] Injury to the knee's ligamentous structures can damage these receptors, impairing proprioception.[21, 22] Rehabilitation programs must include techniques to restore the proprioceptive deficiencies that result from knee injuries.[23, 24]

Although each ligament has its own role in supporting and protecting the knee, some ligaments also provide assistive support to other ligaments (table 19.1). These protective designs are known as primary and secondary restraints. For example, the ACL is the primary restraint protecting the knee against anterior tibial translation, but if it is injured, other structures, such as the capsule, other ligaments, and muscles, act as secondary restraints. Thus joint protection continues in nonsurgical patients in spite of the injury.[25, 26] Sometimes the secondary structures can provide enough stability that surgical repair is not needed, but often they fall short. Instability caused by ACL or PCL insufficiencies is often inadequately supported by secondary structures.[27]

Meniscus

The medial and lateral menisci cushion the joint, deepen the socket, increase joint congruity to better distribute weight-bearing forces, assist in joint lubrication, and provide stability.[28] These structures are commonly referred to as cartilage, although this is a misnomer. They are primarily fibrocartilage (hence the name), but this is certainly not their only component. The knee joint also has articular cartilage, so the term "cartilage" is not only erroneous but sometimes confusing, especially to the patient who has injured articular cartilage, not meniscus.

The medial meniscus is attached to the MCL, the ACL, and the semimembranosus tendon. This arrangement is believed to be one cause for the greater frequency of injury to the medial meniscus.[29] Even though the lateral meniscus is not attached to the LCL, it does connect to the popliteus and PCL. It has more freedom of movement and is not affected by collateral ligament positioning and stresses. When the knee moves through flexion and exten-

TABLE 19.1   Summary of the Most Important Knee Ligaments and Their Functions

Ligament	Function	Notations
Medial collateral ligament (MCL)	Protects against valgus stress. Restricts lateral tibial rotation on femur (or medial femoral rotation on tibia).	Attaches to medial meniscus. Some fibers are taut throughout knee ROM.
Lateral collateral ligament (LCL)	Protects against varus stress. Restricts lateral rotation of tibia on femur (or medial femoral rotation on tibia).	Not attached to meniscus.
Anterior cruciate ligament (ACL)	Protects against anterior translation of tibia on femur. Taut during medial tibial rotation (or lateral femoral rotation).	Some fibers are taut throughout knee ROM. Encased in synovial membrane.
Posterior cruciate ligament (PCL)	Protects against posterior translation of tibia on femur. Restricts knee hyperextension. Taut during medial tibial rotation (or lateral femoral rotation).	Some fibers are taut throughout knee motion. Encased in synovial membrane.

sion within the sagittal plane, the menisci follow the tibial movements.[30] During flexion, the menisci are pulled posteriorly by the semimembranosus and popliteus, and during extension they are pulled anteriorly by the meniscopatellar ligaments.[30] During movement from extension into flexion, the femur slides posteriorly on the tibia during weight bearing so that in a squat position, the weight is borne primarily by the posterior menisci, whereas in extension, the femur is primarily on the anterior menisci.

Compressive forces absorbed by the menisci are up to 50% to 60% of the knee's loads.[29] When the knee is at 90° flexion and the primary force is applied at the posterior aspect of the joint as in a squat position, the meniscal load increases to 85% of the total knee joint compressive forces.[31] Meniscal posterior horn and lateral tears seem to be primarily degenerative tears, whereas anterior horn tears are often traumatic events.[32] Degenerative tears may be related to the increased forces absorbed by the menisci in flexion, as well as to the repetitive activity imposed on the menisci when squatting, stair climbing, and lifting heavy objects.[33] On the other hand, acute tears occur most often during a running or cutting maneuver, when the knee is near extension.[33] A shallower-than-normal joint may also lead to either acute or degenerative meniscal injuries.[34]

The menisci are avascular except for roughly 10% to 33% of their periphery.[35] This has a significant impact on conservative and surgical interventions after injury to the meniscus. This topic is discussed later in the chapter.

Screw-Home Mechanism

The knee joint is a modified hinge joint. This means that although it is similar to a hinge joint, permitting movement in one plane, the bony segments are not entirely congruent throughout. Because the medial aspect of the joint is larger and extends slightly more distally than the lateral side, when the knee moves into extension the lateral joint segments complete their motion before the medial joint segments, so the tibia rotates laterally as the medial tibial plateau completes its motion on the medial femoral condyle in non-weight-bearing conditions. When the knee extends during weight bearing, the femur rotates medially on the anchored tibia. This mechanism, called the screw-home mechanism, occurs in the last 30° of extension and must occur to enable full extension of the knee. This mechanism is accompanied by anterior cruciate ligament tension, and it gives the joint more stability than a pure hinge-joint arrangement would because it provides a kind of locking feature.[36] The popliteus is responsible for unlocking the knee during movement from full extension into flexion.[16] It does this by laterally rotating the femoral condyles with its medial tibial insertion anchored in weight bearing. In non–weight bearing, the popliteus unlocks the knee as it medially rotates the tibia with its proximal insertion stabilized. The importance of this mechanism becomes apparent later in the chapter when we discuss full joint motion and joint mobilization.

Patellofemoral Joint

The patella, the largest sesamoid bone in the body, sits within the femoral groove. Its resting position is knee extension, and its close-packed position is knee flexion. The patella serves to increase the lever-arm length of the quadriceps tendon, adds to the cosmetic appearance of the knee joint, and protects the knee from anterior blows.[37] It is a common site of knee pain and dysfunction.

The quadriceps tendon and its medial and lateral expansions surround the patella. The tendon attachment from the patella to the tibial tubercle is sometimes referred to as the patellar ligament because it travels from bone to bone. This structure is also called the patellar tendon.

Patellar stability is the result of static and dynamic structures. The greatest bony contributor to patellar stability is the femoral sulcus formed by the medial and higher-ridged lateral epicondyles within which the patella sits.[38] Ligamentous stability comes from the patellofemoral and patellotibial ligaments, which help to provide static restraints.[38] Active restraints from the quadriceps provide the greatest dynamic stability.

An examination of patellar alignment occurs in static and dynamic positions. The patella is examined in long sitting for abnormalities in resting. Movement of the patella during quadriceps contraction in long sitting and in weight bearing is also examined because patellar movement in open and closed kinetic chain conditions may differ. A closed kinetic chain position can change the patellar alignment because other factors, such as hip rotation and foot pronation, change the way the patella moves when the quadriceps contract.[39, 40]

Superior Tibiofibular Joint

This joint is not actually a joint of the knee because it is distal to the knee joint, but it can affect the ankle and knee joints. There are no physiological movements in this joint, but it must have full accessory motion for full ankle range of motion to occur.[41] The tibiofibular joint can cause lateral knee pain.[42]

Muscles

The quadriceps and hamstrings have been the most commonly addressed muscles because of their prominence in knee control. Both groups also influence the hip, and because they do, positioning of the hip must always be a consideration when one is exercising the muscles at the knee.

The quadriceps provides the most dynamic restraint for the knee.[43] The rectus femoris is the quadriceps component that also assists in hip flexion. Hip positioning determines where in the motion the rectus femoris contributes the most at the knee.[44] In a supine straight-leg raise, it works throughout the motion, but in sitting, the rectus femoris works only in terminal knee extension.[45]

Because of the angle of their pull and tendon insertions, the hamstrings produce not only knee flexion but also tibial rotation. The biceps femoris produces lateral tibial rotation, and the semimembranosus and semitendinosus produce medial tibial rotation, especially with the knee flexed. They also protect against anterior subluxation, dynamically assisting the ACL;[43] therefore, they should be trained to become more prominent in this role in ACL-deficient knees.

Rehabilitation of isolated hamstring muscles should include the additional movements of tibial rotation along with posterior pelvic rotation and knee flexion. Eccentric and concentric activities for all their motions would most appropriately strengthen the hamstrings throughout all their functions.

Biomechanical and Physiological Concepts

Biomechanical and physiological concepts should help guide the rehabilitation clinician in choosing rehabilitation exercises for various knee injuries. They also help the rehabilitation clinician to understand the indications and precautions. These concepts are briefly reviewed in this section.

Patellofemoral and Tibiofemoral Relationship

When the knee extends, the patella glides superiorly, and during flexion it glides inferiorly for a total excursion of 5 to 7 cm (2.0 to 2.8 in.). The patella must glide freely for full knee motion to be possible.

In normal relaxed extension, the patella's inferior pole is at the knee joint's margin and lies on the supratrochlear fat pad. A patella that lies superior to this position is called patella alta, and one that is inferior to the normal position is called patella baja. Either abnormal position restricts full range of motion of the knee.[46] Injuries of the patellar tendon, including ACL reconstructions that use the patellar tendon, may develop patella baja. Injuries such as repaired quadriceps ruptures have some risk of causing changes in patella positioning.[47] Patella baja or alta requires aggressive patellar mobilization and soft-tissue-stretching techniques. These techniques are discussed in detail later.

During knee flexion and extension, the patella glides within the femoral groove and makes contact with the femoral condyles. When contact between the patella and femur occurs as the knee moves into flexion, compressive forces develop between the posterior patella and anterior femur and affect primarily the lateral patella.[48] These compressive loads during daily functional activities are more than six times body weight.[48] Since the patella rests on the fat pad in

full knee extension, it is not in direct contact with the femur in this position. The area of contact between the posterior patella and the femoral groove migrates from the patella's inferior pole to its superior aspect as the knee moves from about 10° to 20° of flexion to 90°.[49] The area of contact is fairly uniform across the breadth of the patella.[50] Once the knee approaches the end of flexion, however, the contact is on the odd facet medially and the lateral–superior aspect of the patella (figure 19.1) until the patella rests on the top of the lateral condyle in full flexion.[51]

Of significance with this change in points of contact between the patella and femur is the fact that as the knee moves into flexion, the amount of contact pressure and the area of contact both increase.[52] Contact pressure is a ratio between the patellofemoral joint reaction force and the contact area. Joint reaction force is a compressive force equivalent to the resultant vector force (of the patellofemoral quadriceps vector force and patellar tendon vector force). This vector force is perpendicular to the patella's contact surface with the femur, so the force essentially compresses the patella against the femur. Stress to the patellofemoral joint is the force per area of contact. In a closed kinetic chain activity, the joint reaction forces and the area of contact both increase as the knee moves from extension to 90°, but the force applied is greater than the area of contact, so joint compressive stress increases as the knee moves into flexion to 90°.[53-55] As the knee moves from 90° toward 120°, the force decreases and the surface area of contact remains the same, so the stress per unit of surface area decreases. The greatest compressive forces occur in the 60° to 90° positions.[52-55] If a patella is not in good alignment within the femoral groove, the congruency between the two bones is altered;[52] as a result, compressive forces are distributed over a smaller area of contact, increasing the amount of compression per unit of surface area. This may be one reason why malalignment of the patella results in increased pain and irritation of the patellofemoral joint.

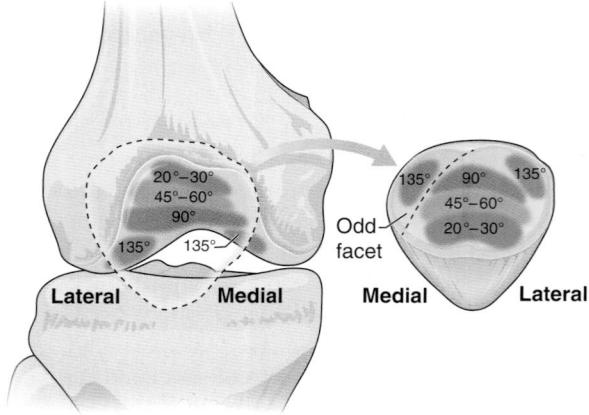

Figure 19.1   Patellofemoral contact patterns on posterior patella of a right knee.

In an open kinetic chain activity, the joint stress is lowest at 90° and greatest at 0°.[53, 54, 56] Although there may be some individual variations, open kinetic chain exercises are least irritating when performed from 45° to 90°, while closed kinetic chain exercises cause the least patellofemoral joint irritation in the ranges of 0° to 45° and greater than 90°.[53, 54, 57]

During closed kinetic chain activities such as the weight-bearing phase of gait, patellofemoral compressive forces of about one-half of body weight are produced, while stair climbing produces about three times body weight and squatting produces compressive forces of over seven times body weight.[58, 59] During open kinetic chain activities, the amount of compressive force changes with the type of activity and the angle at which it occurs.[60] If knee extension is performed with a weight attached to the end of the extremity, compressive forces reach their peak at 35° to 40°, but if the force is applied by a machine arm at right angles to the ankle such as in an N-K table or isokinetic machine, the peak compressive forces occur at 90° and decrease as the knee extends.[55, 59] Based on mathematical formulas, it is estimated that isokinetic exercises reach a peak patellofemoral compressive force of about five times body weight.[58]

Many functional activities are performed in the 0° to 95° range of motion.[61] It is important when you are treating patients with patellofemoral pain to avoid painful arcs of motion. Generally, closed kinetic chain exercises from 0° to 40° of flexion provide less medial–lateral patellar movement and less patellofemoral stress than open kinetic chain exercises, and open-chain exercises in positions greater than 50° of flexion are less stressful.[54, 62]

These numbers may seem confusing, but you need to understand their significance when treating patients with patellofemoral stress injuries. Several points are important to remember. The greatest amount of patellofemoral stress in open-chain exercises occurs in the first 30° of motion, and the least stress occurs in the range of 45° to 90°.[56] The least patellofemoral stress in closed-chain activities occurs in the first 45° of motion, and the greatest amount of stress occurs in the range of 45° to 90°.[56] The more painful the patellofemoral joint is, the more limited are the pain-free ranges of motion through which the patient can exercise without pain to strengthen the quadriceps. Patients with

Factors Influencing Postinjury Strength

We know that injury and surgery weaken the knee muscles. Other factors, however, influence knee strength and function. Some are seldom considered, but all affect knee function and are important for that reason.

These factors—edema,[73] pain,[74] and abnormal ambulation[75]—lead to impaired muscle function. Reduced function leads to atrophy and weakness of the muscle.[76] Muscle weakness leads to reduced function and control of the body segment.[77] The rehabilitation clinician must pay attention to these factors when examining a patient before starting a rehabilitation program.

Edema

One of the important goals of first-aid treatment for musculoskeletal injuries is minimizing edema. Once edema forms, efforts should be made to relieve it as quickly as possible. One reason this is a priority is that studies have demonstrated that swelling in the knee joint causes a reflex shutdown of the quadriceps.[73, 78, 79] Other researchers have injected plasma or saline in small quantities (20 to 30 mL) into normal knees and recorded a profound inhibition of quadriceps activity to levels 60% below normal.[79-81] As fluid quantity increases, quadriceps activity decreases.

Pain

It is commonly understood that pain causes a reflex inhibition of muscle activity.[74, 81, 82] Pain affects both the autonomic and the conscious pathways. The reflex response in the presence of pain is to withdraw. The conscious response is to refrain from activity that produces pain. If pain persists after an injury, the patient's ability to perform active muscle contraction is impaired. The use of electrical stimulation and other modalities to control pain before therapeutic exercise may result in improved strength-output levels during exercises.[83] This can ultimately reduce the patient's rehabilitation time by enhancing strength gains.

Ambulation

Normal ambulation uses the right and left lower extremity equally, applying weight-bearing and propulsive forces equally to and by both extremities. Weakness results when a patient sustains a lower-extremity injury that causes him or her to favor the injured extremity. An unequal gait produces subnormal stresses on the extremity as the patient spends less weight-bearing time on it and applies less stress to it. An antalgic gait produces weakness not only in the injured segment but also throughout that entire lower extremity.[84] Therefore, it is important to examine the entire lower extremity after an injury and to correct postural position and secondary weaknesses that develop in the extremity's noninjured segments.

hyperextended knees may experience pain at and near the range of full extension. For each patellofemoral pain patient, it is important to find pain-free motion within which to strengthen the quadriceps. As strength improves within this available range of motion, the range itself widens, allowing for progressive strengthening throughout a larger range of motion.[63]

Full squat exercises and full range-of-motion exercises with weight boots or cuff weights attached to the ankle should be avoided by patellofemoral patients until later in the treatment program when pain is reduced and strength has improved enough for the patellofemoral joint to tolerate the greater stresses of these activities.[54] It is logical to include a slow progression in range of motion as symptoms decrease and strength increases. Shortening the moment-arm length on weight machines will reduce the compressive forces, but the primary guide to use for program adjustments is the patient's pain. In summary, your rule of thumb is this: If patellofemoral pain occurs with an exercise, reduce either the range of motion or the resistance to create a pain-free exercise to increase strength.

Lower-Extremity Alignment

Excessive rearfoot pronation influences the patella's alignment because it increases tibial medial rotation and changes the quadriceps tendon pull on the patella.[64] Similarly, an anterior or posterior pelvic tilt generates obligatory medial or lateral femoral rotation due to the roll and glide mechanics of the acetabulum on the femur.[65, 66] You should evaluate other lower-extremity alignments during a knee examination because abnormal orientations can increase stress levels on various knee structures. For example, increased hip medial rotation, squinting patellae, genu recurvatum, patella alta, tibial varum, medial tibial rotation, heel height, and compensatory pronation are malalignments that can contribute to patellofemoral pain.[67-70] Because the lower extremity is a closed kinetic chain during most of its functions, we know that malalignment in one segment results in compensatory changes in another segment. Changes at the hip or at the foot cause compensatory changes and increase knee stress.[71, 72] Compensatory pronation and hip medial rotation with resulting medial tibial rotation are two malalignment problems that should be investigated in patients with patellofemoral pain.

CLINICAL TIPS

The quadriceps' ability to provide optimal muscle output decreases significantly in the presence of either pain or edema. Clinicians must control these secondary effects of injury so that rehabilitation can produce the best results.

Rehabilitation Factors

In addition to the routine concepts that guide the development of any rehabilitation program, special factors enter into knee rehabilitation. Clinicians must address them all. The following sections deal with the special factors that have the most influence.

Extensor Lag

The condition in which full passive motion is present but active terminal knee extension does not occur is an **extensor lag**. In other words, the clinician can move the knee into normal extension, but when the patient contracts the quadriceps, the knee does not voluntarily move through the terminal part of its motion. This extensor lag may occur because of edema, pain, stiffness, or weakness.[85] We know that pain and edema result in less quadriceps activation, so if these conditions exist, they may be contributing to active terminal extension loss. If joint or muscle stiffness is present, then passive motion is also going to be less than normal; therefore, when an extensor lag exists, we know by the definition of extensor lag (full passive motion but less than normal active motion)[86] that joint or muscle stiffness is not a likely contributor.

On the other hand, if the quadriceps muscle is weak, it may have inadequate strength to fully extend the knee. Terminal extension to 0° can be difficult for a weakened quadriceps. There is long-standing debate—still unresolved—between those who identify the quadriceps as different muscles with different activations and different functions and those who believe that, although the four muscles have different heads, they activate as one muscle.[87] Some researchers maintain that because of its fiber alignment, the function of the vastus medialis oblique (VMO) is to maintain medial patellar alignment, providing dynamic restraint for the patella.[88] Other investigators indicate that the VMO does not exert any more effort than any of the other quadriceps muscles during terminal extension.[89] It has been demonstrated that the force required of the quadriceps to produce the last 15° of extension is twice as great as it is to produce movement in the other ranges of knee motion.[86] The quadriceps' loss of mechanical advantage (decreased moment-arm length) as the knee approaches its end range means that a much greater effort is needed from the entire quadriceps to complete the movement, not just from the VMO.

Some of the often-used open kinetic chain exercises for strength gains are the quad set, the straight-leg raise, and the short-arc quad. Among these, the quad set is the most effective in producing total quadriceps activity.[90] The rectus femoris works more during the straight-leg raise and the short-arc quad exercises.[90] Vastus medialis activity is most apparent during a quad set. As would be expected, the quadriceps muscles work more during a knee-extension exercise than during a straight-leg raise.[91] Open kinetic chain exercises are an important tool in restoring isolated quadriceps strength, so these exercises are key elements in a therapeutic exercise program for a patient with quadriceps weakness.[92]

Arthrogenic Muscle Inhibition

In more recent years, the term **arthrogenic muscle inhibition (AMI)** has been used to identify reduced quadriceps activation after injury.[93] It is thought to be inhibition of a protective reflex the body uses to reduce stress that would otherwise be applied to the injured knee joint by the strong quadriceps.[94] Quadriceps AMI contributes to delayed treatment response since it inhibits quadriceps activity and can retard effective strengthening efforts because neurogenic muscle inhibition prevents the quadriceps from activating properly.[95] If quadriceps weakness persists because of AMI, knee stability, function, and optimal performance are impaired, and this increases the risk of reinjury if not resolved.[95]

Arthrogenic muscle inhibition is most apparent soon after a joint injury. It has been shown that muscle output is diminished by 50% to 70% within the first few hours after surgery and continues to advance to 80% to 90% inhibition within 1 day.[96] There is slight recovery to a 70% to 80% loss of output by the time the injury moves into the proliferation phase of healing, 3 to 4 d after surgery.[96] Studies have demonstrated that over the first 6 months after injury, there is a plateauing of AMI that is followed by a very slow reduction in AMI over the next several months, lasting up to an average of 4 years.[95]

While the main causes of AMI include pain, effusion, and joint damage, a very powerful influence on quadriceps AMI is joint swelling.[97] Studies have shown that it does not take much joint swelling to inhibit normal quadriceps activity. Wood and colleagues[98] found that only 10 mL (about 1/3 oz) of knee joint effusion caused quadriceps inhibition. Additional studies have found that swelling of 20 to 60 mL decreased quadriceps strength by 30% to 40% of its pre-effusion output.[98, 99] Although the exact mechanisms are not clear, it is evident that neural inhibition at least at the spinal cord levels and perhaps higher cortical levels is a source of this quadriceps response to joint effusion.[95] More recent investigations have demonstrated that the likely source of quadriceps inhibition in the presence of joint effusion is a spinal reflex inhibition of the muscle's alpha motoneuron pool, and not higher central nervous system cortical levels.[97] However, the study's investigators admit that additional studies are needed before such statements may be made with certainty.[97]

A primary concern for knees with AMI is that patients may return to normal activity before the quadriceps has enough strength to provide optimal protection to the knee joint.[100] One study revealed that persons with AMI secondary to joint effusion had greater ground reaction forces imparted to the joint during landing activities.[100] This occurred presumably because those people landed with less knee flexion, so normal shock absorption provided by knee flexion was lacking. When higher ground reaction forces are applied to the joint, there is a higher risk that the person will develop osteoarthritis.[101]

Effective treatment of AMI focuses heavily on prevention. Aggressive treatment of joint effusion in the early days after injury is important. Since poor rehabilitation outcomes reflect greater arthrogenic muscle inhibition,[102] the contrary may be presumed: If less joint effusion results in less AMI, then minimizing joint swelling is important to optimal treatment outcomes. A recent study investigated various ways to increase quadriceps activation and found that the most effective method was transcutaneous electrical nerve stimulation.[103] Other studies have identified additional treatments that produced increased quadriceps activation. These studies used techniques such as cryotherapy,[104] transcutaneous electrical nerve stimulation,[103] local muscle vibration,[105, 106] and total body vibration.[106] When you consider that AMI is thought to result mainly from inhibition of the muscle's alpha-motoneuron pool, it makes intuitive sense that correcting AMI requires facilitation of those receptors being inhibited. Although most of these studies demonstrate early but promising results, an established, effective intervention is yet to emerge.

Open and Closed Kinetic Chain Exercises

Open and closed kinetic chain exercises each have their advocates when it comes to including them in a knee therapeutic exercise program. Some investigators support the use of closed-chain exercises for ACL injuries and reconstructions.[92, 107, 108] More recently, research has indicated that a combination of open and closed kinetic chain exercises begun early in the therapeutic exercise program is beneficial in ACL rehabilitation.[109-111] Results of these studies indicate that better quadriceps strengthening results with earlier use of open-chain exercises for the muscle.

It has been assumed that closed kinetic chain exercises recruit a co-contraction of hamstrings and quadriceps to provide stability; this assumption remains controversial and inconclusive. For example, investigators have demonstrated that the lateral step-up exercise, thought to recruit co-contraction of hamstrings and quadriceps, actually recruits the vastus lateralis and vastus medialis components of the quadriceps significantly but does little to recruit the hamstrings.[112] On the other hand, it has been demonstrated that a squat exercise generated twice as much hamstring activity as a leg press.[113] Additional investigations are needed to determine how much co-contraction actually occurs between hamstrings and quadriceps during weight-bearing exercises.

Shear Stress

We know that shear forces are the most destructive forces applied to joints. Both open and closed kinetic chain exercises can apply shear stresses to the knee joint; however, the range of motion within which these shear forces are applied is different for open- and closed-chain exercises. In an open kinetic chain exercise, as indicated in figure 19.2, less anterior shear stress is applied to the ACL in knee extension resistive exercises from 60° to 90° flexion, and more is applied in terminal-extension ranges of motion.[114] Although investigators report open kinetic chain activity's greatest shear stress on the ACL occurring at different ranges of motion, either 0° to 40° of flexion[114] or 15° to 30° of flexion,[115] clinicians should be wary of positioning patients in resisted open-chain exercises at less than 40° of flexion after recent ACL injury or surgical repair. Resistance added during open-chain activities increases these shear forces.[116]

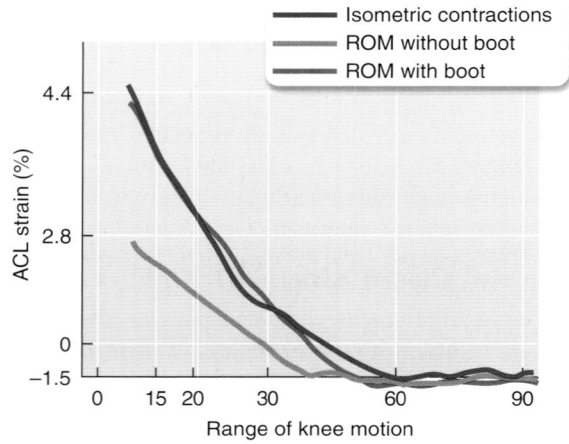

Figure 19.2 ACL strain with open kinetic chain activities. Comparing this figure with 19.3, we can notice similar declines in the stresses applied in open-chain activities as the knee moves from full extension to 90° of flexion.

Adapted from Beynnon et al. (1995).[114]

Since shear stress increases with greater moment-arm lengths, it stands to reason that if manual resistance is used, especially in the early phases of therapeutic exercise, it should be applied immediately distal to the knee joint to reduce excessive shear-force applications. Likewise, exercises using machine resistance in open-chain exercises should have their resistance arms applied close to the knee rather than at the ankle.

Less stress is applied to the ACL in closed kinetic chain activity during these early degrees of motion, but stress to the ACL increases during closed kinetic chain activities when the knee moves beyond about 45° of flexion (figure 19.3).[114] There is less anterior shear stress (and less subsequent ACL strain) in weight-bearing activities that are performed in 0° to 60° of knee motion.[117]

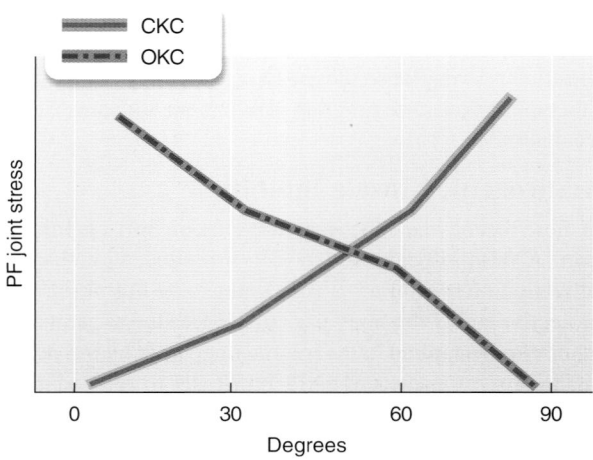

Figure 19.3 Patellofemoral joint stress at different angles. Similarities in stresses during open-chain activities allow complimentary exercises if an ACL patient also has patellofemoral pain.

Based on Steinkamp et al. (1993).[54]

In summary, the least amount of anterior displacement in an anterior cruciate–deficient knee during a closed-chain exercise occurs at 60° and less, while the least displacement in an open-chain exercise occurs at 40° and more.[117] Joint compressive forces that occur during weight bearing may be responsible for reducing the shearing forces and anterior translation that occur in open kinetic chain activities.[118]

Isokinetic exercise is not used until the later phases of rehabilitation because it is open chain; its lever arm can be shortened, but it still applies significant shear stresses. When isokinetic exercise is first used, the slower speeds should be avoided because slower speeds produce a greater torque that can increase anterior tibial displacement and ACL strain. Isokinetic exercises are usually not added to the therapeutic exercise program until the patient enters the latter half of the resistive phase.

Bracing

Perhaps more than any other joint, the knee is a frequent site for braces. There are three types of braces: prophylactic, rehabilitative, and functional. The prophylactic brace is used to prevent or reduce the severity of an injury,[119] the rehabilitative brace restricts motion of an injured joint, and a functional brace improves the stability of an unstable joint.[120] A functional brace can also be a prophylactic brace.

There are custom-made braces and off-the-shelf braces. Custom-made braces are more expensive and can cost several hundred dollars or more. Off-the-shelf braces are similar in construction to the custom-made braces but come in generic sizes, usually ranging from extra small to extra large.

The use of braces after ACL injuries is widespread.[121] Braces provide anterior stability during low-stress loading but have not shown adequate stability during more functional athletic load applications.[122] Although several reports indicate there is no difference whether postoperative ACL patients wear braces or not,[121, 123] other evidence indicates that braces do seem to provide some proprioceptive feedback, so they may be of value for this reason.[124]

Patients who have patellofemoral pain often use knee sleeves. Once again, the proprioceptive benefit as reflected in subjective reports of decreased pain may be the primary advantage. The sleeves do not alter patellar glide or protect the knee from external stress, but there is some evidence to indicate a sleeve has some value.[125] Even considering the evidence, one cannot dismiss the psychological benefits of increased confidence and assurance that using a sleeve may give the patient.[126]

Program Progression

Tissue healing and the injury's response to exercise are primary factors that dictate the rate of progression of a knee rehabilitation program. Range of motion, strength and endurance, balance and agility, and functional performance are advanced as with rehabilitation programs for other body segments. Careful observation by the rehabilitation clinician, as well as reliance on the patient for accurate feedback about responses to exercise, is essential for steady progress.

As with other rehabilitation program progressions, protecting the injury, reducing pain and edema, and maintaining current levels of conditioning are all included in phase I (inactive phase) of knee rehabilitation. Flexibility exercises, joint mobilization, and soft-tissue mobilization are all techniques that usually begin in phase II (active phase); the specific area involved in new tissue formation will dictate whether these techniques may be more appropriate in phase II or in phase III. Early strength and endurance exercises begin in phase III (resistive phase) and encompass a variety of activities that advance from static to dynamic and from isometric to isotonic, and eventually in later phase III or even phase IV (advanced phase), to isokinetic exercises. The tools used to improve strength depend on the timing of the program, the patient's response, the availability of equipment, and the rehabilitation clinician's preference. Isometric exercises are used more often in later phase II, when the knee is immobilized, when range-of-motion exercises are too painful for the patient, and when the aim is to isolate weak ranges of motion. In most cases, a combination of open and closed kinetic chain exercises is beneficial in phase III and sometimes in later phase II to improve strength.

Balance and agility exercises begin with double-support weight-bearing activities in phase III or late phase II and progress to single-limb static balancing on a stable surface. Initial double-support activities might be as simple as gait training with correct weight transfer from the right to the left extremity. From there the activities advance to single-limb stance on a stable surface, then on an unstable

surface in phase III. Balance activities begin at a low level when the patient can bear weight on the extremity in phase II. Once the patient can place total body weight on the injured extremity, single-limb stance activities can begin. For these activities, the patient must be able to correctly shift weight without trunk lean onto the involved extremity. A trunk lean not only does not permit accurate bodyweight transfer onto the extremity, but it also promotes bad weight-bearing habits during gait and other activities that can become difficult to overcome.

Agility activities advance in later phase III from the balance and coordination exercises used in earlier phase III rehabilitation. Prerequisites for a progression to agility exercises are an intact neuromuscular response system and enough strength and motion to return the body's center of mass to its base of support when balance is disturbed.[127] Agility exercises also demand appropriate coordination and muscle power, so they are the next logical step in the rehabilitation progression before functional and performance-specific exercises. Agility exercises are dynamic; they may begin with no-impact activities and progress to high-impact activities according to the patient's ultimate needs. The lower-level agility exercises are unidirectional, and more advanced agility exercises are multidirectional. Agility activities begin at reduced speeds and advance to full speed as the patient progresses in late phase III.

When adding a new agility exercise to a program, it is best to include it early in the exercise session before the patient becomes fatigued; there is evidence to demonstrate that fatigue reduces the knee's proprioceptive function.[128] An agility activity requires proprioceptive feedback for proper execution.[129] Therefore, if fatigue reduces proprioceptive function, the execution will not be performed as well as it should be, and the application is undesirable because of the risk of engramming an incorrect execution.

Once the patient has mastered the agility exercises, the final steps—functional, and then performance-specific exercises—prepare the person physically and psychologically for return to full participation. The program advances to phase IV when the injury exhibits no evidence of postexercise pain or edema and when the injured knee has full range of motion and good balance. Strength needs differ for different activities; the patient should have 70% to 75% normal strength for running, 80% normal strength for submaximal agility activities, and 85% normal strength for performance-specific exercises.[130] As with other rehabilitation programs, functional activities lead up to specific performance-related drills that mimic the patient's normal activities. Performance-specific exercises are designed to come as close to normal participation demands as possible. They may begin at reduced stress levels, but as the patient's skills and confidence return and goals are met, the stress of the activity should be akin to the stress he or she will experience on returning to full participation.

The final examination to determine the patient's readiness for return to full participation should mimic the patient's activity skills and demands. The rehabilitation clinician examines the patient for accurate execution of normal activities, an ability to use both lower extremities equally and without hesitation or any inclination to favor the previously injured extremity, and the ability to perform all motions with confidence.

Rehabilitation Interventions

Among the initial interventions commonly applied to knee injury and pathology are modalities to reduce the signs and symptoms of inflammation. Since they are presented in chapter 9, they will not be repeated in this chapter. Here we discuss the specific applications of the manual techniques and rehabilitation exercises that are commonly used for the knee.

Soft-Tissue Mobilization

Pain in the soft tissue surrounding the knee can result from injury to the local tissue or to distant tissue. The foot and hip can refer pain into the knee.[131] You should examine these areas as possible sources of knee pain if there has been no frank injury. With injuries to other segments, assessment of the hip and knee segments may also be needed to rule out referred pain. You must make a differential diagnosis to eliminate other sources of pain to provide appropriate rehabilitative care for the patient.

Muscles surrounding the knee create their own pain-referral patterns. They can refer pain if they suffer an injury, if they have associated soft-tissue adhesions with restrictions of normal tissue mobility, or if they suffer a loss of flexibility and experience increased stress during activity. Trigger points become active when subjected to abnormal or excessive stresses. These issues are discussed in chapter 11.

Soft-tissue mobilization techniques listed in table 19.2 are discussed in more detail in chapter 11 and include the more common pain-referral patterns and trigger point release techniques identified and advanced by Travell and Simons.[131] For additional trigger points within other knee

TABLE 19.2 Trigger Points Commonly Seen in the Knee Muscles

Knee segment	Muscles with trigger points
Knee flexor	Hamstrings
	Popliteus
Lateral stabilizer	Tensor fasciae latae

muscles, refer to the Travell and Simons text.[131] Other techniques such as deep-tissue massage for relief of scar tissue adhesions and cross-friction massage for tendinopathy around the knee are presented here.

Hip muscles that cross the knee joint or affect knee movement are included in this chapter. Other hip muscles were addressed in chapter 18. For the most part, soft-tissue referral pain in the anterior aspect of the knee and thigh originates from the anterior thigh and hip muscles.

Two areas of the knee and thigh typically require deep-tissue massage: the patellar tendon portion of the quadriceps tendon and the iliotibial band (ITB). When the quadriceps tendon is painful because of excessive stress, irritation, or tendinopathy, cross-friction massage is often used to relieve scar tissue adhesions that can occur secondarily to these conditions. The tendon fibers are cross-frictioned in the manner described in chapter 11. Because the tendon fibers run vertically from the patella to the tibial tuberosity, the cross-friction technique is applied horizontally, across the fibers. It is important that the clinician pull the skin taut with one hand while applying the cross-friction technique with the other hand to the tendon; otherwise there is a risk that the cross-friction massage just moves the skin against the tendon and does not affect the tendon.

Cross-friction massage is also used on surgical scars to prevent or reduce adhesions of skin to underlying adjacent tissues. Even the portal sites of arthroscopy should be examined and treated as needed to prevent adhesions and to promote good tissue mobility after surgery.

The tensor fasciae latae and its long, thick tendon are frequent sites of adhesions, especially after injury or prolonged pathomechanical stresses such as those seen with genu valgus. These areas along the ITB are relieved by deep-tissue massage. The rehabilitation clinician flexes his or her hand's metacarpophalangeal and proximal interphalangeal joints and extends the distal interphalangeal joints so the finger pads rest in the palm. With the hand in this position, the rehabilitation clinician uses posterior surfaces of the middle and distal phalanx to apply an even pressure throughout the hand's contact on the patient's thigh while guiding the hand along the patient's lateral thigh from the knee moving toward the hip. Soft-tissue restrictions are palpated as "sticking points" as the hand moves along the lateral thigh. The rehabilitation clinician repeats the deep-tissue massage strokes several times, spending additional time on the more-restricted regions. It is important to maintain soft-tissue mobility gains by having the patient actively stretch the muscles after the manual treatment is completed.

Several commercial tools are now available to help release soft-tissue adhesions such as those seen in large muscles like the quadriceps and hamstrings or in tendinous regions like the ITB. These tools include Graston, the Stick, the Knobble, and several others. When used properly, they can be effective on soft-tissue restrictions around the knee and can help reduce stress on the rehabilitation clinician's hands.

As the restrictive areas release with treatment, tissue mobility improves, and the patient reports less tenderness with the massage. The range of motion of any joint affected by these soft-tissue restrictions also improves.

In an alternative technique for a home program, the patient applies self-massage using a foam roller or massage roller. If using a foam roller, the patient lies on the involved side, with the weight on both hands and the thigh on the foam roller (figure 19.4). He or she rolls from knee to thigh on the foam roller, initially locating those areas that are most tender and restricted. Then the patient moves back to those areas that are most tender and spends time on each one until the tenderness subsides or reduces. The patient repeats the process at each tender region until the areas of tenderness are treated. This technique should not produce tenderness in normal tissue, but tenderness will occur in areas of soft-tissue restriction. If using a massage roller stick, the patient applies firm pressure with each hand on the ends of the roller as it is moved along the restricted soft-tissue region.

The foam roller can also be used to massage the quadriceps muscle if its fascia is restricted from immobilization or injury (figure 19.5). The patient lies prone with the body weight on both forearms and with the anterior thighs on the foam roller. He or she uses the arms to move the lower extremities from the hips to the knees on the roller, spending more time over the tender sites in a manner similar to that explained for the ITB. The patient makes small back-and-forth motions on the roller until one area of pain is relieved, then moves along the muscle to the next area of tenderness and repeats the treatment at that site. This procedure is used on the entire muscle.

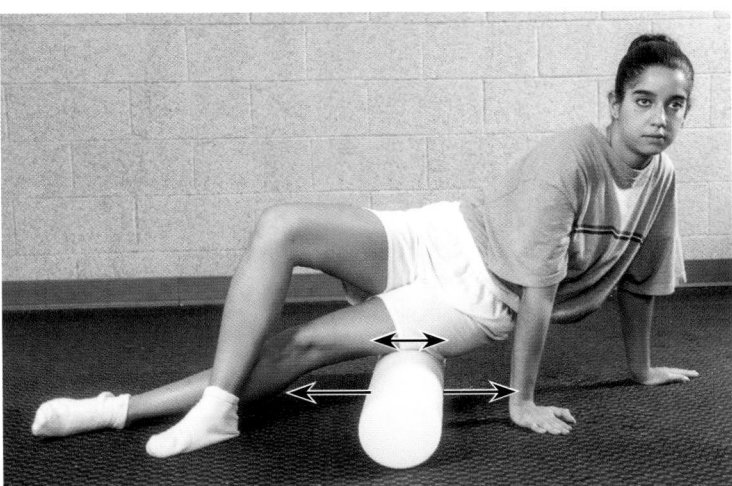

Figure 19.4   Iliotibial band foam roller self-massage.

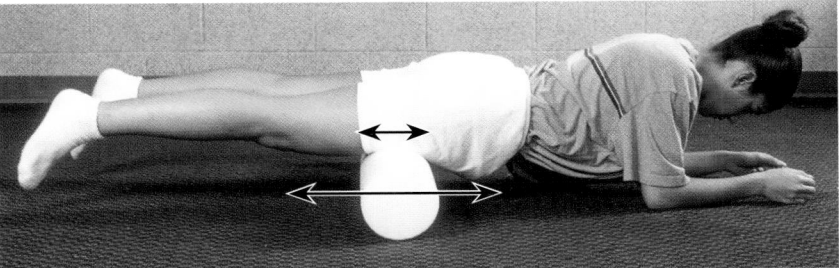

Figure 19.5   Quadriceps foam-roller massage. The application is similar to that for the ITB.

Joint Mobilization

Injury, surgery, edema, and immobilization can lead to reduced joint mobility involving the patellofemoral joint,[70] tibiofemoral joint,[132] and proximal tibiofibular joint.[133] Although the proximal tibiofibular joint is not actually part of the knee, if it develops reduced mobility it can refer pain to the knee and also affect ankle mobility. For this reason, you should assess the tibiofibular joint for restriction during your rehabilitation examination. The following sections describe some of the most commonly used joint mobilization techniques for the knee joints. Keep in mind that the indications listed for each technique use grade III and IV mobilizations, but these techniques can also be used to relieve pain when applied using grade I and II mobilizations.

Proximal Tibiofibular and Patellofemoral Mobilizations

These joints should be assessed after surgery, edema, and immobilization. Full knee range of motion requires normal mobility of the tibiofibular and patellofemoral joints. Knee examinations before the start of a therapeutic exercise program should include assessments of these joints. The resting position for the proximal tibiofibular joint is 25° of knee flexion with 10° of ankle plantar flexion, while its close-packed positions are full dorsiflexion and weight bearing.

Tibiofibular Joint Anterior and Posterior Glides

Joint: Proximal tibiofibular joint.

Resting Position: 25° of knee flexion with 10° of ankle plantar flexion.

Indications: Restricted motion of the knee, ankle, or both.

Patient Position: Supine with hip and knee flexed and foot resting on the tabletop.

Rehabilitation Clinician and Hand Positions: The rehabilitation clinician stands at the side of the treatment table near the knee being treated and grasps the fibular head with pads of thumb anteriorly and index and middle fingers posteriorly.

Mobilization Application: Fibular head is moved anteriorly, then posteriorly (figure 19.6).

Notations: The weight of the leg anchored with the foot on the table stabilizes the tibia.

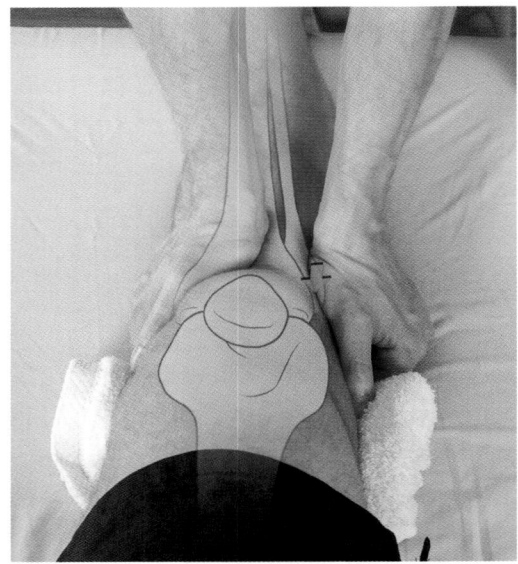

Figure 19.6

Reprinted by permission from R.C. Manske, B.J. Lehecka, M.P. Reiman, and J.K. Loudon, *Orthopedic Joint Mobilization and Manipulation* (Champaign, IL: Human Kinetics, 2019), 190.

Patellofemoral Joint Mobilization

The patella often suffers restricted mobility after injury, joint effusion, or immobilization. Normal patella mobility must be restored to permit full knee range of motion. The rehabilitation clinician should always assess the patella's mobility in all directions before beginning mobility and stretching exercises for the tibiofemoral joint.

Lateral Glides

Joint: Patellofemoral.

Resting Position: Knee extension.

Indications: Restricted medial–lateral motion of the patella.

Patient Position: The patient lies supine, and a rolled towel is placed under the knee for knee comfort and support.

Rehabilitation clinician and Hand Positions: The rehabilitation clinician stands at the side of the treatment table near the knee being treated, and the rehabilitation clinician's thumb pads are on the medial aspect of the patella.

Mobilization Application: Thumbs move the patella laterally (figure 19.7). Care must be taken to apply a lateral force, not a downward or compressive force, on the patella.

Notations: Patellar mobility is necessary for full knee flexion–extension motion and tibial rotation.

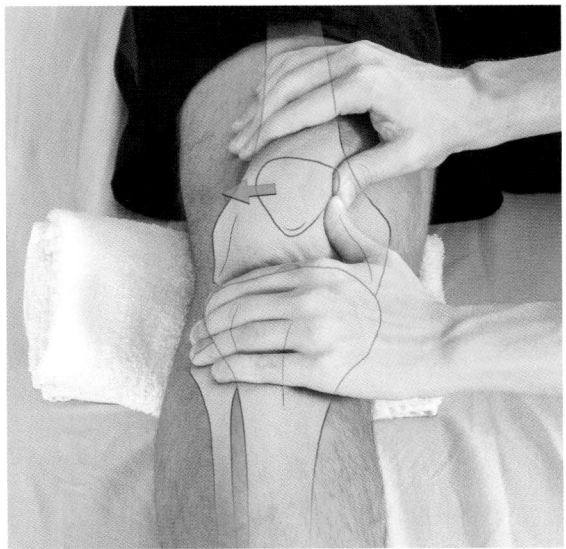

Figure 19.7

Medial Glides

Joint: Patellofemoral.

Resting Position: Knee extension.

Indications: Restricted medial–lateral motion of the patella.

Patient Position: The patient lies supine, and a rolled towel is placed under the knee for comfort and support.

Rehabilitation Clinician and Hand Positions: The rehabilitation clinician stands at the side of the treatment table near the knee being treated. The rehabilitation clinician's index finger pads are on the lateral aspect of the patella.

Mobilization Application: Finger pads move the patella medially (figure 19.8). Care must be taken to apply a medial force, not a downward or compressive force, on the patella.

Notations: Patellar mobility is necessary for full knee flexion–extension motion and tibial rotation.

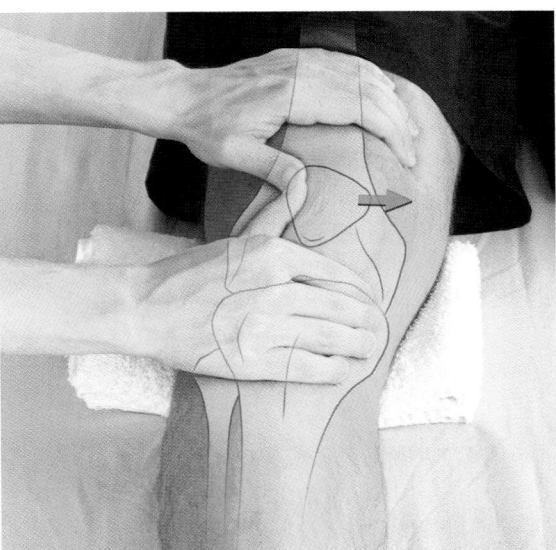

Figure 19.8

Inferior Glides

Joint: Patellofemoral.

Resting Position: Knee extension.

Indications: Restricted inferior motion of the patella.

Patient Position: The patient lies supine, and a rolled towel is placed under the knee for knee comfort and support.

Rehabilitation Clinician and Hand Positions: The rehabilitation clinician stands at the side of the treatment table near the knee being treated. The rehabilitation clinician's thumb and index finger are placed around the superior rim of the patella.

Mobilization Application: The rehabilitation clinician glides the patella distally in an inferior direction toward the toes, being careful not to compress the patella on the femur (figure 19.9).

Notations: Patellar mobility is necessary for full knee flexion–extension motion and tibial rotation.

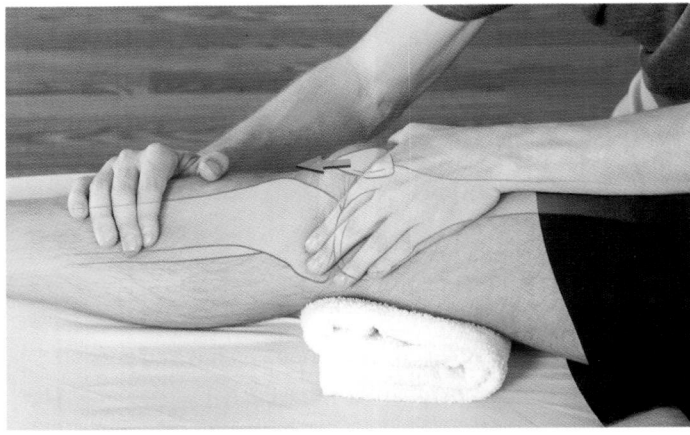

Figure 19.9

Superior Glides

Joint: Patellofemoral.

Resting Position: Knee extension.

Indications: Restricted superior motion of the patella.

Patient Position: The patient lies supine, and a rolled towel is placed under the knee for knee comfort and support.

Rehabilitation Clinician and Hand Positions: The rehabilitation clinician stands at the side of the treatment table near the knee being treated. The rehabilitation clinician's thumb and index finger are placed around the inferior rim of the patella.

Mobilization Application: The rehabilitation clinician's thumb and index finger exert a cephalic force on the patella, avoiding compression of the patella on the femur (figure 19.10).

Notations: Patellar mobility is necessary for full knee flexion–extension motion and tibial rotation.

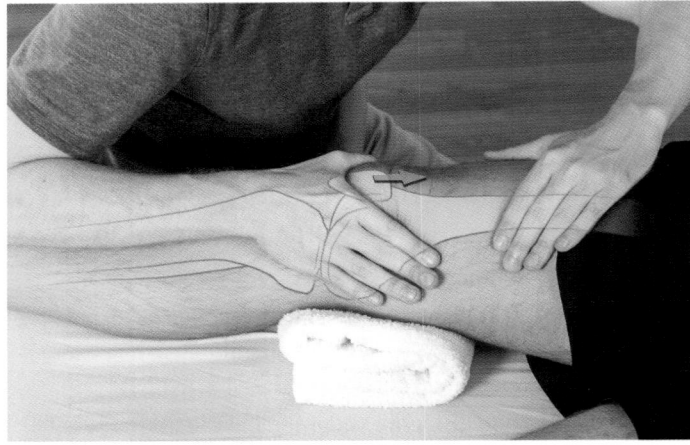

Figure 19.10

Tibiofemoral Mobilizations

This is the joint most often mobilized to improve knee range of motion. Although the patellofemoral and superior tibiofibular joints also can affect total range of motion, the tibiofemoral joint has the greatest impact. Some of the more commonly applied mobilizations for the tibiofemoral joint are included here.

Distraction

Joint: Tibiofemoral joint.

Resting Position: 20° to 25° flexion.

Indications: General restriction or general relaxation.

Patient Position: Supine or seated with knee supported in resting position.

Rehabilitation Clinician and Hand Positions: The femur is stabilized with one hand proximal to the knee, and the mobilizing hand is placed proximal to the ankle joint. If the patient is sitting at the edge of a table, both of the rehabilitation clinician's hands grasp the proximal tibia.

Mobilization Application: The tibia is pulled distally by the mobilizing hand while the stabilizing hand secures the thigh. If the patient is seated, the rehabilitation clinician distracts the tibia distally with both hands (figure 19.11).

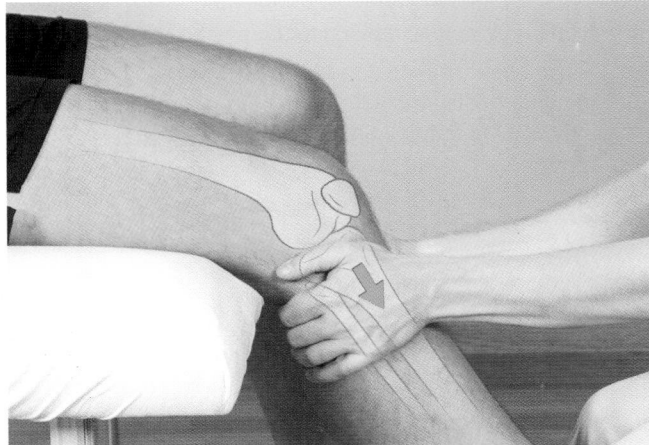

Figure 19.11

Notations: This technique is often used both before and after using grade III and IV mobilizations.

Anterior Glides

Joint: Tibiofemoral joint.

Resting Position: 20° to 25° flexion.

Indications: To increase knee extension.

Patient Position: Prone. The knee is flexed with the thigh supported on the table and the patient's leg resting on the rehabilitation clinician's shoulder. A pad under the distal thigh will make the position more comfortable for the patient and align the thigh more appropriately for the glide.

Rehabilitation Clinician and Hand Positions: With the rehabilitation clinician at the foot of the table, the patient's distal leg is supported on the rehabilitation clinician's shoulder. The rehabilitation clinician clasps his or her hands around the proximal leg near the posterior knee and glides the tibia anteriorly on the femur (figure 19.12a).

Mobilization Application: The glide force must be parallel to the plane of the joint surface. When the knee is moved out of the resting position for mobilizations, the angle of force will also change since the force must always be parallel to the tibia's joint surface.

Notations: The hamstrings should remain relaxed to produce the most effective results.

An alternative posterior-to-anterior mobilization technique is performed with the patient prone and the rehabilitation clinician standing along

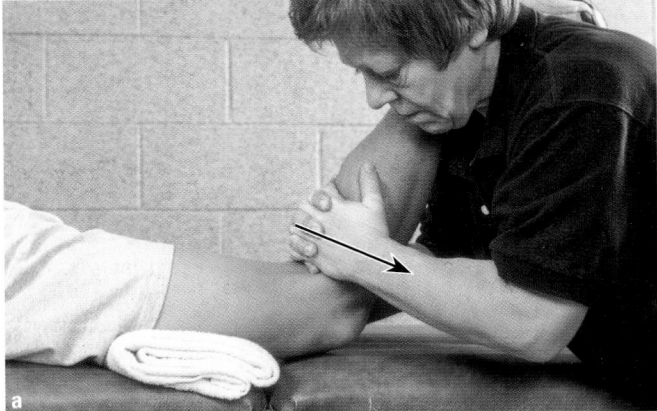

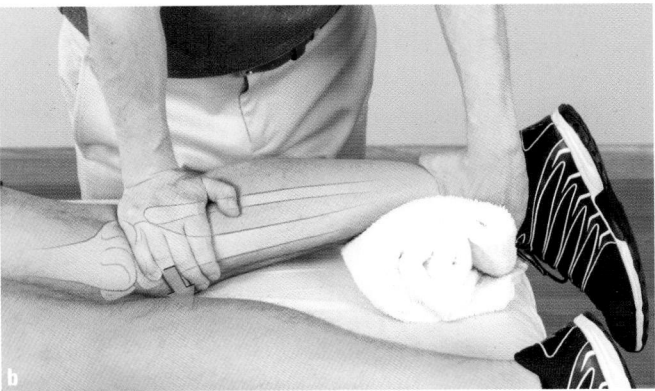

Figure 19.12 Two different positions to achieve a tibiofemoral joint anterior glide.

>*continued*

Anterior Glides >*continued*

the table's side at the level of the patient's knee and rotated to face the patient's foot. The rehabilitation clinician supports the distal tibia with the knee at 30° flexion with the stabilizing hand. An anterior force is applied by the mobilizing hand just distal to the posterior knee joint (figure 19.12*b*).

An anterior glide can also be performed with the patient sitting with the thighs on the table and the legs freely hanging over the side. The rehabilitation clinician sits on a treatment stool facing the patient and secures the patient's leg between his or her knees to place the knee in a resting position and places both hands over the posterior proximal leg just below the knee.

Posterior Glides

Joint: Tibiofemoral joint.

Resting Position: 20° to 25° flexion.

Indications: To increase knee flexion motion.

Patient Position: Patient is supine or seated with a pad under the thigh to keep the joint in a resting position.

Rehabilitation Clinician and Hand Positions: The rehabilitation clinician stands near the treated knee and places the heel of one hand on the anterior proximal tibia, with the other hand stabilizing the distal femur.

Mobilization Application: Posterior glide parallel to the tibia's joint surface (figure 19.13).

Notations: In an alternative position, the patient is sitting with the knee over the edge of the table with a towel roll under the distal

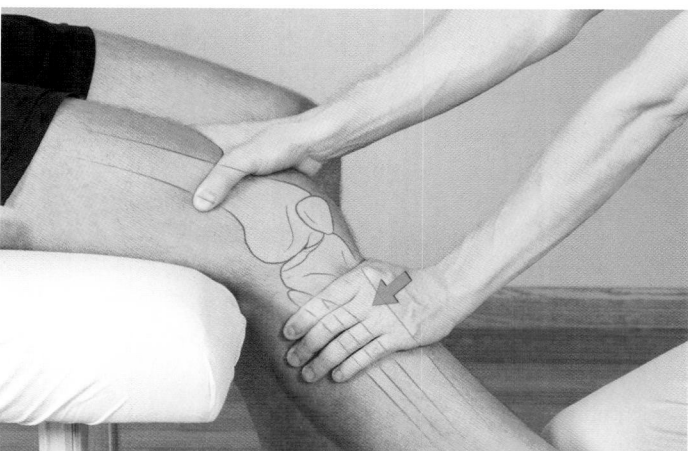

Figure 19.13

thigh for support. The rehabilitation clinician sits on a treatment stool facing the patient and secures the patient's leg between his or her knees to place the knee in a resting position. The rehabilitation clinician applies a posterior glide at the tibial condyles.

Rotational Glide: Anterior Glide of the Medial Tibial Condyle

Joint: Tibiofemoral joint.

Resting Position: Resting position is 20° to 25° flexion, but this technique is often performed in an end-range position.

Indications: Used to gain lateral tibial rotation in terminal knee extension.

Patient Position: Prone with a pad under the distal femur for comfort.

Rehabilitation Clinician and Hand Positions: The heel of one hand is on the posterior medial tibial plateau.

Mobilization Application: A posterior-to-anterior (PA) glide of the medial posterior tibia on the femur to produce the screw-home rotation for full knee extension (figure 19.14).

Notations: This technique is used to gain the last few degrees of extension in a knee.

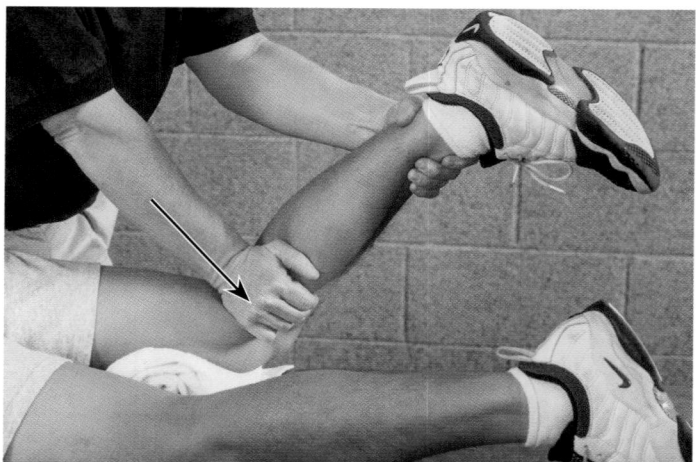

Figure 19.14

Rotational Glide: Posterior Glide of the Medial Tibial Condyle

Joint: Tibiofemoral joint.

Resting Position: Resting position is 20° to 25° flexion, but this technique is often performed in an end-range position.

Indications: Used to gain medial tibial rotation and knee flexion.

Patient Position: Patient is supine with the knee in flexion.

Rehabilitation Clinician and Hand Positions: Rehabilitation clinician places the heel of the hand on the medial tibial condyle anteriorly.

Mobilization Application: An anterior–posterior (AP) force is applied to the medial tibial condyle (figure 19.15).

Notations: This technique may be used to acquire the last few degrees of knee flexion.

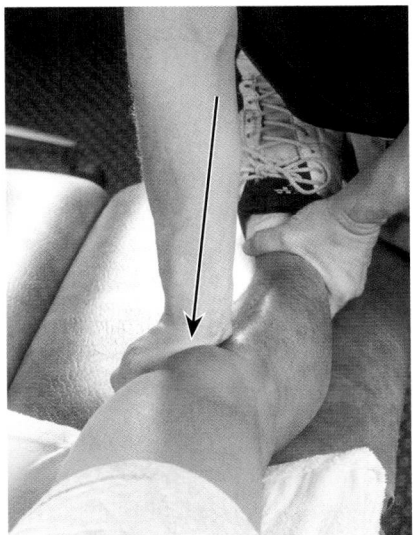

Figure 19.15

Flexibility Exercises

Flexibility exercises for the knee can be active or passive. The techniques used depend on the type of tissue being stretched and how recent the injury is. As a general rule of thumb, healing soft tissue occasionally requires time for immobilization to protect newly forming tissue, but after this immobilization period, movement produces a better result of healing than prolonged immobilization.[134] Very new and developing scars of severe muscle, ligament, and tendon tissue injuries may need up to 3 weeks of immobilization, but controlled motion after this period of immobilization will enhance the new tissue's strength.[134] Mildly injured soft tissue may not need as long an immobilization and may be able to tolerate mild passive stretches, but this must be carefully determined. As scar tissue continues to mature in the later proliferation phase and early remodeling phase, it may be effectively stretched with active and short-term stretches, but this depends on the injury's severity and location. Very adherent scar tissue in its late remodeling phase or later requires a combination of scar tissue massage and stretching to loosen adhesions; if it is very mature, long-term stretches may be the best way to increase mobility by affecting the tissue's plastic element.[135]

After surgical repair of the knee or total knee arthroplasty, orthopedic surgeons often have the patient's knee placed in a continuous passive motion (CPM) machine or begin early active motion.[136] Although not used as often as they were a few years ago, CPMs are beneficial in reducing pain and edema and encouraging the restoration of range of motion in the short term;[137] however, studies have shown no significant long-term differences between patients using CPMs and those not using them.[138]

The exercises presented in the following sections are divided into prolonged and active stretches. The active stretches include some exercises that use assistive equipment and some that need only the patient's active motion. During active stretches, it is important for the patient to contract the opposing muscle whenever possible to enhance relaxation of the stretched muscle and achieve a more effective stretch.

Prolonged Stretches

These stretches are used when scar tissue that is limiting motion is mature or is becoming mature and short-term stretches would be ineffective in improving tissue flexibility or mobility. Although healing timelines vary from structure to structure, as a general rule, prolonged knee stretches are more effective than short-term stretches when scar tissue is more than 30 weeks old since this is when levels of Type III collagen are comparable to those of normal ligament tissue.[139] Healing tissue continues to mature beyond a year,[140] so tissue becomes more rigid as the healing process continues past 30 weeks. Therefore, when determining the time for prolonged stretching, the clinician must account not only for the patient's tolerance but also for the scar tissue's age.

When using prolonged stretches, the rehabilitation clinician must tell the patient that the knee will feel stiff once the stretch is released but that the stiffness should resolve quickly. It may be difficult for the patient to take the first few steps after a prolonged stretch. A prolonged stretch is more effective the longer it is applied, but it is also more difficult for the patient to tolerate. When the force is first applied, the patient may not feel that a stretch is occurring, but as time passes, he or she will feel the stretch. A patient may not be able to tolerate a prolonged stretch for more than 5 min initially. If this is the case, and a weight is being used, the stretch weight should be decreased or removed to make a longer stretch tolerable.

As the patient begins to better tolerate the stretch, either a weight can be applied or the stretch time can be increased.

It is better to increase stretch duration than weight. If the stretch parameters are appropriate and the patient's tolerance adjusts, the patient may be able to eventually tolerate a 10 to 15 min stretch. These prolonged stretches may be used as clinical treatments, home exercise programs, or both. In the case of severe restrictions, using prolonged stretches in both the clinic and the home to increase application frequency may be beneficial.

Prolonged Flexibility Exercises for the Knee

Prolonged stretches are indicated if the knee's end-feel is hard rather than firm. Such an end-feel indicates that the surrounding scar tissue is of sufficient strength that short-term stretches will not be as effective as prolonged stretches. It is better to apply a low-level force for a longer time than a more intense stretch force for a shorter time. If the stretch has sufficient force, the patient may not feel a stretch when the prolonged stretch is initially applied, but as the stretch continues, the patient will report feeling it.

Prolonged Knee Extension in Prone

Body Segment: Knee.

Stage in Rehab: Resistive phase and beyond with a recent injury; active phase if it is an older injury.

Purpose: Increase knee extension motion.

Positioning: Patient is prone with a pad under the distal thigh and the leg hanging off the table (figure 19.16).

Execution: The patient relaxes the leg and maintains this position for 10 to 15 min.

Possible Substitutions: Hip flexion or rotation or pelvis flexion. If substitution occurs, a strap placed across the hips and thighs and around the table will secure the extremity in position.

Notations: The prone stretch relaxes the hamstrings at its proximal end, so this position concentrates more on the joint and its capsule. A weight on the ankle will increase the stretch force, but the weight should start light and increase only as the patient tolerates. The hip and thigh should be secured as necessary to prevent pelvis motion or thigh rotation during the stretch.

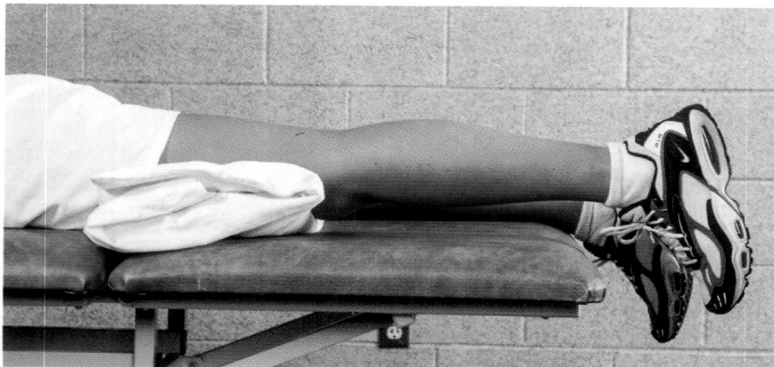

Figure 19.16

Prolonged Knee Extension in Long Sitting

Body Segment: Knee.

Stage in Rehab: Resistive phase and beyond with a recent injury; active phase if it is an older injury.

Purpose: Increase knee extension motion.

Positioning: The patient is sitting with the heel of the foot placed on another chair seat or table. The calf is unsupported (figure 19.17).

Execution: The patient relaxes the lower extremity and allows gravity to pull the knee down. A weight may be applied to the distal and proximal knee to increase gravitational forces.

Possible Substitutions: Hip lateral rotation and knee flexion.

Notations: Applying hot packs before and during the stretch may improve tolerance for the stretch. Because of the hip position, the hamstrings may be stretched as well as the capsule.

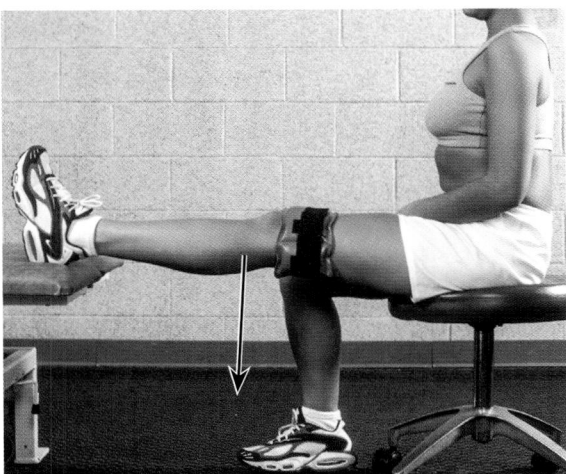

Figure 19.17

 Go to HK*Propel* and watch video 19.1, which demonstrates a prolonged knee stretch.

Prolonged Knee Flexion Stretch

Body Segment: Knee.

Stage in Rehab: Resistive phase and beyond with a recent injury; active phase if it is an older injury.

Purpose: Increase knee flexion motion.

Positioning: Patient is sitting in a chair with a pad around the distal leg and secured with a strap (figure 19.18).

Execution: The strap is anchored to the back chair leg. The strap is attached around the patient's ankle and controlled by the patient's pulling on the strap. The patient is instructed to pull the leg back to a point that feels tight but not painful. He or she holds this position for several minutes before trying to increase flexion further.

Possible Substitutions: Rotating the leg and thigh; not holding the stretch long enough. A timer may need to be used.

Notations: An alternative method is for the patient to sit on the floor with the foot against the wall. The patient moves the buttocks toward the wall until a stretch is felt in the anterior knee. This position is maintained for 2 to 3 min

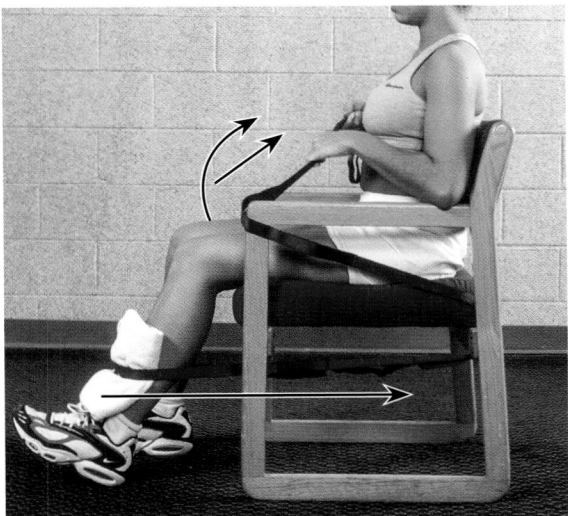

Figure 19.18

before the patient moves the gluteals closer to the wall, then holds that position for several minutes. The total time for the exercise is 10 to 15 min. With the patient in sitting, the stretch force is applied to the joint and its capsule, not the muscle crossing it.

Once the knee flexes to 100° but still needs a prolonged stretch, the patient can be positioned prone on a treatment table with a strap around the pelvis and another one around the mid-thigh. A rolled towel is placed in the posterior knee and a strap is secured around the ankle. The knee is flexed to its end-flexion position and secured with the ankle strap to prevent the knee from moving into extension. With the hip in extension, the quadriceps is being stretched. Start the patient with a 5 min stretch and slowly increase the time as the patient's tolerance improves.

Active Stretches

A number of active stretches are available to gain knee flexibility. The important point to remember for each stretch is to position the muscle so that it is not working during the stretch. A hamstring stretch that many athletes use, standing and bending over to touch the floor, is a good example of what *not* to do. The hamstrings hold the body upright in this position to prevent the person from falling forward; therefore, stretching the muscle in this position is futile because the muscle is contracting to maintain balance while it is being stretched.

Active stretches are repeated several times throughout the day. As discussed previously, either a 15 s hold for about four repetitions or one 30 s stretch is recommended. When possible, the opposing muscle should relax the stretched muscle and produce a more effective stretch on the intended muscle. Common active stretches are presented in the following sections.

Active Flexibility Exercises for the Knee

Wall Slides

Body Segment: Knee (quadriceps).

Stage in Rehab: Active phase.

Purpose: Increase knee flexion motion, especially if the patient is non–weight bearing (NWB).

Positioning: Patient is supine with buttocks about 60 cm (2 ft) or less from a wall. A towel is placed under the foot that is resting on the wall.

Execution: The patient slides the foot down the wall, bending the knee as far as possible (figure 19.19). The uninvolved extremity helps to return the foot to the starting position. As motion improves, the buttocks are moved closer to the wall.

Possible Substitutions: Rotating the hip laterally and hip abduction. The hip, knee, and ankle should remain in good alignment with each other throughout the exercise.

Notations: If the patient can tolerate more movement, he or she can encourage more flexion by using the uninvolved extremity to push on the top of the involved extremity at the ankle.

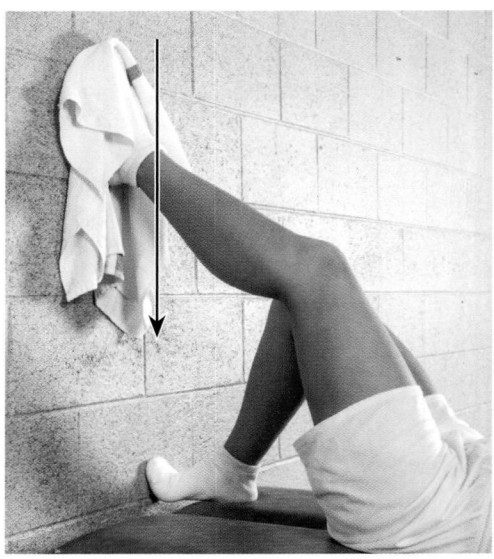

Figure 19.19

Seated Knee Flexion

Body Segment: Knee (quadriceps).

Stage in Rehab: Active phase.

Purpose: Increase knee flexion after achieving 50° of flexion.

Positioning: Patient is sitting in a chair with both feet resting on the floor. The uninvolved foot is placed on top of the involved limb's ankle.

Execution: The uninvolved extremity pushes the involved knee into flexion as far as possible (figure 19.20).

Possible Substitutions: Laterally rotating the hip, extending the hip, abduction of the hip. The knee, hip, and ankle should all remain in the same plane.

Notations: This exercise is used throughout the day to improve knee flexion.

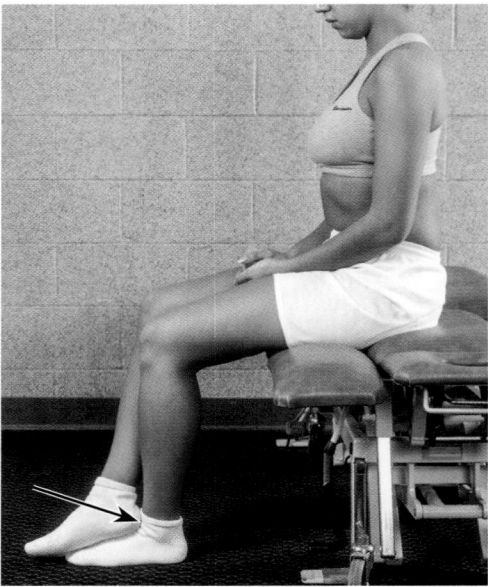

Figure 19.20

Standing Knee Flexion

Body Segment: Knee (quadriceps).

Stage in Rehab: Active phase.

Purpose: Increase knee flexion once near-normal motion is achieved.

Positioning: Patient stands near a wall or table to use as support.

Execution: The patient grasps the foot behind the back and pulls it toward the buttocks (figure 19.21). The knee should point vertically downward to the floor during the stretch.

Possible Substitutions: Forward trunk flexion, hip extension or abduction, and lateral rotation of the tibia. Provide verbal cueing to correct for improper execution.

Notations: If the patient cannot reach the foot because of insufficient flexibility, he or she can use a stretch strap in standing. The strap is wrapped around the ankle and grasped behind the back. The strap is pulled to move the foot toward the buttock. An erect posture must be maintained for this exercise.

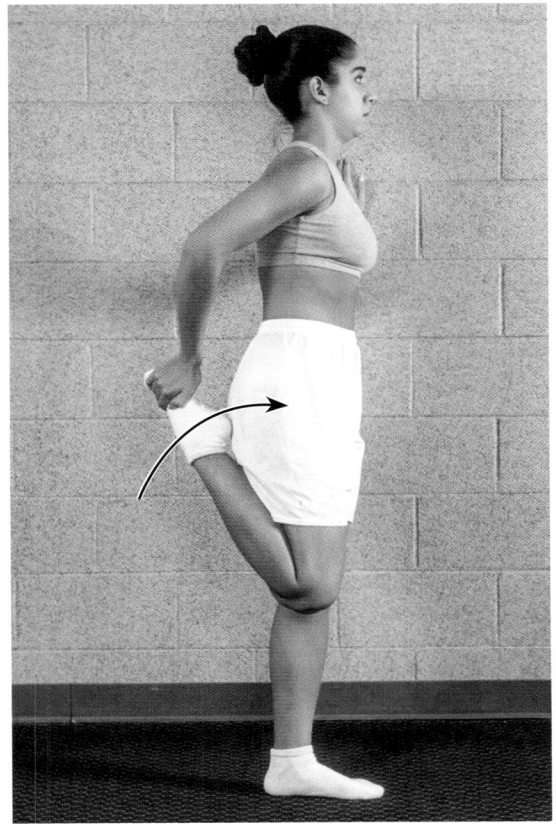

Figure 19.21

Stationary Bike

Body Segment: Knee (quadriceps).

Stage in Rehab: Active phase.

Purpose: Increase knee flexion motion. This exercise is especially good once the patient has 90° of flexion and is at least partial weight bearing (PWB).

Positioning: Feet are secured on foot pedals with straps. The height of the seat should be such that at the bottom of the crank position, the knee is near full extension (figure 19.22).

Execution: The patient uses the uninvolved extremity to guide and control the involved extremity during pedaling.

Possible Substitutions: Ankle plantar flexion, hip hiking, or shifting body weight to uninvolved side. Provide verbal cueing to correct technique.

Notations: It is best to begin with a backward motion because it is easier to achieve a full circle going backward than it is forward. Once the patient is moving the pedals smoothly in reverse, he or she can do forward cycling.

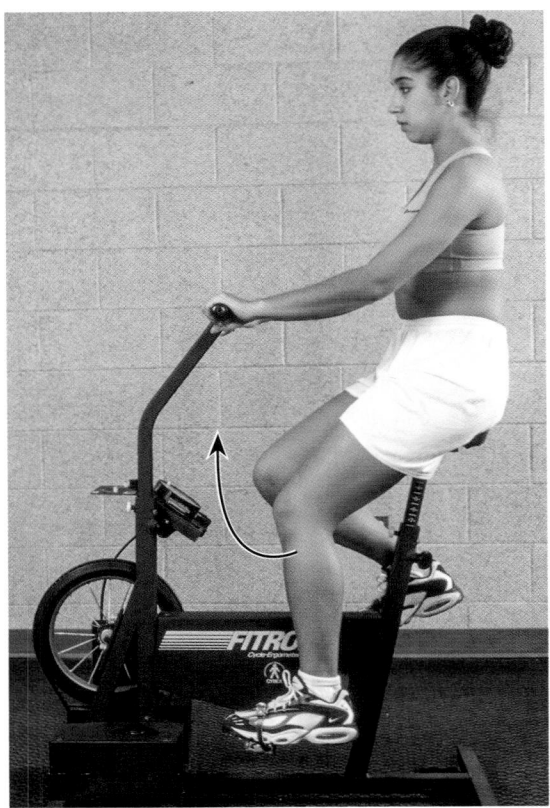

Figure 19.22

Supine Hamstring Stretch

Body Segment: Knee (hamstrings).

Stage in Rehab: Active phase.

Purpose: Increase knee extension motion.

Positioning: The patient lies supine with the uninvolved extremity extended.

Execution: The involved knee is brought toward the chest, and the hands are clasped behind the thigh. The knee is then actively extended as far as possible so that a stretch is felt behind the knee or in the thigh.

Possible Substitutions: Rotating the pelvis posteriorly. To prevent this from occurring, have the patient keep the uninvolved hip and knee in extension during the stretch.

Notations: A stretch strap can be used around the foot if it is too difficult for the patient to reach the thigh. Another alternative is to have the patient lie supine in a doorway with the uninvolved extremity extended into the doorway and the involved foot on the wall (figure 19.23). The stretch is released by bending the knee. As the patient's flexibility increases, the buttocks are moved closer to the doorframe.

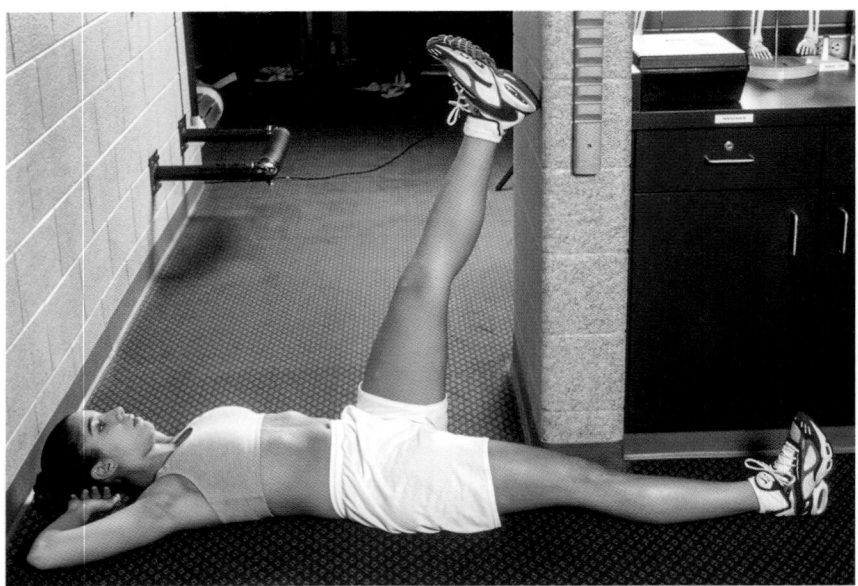

Figure 19.23

Standing Hamstring Stretch

Body Segment: Knee (hamstrings).

Stage in Rehab: Active phase.

Purpose: Increase knee extension motion.

Positioning: The standing limb is positioned with the foot facing forward. The involved knee is kept extended during the stretch, with the foot facing the ceiling.

Execution: The patient bends forward from the hips, not the back, and tries to reach toward the toes with the opposite hand (figure 19.24). As the patient reaches forward with the opposite hand, the motion occurs at the hips with the chest up and the back straight. The standing foot should face forward. Both knees should be straight.

Possible Substitutions: Using the same-side arm to reach forward, flexing from the back rather than the hip, rotating the standing limb, flexing the standing knee or the stretch knee. Reaching forward with the same hand allows trunk rotation. The back should remain straight by keeping the chest raised and core muscles tense as the patient leans forward from the hips during the stretch.

Notations: Standing hamstring stretches ensure stabilization of the pelvis because the supporting extremity remains in extension during the stretch. The height of the surface on which the involved extremity is placed depends on the patient's flexibility. With very tight hamstrings, it may be best to begin the stretch with the foot on a footstool or chair seat. As the patient's flexibility improves, the height of the supporting object can be raised. If flexibility is normal, a person should be able to touch the toes of the foot elevated to hip height with the opposite hand. The patient should not bounce during this exercise. Contraction of the quadriceps improves the flexibility during the stretch.

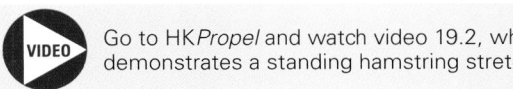
Go to HK*Propel* and watch video 19.2, which demonstrates a standing hamstring stretch.

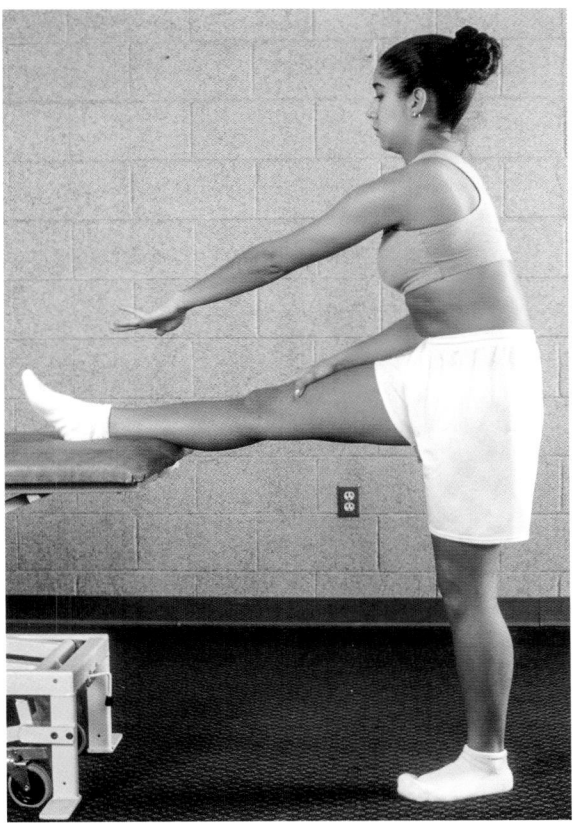
Figure 19.24

Strengthening Exercises

Strengthening exercises can begin early in a therapeutic exercise program even if the knee is immobilized or the patient is non–weight bearing. Isometrics help increase strength and reduce pain.[141] Once active motion is permitted, isotonic activities against gravity can progress to exercises against resistance in the form of free weights, manual resistance, machine resistance, body weight when weight bearing is permitted, and finally, isokinetic exercises, if available and appropriate.

The rehabilitation clinician must bear in mind that some hip muscles and ankle muscles cross the knee joint and must also be included in the rehabilitation process. The hip and lateral thigh muscles act as stabilizers for the knee and are important for knee control.[142] Trunk muscles also are important for knee stability,[143] so exercises for these muscles are included in knee rehabilitation. Although exercises for the trunk, hip, and ankle are not discussed here, they should be included as part of the total rehabilitation program for a knee injury.

Strengthening exercises should not cause pain or swelling, either during or after the exercise. The rehabilitation clinician must solicit routine feedback from the patient about how the knee responds to exercises throughout the program, especially during the initial treatment phase and whenever there are increases in the program. Increased pain and swelling indicate that the exercises are too severe. In the presence of these signs, the exercise intensity or severity must be reduced. It is important not to provide too many new exercises for the same structure at the same time; if the patient experiences increased edema or pain, you will not know which new exercise caused the problem.

In the early phases of a rehabilitation program, it is better to provide a balance of exercises that include perhaps one or two strengthening exercises for various deficient areas rather than to emphasize only the quadriceps or only the hamstrings. For example, the first treatment session's strengthening exercises may include short-arc quads; manual resistance to hip abduction, adduction, and extension; and hamstring curls. In this case, if the patient returns with more anterior knee pain, the short-arc quads probably caused the irritation. If the patient had received short-arc quad exercises along with full-arc quad and standing squat exercises, it would be hard to determine what caused the patient's pain. Once you have established the cause of the knee's reaction, it is easier to decide what exercises are appropriate.

Isometrics

Instructions for 10 s isometric exercises should emphasize a 2 s buildup of the muscle contraction to a maximum level, a hold at the maximum level for 5 to 6 s,[144] and then a 2 s decline to full relaxation before the next repetition. A sudden contraction to maximal levels can cause discomfort and yield a less-than-optimal result. You should also instruct the patient to repeat the exercise in sets of at least 10 several times throughout the day. The following sections provide some suggestions for common isometric exercises. Other exercises in these sections progress from non-weight-bearing to weight-bearing exercises.

Strength Exercises for the Knee

Since normal knee function involves a combination of open- and closed-chain activities, rehabilitation exercises for the knee should also include both types. However, you must be aware of the different types of stresses within the knee's range of motion that are applied by open- and closed-chain activities. There are some injuries for which you should avoid resistance in specific ranges of open and closed motion in the earlier phases of a rehabilitation program. Examples of these include anterior and posterior cruciate ligament injuries and patellofemoral injuries.

Open Kinetic Chain (OKC): Isometric Quad Set

Body Segment: Quadriceps.

Stage in Rehab: Active phase.

Purpose: Strengthen quadriceps during early rehab when the quadriceps is very weak and the patient is NWB.

Positioning: Patient is sitting or supine with the knee extended and the uninvolved knee flexed to relieve back stress.

Execution: The patient tightens the quadriceps, trying to push the posterior knee into the table.

Possible Substitutions: Lateral hip rotation, knee flexion, knee abduction. Verbal cueing will correct these substitutions.

Notations: Placing the hand on the quad to palpate for muscle tightening also helps facilitate a contraction.[145] If the patient cannot feel a contraction, have the person perform the exercise with the uninvolved quadriceps to feel a normal contraction before performing the isometric with the involved knee. If the patient still cannot facilitate a quad contraction, you can lift the heel of the involved limb off the table about 15 cm (6 in.) and instruct the patient to hold this position as you reduce hand support. You should not completely remove your hand, though, because the patient will probably not be able to hold the position independently. A patient who has difficulty producing a quad set in supine can use an alternative position. The patient lies prone with a rolled towel under the ankle, then tries to push the ankle into the towel roll to facilitate quadriceps activation (figure 19.25). The rehabilitation clinician should palpate the quadriceps to monitor active contractions during the exercise. Electrical stimulation can also be useful for quadriceps facilitation if the patient cannot produce a good quad contraction with an active exercise.

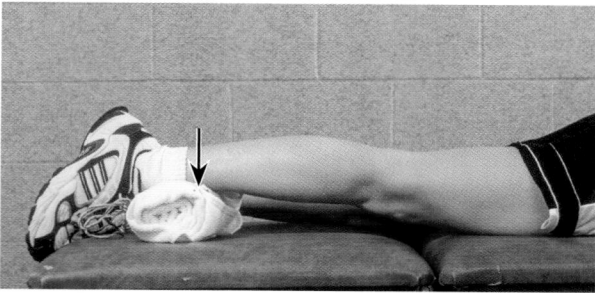

Figure 19.25

OKC: Straight-Leg Raise

Body Segment: Quadriceps.

Stage in Rehab: Active phase.

Purpose: Strengthen the quadriceps.

Positioning: The patient is supine with the uninvolved knee flexed and the involved knee extended.

Execution: The patient first contracts the quadriceps muscle, then raises the involved extremity off the table about 20 cm (8 in.) and holds the limb at that level for about 5 s (figure 19.26). The extremity is then slowly lowered, and the quadriceps muscle is not relaxed until the extremity is on the table.

Possible Substitutions: Hip rotation, hip abduction, knee flexion.

Notations: The straight-leg raise is a hip exercise, but because it requires the quadriceps to hold the knee in extension, it is essentially an isometric exercise for the quadriceps, with the exception of the rectus femoris, which also acts at the hip. The exercise becomes more difficult if the patient is in a long-sitting position rather than supine. It also is more difficult if the hip is laterally rotated during the lift rather than in a neutral position. Weights can also be used to increase the difficulty of the exercise, but whether or not weight is used depends on the injury being treated. Positioning the opposite extremity with the foot flat on the table reduces stress on the lumbar spine. The patient can sit upright to make the exercise more difficult than in the supine position since the rectus femoris cannot work with the other quadriceps muscles.

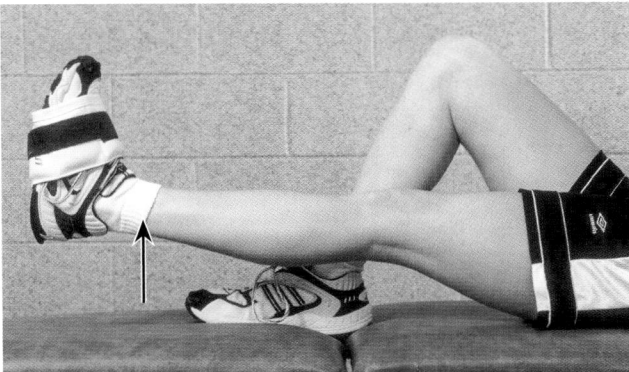

Figure 19.26

OKC: Hamstring Sets

Body Segment: Hamstrings.

Stage in Rehab: Active phase.

Purpose: Increase hamstring strength during NWB and immobilization of the knee.

Positioning: Patient is either sitting or supine with the knee in some flexion.

Execution: If in sitting, the patient places the uninvolved foot behind the distal involved extremity at the ankle and pushes the involved leg against the uninvolved leg, maintaining maximum resistance for 5 s. If in supine, the patient digs the heel of the involved limb into the tabletop, trying to flex the knee but not changing the knee position.

Possible Substitutions: Hip rotation or hip extension.

Notations: If the knee is not immobilized, the exercise may be performed at different points within the range of motion. Whether or not the patient is permitted to perform this isometric at different flexion positions depends on the injury being treated.

Non-Weight-Bearing Isotonic Exercises

Some of these exercises may sometimes begin late in the active phase and certainly occur during the early resistive phase (III) of the therapeutic exercise program, even though the patient is non–weight bearing or partial weight bearing. Open kinetic chain exercises can be useful for strengthening in early resistance activities. The following sections include some suggestions for these exercises.

OKC: Short-Arc Quadriceps Exercise (SAQ)

Body Segment: Quadriceps.

Stage in Rehab: Late active phase or early resistive phase.

Purpose: Strengthen the quadriceps in terminal knee extension.

Positioning: A roll is placed under the knee to position the knee in partial flexion. The patient is supine to use the rectus femoris or is sitting to increase the difficulty of the exercise by shortening the rectus femoris.

Execution: With the uninvolved knee flexed, the limb of the involved knee is lifted to position the knee in full extension, and then returned to the starting position (figure 19.27). The patient holds the position in full extension for about 6 s.

Possible Substitutions: Hip rotation or moving the knee through incomplete extension. Also, moving through the range of motion too quickly uses momentum rather than muscle force.

Notations: This exercise applies a significant stress to the ACL; therefore, this exercise should not be used early in rehabilitating an ACL injury or reconstruction. A weight or manual resistance can be applied to the ankle to increase the difficulty of the exercise. The size of the roll can vary, depending on how much of an arc is desired.

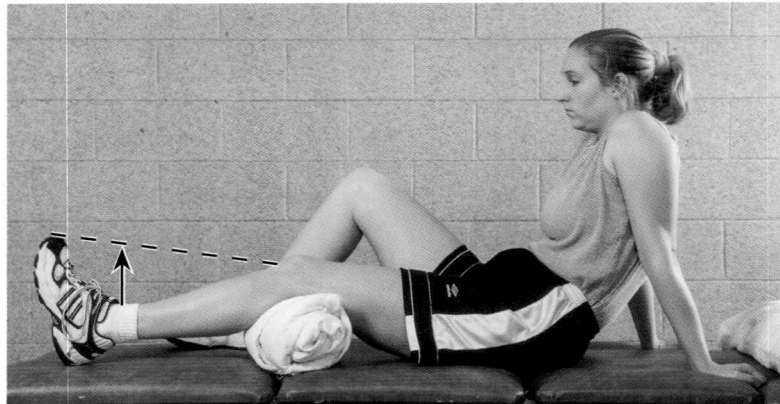

Figure 19.27

OKC: Full-Arc Quad Exercise

Body Segment: Quadriceps.

Stage in Rehab: Late resistive phase and into advanced phase.

Purpose: Strengthen the quadriceps.

Positioning: The patient sits in a chair or on the edge of a table with the knees over the edge.

Execution: The foot is lifted slowly upward to fully extend the knee (figure 19.28). As long as there is no pain and it is not contraindicated because of the injury, manual resistance, ankle weights, or rubber-band resistance can be used to increase the difficulty of the exercise.

Possible Substitutions: Using the hip to move the knee through its range of motion; moving the extremity through its motion too quickly so that momentum rather than muscle strength moves the limb.

Notations: This exercise is used with caution in early phase III. The patellofemoral joint may be painful during the exercise; this is especially the case during the range of motion from 0° to 60° of flexion because this range places more joint reaction force on the patellofemoral joint. The ACL is also stressed during the 0° to 60° arc of motion, so this exercise is inappropriate for recent ACL injuries.

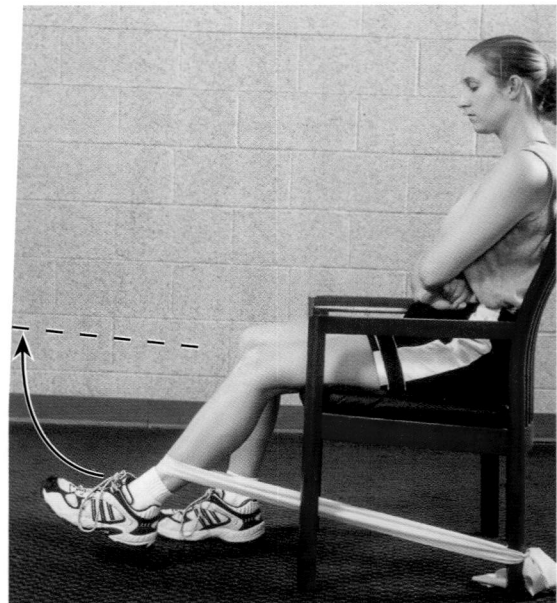

Figure 19.28

OKC: Hamstring Curls in Prone

Body Segment: Hamstrings.

Stage in Rehab: Late resistive phase and into advanced phase.

Purpose: Strengthen hamstrings.

Positioning: The patient lies prone with the foot over the edge of the table and the knee in full extension.

Execution: The knee flexes against gravity, manual resistance, a cuff weight, or a resistance band.

Possible Substitutions: Hip flexion or moving the muscle through a partial range of motion.

Notations: Maximal resistance in this exercise occurs at the beginning of the motion, when the muscle is strongest. This exercise is used with caution in early PCL rehabilitation.

OKC: Hamstring Curls in Standing

Body Segment: Hamstrings.

Stage in Rehab: Resistive phase and into advanced phase.

Purpose: Strengthen hamstrings.

Positioning: The patient stands and is supported by the uninvolved extremity and by the hands, which grasp a stable object.

Execution: The knee is flexed against cuff weights (figure 19.29*a*), manual resistance, resistance bands (figure 19.29*b*), or pulleys, moving through a full range of motion.

Possible Substitutions: Hip flexion and moving through a partial range of motion.

Notations: In this position, maximum resistance occurs at the end of the knee motion, where the hamstring is at its physiologically weakest position. This exercise is used with caution in early PCL rehabilitation.

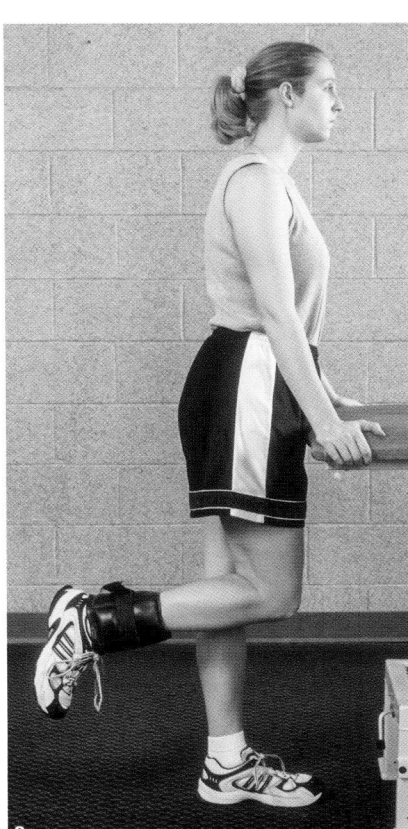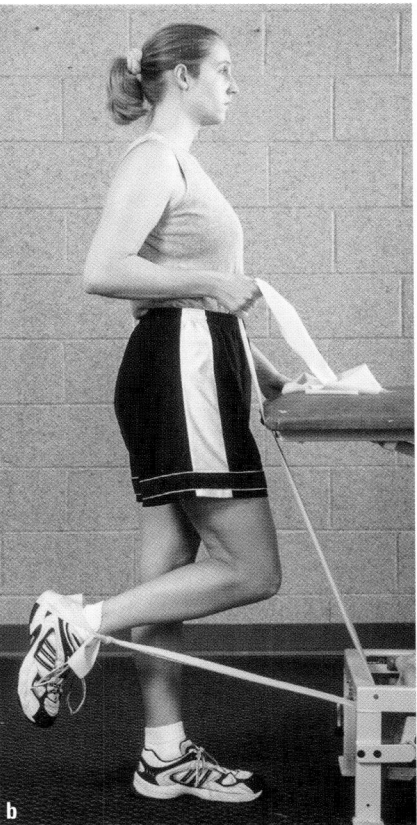

Figure 19.29

Closed Kinetic Chain (CKC): Terminal Knee Extension

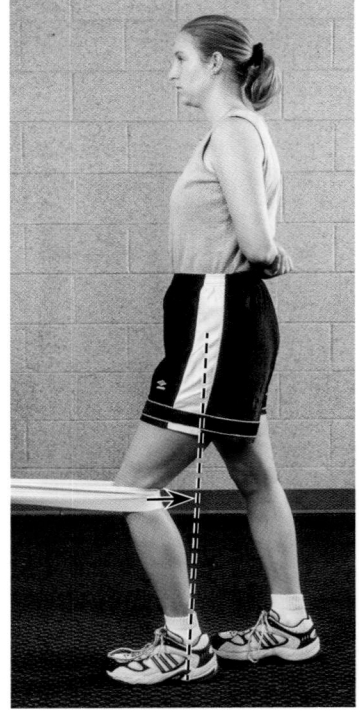

Body Segment: Knee.

Stage in Rehab: Resistive phase.

Purpose: Increase weight-bearing strength of the quadriceps in the final degrees of knee extension.

Positioning: A rubber band is anchored around a stable object such as an upright bar, doorjamb, or table leg. It is placed around the knee. A pad or towel roll between the posterior knee and band will enhance comfort. The patient stands facing the doorjamb or table with the knee slightly flexed to 30° to 45°. The amount of body weight on the involved extremity is as much as is needed to keep the foot flat on the floor; most body weight is on the uninvolved lower extremity. The band is taut at the start of the exercise.

Execution: The quadriceps muscle is tightened to straighten but not lock the knee (figure 19.30). The position is held for up to 6 s and then slowly released. Patient repeats several times.

Possible Substitutions: Common substitutions for this exercise include lifting the heel off the floor, rotating the hips, and bending the trunk.

Notations: If a four-way hip machine is available, it can be used for this exercise with the resistance bar placed behind the distal thigh; the patient's position is otherwise the same. A pulley system can also be used in place of the rubber band.

 Go to HK*Propel* and watch video 19.3, which demonstrates substitutions for CKC terminal extension.

Figure 19.30

Weight-Bearing Resistive Exercises

Once the patient can bear weight on the injured knee, weight-transfer activities and gait training may be needed if the person has been on crutches, has been non–weight bearing or partial weight bearing, or demonstrates an improper gait pattern. These activities, discussed in chapter 7, include weight-transfer exercises on a scale, gait-training activities, and the use of a mirror to facilitate weight transfer and proper gait. Other weight-bearing exercise suggestions are presented in the following sections.

One note about the wall squat exercise described later: Some clinicians place a ball between the knees during this exercise to facilitate an increased response from the vastus medialis, a result of this exercise that was reported by an early investigation.[146] Later investigations, however, discount these findings and show evidence that hip adduction activity during a squat does not produce an isolated increase in VMO activity[147] or any increase in quadriceps activity.[148] This discussion has been expanded by other investigators, who demonstrate an increase in the activity of the entire quadriceps when a ball is placed between the knees to facilitate hip adduction during a squat[149] and during a leg press.[150] Data reveal that it is not possible to isolate VMO activity from that of other muscles within the quadriceps,[151] but if an increase in quadriceps activity is desirable, then hip adduction activity used simultaneously with squat

exercises may increase quadriceps output.[149] Controversy exists on this point because it has also been shown that activated hip muscles do not influence quadriceps activation if analysis is performed using fine-wire electrodes, but changes are observed when surface electrodes are used;[152] these results indicate that perhaps changes seen with surface electrodes are actually due to cross talk from hip adductors rather than increased quadriceps activity.[152]

In summary, the research community continues to debate whether activation of hip adductors simultaneously with quadriceps contraction produces greater quadriceps activity[146, 153, 154] or has no impact on quadriceps output.[148, 155-158] Since there is disagreement among investigators on this point, additional research must be completed before the benefit of hip adduction activity during a squat can be considered indisputable.

Reciprocal Training A machine such as a stationary bike, a treadmill for gait training, a step machine, or a ski machine can be useful once weight bearing is permitted. The stationary bike produces about half as much stress on the tibiofemoral joint as does walking;[159, 160] it can also be used for strengthening and cardiovascular conditioning. Step machines used with controlled degrees of knee motion, and the ski machine, facilitate strength, motion, reciprocal motion between the right and lower extremities, and cardiovascular conditioning.

CKC: Leg Press

Body Segment: Knee and hip; possibly ankle.

Stage in Rehab: Resistive phase.

Purpose: Strengthen quadriceps and gluteus maximus. May also strengthen plantar flexors if plantar-flexion motion is incorporated.

Positioning: Depending on the specific brand of machine, patient is sitting, semireclined, or fully reclined with feet on a platform; knees and hips begin in flexed positions.

Execution: Patient pushes the platform with the lower extremities, extending the

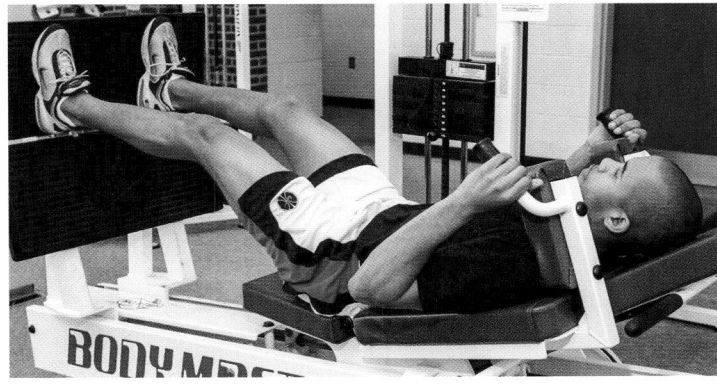

Figure 19.31

hips and knees (figure 19.31). If also strengthening plantar flexors, the patient pushes the platform with the feet to move the ankles into plantar flexion. If the machine is to be used only for plantar flexors, the patient begins the exercises with the knees extended.

This machine can be used in a variety of ways:

1. In the supine or seated position, this exercise can provide resistive concentric and increased eccentric activity if the patient pushes off the platform and catches him- or herself as the feet return to the platform. The speed of this exercise depends on the force with which the patient pushes off the platform and the amount of resistance used.

2. If the patient is in a prone tripod position on elbows and knees with the involved foot on the platform (in a position reverse to the normal position on the machine), the foot is placed high on the platform to facilitate the quads and hip extensors. In this position, the patient performs a slow and controlled motion with special attention given to gaining full knee extension.

In the prone tripod position, the patient can also perform a rapid push-off and eccentric catch; however, the faster speed is more difficult and should be used with caution only after the patient has demonstrated proficiency with the slower exercise.

Possible Substitutions: Collapsing the knee into a valgus position, not moving through a complete range of motion, rotating the hip, or moving the machine too quickly using momentum rather than muscle force. The hip, knee, and ankle should remain in alignment with each other throughout the exercise.

Notations: The patient performs the exercise using both lower extremities or using just the involved limb to isolate the involved extremity. To reduce patellofemoral stress, the foot should be positioned on the platform so the knee is flexed no more than 90° in the starting position.

CKC: Wall Squats

Body Segment: Quadriceps.

Stage in Rehab: Resistive phase.

Purpose: Strengthen quadriceps.

Positioning: The patient stands with the back to the wall and the feet in front of the body.

Execution: Patient squats to bend at the hips and knees, but the knees should remain behind the ankles so the leg does not go beyond a line perpendicular to the floor. The patient can hold this position in an isometric hold for several seconds or move up and down without pausing in the low position. A Swiss ball placed between the wall and the patient allows the patient to perform a smoother squat motion and prevents dye in the patient's shirt from rubbing off on the wall.

Possible Substitutions: Common errors with this exercise include positioning the feet too closely to the wall so that knee flexion goes beyond 90°, placing more weight on the uninvolved extremity, and hiking the hip so that the knee does not flex as much.

>continued

CKC: Wall Squats *>continued*

Notations: If the patient is reluctant to bear weight equally on left and right extremities, a small platform placed under the uninvolved foot can facilitate increased weight bearing on the involved extremity. If the knee flexes to more than 90°, patellofemoral stress increases, and pain may result. The deeper the squat, the farther away from the wall the feet are positioned, so the knee is never flexed more than 90° in the maximum squat position. This exercise can be advanced by increasing the repetitions or sets, increasing the depth of the squat (as long as the knee does not move in front of the ankle in the end-squat position), or having the patient perform the exercise with only one extremity (figure 19.32), placing the uninvolved extremity on a stool or step. The tibia should be perpendicular to the floor at the patient's lowest position. As the patient squats deeper, the feet must be moved farther from the wall. The rehabilitation clinician should watch for substitutions and correct as necessary to ensure correct performance of this exercise.

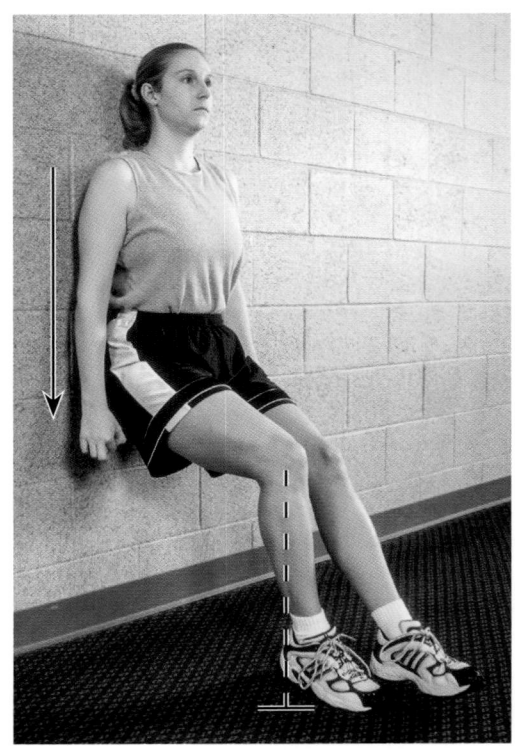

Figure 19.32

CKC: Plié

Body Segment: Quadriceps.

Stage in Rehab: Resistive phase.

Purpose: Strengthen the quadriceps.

Positioning: The patient stands with the feet in a wide stance with the hips and feet turned outward about 45°.

Execution: The buttocks are squeezed as the patient slowly bends the knees, keeping the knees in line with the second toes (figure 19.33).

Possible Substitutions: Not aligning the knees over the second toes; allowing the knees to move into a valgus position; not keeping the weight evenly distributed over right and left lower extremities; and not keeping the back straight.

Notations: The back should remain straight so that as the patient flexes the knees and hips, the trunk leans forward; the pelvis should not be allowed to move into a posterior tilt.

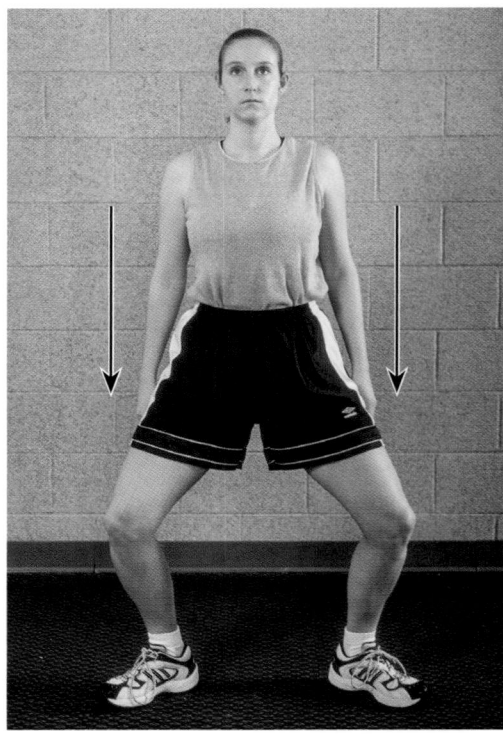

Figure 19.33

CKC: Lunge

Body Segment: Quadriceps and hip extensors.

Stage in Rehab: Resistive phase.

Purpose: Strengthen quadriceps and gluteals.

Positioning: The patient stands with the feet in a forward–backward stance with the involved extremity in front.

Execution: The quadriceps and buttocks are tightened, and the weight is shifted to the front extremity as the patient bends the knee (figure 19.34). This position can be held for several seconds, or the patient can be instructed to walk across the floor in this manner. As the patient moves forward, the body weight is lifted toward the front foot by the front limb, not pushed forward by the back limb.

Possible Substitutions: Common errors are to allow the arch to depress and the knee to move into a valgus position. The knee should not move forward ahead of the foot. The leg position with the floor is no more than perpendicular to the floor. How this exercise is specifically performed (regarding the knee angle) is determined by the type of injury and the phase of healing it is in.[161]

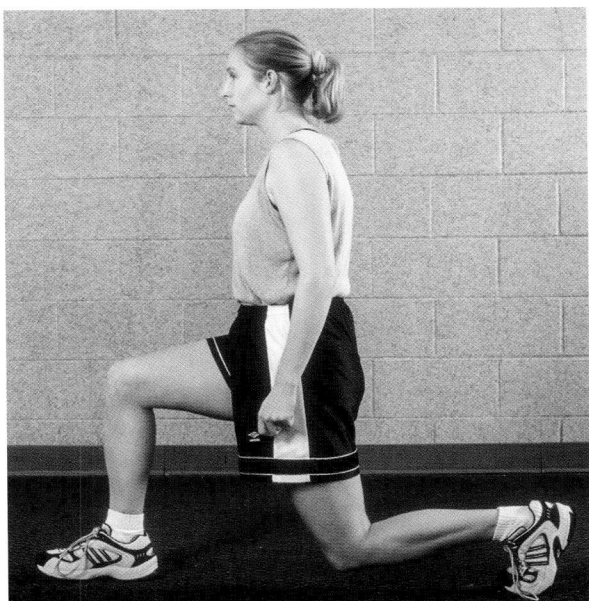

Figure 19.34

Notations: Weights placed in the hands increase the resistance of this exercise. Performing the exercise on an incline also alters the resistance. The back should remain straight with the patient in a pelvic neutral position throughout the exercise. Correct execution is needed to produce the desired results and to avoid putting excessive stress on injured knee structures.

CKC: Mini-Squats

Body Segment: Quadriceps and gluteals.

Stage in Rehab: Resistive phase.

Purpose: Strengthen the quadriceps and gluteals.

Positioning: The patient stands with feet shoulder-width apart and toes turned slightly outward.

Execution: Keeping the weight equally distributed, the patient squats to a comfortable position, keeping the knees in alignment with the second toes. The back remains straight as the patient squats, so the hips flex and move posteriorly and the pelvis remains in neutral throughout the exercise.

Possible Substitutions: Common errors are valgus movement of the knees, trunk flexion, and hip hiking on the involved side to reduce knee flexion. If genu valgus is observed, the patient should be instructed to keep the knees over the second toes and to arch the foot; trunk flexion is corrected with verbal cueing for a straight back with chest up and instructions to push the hips back and to keep the chest up; hip hiking is corrected with instructions to bend the knee more and keep the hips level. Using a mirror to provide the patient with additional feedback is often beneficial.

Notations: In a progression of this exercise, the patient grasps a band that is anchored under the feet to increase resistance for home exercises. Holding weights in the hands increases eccentric and concentric resistance. Performing the exercise on only one extremity increases the difficulty (figure 19.35).

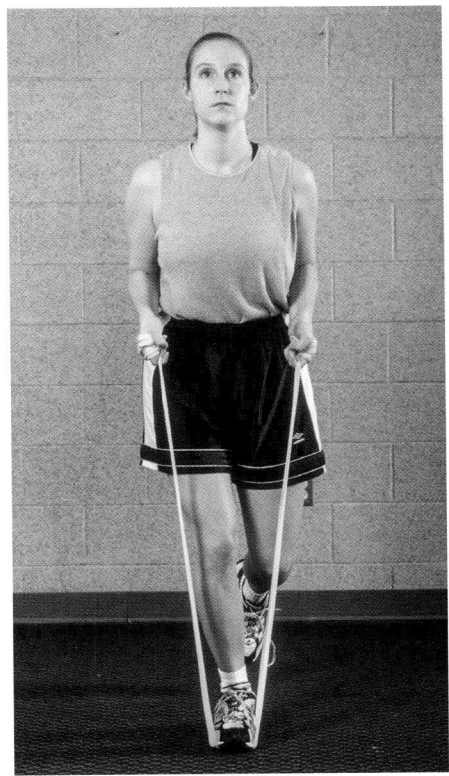

Figure 19.35

CKC: Sit-to-Stand

Body Segment: Quadriceps and gluteals.

Stage in Rehab: Resistive phase.

Purpose: Strengthen quadriceps in midrange and gluteals.

Positioning: The patient sits in a chair with both feet on the floor under the knees.

Execution: Without using arms for assistance, the patient moves in a slow and controlled manner from the sit position to standing and then returns to the chair. The knees should remain in line with the second toes, weight should be equally distributed over the right and left extremities, and the spine should retain normal spinal curves.

Possible Substitutions: Common errors in this exercise include shifting the weight to the uninvolved side, hip hinging, jerking up, and dropping down into the chair. Correction techniques are verbal cueing, using a mirror for visual feedback, or using a higher chair or placing a pad in the chair and later advancing to a lower seat height as strength improves.

Notations: Once the patient meets the goals of this exercise, he or she can advance to a single-limb exercise.

CKC: Good Mornings

Body Segment: Hamstrings and gluteals.

Stage in Rehab: Resistive phase.

Purpose: Strengthen the hamstrings and gluteals.

Positioning: The patient stands with feet shoulder-width apart facing a pulley or wall anchor for rubber tubing. The handle for the pulley rope or rubber tubing is held by the hand on the unaffected side. The pulley or wall anchor is in a low position, and the patient stands with the elbow extended and the arm away from the side with the tubing taut.

Execution: Keeping the elbow extended, the patient leans forward by flexing the hip until the trunk is parallel to the floor as the unaffected lower extremity is raised in hip extension so the limb remains in the same plane as the trunk. The chest remains elevated so the back does not flex as motion occurs from the hip, using the gluteals and hamstrings eccentrically to flex the hip (figure 19.36).

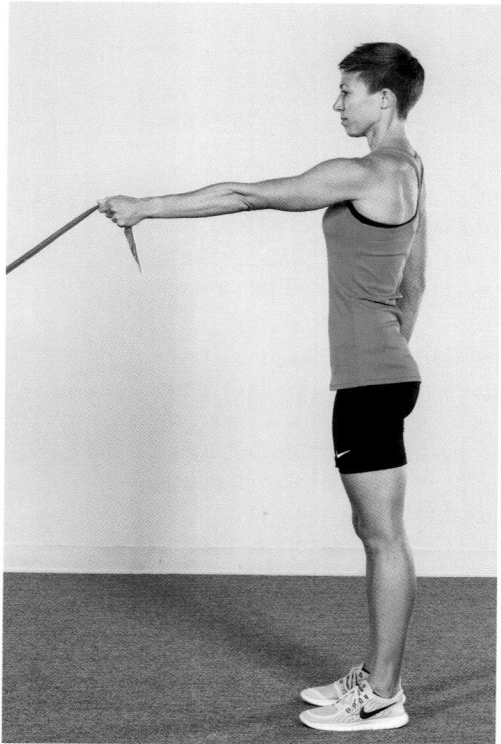

Figure 19.36

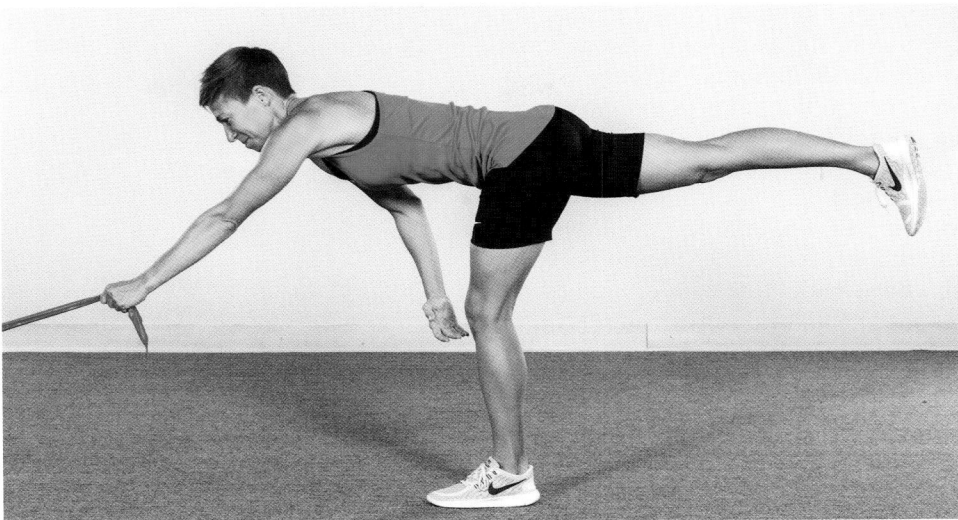

Figure 19.36 *>continued*

Possible Substitutions: Common errors are flexing the back rather than the hip, not flexing the hip far enough, laterally rotating the hip, placing the handle in the same-side hand so the trunk rotates, or not elevating the uninvolved lower extremity high enough as the trunk is lowered.

Notations: In a progression of this exercise, the resistance or repetitions are increased. The patient may have difficulty with balance during the early attempts at this exercise, but as balance and strength improve, stability during this exercise also improves.

Variations of this exercise include other exercises such as picking up cups or cones from the floor. In this exercise, paper cups or cones or other objects are placed around the patient on the floor. The patient reaches down to pick them up, flexing from the hip while keeping the back straight and extending the uninvolved lower extremity posteriorly during the hip flexion motion to make the activity a single-limb stance activity and to provide counterbalance as the patient picks up the object.

Step Exercises The patient should not try these exercises until he or she can bear weight on the involved extremity in a single-limb stance position. Proper weight transfer is also a prerequisite for these exercises. The step height may begin at a low level, around 10 cm (4 in.), and increase to 20 cm (8 in.) as the patient gains strength and knee control. The rehabilitation clinician watches the patient perform the exercise and corrects errors as needed. The patient performs the exercise in a slow and controlled manner. As with other weight-bearing resistive exercises, the knee remains in line with the second toe throughout the motion. The knee should achieve extension at the top of the exercise, but it should not lock in extension. During initial performance of these exercises, patients often demonstrate poor knee control, evidenced by wobbling of the knee as the person raises and lowers body weight. With strength gains, knee movement becomes steady with no lateral knee motion.

Common errors for these exercises include several mistakes for which the clinician observes and corrects, as indicated. These errors include flexion at the hip and trunk to reduce the amount of quadriceps activity required, locking the knee in the extension position to reduce the need for muscular control, hip hiking to reduce the amount of knee flexion in the lowered position, jerking up and dropping down rather than maintaining a smooth and controlled motion, moving the knee into a valgus position and flattening the foot's longitudinal arch, and pushing off with the uninvolved limb. Usually, corrections for these errors require verbal cueing and placing the patient in front of a mirror for visual feedback during the exercise. If pushing off with the uninvolved limb, dropping down or jerking up, and trunk and hip flexion are not corrected with these cues, the height of the step may be too great for the patient's strength limitations; in this case, it is better to use a lower step.

These exercise goals are advanced by increasing the numbers of repetitions and sets, increasing the depth of the step, and adding weights to the hands.

- *Forward Step-Up*. This exercise strengthens the quads. The patient stands facing a step with the involved extremity on the higher step. The patient shifts the weight to the involved extremity and moves the uninvolved extremity up onto the step, straightening the involved knee to lift up the body onto the step. The patient should not push off with the uninvolved limb (figure 19.37). He or she then reverses motion to return to the starting position, stepping back and down to the floor, controlling the rate of descent with the involved extremity.

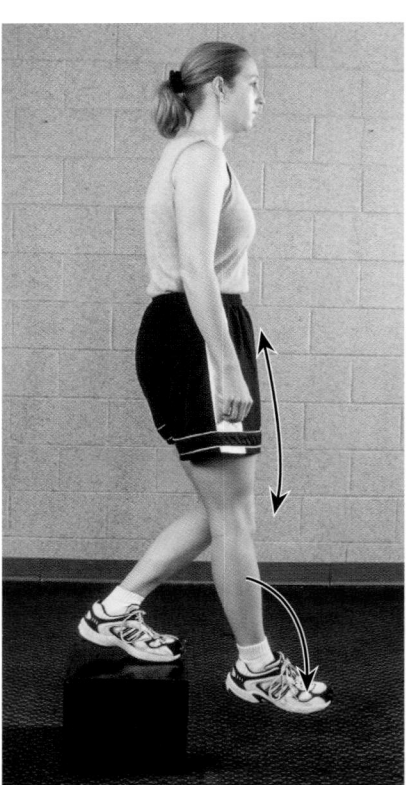

Figure 19.38 Forward step-down.

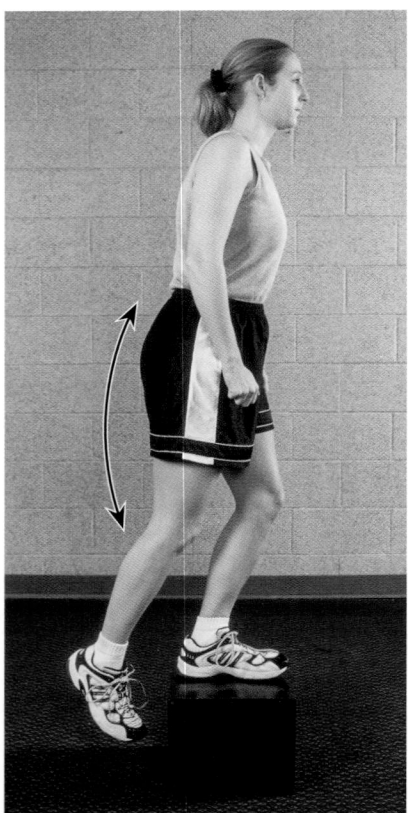

Figure 19.37 Forward step-up.

- *Forward Step-Down*. This exercise strengthens the quads and gluteal muscles. This exercise emphasizes the eccentric portion of the step activity. It stresses the knee more than the step-up exercise does because the patient is moving forward on the extremity, and the knee must move in front of the foot. If the exercise causes knee pain, the patient should perform the exercise on a lower step, but if pain also occurs on the lower step, the exercise should be deferred until knee control and strength increase. The patient stands on a step and slowly lowers the uninvolved extremity to the floor so the heel touches the floor first (figure 19.38). The patient then returns to the start position, lifting the body up and backward. The patient should

not push off with the uninvolved extremity or use the hands except for balance.

- *Lateral Step-Up*. This exercise strengthens the quads and isolates the quads more than the other step exercises. The patient stands sideways on a step, with the involved extremity on the step and the uninvolved extremity on the ground. Only the heel of the uninvolved extremity is in contact with the ground; the toes remain off the ground throughout the exercise. The patient lifts the body up to the step by tightening the quads and gluteals (figure 19.39). The patient then slowly returns the uninvolved extremity's heel to the floor. If the patient flexes at the trunk, the hamstrings are working rather than the quadriceps, so the patient is instructed to maintain an erect trunk or to tighten the gluteals during the exercise. If the patient feels the exercise more in the lateral hip than in the quadriceps, the patient is using the gluteus medius muscle to lift the body rather than the quadriceps; in this case, instruct the patient to flex the knee more and keep the hips level as the uninvolved extremity is lowered to the ground.

 Go to HK*Propel* and watch video 19.4, which demonstrates substitutions for lateral step exercises.

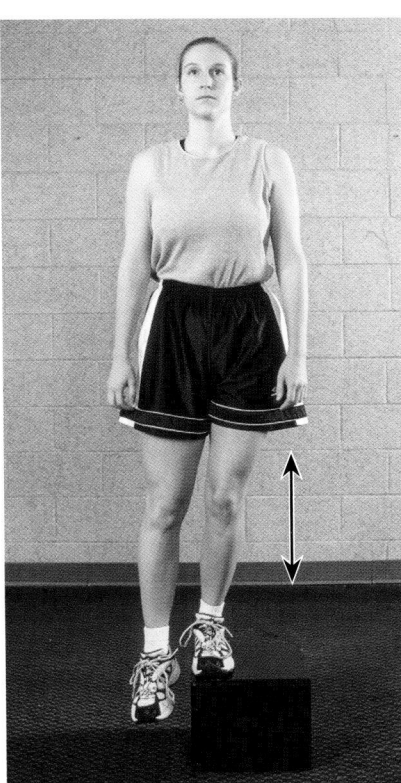

Figure 19.39 Lateral step-up. Careful observation is important to ensure proper execution of this exercise.

You can provide additional overload by requiring the patient to land the heel of the uninvolved extremity away from the step, abducting the involved hips as the extremity lowers to the floor. Increasing the step height is another way to increase the difficulty of the exercise.

Machine Exercises

A number of machine and weight exercises are available for strengthening the knee. These units vary in features or style from one brand to another, but they have underlying similarities and exercise the same muscles or muscle groups. Available equipment varies from one facility to another according to budget, space, and staff preferences. Whatever equipment is used, the rehabilitation clinician must be familiar with the machine, with the instructions for use and the indications, and with the precautions and dangers before using it with patients. The following sections describe exercises with a few of the more commonly used machines.

Knee Extension This machine is used with caution because of its potential for injuring the patellofemoral joint and ACL. It provides an open kinetic chain exercise that produces patellofemoral compression forces that progressively increase from lower levels at full extension to increasing levels as the knee moves to 90° of flexion.[162]

Open kinetic chain exercises place the greatest shear stress on the ACL at 15° to 30° of knee flexion.[114] It is essential that if an open-chain knee extension machine is used, it is used cautiously and in limited degrees of motion. Patients' pain and your knowledge of joint stresses are your primary guidelines when using this machine. As a general rule of thumb, if pain occurs during a machine exercise, either the motion through which it is used should be restricted or the weight should be reduced. If pain still occurs with these changes, the machine should not be used.

The knee extension unit is mentioned here not to advocate for its use, but because many facilities have such a unit, so it is important for rehabilitation clinicians to be aware of it and its potential hazards. It can be effective if used properly.

The patient sits on the knee extension machine with the ankle behind a weighted bar. To facilitate the rectus femoris, the patient inclines backward with the weight on the hands behind the hips. Some machines have the backrest positioned so that the patient is naturally reclined. The patient then extends the knees (figure 19.40).

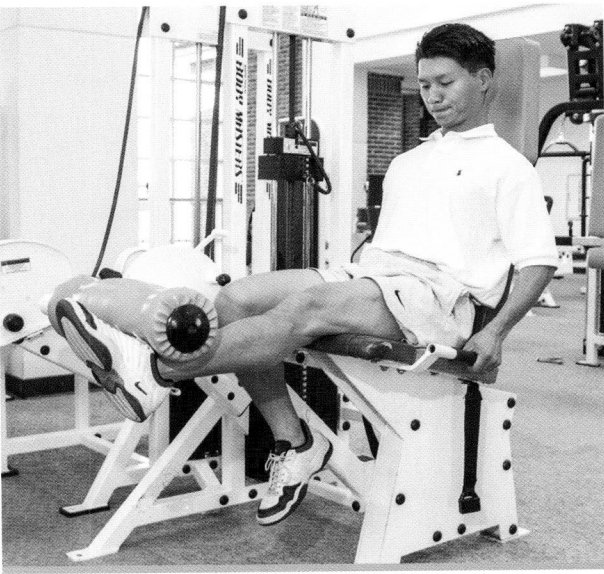

Figure 19.40 A knee extension machine can be an effective therapeutic exercise tool if used correctly.

Squat This exercise strengthens the quads and hip extensors. It is an advanced exercise that is not performed until a patient has demonstrated good strength and knee control with the step exercises and other closed-chain activities previously outlined. It is commonly placed in the latter part of the resistive phase.

With the feet about shoulder-width apart, the weight is placed on the patient's shoulders. Keeping the back straight, the patient squats to no more than a 90° angle at the hips and knees (figure 19.41). The knees should remain in line with and behind the second toe. Figure 19.41

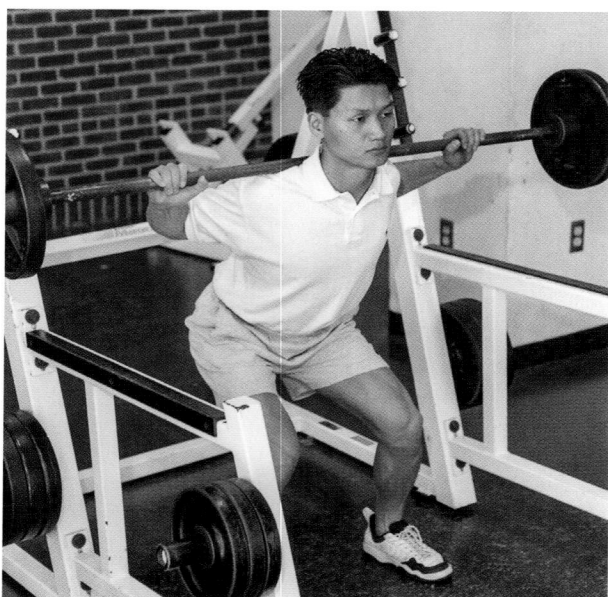

Figure 19.41 Squat exercise can be performed on a variety of equipment types, including a bench-press or calf-raise unit if a squat machine or squat rack is not available.

demonstrates the exercise with a barbell, but the exercise can also be performed with adaptable machines such as a bench-press or heel-raise unit.

Hamstring Curl   This exercise strengthens the hamstrings. Depending on the machine, the patient may lie prone, stand, or sit on the unit with the machine secured around the posterior ankle. The knee begins in an extended position, and the patient flexes the knee (figure 19.42). Since a common substitution with this exercise is flexing the hips to gain additional length for the hamstrings, the rehabilitation clinician should provide verbal cues if substitution occurs.

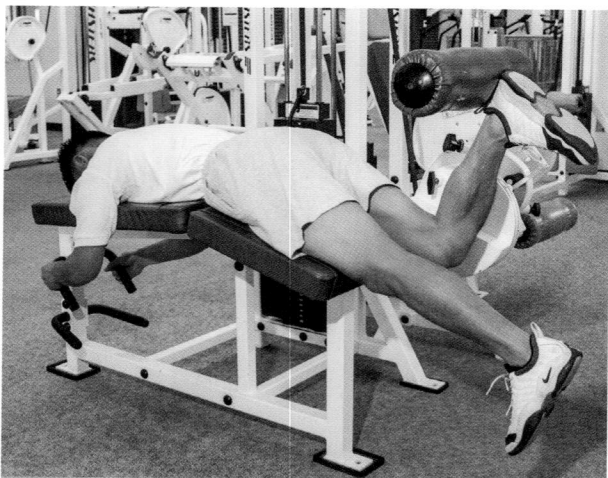

Figure 19.42   Machine hamstring curl.

Isokinetic Exercises

Isokinetic exercises for the quads and hamstrings usually begin after the patient has demonstrated control in isotonic exercises and the injured tissue is strong enough to tolerate the stresses applied with isokinetic activities. Hamstrings and quadriceps can be exercised isokinetically, isometrically, or eccentrically on isokinetic machines. If facilitation of the rectus femoris is desired, the seat back should be reclined to extend the hip (figure 19.43). The hamstrings can be exercised in a seated position to maximize output at the knee or in prone. Many clinics do not have isokinetic equipment; they are not essential to a successful rehabilitation program, but when available, they are useful tools for both testing and strengthening.

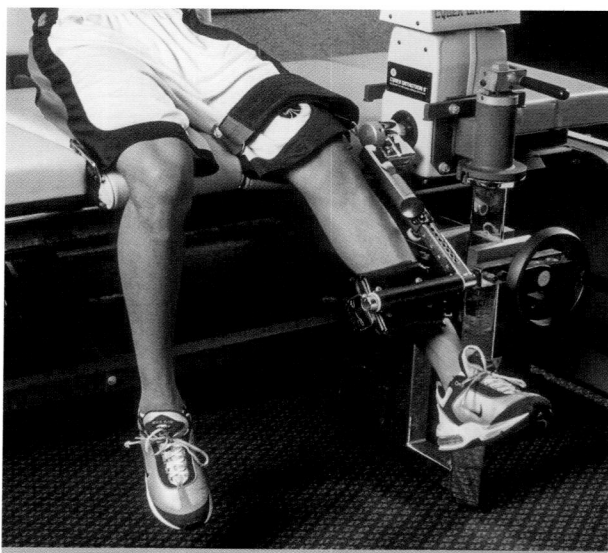

Figure 19.43   Isokinetic machine setup for knee exercises.

Proprioception Exercises

As with other injured areas, balance, agility, and coordination must be restored after knee injury or surgery. Proprioception is basic to these attributes. Early proprioception exercises in phase II before weight bearing can include a variety of activities. For example, with eyes closed, the patient can move the involved knee to mimic the uninvolved knee's position, or with eyes closed, the patient can position the knee at a designated angle. In the latter activity, the rehabilitation clinician measures the angle to determine the patient's ability to produce it.

Weight-bearing proprioception exercises are similar to those discussed for the ankle in chapter 20. The patient performs stork standing (single-limb stance) on the floor with eyes open (figure 19.44*a*), eyes closed, and with eyes open while rotating the head to left and right before advancing to stork standing on unstable surfaces such as the BAPS board (figure 19.44*b*), trampoline (figure 19.44*c*), or foam roller.

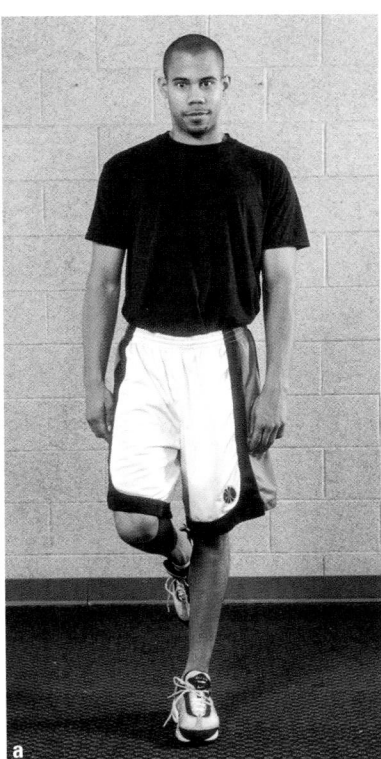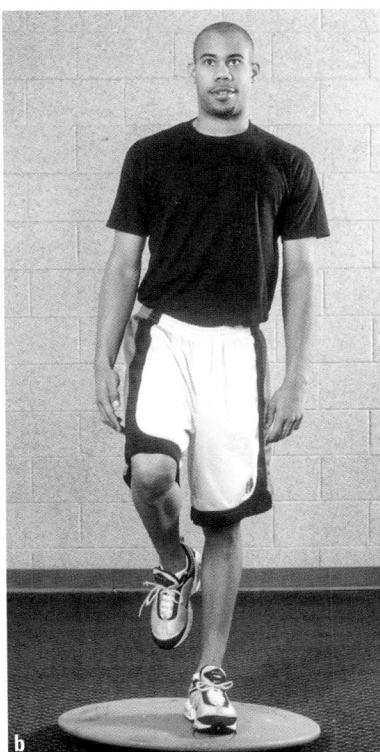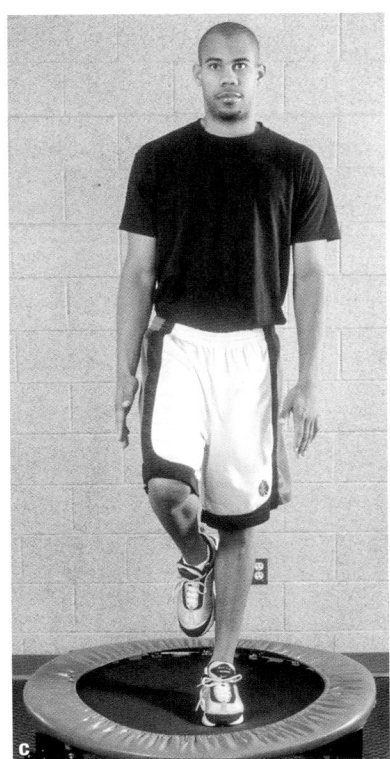

Figure 19.44 Single-limb stance balance progression: *(a)* on ground, *(b)* on BAPS, *(c)* on trampoline.

The next progression is to make the balance activity more challenging and to help it to become a subconscious activity. For example, the patient performs a distracting activity while balancing on an unstable surface, such as standing on a foam roller while using a B.O.I.N.G., Body Blade, or other upper-extremity device (figure 19.45).

Other balance and proprioception exercises include activities on balance boards, the Fitter, and slide boards. Activities that develop agility, coordination, and balance include jumping activities against a resistance band with both lower extremities and then with just the involved extremity; treadmill activities such as retro-walking, side shuffle, and cariocas; and bilateral and unilateral hopping and jumping activities. Plyometric exercises with boxes develop agility and power in preparation for functional exercises. These plyometric exercises are discussed in chapter 20.

During all of these proprioception activities, the rehabilitation clinician

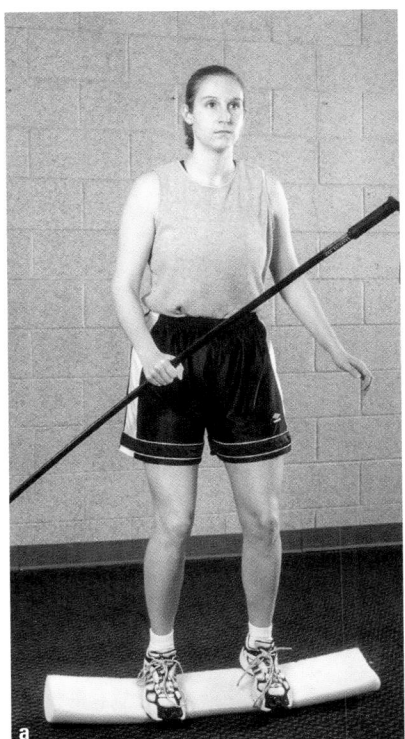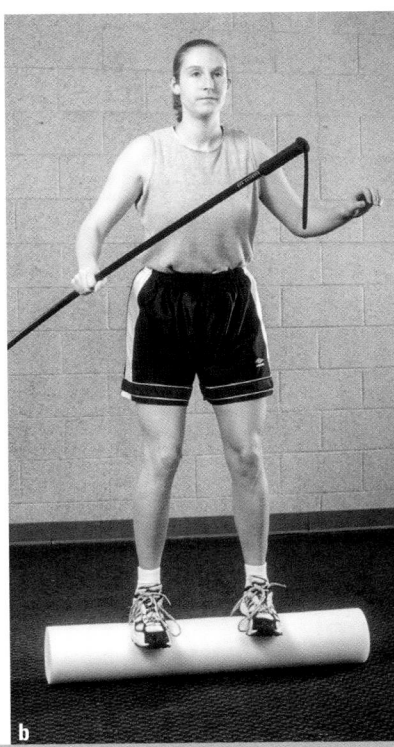

Figure 19.45 Beginning- and advanced-level distracting balance activities *(a)* on a half foam roller and *(b)* on a foam roller.

monitors and corrects the patient's performance. For example, if the patient does not keep the body's center of mass over its base of support, this indicates poor core control, so core control must be addressed before the patient progresses. If the patient cannot perform accurate jumping activities on targets, then the targets should be closer together so that the patient can perform the activity correctly. If the patient does not maintain balance during a single-limb stance on an unstable surface, then the rehabilitation clinician provides the patient with verbal cues that will improve balance; for example, "tighten your quads and your glutes," or "focus on one object in front of you."

Functional and Performance-Specific Exercises

Many of the functional and performance-specific exercises used for the knee are similar to those discussed in chapter 20 for the ankle. The exercises vary more according to the patient's activity demands than the specific injury because a safe return to full participation depends on the entire lower extremity's ability to withstand stresses and perform properly, regardless of the segment injured.

Functional activities include single, double, and triple hops; zigzag runs with sudden changes in direction; backward running with sudden changes to forward running; sprinting; running circles in clockwise and counterclockwise directions; 90° cuts to the left and to the right; and sport-specific drill and skill activities. Performance-specific drill and skill activities are dictated by the patient's specific sport or work-activity requirements. Because running, rapid direction changes, and reliance on both lower extremities are vital to most sport participation, the running and hopping activities are universal and should be a part of most rehabilitation programs. These are discussed in detail in chapters 15 and 20.

Before returning to full participation, the patient must undergo an examination of performance-specific activities. This examination uses many of the exercises and activities the patient has been performing in the advanced phase of the rehabilitation program. The patient should be able to perform all of these activities without psychological or physical impediment and should demonstrate equal use and performance with both lower extremities in all tests performed.

Special Rehabilitation Applications

This section deals with specific injuries to the knee and thigh. The more common knee injuries and their rehabilitation programs are discussed. Before developing a rehabilitation program for any knee injury, you must first perform an examination to identify the patient's problems,

deficiencies, needs, desires, and goals; a clinical diagnosis must be made. To make an accurate clinical diagnosis, you will use various special tests in the examination process.

Special Tests for the Knee

An assessment of the knee's integrity is an important first step in the rehabilitation process. Understanding which structures are involved in a patient's injury helps the clinician to better design a rehabilitation program that addresses each patient's needs. Table 19.3 lists a few of the more common knee ligament tests and their sensitivity and specificity.

Ligament Sprains

Any knee ligament can be injured if the stresses applied are sufficient to exceed the ligament's tensile strength limits. Depending on the magnitude and direction of the forces applied, a single ligament or multiple structures can incur injury. For the sake of simplicity, this discussion focuses primarily on injuries to individual ligaments.

Anterior Cruciate Ligament Sprains

The anterior cruciate ligament (ACL) is the knee ligament that is most often sprained.[172] Considerations unique to this ligament are discussed here, and then a case study is presented.

Although daily activities apply around 454 N (~102 lb) of stress to the ligament, it can tolerate up to 1,730 N (~389 lb) before it ruptures.[173, 174] It is in a position of maximum stress when the knee is either in about the last 30° of extension or experiencing multiplanar loading.[175] The ACL is most commonly injured during a noncontact event when the knee is in slight flexion and experiences a valgus rotation in a foot-planted position as the athlete decelerates.[176] The athlete is often performing a cutting maneuver, and the injury can occur with or without contact with another person. Sudden hyperextension with rotation, moving the knee into a valgus position, is another mechanism of ACL injury.[177] Although it is likely to be a multifactorial issue,[176] there is evidence to demonstrate that females have more ACL injuries than males because females use different landing strategies during jumping than do males.[178, 179] It has been observed that women use less knee and hip flexion than men during landing and stop-jump activities, causing greater activation of the quadriceps than the hamstrings and increasing ACL stress.[180] These studies provide interesting if not compelling evidence for the need to alter women's conditioning programs and muscle activation strategies to prevent or reduce ACL injuries.

When the ACL is injured, it is often only one of the structures injured.[181] In these cases, the surgical repair is usually delayed.[182] When more than one structure is injured, the rehabilitation process becomes more compli-

TABLE 19.3 Commonly Used Special Tests for the Knee

Site/structure tested	Test	Sensitivity	Specificity
Anterior cruciate ligament integrity	Anterior drawer	22% acute; 54% chronic (under anesthesia)[163] 56%[164] 92%[165]	>97% acute and chronic (under anesthesia)[163] 92%[164] 91%[165]
	Anterior Lachman	85% (under anesthesia)[163] 63%[164] 86%[165]	95% (under anesthesia)[163] 90%[164] 92%[165]
Anterolateral instability	Lateral pivot shift	98% (under anesthesia)[163] 31%[164] 22%[165]	>98% (under anesthesia)[163] 97%[164] 99%[165]
	Slocum anterolateral rotary instability	Unknown	Unknown
	Hughston's jerk	Unknown	Unknown
Posterior cruciate ligament integrity	Posterior drawer	90%[166]	99%[166]
	Reverse Lachman	63%[166]	89%[166]
	Godfrey's test for PCL (posterior sag)	79%[166]	100%[166] 100%[167]
	Quadriceps active test for PCL	98%[167] 54%[166]	97%[166]
Posterolateral instability	Reverse pivot shift	26%[166]	95%[166]
Medial collateral ligament integrity	Valgus stress	86%[168]	Not reported
Lateral collateral ligament instability	Varus stress	25%[168]	Not reported
Meniscus integrity	McMurray	16%[169] 29%[170] 37%[171]	98%[169] 95%[170] 77%[171]
	Apley grind	16%[170] 13%[171]	80%[170] 90%[171]
Anteromedial instability	Slocum anteromedial rotary instability	Unknown	Unknown

cated because it must address considerations besides those related to the ACL.

A person with an ACL injury must decide about surgery. There is currently no system for determining a patient's candidacy for ACL reconstruction.[183] The factors usually considered include age, activity level, desire to return to full participation, and knee instability.[184] Long-term comparisons between surgically repaired and non–surgically repaired ACL ruptures indicate no differences in osteoarthritis and functional abilities, but those patients who did not undergo surgical reconstruction developed meniscal damage and instability.[185] Until more definitive

and universal criteria are established, these results seem to indicate that active persons would benefit from surgical repair of a ruptured ACL.

Studies have demonstrated that surgical repair produces the best outcomes when performed after the inflammation has subsided and full range of motion has been restored.[186, 187] Most surgeons perform ACL reconstruction surgery within 3 to 6 weeks after injury.[186] If a patient elects to have reconstructive surgery, the best results in terms of recovery of motion and return to participation occur when surgery is delayed by this amount of time.

Over the years, many types of reconstructive surgeries for the ACL have been tried. Surgical techniques continue to evolve, but currently the most common reconstructive procedures use either an autograft from the patient's patellar tendon or medial hamstring tendons, or an allograft.[188] There are proponents for each technique, but the evidence indicates there is essentially no difference in long-term outcomes between any of the three techniques.[189-191] Surgeon preference may be the primary factor in the choice of technique.[192]

The patellar tendon graft technique, which uses the central third of the patellar tendon with bone-plug ends from the patella and tibial tuberosity, is known as the BPTB, or bone–patellar tendon–bone technique, and it is considered the gold standard for anterior cruciate ligament reconstructions.[189] Parts of this technique are performed arthroscopically, and it involves either one or two surgical incisions. In the hamstring tendon procedure, the semitendinosus and gracilis are used; this is also a combined open and arthroscopic procedure. Advocates of the hamstring tendon graft procedure contend that subjects who receive hamstring tendon grafts have fewer donor-site complications and regain quadriceps strength more quickly.[193] Of the hamstring grafts, the double-bundle grafts are better than the single-bundle grafts.[194] An allograft may be the graft of choice if the reconstruction is on a young patient or the procedure is a repeat surgery with the patient reinjuring a previously replaced ACL.[189] Allografts have been shown to heal more slowly than autografts, but 1 year after surgery, there is no significant difference between allografts and autografts.[195] More than graft selection, the choice of anchor systems for the graft appears to be most important.[191]

Regardless of the surgeon's choice of graft and anchor system, the rehabilitation clinician is responsible for returning the patient to optimal performance levels. Rehabilitation after ACL reconstruction follows two schools of thought, one for delay and the other for acceleration; the better course of action remains controversial.[196] Some clinicians advocate using the accelerated program with competitive and serious recreational athletes but a more conservative program with less serious recreational athletes.[197] Both of these camps commonly prefer weight bearing to tolerance after surgery.[186] Those in the delayed-program camp are concerned about the vulnerability of new tissue and believe that stressing the tissue too soon will risk detachment at the graft site, compromise the graft, and destabilize the joint. A conservative program restricts running until about the fifth or sixth month, with full return to activities occurring 6 to 9 months after surgery.

Those advocating the accelerated program for ACL reconstructions believe that there are fewer complications from the surgery when such a program is used.[198] In the accelerated program, running activities begin after 12 weeks, and the patient can return to full participation in 5 to 6 months. Although the accelerated rehabilitation patients are stronger at 3 months postoperatively, long-term results demonstrate no differences overall between the two groups.[199]

Histologically, the ACL graft undergoes necrosis and remodeling once it is transplanted. Initially it is avascular, but revascularization occurs at 6 to 8 weeks and is completed around 12 weeks postoperatively.[200] Once the graft is inserted, it goes through a process of necrosis and disintegration followed by tissue rebuilding. Because of this process, regardless of the graft material used, the ACL replacement is weakest during the first 6 weeks after reconstructive surgery.[195] As part of the healing process, new collagen is formed around the existing matrix of the graft, maturing the graft site and allowing it to manage progressively greater applied stresses. It may take at least a year for the graft to appear histologically normal, but it never regains normal tensile strength.[201] Although the precise load-tolerance levels of ACL grafts are not known, it is agreed that some mechanical stress is beneficial to the healing graft.[200] For this reason, most surgeons encourage weight bearing, either full or limited, immediately after ACL reconstruction.

If the medial meniscus is injured along with the ACL, it must be repaired to ensure that the ACL reconstruction is successful.[185] This repair is important because the meniscus provides stability to the knee; when the meniscus is injured, the knee joint's stability is compromised. An unstable knee will damage the reconstructed ACL, placing undue stress on it and promoting osteoarthritis within the joint.[185] Therefore, before performing an ACL reconstruction, the surgeon will repair the meniscus; in these cases, postoperative weight bearing may be limited or delayed in order to protect the meniscal repair.[202]

When you design a specific ACL rehabilitation program for a patient who has undergone reconstructive surgery, key considerations must include the type of graft and fixation used, the type of surgery performed, the surgeon's rehabilitation preferences, and other injuries present. Although exercise timing is different in delayed and accelerated programs, the exercises and the progression are essentially the same.

Two program timing progressions are provided here as examples of an accelerated and a delayed ACL program. In practice, a patient's program may be accelerated or delayed or may combine the two approaches. Communication with the physician about the patient's progression is crucial to a safe and successful rehabilitation outcome. You must assess the patient at the start of each treatment session and during the session to determine the appropriateness of the activities. Advancement is based on achieving the goals that have been set, so you must assess the patient to determine when these goals are achieved.

If the patient reports pain with any exercise, the clinician must not only identify where the pain is located but the cause of it. Sometimes patients report pain when they are actually experiencing the burning sensation of muscle fatigue. If a patient has pain with a specific exercise, the rehabilitation clinician should first assess the patient's performance in case incorrect execution is causing pain. If the patient performs the exercise correctly, the next step is to either reduce the intensity of the exercise or remove it from the program until the patient can tolerate it.

Accelerated Post-Op ACL Reconstruction Program

In an accelerated program, the patient ambulates with crutches, weight bearing to tolerance with full knee extension, immediately after surgery. Two days after surgery, passive knee extension to 0°, active hip exercises including straight-leg raises, and ankle range-of-motion exercises begin. The patient may wear a knee brace, but it is set at 0° extension.

During the second week, active range-of-motion exercises for the knee begin, as do patellar mobilization and soft-tissue mobilization. By the end of the second week, the patient should be ambulating without crutches, but he or she continues to use the brace that is now unlocked to allow 0° to 120° of motion.[203] Gait training for proper heel-toe ambulation may be needed. The brace is worn for about 3 weeks and then discarded.[203] In either case, the patient is not allowed to ambulate without the brace until he or she has full active knee extension; allowing the patient to ambulate with a partially flexed knee increases meniscal stress and accelerates joint degeneration.[204] Closed kinetic chain activities such as mini-squats and stationary-bike exercises with minimal tension begin during the second week. Hamstring curls, toe raises, and range of motion to 105° are included at this time.

By the third week, the brace may be removed if the patient has full knee extension and the physician's protocol indicates it. The patient can exercise in the pool; can add other exercise equipment, such as the ski machine and the stepper with no more than a 10 cm (4 in.) step height; and can leg-press through a 45° range of motion. Other exercises include half squats to 45° and hamstring curls. The patient can do stork standing if weight transfer during ambulation is correct. If weight transfer is not correct, then using the weight scale for weight-transfer training is beneficial. By the end of the first month, the patient should have 115° of flexion and full extension. Tibiofemoral joint mobilizations are used at this time if capsular tightness and restriction are evident. The patient is now using the stepper machine and performing wall squats, heel raises, lunges, lateral step-ups, and forward step-ups. None of the exercises should produce pain or edema or give the patient the sensation of increased knee laxity.

During weeks 6 to 8, if the patient has full active extension and flexion to 115° to 120° along with good isometric quadriceps strength, he or she should ambulate without the brace if it has not yet been discontinued. Active knee extensions within 100° to 30° and a treadmill walking program are implemented during this time. Research has demonstrated that a treadmill set at an incline slightly greater than 12% reduces ACL strain and patellofemoral strain but recruits greater quadriceps activity, and thus may be beneficial for ACL and patellofemoral rehabilitation programs.[205]

During the weeks leading up to the third month, the exercises that the patient has done so far continue, progressing in weights, sets, or repetitions as tolerated, provided they do not produce pain or edema. Plyometric exercises begin by week 12 along with jogging activities. By the third to fourth month, the patient progresses to running and sprinting. During this time the patient advances to agility drills, more aggressive plyometrics, and performance-specific drills, provided that full range of motion is present, strength is about 80% of that of the uninvolved knee, and proprioception is good in static and dynamic balance activities.

During the fifth to the sixth month, the program continues into phase IV with strengthening and flexibility exercises and advances to more functional activities as the patient prepares to return to full sport participation or normal work activities. Because the physician often relies on the rehabilitation clinician for the information needed to determine the patient's readiness to return to full participation, the rehabilitation clinician performs an appropriate examination before consulting with the physician. Before returning, the patient must pass all aspects of the performance-specific examination; have full motion, full strength, and normal proprioception; and be pain free without edema after exercise. This program is condensed into a timeline in figure 19.46.

Conservative Post-Op ACL Reconstruction Program
A delayed program has the same progression of exercises, but they are introduced in the program at a slower rate. Weight bearing progresses from weight bearing as tolerated to full weight bearing with the brace locked in extension for 1 week. The brace is used to perform straight-leg raises. The brace is unlocked after 1 week, but the patient remains on crutches. During the first 2 weeks, hip exercises with the brace on, heel raises, and quad sets are the strength exercises with which the patient starts. The patient can remove the brace to perform wall slides to 45°, heel slides, and prone hangs with the foot over the edge of the table for range of motion. When the patient can perform a quad set with good quadriceps control in full extension, the crutches are removed, but the brace must be worn throughout the first 6 weeks. Patellar mobilization starts during week 2, and electrical stimulation and modalities for pain and edema begin during the first week. During the first week, stretching exercises for the hamstrings, gastrocnemius, ITB, and quad sets occur. Cardiovascular activities are limited to an upper-body ergometer or unilateral stationary cycling using only the uninvolved extremity.

ACL Reconstruction, Accelerated Rehabilitation Program

Stage I: Inactive phase	
0-3 weeks	**Inflammation phase: Inactive rehabilitation phase**
Goals	Relieve pain. Reduce edema, ecchymosis. Relieve spasm. Protect surgical repair. Prevent deconditioning of unaffected body segments.
Treatment guidelines	Electrical stimulation for pain, muscle spasm Compression and elevation for edema If brace is used, maintain locked brace at 0° extension After day 2: Active hip exercises while wearing knee brace Ankle ROM exercises Week 2: Begin active ROM of knee; patellar mobilization; soft-tissue mobilization End of second week: ambulate without crutches and brace set at 0° to 120°; gait training PRN Exercises for unaffected body segments HEP for pain, edema, and AROM
Precautions	Weight bearing status: FWB or WBAT. Encourage proper gait. No resistive exercises to knee. No passive ROM.
Stage II: Active phase	
3-9 weeks	**Early proliferation phase: Active rehabilitation phase**
Goals	No pain, edema, spasm. Weeks 6-8: Achieve full knee range of motion. Increase strength of all deficient muscles and muscle groups. Restore normal gait.
Treatment guidelines	End of third week: Discard brace; gait training PRN; aquatic exercises; stationary bike; ski machine, stepper on short step; leg press 0° to 45°; half squats to 45°; hamstring curls if ACL graft is not hamstrings; single-limb stance and other balance activities. End of fourth week: Use joint mobilizations for motion PRN; treadmill walking at an incline; resisted ankle and hip exercises. Week 6: Begin hamstring strengthening if hamstring graft was used; otherwise hamstring strengthening begins after week 3. Initiate early active balance exercises as precursor to agility exercises. Week 8: Increase step height for step-up exercises. HEP for strength gains; ROM maintenance.
Precautions	Use weight-scale exercises if weight transfer is incorrect. Know what type of graft has been used for ACL repair; hamstring stretching and strengthening exercises will be delayed if hamstring graft has been used. Correct exercise execution PRN. Do not repeat home exercises during treatment sessions.

Figure 19.46   Example of an accelerated ACL reconstruction program.

Stage III: Resistive phase	
9-18 weeks	**Late proliferation phase: Resistive rehabilitation phase**
Goals	Maintain normal ROM. Achieve 85% to 90% normal strength. Restore normal running gait.
Treatment guidelines	Continue with strength progression, all muscle groups. Perform progressive agility exercises. Include multiplanar exercises. Weeks 8-12: Begin forward jogging. Week 12: Begin hopping activities and other plyometric exercises. Weeks 12-16: Begin running/sprinting backward, cutting, cariocas.
Precautions	Observe and use verbal cues to correct for execution of all exercises. Avoid pain and joint swelling.

Stage IV: Advanced phase	
20-36 weeks	**Remodeling phase: Advanced rehabilitation phase**
Goals	Maintain normal strength of all muscles. Maintain normal ROM of all joints. Restore normal sport and work performance.
Treatment guidelines	Functional exercise progression Performance-specific exercises and drills progression
Precautions	Correct performance PRN.

ROM = range of motion; FWB = full weight bearing; WBAT = weight bearing as tolerated; LE = lower extremity; PRN = as needed; HEP = home exercise program.

Figure 19.46 >continued

Other exercises are not added until week 6, when the patient can remove the brace and has good quadriceps control in knee extension. The patient continues stationary-bike exercises with both lower extremities, wall squats to 45°, leg press to 45°, lateral step-ups, forward step-ups, backward step-ups, heel raises, and static balance activities. Pool walking and jogging may begin at this time because his incision is well healed.

From 6 to 8 weeks to 5 months, the patient achieves normal gait and full range of motion in the knee. Leg press exercises advance to 60° flexion, and the patient can progress to the stepper and elliptical trainer. At 2 to 3 months, the patient begins fast walking.

Running is not permitted until about 4 to 6 months postoperatively. Cutting and lateral movements are permitted after the sixth month. A progression of plyometrics, agility exercises, and functional and performance-specific exercises is gradually incorporated into the program.

During the sixth through the 12th month, once the patient has passed the same tests as in the accelerated program, return to full sport or work participation is permitted.

Recovery from ACL reconstruction can be a slow process whether the patient follows an aggressive or a conservative rehabilitation program. In a prospective study, patients who underwent ACL reconstruction took anywhere from 1 to 2 years to regain full muscle function and pain relief.[206, 207] The clinician must always consider the tissue healing timeline and coordinate the intensity levels of rehabilitation activities with the timeline. The best outcomes occur when these factors are respected.

Posterior Cruciate Ligament Sprains

Stability provided by the posterior cruciate ligament (PCL) is actually the combined result of the posterior cruciate ligament and the posterior corner structures.[208] These posterior corner structures include an array of ligamentous and musculotendinous elements, such as the popliteus complex and the lateral collateral ligament, which restrict lateral tibial rotation and varus stress.[209] The PCL has two components, an anterolateral bundle that is the largest portion and becomes taut with knee flexion, and the posteromedial bundle that resists posterior tibial translation

Case Study

A 16-year-old male soccer forward suffered a right ACL injury that was repaired 2 d ago. His physician wants the patient to begin rehabilitation using an accelerated program. The patient is using crutches and bearing about 50% of his weight on the right lower extremity. He has a rehabilitative brace on the knee, with the knee joint set at 0° extension and 90° flexion. He is allowed to remove the brace for passive activities only. The knee has minor edema and some ecchymosis around the knee and into the proximal half of the leg. The surgical repair used a patellar tendon graft; the patient has two scars, one over the patellar tendon and one over the distal lateral thigh, in addition to portal scars from the arthroscopy. The surgical scars are healing well but still have sutures that will be removed next week. There are some soft-tissue adhesions around the knee, especially surrounding the surgical incision sites and the suprapatellar area.

The patient reports only minor postoperative pain. Patellar movement is about 50% of normal in all planes, but the patient does not report pain with patellar mobilization tests. Alignment of the patella is normal, without the presence of patella alta or baja. The patient struggles to perform a straight-leg raise and cannot lift the limb against any resistance to the motion. Hip adduction is 3+/5, hip abduction is 4–/5, and hip extension is 4–/5. Knee flexion and extension resistance tests are deferred at this time because the surgery was less than 7 d ago. He reports some pain with attempts at full weight bearing and admits that he is very apprehensive about putting full weight on the extremity.

Questions for Analysis

1. What are his problems and your long-term goals? List them in order of priority.
2. What will your first treatment for this patient include today?
3. What will your goals for this first treatment today be?
4. What pre-gait activities will you use to encourage the patient to put more weight on the right lower extremity?
5. What home instructions will you give him before he leaves today?
6. What exercises will you include in his program over the next 2 weeks?
7. Over the next 6 weeks, what exercises will you assign, and what will be your criteria for advancing the exercises during that time?
8. How long do you expect the patient's program to take, assuming that he follows a routine course of events without complications or problems?
9. When will you have him start on a treadmill, and what will be your first exercise on it?
10. Outline a progression from the treadmill to a full running program.
11. List four exercises you will include in the patient's functional activities program.
12. Describe the performance tests you will use before the patient is allowed back to full sport participation.

and becomes taut in knee extension.[210] Restoring stability through reconstructive surgery has included using either a double-bundle PCL to replace the original PCL elements or a combination of a double-bundle PCL with a posterolateral corner reconstruction.[211] Studies have shown that the latter reconstruction restores preinjury stability, but using only a double-bundle reconstruction does not.[211]

Posterior cruciate ligament injuries are much less common than ACL injuries.[210, 212] The common mechanisms of injury are either hyperextension of the knee or falling onto a flexed knee.[210] Injuries to the PCL occur more often in high-contact sports such as American football, soccer, and rugby and less often in sports such as basketball that require more sudden cutting and pivoting activities.[210] Unlike ACL injuries that may occur without player contact, PCL injuries usually involve player contact or collision. Surgical repair is performed if the knee is unstable, if the posterolateral corner is injured, or if other ligaments have been injured in addition to the PCL.[208] Surgical repair of

the PCL without these additional elements present is controversial, with many surgeons opting for a nonsurgical approach.[210]

The choice of grafts for PCL reconstruction surgery is similar to those for ACL reconstruction: single- or double-bundle hamstring grafts, patellar tendon, and allografts. Studies demonstrate that the BPTB graft has better results than the other options.[213-215]

Rehabilitation considerations for PCL reconstructions are different than those for ACL reconstructions because stresses on the PCL are different than those on the ACL. There is a wide range of protocols for rehabilitation of posterior cruciate ligament reconstructions, with non-weight-bearing restrictions ranging from 3 weeks to 3 months, postoperative bracing ranging from none to up to 12 weeks, and delayed hamstring strengthening beyond isometrics ranging from 6 weeks to more than 12 weeks.[216]

It is generally accepted that the PCL experiences a progressive increase in shear stress in a resisted open kinetic chain flexion exercise as the knee moves from extension to flexion. However, the amount of PCL shear stress experienced during resisted knee extension is a bit more controversial. Some investigations have found high PCL shear stresses in the 85° to 100° range of motion (figure 19.47), with less posterior shear as the knee reaches full extension when anterior shear stress increases.[217] In closed kinetic chain exercises, the posterior shear stress becomes progressively greater, going from extension to flexion with the greatest stresses occurring in the 70° to 100° range of knee flexion.[217] It is advisable, then, to keep OKC extension exercises to no more than 60° of flexion, to avoid OKC resisted exercises with greater flexion until the PCL has healed enough to withstand those stresses, and to keep CKC exercises in a range similar to that for the OKC extension exercises, 0° to 60°.[217]

Knees with isolated PCL deficiencies do not generally feel unstable unless the person is walking down an incline because the PCL protects the tibia from posterior displacement on the femur (or anterior femoral displacement on the tibia). Generally, patients with isolated PCL injuries without instability can return to full participation after an appropriate rehabilitation program without surgical reconstruction.[218]

The initial goals of a PCL postoperative rehabilitation program in phase I are to resolve pain and edema and restore range of motion. Once the signs of inflammation have been managed, important new goals include the restoration of strength, control, and normal function. Modalities to treat pain and edema and electrical stimulation for muscular facilitation are used in phase I. In the early active phase of the rehabilitation program, the knee is supported when the patient is in long sitting to prevent posterior sag of the tibia on the femur. Patellar mobilization is performed during this time. Hip extension and knee flexion activities

are avoided during the first 3 weeks, but hip adduction and abduction exercises can be used with resistance applied on the distal thigh. Range-of-motion exercises include active knee extension and passive flexion. Active and resistive hamstring exercises should be avoided because they produce posterior translation of the tibia on the femur. Strong gastrocnemius contractions should also be avoided beyond 30° of knee flexion because of the translational stress applied to the joint and the stress added to the PCL.[219]

Open kinetic chain exercises in the 0° to 30° range of motion can provide good isolated strengthening for the quadriceps, as long as patellofemoral pain is avoided, because OKC knee extension does not create posteriorly directed forces.[216] If patellofemoral pain occurs, the exercises are modified to avoid pain. Modifications can include changing the degrees of motion and the angles of the exercise, reducing the resistance, reducing the lever arm of the applied resistance, and using less weight with more repetitions. These exercises during the active phase include quad sets, straight-leg raises, and quad range-of-motion exercises up to 60° of flexion.

Posterior shear stress on the knee occurs during hamstring activity in ranges of motion greater than 30°;[220] on the other hand, quadriceps activity increases stress on the PCL during exercises at greater than 60° of flexion.[167] Therefore, early rehabilitation exercises for the hamstrings should stay in the 0° to 30° range of motion, and quadriceps exercises should avoid ranges greater than 60° of flexion.

Weight-bearing allowance immediately after surgery can vary; some physicians allow partial weight bearing with the knee in extension,[221] while most others insist on non–weight bearing within a range of 6 to 10 weeks postoperatively.[222] Most often, crutches are used initially for non–weight bearing during the first 3 to 6 weeks, then weight bearing advances to tolerance with gradual progression to full weight bearing (FWB) without assistive devices by 6 to 10 weeks.[222-224] During this FWB time, the patient is encouraged to bear body weight equally on both lower extremities to facilitate co-contraction and thereby reduce the risk of posterior shear forces on the knee.[216]

A rehabilitation brace is applied postoperatively with the knee locked at 0° extension and is worn for 6 to 10 weeks.[222] The brace is removed after the first week for passive exercises only. Around week 5 or 6, the brace is unlocked to allow full motion.[222] A closed kinetic chain exercise in the last 60° of extension with a resistance band can be used to strengthen the hamstrings and produce minimal posterior tibial translation once the patient is partial weight bearing. This exercise would be the reverse of the one seen in figure 19.31 and would position the patient facing the opposite direction and flexing the knee against a band's resistance. The hamstrings can also be strengthened in an open kinetic chain exercise for hip extension if the patient keeps the knee extended to reduce posterior tibial shear stress.

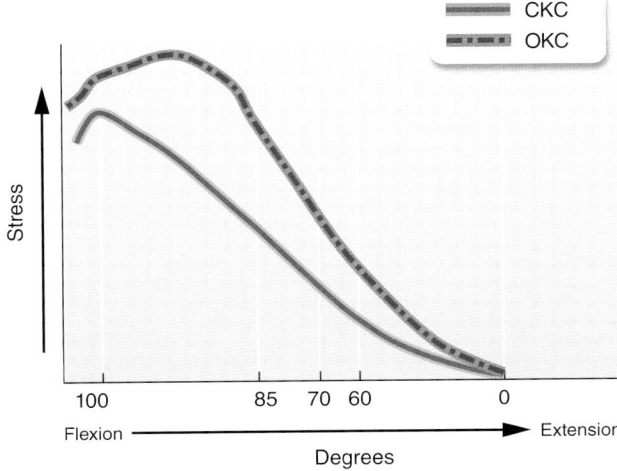

Figure 19.47 Composite of flexion and extension shear stresses applied to the posterior cruciate ligament in open kinetic chain (OKC) and closed kinetic chain (CKC) exercises.
Data based on Wilk et al. (1996).[217]

Once the patient progresses to full weight bearing, other closed kinetic chain exercises begin in the resistive phase. Gait training may be needed if the patient cannot assume a normal gait. Weight transfer activities may be indicated if the patient is reluctant to bear weight on the extremity. Proprioception exercises should emphasize recruiting the quadriceps for posterior translation control, first in static positions and then advancing through dynamic activities. Exercises such as wall squats progressing to standing squats, step-ups, and other CKC exercises are added to the program once the patient is full weight bearing.

By about the eighth to the 10th week, the patient should have full knee extension without an extensor lag and knee flexion to about 90°.[216] Once normal gait is achieved, the patient can walk without assistive devices after the eighth week. At this time, the program can progress to aquatic jogging and running, the leg press, and increased weights with land exercises. Anchoring a weight behind a rolling stool and having the patient sit on the stool, using only the involved extremity to propel the stool, is a good closed-chain hamstring exercise.

By the end of the third month, the patient should have full knee motion. Treadmill walking begins at this time. A more advanced closed kinetic chain hamstring exercise that is performed with the patient kneeling on the table and the clinician anchoring the feet off the table may begin if the patient has enough hamstring strength; as the rehabilitation clinician anchors the legs, the patient leans the trunk forward as far as possible and then returns to the upright kneeling position. The patient may have enough strength for this exercise by the fourth or fifth month. The stepper using small steps or the elliptical trainer is also started at this time.

By the sixth month, the patient enters the advanced phase, jogging on a treadmill with progression to running and then moving into agility exercises, plyometrics (stressing deceleration activities, pivoting, lateral movements, and jumping), and performance-specific exercises. Knee control for posterior tibial translation should be emphasized throughout the program.

Although the rate is much slower, the progression for a surgically reconstructed PCL is the same as for an ACL program, with advancement to agility, plyometric, functional, and performance-specific exercises about the sixth month. The patient can return to full sport participation in an average of 9 months, with an average range of 7 to 12 months.[225] Figure 19.48 provides an example of a rehabilitation progression for a surgically reconstructed posterior cruciate ligament.

Collateral Ligament Sprains

The medial collateral ligament (MCL) can be injured by itself or in combination with other knee structures. Collateral ligament injury treatment is different from cruciate ligament treatment.

Medial collateral ligaments are more often injured than lateral collateral ligaments (LCLs).[226] An MCL injury occurs as the result of a valgus stress, and an LCL injury

Case Study

Last week, an 18-year-old female volleyball player suffered an isolated injury to the left posterior cruciate ligament when landing with the knee hyperextended after jumping to block a ball at the net. The physician will not perform surgery because the knee is stable. He wants you to begin the rehabilitation process with the patient today. Your examination reveals moderate edema around the knee. The patient has a long-leg brace and can bear partial weight on the left extremity. Her range of motion out of the brace is 30° to 60°. Her patellar mobility is limited by about 75%, but her knee is too flexed for you to decide whether the restriction is attributable to the knee position or inadequate patellar mobility. She has pain at 6/10. The edema and ecchymosis surrounding the knee are causing the soft tissue to feel tight from the edema pressure, with restricted mobility during palpation. Her strength is 4–/5 in hip flexors and abductors and 3+/5 in hip extensors and adductors. You have deferred hamstring testing because of the PCL injury and quadriceps testing due to her lack of knee ROM.

Questions for Analysis

1. What will your first treatment with the patient today include?
2. What instructions will you give her to do at home?
3. What exercises will you include in today's session?
4. Outline your expected timeline for beginning hamstring exercises, walking on a treadmill, and stationary cycling. Will you use pool exercises with the patient? If you will use the pool, list three exercises.
5. List four functional exercises and performance skill activities you will include in the last phases of her rehabilitation program.
6. List the performance tests you will use to determine when the patient is ready to return to full sport participation.

Posterior Cruciate Ligament Reconstruction

Stage I: Inactive phase	
0-6 weeks	**Inflammation phase: Inactive rehabilitation phase**
Goals	Relieve pain. Reduce edema, ecchymosis. Relieve spasm. Protect surgical repair. Prevent deconditioning of unaffected body segments.
Treatment guidelines	Electrical stimulation for pain, muscle spasm Compression and elevation for edema Brace remains locked at 0° until week 5-6: then unlock for full motion Progressive WBAT with crutches to FWB by week 6 ROM exercises for hip and ankle muscle groups PROM of knee in prone, 0° to 90° After PWB: Use rubber bands for hamstring resistance, last 60° of extension Patellar mobilization; soft-tissue mobilization PRN OKC exercises: quad set (isometrics) at various positions within 0° to 60°; SLR; hip strengthening; ankle strengthening After week 3: Aquatic exercises and weight shifting, gait training in water Week 2: Stationary bike without resistance for knee ROM only Week 4: Unlock brace for sleeping Exercises for unaffected body segments HEP for pain, edema, and PROM to 90°
Precautions	Encourage proper gait once patient begins some weight bearing. Remove brace for exercises, but otherwise brace remains on in full extension. Limit knee motion to 0° to 90° for first 2 weeks, then progress as tolerated. Avoid knee hyperextension. No hamstring resistance exercises permitted. When performing soft-tissue or joint mobilizations on the patella, place a rolled towel under the knee to prevent hyperextension. Protect surgical repair.
Stage II: Active phase	
6-16 weeks	**Early proliferation phase: Active rehabilitation phase**
Goals	No pain, edema, spasm. Week 6: Full weight bearing. Weeks 8-10: Normal knee ROM. Increase strength of all deficient muscles and muscle groups. Restore normal gait.
Treatment guidelines	Week 6: Discontinue brace and crutches; gait training PRN Week 6: Stepper machine, stationary bike, ski machine, treadmill (walking) Joint mobilizations, PRN FWB balance activities Week 8: Aquatic running, swimming CKC exercises: Mini-squats to 45°, leg press (0° to 60°), wall squats (0° to 60°), heel raises, lunges, hip strengthening OKC exercises: knee extension and hamstring curls, 60° to 0° HEP for strength gains; ROM

>continued

Figure 19.48 Rehabilitation program for posterior cruciate ligament reconstruction.

Stage II: Active phase	
6-16 weeks	**Early proliferation phase: Active rehabilitation phase**
Precautions	Avoid knee pain with exercises. Use weight-scale exercises if weight transfer is incorrect. Do not use home exercises during treatment sessions.

Stage III: Resistive phase	
16-24 weeks	**Late proliferation phase: Resistive rehabilitation phase**
Goals	Maintain normal ROM. Achieve 85% to 90% normal strength. Restore normal gait.
Treatment guidelines	Continue with strength progression, all muscle groups, including CKC hamstring resistance exercises at hip, step-ups, lateral step-ups Progressive agility exercises Include multiplanar exercises Jogging, advancing to running with increase of strength to 85% normal Running or sprinting backward, cutting, cariocas
Precautions	Observe and use verbal cues to correct for execution of all exercises. Avoid pain and joint swelling.

Stage IV: Advanced phase	
24-36 weeks	**Remodeling phase: Advanced rehabilitation phase**
Goals	Maintain normal strength of all muscles. Maintain normal ROM of all joints. Restore normal sport and work performance.
Treatment guidelines	Plyometric exercises Functional exercise progression Performance-specific exercises and drills progression
Precautions	Correct performance PRN.

NWB = non–weight bearing; FWB = full weight bearing; WBAT = weight bearing as tolerated; ROM = range of motion; PROM = passive range of motion; SLR = straight-leg raise; PRN = as needed; HEP = home exercise program.

Figure 19.48   *>continued*

results from a varus stress to the knee. Isolated medial collateral ligament injuries are rarely repaired surgically except when instability results from a combination of ACL and MCL tears. In those situations, the MCL may or may not be repaired even if the ACL is repaired. One reason for this discrepancy may be that the MCL can heal on its own, while the ACL cannot.[227]

The rehabilitation programs are similar for MCL and LCL injuries. Initial treatment includes modalities for pain and swelling. The current philosophy in treating isolated collateral ligament injuries is to use a brace in conjunction with an early rehabilitation program.[228] The patient's injured knee is placed in a functional or rehabilitative brace with limits set at 0° extension and 90° flexion to control ligament stress yet still allow motion. The brace is worn for 3 to 6 weeks, and crutches, with either non–weight bearing or weight bearing to tolerance, are used for 2 to 4 weeks. During this time, active range-of-motion exercises, isometric exercises to retard quad and hamstring atrophy, and hip and ankle exercises are used. Patellar mobilization may be needed if the joint becomes stiff. Cross-friction massage to soft tissues can be helpful in promoting healing and preventing adhesions.[229] In 7 to 10 d, pool exercises are useful for range of motion and strength. After about 2 weeks, the stationary bike can be used if the knee has about 105° of flexion. Before that time, the patient can use the bike as a means of increasing range of motion.

A combination of open and closed kinetic chain exercises is used to increase hamstring and quadriceps strength. These exercises follow the progression outlined for cruciate

Case Study

A 17-year-old male gymnast suffered an excessive valgus stress with subsequent grade II sprain of his right MCL during a rings dismount 3 d ago. The physician wants him started on a rehabilitation program. For the past 3 d he has received ice, elevation, compression, and electrical stimulation for edema control. He is on crutches with a hinged brace set at 0° and 90°. He is bearing about 75% of his body weight on the right extremity when he ambulates. There is moderate swelling with tenderness to palpation along the MCL. His hip and hamstring strength is grossly 4/5. He has an extensor lag of 15°. He reports mild pain unless he tries to bend the knee past 60°; then the pain level becomes moderate. Patellar mobility is normal.

Questions for Analysis

1. List, in order of significance, his problems and your long-term goals for each problem.
2. What will your first treatment for this patient today include? What home program will you give him before he leaves your facility today?
3. Outline the exercise program you will have the patient perform for the next week. How will you determine his progression?
4. List three open kinetic chain and three closed kinetic chain exercises you will have him perform within the next 2 weeks, and list them in the order that you will assign them.
5. What agility exercises will you include in his program?
6. What plyometric exercises will you use?
7. Describe the performance activities you will use in your assessment to determine when the patient is ready to return to full sport participation.

---

ligament injuries and must not produce patellofemoral pain or increase collateral ligament pain. Once the patient is ambulating in full weight bearing, stork standing and other balance activities can begin. Walking on the treadmill with progression to jogging occurs once a normal walking gait has been achieved. Jogging then progresses to running and sprinting as long as pain and edema are avoided.

If full motion is not achieved by around week 5 or 6, joint mobilization techniques and prolonged knee stretches may be needed. The patient progresses in strength and agility exercises as long as there are no deleterious signs. After achieving motion and strength, the patient advances from agility and plyometrics to functional activities and finally to performance-specific exercises. A functional knee brace is often used before and after return to sport. The collateral ligament brace does not need the rotational stability that an ACL brace does, but it should have medial and lateral upright supports to control valgus and varus stress.

A person's tolerance and the severity of the injury will determine the patient's rate of progression. Return to normal function can occur in as few as 3 to 4 weeks or can take as long as 2 to 3 months.

Meniscus Injuries

Among all the rehabilitation programs for knee injuries, the program for meniscal injuries has seen the greatest changes over the past several years. Current trends in treatment allow for a more rapid return to participation than in the past, with fewer deleterious effects.

Surgical treatment of meniscal injuries has evolved in recent years; arthrotomies for complete removal of a damaged meniscus are now a rarity and have been replaced by procedures ranging from partial removal or repair of torn segments to allograft replacements (figure 19.49), all of which are performed through arthroscopes.

Isolated injury to the medial meniscus does not result in instability to the knee, but if a meniscal tear is combined

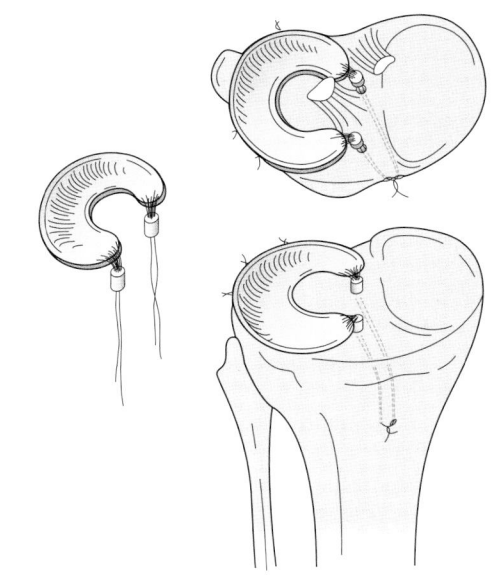

Figure 19.49   Meniscal transplant.

with an ACL rupture, the knee becomes unstable.[230] Isolated meniscal tears tend to be degenerative tears, whereas meniscal tears that accompany ACL injuries are more likely to be acute tears.[231] A stable knee with a meniscal injury may not be a candidate for a meniscal repair, but an unstable knee will become even more unstable if the meniscus is removed or partially removed.[232] We have known for some time that knees that undergo a meniscal repair with an ACL repair do better than knees with an isolated meniscal repair or an isolated ACL repair.[233, 234]

As with any tissue repair, meniscal repairs must have a viable blood supply. The peripheral rim of the meniscus has a blood supply, but most of its inner substance is avascular.[235] Meniscal blood supply can reach inward as far as 6 mm (about 0.25 in.).[236] Therefore, tears that occur over the outer third of the meniscus have the best ability to heal. Tears that extend farther inward than the blood supply do not do well with meniscal repair procedures. Surgeons' preferences vary with regard to the width of the meniscal tears that respond well to repair; width preferences range from 2 mm to 6 mm.[236, 237] Up to 20% of all meniscal tears are repairable.[235] Meniscal repair is preferable to meniscectomy because the meniscus remains, and there is consistent evidence that even partial meniscectomy leads to osteoarthritic changes in the joint.[235] The rehabilitation process, however, is much longer for a meniscal repair or replacement than for a meniscectomy. Whereas a rehabilitation program for a meniscectomy generally requires 4 to 6 weeks, a patient is often restricted from sport participation after a meniscal repair for 4 to 6 months.[238]

The patient who has a medial meniscus and ACL injury that both need surgical repair is a difficult case for the surgeon and rehabilitation clinician. Meniscal repairs do better if performed as soon after the injury as possible.[239] ACL repairs, on the other hand, are most successful when delayed until after the inflammation is resolved. After a meniscal repair, the postoperative care is conservative, with non–weight bearing and limited motion for up to 6 to 8 weeks. ACL repairs require immediate postoperative partial to full weight bearing and motion.

More recently, accelerated programs for the postoperative care of meniscal repairs have been used with success equal to the conservative approach.[202] There is wide variation in the postoperative care of meniscal repairs in such areas as the amount and timing of weight bearing, the use of rehabilitation braces, and the introduction of exercises.[202] The more conservative protocols guard the repair by restricting motion and weight bearing to reduce the shearing and compressive forces that are normally applied to the menisci during walking; the more accelerated programs limit the time on crutches and use partial weight bearing and active motion in the early rehabilitation phase to apply appropriate stresses to healing tissue and to prevent unwanted loss of motion and patellofemoral pain problems.[202] The rehabilitation clinician must communicate closely with the physician to create a feasible rehabilitation program for the patient who has undergone a meniscal repair.

Because of vascular supply, repaired peripheral tears will heal more quickly than complex tears that include the central portions of the meniscus. Factors that may determine whether an accelerated or conservative program is followed include not only the location of the repair but also the type and size of the repair.[235] Conservative rehabilitation follows transplants and complex tear repairs, while more aggressive rehabilitation may be possible for peripheral tear repairs.

Rehabilitation using either a conservative or an accelerated program involves initially protecting the repair or transplant from shear and excessive compression. Patients must be cautioned that deep squats and pivoting will threaten the surgical site's integrity. Activities in a rehabilitation program should not produce increased knee pain or swelling at any time.

Conservative Postoperative Meniscal Repair Rehabilitation Program

A conservative postoperative meniscal repair rehabilitation program includes placing the patient on crutches with the knee in a brace and non–weight bearing on the involved extremity for up to 6 to 8 weeks (figure 19.50). Toe-touch weight bearing is sometimes allowed after 2 weeks, with slowly progressive increases in weight bearing to full weight bearing by 6 to 8 weeks. A rehabilitative brace is used to keep the knee in an extended position at night for the first 3 weeks, but it allows 0° to 90° range of motion during the day for 6 to 8 weeks after surgery. During this time, the patient performs hip and ankle exercises and exercises for the uninvolved body segments. Stretching exercises for the hamstrings, gastrocnemius, soleus, and hips occur during this protective phase. Manual resistance to the hip should be applied above the knee to prevent stress on the knee joint. Quad sets, straight-leg raises, and active knee extension without pain are started within the first 2 weeks. Once the patient demonstrates full active knee extension, the brace is unlocked for night wear. Achieving full knee extension motion and active motion to 90° is the primary concern during the first 3 weeks after surgery. If motion is difficult, it may be necessary to perform patellar mobilizations in all four directions.

After 6 to 8 weeks when the brace is removed, stretching of the quadriceps along with tibiofemoral joint mobilizations can be used to gain additional knee flexion. Crutches are discarded when the patient can walk normally and has adequate quadriceps strength to control the knee. Balance and proprioception activities in weight bearing begin once the patient is full weight bearing. Strengthening the quadriceps and lower extremity with leg press, mini-squats, wall

Meniscal Repair, Conservative Program

Stage I: Inactive phase	
0-6 weeks	**Inflammation phase: Inactive rehabilitation phase**
Goals	Relieve pain. Reduce edema, ecchymosis. Relieve spasm. Protect surgical repair. By week 4: 0° to 90° ROM. Prevent deconditioning of unaffected body segments.
Treatment guidelines	Electrical stimulation for pain, muscle spasm Compression and elevation for edema Brace fixed at 0° to 90° Week 1: NWB; Week 2: TTWB (20% BW); increase weight bearing on involved limb by 20% each week ROM exercises for knee, hip, ankle muscle groups Patellar mobilization; soft-tissue mobilization PRN OKC exercises: quad set; SLR; knee extension; hip strengthening; ankle strengthening After week 3: Aquatic exercises and weight shifting, gait training in water After week 2: Stationary bike without resistance for knee ROM only After week 3: Unlock brace for sleeping Exercises for unaffected body segments HEP for pain, edema, and PROM to 90°
Precautions	Encourage proper gait once patient begins some weight bearing. Maintain brace use except for ROM activities. Protect surgical repair. Brace remains locked in extension at night until patient has good quad contraction in full extension.

Stage II: Active phase	
6-16 weeks	**Early proliferation phase: Active rehabilitation phase**
Goals	No pain, edema, spasm. Week 6: Full weight bearing. Weeks 8-10: Restore normal knee ROM. Increase strength of all deficient muscles and muscle groups. Restore normal gait.
Treatment guidelines	Week 6: Discontinue brace and crutches; gait training PRN Joint mobilizations, PRN Stationary bike FWB balance activities CKC exercises: Mini-squats, leg press (70° to 10°), wall squats, heel raises, hip strengthening OKC exercises: Limited in flexion to 90° and in extension 30° to 90° HEP for strength gains; ROM
Precautions	Avoid knee pain with exercises. Use weight-scale exercises if weight transfer is incorrect. Do not use home exercises during treatment sessions.

>continued

Figure 19.50 Conservative rehabilitation program for meniscal repair.

Stage III: Resistive phase	
16-24 weeks	**Late proliferation phase: Resistive rehabilitation phase**
Goals	Maintain normal ROM. Achieve 85% to 90% normal strength. Restore normal gait.
Treatment guidelines	Continue with strength progression, all muscle groups including CKC hamstring resistance exercises at hip, step-ups, lateral step-ups Progressive agility exercises Include multiplanar exercises Jogging, advancing to running with increase of strength to 85% normal Running and sprinting backward, cutting, cariocas
Precautions	Observe and use verbal cues to correct for execution of all exercises. Avoid pain and joint swelling.
Stage IV: Advanced phase	
24-36 weeks	**Remodeling phase: Advanced rehabilitation phase**
Goals	Maintain normal strength of all muscles. Maintain normal ROM of all joints. Achieve normal sport and work performance.
Treatment guidelines	Plyometric exercises Functional exercise progression Performance-specific exercises and drills progression
Precautions	Correct performance PRN.

NWB = non–weight bearing; TTWB = toe-touch weight bearing; BW = body weight; ROM = range of motion; PROM = passive range of motion; SLR = straight-leg raise; PRN = as needed; HEP = home exercise program.

Figure 19.50   >continued

squats, and open kinetic chain knee flexion and extension exercises occurs at 6 to 8 weeks. Initial ranges of motion are limited in open-chain knee flexion to 90°, in open-chain knee extension 90° to 30°, and in the leg press to 70° to 10° of extension.[239] Pivoting and acceleration–deceleration activities are not allowed for the first 4 to 6 months after surgery. From then on, the patient progresses to functional and performance-specific exercises before returning to sport or normal activities.

Accelerated Postoperative Meniscal Repair Program

Accelerated rehabilitation programs are usually possible after repairs of peripheral meniscal lesions. In an accelerated program, weight bearing is allowed as the patient tolerates it, but the patient uses crutches until he or she can walk normally. Range-of-motion exercises are used during the first postoperative week (figure 19.51). Quad sets and straight-leg raises also begin during the first week. The goal during the first few weeks is to achieve full range of motion without increased edema in the knee. By the end of week 2 or 3, the patient who has good control of knee extension can ambulate normally without crutches; sometimes it may take a patient up to 6 weeks to walk without assistive devices.

In weeks 2 to 4, the patient can use pool exercises and closed kinetic chain exercises, including stationary biking, mini-squats, and a walking treadmill program. By weeks 6 to 9, isokinetic exercises are suitable. Jogging begins around week 8, progressing to running. These running activities are added before lateral and pivoting movements occur in the program. By that time, the patient has at least 85% quad strength. The patient progresses to the advanced phase of rehabilitation when quadriceps strength is 90% and the knee has full motion. Within this phase, multiplanar activities such as cutting, cariocas, and agility activities begin in months 3 to 4. These activities progress to performance-specific exercises, then to full return to normal function with the patient returning to normal activities by weeks 16 to 20.

Meniscal Repair, Accelerated Program

Stage I: Inactive phase	
0-6 weeks	**Inflammation phase: Inactive rehabilitation phase**
Goals	Relieve pain. Reduce edema, ecchymosis. Relieve spasm. Protect surgical repair. By week 2: 0° to 90° ROM; full knee ROM no later than week 6. FWB by weeks 2-6. Prevent deconditioning of unaffected body segments.
Treatment guidelines	Electrical stimulation for pain, muscle spasm Compression and elevation for edema No brace or brace for first 1-2 weeks only Weeks 1-2: TTWB and then WBAT, increasing to FWB by 2-6 weeks ROM exercises for knee, hip, ankle muscle groups Patellar mobilization; soft-tissue mobilization PRN OKC exercises: quad set; SLR; knee extension; hip strengthening; ankle strengthening; core strengthening After week 2: Aquatic exercises and weight shifting, gait training in water After week 2: Stationary bike without resistance for knee ROM only FWB balance activities once patient is FWB Exercises for unaffected body segments HEP for pain, edema, and ROM
Precautions	Encourage proper gait once patient begins some weight bearing. Maintain brace use (if it is used) except for ROM activities. Protect surgical repair.
Stage II: Active phase	
6-12 weeks	**Early proliferation phase: Active rehabilitation phase**
Goals	No pain, edema, spasm. Week 6: Achieve full weight bearing and normal knee ROM. Increase strength of all deficient muscles and muscle groups. Restore normal gait.
Treatment guidelines	Week 6: Discontinue assistive gait devices, if still using them; gait training PRN Joint mobilizations, PRN Stationary bike Jogging at 8 weeks CKC exercises: Mini-squats, leg press (70° to 10°), wall squats, heel raises, hip strengthening OKC exercises: Limited in flexion to 90° and in extension 30° to 90° HEP for strength gains; ROM
Precautions	Avoid knee pain with exercises. Use weight-scale exercises if weight transfer is incorrect. Do not use home exercises during treatment sessions.

>continued

Figure 19.51   Accelerated rehabilitation program for meniscal repair.

Stage III: Resistive phase	
12-15 weeks	**Late proliferation phase: Resistive rehabilitation phase**
Goals	Maintain normal ROM. Achieve 85% to 90% normal strength. Restore normal gait.
Treatment guidelines	Continue with strength progression, all muscle groups including CKC hamstring resistance exercises at hip, step-ups, lateral step-ups Progressive agility exercises Include multiplanar exercises Advance to running with increase of strength to 85% normal Running and sprinting backward, cutting, cariocas
Precautions	Observe and use verbal cues to correct for execution of all exercises. Avoid pain and joint swelling.
Stage IV: Advanced phase	
16-18 weeks	**Remodeling phase: Advanced rehabilitation phase**
Goals	Maintain normal strength of all muscles. Maintain normal ROM of all joints. Normal sport and work performance.
Treatment guidelines	Plyometric exercises Functional exercise progression Performance-specific exercises and drills progression
Precautions	Correct performance PRN.

NWB = non–weight bearing; TTWB = toe-touch weight bearing; WBAT = weight bearing as tolerated; BW = body weight; ROM = range of motion; PROM = passive range of motion; SLR = straight leg raise; PRN = as needed; CKC = closed kinetic chain; OKC = open kinetic chain; HEP = home exercise program.

Figure 19.51   >*continued*

Patellofemoral Injuries

Patellofemoral injuries can be complex and frustratingly slow to respond to treatment. Several factors may contribute to patellofemoral injuries, especially the nontraumatic injuries. This section deals with the most commonly seen patellofemoral injuries.

Patellar Dislocations and Subluxation

Patellar instability is more often seen in women than in men. This is thought to be the result of an increased Q-angle secondary to a wider pelvis, which increases the lateral vector force on the patella.[240] It is surprising to realize that the other strongest predictive factors include age (under 20 years old) and activity level.[241]

The mechanism for patellar dislocation and subluxation is lateral rotation of the thigh with knee flexion on a planted foot. If the patella subluxes rather than dislocates, it often relocates independently or spontaneously. A frank dislocation may or may not relocate on its own. First-time dislocations may not relocate unless they occur in skeletally immature females,[242] but recurrent ones often do relocate

without assistance. Pain and edema are severe, especially in first-time dislocations.

Treatment includes the use of crutches with weight bearing to tolerance. An immobilizer brace may be used at first, but the patient eventually progresses to a functional brace to stabilize the patella. Rehabilitation activities progress to the patient's tolerance. Electrical stimulation to the quadriceps and modalities for pain and edema control are applied during phase I, usually during the first 2 weeks. Increases in pain and edema are avoided throughout the program. Patellofemoral pain can be produced at any time, but especially in the early phases of rehabilitation when the tissues are still inflamed from the initial insult. All rehabilitation exercises should be pain free. If an exercise produces pain, it is delayed until the patient can perform it without pain.

It is important to work on hip stability exercises during phase I. These exercises include strengthening hip extensors and abductors especially. Additionally, core muscle strengthening should be included in any program for the patellofemoral joint, whether it is to manage a dislocation

Case Study

A 20-year-old male ice hockey forward experienced a left knee meniscal tear. He underwent an arthroscopic repair of the meniscus yesterday and comes to you today to begin his rehabilitation program. He is walking PWB with crutches. He reports mild pain and a sensation of tightness around the knee. Your examination reveals swelling of 2.5 cm (1 in.) around the knee's joint margin. The patient's active range of motion is −15° extension and 90° flexion. Passive range of motion is 0° extension and 100° flexion. He can perform a straight-leg raise but cannot tolerate resistance in the motion. Other hip motions are 4/5. Hamstring strength is 4−/5. The patella is slightly restricted in its mobility by about 30%.

Questions for Analysis

1. What will your first treatment with the patient include today?
2. What will you give him as home exercises and instructions before he leaves today?
3. What are your goals with him for the first week of treatment?
4. Preseason hockey practice begins in 2 months. What will you tell the patient when he asks you whether he will be ready by then?
5. When do you expect him to be able to begin full weight bearing? When do you expect him to begin squats with weights?
6. What will you say when the patient asks you why he cannot straighten the knee when he could before the surgery?
7. Present a progression of proprioceptive and neuromotor control exercises that you will include in this patient's rehabilitation program. Discuss the progression of agility exercises you will use. List the performance activities you will include in the final phase of the patient's program.

---

or patellofemoral stress syndrome. As was previously mentioned, hip and core muscles all play important roles in patellofemoral joint stability. See chapters 18 and 17 for hip and core exercises, respectively.

Initial strength exercises in the late active phase and early resistive phase include straight-leg raises and pain-free short-arc exercises with progression into a greater arc of motion as strength gains and pain permit. Rehabilitation exercises are a combination of open and closed kinetic chain activities. Program emphasis should be on quadriceps strength and patellar control during all activities. As strength and knee control improve, exercises in the later program progress to more rapid activities until functional speeds are possible with good patellar control.

Lower-extremity alignment is examined in standing and walking because pronation occurs during ambulation and can increase the risk of patellar instability; feet with excessive pronation may need correction with orthotics.

The duration of the rehabilitation program depends on whether the dislocation or subluxation is a first-time event or a recurring injury. Recovery from an acute subluxation or dislocation can take more time than from a recurring injury. An average expected recovery period is 4 to 12 weeks; recurrent injuries are on the shorter side, and first-time injuries need the longer recovery time.

Patellofemoral Pain Syndrome

Syndromes of the patellofemoral joint can be caused by many factors, individually or in combination. The term for this frustrating injury, "syndrome," demonstrates that the medical community has been unable to identify one specific etiology.

Terminology Patellofemoral pain (PFP) is a common complaint among athletes as well as among the general population. It is often referred to by its generic title, anterior knee pain (AKP), but it has also been identified as chondromalacia, patellofemoral pain syndrome (PFPS), patellofemoral stress syndrome (PFSS), and patellofemoral joint dysfunction (PFJD).[39, 243-245] Chondromalacia is a term that was used in the past to describe anterior knee pain; however, chondromalacia refers to a specific injury that involves softening and degeneration of the patella's posterior articular cartilage and is not an accurate diagnosis for most anterior knee pain conditions. The term most commonly used today to describe anterior knee pain is patellofemoral pain syndrome.[69]

Signs and Symptoms Typical signs and symptoms of PFPS include stiffness after prolonged sitting, pain with activities such as stair climbing and running, and pain after activity.[69] Crepitus is usually present. The patient may experience a giving way of the knee because of reflex inhibition secondary to pain, especially on stairs or ramps. Swelling is usually mild, but the posterior surface of the patella is tender to palpation.

Underlying Factors PFPS is anterior knee pain and irritation caused by abnormal stresses applied to the knee's extensor mechanism. Patellofemoral pain syndrome is a multifactorial condition.[246] Although it can result from direct trauma to the patella, it is more often the result of cumulative stresses in the presence of additional contributing factors, both extrinsic and intrinsic to the joint. These factors are thought to include tightness in the ITB, hamstrings, and gastrocnemius; weakness in the VMO or imbalance of strength between the VMO and vastus lateralis; excessive pronation; increased Q-angle; knee hyperextension; and patellar alignment.[247] More recently, it has been demonstrated that people with PFPS have weak hip muscles compared to persons without the condition.[67, 248] Additionally, the position of the pelvis, due to its influence on the femur, may secondarily affect the patella.[65, 66] Since PFPS is a multifactorial condition, it is likely that a given patient has more than one of these contributing factors. Each element should be evaluated when examining the patient with PFPS because these malalignments must be corrected or compensated for if the PFPS is to be resolved.

Normal function of all body segments relies on a balance between the surrounding structures. This balance includes adequate flexibility and proper strength in the lower quarter so that forces are adequately and appropriately directed to produce the desired motion and applications of force.[66, 249, 250] If hamstring, gastrocnemius, ITB, or lateral connective tissue structures are tight, they apply imbalanced forces to the knee.[251, 252] Tight hamstrings prevent full extension, so the knee is in flexion during activities when it should be extended, increasing compressive forces on the patellofemoral joint. If knee flexion is less than 60°, the need for increased knee flexion during ambulation is compensated for by increased dorsiflexion to clear the toe. Normally 10° of dorsiflexion is needed for ambulation, but if gastrocnemius tightness prevents this motion, or if the hamstrings create a need for more dorsiflexion that is not available, the foot pronates in an attempt to achieve the necessary dorsiflexion. Excessive pronation requires tibial medial rotation, which increases valgus stress on the knee. A tight ITB pulls the patella laterally as the ITB moves posteriorly during knee flexion. In cases of severe distal ITB tightness, the patella is in a lateral tilt position because of the ITB's lateral pull on it.

If the hip muscles, especially the hip extensors and hip abductors, are not strong, the hip will lack the stability needed for normal knee function. A weak hip base for the knee creates an unstable situation for knee function. Instability at the knee makes it difficult to keep the patella in proper alignment during lower-extremity activities. It is not surprising, then, that weak hip muscles have been linked to patellofemoral pain syndrome.[253]

If either the VMO is weak or an imbalance exists between the VMO and the vastus lateralis, the patella moves laterally during quadriceps contractions.[158] This lateral pull causes the patella's lateral rim to ride more on the lateral femoral condyle rather than in the intercondylar groove, where it normally glides during knee motion. If the vastus lateralis is tight, the lateral pull during quadriceps contractions will be exaggerated. Repetitive gliding against the condyle leads to inflammation of the patella's articular surface.

If the knee is hyperextended, the inferior pole of the patella is often tilted inward. This causes the patella to push into the fat pad during full extension, and the patella glides with an inferior tilt during knee motion, changing the relationship between the patella and the femoral groove. The patella has increased contact inferiorly as it glides in the groove, increasing stresses at its inferior pole. Swimmers with hyperextended knees have reported complaints of PFPS.[254]

Any one of these factors by itself may create patellofemoral pain. When more than one of these factors is present, the problem becomes more difficult to resolve.

Patellar Orientation Patellar orientation and alignment are examined in a relaxed long sitting or supine position, and in closed-chain positions in both static and dynamic conditions. Patellar alignment varies from one patient to another; it can also be different from left to right knee in the same person. In a relaxed open-chain position with the knee resting near full extension on a rolled towel and the femur in parallel alignment with the examination tabletop, the rehabilitation clinician assesses the patellar alignment in various planes. The rehabilitation clinician examines for the presence of any of these abnormal positions: lateral glide, lateral tilt, inferior tilt, and rotation. In the relaxed, extended position, the patella should rest near the center of the knee with its inferior pole at the knee's joint margin. If the patella's position is more than a few millimeters to the lateral aspect, it sits in a lateral glide position. A medial glide position is rare. When a finger is placed on top of the medial and lateral poles of the patella, they should be level with each other when observed from eye level; if the lateral finger is lower than the medial finger, the patella is in a lateral tilt. A medial tilt is rare. When a finger is placed on top of the mid-superior patellar surface and another is placed on top of the inferior patellar pole, the fingertips should be level with each other when observed from eye level; if the distal finger sits lower than the proximal finger, the patella sits in an inferior tilt, or posterior tilt. This tilt is also referred to as an AP tilt and is referenced from the location of the patella's inferior pole. Looking from directly above the patella, the superior medial and lateral poles should be in the same plane; if the lateral pole lies more proximally on the knee and the medial pole lies more distally, the patella is laterally rotated. If the medial pole lies more proximally, the patella is medially rotated. A lateral rotation is more common than a medial rotation. These patellar positions are demonstrated in figure 19.52.

Go to HK*Propel* and watch video 19.5, which demonstrates patellofemoral dysfunction during weight bearing.

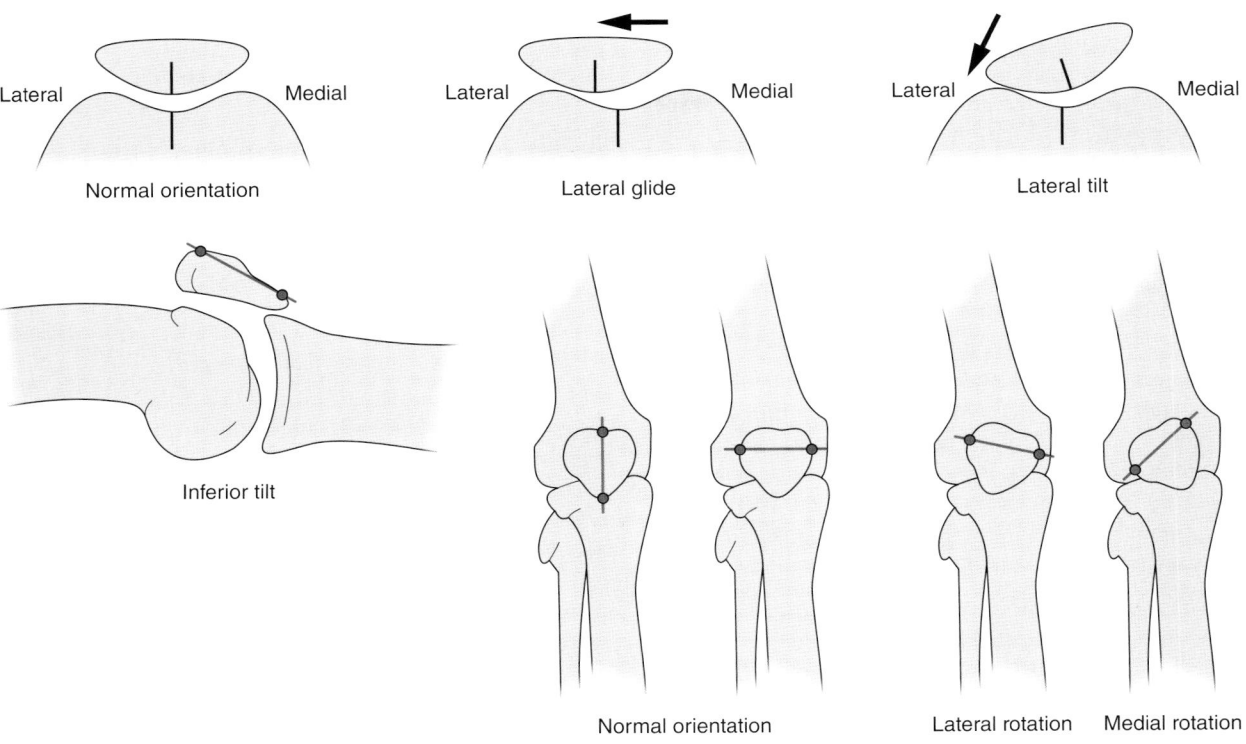

Figure 19.52 Patellar orientation.

The patella's tracking pattern is examined in non–weight bearing. As the patient contracts the quadriceps while in full knee extension, the rehabilitation clinician observes the patella for its movement. Normal patella movement occurs in a pattern similar to an inverted J, so patellar tracking ends with some lateral motion.[255] If lateral structures are tight or the VMO is weak, the patella will move upward in a lateral path from the start of patellar movement. During knee movement into flexion, the patella migrates medially as the Q-angle decreases and the patella becomes centered in the trochlea. Maltracking of the patella is commonly seen in patients with PFPS.[256]

Alignment is also observed in standing, and movement of the patella is observed while the patient performs an activity such as a lunge or step-down. During initial flexion, the patella sometimes moves and tilts laterally but then moves medially by the time the knee reaches flexion at 30°.[257] Changes in patellar alignment and glide during weight bearing can indicate various factors that should be corrected, such as pronation, weakness, incorrect firing patterns, and tightness.

Corrections Common surgical procedures to treat patellofemoral pain and patellofemoral malalignment in the past included a lateral release in which the lateral retinaculum was cut, or the tibial tubercle was advanced medially to produce a better patella alignment. It has been demonstrated, however, that many PFPS patients have

better results with nonsurgical management that consists primarily of exercise.[258]

Determination of the underlying causes dictates what is included in the rehabilitation program. Orthotics may be needed if there is excessive pronation,[259] flexibility exercises and soft-tissue mobilization techniques are needed if tightness and adhesions exist,[260] positioning the pelvis in neutral to properly align the femur will reduce torsional stress on the patella,[66, 261-263] strengthening and improving hip and core control will reduce patellofemoral stresses,[264] and lower-quarter neuromotor reeducation and strengthening exercises, especially for the VMO, are needed with all patellofemoral pain regardless of cause[247] because pain causes an inhibition reflex and weakens the quadriceps.[82]

Patellar Taping Technique A technique developed by Jenny McConnell, an Australian physiotherapist, uses a combination of taping the patella and exercises. Her initial theory stated that the tape corrected patellar alignment to relieve pain and allowed the patient to exercise to regain strength.[265] More recent studies, however, have shown conflicting results on the efficacy of patellar taping. Some have demonstrated that no change in patellar position occurs;[266-269] others have demonstrated that a reduction in pain or minimal short-term changes in alignment do occur with the tape.[270, 271] These studies, however, consistently point out that the effects of taping on patellar position are limited. Patellar position changed only at 10° of knee flexion,[272] and no change occurred in the open-chain position.[271] Changes that did occur lasted less than 15 min after activity began. Empirical evidence persists to support the theory that McConnell taping reduces pain in spite of the now accepted fact that the tape does not change functional patellar alignment. It has been speculated that the tape may provide neural inhibition through neurosensory afferent stimulation of the large A-beta fibers.[273, 274] Similar to McConnell taping, some research indicates that wearing a knee sleeve provides some benefits during activity that are yet to be fully understood;[275, 276] other research indicates that the benefits of a knee sleeve are disputable.[277]

Research has shown that patellar taping facilitates a quicker response of the VMO during step-up activities and delays the onset of vastus lateralis response while increasing the onset of VMO response during a step-down exercise.[278] It has yet to be determined whether this change in muscle response results from improved response secondary to pain reduction or neurosensory facilitation.

Soft-Tissue Mobility   Soft-tissue adhesions and tightness along the distal ITB and into the lateral retinaculum often play a role in patellar malalignment.[279] These structures should be treated with deep-tissue massage, myofascial release, and prolonged stretching in the case of a tight ITB. Deep-tissue massage can be applied by the rehabilitation clinician with the dorsal side of a flat fist (flexed MPs and PIPs, extended DIPs), with pressure delivered over the posterior middle and distal phalanges, as was discussed earlier in this chapter in the section Soft-Tissue Mobilization. Other myofascial techniques using tools such as Graston or The Roller are also effective on these structures. The patient can use a foam roller to perform self-massage techniques (see figure 19.4). The patient can perform manual massage techniques over the distal lateral thigh throughout the day while sitting (figure 19.53).

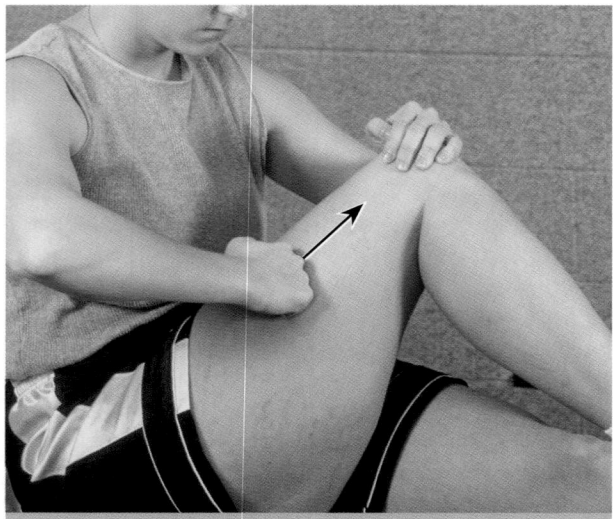

Figure 19.53   Iliotibial band massage.

The patient is instructed to perform stretching exercises for all tight muscle groups and should perform them throughout the day. The muscle groups commonly included are the hamstrings, gastrocnemius, and tensor fasciae latae.

Additional Rehabilitation Exercises   Exercises are a vital part of the total rehabilitation program for patellofemoral pain. Stretching and strengthening exercises can alter patellar tracking to correct alignment.[40, 62, 264, 280] Because muscle imbalance can play a role in PFPS, it is logical to assume that improvement in muscle balances can improve this condition.

As for all extremity programs, exercises for core, pelvic, and hip stabilization should be included in the rehabilitation program.[66, 67, 261, 264, 281, 282] Deficits in the strength of these areas are seen in patients with PFPS.[40, 143, 248] The results of these studies indicate that hip muscles and abdominals, especially lower abdominals, play a key role in providing adequate knee control during closed-chain activities. Trunk and core exercises were presented in chapters 17 and 18 and include strengthening exercises for the abdominal obliques, lower abdominals, and spine extensors. In addition, lateral and posterior hip muscles should be strengthened to provide hip stability during knee activities. Many of these hip exercises are found in chapter 18.

Lower-limb alignment and mechanics have a direct impact on the patellofemoral joint.[69, 283] Muscles in distal and proximal segments must be corrected for imbalances, along with the knee muscles if patellofemoral pain is to be resolved. Muscles that control foot pronation, including the posterior tibialis, anterior tibialis, and peroneals, should be strengthened and reeducated for pronation control and foot stability during closed-chain activities.

Quadriceps strength is crucial to a successful rehabilitation program.[284] Electrical stimulation and biofeedback can be used to facilitate quadriceps activation. These electrical modalities are used in open-chain exercises such as the straight-leg raise and SAQ and in closed-chain exercises for concentric and eccentric activity such as walking, step-downs, and lunges. A combination of open- and closed-chain activities within a pain-free range of motion is part of a total rehabilitation program.

When the patient can perform closed-chain activities in a slow and controlled manner and without pain, and the patient can achieve the goals that have been set, the speed of the activities increases to challenge muscle recruitment patterns and to prepare the patient for agility, functional, and performance-specific exercises. As the patient achieves the goals through gains in strength, control, and flexibility, he or she follows a progression of exercises similar to that for other knee injuries, advancing to increased stress and forces, more challenging coordination and agility activities, functional activities, and finally performance-specific exercises. Return to full participation is possible once the patient is pain free; etiological factors have been corrected;

the patient has normal flexibility, strength, agility, and power; and the patient demonstrates normal execution of performance-specific activities.

Patellar Tendinopathy

Patellar tendinopathy can be related to patellofemoral alignment, so the same factors presented for PFPS should be examined and assessed when the patient has patellar tendinopathy. Patellar tendinopathy is often called *jumper's knee* because jumping activities are the primary precipitating factor. With the energy absorption that occurs when landing from a jump, jumping on hard surfaces and excessive repetitions can overload the tendon beyond its stress-absorbing capabilities. Tissue breakdown then occurs. This stress becomes exaggerated with the presence of muscle imbalances such as weakness or tightness or mechanical malalignments such as foot pronation.

Pain occurs in the patellar tendon between the patella and the tibial tuberosity. Classic activities cause patellar tendon pain: pressure over the tendon, quadriceps tightening (especially eccentric activity), and stair climbing (especially going down). There may be slight edema in the tendon.

Initial rehabilitation goals are to identify and correct the etiological factors and reduce pain. Modalities such as phonophoresis, iontophoresis, ice, and electrical stimulation may be effective. Cross-friction massage across the tendon can help promote healing by improving mobility and reducing soft-tissue adhesions.[285, 286] The rehabilitation clinician applies cross-friction to one tender location on the tendon until the pain is reduced or relieved; he or she then moves to another site on the tendon and repeats the procedure until all tender sites are treated.

Rehabilitation activities include a combination of flexibility and strength. Stretching exercises for the hamstrings, quadriceps, lateral thigh, and calf muscles are taught to the patient and are easily incorporated into a home exercise program. Initial strengthening exercises include primarily eccentric exercises.[287] Eccentric exercises begin slowly and through a relatively pain-free range of motion. Some pain may occur with these exercises, but the pain resolves before the next treatment. Additional exercises include open-chain exercises to isolate the quadriceps and closed-chain exercises for functional stresses. The rate of the program's progression is purely dependent on the patient's response to the exercises. Patients who can do performance-specific exercises without pain or hesitation can return to normal activities.

Quadriceps Tendon Rupture

Quadriceps tendon ruptures occur most commonly in people 30 to 50 years old as a result of a sudden quadriceps contraction; the cause is probably a gradual degeneration, although prior complaints of tendinopathy are not usual.[288] Tendon ruptures occur more often in males than in females. As with Achilles tendon ruptures, the patient

Case Study

A 16-year-old female cross-country runner has had left knee pain for the past month. The pain has progressed so that it now interferes with her workouts and occurs even when she walks. The physician has diagnosed her with PFPS and wants her to begin rehabilitation. Your examination reveals genu valgus and recurvatum with foot pronation in standing. The patient's running shoes have excessive wear on the lateral posterior heel so that the midsole is showing through the outsole. The shoes have a sewn curved last, indicating that the shoe is flexible, providing less stability than a more rigid shoe. The patient's rearfoot and forefoot have excessive mobility. Straight-leg raise is to 70°; ankle dorsiflexion in rearfoot neutral is 0°. She has a positive Ober's test, and deep palpation reveals tenderness along the distal ITB. Her quadriceps strength is 4/5, lower abdominal strength is 3/5, and hip extension strength is 4/5. An assessment of patellar alignment reveals a posterior and lateral tilt. Patellar tracking in long sitting primarily occurs laterally. In standing, lateral patellar tracking is less than in non–weight bearing but continues throughout knee flexion. When the patient performs a step-down exercise, pain occurs, and the knee wobbles. Palpation of the posterior patellar surface reveals tenderness medially and laterally, especially over the inferior aspect.

Questions for Analysis

1. Create a list of the runner's potential etiological factors that have led to her current problem.
2. List her problems in order of priority. Correlate each problem with a long-term goal.
3. What will your treatment for the patient include today? What instructions will you send her home with today?
4. What will you tell her when she asks what she should do about her workouts?
5. Given her signs, in what part of the range of motion would you expect the patient to have the most pain?
6. List two elements you will use to strengthen the VMO during the first week.
7. What are your short-term goals for the next 2 weeks for the patient?

feels as though he has been hit or kicked in the knee. The patient cannot bear weight on the extremity. The rupture can occur from either the tendon attachment between the patella and tibial tuberosity (patellar tendon rupture) or the tendon between the patella and quadriceps (quadriceps tendon rupture). Complete ruptures are surgically repaired, with the knee kept either locked in extension with a brace or on a CPM machine for the first few weeks.

There are two general approaches to rehabilitation: the conservative approach, which includes a long-leg cast or brace with limited weight bearing and motion restricted to 40° of knee flexion for 6 weeks, and an approach that favors early functional activities, which include full weight bearing postoperatively with a gradual progression of increasing knee flexion.[289] In either case, weight bearing is restricted initially and then advanced to weight bearing as tolerated in the brace. One recent study permitted full weight bearing in an extension-locked brace 1 week after surgery with removal of the brace to allow ROM to 55° of knee flexion.[290] At 6 weeks, the patients were allowed to discard the brace and push for full knee motion.[290] It is interesting to note that none of their patients suffered re-ruptures, and in long-term follow-up, the patients were satisfied with their results.[290]

In terms of strength progression after patellar tendon repairs, straight-leg raises, quad sets, and hip exercises are used during the first 10 d to 2 weeks. Patellar mobilizations are used to maintain patellar mobility. After about 3 to 6 weeks, exercises begin out of the brace and follow a progression similar to that for other surgical repair programs. The period until return to full activity is 4 to 9 months.

Strains and Contusions

The severity of a strain determines the length of recovery. Ecchymosis indicates at least a grade II strain and necessitates a longer recovery time than a strain that does not produce bleeding. Ecchymosis is often distal to the site of a muscle tear because gravity pulls the blood caudally. Lack of normal flexibility, fatigue, incoordination, and a sudden violent contraction or stretch of a contracting muscle can all be frequent precipitating factors in muscle strains.

Remember that rehabilitation progression must coincide with tissue healing. Initial treatment goals in phase I include relieving pain, swelling, and spasm. Pulsed ultrasound is effective in promoting the absorption of ecchymosis. Electrical stimulation is useful in relieving pain and spasm. Stretches with activation of the antagonists help to relieve muscle spasm and regain range of motion beginning in phase II.

If the patient cannot ambulate normally, assistive devices are used with weight bearing to tolerance. Strength exercises are incorporated into the program during late phase II or early phase III as the patient tolerates them. Active range-of-motion exercises against gravity may be all that is tolerated initially, but progression to resisted open- and closed-chain exercises occurs within a few days. A variety of activities, including proprioceptive neuromuscular facilitation, manual resistance, aquatic exercises and gait training, stationary-bike exercises, co-contraction exercises, and unilateral weight bearing can begin within 1 to 3 d once spasm and pain have subsided.

The program advances as tolerated to eccentric and isokinetic exercises. Eccentric exercises are important for muscle strains because athletic activity places high eccentric demands on lower-extremity muscle groups.[291] Agility activities requiring more rapid muscle responses are introduced into the program late in the resistive phase as the patient gains strength, coordination, and balance control. After the patient moves into the advanced phase IV and can perform functional and performance-specific exercises, he or she is ready to be tested functionally for return to full work or sport participation.

Hamstrings

As with other strains, hamstring strains most commonly occur at the musculotendinous junction; hamstring strains occur either near the ischial tuberosity, involving the semimembranosis,[292] or more toward the mid-lateral or distal aspect of the muscle, where the biceps femoris tendon inserts more distally.[293] Hamstring strains often occur during high-speed activities such as sprinting or during sudden changes in muscle activity.

A proper rehabilitation program is important after hamstring strains. Stretching exercises begin within 2 to 4 d after an injury in the active phase, phase II. Also during this time, the patient can perform exercises for core muscles and other muscles and body segments not affected by the injury. Single-leg balance activities can also be added during this time. Home exercises will assist in the patient's progression. The rehabilitation clinician should continue with the usual assessment before each treatment session and each activity to ensure optimal progress.

Passive hamstring stiffness is often a predisposing factor in strains.[294] After an injury, additional loss of flexibility occurs. Appropriately timed deep and cross-friction massage to the injury site will promote healing and reduce scar tissue adhesions that will otherwise restrict hamstring mobility. Hamstring strains often recur.[295] Scar tissue that was not adequately treated during the rehabilitation of a hamstring strain may lead to reinjury once the patient returns to normal activities.[296, 297] Therefore, the first time a patient suffers a hamstring strain, the rehabilitation clinician must locate the area of injury and use these deep-tissue techniques to create sufficient scar tissue mobility to reduce the chances that the patient will suffer injury after returning to normal activities. These techniques may be initiated about 3 to 6 weeks after injury, in phase III, once the tissue's collagen develops.

In addition to restoring muscle flexibility and soft-tissue mobility, strength must be restored. As with other injuries, strength exercises begin in phase III. Eccentric exercises have proven to be beneficial for hamstring strain injuries.[298] Other strength exercises can include activities such as bridging, hamstring curls within a pain-free range, lunges, deadlifts, good mornings, step-ups, leg presses, slide board, resisted hip exercises in all directions, and heel raises.

Once the patient's strength is 90% of normal and full motion is restored, the patient enters phase IV, where plyometrics and multiplanar exercises advance to functional and then performance-specific exercises. Before the return to normal activities, the rehabilitation clinician has the patient complete a number of sport- or work-specific tests. When he or she passes these tests and has been released by the physician, the patient can return to normal activities.

Quadriceps

Two-joint muscles that act in jumping or sudden changes in direction during eccentric activities are susceptible to strain injuries;[300] for this reason, the rectus femoris is the muscle of the quadriceps group that is most often strained. The treatment course for this injury follows the same routine and phases as for hamstring strains. The initial rehabilitation phase includes treatment techniques to relieve pain, swelling, and spasm. Stretching activities begin on days 2 to 4 in the active phase and are accompanied initially by isometric exercises as tolerated. Aquatic exercises and gait training, proprioceptive neuromuscular facilitation, passive stretching, and stationary-bike exercises are used early in the program. In the resistive phase (III), isometric exercises are replaced with eccentric activities and progress to other resistive exercises as tolerated. In the advanced phase, isokinetic, agility, plyometric, and functional and performance-specific exercises progress as previously mentioned for other knee rehabilitation programs.

Iliotibial Band Syndrome

Iliotibial band syndrome is an overuse syndrome that results from friction between the ITB and the lateral femoral epicondyle. It is seen most often in middle- and long-distance runners. Friction is thought to take place at 30° of knee flexion when the ITB is pulled over the lateral femoral epicondyle, and it occurs during running when the tensor fasciae latae and gluteus maximus, the muscles attaching to the ITB, are active and are pulling on the band during the initial stance phase.[301, 302] During downhill running, more time is spent in flexion, increasing ITB stress.

Predisposing factors may include leg-length discrepancy, pelvic position, increased Q-angle, genu valgus, and foot pronation. Running hills and increased running distances can also lead to ITB syndrome.[303]

The patient complains of pain along the ITB (especially over the lateral femoral epicondyle), increased pain with walking or running (especially down hills), edema, and crepitus. Snapping can sometimes be felt over the lateral femoral epicondyle.

Rehabilitation must involve correction of predisposing factors, stretching, and strengthening. Modalities to relieve the inflammation and a workout modification are useful in phase I. Running at a faster speed may reduce ITB pain—during faster running, the knee is at more than 30° of flexion in the early weight-bearing phase.[304] When pain is relieved, strengthening exercises for deficiencies should proceed in the resistive phase with the inclusion of open and closed kinetic chain exercises, concentric and eccentric closed-chain activities, and a progression as previously presented for return to full sport participation.

Evidence in Rehabilitation

Hamstring strains are common in many sports. Perhaps one reason for this is that the causes of hamstring strains are multifactorial. As with other injuries that have many varied combinations of causes, hamstring injuries are difficult to prevent. A recent investigation focused on potential causes and interventions.[299] Based on evidence in the literature, the authors concluded that hamstring strains occurred during eccentric contraction of the muscle. It is interesting to note that sports that do not feature eccentric hamstring activity, such as swimming and cycling, do not see hamstring injuries. Another contributing factor may be an excessive anterior tilt to the pelvis since this stretches the hamstrings so that they are stressed before they are activated.

A history of previous hamstring strains increases one's risk for another hamstring strain; the authors theorize that the scar tissue formation may reduce both hamstring strength and flexibility. They also point out that other investigators have identified a proliferation of scar tissue adhesions to adjacent muscle fibers, which further restricts mobility and increases the muscle's susceptibility to damage during eccentric activity. Weakness in the hamstrings after injury creates an imbalance between quadriceps and hamstrings on the ipsilateral limb and an imbalance between left and right hamstrings; both factors increase the risk of reinjury. Finally, muscle fatigue creates incoordination and weakness, further increasing the person's risk of reinjury. Since most hamstring injuries occur during eccentric activity, the authors advocated the use of eccentric exercises as part of the rehabilitation program. Flexibility exercises, neuromuscular coordination activities, and scar tissue management techniques are all recommended to reduce the recurrence of hamstring strains.

Osteochondral Considerations

Fractures of the knee bones can be traumatic or stress related. Femur fractures are not common, but tibial fractures are seen more often. Unfortunately, osteochondral injuries are common in young athletes,[305] and if managed poorly, they can be a source of pathology for years.[306] Before delving into osteochondral injuries, we'll briefly address fracture rehabilitation.

Bone Fractures

Fractures of the knee result from direct blows and impact forces, torsional and traction stresses, or compression loads. A patellar fracture usually occurs as the result of a direct blow, but a tibial fracture occurs most often because of torsional or compression forces. Epiphyseal plate injuries of the proximal tibia or distal femur occur in adolescent patients whose growth plates have not yet matured. Damage to these sites can alter bone growth.[307] Displaced fractures require open reduction and internal fixation (ORIF). Fractures repaired with ORIF procedures become more stable more quickly and can sometimes undergo a more accelerated therapeutic exercise program. Tibial plateau fractures require non–weight bearing after surgery. Rehabilitation of these fractures follows courses similar to those of other lower-extremity fractures. As with any fracture of any segment, rehabilitation activities follow closely with the tissue's healing progression, using the patient's pain and other responses to exercises as a guide to specific exercise application.

Osteochondral Injuries

Articular cartilage covering joint surfaces is a very unique type of cartilage, unlike most other types in the body. Its characteristics along with unique concerns about healing and treatment options after injury are presented in chapters 2 and 3.

Repair Options Osteochondral injuries are articular cartilage defects that occur as a result of trauma to the articular surface, often a direct impact, including bone bruises.[306] These lesions occur most often in young adults.[306] The lesions often develop into localized areas of degeneration. Several treatment options are available for these isolated degenerative changes in the knee. As was mentioned in chapter 2, there are three main surgical options: debriding the chondral surface, resurfacing the chondral defect, and a more recent technique called the *osteochondral autologous transfer system (OATS)*. An abrasion arthroplasty is a debridement technique, while subchondral drilling and creation of microfractures stimulate bleeding to introduce stem cells into the area and are examples of resurfacing techniques. Subchondral drilling uses multiple drill holes to expose subchondral bone, allowing bone marrow blood to move into the injured site.[308] The microfracture technique also accesses the subchondral blood supply but uses a small pick rather than a drill bit to create microfractures around the articular cartilage defect.[309] The debriding, drilling, and microfracture techniques all introduce stem cells into the area via introduction of the marrow blood supply.[310] The initial tissue produced through these techniques is hyaline-like cartilage.[311] Unfortunately, the hyaline-like cartilage is replaced by fibrocartilage within 2 to 3 years.[310] The OATS procedure consists of obtaining a small fragment of bone along with its articular cartilage from a portion of the non-weight-bearing joint surface and inserting it into the articular defect site.[311] Although the OATS procedure is the newest surgical technique for articular cartilage, it also shows the most promise in initial study results. It has been reported that 93% of patients undergoing the OATS procedure were able to return to sports activities, while only 52% of microfracture patients returned to sports activities.[312]

Osteochondral Postoperative Rehabilitation A successful postoperative outcome after osteochondral surgery depends on a good rehabilitation program.[313] The rehabilitation clinician must be aware of the precautions for postoperative care. Issues of concern include providing an environment that is optimal for graft protection and healing. This means providing some stress to allow tissue to heal with optimal strength but not overstressing it to damage the graft. Early controlled loading and motion have been shown to be beneficial.[314] Studies have also demonstrated that cyclic loading increases chondrocyte synthetic activity,[314] so periodic weight bearing and range-of-motion activities may actually stimulate articular cartilage repair. On the other hand, there is a limit to how much weight should be applied since bearing too much weight or bearing it too soon may hinder articular cartilage repair.[315] Therefore, the rehabilitation clinician's goal must be to provide enough stress to create strong tissue but not to overstress the healing tissue.

It is important for the rehabilitation clinician to know where the chondral repair is within the joint and to realize where within the range of motion the patella and femur are in contact to stress that repair. A knowledge of patellofemoral contact areas throughout the knee's range of motion is vital to understanding range-of-motion restrictions placed on the patient, especially during the first several weeks of rehabilitation when contact pressure and stress should be minimized.

Osteochondral rehabilitation is slightly different for repairs of the patella than for repairs of the femoral condyles. Rehabilitation of a patellar graft allows weight bearing immediately after surgery, but motion is limited to the 0° to 30° range, and no open-chain exercises are permitted for the first 3 weeks.[316] Rehabilitation for femoral condylar repairs allows partial weight bearing only after the second week, but open-chain range-of-motion exercises can begin immediately to enhance lubrication and nutrition at the surgical site.[316] The duration of partial weight bearing is determined by the number of plugs used to repair the lesion; for three or fewer plugs, the time of partial weight bearing is 2 weeks, but with each additional plug inserted, one more week of partial weight bearing is required up to a maximum of 8 weeks.[317]

For either the patellar or femoral condylar procedure, a brace locked in extension is used during ambulation to reduce shear stress on the lesion site. Shear stress is among the most damaging of all stresses applied to the joints.[318] Normal ambulation places shear stresses on the knee.[319] Therefore, using a straight-leg brace with no weight bearing for the first 2 weeks protects the surgical site from stresses it would otherwise experience. The brace is often worn at night for the first 2 to 4 weeks, locked in extension.

Early range-of-motion activity occurs using either a CPM machine several hours a day, passive ROM activities, or a combination of both. Recall that the goal during this initial period is to stimulate chondral formation without applying excessive loads to the lesion site. Electrical stimulation, submaximal isometric exercises, and other unresisted open-chain exercises occur after the first week in femoral condylar repairs. Hip, ankle, and core exercises are also used at this time. Biofeedback for muscle reeducation is useful for quadriceps facilitation and control. It is appropriate to add aquatic exercises in deep water for range-of-motion activities after the surgical wounds are well healed.

Patellar mobilization and soft-tissue mobilization are begun in the second post-op week. By the end of the second week, the patient should have 90° of flexion with full extension. By the end of the second week, the brace is unlocked to 20° with increases in motion as the quadriceps gains strength. A stationary bike without resistance for range-of-motion gains is used after the third week. Active-assistive range-of-motion exercises, progressing to active range-of-motion exercises, are also used then. By week 3 or 4, the patient should be able to demonstrate good quad control without an extensor lag and should have near-normal knee range of motion. After the third week, mild resistive aquatic exercises in deep water are suitable.

By 6 to 8 weeks, the knee should have full range of motion. Also at this time, full weight bearing with crutches begins. Crutches are not removed until the patient can ambulate normally, has no extensor lag, and has full motion in knee extension. The brace can also be discontinued by this time. Aquatic exercises can progress from the deep to the shallow end in chest- to waist-high water with progressive weight bearing. Progressive resistive exercises in the open and closed kinetic chain, using small arcs of motion initially and advancing to larger arcs of motion, start after 6 weeks. Exercises such as mini-squats, wall sits, heel raises, and leg presses begin once the patient is full weight bearing. Exercises should remain pain free in all arcs of motion. A ski machine or stepper can also be started. Once the patient can ambulate without crutches, treadmill walking begins. Static balance exercises progress to dynamic balance exercises as tolerated.

A gradual progression from balance exercises to neuro-motor control to coordination exercises to agility exercises takes place as the patient gains strength and improves overall function. Jogging, then running, is allowed at 4 to 6 months postoperatively. Full return to sport participation occurs at 7 to 12 months.

Bone-fracture rehabilitation programs follow the same basic progression, but the timing for return to full sport or work participation is more rapid. A general range of time for return to sport or work after a fracture is 4 to 8 months. The time range varies based on whether the fracture is treated surgically or immobilized without surgery, the location and type of fracture, the age of the patient, and the physician's preference. See figure 19.54 for an outline of progression for rehabilitation.

Osteochondritis Dissecans Osteochondritis dissecans (OCD) is a multifactorial condition that occurs more often in children and adolescents than in adults.[320, 321] A bone flake in juvenile OCD or a bone fragment in adult OCD occurs at various sites of the femoral condyle. Juvenile OCD occurs in youths aged 10 to 20 years.[322] Symptoms include nonspecific knee pain, point tenderness over the site, and quadriceps atrophy. There is minimal effusion, and the patient may experience catching, locking, or giving way during ambulation.

Treatment for adult OCD includes arthroscopic debridement of loose bodies. If the lesion is small, an abrasion arthroplasty or autogenous grafting can also be performed. Arthroscopy is the gold-standard treatment for removing loose bodies in adults with OCD.[322] However, juvenile OCD is more conservative with prolonged rest and immobilization.[323] Non–weight bearing restrictions may extend for 6 to 8 weeks.[320] Studies have shown that juvenile patients do better with nonoperative care using these non–weight bearing and activity restriction strategies as long as the lesion is stable and has an intact cartilage surface.[324]

Rehabilitation for juvenile OCD must try to reverse the deleterious effects of immobilization and inactivity. Cardiovascular exercise using the upper extremities and lower-extremity exercises for the uninvolved segments help to maintain conditioning levels during immobilization. Quad sets, straight-leg raises, and electrical stimulation can help retard atrophy during immobilization as well. Range-of-motion exercises are often permitted during the prolonged time of non–weight bearing. Patellar and soft-tissue mobilizations may also help maintain knee range of motion.

Active exercises are used once knee motion is permitted. Weight-bearing exercises include weight-transfer activities

Chondral Microfracture Rehabilitation

Stage I: Inactive phase	
0-3 weeks	**Inflammation phase: Inactive rehabilitation phase**
Goals	Relieve pain. Reduce edema, ecchymosis, effusion. Relieve spasm. Protect surgical repair. End of week 2: Achieve 0° to 90° knee ROM. Prevent deconditioning of unaffected body segments.
Treatment guidelines	Electrical stimulation for pain, muscle spasm Compression and elevation for edema Brace locked at 0° CPM 6 to 8 h/day Weeks 1-2: NWB; Week 3: TTWB (20% BW); increase weight bearing on involved leg as quad strength improves ROM exercises for hip and ankle muscle groups PROM for knee Biofeedback/electrical stimulation for quadriceps facilitation Patellar mobilization; soft-tissue mobilization PRN OKC exercises: quad set; SLR; hip strengthening; ankle strengthening in knee brace After week 3: Aquatic exercises for ROM Week 3: Stationary bike without resistance for knee ROM only Exercises for unaffected body segments HEP for PROM for the knee often throughout the day
Precautions	Maintain brace use except for ROM activities. Protect surgical repair. Brace remains locked in extension at night first 2 to 4 weeks and until patient has good quad contraction in full extension.
Stage II: Active phase	
3-12 weeks	**Early proliferation phase: Active rehabilitation phase**
Goals	No pain, edema, spasm. Weeks 6-8: Achieve full weight bearing with crutches. Wean from crutches as quad control is achieved. Perform treadmill ambulation without crutches. Week 8: Normal knee ROM. Balance activities once FWB. Increase strength of all deficient muscles and muscle groups. Restore normal gait.
Treatment guidelines	Weeks 6-8: FWB gait training with crutches as needed Joint mobilization, soft-tissue mobilization PRN Stationary bike FWB balance activities CKC exercises: mini-squats, leg press, wall squats, heel raises, hip strengthening OKC exercises: SAQ, hamstring curls Aquatic: cardiovascular conditioning, resistive exercises and gait training PRN HEP for strength gains; ROM

Figure 19.54 Rehabilitation progression after a chondral microfracture.

Stage II: Active phase	
3-12 weeks	**Early proliferation phase: Active rehabilitation phase**
Precautions	Avoid knee pain with exercises. Use weight-scale exercises if weight transfer is incorrect. Do not use home exercises during treatment sessions.

Stage III: Resistive phase	
12-24 weeks	**Late proliferation phase: Resistive rehabilitation phase**
Goals	Maintain normal ROM. Achieve 85% to 90% normal strength. Restore normal gait.
Treatment guidelines	Continue with strength progression, all muscle groups including CKC hamstring resistance exercises at hip: step-ups, lateral step-ups, squats, leg press, lunges Progressive agility exercises Multiplanar exercises Week 16: Jogging, advancing to running with increase of strength to 85% normal Week 20: Running or sprinting backward, cutting, cariocas
Precautions	Observe and use verbal cues to correct for execution of all exercises. Avoid pain and joint effusion.

Stage IV: Advanced phase	
24-52 weeks	**Remodeling phase: Advanced rehabilitation phase**
Goals	Maintain normal strength of all muscles. Maintain normal ROM of all joints. Restore normal sport and work performance.
Treatment guidelines	Plyometric exercises Functional exercise progression Performance-specific exercises and drills progression
Precautions	Correct performance PRN.

ROM = range of motion; CPM = continuous passive motion machine; NWB = non–weight bearing; TTWB = toe-touch weight bearing; FWB = full weight bearing; BW = body weight; SAQ = short-arc quadriceps; CKC = closed kinetic chain; OKC = open kinetic chain; SLR = straight-leg raise; PRN = as needed; HEP = home exercise program.

Figure 19.54 >continued

and gait training. Aquatic exercises with progressive weight bearing can be used, starting in shoulder-high water and moving progressively into shallower water as tolerated. Activities to restore proprioception using a BAPS board and a balance board, as well as single-limb stance balance activities, are helpful.

Rehabilitation after surgical treatment includes immediate weight bearing unless the lesion is large; in this case, weight bearing may be restricted. A gradual progression of exercises that do not produce pain takes place as with other knee lesions. Recovery to full sport participation usually takes about 4 to 6 months.

Total Knee Arthroplasty

A total knee arthroplasty (TKA), usually known as a total knee replacement (TKR), is a very common surgical procedure.[325] While most TKAs are performed as a result of osteoarthritis, and patients are usually older than 65 years, a growing number are performed on those under age 55.[326] While a total knee replacement procedure currently doesn't have as many variations as a total hip replacement (THR) procedure, unicompartmental and cementless procedures are being explored and may become more common in the future.[327, 328]

Rehabilitation programs after a TKA vary and depend upon many factors.[329] However, one parameter observed in nearly all TKA rehabilitation protocols is the need to achieve 90° of knee AROM within the first 2 weeks after surgery.[330] Range-of-motion gains after TKA vary greatly and seldom return to 135° of flexion. Although some patients do gain more than 120°, average knee flexion motions that are achieved are listed in table 19.4.

Although knee flexion ROM does not usually fully recover after TKA, most daily activities do not require 135° of knee flexion to perform them. For example, knee flexion motion needed to perform a proper swing through during ambulation is about 60°, and the amount of knee flexion needed to climb stairs or get up from a chair ranges from 90° to 120°.[61]

Different studies investigating patients undergoing TKA procedures place the average age range of this population from 55 to 68 years.[328] More than one-third of the younger patients return to their sports, which are usually low-impact sports; however, only about 10% of individuals in high-impact sports did return to sports participation.[61] Therefore, although 120° may be adequate knee flexion for most patients after TKA, those who choose to return to their sport or workplace environments may need to acquire more than this level of knee mobility. The rehabilitation clinician must be in tune with the patient's goals at the outset of the rehabilitation program.

Just as these ROM elements differ according to patient needs, specific strengthening and functional tasks also vary greatly, not only in patient expectations but also in

TABLE 19.4 Average Knee Flexion Following TKA

Post-op time	Knee flexion ROM
1-2 weeks[331]	90°
2-3 weeks[331]	95°
3-4 weeks[331]	101°
4-5 weeks[331]	106°
5-6 weeks[331]	108°
6-7 weeks[331]	110°
6 months[332]	116°
12 months[332]	117°

Note: Numbers are recorded to the nearest whole number.

protocol designs. The protocol provided here is only a framework from which you can build an individualized rehabilitation program.

After TKA surgery, the patient usually spends one or two nights in the hospital for observation. Beginning within a few hours after surgery, the early active phase of rehabilitation begins and consists of PROM and AAROM as well as WBAT activities with an assistive device. The customary assistive device used immediately after surgery is a front-wheeled walker; the patient progresses to a cane, and eventually to no assistive device within the next few weeks of the rehabilitation program.

Upon discharge from the hospital, the patient either goes home or to a rehabilitation facility to improve functional strength to perform such tasks as getting dressed and getting in and out of a car. Once the patient is discharged home, he or she begins an outpatient rehabilitation program (figure 19.55).

During the active phase of rehabilitation, which is usually the first 2 to 6 weeks after surgery, knee flexion and extension are the focus as the patient is expected to regain knee motion to improve basic tasks such as walking, standing, and sit to stand. Soft-tissue mobilization and modalities are employed to help improve knee ROM. Research has shown that initiating a program that involves pedaling a stationary bike or similar equipment improves the speed of recovery in this phase of rehabilitation.[333]

As the patient progresses to the resistive phase of rehabilitation in weeks 6 through 12, more challenging activities such as resisted quadriceps, hamstring, and gluteal exercises are introduced. Stair activities begin when knee flexion and quad control are sufficient. Range-of-motion objectives remain, and they may become more vigorous if motion loss continues during this phase since knee stiffness can be a problem in this patient population.[334]

In the advanced phase of rehabilitation, squatting, reciprocal stair use, and upright resisted activities for the lower extremities are possible. More intense range-of-motion activities, such as prolonged stretching, may be needed if the patient continues to demonstrate a lack of appropriate knee extension or knee flexion. The patient advances to proprioceptive and neuromotor exercises, single-leg activities, and functionally specific tasks, with a focus on meeting individual needs as he or she approaches the conclusion of the rehabilitation program.

Total Knee Arthroplasty

Stage I: Inactive phase	
1-3 days	**Inflammation phase: Inactive rehabilitation phase**
Goals	Relieve pain. Reduce edema, ecchymosis. Relieve spasm. Develop proper use of a walker.
Treatment guidelines	Electrical stimulation for pain, muscle spasm Compression and elevation for edema Starting on day 1: WBAT, increasing to FWB by 1-6 weeks ROM exercises for knee, hip, ankle muscle groups, specifically knee flexion and extension Patellar mobilization; soft-tissue mobilization PRN OKC exercises: quad set; SLR; knee extension; hip strengthening; ankle strengthening HEP for pain, edema, and ROM
Precautions	Encourage proper gait once patient begins ambulating. Manage wounds.
Stage II: Active phase	
1-6 weeks	**Early proliferation phase: Active rehabilitation phase**
Goals	No pain, edema, spasm. Prevent deconditioning of unaffected body segments. By week 2: Achieve 0° to 90° ROM; by week 6: 0°-110°. Week 6: Full weight bearing and knee ROM continuing toward 120° of knee flexion. Increase strength of all deficient muscles and muscle groups. Restore normal gait.
Treatment guidelines	Joint mobilizations, PRN Stationary bike FWB balance activities once patient is FWB CKC exercises: mini-squats, leg press (90° to 0°), wall squats, heel raises, hip strengthening OKC exercises: quad, hamstring, and gluteal strengthening with resistance After week 2: Aquatic exercises and weight shifting, gait training in water Core strengthening HEP for strength gains; ROM for knee flexion and extension
Precautions	Do not use home exercises during treatment sessions
Stage III: Resistive phase	
6-12 weeks	**Late proliferation phase: Resistive rehabilitation phase**
Goals	Maintain normal ROM with knee flexion goal of 120°. Achieve 75% to 80% normal strength. Restore normal gait. Execute reciprocal stair use.

>continued

Figure 19.55 Suggested rehabilitation program for a patient after a total knee replacement.

Stage III: Resistive phase	
6-12 weeks	**Late proliferation phase: Resistive rehabilitation phase**
Treatment guidelines	Discontinue assistive gait devices, if still using them; gait training PRN. Continue with strength progression for all muscle groups, including CKC hamstring resistance exercises at hip, resisted side stepping, step-ups, lateral step-ups, and sit to stand. Include multiplanar exercises and lifting objects from the ground. Include functional activities to restore independent daily function.
Precautions	Observe and use verbal cues to correct for execution of all exercises. Avoid pain and joint swelling.

Stage IV: Advanced phase	
12+ weeks	**Remodeling phase: Advanced rehabilitation phase**
Goals	Maintain normal strength of all muscles. Maintain normal ROM of all joints. Restore normal work or daily function.
Treatment guidelines	Single-leg and proprioceptive tasks Functional exercise progression Progress to lifting and carrying tasks
Precautions	Correct performance PRN.

NWB = non–weight bearing; TTWB = toe-touch weight bearing; WBAT = weight bearing as tolerated; BW = body weight; ROM = range of motion; PROM = passive range of motion; SLR = straight leg raise; PRN = as needed; CKC = closed kinetic chain; OKC = open kinetic chain; HEP = home exercise program.

Figure 19.55 >continued

Summary

The knee is positioned between two long lever arms, so it is often the site of injury in any number of activities and sports. The patellofemoral joint is susceptible to pain and dysfunction. Patellofemoral pain syndrome is usually a multifactorial condition, so it is important for the rehabilitation clinician to identify the underlying problems that lead to a patient's condition. Stresses for knee structures change in both open- and closed-chain activities; it is important for the rehabilitation clinician to understand when stresses are high or low so appropriate rehabilitation exercises are used in a patient's program. Trigger point treatment, joint mobilization techniques, and progressive exercises from flexibility to functional activities and performance exercises were included in this chapter. Some of the more common injuries of the knee and thigh were presented along with rehabilitation programs for them.

LEARNING AIDS

Key Concepts and Review

1. Discuss the relationship and alignment between the patella and the femur.

Patellar stability is produced by both static and dynamic structures. The bony configuration, with the patella seated within the femoral sulcus formed by the medial and higher-ridged lateral epicondyles, is the greatest bony contributor to patellar stability. Patellofemoral and patellotibial ligaments help provide static restraints and patellar stability. Active restraints come primarily from the quadriceps. The patella is in various degrees of contact within its groove in the femur during any specific point within the knee's range of motion. A combination of compressive forces and the amount of area of contact determines the stress on the patellofemoral joint.

2. Identify postinjury factors that influence strength output.

Edema and pain both cause automatic withdrawal of quadriceps activity. An abnormal gait, using the injured extremity less than normal, also results in reduced muscle activity. These factors in combination contribute to a further reduction of strength in the injured extremity.

3. Define *quadriceps extensor lag* and *AMI* and explain their significance.

An extensor lag occurs when full passive motion of knee extension is available, but the patient cannot actively achieve full extension. It is an indication of quadriceps weakness. AMI, or arthrogenic muscle inhibition, occurs because of joint swelling, pain, or injury. An inhibition of the muscle's normal motoneuron pool functions inhibits normal activity of the muscle. Quadriceps AMI contributes to delayed response to treatment because it inhibits quadriceps activity and can retard effective strengthening efforts since the neurogenic inhibition prevents the quadriceps from activating properly. This condition may persist for long after the initial injury and can interfere with normal lower-extremity function.

4. Outline a general progression of rehabilitation for a knee.

As with other body segments, specific applications depend on specific deficiencies. Modalities are used to relieve pain, edema, and effusion and to encourage the healing process in phase I. Soft-tissue and joint mobilization techniques may be needed. Range-of-motion activities, active and passive, are used to increase motion in phase II. Easy strengthening exercises can be started late in the active phase or early in the resistive phase within a pain-free range of motion or with isometric exercises. In the resistive phase, manual resistance can progress to machine and body-weight resistances, resistance bands, and isokinetics. A combination of open- and closed-chain exercises are a part of the program once the patient is weight bearing. Weight-bearing proprioception and balance activities begin with something simple like a stork stand and progress to balance activities on unstable surfaces and neuromotor control activities. Once flexibility, balance, and strength have reached appropriate levels, either late in phase III or early in phase IV, plyometric exercises, such as target jumping, lateral jumps, box activities, and depth jumps, can be used. In phase IV, functional activities progress to performance-specific exercises that mimic the patient's sport or work demands before full participation in the patient's sport or work is permitted.

5. Identify three soft-tissue mobilization techniques for the knee.

Three such techniques include foam roller myofascial release to the ITB, trigger point release to the popliteus, and cross-friction massage to the patellar tendon.

6. Identify three joint mobilization techniques for the knee and the purpose of each.

Lateral glides of the patella are used for full flexion–extension range of motion of the knee; posterior glides of the tibia on the femur increase flexion; and rotational glides increase terminal flexion and extension of the knee.

7. Describe three flexibility exercises for the knee, and identify the structures they affect.

Flexibility exercises include standing knee flexion stretch for the quadriceps with the heel behind the buttocks, standing hamstring stretch with the involved extremity on an elevated surface, and the gastrocnemius stretch with the knee straight.

8. Describe three proprioception and balance exercises for the knee.

Exercises for proprioception and balance include stork standing with eyes open, eyes closed, and eyes open with head rotations to the left and right, stork standing on a half foam roller, and standing on a foam roller while catching a ball.

9. Identify three functional activities.

Three functional activities include running and cutting while dribbling a basketball, sprinting forward and then backward with rapid changes in direction, and lateral glides with pivots to left and right.

10. Identify three factors that influence PFPS.

Three such factors are weak quadriceps, weak hip and trunk control, and tight hamstrings.

Critical Thinking Questions

1. In this chapter's opening scenario, how much knee flexion motion would you expect Steve to have after 2 weeks of progress while using an accelerated rehabilitation protocol? What would be the most effective kind of motion exercise he should be able to start on his first day of rehabilitation? What strengthening exercises would you give him for his hip and ankle on his first day of rehabilitation? When you would expect him to have full knee motion? When would you start him on passive stretching exercises for his quads? Justify your timetable.

2. When would you begin patellar mobilization on Steve? When would you begin soft-tissue mobilization to the incision sites? Give your rationale for these timetables.

3. If you had two patients with knee injuries, one with an ACL sprain and the other with an MCL sprain, which one (if either) would you be more cautious with and why? How would their rehabilitation programs differ?

4. If a patient complains of patellar tendinopathy, what structures would you investigate for possible causes? What key items would you include in your history questions? Would you use primarily open- or closed-chain exercises at first, and why?

5. A teenaged patient you have been rehabilitating for weakness after a contusion injury to the anterior knee near the lateral femoral condyle continues to complain of pain in the knee even though his strength is improving. How would you approach the problem, and what would you suspect?

Lab Activities

1. Perform soft-tissue mobilization on your lab partner's ITB. First examine the area for any restrictions, and then apply mobilization to relieve the main restrictive areas. Examine the area after your treatment. What changes do you and your partner (objectively and subjectively, respectively) observe? What do you think has occurred with the treatment? Use a foam roller to perform a soft-tissue mobilization technique on the same area for the same amount of time. Compare the sensory changes between the two techniques. Based on the differences, what would be the advantages and disadvantages of each technique?

2. Locate the trigger points on your lab partner for the muscles listed. As you perform each one, indicate what the pain pattern would be if the trigger point were active.

   A. Popliteus

   B. Medial hamstrings

   Which one was your partner's most sensitive trigger point? Perform a treatment technique on it, and provide your partner with a home exercise for the tender trigger point.

3. Perform grade II and IV joint mobilizations on your lab partner, and identify what restriction would be best treated with each mobilization for the following joints:

   A. Patellofemoral glides
   - Medial glide
   - Lateral glide
   - Superior glide
   - Inferior glide

   B. Tibiofemoral glides
   - Distraction
   - Anterior
   - Posterior glide
   - Anterior glide of the medial condyle

   Are the medial and lateral patellofemoral glide excursions the same? Perform the tibiofemoral glides first in the resting position and then in other open-packed positions. How does the amount of motion change with the different positions? What are the implications of this outcome for treatment?

4. Have your partner perform two different prolonged stretch exercises to increase knee flexion. Is there an advantage to one over the other?

5. Identify short-term stretches you would give a patient to perform at home to improve knee flexion and extension. Identify the position in which you would place a patient to stretch a knee with extension limited to 15° of flexion and the position for another stretch that could be used on a knee with extension limited to 90° of flexion. What factors do you have to consider that are unique to each condition when coming up with an exercise for each situation?

6. Have your partner perform two different exercises (same level of difficulty) to strengthen the quadriceps. How are they different? Why might you use one over the other? Explain your rationale.

7. Have your partner perform a lateral step-up exercise for 20 repetitions on an 8 in. step. What substitution patterns must you watch for, and how would you correct them?

8. Have your partner perform a wall squat using three different ways of doing it so each exercise is a progression of the previous one. Have your partner perform 20 repetitions of each exercise. Does your partner agree that the sequence you created is a progression, or is a later exercise easier than a previous one? What are the substitution patterns you should watch for, and what verbal cues would you give to correct each substitution?

9. Have your partner perform three proprioceptive exercises, each one a progression of the previous exercise. What have you used to determine when your partner can progress to the next exercise (what are your goals for each exercise)?

10. Evaluate your partner's patellar alignment for lateral tilt, lateral shift or glide, inferior tilt, and rotation. What malalignments do you see? Are they bilateral? If there are malalignments, why might your partner have them? What exercises might correct the alignment deficiencies?

11. Have your partner perform a quad set in supine and a lunge in standing or go up and down a step. What differences in patellar tracking do you see between the two positions? How would you correct any deficiencies you noted?

12. You are seeing a patient (a high school basketball forward) for the first time today. She is 2 d postoperative with an ACL reconstruction (patellar tendon graft). List in proper sequence all the exercises you would include in the rehabilitation program. You do not need to identify timing, only the sequence in which you would add the exercises. Also, indicate when you might consider discontinuing an exercise in the program and your rationale for doing so.

20

Foot, Ankle, and Leg

Objectives

After completing this chapter, you should be able to do the following:

1. Discuss normal foot mechanics in ambulation.
2. Identify two foot deformities, and discuss their impact on athletic injury.
3. List the important factors in shoe selection for a pes cavus foot.
4. Describe one joint mobilization technique for improving ankle dorsiflexion.
5. List three stretching exercises for the ankle and extremity, including one that is not mentioned in the text.
6. Identify three strengthening exercises for the ankle and extremity.
7. Describe three agility exercises.
8. Describe three functional exercises for the lower extremity.
9. Provide an example of a rehabilitation program progression for an ankle sprain.

After 2 months of persistent heel pain, cross-country runner Danny felt he could no longer hope the pain would go away on its own, and he decided to seek care for it. After Deena Mare performed her evaluation, she informed Danny that the problem was plantar fasciitis.

Deena concluded from her examination that Danny had a few problems that were contributing to his plantar fasciitis. His excessive pronation would have to be corrected with orthotics; the tight hip rotators were causing altered knee alignment that contributed to increased torsional stress on the plantar fascia and would have to be stretched and corrected, as would the tightness in the iliotibial band and Achilles. The muscle imbalance between Danny's quads and hamstrings was another contributing factor that would be resolved with strengthening activities. Deena also explained to Danny that not only were his shoes too worn to use any longer, they also did not have the proper support that his foot needed. Although there were several problems, Deena was optimistic that they were all correctable with proper rehabilitation and changes in footwear so that Danny would be able to resume his normal running program.

The foot is a masterpiece of engineering and a work of art.

Leonardo da Vinci, 1452-1519,
Italian Renaissance painter, sculptor,
musician, engineer, inventor, writer

The foot is indeed a masterpiece of science and art in its design and function. The foot combines with the ankle to form a complex structure that affects the entire extremity. The foot and ankle form the base through which the rest of the body moves from one location to another. Injuries in the foot and ankle can affect the efficiency and effectiveness of body propulsion, which is the primary function of the lower extremities.

Injuries to the foot and ankle are common.[1] A key responsibility of rehabilitation clinicians is to use their skill and knowledge of the foot and ankle to offer patients appropriate and efficient recovery programs that will permit a return to full participation.

The foot, ankle, and leg, like the hand, wrist, and forearm, are complex structures composed of many bones, joints, and muscles. There are 26 bones and 33 joints in the foot, ankle, and leg, along with several intrinsic and extrinsic muscles.[2] These structures are divided into segments; each segment forms integral relationships with the other segments in the area as well as with more proximal segments such as the knee, hip, and back. There is evidence that substantiates the direct impact that foot position and mechanics have on the knee[3-7] and other body segments.[8, 9] It is important to understand the structure and function of the distal lower extremity so that your rehabilitation programs will return patients to full function without putting additional stresses on other segments.[10-12]

This chapter reviews the basic structure of the leg, ankle, and foot as it pertains to the normal function of those segments as well as the more proximal segments. We will pay specific attention to concepts that directly relate to rehabilitation after injury. The second half of the

chapter addresses the rehabilitation of specific injuries that are most commonly seen in the leg, ankle, and foot, along with case studies.

Special Rehabilitation Considerations

Before discussing foot and ankle rehabilitation programs, we need to review some of the more common terms used to describe these body segments. Some of these terms are unique to the foot and ankle and are often misused, so establishing definitions helps to ensure common understanding and use of terminology.

Terminology

One possible reason for confusion about terms relating to the foot may be that the foot is not in the same plane as the rest of the body; the foot is at roughly a 90° angle to the lower extremity. Another possible reason is that the foot seldom moves in cardinal, or straight, planes. The foot and ankle move in nontraditional planes of motion because the joints are not aligned in straight planes; since their axes are aligned between rather than along the x-, y-, and z-axes of the normal coordinate planes of motion, their motions are essentially multiplanar (figure 20.1). For convenience and ease of discussion, motions around these axes are identified according to the straight-plane axis of the normal coordinate system that is closest to the actual axis of movement; for example, the axis running through the talocrural joint is closest in its alignment to the medial–lateral axis, so the motion around the talocrural axis is referred to as dorsiflexion (flexion) and plantar flexion (extension) since those are the predominant motions that occur around a medial–lateral axis. Keep in mind, however, that as the ankle moves within this plane, it is also going through some amount of inversion and eversion because the joint's actual plane is positioned slightly toward the anterior–posterior axis of motion for those movements.

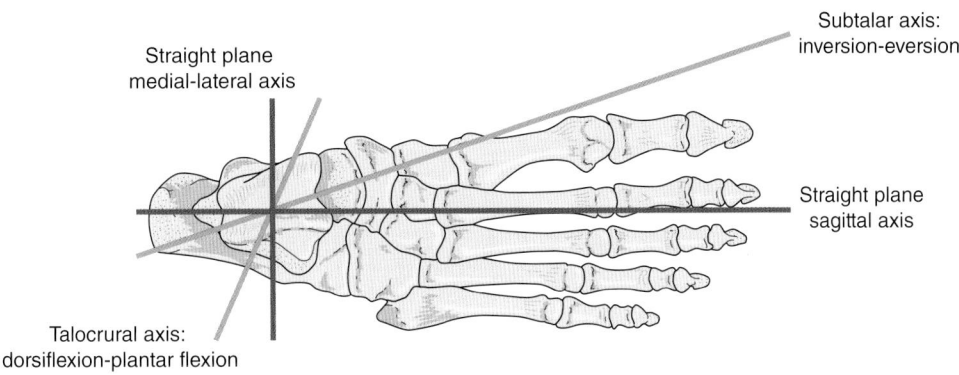

Figure 20.1   Axes of motion of the ankle joints are not in normal straight-plane alignment, so motions around these axes actually involve more than one plane of motion.

Table 20.1 identifies these primary and secondary osteokinematic motions that occur at three of the ankle and foot joints; the movements of these three joints determine the movements of the other foot joints. Table 20.2 lists the predominant plane and axis of motion for each complex movement of the ankle and identifies the direction of each movement. Since none of the joints in the ankle and foot sit in a pure coordinate system plane, this concept of multiplanar movement holds true for the other ankle and foot motions as well. To make for easier discussions, ankle and foot motions are usually described according to the predominant traditional planes of motion in which each movement occurs, even though the motions do not technically occur in them.

TABLE 20.1   Primary Joints of the Ankle and Foot and Their Osteokinematic Motions

Joint	Primary osteokinematic motions	Secondary osteokinematic motions
Talocrural joint	Dorsiflexion–plantar flexion	Abduction–adduction Inversion–eversion
Subtalar joint	Abduction–adduction Inversion–eversion	Dorsiflexion–plantar flexion
Transverse tarsal joint: longitudinal axis	Inversion–eversion	Dorsiflexion–plantar flexion Abduction–adduction
Transverse tarsal joint: oblique axis	Abduction with dorsiflexion–adduction with plantar flexion	Inversion–eversion

Note: These joints guide the motions of the other foot joints. The combined motions of the two axes of the transverse tarsal joint produce supination and pronation; such mobility allows the midfoot to adapt easily to any surface contour on which a person stands.

TABLE 20.2   Common Terminology for Movements of the Ankle Complex

Motion	Plane*	Axis†	Direction
Dorsiflexion (flexion)	Sagittal	Medial–lateral	Foot moves upward to shorten distance between anterior leg and dorsal foot.
Plantar flexion (extension)	Sagittal	Medial–lateral	Foot moves downward to lengthen distance between anterior leg and dorsal foot.
Abduction	Transverse	Vertical	Foot moves away from the body's midline.
Adduction	Transverse	Vertical	Foot moves toward the body's midline.
Inversion	Frontal	Anterior–posterior	Plantar foot rotates to face medially.
Eversion	Frontal	Anterior–posterior	Plantar foot rotates to face laterally.

* Normal coordinate plane of motion. The actual plane of motion is close to but not aligned with this plane of motion.

† Normal coordinate axis of motion. The actual axis of motion is close to but not aligned with this axis of motion.

Rehabilitation of Musculoskeletal Injuries

Pronation and supination are triplanar motions that occur as a result of combined movements in the subtalar and transverse tarsal joints. The precise motions that occur in these joints depend on whether the motion occurs in weight bearing or non–weight bearing. Table 20.3 details the joint motions that make up pronation and supination movement in weight-bearing and non-weight-bearing conditions. Although it may appear that pronation motions are opposite in weight-bearing and non-weight-bearing conditions, a closer examination reveals that they are essentially the same. Figure 20.2 shows that weight-bearing and non-weight-bearing joint motions are principally the same. In the weight-bearing condition, the calcaneus is anchored so the talus moves, while in the non-weight-bearing condition, the talus is the anchored end of the joint and the calcaneus is the moving segment. In either condition of WB or NWB pronation, the calcaneus ends up everting; it everts in the non-weight-bearing condition because it is the moving segment of the joint; in the weight-bearing condition, the position of the plantar-flexed and adducted talus forces the calcaneus to evert.

Pronation is sometimes erroneously referred to as eversion, which is a single-plane motion. Similarly, supination is sometimes erroneously referred to as inversion. Inversion and eversion occur in a single plane at the subtalar joint. Supination (or pronation) result as a combination of inversion (or eversion), adduction (or abduction), and plantar flexion (or dorsiflexion) of the subtalar joint and the midtarsal joints. Since the midtarsal joints include

articulations between the calcaneus and cuboid and the talus and navicular, pronation and supination movements become more complex than inversion and eversion motions of the subtalar joint; pronation and supination involve more than one joint and more than one motion plane.

In closed-chain activities, the calcaneus is anchored by the body's weight, so pronation and supination occur because the talus moves on the calcaneus. Since the motion is closed chain, the tibia's position is also affected by these movements. Therefore, in weight-bearing pronation, the talus moves medially (adducts) and plantar flexes on the calcaneus, causing the calcaneus to evert. In addition, the talus pulls the cuboid and navicular into abduction and eversion. Moving in a closed kinetic chain in the other direction, the tibia medially rotates, the hip flexes and medially rotates, the pelvis moves into nutation, and the lumbar spine extends.

The opposite motions occur in weight-bearing supination. Even though movement occurs at different bones when the foot is weight bearing and non–weight bearing, the *relative* position of these joint segments is the same in either condition. Figure 20.2 demonstrates this concept.

Along with pronation and supination during weight bearing, associated motions take place further up the chain in other joints. Remember from chapter 13 that in closed kinetic chain activities, all weight-bearing joints must move when one joint moves. With pronation, the tibia medially rotates, the knee flexes, the hip flexes and medially rotates, and the pelvis rotates anteriorly.[13] Conversely, with supi-

TABLE 20.3 Talocalcaneal Joint Components of Pronation and Supination Motions in Weight-Bearing and Non-Weight-Bearing Conditions

Motion	NON–WEIGHT BEARING Component movements	Subtalar motions	WEIGHT BEARING Component movements	Subtalar motions
Pronation	1. Dorsiflexion	1. Calcaneus moves on talus in sagittal plane	1. Plantar flexion	1. Talus moves on calcaneus in sagittal plane
	2. Abduction	2. Calcaneus moves on talus in transverse plane	2. Adduction	2. Talus moves on calcaneus in transverse plane
	3. Eversion	3. Calcaneus moves on talus in frontal plane	3. Eversion	3. Calcaneus moves on talus in frontal plane
Supination	1. Plantar flexion	1. Calcaneus moves on talus in sagittal plane	1. Dorsiflexion	1. Talus moves on calcaneus in sagittal plane
	2. Adduction	2. Calcaneus moves on talus in transverse plane	2. Abduction	2. Talus moves on calcaneus in transverse plane
	3. Inversion	3. Calcaneus moves on talus in frontal plane	3. Inversion	3. Calcaneus moves on talus in frontal plane

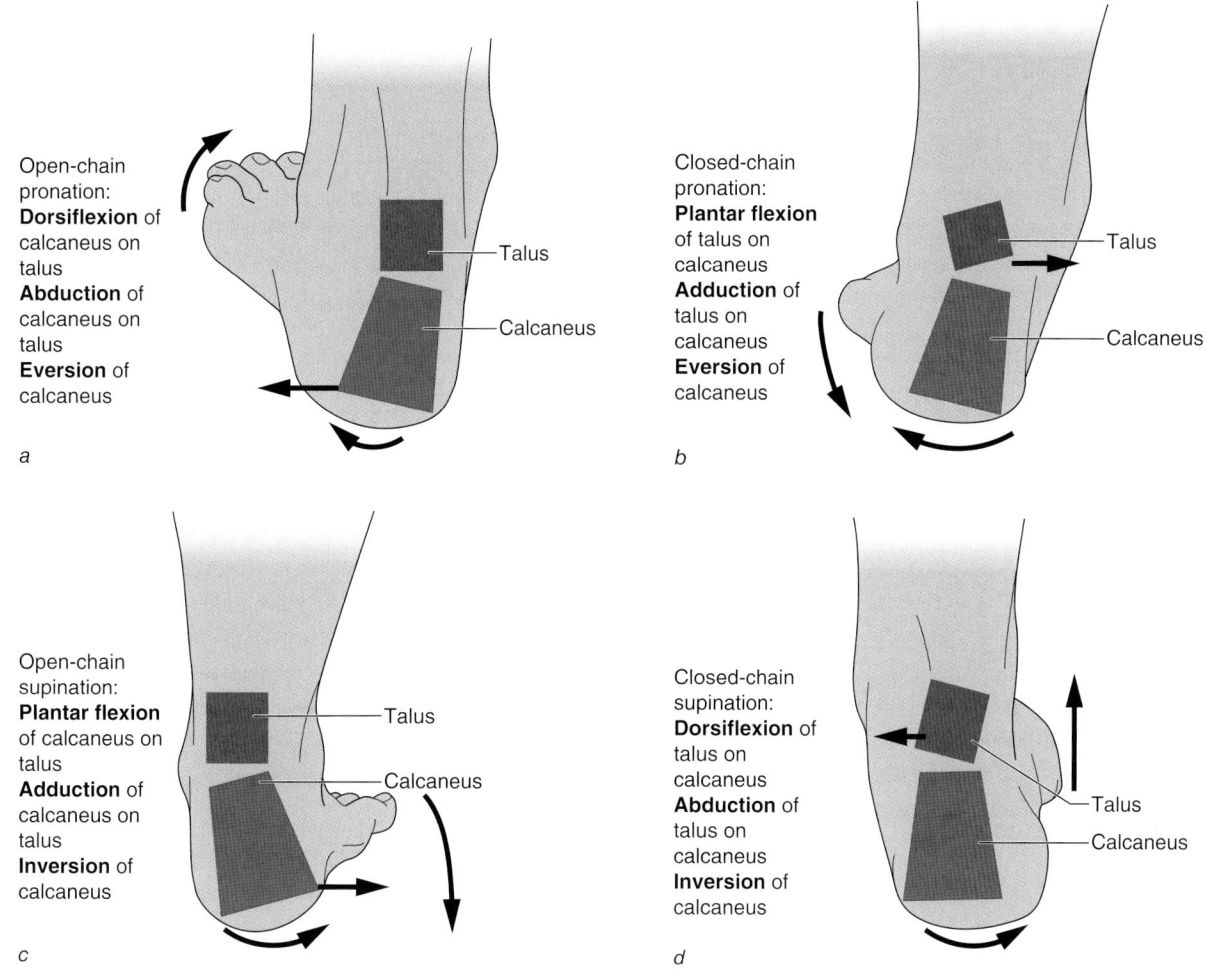

Open-chain
pronation:
Dorsiflexion of
calcaneus on
talus
Abduction of
calcaneus on
talus
Eversion of
calcaneus

— Talus

— Calcaneus

a

Closed-chain
pronation:
Plantar flexion
of talus on
calcaneus
Adduction of
talus on
calcaneus
Eversion of
calcaneus

— Talus

— Calcaneus

b

Open-chain
supination:
Plantar flexion
of calcaneus on
talus
Adduction of
calcaneus on
talus
Inversion of
calcaneus

— Talus

— Calcaneus

c

Closed-chain
supination:
Dorsiflexion of
talus on
calcaneus
Abduction of
talus on
calcaneus
Inversion of
calcaneus

— Talus

— Calcaneus

d

Figure 20.2   In open-chain talocrural motion, the calcaneus moves on the talus, but in closed-chain talocrural motion, the talus moves on the anchored calcaneus. However, the relative position between the talus and calcaneus is the same in open- and closed-chain positions. (These images show the left foot.) *(a)* Calcaneus abducts on a stable talus in open-chain pronation; *(b)* talus adducts on a stable calcaneus in closed-chain pronation; *(c)* calcaneus adducts on a stable talus in open-chain supination; *(d)* talus abducts on a stable calcaneus in closed-chain supination.

nation, the tibia laterally rotates; the knee extends; the hip extends, abducts, and laterally rotates; and the pelvis rotates posteriorly.[14] It has been found, however, that unless supination is sufficient to cause hip medial rotation, the pelvis does not anteriorly rotate.[15]

Because supination and pronation occur primarily in the subtalar joint, this joint is instrumental in foot motion, and it plays a key role in the control of the other joints.[16] For example, if the subtalar joint pronates during weight bearing, the tibia medially rotates, the knee flexes, and the hip medially rotates and flexes. If the subtalar joint stays in pronation when it should be supinating during ambulation, injuries can result either in the foot or in the more proximal body segments when those segments experience increased stresses during the gait cycle because of the subtalar pronation.[17] These injuries are discussed later in this chapter.

Leg, Foot, and Ankle Joints

Specifics of gait analysis are discussed in chapter 7. Reviewing that chapter may help you understand some additional concepts presented here. The first foot structure to hit the ground when walking is the calcaneus. It, along with the talus, forms the subtalar joint, and the talus along with the tibia and fibula form the talocrural joint. Normal function of these two joints permits us to land the foot on the ground and adapt to variations in topography while maintaining balance and a steady gait. The talocrural joint moves mainly in dorsiflexion and plantar flexion. The subtalar joint is responsible for inversion and eversion. Pronation and its component motions loosen the foot and ankle joints to allow the foot to function as a mobile adapter, accommodating for uneven surfaces. Supination moves the foot and ankle joints into congruent positions so that they can become more rigid; this alignment provides for more effective transfer of the propulsive force needed for ambulation.[18] As mentioned in chapter 7, these motions must occur at specific times within the gait cycle to be normal.

The talocrural joint is a mortise joint, with a convex talar dome in contact with a more proximal concave tibial mortise. The lateral malleolus is posterior and distal in its alignment compared to the medial malleolus. This arrangement allows more inversion than eversion to occur in the subtalar joint, and it also causes plantar flexion to occur more in a posterolateral direction and dorsiflexion to occur more in an anteromedial direction.[19] As the ankle goes into plantar flexion, the talus moves anteriorly so that the narrower posterior aspect of the talus sits in the mortise joint.[19] This talus shape and position contribute to instability of the ankle when it is in plantar flexion, and this is one reason why women wearing high-heeled shoes or people landing from a jump with the foot in plantar flexion are especially susceptible to ankle sprains. Conversely, the most stable close-packed position for the talus is with the ankle in dorsiflexion; in this position, the wider anterior talus is wedged firmly into the mortise joint, creating more congruency and stability within the joint.[20, 21] During dorsiflexion, the fibula glides superiorly and rotates medially, and in plantar flexion, it moves inferiorly and rotates laterally.[20] If these fibular motions cannot occur, full ankle dorsiflexion and plantar flexion cannot occur either.

Distal to the talocrural and subtalar joints is the midtarsal joint. This joint is actually a combination of the talonavicular and calcaneocuboid articulations. The midtarsal joint is also known as the transverse tarsal joint or Chopart's joint. The position of the talonavicular and calcaneocuboid joints is determined by the subtalar joint position. The mid-

tarsal joint becomes locked in optimal congruency during supination and unlocked during pronation; this midtarsal joint stability and laxity occur because the axes of its two component joints either oppose each other in supination or are parallel to each other in pronation (figure 20.3). Movements of the midtarsal joint closely follow movements of the subtalar and talocrural joints, and they add to the total supination and pronation motions of the foot, permitting the foot to adapt as it comes in contact with various surfaces.[22] Notice in figure 20.3 that during pronation, the navicular and cuboid bones move medially and inferiorly, and they move laterally and superiorly during supination.[23]

Other intertarsal joints distal to the transverse tarsal joint provide some additional degrees of movement to add to the total supination–pronation motion that occurs throughout the foot. Their primary responsibility is formation of the transverse arch.[24] Additional support and stability of the transverse arch comes from the foot's intrinsic muscles.[25]

The tarsometatarsal joints and their adjacent bony segments are divided into five rays. The first ray includes the first metatarsal, the medial cuneiform, and their shared joint.[26] Although the first ray has triplanar motion because its axis is not aligned in a straight sagittal plane, its movements are generally referred to as plantar flexion and dorsiflexion because its joint is uniaxial.[26] Plantar and dorsal accessory movements of the first ray occur equally in plantar flexion and dorsiflexion, with each movement equivalent to about a thumb's width of motion. The second ray includes the joint and its bones, the second metatarsal, and the middle cuneiform; the third ray includes the third metatarsal and the lateral cuneiform and their joint; the fourth ray is the fourth metatarsal alone; and the fifth ray is the fifth metatarsal alone.[26]

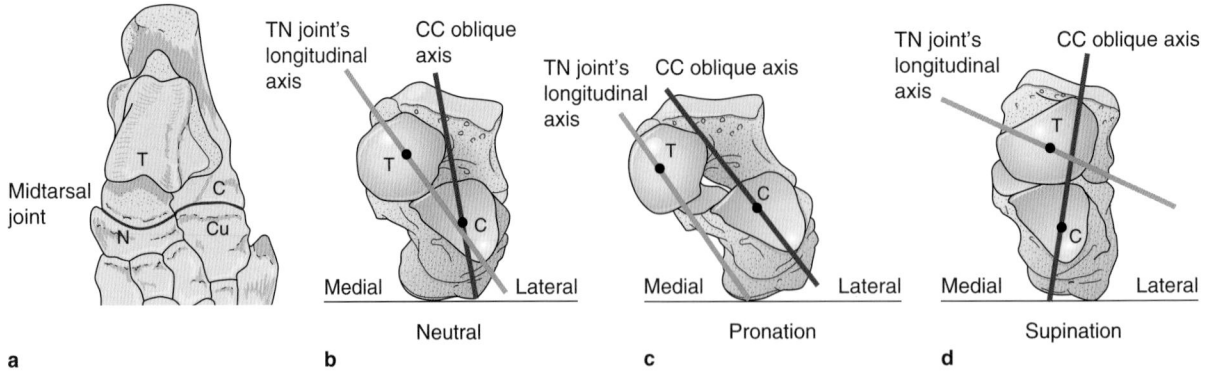

Figure 20.3 Midtarsal (transverse tarsal) joint axes' positions in subtalar neutral, pronation, and supination. *(a)* Superior view of midtarsal joint. *(b, c, d)* Anterior views of a right foot, looking at the talus and calcaneus with the other tarsal bones and foot removed. Notice that in *(b)* neutral and *(d)* supination positions, the axes of the joints comprising the midtarsal joints cross; this position locks them in their alignment. In *(c)* pronation, the axes are parallel to each other, allowing for mobility of the midtarsal joint. Both joints and their axes are dependent on the subtalar joint for their positions. When the subtalar joint pronates, these joints move into pronation with parallel axes to permit maximum mobility of the midtarsal joint; when the subtalar joint supinates, these joints supinate, locking their axes to restrict midtarsal movement. CC = calcaneocuboid joint; TN = talonavicular joint; C = calcaneus; T = talus; Cu = cuboid; N = navicular.

Since metatarsophalangeal (MTP) joints are biaxial, they permit active flexion–extension and abduction–adduction. Similar to the metacarpophalangeal joints, they also have accessory motions of rotation and dorsal–plantar glides. Likewise, the interphalangeal (IP) joints of the toes, like the finger IP joints, are hinge joints, so they permit active flexion and extension with accessory rotation and dorsal–plantar glides. The first MTP joint must have about 65° of hyperextension for normal heel-off and toe-off during gait.[27]

Muscle Function

There are 12 extrinsic muscles and 11 intrinsic muscles of the leg, ankle, and foot. The extrinsic muscles are divided into four compartments or groups: anterior, lateral, superficial posterior, and deep posterior (figure 20.4). The anterior compartment muscles cross the ankle joint anteriorly and provide dorsiflexion, while lateral and posterior compartment muscles cross the ankle posteriorly and are plantar flexors (figure 20.5). The muscles that have the greatest mechanical advantage to produce inversion and eversion because of their positions relative to the anterior–posterior axis are the anterior and posterior tibialis medially and the peroneals laterally.

The posterior leg has a superficial compartment and a deep compartment; the two compartments are separated by deep fascia, the *intermuscular septum*. The superficial muscle group includes the soleus, gastrocnemius, and plantaris. The deep posterior muscles lie closer to the tibia and include the tibialis posterior, flexor hallucis longus, and flexor digitorum longus.

The intrinsic foot muscles are completely contained within the foot itself. Their purpose is to provide stability to the toes, tarsometatarsal joints, and midfoot while extrinsic muscles move the joints.[28] The intrinsic muscles keep the toes on the ground until toe-off during gait and convert the toes to rigid beams for propulsion in gait.[29] These muscles weaken with ankle injuries and must be rehabilitated along with the extrinsic muscles. In a foot that is unstable or hypermobile, such as one that has excessive pronation,

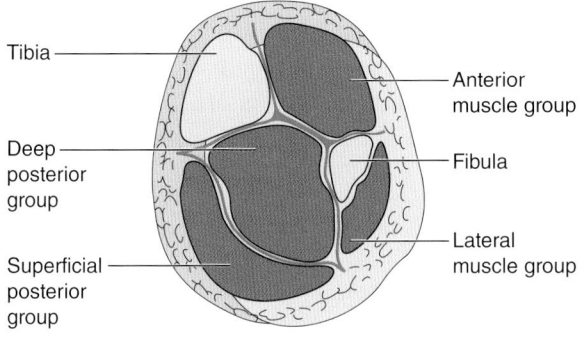

Figure 20.4 Cross section of the right leg muscle compartments.

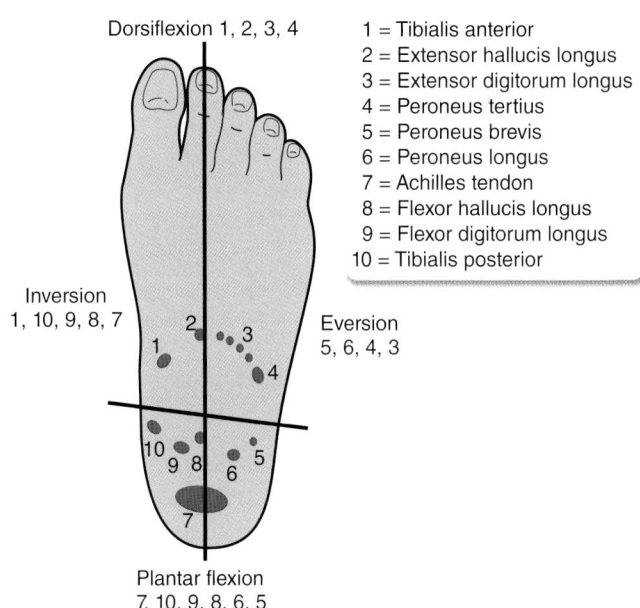

Figure 20.5 Ankle motions. The anterior–posterior axis divides muscles that provide inversion and eversion, whereas the medial–lateral axis divides dorsiflexors from plantar flexors. Muscle numbers in the diagram are listed in order of their mechanical advantage for motion.

the intrinsic muscles are weak yet need to work to provide foot stability.[30] Excessive sweating of these foot muscles and consequent foot odor may be the result of intrinsic muscle overactivity.

Foot Arches

There are three arches of the foot: the medial and lateral longitudinal arches and the transverse arch. These arches result from the architecture of the tarsals and their arrangement with each other, the ligaments, and the supporting muscles.[31] The primary inert tensile supporting structure for the longitudinal arches is the plantar fascia; the peroneus longus supports the transverse arch.[32] The transverse arch protects the underlying blood vessels and nerves,[33] and the longitudinal arches provide an efficient system of support for the body's weight.[29] If the arches cannot maintain a normal configuration, an imbalance occurs, and these abnormal stresses applied to the foot can cause injury. The normal alignment of the longitudinal arches may be determined by **Feiss' line**. In non–weight bearing, a line is drawn from the apex of the medial malleolus to the plantar aspect of the first metatarsophalangeal joint.[34] In weight bearing, the navicular tubercle should lie on the line or near it. A study that looked at changes in Feiss' measurements in arch height from the resting (seated) to weight-bearing (bilateral standing) positions identified ranges for flexible, normal, and rigid feet to be 1.3 to 0.9 cm, 0.9 to −0.1 cm, and −0.1 to −0.6 cm, respectively.[34]

Subtalar Neutral Position

Because the subtalar joint significantly influences the entire lower extremity, the rehabilitation clinician must know what normal subtalar motions and positions are to be able to assess and treat an abnormal subtalar joint.

Subtalar neutral is the position in which the talus is equally palpable from its medial and lateral aspect within the subtalar joint. It is at this point that the talus and navicular are most congruent and the alignment of the subtalar bones is optimal.[37] Subtalar neutral should be assessed in both weight bearing and non–weight bearing.[38]

In non–weight bearing, the patient lies prone or supine with the opposite extremity flexed at the hip and knee and the hip in abduction and lateral rotation to stabilize the pelvis. If the patient cannot hold this figure-4 position because of pain or inflexibility, a rolled towel may be secured under the proximal hip of the extremity being examined to stabilize the pelvis.[39] With the patient's foot and ankle to be examined over the edge of the table, the clinician places the thumb and index finger of the hand medial to the patient's foot on the medial and lateral aspects of the talus. Using his or her thumb, the clinician locates the talus' medial aspect, which is in a depression slightly inferior and anterior to the medial malleolus and just proximal to the navicular. He or she locates the talus' lateral aspect, which is anterior to the lateral malleolus, using the index finger (figure 20.6). As the medial and lateral aspects of the talar dome are palpated with the thumb and index or middle finger of one hand, the other hand grasps the fourth and fifth metatarsal heads between the thumb and fingers and rotates the forefoot in inversion and eversion. When the forefoot rocks inward and upward, the talus inverts so that its lateral border can be more easily palpated by the clinician's finger; when the forefoot rocks outward and upward, the talus everts so that its medial border can be more easily palpated by the clinician's thumb. As the foot is gradually moved into dorsiflexion, it is also rocked back and forth in inversion–eversion with progressively smaller arcs of motion until the talus is centrally positioned and cannot be palpated on either the medial or the lateral aspect or is palpated equally on each side.[40] By the time this

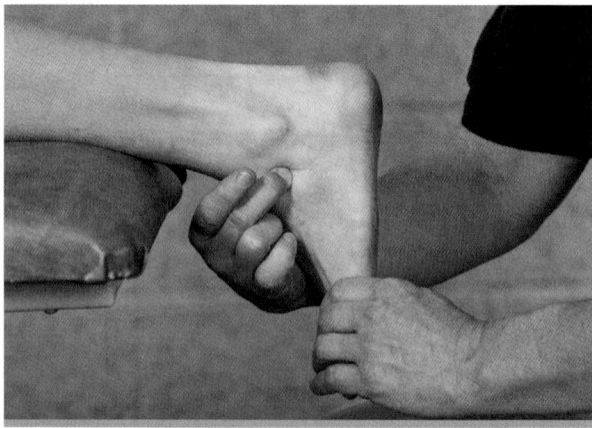

Figure 20.6 Subtalar neutral positioning.

central talus position is located, the ankle is in maximum dorsiflexion; this combined position of subtalar neutral and dorsiflexion locks the rearfoot and forefoot in place.

If subtalar neutral is palpated in weight bearing, the clinician palpates the medial and lateral aspects of the talar dome while the patient elevates and lowers the longitudinal arch as the toes and heel maintain contact with the floor; this motion is performed until the clinician determines that the subtalar joint is in its neutral mid-position.

Go to HK*Propel* and watch video 20.1, which demonstrates finding subtalar neutral and rearfoot–forefoot alignment.

Once you identify subtalar neutral, you assess the range of motion of the rearfoot in this calcaneal position. Normal rearfoot motion in subtalar neutral ranges roughly from 20° to 30°, with one-third of the total motion occurring in eversion and two-thirds in inversion.[41] A perpendicular line bisecting the posterior calcaneus and a line bisecting the posterior tibia are used as reference points. The calcaneus is passively moved into eversion and inversion, and measurements are taken at the end range of each position (figure 20.7).

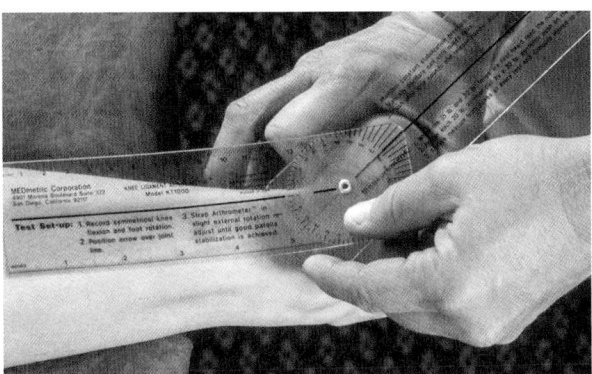

Figure 20.7 Measurement of subtalar range of motion. Lines bisecting the calcaneus and leg are used to define subtalar or rearfoot inversion and eversion range of motion.

Common Structural Deformities

Although the deformities we will consider here are not injuries but structural deviations, they can often lead to injuries. Athletic activities and work activities that involve excessive walking or prolonged standing on concrete surfaces impose greater-than-normal forces on the foot and thereby magnify the impact of a deformity. The rehabilitation clinician must be familiar with these deformities and their impact on the patient to provide appropriate treatment programs.

Pes Cavus

In pes cavus, the foot has an abnormally high longitudinal arch (figure 20.8). The navicular tubercle is above Feiss' line in both weight bearing and non–weight bearing. This is a rigid foot with limited stress-absorption abilities. The foot does not pronate as it should, so rather than being absorbed, impact forces are transmitted up the extremity. Pes cavus feet can lead to fallen transverse arches, hammertoes or claw toes, corns, stress fractures, and other overuse injuries.[42]

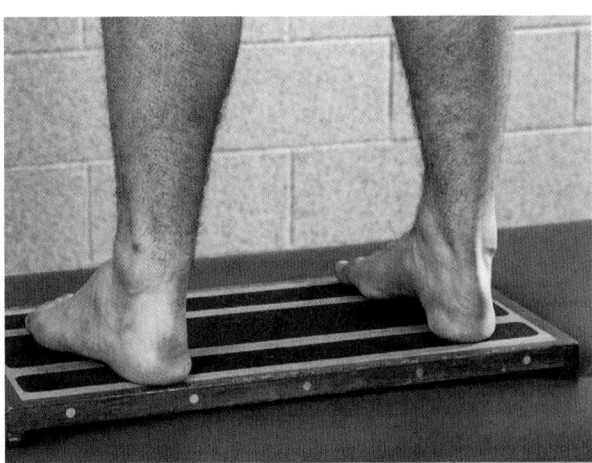

Figure 20.8 Pes cavus.

Pes Planus

In pes planus, the foot has an abnormally low longitudinal arch (figure 20.9). A rigid pes planus has the navicular tubercle below Feiss' line in both weight bearing and non–weight bearing. The more common flexible pes planus foot, however, has the navicular tubercle below Feiss' line in weight bearing but on or near Feiss' line during non–weight bearing. Either rigid or flexible pes planus can lead to injuries. During weight bearing, the foot does not form a rigid lever for propulsion because it remains in a pronated position when it should be supinated. This malpositioning puts additional stresses on more proximal segments of the extremity.[43] During heel-off and just before toe-off, the extremity and hip are laterally rotating; these motions that should occur are opposite to those motions that occur with pathologically prolonged pronation, so torque forces on these segments are exaggerated.[44] This is especially true at the knee, particularly at the patellofemoral joint.[45] The condition also places torsion on the plantar fascia and Achilles tendon[46] because the foot should be supinating, but instead it is pronating. Related terms for pes planus are pronated foot, flatfoot, or pancake arch.

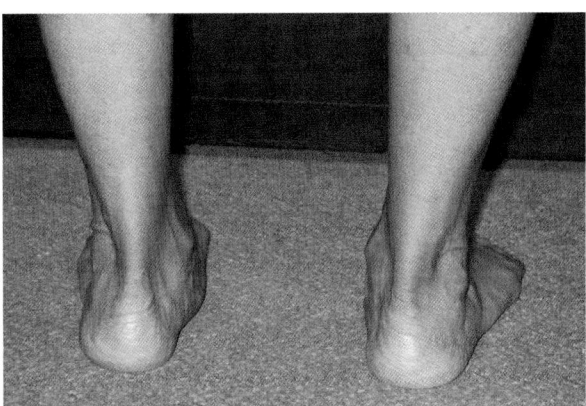

Figure 20.9 Pes planus.

© Peggy Houglum

Hallux Valgus

This condition is also known as a *bunion*. **Hallux valgus** is present when the first MTP joint is in a greater than 10° valgus position with the first toe pointed laterally toward the other toes (figure 20.10).[47] The condition is most commonly seen in feet with excessive pronation. With the foot in pronation, the force at toe-off is transmitted through the medial aspect of the first ray.[47] This increased medial joint stress on the MTP eventually forces the first ray to deviate medially and the phalanx to deviate laterally.[48] A callus is commonly seen on the medial aspect of the great toe resulting from push off forces applied at that point of the toe rather than its plantar aspect.

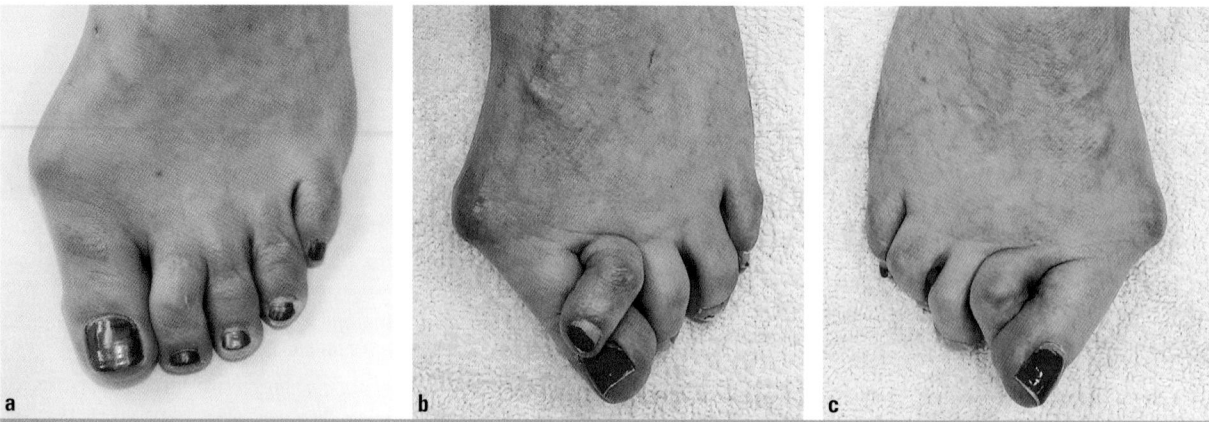

Figure 20.10 Hallux valgus. *(a)* Hallux valgus of number 1 with a number 2 hammertoe; *(b)* hallux valgus with overriding adjacent toe; *(c)* hallux valgus with underriding adjacent toe and hammertoes.

© Peggy Houglum

Tibial Torsion

Tibial torsion is present when the tibia is rotated on its long axis.[49] Normally, the midline of the patella is in line with the first- and second-toe web space.[50] In tibial torsion, the foot is rotated laterally relative to the patella's midline. There are several ways to measure tibial torsion. The more accurate methods include computed tomography, but this is not practical for most clinicians. The technique advanced by Staheli is used by some clinicians.[51] Staheli and Engel[52] advocated the technique in which the patient sits on the edge of a table with the knee flexed to 90° and the anterior thigh directly in line with the hip; with the heel against a flat vertical surface, the clinician passively positions the forefoot so the foot is perpendicular to the vertical surface.[52] A mark is placed over the center point of each malleolus at the broadest portion of the malleolus at the talocrural joint line.[52] With the heel against the vertical surface, the distance of each malleolus mark from the wall is measured, and a conversion chart identifies the patient's tibial torsion.[52]

Staheli and Engel[52] found through their investigations that about 10° is normal. One can also measure a person's tibial torsion with the patient supine and the medial and lateral femoral epicondyles in the transverse plane and the patella facing the ceiling. The rehabilitation clinician measures the angle between the plane of the table and the line between the medial and lateral malleolus (figure 20.11*a*).[53] The normal value is 15°, with a normal range of 2° to 3° in either direction.[52] Another alternative for measuring tibial torsion is with the patient prone and the knee flexed to 90°. The clinician measures the angle between the long axis of the thigh and a line bisecting the medial and lateral malleoli line (figure 20.11*b*).[54]

Patients with tibial torsion have increased stresses at the knee.[55] Tibial torsion may be either excessive lateral rotation or excessive medial rotation of the tibia on the

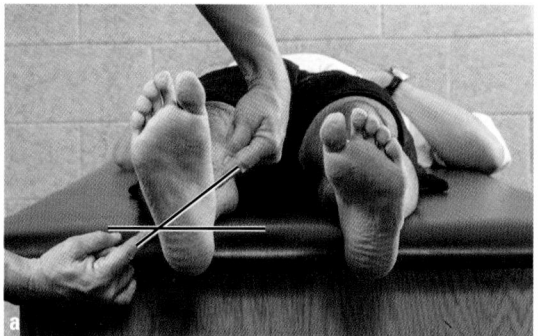

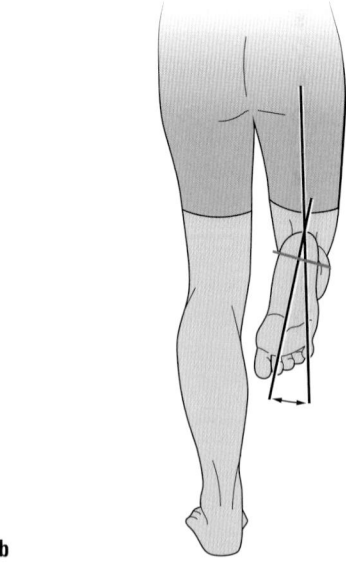

b

Figure 20.11 Measuring tibial torsion using two methods. *(a)* Tibial torsion is the angle formed between the line through the malleoli and the plane of the tabletop when the femoral condyles on the table and the patella are facing the ceiling. *(b)* Tibial torsion using this method is the angle formed between the perpendicular line bisecting the line connecting the medial and lateral malleoli and the line along the long axis of the thigh.

talus; either condition can lead to knee pathologies.[56] Additionally, because the tibia is laterally rotated relative to the patella, an increased torque is applied to the patellar tendon. Lateral rotation of the tibia may also be related to excessive pronation, lateral thigh tightness, and altered patellofemoral alignment.[57]

Tibial Varum

Tibial varum exists when the distal tibia is closer to the mid-line than the proximal tibia.[58] This is measured when the patient is standing. With the patient's feet shoulder-width apart, the rehabilitation clinician places the goniometer's stationary arm on the floor adjacent to the patient's heel and the movable arm aligned with a line bisecting the distal posterior tibia (figure 20.12). The movable arm should be vertical[59] or no more than 4° to 5°; anything greater than that is abnormal.[60]

Tibial varum is usually accompanied by genu varum and coxa valgus. These deformities place exaggerated stresses on the knee, Achilles tendon, and hip.[59]

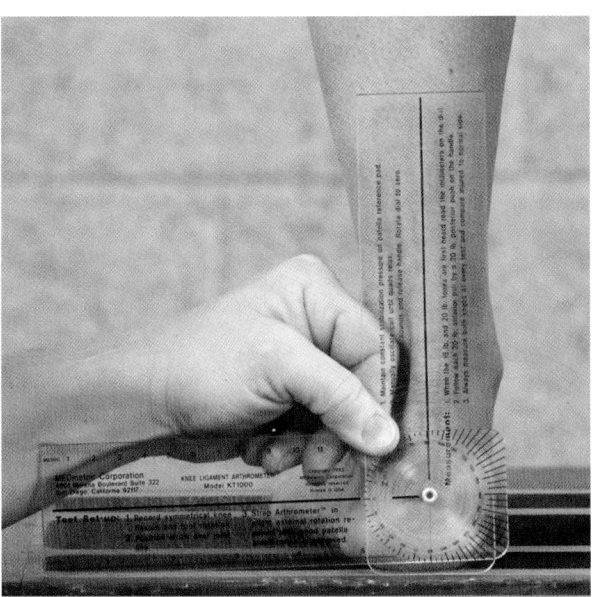

Figure 20.12 Measuring tibial varum. The line bisecting the leg should be vertical or no more than 4° to 5° if tibial alignment is normal.

Rearfoot Varus and Valgus

The rearfoot is composed of the talus and calcaneus, and its pathological alignments are referred to as subtalar varus and subtalar valgus. Rearfoot alignment is determined by the position of the calcaneus relative to that of the leg. Rearfoot varus (figure 20.13b) is present when the calcaneus is inverted relative to the posterior bisection of the distal leg. Rearfoot valgus is present when the calcaneus is everted relative to the distal leg (figure 20.13c). The source

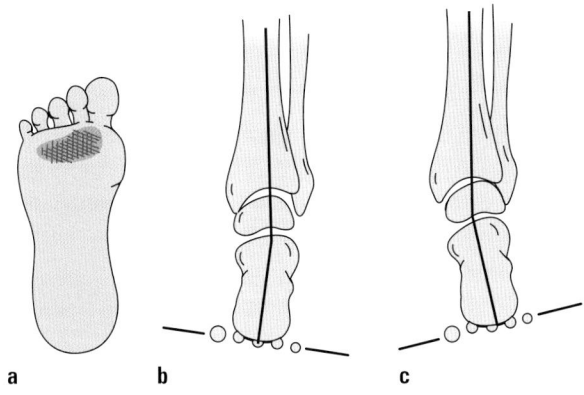

Figure 20.13 Varus and valgus rearfoot deformities: *(a)* callus pattern for compensated subtalar varus, *(b)* rearfoot varus in non-weight-bearing subtalar neutral, *(c)* rearfoot valgus in non-weight-bearing subtalar neutral.

of rearfoot varus is sometimes difficult to ascertain; it may be within the talus, the calcaneus, or both.

Rearfoot valgus is examined in both a relaxed standing position and a subtalar neutral position. Ideally, the results should be the same in the two positions. If a foot has a rearfoot deformity, the body either compensates for it or it doesn't. If it compensates for the rearfoot deformity, the foot usually makes an adjustment in the forefoot so that all toes contact the ground during weight bearing. If the forefoot fails to compensate for a rearfoot deformity, there is no change in the relative position of the rearfoot and forefoot, regardless of the weight-bearing status, similar to the appearance of foot positions seen in figure 20.13*b* and *c*. In an uncompensated forefoot, the lateral foot is in contact with the ground with a rearfoot varus and the medial forefoot is on the ground in a rearfoot valgus. Likewise, if there is a forefoot deformity, the rearfoot either compensates for it or it doesn't, as we will discuss in more detail shortly. Therefore, in a foot that compensates for a rearfoot valgus deformity, the calcaneus is perpendicular to the floor in subtalar neutral or non–weight bearing but is everted when weight bearing at rest.[61] If a foot does not compensate for rearfoot valgus, the calcaneus remains in eversion in both positions,[43] but the amount of eversion is less in subtalar neutral.

With rearfoot varus, the foot remains partially or fully pronated until heel-off during the weight-bearing phase of gait.[30] More pronation than normal must occur to get the inverted heel to the ground. Once the heel is off the ground, the calcaneus rapidly supinates to catch up to the position it should have been in at midstance. This causes a medial heel whip immediately after toe-off, which you can see as you observe the patient posteriorly during gait. This sudden rotation of the heel from eversion to inversion often results in a callus buildup over the posterior calcaneus as the skin rubs against the back of the shoe as it rotates. This callus is known as Haglund's exostosis and is commonly called a *pump bump*;[62] its presence is a good indication that a heel whip occurs during heel-off.

Because the rearfoot remains pronated and does not supinate at the proper times in the gait cycle, hypermobility of the forefoot occurs, and the first ray cannot become fully stabilized for propulsion.[29] This transfers more shear and loading forces to the second metatarsal head, and sometimes to the third and fourth metatarsal heads.[29] This transfer of stress, in turn, causes calluses primarily over the second metatarsal head and secondarily over the third and fourth metatarsal heads (figure 20.13a). The patient's rearfoot position is important to identify because it is a key determining factor for the rest of the foot's posture and function and has a significant impact on knee and hip motion.

Forefoot Varus and Valgus

A forefoot varus is an inversion deformity of the midtarsal joint. It is identified by comparing the plane of the five metatarsal heads with the perpendicular line bisecting the calcaneus. For examination of the forefoot position, the patient lies prone and the rearfoot is passively placed and kept in subtalar neutral by the clinician. Once the subtalar joint is in rearfoot neutral, the forefoot is loaded on the fourth–fifth metatarsal heads, and the ankle is passively moved into dorsiflexion. In the normal forefoot, the line in the plane of the metatarsals and the line bisecting the calcaneus are perpendicular to each other, so the horizontal lines of the forefoot (from medial to lateral toes) and the rearfoot (from medial to lateral plantar calcaneal tubercles) appear parallel to each other (figure 20.14b). In forefoot varus, the medial forefoot is higher than the lateral forefoot (inverted) (figure 20.14a). A related condition is first-ray dorsiflexion.

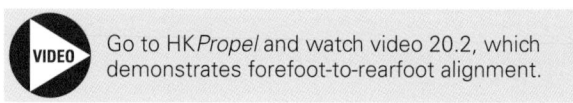
Go to HK*Propel* and watch video 20.2, which demonstrates forefoot-to-rearfoot alignment.

In a patient with a compensated forefoot varus, the subtalar joint pronates to allow the medial toes to touch the ground in weight bearing. This calcaneal pronation persists at a time when the joint should be supinating; however, the rearfoot cannot supinate in time for heel-off and toe-off because the forefoot is still bearing weight and is anchored to the ground, forcing the rearfoot to remain pronated. A

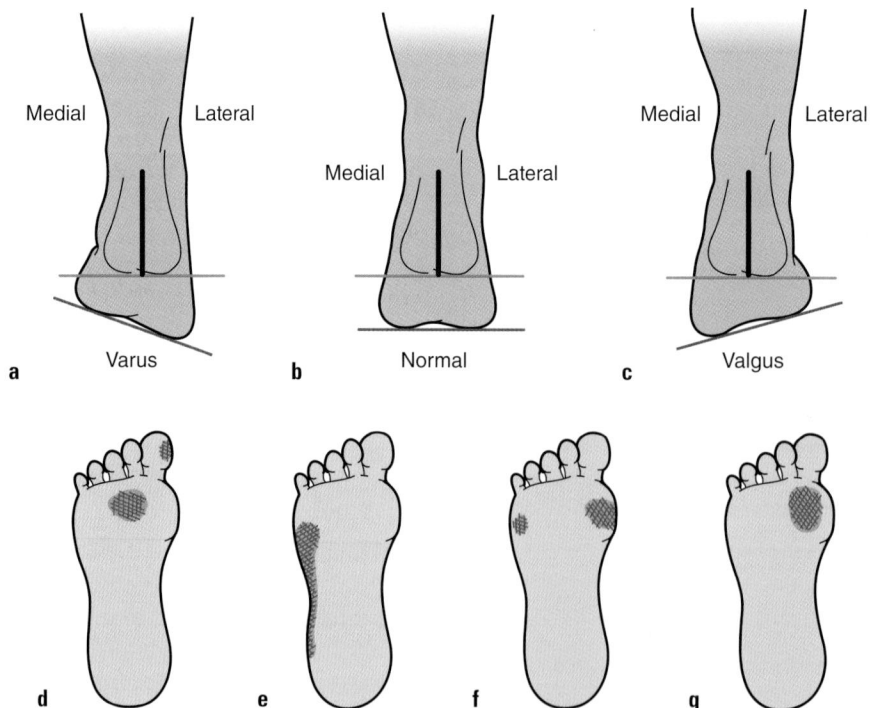

Figure 20.14 Forefoot alignment—varus and valgus deformities with the rearfoot in subtalar neutral. *(a)* Forefoot varus alignment relative to rearfoot is seen when the medial forefoot lies higher than the lateral forefoot in the frontal plane. *(b)* Normal forefoot and rearfoot alignment is seen when the calcaneus and forefoot are parallel to each other. *(c)* Forefoot valgus is present when the lateral forefoot is higher than the medial forefoot in the frontal plane. *(d)* Callus pattern for compensated forefoot varus. *(e)* Callus pattern occurring with an uncompensated forefoot varus. *(f)* Callus pattern for compensated forefoot valgus with a rigid first ray. *(g)* Callus pattern seen with a compensated forefoot valgus and rearfoot varus with a flexible first ray.

slight heel whip may be seen at heel-off, but it usually cannot produce enough supination because the deformity in the forefoot that is causing the compensation keeps the medial forefoot in contact with the ground.

With the rearfoot in pronation throughout propulsion (latter weight-bearing phase of gait), the body's weight is distributed more medially than normal, and the midtarsal joint becomes hypermobile.[47] This causes the first ray to become unstable and incapable of providing an adequate propulsive force.[47] Weight and forces are then transferred from the first to the second and third metatarsal heads, where callus formations appear because of this increased shear and force stress. Since the body's weight is more medially distributed than normal, the foot abducts, and a callus forms on the medial hallux from shearing stresses as the body moves over this aspect of the hallux (figure 20.14*d*).

If the forefoot varus is uncompensated, the person stays on the lateral aspect of the foot and cannot pronate as much as he or she should to provide normal mechanics.[63] The forefoot varus does not permit the rearfoot to pronate during weight bearing, so the calcaneus may appear either erect or slightly inverted. Callus formation in this case occurs over the lateral aspect of the foot and over the fifth metatarsal head[63] because rotation occurs off the fifth metatarsal head, with weight-bearing occurring primarily over the lateral foot (figure 20.14*e*). The rotation is secondary to the rearfoot's failure to go through a full excursion of supination, thereby limiting lateral rotation of the lower extremity; the body tries to abduct the foot so the tibia can tilt to evert the foot to get the propulsive forces delivered from the medial foot, as close to the first metatarsal as possible. Imagine the forces encountered by the tibia, knee, and forefoot joints as the body tries to move the great toe to contact the floor to propel the body forward.

Forefoot valgus is the opposite condition of forefoot varus. The line of the metatarsal heads is higher on the lateral side than on the medial side (everted) when observed from the rearfoot in a subtalar neutral position (figure 20.14*c*). A related condition is first-ray plantar flexion. If the first ray is rigid with little available mobility during ambulation, the first ray will hit the ground too early,[63] and the peroneus longus will assist by moving the weight more medially to prepare for weight transfer to the other foot. In a very rigid first ray, the fifth ray's ability to get to the ground is limited because the foot supinates too early in the mid-weight-bearing phase. With the forefoot in extreme valgus because of the rigid first ray, the forefoot's ability to invert on the rearfoot is severely limited. The rearfoot then tries to compensate by supinating during midstance. This causes the fifth ray to hit the ground suddenly and undergo increased loading before heel-off.[63] In turn, this causes the lateral foot to become unstable; to compensate, the rearfoot moves into pronation at heel-off. Since this foot

is rigid, causing rapid loading rates, it typically produces a loud gait.[63] The pronation imposes increased shearing forces on the forefoot.

Because of the increased shearing forces and the greater amount of time the first ray spends on the ground, there is usually a large callus buildup over the medial first metatarsal head.[63] There is also a callus over the fifth metatarsal head because of the increased friction created during the lateral forefoot activities just presented (figure 20.14*f*).[63]

On the other hand, if the first ray is mobile, the rearfoot will pronate normally, and no problems will be evident because motion occurs close to normal. However, a large callus forms over the first metatarsal head because of the first ray's prolonged contact with the ground in its plantar-flexed position (figure 20.14*g*).

Orthotic Intervention for Foot Deformities

Normal foot mechanics during ambulation include pronation immediately after heel strike and continuing through 25% of the stance phase.[50] During midstance, the rearfoot supinates to a neutral position with the calcaneus erect and all the metatarsal heads in contact with the ground. From that point until toe-off, the rearfoot continues its supination progression as it prepares to convert the foot from a mobile adapter to a rigid lever for propulsion.[64] If the foot does not function this way, stresses increase either within the foot or elsewhere in the extremity.

The purpose of foot orthotics is to make the abnormal foot function more like a normal foot, thus reducing the abnormal stresses imposed on the foot and extremity.[65] Many patients with abnormal foot alignment and function have no symptoms of pathology. For these asymptomatic patients, orthotics may not be indicated; the exception would be if the patient is young and is likely to develop symptoms because of cumulative stresses. Foot orthotics are used to correct or support symptomatic malalignments to reduce stresses on joints and to improve the patient's mechanical efficiency.[65] There is evidence that orthotics affect muscle activity and will therefore affect muscle fatigue and performance.[66] Although a patient may have only one affected extremity, orthotics are always prescribed and worn in pairs.

Premade Orthotics

Several types of orthotics are available. There are premade orthotics and custom-made orthotics. Premade orthotics, the off-the-shelf or over-the-counter (OTC) variety, are less expensive than custom orthotics and in some situations may meet the patient's needs. These needs include items such as heel cushions that help absorb shock at heel strike and can also change rearfoot position when varus or valgus wedges are attached. A variety of pads and inserts can help reduce stress on specific areas of the foot. These include metatarsal pads, arch cookies, heel pads, and other supportive devices. Although most orthotics are used for rearfoot control—so the most important part of an orthotic is the portion from the heel to the midfoot—the top cover is often full length, extending to the toes. These full-length insoles replace the regular sock liners in shoes and further contribute to shock absorption, and in some cases they may provide additional foot support and control.

Custom Orthotics

Custom orthotics are specially designed to satisfy each person's specific needs, either to absorb stress or to correct alignment.[65] Some of the more common types of orthotics are briefly described next.

Three Types of Orthotics

Custom orthotics are either accommodating or functional and are of three basic types: rigid, semirigid, and soft. The more rigid the orthotic, the more exact the measurement must be in order for the device to fit properly and to be most effective. Soft orthotics, often made of soft polyethylene foam, are used for cavus or rigid feet to absorb stresses. They are known as accommodative orthotics; they do not so much correct mechanics as absorb forces and try to relieve symptoms by reducing stresses without altering the foot position.

Semirigid orthotics have proven to be most effective in reducing foot pain.[67] They contain a rigid shell, usually made of acrylic plastic, thermoplastic polymer, or carbon with a soft covering. These are functional orthotics, but they may also have accommodating aspects. Their purpose is to change the position of the rearfoot or forefoot (or both) to improve alignment, reduce shear stresses, reduce shock, and stabilize and support the foot joints.[63] The shell has either intrinsic or extrinsic posts to correct the deformities. These posts are in the rearfoot or forefoot or both, depending on the correction needed. These posts can be made from a variety of materials with varying densities, including ethyl vinyl acetate (EVA), polyethylene, crepe rubber, and polyplastic (figure 20.15). Extrinsic posts are attached to the orthotic device after the shell is constructed. Intrinsic posts are a part of the orthotic shell; they are harder to adjust if changes are needed because they are incorporated into the shell as it is made.

Specialty orthotic devices can also be made for specific performance needs. Special orthotics can be designed to accommodate for the stresses applied in aerobics by providing more control for loading on the anterior foot. Cycling orthotics must be lightweight and must provide control from the anterior foot, which bears the weight during cycling. A variety of low-profile orthotics can be designed to specifically conform to special footwear such as ski boots, soccer shoes, track racing shoes, and dress shoes.

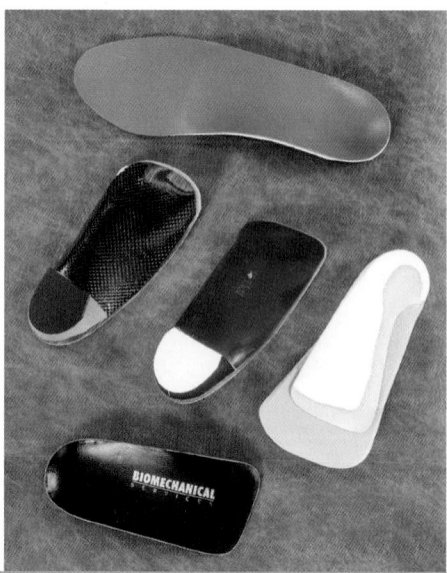

Figure 20.15 Custom orthotics are made from a variety of substances and are either corrective (rigid or semirigid) or accommodative.

Impression Methods

The most common methods of taking foot impressions is to use either plaster casts or foam boxes. With the plaster cast method, the patient is prone or supine as he or she would be if you were finding subtalar neutral. A traditional plaster cast using a double layer of plaster splint material is applied to the plantar foot. While the plaster dries, the foot is passively maintained in a subtalar neutral position. This method is the most useful when a functional orthotic is needed. Although the procedure can be messy, the molds are durable after they dry and can be taken or mailed to an orthotics lab without being damaged.

With the foam-box method, the patient's foot is pushed into a box of foam material much like that used by florists. The foot is actively kept as close to subtalar neutral as possible. This is not an accurate method to use for flexible feet[39] because it can be difficult for a patient with a flexible foot to maintain or find subtalar neutral. A foam box impression is most commonly used for an accommodative orthotic device or for devices that do not require a precision fit.

Both of these methods are being slowly replaced with computers and three-dimensional printers. Digital fabrication of foot orthotics using 3D scanners creates the design, and the computer software converts the scan into a 3D structure that is used to create the orthotic.[68] Computer-assisted orthotics construction has shown promise as not only being more economical in terms of finances and time,[69] but also more precise and accurate than traditional methods.[70]

Regardless of the method used to obtain an impression of the feet, the formed mold is then transformed into a solid replica of the feet. The person's custom-made orthotics are created to fit and correct alignment of these solid feet models.

The more rigid the orthotic, the more accurate the foot's orthotic impression must be. Softer accommodative orthotics tolerate a much larger margin of error in the impressions from which they are made. Both rigid and semirigid orthotics require an accurate impression.

Determining Proper Footwear for Patients

A question clinicians often hear from their patients about footwear is, "What's the best shoe?" There is no single *best* shoe. The *best* shoe is the one that meets the person's specific needs. There are many athletic shoes to choose from, and new models are released by manufacturing companies every six months; the major shoe companies produce equivalent variety of shoes ranging from economy to luxury models. It is more important for clinicians to be aware of general functional concepts and the functions of a shoe's components than it is to know details about specific models. Clinicians can help their patients to choose the correct shoes based on the specific structural designs each person requires in a shoe.

Shoes have many functions, such as protecting the skin and other soft-tissue structures of the feet, providing traction for improved propulsion, reducing impact shock during propulsion activities, increasing foot stability, and accommodating or correcting foot deformities.[71] Companies emphasize styles and fashions to increase the popularity of shoes. Ultimately, a shoe should be chosen on the basis of its structure, function, and fit, not its color, style, or name.

Shoe Structure

All shoes have the same basic structure consisting of an upper section and a lower section. The upper section of an athletic shoe includes the vamp, toe box, saddle, collar, sock liner, and heel counter. The lower section includes the outsole, midsole, wedge, and insole (figure 20.16). The vamp, which covers the toes and forefoot, includes the toe box. Running shoes whose vamp is made of nylon or another fabric usually have a mudguard around the rim of the toe box. The toe box can vary in width and height from one style and company to another. The toe box retains the shape of the shoe's forefoot and provides room for the toes. The saddle, the midsection of the shoe along the longitudinal arch, is usually reinforced by the company's logo or other structure to provide support to the midfoot. The heel counter is an important stabilizer for the rearfoot. A foxing, an additional piece in many athletic shoes, further reinforces the rearfoot and helps to maintain the heel counter's shape. The medial aspect of the heel counter is sometimes extended forward to resist

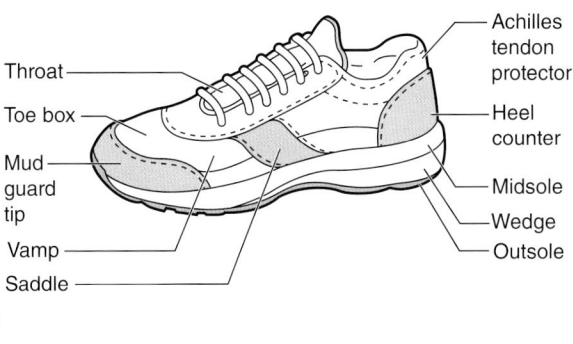

a

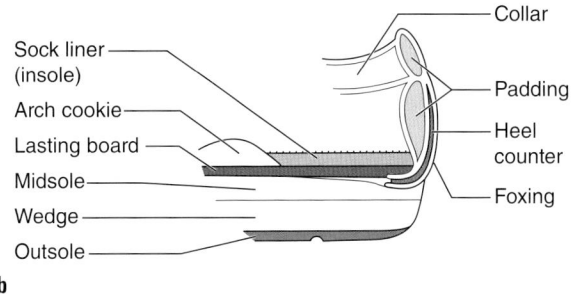

b

Figure 20.16 Shoe anatomy: *(a)* upper section, *(b)* lower section.

pronation. The collar is the top rim of the shoe's heel, often padded to reduce friction on the Achilles. Sometimes the collar is angled inward slightly to fit snugly around the ankle. The board of the insole lies between the upper and lower segments of the shoe and serves as the attachment site for these two segments. A sock liner on top of the insole helps absorb shock and reduce friction. The sock liner may be either glued into the shoe or simply inserted into it for easy removal or replacement. The sock liner usually has a heel cup with raised rim of the sock liner's heel portion to provide additional stability to the rearfoot by seating the calcaneus in place.

The outsole is the portion of the bottom of the shoe that is in contact with the ground. This segment is composed of a durable material and has a variety of designs of ripples, waves, and nubs, depending on the type of surface for which the shoe is designed. The midsole and wedge can be made of a variety of substances, including EVA, gas-filled or gel-filled chambers, and polyurethane. These shoe sections provide shock attenuation, stability, and control. They can include medial wedges to improve stability, varying densities to reduce pronation, and special materials to reduce impact stresses.

The shoe's last is an important component of a shoe. It is what determines the shape, size, and style of the shoe and can be straight, curved, or semicurved (figure 20.17). The straight last, which can be bisected by a lengthwise line that divides the last into two equal parts, has an essentially straight configuration along the medial outsole. It offers the foot the most medial support and is recommended for

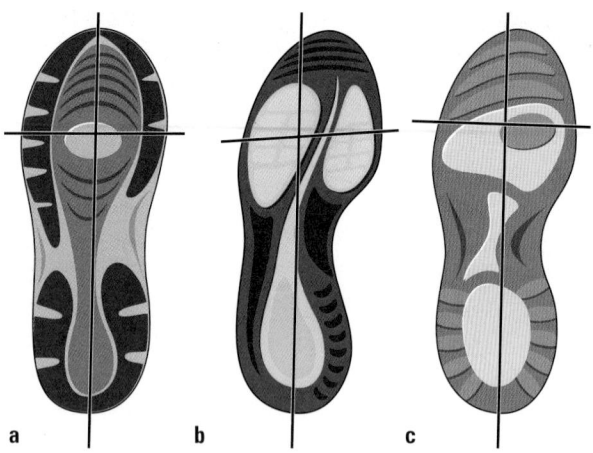

Figure 20.17 Shoe last: *(a)* straight, *(b)* curved, *(c)* semicurved. The last determines the shoe's shape, size, and style.

pronators. Curved lasts are flared inward from heel to toe to varying degrees with the medial outsole curved toward the arch. Curved lasts provide the least medial support and should be avoided by persons who excessively pronate. A curve-lasted shoe is generally more flexible than a straight-lasted shoe and is used by persons with rigid feet. Semicurved lasts are not straight but are less curved than curved lasts; these shoes are for people who need both flexibility and stability in their shoes.

Construction of the shoe around a shoe's slip lasting involves attaching the outsole and midsole to the bottom of the lasting and attaching the heel counter, toe box, and upper section of the shoe to the top of the lasting.

You can easily see the last when you remove the shoe's sock liner. A board lasting is made of a stiff cardboard or fibrous material that provides for a stiff sole and thus adds to the stability of the foot. A slip-lasted shoe looks similar to a sewn moccasin inside the shoe where the lasting and upper-shoe section meet, with the upper section stitched along its bottom to the last. The slip-lasted shoe is appropriate for a more rigid foot and offers more flexibility than a board-lasted shoe. A combination last has a board-lasted rearfoot and a slip-lasted forefoot. This type of last is designed to offer rearfoot stability and forefoot flexibility; forefoot flexibility allows an easy bend in the toe box region to reduce stresses on the plantar fascia and Achilles tendon during heel-off and toe-off.

Shoe Wear

An examination of the patient's worn shoes can give important clues to foot pathologies, helping the rehabilitation clinician to guide the patient toward a more appropriate shoe selection. For example, if the heel counter and medial heel are collapsed to the medial side of the shoe, the patient excessively pronates (figure 20.18). A medial wedge or

a higher-density medial wedge or midsole, along with a strong heel counter, will offer this person more stability. This patient should use a board-lasted shoe.

If the heel counter of the worn shoe has moved laterally over time, the patient has a rigid foot and needs a shoe with slip lasting, a lot of cushion but no medial wedge, and a firm heel counter.

If the patient's hallux has a blackened toenail, the toe box may not be deep enough to accommodate the toes' height. Another reason for a blackened toenail may be that the toe hits the toe box end because the shoe is either too short or too loose if the foot slides forward. If the hallux is wearing through the upper section of the shoe, the patient may have a rigid first ray and may need more shock absorption in the forefoot. The forefoot of the shoe for this type of foot needs to be rigid to protect the first ray.

Although shoe wear is a good indicator of foot pathologies, a shoe that has noticeable wear is one that should be replaced. The life of a shoe depends on the patient, the frequency of use, and the surfaces on which the patient wears them. Footwear varies greatly in longevity.[72] It is important, however, to replace the shoe once a wear pattern develops. A worn shoe changes the mechanics and stresses applied to the foot.[73]

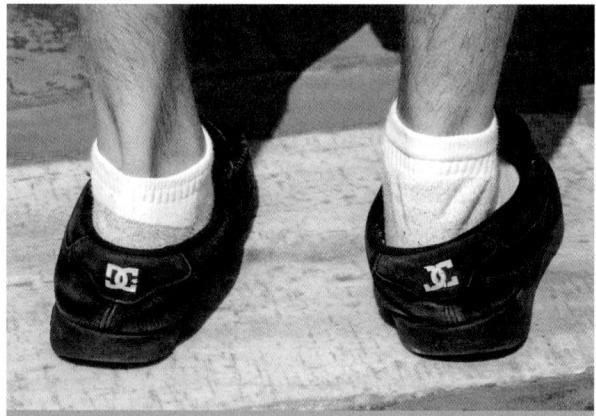

Figure 20.18 Excessive shoe wear provides clues to foot pathologies. This is an example of medial breakdown of a shoe, which indicates excessive pronation.
© Peggy Houglum

Injury History

A profile of the patient's injury history is also useful in determining the correct shoe for that person. For example, if the patient has a history of Achilles tendinopathy, the cause may be either excessive pronation or tightness in the Achilles.[74, 75] This patient should find a shoe that has good heel-counter stability, a straight board or combination last, good forefoot flexibility, and a higher-than-normal elevation in the wedge to relieve Achilles stress.

If the patient has a history of knee pain, excessive pronation may be the cause.[55] A board-lasted shoe with good rearfoot control and a firm heel counter is appropriate for this patient. Plantar fasciitis can also be related to excessive pronation,[76] so a similar shoe would be appropriate for a patient with a history of plantar fasciitis. Table 20.4 provides a quick reference for shoe characteristics that are best for different pathologies.

As a general rule, a foot needs a complimentary shoe. For instance, if the foot is rigid, a flexible shoe is recommended. A person with this type of foot will achieve a better fit with a curved last, sewn to the shoe, and cushion.[63] On the other hand, if the foot is flexible, a more rigid shoe is more appropriate. This person will be most comfortable in a straight board last with good rearfoot control and a firm heel counter.[77]

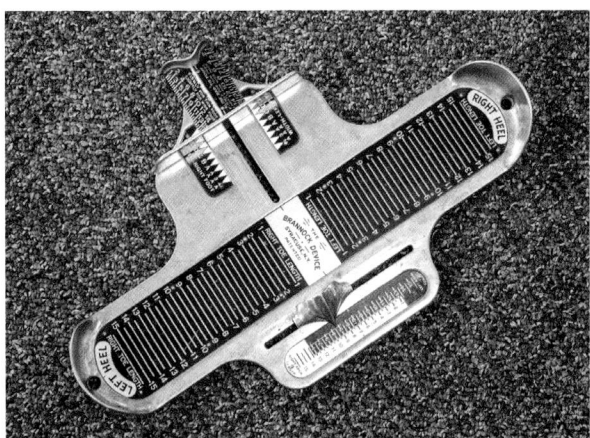

Figure 20.19   Brannock Device foot-measuring device.

Thank you to Body N' Sole Sports of Savoy, Illinois, for providing the Brannock Device for this photo.

Proper Shoe Fit

Once the type of shoe has been determined, the shoe must be fit properly. Shoe size is most easily determined by using the Brannock Device found in shoe stores (figure 20.19). This device determines the width and length of the shoe. The foot is measured in the device with the person standing in the sock to be worn with the shoe being purchased, bearing weight on the foot. A good heel fit is critical for any shoe. The shoe's heel counter should fit snugly to provide adequate support for the rearfoot.[78] There should be approximately one thumb's width (1.3 to 1.6 cm [1/2 to 5/8 in.]) of space between the end of the longest toe and the end of the shoe.[78] The toe box should have adequate depth and width for the forefoot and toes; if the vamp just distal and lateral to the most distal lace eyelets is cloth and can be pinched, the shoe width is appropriate.[78] The bend in the vamp should coincide with the bend of the patient's forefoot, and the first metatarsophalangeal joint should be at the widest part of the shoe.[79] A supportive heel counter should feel firm and should have little or no give when its sides are squeezed together. The vamp should bend easily when you grasp the heel and try to bend the shoe by applying pressure with the index finger of your other hand. If

a shoe has a board last, it should be difficult to wring the shoe or to produce much motion when stabilizing the heel and rotating the vamp.

Shoes should be evaluated before they are purchased to make sure that the heel counter is perpendicular to the sole, the sole is parallel to the floor, and the last is the same on the right as on the left shoe. There should also be no abnormalities in stitching or construction and no unmatched angles from one shoe to the other. Production errors in shoe manufacturing are common. A construction error can cause an injury or aggravate any structural deformity.[80]

Patients should try on shoes in the store, wearing socks of the same type and thickness as those they will use with the shoes. A person should be able to give shoes a good trial in the store on a treadmill or track or be able to run outside before purchasing them. It is best to try on shoes in the later part of the day when foot volume is greater than it is in the morning. Because foot size may vary from right to left,[81] it is advisable to try on both shoes, properly laced. It is a good idea to try on a variety of shoes and compare comfort and fit. The patient should be sure to ask about the store's return policy. The store should stand behind the product

TABLE 20.4   Recommended Shoe Characteristics for Different Pathologies

Shoe characteristic	Tight Achilles or tendinopathy	Flexible foot with excessive pronation	Knee pain	Rigid foot with high arch
Lasting	Board	Board	Board	Sewn
Heel counter	Firm with good control and deep seated heel cup	Firm with good control and deep seated heel cup	Firm with good control and deep seated heel cup	Good control
Last	Straight or combination	Straight or combination	Straight or combination	Curved
Midsole	Elevated heel	Medial wedge	Medial wedge	Soft
Forefoot	Flexible	Flexible	Flexible	Flexible

and permit exchanges if someone who recently purchased a pair of shoes and has used them at home finds that they do not meet specific needs or are uncomfortable; the store owners merely return the shoes to the manufacturer and are reimbursed for their costs.

Barefoot Running

Within the last few years, there has been significant interest in barefoot running. Presumably this is based on claims that fewer injuries occur with barefoot running than with shod running.[82] Others have gone to what is termed *minimalist* running in an effort to create a more natural running pattern.

A minimalist running shoe has a lower profile than a more traditional running shoe. Its sole is very flexible and essentially flat (less than 4 mm rise from forefoot to rearfoot). It lacks the cushioning found in a traditional running shoe, and it has no motion control.[83] The minimalist shoe is believed to offer the benefit of protecting the soles of the feet while lacking the weight and bulk of a traditional shoe, making its use similar to running barefoot.[84]

At this point, long-term studies on barefoot running or minimalist shoe running are very limited.[85] However, a number of studies have looked at both injuries and biomechanical differences between running barefoot, shod in regular running shoes, and shod in minimalist running shoes. For the most part, studies have found that minimalist shoe running and regular shoe running are more biomechanically similar than minimalist shoe running and barefoot running.[83, 86]

Barefoot runners land more on the forefoot than on the heel, and their contact time with the ground is shorter, as are their stride duration and flight time.[86] Because of the shorter stride length, the stride frequency is increased, but the ground reaction forces are decreased in barefoot runners.[87] Barefoot runners have been found to have fewer orthopedic injuries but more injuries overall because of the injuries suffered to the plantar surface of the foot.[88] However, the overall difference in injury frequency between the shod and barefoot runners was statistically insignificant because the barefoot runners had significantly less mileage than the shod runners.[88]

Shoe Types

Since the late 1960s, when research on athletic shoe design began in earnest, the factors that have influenced design include injury prevention, enhanced performance, and comfort.[89] Because different activities place different demands and stresses on the foot, specific requirements for an athletic shoe differ among sports. There are as many types of shoes as there are sports. Patients should not wear shoes intended for use in one sport for a different sport; the shoes are not designed to meet the demands of another sport.

Shoes are made from many different materials. Some of the newer materials for shoe upper elements have improved breathability and durability, while the new materials for lower elements have improved durability and reduced weight. Some shoes, however, are made to satisfy the fashion preferences of the buyer, not the needs of the foot. It is best to buy athletic shoes from athletic shoe stores whose employees have been educated on shoes and know what to seek in a shoe to address each person's needs.

Court Shoes

Court sports such as basketball, volleyball, tennis, racquetball, and squash involve running forward and backward, jumping and landing, sudden stops and changes in direction, and many lateral and sideward movements, so safe participation requires good cushioning, traction control, and medial and lateral support to protect the lateral ligaments and peroneal muscles.[90] Because court sports are played on a variety of surfaces, the outsole should be specific to the surface on which the person plays; for tennis players, the shoe's outsole material should be able to adapt to differing playing surfaces and allow some sliding on the court. A toe guard or reinforcement over the medial toes will prolong the life of the shoe and protect it against toe drag on the serve. In a shoe appropriate for court sports, the heel and toe are at about the same level, whereas a running shoe has an elevated heel to reduce stress on the Achilles. Because placing the foot in a plantar-flexed position makes the ankle susceptible to inversion sprains and because court sports involve lateral movements, a court shoe's sole is flat. Impact stresses secondary to jump-landing activities are reduced by the shoe's midsole.[91] A court shoe also has medial–lateral stability to reduce the risk of rollover into supination during lateral court movements.[89]

Running Shoes

In addition to the elevated heel, a traditional running shoe should be flexible so that the foot does not have to work excessively to bend the shoe during heel-off. Since running is a forward activity, not a lateral one like court activities, there is less risk of ankle sprains that occur when the heel is higher than the forefoot. Running creates a greater risk for Achilles stress than for ankle sprains. A running shoe should have good cushion in the rear and forefoot yet provide stability to the heel. Many traditional running shoes incorporate a dual-density construction in an attempt to absorb forces and control pronation.[89] The firmer midsole on the medial side may include just the heel, or it may extend from the heel to the arch. Makers of distance running shoes have applied the rocker bottom idea used in walking shoes to running shoes to improve muscle efficiency during running; however, investigations into the potential benefits have produced varying results. One investigation found that subjects using rocker bottom running shoes expended more energy, and it identified the increased weight of the rocker shoe as the main reason.[92] Other studies have investigated walking with rocker bottom shoes and found that reduced forces occurred at the ankle but not at other lower-extremity joints.[93, 94]

Although race-running shoes have been in use for a long time, they are in the relatively new category of a minimalist shoe and are designed for speed and not durability. Minimalist shoes is a category that is gaining in popularity because it is thought to mimic barefoot running;[92] however, as mentioned earlier, evidence suggests that minimalist shoe running more closely resembles shod running than barefoot running.[86] Minimalist shoes lack the support that training shoes provide, and their life span is usually only a few races before they must be replaced. Some competitive runners cannot use racing shoes because the shoes lack the support they need. These shoes have also been found to present a greater risk of injury than standard running shoes.[95]

Aerobics Shoes

Aerobics shoes should have good forefoot cushioning, and many have additional cushioning in the sock liner. A reinforced toe box supports the forefoot primarily during forefoot-impact activities. If the shoe does not have good forefoot cushioning in its midfoot section, a viscoelastic insole should be added to the shoe.[96] The forefoot should have good flexibility to allow the foot to bend easily during aerobic activities; in many shoes this flexibility comes from flex bars cut into the sole. There should be good rearfoot stability with a good heel counter for adequate ankle support during medial and lateral activities. Stability is needed for the multidirectional movements in aerobics. Stability straps in the midfoot region can provide medial–lateral stability in the midsole and the upper section. In some shoes, a mid-height upper section provides added medial–lateral support without interfering with plantar flexion–dorsiflexion. Aerobic shoes come in leather and synthetic materials; synthetic material is usually lighter and does not absorb as much moisture as the leather.

Soccer and Football Shoes

A field shoe used in sports such as soccer or American football should have a flexible sole to permit ease in dorsiflexion–plantar flexion motion of the ankle. The cleats should be placed in areas that do not create undue pressure or irritation of the plantar foot; rearfoot cleat placement should be around the heel's perimeter to avoid calcaneal irritation. Cleat design and length vary according to the surface the patient plays on. Short cleats are appropriate for hard turf, whereas long cleats are suitable for softer surfaces[97] such as wet grass. Some soccer shoes are now made in mid-top and high-top styles for additional ankle protection.

Walking Shoes

Walking shoes have many of the same characteristics as running shoes. The heel is slightly raised, but not as much as in a running shoe, and a firm heel counter provides for rearfoot impact stability and midfoot stability.[98] The forefoot is usually more flexible. The outer sole has a rocker bottom (angled rather than squared posterior heel and curved upward at the toes) to provide efficiency and to lessen energy requirements during heel strike and rolling from heel-off to toe-off. The shank portion of the midsole is usually stiffer in a walking shoe to offer better medial–lateral stability over uneven surfaces.[98] Selection of walking shoes should be based on the walkers' age and the type of walking they do.[98] Olympic walkers need flexibility for economy of movement; off-trail walkers need medial–lateral stability and traction for uneven surfaces; and power and fitness walkers need stability and cushioning.

Mountaineering Boots

Requirements for mountaineering boots vary according to the activity involved. Hiking, climbing, and high-altitude climbing each place different demands on the feet and will require different boots. Shoes in this category range from lightweight boots similar to running shoes with uppers made of a fabric–leather combination to heavyweight boots with a steel shank in the sole and an upper made of rigid leather.

Hiking is one of the most popular mountaineering sports. A hiking boot for off-trail hikes should provide stability and should have a good heel counter and midsole for medial–lateral support. Hiking boots should be waterproof or water resistant and should have a very durable outsole. The outsole should have good traction for uneven and rough terrain; commonly, the outsole is made of Vibram and has a waffle pattern for rough terrain.[99] The upper section height should be mid to high for rough terrain and mid to low for easy terrain. A leather upper is often recommended for maximum protection and durability.[99] The tongue is most often padded to permit the laces to be firmly tied yet comfortable. A hiking boot should be lightweight and comfortable, while a mountaineering boot requires a stiff shank and usually has a rocker bottom to compensate for the sole's rigidity;[100] neither boot should have pressure points or a need to be broken in. There is usually a smooth lining in the upper of these boots that both adds to the boot's water resistance and protects the feet, preventing blisters and keeping the feet warm.

Cross-Training Shoes

Cross-training shoes are designed to meet the needs of people involved in multiple activities. The goal is to meet all the needs of all the people all the time. The problem is that these shoes usually do not meet any specific need most of the time. There are various styles of shoes in this category. At this point there have been no substantial investigations comparing cross-trainer shoes with shoes designed for specific activities, so someone who participates in a specific activity may be better off choosing a shoe that meets the demands of that activity.

Work Shoes

The shoe one wears to work depends on the type of work performed. The workplace conditions dictate the shoe requirements. White-collar workers typically wear shoes that have no specific construction requirements; for these workers, appearance and norms of attire most likely guide their shoe selection. Blue-collar workers, on the other hand, must often consider safety in their selection of footwear. This group must protect their feet from both acute injuries and repetitive stresses.

Safety-Toe Shoes Safety-toe shoes, as the name implies, protect the toes from injury. The toe portion of the shoe is reinforced with steel or an alloy or some type of nonmetallic shell that covers the top of that area. This feature protects the toes from falling objects and heavy equipment.

Steel-Insole Shoes Steel-insole shoes are designed for those who spend their workday performing heavy or repetitive activities that demand a lot of work from the foot. These shoes are designed to reduce stresses on the foot joints by stabilizing the foot within the shoe. The steel insole restricts the great toe from bending excessively and increasing repetitive stress on its MTP joint. These insoles can also protect the toes from jamming and from repetitive stresses applied throughout the workday. Workers who ride bikes or who drive heavy trucks or equipment that demands frequent foot pedal activity will seek these types of shoes. They may also be worn by workers who are at risk of stepping on sharp objects such as nails or glass.

Electric Hazard Shoes Electric hazard shoes are worn by those who spend their workdays around high-voltage machines or equipment. They are also used by electricians who engage in repair and installation of electrical wiring, circuits, and power lines. These shoes have soles constructed of non-conductive materials that protect the wearer against the danger of an electrical shock.

Lacing Patterns

Some shoes, especially running shoes, have multiple eyelets that the wearer can select from when lacing the shoe. This arrangement enables the wearer to use a variety of lacing patterns to meet specific needs. It has been demonstrated that lacing patterns do influence biomechanics, comfort, and stability of the foot within the shoe.[101] Alternative lacing patterns can either add to the shoe's support or accommodate for some foot deformities. A person with a narrow foot should use the eyelets farthest from the tongue of the shoe, which will pull the sides of the shoe more closely together (figure 20.20a). People with wide feet should use the eyelets closest to the tongue (figure 20.20b).

Women's feet have a narrower heel than men's feet, which is why women's shoes are not just smaller versions of men's shoes. Women who have a wider forefoot than women's shoe styles account for often prefer to wear men's athletic shoes but find their narrower heel often slides up and down in a men's shoe. These women can adjust the men's shoe fit to accommodate their needs by using two laces, one for the lower eyelets and the other for the higher eyelets, and tying the upper lace more tightly to support the heel (figure 20.20c).

Patients with high arches should avoid lacing a shoe in the traditional crisscross pattern; instead, they should should use a straight-across pattern (figure 20.20d).

People with toe deformities can obtain some relief by using the laces to lift up the forefoot of the shoe. As the shoe is tied, the lace that goes through the eyelet nearest the problem toe is brought directly to an eyelet at the top of the shoe. Pulling on this lace lifts up part of the forefoot (figure 20.20e).

Heel blisters are caused by friction of the shoe over the heel. The wearer can decrease the friction by securing the heel more firmly in the shoe using a loop-through technique at the top of the shoe as seen in figure 20.20f. The lace should be pulled more snugly at the top of the shoe than at the bottom.

A bump on the top of the midfoot can be painful with regular lacing patterns. To relieve pressure on the top of the foot, don't cross the laces; instead, keep the laces on the same side of the shoe and skip the eyelet at the painful level (figure 20.20g).

Sock Selection

One additional topic on foot protection is socks. The science of sock design and construction has improved significantly in the past several years. Athletic socks today are designed to cushion the foot, draw moisture away from the foot, and reduce friction.[102] Some new sock materials are antibacterial, protect against odors, and cushion the foot.[103, 104] Varieties of fibers are used in socks, including cotton, wool, acrylic, nylon, polyester, and CoolMax.[105]

Socks should fit properly to prevent blisters and other similar problems that can occur from improperly fit shoes.[106] Socks should fit properly without bunching up at the toes because they are too large or constricting the foot because they are too short. Sizing systems vary from one manufacturer to another, so the person must be sure the socks fit well before purchasing them.

Wearing proper socks is important, especially in distance events where blisters may result if the athlete is not wearing a proper sock. Blisters are caused by a combination of moisture and friction and can be serious problems in distance events. Socks constructed of synthetic fibers tend to create fewer and smaller blisters than cotton socks.[107] A

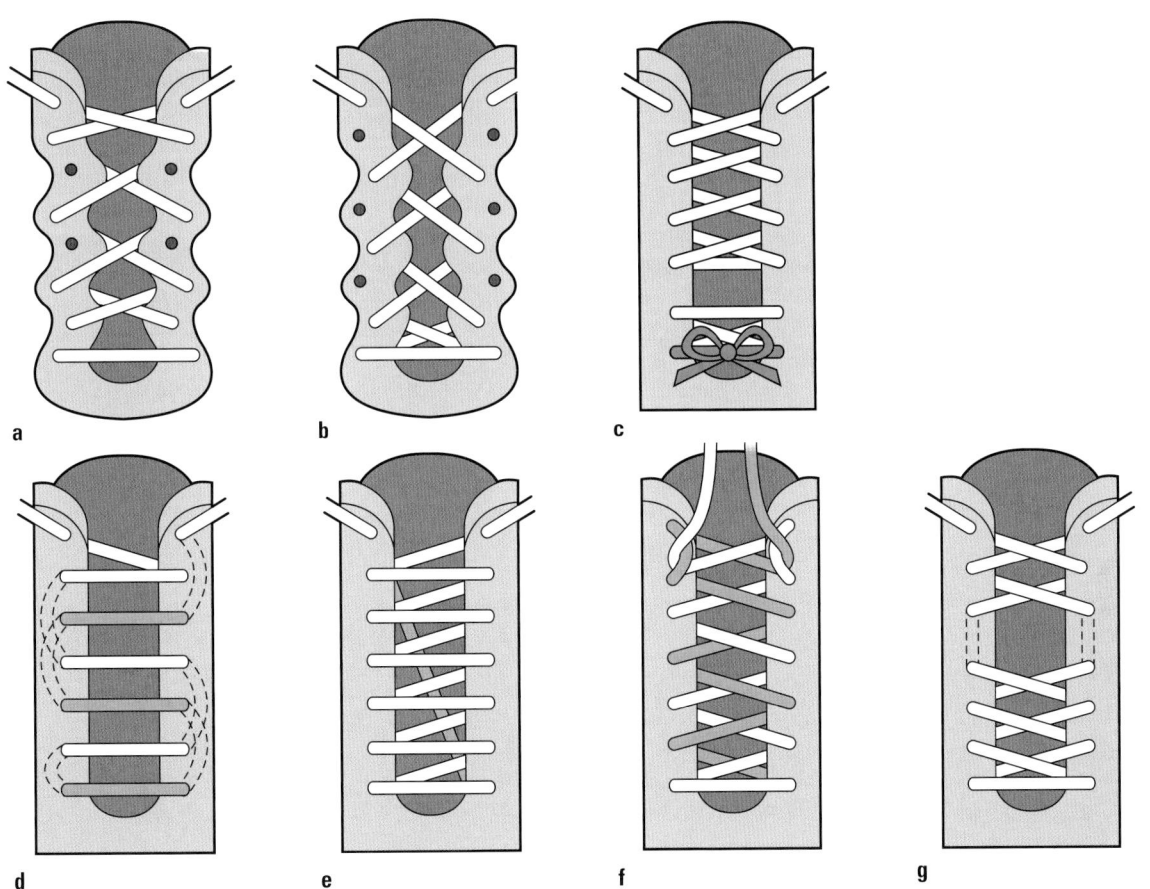

Figure 20.20 Shoe-lacing patterns for *(a)* narrow feet, *(b)* wide feet, *(c)* wide forefoot and narrow heel (using two laces), *(d)* high arches, *(e)* toe problems, *(f)* heel blisters, *(g)* dorsal foot bump.

Copyright 1998 by Carol Frey, MD.

double-layer sock system with a wicking material closest to the skin has been shown to be the best method of preventing blisters.[108]

Socks come in a variety of thicknesses and lengths. The best thickness and length to use depend upon the intended activity. Double-layer socks are used to reduce blister formation. Thicker or padded double-layer socks are worn when padding is needed to reduce impact stresses on the foot, especially the heel. Thinner double-layer socks are used for speed events when the athlete does not want to add weight that may hamper performance. Over-the-calf socks are used to protect the shin and calf from injury. People who participate in activities where the risk of injury to the leg is minimal can use lower-profile socks.

Moisture accumulation is a major problem during any extended activity; for example, athletic events can produce more than 0.5 L (1 pint) of perspiration from each foot. This number includes both the perspiration produced by the feet and that which reaches the feet by moving down the legs from higher up.[109] Therefore, a sock's ability to wick away moisture on the skin's surface is important. A material's wicking ability results from a combination of its fiber structure and compressibility.[109] Cotton socks and wool socks absorb moisture and swell, so they are not good moisture transporters.[109] Synthetic fibers are better able to wick moisture because of their mechanical structure. Synthetic fiber socks also tend to keep their shape better than cotton socks. Although wool socks tend to retain moisture, they also can retain heat; for this reason, they are still the sock of choice for cold-weather outdoor sports.[109] Some manufacturers now combine wool with synthetic materials to reduce the abrasiveness of 100% wool socks and to improve the wicking of moisture.[109] Table 20.5 provides a list of commonly used fibers in sock fabrics.

In short, recent research has demonstrated that sock selection is important in creating an optimal environment for the foot during activities. Socks are made from a variety of materials. Many contain combinations of materials to provide optimal protection and support for the foot. Sock selection is varied and is determined by the activity and the stresses applied to the foot. Table 20.6 lists examples of sock construction and sport applications based on Richie.[109] It is important to recommend appropriate sock selections to patients as well as appropriate shoe selections.

TABLE 20.5 **Fibers Commonly Used in Sock Fabrics**

Fiber	Advantages	Disadvantages	Indications
Cotton	Durable material Soft material for comfort Absorbs moisture Inexpensive	Absorbs moisture but does not wick moisture. Feet are colder because moisture is retained. Can cause friction with prolonged wear. Has no elasticity. Is heavier when wet.	Not recommended for sports Good for everyday wear, especially when blended with other materials
Wool	Absorbs moisture Good insulator	Shrinks. Can be difficult to clean. Will overheat feet in warm weather. Material is bulky.	Hiking Outdoor activities Winter outdoor sports
Bamboo	Great wicking Good thermal regulator in either heat or cold Elastic Dries quickly Breathable Lightweight Soft fabric Comfortable	Expensive	Running Hiking Outdoor activities Most sports activities in general
Acrylic	Good wicking Good cushion Reduces friction Stretchable Retains body heat	May feel bulky or wet. Fabric pills easily when washed. Fabric is flammable.	Running Outdoor activities in cold weather
Nylon	Elastic Some moisture wicking ability Durable Inexpensive Better when blended with other fabrics Can be either thin or bulky	Absorbs moisture. Fabric may pill when washed. Does not breathe well.	Sports activities in general
Polyester	Durable Does not shrink Dries quickly Inexpensive Better when blended with cotton	Retains moisture. Can increase foot temp and sweating. Fabric may pill when washed.	Good for everyday wear
Polypropylene	Strong fiber Great wicking Dries quickly Lightweight	Inelastic. May experience odor buildup. Fabric can occasionally pill when washed.	Winter outdoor sports Hiking Outdoor activities

TABLE 20.6 Sock Selection and Sport Application

Construction	Design or fiber	Sport
Upper design	Over-the-calf	Baseball, basketball, outdoor activities: skiing, snowboarding, soccer
	Mid-calf	Skating
	Slouch	Aerobics
	Crew	Running, golf, tennis, racquetball, hiking
Double layers	Thin	Cycling, race running, skiing
	Thick	Jogging, skiing, hiking, tennis, basketball
Fibers	Acrylic	Golf, tennis, hiking
	Acrylic and wool	Cold outdoor activities
	Acrylic and CoolMax	Warm outdoor activities
	CoolMax	Running, cycling

Adapted by permission from D.H. Richie, Jr., *Socks and Your Feet: Socks: Hosiery—Essential Equipment for the Athlete* (Ocala, FL: American Academy of Podiatric Sports Medicine, 2014).

Evidence in Rehabilitation

Although compressive stockings have been used for years to reduce the risk of deep vein thrombosis after surgery, it has been only recently that long compression socks have attracted the attention of runners and other athletes. Interest in these socks is based on two theoretical benefits of using them in endurance activities: the impact they have on blood flow and the post-activity influence they have on muscle vibration.[110]

It was shown that compression garments promote venous return, so metabolic waste removal and oxygen delivery are more efficient; this efficiency reduces metabolic expenditures, so there is less lactic acid buildup, resulting in less postexercise muscle soreness.[111]

The likely effect of reducing muscle vibration, or oscillation, is to improve muscle efficiency by lowering energy expenditure and reducing muscle damage and fatigue during high-intensity events.[112] This effect reduces post-activity muscle soreness and recovery time.[113] There is also evidence that proprioception improves with the use of long compressive socks;[114] therefore, performance improves through the facilitation of this somatosensory feedback mechanism.[115]

Despite this evidence for the benefits of using long compression socks during endurance activities, there are also studies that show little to no effect with their use.[116-118] Some investigators have proposed that there are no physical benefits from the use of compression socks for endurance activities, but there may be a psychological benefit that cannot be discounted.[119]

Whether one agrees or disagrees that compression socks or other garments are useful, all can agree that the specific mechanisms of those benefits remain elusive. We know that external compression can affect arterial pressure, venous return, and cardiac output.[120, 121] Although Brown and colleagues[122] performed a meta-analysis of current research on compression socks and concluded that their mechanisms of action remain unknown, they also concluded that small but significant benefits on exercise recovery can be achieved when compression garments are used, and the greatest benefits occur with their use during heavy resistance exercises, especially activities such as plyometrics or eccentric exercise. They also recognized that the inconsistencies in protocols, subject pools, and research designs made it difficult to identify consistent results from the investigations included in their study.[122]

Based on the study of Brown and colleagues and the discussions of others, compressive garments, including compression socks, appear to have positive benefits, but additional research is needed before strong conclusions can be made.[122]

Rehabilitation Interventions

Although modalities are included in rehabilitation programs for distal LE injuries, they are discussed in this chapter. Modalities are presented in chapter 9; the choice of modalities depends on the injury and individual patient factors. Not all soft-tissue techniques are included in this chapter since they were covered in chapter 11. Trigger point release is presented for some of the most commonly affected muscles. Descriptions of joint mobilization techniques follow the sections on soft-tissue mobilization. In addition to these manual therapy techniques, a variety of exercises, beginning with flexibility exercises and continuing through to performance-specific exercises, are presented.

Soft-Tissue Mobilization

As with the upper extremity, pain and referred pain in the lower extremity can come from several sources. Sciatica is a common pain-referral source in the lower extremity, with symptoms extending anywhere from the back to the toes. Before the rehabilitation clinician treats pain, he or she must identify its source. If the pain is myofascially based, soft-tissue mobilization techniques can be effective in relieving the pain. Trigger point pain-referral patterns and their treatments presented in chapter 11 are based on the work of Travell and Simons.[123] The most commonly encountered trigger points in the foot, ankle, and leg are presented in table 20.7. Recall that after the trigger point's treatment, the patient should actively move the muscle through its full range of motion several times.

CLINICAL TIPS

The rehabilitation clinician uses a variety of soft-tissue techniques, primarily to relieve pain and secondarily to improve motion resulting from pain relief. In addition to trigger point release, deep-tissue massage of the foot and ankle are effective and can be taught to patients to achieve additional benefits.

Deep-Tissue Massage

Soft-tissue restriction often occurs after a patient has experienced excessive edema or immobilization of the ankle, foot, or extremity. Either the prolonged presence of edema or reduced tissue movement can result in adhesions. Releasing adhesions can improve tissue mobility and restore normal range of motion. Deep-tissue massage techniques, discussed in chapter 11, can help to achieve this. Review that chapter's discussion of the proper way to perform massage techniques before using them. Patients can perform their own deep-tissue massage on intrinsic

TABLE 20.7   Common Trigger Points in the Foot, Ankle, and Leg

Body segment	Muscle with trigger points
Foot	Abductor hallucis
	Quadratus plantae
Leg	Gastrocnemius
	Soleus
	Tibialis posterior

Based on the work of Travell and Simons (1992).[123]

muscles of the foot that are in spasm or have myofascial restrictions. Sitting in a chair, the patient places the bare foot on the side of a ribbed fruit or vegetable can positioned on the floor. Applying some downward force on the knee with the hands, the patient rolls the foot back and forth over the can to provide a self-massage.

Joint Mobilization

Joint mobilization is often needed in the ankle, especially after periods of immobilization. The techniques can be either repeated sustained glides or oscillations. In more restricted joints, sustained glides may be more effective than oscillations. Oscillation may be more comfortable for the patient and is often used in combination with distraction during ankle mobilizations.

To determine whether joint mobilization for improved motion is indicated, the rehabilitation clinician assesses the joint's capsular pattern and motion loss and compares the involved segment with the uninvolved extremity. The capsular pattern for the talocrural joint is more limitation of plantar flexion than of dorsiflexion; in the subtalar joint, inversion is more limited than eversion. The great toe's MTP joint has a capsular pattern that has more limitation of dorsiflexion than plantar flexion. The other toe's MTP joints and all the IP joints have a capsular pattern of more loss of plantar flexion than dorsiflexion. Refer to table 20.8 for this information and for details on close-packed and resting positions for these joints.

As with other joints, precautions and contraindications should be respected. Body mechanics, the direction in which force is applied, and the amount of force should be proper in all manual techniques. The clinician's hands should be as close to the joint as possible, with one hand (usually the proximal hand) acting as the stabilizing hand and the other hand applying the mobilizing force. The convex-on-concave rule determines the direction of the mobilization force. That is, when a convex surface is moved on a concave surface, the force is applied in the direction opposite to that of the bone's movement. Some of the more commonly used techniques for the foot and ankle are presented in the following sections. These techniques are based on Maitland's[124] and Kaltenborn's[125] methods.

Tibiofibular Joint

The tibia and fibula articulate with each other proximally in the distal knee region and distally just proximal to the ankle mortise joint. Both proximal and distal articulations must have normal mobility if ankle dorsiflexion–plantar flexion is to be normal. The resting position for the proximal tibiofibular joint is 25° of knee flexion with 10° of ankle plantar flexion, and the resting position for the distal tibiofibular joint is 10° of ankle plantar flexion with slight inversion.

TABLE 20.8   Capsular Patterns, Resting Positions, and Close-Packed Positions

Joint	Capsular pattern and indications	Resting position	Close-packed position
Proximal tibiofibular	Restricted plantar flexion or dorsiflexion	25° of knee flexion and 10° of ankle plantar flexion	Full dorsiflexion; weight bearing
Distal tibiofibular	Restricted plantar flexion or dorsiflexion	10° of plantar flexion with slight inversion	Full dorsiflexion; weight bearing
Talocrural	Plantar flexion loss is greater than dorsiflexion loss	10° of plantar flexion	Full dorsiflexion
Subtalar	Inversion loss is greater than eversion loss	Midrange of inversion and eversion	Full inversion
Midtarsal (transverse tarsal)	Limited dorsiflexion, plantar flexion, adduction, and medial rotation	Midway between motion extremes	Supination
Number 1 metatarsophalangeal	Dorsiflexion loss is greater than plantar flexion loss	20° of dorsiflexion	Full dorsiflexion
Number 2–5 metatarsophalangeals	Plantar flexion loss is greater than dorsiflexion loss	20° of plantar flexion	Full dorsiflexion
Interphalangeals	Plantar flexion loss is greater than dorsiflexion loss	20° of plantar flexion	Full dorsiflexion

Joint Mobilization of the Foot and Ankle Joints

Since the fibula is part of the ankle, its ability to move in both its proximal and distal tibial joints must be assessed. If the ankle lacks the last few degrees of sagittal plane motion, it may be that one of the tibiofibular joints is restricted. The clinician must assess these joints for their mobility and treat with joint mobilization when normal mobility is lacking.

Anteroposterior (AP) and Posteroanterior (PA) Glides

Joint: Proximal tibiofibular.

Resting Position: 25° knee flexion, 10° ankle plantar flexion.

Indications: Restricted ankle dorsiflexion, plantar flexion, or both.

Patient Position: The patient is positioned to provide the clinician with the best mechanical advantage and ease of force application. For an AP mobilization force, the patient is positioned supine with the hip and knee flexed so the foot is flat on the treatment table. Posteroanterior (PA) mobilization of the proximal tibiofibular joint is performed with the patient side-lying or prone. The weight of the extremity helps with stabilization while the clinician's distal hand stabilizes the proximal tibia.

Clinician and Hand Positions: For an AP mobilization, the tibia is stabilized with the medial hand over the proximal tibia; the fleshy aspect of the thenar eminence of the lateral hand is over the fibular head and the proximal fibula to provide the mobilizing force. For a PA mobilization, the mobilizing hand applies an anterior glide with the thenar pad against the fibular head, while the stabilizing hand prevents motion of the tibia. If the patient is side-lying or prone for the PA mobilization, the clinician uses a mobilizing grip similar to that for the AP technique, but the thenar eminence is placed over the posterior fibular head.

Mobilization Application: For an AP mobilization, a directly posterior force perpendicular to the fibular shaft is applied by the mobilizing hand on the fibular head to produce a posterior glide of the fibula (figure 20.21a). For a PA mobilization, the lateral hand glides the fibular head anteriorly (figure 20.21b).

>continued

Anteroposterior (AP) and Posteroanterior (PA) Glides >continued

Notations: Mobilization of the proximal tibiofibular joint should be performed for any restricted movement of the distal tibiofibular joint or ankle. Normal mobility of this joint allows the fibular head to move anteriorly during knee flexion and posteriorly during knee extension. When performing a PA mobilization with the patient prone, the clinician should place a pad under the distal thigh to prevent the patient's patella from being pushed into the table.

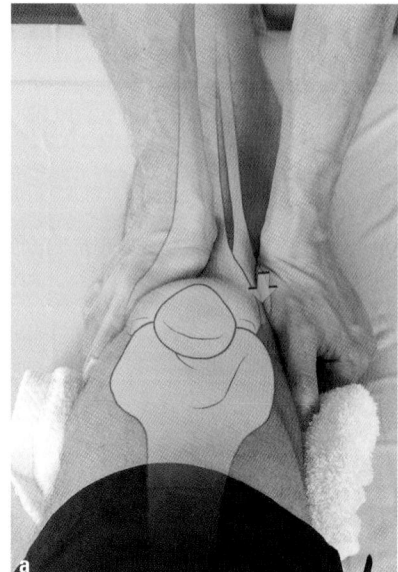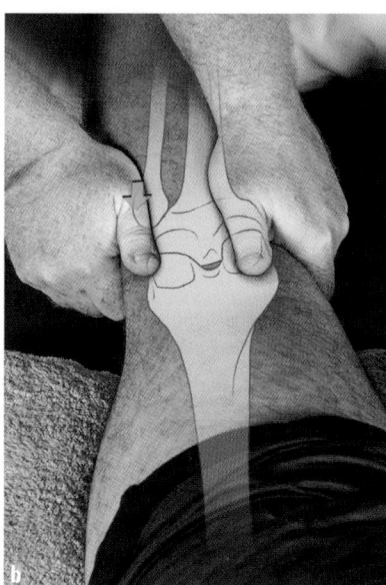

Figure 20.21 *(a)* Posterior glide of proximal tibiofemoral joint; *(b)* anterior glide of proximal tibiofemoral joint.

AP and PA Glides

Joint: Distal tibiofibular.

Resting Position: 10° plantar flexion with slight inversion.

Indications: Restricted ankle dorsiflexion, plantar flexion, or both.

Patient Position: An AP glide is performed with the patient supine. A PA glide is performed with the patient side-lying with a towel or pillow between the patient's two distal extremities.

Clinician and Hand Positions: For an AP glide, the clinician places the medial hand over the medial malleolus and lateral tibia to stabilize the tibia and places the thenar eminence of the lateral hand over the lateral malleolus and distal fibula. For a PA glide, the base of the lateral hand or

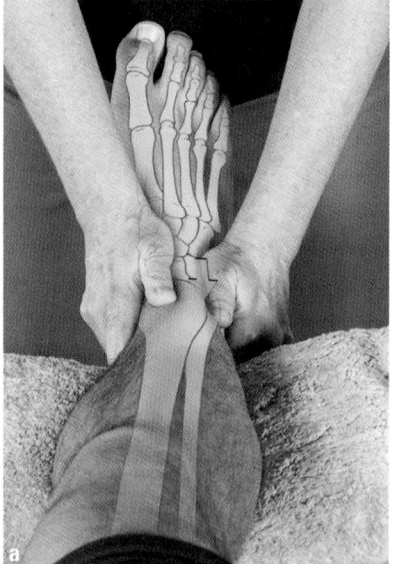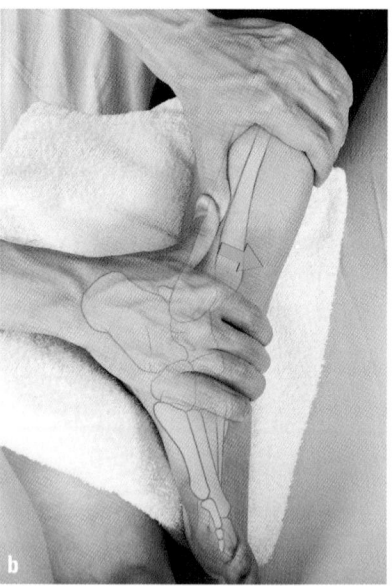

Figure 20.22 *(a)* Posterior glide of distal tibiofemoral joint; *(b)* anterior glide of distal tibiofemoral joint.

the thumbs are placed over the lateral malleolus and distal fibula. The weight of the limb on the table is enough to stabilize the tibia.

Mobilization Application: For an AP mobilization, a posterior glide is performed using a downward movement of the lateral hand (figure 20.22*a*). For a PA mobilization, the anterior force is applied perpendicular to the plane of the distal tibiofibular joint (figure 20.22*b*).

Notations: During ankle dorsiflexion, the distal fibula normally moves superiorly and rotates medially relative to the tibia. During ankle plantar flexion, the distal fibula moves in the opposite directions. Normal ankle motion depends on good fibular mobility. Restriction of joint play between the fibula and tibia may require fibular mobilization in both AP and PA directions to restore normal motion.

Talocrural Joint

There are several joints throughout the ankle and foot. The talocrural joint is the true ankle joint, allowing dorsiflexion (flexion) and plantar flexion (extension) motions. The following sections present some of the most commonly used joint mobilization techniques for this joint.

Distraction

Joint: Talocrural.

Resting Position: 10° plantar flexion.

Indications: To increase general joint play in the ankle joint; can also be used with lower grades of mobilization to relieve pain.

Patient Position: Supine with knee and hip extended.

Clinician and Hand Positions: The rehabilitation clinician stands with the back to the patient's head and faces the foot, grasping the top of the ankle with both hands, intertwining or overlapping the fingers of the two hands around the foot (figure 20.23a).

Mobilization Application: Clinician leans forward to apply a distraction force.

Notations: This technique is also used to assist in relaxation before the application of grade III and IV mobilization techniques. An alternative technique is with the clinician at the foot of the patient, facing the patient. The clinician grasps the foot's dorsum with both hands, again intertwining the fingers and the thumbs on the plantar foot. The clinician leans backward to apply the distraction force (figure 20.23b).

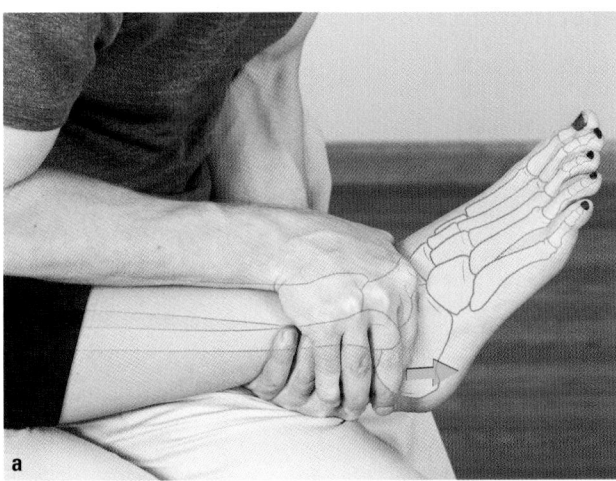 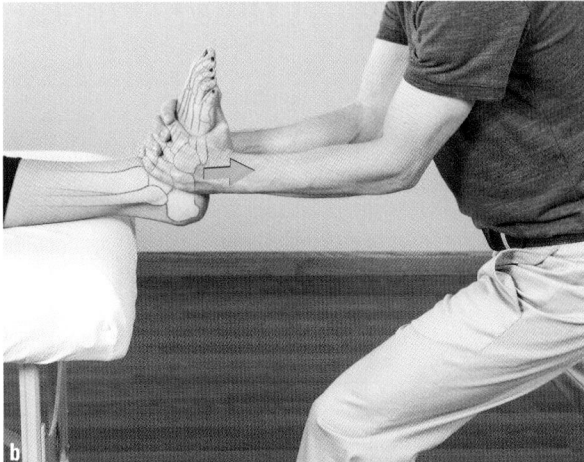

Figure 20.23   Talocrural joint distraction. (a) Joint distraction technique using a pushing force; (b) joint distraction technique using a pulling force.

Anterior Glide

Joint: Talocrural.

Resting Position: 10° plantar flexion.

Indications: Restricted plantar flexion.

Patient Position: Supine with knee extended and ankle over the end of the table.

Clinician and Hand Positions: Clinician faces the foot. The stabilizing hand is placed anteriorly around the distal leg, with the thumb and index finger in contact with the inferior aspect of the adjacent malleoli. The mobilizing hand is placed around the superior aspect of the heel.

Mobilization Application: The talus is glided anteriorly in the plane of the joint (figure 20.24a).

Notations: Also known as a dorsal glide or PA movement. This technique may be performed with the patient prone (figure 20.24b).

>continued

Anterior Glide *>continued*

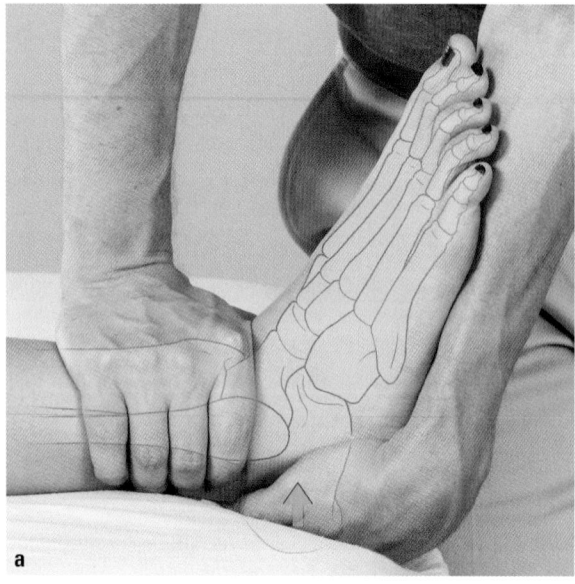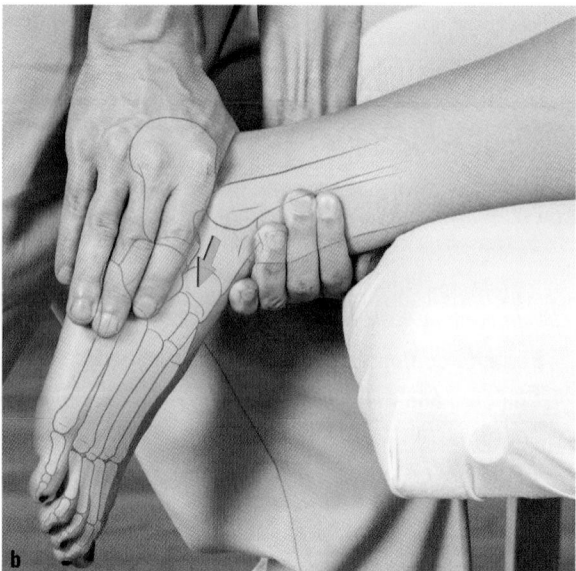

Figure 20.24   Anterior talar glides. *(a)* With the patient supine; *(b)* with the patient prone.

Anterior Glide of Tibia in Weight Bearing

Joint: Talocrural.

Resting Position: 10° plantar flexion.

Indications: Restricted dorsiflexion.

Patient Position: The patient stands in a forward–backward stride position on a treatment table with the treated extremity ahead of the uninvolved extremity. A mobilization strap is secured around the distal tibia and fibula and the clinician's hips, and it is then adjusted for a comfortable length.

Clinician and Hand Positions: Clinician places the web of the thumb and index finger of the stabilizing hands around the anterior ankle joint and stands in a forward–backward stride position.

Figure 20.25

Mobilization Application: With knees partially flexed, the clinician uses the hips to pull the strap forward, moving body weight from front to back leg (figure 20.25).

Notations: This method is an alternative to the one described for figure 20.24. The strap provides additional mechanical leverage. In this technique, the concave mortise is being mobilized over a stabilized convex calcaneus, so the glide and joint movement are in the same direction.

Posterior Glide

Joint: Talocrural.

Resting Position: 10° plantar flexion.

Indications: Restricted dorsiflexion.

Patient Position: Supine with knee extended and ankle over the end of the table with a rolled towel under the distal leg for comfort.

Clinician and Hand Positions: The clinician faces the foot. The stabilizing hand is placed posteriorly around the distal leg at the level of the malleoli, and the mobilizing hand is placed around the proximal dorsal foot with the thumb and index finger adjacent to the distal aspect of the malleoli.

Mobilization Application: The talus is glided posteriorly in the plane of the joint (figure 20.26).

Notations: Also known as a ventral glide or AP glide.

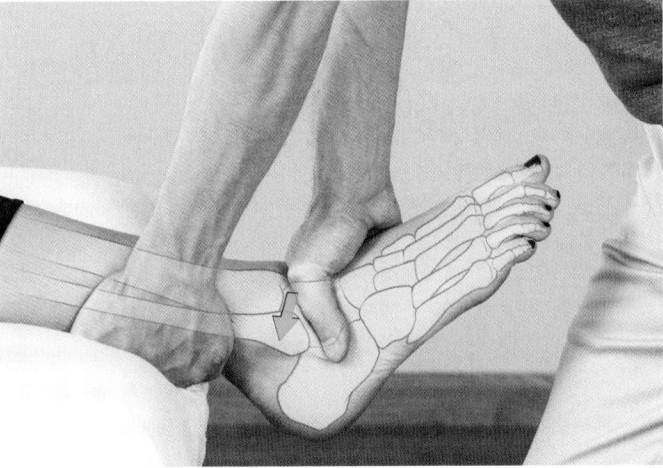

Figure 20.26

Subtalar Joint

The subtalar joint allows for both inversion and eversion movements, which are combined with multiplanar motions of this and other foot joints to permit ambulation on uneven surfaces without injury. Some, but not all, mobilization techniques for the subtalar joint are presented in the following sections. Hand positions for some of these techniques, such as distraction, are only subtly different from those for talocrural mobilization, but these distinctions are important.

Distraction

Joint: Subtalar.

Resting Position: Midway between extreme positions of inversion and eversion.

Indications: To improve general mobility.

Patient Position: Patient is supine or prone with the foot over the end of the table.

Clinician and Hand Positions: Clinician faces the foot. The stabilizing hand grasps the talus anteriorly, and the mobilizing hand cups the posterior calcaneus (figure 20.27).

Mobilization Application: The calcaneus is pulled distally along the long axis of the extremity.

Notations: This technique can be used to relieve pain and is good to use before and after grade III and IV techniques.

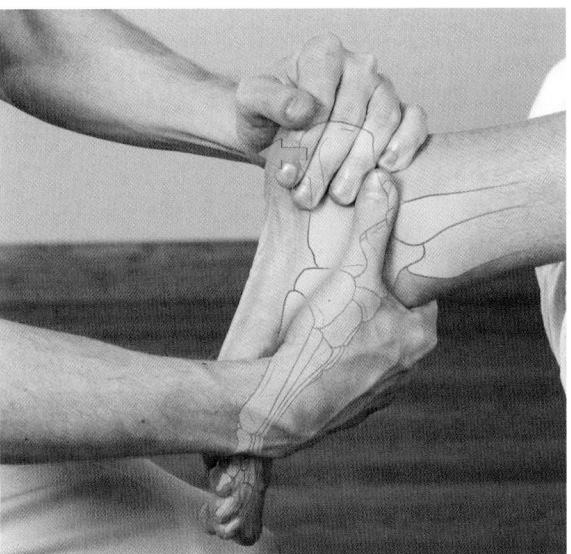

Figure 20.27

Medial Glide

Joint: Subtalar.

Resting Position: Midway between extreme positions of inversion and eversion.

Indications: To increase eversion.

Patient Position: Patient is side-lying on uninvolved extremity. Involved ankle is off the end of the table with a towel roll placed under the distal leg.

Clinician and Hand Positions: The distal leg is stabilized with the cephalic hand over the lateral leg just proximal to the ankle; the caudal hand is cupped around the calcaneus with the fingers and base of the hand on the medial and lateral calcaneus (figure 20.28).

Mobilization Application: A downward medial glide is applied to the calcaneus. Slight traction during the medial glide makes the technique more comfortable for the patient.

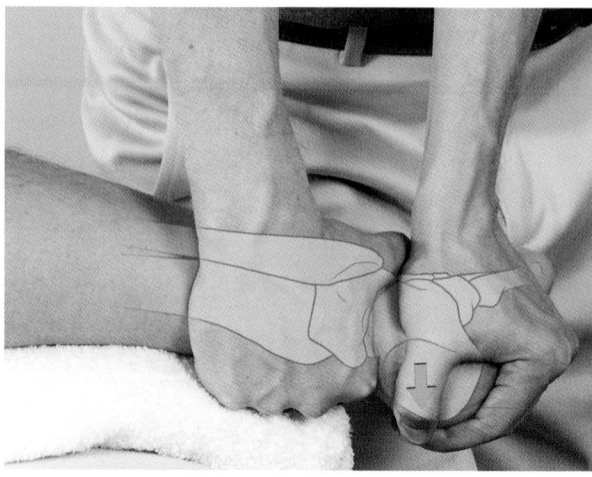

Figure 20.28

Notations: This technique may be applied with the patient in supine, but a downward force on the joint is easier to apply than a lateral-to-medial force that is required with the patient supine.

Lateral Glide

Joint: Subtalar.

Resting Position: Midway between extreme positions of inversion and eversion.

Indications: To increase subtalar inversion.

Patient Position: Patient is side-lying on the involved side. The foot is over the end of the table, and a towel is under the distal leg.

Clinician and Hand Positions: The rehabilitation clinician stabilizes the extremity with the cephalic hand over the medial distal extremity immediately proximal to the malleoli. The mobilizing hand is cupped around the calcaneus with the fingers and base of the hand on the lateral and medial calcaneus (figure 20.29).

Mobilization Application: The force applied occurs directly downward and parallel to the joint surface.

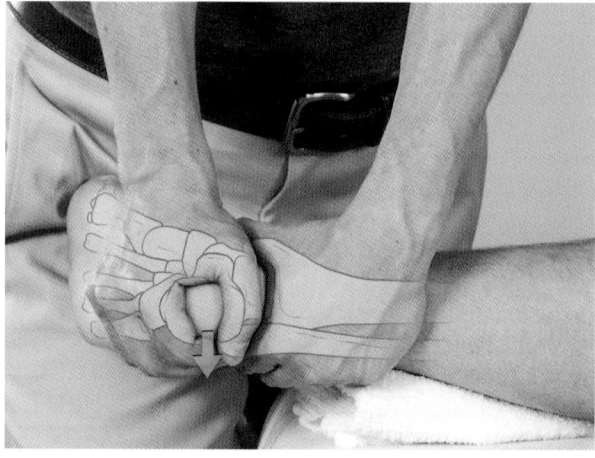

Figure 20.29

Notations: This technique may be applied with the patient in supine, but a downward force on the joint is easier to apply than a medial-to-lateral force that is required with the patient supine.

Intertarsal Joints and Intermetatarsal Joints

Mobilizations can be performed on all intertarsal joints, including the transverse tarsal (talonavicular and calca-neocuboid) and naviculocuneiform joints. Likewise, if restriction between metatarsal joints is apparent, these joints should also be mobilized. Not all of these mobilization techniques will be included in this section, but a couple of examples are presented here.

Anterior Glide

Joint: Talonavicular joint.

Resting Position: Midway between inversion and eversion with 10° plantar flexion.

Indications: To increase midtarsal dorsiflexion and inversion.

Patient Position: Prone with knee flexed to 90°.

Clinician and Hand Positions: Clinician grasps the navicular with the thumb on the plantar surface and the index finger on its dorsal surface. The talus and calcaneus are stabilized with the opposite hand (figure 20.30).

Mobilization Application: The mobilizing hand performs a PA movement of the navicular.

Notations: Weight of the leg helps to stabilize the ankle.

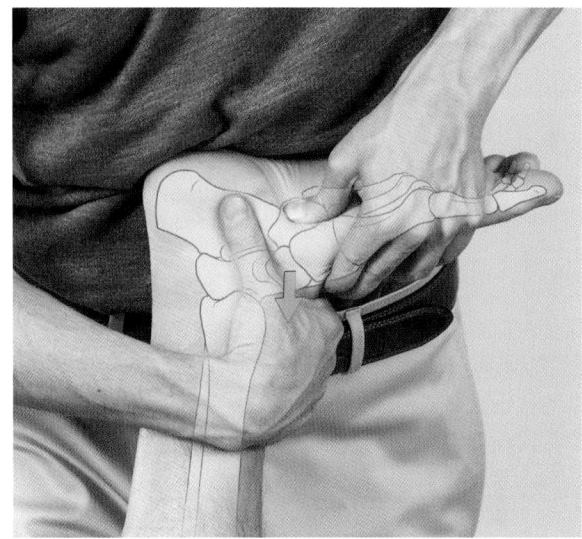

Figure 20.30

Posterior Glide

Joint: Talonavicular joint.

Resting Position: Midway between inversion and eversion with 10° plantar flexion.

Indications: To increase midtarsal plantar flexion and eversion.

Patient Position: Supine.

Clinician and Hand Positions: Clinician stabilizes rearfoot with one hand and places the thumb of the other hand on the navicular's dorsum and the fingers on the plantar aspect of the navicular.

Mobilization Application: Mobilizing hand applies an AP movement in the plane of the joint surface (figure 20.31).

Notations: Placement of the plantar surface of the foot on the table may also be used to stabilize the rearfoot.

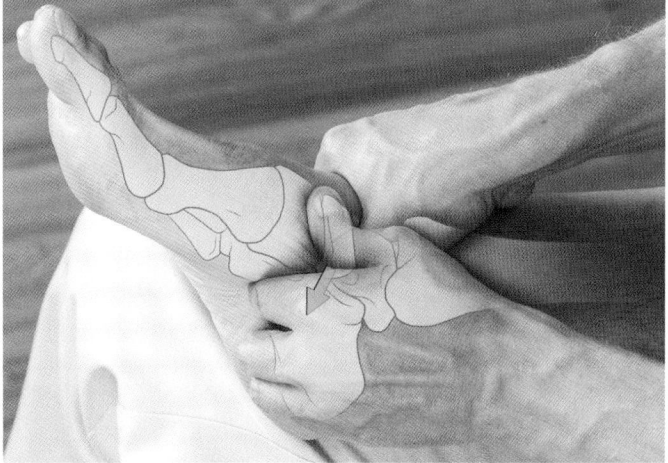

Figure 20.31

Intermetatarsal Joint Anterior and Posterior Glides

Joint: Intermetatarsal joints.

Resting Position: Undefined.

Indications: To increase intermetatarsal mobility.

Patient Position: Supine on the table with foot extended.

Clinician and Hand Positions: The rehabilitation clinician stabilizes one metatarsal and grasps the adjacent one, with the thumb on the dorsum and the fingers on the plantar aspect.

Mobilization Application: Anteroposterior or posteroanterior force is applied to the metatarsal (figure 20.32).

>continued

Intermetatarsal Joint Anterior and Posterior Glides >continued

Notations: A gross AP and PA glide can also be applied to the intertarsal joints: The proximal tarsal row is stabilized, and the distal row is mobilized in either an anterior or a posterior direction.

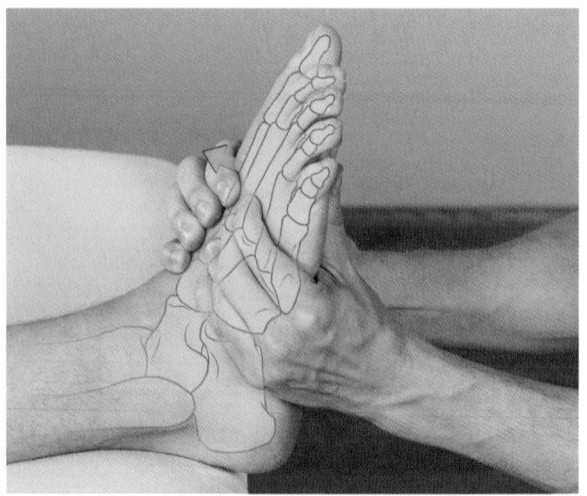

Figure 20.32

Tarsometatarsal, Metatarsophalangeal, and Interphalangeal Joints

Many of the basic hand positions and force applications are the same for these joints, so they are grouped together in the following sections. You must realize, however, that specific finger and hand positions vary according to the joint being mobilized, with the stabilizing fingers on the proximal end of the joint and the mobilizing fingers immediately adjacent to them on the distal bone segment of the joint.

Distraction

Joint: Tarsometatarsal, metatarsophalangeal, and interphalangeal joints.

Resting Position: First toe: 20° dorsiflexion; toes 2 through 5: 20° plantar flexion.

Indications: To enhance general joint mobility and relaxation.

Patient Position: Patient is relaxed, supine on the table with pad under ankle and foot off the end of the table.

Clinician and Hand Positions: Phalanx is grasped with the thumb and fingers while the metatarsal is stabilized with the opposite hand (figure 20.33).

Mobilization Application: Distraction force is applied to the phalanx.

Notations: May also be used before and after grade II and III joint mobilization techniques.

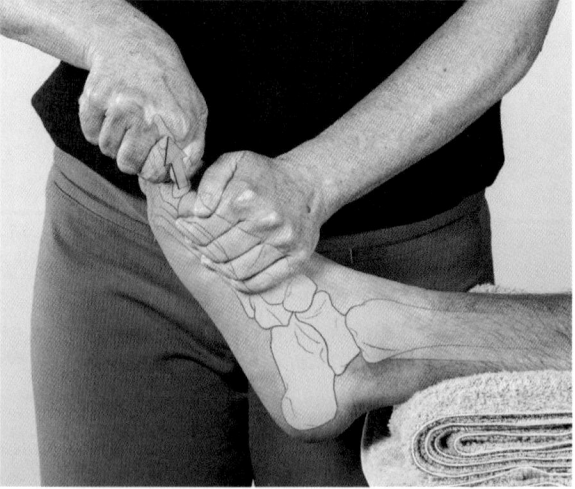

Figure 20.33

Anterior and Posterior Glides

Joint: Tarsometatarsal, metatarsophalangeal, and interphalangeal joints.

Resting Position: First toe: 20° dorsiflexion; toes 2 through 5: 20° plantar flexion.

Indications: Anterior (dorsal) glides increase extension of these joints. Posterior (ventral or plantar) glides increase flexion of these joints.

Patient Position: Patient is comfortable with foot over end of the table and a pad under the distal leg.

Clinician and Hand Positions: For the MTP and tarsometatarsal joints, the metatarsal is stabilized with one hand while the mobilizing hand grasps the proximal phalanx. For the IP joints, the proximal phalanx is stabilized by the clinician's fingers and thumb.

Mobilization Application: For MTP and tarsometatarsal joints, an AP or a PA glide is applied. For IP joints, the mobilizing force is applied to the base of the distal phalanx while the head of the proximal phalanx is stabilized (figures 20.34a, b).

Notations: Slight traction is simultaneously applied to provide more comfort for the patient.

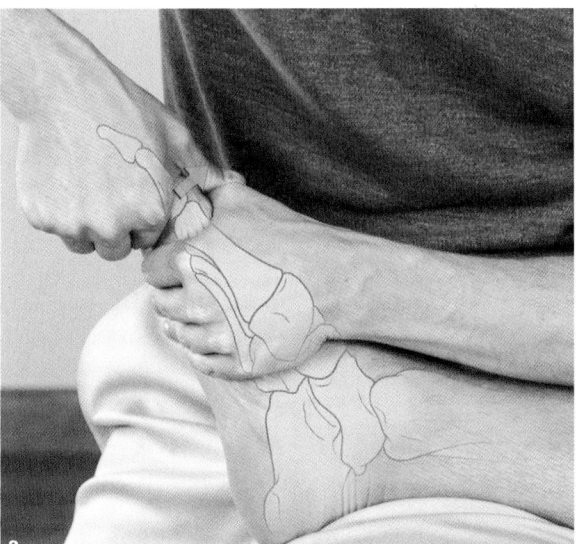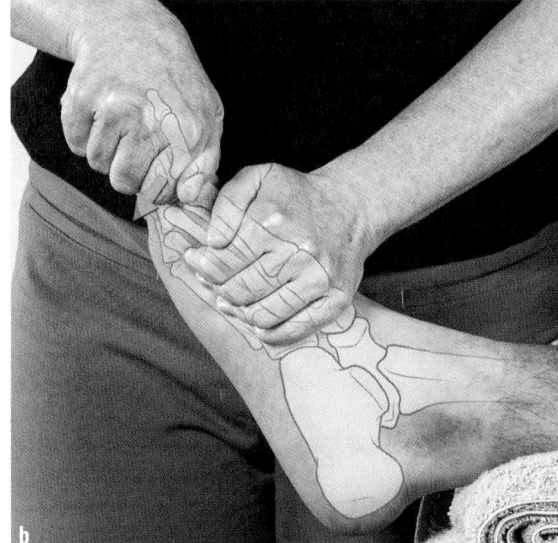

Figure 20.34   *(a)* Anterior (dorsal or PA) glide; and *(b)* posterior (plantar or AP) glide.

Sesamoid Glides

Joint: Sesamoids.

Resting Position: First toe: 20° dorsiflexion; toes 2 through 5: 20° plantar flexion.

Indications: These bones may become restricted in their mobility, resulting in a reduced ability to protect the first MTP from excessive forces while standing on the toes. Excessive or prolonged edema in the foot accompanied by immobilization after foot or ankle injuries may lead to reduced mobility of the sesamoids.

Patient Position: Patient is comfortable in supine, with foot over the end of the table and a pad under the distal leg.

Clinician and Hand Positions: The distal first metatarsal is stabilized with one hand while the mobilizing hand locates the medial and lateral sesamoids just behind the metatarsal head.

Mobilization Application: The clinician applies a distal glide to the proximal end of the sesamoid to move it through its available range of motion (figure 20.35).

Notations: Do not compress the sesamoid into the metatarsal.

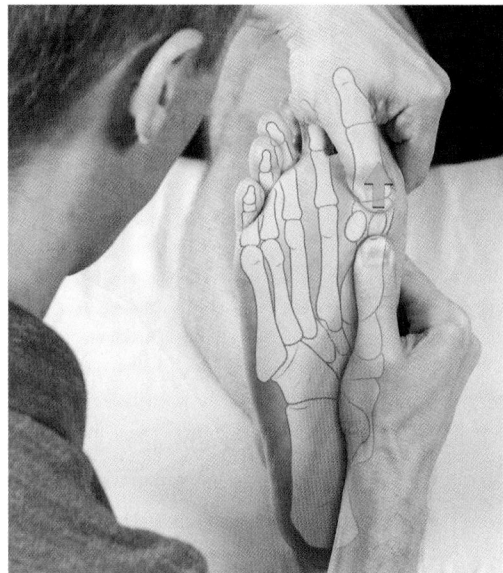

Figure 20.35

Flexibility Exercises

This section includes detailed information on some of the more commonly used techniques for improving ankle and foot flexibility. As with most exercises, the rehabilitation clinician must have knowledge of the body's mechanics, the muscle's function, and the appropriate application of forces to identify effective flexibility exercises for a patient's rehabilitation program.

Although there are some exceptions, based on available evidence that was presented in chapter 12, active flexibility exercises should be held for 10 to 30 s and performed for 1 to 4 repetitions.[126, 127] Patients with less-than-normal flexibility should repeat the exercises often throughout the day.

Flexibility Exercises for the Foot and Ankle

Exercises in this section include a number of stretching exercises. Once the patient can accurately perform the exercises without verbal or tactile cues, they can be included in the home exercise program.

Standing Stretch

Body Segment: Gastrocnemius.

Stage in Rehab: Active phase.

Purpose: Increase flexibility of gastrocnemius.

Positioning: The patient is in a forward–backward straddle position with the extremity to be stretched behind the contralateral extremity.

Execution: The patient places his or her body weight on the hands, which are on the wall and on the front foot, while the back extremity remains extended at the knee. The heels remain in contact with the floor, the hip should be forward of the knee, and the foot should be behind the knee and in a straight line, or the toes may be turned slightly inward (figure 20.36).

Possible Substitutions: Common substitutions are allowing the midfoot to collapse by rotating the foot outward, lifting the heel off the floor, bending the knee, and moving the hip posteriorly.

Notations: Because the gastrocnemius extends from above the knee to the calcaneus, both the knee and ankle joints must be placed on stretch to effectively stretch the muscle.

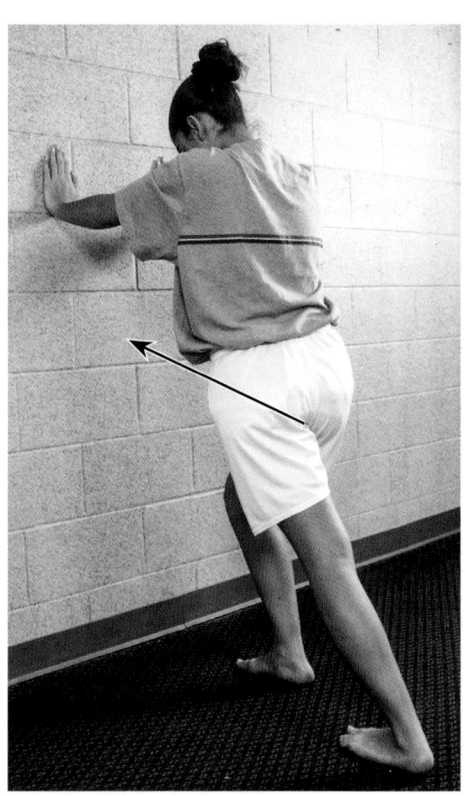

Figure 20.36

Seated Stretch

Body Segment: Gastrocnemius.

Stage in Rehab: Active phase.

Purpose: Increase gastrocnemius flexibility.

Positioning: With the patient in a long sitting position, a stretch strap or towel is hooked around the plantar forefoot.

Execution: Keeping the knee straight, the patient pulls on the strap or towel to dorsiflex the ankle. Additional stretch can be applied with active contraction of the ankle dorsiflexors.

Possible Substitutions: Hip rotation and foot pronation.

Notations: If the patient is non–weight bearing, he or she can use this gastrocnemius stretch to increase flexibility until weight bearing is permitted.

Standing Stretch

Body Segment: Soleus.

Stage in Rehab: Active phase.

Purpose: Increase soleus flexibility.

Positioning: In the standing position, the patient is in a position similar to that described for the gastrocnemius. With the involved extremity behind the uninvolved extremity, he or she keeps the foot flat on the floor with the foot turned slightly inward.

Execution: Patient slowly flexes the knee until a stretch is felt deep in the calf (figure 20.37).

Possible Substitutions: Outward rotation of the foot, knee valgus positioning, and posterior movement of the hip as the knee is flexed.

Notations: Because the soleus does not cross the knee joint, to isolate this muscle the stretch should be applied with the knee flexed. This eliminates the stretch on the gastrocnemius and isolates the stretch to the soleus.

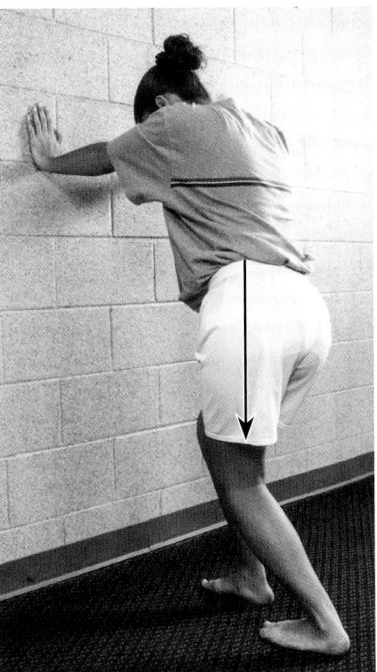

Figure 20.37

Seated Soleus Stretch

Body Segment: Soleus.

Stage in Rehab: Active phase.

Purpose: Increase soleus motion.

Positioning: If partial weight bearing, patient can perform this exercise in sitting with the feet on the floor. Forefoot is on a half foam roller, and the heel is off the roller. If the patient is non–weight bearing, a strap is placed around the forefoot with the knee in partial flexion.

Execution: For the partial-weight-bearing stretch, the patient pushes the heel to the floor until a stretch is felt in the distal calf (figure 20.38*a*). For the non-weight-bearing stretch, the patient pulls on the strap to move the ankle into dorsiflexion until a stretch in the lower calf is felt (figure 20.38*b*).

Possible Substitutions: Increasing knee flexion rather than ankle dorsiflexion and placing the strap too proximal on the foot to apply an effective stretch force.

Notations: Since the soleus does not cross the knee joint, the stretch should be applied with the knee flexed to eliminate the stretch to the gastrocnemius and to isolate the stretch to the soleus.

>continued

Seated Soleus Stretch *>continued*

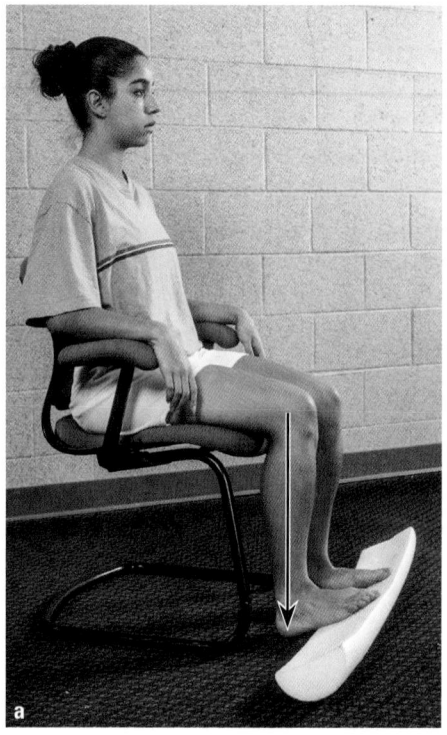

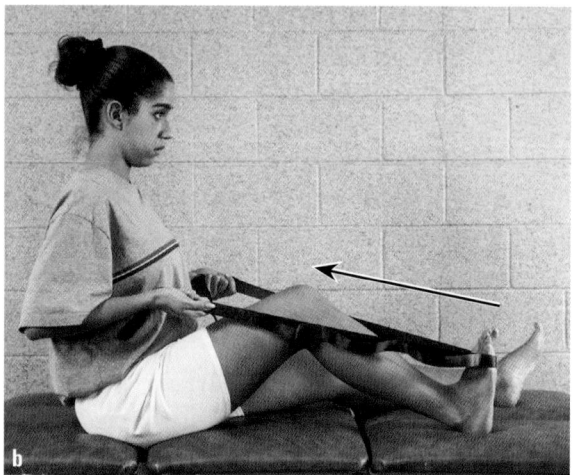

Figure 20.38

Prolonged Achilles Stretch

Body Segment: Achilles.

Stage in Rehab: Late active phase and early resistive phase.

Purpose: Improve mobility of Achilles tendon.

Positioning: The patient stands with the back to a wall. The feet are positioned on an incline (figure 20.39a) or the balls of the feet are placed on the edge of a book or wood block (figure 20.39b), with the heel no more than 2.5 cm (1 in.) from the wall. A towel roll is placed between the posterior knees and the wall to prevent knee hyperextension.

Execution: The patient stands in this position for a prolonged period, at least 5 min and as much as 20 min, if tolerable. It is useful to place a chair next to the patient so that he or she can place the hands on the back of the chair for stabilization and support. The hips should remain in contact with the wall throughout the stretch.

Possible Substitutions: Common substitutions are standing with the feet in pronation, standing too far away from the wall, and hyperextension of the knees. Some people try to stretch the Achilles or gastrocnemius on the edge of a step. This is ineffective because the very muscle that is being stretched is simultaneously contracting to maintain balance.

Notations: The Achilles tendon is the largest and strongest tendon of the body.[128] Collagen, especially Type I collagen, is the main component of any tendon,[129] and it provides the tendon with its durability and strength.[130] Given the size of the Achilles tendon and its collagen content, it would seem that a prolonged stretch would be effective for increasing motion. There have been few studies involving prolonged stretches beyond 90 s to identify the optimal duration of stretch to achieve length gains in the Achilles tendon; however, one study investigating this topic used a prolonged stretch of 10 min to produce an increase in Achilles length.[131] This topic requires additional investigation. When using a prolonged stretch, the clinician should warn the patient that once the stretch is released, the patient commonly feels stiffness in the posterior calf or ankle area, but this should subside quickly.

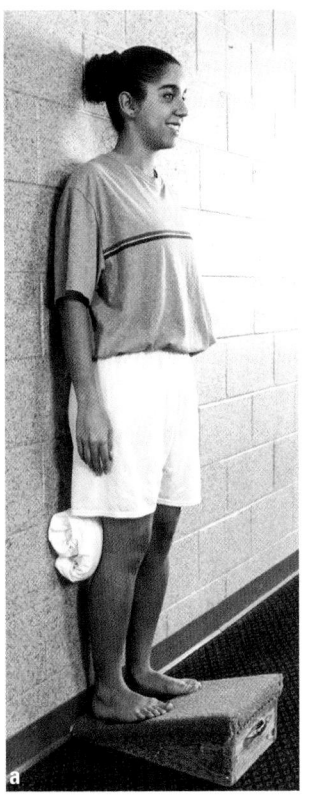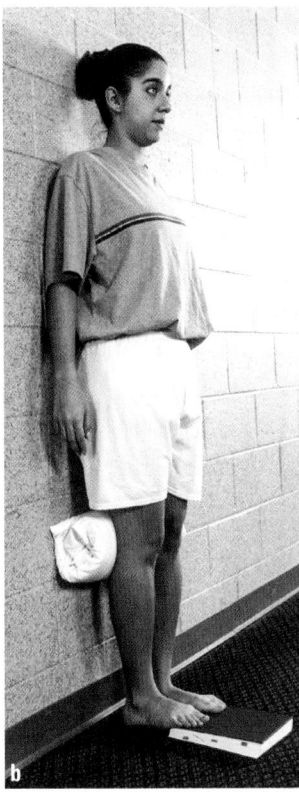

Figure 20.39

Ankle Dorsiflexor Stretch

Body Segment: Ankle dorsiflexors.

Stage in Rehab: Later active phase.

Purpose: Increase ankle plantar-flexion motion.

Positioning: Patient begins in a quadruped position.

Execution: With the dorsum of the feet in contact with the floor, the patient pushes hips back toward heels as far as tolerable. If there are no knee injuries, patient should be able to sit on the ankles. In this position, the anterior ankle should be flat on the floor (figure 20.40).

Possible Substitutions: Keeping the ankle in a flexed position, and rotating the limbs so the feet are not directly in line with the tibias.

Notations: With very tight ankles, full weight bearing onto the ankles in this position may be too uncomfortable. A less aggressive stretch can be performed in standing, using a foam roller. The patient places the dorsum of the foot on the foam roller on the floor and pushes the ankle downward toward the floor. If the patient has a history of knee problems, the sitting position should be avoided.

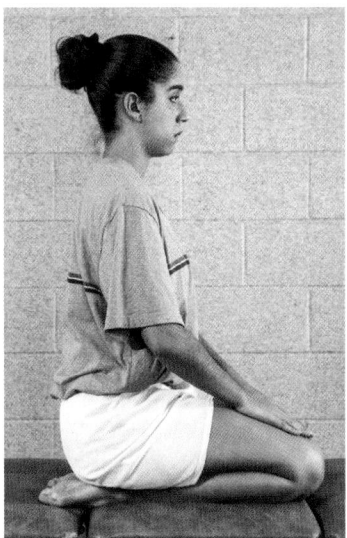

Figure 20.40

Active Ankle Pumps, Alphabet, and Toe Exercises

Body Segment: Ankle, foot, and toes.

Stage in Rehab: End of active phase and early resistive phase.

Purpose: Improve flexibility of ankle, foot, and toes.

Positioning: Patient can perform these exercises in sitting.

Execution: Leaving the heel on the floor for ankle pumps, the patient moves the ankle from plantar flexion to dorsiflexion, going through as much motion as possible with each repetition. In another active-motion exercise, the patient spells the alphabet with the toes and foot while keeping the heel on the floor. These exercises are used as a home exercise program with instructions to perform them throughout the day.

Possible Substitutions: Using the leg or hip rather than the ankle and toes to perform the motions.

Notations: These are general, active exercises that the patient can perform independently throughout the day to increase ankle motion. These exercises can also be performed with the ankle elevated, and they can help reduce edema.

BAPS Board

The BAPS board, or Biomechanical Ankle Proprioception System (Spectrum Therapy Products, Adrian, MI), is used to increase ankle mobility, proprioception, and strength.[132, 133] It consists of a board or platform and various sizes of half-balls to which the platform is attached. The size of half-ball selected for an exercise depends on the patient's range of motion and the goal of the exercise. Patients may begin by sitting in a chair, placing the involved foot on the board, performing active range-of-motion exercises. They can advance to weight bearing on two extremities and then weight bearing on only the involved extremity to perform full range-of-motion exercises with the ankle (figure 20.41). Once the patient has attained full range of motion and control on the BAPS board, you can add weights to the board to provide resistance to specific muscle groups. In an example of using the BAPS board as a proprioception exercise device, the patient stands on

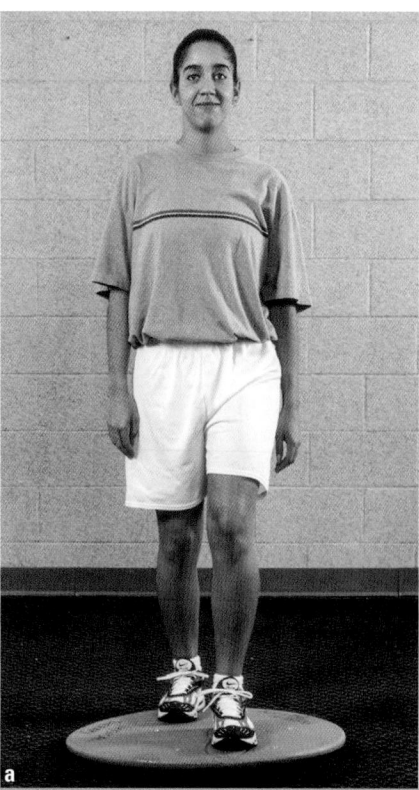
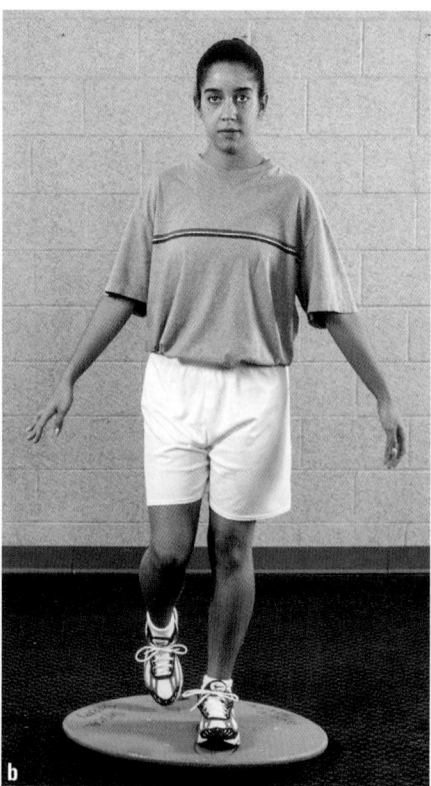

Figure 20.41 BAPS board: *(a)* double-limb support, *(b)* single-limb support.

only the involved limb and slowly performs controlled isolated motions of inversion–eversion or plantar flexion–dorsiflexion.

Additional Active-Motion Exercises

Cardiovascular equipment that can be used to improve ankle range of motion while building cardiovascular fitness includes stationary bikes (figure 20.42) and cross-country ski machines. These types of machines help improve range of motion in the ankle, especially when the patient has

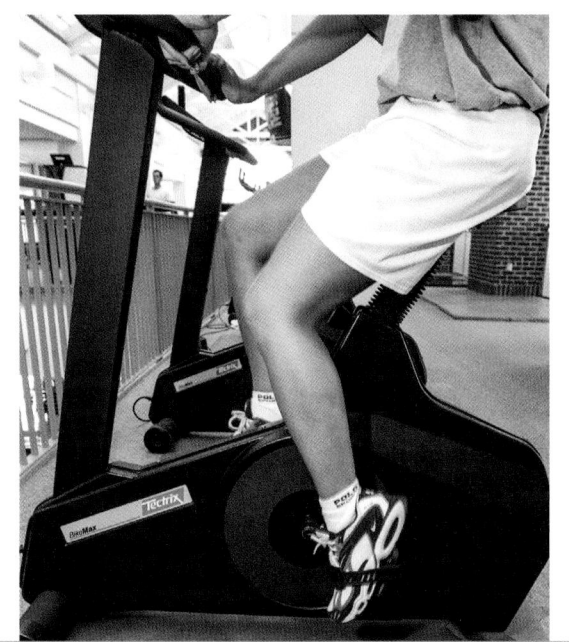

Figure 20.42 A stationary bike is an example of a cardiovascular machine that may be used to promote ankle range of motion.

received careful instruction in performing the exercise properly. You should teach the patient *ankling* on the bike: dorsiflexing the ankle on extremity lift and plantar flexing the ankle on the downstroke. On the cross-country ski machine, the patient should try to push off from the posterior extremity by lifting the heel and bearing weight on the ball of the foot before pulling the extremity and ankle forward and upward.

> ## CLINICAL TIPS
>
> There are many flexibility exercises for the ankle, foot, and leg. Among those often used are gastrocnemius, soleus, and Achilles stretches; ankle exercises the patient can do throughout the day; and BAPS board exercises.

Strengthening Exercises

Strengthening exercises that can be used earliest in a rehabilitation program include isometrics. The patient can perform these even while the foot is in a cast, boot, or immobilizer. Normal strength progression may begin with isometrics and progress to isotonics and then to isokinetics. Isotonic exercises include those that use resistance bands, free weights, machine weights, and body resistance. Isokinetic exercises are usually not included in the rehabilitation program until the patient's foot and ankle have enough strength to control isotonic activities and the patient is near the end of the resistive phase or entering into the advanced phase. The following sections provide examples of a few of the more commonly used strength exercises for the ankle, foot, and toes in the early part of the resistive phase of the rehabilitation program.

Early Strength Exercises for the Foot and Ankle

As with other body segments, strength exercises for the foot and ankle begin with isometric exercises and progress to more difficult exercises as the body segment moves through the healing process. Since the intrinsic muscles of the foot are responsible for stability,[134, 135] a rehabilitation program should include exercises to restore their strength. Intrinsic muscle exercises are performed with high repetitions because of the repetitive functions these muscles perform during lower-extremity activities.[36] Each of the intrinsic exercises listed next should be performed anywhere from 40 repetitions with a 3 s hold[136] to over 100 repetitions throughout the day.[137] As the patient improves, the exercise progression for the intrinsic muscles moves from the patient in a sitting position, to bilateral standing, and finally to unilateral standing to perform the exercises.[138]

    Body Segment: Foot intrinsic muscles.

    Stage in Rehab: Late active to early resistive.

    Purpose: Strengthen foot intrinsic muscles.

    Positioning: Patient sits with involved knee flexed greater than 90° to prevent extrinsic foot muscles from working. Foot rests flat on the floor. Each exercise is performed for 40 to 50 repetitions.

Execution:

1. *Short-foot exercise:* The patient shortens and elevates the medial longitudinal arch by bringing the heads of the metatarsals toward the calcaneus without flexing the toes or contracting the gastroc-soleus (figure 20.43a).

2. *Toe spread exercise:* The patient extends all the toes and spreads them apart and then, while keeping the toes in abduction, the patient pushes the great toe outward and away from the foot so it touches the floor. While holding the toes in this position, the patient then moves the fifth toe outward and down so it touches the floor (figure 20.43b).

3. *Great toe extension exercise:* The patient begins by flexing all metatarsal heads so all toes begin on the floor. The patient then extends the great toe, lifting it off the floor, while flexing the other metatarsal heads to keep the other toes on the floor (figure 20.43c).

4. *Lateral toe extension exercise:* The patient begins by flexing all metatarsal heads so all toes begin on the floor. The patient then extends the four lateral toes, lifting them off the floor, while flexing the first metatarsal head to keep the great toe on the floor (figure 20.43d).

Possible Substitutions: Using the extrinsic muscles to perform the exercises rather than the intrinsic muscles.

Notations: Some of these exercises can be difficult to perform. If the patient cannot perform the exercise correctly, the clinician passively positions the foot and toes and instructs the patient to hold the position for 3 to 5 s. Repetitions of this passively positioned exercise occur until the patient can actively perform the exercise without the clinician's assistance.

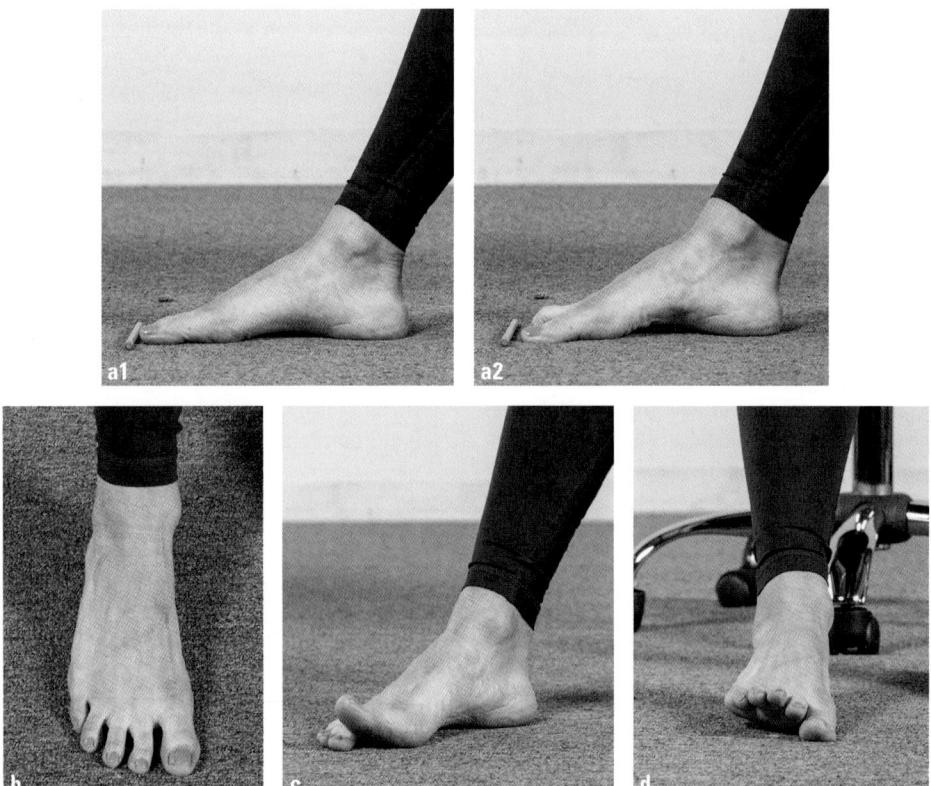

Figure 20.43 Foot intrinsic exercises: *(a)* short-foot exercise *(a1)* start position and *(a2)* end position; *(b)* toe spread exercise; *(c)* great toe extension exercise; and *(d)* lesser toe extension exercise.

Isometric Inversion

Body Segment: Subtalar joint.

Stage in Rehab: Late active and early resistive.

Purpose: Strengthen ankle inverters.

Positioning: Patient sits with the medial aspect of the foot against a table leg.

Execution: Patient pushes the medial foot against the table leg, trying to invert the ankle. The ankle does not move, and the patient should feel muscles working on the medial leg. The patient may also perform the isometric exercise by placing the medial aspects of the feet together and applying an inversion force with the involved foot against the uninvolved foot.

Possible Substitutions: Hip abduction, hip rotation, and tibial rotation.

Notations: Isometrics are held at the maximum contraction for 6 s[139] with a slow buildup and release of the force so that the total contraction is about 10 s long.

Isometric Eversion

Body Segment: Subtalar joint.

Stage in Rehab: Late active phase to early resistive phases.

Purpose: Strengthen peroneals.

Positioning: Patient sits with the lateral aspect of the foot against a table leg.

Execution: Patient pushes the lateral foot against the table leg, trying to evert the ankle. The ankle does not move, and the patient should feel muscles working on the lateral leg. The patient may also sit with the ankles crossed with the involved ankle over the uninvolved ankle, pushing it into eversion against the uninvolved ankle.

Possible Substitutions: Hip abduction, hip rotation, and tibial rotation.

Notations: Isometrics are held at the maximum contraction for 6 s,[139] with a slow buildup and release of the force so that the total contraction is about 10 s long.

Isometric Dorsiflexion

Body Segment: Talocrural joint.

Stage in Rehab: Late active to early resistive.

Purpose: Strengthen dorsiflexor muscles, especially tibialis anterior.

Positioning: Patient sits with uninvolved heel on top of the involved foot.

Execution: The patient pushes the involved foot upward against the top foot, trying to dorsiflex the ankle against the opposite foot (figure 20.44).

Possible Substitutions: Hip flexion and foot eversion.

Notations: Isometrics are held at the maximum contraction for 6 s,[139] with a slow buildup and release of the force so that the total contraction is about 10 s long.

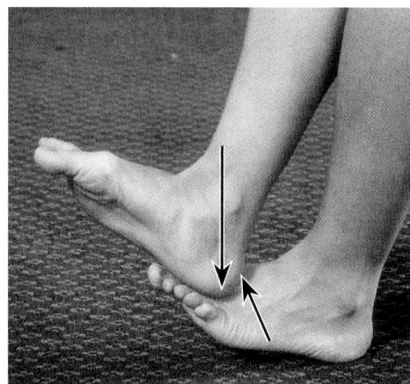

Figure 20.44 Isometric ankle dorsiflexion

Resistance-Band Exercises

Because the various ankle muscle groups have different strengths, you must examine the patient's strength for each exercise before determining which band's resistance is most appropriate to obtain the desired results from the resistive exercise. Normally, ankle plantar flexors are the strongest, and ankle evertors are the weakest.[140] Injured ankles have reduced levels of strength in all motions, but most of the time, the proportional strength remains close to normal.[141] In other words, even though a patient's ankle may have less-than-normal strength, the plantar flexors are still the strongest muscle group and the ankle evertors the weakest. Resistance-band exercises are included in the following sections.

Resistance-Band Eversion

Body Segment: Subtalar joint.

Stage in Rehab: Early resistive phase.

Purpose: Strengthen evertors.

Positioning: The patient sits in a chair, with the band around the forefoot and anchored to a table leg or door jamb at the lateral side of the uninvolved extremity.

Execution: The ankle begins in inversion and is moved against the band into a full range of eversion (figure 20.45a).

Possible Substitutions: Hip abduction and medial rotation and tibial lateral rotation. To eliminate substitutions, you should instruct the patient in the proper technique and caution against moving the knee. Placing the hands on either side of the knee to stabilize the thigh also reduces substitutions.

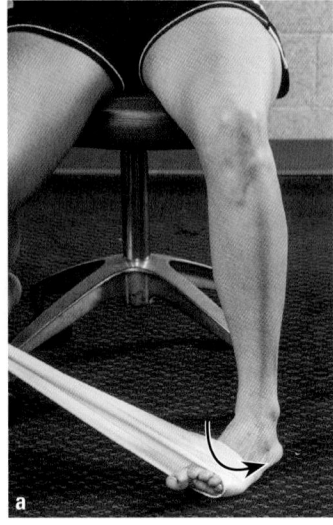
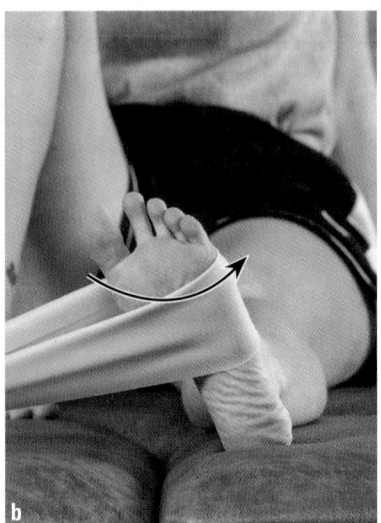
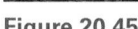

Figure 20.45

Notations: These exercises can also be performed with either manual resistance or pulleys. The patient can perform this exercise in a long sitting position, but it is more difficult to stabilize the thigh and avoid hip substitutions in this position (figure 20.45b).

Resistance-Band Inversion

Body Segment: Subtalar joint.

Stage in Rehab: Early resistive phase.

Purpose: Strengthen ankle inverters.

Positioning: The patient sits in a chair with the band around the forefoot and anchored to a table leg or door jamb lateral to the involved side.

Execution: Patient starts with the ankle in full eversion and moves it into a full range of motion to end-range inversion (figure 20.46).

Possible Substitutions: Hip adduction and lateral rotation and tibial medial rotation. To eliminate substitutions, you should instruct the patient in the proper technique and caution against moving the knee. Placing the hands on either side of the knee to stabilize the thigh also reduces substitutions.

Notations: These exercises can also be performed with either manual resistance or pulleys. The patient can perform this exercise in a long sitting position, but it is more difficult to stabilize the thigh and avoid hip substitutions in this position.

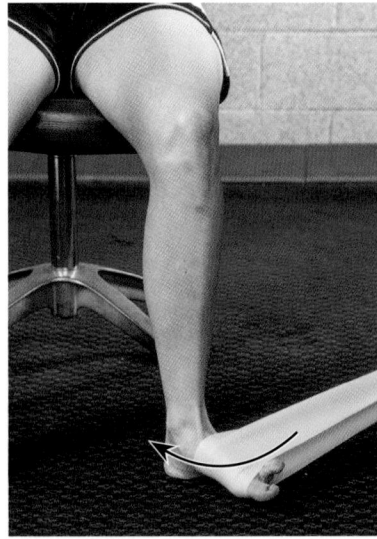

Figure 20.46

Resistance-Band Dorsiflexion

Body Segment: Talocrural joint.

Stage in Rehab: Early resistive phase.

Purpose: Increase strength of dorsiflexors.

Positioning: The patient sits with the band around the forefoot and anchored to a table leg or door jamb, which the patient faces.

Execution: The patient pulls the foot toward the shin, dorsiflexing the ankle (figure 20.47).

Possible Substitutions: Hip or knee flexion is the most common substitution.

Notations: These exercises can also be performed with either manual resistance or pulleys.

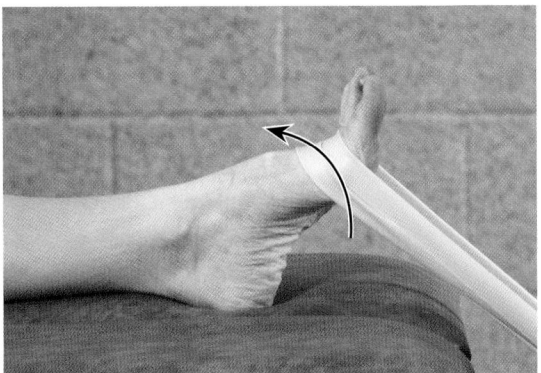

Figure 20.47

Resistance-Band Plantar Flexion

Body Segment: Talocrural joint.

Stage in Rehab: Early resistive phase.

Purpose: Strengthen ankle plantar flexors when patient is non–weight bearing.

Positioning: The patient is in a long sitting position with the band grasped in both hands and wrapped around the plantar foot.

Execution: Patient maintains a firm tension on the band. Starting with the foot in full dorsiflexion, the patient pushes the foot against the band to move the ankle into full plantar flexion (figure 20.48).

Possible Substitutions: Going through an incomplete range of motion.

Notations: This exercise can also be performed with the knee in flexion and the patient sitting on a table with his or her extremity hanging off the table. In this position, plantar-flexion motion isolates and strengthens the soleus muscle. If the patient has good strength in the early ranges of plantar flexion but cannot stand in full plantar flexion, the band can be used to facilitate strength in the weak part of the motion. To do this, the patient places the foot in the weak range of motion and positions the band around the plantar foot. While the patient maintains this ankle position, he or she increases tension on the band by pulling on it with the arms to provide the resistance in the weak position. Keeping good tension on the band, the patient slowly dorsiflexes the ankle to facilitate an eccentric contraction of the plantar flexors. This technique can be used to isolate weak portions of motion in the other positions as well.

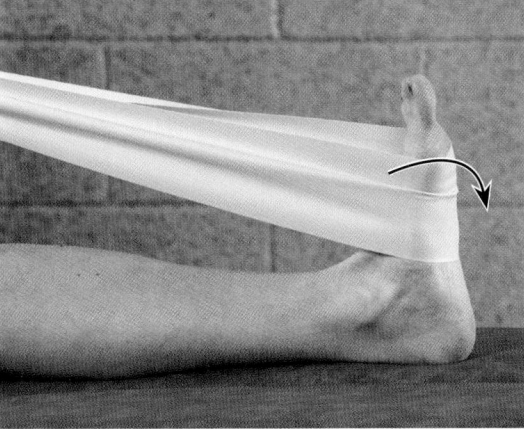

Figure 20.48

Toe Exercises

Strengthening toe muscles helps to restore optimal foot function. Both intrinsic and extrinsic toe muscles are strengthened with these exercises. Since they cross the ankle, the long toe muscles contribute to ankle support.[142]

Intrinsic muscles provide balance and stability.[143] Since both intrinsic and extrinsic toe muscles are important for normal function, some exercises for these muscle groups are presented in the following sections.

Towel Roll

Body Segment: Toes.

Stage in Rehab: Late active phase to early resistive phase.

Purpose: Strengthen toe flexors.

Positioning: The patient sits with a towel placed on the floor in front of the patient's feet.

Execution: Without shoes and socks on, the patient curls the toes of the involved extremity to pull the towel toward the foot (figure 20.49). As the towel bunches under the arch, the patient moves the gathered towel behind the foot until the toes reach the far end of the towel. The thigh and knee should not move during the exercise.

Possible Substitutions: Using the heel to pull the towel or flexing the knee to pull the towel.

Notations: Resistance can be added by placing a weight at the far end of the towel, using a wet towel, or using a newspaper. This exercise should be performed on a smooth surface such as a wood or vinyl floor, not on carpeting.

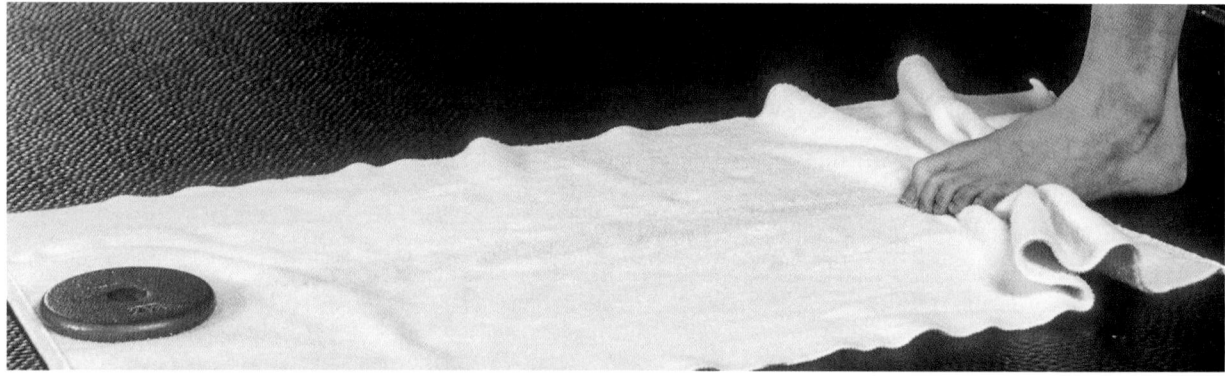

Figure 20.49

Marble Pickup

Body Segment: Toe flexors.

Stage in Rehab: Late active phase to early resistive phase.

Purpose: Strengthen toe intrinsic and extrinsic muscles, facilitate ankle inverters and evertors.

Positioning: Patient is sitting or standing.

Execution: The patient uses the toes to pick up marbles that have been placed on the floor. The marbles are placed in the hand on the same side to facilitate eversion and in the hand on the opposite side to facilitate inversion (figure 20.50).

Possible Substitutions: Not moving the toes or ankle through full motion during the exercise.

Notations: Objects such as a pencil, pieces of paper, or a towel can be used in place of the marbles.

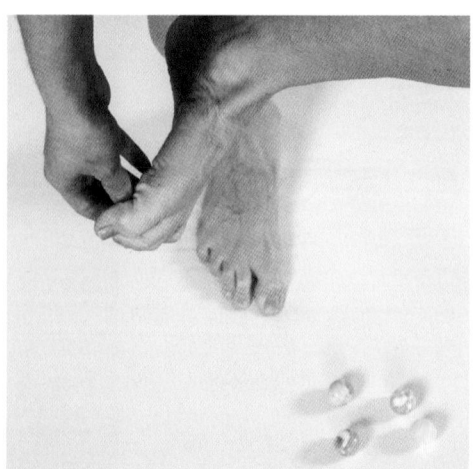

Figure 20.50

Body-Weight Resistance Exercises

Exercises for both the gastrocnemius and soleus are needed for complete restoration of plantar flexion strength. Body weight is an excellent form of resistance that strengthens many body segments, including the ankle and foot. These exercises are introduced during the resistive phase of the rehabilitation program once full weight bearing is permitted.

Heel Raises

This exercise strengthens the calf muscles. With feet about shoulder-width apart, the patient rises up on the toes as high as possible and then returns to feet flat on the floor. This exercise is more difficult when performed through a greater range of motion, such as on an incline (figure 20.51) or on the edge of a stair, and also when it is performed on only the involved extremity. Common substitutions include using the hamstrings by flexing the knees during the heel raise, moving the body forward or rocking rather than moving straight upward, and placing most of the body weight on the uninvolved extremity rather than equally distributing the weight over both extremities.

Weight-Scale Exercise

If the patient has difficulty bearing weight on the involved extremity, or is apprehensive about transferring weight onto that side, a weight scale is an effective tool for teaching weight transfer, helping the patient gain confidence in the involved extremity, and improving strength.

This exercise uses a balance-weight scale and a platform of height equal to that of the scale's foot plate. The platform is placed next to the scale. The patient stands with the uninvolved extremity on the platform and the involved extremity on the scale, and initially stands with most weight on the uninvolved extremity (figure 20.52). The scale balance is moved to a desired weight for the exercise, using either a percentage of the patient's weight or specific poundage. The patient transfers enough weight to the involved side to move the balance arm to the top of the scale, then keeps the balance arm in that up position while performing a heel raise. As the patient's strength improves, the scale's weight is increased until the patient can perform a single-extremity heel raise with full body weight. The most common substitutions during this exercise are shifting the body weight to the uninvolved extremity as the patient begins to go up on the toes, rocking forward rather than moving straight upward, leaning forward, and flexing the knee.

Go to HK*Propel* and watch video 20.3*a*, which demonstrates a weight-transfer exercise, and video 20.3*b*, which demonstrates weight-scale heel raises and squat exercises.

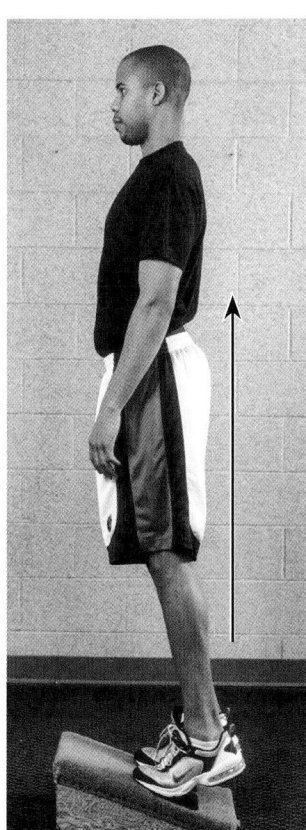

Figure 20.51   Heel raise on an incline.

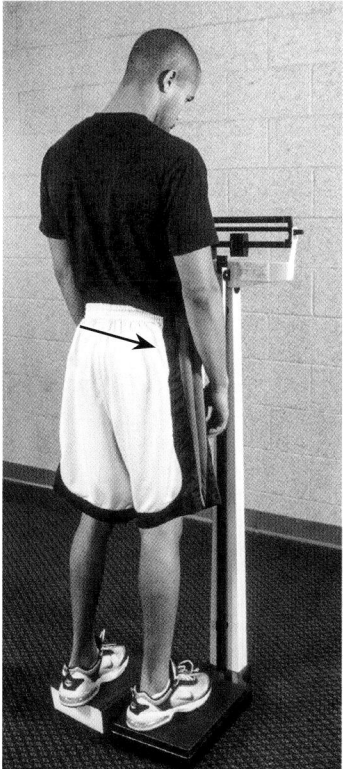

Figure 20.52   Weight-scale exercises are used to teach weight transfer and to increase the strength of the involved extremity.

This exercise is also good for weight-transfer instruction in early gait training. The technique is similar, but the instruction is to shift body weight from the left to the right lower extremity. The scale weight is increased as the patient improves in his or her ability to transfer weight properly. Substitutions during this activity occur commonly if a patient has been non–weight bearing for a while or muscles are very weak in the involved extremity. A common substitution is keeping the weight shifted to the uninvolved side but rotating the trunk toward the involved extremity. Hesitancy and reluctance to shift weight onto the involved extremity are common as well; in these cases, it is better to start with a low percentage, such as 25%, of the person's body weight on the scale. This way, the patient gains confidence that the extremity can tolerate the body weight, and he or she performs the activity correctly.

Toe Raise

This exercise increases the strength of the ankle dorsiflexors. The patient stands on an incline with the heels on the higher aspect of the incline. Keeping the heels in contact with the incline, the patient lifts the toes and forefoot upward and off the incline (figure 20.53). If this exercise is too difficult, the patient first performs the exercise on the floor. Using the incline requires the muscles to work through a greater range of motion and increases the diffi-culty of the exercise. Common substitutions include hip flexion, forward trunk flexion, and body sway. For optimal results, correct improper execution with verbal cueing or tactile stimulation to facilitate proper performance.

> ### CLINICAL TIPS
>
> Strengthening activities for the foot and ankle include isometrics, rubber-tubing activities, body-weight resistance for the ankle and foot, and resistance with equipment. Exercises should also include strength exercises for intrinsic and extrinsic muscles of the foot.

Equipment Resistance

In addition to body weight and rubber tubing or bands, several kinds of equipment can be used to strengthen the ankle and foot. A few of the possibilities are presented here.

Free Weights

Cuff weights can be used to strengthen ankle inversion, eversion, and dorsiflexion. A cuff weight is wrapped around the midfoot, and the patient is positioned so the muscle group exercised works against gravity. For dorsiflexion, the position is sitting (figure 20.54a). For inversion and eversion, the position is side-lying on the involved side and on the uninvolved side, respectively (figure 20.54b).

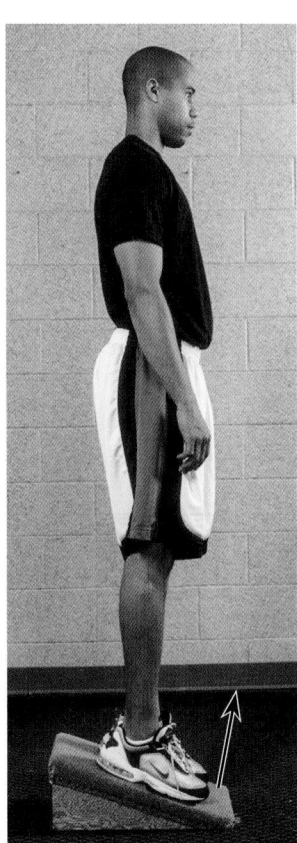

Figure 20.53 Toe raise on an incline.

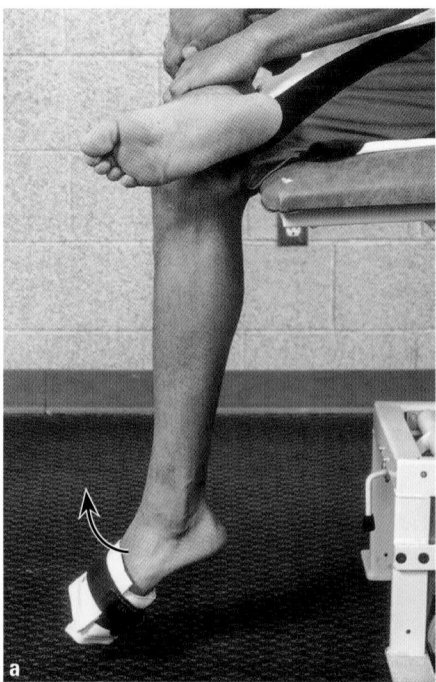

Figure 20.54 Cuff-weight exercises: *(a)* dorsiflexion, *(b)* inversion. The weight is lifted against gravity through a full range of motion.

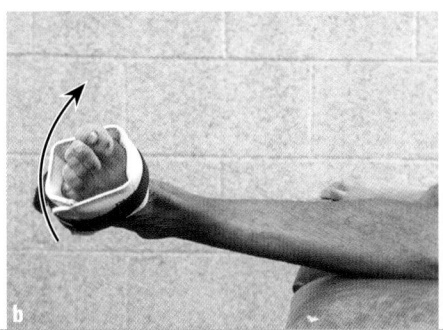

Figure 20.54 *>continued*

Machine Weights

Calf raises in the standing and seated positions using machines strengthen the gastrocnemius and soleus, respectively. Standing calf raises can be performed on machines designed specifically for that exercise, or on machines such as an upright press, bench press, or squat machine that can be modified for use as a calf-raise machine. A seated heel-raise exercise to isolate the soleus muscle can be performed on a unit designed specifically for soleus strengthening or on a hamstring-curl machine.

The difficulty of these exercises is increased by placing an incline board under the foot in the seated heel raise or having the ball of the patient's feet on the edge of a standing heel raise platform. These modifications require the muscle to move through a greater range of motion, increasing the exercise difficulty.

Proprioception and Neuromotor Exercises

Proprioception is fundamental for kinesthesia and balance control.[144] Research shows that deficits in these areas exist after ankle sprains, especially chronic ankle sprains.[145-150] Posture and balance, important factors in controlling ankle stability, can be improved with rehabilitation.[151-153] It is important, then, to include proprioception exercises in an ankle rehabilitation program. If a patient is non–weight bearing, early neuromotor exercises can include mirroring activities with the two ankles, with the patient's eyes closed. The alphabet exercise mentioned earlier can also help improve kinesthetic awareness.

Once the patient is weight bearing, additional proprioception and neuromotor reeducation exercises can be incorporated into the program. One of the beginning weight-bearing exercises is a tandem stance with the involved foot directly behind the uninvolved foot so the front foot's heel touches the back foot's toes. This position should be held for 30 s with no loss of balance. Another beginning exercise is the stork stand, or the single-limb stance (figure 20.55a). The patient stands on the involved extremity while trying to maintain balance for 30 s.[154]

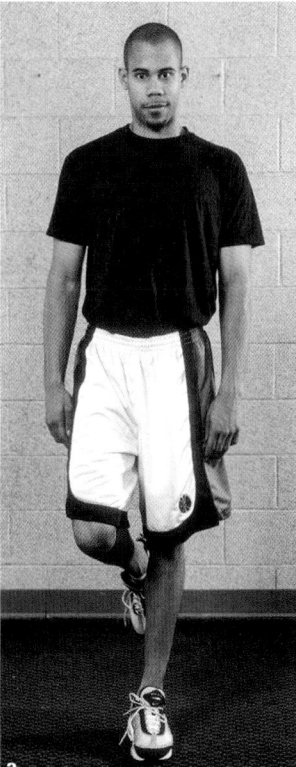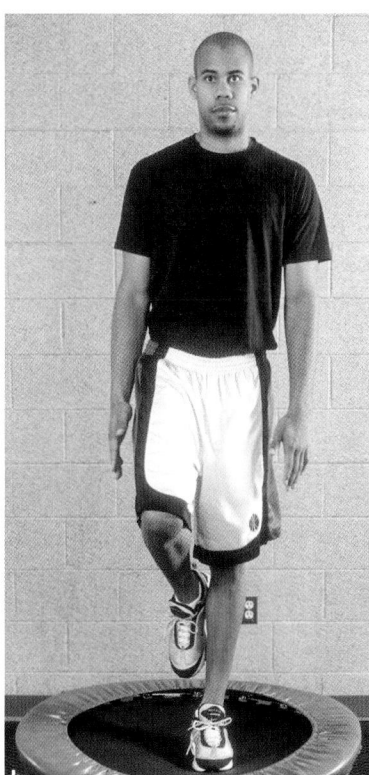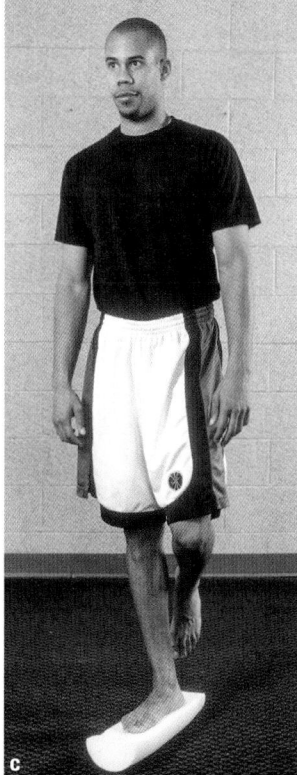

Figure 20.55 *(a)* Stork stand on floor. Advanced stork-stand exercises on unstable surfaces: *(b)* on trampoline, *(c)* on foam roller.

Having mastered this, the patient then performs the exercise with eyes closed (to eliminate the visual component of balance) and then with the eyes open while rotating the head left to right (to eliminate the vestibular component of balance). The next level is to have the patient stork-stand on an unstable surface, such as a trampoline, a foam roller, or a half roller (figure 20.55*b* and *c*).

For more advanced balance activities, patients either try to balance while performing an activity with another body part to divert their attention from balancing, or they perform another activity with the lower extremity while keeping their balance. In other words, they are maintaining balance while performing dynamic activites. For example, a football receiver or a softball or baseball player catches a medicine ball while balancing on a foam roller or trampoline. The ball is thrown at different levels and to different sides of the body so the patient must reach for the ball and still maintain balance. If the patient is a basketball player, bouncing a ball while balancing on an unstable surface is also a good activity (figure 20.56*a*). Setting a volleyball while stork standing on an uneven surface diverts the volleyball player's conscious effort from balance to enhance autonomic responses for balance.

Other neuromotor activities that facilitate balance may be performed on various kinds of balance boards that can be either made or purchased. Wobble boards, circle boards, BAPS boards, or balance boards can be used for various balance activities. A board placed on top of a PVC pipe is a simple balance board. In an exercise with this type of board, the patient tries to keep the ends of the board off the floor (figure 20.56*b*). This exercise becomes more difficult if the patient intentionally rolls the board side to side while keeping the ends of the board off the floor. This exercise also becomes more difficult if smaller-diameter PVC pipes are used because the ends of the board are closer to the floor, so the patient has less time to correct and keep the board ends from touching down.

Once patients can demonstrate good balance, they advance to more complex exercises that require any combination of balance, agility, control, coordination, and strength. These exercises include activities with equipment such as the Fitter, a resistance band, a slide board, and boxes. The Fitter and slide board develop eccentric and concentric strength and proprioception of the intrinsic and extrinsic muscles (figure 20.57*a*). These exercises can also assist in cardiovascular conditioning.

Increased resistance exercises include using bands attached to the waist as the patient begins with left-to-right lateral or forward–backward jumps and progresses to single-extremity lateral and forward–backward jumps (figure 20.57*b*). Resistance-band exercises develop concentric strength, eccentric strength, power, control, coordination, and agility.

Plyometric exercises may use box activities to promote power and agility in the advanced rehabilitation phase. Patients can perform various plyometric exercises created and designed by the rehabilitation clinician. Generic examples of these activities include rapid lateral jumping (figure 20.58*a*), rapid front-to-side agility step-ups (figure 20.58*b*), and multidirectional-change jumps (figure 20.58*c* and *d*). Plyometric jumps can then advance to lateral high jumps (figure 20.58*e*) and box drop-jumps. For additional suggestions on plyometric exercises for the lower extremities, refer to chapter 15.

Treadmill Activities

The treadmill can be used for more than gait analysis, walking, and running. It is useful in identifying subtle differences between the involved and uninvolved extremities during walking and running. Besides using the treadmill to observe walking and running mechanics, you can use it as an auditory tool for defining running abnormalities. Listening to the foot hit the treadmill surface becomes a

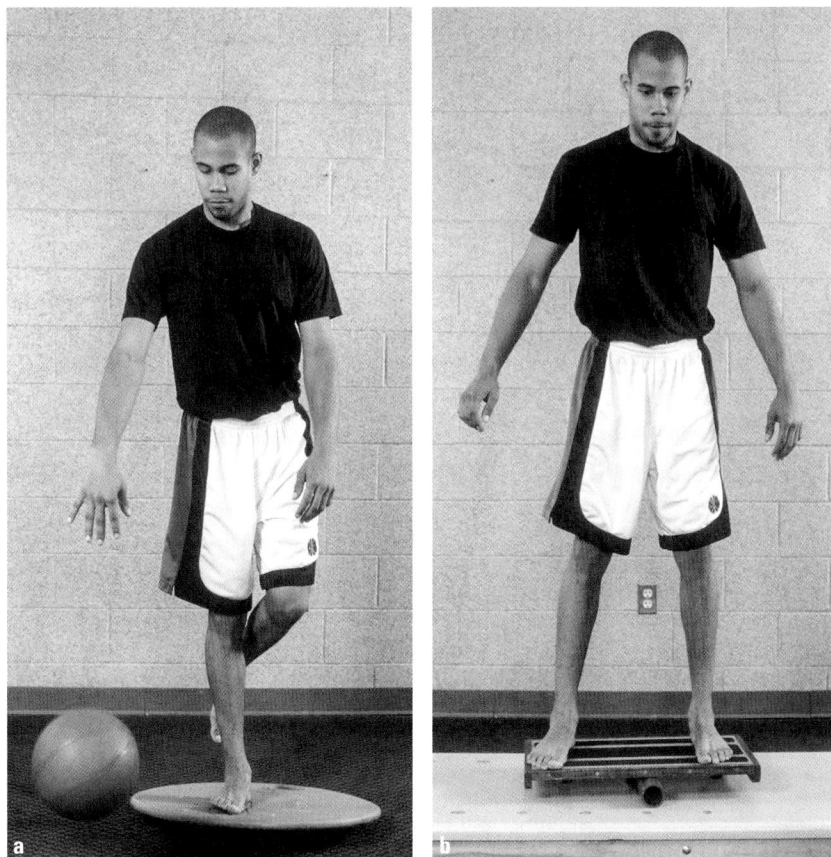

Figure 20.56 Examples of advanced balance exercises: *(a)* sport activity on unstable surface, *(b)* the patient keeps the sides of the board off the ground while maintaining the supporting roller in the middle of the balance board.

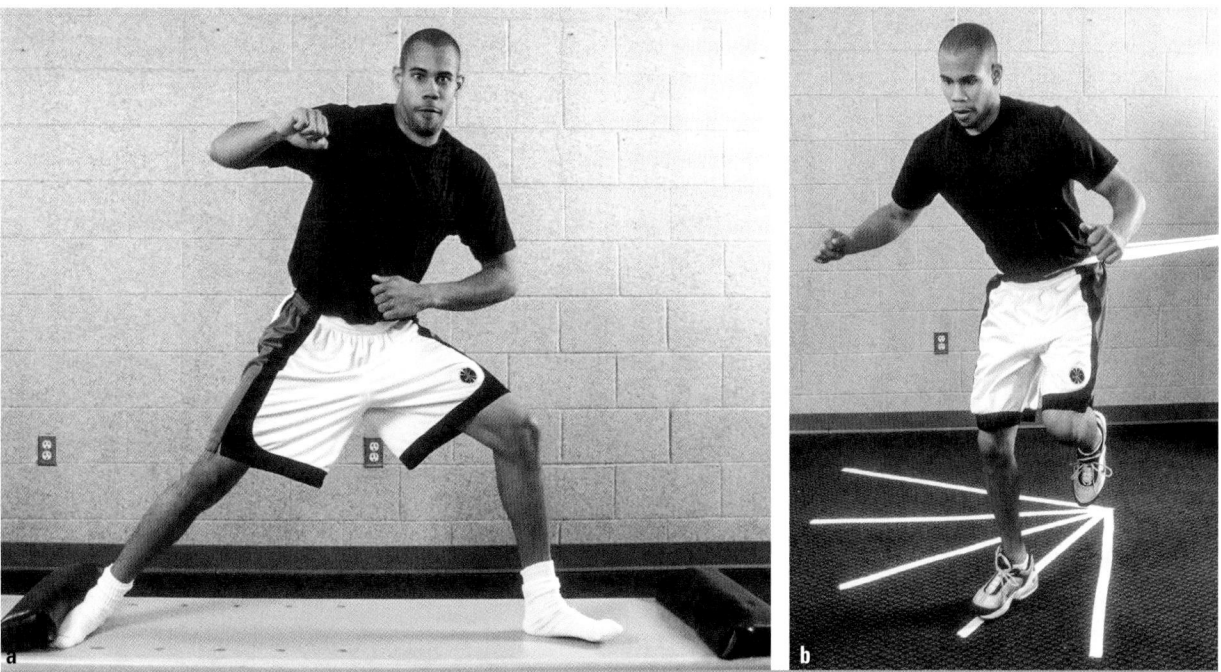

Figure 20.57 Examples of agility exercises: *(a)* slide board, *(b)* tubing exercise—lateral, left-to-right hopping activity.

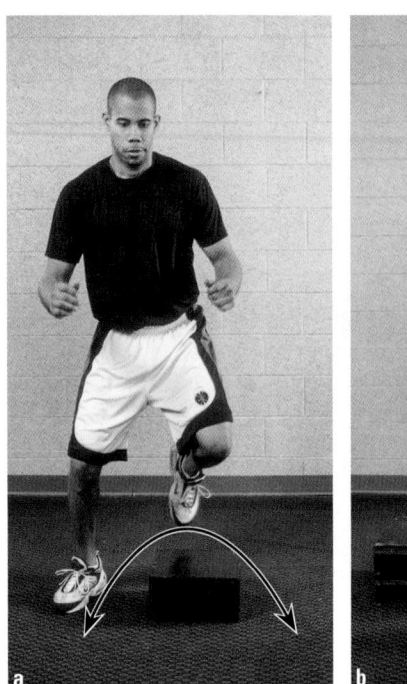 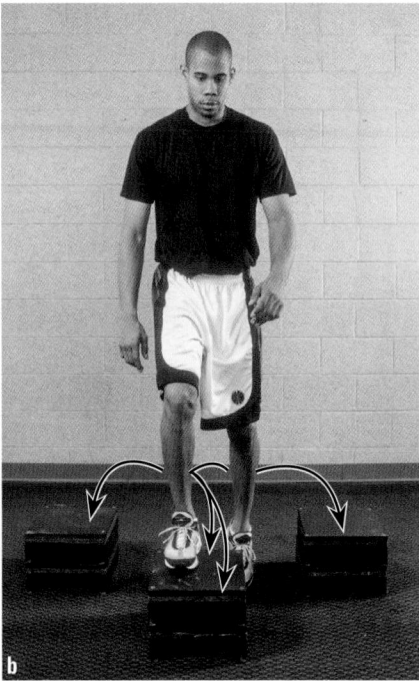 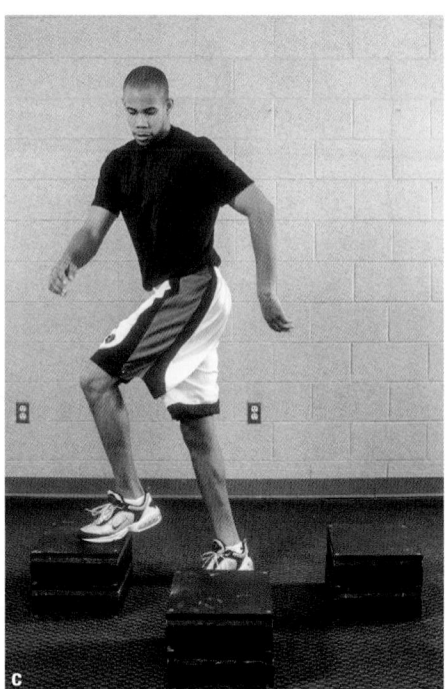

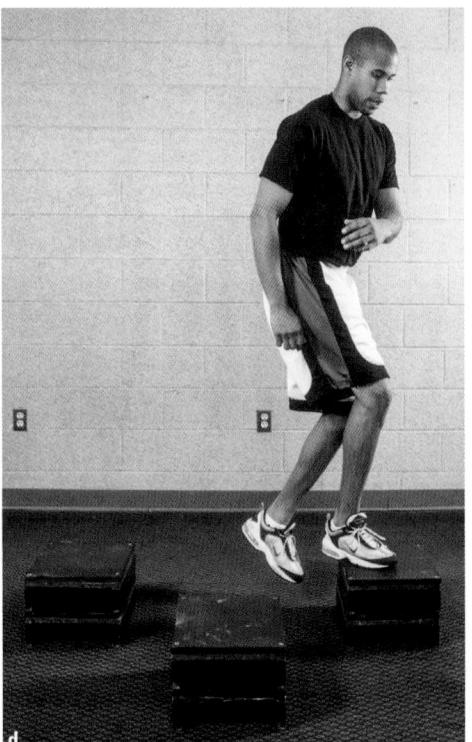 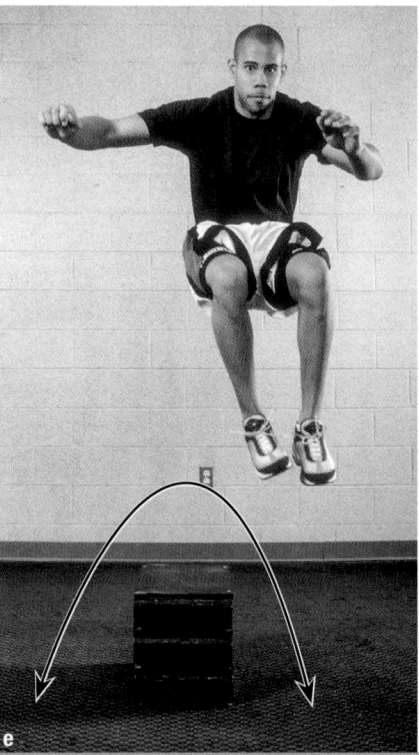

Figure 20.58 Examples of plyometric box activities: *(a)* jump-over side-to-side, *(b)* alternate jumps right side-to-front-to-left side, *(c–d)* rapid sequencing from one box to another, *(e)* lateral high jumps.

comparative tool; if the patient's feet do not sound the same at impact, it is likely that the person has a different pattern between the involved and uninvolved extremities. Increasing the treadmill speed reveals subtle differences from left to right by exaggerating differences in stride, gait, and weight transfer that may not be as noticeable at slower speeds.

The treadmill may also be used for facilitation, range-of-motion, strength, agility, and coordination exercises. Walking backward on a treadmill—retro walking (figure 20.59a)—has been shown to increase range of motion and muscle activity demands on the knee and ankle.[156] In retro walking, the ankle needs more dorsiflexion, greater

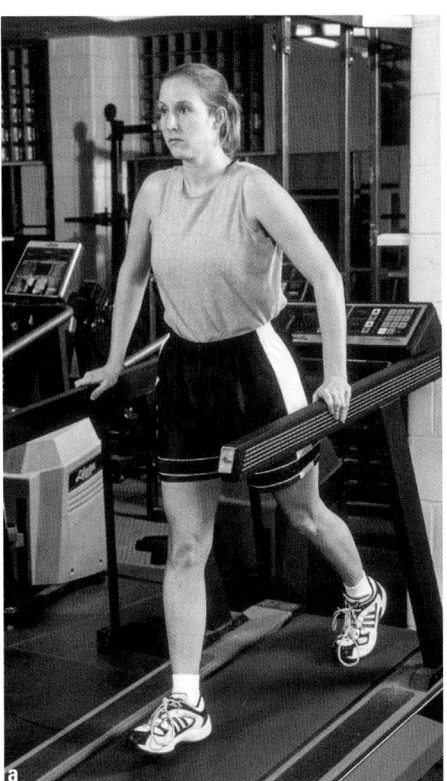 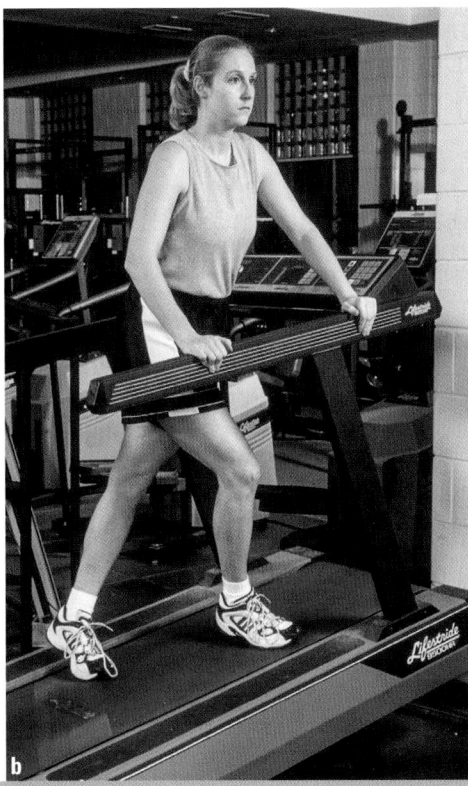

Figure 20.59   Treadmill activities: *(a)* retro walking on an incline, *(b)* carioca on an incline.

eccentric activity is required of the gastrocnemius, and the anterior tibialis is also more active.[156] Many believe that these increased demands help to facilitate the kinesthetic system and that they improve lower-extremity proprioception.[148, 156] Varying the speed of the treadmill also changes demands on the muscles.

Agility and coordination exercises on the treadmill include activities such as side shuffles and cariocas going in left and right directions (figure 20.59*b*). The patient may start with sets of 30 s bouts in each direction and then increase the time on each bout or increase the number of times the bout is repeated as goals are achieved and endurance improves. Requiring the patient to make more rapid changes when performing side-to-side activities on the left side and then the right side increases the agility demands of the exercise. Inclining the treadmill surface or increasing the speed also increases the difficulty.

Hopping Activities

Hopping exercises are often a necessary part of an ankle rehabilitation program because many athletic events include hopping or jumping. These exercises begin on a soft, force-absorbing surface such as a trampoline or mat and then advance to the patient's normal playing-field surface. There are many combinations of hopping activities. Which patterns to choose may depend on the patient's sport or activity requirements, the injured ankle's deficiencies,

and general conditioning capability. Some examples of hopping patterns include box hops, side-to-side hops, forward–backward hops, cross-pattern hops, high hops, long hops, zigzag hops, and circular hops. Some of these are presented as suggestions in figure 20.60. Patients may begin with bilateral limb jumps and advance to unilateral limb hops. They may also alternate extremities or perform hops in combinations, such as two on the left and then two on the right, or two on the injured side and then one on the uninjured side.

CLINICAL TIPS

Proprioception and neuromotor control are important parts of any ankle rehabilitation program. These exercises for posture and balance help improve ankle stability. They are exercises that can begin early in the rehabilitation program and advance to more complex activities during the functional portion of the program during the late resistive and early advanced phases.

Functional and Performance-Specific Exercises

As the patient nears a return to full participation, functional then performance-specific exercises must become a part of the rehabilitation program. As mentioned throughout

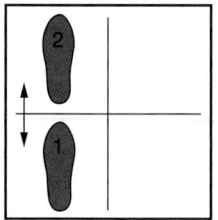

Forward-backward hop: Hop forward and backward between two quadrants.

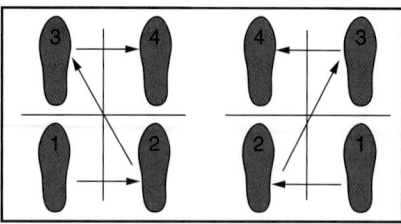

Cross-pattern hop: Hop in an X pattern.

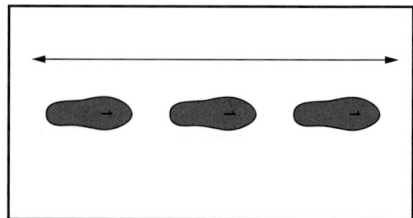

Straight-line hop: Hop forward and then backward along a 15- to 20-ft line.

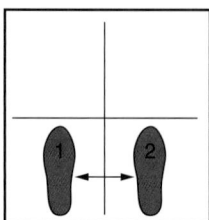

Side-to-side hop: Hop laterally between two quadrants.

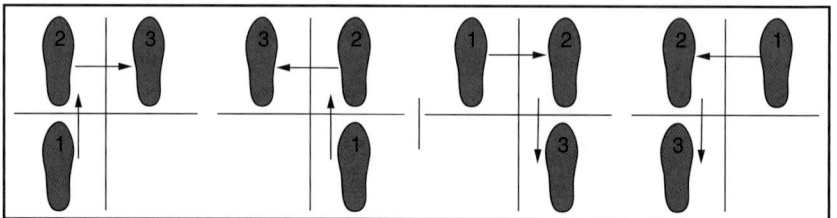

Triangular hop: Hop within three different quadrants. There are four triangles, each requiring a different diagonal hop.

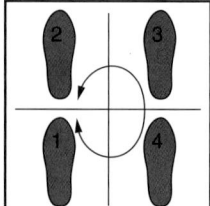

Circular hop: Hop from square to square in a circular pattern. Sets are performed clockwise and counterclockwise.

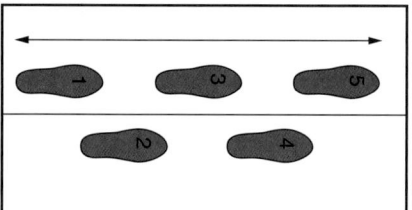

Zigzag hop: Hop from side to side across a 15- to 20-ft line while moving forward and then backward.

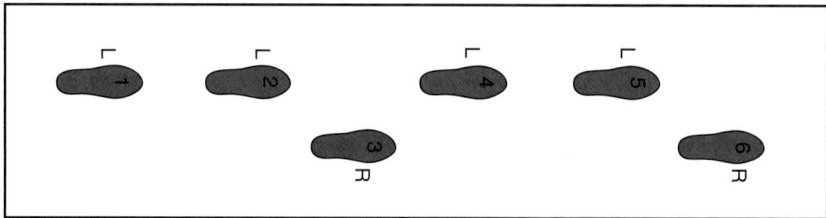

Mixed patterns: Various combination hop patterns can be used, such as two on the injured (i.e., left) side and one on the uninjured (i.e., right) side.

Figure 20.60 Suggestions for hopping patterns. You can design a number of hopping patterns, limited only by your imagination.

this book, functional activities are precursors to performance-specific exercises and are designed to place multiplanar stress on those muscles and joints used in performance-specific exercises. Performance-specific exercises mimic the activities that patients will use after their rehabilitation. Performance-specific exercises (or drills) can also be used to assess the patient's ability to perform normal activities and skills accurately and safely.[157-159]

Functional exercises advance to performance-specific drills and skill activities that are unique to the demands of each patient. You must understand each patient's work or sport activities well enough that you can incorporate the correct drills and exercises into the final phase of that person's rehabilitation program. For example, although tennis and soccer both involve running and cutting, the specific activities and skill drills are different, and athletes returning to these sports will have very different performance-specific exercises during the final phase of their rehabilitation programs. Likewise, an auto-assembly worker and a garage mechanic each work on automobiles, but the specific tasks and demands for each job are very different, so the final phases of their rehabilitation programs must also be very different.

Although performance-specific exercises will vary for patients in lower-extremity sports, running sports often include many of the same functional and even performance-specific activities. These exercises may include single, double, or triple hops; zigzag runs with rapid changes in direction; backward running; sprinting; running circles in clockwise, counterclockwise, backward, and forward directions; 90° cuts to the left and to the right; and running figure-8s. The patient should be able to perform all exercises rapidly and efficiently, without hesitation, smoothly in both directions, and without favoring the involved extremity.

Special Rehabilitation Applications

This section deals with specific injuries to the foot and ankle. Injuries to the extremity, especially the ankle, are among the most common orthopedic injuries.[160, 161] Some—certainly not all—of the more common injuries are discussed in the following sections.

Before we present rehabilitation programs for some of the more common ankle and foot injuries, we must repeat that any rehabilitation program must be preceded by an examination of the injury. Part of that examination includes special tests to help identify the clinical diagnosis for which the rehabilitation program will be designed. Table

20.9 identifies some of the more commonly used special tests for the foot and ankle, along with their sensitivity and specificity findings.

Ankle Sprain or Dislocation

An ankle dislocation and an ankle sprain are on the same continuum since they involve the same structures but differ in severity, so we will consider these two injuries together. As with other sprains, the severity determines the rate at which rehabilitation will progress and the time when various rehabilitation exercises begin. The more extensive the injury and consequent tissue damage, the less aggressive the program is in the initial stages. Clinicians must understand healing concepts and timelines, and they must assess the severity of the injury before proceeding with a rehabilitation program.

Ankle dislocations are the most extreme of ligamentous injuries. Fortunately, they are rare events.[170] They may or may not need surgical repair, but usually the patient receives general anesthesia to at least perform a closed reduction of the injury.[170] The need for surgical repair depends on the type of dislocation and whether other injuries accompany the dislocation.[171] Ankle dislocations will follow a rehabilitation program similar to those for ankle sprains, but the recovery will require longer periods for the first three rehabilitation phases.

TABLE 20.9   Foot and Ankle Special Tests and Their Sensitivity and Specificity Ratings

Site or structure tested	Special test (other name)	Sensitivity[a]	Specificity[a]
Syndesmosis	Cotton test (Clunk test)	29% [162]	71% [162]
	External rotation test (Kleiger test)	50% [162]	0% [162]
	Dorsiflexion maneuver	50% [162]	57% [162]
	Fibula translation test	64% [162]	57% [162]
	Squeeze test	57% [162]	14% [162]
	Dorsiflexion with external rotation test	71% [163]	63% [163]
	Point test (syndesmosis palpation)	92% [163]	29% [163]
Collateral ligaments	Anterior drawer	36% [162]	43% [162]
	Medial talar tilt	50% [164]	88% [164]
	Lateral talar tilt	Unknown	Unknown
Achilles tendon integrity	Thompson test (Simmonds test)	96% [165]	98% [165]
	Matles test	88% [165]	92% [165]
Medial longitudinal arch	Navicular drop test	88% [166]	100% [166]
	Feiss' line	Unknown	Unknown
Vascular status	Homan's sign	21% [167]	33% [167]
Neurologic status	Tinel's sign	30% [b] [168]	81% [b] [168]
	Morton's test	Unknown	Unknown
	Mulder test (Mulder's click)	95% [169]	100% [169]

[a]Numbers rounded to the nearest whole number.

[b]Number is the average of 3 foot and ankle locations on which the test was performed.

We know that discoloration appearing after an injury is the result of bleeding in the area. If no discoloration occurs, the sprain is likely mild, or first degree, and the patient's other symptoms should be consistent with this assessment. If discoloration occurs, at least a second-degree sprain is likely. Instability indicates a possible third-degree sprain of at least one ankle or foot ligament. Recovery from second- and third-degree sprains requires a longer rehabilitation time than do first-degree sprains. A first-degree ankle sprain may restrict the patient from normal activities for up to a week, with return to full participation in 2 to 3 weeks or less, but a second-degree sprain may restrict the patient from participation for 3 weeks and full participation for 4 to 6 weeks.[172] Third-degree ankle sprains vary widely in recovery times, which may depend, at least, on the course of treatment provided.[173] Third-degree sprains can take as little as 6 weeks or as much as 3 or more months to improve before the patient can return to full participation.[173] In essence, the range of recovery times from acute ankle sprains ranges from 4 weeks to 4 months and depends on a number of factors, such as age, severity of injury, pain, and complications that may arise.[174]

Third-degree sprains and dislocations can be treated either conservatively with rehabilitation or with surgery and postoperative rehabilitation. The choice is often made according to the patient's objective and subjective findings, age, and level of sport participation, and the surgeon's preference. Studies indicate that there is no difference in outcomes between the surgically treated and non–surgically treated groups, but there is a more rapid return to function after conservative treatment.[175] Ankle instabilities that do not respond well to conservative treatment are surgically repaired.[176] Studies show that early rehabilitation that features controlled weight bearing with the foot in a boot and early active-motion and rehabilitation yields better results than the more conservative approach of prolonged casting with a later start to rehabilitation.[172, 173, 177]

Recovery from an ankle sprain depends in part on the patient's injury history.[178] The clinician must obtain an accurate history from the patient before beginning a rehabilitation program; previous ankle sprains that received inadequate care can complicate the patient's findings and change the program's requirements.

Chronic ankle sprains also introduce other factors. One of these is additional scar tissue with probable adhesions that limit joint and soft-tissue mobility. Repeated ankle sprains can result in chronic muscle weakness and reduced kinesthetic awareness, making the ankle prone to further injury.[144, 148, 179, 180] Chronic ankle sprains may also lead to compensatory changes in gait, strength, and flexibility, reducing the mechanical effectiveness of the ankle and foot.[181] Because of these additional factors, chronic ankle sprains need more time to properly rehabilitate.[182]

Most ankle sprains are inversion sprains.[183] The specific ligaments and structures involved and the severity of the injury depend on the mechanical forces and the angle of stress applied. Ankle sprains may also involve other structures; for example, there may be an avulsion fracture of the malleoli, peroneal strains or dislocations, or other tendon injuries.[184-186]

Of the ankle ligaments, the anterior talofibular is the most commonly injured ligament, and the calcaneofibular is the next most commonly injured ligament.[187] Occasionally, the tibiofibular ligament is injured. This is known as a syndesmosis ankle sprain, or a "high ankle sprain."[188] This ligament injury requires careful attention. The function of the tibiofibular ligament is to hold the tibia and fibula in alignment and to maintain the ankle mortise joint.[189] When weight is borne on the extremity, the force tends to spread the two long bones apart, but the tibiofibular ligaments hold the joint components in structural alignment.[190] When the anterior tibiofibular ligament is injured, repetitive stress with weight bearing may inhibit the healing process.[191] When this ligament is injured, the patient should be instructed in non–weight bearing (NWB) or partial weight bearing (PWB) on crutches to ambulate pain free until full weight bearing (FWB) does not cause pain. This way, the injury can heal without complications or lasting detrimental results.[192] If this approach is not followed, chronic pain will likely develop, and the condition can become difficult to treat successfully.[193] Syndesmosis sprains generally take much longer to return to normal function than lateral ankle sprains, and the recovery time is directly related to the severity of the injury and the accuracy of diagnosis.[194, 195]

The more typical sprains involving the lateral ligaments permit weight bearing to tolerance.[196] The rule of thumb is that if the patient can ambulate normally, crutches are not needed; however, if pain or dysfunction causes an abnormal gait, crutches are used with either PWB or NWB. In most cases when crutches are needed, weight bearing can be partial, to tolerance.

Control of edema and pain occurs in the inactive rehabilitation phase and is the first priority, as with any injury. Common methods of reducing edema and pain include the use of ice and other modalities, such as electrical stimulation, along with strapping, wrapping, or bracing. Active range-of-motion exercises are instituted early, usually within the first 3 d, to restore ankle range of motion. Joint mobilization and soft-tissue mobilization techniques are used as indicated, based on the pretreatment assessment findings. Grades I and II are used within the first few days to relieve pain, while grades III and IV are used later in the resistive phase to restore joint motion. With chronic sprains, there are usually scar tissue adhesions in the joints and surrounding tissue.[197] Sometimes intertarsal and metatarsal joints become restricted, especially if the patient's ankle was placed in an immobilizer boot or a cast after previous injuries.[198] All areas of potential restriction should be assessed before starting a treatment program.

Non-weight-bearing exercises are used early in the rehabilitation program for early strengthening late in the active phase or early in the resistive phase, depending on the injury's severity. These early strengthening activities include isometric exercises, aquatic exercises, and manual resistance as tolerated. The BAPS board used in a seated position provides AROM when the patient is PWB.

Ankle inversion–eversion strength is important to ankle stability.[199, 200] Exercises for the muscles that control these movements must be included among rehabilitation exercises for a sprained ankle. Isometrics, manual resistance, pulleys, rubber tubing or bands, and aquatic exercises can all provide good strengthening activities for these groups during the resistive phase. Progression to closed kinetic chain exercises for inversion and eversion movements during the resistive phase make strengthening of these motions more functional and enhance neuromotor control and proprioceptive gains.

Once FWB is pain free, gait training and closed kinetic chain exercises produce additional strength and coordination. Balance activities progress from single-leg stance (SLS) on the floor to SLS on a half foam roller, trampoline, or other unstable surface. Initial closed-chain strengthening exercises begin with low resistance, repetitions, and sets and increase to more resistance, repetitions, and sets as the patient's tolerance and abilities progress. Early closed-chain activities are performed slowly and in a controlled manner, but as the patient gains strength and neuromotor control of the ankle, quicker movements requiring more control and strength are added. This progression places demands on muscles for strength and on the neuromotor system for balance, coordination, and agility.

The decision to add plyometrics to a patient's rehabilitation program is based on a number of factors.[201] The patient must have full and pain-free range of motion. The clinician must also consider the patient's age, sex, the ability of the injured segment to withstand plyometric forces, and the patient's competitive level.[201] Plyometrics is not appropriate for all patients; clinicians must use their best professional judgment on whether a patient is a candidate, and if so, when it is appropriate to begin.

The final rehabilitation phase, the advanced phase, includes functional activities, then performance-specific activities before return to full participation. A timeline of rehabilitation progression for a moderate syndesmosis sprain is outlined in figure 20.61.

Syndesmosis Ankle Sprain

Stage I: Inactive phase	
0-2 weeks	**Inflammation phase: Inactive rehabilitation phase**
Goals	Relieve pain. Reduce edema, ecchymosis. Relieve spasm. Protect injured ligament from excessive stress. Maintain conditioning levels (MCL).
Treatment guidelines	Modalities for pain, edema, ecchymosis, and spasm Grade I and II joint mobilization for pain NWB on crutches Maintenance exercises (ME) for conditioning
Precautions	There should be no pain during weight bearing; if patient has pain, crutches with NWB status on the injured limb are required.
Stage II: Active phase	
3-6 weeks	**Early proliferation phase: Active rehabilitation phase**
Goals	Restore range of motion. Achieve early gains in proprioception. Reach early stage of improved muscle endurance. Make early strength gains toward end of this phase. Reduce adhesions resulting from scar tissue or edema toward end of this phase. Progress to FWB as tolerated. No pain, spasm, or edema are present.

>continued

Figure 20.61 Rehabilitation program for moderate syndesmosis ankle sprain.

Stage II: Active phase	
3-6 weeks	**Early proliferation phase: Active rehabilitation phase**
Treatment guidelines	Begin with isometrics for the ankle and progress to isotonics as tolerated toward end of this phase Toe and intrinsic exercises Early proprioception exercises Soft-tissue mobilization Weeks 3-4: Grade III and IV joint mobilization as needed Gait training as indicated Ambulation in pool along with aquatic exercises ME continues with emphasis on hip and knee muscles of involved extremity Modalities as indicated
Precautions	Maintain crutch use and NWB or PWB status as indicated as long as pain occurs with FWB. There should be no pain with any exercises. This phase may take longer than 6 weeks, depending on the injury's severity and patient's pain level.

Stage III: Resistive phase	
6-12 weeks	**Late proliferation phase: Resistive rehabilitation phase**
Goals	Achieve full weight bearing without pain. Achieve full ROM. Regain normal strength. Regain normal proprioception. Restore normal gait. MCL.
Treatment guidelines	Continue with ROM exercises as needed. Perform progressive strengthening exercises for the ankle, foot, and leg. Begin multiplanar exercises when strength is at least 80% normal. Perform balance exercises, progressing to agility as tolerated. Continue with ME.
Precautions	Should have no pain in this phase. Use weight scale for weight-transfer progression if patient is reluctant to bear weight on the involved extremity.

Stage IV: Advanced phase	
8-16 weeks	**Remodeling phase: Advanced rehabilitation phase**
Goals	Perform functional exercises properly. Perform performance- and sport-specific exercises properly. Return to full participation without pain, with normal strength, mobility, agility, and performance.
Treatment guidelines	Plyometrics for LE Advanced functional activities Sport- and performance-specific exercises
Precautions	Observe and correct exercise execution as needed.

MCL = maintain conditioning levels; ME = maintenance exercise; AROM = active range of motion; ROM = range of motion; NWB = non–weight bearing; WB = weight bearing; PWB = partial weight bearing; FWB = full weight bearing; LE = lower extremity.

Figure 20.61 >*continued*

Case Study

A 16-year-old volleyball hitter jumped up for a hit and landed on another player's foot, causing an inversion sprain to the right ankle 3 d ago. She felt a pop and had immediate swelling. She could not bear weight on the ankle at the time. X-rays were negative, but the patient was placed on crutches, with weight bearing to tolerance. Ice, elevation, and taping have been applied periodically for the past 3 d, but the patient comes to you today to start her rehabilitation program.

She denies any previous ankle injury. So far she has performed only alphabet exercises because it was too painful for her to do anything else. She can bear about 11 kg (25 lb) of her body weight on the foot in standing before she complains of pain in the lateral ankle and above the ankle joint. Her pain is located over the anterior talofibular, anterior tibiofibular, and calcaneofibular joints, with most of the pain over the first two ligaments. She has moderate swelling of the ankle, foot, and toes, with ecchymosis over the dorsal surface from the midfoot to the toes. She can wiggle her toes through about 50% of normal motion; it appears that swelling in the toes may be limiting this ROM. Her ankle's AROM is 45° of plantar flexion, 10° of inversion, 10° of eversion, and −10° of dorsiflexion; all motions, especially inversion and dorsiflexion, and weight bearing are painful.

Her ankle strength is restricted by pain on dorsiflexion and inversion. Since she cannot bear weight on the foot, you cannot examine the antigravity strength of the calf; however, you can easily overcome plantar flexion with manual resistance. Eversion strength is 4/5. All resisted ankle motions are painful. Joint mobility is normal but painful at end motions throughout the ankle joints. Soft-tissue mobility is limited by the edema present, but you cannot palpate any abnormal soft-tissue restriction.

Questions for Analysis

1. List, in order of priority, what her problems are, and establish short-term and long-term goals for each of them.
2. What treatment will you provide for the patient today?
3. What home instructions will you give her?
4. What precautions will you give her?
5. What will be your guidelines for deciding when she can begin resistive weight-bearing exercises?
6. List three agility exercises that you will include in the patient's program when she can do them.
7. What will your functional testing include before her return to full sport participation?

Throughout any rehabilitation progression, you must watch for signs of increased inflammatory response, indicating that too much stress has been applied to the ankle. These signs include postexercise swelling and pain either during or after the treatment session. If these signs are present, you should reduce the severity of the program for 1 to 3 d and then try advancing the patient again to the next level of exercise difficulty.

It is advisable to have the patient refrain from wearing a protective brace during in-clinic rehabilitation exercises unless indicated by the physician. During these times, the patient performs activities under controlled circumstances and in a restricted environment, so the risk of injury is low.

However, as patients return to their normal activities at the end of the rehabilitation program, they may feel more comfortable using a supportive ankle device since they are now performing in an unpredictable setting. This kind of environment presents an increased risk of injuring scar tissue that has less-than-maximum tensile strength. Because it may take a year or more for the injured tissue's tensile strength to achieve maximum levels, patients may benefit from the additional protection of ankle supports.

A number of studies have demonstrated that these devices can improve the stability of formerly injured ankles.[202-208]

Peroneal Tendon Dislocation

Peroneal tendon dislocations are often overlooked, probably because they often occur in conjunction with other injuries.[209] Because the tendon usually spontaneously repositions itself after the dislocation, this is an injury that is usually diagnosed some time after the ankle sprain has occurred when the patient continues to complain about lateral ankle pain and perhaps a clicking or snapping in the ankle during movement.[210] It is also frustrating to resolve unless discovered with good examination techniques.

Peroneal tendon dislocation occurs most commonly through one of two mechanisms, ankle dorsiflexion with active peroneal contraction, or an inversion sprain.[211] In an inversion ankle sprain, the peroneal tendons are most susceptible to dislocation with the ankle in 15° to 25° of plantar flexion.[211] This position places the tendons in a tenuous position along the distal fibula. If an inversion ankle sprain occurs with the ankle in less than 15° of plantar flexion, the peroneal retinaculum can be stretched, leading to instability of the peroneal tendons.[212] Skiers are commonly subjected to these injuries. If the ankle is in more than 25° of plantar flexion, the peroneal tendons move into a deep-seated position posterior to the fibular head and are stable in that position with little chance of dislocation.[212]

Peroneal dislocations are usually self-reduced once the ankle is in a nonstressed position.[213] The patient typically complains of a painful, snapping sensation in the posterolateral ankle with walking or performing ankle circumduction.[214] Swelling along the tendon is sometimes observable. Initial intervention includes controlling the inflammation with modalities. Stabilizing the tendons with taping and pad support to prevent the tendon from moving forward on the fibula can sometimes help to relieve the subluxation episodes. If conservative intervention fails to prevent recurrent dislocations, surgical repair is needed.[215] Although several surgical options are possible, deepening the posterior malleolar groove has proven to be a very successful procedure for athletes and allows a safe and rapid return to activity.[210]

Postoperative rehabilitation once the sutures have been removed includes soft-tissue massage around the surgical site to reduce soft-tissue adhesions in the area. Joint mobilization techniques should be used in areas that demonstrate restricted joint mobility. Active range of motion is permitted anywhere from 10 to 21 d postoperatively. Ankle plantar flexion and eversion cause the least disruption of the peroneal tendons and can occur passively fairly early in the program.

Once weight bearing is permitted in the active rehabilitation phase, the exercises and progression mentioned earlier for other ankle and extremity injuries can begin. A weight-scale weight-bearing progression can help the patient gain confidence bearing weight on the injured extremity. Balance activities begin once the patient is fully weight bearing, starting with SLS and progressing to more difficult exercises as strength and neuromotor control improve during the latter part of the active phase and moving into the resistive phase.

Strengthening exercises for the involved structures begin with easy isometrics in the late active phase and progress to isotonics in the resistive phase using techniques such as manual resistance, pulleys or tubing, and progressive standing heel raises. Strengthening of the hip and knee muscle groups starts in the inactive phase and continues into the resistive phase. Because the entire extremity is not used normally after a foot or ankle injury or surgery, the muscles of these other lower-extremity segments diminish in strength; therefore, they too need restoration if the patient is to be returned to optimal function.

When the patient has achieved full range of motion and adequate strength for neuromotor control, dynamic balance exercises in the resistive phase progress to agility exercises later in this phase. Various agility exercises on boxes, jumping with tubing resistance, and lateral movements are included among the final activities in the late segment of the resistive phase before functional and performance-specific exercises begin in the advanced rehabilitation phase.

Achilles Tendon Rupture

In spite of the fact that the Achilles tendon is the largest and strongest tendon in the body,[216] it is also the site of the most common tendinous injuries of the foot and ankle.[217] Perhaps the frequency of injury to this structure is due, at least in part, to the fact that the Achilles must withstand forces that are equivalent to eight times the body's weight during athletic activities.[218] It is no wonder that an injury to the Achilles can be debilitating and can restrict the patient's rapid return to sport participation.[219]

Among the more debilitating injuries to the Achilles tendon is a rupture. Rehabilitation programs for Achilles ruptures have become less conservative in recent years, mainly because better results are seen with early weight bearing and rehabilitation after surgical repair.[220-222]

Achilles ruptures most commonly occur in persons in the third and fourth decades of life.[223] The number of Achilles rupture patients has increased in recent years.[224, 225] This increase is attributed to the growing number of people who continue sport activities well into their adult years.[225] In younger athletes, a rupture occurs when the foot is anchored and the person is thrust forward, producing a sudden stretch on the tendon. For example, a younger athlete in a football pileup may end up with one player on top of his foot when his body is suddenly pushed forward by another player who comes into the pileup.

A more typical history for an Achilles rupture is an event in which a 30- to 50-year-old patient is running or cutting and suddenly feels as though he or she was shot in the calf. Usually, a pop is felt or heard. The pain is intense, and the patient cannot walk on the extremity.

In the past several years, research has produced conflicting results from studies of different management approaches. Some studies have shown similar outcomes for both surgically repaired and nonoperative management of Achilles ruptures,[219, 225, 226] while others have demonstrated higher re-rupture rates among patients treated with nonsurgical approaches.[227, 228] Both nonoperative and operative management of Achilles ruptures seem to have better outcomes if the treatment program features early weight bearing and rehabilitation.[229-231]

Surgical repair includes a variety of techniques, ranging from open repair to less-invasive percutaneous repair, with reapproximation techniques ranging from the use of fibrin glue, autogenous tendon grafts, and acellular dermal grafts to sutures.[221, 232] Of the surgical options, percutaneous repairs have demonstrated effectiveness comparable to open repairs while offering a quicker return to participation.[232, 233]

As with surgical repair, conservative management also includes different techniques ranging from cast immobilization for an extended period to a cast for 1 week followed by progressive reduction in plantar flexion through the use of a boot with adjustable heel elevations.[219, 234] Conservative care with cast immobilization presents the greatest risk of re-rupture.[219] Because of the positive outcomes, recent advances in Achilles rupture management have moved to immediate weight bearing in both surgical and nonoperative treatment protocols.[220, 231, 234]

Initial rehabilitation treatments in the inactive phase include cardiovascular conditioning and exercises for the uninvolved lower-extremity segments (excluding knee flexion exercises) and other body segments. The patient is in a cast or boot immobilizer on the foot and leg. Easy isometric exercises in the immobilization device may be encouraged, but the patient is instructed to perform a slow buildup to maximum with a maximal hold and a gradual release of muscle tension. Goals of treatment during this inactive rehabilitation phase include promoting wound healing through wound care and reducing edema and pain.

If a cast is the immobilizing device, it is removed after 2 weeks and replaced with a walker boot. The boot has a 2 cm[221] to 4 cm[219] elevated heel. The patient can ambulate using the boot with weight bearing as tolerated. Every 2 weeks, the heel elevation is reduced until the ankle is at 0° by weeks 6 to 8.[219, 221, 235] By weeks 6 to 8, the patient should be in a normal shoe with a heel lift as needed for comfort.[219, 235]

Examination of the patient's leg following the presence of excessive edema will determine areas of soft-tissue adhesions and joint restriction secondary to the edema and immobilization. Soft-tissue massage and mobilization around the ankle and distal leg, along with ankle, foot, and tibiofibular joint mobilizations, often begin in the active phase (around weeks 6 to 9) to help restore flexibility and range of motion. Plantar foot massage with a ribbed can, golf ball, or rolling pin is also appropriate during this time.

The boot is removed for rehabilitation exercises except during weight-bearing activities, when the boot is required. Active range-of-motion exercise begins after week 2, with the patient moving the foot and ankle joints in all directions; the caveat here is that dorsiflexion stretching is limited to 0° to prevent overstretch of the recent repair. Resistance exercises using rubber bands or manual resistance occur at this time for all motions except plantar flexion; plantar flexion exercises are limited to easy isometric exercises. Other activities include exercise on a stationary bike, the towel-roll exercise, the four intrinsic muscle exercises explained earlier in this chapter, and marble pickups for extrinsic and intrinsic muscles. Exercises may also include the BAPS board in sitting and may then advance to standing, single-limb balance activities once the patient is FWB on the extremity. Resisted exercises for the hip and knee should also be used during this time as long as no weight is placed on the foot.

By the eighth postoperative week, the patient is walking without the boot. It may be necessary to instruct the patient in a proper gait pattern if bad habits have developed. Resistive gastrocnemius exercises begin, as do stretching exercises into dorsiflexion, but forceful activities are avoided until weeks 12 to 16. Gait training in a pool may be beneficial before this time. Gait training on land is a necessary part of the rehabilitation program once the patient is fully weight bearing and out of the boot.

Patients typically hesitate to immediately bear weight on the involved extremity once they are permitted full weight bearing without the boot. A good way to help the patient develop confidence in the limb is to use a weight scale to progressively transfer increasing amounts of body weight onto the involved limb. It is a good tool for teaching accurate weight transfer onto the involved extremity. The scale can also be used to monitor correct technique in heel-raise exercises. The scale can be especially useful if the surgeon is permitting limited weight bearing on the extremity; for example, if 50% weight bearing is permitted, the scale's balance is positioned at half the patient's weight, and the patient then transfers body weight to the involved extremity until the scale's balance arm moves up, indicating that half the body weight is borne by the extremity. The scale can also be used in full-weight-bearing exercises such as heel raises, and it can be used for monitoring and recording increases in the patient's ability to bear weight on the involved extremity through a full range of motion.

Weight-bearing exercises such as squats and lunges begin after week 8. These exercises are presented in chapters 18 and 19. Other beneficial activities include step exercises, balance and agility exercises, and eventually plyometric exercises, if appropriate, as described earlier in this chapter and in chapter 14. Functional exercises and then performance-specific exercises are part of the advanced phase of the rehabilitation program and are specific to the patient's sport or occupation.

In summary, during the inactive phase of the rehabilitation program, manual-resistance and other NWB exercises for the hip and knee are feasible even when the extremity is immobilized. Trunk and core exercises should also be included in this early phase. Isometrics and manual resistance to the ankle begin once the immobilization brace or cast is off in the later part of the active phase, if the healing tissue is not overstressed and exercises are done cautiously. Weight-bearing exercises are gradually increased as the patient and the healing injury tolerate them. At first, the resistance and repetitions are low, and emphasis should be on correct technique and proper execution more than on the amount of resistance. The patient may tolerate increasing repetitions better than increasing resistance in the early days of the resistance phase.

Resistance exercise beyond body weight is added to the program in the resistive phase when the tissue is well along in the healing process, around 8 to 12 weeks postoperatively. Once the patient has 10° to 15° of dorsiflexion, usually toward the end of the second month or the beginning of the third, jogging activities begin. Straight jogging on a flat surface is permitted until the patient is up to 3.2 km (2 mi). After that, agility drills are appropriate.

A timeline for rehabilitation progression after an Achilles tendon repair is provided in figure 20.62.

Achilles Repair

Stage I: Inactive phase	
0-2 weeks	**Inflammation phase: Inactive rehabilitation phase**
Goals	Protect surgical site. Relieve pain, spasm, swelling. Maintain ROM of all uninvolved segments. Maintain strength of uninvolved body segments. Maintain core and hip strength.
Treatment guidelines	NWB cast or boot × 2 weeks Modalities for pain, swelling, and spasm ROM of toes, knee, hip Resistive exercises for uninvolved muscle groups After week 1: Easy isometric exercises for ankle dorsiflexion (in plantar flexion), inversion, and eversion Core and hip strengthening and stabilization exercises After week 2: Walker boot with elevated heel After week 2: AROM with dorsiflexion limited to 0°
Precautions	Observe surgical wound for proper healing. Uninvolved shoe should be of same height as walker boot. Avoid overstressing ankle beyond 0° dorsiflexion.
Stage II: Active phase	
2-6 weeks	**Early proliferation phase: Active rehabilitation phase**
Goals	Relieve pain to 1-2/10. Achieve gains in ankle ROM. Week 3: Remove cast and replace with walking boot (with 2-4 cm heel lift). Weeks 6-8: Achieve full ROM. Reduce scar tissue adhesions, but take care around surgical scar. Achieve early strength gains. WB to tolerance: Heel of walker boot is 4-6 cm for weeks 2-4 and then 2-4 cm for weeks 4-6. Normal gait pattern with boot; WBAT.
Treatment guidelines	Begin isometrics for plantar flexors Week 3: Manual resistance and rubber band resistance to all motions except plantar flexion Stationary bike Soft-tissue mobilization of edema-produced adhesions Joint mobilization PRN Resistive exercises for inversion–eversion Dorsiflexion resistive exercises to 0° Early proprioception exercises Intrinsic foot muscle strengthening Lunges and squats HEP for self-massage of plantar foot and AROM exercises
Precautions	Remove boot for therapeutic exercises except WB exercises. Avoid pain with exercises.

Figure 20.62   Rehabilitation program for postoperative Achilles repair.

Stage III: Resistive phase	
7-16 weeks	**Late proliferation phase: Resistive rehabilitation phase**
Goals	Experience no pain. Week 8: Achieve active dorsiflexion to 0°. Week 12: Achieve full range of motion in ankle. Restore normal gait without assistive devices. Achieve normal strength of foot, ankle, and leg in straight-plane and multiplanar activities.
Treatment guidelines	Maintenance exercises for range of motion and strength of core and uninvolved segments Decrease heel lift every 2 weeks to none by weeks 6-8 Weeks 8-10: Ambulation in normal shoe Gait training Soleus and gastrocnemius stretches Body-weight resistance exercises for plantar flexors Single-limb stance activities Week 8: Stand on heels and on toes Advance from bilateral heel raise to unilateral heel raise Slide board and other lateral activities Dynamic proprioception exercises Triplanar activities Plyometric exercises Jogging at 12 weeks Early functional exercises
Precautions	Watch patient for weight shift to uninvolved side during weight-bearing exercises; correct as needed or start with weight-scale weight-shift exercises. Patient should perform exercises through full range of motion.

Stage IV: Advanced phase	
16-30 weeks	**Remodeling phase: Advanced rehabilitation phase**
Goals	Maintain normal strength of all muscles. Maintain normal ROM of all joints. Restore normal sport and work performance.
Treatment guidelines	Functional exercise progression Performance-specific exercises and drills progression
Precautions	Correct performance PRN.

PROM = passive range of motion; AROM = active range of motion; ROM = range of motion; CV = cardiovascular; NWB = non–weight bearing; WB = weight bearing; FWB = full weight bearing; LE = lower extremity; PRN = as needed; PF = plantar flexion.

Figure 20.62 >continued

CLINICAL TIPS

As with any injury or surgical repair, progression of the strengthening exercises is determined by tissue healing times, the patient's flexibility and mobility, and his or her tolerance. Pain and swelling are the primary signs to avoid with any exercise. The objective of strengthening exercises is to achieve muscle fatigue without causing pain or swelling. Exercise stress is gradually increased, and the response to any increase in exercise stress—either increased difficulty in an exercise or the addition of new exercises—must be carefully monitored. You must rely on your own observations, as well as on the patient's reports of how the Achilles responds to changes in the rehabilitation program, to gauge the effectiveness of the program. These results dictate whether changes are needed.

Foot, Ankle, or Leg Tendinopathies

As with other body segments, the distal lower extremity is also subject to its share of tendinopathy. Any tendon may experience tendinopathy, although there are specific tendons in each body segment in which the risk of tendinopathy is greater. In the lower limb's distal segment, these tendons include the Achilles, tibialis posterior, and peroneal tendons.[236]

Most tendinopathies are multifactorial in their origin. In other words, there are usually several factors present, each adding to the tendon's compounding stresses. Histopathological changes occur in response to repetitive stress that leads to a degradation of the tendon and an inability to respond sufficiently to repair the tendon.[236]

Therefore, any approach to effectively treat tendinopathies of the leg, ankle, and foot must first identify the causative factors. It is important that the clinician identify all of the potential causative factors so that they may be corrected to minimize the risk of recurrence. If the clinician treats only the symptoms without impacting the cause of those symptoms, the problem is certain to return later.

Of the modalities that are available to treat tendinopathies, ultrasound has been shown to be a very effective one.[237] It now appears to be an accepted concept in the rehabilitation community to utilize eccentric exercises early in a tendinopathy rehabilitation program.[238] There has been evidence to demonstrate that when eccentric exercise is combined in the treatment program with soft tissue mobilization techniques, the outcomes are improved over eccentric exercises alone.[239]

Since the Achilles tendon is the frequent site of tendinopathy, it is discussed by itself in the next section. The other tendinopathies found most commonly in the leg and ankle are grouped into one section after the Achilles tendinopathy discussion.

Achilles Tendinopathy

If not treated correctly, any tendinopathy can be a frustrating and prolonged condition. Causes must be addressed and the condition brought under control before rehabilitation exercises can begin. Achilles tendinopathy is presented here separate from other tendinopathies in the leg, foot, and ankle since it is such a prevalent injury, especially in athletes.[240]

Achilles tendinopathy is usually a gradual-onset injury that originates secondary to overuse. Overuse of the Achilles tendon occurs when the tendon undergoes excessive stresses without enough time between force applications to adjust to those stress levels. Excessive stress can be the result of cumulative forces caused by inherently poor foot mechanics, increased conditioning sessions, improper surfaces and playing fields, inadequate or improper footwear, weakness, or inflexibility.[241, 242] Intrinsic factors such as

Case Study

A 20-year-old tennis player was downhill skiing during winter break with his family. While he was on the slopes, maneuvering to the right, he fell forward and dislocated his left peroneus longus tendon. The injury was surgically repaired. The ankle was placed in an immobilizer boot, and the patient was NWB for 2 weeks. He can now bear partial weight to about 75% on the left and is to start rehabilitation. He presents to you today still NWB on the left. He admits that he is fearful of bearing weight on the extremity. His hip and knee strength is grossly 4/5 throughout all muscle groups. Ankle dorsiflexion and inversion strength is 3/5, and ankle eversion strength is 2+/5. His ankle range of motion is 0° in inversion, 5° in eversion, 40° in plantar flexion, and –5° in dorsiflexion. Joint mobility is moderately restricted in the subtalar and intertarsal joints. The calcaneocuboid and cuboid-metatarsal joints are also restricted. Soft-tissue mobility around the surgical scar, along the lateral foot, and into the posterior ankle is moderately limited. There is mild to moderate swelling around the ankle.

Questions for Analysis

1. What are your patient's problems, and what short-term and long-term goals will you establish to relieve these problems?

2. What will your first treatment today include?

3. What will your goals for today's treatment be?

4. What techniques will you use to encourage him to bear weight on the left lower extremity?

5. What instructions will you give the patient today before he goes home?

6. What do you expect to accomplish in the next 2 weeks of treatment?

7. List precautions that you must respect at this point in the rehabilitation program.

8. List three strengthening exercises that you will use when the ankle is ready, and explain their progression.

9. What agility exercises will you eventually include in the rehabilitation program?

genetics and mechanical factors such as overuse are some of the most common causes of Achilles tendinopathy.[243, 244] As with other tendinopathy conditions, to achieve a full recovery and reduce the risk of reinjury, the causative factor or factors must be corrected.

Achilles tendinopathy can be categorized in different ways, but two of the main categories often discussed are based on the site of pain and are classified as either insertional tendinopathy or noninsertional tendinopathy. *Insertional tendinopathy* occurs over the insertion site of the Achilles on the posterior calcaneus. Insertional tendinopathy is sometimes associated with retrocalcaneal bursitis and the appearance of Haglund's deformity, or a "pump bump."[62] These patients present with pain over the distal 2 cm of the Achilles tendon and usually have swelling over the heel where a bone spur is sometimes palpable.[245] The most tender section of this region is the lateral aspect of the calcaneal swelling. It is thought that the force directed at this location occurs because of compression applied to the deep fibers of the tendon that lie between the retrocalcaneal or superficial Achilles bursa and the posterior surface of the calcaneus.[245]

On the other hand, *noninsertional tendinopathy* is identified with a nodule of swelling and tenderness about 2 to 7 cm proximal to the insertion of the tendon on the Achilles.[62] This tendinopathy is also referred to as mid-portion Achilles tendinopathy or mid-substance Achilles tendinopathy and is occasionally identified as the "main body of the Achilles tendon."[62] This portion of the tendon undergoes more axial tension stresses from the muscle pull of the gastrocnemius and soleus on the anchored tendon, especially during running or jumping activities.[246] Although healthy tendons are essentially avascular, this tender area of Achilles tendinopathy commonly has blood vessels.[247] For this reason, it is thought that the mid-portion Achilles tendinopathy has made attempts at healing but could not complete the process; it may be that repetitive stresses applied to it have interrupted the process.[62]

The Achilles tendon withstands extreme loads during normal activities. During running, for example, the forces applied to it can exceed 12.5 times the runner's body weight.[248] A foot with excessive pronation puts additional stresses on the Achilles tendon.[249]

The Achilles tendon's normal configuration has a medial spiral rotation from its proximal origin in the gastrocnemius–soleus complex, where it begins as a flat, fan-shaped tendon, to its insertion on the calcaneus, where it ends as a rounded cord[250] (figure 20.63). This spiral rotation begins about 12 to 15 cm (4.7 to 5.9 in.) above its insertion, rotating about 90° by the time the tendon attaches to the calcaneus. Most of the tendon's posterior fibers come from the gastrocnemius; as these tendon fibers move distally, they spiral and become the posterolateral portion of the Achilles tendon at its insertion.[251] The tendon fibers from

the lateral gastrocnemius and from the soleus spiral to become the anterior layer of the Achilles tendon.[251] This twist of the tendon is an area where stress concentrates, especially 2 to 5 cm (0.8 to 2.0 in.) above its calcaneal insertion where the rotation is at its greatest. This region is also an area of reduced circulation within the tendon.[252] This site is the most common location for mid-portion tendinopathy in the Achilles.[252]

If the calcaneus is everted when it should be erect, the Achilles tendon suffers an additional torque force. If the Achilles is tight, even more subtalar pronation occurs to create needed ankle dorsiflexion during ambulation.[253] If pronation is prolonged into the heel-off phase of gait and beyond when inversion should be occurring, a wringing of the tendon results, increasing stress on the Achilles at the medial portion of its most vulnerable place.[254] In cases of repetitive stress and prolonged tendinopathy, a nodule of scar tissue from microscopic tears can often be palpated on the tendon 2 to 5 cm (0.8 to 2.0 in.) above its calcaneal insertion. The nodule is usually larger and more tender on the medial aspect, where the tendon incurs more stress.[254]

Common signs of mid-portion Achilles tendinopathy include tenderness along the Achilles, especially in the 2 to 5 cm (0.8 to 2.0 in.) above the calcaneal insertion, where a nodule can often be palpated; other signs include reduced ankle dorsiflexion, swelling, weakness, crepitus to palpation, and pain with unilateral hopping. Inflexibility, weakness, scar tissue adhesions and joint immobility from previous injuries, and changes in footwear should all be assessed and corrected as needed. A good history must include inquiries about recent changes in conditioning or workout sessions that may be overstressing the tendon. Changes in surfaces, such as when a person goes from flat surfaces to hills or from soft to hard surfaces, may be additionally contributing to the problem and must be corrected.

As with other tendinopathies, treatment includes initially correcting the cause of the tendinopathy and reducing pain and swelling. If the cause is excessive pronation, orthotics may be needed. A low-dye strapping technique to stabilize the calcaneus and reduce pronation can be used either alone or in combination with heel cups or medial heel wedges to assess the effectiveness of orthotics. If these devices reduce the patient's pain, the patient will probably benefit from orthotics. Over-the-counter (OTC) orthotics may correct pronation for some patients, while others may need custom orthotics.[255] If the clinician decides that the patient needs orthotics, OTC orthotics are usually tried before custom orthotics are considered.

In extreme cases, the patient may need to stop aggravating the injury by reducing activity until the symptoms are under control. Early intervention techniques that may be helpful include the use of various modalities, such as ultrasound, phonophoresis, iontophoresis, vibration therapy, electrical stimulation, ice, and others presented by

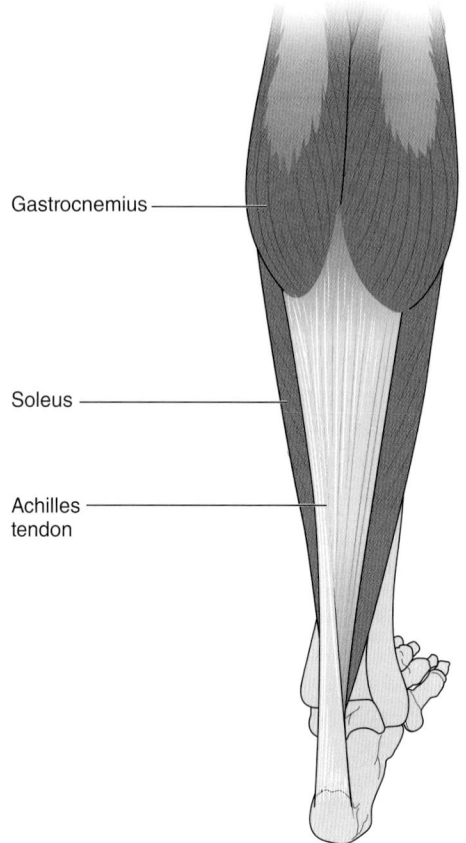

Gastrocnemius

Soleus

Achilles
tendon

a

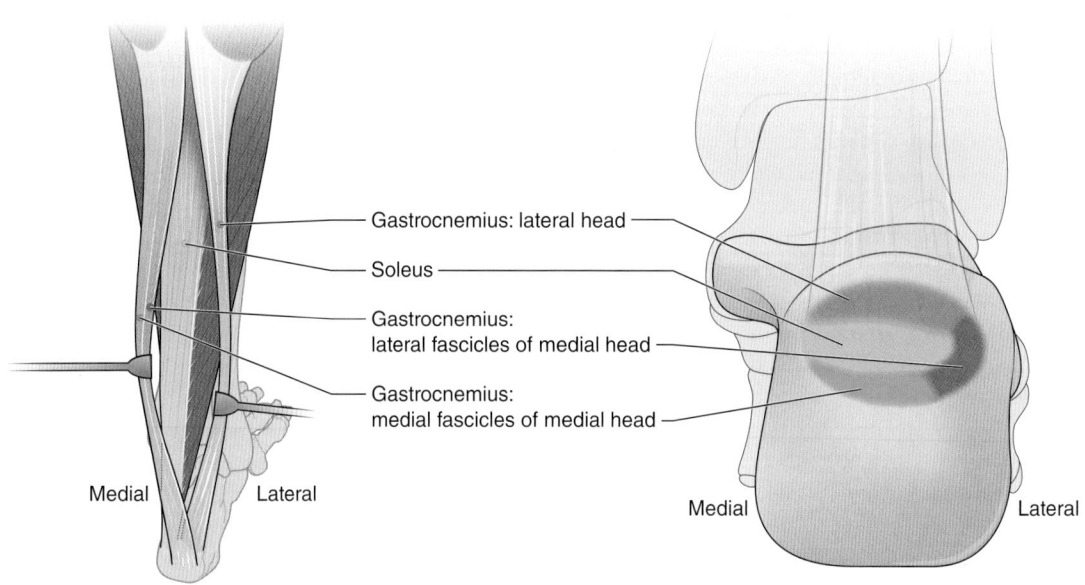

Gastrocnemius: lateral head

Soleus

Gastrocnemius:
lateral fascicles of medial head

Gastrocnemius:
medial fascicles of medial head

Medial   Lateral

Medial   Lateral

b

Figure 20.63 Achilles tendon. *(a)* The tendon has a flat structure proximally and then evolves into a spiral structure as it descends to become oval-like near its distal insertion on the calcaneus. *(b)* A cross-sectional view of the distal Achilles tendon based on the work of Szaro and colleagues.[251] This image shows that the soleus portion of the tendon is in the center and is surrounded by aspects of the medial and lateral gastrocnemius portions. The medial head of the gastrocnemius tendon divides into two fascicles that split but form the posterior Achilles tendon.

Denegar and colleagues.[256] Cross-friction massage over the nodule and other areas of soft-tissue restriction help to mobilize the adherent scar tissue to reduce pain and improve soft-tissue mobility.

Rehabilitation must include stretching and flexibility activities for restricted areas. There is a relationship between hamstring and hip muscle tightness and Achilles flexibility, so these muscle groups should be evaluated and corrected as needed.[257] Gastrocnemius and soleus tightness should also be addressed with the flexibility exercises presented earlier.

Once full weight-bearing, the patient begins eccentric heel raises. A number of eccentric exercise programs have been developed in recent years to address Achilles tendinopathy.[258-263] Of all the treatments available for Achilles tendinopathy, it is generally agreed that eccentric exercises provide the most benefit,[238] to the point that eccentric exercise is considered the "gold standard" because it is the only part of a rehabilitation program that has almost universal acceptance in the treatment of Achilles tendinopathy.[262]

Concentric strength exercises are begun cautiously because it is important to avoid worsening pain. Weight-bearing strength exercises begin when the patient reports pain at around 5/10. Until then, resistance band exercises for ankle inversion, eversion, and dorsiflexion strength are appropriate. The patient can perform rubber band exercises for ankle plantar flexion through a full, pain-free range of motion. Concentric weight-bearing Achilles exercises can include heel raises on a leg-press machine, standing heel raises beginning on a flat surface and progressing to an incline, and heel raises with weights. Other exercises for the lower extremity include squats, lunges, and knee flexion strengthening exercises as tolerated. When the patient's pain level is 2-3/10, agility exercises are suitable. Plyometrics starts once the patient is pain free. At no time in the rehabilitation program should any exercise increase Achilles pain. If an exercise progression results in Achilles pain, the patient should return to previous levels of activity for another one or two treatment sessions, then try again to go to the next level without pain.

Once patients can perform plyometric exercises without pain, they can progress to functional and then performance-specific exercises before returning to normal activities. Throughout the program, patients must communicate with their clinicians about any changes in pain and responses to treatment. You must respect the patient's pain and bear in mind that each person will respond differently to an exercise progression. The key to success is correcting the underlying causes of the Achilles tendinopathy and getting the signs and symptoms under control before advancing the patient in the program.

Retrocalcaneal bursitis is often mistaken for Achilles tendinopathy. Bursitis-related pain occurs over the posterior aspect of the calcaneus where the bursa is located and often accompanies insertional Achilles tendinopathy. This is because bursal pain occurs in the same location as insertional Achilles tendinopathy; therefore, a patient presenting with complaints of pain in this area should be examined for bursitis as well as tendinopathy. As previously mentioned, a "pump bump" is often present because a heel whip occurs as the calcaneus moves toward supination during late stance and heel-off after staying in pronation longer than it should during the stance phase of gait. The bursa and Achilles tendon can both become irritated with friction against the shoe's heel counter, especially with a heel whip. In addition to tending to the Achilles tendinopathy, intervention includes symptomatic relief of the bursal inflammation and correcting the cause of the bursitis. In addition to excessive pronation, other causative factors of bursitis include tight Achilles, tight plantar fascia, and poor shoes.

Other Tendinopathy

Although several tendons in the foot, ankle, and extremity can develop tendinopathy, other common sites are the tibialis posterior and the peroneal tendons.[264, 265] These tendons become irritated most often because of overuse secondary to excessive pronation combined with increased running mileage on hard surfaces.

The tibialis posterior works eccentrically to decelerate subtalar pronation and medial rotation of the tibia at heel strike, and it works concentrically as a supinator and inverter of the subtalar joint and lateral rotator of the tibia during stance. In other words, it is a key active stabilizer and controller of the medial longitudinal arch.[264] The peroneus longus and brevis work as pronators of the subtalar joint and as plantar flexors and evertors of the first ray during the non-weight-bearing phase of gait. In other words, the peroneals are another important ankle stabilizer.[266] During midstance and heel-off, they evert the foot to transfer weight from the lateral to the medial portion. In sum, these lateral and medial muscles both act as stabilizers during weight bearing. The tibialis posterior stabilizes the midtarsal joint, and the peroneus longus stabilizes the first ray to accept the load as it is transferred from the lateral to the medial foot at heel-off.[267] When the foot pronates longer than it should in weight bearing, excessive stresses are placed on these tendons.[268] When a tendon is not given enough time between events that stress it, tendinopathy can occur.[269]

Tibialis posterior tendinopathy results in pain in the posteromedial ankle region or into the tendon's insertion site on the navicular and surrounding tarsals; the pain increases with heel raises.[270] Peroneal tendinopathy pain, located in the posterolateral ankle region, can run along the tendon on the lateral foot.[271]

As with Achilles tendinopathy, the clinician must identify the causes if a treatment program is to have lasting effects. Once you have identified the causes, you must take steps to correct them. If the injury is not severe, it may be possible for the patient to continue normal activities once the causes have been corrected. In severe cases, the patient may need to refrain from full participation until the symptoms subside.

Initial treatment includes the use of pain-relieving modalities that have been discussed already. The patient should be instructed in proper stretching exercises for tight areas.[272] These may include structures close to but not adjacent to the injured area. For example, femoral anteversion may affect the tibialis posterior tendinopathy.[273]

Initial strengthening activities, once pain is under control, include eccentric exercises discussed previously.[274] As the patient improves and progresses in the rehabilitation program, combined concentric–eccentric exercises for all ankle muscles are added, especially for muscles of the injured structures and for those that are deficient in strength or endurance. Antigravity resistance using weights, resistance bands, or manual resistance for inverters and evertors provides additional challenge to those muscles. Neuromotor control activities, such as marble pickups with placement of the marbles in the ipsilateral or contralateral hand, lateral towel roll, and inversion–eversion on a BAPS board or wobble board are important exercises for peroneal and tibialis posterior tendons. Balance activities provide stress to lateral ankle tendons. The Fitter and rolling balance board can also be used for lateral ankle-stressing exercises. Resistive exercises for ankle dorsiflexors and plantar flexors should also be included.

Agility exercises and functional exercises are the same as for other injuries; you should add these to the program once the patient is pain free with activity. Likewise, the final progression for a patient with this injury is similar to other rehabilitation progressions: performance-specific activities that ensure a smooth transition to a preinjury lifestyle.

Medial Tibial Stress Syndrome

Medial tibial stress syndrome is also known as shin splints.[275] More recently, it has also been referred to as exercise-related leg pain.[276] By any name, it is a stress reaction at the periosteal and musculotendinous fascial junctions. The pain is located in the middle and distal third of the extremity with tenderness to palpation along the posterior aspect of the tibia's distal medial ridge.[277] The pain may vary in intensity, from pain that resolves after running to pain that interferes with daily activities.

This condition is usually seen in distance runners and is likely caused by multifactorial problems such as training errors and biomechanical problems.[277, 278] A recent theory indicates that these factors create microfractures in the medial tibia.[279] It appears that excessive pronation produces prolonged eccentric contraction of the soleus that exacerbates the condition.[277] Interventions for rehabilitation include correcting the causes and reducing activity until symptoms are under control.[280] In addition, modalities may be used to relieve pain.[281] The Achilles, soleus, and other tight structures should be stretched throughout the day, and strengthening exercises should be performed for weak muscle groups, hip muscles, and core stabilizers.[278] Soft-tissue release through deep-tissue massage can help to relieve adhesions that increase the patient's pain. Orthotics also often help to reduce pain and to correct the causes of medial tibial stress syndrome.[282]

If "shin splint" complaints occur on the anterolateral leg, the cause is usually an overuse reaction of the tibialis

Case Study

An 18-year-old male sprinter presents to you with complaints of lateral and anterior leg pain that began about 1 week ago. He has started training for the outdoor track season and is distance running to create a cardiovascular base. He reports that he had this pain last year but it went away after a couple of weeks, so he didn't think too much about it; however, this year, his first year as an intercollegiate athlete, the pain seems more intense. He likes the team's shoes, which he started wearing when he began training this year; he had never used the brand before.

Your examination reveals tightness in the Achilles with ankle dorsiflexion to 0°. Hamstring range of motion is 65° in a straight-extremity raise. His new shoes have a stiff sole. He is tender to palpation of the tibialis anterior.

Questions for Analysis

1. What will your first treatment today include?
2. What will you give the patient for a home program?
3. What will be your recommendations about his shoes?
4. What will be your recommendations about his workouts?
5. What are your short-term goals for him?
6. List three exercises you will include in his program.

anterior and extensor digitorum communis, compounded by excessive pronation, hill running, poor shoes, or training errors. It is not technically shin splints, but it is debilitating and painful nevertheless. This condition is usually relieved with changes in shoes, training methods, and orthotics.

Athletes may experience anterolateral leg pain at the outset of preseason conditioning, especially if they have not maintained an appropriate activity level up to that time. In these cases, the pain resolves with time as the patient becomes conditioned. Ice and stretching can provide symptomatic relief in the short term. If symptoms continue beyond normal expectations, the patient should be referred to the physician to rule out anterior compartment syndrome.

Foot Injuries

A number of foot problems both common and uncommon can also arise as either chronic or acute injuries. Some of the more commonly seen conditions are presented here.

Plantar Fasciitis

Of all foot injuries, plantar fasciitis is among the most common.[283] Its cause can be traced to any number of factors, and you must recognize and correct the cause to correct the problem and reduce the risk of reinjury.

The thick aponeurosis that covers the plantar foot from the calcaneus to the MTP joints is the plantar fascia. It is a thick connective tissue structure that protects the structures in the plantar foot, provides flexibility for shock absorption, and creates a windlass mechanism that transforms the foot into a rigid lever for transmitting propulsion forces during push-off.[284] It can become irritated when subjected to abnormal stress, usually during running activities. Patients in any sport involving running can be susceptible to plantar fasciitis.[271] It is also commonly seen in workers whose tasks involve high-impact forces on the foot.[285] High arches and excessive pronation can both be culprits that increase normal stress loads and lead to plantar fasciitis.[284] These inherent structural stresses are usually combined with other factors such as increased workout levels, poor shoes, restricted dorsiflexion from tight Achilles or calf muscles, restricted great-toe dorsiflexion, and workouts on hard surfaces.[255, 286]

The classic symptom of plantar fasciitis is heel pain with weight bearing that occurs upon arising in the morning and after prolonged sitting, and that decreases with continued walking.[287] In more severe cases, pain can occur at rest and can extend into the mid-arch region. The pain is usually unilateral. X-rays often reveal a heel spur; however, the source of pain is not the heel spur but the soft tissue that is irritated because of the stress it is experiencing. Repetitive stresses applied to the plantar fascia at its origin on the calcaneus commonly result in the development of exostosis where the fascia attaches.[288]

Any intervention must include correction of the underlying causes. This often involves flexibility exercises for tight structures, proper shoe selection, orthotics if needed to correct abnormal foot structure, changes in conditioning, and changes in workout surfaces.[289] Rehabilitation may also include modalities such as extracorporeal shock wave to relieve the symptoms.[290] Occasionally, the physician may opt for a cortisone injection into the painful area. Alternative methods that may provide relief to the tender tissues include applying a low-dye strapping technique to the arch to reduce the stress on the plantar fascia, putting heel lifts in the shoes to reduce the stress from a tight Achilles tendon, and providing a heel cup to increase calcaneal stability and provide a cushion to the plantar calcaneus.[80, 291] Wearing a night splint that places a low-level stretch on the Achilles has been shown to reduce pain associated with plantar fasciitis.[289, 292]

Stretching the Achilles and calf must be introduced early in the program so that the heel lift can be discarded as soon as possible; prolonged use of the heel lift can encourage tightness and prevent the restoration of full motion. Calf stretching must be performed with the ankle in subtalar neutral[293] so that the foot does not collapse (pronate) and give a false impression of stretching the calf. Stretching of the plantar fascia and great toe can be performed with the ankle in dorsiflexion and the great toe in hyperextension. Massage with golf balls, a rolling pin, or a ribbed can may provide additional relief.

Before custom orthotics are provided, the rehabilitation clinician should use OTC orthotics or taping to assess whether it provides relief. If either a temporary orthotic or a low-dye strapping technique reduces the patient's pain complaints, this is a good indication that a permanent orthotic is needed.

Once pain is under control and flexibility exercises are a routine part of the rehabilitation program, the patient begins strengthening exercises for the ankle inverters and for the intrinsic and extrinsic toe flexors. These muscles help to support the arch and plantar fascia. Intrinsic strengthening exercises, picking up marbles and dropping them into the opposite hand, and towel-roll, heel-raise, and resisted inversion exercises are all appropriate for plantar fasciitis.

Only in extreme cases will patients need to refrain from normal activities; however, they may need to reduce their activity level for a time. Pain is normally the limiting factor, but because the fascia is weakened, it is susceptible to tears, especially during sudden acceleration or push-off movements. If the plantar fascia ruptures, acute pain and swelling will prevent normal ambulation. A stiff-soled shoe or boot or PWB on crutches for 3 to 7 d may be necessary. Treatment for a plantar fascia rupture follows a course similar to that for plantar fasciitis. Symptom control, flexibility exercises, and the usual progression to strengthening, coordination, agility, and functional activities are normal program components for a ruptured plantar fascia.

Tarsal Tunnel Syndrome

The tarsal tunnel is formed by the medial malleolus, calcaneus, talus, and deltoid ligament's posterior aspect. Tarsal tunnel syndrome is an entrapment of the posterior tibial nerve as it passes under the flexor retinaculum posterior to the medial malleolus along with the tendons of the tibialis posterior, flexor digitorum longus, and flexor hallucis longus (figure 20.64). Excessive pronation, especially with improper shoes, can cause increased tension on the flexor retinaculum to increase compression on the nerve. Dancers, especially tap dancers who wear rigid shoes and sustain high impact forces, are susceptible to tarsal tunnel syndrome.[294] Swelling from trauma or tendinopathy can also cause tarsal tunnel syndrome. Symptoms during weight bearing include a burning pain, tingling, and numbness in the medial and plantar foot.[295] Tinel's sign is often positive. Toe flexor and abductor hallucis weakness and a reduced ability to plantar flex and invert the foot can be noted in more advanced cases.

Only severe cases need cessation of activities or surgery. Most cases can be treated conservatively. Rehabilitation includes orthotics to reduce pronation and posterior tibial nerve irritation, modalities such as phonophoresis or iontophoresis to diminish inflammation, and therapeutic exercises to resolve weakness.[294] Properly fitted shoes and anti-inflammatory medications are also useful. Flexibility exercises and soft-tissue mobilization for release of adhesions can also be beneficial for pain relief. If shoe compression on the medial foot contributes to the problem, inserting a pad to relieve pressure on the nerve can reduce symptoms.

Cases requiring surgical release of the retinaculum may need either a walking boot or a non-weight-bearing posterior splint for about 2 weeks postoperatively.[294] A normal rehabilitation progression introduces jogging at around 6 to 8 weeks and return to full participation at around 10 to 12 weeks after surgery.

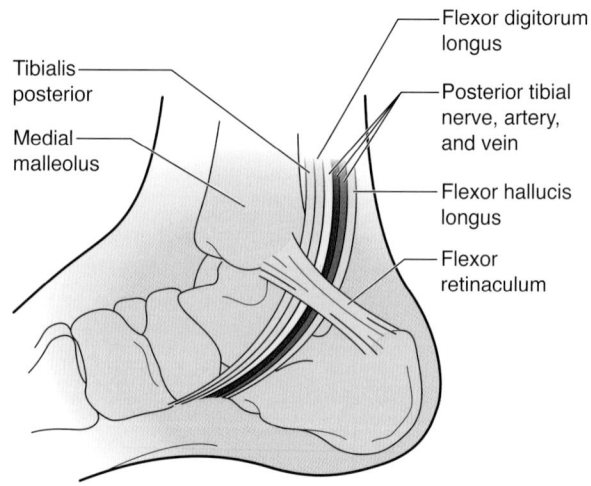

Figure 20.64 The tarsal tunnel is a location where the posterior tibial nerve may become entrapped, which produces pain and dysfunction in the toes and foot.

Sesamoiditis

The two sesamoids under the first metatarsal head enhance the windlass mechanism of the foot for increased propulsion, and they improve the leverage of the great toe flexor tendon and disperse weight-bearing forces.[296] Although they are small, these sesamoids transfer and disperse forces at the final phase of weight-bearing gait that are equivalent to up to 300% of the body's weight.[297] In this way they cushion the first MT head and also protect the flexor hallucis tendon.[298] Therefore, they serve important protective roles in weight-bearing activities.

Case Study

A 19-year-old basketball player has developed right plantar fasciitis over the past month. He has pain when he gets up in the morning and when he stands after sitting in class for an hour. He can perform his workouts without any difficulty, but he has noticed that the pain is worse the morning after a particularly hard workout. Your examination reveals higher-than-normal arches of both feet. Ankle dorsiflexion in subtalar neutral is –5°. Great-toe hyperextension is 50°. There is tenderness to pressure over the plantar medial calcaneus where the plantar fascia inserts. Shoe wear is excessive on the lateral aspect of the shoe.

Questions for Analysis

1. What will your first treatment include?
2. What home exercises will you give the patient before he leaves today?
3. What accommodations will you place in his shoes or on his feet?
4. What strengthening exercises will you give him, and when will you give them?
5. If you decide that the patient needs orthotics, what specifications will you want in them? How will you decide that he would benefit from orthotics?

Sesamoiditis does not actually involve the sesamoids but rather the soft tissue surrounding the bones. Restriction of soft tissue around the sesamoids, a tight Achilles tendon, plantar-flexed first ray, reduced great-toe hyperextension motion, and a restricted midfoot can all be underlying causes of sesamoiditis.[299] Occasionally, poor cleat placement on shoes can increase pressure on the sesamoids and cause soft-tissue irritation. Hyperextension of the first metatarsophalangeal joint to at least 60° is needed for walking activities,[300] and more is needed for running activities. Less hyperextension than that can increase forces imposed on the sesamoid region during propulsion.

The patient complains of pain with running, especially during push-off. Pain is located over the first metatarsal head. Standing heel raises with pressure over the first metatarsal head are painful, as is passive dorsiflexion of the great toe. Palpation reveals tenderness of the sesamoids.

Intervention for rehabilitation includes relieving the symptoms and correcting the underlying cause. Flexibility exercises to correct tight structures are vital. Soft-tissue mobilization is usually needed because the soft tissue becomes adherent around the sesamoids and further restricts great-toe hyperextension motion. A pad or orthotic with a cutout for the first ray and with an extension pad to the second metatarsal head and toe can help to reduce stress on the sesamoids.[299] Placing the foot in a rigid-soled shoe also limits the stress applied to the sesamoids.[48]

This injury is self-limiting and does not usually require patients to cease activity. Modification of shoe wear, correction of the causes, and modifications in activity usually will enable the patient to continue some level of participation. If the patient has had this condition for a while, changes in gait and secondary weaknesses in less-used muscles will develop. Deficiencies should be identified and corrected.

Fractures

The primary concern with a fracture in a young patient is that it may include the growth plates. If it does, further development and bone growth can be severely impaired. Stress fractures and acute fractures are common. Each is treated differently; programs and considerations related to these fractures are outlined here.

Fractures can occur in any of the leg, ankle, or foot bones. Stress fractures result from repetitive stress to the tibia and metatarsal bones, whereas acute fractures result from the sudden application of excessive forces. In younger patients, epiphyseal plate fractures can occur, especially in the distal fibula and tibia. Acute fractures vary greatly in their presentation. Lateral stresses to the ankle can result in malleolar fractures; compression forces from jumping can cause talus, tibia, and metatarsal fractures; crush injuries from having the foot stepped on can cause metatarsal and phalangeal fractures; other phalangeal fractures can occur as a result of stubbing a toe; and torsional stresses can cause spiral fractures of the tibia and foot.

Phalangeal fractures are painful but are seldom casted. The fractured phalanx is commonly buddy taped to an adjacent toe.[301] Metatarsal fractures of the second, third, and fourth metatarsals are commonly placed in a controlled ankle motion (CAM) boot to restrict movement during ambulation. Crutches are sometimes needed if the patient cannot ambulate normally. Fractures of the first metatarsal need special attention because this is a major weight-bearing bone. Fifth metatarsal fractures also deserve special attention because they can cause problems that linger, depending on the fracture's location. Tarsal fractures can be interarticular and involve interarticular ligamentous damage. If the fracture is displaced, surgery is usually indicated. Ankle fractures are often surgically repaired because even minimal displacement of fragments has better outcomes with surgical repair than with conservative management.[302] Fractures in young patients should be referred to an orthopedic surgeon because epiphyseal fractures are serious injuries that can impair normal bone growth.

Because the tibia, talus, calcaneus, and first ray are the primary weight-bearing structures of the foot and leg, fractures to these bones need immobilization and non–weight bearing. The fibula is essentially a non-weight-bearing bone, so walking boots or walking casts are usually used for fractures of this bone. Displaced fractures are surgically repaired, whereas nondisplaced fractures may be immobilized with or without surgery.

Immobilization of fractures of the leg, ankle, or foot must all include immobilization of the ankle. After immobilization, limited joint mobility is one of the greatest debilitating factors.[303] The greater the damage, the more extensive the scar-tissue formation. The risk of scar-tissue formation increases as edema becomes greater and as immobilization is more prolonged. Immobilization and soft-tissue edema with subsequent scar-tissue adhesions combine to produce restricted joint mobility.[304] This joint restriction can occur at the ankle and other regional joints or anywhere in the body where soft-tissue edema with scar tissue adhesions forms. Normal mobility must be restored to these joints to restore full balance of function. If one joint is restricted, an adjacent joint will suffer exaggerated stresses as it compensates for the lost mobility of the restricted joint. Over time, the increased stress can lead to tissue breakdown and injury.

The immobilization time needed to heal a fracture usually leads to capsular restriction, muscle weakness, balance and proprioception deficits, and deficiencies in muscle endurance.[305] Joint motion and soft-tissue mobility must be emphasized in early rehabilitation because the window of opportunity for regaining these elements is narrower than for the other factors such as strength and agility. As scar tissue matures, the opportunity to change its length diminishes. If prolonged immobilization has resulted in extensive scar-tissue formation, prolonged stretches may be the most appropriate way to increase the mobility of shortened tissue and adherent collagen. These concepts were presented in detail in chapter 2.

Foot, ankle, and leg fractures typically require 3 to 6 weeks of immobilization.[306] This time may vary for stress fractures and surgically repaired fractures. Stress fractures are not often casted, but activity is reduced to relieve stress on the fracture site and to provide an optimal healing environment. Fractures that undergo open reduction internal fixation (ORIF) usually advance to weight bearing sooner than conservatively treated fractures. Patients with fractures that involve the primary weight-bearing bones are advanced to partial weight bearing with more caution, and full weight bearing is delayed.

Joint mobilization and soft-tissue mobilization techniques are begun as soon as they can be done safely. Modalities such as heat or ultrasound, when applied before mobilization techniques, can help to prepare soft tissue and lead to better treatment results. Massage is useful in relieving edema. Deep-tissue massage, friction massage, and myofascial techniques are used to improve soft-tissue mobility.

Joint mobilization techniques for pain relief occur early, in the inactive phase, whereas grades III and IV are applied in the later portion of the active phase and into the resistive phase, if necessary. If a joint is very tender, grade III and IV techniques may not be possible until pain is under control. Active stretches, passive stretches, and contract-relax-stretch techniques are useful during the active phase to increase the motion of both joint and soft-tissue structures.

Immobilization and periods of restricted weight bearing may require gait-training instructions once the patient can resume full weight bearing. Before this time, the patient can perform pool exercises in shoulder-high water that place only 10% of body weight on the extremity, and these can be used to address normal gait techniques.[307] For patients who are partial weight bearing, it is important to instruct them in a normal heel-toe gait to encourage proper gait patterning in preparation for full weight bearing. Once the patient is allowed to bear full weight on the extremity, pre-gait instruction, including weight-transfer activities and normal stride reeducation, is usually needed.

Closed kinetic chain exercises for strengthening, as well as static balance activities such as stork standing, begin when full weight bearing is permitted. Rehabilitation

Case Study

A 16-year-old wrestler sustained a lateral malleolar fracture to his left ankle during a wrestling match. He underwent an ORIF the next day and was placed on crutches, non–weight bearing on the L for 2 weeks before advancing to partial weight bearing. It is now 4 weeks after the surgery, and the patient is not yet full weight bearing, although the surgeon instructed him to begin weight bearing to tolerance and to advance to weight bearing without the crutches. The patient admits to you that he is apprehensive about putting weight on the extremity for fear of breaking it again. The extremity had been placed in a cast after surgery until yesterday, when the cast was removed.

On examination, the patient's ankle moves to 10° plantar flexion for maximum dorsiflexion. Other measures include 30° of plantar flexion, 0° of eversion, and 5° of inversion. Ankle strength in these directions is 2+/5 in the available ranges of motion. His hip and knee ranges of motion are normal, but strength is 4–/5 for all of the muscle groups. The surgical scar is well healed, but sloughing skin is present around the ankle, and there are dry scabs over the surgical wound. Palpation reveals stiffness of soft tissue around the ankle and into the foot. The foot is mildly enlarged, but there is no pitting edema. Mobility of the ankle joints is restricted to no more than 30% of normal, and the intertarsal and metatarsal joints are restricted to 50% of normal mobility.

Questions for Analysis

1. What are your goals for today's treatment session?
2. What home program will you send with the patient today?
3. The patient wants to attend a wrestling camp in 10 weeks; what will you tell him when he asks whether he will be able to attend the camp?
4. List your long- and short-term goals for the patient for the next 6 weeks.
5. What will be your criteria for advancing him to closed kinetic chain exercises?
6. List three closed kinetic chain exercises that you will give the patient on the first day to encourage him to bear more weight on the left lower extremity.
7. List three non-weight-bearing exercises that you will give him in the next week.
8. List three agility exercises you will use in the patient's program and the criteria he must meet before they are used.

exercises proceed in the manner discussed earlier in this chapter. Advancement follows a logical progression from light to heavier weights, few to more repetitions, static to dynamic balance and agility exercises, and simple to complex activities until the patient advances to plyometric exercises and finally to functional activities before returning to full activity.

The rate of progression is determined by the tissue-healing timeline, the tissue's response to stresses, and the patient's ability to tolerate the rehabilitation progression. Performance-specific exercises and testing before return to full participation must mimic demands that the patient will encounter during performance. Once all the parameters are restored and the patient passes all tests without any difference in performance between left and right lower extremities, he or she may resume normal participation. Depending on the extent of the injury, the duration of immobilization, the age of the patient, and initial joint and soft-tissue restrictions after immobilization, 3 to 6 months is a reasonable amount of time to expect until resumption of normal participation.

Summary

This chapter discusses the characteristics of a normal foot and deviations from this norm. Variations from normal can increase stresses along the closed kinetic chain. To reduce these stresses, it is important to have a foot that is well aligned. Proper shoes, both in fit and design, will help to optimize foot function. Basic shoe construction and specific designs for various activities were presented. Occasionally, it may be necessary to use an orthotic to correct more profoundly misaligned feet. Either an off-the-shelf or a custom-made orthotic may be needed to reduce stresses caused by poor foot alignment. Trigger point treatment, joint mobilization techniques, and progressive exercises from flexibility to functional activities were included in this chapter. Some of the more common injuries of the foot, ankle, and leg were presented along with rehabilitation programs for these injuries.

LEARNING AIDS

Key Concepts and Review

1. Discuss normal foot mechanics in ambulation.

The first structure to hit the ground during ambulation is the calcaneus. It combines with the talus to form the subtalar joint, and the talus combines with the tibia and fibula to form the talocrural joint. Normal function of these two joints enables us to place the foot on the ground and adapt to varied ground contours and stresses while maintaining a steady gait. The talocrural joint moves primarily in dorsiflexion and plantar flexion. The subtalar joint is responsible for inversion and eversion. Pronation and its component motions convert the foot into a mobile adapter to accommodate to uneven surfaces. Supination causes the foot articulations to become more rigid in order to transfer power and distribute the forces needed for propulsion in ambulation. As the ankle goes into plantar flexion, the talus moves anteriorly so that the posterior, narrower aspect of the talus sits in the mortise joint. During dorsiflexion, the fibula glides superiorly and rotates medially; in plantar flexion, it moves inferiorly and rotates laterally. In addition to the talocrural and subtalar joints, the more distal tarsal bones of the foot form the midtarsal joint. This joint's movements closely follow the subtalar and talocrural joint movements. During supination, the navicular and cuboid bones move medially and inferiorly; during pronation they move laterally and superiorly. The first-ray movement occurs in plantar flexion and dorsiflexion; movement extends about a thumb's width and is equal in each direction. The second ray includes the joint between the second metatarsal and middle cuneiform; the third ray includes the third metatarsal and the lateral cuneiform; the fourth ray is the fourth metatarsal alone; and the fifth ray is the fifth metatarsal alone. Metatarsophalangeal joints permit flexion–extension, abduction–adduction, and accessory rotation and dorsal–plantar glides. The IP joints, which are hinge joints, permit flexion and extension with accessory rotation and dorsal–plantar glides. The first MTP joint must have at least 60° of hyperextension for toe roll-off during gait.

2. Identify two foot deformities, and discuss their impact on athletic injury.

Pes cavus, a rigid foot, limits the ability of the foot to absorb force, causing forces to be absorbed farther up the closed chain and thus risking injury to other structures. Pes planus, or flatfoot, causes the foot to move inefficiently, requiring more effort from, and thus applying more stress to, other structures. It also changes the mechanics of the extremity, increasing stresses applied to structures such as the Achilles, patella, and hip.

3. List the important factors in shoe selection for a pes cavus foot.
Because a pes cavus foot is rigid and has a limited ability to absorb stress, a shoe for someone with this deformity should have as much absorptive capacity as possible. Factors such as a soft midsole, a curved last, and flexibility should be standards in a shoe for a rigid foot.

4. Describe one joint mobilization technique for improving ankle dorsiflexion.
A dorsal glide can be used: The stabilizing hand is placed anteriorly around the distal extremity, and the mobilizing hand is placed around the proximal foot with the thumb and index finger in contact with the malleoli. The talus is glided posteriorly in the plane of the joint.

5. List three stretching exercises for the ankle and extremity, including one that is not mentioned in the text.
Some stretches for these structures are the standing gastrocnemius stretch, the seated soleus stretch with a strap, and standing sideways on an incline board with the ankle positioned in inversion.

6. Identify three strengthening exercises for the ankle and extremity.
Exercises for strengthening the ankle and extremity include calf raises, toe raises, and eversion in side-lying with a weight attached to the ankle.

7. Describe three agility exercises.
Agility exercises the patient can do include lateral jumps, zigzag runs, and rapid change-of-direction maneuvers performed on command.

8. Describe three functional exercises for the lower extremity.
Some functional exercises for the lower extremity are side-to-side sprints; run, stop, and jump exercises; and running and stopping on command.

9. Provide an example of a rehabilitation program progression for an ankle sprain.
Initial treatment in phase I includes modalities for edema and pain relief and reduction of inflammation. Joint mobilization and soft-tissue mobilization may be needed in the active phase if normal movements are impaired. Active and passive range-of-motion exercises are accompanied by mild strengthening exercises, such as isometrics, manual resistance, and rubber band exercises later toward the end of the active phase. If the patient has been non–weight bearing, it may be necessary to use exercises with a weight scale to reintroduce the concept of weight bearing on the extremity as a prelude to gait training. Body-weight resistance exercises and machine-weight resistance exercises are then included as the patient progresses to the resistive phase. Neuromotor control, balance, and proprioception exercises begin with simple stork standing and progress to standing on unstable surfaces, then to moving on one extremity. When strength, flexibility, and balance are restored, plyometric and then functional and performance-specific exercises are used in the advanced phase before return to participation.

Critical Thinking Questions

1. Explain how Deena concluded that Danny's plantar fasciitis was being caused by his pronation, hip tightness, and knee and tibial malalignments. Why would she suspect that Danny's thigh muscle imbalance was also contributing to the plantar fasciitis? What shoe features should Danny look for when he buys his next pair of running shoes?

2. If a patient had a limb-length discrepancy but no other major structural problems, would you expect to see an abnormal wear pattern on the bottom of his or her shoes? If so, what?

3. What activities would you include in an aquatic exercise program for this patient for range of motion, strength, and cardiovascular conditioning? When could you begin this aquatic program?

Lab Activities

1. Perform a deep-tissue massage to your lab partner's leg. Can you locate any areas of restriction? Is that same area also tender when you apply a deep massage to it? Why would this be?

2. Locate the trigger points for the following muscles on your lab partner:

   A. Gastrocnemius

   B. Soleus

C. Abductor hallucis

Where were your partner's most sensitive trigger points? Perform a trigger point technique on each of them, and provide your partner with a home exercise for each tender trigger point.

3. Perform grade II and IV joint mobilizations on your lab partner, and identify what restriction would be best treated with each mobilization for the following joints:

A. Tibiofibular joints

- Superior: AP, PA glides
- Inferior: AP, PA glides

B. Talocrural joint

- Distraction
- Anterior glide
- Posterior glide

C. Subtalar joint

- Distraction
- Anterior glide
- Posterior glide

D. TMT, MTP, IP joints

- Distraction
- Anterior glide
- Posterior glide

4. Have your partner perform a gastrocnemius stretch and a soleus stretch. What are the substitution patterns, and where does your partner feel the stretch for each of the exercises? What verbal cues did you use to correct the errors in performance?

5. Have your partner perform a prolonged Achilles stretch for 3 min. How could she perform the exercise incorrectly so that the stretch would not be optimally effective? When she steps out of the stretch, have her explain what she feels in the calf.

6. Provide your partner with manual resistance to dorsiflexion, inversion, and eversion, 10 repetitions each. Be sure to provide enough resistance to make the motion smooth, accommodating your resistance to match your partner's and still obtain a maximal output through a full range of motion for each exercise. What position did you place him in to provide resistance most efficiently?

7. Now have your partner perform the same exercises as in the previous question with a Thera-Band. First, how will you determine what color of Thera-Band she should use for each exercise? Have her perform an exercise and then describe the differences between the manual resistance and the Thera-Band resistance throughout the range of motion for that exercise. How would these results influence your choice of what kind of exercise to include in a rehabilitation program?

8. Have your partner perform balance exercises that progress from static balance to balance on an unstable surface to balance while performing distracting activities. Evaluate your partner's performance as you would for a chart note. Be sure to include the activity, number of repetitions, and your assessment of performance quality.

9. Have your partner perform one agility drill that you design using tape marks on the floor. Diagram the exercise on paper. Have him perform it first without resistance, then with resistance. Did your partner's ability to perform the activity change with the addition of resistance? If so, how did it change? What performance factors did you watch and correct for, and what were your cues for correction? For which sport would your exercise be most appropriate?

10. Design one plyometric or hopping activity. Describe it, and identify why this is the one you chose. Have your partner perform it. What performance factors did you watch and correct for, and what were your cues for correction? What would be the criteria for your partner to advance to the next level of exercise? Which patients would benefit most from these activities as part of their rehabilitation program?

Shoulder and Arm

Objectives

After completing this chapter, you should be able to do the following:

1. Discuss the importance of stability in shoulder rehabilitation.

2. Explain the role of scapular stabilization in shoulder function.

3. Define *scapular dyskinesis*.

4. Explain how scapular dyskinesis can affect the shoulder's function.

5. List three joint mobilizations for the shoulder.

6. Identify three strengthening exercises for the scapulae and three for the glenohumeral muscles.

7. Discuss the general rehabilitation progression of strengthening exercises for the shoulder.

8. List precautions for a rehabilitation program following a rotator cuff repair.

9. Outline key factors for a program for a biceps tendinopathy.

Logan Jacobs, certified athletic trainer for the local baseball farm team, sees several shoulder injuries each season. He is very familiar with the shoulder rehabilitation process, having successfully treated many players over the years.

His latest patient, Benj "Quickdraw" Charles, is one of the more promising pitchers Logan has seen in recent years. Benj began having shoulder pain as a result of scapular muscle weakness and fatigue. Although he didn't have any shoulder capsular tightness that would have required joint mobilization techniques, he did have the lateral rotator tightness that pitchers often acquire. Logan has provided Benj with a good rehabilitation program that has resolved the shoulder's motion and strength deficits, and Benj is about to begin a plyometric exercise program before beginning throwing activities.

Logan likes to make the rehabilitation program interesting for his baseball players. On different days, he provides different exercises that can produce the same result. He uses elastic resistance bands, manual resistance, and medicine balls instead of machine weights or dumbbells because he feels that his patients find these more interesting and fun than weights.

He hits it long. His shoulders are impressively quick through the ball. That's where he's getting his power from. He's young and has great elasticity.

Nick Faldo, 1957-,
former English professional golfer
and currently an on-air golf analyst

The shoulder girdle is a complex multiplex. Its complexity makes it a challenging region to assess from both a functional and a rehabilitation perspective.[1] Rather than approaching the shoulder complex as an obstacle to our understanding, we will identify its parts and how they function so that you can learn to identify problems and confidently address them in a rehabilitation program. This chapter will help you to understand the shoulder's complexity and appreciate rather than fear it.

The shoulder's most elementary and most important role is to position the hand for function.[2] The shoulder girdle provides the impetus for propelling objects from the hand; it also places the hand in a position that enables you to catch, throw, or touch. Just as Mr. Faldo's observations of the golfer's swing imply, the entire shoulder complex, including its joints and muscles, must operate with precise timing, intensity, positioning, and speed of movement if the shoulder is to perform to its full potential.

The shoulder has more mobility than any other joint in the body. In terms of primary increments, there are approximately 16,000 possible shoulder positions.[3] The shoulder is designed for large ranges of motion, making thousands of hand placements possible. People who participate in overhead sports such as baseball, softball, golf, football, swimming, volleyball, racket sports, and field events including javelin, discus, and shot put likely take it for granted as they use the shoulder's expansive mobility each day during practice and competition. Overhead sports require tremendous forces to produce great upper-extremity

velocity. During the acceleration phase of pitching, for example, arm movement has been recorded at a velocity of around 7500°/s.[4] Rotational velocity in a tennis serve is 1500°/s, and hand speed at ball impact has been clocked at 75.6 kph (47 mph).[5] These velocities are generated from the shoulder starting essentially at rest in the cocking phase of a movement, accelerating to these top speeds, and then suddenly decelerating in the follow-through, all in the space of milliseconds of time. No manmade machine can accelerate to those speeds from 0 mph and decelerate back to 0 mph in that brief amount of time. For the shoulder to withstand these repeated stresses, the joints and muscles must work together as a highly synchronous, well-balanced unit. If a joint fails to move correctly or the muscles are imbalanced, an injury is sure to occur.[6]

The risk of injury makes it vital for the rehabilitation clinician to understand the mechanics of normal shoulder motion and to have the knowledge, skill, and good judgment to provide an appropriate rehabilitation progression. Before presenting specific rehabilitation programs for the shoulder, this chapter introduces basic considerations that are unique to the shoulder. As a clinician, you must understand these factors to design appropriate functional and performance-specific elements of a shoulder rehabilitation program.

Special Rehabilitation Considerations

The shoulder complex is a unique area composed of several joints: the sternoclavicular, acromioclavicular, scapulothoracic, and glenohumeral joints. Not only must these joints have extensive mobility while providing stability, but the muscles that surround and control them must all work together to provide normal shoulder function and essential timing of movement. Several adjacent structures have a profound influence on the shoulder complex, both in position and in function. Whenever a rehabilitation clinician treats a shoulder patient, these elements and their influence must be considered. Each of them is presented in this section.

The interdependence of the structures of the shoulder complex produces smooth, complete motion. The scapula not only provides the socket portion of the shoulder joint but also the attachment point for the rotator cuff muscles. When the shoulder is elevated, the scapula rotates to minimize changes to the relative lengths of the rotator cuff muscles through the higher ranges of motion. This rotation of the scapula during shoulder elevation maintains the length–tension relationship of these muscles, so they continue to provide glenohumeral stability even at the farthest extent of shoulder elevation.[7] By keeping the humeral head directly aligned with the glenoid fossa, the rotator cuff increases the joint's congruency to provide additional stability when the shoulder is in an overhead position.[8]

When the glenohumeral joint of the shoulder complex moves, all of the joints move. When motion is deficient in one of these joints, glenohumeral motion is restricted.[9] Even the anatomical architecture contributes to glenohumeral motion; the crank-like shape of the clavicle provides for greater elevation of the shoulder than would otherwise be available if the bone was straight.[10, 11] The combined motions of sternoclavicular and acromioclavicular joints enable the scapulothoracic motions to occur.[12, 13] During the first 30° of elevation, glenohumeral motion is the predominant motion, and the scapula is in what some refer to as the "setting phase."[14] As the shoulder continues to move to the end of glenohumeral elevation, the scapula and clavicle both move to provide what we know of as full flexion or abduction of the glenohumeral joint. The clavicle and scapula each move in three planes of motion in a coordinated manner, although the precise manner appears to vary from person to person.[15-18]

Stability

Stability is fundamental to any normal joint function. When an injury occurs, normal joint stability is compromised, and full recovery is threatened unless stability is restored.[19] Joint stability is provided by static and dynamic factors. Static stability is provided by the inert structures. In the shoulder joint, these inert structures include the joint capsule, ligaments, and glenoid labrum. Dynamic stability is the responsibility of the nerves and muscles; the neurological system sends input from the afferent receptors into the central nervous system to impart timely support through balanced muscle activity.[20] This neuromotor process was discussed in chapter 14. When the joint's ligaments are injured, the afferent receptors in those ligaments provide inadequate sensory input,[19] which leads to insufficient neural input and, in turn, inappropriate muscle responses. The result is a deficiency in static stability because of the

injury itself and a secondary dynamic instability caused by the damage to the afferent receptors.[19] These conditions produce a continuous injury cycle in which dynamic and static instability cause functional instability. This cycle leads to progressive injury, neuromotor imbalances, and chronic functional deficits (figure 21.1).

Dynamic instability occurs when muscles surrounding the shoulder are imbalanced. The imbalance of agonists and antagonists causes a loss of accurate proprioceptive and kinesthetic information, leading to dynamic instability.[21] Muscle imbalances in flexibility, strength, and function, if not corrected, can be the primary cause of shoulder injury, perpetuating the joint instability cycle.[22]

The rehabilitation clinician can break this cycle with a rehabilitation program to restore dynamic stability. Rehabilitation programs include reeducation of the neuromuscular system and exercises that reestablish balance between agonists and antagonists. Sometimes this is enough to restore the patient to normal function. When static instability is too great to be controlled conservatively, surgical intervention is needed. Rehabilitation for the restoration of dynamic stabilizers is just as important after surgery as it is in cases without surgery. This rehabilitation program is presented later in this chapter.

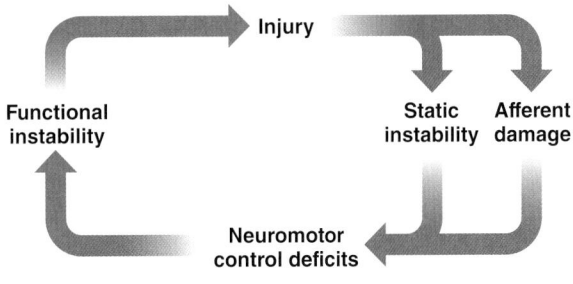

Figure 21.1 Joint instability cycle.

Scapular Muscles

Fundamental to all shoulder rehabilitation programs is rehabilitation of the scapular stabilizers.[23] These muscles control scapular motion. Their strength and control are crucial to the shoulder because the scapula serves as a platform upon which the shoulder moves.[24] Weak scapular muscles create an inadequate base for shoulder movement. The difference between a stable and an unstable scapula is similar to the difference between running on firm ground and running on a suspended wood-and-rope footbridge. The ground enables a runner to move smoothly and efficiently. An unstable footbridge places high energy demands on the runner's muscles, causes inefficient movement, and increases the risk of injury. So, too, a shoulder with an unstable scapula moves inefficiently and is at risk for injury. An unstable scapula can lead to injuries such as glenohumeral impingement and biceps or rotator cuff tendinopathy.[25-27] It is therefore essential that all rehabilitation programs for the shoulder include exercises for the scapular stabilizing muscles.

Scapular muscle fatigue can also affect shoulder motion and performance.[28] The scapular muscles' role as stabilizers is disrupted when these muscles fatigue. This disruption occurs because changes in normal scapulohumeral rhythm accompany scapular muscle fatigue, as shown by McQuade and colleagues.[29] The results of their study point to the importance of scapular muscle endurance activities in a rehabilitation program. It is advisable to use high-repetition, low-resistance exercises for scapular muscles, especially for patients who will be returning to activities that require high endurance levels from the lower trapezius and serratus anterior muscles. Athletes who must perform extended muscle activity of this type include repetitive throwers such as baseball and softball pitchers and catchers; swimmers, especially distance swimmers; gymnasts, especially those on upper-body apparatus; volleyball hitters; oarsmen; and tennis players and other racquet sport athletes. In the workplace, both white collar and blue collar workers are susceptible to scapular muscle fatigue;[30, 31] rehabilitation programs for workers who perform sustained or highly repetitive activities with their shoulders must likewise include endurance activities for the scapular muscles.

Because scapular muscle strength is so important to the function and stability of the shoulder, exercises for these muscles begin early in the rehabilitation program, even if the injury involves surgical repair.[23] Strengthening exercises for these muscles can start early since, by the use of manual resistance, they can be exercised without stressing the glenohumeral joint. Often the upper trapezius and levator scapulae muscles are not weak; although the other scapular muscles are not as weak, they are usually weaker than they should be, so all scapular muscles need both reeducation and rehabilitation.[32] Scapular depression, protraction, retraction, and upward and downward rotation are all motions that can and should be manually resisted as early as is safely possible in the rehabilitation process.

If the upper trapezius and levator scapulae are weak, of course, these muscles must be strengthened. More often than not, however, these two muscles are strong and overpower weaker shoulder muscles during scapular rotation movements, so their greater strength is often a contributing factor to scapular muscle imbalances.[33] If the rotator cuff is weak, the upper trapezius commonly substitutes for the rotator cuff and works with the deltoid to elevate the shoulder, further encouraging muscle imbalances and incorrect firing-sequence patterns and perpetuating the shoulder injury.[34-36] Two techniques that can control and retrain the upper trapezius are biofeedback and taping.[37, 38] Biofeedback can be used to either facilitate rotator cuff

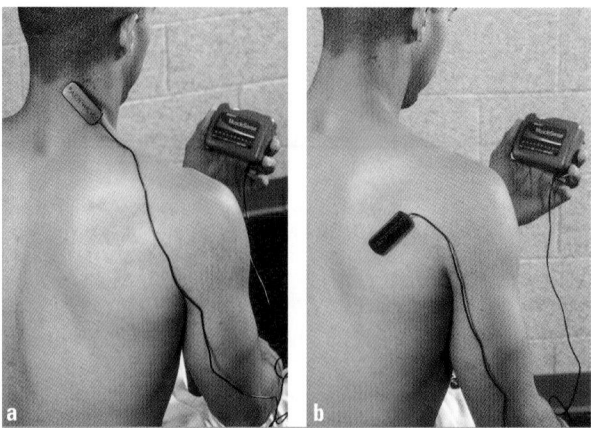

Figure 21.2 Biofeedback: electrode placement *(a)* for upper trapezius inhibition to decrease activity, and *(b)* for infraspinatus facilitation to increase activity.

activity or reduce upper trapezius activity during shoulder elevation exercises (figure 21.2). The specific application depends on the electrode placement, machine settings, and motions desired. Refer to Denegar and colleagues[39] for specific modality applications.

Scapular taping can be useful in cases of secondary impingement in which faulty positioning of the scapula during overhead movements causes impingement of the rotator cuff tendons.[40] The taping must be accompanied by retraining exercises to reeducate the scapular muscles so that they position the scapula correctly during shoulder motions. The taping technique was introduced by Jenny McConnell, an Australian manipulative physiotherapist. Limited research by McConnell has demonstrated that tape application inhibits upper trapezius activation and facilitates lower trapezius activation.[41] This response can improve scapular stability by improving muscle balance to permit arm movement without impingement pain; it can also enhance neuromotor reeducation for normal scapular muscle timing and scapular positioning.[42, 43] Different tapes and taping techniques have recently been developed and their effectiveness demonstrated for lower trapezius facilitation or inhibition of upper trapezius activity or both.[43-49] Although applying therapeutic tape to the shoulder is generally believed to have beneficial effects, the mechanism that makes it so is not yet fully understood. Different hypotheses have been advanced, but as yet, they remain hypotheses.[50] Figure 21.3 provides two examples of therapeutic taping of the scapular muscles.

 Go to HK*Propel* and watch video 21.1, which demonstrates scapular taping support to improve lower trapezius facilitation.

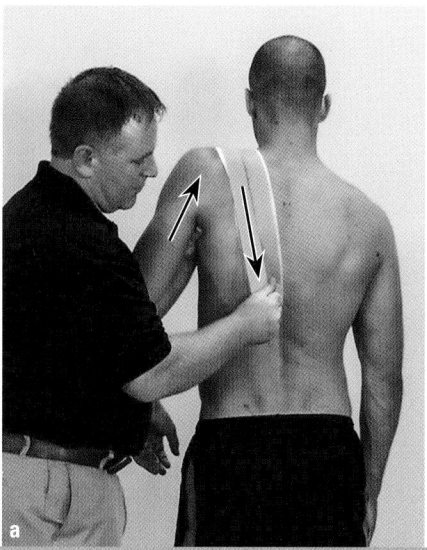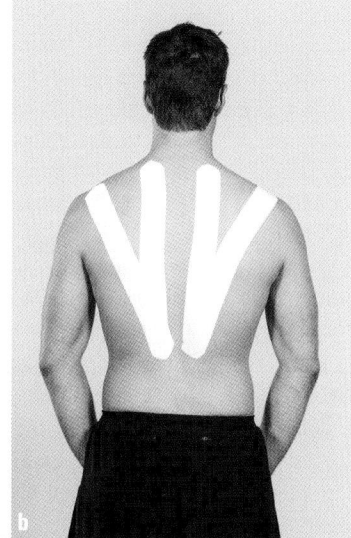

Figure 21.3   Examples of different taping techniques to facilitate scapular muscle activity. *(a)* McConnell taping to improve lower trapezius activity. *(b)* Alternative taping to facilitate lower trapezius activity.

Force Couples

Force couples are two equal forces that act in opposite but parallel directions to produce rotatory motion. The shoulder complex has several force couples that function during shoulder motion. The muscles within each of these force couples should be balanced if the force couple is to work properly. The shoulder complex has four force couples, two for the glenohumeral joint and two for the scapulothoracic joint.

In the glenohumeral joint, the infraspinatus and teres minor form a force couple with the subscapularis to produce downward translation of the humeral head in the glenoid.[51] This movement prevents compression of the humeral head against the coracoacromial arch and allows for greater motion during overhead activities. The second glenohumeral force couple is between the entire rotator cuff and the deltoid.[52] The anterior and posterior rotator cuff muscles (subscapularis, infraspinatus, and teres minor) depress the humeral head.[53] The supraspinatus assists in this depression and compression force on the humeral head into the glenoid as the deltoid elevates the humerus.[54] The rotator cuff depression and deltoid elevation work together to create humeral head rotation within the glenoid.

One scapular force couple includes the upper and lower trapezius and the serratus anterior. These muscles work together to rotate the scapula upward.[14] The other scapular force couple includes the pectoralis minor, levator scapulae, and rhomboids; these muscles work together to downwardly rotate the scapula against resistance.[14]

The muscles within each force couple must work cooperatively, both in timing and in intensity, to produce the desired activity, or injury can result. For example, if the deltoid overpowers the rotator cuff, the humeral head elevates in the glenoid, and impingement of superior glenohumeral soft tissues occurs. If the upper trapezius is stronger than the lower trapezius and serratus anterior, the scapula is not positioned correctly during arm elevation, and impingement of the rotator cuff occurs.[55]

Relationship Between the Trunk, Hip, and Shoulder

Just as scapulothoracic stability, strength, and endurance are important for glenohumeral function, trunk and lower-extremity stability and strength are important for scapular function. The trunk must have the strength to maintain a stable base for the scapula to function effectively.[33, 56] The legs and trunk provide 51% to 55% of the total kinetic energy and total force for overhead shoulder activities, while the shoulder contributes only 13% to the total energy production and 21% of the total force.[5] For these reasons, exercises for hip rotators, extensors, and abductors, as well as the trunk core muscles, should all be included in a shoulder rehabilitation program.

The forces generated from the legs, hips, trunk, shoulder, and arm are delivered through summation via the body's kinetic chain and are ultimately delivered to the hand and transferred to the object within the hand.[57] These forces must be timed, directed, and applied in a specific sequence.[58, 59] In other words, normal neuromotor function and desired performance require a balance of muscle strength and timing through all the segments involved.

Posture

Any patient with a shoulder injury should have a posture examination. Correct posture is crucial to shoulder balance and function. As we learned in chapter 17, a patient with a forward-head posture and thoracic kyphosis also has protracted scapulae with shoulders that are drawn forward and medially rotated (figure 21.4). This is a scapular posture of protraction, elevation, and anterior tilt with medial rotation of the humerus.[60] This posture is essentially the upper crossed syndrome described in chapter 17, which creates a kyphotic posture that results in secondary weakness of the scapular retractors and shoulder lateral rotators, and tightness of the scapular protractors and shoulder medial rotators. These postural changes prevent full elevation of the glenohumeral joint and lead to subacromial impingement and rotator cuff tendinopathy.[60] In short, muscle imbalance develops within the shoulder complex, with a shortening of the anterior muscles along with weakness and lengthening of the posterior muscles. Posture must be corrected if the shoulder rehabilitation program is to succeed.

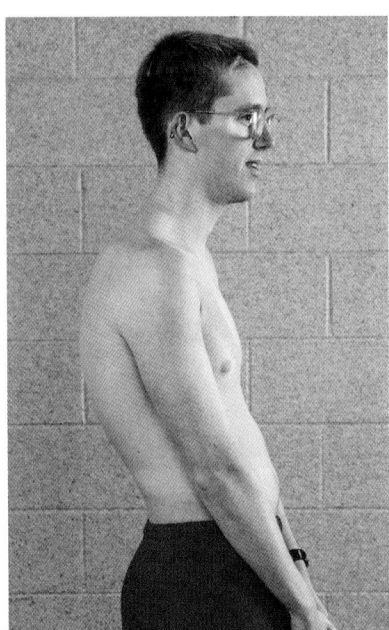

Figure 21.4   Forward-head, kyphotic posture creates pathological positioning of the shoulder complex, also referred to as an upper crossed syndrome.

Cervical Influence

There is an intimate relationship between the cervical spine and shoulder that goes beyond posture. Patients who complain of shoulder pain without a frank shoulder injury should be examined for cervical involvement. Cervical disc pathology can refer pain along the medial border of the scapula, into the shoulder joint, or down the arm.[61] If shoulder symptoms increase with movement, palpation, or joint mobilization of the spine, the cervical spine is likely the source of shoulder pain. It is sometimes difficult to determine whether the cervical spine or the shoulder is the primary source of pain.[62]

A quick range-of-motion test can often rule out the possibility of cervical involvement. The patient performs active range of motion of the cervical spine; if the patient reports no pain, gentle and gradual overpressure by the clinician is applied in each end-motion position. If range of motion or overpressure in any position produces pain, a more thorough examination of the cervical spine is indicated.[63] If range-of-motion and overpressure tests are negative, the shoulder rather than the neck may be the source of pain; however, if the patient does not respond to shoulder treatment after 3 to 5 treatments, reassessment of the cervical spine is in order. Reproducing the patient's pain is a key component of the rehabilitation examination when determining the origin of the patient's complaints.

Thoracic Influence

Shoulders that lack full range of motion may have restricted joint mobility in the ribs or thoracic spine.[64] If a patient lacks the last few degrees of full glenohumeral joint elevation, the thoracic spine and costothoracic joints should be examined for hypomobility. Restricted costothoracic and thoracic spine mobility can restrict the shoulder's movement by limiting the expansion of the trunk needed for full shoulder motion.[65] This is especially true if the patient has habitually poor thoracic or cervical posture. Posterior–anterior mobilization of the thoracic spine or rib mobilization techniques, or both, should restore normal shoulder mobility when thoracic hypomobility is a factor in a patient's difficulty achieving the last few degrees of glenohumeral motion.[64, 66, 67] If poor posture is contributing to the reduced thoracic motion, it must be corrected with stretching of this area's tight soft-tissue structures and strengthening of the weak structures, as was discussed in chapter 17.

Scapular Plane

It is important to exercise the rotator cuff in the scapular plane.[68] This position is approximately 30° forward of the coronal plane. Elevation in this plane is sometimes called *scaption*, a term coined by Dr. Jacqueline Perry.[2] In the scapular plane, arm elevation occurs in line with the scapula's position as it lies on the ribs. It is the functional position for the rotator cuff and glenohumeral joint that allows for better joint congruity than occurs in the frontal plane and is the position in which functional motion occurs.[69] If rotator cuff exercises are performed in the coronal plane, they are usually too uncomfortable for the rotator cuff because their tendons are impinged in that plane of elevation. Placing the shoulder in the scapular plane reduces this possibility and is functional, practical, and more comfortable. Additionally, the scapular plane places the rotator cuff muscles in an optimal length–tension position for maximal output from the muscles that elevate the shoulder,[68] so better performance occurs as a result.[70]

It is interesting to note that during the late 1970s, Dr. Perry[3] theorized that the various fiber arrangements of the subscapularis on the anterior scapula and the different innervations between the upper and lower portions of the muscle were indicative of varied functions of the muscle. Only recently have electromyographic studies given credence to this idea. Wickham and colleagues[72] studied the upper and lower subscapularis segments during a variety of shoulder activities. Their results demonstrated some similarities and even more differences. They found that both (upper and lower) subscapularis segments activated similarly during resistance to medial and lateral rotation; on the other hand, they discovered that not only is there a significant difference in activity between the two segments of the muscle during shoulder elevation, but their onset and timing also differ. They found that the lower subscapularis muscle was much more active during elevation, presumably to facilitate humeral head depression within the glenoid fossa. They also found that the lower subscapularis provided anterior–posterior stability to reduce anterior translation when the shoulder was in mid-abduction ranges of motion. Since the lower subscapularis activates before the upper subscapularis during shoulder abduction, the authors suggested that the lower subscapularis activates first to resist the shear forces created by the deltoid during elevation.

From a clinician's perspective, these findings provide important rehabilitation information. Specific recruitment of the lower subscapularis may be needed to stabilize the glenohumeral joint after injury, especially anterior instability injuries. Lower subscapularis strength is needed if an injured patient is to perform safe elevation activities after any injury where subscapularis weakness is evident. On the other hand, the upper subscapularis must be included in rehabilitation for strengthening rotation motion.

When glenohumeral medial and lateral rotation exercises are performed, a towel roll should be placed between the arm and the ribs (figure 21.5). Using a towel in this manner places the shoulder in a scapular plane. This position also reduces the tension on the supraspinatus tendon, lessening irritation to the tendon.[71] This position may also improve the subscapularis alignment to more effectively depress the humeral head during shoulder elevation.[72]

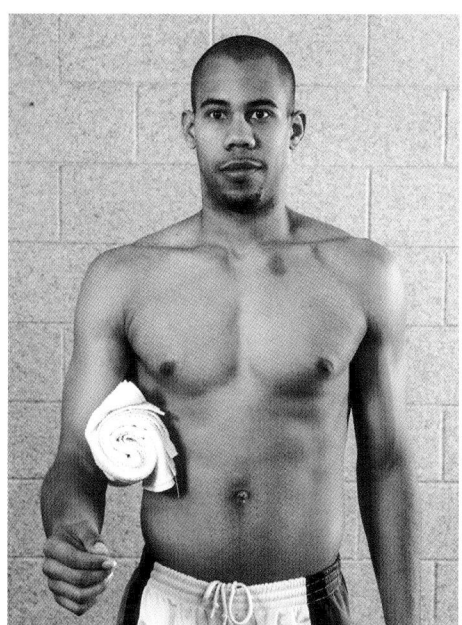

Figure 21.5 Using a rolled towel under the arm helps to reduce supraspinatus tendon stress and better align the subscapularis during glenohumeral medial and lateral rotation exercises.

Progression in the Exercise Plane and Rehabilitation Height

Strength exercises may begin as isometrics when shoulders are very weak or restricted in their motion, and they may progress to concentric and eccentric exercises as mobility and healing allow. When agonists are weak and are out of balance with their antagonists, the exercises should first be performed in straight-plane motions.[73] As strength and control of motion improve, the exercises progress to diagonal, multiplane, functional motions and more dynamic, performance-specific activities.[74] Strength exercises start in single-plane motions to target the weak muscles while minimizing the risk that stronger muscles will perform the exercise or that erroneous muscle firing patterns will continue. Straight-plane exercises focus on the muscles that need to be strengthened. Once these muscles gain strength, multiplanar exercises are added to encourage proper sequential muscle activation as the patient continues to progress toward normal activities.

The exception to this progression from single-plane to multiplanar exercises is when neuromotor development is used to reeducate muscle timing sequences. In these cases, the patient is instructed in motor pattern execution without the use of weights until muscle timing throughout the activity is correct.[75] This technique is becoming more popular for correcting shoulder pathologies that occur mainly because of scapular dysfunction.[76]

Scapular muscles have multiple roles during functional activities: Not only must they stabilize the scapula for shoulder activity, but they must also move the scapula as the shoulder moves to position the hand for highly complex and often rapid shoulder movements. As the shoulder moves higher, more demands are placed on the scapula's upward rotators, especially the serratus anterior and lower trapezius.[77] For this reason, shoulder position during strengthening exercises should be kept below 60° of elevation during the initial strengthening stage; since little scapular motion occurs in the first 60° of glenohumeral motion, scapular muscles exercised below 60° work primarily as stabilizers, not as scapular movers.[78]

Glenohumeral elevation higher than 90° is an unstable position for the glenohumeral joint, and scapular muscles in the early resistive phase lack the strength to keep the shoulder stabilized. As with any muscle, weakened scapular muscles naturally lose strength as they shorten (in higher elevations), and because they are weaker to begin with, they cannot provide the scapular stabilization needed for glenohumeral motion above 60° of elevation.[78] Once scapulothoracic and glenohumeral muscles have enough strength to control shoulder complex motion and provide the stabilization needed for activity at 80° to 110°, the rehabilitation clinician can progress the exercises to the fully elevated ranges. In the terminal elevation range, the scapular rotators are not only at their shortest length but also must meet their highest demands and produce the most control;[79, 80] therefore, strengthening exercises at higher levels of elevation are introduced only after lower-elevation strength is developed.

Rehabilitation Intervention Techniques

Manual therapy techniques, including soft-tissue mobilizations and joint mobilizations, are presented in this section. This is followed by a discussion of various exercises that may be included in rehabilitation programs for the shoulder complex. Manual therapy techniques are presented ahead of the exercises since those usually precede exercises in a treatment session. The exercises also follow a typical sequence, starting with flexibility and ending with performance-specific exercises.

Soft-Tissue Mobilization

Because of the intimate relationship between the cervical spine and the shoulder, some of the muscles discussed in chapter 17 are also relevant to the shoulder. Table 21.1 presents the most commonly seen trigger points in the muscles surrounding the shoulder. Refer to chapter 11 for details on soft-tissue mobilization theory, application, and interventions.

Supraspinatus friction massage is used to treat supraspinatus tendinopathy. The patient sits with his or her hand behind the back to expose the supraspinatus tendon just anterior and inferior to the acromion. The rehabilitation clinician's index finger is reinforced by the middle finger and placed on top of the tendon on the anterior shoulder about two finger widths inferior to the acromion. Cross-friction

TABLE 21.1 Trigger Points Most Commonly Found in Shoulder Complex Muscles

Shoulder segment	Muscle with trigger points
Glenohumeral stabilizers	Supraspinatus
	Subscapularis
	Teres minor
	Infraspinatus
Scapular stabilizers	Rhomboids
	Upper trapezius
Large glenohumeral muscles	Teres major

pressure is applied to the tendon for 1 to 2 min or until the tenderness subsides (figure 21.6). Once the pain subsides where the massage is applied, the clinician moves the finger slightly until the patient reports another area of tenderness; cross-friction is applied to this location. The clinician repeats the procedure until there are no areas of tenderness along the tendon. Although cross-friction technique is presented here only as a treatment for the supraspinatus tendon, the same techniques may be applied to any other area that is superficial enough to be affected by this intervention, such as the long head of the biceps.

Joint Mobilization

Joint mobilization can be performed on all joints of the shoulder complex. The findings of your initial examination will indicate which joints need mobilization. Glenohumeral joint mobility is also influenced by the mobility of the ribs and thoracic spine.[67] As mentioned earlier in this chapter, if a shoulder lacks full range of motion but has good mobility in its joints, an examination of rib and thoracic spine mobility may reveal a restriction of these joints. If this proves to be the case, thoracic and rib mobilization

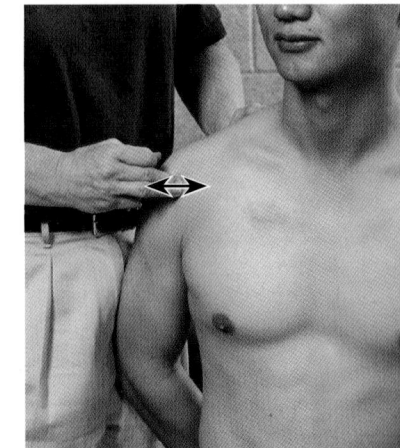

Figure 21.6 *Cross-friction massage to supraspinatus tendon.*

techniques discussed in chapter 17 for these areas may help to restore full shoulder motion.

Capsular restriction of the glenohumeral joint follows a unique capsular pattern: more restricted motion in lateral rotation than in abduction and more restricted motion in abduction than in medial rotation.[81] For example, if a patient's shoulder has 70° of medial rotation, 90° of abduction, and full lateral rotation, the joint capsule is not the primary structure limiting full motion. However, if the joint measures 70° of medial rotation, 90° of abduction, and 50° of lateral rotation, the joint capsule is probably restricting full motion. When a capsular pattern exists, joint mobilization is needed to restore glenohumeral motion. If a shoulder does not demonstrate loss of motion with this capsular pattern, capsular restriction is not the primary cause of motion loss. However, the clinician must still inspect the capsule to eliminate any adhesions that would require joint mobilization.

Glenohumeral mobilizations are initially applied with the joint in its resting position—55° flexion and 20° to 30° horizontal abduction. If additional motion is gained but full mobility is still lacking, the joint may need to be mobilized out of its resting position and in other loose-pack positions. The extreme close-packed position for the glenohumeral joint is full abduction with full lateral rotation; in that position, the joint is in its most congruent position with the greatest contact between the two joint surfaces.

While applying joint mobilization, the rehabilitation clinician always uses proper body mechanics. The hand applying the force is positioned as close to the joint as possible. The mobilization force comes from the legs transmitting the force through the trunk to the upper extremities; the arms do not provide the force.

The rehabilitation clinician must remember the principles of glide, roll, and spin so that the force is applied to achieve the desired motion gains. Since the humeral head is a convex surface moving on the glenoid fossa's concave surface, the convex-on-concave rule applies. The joint mobilization techniques presented here are those most commonly used. As with any joint mobilization procedure, the clinician should visualize the joint surfaces and apply the mobilization force parallel or perpendicular to the plane of the surface. As the shoulder is moved into different positions, the plane position of the glenoid changes; you must consider this as you determine the angle at which you apply the mobilization force.

Precautions and contraindications are always respected. The timeline for tissue healing and the status and strength of new tissue must be considered when one is deciding whether to apply joint mobilization and how much force to use. Joint mobilizations applied at a grade III or IV level to hypermobile joints can worsen instability and cause further damage, and they are contraindicated. Improper technique, incorrect application of force, excessive force, and inappropriate timing of application can all create discomfort for patients and yield ineffective results.

Glenohumeral Joint

During some mobilization techniques for the glenohumeral joint, a sustained joint distraction force is applied in addition to the mobilization force. A **joint distraction force** is an application in which the clinician applies long-axis traction to move the two joint ends apart. This application may be used alone to produce joint mobility, relaxation, or pain relief, or it may be used with another joint motion such as an anterior–posterior mobilization technique. The techniques are usually named according to the direction of the mobilization force. The following section provides instructions for mobilization of the glenohumeral joint.

Mobilization of the Glenohumeral Joint

Oscillation

Shoulder Position: 55° flexion and 20° to 30° horizontal abduction.

Mobilization Technique: Oscillation of the shoulder.

Indications: For general relaxation of the shoulder muscles before and after other joint mobilization techniques.

Patient Position: Supine and relaxed with shoulder near edge of table.

Clinician and Hand Positions: Clinician stands on the side of the patient, facing the patient's shoulder, and grasps the patient's distal forearm and wrist with both hands.

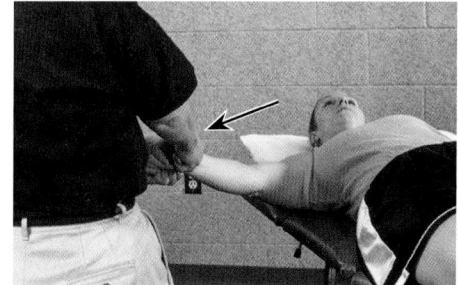

Figure 21.7

Mobilization Application: Mild distraction force perpendicular to the glenohumeral joint plane as oscillations are performed (figure 21.7).

Notations: Distraction force is applied by the clinician's body weight on the back foot while the clinician gently pulls on the shoulder with the hand grasping the forearm and wrist.

Distraction

Shoulder Position: 55° flexion and 20° to 30° horizontal abduction.

Mobilization Technique: Longitudinal distraction.

Indications: To improve inferior capsular mobility.

Patient Position: Supine with the involved shoulder as close to the side edge of the table as possible.

Clinician and Hand Positions: For a right shoulder, the rehabilitation clinician places his or her right hand in the axilla to stabilize the glenoid. The left hand grasps the lateral mid-humerus.

Mobilization Application: A distraction force is applied to the humerus (figure 21.8).

Notations: Good initial technique. A prolonged force is more effective, but oscillation combined with distraction can also be used.

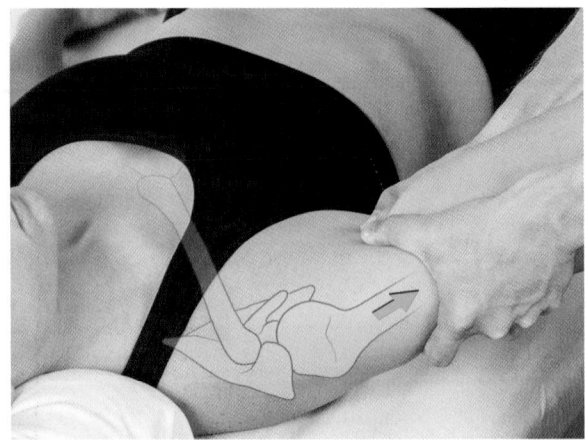

Figure 21.8

Inferior Glide

Shoulder Position: 55° flexion and 20° to 30° horizontal abduction.

Mobilization Technique: Inferior capsule glide or caudal glide.

Indications: To improve inferior capsular mobility and glenohumeral abduction.

Patient Position: Supine with involved shoulder as close to the side edge of the table as possible.

Clinician and Hand Positions: The mobilizing hand is on the superior lateral aspect of the humerus as close as possible to the glenohumeral joint, and the stabilizing hand is on the middle to distal humerus proximal to the elbow. The mobilizing hand web space should be over the superior humeral head just off the acromion.

Mobilization Application: The stabilizing hand holds the shoulder in its resting position while applying some distraction as the mobilizing hand applies a glide force in a caudal direction parallel to the joint's surface (figure 21.9a).

Notations: If the supine body's weight on the scapula is insufficient to stabilize the scapula, a stabilization belt around the patient's chest may be used to stabilize the scapula. The patient can be sitting with the shoulder abducted to the point of restriction as shown in 21.9b; however, initial glides should be performed in the resting position. Once approximately 120° of flexion is achieved, an inferior glide can be performed with the arm in an overhead position as shown in figure 21.9c. Keep in mind that as the shoulder's position changes, the glenoid joint surface position also changes. Likewise, the direction of the mobilization force changes as the joint plane changes: The force is directed inferiorly in any of these positions, but the specific plane must be in the plane of the joint's surface.

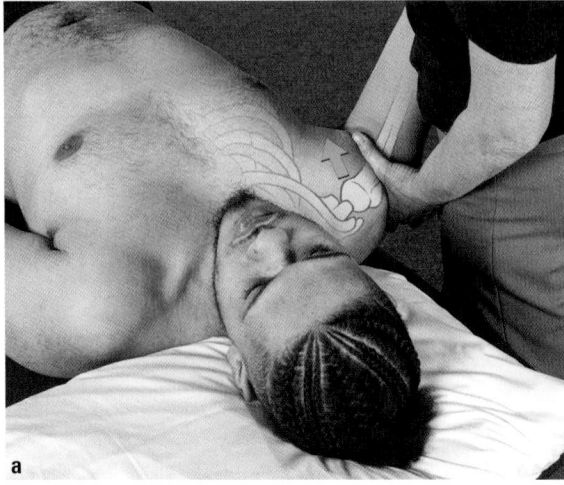
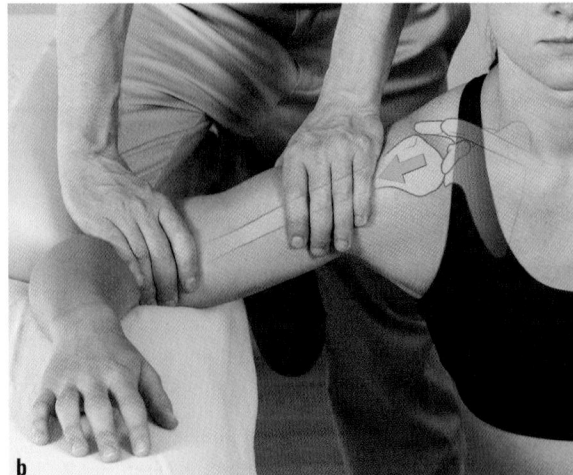

a b

Figure 21.9

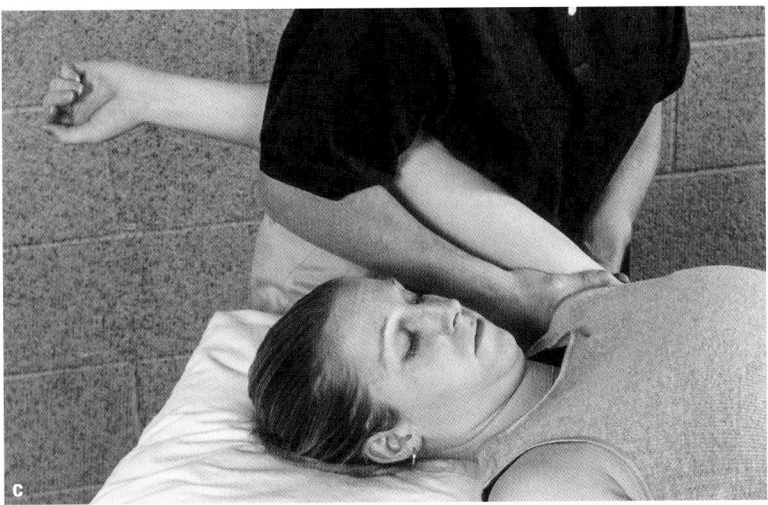

Figure 21.9 >*continued*

Alternative Inferior Glide

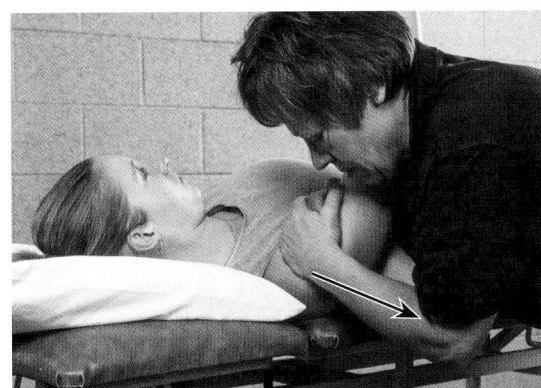

Shoulder Position: Shoulder flexion to 90°. The patient's humerus rests on the clinician's shoulder.

Mobilization Technique: Inferior capsule glide or caudal glide.

Indications: To improve inferior capsular mobility and glenohumeral abduction.

Patient Position: Supine with involved shoulder as close to the side edge of the table as possible.

Clinician and Hand Positions: Both of the rehabilitation clinician's hands grasp the humerus as close as possible to the shoulder joint with the patient's arm resting on the rehabilitation clinician's shoulder.

Figure 21.10

Mobilization Application: An inferior force is applied to the proximal humerus as the clinician uses her front leg to push her body away from the patient's shoulder joint (figure 21.10).

Notations: A sustained mobilization or oscillation technique can be used.

Lateral Distraction

Shoulder Position: 90° flexion with some horizontal adduction.

Mobilization Technique: Lateral distraction.

Indications: To stretch the posterior and superior capsule of the glenohumeral joint.

Patient Position: Patient is supine with involved shoulder as close to the side edge of the table as possible.

Clinician and Hand Positions: The clinician faces the patient at shoulder level and grasps the patient's humerus with the medial hand as proximal to the joint as possible with the patient's shoulder flexed to 90° and the other hand on the distal lateral humerus.

Mobilization Application: Lateral force is applied to the proximal humerus while the distal hand provides some joint distraction (figure 21.11).

Notations: The clinician should use proper body mechanics, keeping the back straight and using the legs.

>*continued*

Lateral Distraction >*continued*

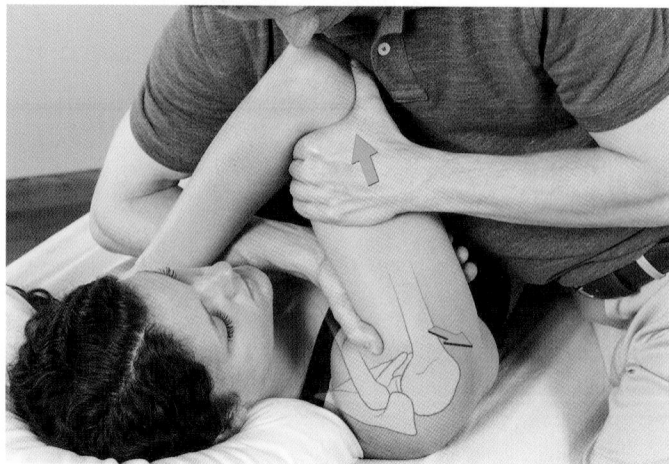

Figure 21.11

Posterior Glide

Shoulder Position: 55° flexion and 20° to 30° horizontal abduction.

Mobilization Technique: Posterior glide or dorsal glide.

Indications: To improve shoulder flexion and medial rotation by improving posterior capsular mobility.

Patient Position: Supine with shoulder as close to the side edge of the table as possible. A towel roll or wedge can be placed under the scapula for stabilization.

Clinician and Hand Positions: The clinician abducts the patient's arm to the resting position and stands between the patient's arm and trunk; the clinician places the stabilizing hand proximal to the elbow and the mobilizing hand on the proximal humerus just past the acromion.

Mobilization Application: The mobilizing hand applies a downward and slightly lateral force, while the stabilizing hand applies slight traction to the patient's glenohumeral joint at the patient's elbow (figure 21.12*a*).

Notations: An alternative technique is performed with the patient's shoulder in medial rotation to gain additional motion in that direction (figure 21.12*b*). An advanced flexion technique can be performed with the patient's shoulder flexed to 90° and horizontally adducted with the elbow flexed. In this position, the rehabilitation clinician stabilizes the scapula with a hand under the scapula. A posterior and slightly laterally directed mobilization force is applied with the mobilizing hand on the patient's elbow and the clinician's forearm in line with the patient's arm (figure 21.12*c*).

A final alternative application occurs with the patient's shoulder and the clinician positioned as in 21.12*b*, but the stabilizing arm is positioned so the clinician's medial forearm stabilizes the scapula with pressure over the inferior aspect of the anterior deltoid and the mobilizing hand is on the patient's distal forearm. The mobilizing force is an oscillation of the patient's shoulder in end-range medial rotation (figure 21.12*d*).

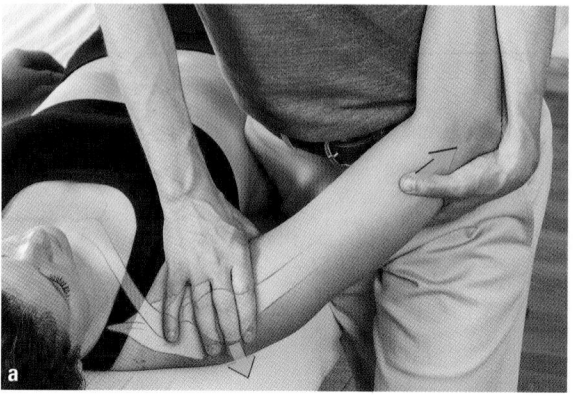
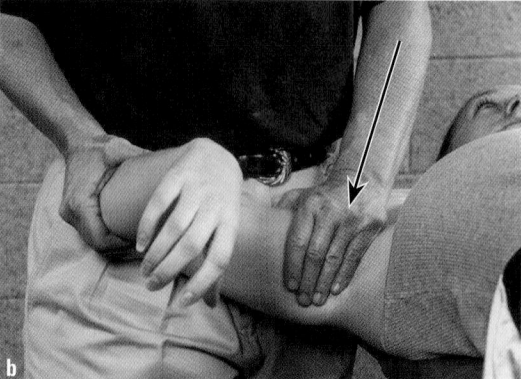

Figure 21.12

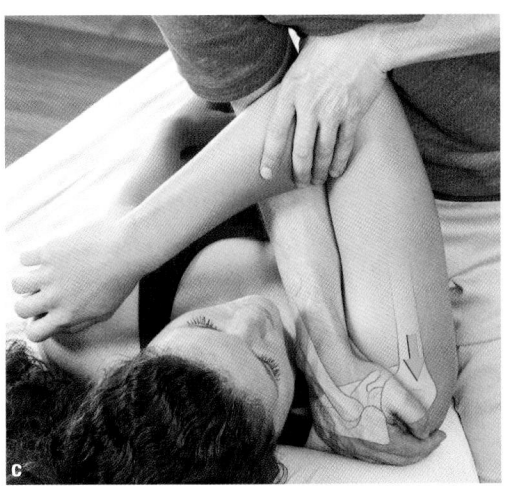
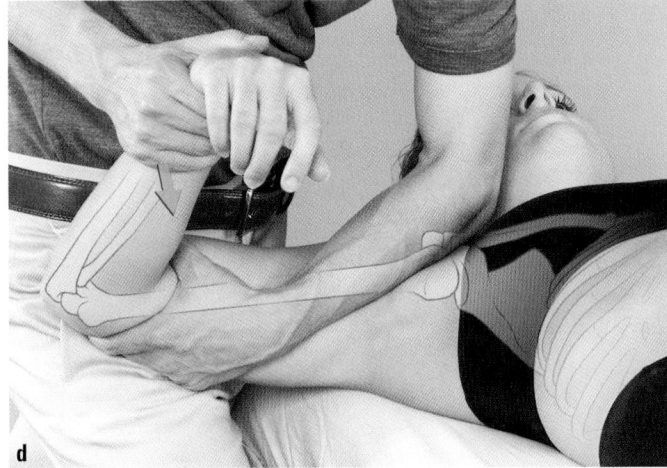

Figure 21.12 >continued

Anterior Glide

Shoulder Position: 55° flexion and 20° to 30° horizontal abduction.

Mobilization Technique: Anterior glide or ventral glide.

Indications: To increase anterior capsule mobility so that glenohumeral extension and lateral rotation improve.

Patient Position: Prone with a towel or wedge support under the anterior clavicle and coracoid process to stabilize the shoulder. The glenohumeral joint is off the side edge of the table, and the shoulder is placed in its resting position.

Clinician and Hand Positions: The rehabilitation clinician stands between the patient's arm and side, facing the shoulder, and places the stabilizing hand on the distal humerus and the mobilizing hand on the posterior aspect of the humeral head just distal to the acromion.

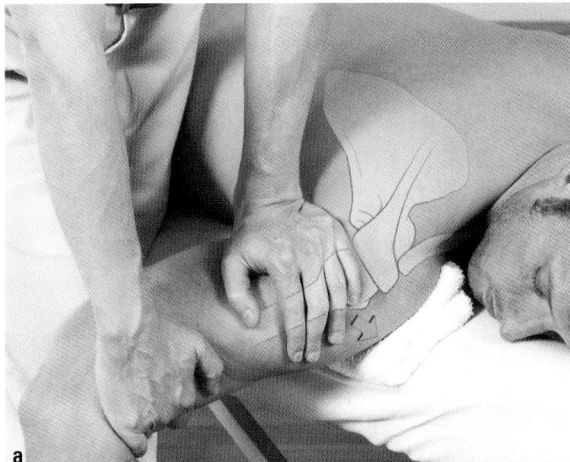

Mobilization Application: As the stabilizing hand applies a distraction force, the proximal mobilizing hand applies an anterior and slightly medial mobilization force (figure 21.13a).

Notations: If additional motion is achieved but restriction in the anterior–inferior capsule remains, an alternative position for mobilization is with the arm more elevated. An alternative technique can be used to increase lateral rotation by positioning the arm in additional lateral rotation during the mobilization; however, in this position there is a tendency for the clinician to extend the shoulder with the patient in a prone position (figure 21.13b). An anterior glide can also be performed with the patient in supine, but emphasis is more on lateral rotation: The patient is supine and the clinician applies the mobilization force at the distal forearm with the elbow flexed. The stabilizing hand stabilizes the scapula while the

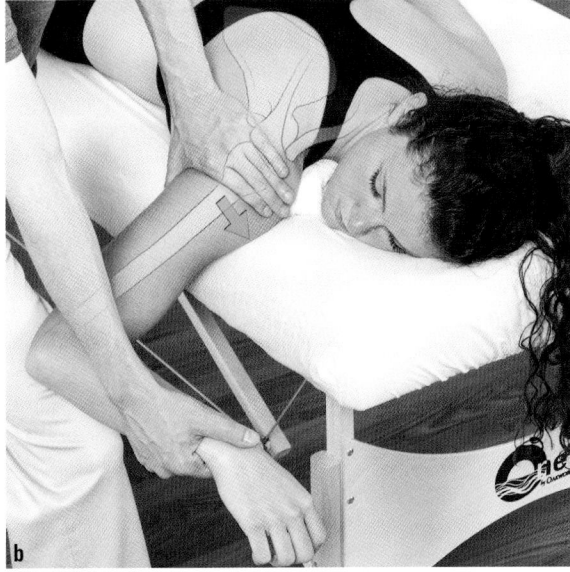

Figure 21.13

Anterior Glide >*continued*

mobilizing hand oscillates the humerus into its end ranges of lateral rotation (figure 21.13*c*). The resting position of the joint should be maintained throughout the treatment, regardless of the patient's resting position until later phases of rehabilitation when full motion is not yet achieved but tissue tolerance is improved.

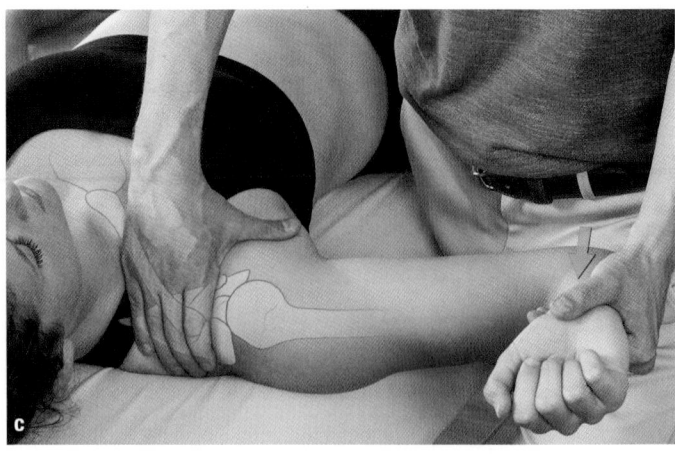

Figure 21.13 >*continued*

Scapulothoracic Joint

The mobilization techniques described in the following sections are possible only if the patient remains relaxed.

If a patient is not relaxed, the rehabilitation clinician will not be able to position his or her hands between the scapula and the ribs to apply these techniques.

Mobilization of the Scapulothoracic Joint

Scapular Distraction

Resting Position: The scapula is resting against the thoracic cage.

Mobilization Technique: Distraction of the scapula from the thorax.

Indications: To improve movement between the scapula and the thoracic ribs.

Patient Position: Side-lying with the involved arm on top.

Clinician and Hand Positions: Clinician faces the patient at chest level. Clinician's arm closest to the patient's head approaches the patient's scapula from over the top of the shoulder. Clinician's arm most distant from the patient's head is placed between the patient's arm and rib cage, and the clinician positions the fingers of both hands along the scapula's anterior vertebral border. The hand closest to the patient's head grasps along the scapula's upper vertebral border, while the other hand grasps under the inferior aspect of the vertebral border.

Mobilization Application: For personal comfort and professional consideration, a pillow should be placed between the patient and the clinician. As the shoulder is moved into retraction by the clinician's abdomen against the pillow positioned anteriorly to the patient's anterior shoulder and upper trunk, the fingers of both hands apply a force to tilt the vertebral border of the scapula posteriorly away from the ribs (figure 21.14*a*).

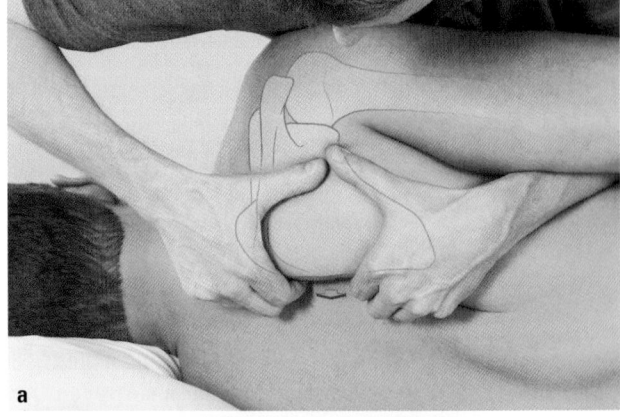

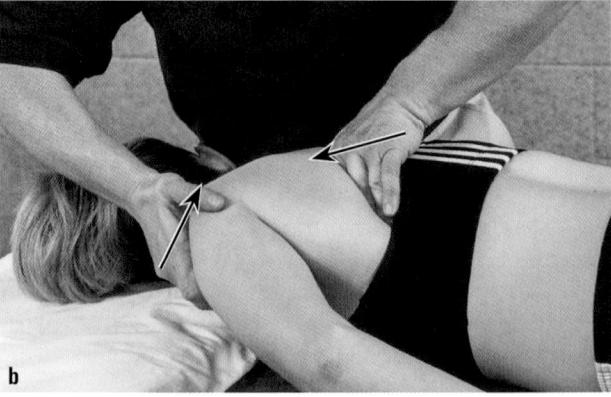

Figure 21.14

Notations: An alternative position is with the patient prone. The patient's arm is extended alongside the body, supported on the table. The clinician stands beside the patient, facing the patient's head, cups one hand around the anterior humeral head, and places the other hand under the inferior angle of the scapula as shown in figure 21.14*b*. The hands are moved simultaneously toward each other, the hand under the anterior shoulder lifting upward and medially and the hand under the scapula moving superiorly and pushing to gain access under the scapula.

Inferior Glide

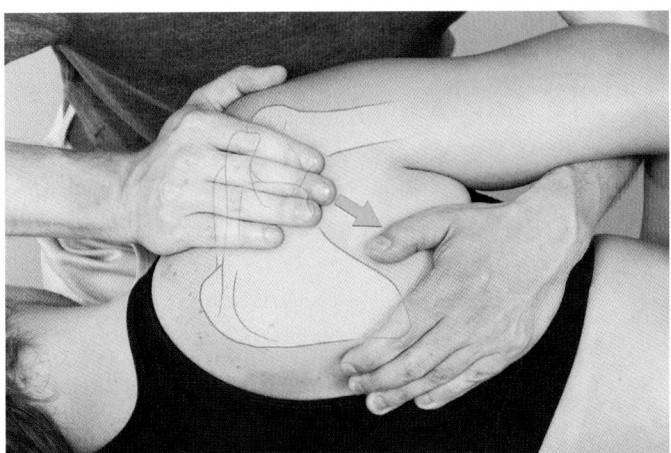

Resting Position: The scapula is resting against the thoracic cage.

Mobilization Technique: Inferior glide or caudal glide of the scapula.

Indications: To improve scapular mobility on the thorax.

Patient Position: Side-lying with the involved arm on top.

Clinician and Hand Positions: The clinician's cephalad hand is placed over the superior scapular border, and the caudal hand is positioned with the web space and lateral index finger cradling the inferior angle of the scapula.

Figure 21.15

Mobilization Application: As the superior hand pushes the scapula in a caudal direction, the index finger of the inferior hand pushes in a cranial direction to gain access under the inferior angle of the scapula (figure 21.15).

Notations: The patient must be relaxed for this technique to succeed.

Clavicular Joints

Because clavicular motion contributes 60° to glenohumeral motion,[14, 16] it is important for acromioclavicular and sternoclavicular joint mobility to be normal. After a period of shoulder immobilization, these joints may become restricted if the glenohumeral joint is hypomobile.

Four mobilization techniques are used at the sternoclavicular (SC) and acromioclavicular (AC) joints: inferior (caudal), superior (cranial), anterior (ventral), and posterior (dorsal) glides. The force is applied with the thumb pad

of one hand, reinforced by the other thumb. Mobilization techniques for these joints are described in the following section.

The resting position for the AC and SC joints is called the physiological position; it is the position the joints are in when the arm is resting at the side. The close-packed position for the SC joint is with the arm in full elevation overhead. The close-packed position for the AC joint occurs with the arm abducted to 90°.

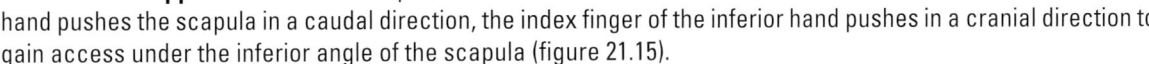

Mobilization of the Clavicular Joints

Acromioclavicular Inferior Glide

Resting Position: Joint is in its physiological position with the arm at the side.

Mobilization Technique: Inferior or caudal glide.

Indications: Hypomobility of the AC joint.

Patient Position: Supine with the arm relaxed at the side.

Clinician and Hand Positions: Clinician stands at the patient's head. The clinician's thumb is positioned on the superior aspect of the acromion.

>continued

Acromioclavicular Inferior Glide >*continued*

Mobilization Application: A superior-to-inferior mobilization force is applied to the distal acromion. Force is applied parallel to the joint plane.

Notations: This technique may also be performed with the patient sitting. In this position, the arm is supported to relieve stress on the AC joint, and the clinician faces the seated patient.

Acromioclavicular Posterior Glide

Resting Position: Joint is in its physiological relaxed position with the arm at the side.

Mobilization Technique: Posterior, dorsal, or anterior-to-posterior (AP) glide.

Indications: Hypomobility of the AC joint.

Patient Position: Supine with the arm relaxed and supported at the side.

Clinician and Hand Positions: When the patient is supine, the clinician stands at the head for inferior glides and at the side for anterior and posterior glides. One thumb is reinforced by the clinician's other thumb over the distal acromion while the fingers are used as buttresses to support thumb motion on the AC joint.

Mobilization Application: An anterior-to-posterior mobilization force is applied to the anterior aspect of the most lateral acromion. Force is applied parallel to the joint plane (figure 21.16).

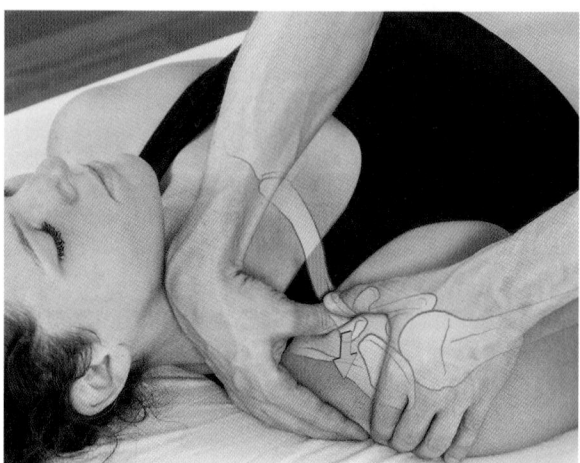

Figure 21.16

Notations: This technique may also be performed with the patient sitting and the clinician facing the patient to perform posterior and inferior glides or behind the patient to perform anterior glides.

Acromioclavicular Anterior Glide

Resting Position: Joint is in its physiological position with the arm at the side.

Mobilization Technique: Anterior, ventral, or posterior-to-anterior (PA) glide.

Indications: Hypomobility of the AC joint.

Patient Position: Seated with the arm relaxed and supported at the side.

Clinician and Hand Positions: Clinician stands behind the patient. The clinician's thumb is positioned on the posterior aspect of the most lateral acromion.

Mobilization Application: A posterior-to-anterior mobilization force is applied at the lateral end of the posterior acromion. Force is applied parallel to the joint plane (figure 21.17).

Notations: This technique may also be performed with the patient supine.

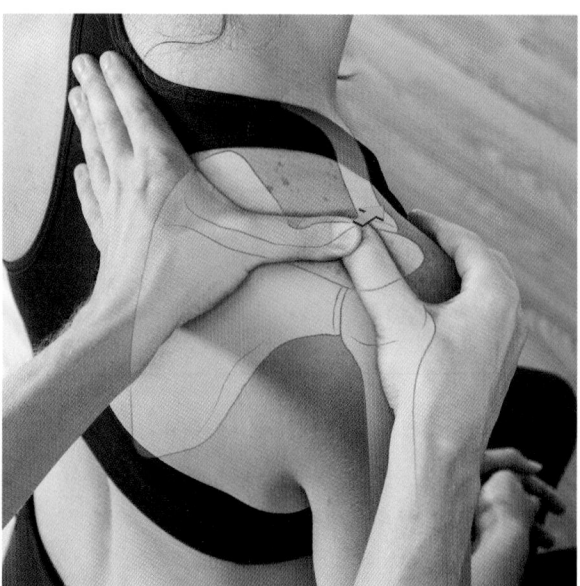

Figure 21.17

Sternoclavicular Inferior Glide

Resting Position: Arm is relaxed at the side of the body.

Mobilization Technique: Inferior or caudal glide.

Indications: Hypomobility of the SC joint or reduced clavicular rotation.

Patient Position: Supine.

Clinician and Hand Positions: Clinician's thumb is placed on the proximal clavicle just lateral to the manubrium at the clavicle's superior aspect.

Mobilization Application: Force is applied inferiorly toward the patient's waist (figure 21.18).

Notations: Force is applied parallel to the joint surface.

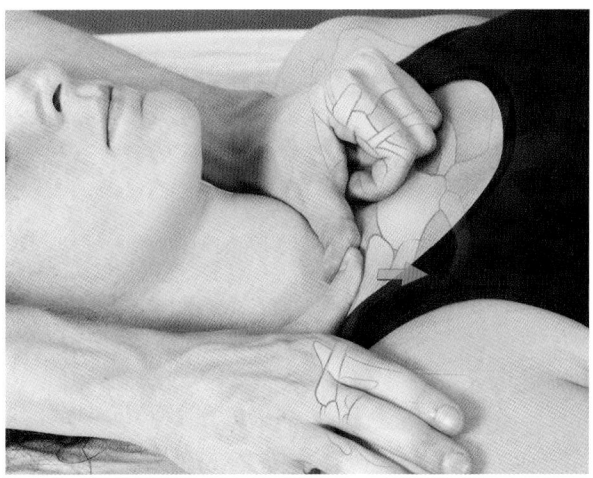
Figure 21.18

Sternoclavicular Posterior Glide

Resting Position: Arm is relaxed at the side of the body.

Mobilization Technique: Posterior, dorsal, or anterior-to-posterior (AP) glide.

Indications: Hypomobility of the SC joint or reduced clavicular rotation.

Patient Position: Supine.

Clinician and Hand Positions: Clinician's thumb is placed on the proximal clavicle on its anterior aspect just lateral to the manubrium.

Mobilization Application: Force is applied posteriorly down toward the table (figure 21.19).

Notations: Force is applied parallel to the joint surface. Clinician may also stand at the patient's side.

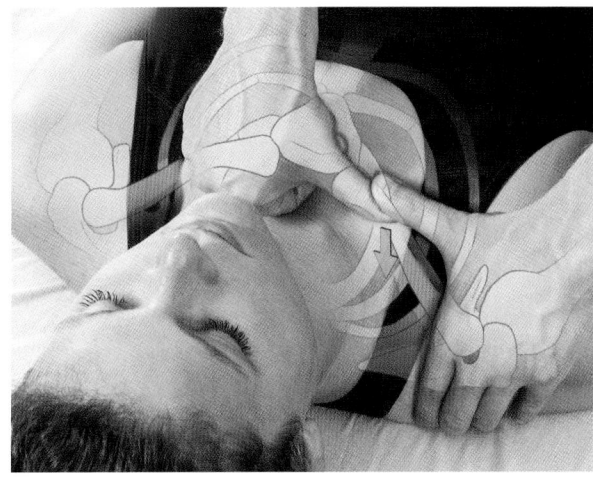
Figure 21.19

Sternoclavicular Superior Glide

Resting Position: Arm is relaxed at the side of the body.

Mobilization Technique: Superior or cranial glide.

Indications: Hypomobility of the SC joint or reduced clavicular rotation.

Patient Position: Supine.

Clinician and Hand Positions: Clinician stands at the patient's side near the waist, facing the patient's head. Clinician's thumb is placed on the proximal clavicle along its inferior aspect just lateral to the manubrium (figure 21.20).

Mobilization Application: Force is applied superiorly.

Notations: Force is applied parallel to the joint surface.

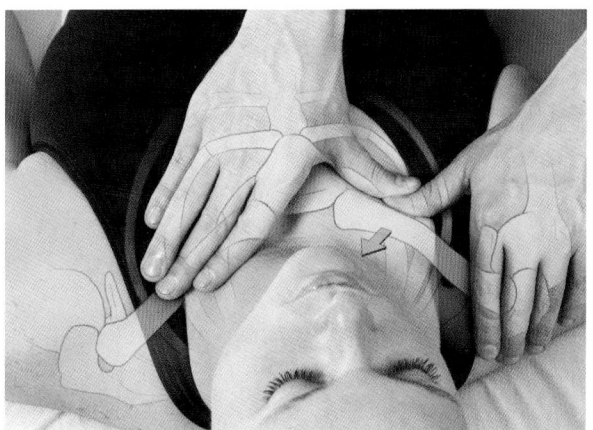
Figure 21.20

Flexibility Exercises

The stretch force for all flexibility exercises should be sufficient to produce a stretch sensation without pain.[82] Pain indicates that the stretch force is too aggressive; it should be reduced because pain will cause a withdrawal reflex to reduce the stretch's effectiveness.[83] Stretches can be either short-term or prolonged; recent injuries may respond to short-term stretches, while older, more mature injuries likely will need more prolonged stretches.[84] As was mentioned in chapter 12, the most effective repetitions and durations of stretches have not been determined for recent acute injuries; recommendations are based on research with normal subjects. Unfortunately, these recommendations conflict with one another: one or two 30 s stretches have demonstrated effective flexibility changes,[85] while two to four stretches for 10 to 30 s have also demonstrated positive flexibility changes.[86] How these data translate to effectiveness in regaining motion after injury is yet to be determined.

Injuries that occurred several months before rehabilitation and contain more mature scar tissue will benefit from prolonged stretches to improve flexibility and mobility. The following is by no means an exhaustive list of flexibility exercises for the shoulder complex, but the exercises presented here provide a beginning list to which you can add as you gain more experience in shoulder rehabilitation.

Active Stretches

Selection of these stretches is based on the ranges of motion that are restricted. These exercises are often used in conjunction with joint mobilization.

Active Shoulder Flexibility Exercises

Before you allow patients to perform these exercises as part of the home exercise program (HEP), they should demonstrate correct performance without verbal cueing or assistance. In any HEP, the clinician instructs the patient about how long to hold the stretch and numbers of repetitions and sets to perform each day.

Pendulum Exercises or Codman's Exercises

Passive motion of the shoulder occurs when weight transfers back and forth between the left and right lower extremities while the upper extremity remains relaxed.

Body Segment: Glenohumeral joint.

Stage in Rehab: Inactive and active phases.

Purpose: Gain early motion, relax muscles, distract the glenohumeral joint, modulate pain.

Positioning: The patient is flexed forward at the waist with the involved arm hanging in a resting position away from the body; the body weight is supported by the uninvolved arm on a table.

Execution: Involved shoulder motion occurs because of lower extremity motion, not shoulder motion. The entire arm remains relaxed throughout the motions. Passive flexion–extension motion of the shoulder occurs with the patient's lower extremities in a forward–backward straddle position; body weight is transferred from the front to the back limbs to provide momentum for arm movement (figure 21.21a). Horizontal flexion–extension movement

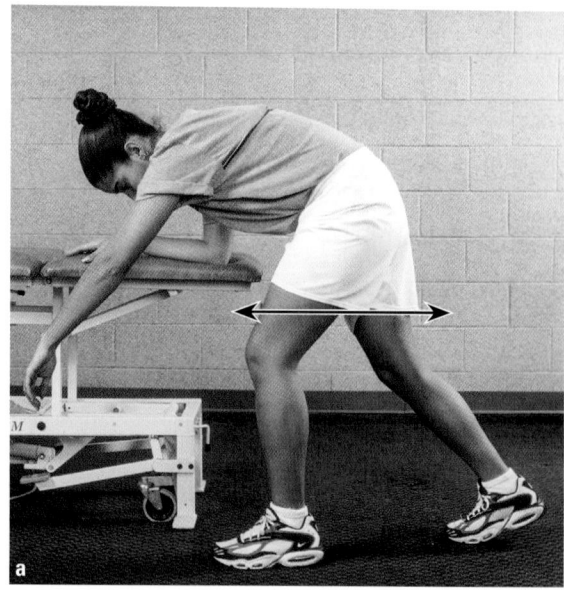

Figure 21.21

occurs with the patient standing in a side-to-side straddle position; body weight is transferred from the left to the right lower extremities to produce sideward arm motion (figure 21.21*b*). Circular motion of the shoulder is produced by the hips as the patient moves the body in a circular direction while the arm hangs passively, swinging with momentum produced from the hips. Circular motion can occur in a clockwise or counterclockwise direction.

Possible Substitutions: Using shoulder muscles to move the upper extremity rather than hip and leg muscles.

Notations: Because this is a passive exercise, the patient must not use shoulder muscles to move the arm; motion comes from the lower extremities. If a weight is used for additional joint distraction, it should be a cuff weight, not a dumbbell weight, so that the upper extremity muscles remain relaxed.

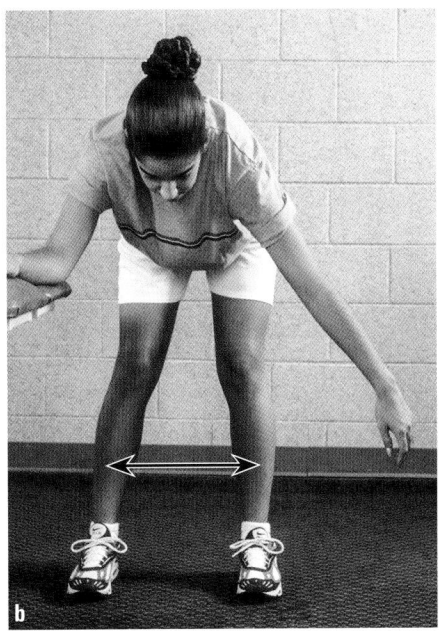

Figure 21.21   *>continued*

Inferior Capsule Stretch

Body Segment: Glenohumeral joint.

Stage in Rehab: Active phase through advanced phase until desired inferior capsular mobility is achieved.

Purpose: Increase mobility of the inferior capsule to improve shoulder elevation.

Positioning: The patient positions the elbow overhead and flexed with the forearm behind the head and the arm next to the ipsilateral ear.

Execution: The uninvolved hand, placed on the elbow, pulls the elbow behind the head (figure 21.22).

Possible Substitutions: A common substitution with this exercise is lateral trunk lean away from the shoulder being stretched. If this occurs, the patient should perform the exercise in front of a mirror to monitor and correct the trunk position. The patient should not shrug the shoulder as it is stretched.

Notations: This exercise is an active stretch.

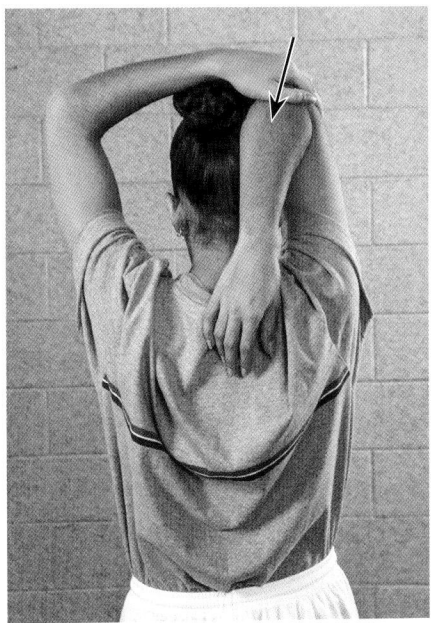

Figure 21.22

Posterior Capsule Stretch

Body Segment: Glenohumeral joint.

Stage in Rehab: Active phase through advanced phase until desired posterior capsular mobility is achieved.

Purpose: Gain medial rotation and horizontal flexion of the glenohumeral joint and stretch the posterior capsule.

Positioning: The patient positions the involved arm at shoulder level and grasps the elbow with the opposite hand.

Execution: The patient pulls the arm across the body, trying to place the hand of the involved shoulder behind the opposite shoulder and the elbow close to the chin (figure 21.23).

Possible Substitutions: A common error is to rotate the trunk rather than pulling the arm across the body. The patient may also tend to lower the elbow below shoulder level. The clinician uses verbal cueing to correct for proper execution. The patient can also stand in front of a mirror for visual feedback.

Notations: If the exercise is not performed correctly, stretch results will not be optimal.

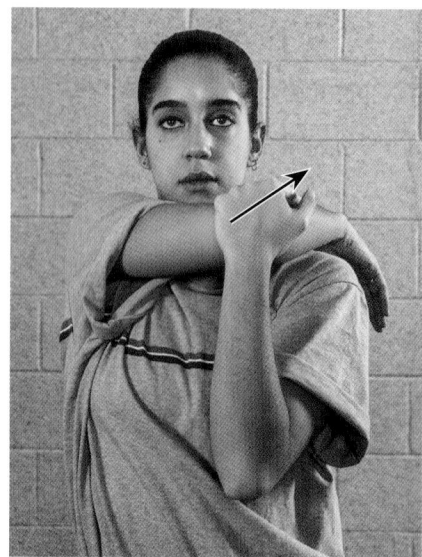

Figure 21.23

Anterior Capsule Stretch

Body Segment: Glenohumeral joint.

Stage in Rehab: Active through advanced phases until desired anterior capsular mobility is achieved.

Purpose: Gain horizontal extension and lateral rotation. This exercise stretches the anterior capsule and pectoralis major.

Positioning: The patient stands in the middle of a doorway with the elbows and forearms on either side of the doorjamb.

Execution: To stretch the upper pectoralis fibers and upper anterior capsule, the elbows are positioned below the shoulders (figure 21.24a). To stretch the middle fibers of the muscle and midanterior capsule, the elbows are positioned at shoulder level. To stretch the lower fibers of the muscle and inferior-anterior capsule, the elbows are positioned above the shoulders (figure 21.24b). With one foot placed in front of the other, the patient pushes from the back foot to lean through the doorway and feel a stretch in the anterior chest and shoulder areas.

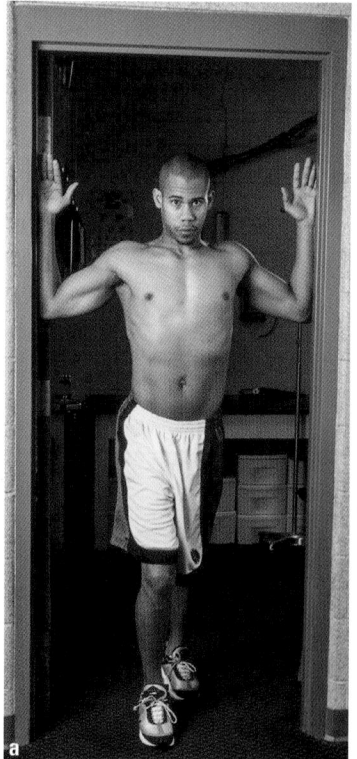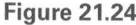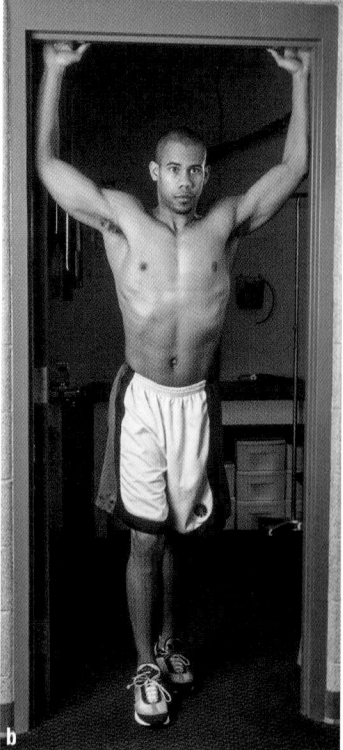

Figure 21.24

Possible Substitutions: Common substitutions include arching the back, moving the elbows off the doorjamb, and keeping the involved shoulder behind the uninvolved shoulder so that the trunk is at an angle toward the involved shoulder. Verbal cueing for proper technique should be used to correct these substitutions.

Notations: This stretch can also be performed in a corner, but it is often difficult to find an available corner that is not occupied with furniture or other difficult-to-move objects.

Superior Capsule Stretch

Body Segment: Glenohumeral joint.

Stage in Rehab: Active through advanced phases until desired superior capsular mobility is achieved.

Purpose: Increase superior capsule mobility and shoulder extension.

Positioning: In standing, the patient places a rolled towel under the axilla and positions the elbow next to his or her side.

Execution: With the uninvolved hand, the patient pulls the elbow toward the side (figure 21.25).

Possible Substitutions: A common error is to use a roll that is not large enough to provide adequate stretch.

Notations: Applying the stretch force too high on the humerus delivers less stretch force.

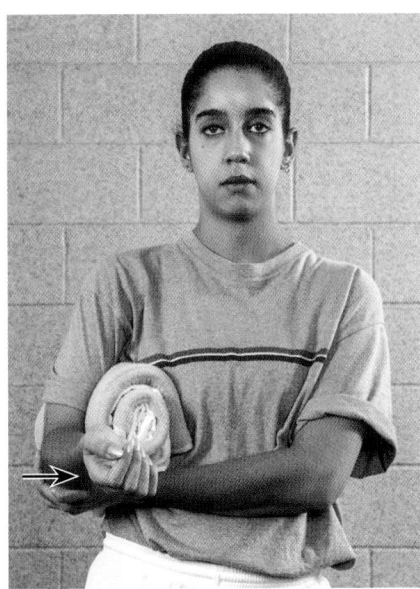

Figure 21.25

Medial Rotation Stretch

Body Segment: Glenohumeral joint.

Stage in Rehab: Active through advanced phases until desired medial rotation motion is achieved.

Purpose: Increase medial rotation and stretch the glenohumeral joint capsule.

Positioning: Patient stands with hands behind the back and grasps the countertop with both hands. The feet are shoulder-width apart.

Execution: Patient squats down while grasping the countertop (figure 21.26).

Possible Substitutions: The most common substitutions are bending over at the waist, looking down at the floor, and flexing the wrist. The wrist should remain straight, and the patient should stay erect. Giving the patient a verbal cue to keep the head up or to look at the ceiling will help correct the posture.

Notations: The hands may start in a shoulder-width grip, but the patient should move the hands closer together as flexibility is gained until one hand is on top of the other.

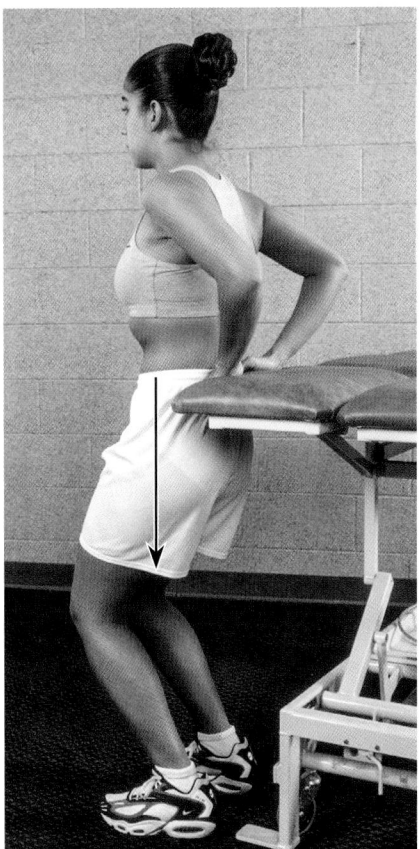

Figure 21.26

Rhomboid Stretch

Body Segment: Scapula.

Stage in Rehab: Active through advanced phases.

Purpose: Improve rhomboid flexibility and posterior capsule mobility.

Positioning: Patient stands facing the edge of an open door, with the feet placed on either side of the door and the hands on the doorknobs.

Execution: The patient pushes the hips backward into flexion while keeping the knees extended. The elbows remain extended and the upper extremities relaxed as the body weight moves backward (figure 21.27).

Possible Substitutions: A common error is not allowing the body weight to stretch the shoulders. If this error occurs, instruct the patient to relax the arms and let the hips move backward and downward, trying to sit on the floor while the knees are kept straight.

Notations: Keeping the shoulders relaxed allows for a better stretch.

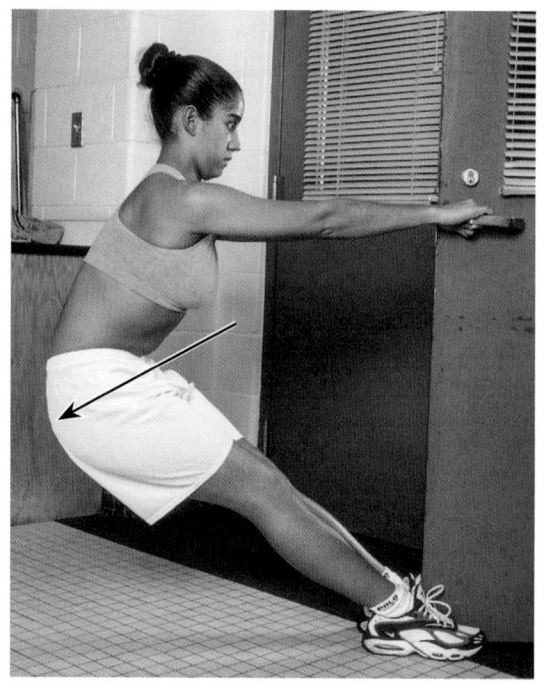

Figure 21.27

Supraspinatus Active Stretch

Body Segment: Glenohumeral joint.

Stage in Rehab: Active through advanced phases.

Purpose: Increase supraspinatus flexibility and superior capsular mobility.

Positioning: The patient positions the involved arm behind the body with the elbow flexed and grasps a chair back with the hand.

Execution: The patient leans sideways away from the hand.

Possible Substitutions: Twisting the body and bending the trunk rather than leaning.

Notations: An alternative technique is to grasp the hand behind the back with the opposite hand and pull the involved arm toward the uninvolved side (figure 21.28).

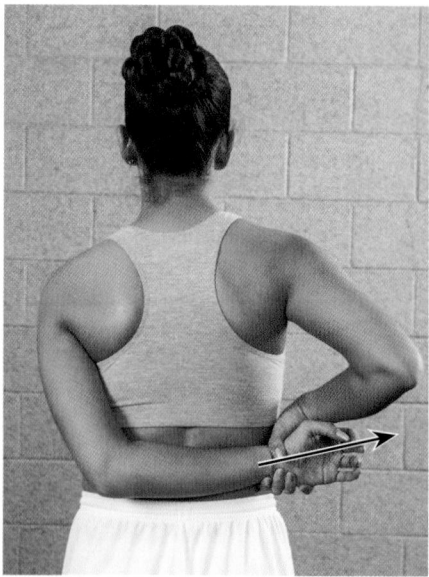

Figure 21.28

Assistive Stretches

Most of these stretches need the clinician's assistance. These stretches may be combined with contract-relax-stretch techniques to give the stretch a proprioceptive neuromuscular facilitation (PNF) element. Improper technique and substitutions should be corrected so that the intended structures are appropriately stretched. The PNF techniques are described in later sections.

If PNF is not used for active stretch exercises, the shoulder is brought to the end range and held in that position for 10 to 30 s for 2 to 4 repetitions. Regardless of the hold time selected, these exercises should be repeated 2 to 4 times throughout the day in the early rehabilitation phases.

Once the desired range of motion is achieved, the exercise is continued 2 to 3 d a week to preserve it.[87]

Most of these stretches will begin in the active phase of the rehabilitation program. There are exceptions, however, depending on the injury or surgical repair. For example, a recent Bankart repair is a contraindication for stretches to the anterior capsule and subscapularis, while posterior capsule, infraspinatus, and teres minor stretches are contraindicated when a patient has recently undergone a reverse Bankart repair. The clinician must be aware of the patient's diagnosis and the precautions and contraindications that accompany each diagnosis.

Assistive Stretches for the Shoulder

Supraspinatus Stretch

Body Segment: Supraspinatus.

Stage in Rehab: Start in the active phase and continue as maintenance once full motion is achieved.

Purpose: Increase supraspinatus motion and improve superior capsular mobility.

Positioning: Patient stands with the involved arm behind the back. The uninvolved hand grasps the wrist of the involved arm.

Execution: Patient pulls the arm across the back to bring the involved hand to the opposite side of the body. The patient maintains medial rotation of the shoulder.

Possible Substitutions: Lateral flexion of the trunk and trunk rotation.

Notations: This can also be performed with the clinician providing the stretch.

Infraspinatus Stretch

Body Segment: Infraspinatus.

Stage in Rehab: Start in the active phase and continue as maintenance once full motion is achieved.

Purpose: Increase infraspinatus flexibility and improve posterior capsular mobility.

Positioning: Patient sits and places the involved arm in front of the body in medial rotation with the elbow flexed.

Execution: The clinician grasps the elbow or wrist and pulls the arm across the body while maintaining medial rotation (figure 21.29).

Possible Substitutions: Trunk lean and trunk rotation. Place a hand on the patient's shoulder to stabilize the trunk, or have the patient perform the exercise in front of a mirror to self-monitor performance.

Notations: If the patient performs the stretch without assistance, the uninvolved hand is placed on the elbow to pull the arm across the body.

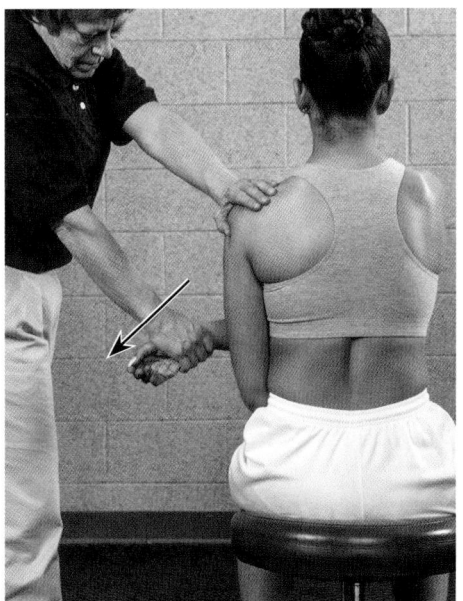

Figure 21.29

Subscapularis Stretch

Body Segment: Subscapularis.

Stage in Rehab: Start in the active phase and continue as maintenance once full motion is achieved.

Purpose: Increase subscapularis flexibility and improve inferior capsular mobility.

Positioning: Patient is supine. Shoulder is abducted to about 90° and the end of lateral rotation; the elbow is flexed to 90°.

Execution: Clinician applies a stretch force into lateral rotation (figure 21.30).

Possible Substitutions: Arching the low back is a common substitution. Verbally cueing the patient and flexing the hips and knees will prevent the back from arching, or else have the patient perform the exercise with both knees pulled toward the chest.

Notations: Since the clinician has a distinct advantage at the elbow when this stretch is applied, extreme care must be taken to avoid excessive elbow stress during the stretch.

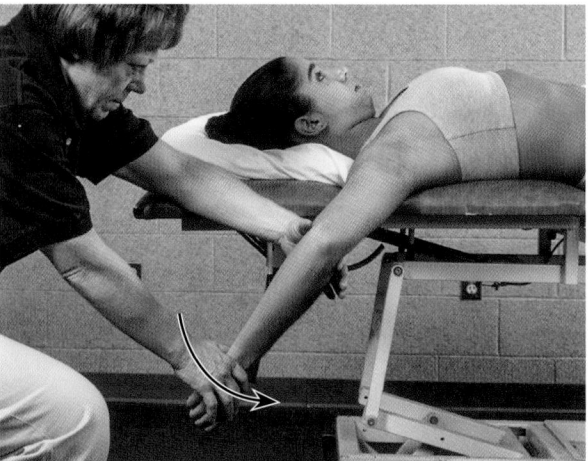

Figure 21.30

Teres Minor Stretch

Body Segment: Teres minor.

Stage in Rehab: Start in the active phase and continue as maintenance once full motion is achieved.

Purpose: Increase teres minor flexibility and stretch the inferior capsule.

Positioning: Patient is seated with the shoulder in abduction and medial rotation and the elbow flexed about 90°.

Execution: Clinician stabilizes the scapula to isolate teres minor and then applies a medial rotation stretch (figure 21.31).

Possible Substitutions: Scapular rotation may occur if the scapula is not stabilized.

Notations: An alternative position can be used with the arm overhead in end-range shoulder abduction with medial rotation; the scapula must be stabilized by the clinician in this stretch. Any time a stretch is applied distally on the extremity with the elbow flexed, the clinician must take particular care to avoid overstressing the elbow because it is in a vulnerable position relative to the forces applied.

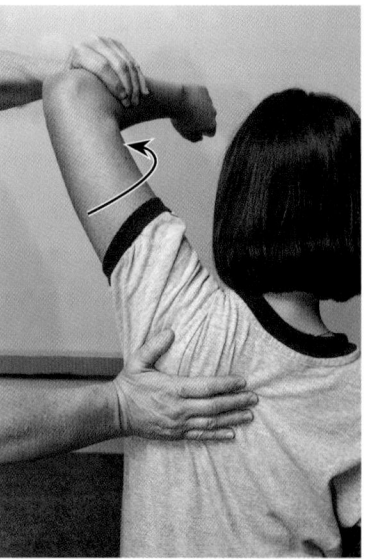

Figure 21.31

Teres Major Stretch

Body Segment: Teres major.

Stage in Rehab: Start in the active phase and continue as maintenance once full motion is achieved.

Purpose: Increase teres major flexibility.

Positioning: Patient is supine with the arm overhead in shoulder flexion and lateral rotation. The elbow may be either flexed or extended.

Execution: Clinician applies the stretch force, moving the shoulder gradually into additional flexion and lateral rotation as the patient tolerates (figure 21.32).

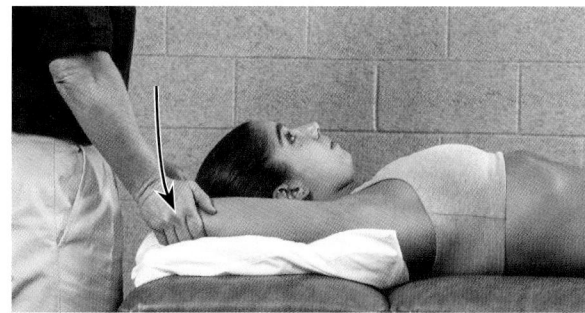

Figure 21.32

Possible Substitutions: The lumbar spine should not rise off the table. Instruct the patient to lie with the hips and knees flexed, with the back flat on the table, to prevent lumbar hyperextension.

Notations: Clinician may stand either at the head or at the side of the patient. Active contraction of shoulder extensors against isometric resistance followed by relaxation before stretching may enhance the effect of this stretch.

Latissimus Dorsi Stretch

Body Segment: Latissimus dorsi.

Stage in Rehab: Start in the active phase and continue as maintenance once full motion is achieved.

Purpose: Increase latissimus dorsi flexibility.

Positioning: Patient lies prone with the arm overhead.

Execution: Clinician grasps the forearm and then distracts the shoulder and laterally rotates the shoulder as the arm is lifted toward the ceiling (figure 21.33).

Possible Substitutions: Trunk rotation and elbow flexion are substitutions.

Notations: If the patient has a history of elbow or wrist injury, the force is applied just proximal to the elbow joint.

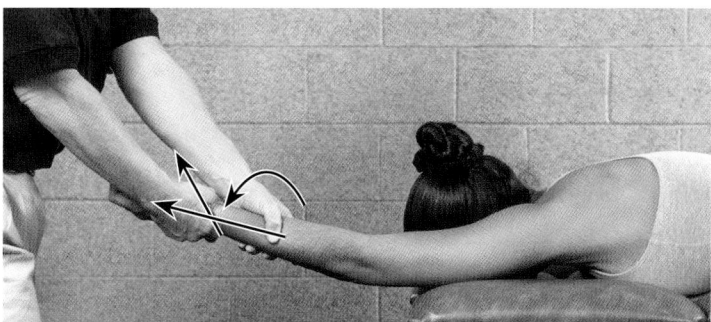

Figure 21.33

Wand Exercises

The following exercises are performed with a wand using the uninvolved contralateral arm to provide the stretch force. Commercial wands and T-bars are available, but dowels (2.5 cm [1 in.] in diameter), broom handles, canes, PVC pipe, and other similar items are readily available, inexpensive, and just as effective.

The patient uses the uninvolved arm to guide the wand in the desired direction to provide the stretch force needed to increase motion. He or she holds the end position 5 to 10 s and repeats each motion several times. The advantage of these exercises is that the patient can perform them independently several times throughout the day as part of the HEP. These exercises are detailed in the following sections.

Wand Exercises for the Shoulder

Wand exercises may be performed with either an improvised device or a wand specifically designed for upper-extremity exercises. These exercises may become part of the HEP once the patient can perform them correctly without verbal cueing or assistance from the clinician. Some of the more commonly used exercises are listed here.

Wand Flexion Stretch

Body Segment: Shoulder flexion.

Stage in Rehab: Early active phase.

Purpose: Increase glenohumeral flexion motion.

Positioning: Patient may be sitting, standing, or supine.

Execution: Patient grasps the wand in each hand, with the hands shoulder-width apart. He or she moves the arms overhead as far as possible without pain, keeping the elbows straight throughout the exercise (figure 21.34).

Possible Substitutions: Arching the back, bending the elbows, and hyperextending the wrists.

Notations: The exercise should begin in a supine position to eliminate the need for strength in later ranges of motion.

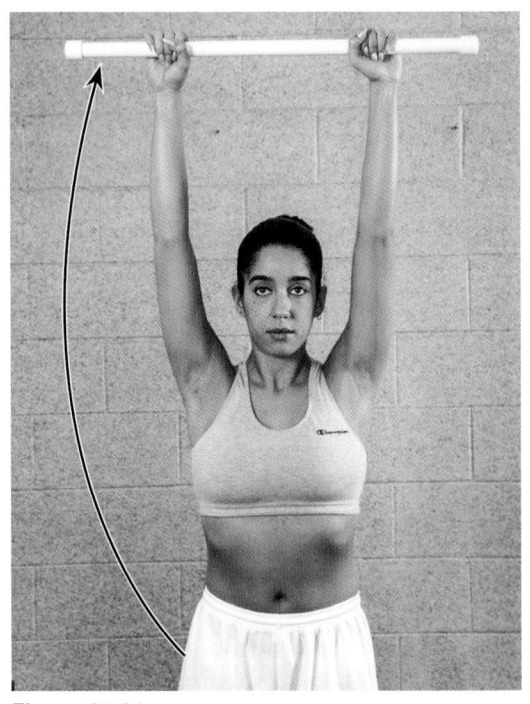

Figure 21.34

Wand Abduction Stretch

Body Segment: Shoulder abduction.

Stage in Rehab: Early active phase.

Purpose: Increase glenohumeral abduction motion.

Positioning: Supine or standing. Patient grasps the end of the wand with the involved hand and places the uninvolved hand toward the other end of the wand.

Execution: The uninvolved arm pushes the involved shoulder upward into abduction (figure 21.35).

Possible Substitutions: Leaning sideways, moving the shoulder into the flexion plane, shrugging the shoulder, and flexing the elbow.

Notations: Placing the involved hand in an underhand grasp may reduce shoulder soft-tissue impingement in higher elevations.

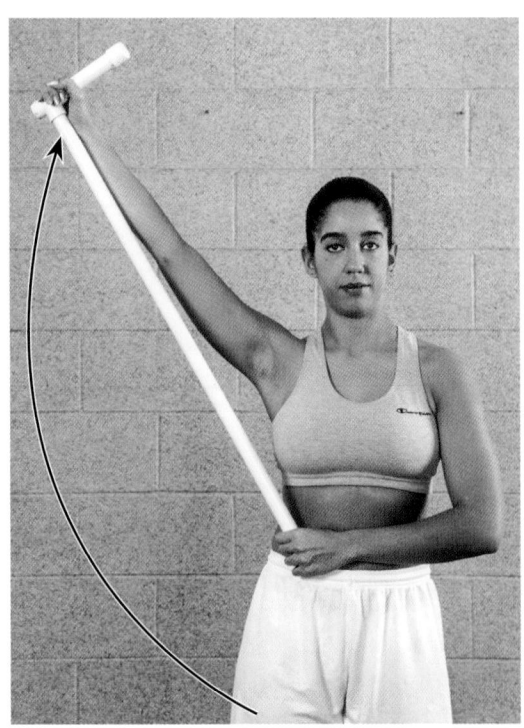

Figure 21.35

Wand Lateral Rotation Stretch

Body Segment: Shoulder lateral rotation.

Stage in Rehab: Early active phase.

Purpose: Increase glenohumeral lateral rotation motion by stretching medial rotators.

Positioning: The patient lies supine with the involved hand on one end of the wand and the uninvolved hand toward the other end. The involved elbow is kept next to the side at 90° flexion throughout the exercise.

Execution: Using the uninvolved hand on the wand, the patient pushes the involved hand away from the body to laterally rotate the shoulder (figure 21.36a).

Possible Substitutions: Extending the elbow as the wand is pushed laterally and abducting the involved shoulder.

Notations: A more advanced lateral rotation exercise can be performed with the hands shoulder-width apart on the wand. The patient raises the wand overhead and then bends the elbows to try to place the wand behind the neck (figure 21.36b). Neck flexion, trunk flexion or rotation, shoulder horizontal adduction, elbow extension, and wrist hyperextension are common substitutions with this exercise.

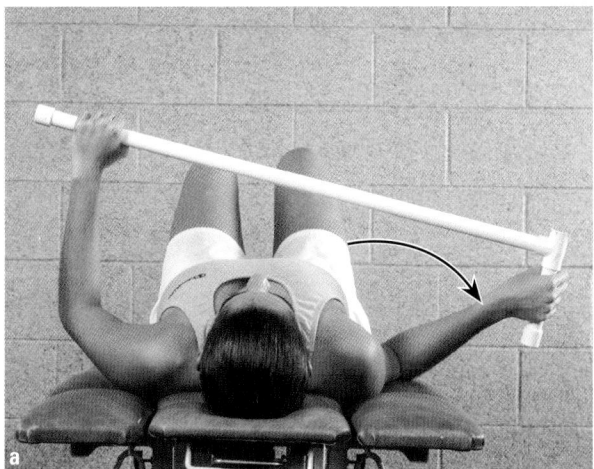
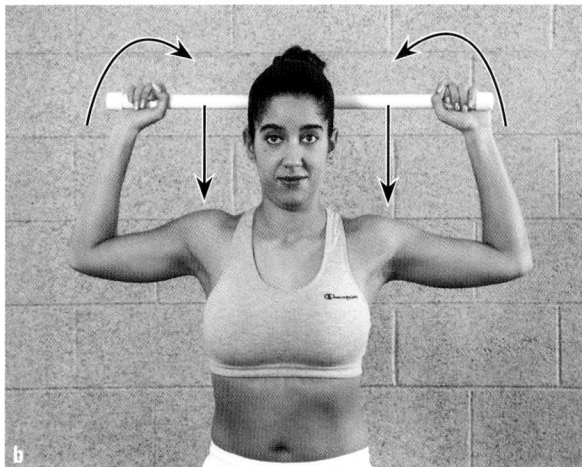

Figure 21.36

Wand Medial Rotation Stretch

Body Segment: Shoulder medial rotation.

Stage in Rehab: Early active phase.

Purpose: Increase glenohumeral medial rotation by stretching the lateral rotators.

Positioning: The patient stands with the wand behind the waist; hands are placed shoulder-width apart.

Execution: The wand is raised along the back as high as possible (figure 21.37a).

Possible Substitutions: Excessive wrist flexion and trunk lean.

Notations: An alternative stretch is with the wand placed vertically behind the back. The involved hand is behind the waist, and the uninvolved hand is at the top of the wand near the ipsilateral shoulder. The wand is pulled upward with the

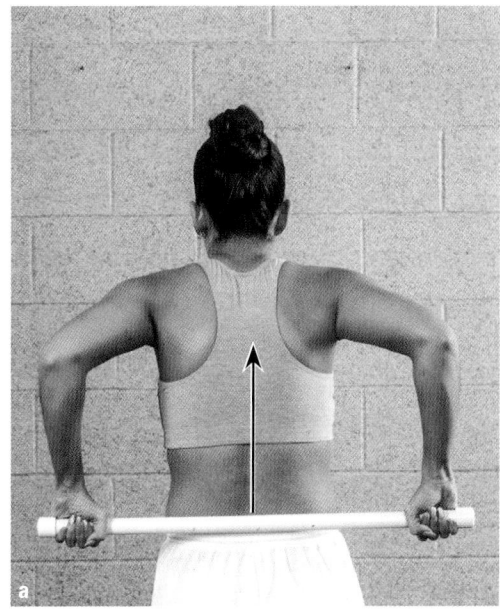

Figure 21.37

>continued

Wand Medial Rotation Stretch *>continued*

top hand (figure 21.37*b*). Trunk flexion is a common substitution with this alternative stretch. If the patient reverses the hands and pulls the wand with the uninvolved arm's hand downward, the patient stretches the involved shoulder's medial rotators.

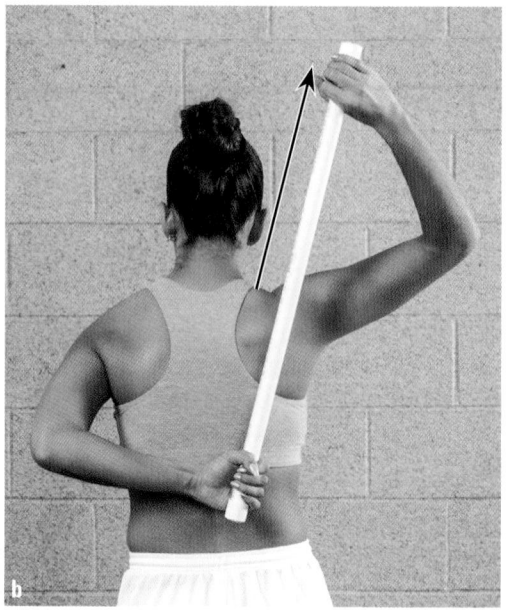

Figure 21.37 *>continued*

Wand Glenohumeral Horizontal Flexion–Extension Stretch

Body Segment: Shoulder horizontal flexion and extension.

Stage in Rehab: Early active phase.

Purpose: Increase horizontal motions by stretching the pectoral muscles and anterior capsule.

Positioning: The patient lies supine with the hands overhead, shoulder-width apart on the wand, and the elbows straight.

Execution: The uninvolved arm pushes the involved arm away from the body as far as possible, and then pulls the arm across the body as far as possible (figure 21.38).

Possible Substitutions: Elbow flexion, trunk rotation, moving the shoulders into extension, and shoulder rotation.

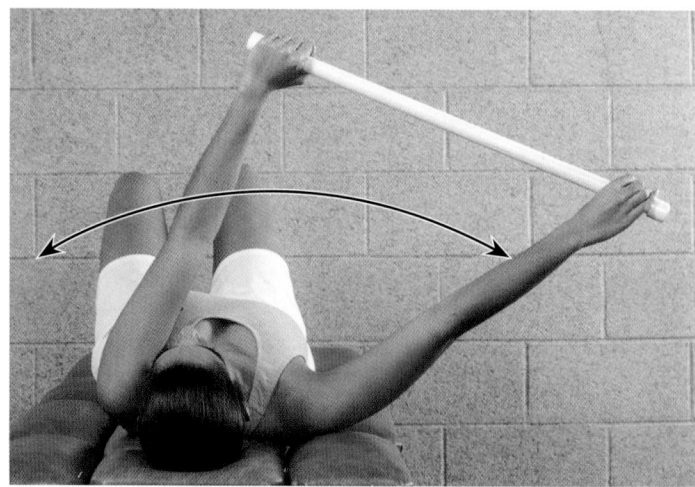

Figure 21.38

Notations: Throughout the exercise, the hands remain at shoulder level and the elbows remain straight.

Sleeper Stretches

Throwers' shoulders tend to develop posterior capsular tightness and anterior laxity.[88, 89] One of the effects of this posterior tightness is secondary glenohumeral impingement.[90] To prevent injury to throwing shoulders, there is a series of stretches called "sleeper stretches" and "rollover sleeper stretches."[24] Although there is controversy over their effectiveness,[91, 92] clinicians often apply these stretches to throwing athletes.

Modifications to the sleeper stretches have been suggested recently because there have been some reports of pain with their use,[92] and they present the potential for subacromial impingement.[93] One modified stretch technique is the horizontal adduction stretch; unfortunately, this stretch does not stabilize the scapula, so the stretch does not effectively isolate its force to the posterior glenohumeral capsule as intended.[94] Another modified version of the sleeper stretches involves stabilization in the scapular plane to allow a more focused application of stretch to the posterior capsule with less risk of pain.[94] All of these stretches are included in this section so that you may make your own clinical determination about their effectiveness for your patients.

Sleeper Stretch[24]

Body Segment: Posterior shoulder capsule.

Stage in Rehab: Active phase or early resistive phase, then continued for maintenance of posterior capsule mobility.

Purpose: Increase mobility of the posterior capsule.

Positioning: The patient is side-lying on the dominant (involved) side with the hips and knees flexed to stabilize the body in a position perpendicular to the tabletop. The dominant shoulder and elbow are each flexed to 90°. The top hand is placed on the distal forearm of the dominant arm.

Execution: The top hand pushes the involved forearm down toward the tabletop until a stretch in the posterior shoulder is felt (figure 21.39a). Some people change the position of the dominant shoulder to stretch other portions of the posterior capsule. Figure 21.39b demonstrates stretch of the upper posterior capsule with the shoulder positioned at about 60° of flexion. Figure 21.39c shows a stretch of the inferior posterior capsule with the shoulder flexed to about 120° of flexion.

Possible Substitutions: Elbow extension, moving the shoulder into extension, and shoulder rotation.

Notations: The stretch is held for 30 s.

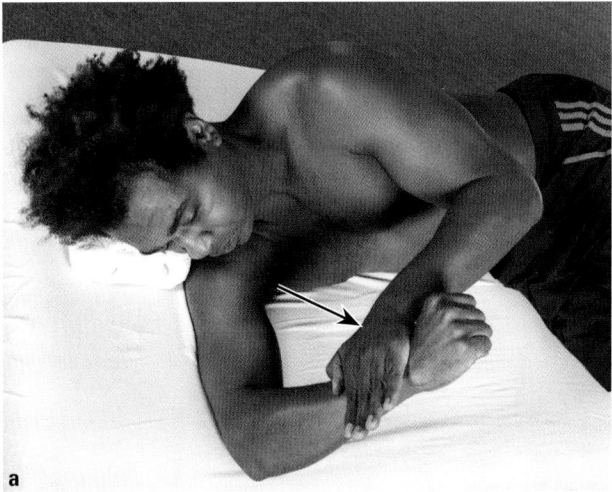

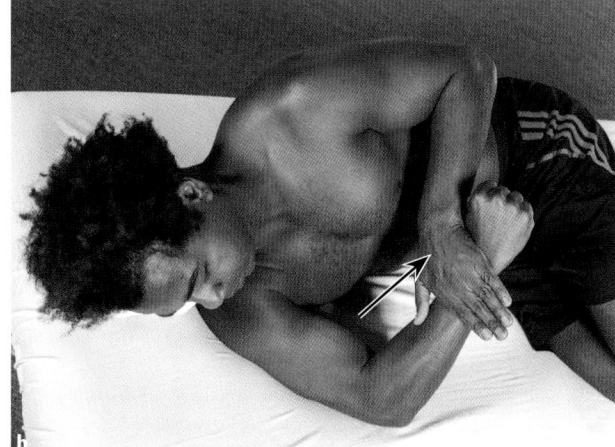

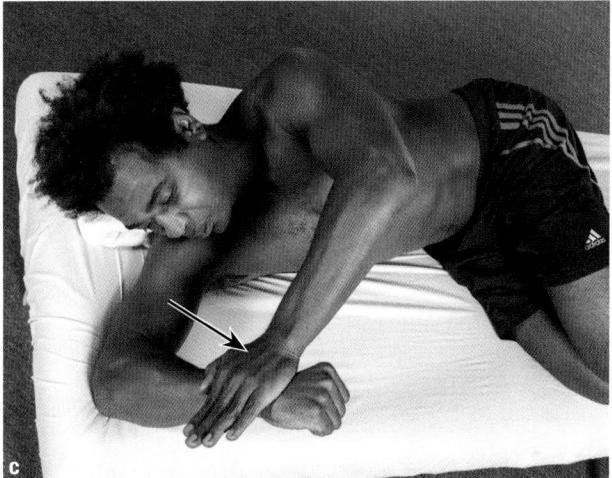

Figure 21.39

Rollover Sleeper Stretch[24]

Body Segment: Posterior shoulder capsule.

Stage in Rehab: Active phase or early resistive phase and then continued for maintenance of posterior capsule mobility.

Purpose: Increase horizontal adduction and mobility of the posterior capsule.

Positioning: The patient is side-lying on the dominant (involved) side with the hips and knees flexed to stabilize the body. The dominant shoulder is flexed to 50° to 60°, and the elbow is flexed to 90°. The top (nondominant) hand is placed on the dorsal distal forearm of the dominant arm.

Execution: The uninvolved hand pushes the involved forearm down toward the tabletop until a stretch in the posterior shoulder is felt (figure 21.40). While holding this stretch position, the patient rolls forward 30° to 40° from the initial perpendicular position.

Possible Substitutions: Elbow extension, moving the shoulder into extension, and shoulder rotation.

Notations: The stretch is held for 30 s.

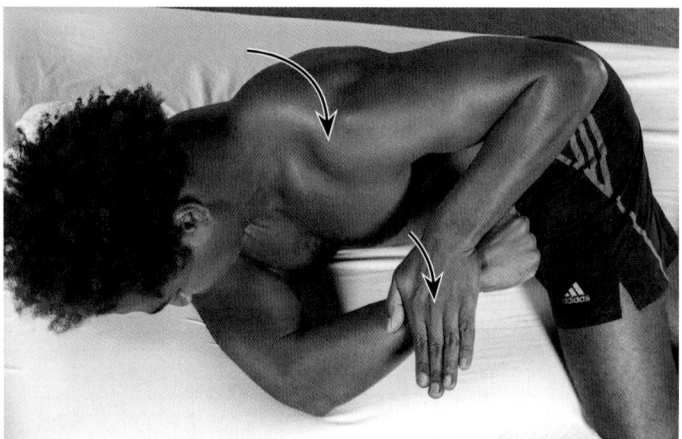

Figure 21.40

Cross-Body Stretch[92]

Body Segment: Posterior shoulder capsule.

Stage in Rehab: Active phase or early resistive phase and then continued for maintenance of posterior capsule mobility.

Purpose: Increase mobility of the posterior capsule.

Positioning: The patient sits or stands and elevates the involved shoulder to 90° of flexion. The uninvolved hand grasps just proximal to the involved arm's posterior elbow.

Execution: The uninvolved hand pulls the involved humerus across the body until a stretch in the posterior shoulder is felt (figure 21.41).

Possible Substitutions: Shoulder moves toward extension, the shoulder rolls toward lateral rotation, or the trunk rotates.

Notations: The stretch is held for 30 s.

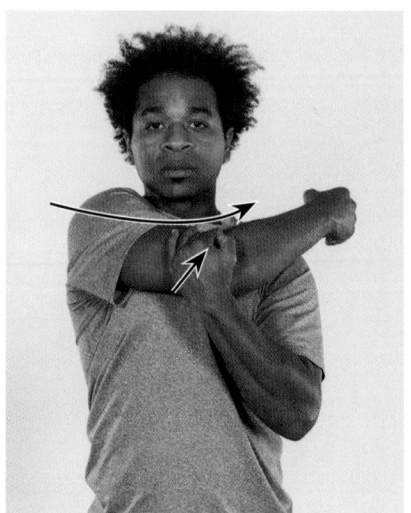

Figure 21.41

Modified Sleeper Stretch[94]

Body Segment: Posterior shoulder capsule.

Stage in Rehab: Active phase or early resistive phase and then continued for maintenance of posterior capsule mobility.

Purpose: Increase mobility of the posterior capsule.

Positioning: The patient is side-lying on the involved extremity with the trunk rolled posteriorly about 20° to 30° from the vertical y-axis. The involved shoulder is flexed to 90°, and the hand of the uninvolved extremity is placed proximal to the wrist of the extremity being stretched.

Execution: The hand of the uninvolved arm moves the involved shoulder into medial rotation, pushing the forearm toward the tabletop until a stretch in the posterior shoulder is felt (figure 21.42a).

Possible Substitutions: Involved shoulder or elbow moves toward extension or trunk rotates as shoulder is stretched.

Notations: An additional stretch to the infraspinatus may be provided by placing a towel under the humerus (figure 21.42b). Perhaps this is an exercise that Logan used in the opening scenario to improve the flexibility of the lateral rotators of his pitcher, Benj. Whether using the towel or not, the patient must hold the trunk position that keeps the humerus in the scapular plane during either of these techniques.

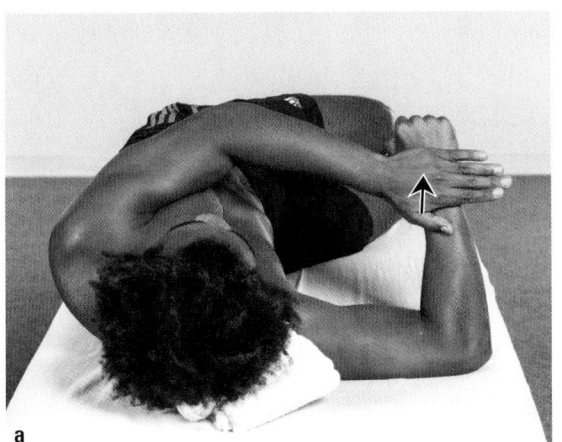 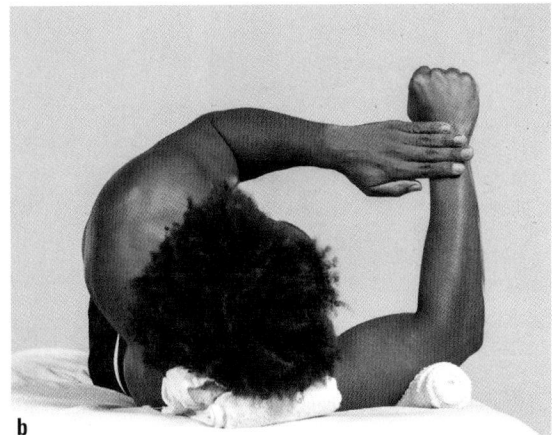

a   b

Figure 21.42

Pulley Exercises for Range of Motion

These exercises can be performed with a pulley, rope, or stretch strap. They are easy to incorporate into a HEP that the patient can perform independently. The patient must avoid driving the humeral head into the glenoid socket, especially when using the pulleys for frozen-shoulder exercises. The patient is instructed to keep the scapula in a depressed position throughout glenohumeral motion.

Shoulder Flexion   For this exercise, an overhead rope and pulley or a stretch strap and hook are attached overhead in a doorway or on a wall. The patient sits with his or her back to the door or wall. The uninvolved arm pulls the rope or strap down to elevate the involved shoulder into flexion as high as possible. The involved arm is lowered using the uninvolved arm's control on the rope, and the motion is repeated several times. Moving the patient's chair more forward of the pulley creates greater elevation potential for the shoulder.

One alternative stretch uses a stretch strap placed over the top of a door. The patient reaches up as high as possible on the strap and then bends the knees to lower the body to stretch the shoulder. Another alternative position is with the patient supine and the pulley attached lower on the wall or in a doorjamb (figure 21.43a).

Shoulder Abduction   This exercise is similar to the shoulder flexion exercise except that the arm is raised in abduction from the side of the body. The hands should have an underhand grip on the handles (figure 21.43b); if they do not, impingement may occur when the shoulder is in full abduction. The patient tries to move the involved extremity as close as possible toward the head, working to increase abduction motion, using the uninvolved extremity as the moving force.

Shoulder Medial Rotation   This exercise is performed while standing. The pulley is in the same position as in the other two reciprocal pulley exercises. The hand

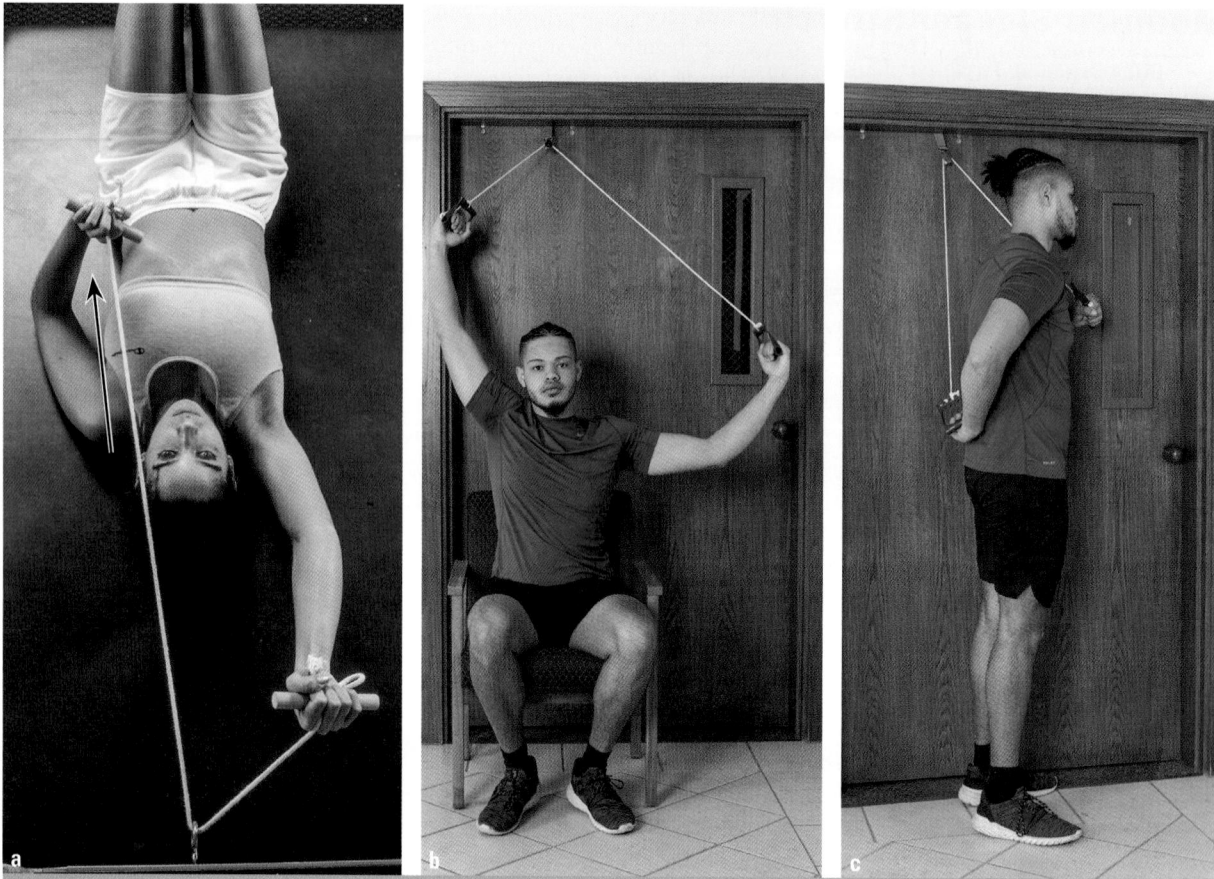

Figure 21.43   Reciprocal pulleys for: *(a)* shoulder flexion; *(b)* shoulder abduction; and *(c)* shoulder medial rotation.

of the involved extremity grasps the handle behind the patient near the hip, and the uninvolved extremity grasps the elevated handle in front. With the involved extremity kept behind the back, the uninvolved extremity then pulls the pulley to move the involved extremity's hand up the back, increasing the shoulder's medial rotation motion (figure 21.43*c*).

> ## CLINICAL TIPS
>
> Flexibility exercises for the shoulder include pendulum exercises, sleeper stretches, active and assistive stretches, wand exercises using the uninvolved extremity, and pulley exercises.

Strengthening Exercises

These exercises incorporate a broad spectrum of both difficulty and stresses for the shoulder. They are presented here from easiest to more advanced exercises, beginning with early resistive phase isometric exercises that, in some cases, may begin in the latter part of the active phase, progressing to later resistive phase plyometric exercises. As the patient's strength improves, the exercises become more difficult and also advance from straight-plane to diagonal exercises. The rehabilitation clinician should correct any substitution patterns seen in the patient's performance to ensure that the intended muscles achieve optimal strength gains and that appropriate neuromotor patterns are supported.

Isometrics

Isometrics begin early in a rehabilitation program when the patient is weak and motion is limited by either reduced mobility or postinjury precautions. These exercises help minimize atrophy during times when use or motion of the shoulder is limited or constrained. They are performed in pain-free positions and may be performed at multiple angles of a motion, if motion is permitted. Whether motion is limited or not, the exercises are performed in nonaggravating positions.

Each isometric exercise builds during the first 2 s to a maximum contraction. The muscle's tension is held at that maximum for 6 s, and then it decreases over 2 s until the muscle is fully relaxed before the next repetition begins. The patient is instructed to avoid sudden maximal contractions to avoid injury or undue strain. Pain is avoided during isometric contractions. If pain occurs, effort is limited to a submaximal contraction until a maximal effort is nonirritating. To allow for the buildup to and decline from the maximal contraction, each isometric is held for 10 s and repeated 10 times. These exercises are performed often throughout the day. The following section describes these exercises.

Isometric Exercises

Isometric exercises are the most basic strengthening exercises. Since they provide tension in the muscle without movement, they are often used after severe injury or surgery when little or no motion of the shoulder is permitted.

Isometric Shoulder Flexion

Body Segment: Glenohumeral joint.

Stage in Rehab: End of active phase or beginning of resistive phase.

Purpose: Prevent deconditioning or strengthen shoulder flexors.

Positioning: Patient stands facing a doorway or wall; the involved arm is slightly forward with the radial hand on the doorframe or wall.

Execution: Patient tries to move the shoulder into flexion while pushing the hand against the doorframe or wall (figure 21.44).

Possible Substitutions: Elbow flexion, trunk extension.

Notations: The patient should keep the elbow straight and the trunk stable. If the hand is uncomfortable from the pressure, he or she should place a towel between the hand and the wall.

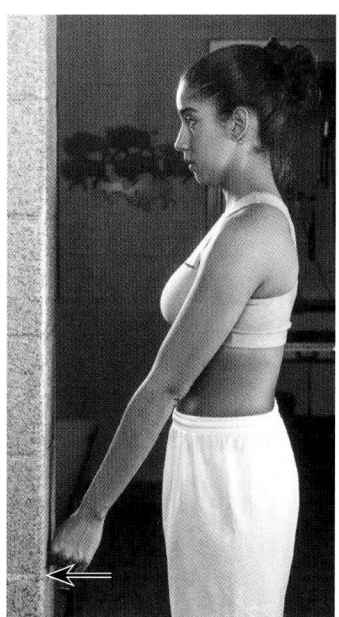

Figure 21.44

Isometric Shoulder Abduction

Body Segment: Glenohumeral joint.

Stage in Rehab: End of active phase or beginning of resistive phase.

Purpose: Prevent deconditioning or strengthen shoulder abductors.

Positioning: Patient stands with the involved side facing a wall or doorway. The shoulder is positioned in slight abduction with the dorsum of the hand against the wall.

Execution: The patient keeps the elbow extended and pushes the hand against the wall, trying to move the shoulder into abduction.

Possible Substitutions: Elbow flexion, shoulder flexion, and trunk leaning away from wall.

Cues and Notations: The patient should keep the arm in line with the body's frontal plane rather than forward of it. If the hand is uncomfortable from the pressure, the patient should place a towel between the hand and the wall.

Isometric Shoulder Extension

Body Segment: Glenohumeral joint.

Stage in Rehab: End of active phase or beginning of resistive phase.

Purpose: Prevent deconditioning or strengthen shoulder extensors.

Positioning: Patient stands with the back to the wall and positions the arm slightly behind the body, with the ulnar hand against the wall.

Execution: The patient pushes the hand backward to the wall, keeping the elbow extended (figure 21.45).

Possible Substitutions: Elbow flexion and trunk lean.

Cues and Notations: The patient should keep the body upright and the elbow extended. If the hand is uncomfortable from the pressure, a towel may be placed between the hand and the wall.

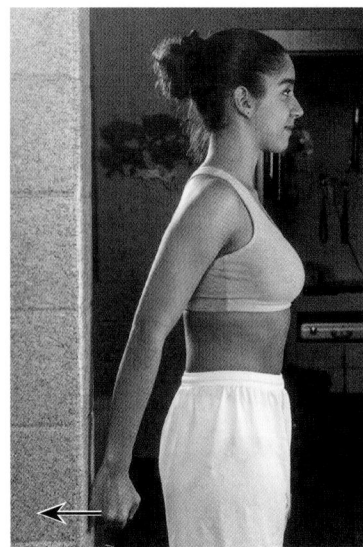

Figure 21.45

Isometric Shoulder Medial Rotation

Body Segment: Glenohumeral joint.

Stage in Rehab: End of active phase or beginning of resistive phase.

Purpose: Prevent deconditioning or strengthen medial rotators.

Positioning: The patient stands facing a doorway with the elbow flexed to 90° and the anterior distal forearm placed against the surface of the doorframe.

Execution: Patient tries to roll the forearm inward toward the abdomen.

Possible Substitutions: Elbow extension and shoulder abduction.

Cues and Notations: Patient should keep the elbow at his or her side.

Isometric Shoulder Lateral Rotation

Body Segment: Glenohumeral joint.

Stage in Rehab: End of active phase or beginning of resistive phase.

Purpose: Prevent deconditioning or strengthen lateral rotators.

Positioning: Patient stands facing a doorway with the elbow flexed to 90° and the posterior distal surface of the forearm against the doorframe.

Execution: Patient tries to roll the forearm outward (figure 21.46).

Possible Substitutions: Elbow extension and shoulder flexion or shoulder adduction.

Cues and Notations: Patient should keep the elbow at his or her side.

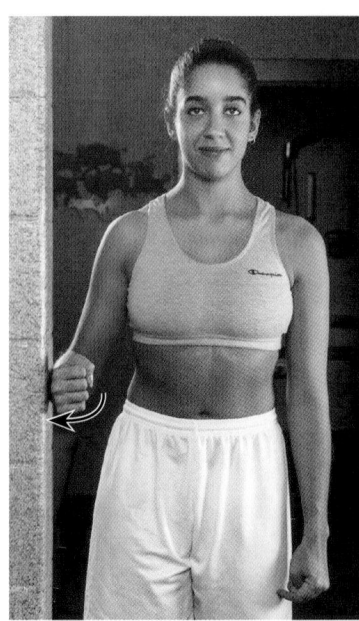

Figure 21.46

Isolated-Plane Isotonic Exercises

As mentioned previously, initial strengthening exercises should include primarily straight-plane activities. Once strength is sufficient to control the joint during motion, multiplanar and diagonal exercises can begin. Here we look first at straight-plane exercises and then move to multiplane exercises. This section includes many of the commonly used exercises, but the listing here is far from exhaustive.

Although functional shoulder motion requires active contributions from both scapulothoracic and glenohumeral muscles, patients can and should perform isolated exercises of these muscles until they have enough strength to control their individual joints during functional shoulder complex motions. To make it easier to identify specific exercise functions, the straight-plane exercises for the scapulo-thoracic and glenohumeral muscle groups are presented separately in the following sections. The exercises are presented from easiest to most difficult.

Scapulothoracic Exercises

If the patient has shoulder pain with movement into elevated positions, it is best to provide manual resistance to the scapular muscles with the shoulder positioned in the lower planes of motion. An advantage of offering manual resistance to the scapulothoracic muscles is that these exercises can be performed without affecting the glenohumeral joint, so they may begin very early in the rehabilitation program. Although the serratus anterior and lower trapezius muscles are the most important scapular stabilizers,[95] any weak scapular muscle should be strengthened.

Isotonic Strength Exercises

Straight-plane exercises are presented first. Single-plane movements isolate the weak muscle and prevent other stronger muscles from producing the desired movement.

Manual Resistance to Scapular Retractors and Protractors

Body Segment: Scapulothoracic.

Stage in Rehab: Resistive phase. The exercise may occur during the later active phase if the injury is to the glenohumeral joint or muscles and not to the scapulothoracic joint or muscles.

Purpose: Strengthen scapular retractors and protractors.

Positioning: Patient is side-lying on the uninvolved side. The involved arm rests on the body's side. The clinician faces the patient and places his or her hand closest to the patient's head on the anterior shoulder. The other hand is placed on the posterior scapula with the clinician's arm between the patient's involved arm and ribs. The patient's arm may rest on the clinician's arm to keep the shoulder in the scapular plane (figure 21.47a and b).

Execution: Patient is instructed to squeeze the scapulae together as the clinician resists the motion with the hand on the posterior scapula. The patient is then instructed to protract the scapula as the clinician resists scapular retraction by pressure over the anterior shoulder. This sequence is repeated until either the repetition and set goals are achieved or the patient's muscle fatigue prevents additional repetitions through a full range of motion.

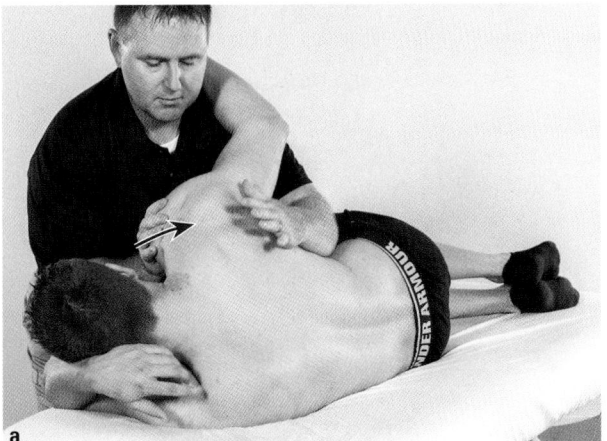 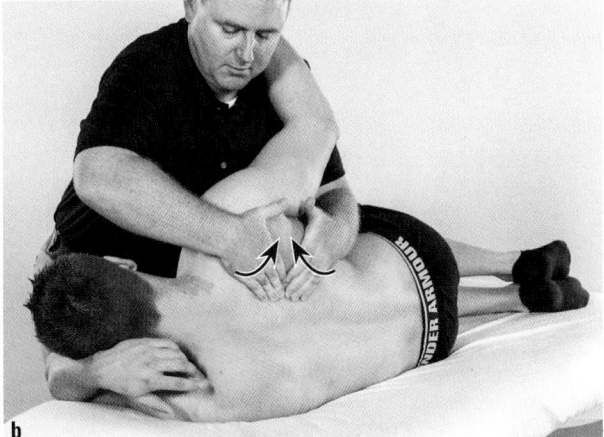

Figure 21.47

>continued

Manual Resistance to Scapular Retractors and Protractors >*continued*

Possible Substitutions: Trunk rotation.

Cues and Notations: Remind the patient to keep the scapula "pulled down and toward your back pocket" throughout the exercise. A pad may be placed between the anterior shoulder and the clinician's hand if the patient reports pressure discomfort from the clinician's hand during protraction. The clinician's pressure should enable the patient to perform a full range of protraction and retraction motion throughout a smooth, full range of scapular motion; as the patient fatigues, the clinician may need to reduce the amount of force applied to allow for a smooth motion through the full ROM to continue. Pain should not occur with any portion of the exercise.

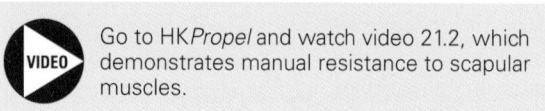
Go to HK*Propel* and watch video 21.2, which demonstrates manual resistance to scapular muscles.

Manual Resistance to Scapular Depression

Body Segment: Scapulothoracic.

Stage in Rehab: Resistive phase. The exercise may occur during the later active phase if the injury is to the glenohumeral joint or muscles and not to the scapulothoracic joint or muscles.

Purpose: Strengthen scapular depressors: the lower trapezius and latissimus dorsi.

Positioning: Patient is side-lying on the uninvolved side. The involved arm is along the side of the body. The clinician faces the patient and places his or her hand closest to the patient's head over the shoulder section of the upper trapezius. The other hand is placed in contact with the scapula's inferior angle with the clinician's arm between the patient's involved arm and ribs. The patient's arm may rest on the clinician's arm to keep the shoulder in the scapular plane (figure 21.48*a*).

Execution: The patient's scapula is passively shrugged by the clinician's hand at the scapula's inferior angle. The patient is instructed to depress the scapula ("pull your shoulder blade down to your back pocket") as the clinician resists and controls the scapular motion with resistance at the inferior angle (figure 21.48*b*). The scapula is then passively positioned in the start position, and the motion is repeated.

Possible Substitutions: Trunk extension or rotation.

Cues and Notations: Resistance to elevation is often not needed because the upper trapezius is much stronger than the lower trapezius, causing an imbalance of the scapular upward rotators. The clinician's pressure should allow the patient to perform a full range of smooth protraction and retraction motion throughout the exercise, so as the patient fatigues, the clinician may need to reduce the amount of force provided. Pain should not occur with any portion of the exercise.

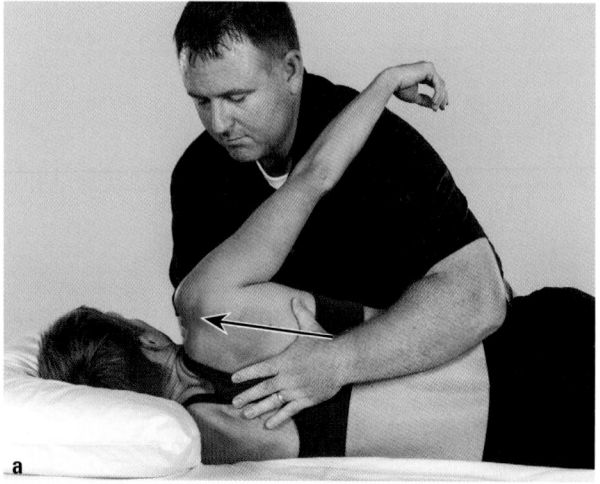 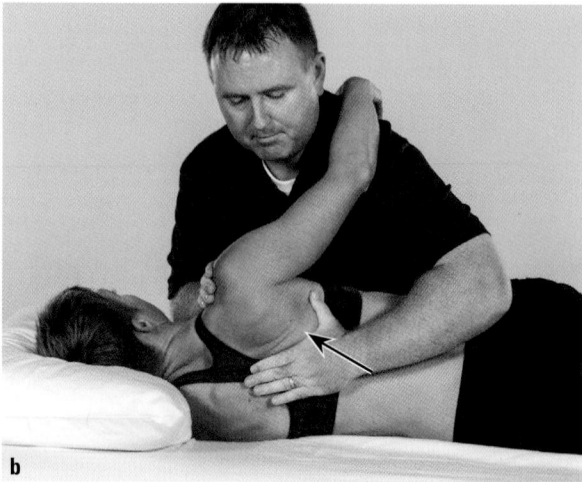

a b

Figure 21.48

Manual Resistance to Serratus Anterior

Body Segment: Scapulothoracic.

Stage in Rehab: Resistive phase.

Purpose: Strengthen serratus anterior for glenohumeral elevation stability.

Positioning: Patient lies supine with the arm flexed to 120° to 150° and the elbow extended.[96]

Execution: The hand is pushed toward the ceiling, with the movement coming from the scapula as it rolls forward and anteriorly around the ribs. This motion can be resisted manually (figure 21.49), with a dumbbell in the hand, or on a bench-press machine with the bar lifted into position by the clinician.

Possible Substitutions: Incomplete range of motion, shoulder extension, trunk rotation, use of upper trapezius to hold arm above 90°.

Cues and Notations: Patients are instructed to "keep the shoulder blade pulled down toward your back pocket." This exercise should not be performed until the shoulder joint has more than 120° of flexion and the glenohumeral joint can withstand the stress applied to it.

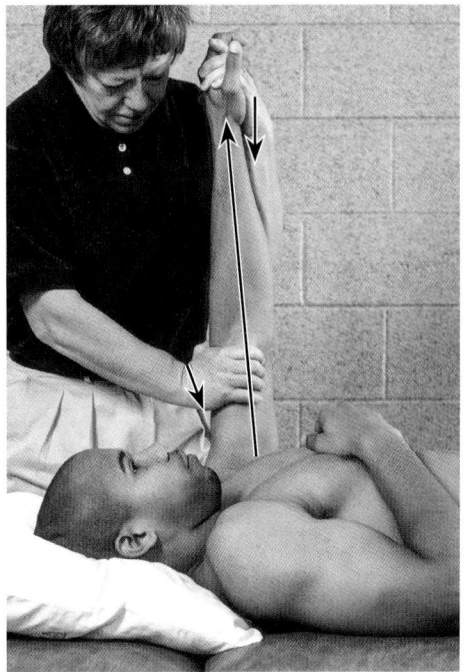

Figure 21.49

Push-Up Plus

Body Segment: Scapulothoracic.

Stage in Rehab: Resistive phase.

Purpose: Facilitate serratus anterior strength.

Positioning: This exercise starts in push-up position with the hands shoulder-width apart, the elbows flexed, and the hands above shoulder level on the wall. The feet are far enough from the wall that the patient leans forward with trunk and hips extended to reach the wall with body weight borne as much as possible on the hands.

Execution: Patient pushes the body away from the hands by extending the elbows and rolling the scapulae anteriorly along the ribs while maintaining hand contact on the surface and body alignment as in the start position. The scapulae slide forward on the rib cage (figure 21.50). From a wall push-up, the patient progresses to an incline push-up with feet on the floor and hands on a tabletop, to a modified push-up on the floor, then a regular push-up, and finally to a decline push-up position with the feet higher than the hands. With the feet higher than the hands, the serratus anterior and the upper trapezius are especially engaged.[97]

Possible Substitutions: Trunk forward lean toward the wall, elbow flexion, hands close together, shoulder shrug rather than scapular protraction, hands too low on the wall.

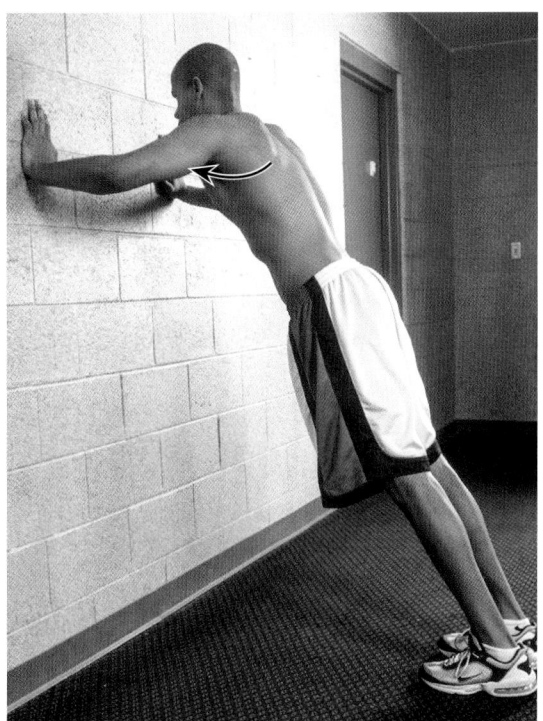

Figure 21.50

Cues and Notations: Patients with anterior instability or those who have had recent anterior shoulder surgery should avoid lowering the body to the point where the shoulders move in front of the plane of the elbows during push-ups. This exercise is contraindicated for those with posterior instability or posterior repair.

Scapular Protraction With Resistive Pulleys or Bands

Body Segment: Scapulothoracic.

Stage in Rehab: Resistive phase.

Purpose: Strengthen serratus anterior.

Positioning: Elastic bands or pulleys are anchored just below shoulder level, and the patient stands or sits with his or her back to the anchor. The elbow begins the exercise in flexion with the upper extremity next to the body and the hand near the shoulder (figure 21.51a).

Execution: The patient pushes the band forward and slightly upward, reaching as far as possible, extending the elbow and punching the scapula forward so the shoulder ends in 120° to 150° of elevation (figure 21.51b).

Possible Substitutions: Using the trunk to rotate the arm forward rather than using the serratus anterior to punch the scapula forward, extending the elbow without protracting the scapula, flexing the trunk, moving the shoulder below 120° of elevation.

Cues and Notations: An alternative exercise using rubber tubing or a resistance band can be performed with the patient supine and the tubing or band under the shoulders and back area. The patient grasps the ends of the tubing or band and starts with the elbows extended and the shoulders flexed to 120° so that the hands are toward the ceiling and the tubing or band is taut. The patient punches the hands toward the ceiling, protracting the scapulae.

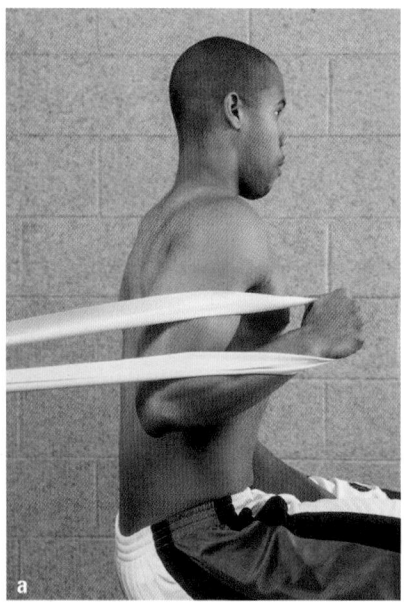 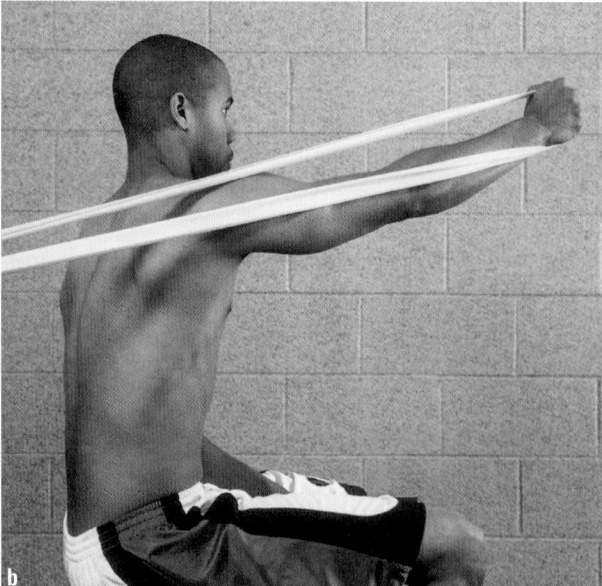

Figure 21.51

Dynamic Hug With Pulleys or Resistance Bands

Body Segment: Scapulothoracic.

Stage in Rehab: Resistive phase.

Purpose: Strengthen serratus anterior.

Positioning: The band is wrapped around the patient's back with the patient grasping one end with each hand. The elbows are partially flexed. If using a resistive pulley system, the pulleys are anchored just below shoulder level, and the patient stands or sits with his or her back to the anchors, grasping a handle with each hand. The shoulders are at 60° of elevation with the elbows slightly flexed (figure 21.52a).

Execution: The patient pushes the band forward, reaching as far as possible, as if hugging a small tree (figure 21.52b).

Possible Substitutions: Arching the back rather than using the serratus anterior to punch the scapula forward, extending the elbow without protracting the scapula, flexing the shoulders above 60°.

Cues and Notations: It is not a large motion since most of it comes from scapular protraction. Patients often try to make the motion larger than it needs to be by using the substitution techniques. When using pulleys, it may sometimes be easier to perform the exercise with only the affected extremity if the correct handle attachments do not allow the simultaneous use of both upper extremities.

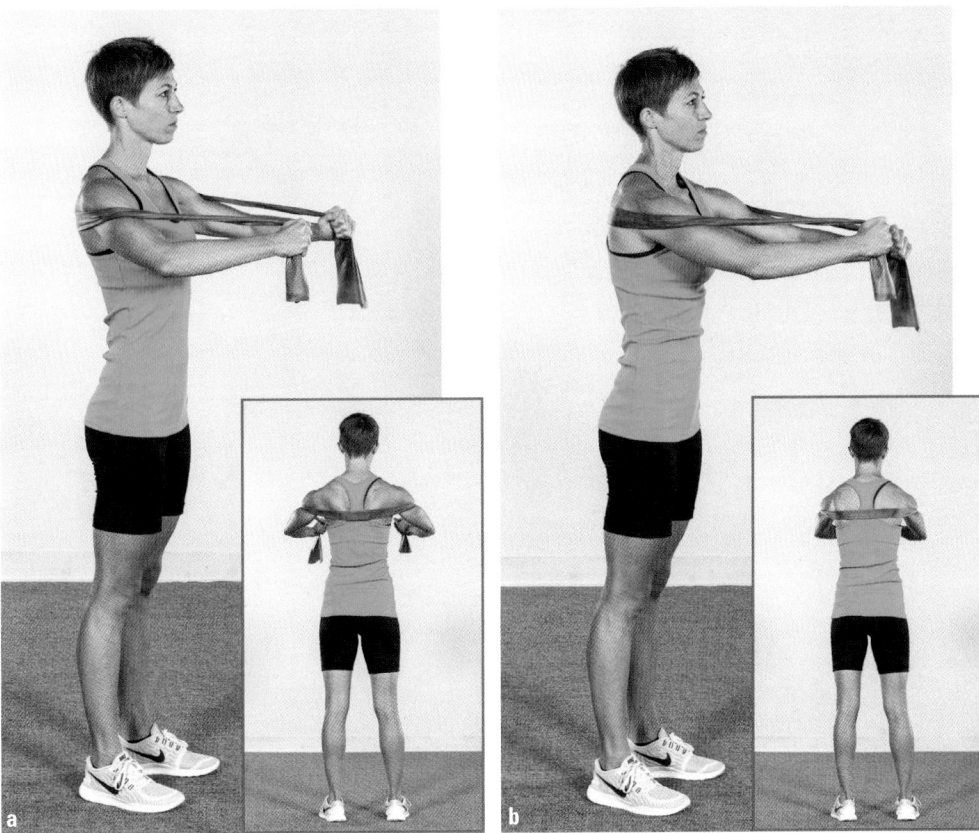

Figure 21.52

Wall Slide

Body Segment: Scapulothoracic.

Stage in Rehab: Resistive phase once full elevation is possible.

Purpose: Strengthen serratus anterior.

Positioning: The patient stands facing the wall with the feet parallel and about 2 to 3 in. from the wall. The ulnar aspects of both forearms contact the wall shoulder-width apart with shoulders and elbows flexed to 90° and the scapulae retracted (figure 21.53a).

Execution: As the scapulae are retracted and depressed, the patient slides the forearms upward along the wall, reaching as far as possible, and then lowers the forearms as far as possible while maintaining contact with the wall (figure 21.53b).

Possible Substitutions: Arching the back rather than using the scapular rotators to move the scapula, using the upper trapezius to elevate the scapula rather than allowing the serratus anterior and lower trapezius to rotate it, extending the elbow without protracting the scapula, flexing the shoulders above 60°.

Cues and Notations: The patient should concentrate on keeping the scapulae depressed throughout the movement. Instruct the patient to tighten the abdominals if the back arches when the forearms move up the wall. An advanced form of the exercise is performed by having the patient move the arms into a Y-configuration as the forearms move up the wall. Another advanced exercise requires that the patient use a looped elastic band around the two forearms and push them away from each other as the forearms move up the wall.

>continued

Wall Slide *>continued*

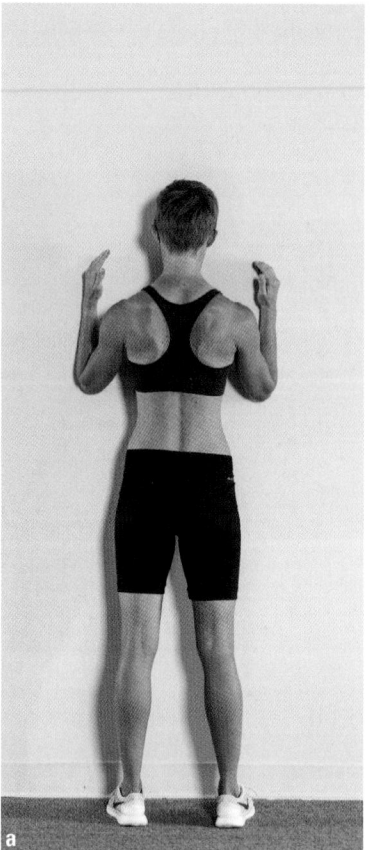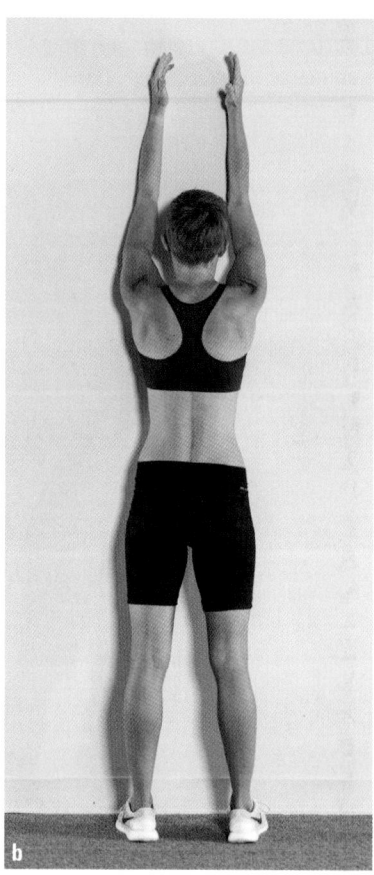

Figure 21.53

Scapular Squeeze

Body Segment: Scapulothoracic.

Stage in Rehab: Active phase and early resistive phase.

Purpose: Strengthen rhomboids and middle trapezius.

Positioning: Patient sits with elbows at the sides.

Execution: Patient squeezes the scapulae together, keeping the elbows at the sides, and holds for 5 to 10 s at the end of the range of motion.

Possible Substitutions: Extending the back, shrugging the shoulders, and extending the shoulders without retracting the scapulae. Provide verbal cues to correct execution, such as "tighten your core to prevent your back from arching," "keep your shoulder blades pulled down and back," and "squeeze your shoulder blades together."

Cues and Notations: This is the first level of exercise for retractors. The next three exercises are progressions of this one.

Wings

Body Segment: Scapulothoracic.

Stage in Rehab: Resistive phase.

Purpose: Strengthen rhomboids and middle trapezius.

Positioning: Patient is seated or standing with elbows flexed to 90° and at the sides. Patient grasps rubber tubing in both hands and makes it taut and parallel to the floor (figure 21.54*a*).

Execution: While keeping the elbows at the sides and forearms parallel to the floor, the patient squeezes the scapulae together as the shoulders move simultaneously into lateral rotation as far as possible (figure 21.54*b*).

Possible Substitutions: Glenohumeral extension, shoulder lateral rotation without scapular retraction, moving the elbows away from the sides.

Cues and Notations: Patient is instructed to "squeeze the shoulder blades together" while "moving the forearms away from each other." The forearms must remain parallel to the floor throughout the exercise. This exercise is contraindicated in patients with recent anterior shoulder repairs of either the capsule or the rotator cuff until normal lateral rotation motion is permitted.

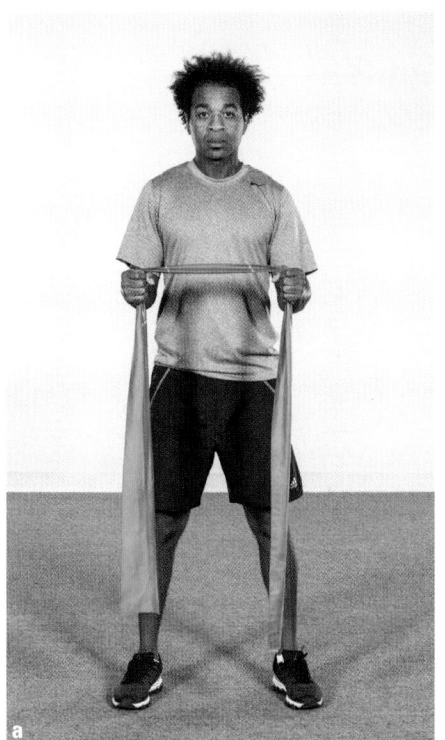
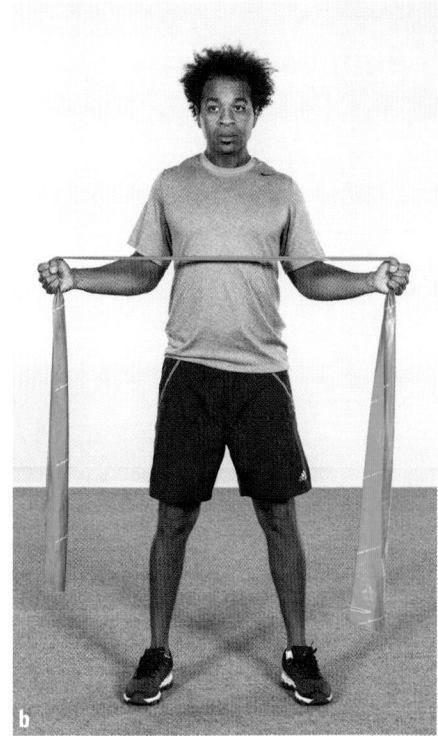

Figure 21.54

Prone Horizontal Abduction at 90° With Full Lateral Rotation (Prone Flys or Reverse Flys)

Body Segment: Scapulothoracic.

Stage in Rehab: Resistive phase.

Purpose: Strengthen rhomboids and middle trapezius.

Positioning: Patient is prone with the arms elevated to 90° and hanging over the end of the table.

Execution: With the shoulders in full lateral rotation, the patient lifts a weight in horizontal abduction as the scapulae are squeezed together in retraction. The elbows remain extended but not locked throughout the movement (figure 21.55). Although the patient need perform the exercise with only the involved extremity, a greater facilitation of the muscles occurs if both arms perform the exercise simultaneously.[98, 99]

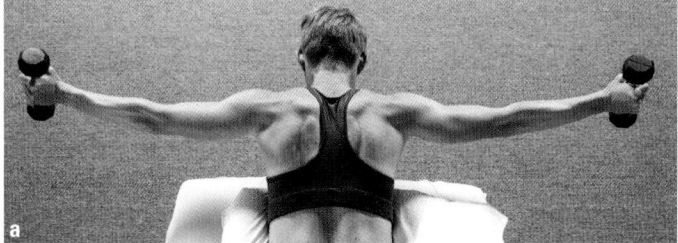
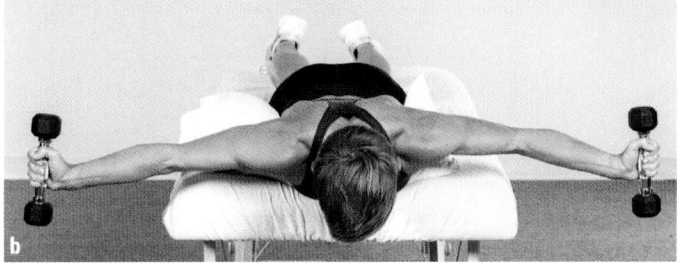

Figure 21.55

>continued

Prone Horizontal Abduction   >*continued*

Possible Substitutions: Shoulder horizontal extension without scapular retraction, dropping the shoulders below 90°, not maintaining full lateral rotation throughout the exercise.

Cues and Notations: A modification of this exercise is performed with the arms at 125° of elevation with the shoulders in full lateral rotation to facilitate the lower trapezius as well as the middle trapezius. If the patient lacks sufficient strength or flexibility, an alternative exercise is to allow the elbows to flex as the scapulae are retracted, but the shoulders should remain at 90° and in lateral rotation.

Rows With Pulleys or Resistance Bands

Body Segment: Scapulothoracic.

Stage in Rehab: Resistive phase.

Purpose: Strengthen rhomboids and middle trapezius.

Positioning: In sitting or standing, the patient faces resistance bands or pulleys that are anchored to a door or wall at or slightly below shoulder level. The patient tightens the abdominals to keep the back from arching (figure 21.56*a*). If sitting, the hips and knees are at 90°; if standing, the hips and knees are slightly flexed to reduce stress on the back during the exercise.

Execution: Maintaining proper trunk position with abdominal muscle tension, the patient pulls to retract the scapulae, squeezing them together while keeping the elbows at the sides (figure 21.56*b*).

Possible Substitutions: Extending the trunk and hips; using shoulder extensors without retracting the scapulae.

Cues and Notations: Patient may sit on a Swiss ball to make the exercise more challenging. Some weight machines also provide this exercise.

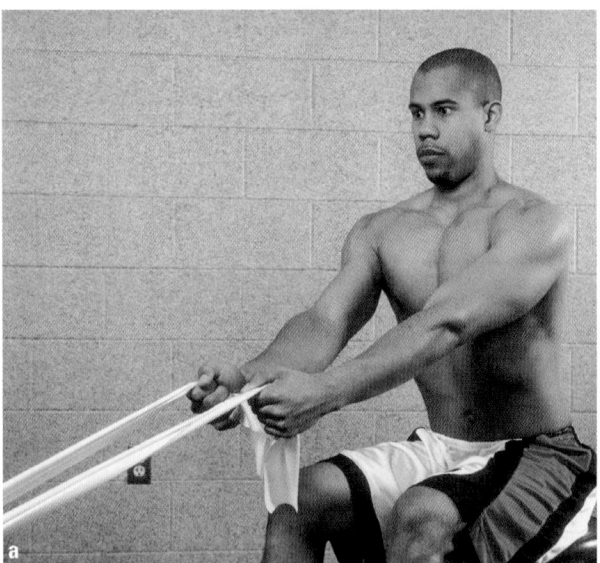 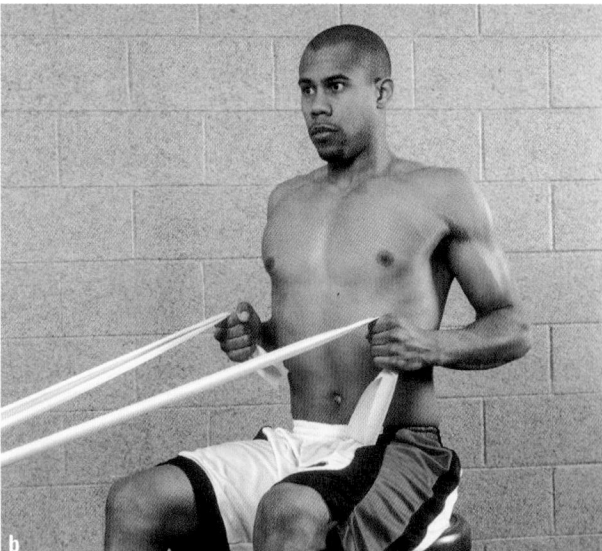

Figure 21.56

Seated Push-Up

This exercise is sometimes called a press-up or a press-down.

Body Segment: Scapulothoracic.

Stage in Rehab: Later resistive phase.

Purpose: Strengthen lower trapezius and pectoralis minor. Latissimus dorsi is also strengthened.

Positioning: Patient is seated with hands alongside the hips on the chair seat. If patient has sufficient strength and the chair has arms, the hands may be placed on the chair arms.

Execution: The patient pushes down to lift the hips off the chair (figure 21.57). The elbows must extend, and then the patient pushes down further to depress the scapulae.

Possible Substitutions: Using legs to lift body up, leaning forward to tilt trunk forward.

Cues and Notations: If the patient complains of shoulder joint pain, the rotator cuff muscles are not strong enough to stabilize the glenohumeral joint during this exercise. In this case, begin with the exercise listed next and return to this exercise once the patient gains additional rotator cuff stability and strength.

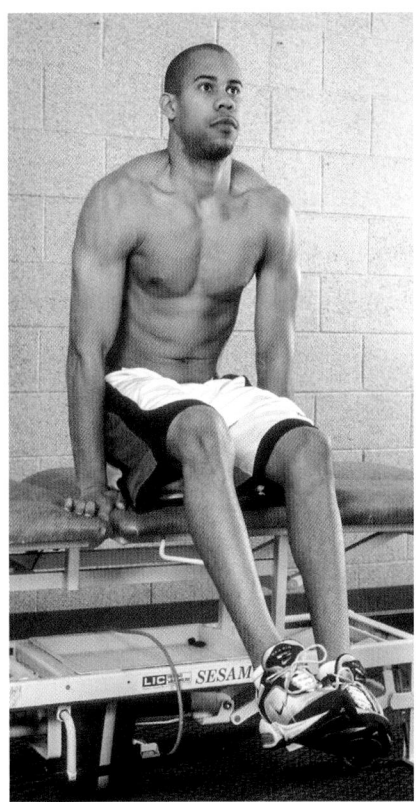

Figure 21.57

Press-Downs Using Pulleys or Resistance Bands

Body Segment: Scapulothoracic.

Stage in Rehab: Later resistive phase.

Purpose: Strengthen scapular depressors.

Positioning: The pulley or band is positioned high overhead, and the patient grasps the handle or band with an extended elbow and with the shoulder in full elevation (figure 21.58a).

Execution: While keeping the shoulder and elbow joints in their start positions throughout the exercise, the patient actively contracts the lower trapezius to depress the scapula as far as possible, and then relaxes the muscles to allow the shoulder to shrug to its start position.

An alternative exercise uses a latissimus bar: Using both hands—the involved hand positioned at the end of the bar and the uninvolved hand grasping closer to the middle of the bar—the patient begins with the elbows extended and both shoulders in full elevation overhead. The motion comes only from the scapula's depressor muscles as the patient contracts them to move the scapula through a full motion of depression; the elbow and glenohumeral joint positions do not change.

Possible Substitutions: Lateral trunk lean, going through a partial range of motion, extending the shoulder, flexing the elbow.

Cues and Notations: An alternative for this exercise can be performed with the resistance device anchored to the shoulder rather than with the patient grasping the handle; in this position the shoulder is not placed in an elevated position (figure 21.58b). This exercise isolates the depressors and does not put stress on the glenohumeral joint, so the exercise may begin earlier in the resistive phase.

>continued

Press-Downs Using Pulleys or Resistance Bands *>continued*

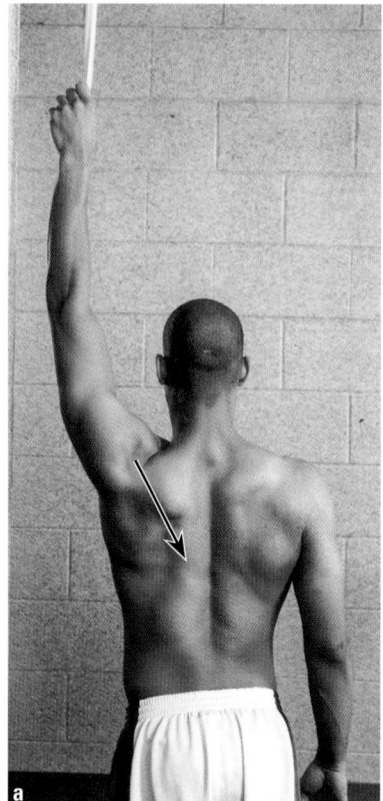 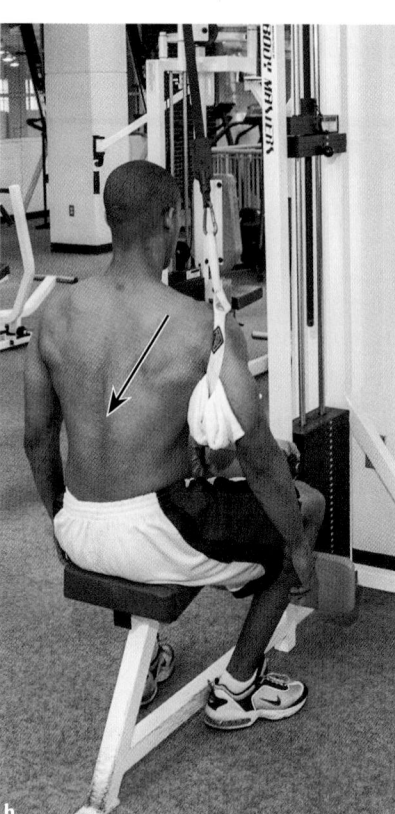

Figure 21.58

Bouhler Exercises

Body Segment: Scapulothoracic.

Stage in Rehab: Resistive phase once full elevation is achieved.

Purpose: Strengthen lower trapezius as an upward rotator.

Positioning: Patient stands with the back and buttocks to the wall and the heels about 1 in. (2.5 cm) from the wall.

Execution: With the abdominal muscles tightened to prevent the back from arching, the patient fully elevates the shoulders overhead with the elbows extended and close to the ears. In the first exercise, the thumbs face the wall and are pushed to the wall (figure 21.59a). In the second exercise, the arms are in the same position as in the first exercise, but the shoulders are rotated medially so the thumbs face each other as the arms are moved to the wall (figure 21.59b). In the last exercise, the arms are positioned at a 45° angle from the body and are moved to the wall as the scapulae retract (figure 21.59c). In each exercise, the patient holds the position for 5 to 10 s and repeats several times.

Possible Substitutions: Arching the back, standing farther away from the wall, moving the elbows away from the head, flexing the elbows.

Cues and Notations: It may be necessary to add one of these exercises at a time on separate days since the lower trapezius may fatigue quickly. To perform these exercises at a more advanced level, the patient lies prone on either a table or a Swiss ball. Weights can be added to the hands for additional resistance (figure 21.59d).

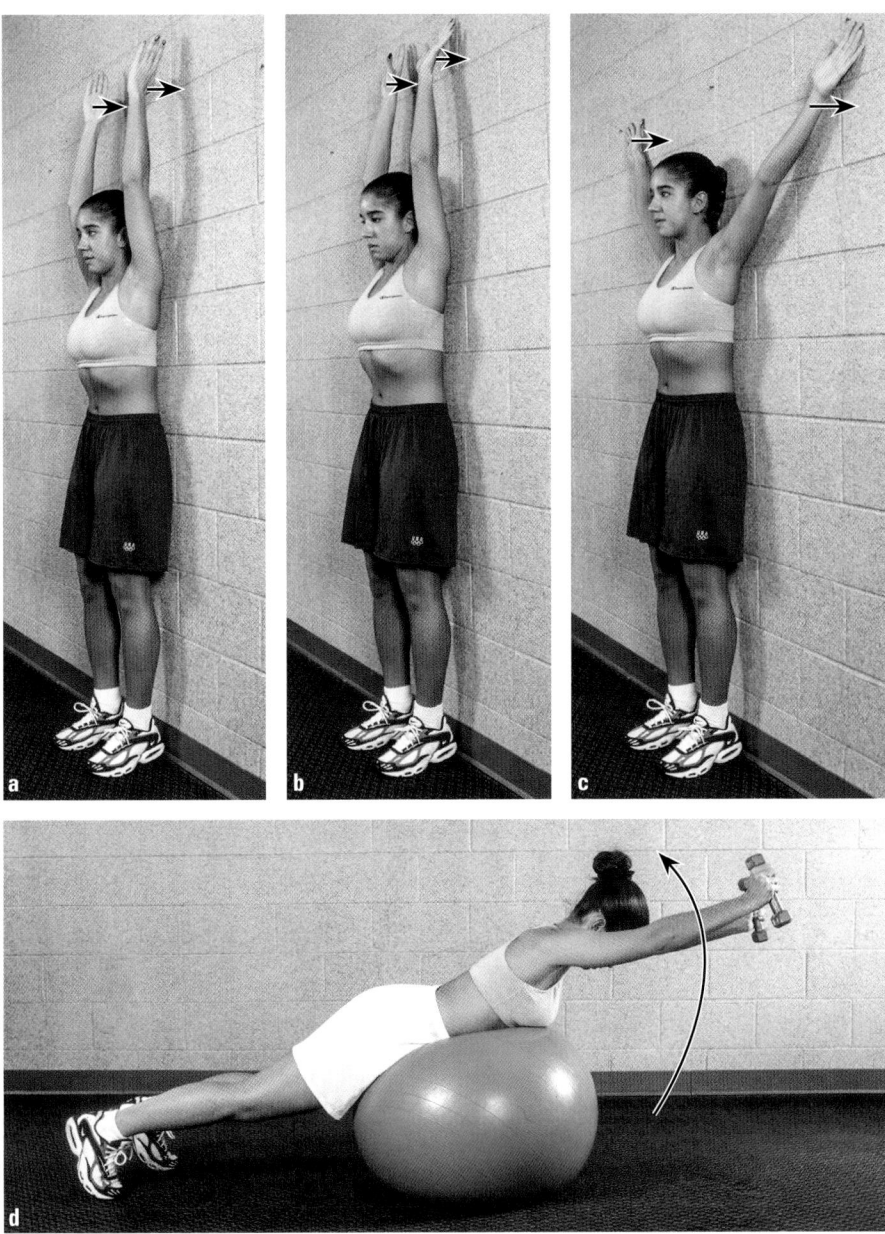

Figure 21.59

Lawnmower Exercise[100]

Body Segment: Scapulothoracic neuromotor reeducation.

Stage in Rehab: Early resistive phase.

Purpose: Strengthen lower trapezius and serratus anterior and facilitate proper neuromotor activation.

Positioning: Patient stands flexed at the hips and knees with the upper torso rotated toward the outer aspect of the thigh that is contralateral to the involved shoulder. Patient grasps a pulley handle or band that is attached to the wall near the floor near the contralateral foot, or else the patient stands on the band with the contralateral foot to anchor it (figure 21.60a).

>continued

Lawnmower Exercise[100] *>continued*

Execution: As the hips and knees extend to stand upright, the hips also rotate while the involved arm's elbow flexes, the forearm moves next to the ribs, the shoulder extends, and the scapula retracts (figure 21.60*b*).

Possible Substitutions: Using the back to flex and extend rather than the hips and knees, failing to retract the scapula, horizontally abducting the shoulder rather than extending it, elevating the scapula, performing the sequence out of order.

Cues and Notations: Instruct the patient to keep the chest up and the back straight in the start position so that the hips and knees do the moving. Keep the elbow to the side, pulling it toward the spine. Squeeze the shoulder blades as you stand erect. Keep your abdominals tight so you do not arch your back. Providing more resistance increases the difficulty of the exercise. Since these muscles must work for prolonged periods during upper-extremity activities, high repetitions are used to improve their endurance. This exercise may also be performed using kettle balls. This exercise is advocated by its authors because it is a multisegment exercise that facilitates normal activation patterns, thereby producing efficient, stable joint positions throughout the movement.[100]

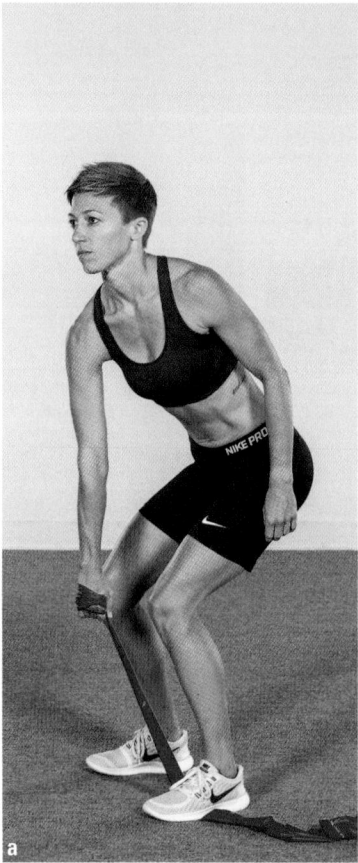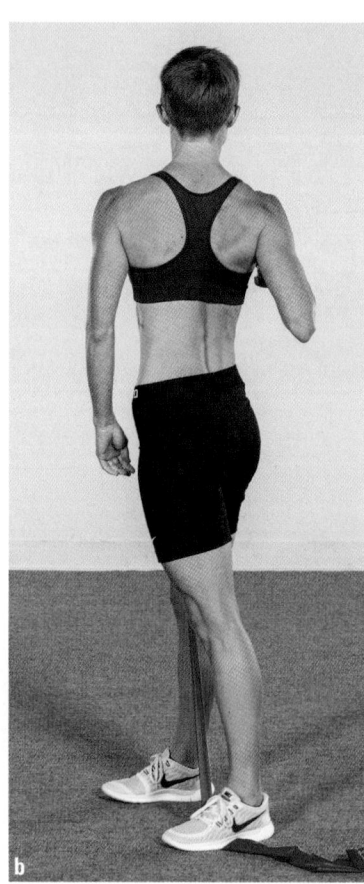

Figure 21.60

Robbery Exercise[100]

Body Segment: Scapulothoracic neuromotor reeducation.

Stage in Rehab: Early resistive phase.

Purpose: Strengthen middle trapezius, rhomboids, and lower trapezius and facilitate proper neuromotor activation.

Positioning: Patient stands flexed at the hips and knees with back straight. Trunk is positioned about 40° to 50° from erect with the feet about shoulder-width apart and arms relaxed, hanging in front of body with hands facing thighs (figure 21.61*a*).

Execution: As the hips and knees extend to move the body upright, the shoulders move into extension as the elbows flex while staying close to the body, the wrists extend to face the palms forward and away from the body, and the scapulae retract into the back pockets. This position is held for 5 s (figure 21.61*b*).

Possible Substitutions: Flexing and extending from the back rather than the hips and knees, failing to keep the arms next to the sides, shrugging the shoulders.

Cues and Notations: Instruct the patient to keep the chest up and the back straight in the start position so the hips and knees do the moving. Keep the arms close to the sides. Pull the scapulae down as you squeeze them together. This exercise is advocated by its authors because it is a multisegment exercise that facilitates normal activation patterns, thereby producing efficient, stable joint positions throughout the movement.[100] This exercise does not facilitate as much effort from the muscles as other exercises,[101] but it may help to begin strengthening in the early resistive phase before the patient has regained full glenohumeral motion.

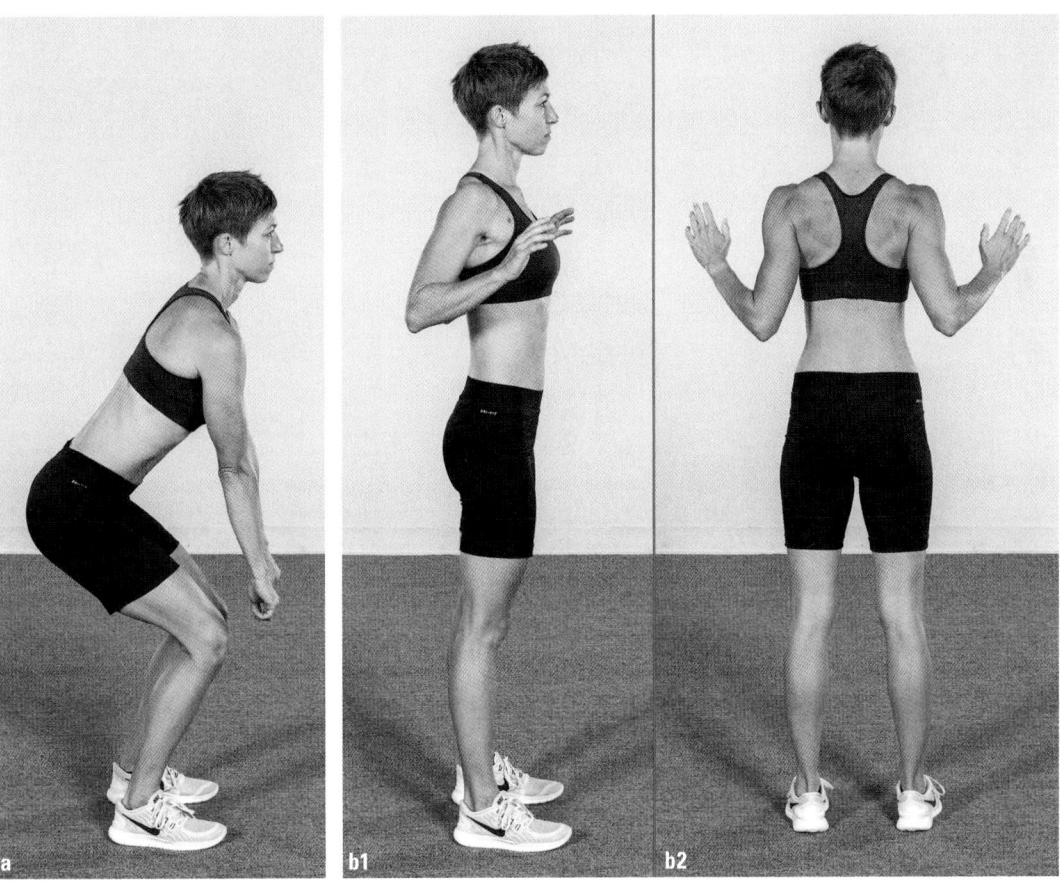

Figure 21.61

Low Row Exercise

Body Segment: Scapulothoracic neuromotor reeducation.

Stage in Rehab: Early resistive phase.

Purpose: Facilitate proper neuromotor activation of scapular stabilization muscles.

Positioning: Patient stands with involved side next to a treatment table in a forward-backward straddle; the ipsilateral leg is ahead of the contralateral leg and the body weight is primarily on the back leg. The involved extremity's hand is placed with the palm on the tabletop (figure 21.62a).

Execution: As the patient transfers body weight, pushing off from the back to the front leg, he or she pushes down on the involved hand as the arm accepts the body's weight and the scapula is depressed (figure 21.62b).

Possible Substitutions: The patient does not bear weight on the involved upper extremity, the weight transfers more to the contralateral leg than the upper extremity, the elbow flexes, the scapula is not depressed.

Cues and Notations: This is an early closed kinetic chain exercise that applies less stress than open-chain exercises and facilitates lower trapezius and serratus anterior activation while depressing upper trapezius activation.[102]

This exercise can be modified and performed against resistance as seen in figure 21.62c. Rather than moving the body, the patient stands still and pulls a resistance band or rope toward and past the hip, retracting the scapula as the arm moves into extension.[103]

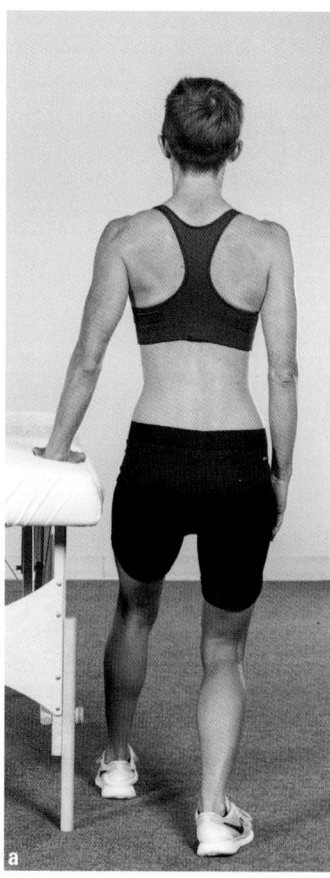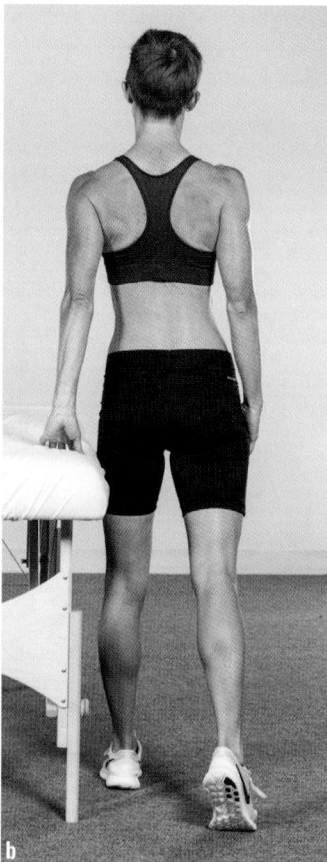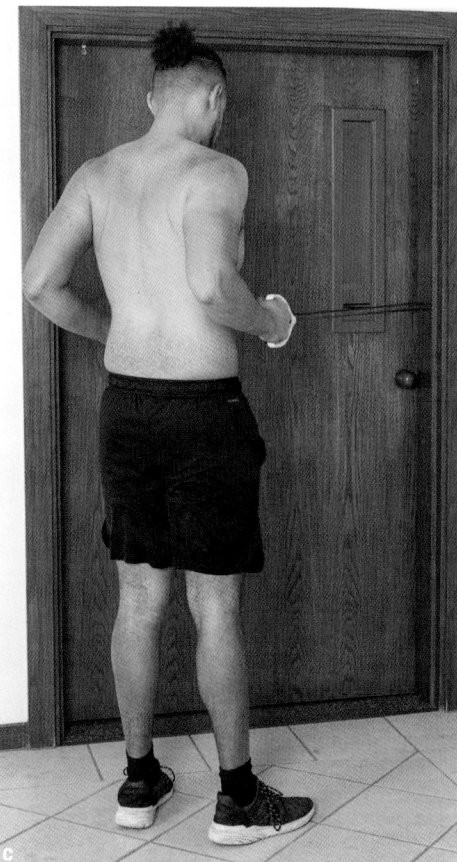

Figure 21.62

Scapular Elevation

This exercise is also known as shoulder shrugs.

Body Segment: Scapulothoracic.

Stage in Rehab: Resistive phase.

Purpose: Strengthen upper trapezius and levator scapulae muscles.

Positioning: Patient stands with arms at sides.

Execution: Patient shrugs shoulders up to the ears.

Possible Substitutions: Cervical extension, scapulae protraction.

Cues and Notations: These muscles are normally strong and often overpower their synergists and antagonists, resulting in a muscle imbalance, so they may not need strengthening; your examination will determine their status. They are often used incorrectly during shoulder elevation as a substitution for weak rotator cuff muscles, contributing to faulty mechanics, further muscle imbalances, and prolonged recovery from injury. In patients who have weakness of these muscles, initial strengthening can include shoulder shrugs and manual resistance to shrugs. A more advanced exercise uses dumbbell weights during shrugs.

Upright Press

This exercise is also known as the overhead press or military press.

Body Segment: Scapulothoracic.

Stage in Rehab: Starts during the last half of the resistive phase.

Purpose: Strengthen upper trapezius and levator scapulae. Also strengthens glenohumeral deltoid muscles.

Positioning: Patient stands, elbows flexed, with weights in hands. Hands are at shoulder level.

Execution: Patient pushes weights straight overhead to end with hands above the head and elbows fully extended but not locked.

Possible Substitutions: Arching the back, using momentum to lift the weight by swinging the weights upward.

Cues and Notations: This is a later exercise that is not always included in rehabilitation because of the stress it may place on the glenohumeral joint. The upper trapezius is seldom deficient and may not need strengthening. Scapular upward rotator (lower trapezius and serratus anterior) muscles and glenohumeral rotator cuff muscles should have good strength before this exercise is used.

Scapular Upward Rotation

Body Segment: Scapulothoracic.

Stage in Rehab: Starts during the last half of the resistive phase.

Purpose: Strengthen scapular upward rotators. The exercise is also used to strengthen deltoid and pectoralis major muscles of the glenohumeral joint.

Positioning: Patient stands with arms relaxed at sides. With weight in hand, the thumb faces forward.

Execution: The elbow is kept in extension but not locked, and the upper extremity is elevated in the scapular plane, moving through a full range of motion and then returning to the start position (figure 21.63). The patient must maintain scapular control and correct glenohumeral positioning.

Possible Substitutions: Hyperextending the back, shrugging the shoulder to initiate movement.

Cues and Notations: Full range-of-motion exercise for scapular rotation also includes glenohumeral motion, so the rehabilitation clinician must be sure that rotator cuff strength and glenohumeral joint stability are adequate before including these full-motion scapular activities in the rehabilitation program.

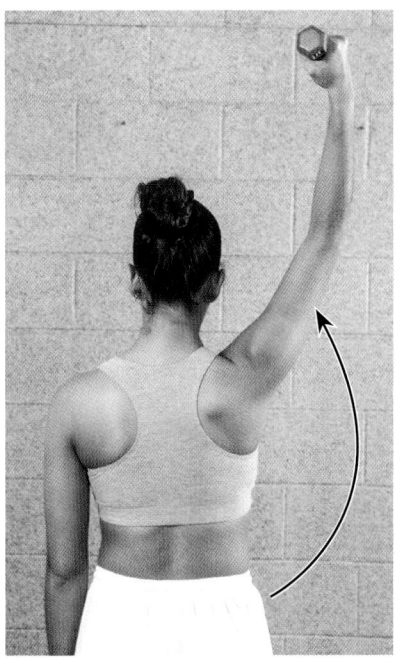

Figure 21.63

Scapular Downward Rotation

Body Segment: Scapulothoracic.

Stage in Rehab: Starts in later resistive phase.

Purpose: Strengthen downward rotators of the scapula.

Positioning: Patient is prone with the shoulder over the edge of the table, and humerus is perpendicular to the floor. Weight is in the hand, and the wrist is in a functional position.

Execution: Keeping the scapula depressed, the patient moves the upper extremity into full hyperextension at the shoulder (figure 21.64).

Possible Substitutions: Elbow flexion, shoulder shrugging.

Cues and Notations: The seated or standing latissimus pull-down exercise using a machine or pulley bar is an advanced resistance exercise for downward rotation. The hands are shoulder-width apart on the overhead latissimus bar, and the elbows are kept extended but not locked throughout the exercise. The patient "sets" the scapulae and then pulls the bar toward the anterior thighs.

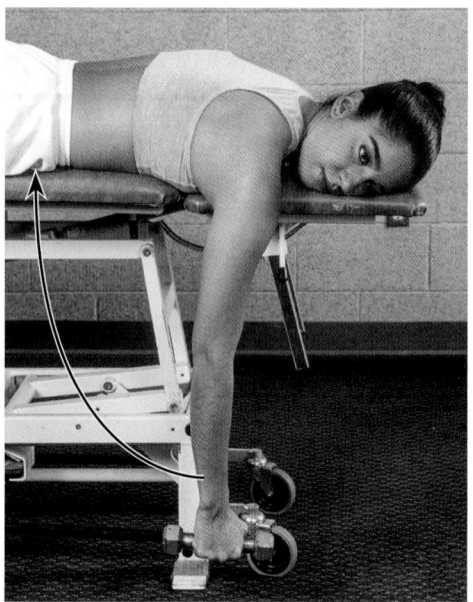

Figure 21.64

Glenohumeral Exercises   As you may have noticed in the previous group of strengthening exercises for the scapulothoracic muscles, as the range of motion of the activity expands, the connectedness of the structures within the glenohumeral complex becomes more apparent. You realized that when the scapula moves through its full range of upward rotation, the glenohumeral muscles also work to perform humeral motion. Because of the close relationship between the segments of the shoulder complex, it is difficult to isolate them when full motion occurs within an exercise or activity. For this reason, the clinician must understand the shoulder complex elements and their functions, both in isolation and as part of a unit with the other components. For example, a patient's rotator cuff injury might not limit the motions of the scapulothoracic muscles, but moving the scapula through its entire range of motion is contraindicated for a new rotator cuff repair.

The exercises in this glenohumeral muscle section are divided into two subsections. The first subsection deals with muscles that stabilize the glenohumeral joints, and the second subsection covers the movers of the joints. Although the rotator cuff muscles can move the glenohumeral joint, they are also the joint's stabilizers; therefore, their strength is important to the normal function of the shoulder complex. The other glenohumeral muscles include the large muscles that are often considered the "movers" or "prime movers" of the shoulder; these muscles include the deltoid, pectoralis major, and latissimus dorsi.[104]

Although we do not provide detailed exercise suggestions for the prime movers of the glenohumeral joint, they remain important muscles to strengthen whenever an examination reveals deficiencies in them. Most clinicians are already familiar with strengthening activities for these large muscles; on the other hand, the rotator cuff muscle exercises may be less familiar, so they are therefore presented here. Some of the rotator cuff strengthening exercises included here will also strengthen the prime movers, especially when the exercise is performed in the alternative positions presented.

Rotator Cuff Exercises

As you will notice, the exercises in this section are primarily used to strengthen the rotator cuff muscles. Because it is difficult to isolate the rotator cuff muscles completely, some of the larger muscle movers of the shoulders are also impacted by these exercises.

Glenohumeral Lateral Rotation

Body Segment: Glenohumeral joint.

Stage in Rehab: Resistive phase.

Purpose: Strengthen teres minor, infraspinatus, and posterior deltoid.

Positioning: This exercise may be performed in different positions either to accomplish different goals or to provide maximum resistance at different points within the range of motion.

1. In side-lying on the uninvolved side with a towel roll placed between the humerus and lateral ribs, the patient positions the elbow at 90° (figure 21.65a).
2. The patient is prone with the shoulder at 90° abduction (figure 21.65b).
3. The patient stands and grasps an elastic band or rubber tubing that is attached to a wall and runs parallel in front of the patient. The involved elbow is at the side and flexed to 90°. The forearm is near the abdomen (figure 21.65c).

In all positions, a rolled towel is placed between the distal humerus and the side.

Execution:

1. For 1 above, patient lifts the weight upward until the forearm is parallel to the floor. As motion improves, the weight may be lifted toward the ceiling.

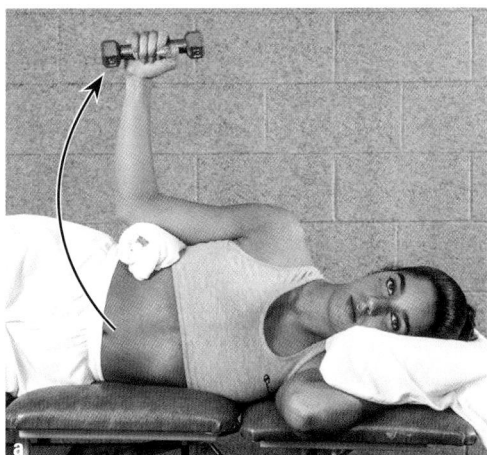
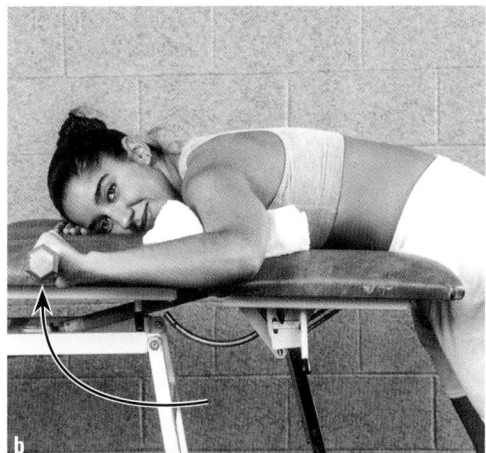
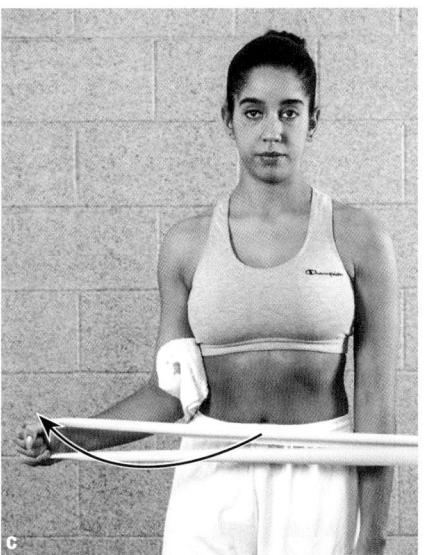
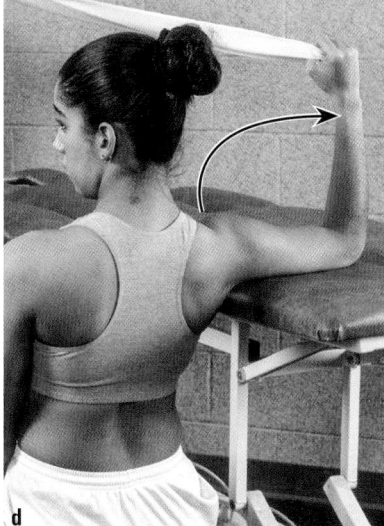
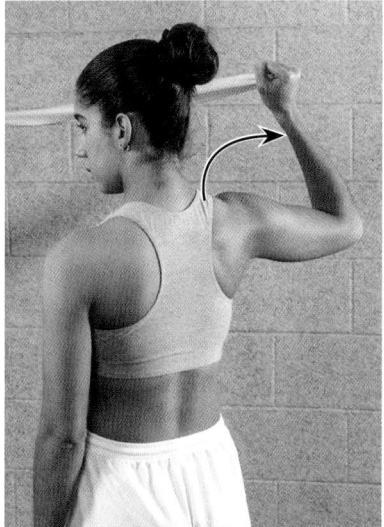

Figure 21.65

>continued

Glenohumeral Lateral Rotation >*continued*

2. For 2 above, patient lifts the weight toward the ceiling while holding the humerus at 90° of abduction.

3. For 3 above, patient laterally rotates the shoulder by pulling the band away from the abdomen while keeping the upper arm parallel to the floor.

Possible Substitutions: Elbow extension or shoulder extension in positions 1 and 3, elbow flexion or shoulder horizontal extension in position 2; rolling the trunk in all three positions.

Cues and Notations: Exercise should be performed in the scapular plane. Once scapular stability is achieved, this exercise can be performed with the shoulder elevated to 90° in the scapular plane. At first, it may be necessary to support the elbow (figure 21.65*d*), but as strength improves, elbow support becomes unnecessary (figure 21.65*e*). In the elevated position, the shoulder is kept at 90° abduction without horizontal adduction, and the elbow remains level with the shoulder.

Medial Rotation of the Glenohumeral Joint

Body Segment: Glenohumeral joint.

Stage in Rehab: Resistive phase.

Purpose: Strengthen subscapularis. This exercise also strengthens the teres major, latissimus dorsi, anterior deltoid, and pectoralis major.

Positioning: The patient can be side-lying on the involved side or supine. In either position, the elbow is flexed to 90°. If the patient is supine, the arm is abducted slightly. If the patient is side-lying, the elbow is on the table with the shoulder in slight flexion. When using elastic resistance, the patient stands and grasps an elastic band or rubber tubing that is attached to a wall and runs parallel to the

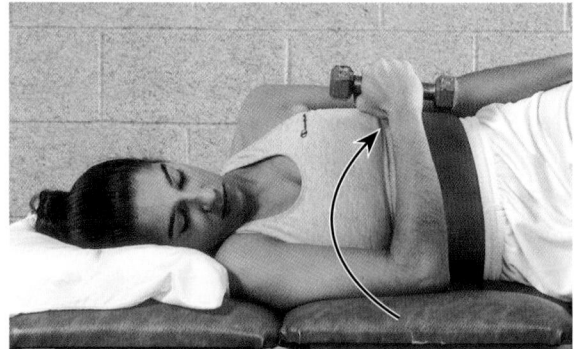

Figure 21.66

floor. The involved elbow is at the side and flexed to 90°. This exercise is just the reverse of the image shown in figure 21.65*c*, so the forearm begins away from the patient and moves toward the patient's abdomen as the patient performs the exercise. In this exercise, instead of the band being anchored near the uninvolved side, it is anchored closer to the involved side.

Execution: In all positions, a rolled towel is placed between the distal humerus and the patient's side, and the movement that occurs is the shoulder rolling into medial rotation so that the hand moves toward the abdomen (figure 21.66).

Possible Substitutions: Elbow flexion to 90° is not maintained throughout the motion. Other substitutions include rotating the trunk and flexion of the shoulder.

Cues and Notations: If the patient lacks full lateral rotation so that the forearm cannot contact the table, a rolled towel may be placed where the forearm contacts the surface to limit lateral rotation. As with the previous exercise, once scapular stability is achieved, this exercise can be performed with the arm abducted to 90°. At first, it may be necessary to support the elbow as shown in figure 21.65*d* for medial rotation, but as strength improves, elbow support becomes unnecessary. In the elevated position, the shoulder is held at 90° of elevation, and the elbow stays level with the shoulder.

Glenohumeral Abduction in the Scapular Plane

Body Segment: Glenohumeral joint.

Stage in Rehab: Resistive phase.

Purpose: Increase supraspinatus strength.

Positioning: Patient stands or sits with a weight in the hand (figure 21.67*a*).

Execution: The arm is raised in the scapular plane to 90°.

Possible Substitutions: Shoulder flexion, trunk lateral flexion to the opposite side, trunk extension, shoulder shrugging, elbow flexion.

Cues and Notations: Patient control of the glenohumeral joint is paramount throughout this exercise. If the patient cannot control the glenohumeral joint to 90°, the exercise height is limited to the first 30° to 60° of elevation, or the patient is positioned in side-lying on the uninvolved side to perform the exercise. The exercise begins with the patient performing it in only the first 30° of elevation in the scapular plane. As scapular control improves, the shoulder moves next to 60° to 90°, and then as glenohumeral control occurs at that level, the patient moves the shoulder through a full range of scapular plane elevation (figure 21.67b). A verbal cue to "pull the scapula down toward your back pocket" while elevating the shoulder may be helpful.

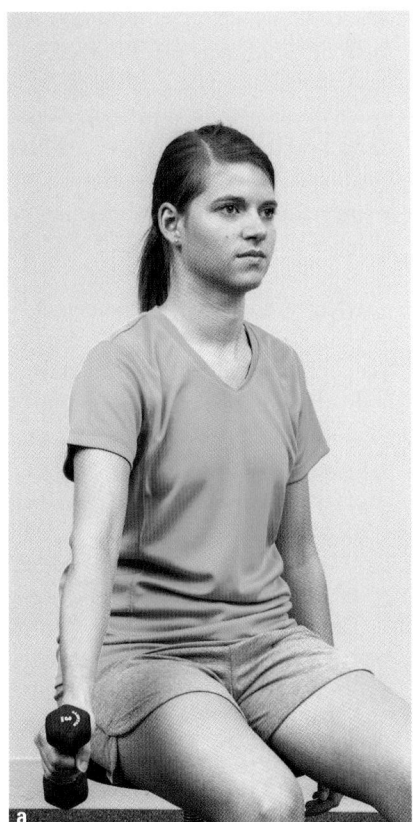 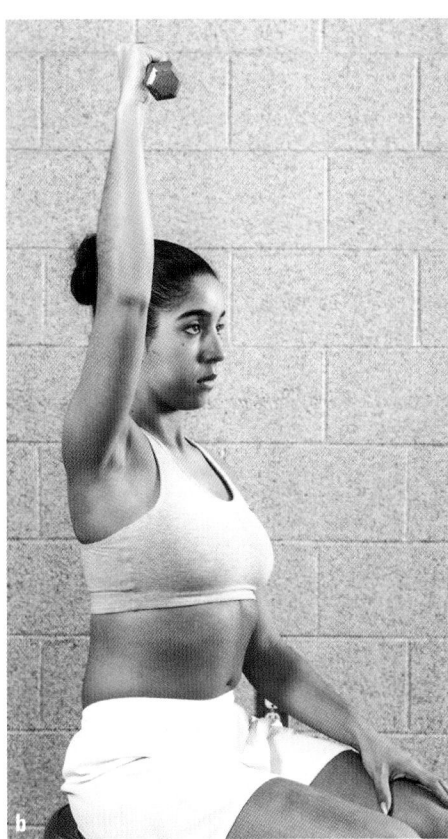

Figure 21.67

 Go to HK*Propel* and watch video 21.3, which demonstrates maintaining scapular position during shoulder elevation in the scapular plane.

Horizontal Abduction or Horizontal Extension

Body Segment: Glenohumeral joint.

Stage in Rehab: Resistive phase.

Purpose: Strengthen teres minor and infraspinatus muscles. This exercise also strengthens posterior deltoid and scapular stabilizers.

Positioning: Patient lies prone with the arm over the edge of the table. Weight is in the hand.

Execution: The arm is lifted toward the ceiling into horizontal extension (abduction) with the shoulder in lateral rotation (thumb facing the ceiling when at end range).

Possible Substitutions: Rolling the trunk rather than lifting the arm, moving out of the plane of motion, placing the hand closer to the hip, flexing the elbow.

Cues and Notations: This is similar to the prone fly but concentrates more on the rotator cuff lateral rotators than on scapular retraction.

Prime Mover Exercises As the shoulder moves through larger arcs of motion, the prime mover muscles become involved in the activity. Many strengthening exercises for the prime movers simply involve moving the shoulder complex muscles that have already been presented through greater ranges of motion. Here we present a brief discussion of important considerations to keep in mind during full shoulder complex motion activities.

Most shoulder exercises performed in the lower levels of shoulder elevation emphasize the glenohumeral muscles. Once the shoulder muscles move the arm into elevation, scapular muscles also contract during the movement to maintain the glenoid position relative to the humeral head. Since scapular muscles play a vital role in positioning the shoulder, early strengthening of shoulder muscles starts with exercises performed in the lower levels of elevation (first 60°) until there is enough scapular muscle strength to stabilize the shoulder in its correct position; as previously mentioned, in activities below 60°, scapular muscles contract isometrically to "set" the scapula.[14] We divide shoulder rehabilitation exercises into three divisions, or levels: below 60°, 60° to 120°, and above 120°. As shoulder elevation positions in these exercises increase, scapular muscles must work harder both to stabilize and to move the scapula at the same time.[16] Scapular stabilization is required for good glenohumeral motion and control throughout shoulder elevation,[105] so scapular muscle strength is achieved in the low ranges of elevation first in a rehabilitation program and then in the middle and end ranges of elevation motion as strength increases.

Glenohumeral abduction motion occurs through force-couple activity of the deltoid with the supraspinatus.[53] The other rotator cuff muscles also play an important role during shoulder abduction and flexion as they co-contract during abduction to depress the humeral head into the glenoid.[106] Thus, the rotator cuff and deltoid collectively stabilize the glenohumeral joint during elevation activities.[107] The scapular muscles must also work to position the scapula during shoulder abduction, thereby providing stability to the glenohumeral joint.[108] The degrees of elevation through which the scapular muscles provide glenohumeral joint stability range from the first 30°[15] of elevation to 60°[14] to 90°.[109]

In the early strengthening stages, the patient may need reminders to fix or "set" the scapula by tensing the lower

trapezius and serratus anterior before moving the humerus so that proper neuromotor activation occurs. As part of Logan's routine program for his pitchers in the opening scenario, the position at which rotator cuff exercise is performed is determined primarily by the pitcher's scapular control. In other words, as scapular muscle strength improves, Logan advances the height at which the rotator cuff exercises are performed, starting below 60° of elevation, then advancing to mid-range elevation exercises and finally to end-range elevation activities.

Abduction can be performed in the coronal plane, but the recommendation is to perform elevation in the scapular plane, approximately 30° forward of the frontal plane. This position is best for facilitating the rotator cuff muscles.[110] As previously mentioned, glenohumeral motion in this plane of the scapula is called **scaption**.[111, 112]

Studies have demonstrated that the best position from which to strengthen the supraspinatus is with the hand in a full-can position rather than an empty-can position.[107, 113, 114] The full-can exercise is commonly performed with the body in one of two positions, prone or standing. However, the posterior deltoid muscle works more when the patient lies prone than when the patient stands,[113] so the best position in which to isolate and strengthen the supraspinatus is in a standing position using the open-can hand position.[113] The elbow is held in an extended but not locked position as the arm elevates in the scapular plane.

The empty-can exercise is performed in the scapular plane as with the open-can exercise, but the shoulder is medially rotated. Although this position facilitates the supraspinatus and deltoid, it may also aggravate the supraspinatus tendon by impinging it if the rotator cuff is not strong enough to counterbalance the deltoid.[113]

Key Shoulder Strengthening Exercises

For several years, clinical researchers have investigated various exercises to identify which of them are best at strengthening shoulder and scapular muscles. Because there are so many muscles and even more exercises, most investigators can focus on only a few muscles within any one study. Hence, many investigations are needed before we have all the answers to the question of which exercises are most effective. Occasionally, research results conflict because of the different variables used in different studies. Changes in protocols, methods of performing the exercise, body position during the exercise, number of subjects studied, healthy or injured subjects, age and sex of subjects, and any number of other variables can affect the results. Table 21.2 provides a summary of the results from several investigations.[96, 100, 113, 115-131]

TABLE 21.2 Summary of Optimal Shoulder Rehabilitation Exercises

Shoulder complex segment	Muscle	Exercises for optimal strength results
Scapula	Serratus anterior	Push-up plus Scaption elevation Dynamic hug Shoulder abduction Seated rowing Lawnmower Inferior slide
	Lower trapezius	Press-up Prone horizontal abduction at 90° with full lateral rotation Prone horizontal abduction at 100° to 125° Abduction with full lateral rotation Prone lateral rotation at 90° abduction with elbow at 90° flexion Bilateral scapular retraction Scaption elevation Seated rowing Shoulder abduction especially in 90° to 125° range Lawnmower Inferior slide
	Middle trapezius and rhomboids	Prone horizontal abduction at 90° with thumb up Prone horizontal abduction at 100° to 125° abduction with full lateral rotation Seated rowing
	Upper trapezius	Scaption elevation Seated rowing
	Pectoralis minor	Push-up plus Scaption elevation Press-up
Humerus: rotator cuff	Supraspinatus	Scaption elevation Horizontal abduction at 100° in prone Military press
	Infraspinatus and teres minor	Lateral rotation in side-lying Prone horizontal abduction at 90° with full lateral rotation Prone lateral rotation at 90° abduction with elbow at 90° flexion Scaption elevation Abduction (bilaterally) Weight-bearing exercises (infraspinatus)
	Subscapularis	Medial rotation Scaption elevation

>continued

TABLE 21.2 *>continued*

Shoulder complex segment	Muscle	Exercises for optimal strength results
Humerus: large movers	Anterior deltoid	Scaption elevation
		Military press
		Shoulder abduction
	Middle deltoid	Scaption elevation
		Seated rowing
		Shoulder abduction
		Military press
	Posterior deltoid	Seated rowing
		Horizontal abduction
		Shoulder extension
	Pectoralis major	Press-up
		Push-up
	Latissimus dorsi	Press-up

Based on data from several investigations: [96,100,113,115-131]

Stabilization, Proprioception, and Neuromotor Exercises

The importance of stability during shoulder motion cannot be overstated. As previously discussed, trunk, or core, stabilization must provide a firm base from which the scapula operates. Likewise, the scapula must provide a firm foundation for shoulder movement.[132] Rotator cuff stabilization enables the humerus to undergo smooth, synchronous glenohumeral motion for functional upper-extremity activity.[133]

Trunk stabilization exercises are discussed in chapter 17. A few will be mentioned later in this chapter, but only as they relate to shoulder exercises. Refer to chapter 17 for specific trunk stabilization exercises.

Beyond strengthening the shoulder, stabilization exercises help in performance recovery. They also facilitate proprioception and neuromuscular reeducation of the shoulder; they stimulate the afferent receptors to provide appropriate feedback into the central nervous system, reeducate and reactivate the proprioceptive pathways, and promote correct muscle firing sequence patterns that will eventually lead to proper functional performance.[134-136]

Although some of these exercises are open kinetic chain activities, many are closed kinetic chain activities. One can argue that because most people involved in physical activity do not perform upper-extremity closed kinetic chain activities, the use of closed kinetic chain exercises for the upper extremities is not useful in a rehabilitation program. However, closed kinetic chain exercises are useful for the upper extremity for a couple of reasons. In a closed-chain position, the shoulder has more stability because of increased joint congruity; less stress is applied to the ligaments, and joint proprioceptors are stimulated.[93] Closed kinetic chain exercise also facilitates the co-contraction of muscles around the joint.[137] This co-contraction during closed kinetic chain exercises permits stabilization activities to begin with less shear force applied to the static structures, and it also promotes dynamic joint stability.[138]

Not every exercise must mimic functional motions. In fact, in the early and middle stages of rehabilitation, it is important to improve muscle strength in single-plane motions before functional movements in multiplanar dimensions are begun. Neither straight-plane exercises nor pure closed kinetic chain exercises are necessarily functional since most of them do not mimic the shoulder's functional movements. They are crucial in a rehabilitation program, though, in that they facilitate, develop, and improve specific muscle activity that permits eventual progression to functional shoulder movement.[103, 139]

Scapular Stabilization

Because scapular stability is vital to functional shoulder motions, scapular stabilization exercises should begin early in the rehabilitation program. Depending on the exercise, the injury, and motion and activity restrictions, these exercises may start anywhere from the early active phase to the early resistive phase.[140] A variety of scapular stabilization exercises are described in the following sections.

The progression begins with isometric stabilization exercises and advances to stabilization activities during arm movement, first in simple planes and then in diagonal planes. The progression also begins with movements in the lower shoulder positions (30° to 60° elevation), where the scapula has relatively little motion and its muscles work mainly to position, or set, the scapula in preparation for glenohumeral motion.[141] The progression advances to middle-range positions of shoulder elevation (60° to 120°), where the scapular muscles must stabilize and rotate the scapula simultaneously.[121] Rehabilitation exercises at higher shoulder elevations are begun only after strength and neuromotor control in the lower ranges are achieved; as previously mentioned, it is in the higher ranges of motion that the scapular muscles are most stressed. This stress increases because these muscles must continue to provide glenohumeral stability while also moving the scapula in its final degrees of motion where the muscles are at their shortest and weakest positions.[121] In the final stabilization exercises, movements include a combination of high and low joint positions, increased resistance, and greater speed. These activities then advance to be more functionally based.

CLINICAL TIPS

The progression of shoulder resistance exercises should begin with the scapula in its "set" position and stay within the first 30° to 60° of glenohumeral elevation. In this range of motion, scapular muscles work mainly to stabilize the scapula in preparation for glenohumeral motion. This is the first level of resistance for these muscles. As the scapular muscles and rotator cuff muscles become stronger and can perform their respective tasks of scapular and glenohumeral stabilization, exercises progress to mid-shoulder elevation ranges of motion, 60° to 120°. At this level, the scapular muscles rotate the scapula to continue to give the rotator cuff an advantageous moment arm length, and they also continue to stabilize the scapula. Exercises in the highest elevation of shoulder motion, above 120°, do not occur until the scapular stabilizers have achieved enough strength and control in the mid-ranges of motion to withstand the stresses that will be placed on them at the highest glenohumeral positions, where the scapular muscles are at their shortest and weakest.

Scapular Stabilization, Proprioception, and Neuromotor Exercises

Every body segment must function upon a firm foundation. The shoulder is no exception. The glenohumeral joint relies on a stable scapula to provide the base from which it performs. Some of the scapular stabilization exercises are presented here.

Swiss Ball Stabilization

Body Segment: Scapula.

Stage in Rehab: Early resistive phase.

Purpose: Basic exercise to improve scapular stability early in rehab.

Positioning: The Swiss ball is placed on a table or on the floor.

Execution: Patient bears weight through the shoulder as the ball is moved from side to side, forward and backward, and in circles. If the patient does not have 90° of shoulder motion, the patient can begin in lower degrees of motion and moving it within the available shoulder motion. The patient bears weight on the upper extremity and rolls the ball in varying patterns.

Possible Substitutions: Using the trunk or hips to move the ball rather than the shoulder.

Cues and Notations: The patient should move his or her body from forward to back and from side to side on the ball while weight bearing through the upper extremities (figure 21.68a).

A more advanced weight-bearing exercise with the Swiss ball has the patient's lower body on a table

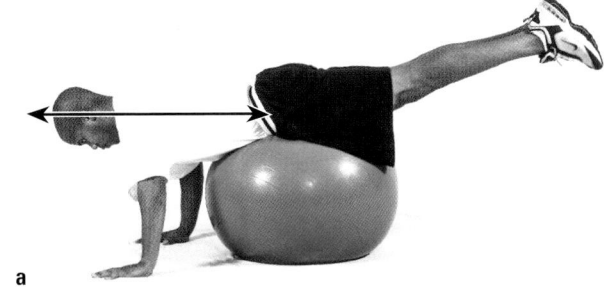
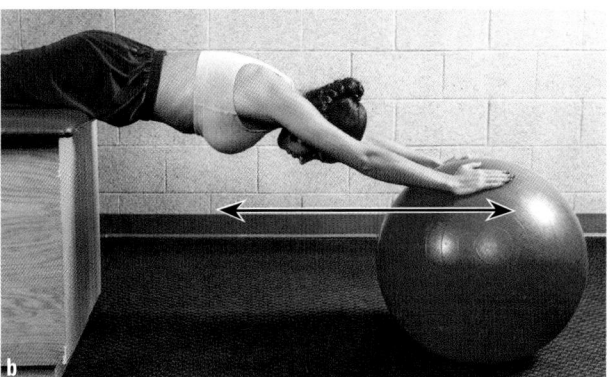

Figure 21.68

and the hands placed on the ball while the upper body is over the edge of the table. The patient moves the ball out and away from the body as far as possible, then moves the ball closer (figure 21.68b).

Rhythmic Stabilization 1

Body Segment: Scapula.

Stage in Rehab: Early resistive phase.

Purpose: Reeducate the proprioceptors and improve neuromotor function.

Positioning: Patient is supine with the arm in a scapular plane and elevated to 90° to 100°.

Execution: The patient holds a weight in the hand with the shoulder in a specific position, maintaining the angle with the eyes closed (figure 21.69a, open kinetic chain). As an alternative, the clinician can offer manual resistance in different directions while the patient provides an isometric resistance to the movements.

Possible Substitutions: Flexing the elbow, lowering the shoulder to below the start position.

Cues and Notations: The exercise can be repeated with the arm placed in different positions, each time requiring the patient to maintain the designated position of the shoulder with the eyes closed. Figures 21.69b through h demonstrate progressive variations of closed kinetic chain positions in which this exercise may be performed: (b) weight bearing in standing, (c) quadruped weight bearing, (d) tripod weight bearing, (e) bipod weight bearing, (f) with a resistance band providing resistance to the uninvolved extremity, (g) with proprioceptive neuromuscular facilitation manual resistance to the uninvolved extremity, (h) unilateral weight bearing. Each progressive exercise is described next.

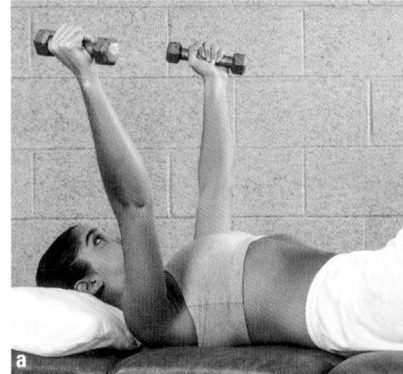
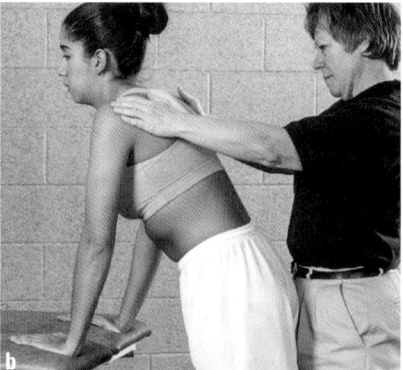
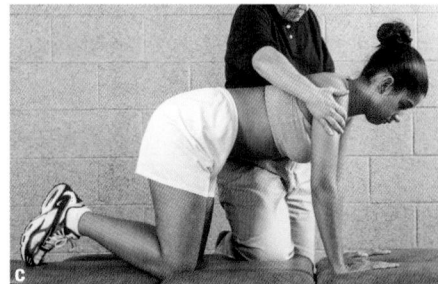
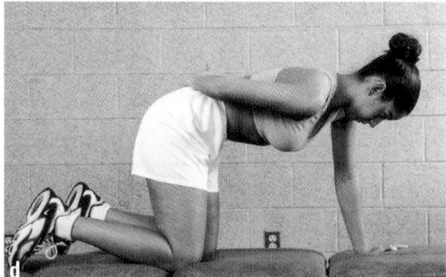
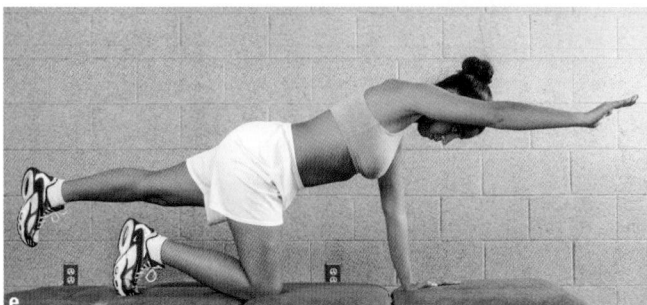
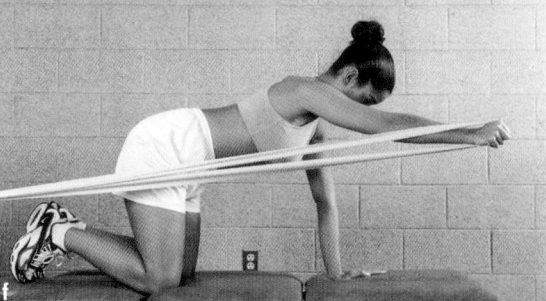

Figure 21.69

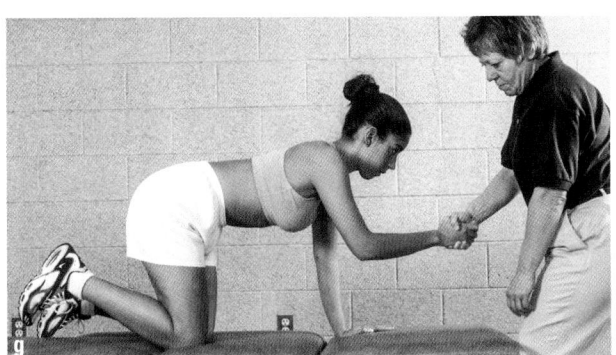 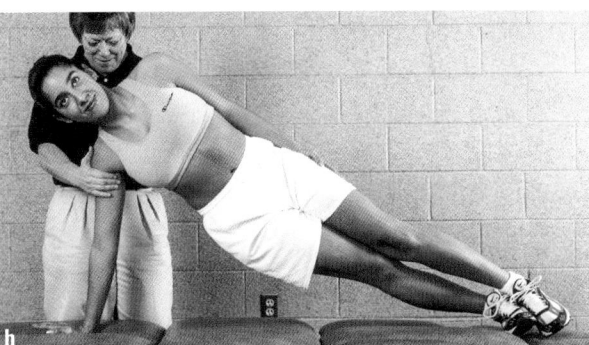

Figure 21.69 *>continued*

 Go to HK*Propel* and watch video 21.4, which demonstrates a closed kinetic chain shoulder stabilization exercise in tripod and bipod positions.

Rhythmic Stabilization 2

Body Segment: Scapula.

Stage in Rehab: Early resistive phase.

Purpose: Reeducate the proprioceptors and improve neuromotor function.

Positioning: Patient stands on the floor, bearing body weight on the arms on a tabletop.

Execution: The clinician provides resistance to the patient as the patient shifts weight from one arm to the other, trying to move the patient off balance (figure 21.69*b*).

Possible Substitutions: Using the legs more than the arms to provide stability.

Cues and Notations: Progression can advance to using only the involved upper extremity on the table.

Rhythmic Stabilization in Quadruped 3

Body Segment: Scapula.

Stage in Rehab: Resistive phase.

Purpose: Reeducate the proprioceptors and improve neuromotor function.

Positioning: In a quadruped position, the shoulders are directly over the hands, and the hips are slightly forward of the knees so the weight is primarily on the upper extremities.

Execution: The simplest exercise is to have the patient shift weight from the left to the right arm. As the patient tries to stabilize in the quadruped position, the clinician offers manual resistance, trying to move the patient off balance (figure 21.69*c*). Once the patient can stabilize, he or she balances in a tripod position with the uninvolved arm off the table (figure 21.69*d*). From this exercise the patient can advance to a bipod position, with the involved arm and the opposite leg bearing the weight (figure 21.69*e*).

Possible Substitutions: Using the legs more than the arms to stabilize the trunk, moving the hips and shoulders posteriorly, flexing the elbows.

Cues and Notations: If the patient cannot hold this position, the hips may be positioned directly over the knees to equalize weight distribution between the upper and lower extremities. The patient must be able to bear weight on the shoulder and accept posterior capsule stress to perform this exercise.

For an additional challenge, you can provide a push–pull resistance to the uninvolved arm using a pulley, resistance band, or manual resistance at various angles while the involved arm maintains balance (figure 21.69*f-g*).

Rhythmic Stabilization 4

Body Segment: Scapula.

Stage in Rehab: Resistive phase.

Purpose: Reeducate the proprioceptors and improve neuromotor function.

Positioning: Patient is in a side-lying position. The involved upper extremity and its ipsilateral lower extremity are on the floor with the patient's lower extremities in full extension and stacked one on top of the other. The patient then lifts the body upward into a side-bridge position so the body's weight is on the involved upper extremity's hand and the ipsilateral foot (figure 21.69*h*).

Execution: The clinician provides manual resistance at the shoulder as the patient tries to maintain balance.

Possible Substitutions: Flexing or rotating the trunk, placing the knees on the floor, flexing the hips or knees.

Cues and Notations: This is a difficult exercise that may not be indicated for all patients.

Stabilizing Distal Movement These activities involve movement of the distal upper extremity, requiring shoulder neuromotor control, strength, and stability. You must have the patient maintain correct scapular position throughout each of these exercises. Verbal cueing may be needed as a reminder to maintain proper scapular positioning. In one activity, the patient lies prone with a roller stool under the hips or pelvis; feet are off the floor and hands are on the floor. The patient then moves across the floor, using only the arms to move the roller stool (figure 21.70*a*).

Another distal movement activity is performed with a weighted ball in the hand. The patient stands or sits with the arm outstretched at from 60° to 110° elevation in the scapular plane. In this position, the patient spells out the alphabet with the ball (figure 21.70*b*). Heavier balls provide additional resistance. The clinician should observe for

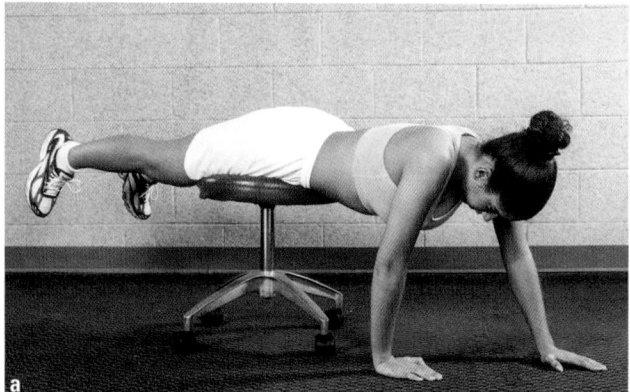
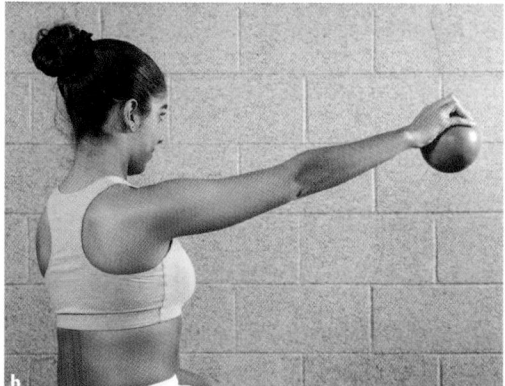
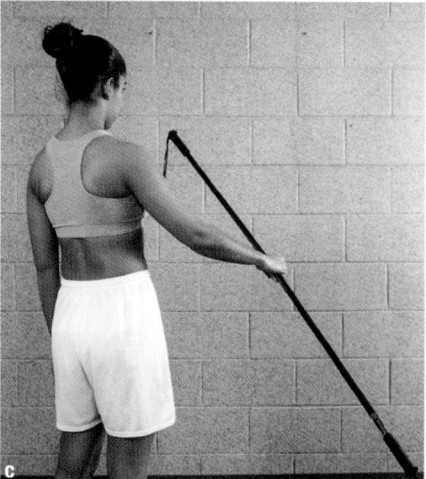

Figure 21.70   Distal movement stabilization exercises: *(a)* walk on hands while prone on roller stool, *(b)* alphabet with distal weight, *(c)* rhythmic wand.

scapular control during arm motions and provide verbal or tactile cues as needed for the correct exercise execution.

The Bodyblade (Hymanson, Inc., Los Angeles, CA), B.O.I.N.G. (Body Oscillation Integrates Neuromuscular Gain) (exclusively distributed by OPTP, Minneapolis, MN), and other commercially available rhythmic-wand equipment are useful in rhythmic stabilization exercises.[142, 143] They can be used in different positions, beginning in the scapular plane at 30° elevation (figure 21.70c) and advancing to overhead and diagonal positions as strength improves.

Upper-body ergometers or using the upper extremities on stepper machines or treadmills are other ways to offer distal movement and proximal stabilization. These machines also provide cardiovascular exercise.

Proprioceptive Neuromuscular Facilitation Proprioceptive neuromuscular facilitation (PNF) is useful in shoulder rehabilitation. The advantages to using PNF were discussed in chapter 11. There is no cost because this form of exercise uses the clinician's manual resistance; PNF is appropriate throughout most of the program. In the early rehabilitation stages, PNF can enhance proprioception and neuromuscular control, and at later stages it can improve strength and coordination of muscle firing.[144] Techniques include isometrics, concentrics, eccentrics, and rhythmic stabilization.[145] PNF incorporates functional positions because it uses multiplane motions.

In the early rehabilitation stages, PNF is commonly used for rhythmic stabilization (figure 21.71). This helps in the reeducation of synchronous muscle firing and helps provide joint stability.[145] Moving through functional patterns can stimulate neuromuscular control for stability and synchronous patterns of movement.[146, 147] The rehabilitation clinician provides isometric resistance at points in the range of motion that are weak.[145]

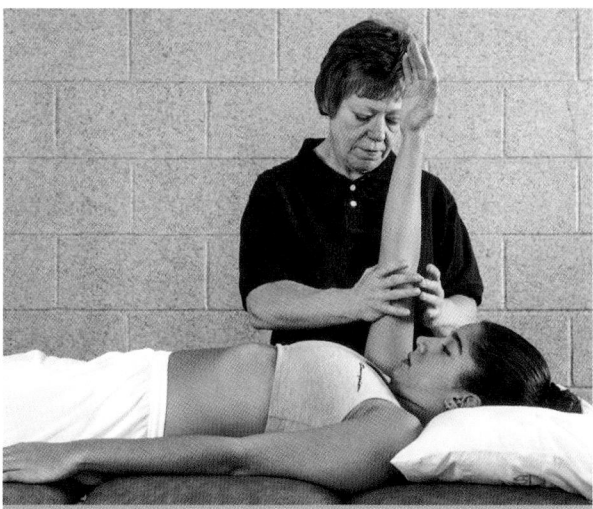

Figure 21.71 Proprioceptive neuromuscular facilitation: rhythmic stabilization.

In later rehabilitation stages, PNF can increase coordination by the use of eccentric resistance in functional planes and by combining eccentric with concentric and isometric resistance as the arm moves through its motion patterns. In this activity, the patient tries to move the arm through either a D1 or D2 flexion–extension pattern at a constant rate of speed as the rehabilitation clinician provides various types of resistance—eccentric, concentric, and isometric.

Advanced Open-Chain Exercises

These exercises can incorporate various types of equipment. They are performed unsupported, first in straight-plane and then in diagonal motions. The unsupported motion is the primary distinction between these and earlier exercises. The unsupported motions require more effort for control and stability from both scapular and glenohumeral muscles.

Open-Chain Elastic-Band Exercises Elastic-band or rubber-tubing activities in an OKC provide another type of resistive exercise to challenge the patient. The challenge is to maintain stability during resisted shoulder movement. This is the next step after CKC stabilization exercises. The patient must now perform resistive exercises without the feedback of the clinician as in PNF and without the feedback of joint compression that closed kinetic chain activities provide. These exercises include a combination of concentric and eccentric resistance. The need for dynamic stabilization during these exercises more closely resembles functional activity demands, and these exercises prepare the shoulder for the next level of resistive exercises, plyometrics.

Straight-Plane Exercises By the second half of the resistive phase, the patient should be able to maintain joint stability with the arm in 60° or more of elevation. Straight-plane exercises include medial and lateral rotation with the elbow at shoulder level and the shoulder in the scapular plane. As control is achieved, the shoulder is elevated to higher levels (figure 21.72). You must correct errors in execution. Common errors include dropping the elbow, horizontally abducting the shoulder during lateral rotation and horizontally adducting it during medial rotation, and extending the elbow during lateral rotation and flexing it during medial rotation. It is important to maintain scapular control while performing these exercises.

Diagonal-Plane Exercises These exercises are performed once the patient demonstrates proper stabilization and adequate strength in straight-plane exercises. PNF movements in D1 and D2 flexion and extension patterns are used (figure 21.73). It is important for the patient to execute the motion correctly and to maintain appropriate joint stability throughout these motions. Joint stability is not maintained if the patient shrugs the shoulder during

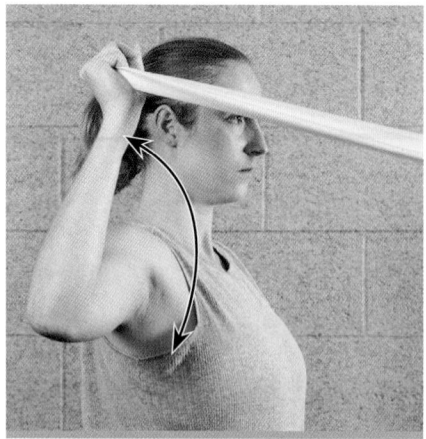

Figure 21.72 Open kinetic chain straight-plane lateral rotation using elastic-band exercises.

activity or initiates the activity with a shoulder shrug. In these cases, verbal cues to "keep the shoulder blade pulled down into your back pocket" or tactile cues such as tapping or stroking the skin over the lower trapezius will help patients to correct their execution.

Plyometric Exercises

Once patients gain adequate strength and achieve static and simple dynamic stabilization control, they progress to plyometric exercises before performing functional activities. Plyometrics are the most demanding exercises thus far introduced into the rehabilitation program because they require maximum strength and optimal joint stabilization, agility, and coordination during high-level dynamic activities. The following sections provide some examples of plyometric exercises for the shoulder girdle.

Medicine-ball exercises begin with a lightweight ball—approximately 0.9 kg (2 lb)—and progress as the patient can control higher weights and still perform the exercise correctly.

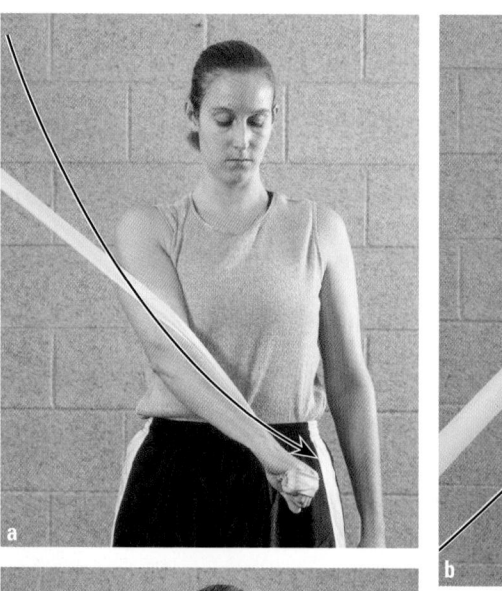
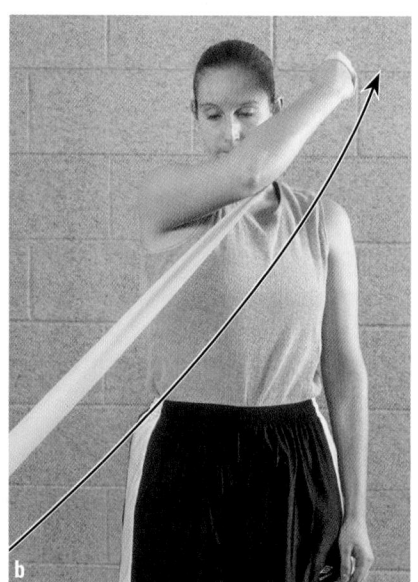
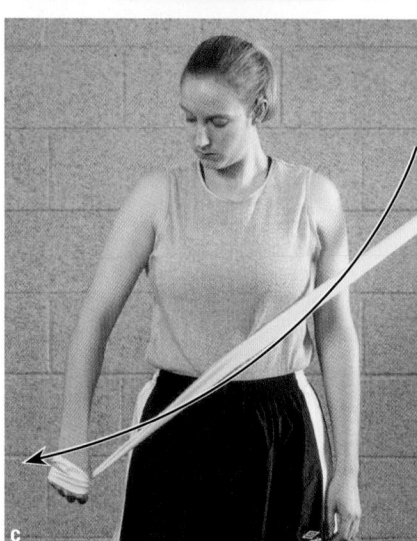
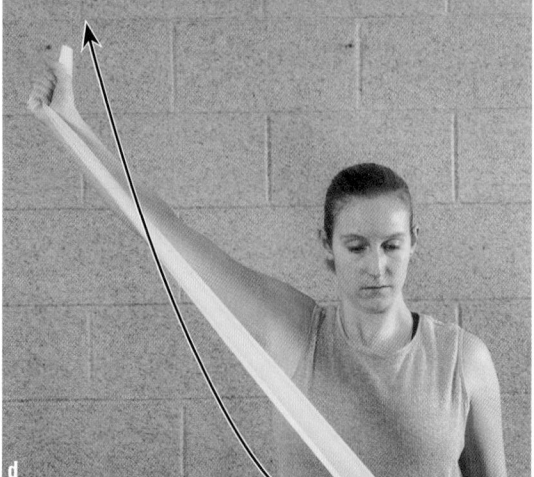

Figure 21.73 Diagonal-plane exercises using rubber-band resistance: *(a)* D2 extension, *(b)* D1 flexion, *(c)* D1 extension, *(d)* D2 flexion.

Plyometric Exercises for the Shoulder Girdle

Not all patients will have plyometric exercises included in their rehabilitation programs. Clinicians decide what to include based on such patient factors as age, weight, competitive level, and the demands of returning to optimal function.

Dynamic Stabilization on Unstable Surfaces

Body Segment: Upper extremity.

Stage in Rehab: Advanced phase.

Purpose: Challenge muscles to provide shoulder stability during motion.

Positioning: A slide board, Fitter, Swiss ball, or other apparatus may be used to challenge balance.

Execution: Patient places the hands on the surface of the slide board, Fitter, Swiss ball, or other apparatus and tries to maintain balance while moving the arms (figure 21.74a through c). Depending on the apparatus used, shoulder motions may include lateral, up-and-down, or circular motions.

Possible Substitutions: Using the trunk to move the shoulders or the hips to control the motion.

Cues and Notations: One progression includes having the patient move from weight bearing on the knees to weight bearing on the feet, and a more difficult progression consists of making both the hand surface and the lower-extremity surface unstable. Instructing the patient to incorporate the core and pull the scapula into the back pocket may improve performance.

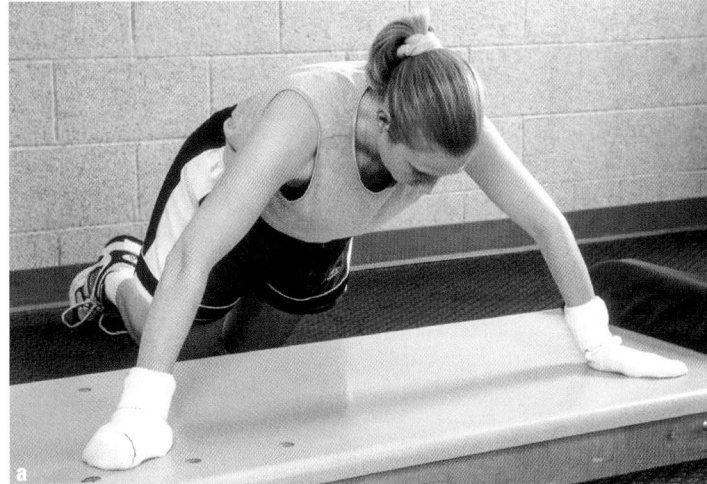

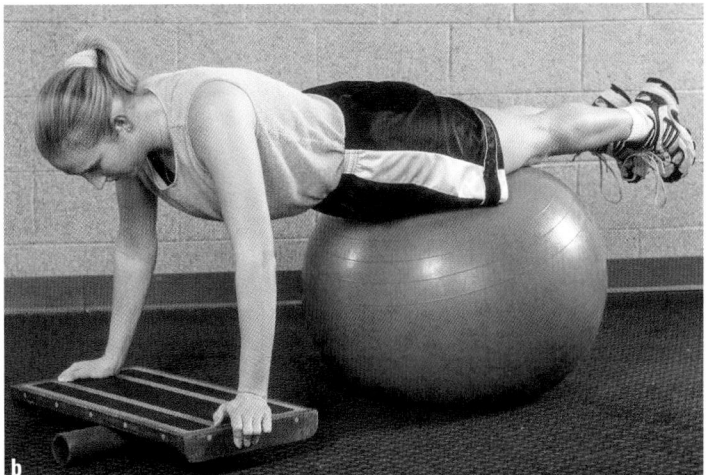

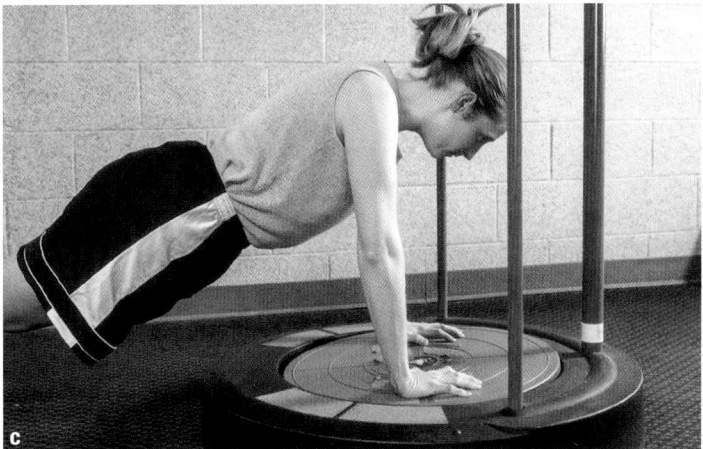

Figure 21.74

Plyometric Push-Ups

Body Segment: Upper extremity.

Stage in Rehab: End of resistive phase through advanced phase.

Purpose: Prepare muscles for functional activity with sudden eccentric–concentric exercises while maintaining shoulder control.

Positioning: The progression of plyometric push-ups begins with a wall push-up. This aspect of the exercise begins in the resistive phase. The patient stands farther than an arm's length from the wall and places the hands at shoulder level on the wall. Elbows start in a flexed position but are anterior to the shoulders, and scapulae are retracted.

Execution: The patient pushes away from the wall with enough force to remove the hands from the wall. When the patient's hands come off the wall, the rehabilitation clinician pushes the patient back toward the wall, and the patient stops the movement toward the wall by "catching" him- or herself with both hands on the wall. The impact force is absorbed by eccentric control of triceps and scapular protractors as the elbows flex and the scapulae retract, returning the body to the starting position. This exercise progresses to an incline push-up. The patient pushes off the incline support, such as a tabletop or counter, to lose hand contact and is pushed back to the start position by the clinician, similar to the wall push-ups.

An additional progression in the advanced phase involves having the patient perform a regular or modified push-up, first with the uninvolved hand on a medicine ball and the involved hand on the floor, then with both hands on the ball (figure 21.75a and b).

Possible Substitutions: Flexing at the trunk, not flexing the elbows to absorb the force, using the back and legs to move away from the wall, not standing far enough from the wall to perform a good plyometric exercise.

Cues and Notations: Plyometric push-ups can also be performed on a trampoline. With the patient in a regular push-up position and the hands on the trampoline, the patient "jumps" the hands off the trampoline and lands them laterally toward the trampoline rim, then "jumps" them back to the center on the next push-up movement; this exercise looks like a jumping jack for the upper extremities. The most difficult plyometric push-up is performed with boxes (figure 21.75c). Two boxes of the same height are placed on either side of the patient. The recommended starting height is 10 to 15 cm (4-6 in.). The patient begins with the hands on the floor in either a modified or a regular push-up position and pushes up and away from the floor to jump each hand onto the adjacent box. Progressions include having the patient move his or her lower-extremity support from the knees to the feet and making both the hand surface and the lower-extremity surface unstable.

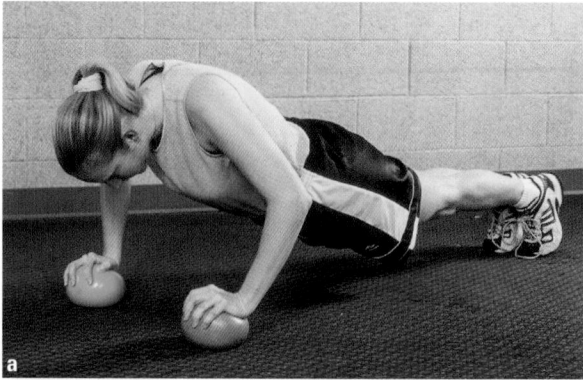

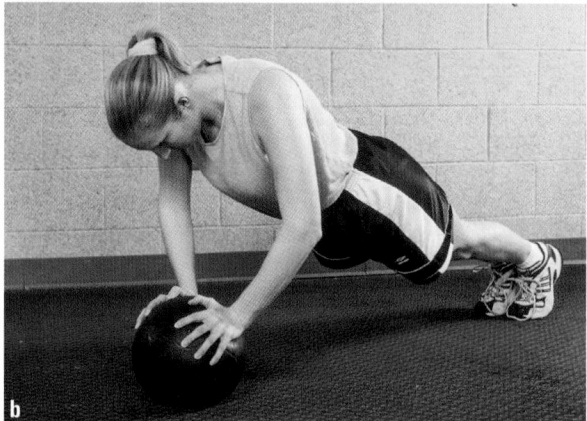

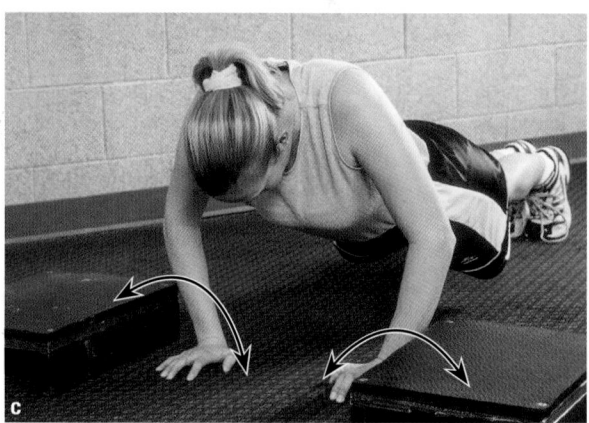

Figure 21.75

Resisted Movements in Weight Bearing

Body Segment: Upper extremity.

Stage in Rehab: Advanced phase.

Purpose: Facilitate neuromotor control and muscle endurance.

Positioning: The patient kneels on the floor at the end of the treadmill with hands on the treadmill's belt.

Execution: The patient "walks" the hands as the treadmill belt or stair machine steps move (figure 21.76*a* and *b*).

Possible Substitutions: Shoulder shrugging or trunk rotation to move the arms.

Cues and Notations: A stair machine, treadmill, or step machine may be used. The speed of the machine depends on the patient's abilities. It is recommended that a manual setting at no more than 2 mph be used initially, but a random setting may be appropriate as the patient progresses. Bouts of 30 s to 1 min provide ample challenge at first. As the patient improves, speed, time, and resistance may be increased. The patient may also move from a modified push-up position to a regular push-up position. Wearing gloves during the exercise will protect the patient's hands.

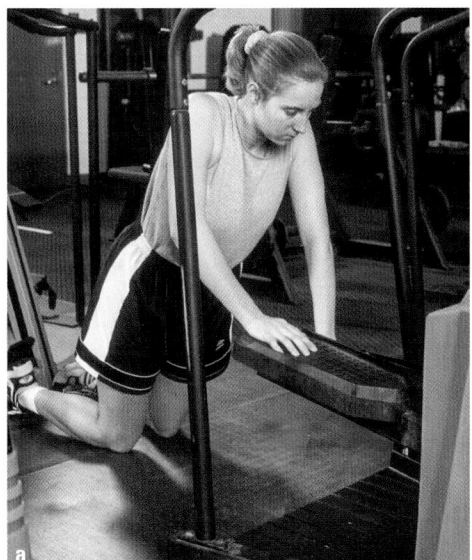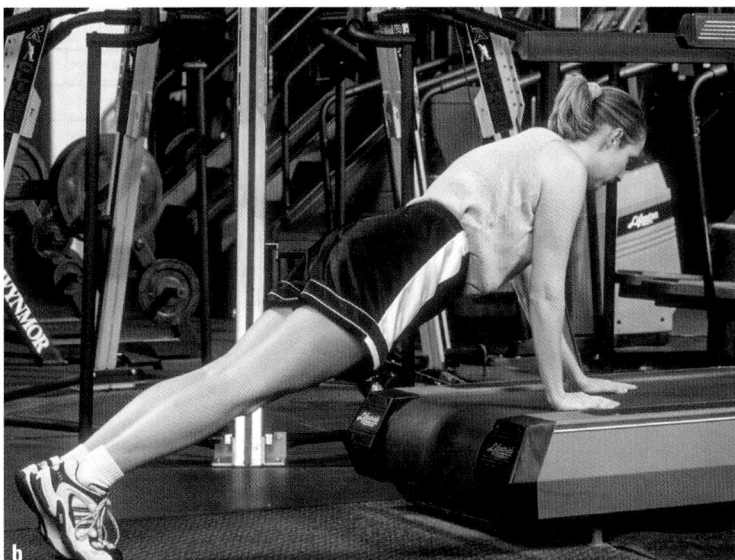

Figure 21.76

Medicine-Ball Rotation Progression

Body Segment: Upper extremity.

Stage in Rehab: Advanced phase.

Purpose: Progress eccentric and concentric activity of medial rotators and scapular stabilizers from a supported to an unsupported position.

Positioning:

1. The patient is supine on a table with the shoulder at 90° abduction and laterally rotated; the entire extremity is supported by the table. The forearm support prevents excessive lateral rotation during the initial phases of this exercise.

2. The patient is in the same position as described for 1.

3. The patient is in the same position as in 2 but moves to the side of the table so the upper extremity is unsupported by the table during the catching-tossing maneuver; the table does not limit lateral rotation motion, so the patient must use greater eccentric control of the medial rotators while catching and greater concentric effort during tossing.

>continued

Medicine-Ball Rotation Progression >*continued*

4. The patient sits on a Swiss ball or stands or kneels on the floor. The patient must maintain an elevated elbow at 90° of shoulder abduction and elbow flexion.

Execution: Each number here corresponds to a number identifying the patient's position for the exercise.

1. The medicine ball is dropped from the level of the rehabilitation clinician's shoulder to the patient's hand. Initially the patient only catches the ball, but he or she should quickly advance to catching and tossing the ball back to the clinician (figure 21.77*a*).

2. The clinician stands away from the patient near the patient's feet and tosses the ball to the patient. The patient catches the ball and returns the toss, keeping the shoulder at 90° abduction and allowing the shoulder to laterally rotate as the ball is caught. The shoulder moves into medial rotation when the ball is thrown back to the rehabilitation clinician (figure 21.77*b*).

3. Tosses continue without support to the upper extremity. Motion is a smooth transition from eccentric external rotation as the ball is caught to concentric external rotation when the ball is tossed back to the clinician without pausing or stopping between catching and tossing.

Possible Substitutions: Flexing the elbow, dropping the elbow, moving the shoulder in front of the body.

Cues and Notations:

1. When the person can perform this exercise for the desired number of sets and repetitions, the next level of exercise begins.

2. Good control and a smooth transition without pausing from lateral to medial rotation are important.

3. The patient must maintain an elevated elbow at 90° of shoulder abduction and elbow flexion throughout each exercise progression. Dropping the elbow is an indication of fatigue in the scapular or glenohumeral muscles; verbal cues may correct the position unless the patient's muscles are too fatigued to continue with proper execution.

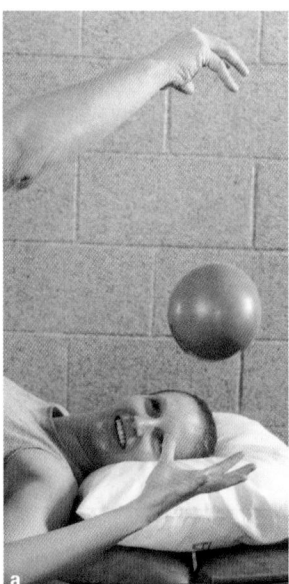
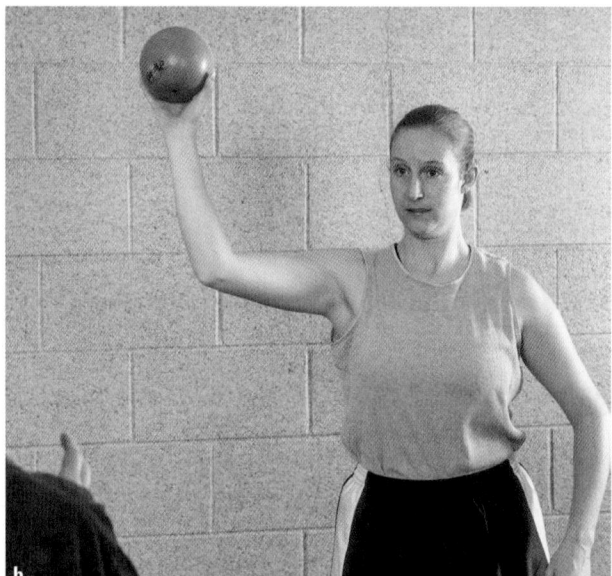

Figure 21.77

Medicine-Ball Rotation

Body Segment: Upper extremity.

Stage in Rehab: Advanced phase.

Purpose: Eccentric–concentric activity for the shoulder lateral rotators.

Positioning: The patient sits on a Swiss ball or stands or kneels on the floor with his or her back to the clinician. The patient must maintain an elevated elbow at 90° of shoulder abduction and elbow flexion. The patient rotates the neck to look over the shoulder for the ball's approach.

Execution: The clinician tosses the medicine ball to the patient; the patient catches the ball with the shoulder in some lateral rotation, and then allows the weight of the ball to pull the shoulder into medial rotation before throwing the ball back to the clinician (figure 21.78). The patient then tosses the ball back to the clinician using a concentric contraction of the lateral rotators while keeping the elbow elevated.

Possible Substitutions: Dropping the shoulder, twisting the body too much, using too much elbow flexion.

Cues and Notations: Increasing the distance and repetitions increases the difficulty of the exercise. The patient must maintain an elevated elbow with the shoulder at 90° of abduction. Dropping the elbow is an indication of muscle fatigue in the scapular or glenohumeral muscles.

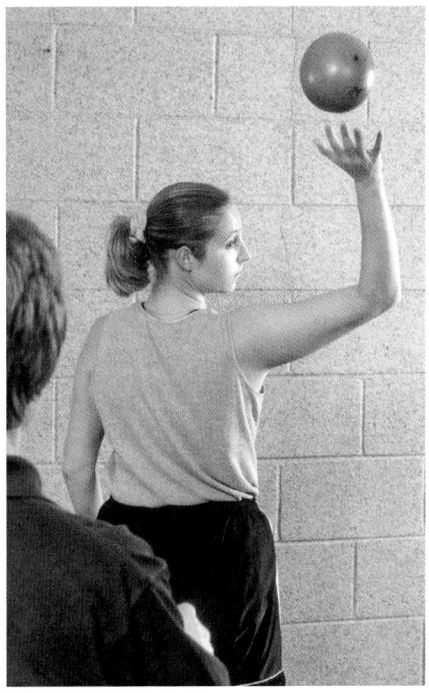

Figure 21.78

Rotational Tosses

Body Segment: Upper extremity and trunk.

Stage in Rehab: Advanced phase.

Purpose: Neuromotor control of the trunk and shoulder.

Positioning: Patient stands away from the wall with the back to the wall. The arms are held at a low level initially (figure 21.79a), then raised as shoulder strength and control improve.

Execution: Standing far enough from the wall, the patient tosses the ball to the wall as trunk rotation occurs. He or she catches the ball and winds the trunk away from the wall, then repeats the toss.

Possible Substitutions: Stopping between trunk rotation and ball toss to create two separate motions rather than one.

Cues and Notations: As strength improves, the arms are raised higher (figure 21.79b). Overhead toss exercises can be performed while standing or kneeling.

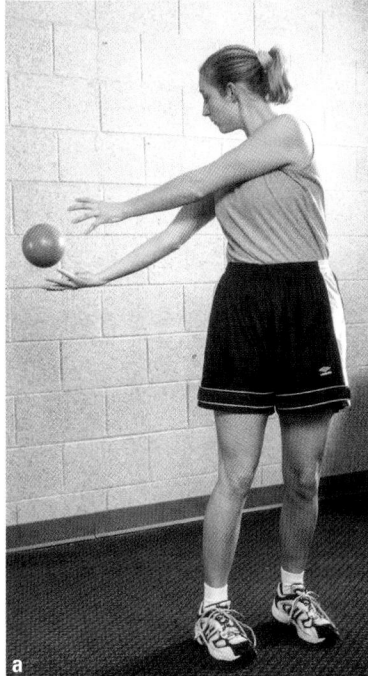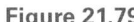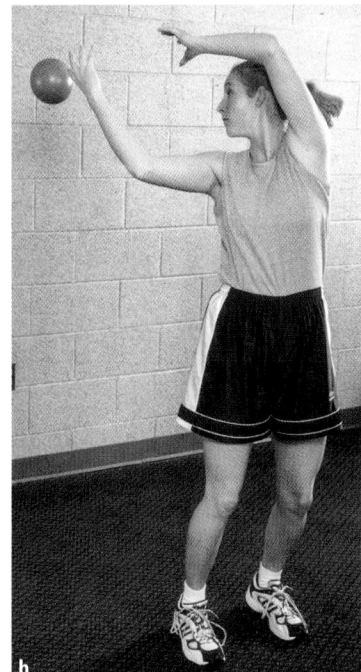

Figure 21.79

Overhead Tosses

Body Segment: Upper extremity and trunk.

Stage in Rehab: Advanced phase.

Purpose: Enhance trunk and shoulder neuromotor control and strength.

Positioning: Patient is supine on the floor with the knees and hips flexed. The hands are overhead.

Execution: The patient tosses the ball to the clinician and moves into a partial sit-up position as the ball is released. The patient stays in the partial sit-up position until the clinician tosses the ball back, aiming overhead so that the patient must reach overhead to catch the ball. The patient simultaneously catches the ball and returns to the start position in one smooth motion (figure 21.80).

Possible Substitutions: Using the legs to curl up rather than the abdominal muscles; the trunk and shoulders move as two separate entities rather than together in one smooth motion.

Cues and Notations: Verbal cues to engage the core before tossing or catching the ball may be needed if the patient arches the back or loses trunk control during the activity. Trunk rotation can also be incorporated by having two people, one on either side of the patient (about 30° to 45° to the side), catch the ball. The patient tosses to one and receives the ball, then tosses to the other.

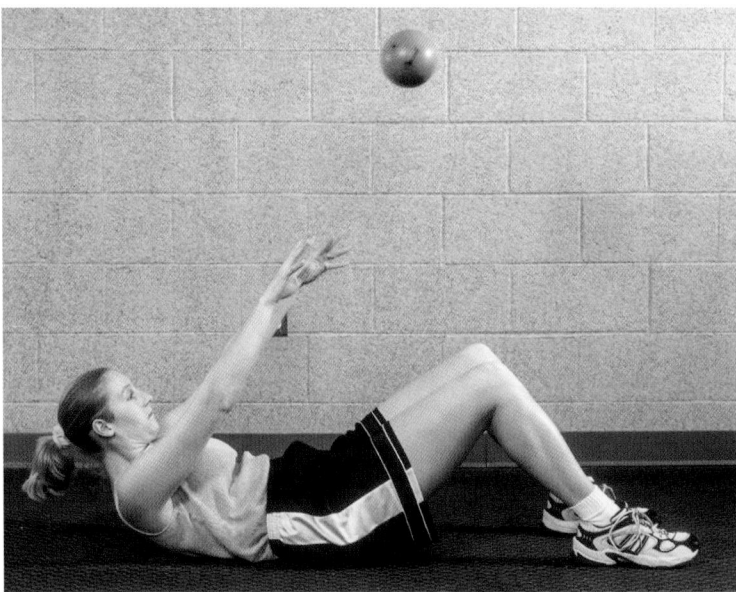

Figure 21.80

Functional and Performance-Specific Exercises

By the time functional activities are the emphasis of a rehabilitation program, the exercises are dictated by the demands of the patient's normal activity. Regardless of the sport or activity to which patients will return, the progressions all build on gains made by patients as they move through this final rehabilitation phase. As with the other phases, goals are set for each segment within this phase, and the patient moves from one segment to the next only after those goals are achieved.

The functional and performance-specific activities can be divided into five segments, each building upon the previous segment: (1) linear and balanced activities, (2) multiplanar activities, (3) simple specific drills, (4) complex specific drills, and (5) simulated activities.[148] Table 21.3 identifies the provisions of each of these steps.

If a patient participates in a throwing sport, during the plyometric exercise phase he or she can begin throwing a foam rubber ball or knotted sock toward a mirror, watching for form and motion patterns (figure 21.81). A tennis player can begin forehand and backhand strokes in the same manner in front of a mirror. This helps to improve proprioception and appropriate neuromotor activation through the additional afferent feedback that comes from the visual system.[149]

TABLE 21.3   **Functional and Performance-Specific Segments in the Final Rehabilitation Phase for the Shoulder**

Sequential segments	Activities included in each
1. Linear and balanced activities	Activities demonstrate balanced performance between L and R extremities. Bilateral upper extremity activities are accurate and unimpaired. Acceleration and deceleration activities, balance, endurance are functional.
2. Multiplanar activities	Underhand and overhand tossing and throwing, lobbing, target hitting, and fast throwing for technique.
3. Simple specific drills	Early sport- or work-specific drills and basic skills are used and performed with accuracy and endurance. These skills begin at a basic level and become more complex as the goals for each skill are met.
4. Complex specific drills	Compound and complex skills are executed with precision and proper speed as would normally be expected during performance. Speed, accuracy, endurance, intensity, and overall demands increase to adjust to the patient's performance.
5. Simulated activities	Activities simulate the patient's demands during normal sport or work performance with realistic demands in all aspects of performance.

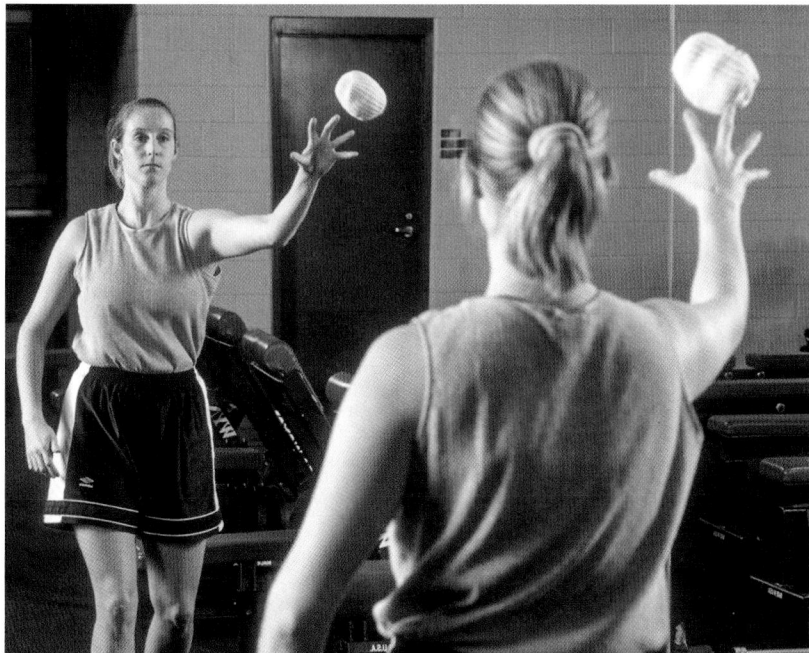

Figure 21.81   Mirror feedback is helpful in regaining control and accuracy.

Chapter 15 covers progressive functional and performance-specific programs, outlining sequences of exercises as a guide to preparing patients to return to full activity. The point to remember is that the performance-specific activities should demand skills that match the patient's abilities. Skill demands begin at an easy level, then progress to higher levels, then progress to combinations of skills until the patient executes all the skills smoothly and at a level of performance comparable to preinjury levels.

One activity element is increased at a time to allow the body to adjust to new stresses. For example, if a pitcher increases throwing speed from 50% to 75% of normal speed, the distance of throws and the number of repetitions remain unchanged for the session. An increase in the program is usually added only every third day of activity, so after the third day of increased speed, the pitcher's throwing distance can increase. This gives the body the time it needs to adapt to new levels of stress before moving up to additional levels. So if a golfer performs a full swing with the long irons in today's treatment session, it will be three sessions before he or she advances to using the woods.

In overhead events, the patient progresses through a program of low- and medium-height movements and tries high movements last. For example, a tennis player begins tennis activities with forehand and backhand ground strokes. Only when the player can perform full-distance and full-force hits with these strokes does he or she progress to overhead strokes. Because serves are the most strenuous overhead activity, they are the last stroke the patient resumes. Partial force is used in the initial stages of serve activities, with progression to normal serves.

Special Rehabilitation Applications

As with any other body segment, before a rehabilitation program can be developed, the clinician must first perform an examination to identify the patient's problems and develop goals based on those problems. The rehabilitation program is then developed from these goals and identified problems. Special tests are used during this examination as part of the process to ascertain a clinical diagnosis. Some of the more commonly used special tests for the shoulder, along with their sensitivity and specificity, are provided in table 21.4. This list of special tests is by no means an exhaustive one. Not all of the tests listed have high sensitivity or high specificity, but some lower-scoring tests are included to show how they compare with other tests with higher sensitivity and specificity. Some tests are not listed in table 21.4 because they are low in both sensitivity and specificity.

The combination and progression of exercises used in each rehabilitation program are based on the needs of the patient and the injury. Some injuries raise special concerns. Some of these injuries and the concerns unique to them are addressed here.

TABLE 21.4 Special Tests Commonly Used in a Shoulder Examination

Site or structure tested	Condition tested	Special test (other name)	Sensitivity	Specificity
Glenohumeral joint	Anterior instability	Anterior apprehension test	66%[150] 53%[151]	95%[150] 99%[151]
		Relocation test (Jobe's relocation test; Fowler's sign)	65%[150] 57%[152] 44%[153]	90%[150] 100%[152] 87%[153]
		Surprise test (anterior release test)	82%[150] 92%[152]	86%[150] 89%[152]
		Anterior load and shift	50%[152]	100%[152]
	Posterior instability	Posterior load and shift	14%[152]	100%[152]
		Posterior drawer	Unknown	Unknown
		Posterior apprehension test	Unknown	Unknown
		Jerk test	90%[154]	85%[154]
		Jerk test with Kim test	97%[154]	Unknown
	Inferior instability	Sulcus sign, >1 cm	72%[152]	85%[152]
		Sulcus sign, >2 cm	28%[152]	97%[152]
Subacromial space	Subacromial impingement	Neer sign	89%[155] 83%[156] 68%[157]	32%[155] 51%[156] 69%[157]
	Impingement	Painful arc test	32%[155] 74%[157]	82%[155] 81%[157]
	Subacromial impingement	Hawkins' test (Hawkins-Kennedy test)	88%[156] 72%[157]	43%[156] 66%[157]

Site or structure tested	Condition tested	Special test (other name)	Sensitivity	Specificity
Biceps	Biceps tendinopathy	Yergason's test	32%[158]	78%[158]
			41%[159]	79%[159]
Acromioclavicular joint	Acromioclavicular pathology	O'Brien's test	100%[160]	97%[160]
Glenoid labrum	Labral tear	O'Brien's test	100%[160]	99%[160]
			67%[150]	37%[150]
			54%[161]	31%[161]
			63%[153]	73%[153]
		Crank test	46%[161]	56%[161]
			91%[162]	93%[162]
	SLAP lesion	Pain provocation test	100%[163]	90[163]
		Speed's test	38%[157]	83%[157]
			54%[159]	81%[159]
		Biceps load test I	91%[164]	97%[164]
		Biceps load test II	90%[165]	97%[165]
		Anterior slide	78%[166]	92%[166]
Rotator cuff	Infraspinatus integrity	Lag sign at 0°	10%[167]	98%[167]
		Hornblower's sign	17%[167]	96%[167]
	Subscapularis integrity	Lift-off test	22%[167]	94%[167]
			18%[168]	100%[168]
		Bear hug	60%[168]	92%[168]
			79%[159]	60%[159]
	Supraspinatus integrity	Drop arm test	27%[157]	88%[157]
			24%[167]	96%[167]

Note: Sensitivity and specificity values rounded to the nearest whole number. Remember that a high sensitivity means that it is a good test to use to confirm the presence of a condition, while a high specificity means it is a good test to use to confirm that the patient does not have the condition.

Scapular Dyskinesis

Scapular dyskinesis is a term that has been used in orthopedic terminology and diagnosis since the mid-1990s.[5] The term is actually part of an acronym that describes the visually observed pathology of the condition: SICK scapula. This acronym stands for **S**capular malposition, **I**nferior medial border prominence, **C**oracoid pain and malposition, and dys**K**inesis of scapular movement.[169] The term *scapular dyskinesis* was first applied to throwing athletes who developed shoulder pain secondary to muscle fatigue,[103] but it has now become an accepted term for anyone who displays the signs and symptoms of SICK scapula.[170] SICK scapula, or scapular dyskinesis, is not a condition as much as it is a group of signs and symptoms. When signs and symptoms occur together to create a consistent pattern or profile that together are characteristic of a condition, complaint, or infirmity, they are often referred to as a **syndrome**.

Scapular Dyskinesis Syndrome

The key features of this syndrome include the following: the inferior angle of the scapula is prominently posterior; the scapula is protracted and medially rotated; the shoulder appears lower on the involved side; and the coracoid tilts inferiorly and is tender when palpated. In addition, when raising and lowering the arms with a light weight (3 to 5 lb) in flexion and in abduction for 3 to 5 repetitions in each motion,[171] the involved scapula rotates more quickly than the uninvolved one during eccentric lowering of the arms; when moving during concentric shoulder flexion or abduction, the scapula elevates or shrugs.[172, 173] It is visually obvious that scapular motion is not smooth, coordinated, or correctly timed with full shoulder flexion or abduction when the arm is raised or lowered.[173] In more advanced cases, the medial scapular border may appear more posteriorly prominent than in the uninvolved shoulder (figure 21.82).[103]

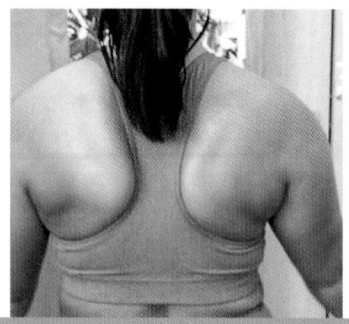

Figure 21.82   Patient with scapular dyskinesis. Notice the left scapula with its prominent posterior inferior angle, and note that the scapula is protracted and medially rotated. The shoulder appears lower on the left side, and the medial border is more prominent than that of the right scapula.

© Peggy Houglum

Go to HK*Propel* and watch video 21.5a, which demonstrates a patient's scapular motion with dyskinesis, and video 21.5b, which demonstrates the same patient's scapular motion after performing a scapular dyskinesis rehabilitation program for 3 weeks.

Patients with scapular dyskinesis often complain of anterior shoulder pain, but pain may also be present in the superior-posterior scapula or superior shoulder.[103] Referred pain may also occur proximally into the lateral neck or into the distal upper extremity.[103]

There are many potential causes for scapular dyskinesis. Occasionally, an injury to any part of the shoulder complex or to its adjacent bony, neurological, or soft-tissue structures may cause scapular dyskinesis.[174] More often, however, the cause is related to inflexibility of soft-tissue structures, which results in associated limitations of glenohumeral motions, increased scapular protraction, serratus anterior and lower trapezius weakness and dysfunction, upper trapezius hyperactivity, and altered timing of scapular rotation.[172] With these changes, scapular dyskinesis creates abnormal kinematics of the scapula and therefore abnormal clavicular motion. Scapular dyskinesis is essentially an unstable scapula that functions pathologically.[174] Research has demonstrated that pathologic function of the scapula and clavicle result in a number of shoulder problems, including glenohumeral instability,[175, 176] subacromial impingement,[177, 178] rotator cuff tendinopathies,[179, 180] and rotator cuff tears.[181, 182]

Although scapular dyskinesis may not be an injury or condition, it certainly may either contribute to a pathological condition or result from pathology.[183] Therefore, the rehabilitation examination should include an assessment for the presence of scapular dyskinesis in patients who present with shoulder pain.[184] The clinician should observe the patient anteriorly, laterally, and posteriorly for postural malalignments. The active test (concentric–eccentric arm raising–lowering test) described previously has been a reliable diagnostic tool for scapular dyskinesis.[171]

Discounting acute injuries of the shoulder complex, pathological posture is an important factor that leads to scapular dyskinesis.[132] Over time, postural changes affect soft-tissue length and balance, leading to pathological function as these soft tissues adapt to stresses imparted to them by developing low-level, persistent postural changes.[23] Eventually, scapular dyskinesis develops and establishes a domino effect of other shoulder complex pathologies. Figure 21.83 shows this progression of events.

Scapular dyskinesis leads to instability of the glenohumeral joint;[175] either alone or in combination with glenohumeral instability, scapular dyskinesis can create secondary impingement of subacromial soft-tissue structures within the glenohumeral joint.[178] Scapular instability provides an unstable platform for the glenohumeral joint, so the rotator cuff has a difficult time creating glenohumeral joint stability during shoulder activities. It would be like the difference between walking on terra firma and walking on a rope bridge; with the unstable rope bridge, muscles have a much more difficult time creating a stable gait. Likewise, if the scapula is not stable, the rotator cuff muscles have a harder time doing their job. Because of pathological scapular positioning and function, the subacromial space narrows.[185] Glenohumeral instability adds to this narrowing.[186] Ultimately, secondary impingement occurs, and as a result of this impingement, rotator cuff pathology develops.[179] When unchecked, rotator cuff tendinopathy progresses to a rotator cuff tear.[181]

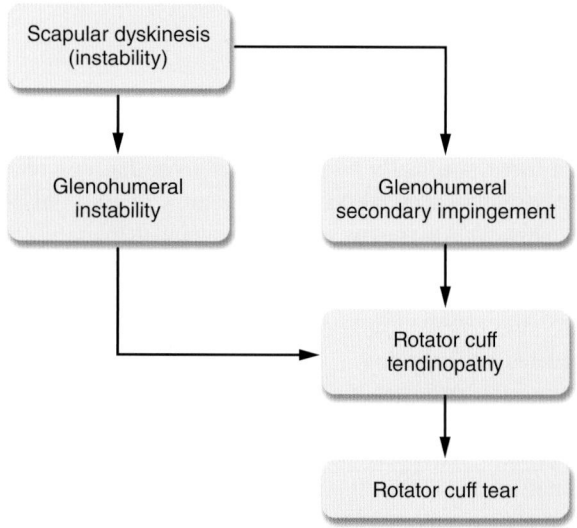

Figure 21.83   Paradigm of shoulder pathology secondary to scapular dyskinesis.

Scapular Dyskinesis Rehabilitation

Scapular dyskinesis usually develops over time until the patient finally seeks care because the pain interferes with function. Scapular dyskinesis is multifactorial in presentation and includes three main areas of deficiency: a loss of soft-tissue mobility, a lack of sufficient muscle strength and endurance, and muscle dysfunction during recruitment.[187] Each of these deficiencies must be identified and addressed before normal scapular and glenohumeral function can return without pain.

Resolving scapular dyskinesis requires time and patience. Most patients have developed dyskinesis after many, many repetitions of activities deficient in flexibility, strength, and activation timing, so changing the resulting patterns and compensatory mechanisms requires consistent and prolonged rehabilitation.[173] Clinicians must be patient and persistent. You must watch and correct for proper execution of exercises to ensure correct muscle performance.

Since poor posture with a forward head, protracted scapulae, and medially rotated humerus is the common profile of a patient with scapular dysfunction, the clinician must include patient education and instructions for restoring proper posture, as has been outlined in previous chapters. The patient's home exercise program should feature frequent reminders to correct posture; these reminders can include any number of previously mentioned cues such as a rubber band around the wrist or a painted dot on the hand. Flexibility exercises should also be included in the home exercise program.

Shoulder posture cannot change without appropriate adjustments in adjacent supporting structures. Since thoracic kyphosis and a forward head posture are often associated with protracted scapulae, an assessment of spinal posture is an important part of the examination. Poor thoracic and cervical posture is likewise related to insufficient control of the pelvis, lumbar spine, and hips. Therefore, an assessment of trunk and hip stability is also included in the patient's examination; if there are deficiencies, these must be addressed early in the rehabilitation program. The inclusion of trunk activities with kinetic chain exercises for the shoulder has beneficial effects on muscle activation and timing.[188] Applying tape to the back provides tactile stimulation that has the dual effect of improving trunk posture and improving shoulder motion.[189] Taping variation examples are shown in figure 21.3.

There may be a loss of soft-tissue mobility in the glenohumeral capsule, scapular muscles, and glenohumeral muscles. Based on the clinician's findings on examination, any one or more of these structures may need treatment. Typically, the posterior and inferior aspects of the glenohumeral joint capsule are tight, as are the levator scapulae and anterior chest muscles, including the pectoralis major and pectoralis minor.[190] Glenohumeral medial rotators (i.e., subscapularis and latissimus dorsi) are often restricted in

their range of motion as well.[170, 190] Joint capsular treatments include joint mobilization, while restricted muscles may need a combination of fascial release techniques and stretching. Stretching exercises may include active stretches, passive stretches, and assistive stretches. Flexibility exercises and capsular stretches presented earlier in this chapter are effective for increasing motion in patients with scapular dyskinesis. Treatments to improve mobility should be included in both clinic treatments and the patient's home exercise program. Active or latent trigger points in the shoulder complex muscles may cause pain in the distal upper extremity and a loss of motion in the glenohumeral joint; trigger points and tender points should be examined and treated if present.[191]

In patients with scapular dyskinesis, the serratus anterior and lower trapezius muscles are hypoactive and weak, while the upper trapezius is hyperactive and strong;[59, 192] this pathology results in a shrugging of the scapula rather than a smooth upward rotation during shoulder elevation activities. These deficiencies and imbalances in muscle strength and muscle endurance are approached using a number of techniques.

Strengthening exercises can incorporate reeducation techniques through the use of verbal and tactile cues during the exercises.[170] One important verbal cue is to "squeeze the shoulder blades and pull the shoulder blade downward toward the back pocket" during any shoulder exercise; it has been demonstrated that conscious correction of scapular positioning immediately before shoulder motion improves muscle responses.[100, 193] The taping technique shown in figure 21.3 can also help to correct motor activation: Evidence indicates that it reduces upper trapezius activation and facilitates lower trapezius activation during shoulder elevation activities.[41] Patients who respond well to verbal or tactile cues in repositioning the scapula would likely respond well to taping.[194]

Rehabilitation for patients with scapular dyskinesis produces the best results when the focus is on reducing areas of tightness and strengthening weak muscles. The weak muscles are exercised in single-plane motions against resistance to achieve strength gains and in multiplanar motions without resistance to encourage the reeducation of neuromotor activation patterns.[103, 195] The most restricted areas of tightness in a dyskinetic shoulder are the pectoralis minor and the posterior-inferior capsule.[103] These areas are most effectively stretched with the patient lying longitudinally on a foam roller while having a passive downward force applied to the shoulders. The posteroinferior capsule is stretched with the sleeper stretches that were described earlier in this chapter.[103]

The most important scapular stabilizers include the serratus anterior and lower trapezius.[195] When strengthening these muscles, it is important to use exercises that focus specifically on the motions these muscles produce and avoid recruiting muscles that perpetuate compensatory patterns.[103] The clinician should monitor the patient throughout the session to ensure proper execution of the exercise using the desired muscle. Sometimes verbal cues may be needed to correct a patient's performance; at other times, tactile stimulation such as tapping the muscle or stroking the length of the muscle's fibers during the motion may facilitate an improved response.

Early in the process of strengthening scapular stabilizers, weight-bearing exercises without resistance are used to promote scapular control.[103] These are used as early strengthening exercises because they need less output from the weak muscles. Such activities can include standing with the hands on a tabletop or on the wall and moving through scapular retraction–protraction motions, or moving a Swiss ball on the wall with an outstretched arm or a partially flexed elbow. Other early exercises can include total body activities to encourage neuromotor activation for proper muscle sequencing in nonresistive activities such as the robbery and lawnmower exercises.

As patients gain scapular muscle strength and control in their rehabilitation progression, they advance to multiplanar motions.[101] These exercises are first performed without weights to enable the patient to relearn movements through the proper sequential timing of muscle activation. These exercises incorporate hip and trunk motions as well as shoulder and other upper-extremity segment movements.

During these multiplanar exercises, clinicians should observe and correct compensations made by inappropriate muscles. For example, if a patient was going through the motions of the low row and lawnmower exercises listed earlier in this chapter, the clinician would provide verbal cues to facilitate the activation of the lower trapezius, diminish the activity of the upper trapezius, and promote scapular retraction with scapular depression. Tactile cues such as tapping the skin over the lower trapezius as the patient performs the exercise will facilitate its activation.[196] Clinicians should correct their patients whenever they see incorrect muscle performance. For example, if the patient shrugs the scapula when he raises his arm to put on a jacket at the end of a treatment session, the clinician should remind him to "squeeze and pull the shoulder blade down into the back pocket" when the shoulder elevates.

As the patient's neuromotor activation and strength progress, the clinician introduces activities and resistance exercises that are performed at progressively higher planes of motion and with greater resistance. After these activities are performed with full motion and adequate strength and neuromotor control, the next step is functional activities and finally performance-specific exercises that were introduced in chapter 15.

Figure 21.84 presents a rehabilitation program for patients with scapular dyskinesis. This is a generic program; most patients may follow a progression of similar exercises, but individual programs may vary in timing and rate of progression. You will notice that the rehabilitation program for scapular dyskinesis starts with the second phase rather than the first phase. Since scapular dyskinesis is a progressive condition that does not necessarily produce symptoms until it is advanced, there usually is no acute

Scapular Dyskinesis

Stage I: Inflammation phase: Inactive rehabilitation phase

Since scapular dyskinesis is not identified until the condition has progressed to a subacute condition, the rehabilitation program does not deal with an inflammation phase.

The timeline for treatment progression varies according to how advanced the dyskinesis is and its duration before the onset of rehabilitation; the longer the time until rehabilitation, the longer the rehabilitation program will take to restore the patient's shoulder to normal function. For this reason, time ranges are not set for this condition; the clinician advances the patient to the next phase once the goals have been achieved.

Stage II: Active phase

Goals	Relieve pain.
	Correct posture.
	Restore neuromuscular coordination.
	Activate lower trap and serratus anterior.
	Regain motor control and function.
	Restore soft-tissue mobility.
	Restore joint mobility.
	Restore full range of motion.
	Restore normal proprioception.

Figure 21.84 Rehabilitation progression for scapular dyskinesis.

	Stage II: Active phase
Treatment guidelines	Modalities PRN for pain Joint mobilization to increase posterior and inferior glenohumeral capsule mobility Soft-tissue mobilization for infraspinatus, subscapularis, pectoralis minor, levator scapulae Flexibility exercises to gain soft-tissue and joint motion Instruction in proper posture Core and hip muscle strengthening for posture Exercises to isolate and strengthen lower trapezius, middle trapezius, rhomboids, serratus anterior Weight-bearing exercises (wall or tabletop) Nonresistive functional patterns (e.g., low row, lawnmower, robbery exercises) for lower trapezius and serratus anterior facilitation, coordination, and motor control Taping for posture correction and correct muscle facilitation
Precautions	Do not tape for posture correction too early, or the patient will be unable to tolerate the sustained position; patient's muscles must have gains in flexibility and strength before applying tape. Use tactile cues by tapping lower medial aspect of scapula (lower trapezius, middle trapezius), and use verbal cues such as "pull your shoulder blade down toward your back pocket" or "squeeze your shoulder blades together slightly" before the patient engages in exercise to encourage scapular positioning and awareness.

	Stage III: Resistive phase
Goals	Achieve normal scapular muscle strength and endurance. Restore scapular control throughout all degrees of glenohumeral elevation. Restore normal scapulothoracic motion during all diagonal and triplanar activities. Regain normal posture 80% to 90% of the time.
Treatment guidelines	Offer resistance to scapular muscles first in isolated motions and then in multiplanar motions. Begin in lower levels of humeral elevation. Progress to mid-level humeral elevation. Advance to high-level humeral elevation. Proceed to make normal gains in muscle strength and muscle endurance with increased resistance and repetitions, respectively. Correct posture as needed. Offer early functional exercises.
Precautions	Provide verbal cues to correct patient's scapular position.

	Stage IV: Advanced phase
Goals	Regain normal performance of functional skills. Regain normal performance-specific activation. Experience no pain with any activities. Eliminate scapular dyskinesis signs and symptoms. Return to full participation in normal activities.
Treatment guidelines	Late functional activities Advance to performance-specific exercises and drills as goals are met
Precautions	Watch for incorrect scapular motion during activities; use verbal cues as needed.

PRN = as needed.

Figure 21.84 >continued

inflammatory phase. Therefore, exercises may begin at the start of the rehabilitation program.

Shoulder Instability

The shoulder has two systems of stability, **static restraints** and **dynamic restraints**. The static restraints include the ligaments, capsule, and glenoid labrum. The dynamic restraints are the neuromuscular components. If the static restraints are damaged by joint sprains, subluxations, or dislocations, the neural input from proprioceptors in these static structures is compromised.[19, 21] Damage to static restraints results in muscle function changes.[197] Instability occurs when shoulder restraints are deficient.[198, 199] Two of the most common sources of instability are a sudden traumatic injury and chronic stresses on the joint.[200] The sudden traumatic event occurs when the joint receives an external force that moves the humeral head beyond its normal mobility range, while chronic stresses accrue over time until support from soft-tissue structures begins to decline. A third cause of glenohumeral instability is genetic laxity; excessive laxity in several joints can be an inherited condition. These patients have multidirectional instability that may lead to frequent joint injuries if they participate in sports or other strenuous activities.[201]

Joint laxity and instability lie on a continuum. At one extreme is complete dislocation of the joint, while at the other extreme, the joint simply has greater-than-normal movement. Dislocations are usually caused by a sudden extreme force on the joint. Laxity of shoulders without frank dislocations or subluxations usually results from a gradual, repetitive application of stresses to the joint. The laxity may be minor at first, but with repeated activity, glenohumeral laxity can move toward the middle of the instability continuum. Eventually the patient experiences pain secondary to impingement or other injuries secondary to the progressive laxity. Baseball pitching is a good example of repetitive stress that may eventually produce glenohumeral joint laxity and other injuries.

If instability is not corrected either by surgery or by rehabilitation, or both, the joint continues to be reinjured until it becomes so unstable that it may repeatedly sublux or dislocate and the impinged soft tissues break down and tear (figure 21.85). A secondary problem that can result from chronic instability is rotator cuff tendinopathy, which can lead to rotator cuff tears with repetitive impingement and breakdown.[182] The long head of the biceps is also at risk of tendinopathy secondary to glenohumeral instability.[202] It is therefore important that the rehabilitation clinician be aware of the potential causes of instability and of the fact that if glenohumeral instability is not identified early, it may lead to other more serious injuries.

Figure 21.86 shows that although there may be initial differences in the mechanism, both causes of laxity may eventually require surgical correction.[203] An acute dislocation or subluxation may result in acute injuries to other joint elements and surrounding structures, but chronic laxity

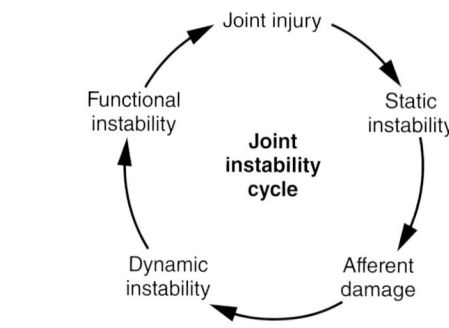

Figure 21.85 Glenohumeral instability occurs when either static or dynamic restraints are damaged. Unchecked, a cycle of perpetual instability develops as static structures, neurological input, and dynamic support become more and more deficient.

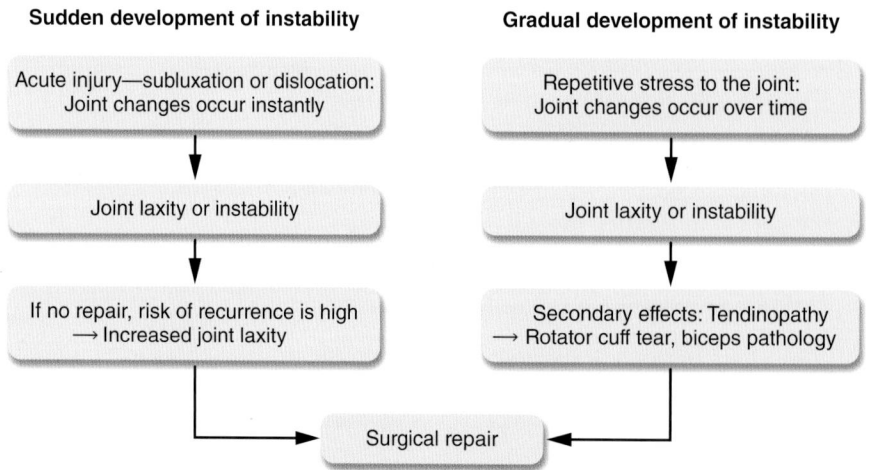

Figure 21.86 Acute and chronic development of glenohumeral instability.

usually involves changes in the rotator cuff and biceps, for the gradual progression of laxity causes secondary injury to the active structures protecting the glenohumeral joint.[182]

Before you design a rehabilitation program for a patient with shoulder instability, you must know the type of instability and the precautions related to it. As you may recall, the most common instability is anterior instability, which occurs when anterior structures become damaged. Inferior instability is the rarest type and is the result of injury and laxity of the inferior capsule and support structures. Posterior instability, which is less common than anterior instability but more common than inferior instability, occurs with damage to the posterior joint structures.

There is also a classification of instability based on whether the condition is genetic or the result of trauma. Two acronyms, AMBRI and TUBS, indicate the differences between congenital and traumatic shoulder instability and present guidelines for treatment. The acronym **AMBRI** stands for "**A**traumatic, **M**ultidirectional, **B**ilateral, responds well to **R**ehabilitation, but if surgery is needed an **I**nferior capsular shift is indicated."[204] Patients with this congenital condition usually have bilateral shoulder laxity as well as hypermobility in most joints. Multidirectional instability (MDI) usually responds well to the conservative treatment of rehabilitation.[205] Conservative treatment includes patient education and modification of activities to prevent joint subluxation or dislocation.[206] Conservative treatment also includes proprioception activities and progressive strengthening exercises for scapular stabilizers, rotator cuff, and deltoid muscles.[206] It may take 6 months for a full recovery.[207]

If surgery is required, an anterior-inferior capsular shift is usually the procedure of choice since it produces better results than an anterior tightening.[208] Although research outcomes have been conflicting, some surgeons in the past few years have used an electrothermally assisted capsular shift to relieve multidirectional instability.[209-211] Surgical repair of MDI using either arthroscopic or open procedures is usually followed by sling immobilization for 6 weeks, after which the patient begins a progressive restoration of range of motion and a return to normal strength.[206] Similar to the conservative approach, it may take the patient at least 6 months to return to normal activities.[206]

Some surgeons like the shoulder to be immobilized in a sling for 3 to 6 weeks whether the shoulder has been surgically repaired or not.[212, 213] Immobilization after acute dislocation, however, is controversial; some physicians have reported that their patients do better without it.[214] Older patients should be the exception to extended immobilization. Patients over 30 years old should begin early postoperative exercise, regardless of the surgical procedure performed, because a frozen shoulder is a common complication if the shoulder remains immobilized for extended times after any surgical procedure.[213]

The time needed to complete a rehabilitation program varies depending on a number of factors, such as whether the instability is chronic or acute, whether there was surgical repair, the amount of instability, the patient's age, the patient's activity level, the presence of other pathologies, and the patient's goals.[215] Patients in overhead sports such as tennis, baseball, or volleyball, where demands on the shoulder are greater, may need a longer rehabilitation process than those whose shoulder demands are minimal, such as soccer players. An average program may take anywhere from 6 to 9 months.[216]

The rehabilitation processes for surgically corrected instability and nonrepaired acute instability are similar. A nonrepaired shoulder may need little or no time in a sling and less total rehabilitation time, but the types of exercises in postoperative and nonoperative programs are similar. Other differences include mainly precautionary factors. For example, surgical repairs and sudden dislocations without surgical repair may both require a sling, while a chronically unstable shoulder will not. Healing tissue must be protected in shoulders with either surgical repair or sudden dislocation, whereas chronically unstable shoulders do not usually need extensive restrictions. Surgically repaired shoulders will also have more severe range-of-motion limitations in the first 6 to 8 weeks of rehabilitation.

Table 21.5 identifies the differences between treatment programs for repaired and nonrepaired unstable shoulders. The differences are largely based on the need to protect newly formed tissue until it is mature enough to withstand tension within the range of motion. Chronically unstable shoulders do not have this newly forming tissue, so the clinician can provide a rehabilitation progression without those concerns.

Anterior Instability

Shoulders with **TUBS** (**T**raumatic, **U**nilateral, **B**ankart lesion, **S**urgery required)[204] have suffered a traumatic dislocation. A **Bankart lesion**, or tear of the anterior capsulolabral complex, requires surgery to correct it.

In addition to congenital and traumatic injuries, chronic stress on the glenohumeral joint can also result in instability. Patients in overhead-throwing sports commonly experience anterior instability because the throwing motion places repetitive stresses on the anterior joint structures, especially when the object thrown is released (during the deceleration, or follow-through, phase).[217] This problem is often accompanied by tightness in the posterior capsule and medial rotators.[218] In these patients, the rehabilitation program for instability should include stretching these structures.

Surgical patients undergoing an anterior capsulolabral reconstruction (ACLR) repair have one of two options: an open procedure or an arthroscopic procedure. In the open procedure, an axillary incision over an inch long is made,

TABLE 21.5 Differences in Rehabilitation of Shoulders With Acute Dislocations, Surgical Repairs, and Chronic Instability

Rehabilitation factors	Surgical repair	Acute dislocation without surgical repair	Chronic instability without surgical repair
Sling	Sling is worn 3-6 weeks	If used, a sling may be worn anywhere from 3 days to 3-4 weeks	No sling
Tissue healing	Protect healing tissue	Variable concerns of scar tissue formation in terms of allowing use of the shoulder	No scar tissue or healing tissue concerns
Range of motion	Motion that stretches repaired tissues (rotation and rotation with elevation) is limited or prevented for 1-2 weeks, then gradually progresses to normal by 8-10 weeks postoperatively. Exercises start as passive and progressive to active-assistive. Active stretching starts about week 6.	Motion is primarily restricted by patient's complaints of pain. Exercises start as active-assistive and progress to active stretches more rapidly than surgical repairs.	No limitations as long as patient moves pain free. Exercises start as active and progress as patient is able.

and the muscles are separated rather than cut to view and repair the glenohumeral joint structures,[216] so there is more postoperative pain with the open repair than with the arthroscopic repair.[219] Fortunately, most shoulder surgeries are now performed using **arthroscopy** rather than open procedures because of advancements in techniques, technology, and instrumentation.[220] In the arthroscopic procedure, the redundancy in the capsule is taken up, and the capsule is usually tightened by overlapping the redundant capsular portions and securing them with sutures.[219, 221]

A commonly used repair for anterior instability with labral tear using either the open method or arthroscopy is the Bankart repair.[204] With advances in the arthroscopic repair of anterior shoulder instability, both open and arthroscopic repairs are effective in treating instability, but the arthroscopic procedure is used more often.[219, 222] Arthroscopic Bankart repairs have shown better short-term and long-term results with less surgical invasiveness than the open repairs.[221, 223, 224] Although the Bankart repair is considered the gold standard for repair of anterior instability,[225] when there is accompanying glenoid bone loss with recurrent anterior shoulder instability, the Latarjet procedure is becoming a popular and effective surgical option.[226] In this surgery, the coracoid process with its attached tendons (biceps and coracobrachialis) is resected and attached to replace the damaged glenoid to serve as a bone block and strut to restore stability to the glenohumeral joint.[227]

The rehabilitation program presented here deals with the arthroscopic Bankart repair since this the preferred procedure for anterior instability. There are no active exercises for the glenohumeral joint in the first week after Bankart

repair surgery, and the shoulder remains in an abduction sling during this time.[228] Pendulum exercises, however, are used once postoperative pain subsides by the end of the first postoperative week.[229] Exercises for the other upper extremity joints, including manual resistance to the scapular muscles and ROM exercises for the elbow, forearm, wrist, and hand can occur within the first postoperative week.[203] Although the arm is removed from the sling to perform these exercises, it remains in the abduction sling for 3 to 4 weeks.[203, 229, 230] During this time, the clinician's efforts focus on relieving pain, spasm, and swelling with appropriate modalities.

Shoulder range-of-motion activities begin at the third week.[230] The shoulder is removed from the sling to permit passive or active-assistive range of motion in straight-plane motions. Gentle, passive motion is restricted to 0° lateral rotation with the elbow at the side. Progressive abduction to 30° and progressive flexion to 90° are also permitted with these limits.[216] Home exercises should include flexibility exercises. Submaximal isometrics in nonstressful and nonpainful positions may be permitted after the first week, providing there is no pain with these range-of-motion exercises.[230] Care must be taken during the first 6 weeks to avoid lateral rotation greater than 20° to 30° and abduction greater than 30° to 40°. The anterior shoulder joint should be minimally stressed during the first 3 weeks. Manual resistance to scapular stabilizers while avoiding stress to the glenohumeral (GH) joint should continue until the patient is allowed to begin resistance exercises for the glenohumeral joint. The most stressful position for the anterior glenohumeral joint is lateral rotation in

90° of abduction; this position is avoided for the first 5[230] to 10[229] weeks.

During the first 2 weeks, grade I and II joint mobilization techniques to the GH joint in its resting position may provide pain relief.[231] Simple, mild distraction with oscillation may be beneficial.

While the patient is wearing a sling, he or she may develop trigger points in the upper trapezius and levator scapulae as well as in other neck and shoulder muscles.[232] These trigger points are identified and treated during this time.

By the end of the second week, elevation in the scapular plane is approximately 110° to 135°, and by the fourth week, passive shoulder flexion range of motion should be normal or nearly normal.[225] By the sixth week, passive lateral rotation should be approximately 50° to 60° with the elbow at the side. By the eighth to tenth week, full passive range of motion should be present in all motions except lateral rotation, which should be at approximately 75°. Between weeks 10 and 12, full passive motion should be possible in all movements.[225, 229]

After the third week, gentle, active-resistive isotonic exercises for medial rotation, lateral rotation to about 20° to 30° with the elbow near the side, and abduction to 20° can begin in a scapular plane.[230] Scapular exercises should advance as tolerated without the imposition of additional stress on the glenohumeral joint. By the fourth week, horizontal abduction exercises begin.

Immobilization may lead to adhesive capsulitis in some patients.[233] If this occurs, grade III joint mobilizations can begin between the fourth and sixth week.[234] These mobilizations should occur in the resting position. If a capsular pattern is present, the clinician should identify those positions of the capsule that are restricted and perform joint mobilizations to improve mobility in the appropriate ranges. Joint mobilization stress to the anterior capsule should be mild and should start at grade III.

By the end of the third to sixth week, the shoulder sling is removed.[203, 229] This can be a time of apprehension for the patient. The lack of shoulder support can also be initially fatiguing for the shoulder muscles. The patient should be encouraged to support the extremity throughout the day by placing the forearm on top of a table or desk while sitting, and by putting the hand in a pocket when standing. This will allow muscles to rest. With increased muscle demands, trigger point treatment during this time may be effective if trigger points are a source of the patient's discomfort.

By the seventh to tenth week, rotator cuff strength exercises can progress through increased ranges of motion as long as the anterior joint is not excessively stressed.[235] The program should continue with low weights and high repetitions. The elbow is kept near the side to keep shoulder motion in the scapular plane, and lateral rotation progresses to 45° to 60°. Mild isokinetic exercises with the shoulder stabilized can begin during this time.

Joint mobilization by the eighth week can be any grade. By this time, repaired structures have enough strength to withstand joint mobilization forces. The clinician should emphasize attaining full range of motion in all planes by this time. If necessary, the clinician may apply joint mobilization in other loose-pack positions besides the resting position. Home exercises for range-of-motion gains can also be more aggressive at this time.

When the patient has full lateral rotation, eccentric exercises for the rotator cuff muscles begin. These start with the shoulder at a low elevation, less than 60°, and progress to higher positions as tolerated. Once the patient has achieved adequate strength and control of the joints during motion, overhead activities, plyometrics, and functional activities followed by performance-specific exercises are added in the final phase of the rehabilitation program. By weeks 20 to 32, the patient should be able to return to sport or work activities at a normal level.[225, 228]

In summary, active-assistive ROM exercises that do not stress the anterior capsule begin 2 weeks after surgery, contingent on the patient's tolerance and the physician's instructions. Scapular exercises that do not stress the glenohumeral joint are also incorporated early in the program. Progressive scapular strengthening that does not stress the glenohumeral joint continues through this time. Isotonic exercises are well ingrained in the program by the third month, when the patient should have about two-thirds normal strength in the shoulder. Once the involved shoulder has about 75% of the strength of the contralateral extremity, functional and then sport- or performance-specific activities are added to the program.

Throughout the program, the clinician must receive feedback from the patient about the shoulder's response to activity. Pain should not occur with any activities. The scapula must be stable before the patient advances to activities that place the arm above shoulder level. If this principle is ignored, rotator cuff tendinopathy may occur and delay the patient's return to normal activities.

Performance-specific progressions are included in the final rehabilitation phase and will depend on the sport, job, or other activity to which the person will return. Patients who perform sport activities such as throwing, pitching, golf, swimming, tennis, or volleyball or who do work such as automobile repair, painting, drywall installation, and other overhead tasks will need to start performance-specific activities at lower and middle levels and finish with overhead activities. For example, tennis players start with ground strokes in both forehand and backhand motions and progress to performing overhead hits and serves.

Speed or force, distance, repetitions, and types of throws or hits are all variables that change as patients progress in their performance-specific programs. Every session should include a warm-up and cool-down of easy performance activities. Stretching exercises are performed at the end of the session. Speed or force is usually the last factor to increase after pain, mobility, strength, and neuromotor goals have been reached. Patients typically return to full function by the sixth to ninth month after surgery.[216]

Posterior Instability

Traumatic posterior dislocation usually occurs from a fall on an outstretched, adducted, and medially rotated shoulder. Impact forces are directed through the extremity, forcing the humeral head posteriorly. Football linemen, swimmers, pitchers, rowers, and tennis players are especially susceptible to chronic posterior instability problems because of the repeated anterior-to-posterior forces their shoulders sustained during play.[236, 237]

After an acute posterior dislocation or subluxation, positions that put stress on the posterior capsule are avoided at first; these include flexion with adduction and medial rotation and weight bearing on the upper extremity. Rehabilitation after surgical repairs for posterior instability follows a routine similar to that for the surgical repair of anterior instability, but different motions are restricted. Excessive medial rotation and horizontal adduction are performed carefully after the first 3 to 4 weeks, but active assisted lateral rotation and abduction can begin on post-op day 3 to 7, depending on the physician's preference. Isometric exercises for shoulder flexion, extension, abduction, adduction, and lateral rotation can begin after post-op day 7. Weight-bearing activities in a quadruped position are avoided at first. This position puts too much stress on the posterior capsule. Other exercises that are modified or avoided because of the posterior capsule stress they impose include chest flys, bench press, and push-ups. These activities are added to the program carefully, and not until the later stages of the rehabilitation program.

In the active phase, exercises are performed with the shoulder in some lateral rotation and abduction. Glenohumeral lateral rotation exercises begin with the patient supine and progress to the patient sitting. Joint stability is harder to maintain in sitting than it is in supine. Seated weight-bearing exercises, such as press-ups, do not stress the posterior capsule, so they can occur earlier in the resistive phase of the program than quadruped weight-bearing exercises. Medial rotation exercises are performed from full lateral rotation to neutral in the early phases. Horizontal adduction exercises are avoided early in the resistive phase. When added later, they begin with horizontal adduction limitations to approximately 45° forward of the frontal plane. Gradually, full horizontal adduction is introduced in the later stages.

Quadruped weight-bearing exercises for the shoulder begin in the later part of the resistive phase only after the patient has achieved stabilization and adequate strength, and after enough time has passed for tissues to heal. When the bench press is begun, also later in this phase, it is performed with a wide grip so that the shoulders are in abduction and horizontal extension.

In summary, the timeline used for posterior shoulder instability repair is similar to that outlined for anterior instability repair. As with any injury, pain should be avoided with exercise. Full motion is expected at around 2 months. Once the involved shoulder has 75% strength compared to the contralateral limb, functional exercises begin and progress to performance-specific activities.

Case Study

A 16-year-old basketball player was seen by the physician after experiencing a right shoulder subluxation. The injury occurred as he was going under the basket for a layup and his arm was caught by an opponent and pulled into horizontal extension with lateral rotation. He has no history of prior injury. The physician has placed the arm in a sling and instructed you to begin a rehabilitation program for this patient. It has been 1 week since the injury.

The patient reports some difficulty sleeping at night; he cannot get comfortable because of the pain. He reports that he wears the sling all the time except for showers, as the physician has instructed. On examination, you find some discoloration in the upper arm, but the swelling of last week is gone. There is some muscle spasm and tenderness to palpation of the infraspinatus, supraspinatus, teres minor, rhomboids, upper trapezius, and levator scapula. You notice that atrophy of the supraspinatus is already evident after 1 week. Range of motion of the shoulder is 20° medial rotation, 20° abduction; the patient cannot move into lateral rotation by 10° from neutral (his shoulder cannot get to neutral by 10°, so end lateral rotation remains in medial rotation).

Questions for Analysis

1. What will be your initial treatment?

2. Outline the exercises you will use for this patient during the first week of treatment.

3. What precautions must you take with his treatments?

4. Give a general outline of progression for his rehabilitation program, specifying what guidelines you will use to move from one stage to the next.

Inferior Instability

Shoulder inferior instability is treated in a manner similar to anterior and posterior instability. The only caveat is that it is common to have multiplanar instability when inferior instability is present. In these cases, the clinician must be aware of all the positions and movements that may put the shoulder joint at risk and avoid these positions, especially in the early phases of rehabilitation.

Initial positions to avoid with inferior instability injuries include placing the arm overhead and allowing it to hang at the side unsupported. The upright press and shrugs are exercises that the patient should avoid until later in phase III because of the stress they place on the inferior capsule.

Subacromial Impingement

Subacromial impingement is associated with unique factors that you must consider in developing and executing a rehabilitation program. These are discussed as program considerations before the case study is presented.

The subacromial space is not a large area—a little wider than a pencil's width.[238] Because the space is small, even a slight change in its normal structures can have significant consequences, especially for a patient who places great stress on the joint throughout daily activities.

Subacromial impingement is considered a syndrome because its diagnosis is established on the presence of consistent signs and symptoms. Subacromial impingement syndrome (SAIS or SIS) has been more recently divided according to its mechanisms; one camp identifies those mechanisms as either intrinsic or extrinsic, while another camp uses the terms primary and secondary impingement. The extrinsic–intrinsic classification recognizes that repetitive compression and microtraumatic degeneration of the rotator cuff tendon occurs, either because of tension applied to the rotator cuff tendon at a place of compromised circulation (intrinsic impingement)[239] or because of the stress-induced formation of a spur on the acromion's underside (extrinsic impingement).[240]

The primary–secondary classification divides impingement etiology between structural and functional pathology sources. Primary impingement is the result of structures in the subacromial space that narrow the normal size of the space to compromise the soft-tissue structures within it—the rotator cuff tendons (primarily supraspinatus, infraspinatus, and subscapularis), biceps tendon, and subacromial bursa. Among these structural factors are a congenital anomaly of the acromion structure, an osteophyte on the distal acromion, a narrower-than-normal subacromial space, and a larger-than-normal tendon or bursa.[241] All these structural variations narrow an already small space and cause the soft-tissue structures to become impinged. Most often, the cause of primary impingement is either a congenital anomaly in the distal acromion configuration or a bone spur.[242-244] For consistency and convenience, we will present impingement dysfunction on the basis of primary and secondary impingement pathology.

Acquired, or secondary, impingement reduces the subacromial space because of changes in the shoulder's function that lead to a functional narrowing of the space. These factors can include capsular laxity or tightness,[245] postural deviations,[246] rotator cuff weakness or pathology,[247] and scapular rotator muscle imbalances, including dyskinesis.[103] Cervical radiculopathy can also result in impingement if muscle weakness occurs,[248] resulting in muscle imbalances during shoulder motion. If the capsule is loose, the humerus moves forward during the follow-through of throwing motions, reducing subacromial space and increasing rotator cuff stress.[249] If the posterior capsule is tight, it tends to push the humerus up and into the anterior joint during shoulder motions and rotate the scapula anteriorly, narrowing the subacromial space.[250]

Normally the rotator cuff depresses the humeral head when the shoulder is elevated to maintain adequate subacromial space,[106] but if the rotator cuff is weak, the humeral head rides higher than it should in the glenoid, causing impingement.[133] When the scapular rotator muscles are imbalanced, the upper trapezius and levator scapulae usually overpower the weaker lower trapezius.[126] This strength imbalance causes poor scapulohumeral rhythm and narrows the subacromial space under the coracoacromial arch during shoulder motion because normal scapular elevation and upward rotation do not occur with shoulder elevation.[251]

Poor posture causes the shoulders to round forward so that the greater tubercle is more directly under the acromial arch, causing impingement earlier in the range of motion.[252] Related to posture is the position of the scapula on the thorax; those with impingement show more of an elevated and protracted scapula with less of a posterior tilting angle.[60] If shoulder medial rotation is lacking, the scapula's protracted position is such that impingement occurs at the end of medial rotation.[250] Finally, if the scapular stabilizers become fatigued, the biomechanics of the glenohumeral joint are altered, leading to impingement of the glenohumeral soft-tissue structures under the coracoacromial arch.[253]

All of these secondary impingement causes can be placed into four categories, with some of them closely related. These include (1) the scapula's position on the thorax, (2) changes in glenohumeral range of motion, (3) deficiency of rotator cuff muscles, and (4) dysfunction of scapular stabilizers. The association among these categories centers on the function and position of the scapula; if the scapula is not properly positioned because of injury or bad posture, it changes the relationship between muscles and all other joints of the shoulder complex. For example, if the patient has rounded shoulders with a forward head posture, the scapulae are protracted and anteriorly tilted. This scapular position permits less glenohumeral elevation, with the result that the rotator cuff is less able to maintain its mechanical advantage with scapular rotation.[254] Likewise, a protracted scapular position leads to tightness of the pectoralis minor and lengthening of the rhomboids; these length changes affect muscle strength as well as muscle function.[255] When muscle strength and function change, muscle timing and the sequencing of muscular activities are negatively affected.

Figure 21.87 graphically displays the sources of secondary impingement and how they evolve to produce impingement. As figure 21.87 indicates, each of these secondary problems can result in subacromial impingement. Uncorrected secondary impingement leads to a gradual, progressive shredding of the rotator cuff tendon and ultimately results in rotator cuff tears. Although the problem may begin at a young age, manifestations of secondary impingement and rotator cuff tears are more common in athletes over the age of 35 than in those who are younger.[256]

Secondary and primary impingement both result in inflammation of the soft-tissue structures in the subacromial space. This inflammation most commonly includes the supraspinatus tendon.[257] The infraspinatus tendon and subscapularis tendon can sometimes be affected as well. The subacromial bursa and biceps tendon can also be involved. Impingement, then, causes tendinopathy or bursitis. Irritation of the rotator cuff tendons weakens the tendons and can lead to tendon rupture if the condition is poorly managed or untreated.[258]

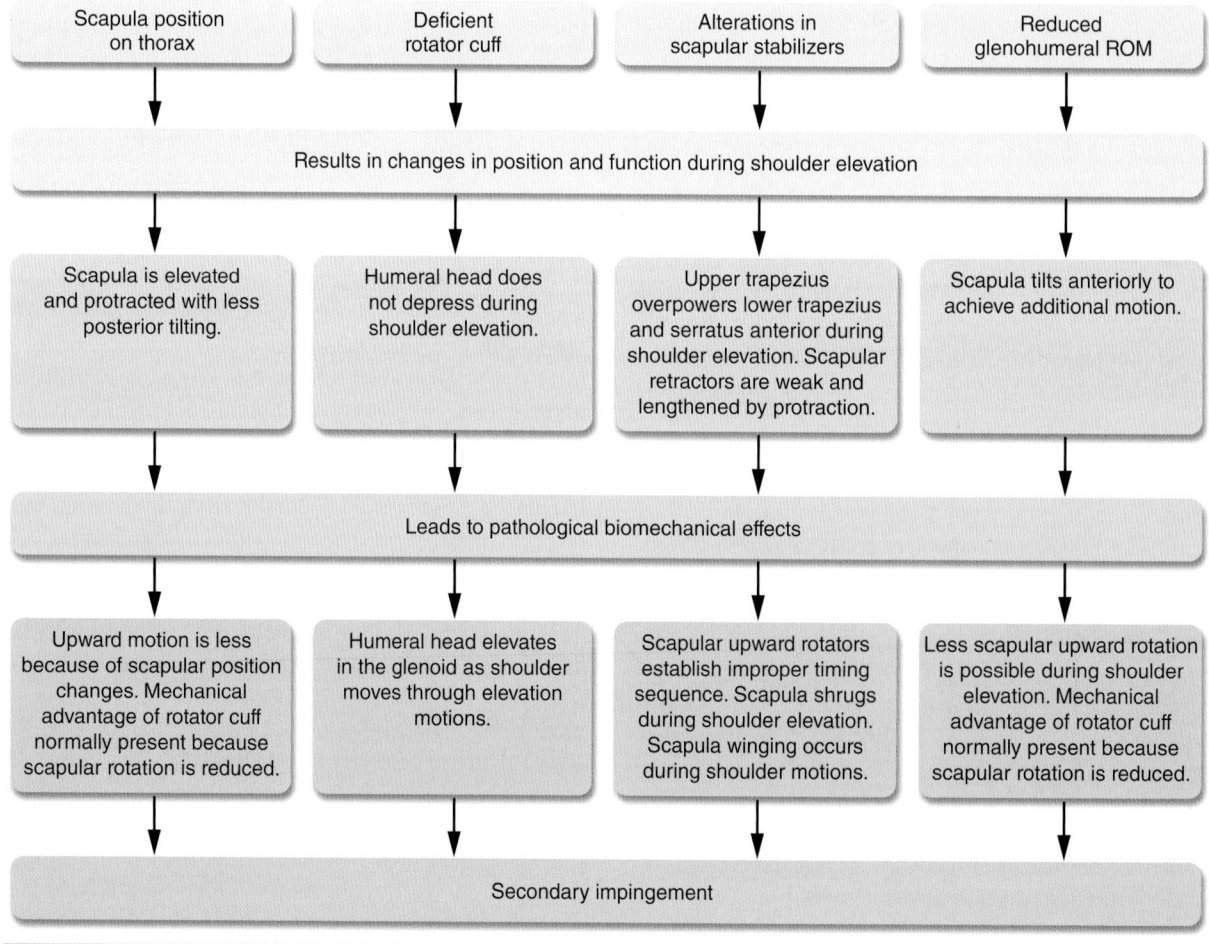

Figure 21.87 Sources of secondary subacromial impingement.

Secondary impingement can be resolved with a conservative approach if the cause of the impingement is corrected. Factors associated with secondary impingement, such as muscle imbalances with length or strength changes, asynchronous shoulder motion, and poor posture, must be assessed and treated if present. Both primary and secondary problems should be treated conservatively with rehabilitation first, whether surgery is performed later or not.[239] Assuming no rotator cuff damage, the most common surgical corrections include osteophyte removal (if present), anterior acromioplasty, and bursectomy.[259] These procedures relieve compression beneath the coracoacromial arch and have a successful history of relieving primary impingement.[260]

Early rehabilitation in the inactive and active phases emphasizes control of the inflammation, correction of secondary causes, and restoration of normal shoulder function. Initially, the focus is on pain and inflammation control and regaining full range of motion. Placing the shoulder in a resting position with the arm slightly abducted and flexed helps to create an environment for optimal circulation to the tendons.[261] We know that gentle grade I and II mobilizations are helpful in relieving pain. If inferior capsule tightness is present, inferior glenohumeral glide mobilizations will increase general capsule mobility. Gaining inferior capsule mobility allows the rotator cuff to perform its task of positioning the humeral head caudally in the glenoid during arm elevation. The rehabilitation clinician can massage the supraspinatus tendon at its insertion on the greater tubercle by placing the patient's hand behind the hip to expose the anterior humerus and providing deep cross-friction massage to the tender area until the pain subsides (see figure 21.6).

Posture correction and instruction includes giving the patient information about normal posture and pointing out how the patient's posture differs from normal. Patient education and home instructions are then provided on how to improve posture. The patient must be reminded that posture change occurs by using two tactics: (1) making conscious changes throughout the day to establish new habits and (2) improving the strength of weak muscles and stretching tightened muscles. Improving posture is a slow process that requires persistence. The patient's home program also includes stretching exercises and adds strength exercises when appropriate.

Strengthening exercises for scapular stabilizers can begin early without stressing the painful rotator cuff tendons. Early on, the program incorporates simple neuromotor reeducation techniques for proprioception and improved kinesthetic awareness of the scapular rotators for correct scapular positioning during shoulder movement. Rotator cuff exercises in a pain-free range of motion are important at this time as well. Most rotator cuff exercises are performed in the lower positions (below 60°), where the scapula is in a "set" position.[14] The "set" position is achieved with simple instructions to the patient: "pull your shoulder blades together and down toward your back pocket." Resistive exercises begin with high repetitions and lower weights. These exercises for the scapular and rotator cuff muscles are listed earlier in this chapter. See figure 21.88 for an outline of this program.

Case Study

A 40-year-old competitive tennis player reports to you that she has had right dominant shoulder pain since the first half of the tennis season. Now she cannot serve without pain. She has pain in the beginning of her warm-ups, but before a match begins, the pain goes away. About 2 h after a match, her pain is significant. She reports that her pain is located in the deltoid insertion area. The physician has ruled out primary impingement but feels that a course of rehabilitation is needed before the patient returns to tennis. On examination, this patient has full range of motion except that she is lacking about 10° in elevation. Pain occurs in the end ranges of movement and in the painful arc within midrange shoulder elevation. She has a forward-head, round-shouldered posture. Her glenohumeral rotators and abductors are weak and painful. She has weakness in the lower trapezius, serratus anterior, and rhomboids. As she lowers her arms from full abduction, you observe that the right scapula does not move smoothly, and when her arms are resting at her sides, the right shoulder is more elevated than the left.

Questions for Analysis

1. What is the cause of her secondary impingement?
2. What will you do to relieve the causes?
3. What will your first treatment include?
4. How will you help the patient to progress in her rehabilitation program?
5. What guidelines will you use for her progression?
6. What functional program will you use to prepare her for her return to tennis?

Progression of exercises is based on the patient's pain and strength. Exercises that produce pain are avoided. In the early stages, these exercises include activities that place the arm above 60° to 90° or behind the back, and diagonal-plane motions. As the pain subsides and the patient achieves scapular control and strength, she performs glenohumeral exercises at higher shoulder positions, and more challenging exercises are added to the rehabilitation

Subacromial Secondary Impingement

Stage I: Inactive phase	
Since secondary subacromial impingement is a subacute condition, the inactive phase is not part of the therapeutic exercise program. Timeline for treatment progression varies according to how advanced the condition is and its duration prior to onset of rehabilitation; the longer the time until rehabilitation starts, the longer the rehabilitation program will take to restore the patient's shoulder to normal levels. For this reason, time ranges are not set for this condition; the clinician advances the patient to the next phase once the goals have been achieved.	

Stage II: Active phase	
Goals	Relieve pain. Improve posture. Restore shoulder complex ROM. Maintain ROM of elbow, wrist, and hand. Maintain strength of all other UE segments. Retrain muscles for proper timing during motions. Maintain core and hip strength.
Treatment guidelines	Modalities for pain Trigger point treatment PRN Soft tissue and joint mobilization PRN Proper posture instruction ROM and strength exercises for other UE segments PROM and AROM for tight muscles and joints such as wand exercise, pulley exercise, wall-stretch exercise, or foam roller stretches Weight-bearing and weight-shifting exercises on tabletop or Swiss ball Multiplanar activities without resistance for proper muscle activation such as robber and lawnmower exercises Manual resistance and mild strength exercises for scapular retraction, protraction, depression Core and hip strengthening and stabilization exercises

Stage II: Active phase	
Precautions	Observe and correct for scapular dyskinesis; if present, use tactile cues by tapping lower medial aspect of scapula, and use verbal cues such as "pull your shoulder blade down toward your back pocket" or "squeeze your shoulder blades together slightly" before the patient engages in exercise to encourage scapular positioning and awareness. Avoid shoulder joint pain during activities.

Stage III: Resistive phase	
Goals	Restore proper muscle activation for functional activities. Restore strength of shoulder complex muscles. Recover proprioception. Maintain normal ROM. Achieve normal posture. Maintain core and hip strength.

Figure 21.88   Rehabilitation progression for subacromial secondary impingement.

	Stage III: Resistive phase
Treatment guidelines	Progressive scapular strengthening and endurance exercises from single-plane to multiplanar with proper muscle execution using pulleys, weights, or bands Progressive rotator cuff muscle and large muscle strengthening and endurance exercises using dumbbells, pulleys, or bands, starting at lower levels of elevation and progressing to overhead motions as scapular control and proper humeral head positioning are achieved Dynamic proprioception exercises such as balance board, slide board, or manual resistance exercises Maintenance ROM exercises for HEP Modalities PRN Continued posture instruction and reminders to maintain proper posture Maintenance program for core and hip strength
Precautions	Advance to higher shoulder elevation levels only as patient's strength and control (ability to maintain humeral head in its proper glenoid position) improve.
	Stage IV: Advanced phase
Goals	Maintain normal strength of all muscles. Maintain normal ROM of all joints. Restore normal sport or work performance.
Treatment guidelines	Plyometric exercise progression Functional exercise progression Performance-specific exercises and drills progression
Precautions	Observe for incorrect humeral shrugging during all activities; use verbal cues as needed.

ROM = range of motion; AROM = active range of motion; PROM = passive range of motion; PRN = as needed; UE = upper extremity.

Figure 21.88 *>continued*

program. Finally, the plyometric and functional exercises are incorporated into the program before performance-specific exercises. Once the patient has completed this series of exercises, the patient returns to full activity. Figure 21.88 provides an outline of progression for the rehabilitation of secondary impingement that you may consider using as a guide in this patient's rehabilitation program.

Traumatic Rotator Cuff Conditions

Traumatic rotator cuff injuries are different from degenerative tears that usually occur in older patients. You must take into account several unique factors associated with traumatic rotator cuff injuries before developing a rehabilitation program for a patient with this type of injury.

Traumatic rotator cuff conditions include a spectrum of conditions that includes acute rotator cuff strains, partial tears, complete tears, and post-surgical conditions. Although rotator cuff tears are more commonly seen in older people, patients now begin sport participation at an earlier age and at a greater level of intensity than earlier generations did, so rotator cuff tears are increasingly seen in patients as young as 35.[256] A sudden traumatic event

such as a shoulder dislocation or a fall on the outstretched, laterally rotated arm can cause a rotator cuff tear at almost any age, and it may occur in a healthy rotator cuff or in one with minor asymptomatic changes. More often, however, rotator cuff injuries and tears occur as a result of repetitive stresses, even in younger athletes.[262] These rotator cuff pathologies are associated especially with overhead physical activities in which the musculotendinous unit has encountered chronic stress and tissue fiber damage.[263]

Surgical repair of rotator cuff tears includes open repair, arthroscopic repair, and a combination of arthroscopic and open repair, which is called a mini-open repair.[264] The mini-open repair uses the arthroscope to perform the subacromial decompression and prepare the rotator cuff for repair by extending the arthroscopic puncture wound to a large enough opening to split the deltoid and repair the rotator cuff tear.[264] Open repairs are used more often for large rotator cuff tears where viable tissue may be minimal and damage is extensive.[264] Although an open repair was formerly the repair of choice, arthroscopic repair has proven to be effective in allowing a return to sports, and open repairs are now infrequent.[265] Studies have shown either no difference in results between open and arthroscopic rotator cuff repairs[266] or they have found better results from arthroscopic repairs in terms of postoperative pain and long-term range of motion results.[267]

Even though surgeons may differ in their arthroscopic repair techniques, postoperative rehabilitation often follows a similar course regardless of the technique used. After arthroscopic surgical repair, the starting point, duration, and progression of rehabilitation depend on the size of the tear, the repair procedure, the extent of the surgical repair, the integrity of the deltoid (whether it was cut or preserved in surgery), and the patient's age.[268] If the biceps tendon was involved in the surgical repair, undergoing either a tenodesis or tenolysis, rotator cuff rehabilitation may begin at the usual time, but biceps strengthening is likely to be delayed.[269]

A sling with an abduction brace to avoid extreme adduction and medial rotation is often used immediately after surgery and continued for about 4 to 6 weeks.[270] After 7 to 10 d of immobilization, mild passive and active-assistive range-of-motion exercises may be possible, but this depends on the surgeon's preference.[271] Since repair was performed on active tissue, early active exercises that engage this repaired tissue are usually contraindicated. Until the tissue is strong enough to tolerate stress, early exercises include primarily passive (and occasionally active-assistive) elevation and lateral rotation, extension, and medial rotation. Passive pendulum exercises are also appropriate early in rehabilitation and can be part of the home exercise program. Joint mobilization for pain relief (grades I and II) can be used early as well.[234] With the patient side-lying on the uninvolved shoulder, manual resistance to scapular rotators with the involved arm at the side also begins early in the program.[271]

Some physicians allow mild isometric exercises using a gradual buildup to a desired contraction level of medial and lateral rotators during this time.[271] Trigger point treatments for scapular muscles and rotator cuff muscles may be needed, as indicated by the patient's signs and symptoms. Distal joint motions for elbow, forearm, wrist, and fingers and ball squeezes are performed to increase range of motion in the distal segments. Resistance exercises using manual resistance or dumbbells for these segments can also be started as long as stress is not applied to the shoulder. At the end of the first 3 weeks, rhythmic stabilization with the shoulder at about 90° of flexion begins.[272]

The time to start active exercises depends on the size of the tear and the type of repair, but an average time is approximately 4 to 8 weeks after the surgery.[271, 273] By about week 4 or 5, active ranges of motion in lateral and medial rotation are performed with the elbow at the side.[234] By around week 6 to 8, resistive exercises for the rotator cuff and other shoulder muscles begin.[234, 271] Active range of motion is performed in the scapular plane and is accompanied by isometric exercises in different arm positions as long as the motion is pain free. Resistive exercise with a resistance band or manual resistance can begin for the rotator cuff with the arm kept at the side. By week 8, joint mobilization for increased mobility (grades III and IV) can begin. Biceps and triceps exercises are performed against resistance. Antigravity shoulder extension, supine fly, and prone fly to no more than a horizontal neutral position, as well as weight-bearing scapular stabilization exercises, are suitable at this time. Exercises are performed in a straight plane.

At 10 to 12 weeks, the patient should have nearly full range of motion. More vigorous stretching exercises, such as overhead hangs, are permissible if full motion has not been regained. Exercises should remain in a pain-free range. Medial and lateral rotation exercises start with the shoulder elevated to 90° if scapular control exists. Isokinetic exercises in the scapular plane are appropriate once the patient has enough single-plane strength in the rotator cuff and scapular stabilizers. PNF patterns for strength can be used at this time.

After 12 weeks, the scapular stabilizers should have adequate strength to control the scapula in all levels of elevation. The shoulder should be able to tolerate an advanced strengthening program.[234] Resisted diagonal movements begin in the lower levels, progress to shoulder level, and then progress to above-shoulder levels. Plyometrics such as medicine-ball exercises are started at this time.

At 15 to 18 weeks, resisted rotation exercises with the arm at 90° of abduction can be performed, as can advanced resistive exercises for all shoulder muscle groups. Toward the end of this time, once the patient has full pain-free motion, normal strength of all shoulder muscles, and normal scapulohumeral muscle timing, a progression of functional exercises is begun. By 21 to 26 weeks, the patient should be able to return to full participation. Figure 21.89 provides an outline of this progression from postoperative day 1 to full return to normal activities.

The differences in rehabilitation between a conservatively managed rotator cuff tear and postoperative rotator cuff repair lie primarily in the initial treatment and the progression rate. In conservative (nonoperative) treatment, the inflammation after injury must be initially treated with modalities and modification of activities. Isometric exercises begin earlier for conservatively treated injuries, and active motion can be initiated early as long as the shoulder remains pain free and scapular strength is sufficient to maintain proper scapular stabilization during shoulder motion. Early shoulder medial and lateral rotation exercises are performed with the elbow near the side in a scapular plane. Shoulder elevation can occur to 90° as long as the shoulder is pain free and scapular stabilization is maintained. Resistance exercises begin with high repetitions and low resistance and progress to higher resistance with increased scapular and glenohumeral control.

Rotator Cuff Tear With Surgical Repair

Stage I: Inactive phase	
0-3 weeks	**Inflammation phase: Inactive rehabilitation phase**
Goals	Relieve pain, spasm, swelling. Protect surgical repair. Maintain ROM of elbow and wrist. Strengthen scapular stabilizers without jeopardizing surgical repair. Maintain core and hip strength.
Treatment guidelines	Sling with abduction pillow 4-6 weeks during day Sling at night for 1 month Modalities for pain, swelling, and spasm Grade I and II joint mobilization for pain relief Trigger point treatment PRN Passive pendulum exercises AROM of elbow, wrist, hand Manual resistance to scapular retraction, protraction, depression Core and hip strengthening and stabilization exercises
Precautions	Protect surgical site. Check surgical scars for healing status. Restrict ROM. Follow surgeon's protocol about ROM advances.
Stage II: Active phase	
3-12 weeks	**Early proliferation phase: Active rehabilitation phase**
Goals	Improve glenohumeral range of motion to normal levels. Achieve strength gains of glenohumeral muscles. Recover proprioception. Restore normal strength to distal UE without stress to GHJ.
Treatment guidelines	Progressive scapular strengthening exercises Weeks 2-4: Standing UE weight-bearing activities for stabilization, proprioception exercises Passive and active-assistive range of motion with elbow at side Weeks 3-4: Begin isometric exercises to rotator cuff Weeks 5-8: Start isotonic exercises for GHJ Week 8: Grade III and IV joint mobilization and soft-tissue mobilization PRN Modalities PRN
Precautions	Avoid pain with any strength exercises. Follow surgeon's protocol about motion and strength gains. Provide verbal and tactile cues for proper glenohumeral and scapular motion during exercises and activities.
Stage III: Resistive phase	
12-20 weeks	**Late proliferation phase: Resistive rehabilitation phase**
Goals	Maintain full range of motion. Maintain normal scapular muscle strength and endurance. Achieve normal glenohumeral joint muscle strength. Achieve normal proprioception.

>continued

Figure 21.89 Rehabilitation progression for rotator cuff tear with surgical repair.

Stage III: Resistive phase	
12-20 weeks	**Late proliferation phase: Resistive rehabilitation phase**
Treatment guidelines	Maintenance exercises for range of motion Maintenance exercises for scapular muscle strength and endurance Progressive exercises to strengthen rotator cuff and large GHJ movers (deltoid, pectoralis major, etc.) Dynamic proprioception exercises Isokinetic exercises
Precautions	Avoid shoulder pain with strength exercises. Follow surgeon's protocol. Provide verbal cues for proper shoulder complex positioning during activities.

Stage IV: Advanced phase	
18-36 weeks	**Remodeling phase: Advanced rehabilitation phase**
Goals	Maintain normal strength of all muscles. Maintain normal ROM of all joints. Normal performance in all activities.
Treatment guidelines	Plyometric exercise progression Functional exercise progression Performance-specific exercises and drills progression
Precautions	Observe and correct for proper glenohumeral and scapular function (avoid shoulder shrugging during activities).

ROM = range of motion; AROM = active range of motion; GHJ = glenohumeral joint; PROM = passive range of motion; PRN = as needed; UE = upper extremity.

Figure 21.89   >continued

Evidence in Rehabilitation

Although arthroscopic rotator cuff repairs are commonly performed to provide the patient with a functional shoulder, about half of those repairs do not heal properly.[274] As a result, efforts have been made to biologically improve these outcomes. Orthobiologics is a relatively new term that defines this process. Although the term may be new, the concept is not. **Orthobiologics** is defined as the use of biological substances to enhance the healing process of musculoskeletal injuries.[275] Often these biological substances are from the patients themselves. These substances may include bone grafts, platelet-rich plasma, or stem cells.[275] Bone grafts move bone from one location and attach it to another within the patient's body. Platelets, not red or white blood cells, contain several growth factors that the body uses in tissue growth and repair. Autologous platelet-rich plasma injections deliver human growth hormones into areas with pathology such as rotator cuff tendinopathy to promote healing.

Of these orthobiologics, one of the more interesting and perhaps promising advances is the use of stem cells in shoulder surgery and other orthopedic treatments.[276] Although embryonic stem cells are found only in embryos, mesenchymal stem cells are the type most often used in orthopedics. Mesenchymal stem cells are found in human tissue such as bone marrow, fat tissue, umbilical cords, and amniotic fluid.[277] Among other things, mesenchymal stem cells differentiate into tendon cells. For this reason, some investigators have used stem cells in an attempt to create better results for rotator cuff repairs.[274, 278, 279] Although promising results have been seen from their procedures,[280-282] the process is very controversial.[283, 284] Most concerns center around inconsistent results, inadequate details in reports that limit other investigators' opportunity to reproduce the results, and ethical concerns about potential abuse and misuse of the technology.[283, 284] This is a topic that is sure to become more prominent in the near future.

Arthroscopic Decompression

The continued development of arthroscopic procedures to improve subacromial arch space has improved recovery times after surgery to relieve subacromial impingement.[285] Simple debridement without the need for repairs allows for an uncomplicated and relatively rapid post-surgical process.

Debridement of rotator cuff tendons and decompression of the subacromial space via an **arthroscopy** permits early rehabilitation because there has been no disruption of the deltoid, and the surgical insult is less than with open surgical repairs. A decompression relieves primary impingement, and debridement relieves chronic tendinopathy.

Rehabilitation after arthroscopic decompression can begin immediately after surgery.[286] The first week or two mostly involves modulation for pain and swelling and passive range-of-motion exercises.[286] Grade I and II joint mobilization can be used to achieve pain relief. Early motion exercises can include Codman's exercises and active-assistive range-of-motion exercises with a wand, pulley, or the rehabilitation clinician. Home exercises for motion gains are also beneficial. Medial and lateral rotation exercises start with the elbow near the side with a towel roll between the side and the elbow; they progress to positioning the shoulder at 45° and then 90° of abduction during rotation exercises. Motion activities also include capsular stretches and joint mobilization. Submaximal isometric exercises begin in the first 2 postoperative weeks. Scapular stabilization exercises and biceps and triceps exercises are important in the early program as well. Early neuromuscular control exercises such as proprioception drills for glenohumeral positioning with eyes closed are started early.

Once pain is relieved and near-full motion is possible, straight-plane resistive exercises are added, first below 60° in the scapular plane. As scapular control improves, lateral and medial rotation are performed at 90° of abduction, first with the arm supported, and then with the arm unsupported during exercise. Isokinetics in the scapular plane begin once the patient can perform unsupported and elevated rotation exercises. Full range of motion and good capsular mobility should be present before the patient moves to the next step of the progression. Once scapular stabilization and straight-plane strength goals are achieved, multiplanar exercises using pulleys or resistance bands can be added. These are followed by first low-level, then higher-level (about 90°), and finally overhead medicine-ball activities. Plyometrics are followed by functional exercises, then by performance-specific exercises before the patient returns to normal activities. The entire rehabilitation process may average 3 to 5 months. Figure 21.90 outlines a progressive rehabilitation program for an arthroscopic subacromial decompression.

Arthroscopic Subacromial Decompression

Stage I: Inactive phase	
0-2 weeks	**Inflammation phase: Inactive rehabilitation phase**
Goals	Relieve pain, spasm, swelling. Protect surgical site. Maintain ROM of elbow and wrist. Use PROM for pain relief. Strengthen scapular stabilizers without jeopardizing surgical site. Maintain core and hip strength.
Treatment guidelines	Sling PRN Modalities for pain, swelling, and spasm Grade I and II joint mobilization for pain relief Trigger point treatment PRN Passive pendulum exercises AROM of elbow, wrist, hand Manual resistance to scapular retraction, protraction, depression Core and hip strengthening and stabilization exercises
Precautions	Monitor surgical wounds for proper healing. Refrain from AROM exercises for first 3 days postoperative.

>continued

Figure 21.90 Rehabilitation progression for arthroscopic subacromial decompression.

Stage II: Active phase	
2-6 weeks	**Early proliferation phase: Active rehabilitation phase**
Goals	Achieve full glenohumeral range of motion. Achieve strength gains in glenohumeral muscles. Recover proprioception. Restore normal strength to distal UE and scapular stabilizers.
Treatment guidelines	Progressive scapular strengthening exercises UE weight-bearing activities for stabilization, proprioception exercises Active and active-assistive range of motion of shoulder as tolerated Start with isometric exercises to glenohumeral muscles and progress to isotonic exercises as tolerated Quadruped exercises for stabilization and proprioception Grade III and IV joint mobilization and soft-tissue mobilization PRN
Precautions	Avoid pain over surgical site during exercises. Continue with modalities as needed for pain, edema. Observe for proper glenohumeral and scapular motions during AROM (avoid shoulder shrugging during elevation activities).
Stage III: Resistive phase	
6-12 weeks	**Late proliferation phase: Resistive rehabilitation phase**
Goals	Maintain full range of motion. Maintain normal scapular muscle strength and endurance. Achieve normal glenohumeral joint muscle strength. Achieve normal proprioception.
Treatment guidelines	Maintenance exercises for range of motion Maintenance exercises for scapular muscle strength and endurance Progressive multiplanar exercises Eccentric rotator cuff exercises with shoulder at 90° elevation Dynamic proprioception exercises Isokinetic exercises
Precautions	Continue to monitor for glenohumeral shrugging during elevation activities. Exercises should be performed through a full range of motion.
Stage IV: Advanced phase	
12-20 weeks	**Remodeling phase: Advanced rehabilitation phase**
Goals	Maintain normal strength of all muscles. Maintain normal ROM of all joints. Restore normal performance.
Treatment guidelines	Plyometric exercise progression Functional exercise progression Performance-specific exercises and drills progression
Precautions	Provide verbal cues for correct execution as needed.

ROM = range of motion; AROM = active range of motion; PROM = passive range of motion; PRN = as needed; UE = upper extremity.

Figure 21.90 >*continued*

Case Study

A 19-year-old volleyball player underwent an arthroscopic decompression of her right-dominant shoulder after an 8-week course of rehabilitation failed to alleviate her shoulder pain. The surgery was 2 d ago. The surgeon wants her to begin a rehabilitation program today. On examination she reports normal postoperative shoulder pain, but no more rotator cuff pain. There is minimal ecchymosis around the shoulder. The surgical portal sites are covered with adhesive suture strips. There is some spasm in the rotator cuff muscles and upper trapezius. Range of motion of the shoulder is 150° flexion, 100° abduction, 80° lateral rotation, and 90° medial rotation. Her strength has diminished from preoperative levels and is now 3/5 in the rotator cuff muscles, 3–/5 in shoulder abduction, 3/5 in shoulder flexion, and 4–/5 in the scapular rotators. The patient tends to shrug her shoulder when she elevates the arm. She has a forward head posture with rounded shoulders. You also observe that she has protracted scapulae bilaterally.

Questions for Analysis

1. What do you suspect is the reason she developed a subacromial spur that required her decompression surgery?
2. Given this problem, what will you need to include in her rehabilitation program to correct it?
3. What will you include in your treatment today?
4. What instructions will you give the patient today?
5. What will the next three treatment sessions include?
6. Explain what you will use as guidelines to determine when she is ready to progress from straight-plane to diagonal-plane exercises, from diagonal-plane to plyometrics, and from plyometrics to functional exercises.
7. List four exercises for each exercise level, and justify their inclusion.
8. Describe the functional and performance-specific programs you will use before the patient's return to volleyball.

Glenoid Labral Tears and SLAP Lesions

Glenoid labral tears are difficult to identify. Nevertheless, when they are diagnosed, and whether an anterior or posterior tear is present, special considerations are warranted in designing a rehabilitation program. We look at these considerations first and then at a case study and rehabilitation progression.

Although they are different, glenoid labral tears and SLAP lesions are similar. Glenoid labral tears are a detachment of the labrum from the glenoid. Detachment can occur anywhere on the labrum and can include a range from small to large tears, depending on the forces and mechanisms causing the injury. Labral tears are commonly caused by either sudden forces—such as those associated with dislocations and subluxations—or repetitive stresses on the glenohumeral joint, as is seen with posterior tears in football linemen or anterior tears in throwing athletes.[287, 288] A **SLAP lesion**—**S**uperior **L**abrum tear **A**nterior and **P**osterior in location—also includes tears of the labrum, but it is related to the biceps tendon's insertion on the superior rim of the labrum, not the anterior–posterior glenohumeral stresses seen in frank labral tears.

Evidence indicates that glenoid labrum tears and SLAP lesions are common in other overhead sports such as tennis[289] and in contact sports.[290] Labral tears are the bane of throwing athletes.[291] SLAP lesions also may occur

either as frank injuries or as a result of repetitive stresses.[292] Acute lesions may occur from falling on an abducted arm, causing compression of the joint.[293, 294] In throwers, they often occur secondary to excessive stress applied by the long head of the biceps tendon at its attachment on the rim of the superior glenoid labrum.

Various theories regarding etiology identify the biceps tendon's attachment to the glenoid labrum as a primary contributing factor to SLAP lesions. One theory indicates that during the overhead throwing motion, the biceps' attachment on the glenoid is twisted at the end of the wind-up with the shoulder in abduction and maximal lateral rotation; this position places torsional stress on the tendon's attachment to the labrum.[103, 295] Another theory supports the idea that deceleration stresses of the biceps during release and follow-through apply tension forces on the biceps tendon's insertion and, over time, cause the labrum to tear away from the glenoid fossa.[296] There are others who contend that the presence of SLAP lesions is secondary to glenohumeral instability.[289, 297] Of these theories, the most popular is the one that indicates that SLAP lesions occur because of the tremendous throwing deceleration forces applied in this area when the long head of the biceps tendon strains its insertion site on the labrum as it works to simultaneously decelerate both the shoulder and the elbow.[298] The posterior-superior lesions are thought to occur because of glenohumeral joint instability. If a glenoid labrum tear is present, instability is often an accompanying problem and should be examined and treated as part of the total rehabilitation process.[299]

Labral tears often involve the long head of the biceps, especially when they occur during the wind-up or deceleration and follow-through throwing phases. When the biceps–labral complex is involved, SLAP lesions occur, the labrum can be torn from the superior aspect of the glenoid, and the biceps tendon can be either avulsed with the labrum or suffer a partial tear at its proximal insertion. One surgeon's group noted that 83% of labral tears also involved the biceps–labral complex.[296]

It is important to distinguish between labral tears and SLAP lesions because rehabilitation involves more precautions when the biceps tendon is involved, especially after surgical repairs. Most repairs for both conditions are performed via arthroscopy and involve using sutures to anchor the labrum to the glenoid. Since SLAP lesions include the biceps, postoperative restrictions on elbow flexion and forearm supination must be included with shoulder elevation restrictions during the first few weeks after surgical repair. The following rehabilitation programs for labral tears and SLAP lesions provide progressions that include this constraint.

Labral Tear Rehabilitation

Whether or not instability is present, the usual treatment choice is to try a conservative approach with rehabilitation first. If this is unsuccessful, arthroscopic repair is the most commonly performed surgical technique.[300] A variety of surgical repairs are used for this problem, including Bankart repair and capsulolabral reconstruction.[301, 302]

Given the current advances in arthroscopic surgery, most surgeons opt to repair the glenoid labrum using arthroscopic techniques.[302] If an open repair is needed, the rehabilitation process will be delayed because of the additional time required for immobilization; the rehabilitation program proceeds more slowly and cautiously because of the greater shoulder area involved and the risk of damaging the surgical repair if the rehabilitation is too aggressive. An open repair damages more proprioceptors than an arthroscopic procedure, so rehabilitation for these procedures should emphasize proprioceptive activities once active motion is possible.[303] The open surgical cases will more closely follow the timeline outlined for the rotator cuff repair program discussed previously; refer to that program for guidelines on procedures and timelines.

SLAP Lesion Rehabilitation

SLAP lesions are placed into four categories, depending upon the amount of injury to the biceps tendon and the glenoid labrum to which it attaches.[289] Snyder and colleagues,[293] the first group to use the term *SLAP lesion*, also classified them, and although their initial SLAP classification system has undergone a few revisions, it remains the reference by which SLAP lesions are discussed.[304] A type I lesion has fraying of the superior labrum where the biceps attaches, but the labrum and biceps tendon remain intact (table 21.6). A type II lesion has both the superior labral fraying and some detachment of the glenoid labrum and biceps tendon from the glenoid neck. Type II lesions are further subdivided into three categories: anterior, posterior, and a combination of anterior and posterior (anteroposterior) involvement. Since the glenoid labrum provides stability to the shoulder joint, if it is partially disrupted, instability ensues, requiring surgical fixation to restore stability.[292] In type III lesions, the biceps tendon and labrum remain attached at their peripheral margins on the fossa, but there is a bucket-handle tear of the central section of the labrum. In type IV lesions, there is both a bucket-handle tear of the labrum and a tear of the biceps tendon at its attachment site, so portions of the labrum and tendon appear as a flap that may shift within the joint. Arthroscopic fixation is usually performed on type III and type IV lesions, while arthroscopic debridement is the usual treatment for type I and II SLAP lesions.[289] If there is a substantial biceps tendon tear of more than 30% of its substance in a type IV lesion, the surgeon will use sutures in an arthroscopic repair of the tendon along with fixation of the tendon and labrum to the glenoid.[305]

A few years after Snyder's group developed the four classifications of SLAP lesions, Maffet and his associates[306] found shortcomings with the Snyder system and created three additional types of SLAP lesions. Their revision was based on the fact that they found that their SLAP lesion patients often had additional conditions that had to be considered in their diagnoses and treatment.

The rehabilitation of SLAP lesions is unique since the biceps is important to the function of both the shoulder and the elbow. In addition, as indicated in table 21.6, various lesions and degrees of lesions can occur, so the severity of injury and the physician's choice to approach the problem surgically or nonsurgically further complicate rehabilitation choices. In addition to complex SLAP lesion classifications, other shoulder lesions such as rotator cuff tears, Hill-Sachs lesions, chondral lesions, and instability also occur with SLAP lesions,[298] making the treatment process even more challenging for rehabilitation clinicians. If any of these conditions are also present, the rehabilitation program may need more than the average amount of time for full recovery.

Specific rehabilitation techniques and their rates of progression depend upon the extent of the injury and the surgery performed. As you would expect, rehabilitation after a debridement is much more aggressive and faster than rehabilitation after a surgical repair. In the rehabilitation examination, the clinician identifies precautions based on the mechanism of injury. For example, if the patient's injury involved a traction-type mechanism such as that which occurs with deceleration forces, the patient should avoid eccentric and higher-weight exercises until the surgical site can tolerate the stresses. On the other hand, if the patient's injury was caused by compression of the joint, which often occurs in rugby players or football linemen,[308] then weight-bearing exercises should be avoided until the area is sufficiently healed. These precautions should be observed regardless of the type of surgical correction the patient has undergone.

Rehabilitation of SLAP Lesion Debridement

When conservative care has not resolved the patient's problem, debridement is the surgical option used to manage type I and II SLAP lesions.[304] Rehabilitation for

TABLE 21.6   Types of Biceps Tendon–Glenoid Labrum (SLAP) Lesions and Their Treatment

Type of lesion	Visual representation	Description	Surgical treatment
Type I		Fraying of superior labrum at site of long head of the biceps attachment	Arthroscopic debridement Biceps tenodesis or tenotomy if frayed, hypertrophied, or synovitic
Type II		Fraying present in type I along with some degree of labral and biceps tendon detachment off glenoid rim Type IIa: superior-anterior detachment Type IIb: superior-posterior detachment Type IIc: combined superior-anterior and superior-posterior detachment	Arthroscopic repair with instability or persistent pain
Type III		Bucket-handle tear of the superior attachment of the labrum and biceps tendon with peripheral margins intact with the glenoid rim	Arthroscopic repair of glenoid labrum to glenoid rim Biceps tenodesis or tenotomy if frayed, hypertrophied, or synovitic

>continued

TABLE 21.6 >*continued*

Type of lesion	Visual representation	Description	Surgical treatment
Type IV		Bucket-handle tear of the labrum and biceps tendon from the rim along with detachment of the biceps tendon from the labrum	Arthroscopic repair of biceps tendon and glenoid labrum to glenoid rim
Type V		Additional pathology: Bankart lesion in anterior capsule and its attachment to anterior labrum	Arthroscopic repair of both pathologies
Type VI		Avulsion of biceps tendon from glenoid rim and glenoid labrum along with superior anterior–posterior labral tear off the rim	Arthroscopic repair of all pathologies unless open repair is indicated
Type VII		Tear of glenoid labrum from superior anterior rim and inferiorly far enough to affect middle glenohumeral ligament	Arthroscopic repair of all pathologies unless open repair is indicated

Based on Snyder et al.[293] with revisions by Maffet et al.;[306] Some surgical recommendations based on Michener et al.[307]

a SLAP lesion debridement begins within the week after surgery. The patient likely wears a sling for the first 3 d or so, primarily for discomfort that immediately follows surgery. Thereafter the patient often finds that the sling is not needed. Although it may be uncomfortable, passive and active range-of-motion exercises may begin within a day of the surgery. Sometimes patients find that moving the shoulder actually reduces the normal postoperative discomfort.[230] Motion activities are more comfortable when performed in the scapular plane. Full range of motion in all planes should be normal within 2 weeks.

Strengthening exercises begin early when only debridement has been performed. During the first week, the clinician can introduce pain-free isometrics for the glenohumeral muscles and scapular muscle strengthening using manual resistance to the scapular rotators.[309] Neuromotor and proprioception exercises for the glenohumeral joint begin with early joint position sense activities. After the first week, isotonic exercises with resistance begin

for the glenohumeral muscles.[309] More active neuromotor and proprioception exercises, including weight-bearing activities, begin after the first week as well. As with other shoulder rehabilitation programs, elevation of the shoulder against resistance occurs in a progressive manner as the patient becomes able to maintain good glenohumeral position and stability through scapular muscle control during glenohumeral activities.

Between weeks 4 and 6, plyometric exercises using medicine balls begin.[309] By this time, the patient has good control of the glenohumeral joint and can appropriately recruit the scapular muscles, so there is no impingement or hyperactivity of the upper trapezius. The last phase of rehabilitation occurs in the third to fourth months.

Rehabilitation of SLAP Lesion Repair

A rehabilitation progression for a SLAP lesion repair is shown in figure 21.91. The program's rate of progression will vary depending on the location and extent of the repair.

Type II SLAP Lesion Repair

Stage I: Inactive phase	
0-3 weeks	**Inflammation phase: Inactive rehabilitation phase**
Goals	Relieve pain, spasm, swelling. Protect surgical repair. Maintain ROM of elbow, wrist, and hand. Strengthen scapular stabilizers without jeopardizing surgical site. Maintain core and hip strength. Achieve early gains in proprioception.
Treatment guidelines	Sling 3-4 weeks Modalities for pain, swelling, and spasm Grade I and II joint mobilization for pain relief Sling removed for PROM for pain relief after week 1 Trigger point treatment PRN Passive pendulum exercises after week 1 AROM of elbow, wrist, hand Manual resistance to scapular retraction, protraction, depression Core and hip strengthening and stabilization exercises Mild isometrics of rotator cuff toward the end of week 1 Week 2: Rhythmic stabilization and co-contraction for proprioception
Precautions	Follow surgeon's protocol. Monitor surgical wound for proper healing. Refrain from AROM exercises for first 3 days postoperative. Avoid pain with exercises. Avoid active engagement of biceps or stress to glenoid labrum during manual scapular exercises. Week 2: PROM is limited to no more than 90° of elevation in the scapular plane; rotation occurs with elbow near the side in the scapular plane: 0° lateral rotation and medial rotation to the abdomen. Week 3: Achieve lateral rotation to 15°.

>continued

Figure 21.91   Rehabilitation progression for type II SLAP lesion repair.

Stage II: Active phase	
2-12 weeks	**Early proliferation phase: Active rehabilitation phase**
Goals	Achieve full glenohumeral range of motion. Achieve strength gains in glenohumeral muscles. Recover proprioception. Restore normal strength to distal UE and scapular stabilizers.
Treatment guidelines	Progressive scapular strengthening exercises Active and active-assistive range of motion of shoulder as tolerated Start with isometric exercises to glenohumeral muscles and progress to isotonic exercises as tolerated Quadruped exercises for stabilization and proprioception Grade III and IV joint mobilization and soft-tissue mobilization PRN Week 6: Begin easy biceps strength exercises Weeks 7-8: Begin posterior capsular stretches
Precautions	Avoid pain during exercises. Until week 6: Avoid biceps activity or glenoid stress during scapular muscle exercises. By week 6: Achieve full ROM in all motions except lateral rotation. By weeks 8-10: Achieve full ROM in all motions.
Stage III: Resistive phase	
12-20 weeks	**Late proliferation phase: Resistive rehabilitation phase**
Goals	Maintain full range of motion. Maintain normal scapular muscle strength and endurance. Achieve normal glenohumeral joint muscle strength. Achieve normal proprioception.
Treatment guidelines	Maintenance exercises for range of motion Maintenance exercises for scapular muscle strength and endurance UE weight-bearing activities for stabilization, proprioception exercises Week 12: Aggressive biceps strength exercises begin Progressively higher-motion resistance exercises as patient gains strength and control at lower levels of ROM Progressive multiplanar exercises Eccentric rotator cuff exercises with shoulder at 90° elevation Dynamic proprioception exercises Isokinetic exercises
Precautions	Continue to monitor for glenohumeral shrugging during elevation activities. Raise height of resistance during elevation exercises only as patient gains strength and maintains shoulder control. Exercises should be performed through a full range of motion.
Stage IV: Advanced phase	
20-36 weeks	**Remodeling phase: Advanced rehabilitation phase**
Goals	Maintain normal strength of all muscles. Maintain normal ROM of all joints. Restore normal sport and work performance.

Figure 21.91   *>continued*

Stage IV: Advanced phase	
20-36 weeks	**Remodeling phase: Advanced rehabilitation phase**
Treatment guidelines	Plyometric exercise progression Functional exercise progression Performance-specific exercises and drills progression
Precautions	Provide verbal cues for correct execution as needed.

ROM = range of motion; AROM = active range of motion; PROM = passive range of motion; PRN = as needed; UE = upper extremity.

Figure 21.91 >continued

Given this variability, a SLAP repair rehabilitation progression is more conservative than that for a debridement.

A big consideration is the status of healing tissue. The effects of the program should be to move the patient in an efficient and progressive manner to normal activities without disrupting the healing tissues. Postoperatively, the patient's arm is placed in a sling for 3 to 4 weeks, and the sling is removed only for bathing.[24] During this time, the clinician controls inflammation, swelling, and pain with modalities and manual techniques effective for those purposes. The patient is given a rubber ball or sponge ball to perform squeezes throughout the day.

After 1 week, the arm is removed from the sling for exercises.[24] These exercises are initially passive range of motion and are limited to no more than 90° of elevation in the scapular plane; rotation is performed with the elbow near the side in the scapular plane: 0° of lateral rotation and medial rotation to the abdomen. The patient can also start pendulum exercises a few times a day and can perform elbow and forearm active range-of-motion activities. After the first 2 weeks, passive lateral rotation to 15° is permitted.[292]

Strength activities begin as isometrics in the first week but should not be painful. Scapular stabilization is also started in the first week using manual resistance to scapular protractors, retractors, and depressors with the shoulder in a comfortable resting position. Rhythmic stabilization for proprioception and co-contraction is started during the first 2 weeks.[292]

During weeks 3 to 6, the patient continues to work on scapular stabilizer muscles and rhythmic stabilization exercises for proprioception and strength training as long as the exercises do not stress the glenoid or biceps. Resistance-band exercises for medial and lateral rotation with the elbow at the side, shoulder extension, shoulder flexion to 90°, and shoulder abduction to 45° in the scapular plane can begin as long as the exercises are pain free.[310]

By the sixth week, the shoulder should have full motion except in lateral rotation, which should be about 45°. Full lateral rotation should be achieved without pain by weeks 8 to 10.[311] Early biceps strengthening exercises can start at weeks 6 to 8, but aggressive biceps strengthening is avoided for another 6 weeks.

Posterior capsular stretches begin between weeks 7 and 8. Strengthening exercises using weights for the rotator cuff, deltoid, pectoralis major, and scapular muscles begin at this time as well. This is when weight-bearing exercises are introduced for the first time. The caveat is that these exercises must be pain free. Strengthening of the muscles surrounding the shoulder continues to progress as tolerated during this 8- to 12-week time frame.[292] As long as the scapular muscles can control the glenohumeral position, the arm can also be raised overhead for full-motion resistance exercises at this time, and exercises can also occur for medial and lateral rotation with the shoulder elevated to 90°.[311] By 12 weeks, the biceps is stable enough to tolerate more aggressive resistance and exercises, so the bench press, military press, and latissimus pull-downs are added at the 3-month mark.[292] During this 3- to 4-month period, stretches continue to preserve full motion, and exercises become more specific to the patient's needs. For example, if the patient needs power and strength, then a program is designed with high resistance and fewer repetitions, but if the patient will return to an endurance activity, then low resistance is used with higher repetitions.

By 4 to 5 months, the patient progresses to functional activities, once goals for flexibility, strength, endurance, and neuromotor control are met.[292] The transition from the functional phase of the program to the performance-specific phase depends upon the patient's response to the exercises and the surgeon's objectives. Throwers usually begin easy throwing during the fourth postoperative month. A progressive program of performance-specific routines must be monitored for gradual progression without pain or other deleterious effects from the activities. It may take a patient 6 to 8 months to fully recover and 9 to 12 months to resume normal activities after a SLAP lesion repair.[292]

Post-rehabilitation outcomes following SLAP lesion treatments vary widely, whether the treatments are surgical or nonsurgical.[312, 313] Variables that influence the outcome include factors such as the patient's age, the severity of the injury, comorbidities involved, impairments, and physical demands.[307, 312] Some patients may not fully return to preinjury performance levels, while others have been able to return to their former activities and perform even better.[307] Patients and clinicians should understand the possibilities—patients, so they can make more informed decisions about their treatment, and clinicians, so they can try to provide optimal rehabilitation experiences for their patients.

Adhesive Capsulitis

Adhesive capsulitis is more commonly seen in patients over age 35 than in younger patients, but it does occur in younger age groups, especially in those with some endocrine disorders.[314] Understanding the condition is essential to designing an appropriate rehabilitation program.

Adhesive capsulitis is commonly referred to as a *frozen shoulder*. The condition was first described by Codman in 1934. After investigating the glenohumeral joint's synovial changes in 1945, Neviaser identified the condition as "adhesive capsulitis."[315] The generic term for adhesions in the capsule is arthrofibrosis. Adhesive capsulitis is divided into two subcategories based on the etiology: idiopathic and secondary.[316] Idiopathic adhesive capsulitis is also primary adhesive capsulitis and is the diagnosis used when no etiological condition or cause can be identified.[316] Idiopathic frozen shoulder occurs spontaneously. Idiopathic frozen shoulder occurs predominantly in middle-aged patients, in females more than males, usually between 35 and 70 years old.[317] This condition occurs gradually, so patients do not usually seek medical attention until they find themselves unable to perform daily activities. Women commonly report not being able to attach their bra behind them, and men complain that they cannot remove their wallet from a back pocket. Secondary adhesive capsulitis occurs when there is an underlying cause or medical condition or a history that may lead to a frozen shoulder.[316] These conditions or histories can include surgery that changes the biomechanics of the shoulder, prolonged immobilization of the shoulder, scar tissue adhesions in the capsule or ligaments surrounding the shoulder, and prolonged inflammation of the tendons, bursa, and other soft tissue around the shoulder.[318, 319] Other non-injury-related conditions that have been associated with adhesive capsulitis include diabetes mellitus, thyroid pathologies, and hypoadrenalism.[316, 318]

Immobilization causes adhesions in connective tissue that can reduce muscular tissue mobility. Reduced muscle tissue mobility decreases the number of sarcomeres in the muscle.[320] The additional changes that occur with immobilization in muscle, joints, and supportive tissue were discussed in chapter 2. When the glenohumeral joint capsule is affected, loss of motion is most notable in lateral rotation, abduction, and flexion of the shoulder. A capsular pattern of motion loss in the glenohumeral joint is evident with lateral rotation more limited than abduction, abduction more limited than flexion, and flexion more limited than medial rotation.[81] Because these changes occur after injury or immobilization, secondary adhesive capsulitis may occur in persons under age 35.[314]

Reeves[321] identifies three stages through which patients with adhesive capsulitis progress before resolution, and Neviaser[322] identified four stages. The primary difference between Reeves and Neviaser is that Neviaser divided stage I into two different stages to delineate changes in patient pain reports and histology within the capsule. To keep concepts simple, we will discuss Reeves' three stages of adhesive capsulitis. Table 21.7 provides a summary of

TABLE 21.7   Stages of Adhesive Capsulitis

Stage	Histology	Duration	Signs and symptoms	Treatment
I: Freezing stage	Inflammatory agents present	6 weeks to 9 months	Pain is greatest problem; achy pain with rest, sharp pain with motion; nocturnal pain; loss of motion in flexion, abduction, and rotation, especially lateral rotation	Modalities for pain relief; grades I–II joint mobilizations; AROM; avoid stretching
II: Frozen stage	Fibrosis of capsule evident	6 months	Loss of motion is most evident and is the greatest problem; pain at ends of motion; minimal nocturnal pain	Ultrasound prior to other treatments; grades III–IV joint mobilization; active stretches; strengthening to maintain motion gains
III: Thawing stage	Evidence of chronic inflammation; presence of inflammatory agents with fibrosis of capsule	6 months to 2 years	Motion gains have occurred; pain minimal at the ends of motion	Continued joint mobilizations and stretching exercises to preserve motion gains; strengthening scapular rotators, rotator cuff, and large glenohumeral muscles to achieve normal function

these three stages. Stage I is the "freezing stage," when pain is the primary problem; stage II is the "frozen stage," when the pain has subsided but range-of-motion loss is predominant; and stage III is the "thawing phase" with the recovery of motion.[321] The entire process without treatment intervention may take up to 3 years.[323]

As shown in figure 21.92, when adhesive capsulitis is in stage I, hallmark signs include shoulder pain, pain at the end ranges of movement, difficulty sleeping on the shoulder, and progressive loss of motion. The pain is achy at rest and sharp with movement.[324] It is during this stage that the capsule shows signs of inflammation with the presence of inflammatory cells in the area.[325] Lateral rotation demonstrates the greatest loss of available motion, with movements of flexion, abduction, and medial rotation showing less loss. This stage may last anywhere from 2 to 9 months.[317] The most effective treatment at this time is active and active-assistive range-of-motion exercises within the tolerated ranges.[326] Joint mobilization should not be painful and should be oriented more toward pain relief (grades I and II) than mobility gains.[327] Stronger mobilization grades only aggravate the capsule and may promote an inflammatory response or cause a reactive muscle spasm that will increase pain. Active range-of-motion and AAROM exercises maintain muscle length. Attempts at stretching the capsule at this time cause pain but little change in mobility. The goals during the freezing stage are to reduce the pain and the inflammatory response of the shoulder.[324]

By the frozen stage (II), adhesive capsulitis has become evident both in motion and arthroscopically.[328] The glenohumeral joint has lost its normal mobility, so the shoulder is very stiff; this is the primary complaint. There is pain at the end of available motion. Pain overall is less than it was during the freezing phase, and with the shoulder at rest or during sleep, pain is minimal. The patient may complain of pain in the elbow and of being unable to lie on the shoulder. This stage lasts about 6 months.

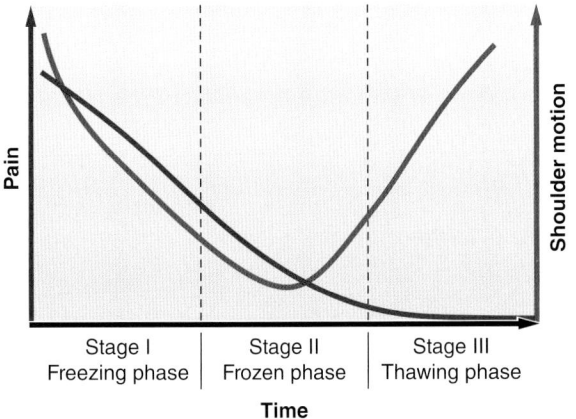

Figure 21.92 Intensity of pain and amount of range of motion during the different phases of adhesive capsulitis.

CLINICAL TIPS

If patients with adhesive capsulitis are treated while they are still in stage I of the injury, treatment to regain motion will not be effective, and there will be a greater risk of increasing pain and reducing motion. It is better to wait until patients are in the frozen phase to begin treatment. Once the rehabilitation program is completed, patients will likely regain full functional motion and ability, but they will not have 100% of normal shoulder motion.

At this time, more aggressive joint mobilization is used as long as it does not produce an inflammatory response. Joint mobilization has been shown to be effective in reducing pain and improving motion during this phase.[329] Continued active stretches are also used. Strengthening exercises in the available ranges are a part of the program. Although there is some conflict in the literature, applying ultrasound before joint mobilization may improve results from the mobilization.[330, 331] Modalities and exercises during this phase are designed to reduce pain and restore range of motion. Joint mobilizations and home exercise programs are also part of the rehabilitation program.[323]

In the final, thawing stage, the patient's pain is minimal, and motion gains are evident.[332] The primary area of pain is distal on the arm, not in the shoulder. There is pain at rest as well as during activity. It may take up to 3 years to complete this phase.[323] At this stage, there is evidence of chronic inflammation within the capsule.[333] Histological and cellular studies indicate an ongoing inflammatory process with the presence of agents that create chronic inflammation and the development of a fibrotic capsule that is seen clinically when passive range-of-motion assessment demonstrates a hard, leathery end-feel with more profound motion loss in a capsular pattern.[333] Scapulohumeral rhythm is lost because glenohumeral capsular restrictions prevent normal motion between the scapulothoracic and glenohumeral joints. Because glenohumeral rhythm is lost, shoulder elevation is replaced with shoulder shrugging, and the scapula moves at the same time and rate as the humerus.

Grade III and IV joint mobilizations are used at this time.[327] Continued range-of-motion exercises and active stretches as part of the home exercise program are performed throughout the day to promote mobility gains. Self-mobilization techniques are taught and are included in the patient's home program. Strength exercises for the scapular rotators, rotator cuff, and large glenohumeral muscles (deltoid, pectoralis major, teres major, and latissimus) are included in a progressive program.[326] Since scapular dyskinesis often accompanies adhesive capsulitis, exercises to restore proper muscle timing are needed as part of the rehabilitation process.[334] If the patient is not treated until the glenohumeral joint is in the third stage, a 3- to 6-month treatment program may be needed to resolve the condition.

Rehabilitation of adhesive capsulitis can be a prolonged process. Patients usually do not recover full motion after having this condition, but they recover enough motion to perform functional activities.[335] It has been demonstrated that patients with frozen shoulders do better when rehabilitation techniques are combined with cortisone injections.[336] Most patients with adhesive capsulitis recover well enough with rehabilitation techniques and do not need surgery.[337]

Acromioclavicular Sprain

Although first-degree sprains are not usually difficult to manage, the treatment approach for more severe acromioclavicular (AC) sprains is more complex.

Acromioclavicular sprains were first classified into three categories, based on their degree of instability.[338] A couple of decades later, this classification was expanded to include another three groups.[339] These six categories are provided in table 21.8. As with most classifications, these range from slightest to greatest injury.

Most AC sprains fall into the lesser injury classifications and are not surgically repaired but are treated conservatively.[341] Surgery is the treatment of choice in cases where the person's injury remains painful or demonstrates persistent joint instability.[342] The speed with which conservative care is advanced depends on the severity of the injury and the patient's response to treatment.

In sprains treated conservatively without surgery, the shoulder may be immobilized in a sling for a few days to relieve the traction discomfort caused by the weight of the arm pulling on the AC joint.[343] Modality use relieves pain, swelling, and muscle spasm. Pain-free active and active-assistive range-of-motion exercises are initiated on day 1 or 2 after the injury. Isometrics to tolerance also begin immediately.[343] Once full motion is restored, a progression of strengthening exercises is used until the patient has full function without pain, has normal motion and strength, and can return to full sport participation unimpeded.

In type II and III sprains, the AC ligament is torn. In type II sprains the coracoclavicular ligament is intact, but in type III sprains it is not.[338] Some deformity is present in both type II and type III sprains.[338] Attempts at restoring alignment often fail because of the discomfort and restriction of the immobilizing device and the difficulty in stabilizing the AC joint. The benefits of surgical repair for type III sprains are disputable.[344] Some surgeons opt for a 6- to 12-week trial of rehabilitation to determine whether surgery would be beneficial; if there is little or no response to conservative treatment, surgery is indicated.[345] If nonsurgical treatment is selected, a sling is used to relieve the distraction force of the weight of the arm on the AC joint, and then the rehabilitation process is begun. Some deformity usually persists, but this is a cosmetic issue and does not interfere with activity or shoulder function. The more severe injuries (types IV, V, and VI) are surgically repaired, especially in overhead throwing athletes, because of the significant damage to both static and dynamic structures

TABLE 21.8   Classification of AC Sprains

Classification	Frequency[340]	Description[340]	Treatment course
Type I	Very common	Isolated sprain of AC ligaments; no instability; no deformity; no disruption of the joint	Conservative with rehabilitation
Type II	Very common	Complete tear of the AC ligaments with sprain of the coracoclavicular (CC) ligaments; some AC instability; mild deformity with minimal displacement of the clavicle superiorly	Conservative with rehabilitation
Type III	Common	AC joint dislocation with tear of AC and CC ligaments; obvious deformity with superior positioning of distal clavicle relative to acromion; distal clavicular instability vertically and horizontally	Either conservative care with rehabilitation or surgical repair
Type IV	Unusual	Posterior dislocation of distal clavicle; may also have SC injury or dislocation; AC ligament disruption and usually CC ligament disruption, but not always	Surgical repair
Type V	Rare	Dislocation as in type III but additional damage to deltoid and upper trapezius muscles; obvious deformity with tent appearance of soft tissue over AC area	Surgical repair
Type VI	Very rare	Inferior dislocation from high-energy trauma; clavicle is forced inferiorly; associated with other severe injuries	Surgical repair

AC = acromioclavicular; CC = coracoclavicular; SC = sternoclavicular.

Based on Tossy et al.;[338] Rockwood et al.[339]

around the joint.[346] Surgical patients do not begin isotonic exercises until week 12, but isometrics begin after weeks 1 or 2. Pain-free scapular manual resistance exercises can also begin early since they will not stress the AC joint. Since motions of full elevation, medial rotation, and horizontal adduction compress the AC joint, these motions are delayed for the first few weeks and permitted only if they are pain free. Weight-bearing exercises without pain are also used about weeks 6 to 8. As with most other shoulder conditions, the patient should have full shoulder range of motion by about weeks 10 to 12.

In the type II and III injuries, the shoulder may be immobilized for 1 to 2 weeks. Active-assistive range-of-motion exercises for the glenohumeral joint may begin early and include closed-chain exercises.[345] If proprioception is deficient, basic exercises to restore it can begin early in the program and advance as pain subsides and motion and strength improve. Strengthening exercises (below 60°) follow a normal shoulder rehabilitation progression from stabilization and weight-bearing, straight-plane, and low-level elevation exercises to higher-level elevation exercises and diagonal movements.[345] Plyometric exercises are followed by functional exercises. Normal progression to heavy lifting occurs at about 8 to 12 weeks postinjury, and the patient returns to full participation after having performed functional exercises correctly.

By now, you should notice a pattern within rehabilitation programs. Consideration for the healing process is a primary factor in deciding when to make activities more difficult. The clinician must be very aware of exactly what tissues are involved in the injury or surgical repair and should protect those elements, especially early in the rehabilitation process. Once the injury enters the proliferation healing phase, especially the latter half of that phase, there is less concern for protecting the tissue and more concentration on building and restoring deficient factors. The clinician is always alert for substitutions and uses the patient's complaints of pain as a guiding factor in providing exercises and progressions. If you look at each of the rehabilitation programs provided for the shoulder in this chapter and take away the unique factors for each injury, the progression of rehabilitation varies only slightly and is based on how well the tissue heals.

Biceps Tendinopathy

Although it might seem appropriate to deal with the biceps tendon in the elbow chapter, the long head of the biceps plays an important role in shoulder stabilization;[347] therefore, it is presented in this chapter. Since the most common injury seen in the biceps tendon is tendinopathy, we will address that injury here. Bicipital tendinopathy occurs primarily in the long head tendon and usually occurs as a result of shoulder instability, impingement, rotator cuff pathology, or overuse of the shoulder.[202, 348] The patient reports tenderness in the bicipital groove. Cervical pathology can refer into the arm and biceps area and must be ruled out if no frank injury has occurred to cause the pain.[349]

Rehabilitation treatment must include an examination of the rotator cuff because its pathology is often related to biceps and anterior arm pathology.[232] As with any pathology that develops over time, the underlying causes for it must be identified and corrected. Control of pain, swelling, and inflammation is an initial goal of treatment. The use of modalities, pain medication, and rest initially may be beneficial. Rest is usually accompanied by active-assistive range-of-motion exercises. Initial resistance exercises primarily include eccentric exercises for the biceps.[350] Pain is an important guide in determining when to start an exercise and when to progress it. Any biceps rehabilitation program should also include supination and elbow flexion exercises.

Total Shoulder Arthroplasty

As with other joint replacements, total shoulder arthroplasty is a last-resort surgery for people with severe shoulder osteoarthritis (OA). Unfortunately, people under age 65 are often affected with disabling OA. For these patients, the best option may be a resurfacing of the joint or a hemiarthroplasty, a surgical procedure that usually involves replacing the humeral head. The best results, however, have occurred with TSA rather than with the hemiarthroplasty[351] or other interventions for pain relief and restoration of function.[352] Patients who receive TSAs are younger than those who receive either the THA or the TKA.[351]

There are two major types of TSA—the traditional type with the humeral head and glenoid fossa (figure 21.93a), and the reverse total shoulder arthroplasty (rTSA), or reverse shoulder arthroplasty (RSA), in which the convex portion of the joint is the scapular component and the concave portion is the humeral component (figure 21.93b). Patients considered good candidates for a TSA have intact rotator cuffs. If a TSA is the only option remaining, but the rotator cuff is neither repairable nor viable, a rTSA may be the best option;[353] investigations show a significant reduction in function 6 years after implantation if the anatomic TSA is used in patients with damaged rotator cuffs.[353, 354] However, it is unclear whether this accelerated deterioration occurs because of faulty design of the prosthesis; because the patients had very deficient, damaged shoulders before the surgery; or because the rotator cuff's center of rotation is changed, causing increased stresses on the scapular component.[351]

Although the rTSA has been available in Europe since 1994, it has been used in the United States only since 2003.[355] Even after such a short time, the benefits of the rTSA have become apparent for those whose rotator cuffs are nonfunctional. Postoperatively, these patients have better shoulder elevation and overall function than those whose rotator cuffs are torn and have the anatomic

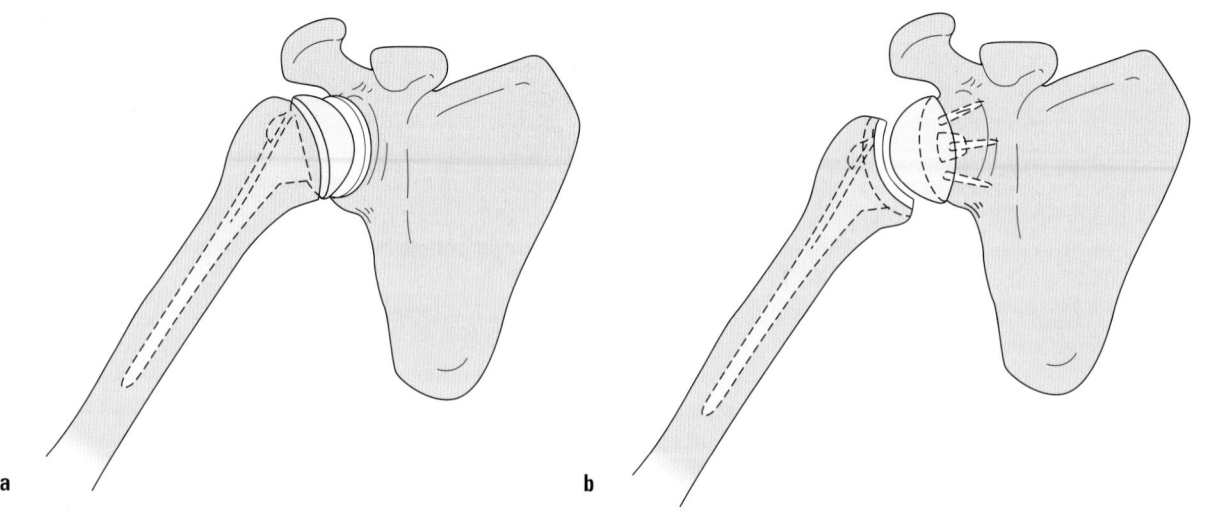

Figure 21.93 Total shoulder arthroplasty (TSA). *(a)* Traditional TSA; *(b)* reverse TSA.

TSA procedure.[356] By reversing the convex and concave surfaces, the deltoid can take over functions of shoulder elevation that have been lost by the damaged rotator cuff.[357] Reverse total shoulder arthroplasty patients achieve around 120° of elevation, while the rotator cuff–damaged patients who undergo anatomic total shoulder arthroplasty achieve around 60° of elevation.[358]

The TSA surgical procedure varies somewhat, but the basic technique involves an anterior incision from a point lateral to the coracoid process and inferiorly toward but not to the axilla.[359] The pectoralis tendon is detached, as is the subscapularis tendon, and the humeral head is then excised.[359] The humeral head replacement is either cemented in or placed in the humeral medullar canal without cement.[359] The cementless technique relies on bone ingrowth to secure the prosthesis.[360] The glenoid is then prepared for its prosthesis, and the artificial glenoid is cemented in place.[357] The detached tendons are then reattached and the surgical site is closed by layers. Staples or Steri-Strips hold the skin layer in place.

Postoperatively, the patient may have the arm in a sling or an immobilizer with the shoulder positioned in medial rotation, adduction, and some forward flexion.[361] If other procedures such as a rotator cuff repair were also performed during the TSA, other postoperative restrictions may also be indicated. The rehabilitation clinician must communicate with the surgeon so that appropriate follow-up rehabilitation may be provided.

Although there is no consensus on postoperative rehabilitation, there is good agreement on common movement restriction recommendations for lateral rotation for the first 3 to 6 weeks.[361, 362] Although most clinicians agree that the shoulder should be removed from the sling for PROM exercises, the amount of early movement advised varies from one investigator to another.[361] Since the subscapularis is cut during preparations to dislocate the joint before osteotomy, some authors recommend limiting lateral rotation

to neutral, while others indicate that it is safe to allow 30° or 40° of lateral rotation.[361] Other passive PROM limits may include flexion and abduction restrictions to 90° for the first 3 weeks because the pectoralis major is the other muscle that is detached and reattached during the surgical procedure.[362] Therefore, these motion restrictions protect the anterior capsule and subscapularis and pectoralis tendons that were reattached during the implant surgery. Some surgeons find it beneficial to have their patients use a continuous passive motion machine during the first few early postoperative weeks.[363]

To protect the repaired rotator cuff muscles, patients are often instructed to avoid moving their shoulders past the midline into extension and to avoid the combined motions of medial rotation, adduction, and extension since that position puts the joint at risk for dislocation.[364] These patients are usually advised during the first 6 to 8 weeks to keep their shoulders positioned so they can see their elbows. The progression of rehabilitation for rTSA provided in figure 21.94 provides average recommendations for precaution, motion, and strength progressions. Any clinician who is rehabilitating a total shoulder replacement patient must obtain a copy of the rehabilitation protocol that the physician prefers to use for his or her post-op patients.

Immediately after surgery, the patient's arm is kept in a sling for 3 to 6 weeks and taken out of the sling only for exercises and showering.[352] Early exercises, which are passive, include pendulum exercises and tabletop exercises. The tabletop exercises are performed with the patient's hands in a weight-bearing position on the table. In this position, the patient's body moves from side to side to allow the shoulders to move into horizontal abduction and adduction; trunk flexion moves the shoulders into flexion; and with only the hand of the involved side on the table, the patient rotates the body toward and away from the hand to provide medial and lateral rotation at the shoulder (figure 21.95).

Total Shoulder Arthroplasty

Stage I: Inactive phase	
0-3 weeks	**Inflammation phase: Inactive rehabilitation phase**
Goals	Control and treat pain, spasm, and swelling. Protect the surgical site. Protect the subscapularis. Maintain proper immobilization of the repair site via sling or immobilizer. PROM: flexion and abduction 90°; lateral rotation 0°-45°. Maintain core and hip strength. Maintain independence in self-care.
Treatment guidelines	Day 3: Remove bulky surgical dressing, inspect and care for surgical site Week 1: Arm elevation to reduce edema Use immobilization device and sling Grade I and II joint mobilizations for pain Modalities for pain, swelling, and spasm PROM to shoulder in scapular plane Codman's exercises AROM for elbow, wrist, and hand Trigger point treatment PRN Week 2: Isometrics for scapular muscles Core and hip strengthening and stabilization exercises
Precautions	Monitor surgical site for proper healing. Wear sling unless otherwise instructed. Use a support pillow behind the shoulder and elbow to prevent shoulder extension when lying supine. Do not drive for 3 weeks after surgery. Follow surgeon's protocol.
Stage II: Active phase	
4-7 weeks	**Early proliferation phase: Active rehabilitation phase**
Goals	Relieve pain to 0–2/10. Increase shoulder ROM: flexion to 135°; abduction to 135°; LR to 45°- 60°. Improve dynamic stability of shoulder.
Treatment guidelines	Continue modalities PRN Continue TrP release PRN Week 4: Begin AAROM Joint mobilization Wand exercises and reciprocal pulleys Submaximal isometrics for rotator cuff Deltoid isometrics Aquatic exercises Manual resistance and other early stabilization exercises for scapular muscles, especially protraction, retraction, and depression without glenohumeral motion Early CKC proprioception exercises Week 6: Begin easy weight-bearing exercises Week 6: Resistance band exercises for medial and lateral rotation
Precautions	Respect healing tissues. Avoid pain. Follow surgeon's protocol.

>continued

Figure 21.94 Rehabilitation of total shoulder arthroplasty.

Stage III: Resistive phase	
8-16 weeks	**Late proliferation phase: Resistive rehabilitation phase**
Goals	Avoid pain. Achieve full AROM, all planes. Strengthen muscle groups. Week 12: Resume driving.
Treatment guidelines	Remove sling Exercises for full ROM in all planes Joint mobilization PRN Biceps and triceps resistance exercises Scapular resistance exercises Rotator cuff resistance exercises Weight-bearing exercises
Precautions	Avoid sudden jerking, lifting, or twisting shoulder motions. Avoid resistance exercises above level where scapular control is lost. Avoid shoulder pain with strength exercises. Follow surgeon's protocol. Provide verbal cues for proper shoulder complex positioning during activities.

Stage IV: Advanced phase	
16-24 weeks	**Remodeling phase: Advanced rehabilitation phase**
Goals	Maintain normal strength of all muscles. Maintain normal ROM of all joints. Achieve normal sport and work performance.
Treatment guidelines	Plyometric exercise progression Functional exercise progression Performance-specific exercises and drills progression
Precautions	Observe and correct for proper glenohumeral and scapular function (avoid shoulder shrugging during activities).

ROM = range of motion; PROM = passive range of motion; AAROM = active-assistive range of motion; AROM = active range of motion; PRN = as needed; LR = lateral rotation; CKC = closed kinetic chain.

Figure 21.94 >continued

Weight-bearing exercises for the shoulder facilitate proprioception, reduce pain, and stabilize the joint by recruiting co-contraction activity of the agonists and antagonists.[188] Passive rather than active motion is used during early rehabilitation to reduce stresses to the deltoid, subscapularis, and joint. Passive lateral rotation and active medial rotation are restricted in the first several weeks to reduce the pull on the subscapularis tendon. Active exercises for the elbow, wrist, and hand are performed often throughout the day.

When the patient is not exercising, the arm is in a sling. At night, the patient should lie supine with a support (such as a pillow) placed posterior to the humerus and elbow, and the sling should be worn throughout the night so that the shoulder does not move into hyperextension.[365] Sometimes patients find it more comfortable to sleep in a recliner chair, but they should still place pillows behind the shoulder and elbow.

The patient may begin rehabilitation exercises within a week or two after surgery. It is important to work on motion gains rather than strength gains during the first month. By the end of the third week, the patient should have about 130° of passive flexion and around 25° of passive lateral rotation.[366] These desired motions may vary from one surgeon to another, so the clinician must know the specific goals physicians set for their patients and work

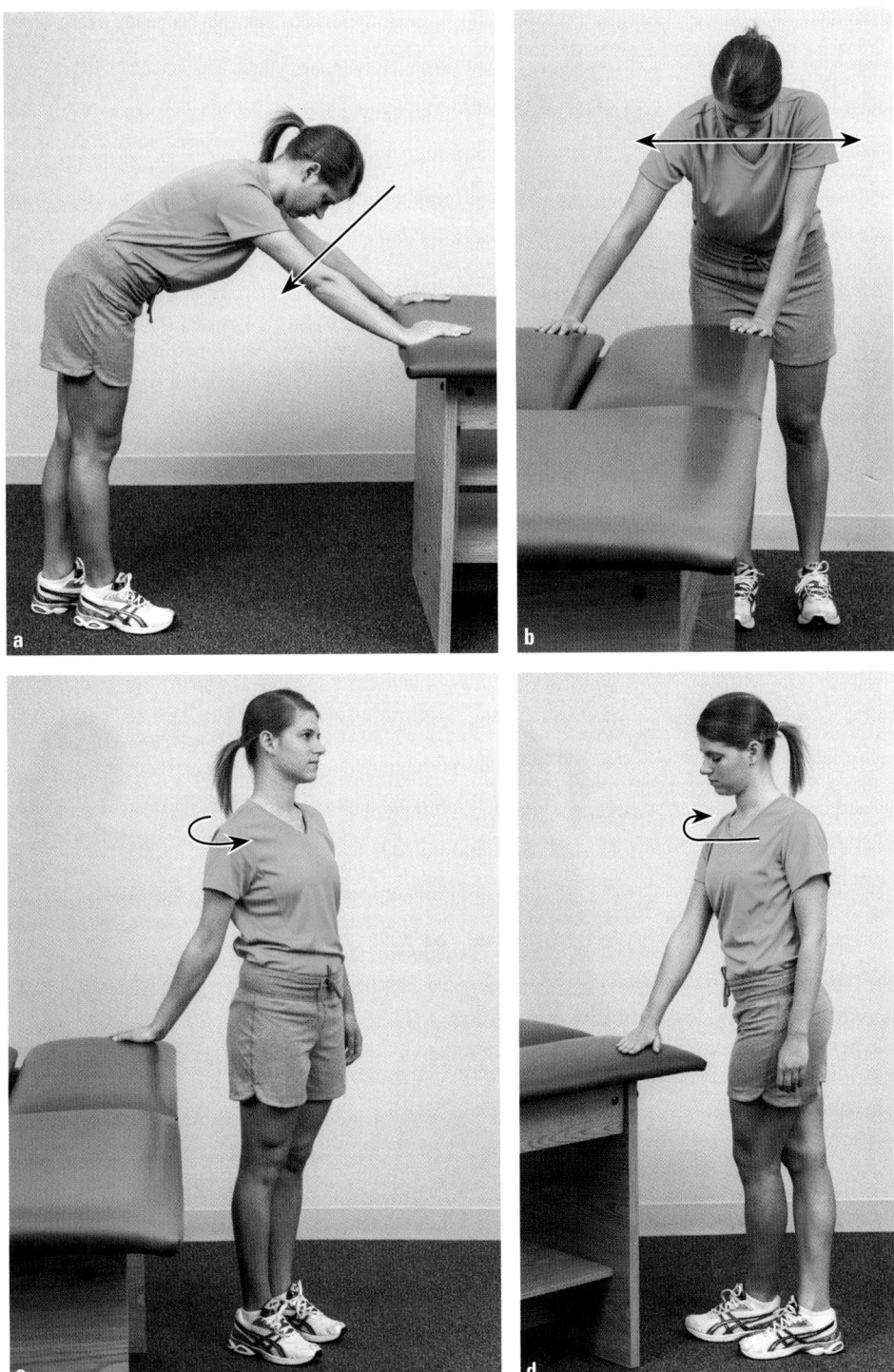

Figure 21.95 Weight-bearing exercises for range of motion for total shoulder arthroplasty patients. *(a)* Patient anchors hands on table and leans forward to move shoulder into flexion. *(b)* With hands anchored on table, patient moves the body side to side. *(c)* Patient anchors hand and rotates body away from arm to move shoulder into lateral rotation. *(d)* Patient anchors hand and rotates body toward arm to move shoulder into medial rotation.

to achieve them. Rotation and abduction motions should be performed in the scapular plane because there is less risk of subacromial impingement in this plane than in the sagittal plane.[367]

Although strength exercises for the rotator cuff and other glenohumeral muscles are essentially avoided during the first 6 to 8 weeks after surgery, scapular muscles can be strengthened during this time. Manual resistance applied directly to the scapula can strengthen scapular muscles in motions of elevation, depression, protraction, and retraction without stressing the glenohumeral joint. Wrist and hand resistance exercises with light to medium weights can be started around the third post-op week.

By the eighth to tenth week, the patient begins light-resistance, high-repetition exercises for the shoulder muscles, including the rotator cuff and deltoid. Light dumbbell weights and elastic resistance or rubber tubing exercises may be used at this time. The patient can also remove the sling around this time. Rotation and abduction are performed in the scapular plane. Full shoulder motion should be present sometime between weeks 8 and 12. Sudden jerking, lifting, or twisting motions of the shoulder are avoided to reduce the risk of dislocation. Activities such as Swiss ball proprioception motion circles, low-elevation (less than 60° elevation) resistance exercises, and weight-bearing resistance exercises are used to improve both glenohumeral and scapular muscle strength. After weeks 12 to 16, the patient should increase strength, making gains similar to those experienced by a rotator cuff repair patient.

The patient progresses in the rehabilitation program to functional and performance-specific exercises by the fourth to sixth month before resuming normal activities. Depending on the specific shoulder joint arthroplasty used, the patient will regain functional but not necessarily normal range of motion; final flexion range of motion may vary from 80° to 120° with rTSA[365] and to 157° with TSA.[368]

Summary

The shoulder undergoes tremendous stresses during use, especially in upper-extremity sport activities such as throwing and sustained overhead work activities such as auto repair. Shoulder area trigger point treatments were outlined, and joint mobilization techniques were presented. Rehabilitation program elements from flexibility to activity-specific exercises were presented in a progressive manner throughout the chapter. Of special concern in the shoulder area is scapular dyskinesis; this pathological condition is usually slow in onset but results in a number of secondary problems of the shoulder. Glenohumeral stability during normal activities is also a common malady of the shoulder complex that must be identified and treated if the patient's upper extremity is to function without difficulty. Two primary muscle groups provide glenohumeral stability: (1) scapular muscles, which anchor the glenohumeral joint to the trunk to provide a stable platform from which the joint functions, and (2) the rotator cuff, which provides glenohumeral stability so the larger "mover" muscles such as the deltoid, pectoralis, and latissimus can perform their functions at the shoulder. Some of the more common injuries seen in rehabilitation of the shoulder complex were presented with suggested rehabilitation progressions.

LEARNING AIDS

Key Concepts and Review

1. Discuss the importance of stability in shoulder rehabilitation.
The stability of the glenohumeral and scapulothoracic joints is crucial to performance and to reducing the risk of shoulder injuries. The glenohumeral joint is stabilized by strong scapular muscles that move and hold the scapula in positions that are advantageous for glenohumeral function. Studies have demonstrated the significance of good stabilization of these joints and the importance of good therapeutic exercise programs to restore stability to these areas.

2. Explain the role of scapular stabilization in shoulder function.
Scapular stabilization is basic to shoulder function. Scapular muscles serve as the foundation upon which the shoulder moves, so when scapular muscles do not function properly because of weakness, loss of motion, or limited endurance, the shoulder is at great risk of injury.

3. Define *scapular dyskinesis*.
Scapular dyskinesis is an orthopedic term used to define the condition in which the scapula is malpositioned on the thorax with a posteriorly prominent inferior medial border and does not move properly during shoulder elevation. It is sometimes referred to as SICK scapula.

4. Explain how scapular dyskinesis can affect the shoulder's function.
Scapular dyskinesis creates abnormal kinematics of scapular and clavicular motions because of its pathological position on the thorax and its dysfunctional muscle activation during shoulder elevation. Scapular dyskinesis creates an unstable scapula that functions pathologically. Pathologic function of the scapula and clavicle result in a number of shoulder problems, including glenohumeral instability, subacromial impingement, rotator cuff tendinopathies, and rotator cuff tears. Without a stable scapula, the glenohumeral joint functions from an unstable base, causing a chain of dysfunctional events throughout the shoulder complex, all of which place it at risk for injury.

5. List three joint mobilizations for the shoulder.
Shoulder joint mobilization techniques target the restricted joints. If the AC joint is restricted, PA, AP, and inferior glides can be used. If the scapula is restricted, scapular distraction is appropriate. If the glenohumeral joint is restricted, an arm pull is a gross technique, and an inferior glide is a more specific technique for improving joint mobility. Joint mobilization must be performed in grades III and IV to improve motion.

6. Identify three strengthening exercises for the scapulae and three for the glenohumeral muscles.
Scapular muscle strengthening exercises can include maneuvers such as the push-up plus, prone fly, and Bouhler exercises. Glenohumeral muscle strengthening exercises can include medial and lateral rotation exercises starting with isometric exercises and moving to resistance-band and free-weight exercises, as well as abduction in the scapular plane.

7. Discuss the general rehabilitation progression of strengthening exercises for the shoulder.
The specific progression depends on the injury and its severity. A general progression of strengthening exercises begins with scapular stabilization exercises and isometric rotator cuff exercises. Manual resistance to the scapular muscles can begin early in the program. From there, the exercises include active-resistive exercises in the lower third of shoulder motion until the scapular muscles are strong enough to provide control in the middle ranges of motion, and finally in motion over 100°, so overhead exercises can be performed with scapular and glenohumeral positioning in control. Eccentric exercises for the rotator cuff using resistance bands, medicine balls, and even manual resistance begin in straight planes and progress to diagonal planes. Exercises in both weight bearing and non–weight bearing are used for stabilization and strengthening. Plyometric activities begin slowly and progress as the patient gains proficiency. Functional exercises using sport equipment such as a tennis racket or golf club then follow, at first in low ranges of motion with reduced force until control and proficiency have been demonstrated. Exercises then progress to greater ranges of motion and begin to mimic the actual activity. Functional overhead activities advance to performance-specific exercises; they are the last item to be added to the rehabilitation program. In addition to the shoulder, the biceps, triceps, and core muscles must also be included in the rehabilitation program.

8. List precautions for a rehabilitation program following a rotator cuff repair.
Care must be taken to allow tissue healing before exercises begin. Range of motion usually begins at 7 to 10 d. If immobilization continues for an extended period, there can be complications such as adhesive capsulitis, especially in patients over 30 years old. Range-of-motion exercises begin with activities such as Codman's and must progress on the basis of the status of the healing tissues. Strength exercises begin slowly with high endurance and low resistance, progressing as the patient gains control and strength. Scapular exercises can be initiated early, but rotator cuff exercises begin with submaximal isometrics. Range-of-motion gains in lateral rotation occur slowly and cautiously.

9. Outline key factors for a rehabilitation program for a biceps tendinopathy.
Early identification and correction of root causes for the condition is essential to prevent a recurrence of the pathology. Active range of motion for shoulder, elbow, and forearm is followed by strengthening exercises for motions including elbow flexion, supination, and shoulder flexion and extension. Early strengthening exercises for the biceps are limited to eccentric exercises and progress to concentric as the biceps responds to treatment. The progression of exercises follows a pattern similar to that for other shoulder programs, with considerations for pain, control, and tissue healing occurring early in the program and aggressive exercises at the end.

Critical Thinking Questions

1. If you were Logan in the opening scenario for this chapter, what techniques would you have used to relieve Benj's posterior shoulder tightness and the scapular muscle weakness? What plyometric exercise progression would you have used to advance him to functional activities? What criteria would you have used to begin his functional activities, and what would your throwing progression have been?

2. If an injured wrestler who experienced an anterior shoulder dislocation 2 weeks ago comes to you to begin rehabilitation, what must your most important precaution be? Into how much elevation can you safely have the patient move his shoulder, and why? What exercises should you be able to do with him at 2 weeks postinjury?

3. If one of your baseball pitchers has undergone an arthroscopic Bankart repair, when can you begin to rehabilitate this player? Based on your knowledge of healing and the shoulder, what precautions should be taken, and what exercises can you perform in the first 3 to 6 weeks postoperatively?

4. Recall the case of the 40-year-old tennis player presented in the section on impingement in this chapter. Have you figured out the cause of her problem? If posture is a primary contributing factor, what instructions will you give her to improve her posture? What exercises will you give her to change her posture? If her posture has been incorrect for some time, what soft-tissue changes will need to be treated?

5. If you have a patient whose rule-out diagnoses have been narrowed down to rotator cuff tendinopathy, shoulder instability, shoulder impingement, capsulitis, and cervical radiculopathy, how will you determine which diagnosis is correct? What tests will you use to differentiate between these diagnoses? Would the rehabilitation program change with different diagnoses? Why or why not?

6. A sophomore softball pitcher is diagnosed with a type II SLAP lesion. She is scheduled to have surgery tomorrow. She wants you to outline for her what she will be doing and how long her rehabilitation will take. She knows that the surgeon has already spoken with you and wants you to start her on rehabilitation 2 d after surgery, but she is concerned that she will be too sore and painful to do anything. She has never had an injury before that has required surgery, so she is apprehensive about the surgery and concerned that she will not be able to pitch again. What will you say to her, and how much will you outline of what lies ahead for her? What will you say to reduce her fears about the surgery and her pitching career?

7. As a clinician working in a sports medicine clinic, you have a new patient who is a 45-year-old downhill skier who had a total shoulder arthroplasty 1 week ago. You have the physician's rehabilitation protocol and are familiar with this surgeon's work because you have treated patients of hers in the past. What restrictions will you have in your evaluation of this patient today? In other words, what will you not be able to do with this patient that is part of your normal shoulder examination? What potential problems do you expect this patient to express to you today? How will you manage them during his first treatment? What items will you include in your explanation of the plans you will have for his rehabilitation program? You suspect that he is having problems sleeping because of his recent surgery; what suggestions will you give him that might make it easier for him to sleep?

Lab Activities

1. With your lab partner as a patient, perform grade I, II, III, and IV joint mobilizations on all shoulder complex joints. For the glenohumeral joint, apply an inferior glide to determine joint mobility. Identify how large the movement is for each of the grades as you go through the joint's total mobility range. Now repeat the examination on another person. How does the range of mobility of each joint compare between the individuals?

2. Apply the following joint mobilization techniques on your partner. While applying each technique, notice where the resistance to movement occurs and where movement stops. Why are these items important to assess for each motion and joint?

   A. Glenohumeral anterior glide

   B. Glenohumeral posterior glide

   C. Glenohumeral lateral glide

   D. Scapulothoracic glides

   E. Acromioclavicular inferior glide

   F. Acromioclavicular anterior–posterior glides

   G. Sternoclavicular AP glide

   H. Sternoclavicular PA glide

3. Locate the trigger points for the following muscles on your lab partner:

   A. Subscapularis

   B. Supraspinatus

   C. Infraspinatus

   What muscles contained your lab partner's most sensitive trigger points? Perform a treatment on the most sensitive areas after you have examined the muscle's active range of motion. After the treatment, have your partner repeat the active ROM so you can determine the effectiveness of your treatment. How did the AROM change from before to after the treatment? Why?

4. If your partner has a tight anterior and inferior capsule, list the shoulder motions that will be restricted and the flexibility exercises you would give him. Have your partner go through them and tell you where he feels the stretch.

5. If your partner has a tight posterior capsule, identify the motions that will be restricted and list the flexibility exercises you would give her. Have your partner perform each exercise and tell you where she feels the stretch.

6. Teach wand exercises to increase shoulder flexion, abduction, horizontal abduction, and lateral rotation to your partner and have him perform each one. List all possible substitution patterns he performs and the verbal cues you use to correct these patterns.

7. Perform isolated scapular exercises using manual resistance on your partner to protraction, retraction, and depression in side-lying and supine. How many repetitions for each exercise could she perform before fatigue occurred? How could you identify when she fatigued? Based on your findings, set a goal for her next treatment session's exercise.

8. Have your partner perform a progression of push-up exercises, beginning with wall push-ups and ending with box jumps on the floor (use footstools). List the progression you used and the number of repetitions your partner could do. What are you looking for in terms of his or her performance? How are you determining when your partner has performed enough repetitions to reach adequate fatigue levels?

9. Have your partner perform one exercise each for the lower trapezius, middle trapezius, serratus anterior, and rhomboids. List the exercise and how many repetitions your partner could perform correctly. What would be a progression for each exercise, and when would you advance your partner to the next level?

10. Have your partner perform one exercise for each of these shoulder muscle groups: abductors, MR, and LR. Describe the exercise you have chosen, why you have chosen it, how many repetitions your partner could do, possible substitution patterns to watch for, and your next progression for each exercise.

11. Have your partner perform any two of the scapular stabilization exercises in this chapter. What muscle did your partner feel working while executing the exercise, and what possible substitution patterns could have been used?

12. Have your partner perform any two of the plyometric or functional exercises in this chapter. What purpose do they serve (goals for the exercise), and what substitution patterns could be used for each? How will you determine when she should advance to the next level of exercise (what are your goals)? Can you think of another plyometric or functional exercise that is not in this chapter?

22

Elbow and Forearm

Objectives

After completing this chapter, you should be able to do the following:

1. Discuss why you should avoid overstretching the elbow, especially during the inflammation phase of healing.
2. Describe the convex-on-concave rules for the various elbow joints.
3. Identify the resting positions for the elbow joints.
4. List three joint mobilizations for the elbow, and identify why they would be used.
5. Explain three strengthening exercises for the elbow and their purpose.
6. Discuss the general progression of strengthening exercises for the elbow.
7. Outline a rehabilitation program for epicondylopathy.
8. Indicate precautions to consider in a Little League elbow rehabilitation program.
9. List precautions for a rehabilitation program following an ulnar nerve transposition.
10. Explain the differences between rehabilitation programs for an arthroscopic elbow debridement and a medial collateral ligament reconstruction.

Brian has worked as the certified athletic trainer in the local high school for the past 10 years. Occasionally a parent brings a preteen athlete to him, knowing that he has worked successfully with the child's older sibling. He normally provides an examination of the youngster's injury and makes recommendations to the parents for first-aid treatment or referral to the family physician.

Today, he is visited by a parent who is familiar to Brian because she has had two teenagers pass through Brian's athletic training facility during their high school careers. Mrs. Daisy reports that her youngest son, 10-year-old Abraham, developed medial elbow pain while pitching in a Little League baseball game last week. Although it had been bothering him for a couple of weeks before last week's game, Abraham hadn't complained about it until the pain became too intense.

From his past experience, Brian suspects Little League elbow. But he knows he should not assume anything and should perform an examination with an open mind before he identifies his differential diagnosis.

All the forces in the world are not so powerful as an idea whose time has come.

Victor Hugo, 1802-1885, French poet, novelist

Like the shoulder, the elbow has special and distinct characteristics that must be considered when developing rehabilitation programs for elbow injuries. As the joint between two long moment arms, the elbow can experience large applications of force from its proximal and distal arms. Open-chain activities apply large velocities with sudden acceleration and deceleration forces from the proximal arm of the joint, while closed-chain activities apply compressive stresses and torsional forces from the distal arm. The differences in the effects of these forces are important in the elbow and are discussed later in this chapter. Elbow muscles must work synchronously with adjacent muscles, and the joints and muscles must have the mobility, flexibility, and strength they need to withstand these forces.

Because the elbow lies between the shoulder and wrist, some muscles that traverse the elbow also affect either the shoulder or the wrist. It is difficult to separate these, and thus it was difficult to decide which chapter some of the techniques and exercises should be discussed in. It may seem that some of the techniques and exercises discussed here would be better suited to the shoulder or wrist chapter, but how best to classify an exercise depends on the injury. For example, if a patient has a tennis elbow injury, exercises and techniques for wrist extensor muscles are appropriately discussed in the context of the elbow. However, if a patient has a wrist sprain, those same techniques and exercises for wrist extensor muscles are best addressed in a discussion of wrist injuries. For this reason, some of the techniques and exercises you read about in this chapter are also mentioned in chapter 23 on the wrist and hand.

This chapter outlines basic considerations for elbow rehabilitation and then presents specific rehabilitation applications. A list of soft-tissue techniques, joint mobilization techniques, flexibility exercises, strength exercises, and plyometric and functional considerations are then presented. Considerations for some of the more commonly seen elbow injuries are discussed, and case studies for some of these injuries are presented so that you can problem-solve and devise your own rehabilitation programs.

Special Rehabilitation Considerations

The rehabilitation clinician must understand the distinctive characteristics of the elbow to properly design and execute a rehabilitation program for it. You should also appreciate how the design and function of the elbow add to the mobility and function of the hand. The following sections focus on these characteristics.

Relationship Between the Scapula, Shoulder, and Hand

As in the lower extremity, there is a kinetic chain relationship between the joints of the upper extremity. Chapter 21 addresses the importance of scapular stability for shoulder function. Both scapular stability and optimal shoulder function are equally important for elbow function. There must be a stable base proximally for the elbow to effectively and efficiently place the hand in space. At the same time, the mobility and stability of the elbow and forearm allow for optimum use of the hand for functional tasks. Flexion and extension of the elbow, rotation of the forearm, and adequate muscular control all enable functional activities of the hand such as dressing, grooming, eating, reaching, using tools or utensils, catching, throwing, and hitting. When you treat elbow injuries, the scapula and shoulder must be included in the rehabilitation program to ensure that the upper extremity works at its best. Depending on the patient's goals, it may also be necessary to incorporate trunk stability and lower-quarter strengthening into the rehabilitation program.

Joint Stresses

As mentioned in chapter 21, overhead motions are actually total body movements that include a summation of forces and properly timed execution of movements that start in the lower extremities and trunk and transfer forces to the shoulder, elbow, and hand. As the summation of forces accelerates the extremity in throwing sports, the elbow and forearm velocity must reach high rates to successfully propel the hand or the object it holds at the desired speed. Researchers have reported different angular velocities for different sports. Baseball pitching produces the highest velocity, at 2300°/s.[1, 2] Javelin throwers produce an angular velocity of 1900°/s,[3] the tennis serve has been recorded at 982°/s,[4] and in fast-pitch softball, 680°/s velocities have been recorded.[5]

Most of these overhead motions place additional valgus or varus stress on the elbow. The greatest applications of force occur during either the late cocking and early acceleration or the deceleration phase of a throw.[2, 6] At the elbow, high demands are placed on the biceps, brachioradialis, and brachialis during deceleration to slow forearm motion and prevent overextension and injury to the elbow. During acceleration, the elbow experiences compressive forces laterally and distraction forces medially. In part, this is because of the anatomical design of the distal humerus, which has a more distally positioned medial condyle (trochlea) than its lateral condyle (capitulum). In the anatomical position, we can easily see the valgus angulation of the forearm to the humerus (carrying angle) that occurs because of the anatomy of the proximal elbow joint segment. Valgus torque on the elbow increases significantly during flexion activities such as cocking and early acceleration, and there are large compressive forces on the lateral elbow during rapid extension activities such as those seen in throwing[7, 8] (figure 22.1).

Since the medial elbow is stretched during flexion activities, the stresses placed on this part of the elbow are tension stresses. Excessive or repeated tension stress can result in injuries such as neuritis, tendinopathy, and medial joint sprains and muscle strains.[8, 9] Since the lateral elbow is compressed during extension activities, lateral compressive stresses are applied to this aspect of the elbow and can cause compression injuries to the bones; these injuries include osteochondritis dissecans in young athletes and bony osteophytes, loose body formations, articular damage, and degeneration in older athletes.[8, 9]

It is common for athletes with a lengthy throwing career to develop flexion contractures because of articular and muscular changes. As these changes occur, elbow biomechanics adapt, and joint stresses become magnified. Proper mechanics, timing, and balanced joint and muscle function are crucial in the prevention of elbow injuries. It is important to remember that the forces applied to the elbow during pitching and other throwing activities

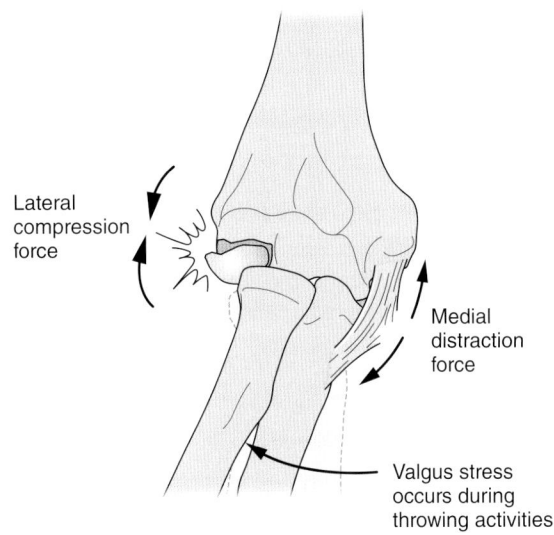

Figure 22.1 The elbow has compression forces applied to the lateral joint and distraction forces applied to the medial aspect during throwing and throwing-like activities.

include a valgus distraction stress medially with a lateral compressive force.[8, 10]

Tennis produces stress over the lateral epicondyle during the backhand stroke, and it produces medial epicondyle distraction stresses during overhead serves and late-hit forehand strokes.[11] Gymnastics, an upper-extremity weight-bearing sport, places excessive lateral compressive stress on the joint because of the elbow's normal valgus position. Golfers with incorrect mechanics can place excessive medial distraction force on the trailing elbow or excessive lateral compressive force on the leading elbow.[12] Pitchers with inflexibility in the hips, trunk, or shoulder open up too soon during their delivery and increase the elbow's medial joint distraction stress. If shoulder tightness, weakness, or fatigue causes the elbow to drop, increased medial joint stresses are placed on the elbow during the cocking phase in pitching.[13] In tennis, increased lateral compressive stress is placed on the elbow when the player leads with the elbow on the backhand, and increased medial distraction stress is applied on the forehand stroke when the ball is hit late.[14]

It is important for the rehabilitation clinician to understand these stress and torque applications because at some point during the rehabilitation program, the clinician must examine how the patient executes skills. Incorrect techniques may be the underlying cause of the patient's problem, and the program must include correction of those techniques to prevent a recurrence of the injury.

Unique Structure

The elbow has unique anatomical characteristics that create advantages and disadvantages. There is a high degree of congruency within the humeroulnar joint. That design makes it stable. The brachialis muscle traverses the joint and inserts onto the ulna. The biceps brachii's short head and long head tendons merge into the muscle proximally, and distally its tendon not only attaches to the radial head but also extends fibers that form the bicipital aponeurosis, blending with the fascia that covers the medial proximal forearm muscles. This aponeurosis is believed to help stabilize the medial forearm muscles.[15] Cadaveric studies have revealed that many people have two separate biceps brachii muscle bellies, rather than one, with two separate tendon attachments to the radial tuberosity.[16] This variation in biceps anatomy, however, does not seem to change biceps function at the elbow.

Stiffness and reduced motion can easily occur in the elbow after injury or surgery.[17, 18] Basic science research has found that after injury or surgery, the elbow capsule becomes thicker than normal and contains large numbers of myofibroblasts, factors that lead to capsule stiffness and contracture.[19] Animal studies have shown that capsular restriction occurs 2 to 4 weeks after injury;[20] such findings indicate the need for early elbow mobilization. Immobilization must be used cautiously, and extended periods of immobilization should be avoided.[21] Based on these findings, immobilization for more than 2 weeks can cause elbow mobility restrictions.

Adhesions occur rather easily in the elbow, but the joint's anterior capsule is normally rather thin, so it can easily incur damage if stretched too aggressively, resulting in additional scarring. For this reason, it is important that aggressive, high-intensity stretching at the elbow be avoided. This is especially crucial during the inflammation phase, when the area is weaker and more easily aggravated than it will be later.[22] Soft-tissue tearing, scarring, and loss of joint motion can occur with passive overstretching. Early stretching techniques should mainly feature active stretches, not passive stretches. Passive range-of-motion exercises are permissible, but they should be pain free and performed in controlled and monitored situations.

CLINICAL TIPS

Throwing activities focus great forces on the elbow, with medial valgus torque occurring primarily during late cocking and early acceleration. This can place excessive tension stress on medial structures. As the elbow extends during acceleration, the lateral elbow has forces up to 500 N (112.4 lb) compressing it.[7] With these high forces delivered repetitively, injuries common to the elbow include medial-tension injuries such as ligament sprains, muscle strains, neuritis, and tendinopathy, while the lateral-compression injuries include osteochondritis dissecans in young athletes and bony osteophytes, loose-body formations, articular damage, and degeneration in older athletes.

Joint Mobility

The elbow has three joints that should be examined for mobility: the humeroulnar, humeroradial, and radioulnar joints. Each elbow joint has different **resting** and **close-packed positions** that are important to know when performing mobilization techniques. The humeroulnar joint's resting position is at 70° of elbow flexion with 10° of supination, and its close-packed position is full extension. The humeroradial joint's resting position is at full extension and full supination, and its close-packed position is at mid-flexion with mid-pronation. The radioulnar joint's resting position is at 70° of elbow flexion with 35° of supination, and its close-packed position is full pronation or full supination. Joint mobilization is initially performed in the resting position, where the capsule has the greatest mobility. In later rehabilitation phases, it may be necessary to move the joint into other loose-packed positions to perform mobilizations in an effort to regain full motion. The close-packed position can also be used as an exercise position for unstable joints to provide increased stability during resistance activities.

Because the humeroulnar and humeroradial joints have a concave ulna and concave radius moving on a convex humerus, the concave-on-convex rule applies for mobilization techniques to these joints. Therefore, the application of mobilization force should be in the same direction as the restricted movement. Joint distraction applied in a resting position will stretch the anterior and posterior capsule. If the elbow is placed in flexion, and distraction is applied, the posterior capsule is stretched to increase elbow flexion, but if distraction is applied with the joint in extension, the anterior capsule is stretched to increase elbow extension.

The radius and ulna are connected by two joints, the proximal radioulnar joint immediately distal to the elbow and the distal radioulnar joint just proximal to the wrist. Both joints must have normal movement to produce full forearm supination and pronation. The proximal joint is formed by the convex radial head in the ulna's concave radial notch. This joint abides by the convex-on-concave mobilization rule. Therefore, the mobilization force is applied in the opposite direction from restricted movement. For example, to improve supination, the force is applied posterior-to-anterior; to improve pronation, the force is applied anterior-to-posterior. The distal radioulnar joint is presented in chapter 23.

Force Applications

Depending on the injury, the clinician may need to take special precautions with some strength exercises. Stresses applied to the elbow during strengthening can be excessive, depending on the arm position and the weight lifted. Lifting weights with the elbow extended places more stress on the anterior elbow, while lifting weights with the elbow flexed places more stress on the posterior elbow. Because of moment-arm lengths, a resultant force of up to three times body weight occurs when the elbow is flexed 30°.[5] Lighter weights or cuffs attached to the mid-forearm reduce these stresses and should be used, especially with earlier strengthening exercises.

A weight-bearing exercise such as a push-up delivers stress to the elbow, but the arm position determines the degree of stress. In a normal push-up position, the greatest compression force at the elbow is 45% of body weight, but the compression force is decreased if the hands are moved farther apart.[23] When the hands are placed in a superior position, the compression force decreases in the elbow, but the valgus torque increases by 54%.[5] Progressing a push-up from a wall to a table, to kneeling, and then to a normal push-up position will help reduce stresses to the elbow until the injury can tolerate the stress of a regular push-up.

Low-resistance, high-repetition strength exercises are used in the early phases of elbow rehabilitation to reduce excessive joint stresses. Once tissue healing has progressed and neuromuscular control and strength gains permit good joint control, higher weights with lower repetitions can be used.

Rehabilitation Interventions

Although modalities are included in rehabilitation programs for elbow injuries, they are not included in this section. These modalities are presented in chapter 9; the selection of modalities for elbow injuries depends on the injury and the patient. The soft-tissue techniques for the elbow covered in this section are complementary alternative medicine applications. These techniques include trigger point release, soft-tissue massage, myofascial release techniques, and instrument-assisted soft-tissue mobilization (IASTM). Descriptions of joint mobilization techniques follow the sections on soft-tissue mobilization. In addition to these manual therapy techniques, a variety of exercises, beginning with flexibility exercises and continuing through to performance-specific exercises, are presented.

Soft-Tissue Mobilization

Recall from chapter 11 that trigger points are a common cause of muscle pain.[24] The trigger point referral patterns and trigger point releases are based on the work of Travell and Simons.[25] The most common ones are described in chapter 11 and are listed for your convenience in table 22.1.

It is important to note the locations of the patient's pain. Pain assessment includes either eliminating or confirming trigger points, neurological pathology, and localized injury as the source of the pain. If pain is not neurologically based, trigger points may often be the source, especially when the site of injury differs from the location of pain and the pain

TABLE 22.1 Trigger Points Most Commonly Found in Elbow Complex Muscles

Elbow segment	Muscles with trigger points
Elbow flexor	Biceps brachii
	Brachioradialis
Elbow extensor	Triceps brachii

complaints do not align with typical neurological symptoms. Trigger point pressure release and spray-and-stretch techniques are used to treat symptomatic trigger points.

Soft-tissue massage techniques can be used to address musculotendinous symptoms. Refer to chapter 11 for a thorough review of soft-tissue massage techniques. Effleurage (superficial) and pétrissage (deep) are used to treat symptomatic muscles in the elbow and forearm. Cross-friction massage is usually performed over the lateral or medial epicondyle at the tendon and junction of the common wrist extensors and common wrist flexors as part of the treatment for tendinopathy. It may help relieve pain and enhance the mobilization of connective tissue restrictions.[26] The area of tenderness is identified and isolated for treatment with a finger or thumb pad. Pressure over the area is maintained while deep friction is applied to the area. The finger or thumb moves the overlying soft tissue against the underlying bone in a direction perpendicular to the fiber direction. Figure 22.2 shows application over the lateral epicondyle. Sometimes it may be necessary to pull the skin taut with the other hand while applying the cross-friction massage to maintain pressure over a small, isolated area. When the skin and subcutaneous tissue are very mobile, the finger or thumb can easily move off the treatment site.

Myofascial release techniques can be used to address myofascial restrictions in the elbow and forearm. Chapter 11 provides detailed information about myofascial release. Wringing, J-stroke, and oscillation (table 11.2) are exam-

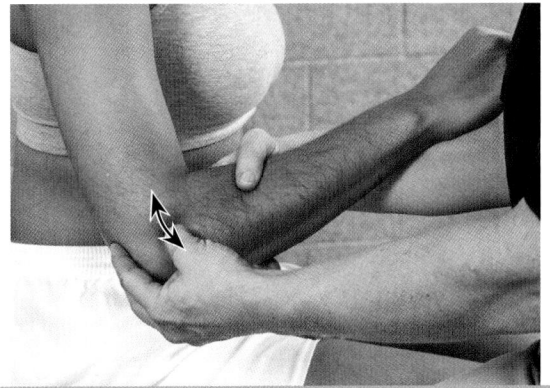

Figure 22.2 Transverse cross-friction massage.

ples of techniques that can be easily applied to the elbow and forearm. The combination of pressure and stretch may help to relieve pain and improve restricted myofascial mobility resulting from elbow injury.

Instrument-assisted soft-tissue mobilization may be used to decrease pain, facilitate tissue healing, and promote soft-tissue mobility by breaking down scar tissue, adhesions, and fascial restrictions. Refer to chapter 11 for details on IASTM. A superficial feathering or scrapping technique is used to decrease pain where a deeper chopping technique is used to facilitate tissue mobility. Either technique can be used as part of the treatment for tendinopathy. Figure 22.3 shows an application for wrist extensor tendinopathy.

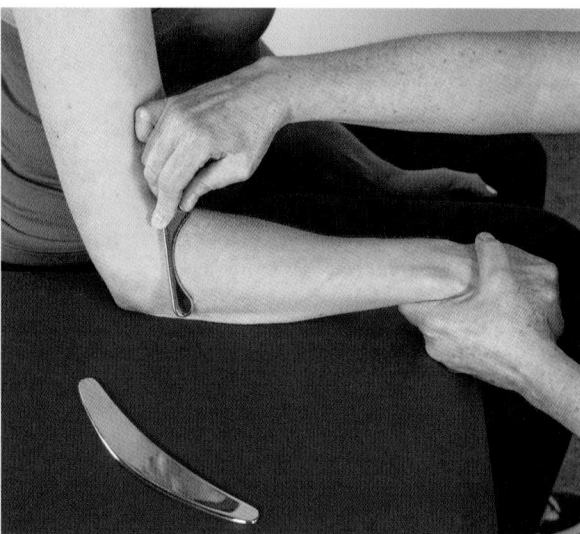

Figure 22.3 IASTM for wrist extensor tendinopathy.

Joint Mobilization

Post-traumatic elbow stiffness is a common impairment after an elbow injury.[27] Loss of elbow motion can lead to many functional limitations, such as difficulty reaching, eating, grooming hair, and throwing. In this section, we address joint motion related to capsule mobility.

With capsular tightness in the elbow and forearm, flexion is more limited than extension, and supination and pronation are equally limited. A patient who presents with this type of motion loss can be effectively treated with joint mobilization. Since three joints are enclosed in one capsule, capsular restriction may affect all of the joints.

If the elbow is very irritated, initial joint mobilization techniques are mild (grades I and II) for pain relief. Appli-

cation of more aggressive grades (III and IV) is postponed until the elbow pain is under control. Aggressive techniques applied too soon may cause additional damage to a weak joint capsule.

Joint mobilization is performed in the resting position when grades I and II are applied and during the initial application of the more aggressive grades. This position maximizes the effects of the mobilization techniques without aggravating the joint. If joint mobilization techniques are needed to gain motion, other open-packed positions may be used as motion improves.

The clinician should always use good body mechanics when applying joint mobilization. The hand applying the force should be positioned as close to the joint as possible. Keep in mind the principles of glide, roll, and spin so that you apply forces properly. Both the radial head and the ulna are concave surfaces that move on a convex capitulum and convex trochlea, respectively, so mobilization force is applied in the same direction as the restricted movement. In the proximal radioulnar joint, however, the force is applied in the direction opposite the restricted movement; the convex-on-concave rule applies at this joint because the convex radial head moves in the concave radial notch of the ulna with forearm pronation and supination.

The joint mobilization techniques presented here are those most commonly used for the elbow. As with any joint mobilization procedure, you should visualize the joint surfaces and apply the mobilization force parallel to those surfaces. You must respect precautions and contraindications, and you must consider the healing timeline and the new tissue's tensile strength when deciding whether to apply joint mobilization and how much force to use. As always, joint mobilization is contraindicated for hypermobile joints. Improper technique, excessive force, and inappropriate timing of application can all result in unnecessary injury. You must understand the appropriateness of accessory and physiological joint mobilization before you decide to use the techniques.

Humeroulnar Joint

Since most joint names include the more proximal segment first, this joint is less commonly referred to as the ulnohumeral joint. Although the elbow has three joints, the humeroulnar joint is often considered the primary elbow joint. Even though all three joints lie within the same capsule, joint mobilization for each joint can produce significant range-of-motion gains. The resting position for the humeroulnar joint is 70° of flexion with 10° of supination.

Joint Mobilization of the Elbow and Forearm Joints

With any elbow injury, forearm mobility should be examined and treated when deficient. Drawing a movement diagram may help you to visualize joint movement restrictions and pain. The three separate joints in this region all fit within one capsule, so a deficiency in the mobility of any of these joints should be assumed to affect the other two until it is ruled out.

Distraction

Joint: Humeroulnar joint.

Resting Position: 70° flexion with 10° supination.

Indications: To relieve pain, generally increase motion.

Patient Position: Supine with elbow in resting position.

Clinician and Hand Positions: The rehabilitation clinician faces the supine patient. The patient's wrist and distal forearm rest against the clinician's shoulder. The humerus is fixed using a stabilization strap, an assistant, or the rehabilitation clinician's hand. The stabilizing hand grasps the patient's proximal humerus on the dorsal side. The mobilizing hand is placed just distal to the elbow joint on the ventral side of the ulna as seen in figure 22.4.

Mobilization Application: The clinician applies a distraction force to separate the humeroulnar joint by leaning backward.

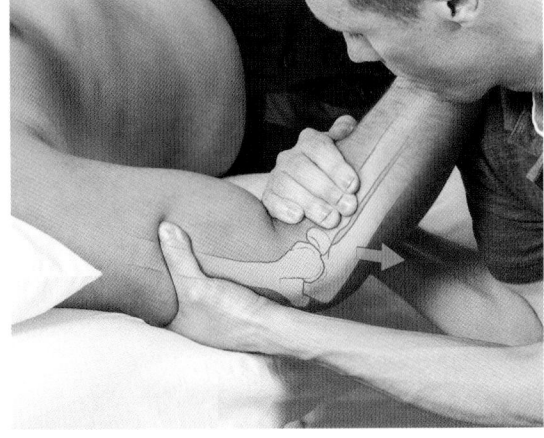

Figure 22.4

Notations: The clinician's weight transfer from the front to the back foot provides the distraction force; the clinician's arms should be relaxed. The fingers are together, using the hands as a "paddle" to apply traction force over a larger area than if the fingers were spread apart. An alternative placement for the stabilizing hand is over the anterior distal humerus.

Medial Glide

Joint: Humeroulnar joint.

Resting Position: 70° flexion with 10° supination.

Indications: To relieve pain, improve elbow flexion or extension.

Patient Position: Patient is supine or sitting.

Clinician and Hand Positions: The rehabilitation clinician faces and stands alongside the patient. The patient's elbow is positioned in the humeroulnar joint's resting position, and the distal forearm and wrist are placed between the rehabilitation clinician's lateral rib cage and medial humerus. The rehabilitation clinician's stabilizing hand is placed against the medial distal humerus. The mobilizing hand is placed on the proximal ulna at the lateral forearm near the elbow joint.

Mobilization Application: The mobilizing hand and the clinician's lateral-to-medial weight shift apply a medial glide

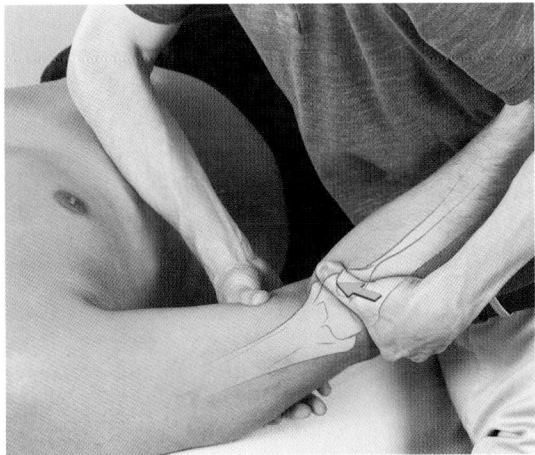

Figure 22.5

against the proximal ulna that indirectly glides the radius medially (figure 22.5).

Notations: The pressure against the medial elbow from the stabilizing hand may cause discomfort or injury to the ulnar nerve, so it must be applied with caution or with the use of a towel for padding.

Lateral Glide

Joint: Humeroulnar joint.

Resting Position: 70° flexion with 10° supination.

Indications: To reduce pain, improve elbow flexion and extension.

Patient Position: Patient is supine or sitting, similar to the medial glide position.

Clinician and Hand Positions: The clinician's hand placement is reversed from the positions for the medial glide, so the stabilizing hand is on the patient's distal lateral humerus and the mobilizing hand is on the medial forearm immediately distal to the joint. The patient's distal forearm and wrist are secured between the clinician's lateral ribs and humerus.

Mobilization Application: The clinician shifts weight in a lateral direction as the mobilizing hand applies a lateral glide against the proximal ulna from the medial forearm (figure 22.6).

Notations: The clinician's weight shift provides the force for the lateral glide.

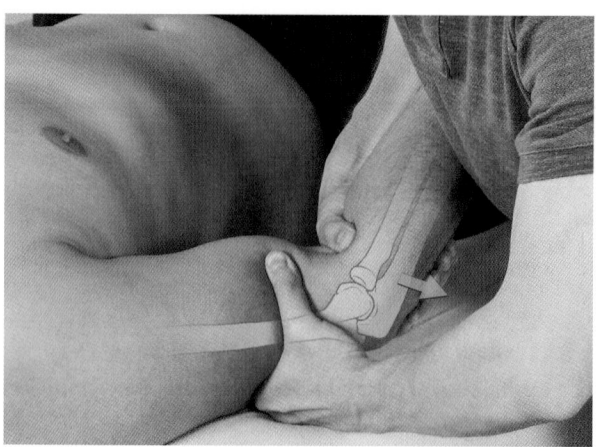

Figure 22.6

Humeroradial Joint

The humeroradial joint is also less commonly referred to as the radiohumeral joint. The humeroradial joint lies lateral to the humeroulnar joint and should not be ignored when there is capsular restriction in the elbow. Mobilization of this joint can make a significant difference in overall elbow mobility. The resting position for the humeroradial joint is full extension with full supination.

Distraction

Joint: Humeroradial joint.

Resting Position: Full extension with full supination.

Indications: To reduce pain, improve overall humeroradial mobility of elbow flexion and extension and forearm pronation and supination motion.

Patient Position: Supine or sitting in a chair with the arm slightly abducted and supported on the table.

Clinician and Hand Positions: Rehabilitation clinician stabilizes the arm with the proximal hand on the distal humerus. The mobilizing hand is placed around the lateral-side distal radius but not on the distal ulna.

Mobilization Application: The mobilization force is applied with a weight shift when the clinician moves his or her body weight to the back foot; the clinician's body is used to distract the radius in a distal direction.

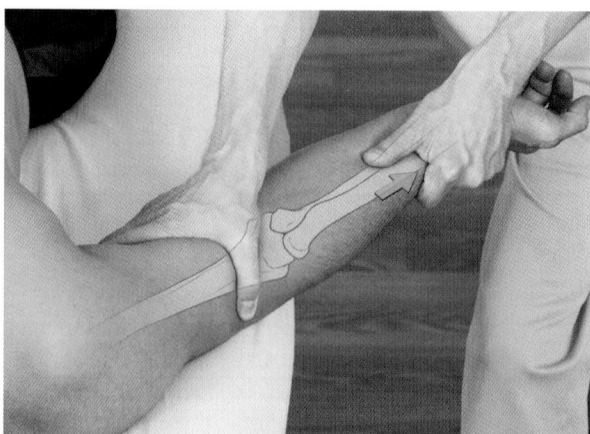

Figure 22.7

Notations: The clinician uses body weight transfer from the front to the back foot rather than arm force to deliver the joint distraction (figure 22.7).

Anterior Glide

Joint: Humeroradial joint.

Resting Position: Full extension with full supination.

Indications: To reduce pain or increase elbow flexion and forearm supination.

Patient Position: Supine with the elbow in extension and forearm in neutral pronation and supination position.

Clinician and Hand Positions: The rehabilitation clinician places the stabilizing hand on the distal humerus and the mobilizing hand on the proximal radius as shown in figure 22.8.

Mobilization Application: The mobilizing hand glides the proximal radius in a posterior-to-anterior direction.

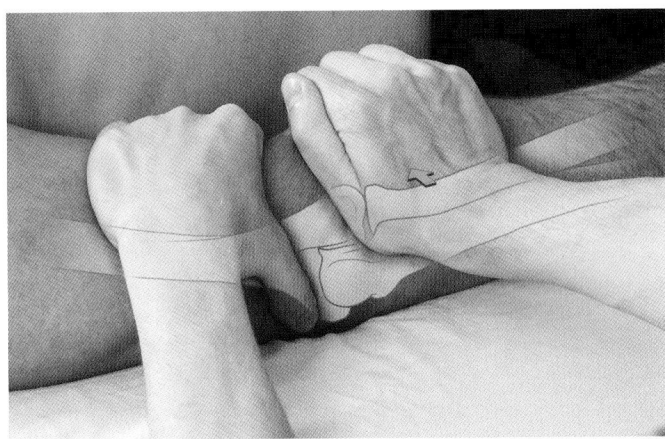

Figure 22.8

Notations: Also called ventral glide, posterior–anterior glide, or PA glide. In addition to the mobilizing hand gliding the radial head in an anterior direction, the clinician's weight shift forward provides the force for the mobilization.

Posterior Glide

Joint: Humeroradial joint.

Resting Position: Full extension with full supination.

Indications: To reduce pain or increase elbow extension and forearm pronation.

Patient Position: Supine with arm supported on the table.

Clinician and Hand Positions: The rehabilitation clinician places the stabilizing hand on the medial distal humerus and the mobilizing hand on the proximal radius, with the fingers on its posterior aspect and the thenar eminence on its anterior aspect (figure 22.9).

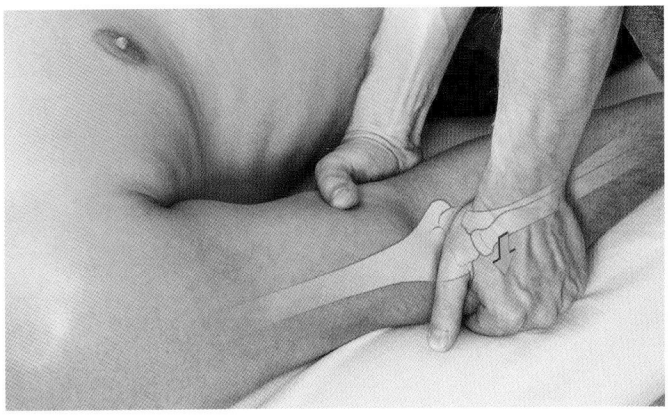

Figure 22.9

Mobilization Application: The thenar eminence on the anterior radius glides the radial head posteriorly.

Notations: Also called a dorsal glide, an anterior–posterior glide, or an AP glide. In addition to the thenar eminence gliding the radial head in a posterior direction, the clinician's weight shift forward assists the mobilization.

Proximal Radioulnar Joint

Although this joint is not actually part of the elbow's flexion–extension joint, the fact that it lies within the same capsule as the two elbow joints means that it is part of the elbow. In fact, restriction of this joint can affect overall elbow movement and should not be ignored.

Dorsal Glide

Joint: Proximal radioulnar joint.

Resting Position: 70° flexion with 35° supination.

Indications: To reduce pain or improve forearm pronation.

Patient Position: Sitting or supine with arm supported on the table.

Clinician and Hand Positions: The rehabilitation clinician faces the patient. The proximal ulna is stabilized by the medial hand, and the mobilizing hand is wrapped around the radial head with the thenar eminence and thumb pad on the anterior aspect and the finger pads on the posterior radius. If the clinician cannot maintain the resting position with the stabilizing hand, the patient's forearm and wrist may be supported with a rolled towel or pillow.

Mobilization Application: A downward pressure is exerted from the rehabilitation clinician's shoulder down through the mobilizing hand to glide the proximal radius in a posterior (dorsal) direction (figure 22.10).

Notations: Also called an anterior–posterior glide, posterior glide, or AP glide.

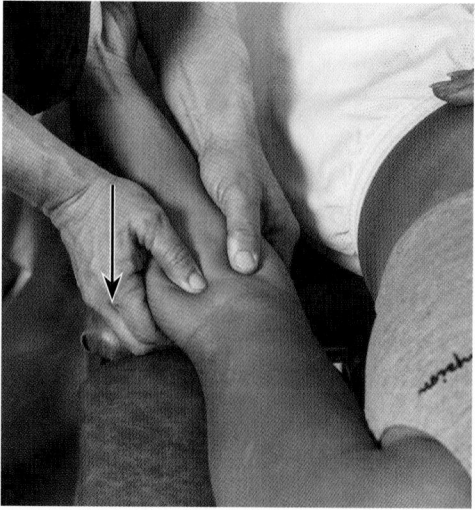

Figure 22.10

Ventral Glide

Joint: Proximal radioulnar joint.

Resting Position: 70° flexion with 35° supination.

Indications: To reduce pain or improve forearm supination.

Patient Position: Sitting with forearm supported on the table.

Clinician and Hand Positions: The stabilizing hand is placed around the proximal ulna at the olecranon process, and the mobilizing hand is placed around the proximal radius with the palm on the dorsal surface and the fingers anteriorly positioned.

Mobilization Application: Radial head is glided in an anterior (ventral) direction, using the heel of the hand (figure 22.11).

Notations: Also called an anterior glide, posterior-to-anterior glide, or PA glide. The elbow can be placed either in the resting position in early treatments or closer to the close-packed position for a more aggressive application in later treatments.

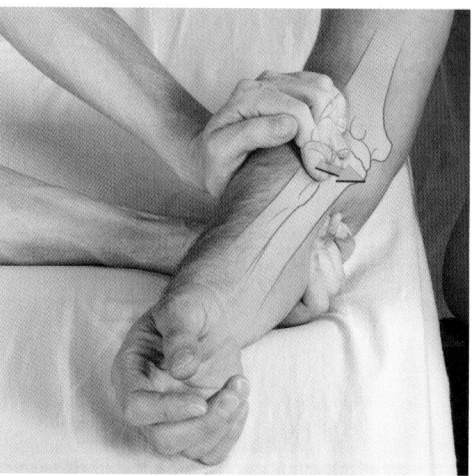

Figure 22.11

CLINICAL TIPS

Joint mobilization for the elbow addresses the humeroulnar joint, the humeroradial joint, and the proximal radioulnar joint. Since all three joints are within the same capsule, each must be evaluated for potential capsular tightness when one of these joints has reduced mobility.

Flexibility Exercises

The best way to achieve normal elbow flexibility is to prevent loss of motion. This can be done with the use of continuous passive motion (CPM) machines, early mobilization and stretching after injury or surgery, progressive static splinting, and abbreviated periods of immobilization when appropriate.[27-30] Physicians are often torn between letting the elbow heal and preventing stiffness and loss of motion in the joint after immobilization.[31] When there is a loss of normal motion, a variety of methods can be used to regain it. The elbow heals as other areas of the body do, producing collagen that becomes scar tissue, but it also differs from other joints in that it produces more scar tissue than most.[19] As the collagen matures, stretching techniques and forces must change to influence the collagen arrangement and ultimately its strength. Short, active stretches can be used early to improve flexibility and motion, but prolonged stretches are needed later when the collagen matures. These principles and guidelines are discussed in chapters 2 and 12.

Prolonged Static Stretches

Prolonged static stretches to the elbow must be applied with caution. Light forces are applied to improve range of motion without disrupting the anterior capsule. Prolonged static stretches are used after 6 weeks[27] only after active stretches have failed to restore elbow motion.

Progressive Splinting For patients in whom motion gains are difficult to achieve or for whom other methods have not succeeded, progressive splinting can provide prolonged, low-level forces to increase connective tissue lengthening.[30, 32] There are three methods of prolonged splinting that can be used for stiff elbows: static progressive splinting, dynamic progressive splinting, and serial casting. Each method uses the concept of creep (see chapter 12) to elongate tissue. There are pros and cons with each method. The inconvenience and cost of making a new cast each time motion gains are achieved make serial casting the least used option in normal populations. Similar outcomes have been achieved with either static or dynamic progressive splinting.[32, 33] The main difference between the two progressive splinting methods is that the dynamic splints have moving parts and the static splints do not. Some patients find the dynamic splint painful or uncomfortable and choose not to wear it.[34, 35] Static progressive splinting can be used instead, and it has demonstrated good results.[30]

A static progressive splint is an adjustable splint that positions the joint at its soft tissue's maximum tolerable end range without adding stress beyond that length.[36] As the tissue responds to this low-load stress and lengthens, the splint is adjusted to the tissue's new length until the desired motion is achieved.[36] The length of time the patient wears the splint varies depending on the joint restriction; if the joint's restrictive tissue has a soft, springy end-feel, it is worn 3 to 4 h a day, but if it has a hard end-feel, the brace is worn 23.5 h a day and is removed only for bathing.[36] The longer the brace is worn, the more effective the increases in motion will be, and the more rigid the scar tissue is, the longer the brace needs to be worn before tissue lengthens. Therefore, the brace must be comfortable or the patient will not use it. The force and angle of the brace can be adjusted to meet the patient's needs, ensuring that it fits well and is comfortable. It may take a few days for the patient to adjust to the brace; however, continued wear, if tolerated, can significantly improve range of motion. The patient should be instructed to remove the splint every hour to move the elbow joint so that motion is not lost in other directions. For example, if a splint is worn to improve elbow extension, instruct the patient to remove

the splint every hour and perform 10 reps of elbow flexion and forearm pronation and supination.

Equipment Stretches Although they are not performed for as long as the progressive splint is worn, the stretches described in this section are prolonged stretches. The use of equipment increases the risk that they may be applied too aggressively. Therefore, you should use less force than you think is needed because a longer stretch has significantly more impact on tissues than a brief stretch that uses the same force.[37] Rather than applying too much force and risking capsular damage, you should begin with a force lighter than you think you need and increase it if the results and patient response warrant.

It is important to watch for substitution patterns or errors in the execution of these stretches. Substitutions occur if patients cannot relax, are not properly stabilized, or are trying to produce as much motion as possible. If you see substitution patterns, you should correct them because they can result in an ineffective stretch.

- *Flexion–Extension Stretches.* Often a variety of machines are available in the clinic to provide a prolonged stretch. These can be applied for at least 10 to 15 min and longer, if the patient can tolerate them.[38, 39] A few pounds of force are applied to stretch the elbow in either flexion or extension while the shoulder is stabilized. An isokinetic machine can be used to position the elbow on stretch in either flexion or extension with the speed set at zero to maintain the desired angle. An Iso-quad exercise unit can also be used to apply a prolonged stretch. If neither of these machines is available, the patient can use free weights in the supine position: a 4.5 kg (10 lb) weight at the shoulder to prevent the shoulder from rising off the table, and no more than a 1.8 kg (4 lb) weight attached to the wrist. The distal arm should have a towel roll under it to protect the elbow from excessive posterior pressure on the table (figure 22.12).
- *Pronation–Supination Stretches.* A weighted bar can be used to increase either supination or pronation. The patient sits with the elbow supported on a table; the elbow is positioned directly under the shoulder. The patient grasps a bar, wand, or broom handle with the forearm positioned at the end range in either supination or pronation (figure 22.13). The stretch is more effective if the bar is strapped to the hand; this allows muscles to relax to improve the stretch results.

Active Static Stretches

Patients can perform active static stretches throughout the day. They do not need a great deal of equipment, so the exercises are convenient and easy to perform. Active

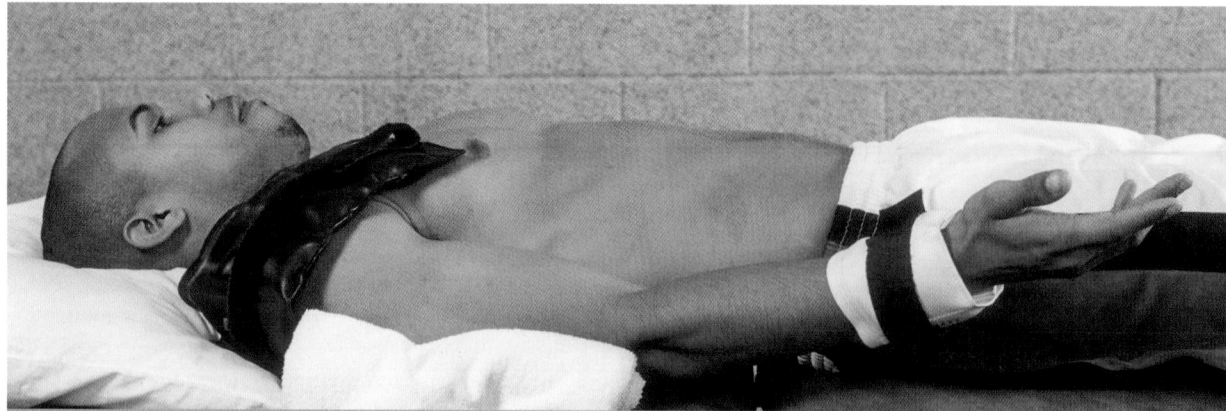

Figure 22.12 Extension equipment stretch using a free-weight with 4.5 kg (10 lb) at the shoulder to stabilize it and no more than 1.8 kg (4 lb) at the wrist to produce the stretch.

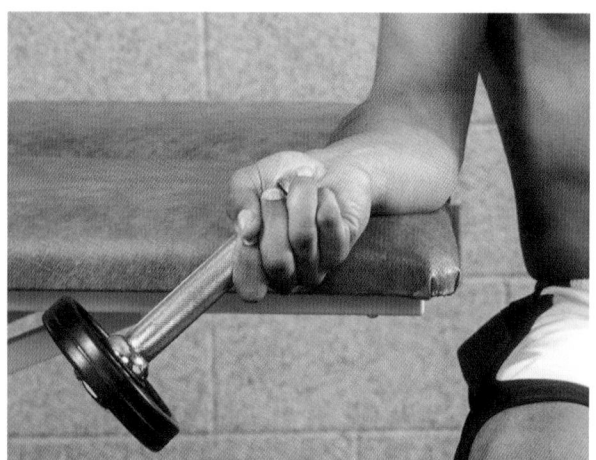

Figure 22.13 Supination equipment stretch.

stretches can affect both muscle and joint structures. Unless otherwise indicated, the stretch is performed often throughout the day with 1 to 4 repetitions at each session; the shorter the hold, the more repetitions performed. If a 30 s hold is used, 1 to 2 repetitions is sufficient,[40-42] but if a 15 s hold is used, the exercise is repeated 4 times.[43, 44] Refer to chapter 12 for additional information on stretching. Again, substitution patterns should be avoided and corrected immediately. Active static stretches are explained in the following sections.

Static Flexibility Exercises for the Elbow and Forearm

Stretching exercises for the elbow should be applied with care. Overstretching the joint with too much force can be detrimental.

Active Elbow Flexor Stretch

Body Segment: Elbow.

Stage in Rehab: Active phase and into resistive phase if necessary.

Purpose: Increase elbow extension motion.

Positioning: Patient is supine or sitting with the uninvolved forearm across the abdomen and the hand's dorsum placed just proximal to the involved elbow's posterior joint.

Execution: With the forearm supinated and held in this position, the patient extends the elbow actively as much as possible (figure 22.14).

Possible Substitutions: Scapular protraction, forward trunk lean, shoulder extension, and an active inferior glenohumeral glide or distraction.

Notations: If the patient has difficulty stabilizing the scapula, the supine position is more effective.

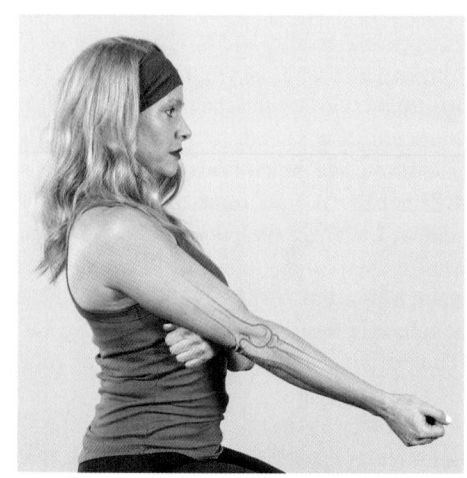

Figure 22.14

Active Elbow Extensor Stretch

Body Segment: Elbow.

Stage in Rehab: Active phase and into resistive phase if necessary.

Purpose: Increase elbow flexion motion.

Positioning: Patient is supine or sitting. The involved distal forearm is held by the contralateral hand. The elbow is stabilized next to the side or on a tabletop.

Execution: Patient pulls the involved forearm toward the shoulder with the contralateral hand (figure 22.15).

Possible Substitutions: Shoulder extension and scapular retraction.

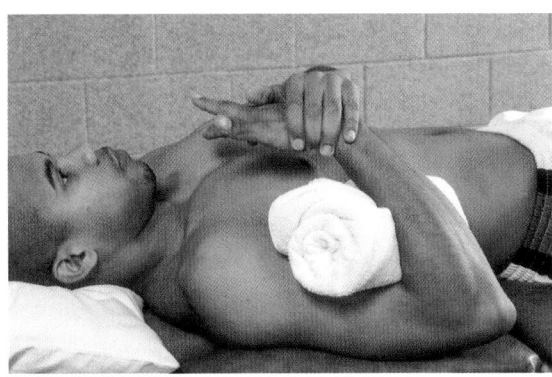

Figure 22.15

Notations: This stretch can be made more effective and more comfortable if a rolled-up towel or pad is placed in the antecubital fossa; the pad provides a distraction on the joint during the stretch.

Active Pronator Stretch

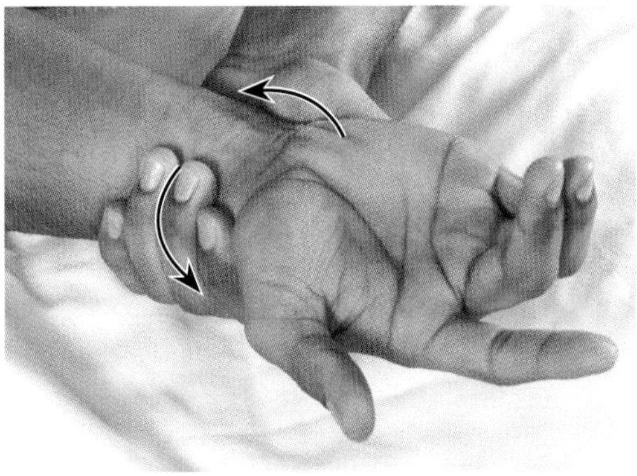

Body Segment: Forearm.

Stage in Rehab: Active phase and into resistive phase if necessary.

Purpose: Improve supination by stretching the pronators.

Positioning: The patient sits with the elbow flexed to 90° and stabilized next to the ribs. The forearm is positioned in as much supination as possible. The uninvolved hand is placed in an underhand grasp on the distal forearm so that the finger pads are on the volar aspect of the radius and the base of the hand is on the dorsal aspect of the ulna.

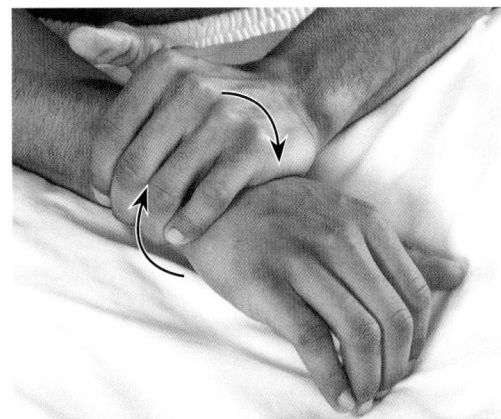

Figure 22.16

Execution: The finger pads rotate the radius downward as the base of the hand rotates the ulna upward into further supination (figure 22.16).

Possible Substitutions: Shoulder adduction, and trunk lean toward the arm.

Notations: The humerus should be placed securely against the ribs to prevent extraneous movement during the stretch.

Active Supinator Stretch

Body Segment: Forearm.

Stage in Rehab: Active phase and into resistive phase if necessary.

Purpose: Increase pronation by stretching the supinators.

Positioning: The patient sits with the elbow stabilized next to the ribs and flexed to 90°. The forearm is actively positioned in as much pronation as possible. The patient grasps the distal forearm with the uninvolved hand in an overhand grasp by placing the finger pads around the ventral aspect of the ulna and the base of the hand on the dorsal aspect of the radius.

Execution: The finger pads are pulled upward as the base of the hand is pushed downward (figure 22.17).

Figure 22.17

Possible Substitutions: The elbow moves away from the side as the shoulder abducts, and the trunk leans away from the arm. The elbow must remain in contact with the lateral trunk.

Notations: Instruct the patient to relax the shoulder and perform only to the point that he or she feels a stretch without pain.

Clinician-Assisted Stretches

With clinician-assisted stretches, the clinician provides the stretching force. The stretch is typically held for 15 to 30 s and applied for 2 to 4 reps. The clinician should use caution in applying any stretch to the anterior joint. Overstretching this area can result in more adhesions or capsular injury.[5] Patient positioning and proper execution of the stretch are important. Contract–relax PNF stretch techniques with active contraction of the antagonists can be used in assistive stretches.

Assistive Stretch to the Elbow Extensors

Body Segment: Elbow.

Stage in Rehab: Active phase and into resistive phase if necessary.

Purpose: Increase elbow flexion motion.

Positioning: The patient is sitting or supine. The clinician stabilizes and supports the elbow and places the other hand on the patient's wrist.

Execution: The clinician moves the patient's hand toward the patient's shoulder (figure 22.18).

Possible Substitutions: If not properly stabilized, the shoulder can elevate to give a false impression of improved range of movement.

Notations: Placing the clinician's other hand or a rolled-up towel in the antecubital fossa provides joint distraction to make the stretch more comfortable and more effective since the towel helps distract the joint. To stretch the long head of the triceps, the elbow is flexed by the clinician's hand on the distal forearm. The shoulder is then flexed overhead by the other hand on the patient's elbow.

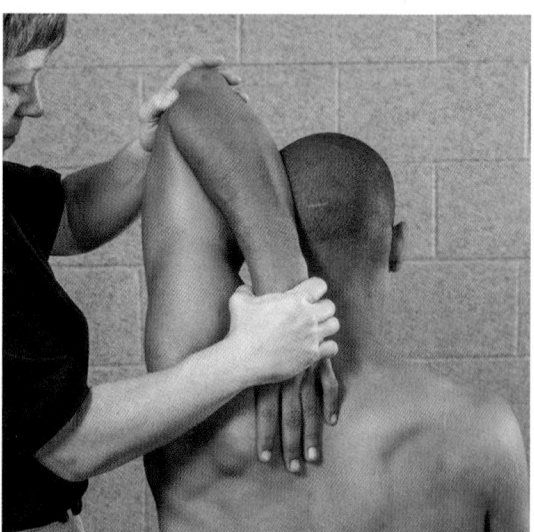

Figure 22.18

Assistive Stretch to the Elbow Flexors

Body Segment: Elbow.

Stage in Rehab: Active phase and into resistive phase if necessary.

Purpose: Increase elbow extension motion.

Positioning: The patient is sitting or supine. The clinician supports the elbow.

Execution: The clinician applies the stretch as the elbow is extended and the shoulder is moved into hyperextension (figure 22.19). This stretches the biceps and other anterior elbow structures.

Possible Substitutions: Scapular protraction, scapular tilting.

Notations: The biceps is maximally stretched when the forearm is in pronation, but the stretch should also be applied in supination.

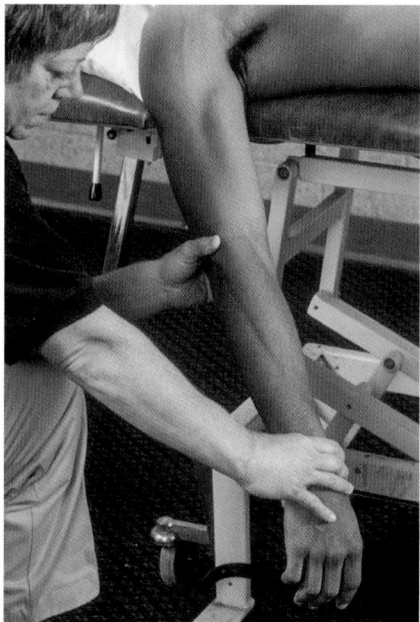

Figure 22.19

Assistive Forearm Stretches

Body Segment: Forearm.

Stage in Rehab: Active phase and into resistive phase if necessary.

Purpose: Increase forearm supination and pronation.

Positioning: Patient is sitting or supine, and the elbow is flexed to 90°. Clinician grasps the distal humerus to stabilize it and places the stretch hand on the patient's wrist.

Execution: The radioulnar joints are moved to their end range with overpressure in supination and then in pronation (figure 22.20).

Possible Substitutions: Shoulder abduction with pronation and shoulder adduction with supination. The force is applied to provide the stretch at the radioulnar joints, not twisting the hand.

Notations: It is more comfortable if this stretch is performed with the forearm submerged in warm water. Results are better if all supination stretches are performed and then all pronation stretches are performed, as opposed to alternating.

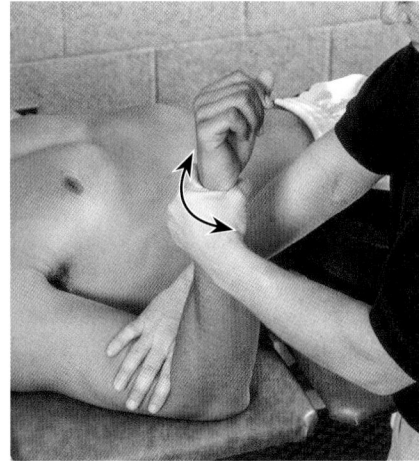

Figure 22.20

CLINICAL TIPS

Elbow stiffness and loss of motion are common problems after injury or surgery. After an injury, the elbow should be immobilized for only as long as necessary to protect the healing tissue. Early active exercises, if permitted, may reduce the risk of elbow motion loss. Prolonged stretches are often needed to restore the normal flexibility of the elbow. Assisted stretching using either a machine or a clinician will also help in regaining motion.

Strengthening Exercises

As with other joints, the most basic elbow strengthening exercises include isometrics. From isometrics, the strengthening program progresses to isotonic exercises in straight-plane motions. Once muscle activation and timing are corrected and the weak muscles are sufficiently improved, diagonal-plane strengthening exercises begin. When the patient demonstrates strength and neuromotor control in diagonal patterns, he or she is ready for plyometric exercises. The final piece of the rehabilitation program includes functional exercises and performance-specific exercises before the patient returns to normal activities.

Isometric Resistance Exercises

The patient can perform isometric resistance exercises independently and often throughout the day. Each exercise is held for 6 s[45] and is usually repeated 10 times each session. The number of repetitions and the frequency of the exercise depend on the condition of the muscle, the ability of the body part to move, and the phase of the healing process. On either side of the 6 s maximum hold is 2 s for a gradual buildup and 2 s for relaxation to avoid sudden, painful muscle contractions.

Begin with submaximal contractions and progress toward more maximal recruitment as the patient tolerates. It is important to caution patients to avoid a Valsalva maneuver during isometric exercises. Correct posture and scapular positioning are needed for proximal control and proper execution of isometric exercises for the upper extremity. The patient should be able to perform the exercises correctly before they are added to the home exercise program.

Elbow Flexion The involved elbow is flexed, and the patient's contralateral hand is placed on the distal forearm. The patient tries to move the elbow into flexion while using the opposing hand to resist the movement (figure 22.21). This exercise should be performed in supination,

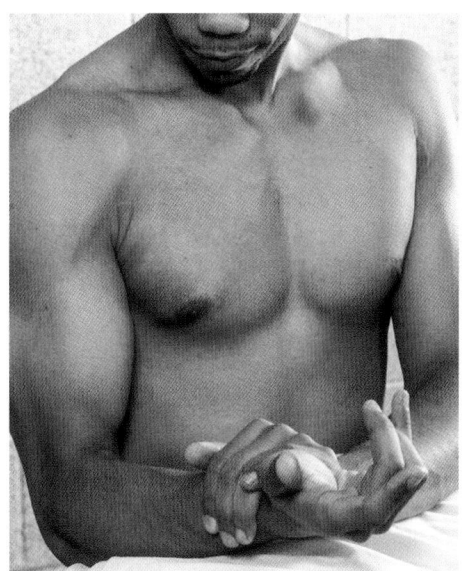

Figure 22.21 Isometric flexion.

pronation, and neutral, as well as at several different angles of elbow flexion.

Elbow Extension   For this exercise, the resistance is applied to the distal forearm as the patient tries to extend the elbow. This exercise should be performed at several different positions in the range of motion.

Forearm Pronation–Supination   In this exercise, resistance is applied to the distal forearm as the patient tries to pronate or supinate the forearm. This exercise should be performed at various positions in the range of motion of elbow flexion–extension and forearm pronation–supination.

Manual-Resistance Exercises

Straight-plane manual resistance is provided by the rehabilitation clinician. The elbow must move through the full range of motion during these exercises. The movement should be smooth, so the clinician must adjust his or her resistance force to follow the changes in the patient's strength as the elbow moves through its range of motion. If there is a point of weakness within the range of motion, the rehabilitation clinician may offer an isometric resistance at that point before proceeding through the remaining motion. If you decide to use this approach, tell the patient beforehand that you will provide an isometric resistance when you detect a point of weakness. You can begin manual resistance early and use it throughout the rehabilitation program because you can easily change the resistance to meet the patient's abilities and still respect tissue-healing precautions. It is important to provide proper stabilization when applying manual resistance to ensure that you are isolating the intended muscle or muscle group.

Elbow Flexion–Extension   The best position for elbow manual-resistance strengthening exercises is with the forearm in an antigravity position. This position uses the weight of the forearm as additional resistance. For elbow flexion, the patient is sitting or supine. Supine position is preferred with manual-resistance exercises because the elbow is more easily stabilized and can go through a full range of motion. The rehabilitation clinician stabilizes the shoulder with one hand and resists elbow flexion with the other hand over the distal forearm (figure 22.22a). To resist primarily the biceps, the forearm is supinated. To eliminate the biceps and resist primarily the brachialis, the forearm is pronated. To add more resistance to the brachioradialis, the forearm is in neutral. Common substitutions in this exercise include shoulder flexion, shoulder shrugging, and scapular retraction.

Elbow extension is performed with the patient in a prone position to maximize gravity's effect at end-range extension. The humerus is abducted and supported on the table, with the forearm hanging over the side. A towel support is placed under the distal arm to increase patient comfort and to raise the humerus to a position parallel to the floor. The rehabilitation clinician stabilizes the distal humerus with one hand and provides resistance to elbow extension at the distal forearm with the other (figure 22.22b). This exercise can also be performed with the patient sitting with the shoulder fully elevated and the elbow overhead, next to the ear. This position provides maximal gravitational resistance in the middle of the range of motion, and because the long head of the triceps is on stretch in this position, it will enable the triceps to produce greater force. A common substitution in triceps resistance exercises is scapular protraction.

Forearm Supination–Pronation   This exercise can be performed with the patient sitting or supine. The elbow is flexed to 90°, and the rehabilitation clinician places both hands around the patient's distal forearm. As the patient supinates the forearm, the rehabilitation clinician resists

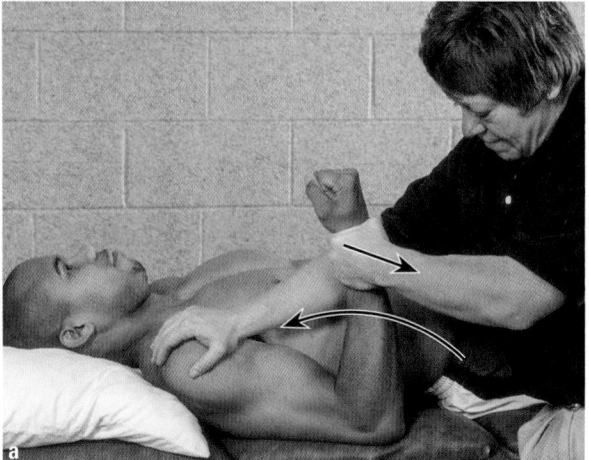
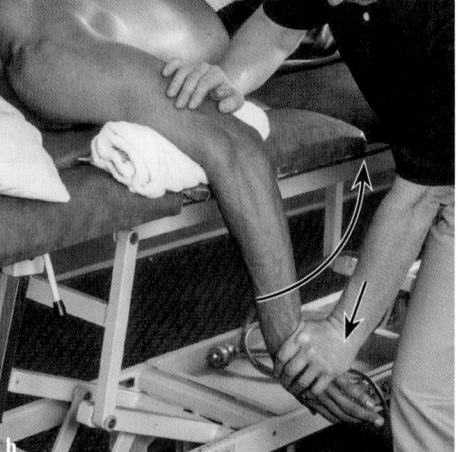

Figure 22.22   Manual resistance: *(a)* resisted elbow flexion in supination, *(b)* resisted elbow extension.

the movement. Resistance by the opposite hand occurs in the opposite direction for pronation (figure 22.23). The elbow is secured at the patient's side or on the table to prevent shoulder abduction with pronation and adduction with supination.

Straight-Plane Resisted Exercises

Before beginning straight-plane resisted exercises, it is critical that the patient start in good posture with the core set and the scapula stabilized. Patients should perform these exercises through a full range of motion in a slow and controlled manner. Straight-plane resistance exercises are described in the following sections.

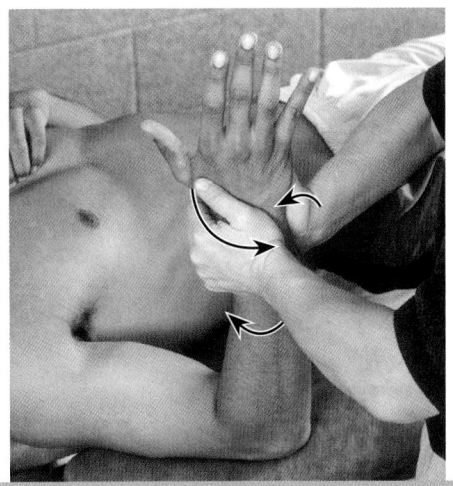

Figure 22.23   Manual resistance to supination and pronation.

Strength Exercises for the Elbow and Forearm

A variety of exercises can be used to strengthen the elbow and forearm. Only a few examples are provided here.

Elbow Flexion

Body Segment: Elbow.

Stage in Rehab: Resistive phase.

Purpose: Strengthen elbow flexors.

Positioning: The patient stands with the uninvolved hand behind the involved distal humerus just above the elbow. The weight is held in the hand in a supinated, pronated, or neutral position as the patient slowly flexes the elbow (figure 22.24a).

Execution: Elbow flexion occurs in a smooth, controlled motion.

Possible Substitutions: The contralateral hand is positioned behind the involved arm to stabilize the humerus and prevent the shoulder from lifting the weight, the most common substitution in this exercise. Another substitution is to heft the weight up with a sudden shrug movement of the shoulder, hyperextending the trunk, or using momentum. If any of these substitutions occurs, lower the resistance.

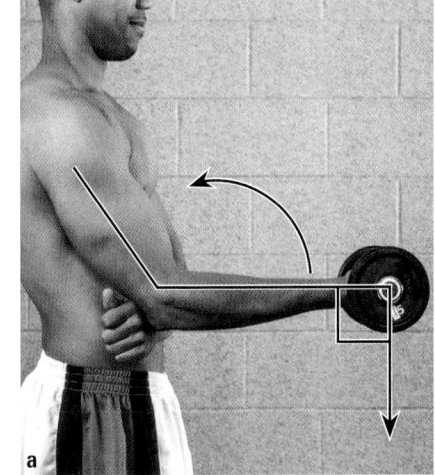

Figure 22.24

Notations: Depending on the forearm position, the biceps, brachialis, or brachioradialis (or more than one of these) is strengthened. Supination emphasizes the biceps, pronation emphasizes the brachialis, and neutral works the brachioradialis. An alternative position is with the shoulder flexed to 90° and the humerus supported to hold this position while the elbow is flexed against resistance (figure 22.24b). This position provides maximum resistance in the beginning of the exercise but reduces the biceps' ability to provide force at the elbow since it is already shortened at the shoulder. Elbow flexion can also be performed with resistance bands or pulleys. The pulley or band is anchored low, near the ground, to have maximum resistance occur at midrange. Changing the anchor position changes the point in the motion where maximum resistance occurs. Refer to chapter 13 for additional information on joint positions and maximum resistance. It is important to stabilize the humerus by placing the opposite hand behind the upper arm, as seen in figure 22.24c.

>continued

Elbow Flexion >*continued*

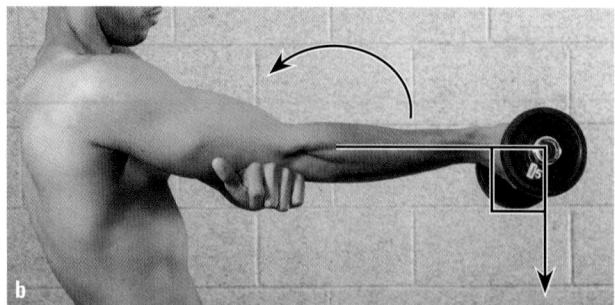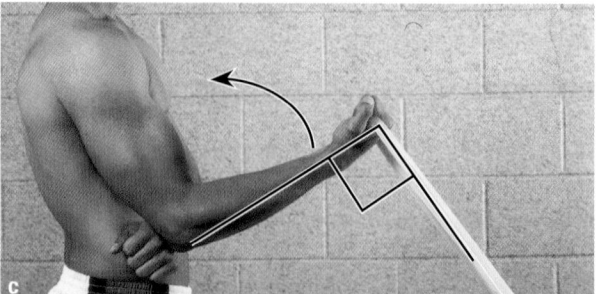

Figure 22.24 >*continued*

Elbow Extension

Body Segment: Elbow.

Stage in Rehab: Resistive phase.

Purpose: Strengthen triceps and anconeus.

Positioning: The shoulder is elevated with the elbow directly over the shoulder.

Execution: The elbow extends while maintaining its position overhead. The contralateral hand maintains the elbow position with support on the posterior humerus (figure 22.25a).

Possible Substitutions: Shoulder flexion, shoulder abduction, trunk extension.

Notations: If the long head of the triceps is to be emphasized less, the exercise can be performed with the patient supine (figure 22.25b). To emphasize resistance at end range, the patient leans over at the waist in standing or lies prone on a table with the arm parallel to the floor and the elbow flexed; the elbow is extended to place the forearm alongside the body (figure 22.25c). Equipment such as the latissimus pull-down bar can also be used to strengthen elbow extensors (figure 22.25d). The patient positions the bar so that the elbows are at the sides and flexed. Maintaining this humerus position, the patient lowers the bar by extending the elbows (figure 22.25d).

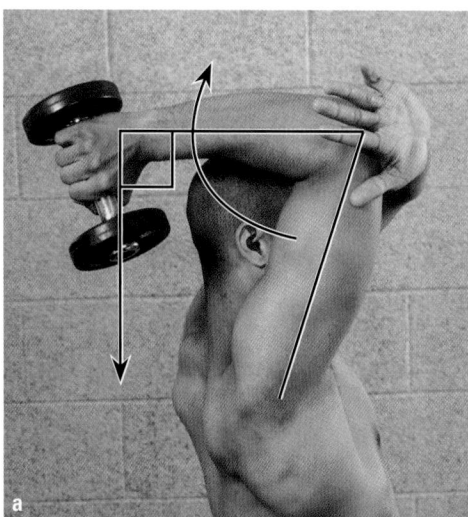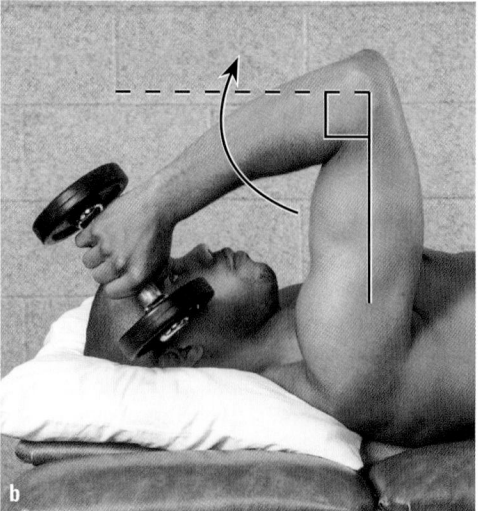

Figure 22.25

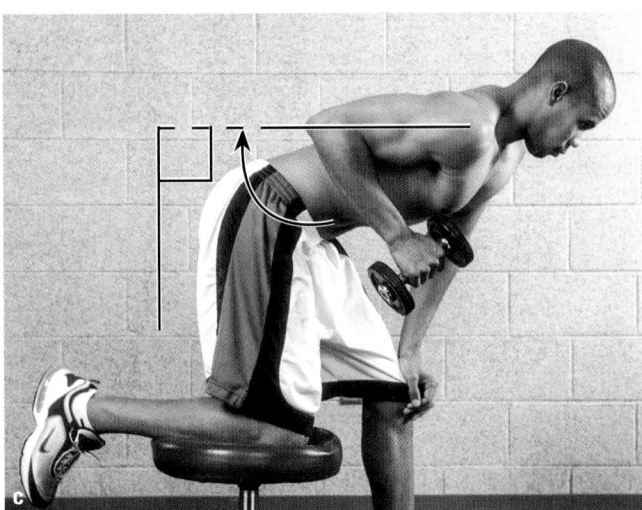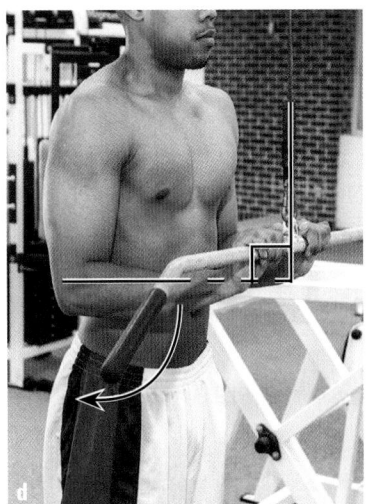

Figure 22.25 >continued

Supination

Body Segment: Forearm.

Stage in Rehab: Resistive phase.

Purpose: Strengthen forearm supinators.

Positioning: This exercise is performed with the patient sitting and the forearm supported on the table and the wrist over the end of the table. A weighted bar is held at one end with the forearm in pronation.

Execution: The patient rotates the bar upward until the bar is pointing toward the ceiling for a concentric exercise (figure 22.26).

Possible Substitutions: Letting the weight fall rather than controlling its movement and speed, shoulder adduction, and elbow extension.

Notations: To perform an eccentric exercise, the patient slowly returns the bar to the start position with the palm turned down. Resistance for supinator muscles is usually less than for pronator muscles.

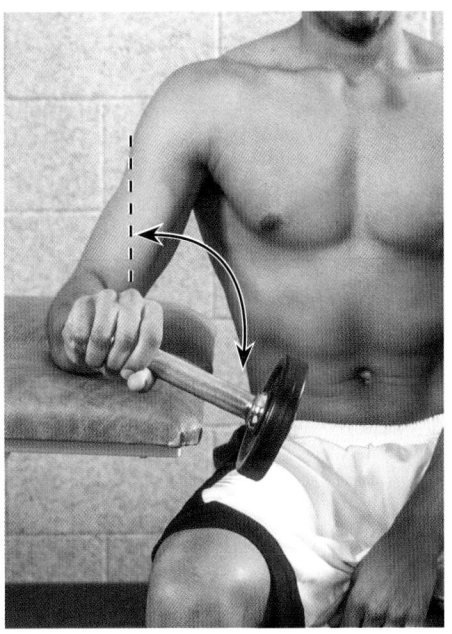

Figure 22.26

Pronation

Body Segment: Forearm.

Stage in Rehab: Resistive phase.

Purpose: Strengthen forearm pronators.

Positioning: The patient is seated as in the supination exercise just described, but the forearm is positioned in full supination this time.

Execution: The patient rotates the bar from full supination to the mid-position until the bar is vertical to the floor for a concentric exercise and then returns to full supination for an eccentric exercise (figure 22.27). The patient should

>continued

Pronation >*continued*

not go beyond the vertical position with the bar since the supinators will be eccentrically resisted as the bar is lowered into full pronation. Since supinators are weaker than pronators,[46] the weight would have to be less than optimal for the pronators to perform this exercise beyond the vertical position to full supination; lowering the weight to perform a full range of motion means the pronators would not be resisted maximally.

Possible Substitutions: Shoulder abduction, elbow flexion.

Notations: The weight should be controlled throughout the range of motion. It is incorrect to use a dumbbell to perform this exercise and the supination exercise because one end of the dumbbell will act as a counterbalance force for the other end, making the exercise ineffective.

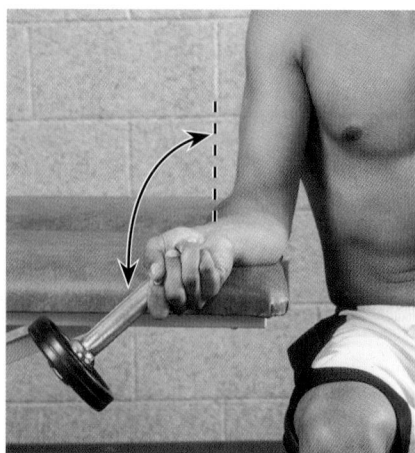

Figure 22.27

Diagonal-Plane Exercises

The body functions in the context of a kinetic chain. With that in mind, you must address scapular and proximal control when rehabilitating any upper-extremity injury that includes the elbow, wrist, and hand. Patients who demonstrate proper proximal (scapular) stabilization and adequate strength in the elbow straight-plane exercises can progress to diagonal-plane exercises. Proprioceptive neuromuscular facilitation (PNF) D1 and D2 flexion and extension patterns are used to strengthen the elbow in diagonal planes of motion. Refer to chapter 11 for information on PNF and to chapter 21 for upper extremity diagonal-plane PNF pattern exercises.

Plyometric Exercises

Once the patient demonstrates proximal stability and has gained strength and control in straight-plane and diagonal-plane patterns, he or she can progress to plyometric exercises. Plyometric exercises combine maximum strength and joint stabilization with high-level dynamic activities that require agility and coordination. Plyometric exercises were introduced in chapter 15. You must determine if plyometric exercises are appropriate for each patient. Gymnasts, wrestlers, carpenters, and heavy machine operators would benefit from upper-extremity plyometric exercises because they need power, endurance, and strength in their upper extremities to perform well. Plyometric exercises may not be needed for someone who leads a sedentary lifestyle or who does not perform power- or speed-related activities.

Carryover Shoulder Exercises

As we have already indicated, many of the exercises discussed in chapter 21 are appropriate for the elbow. Instead of repeating details here, we suggest that you refer to

chapter 21 for a listing and for information about the progression of these exercises. The push-up, seated push-up, Swiss ball weight-bearing exercises, rhythmic stabilization activities, and distal movement stabilization exercises are all appropriate for the elbow.

Resistance-band diagonal patterns in D1 and D2 flexion and extension can incorporate elbow movements of flexion or extension or they can keep the elbow stationary. Which pattern to use depends on the patient's sport or work activities. For example, pitchers, tennis players, and automobile mechanics should use D2 flexion and extension patterns because those patterns most closely mimic the motions in their activities. A breaststroke swimmer, on the other hand, should use D1 flexion and extension patterns.

Unstable-surface activities as discussed in chapter 21 are recommended for mid-resistive phase elbow rehabilitation. Resisted movements using the treadmill or stair machine, and medicine-ball exercises and their progressions, are applicable for elbow therapeutic exercise progressions in the advanced phase.

CLINICAL TIPS

Strengthening exercises for the elbow use isometric resistance, manual resistance, straight-plane resistance, multiplanar resistance, plyometrics, carryover shoulder exercises, and isokinetics in a careful progression. Isokinetic exercises are not a required part of a rehabilitation program, but performance-specific exercises should always be included.

Functional and Performance-Specific Exercises

When tissue healing has progressed sufficiently and the patient demonstrates adequate strength, coordination, and neuromotor control, the emphasis of the rehabilitation program shifts to function and performance-specific exercises. Many of the functional programs discussed in chapters 15 and 21 can be used very appropriately for the elbow. Of course, once the patient qualifies to move on to performance-specific challenges, specific applications depend on the patient's ADLs, sport, or work activity and demands.

Although specific exercises in this phase are individually determined, there is general information that applies to any patient at this point in the rehabilitation progression. Functional exercises and performance-specific challenges should include warm-up and cool-down activities. Overhead activity progressions for both groups of exercises should begin with easy activities at diminished distances, forces, and speeds and should gradually increase only one of these factors at a time until the patient can perform all activities at normal performance levels. Progression occurs only every third exercise session to give the body time to adapt to the increased stress levels. Patients who experience pain with any increase should return to the previous level of exercises for an additional 3 d before trying the next level again.

Examples of functional activities might include medicine ball tossing for a javelin thrower, plyometric push-ups for a football guard, resistance-band pull activities for a swimmer, or hammering nails for a drywall installer. Rather than repeating other programs that have already been described, we suggest that you refer to chapters 8, 15, and 21 for details on programs, their progressions, and the precautions that guide those progressions.

Special Rehabilitation Applications

We will now look at rehabilitation programs for some of the more common elbow injuries. For each injury, specific aspects unique to that injury and the rehabilitation program for that injury are presented. Some of these discussions are followed by a case study that will enable you to apply your new knowledge of elbow rehabilitation.

As we discuss each rehabilitation program, you should notice a couple of consistent factors. All programs consider where in the healing process the patient is to determine the program's progression. In rehabilitation phase I, the inactive phase, the goals are to calm the injury site, reduce pain and swelling, and prevent deconditioning of the nonaffected segments. In phase II, the active phase, the focus is mainly on regaining normal motion; toward the end of this phase, easy nonresistive strengthening and static proprioception exercises may begin. In phase III, the resistive phase, the focus is on restoring normal proprioception and strength, including strength in multiplanar motions. By phase IV, the advanced phase, the patient is preparing to return to normal function, so activities in this phase include all exercises that mimic the demands the patient will experience once he or she returns to normal activities.

You must do an examination before you can establish a rehabilitation program. Special tests are part of the examination process. Table 22.2 provides examples of common special tests that may be included in the examination of the elbow. More than one special test is usually used to further justify the clinical diagnosis that is made.[47]

TABLE 22.2 Common Diagnostic Special Tests for the Elbow With Their Sensitivity and Specificity Ratings

Site or structure tested	Special test (other name)	Sensitivity*	Specificity*
Neurologic status	Median nerve ULTT	94%-97%[48]	22%[48]
	Radial nerve ULTT	72%-97%[48]	33%[48]
	Ulnar nerve ULTT	Unknown	Unknown
Cubital tunnel	Tinel's sign	68%-70%[49]	76%-98%[49]
	Elbow flexion test (pressure flexion test)	89%-98%[49]	95%-98%[49]
Median nerve compression	Pronator stress test	Unknown	Unknown
Lateral instability	Varus stress test	Unknown	Unknown
Lateral tendinopathy	Cozen's test	84%[50]	0%[50]
	Maudsley's test (extensor digitorum test)	Unknown	Unknown
	Mill's test	Unknown	Unknown
Medial instability	Valgus stress test	63%-66%[51]	60%[51]
	Moving valgus stress test	100%[51]	75%[51]
Medial tendinopathy	Medial epicondyle passive test	Unknown	Unknown

*Numbers rounded to the nearest whole number.

ULTT = Upper limb tension test

Epicondylopathy

Epicondylopathy, or **epicondylalgia**, is commonly seen in the elbow. A **tendinopathy** is a condition of a tendon that demonstrates signs and symptoms of pain, swelling, and reduced function.[52] An important part of treating these types of conditions is discovering and correcting the cause of the problem. If you do not correct the cause of the injury, there is a very high risk that it will recur. Because elbow motion applies torsion stress to the medial elbow, it is susceptible to tendon pathology, especially when the forces applied are exaggerated because of poor technique.

Lateral epicondylopathy is often referred to as "tennis elbow," and medial epicondylopathy is commonly known as "golfer's elbow," although many people with these conditions do not play either sport.[53, 54] In fact, lateral epicondylopathy is a common occupational disorder.[55] The lateral elbow is affected more often than the medial elbow, which is probably why there have been fewer studies of medial epicondylopathy.[56] These conditions both come under the general heading of tendinopathy or epicondylalgia and usually result from cumulative trauma.[57-59]

Etiology and Complaints

Lateral epicondylopathy commonly involves the extensor carpi radialis brevis.[59] In tennis players, it is likely the result of various improper backhand techniques such as hitting the ball too late, leading with the elbow, or flipping the wrist into extension.[60] Occupational or recreational activities that involve repetitive loading of the tendon by twisting motions and forceful gripping may lead to lateral epicondylopathy.[59, 61] Medial epicondylopathy is seen in golfers secondary to overuse or poor technique.[56] Others who commonly experience epicondylopathy include javelin throwers, gymnasts, and those who do repetitive wrist flexion or extension activities.[54, 62]

In either medial or lateral epicondylopathy, the patient usually experiences a gradual, progressive onset of epicondylar pain. It may begin with pain only after activity. Then it may progress to some pain at the start of activity that resolves as the activity continues but returns after activity. Eventually, pain occurs with daily activities and then at rest. Grasping objects and shaking hands are painful. Extending the wrist against resistance with lateral epicondylopathy and flexing the wrist against resistance with medial epicondylopathy are painful. The pain is localized to the involved epicondyle, but if left untreated, it can extend more distally on the forearm.[59] Pronation or supination activities can become painful. Grip strength weakens, as does wrist flexion and extension, primarily from pain.[63, 64] Pain can restrict the full range of wrist motion, especially when it is combined with elbow extension in lateral epicondylopathy and with elbow flexion in medial epicondylopathy.

Conservative Rehabilitation

As with other tendinopathy treatments, the cause of the injury must first be determined and corrected to reduce the risk of reinjury. If you are not familiar with the skills of the patient's sport or activity, it is best to have a coach or supervisor help in skill analysis when you suspect poor execution. You should also inspect the fit and weight of hand implements that are used in the sport or work environment.

During the first phase of rehabilitation, goals include not only finding the source of epicondylopathy but relieving the pain it is producing. Although there is no consensus on the most effective modalities, there is some evidence for the effectiveness of shock wave therapy, radiofrequency, laser therapy, ultrasound, electrical stimulation, and ice.[55, 58, 64-66] Manual therapy interventions have also proved beneficial. Once pain intensity decreases, cross-friction massage to the tender teno-osseus junction of the epicondyle areas can help to reduce tissue adhesions and increase local circulation.[64] Joint mobilization techniques directed at the elbow can have a positive effect on both pain and functional grip ability.[67] A forearm, or tennis elbow, strap is sometimes used to reduce forearm muscle activity, thereby reducing stress on the muscle's tendinous insertions on the epicondyle and allowing it to heal.[68, 69]

Flexibility exercises should be within the patient's pain tolerance and should include all muscles from the shoulder to the hand. A variety of exercises can be used to maintain or return normal ranges of motion to the shoulder, elbow, wrist, finger flexors and extensors, and forearm pronators and supinators. If joint motion presents with a capsular pattern, joint mobilization techniques are indicated. End-range stretches and mobilizations should not be aggressive, especially in the early rehabilitation phases when pain is significant. Patients who are long-term participants in tennis or throwing sports may have flexion contractures and valgus deformities.[10] These occur from repetitive microtears, scarring, and possible ossification of the flexor muscles and anterior capsule or hypertrophic bone changes.[5] In the presence of these ossification changes, attempts to stretch the elbow are frustrating and are not advised. During the active phase and early resistive phase of rehabilitation, stretching exercises should be active and within the patient's comfort range.

If the patient still lacks normal range of motion in the resistive phase, you should introduce mobilization and more aggressive flexibility techniques. If a bony end-feel is palpated at less than normal extension, the patient may have structural changes or loose bodies that prohibit full extension.[70] If the end-feel is capsular, however, joint mobilization techniques are indicated. In addition to elbow-joint mobilization, joint mobilizations for the wrist and forearm should be considered for epicondylopathy treatment because muscles that originate on the epicondyle affect the movement of these segments. Specific wrist joint mobilizations and flexibility exercises are discussed in chapter 23. In addition to mobilization techniques, active-assistive and passive stretching exercises can be used to improve wrist, forearm, and elbow motion in the active and resistive phases. Contract–relax and hold–relax stretching techniques[71] have proven beneficial for improving range of motion and decreasing pain in lateral epicondylopathy.

Strength exercises include isometrics, eccentrics, concentrics, and plyometrics, each provided in a logical progression. Isometrics are used in the early rehabilitation phase either when it is too early for more resistive activities or when other resistive exercises are too painful. Effective strengthening exercises for tendinopathy include an eccentric exercise program.[59, 63, 72, 73] Such a program is also used for epicondylopathy; it starts with submaximal eccentric exercises using weights or resistance bands and progresses to more aggressive use of heavier weights with increased speeds as tolerated by the injury. A systematic review with meta-analysis performed by Chen and Baker[59] concluded that 3 sets of 10 to 15 reps with pain no higher than 5/10 on VAS is the best eccentric program for lateral elbow tendinopathy. Their study also indicated that the eccentric program should be carried out for a period of at least 6 weeks.[59] Shoulder and trunk strength exercises should be included in the active phase to maintain conditioning levels in these areas and to provide a stable base from which the arm can function.

The resistive phase begins with eccentric exercises and progresses to concentric exercises, diagonal motions, and more functional patterns of movement toward the end of this phase to prepare the injury for plyometric exercises. Other exercises in this phase are those listed in the shoulder rehabilitation program in chapter 21. Exercises begin in a slow and controlled manner and progress to faster movements while the patient maintains control of the scapula and the entire upper extremity throughout the motion. Closed kinetic chain exercises and neuromuscular facilitation exercises are used in this phase as well. If available, isokinetic exercises may be used; however, some clinicians do not use them because the evidence for their benefits with epicondylopathy is weak.[74] All exercises should remain pain free with no associated post-exercise discomfort.

Plyometrics transitions the patient from the resistive phase to the advanced phase. These exercise progressions are mentioned in chapter 21. The progression is the same as that presented for the shoulder, beginning with easier plyometrics and advancing to higher speeds and more resistance as the injured segment adapts and the patient can tolerate higher stresses.

Performance-specific exercises are based on each patient's needs. Guidelines for these performance-specific progressions are based on the patient's response to the exercises. As a rule, increases are introduced every third day at most. Only one parameter is increased at a time. So if a pitcher increases throwing distance on a particular day, the speed of the throw is not increased at the same time. In fact, it may sometimes be prudent to reduce the throwing speed when increasing distance and to gradually return it to the previous level; however, this is individually determined. Patients who have pain with any step up in the program should return to the immediately preceding level for another three sessions before advancing again. Figure 22.28 provides an outline of a rehabilitation progression for patients with either medial or lateral epicondylopathy.

Bracing may help the patient to have pain-free performance. A counterforce brace is approximately 5 cm (2 in.)

Nonsurgical Epicondylopathy

Stage I: Inactive phase	
This phase is included for tendinopathy treatment only in extreme cases where pain is sufficient to limit any motion. In most cases, there is no stage I phase, and modality use is incorporated into stage II, the active phase.	Inflammation phase: Inactive rehabilitation phase
Goals	Relieve pain, spasm, swelling. Maintain ROM of all UE segments. Maintain strength of shoulder and scapular muscles. Maintain core and hip strength. Correct postural deficiencies. Maintain CVL.

>continued

Figure 22.28 Rehabilitation program for nonsurgical epicondylopathy.

Stage I: Inactive phase	
This phase is included for tendinopathy treatment only in extreme cases where pain is sufficient to limit any motion. In most cases, there is no stage I phase, and modality use is incorporated into stage II, the active phase.	**Inflammation phase: Inactive rehabilitation phase**
Treatment guidelines	Modalities for pain, swelling, and spasm Use of elbow or wrist extension brace to reduce elbow stress Cross-friction massage over epicondylar area of pain once pain intensity decreases Trigger point, STM, MFR, and IASTM techniques PRN AROM and PROM of elbow, forearm, wrist, hand Resistive exercises for shoulder and scapula that do not cause elbow pain Core and hip strengthening and stabilization exercises CV exercises
Precautions	Shoulder and forearm trigger points may refer to the epicondyle and should be checked before treatment. Several locations on the epicondyle may need cross-friction massage for pain relief; the entire epicondylar area should be investigated for possible painful segments. Pain should not exceed 5/10 on VAS. Use HEP to facilitate treatment gains.

Stage II: Active phase	
Time and duration vary, depending on injury severity and treatment response.	**Early proliferation phase: Active rehabilitation phase**
Goals	Achieve pain relief to 2-3 on a scale of 10. Achieve full ROM of elbow, wrist, and hand. Achieve normal proprioception. Achieve strength gains to at least 75% of normal for elbow and forearm muscles. Develop good postural strength. MCL.
Treatment guidelines	UE weight-bearing activities for stabilization and proprioception AROM and PROM exercises for elbow, forearm, wrist, and hand Eccentric exercises for involved elbow, wrist, and forearm muscles Concentric–eccentric exercises for elbow, wrist, and hand muscles not involved in epicondylitis without pain in affected muscles Grade III and IV joint mobilization and soft-tissue mobilization PRN Continue to progress core and hip strengthening and stabilization exercises Progress postural strengthening exercises CV exercises

Figure 22.28   >*continued*

Stage II: Active phase	
Time and duration vary, depending on injury severity and treatment response.	**Early proliferation phase: Active rehabilitation phase**
Precautions	Patient may experience mild discomfort after the second set of eccentric exercise and more discomfort after the third set, but this is normal and should not deter the use of eccentrics; however, if the patient reports increased pain after the treatment session, then the eccentric exercise intensity should be reduced. Concentric exercises are not included as part of the rehabilitation program for the involved muscle group until eccentric exercise series is completed. Use HEP to facilitate treatment gains.

Stage III: Resistive phase	
Time and duration vary, depending on injury severity and treatment response.	**Late proliferation phase: Resistive rehabilitation phase**
Goals	Become pain-free. Achieve full range of motion in elbow, wrist, and hand. Maintain normal scapular muscle strength and endurance. Achieve normal strength of elbow, wrist, and hand muscles. Restore pain-free functional use in ADLs.
Treatment guidelines	Maintenance exercises for range of motion Maintenance exercises for shoulder complex strength and endurance Begin concentric exercises for involved muscles of elbow, wrist, and hand Progress to multiplanar exercises after concentric exercise strength is 80% Dynamic proprioception exercises
Precautions	Proper sequencing of muscle activation is important for all exercises; the clinician should watch to ensure that exercises are done correctly and should correct errors using verbal and tactile cues as necessary. Use HEP to facilitate treatment gains.

Stage IV: Advanced phase	
Time and duration vary, depending on injury severity and treatment response	**Remodeling phase: Advanced rehabilitation phase**
Goals	Maintain normal ROM of all joints. Maintain normal strength of all muscles. Restore normal sport and work performance.
Treatment guidelines	Plyometric exercise progression Functional exercise progression Performance-specific exercises and drills progression
Precautions	Correct execution of all activities should be observed.

ROM = range of motion; UE = upper extremity; PRN = as needed; MCL = maintain cardiovascular level; IASTM = instrument-assisted soft-tissue mobilization; HEP = home exercise program; CV = cardiovascular; AROM = active range of motion; PROM = passive range of motion; VAS = visual analog scale; ADLs = activities of daily living.

Figure 22.28 >continued

wide or slightly larger and is made of nonelastic strapping, usually secured with Velcro (figure 22.29). Its purpose is to reduce wrist extensor activity to lessen the stresses applied to the extensor tendons, thereby allowing them to heal.[68, 69] The brace is worn during the treatment phase and also when the patient returns to normal participation. Although both are effective, there is evidence to indicate that a wrist extension splint is more beneficial in reducing epicondylar pain than the forearm strap.[75] It is believed that one reason the wrist extension splint provides better pain relief is that less stress is applied to the epicondyle with the wrist extensors passively positioned in extension.[75]

Before racket-sport patients begin performance-specific activities, their equipment should be examined for appropriateness. Racket weight, stiffness, and size should be evaluated. A heavy racket requires more strength, energy, and muscle endurance than a light one. A stiff racket enables the patient to put more power on the ball, but it also absorbs less impact stress and transfers the unabsorbed force to the patient's upper extremity. A tightly strung racket also increases impact-stress transfer to the upper extremity; therefore, a patient returning to participation may be advised to reduce the string tension slightly. A less stiff racket with less string tension absorbs more force because the ball is in contact with the racket longer (Newton's second law of motion). The impact force is reduced because it is spread out over a longer period of time.

Grip size is another factor that requires assessment before the patient uses a racket. A grip that is too large or too small may require more strength or more muscle shortening to maintain a grasp, adding stress to the epicondyles and increasing forearm muscle fatigue. To measure grip size, place the hand flat on a tabletop with the palm facing up and fingers extended. Extend a tape measure from the proximal palmar crease in the palm to the end of the fourth finger (figure 22.30). This distance to the nearest 3 mm (1/8 in.) between the proximal palmar crease and the end of the fourth fingertip is the person's grip size.[78]

Post-Surgical Rehabilitation

Although most cases respond well to conservative treatment,[54, 58] surgery is occasionally needed to completely

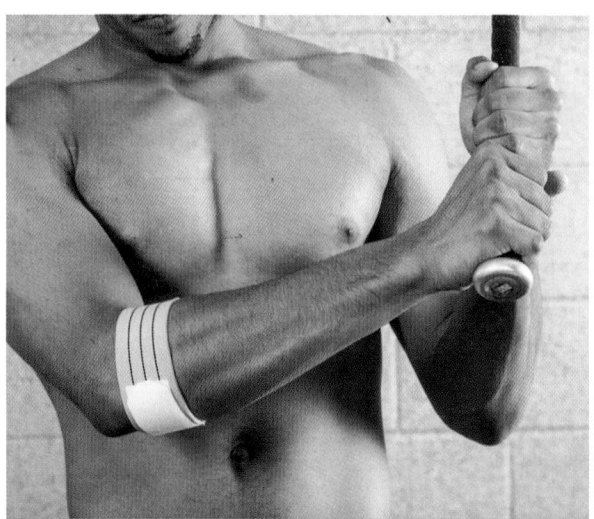

Figure 22.29 Counterforce brace.

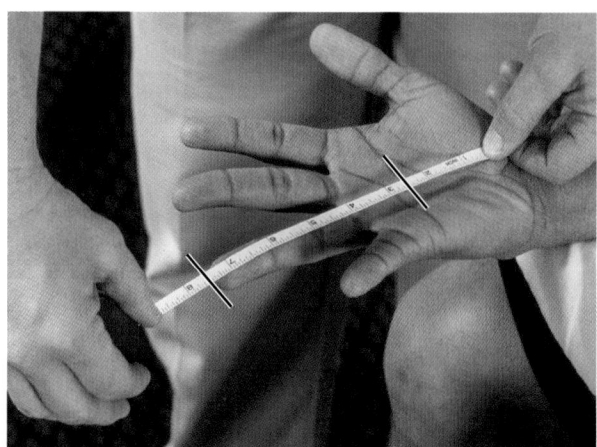

Figure 22.30 Racket-grip measurement.

Evidence in Rehabilitation

Two studies demonstrate a significant reduction in pain for patients who wore elbow counterforce braces.[76, 77] Both studies looked at the immediate effects of counterforce bracing and came to similar conclusions: Counterforce braces for elbow epicondylopathy are effective for immediately reducing pain. Interestingly, the Yoon and Bae study[77] concluded that the counterforce brace concentrated its compression on a focal area of the proximal forearm to relieve the pain by reducing the muscle's electromyographic output.

Recently, Kroslak and colleagues[69] compared counterforce bracing to placebo bracing and concluded that the counterforce brace provided a significant reduction in pain in the short term (2-12 weeks), in addition to significant improvement in overall elbow function at 26 weeks. These data support the use of counterforce bracing in the treatment of acute lateral epicondylopathy.

Although the precise mechanism by which counterforce braces relieve epicondylopathy pain is unknown, it is generally accepted that they are effective. Perhaps the mechanism may be identified as studies continue. Once we understand the physiological mechanisms in play, we may be able to develop other successful treatments.

resolve more persistent cases of epicondylopathy. The primary source of pathology in lateral epicondylopathy is the extensor carpi radialis brevis tendon; in medial epicondylopathy the flexor carpi radialis and pronator teres portions of the conjoined flexor tendon mass form the most common site of pathology.[56] In both conditions, either a small surgical incision about 2.5 cm (1 in.) long or an arthroscopic procedure is used to visualize the pathologic tissue, which is then removed from the region.[56, 79] Investigations have shown that both open and arthroscopic procedures produce successful results,[55, 79] but the arthroscopic method has fewer complications.[55]

Postoperative rehabilitation is similar to the nonoperative routine except that the initial 1 to 2 weeks includes postoperative concerns. Once the patient's elbow is into the end of the proliferation phase, rehabilitation care closely follows the nonoperative routine. If the open approach is used, an elbow immobilizer is applied immediately after surgery and continues to be worn about 2 d; the immobilizer positions the elbow at 90° with the forearm in neutral.[56] After the first two postoperative days, the immobilizer is continued only as the patient's comfort dictates until 1 week after surgery.[56] After the first week, a counterforce brace may be used as a protective device until the extremity regains normal strength.[56]

When the wrist and hand are free of the immobilizer, active range-of-motion exercises for the wrist and fingers can start after surgery, although the patient will probably not want to begin these until at least the second postoperative day. Gentle active and active-assistive range of motion of the elbow can begin around day 5. By the third week, the patient should have full range of motion.

At 2 weeks, active exercises against gravity without resistance can begin, as can squeezing a soft ball. Pronation and supination motion exercises for the forearm, as well as flexion and extension range-of-motion exercises for the wrist and elbow, should continue.

The patient is at the end of the active phase and into the early resistive phase by 3 weeks after surgery, so the patient progresses from isometrics to low-resistance, low-repetition exercises in straight-plane motions. The patient should have full motion by this time. The patient progresses as tolerated into higher-repetition exercises before moving into heavier weights.

Diagonal-plane exercises begin at 4 to 8 weeks, depending on the patient's pain tolerance and strength. Once the patient displays good strength and control without pain in diagonal motions, it is appropriate to begin plyometrics at the end of the resistive phase.

By 3 to 4 months, functional activities can begin if there is no pain with plyometrics and if the patient has normal strength, muscle endurance, and flexibility. Patients undergoing medial or lateral epicondylar open releases may not be able to return to full participation for 3 to 6 months, but those who undergo arthroscopic procedures may be able to return to normal participation earlier.[55, 80, 81]

Little League Elbow

Little League elbow is another chronic condition of the elbow, but it is unique because it occurs only in young athletes. Its name comes from the population it most often affects, pitchers in Little League baseball. It has been a common enough problem that youth league governing bodies now regulate pitching for their players, but the problem remains. We will discuss the special issues with this injury and present a case study for you to solve.

Little League elbow is unique to the preadolescent population. It involves a number of conditions that have the common thread of elbow pathology secondary to pitching. The most common site of pathology is the medial elbow because of the excessive traction forces on the medial epicondyle epiphyseal plate during the late cocking phase.[82] The rotation of the humerus during this phase places excessive torque on the elbow by producing either humeral retrotorsion or proximal humeral epiphysiolysis after many repetitions.[82] Curves and breaking pitches are thought to increase the demands on wrist flexion and pronation, thereby increasing the medial epicondyle stresses; however, this premise continues to be disputed because no current studies show a definitive result.[83] Pitch velocity has been associated with increased medial elbow pain. A study by Kurokawa and colleagues[84] concluded that pitch velocity was significantly associated with abnormal findings of the medial epicondyle and medial elbow pain. It is thought that injury to the inherently weak epiphyseal plate may begin as an inflammation and progress to an avulsion of the plate if repetitive trauma persists.[85] In severe cases, osteochondritis dissecans of the radioulnar joint can also occur.[85]

Less often, the lateral, anterior, or posterior elbow is affected by excessive stresses applied during throwing. Osteochondritis dissecans of the humeral capitellum results from increased valgus stress causing lateral elbow compression.[86, 87] The pronator teres suffers greater stresses laterally during extreme pronation, and increased hyperextension forces during deceleration after ball release can increase anterior and posterior joint stresses.[10, 88] Interestingly, the stiffness of the pronator teres has been noted in the throwing arms of young athletes with elbow pain.[88]

In the more common medial Little League elbow, the athlete experiences progressive medial elbow pain with activity, pain with end-motion finger and wrist extension, tenderness to medial epicondyle palpation, and pain and weakness with resisted wrist and finger flexion. Swelling and, in more severe cases, ecchymosis can be present over the medial epicondyle.

Common causes for Little League elbow are improper warm-up or lack of warm-up, improper or insufficient conditioning, poor pitching mechanics, inadequate rest between games, and pitching too many innings.[89] Adequate conditioning programs and proper warm-up and cool-down procedures should be included in a team's program, and Little League Baseball pitching rules should be enforced for practices as well as games.[90] Little League Baseball[91] regulations and USA Baseball[92] and MLB Pitch Smart[93] recommendations use ball count and required rest periods as a method of restricting youth league pitchers' participation. See table 22.3. These recommendations and regulations are based on the number of pitches and the amount of rest between games; they were established to help prevent the occurrence of Little League elbow in young baseball pitchers.[94]

Recent evidence suggests that abnormal MRI findings of distal humeral physeal widening, loss of shoulder medial rotation, and medial elbow pain are common in Little League baseball players who comply with the Little League throwing guidelines; however, they are usually associated with youngsters who play year-round.[95,96] These findings highlight the strong correlation between elbow pathology and single-sport specialization in youth baseball. They demonstrate the importance of taking time off from throwing for at least 4 months per year.

Several risk factors have been associated with the increased incidence of elbow pain and injury in baseball players; these include altered shoulder range of motion, decreased elbow extension mobility, increased posterior shoulder tightness, rotator cuff weakness, and scapular dysfunction.[98-100] Recent studies have examined the regional interdependence and the role of the lower quarter in elbow injuries in youth baseball players. Lower-extremity muscle tightness, decreased hip medial rotation, deficits in single-leg standing balance, and low back and knee pain were found to be independent risk factors for elbow pain and injury in throwing athletes.[101-103] In addition to time off from throwing, a prevention program aimed at improving overall physical function can prevent medial elbow injury in youth baseball players.[103]

If growth plate damage is evident with the elbow injury, the athlete should be advised to stop pitching and rest until the injury is resolved.[104] Early inactive phase treatment for Little League elbow includes rest, ice, and in advanced cases, immobilization. Active range-of-motion exercises to tolerance are encouraged. Pain and passive stretches should be avoided. Because of the age of the patient, using heavy weights is contraindicated because they can aggravate sensitive growth plates.

Exercises are neither as aggressive nor as intensive as they are for adult patients, but a young patient's epicondylopathy program should follow the same progression as that of an adult. This progression emphasizes pain relief in the inactive phase, pain-free motion and shoulder and hip flexibility in the active rehabilitation phase, advancement to a progressive strengthening program in the late active and resistive phases, and finally functional and performance-specific activities in the advanced phase. Proximal scapular stabilization and rotator cuff strengthening, along with core and lumbopelvic stability, must also be included

TABLE 22.3   **USA Youth Baseball Pitching Recommendations and Restrictions**

Pitching limits	7-8 years old	9-10 years old	11-12 years old	13-14 years old	15-16 years old	17-18 years old
Max pitches/game	50	75	85	95	95	105
Required rest (pitches): 0 d	1-20	1-20	1-20	1-20	1-30	1-30
Required rest (pitches): 1 d	21-35	21-35	21-35	21-35	31-45	31-45
Required rest (pitches): 2 d	36-50	36-50	36-50	36-50	46-50	46-50
Required rest (pitches): 3 d	N/A	51-65	51-65	51-65	61-75	61-75
Required rest (pitches): 4 d	N/A	66+	66+	66+	76+	81+
12-month combined inning tally	60	80	80	100	100	100
Time off throwing in 12 months	At least 4 months with at least 2-3 being continuous for all age groups					

Note: Based on Little League Baseball,[91] USA Baseball,[92] and American Sports Medicine Institute.[97]

Case Study

A 12-year-old baseball pitcher is in the middle of his season. For the past month he has experienced progressive medial elbow pain in his left throwing elbow. He is the team's top pitcher and usually pitches 3 d a week. An invitational tournament is planned for next weekend, and he wants to pitch. His parents are reluctant to allow him to do so, but they want your opinion. He has full range of motion of the elbow, but wrist extension is painful in the last 10°. Resisted pronation and wrist flexion are weak and painful. The medial epicondyle is tender to palpation and edematous.

Questions for Analysis

1. What will be your recommendation to the patient about the weekend invitational tournament?
2. What will be your recommendations on future pitching?
3. What treatment procedure will you recommend he follow to reduce the pain and inflammation? Given his age, what precautions must you consider?
4. What will be your instructions about exercises he should perform?
5. How much information will you give the patient's parents about the injury and potential harm?

in the rehabilitation program. Valgus stress is avoided until it does not cause pain. A gradually progressive throwing program is included when the elbow is pain free and has full range of motion with normal muscle strength and endurance.

Sprains

Sprains in the elbow commonly occur as hyperextension or medial collateral ligament injuries.[105] In addition to ligament involvement, the capsule of the elbow can be disrupted with a ligamentous injury. Capsular injury of the elbow can be frustrating if not treated correctly at the outset. Special considerations relating to hyperextension and medial collateral ligament injury are presented, followed by a case study.

Etiology and Complaints

Elbow sprains usually occur as either hyperextension injuries or ulnar (medial) collateral ligament (UCL) sprains.[105] A hyperextension sprain can occur in football when an opponent runs into and past an outstretched arm, when a gymnast does a handstand with a locked elbow, or when a person falls onto an outstretched hand with the elbow locked in extension. In a hyperextension injury, the anterior capsule is injured, and it may also involve the medial collateral ligament or the lateral collateral ligament.[106] Any sudden valgus force, such as a sidearm throw by a shortstop or a wrench of the elbow by a wrestling opponent, can cause a sprain to the UCL. When valgus overstress occurs—such as in handball, tennis, volleyball, javelin, or baseball—the medial (ulnar) collateral ligament, which is the primary stabilizing unit for the elbow, is injured.[107, 108] Ulnar collateral ligament injuries have increased exponentially in recent years and are affecting athletes at younger ages.[109] Conte and colleagues[110] reported that 25% of major league pitchers and 15% of minor league pitchers have a history of

UCL surgery. In major league athletes, the injury is related to extensive ligament damage due to repeated microtrauma from years of throwing.[109] In younger patients, the injury is usually related to a proximal partial tear or sprain.[109]

Hyperextension injuries cause pain in the anterior and medial joint. Sudden, forceful hyperextension stress can also cause a bone contusion and pain from the olecranon or olecranon fossa. Ulnar collateral ligament sprains cause medial joint pain. Isolated injuries to the UCL occur most often in overhead throwing athletes, who will report medial elbow pain in the acceleration phase of throwing.[111]

Conservative Rehabilitation

For either hyperextension or medial joint injuries, a support brace may be used during the first couple of weeks after injury to support and protect the area. Typically, a functional elbow brace is used to allow for controlled motion.[112] Initial inactive phase rehabilitation includes treatment to relieve pain and swelling. Active and active-assistive ranges of motion are used in the late inactive phase and into the early active phase of rehabilitation. Easy strength exercises may begin during the active phase, but pain with any activity is avoided. During this phase, it is appropriate to address scapular strengthening and core and lumbopelvic stability as long as it does not cause elbow symptoms.

Strengthening exercises start in earnest in the resistive phase and should include the biceps and triceps, as well as shoulder complex muscles, wrist and finger flexors and extensors, and forearm pronators and supinators. After hyperextension or medial collateral ligament injuries, the elbow must rely on dynamic stability from the muscles to substitute for damaged ligamentous and capsular tissues; the main dynamic stabilizers for the elbow after sprains are the medial flexor–pronator muscles coming off the medial epicondyle.[88, 113] Of this group, the flexor carpi ulnaris makes the greatest contribution to elbow stability.[113, 114]

Therefore, resistance to the flexor carpi ulnaris may over-stress medial joint and hyperextension injuries in early rehabilitation, and such exercises should be deferred until the resistive phase of rehabilitation. Any flexibility issues in the shoulder and hip can be addressed during this phase.

By the end of the active phase, the elbow should have full range of motion. Strengthening exercises occur in the next phase for the flexor carpi ulnaris in wrist flexion and ulnar deviation. Straight-plane exercises isolate and focus on the weak muscles, and their resistance and repetition levels increase as progress is made. Eccentric and concentric exercises are used. By the end of phase III, diagonal-plane movements begin with PNF stabilization activities and closed kinetic chain exercises; multiplanar resistance-band exercises are added as long as the stresses do not cause pain either during or after the exercise. Isokinetics are appropriate in this phase if they are available, beginning with straight-plane movement and progressing to diagonal planes of movement. Scapular stabilization, rotator cuff strengthening, and core and lumbopelvic stabilization exercises are continued and progressed through all phases of rehabilitation.

In the late resistive phase, plyometric exercises begin. These are the same exercises as those described for epicondylopathy. Functional planes of movement are used during these exercises as the patient prepares to advance to the final rehabilitation phase. The patient should be able to maintain good proximal control and elbow joint stability during all activities. Cross-friction massage to adherent scar tissue can relieve pain that occurs with motion; it may also improve motion if the joint still lacks normal mobility. The goal of this phase is to prepare the injury site for performance-specific exercises in the advanced phase of rehabilitation. If the patient is a throwing athlete, throwing programs begin during this final phase.

The use of biologic treatments for UCL injuries is increasing. In a survey of the American Shoulder and Elbow Surgeons performed by Hurwit and colleagues,[115] 36.3% of respondents used platelet-rich plasma (PRP) injections to manage UCL injuries. Recent studies have reported a greater than 70% return-to-sport rate after PRP injections coupled with rehabilitation in athletes with UCL tears.[116, 117]

Ulnar Collateral Ligament Repair and Reconstruction

The elbow is usually unstable after a severe injury to the UCL, especially the anterior portion of the ligament.[111] As a result, the elbow has posterolateral rotatory instability.[7] In these cases, surgical intervention is usually needed, especially if the patient wants to continue normal activities. Surgical management is usually performed using either a ligamentous repair or a tendon graft ligament reconstruction.[111, 118, 119] The tendon graft most often used

is the palmaris longus tendon.[111, 119, 120] Both the repair and the reconstruction method have comparable outcomes.[120]

Although UCL reconstruction is the gold standard in the treatment of symptomatic UCL injuries in competitive overhead athletes, UCL repair with internal brace augmentation, using collagen tape, has proven beneficial with avulsion injuries and permits an earlier return to sport than UCL reconstruction.[111, 121] The UCL must demonstrate good to normal ligament quality for a repair to be a consideration.[111] Long-term data on the success of surgical repair are lacking;[122] on the other hand, short-term results indicate a high return-to-play rate following surgery: anywhere from over 80%[123] to up to 97%.[124] Since Jobe[125] first developed a surgical reconstruction method that allowed athletes to return to sport participation after surgery, advances in reconstruction methods have made successful surgical reconstructions commonplace rather than the exception they once were.[111, 126] This surgical procedure is often referred to as the "Tommy John surgery" because this baseball pitcher from the Los Angeles Dodgers was the first patient on whom Jobe performed his reconstruction technique in 1974.[127]

After UCL reconstruction surgery, the elbow is locked at 90° in an adjustable elbow flexion splint or brace for the first week.[111, 121] During this time, the patient performs active shoulder, wrist, and finger motion exercises. Submaximal isometric exercises for the biceps and the shoulder occur as long as the patient avoids lateral rotation of the shoulder, a motion that increases valgus elbow stress. The patient can also squeeze a ball.

By the end of the second week, the brace's motion-stop pegs are positioned to permit elbow motion to 30° from extension and 100° of flexion.[111] Submaximal wrist and elbow isometrics can start after the second week. The patient now starts to actively move the elbow within the restricted range of motion allowed by the brace. The brace is adjusted each week to increase motion in both flexion and extension until it is set to full motion by the fourth week. With each change in brace positions, the patient's active motion also improves through active exercises.

After 3 weeks, a gradual progression of strength exercises is added to the program. These exercises include mild resistance to wrist and elbow flexion and extension and forearm pronation and supination. Early proprioception exercises for joint-position sense with eyes closed is appropriate, but valgus stress to the elbow is avoided. Proprioceptive exercises that avoid valgus stresses advance as tolerated. Shoulder exercises, with the exception of lateral rotation motions, are performed as well. Shoulder lateral rotation exercises start after the sixth week. Concentric, eccentric, and mild isokinetics are used in straight-plane movements to isolate and strengthen the weak muscle groups. Co-contraction exercises for the biceps and triceps are also started as long as valgus stress is avoided. Closed

Case Study

A 30-year-old right-handed golfer injured his right elbow when he hit a divot and tore his ulnar collateral ligament. He tried to continue playing through the season, but pain persisted. Since the physician diagnosed him with posterolateral rotatory instability, he underwent a medial collateral ligament reconstruction. The surgery was 10 d ago, and he has been instructed by the surgeon to begin rehabilitation. The elbow is in a functional brace with motion blocks that are at 30° from extension and 100° flexion. Supination is possible to neutral. Your examination reveals mild discoloration still present in the forearm and distal upper arm medially. There is spasm in the upper trapezius and biceps. Active range of motion out of the brace is limited to 60° from extension and 100° into flexion. Wrist extensors have 4/5 strength, the shoulder complex grossly has 4–/5 strength, the biceps and triceps are also 4–/5, and the wrist flexors are 3–/5. You notice weakness in the lumbopelvic region with single-leg squat. There are active trigger points in the forearm on the flexor and extensor surfaces.

Questions for Analysis

1. What will your first treatment session include?
2. What precautions will you give the patient?
3. When will you start pronation and supination motion activities? What must be considered before these exercises are added?
4. What strengthening exercises will you include in the first week, and how will you advance them (what will your criteria be)?
5. At what motion limits will you set the brace in week 5?
6. When will you start shoulder external-rotation exercises?
7. What functional-exercise program will you establish for the patient, and when will you start it?

---

kinetic chain exercises and other stabilization exercises are permissible once the patient has strength and control of the elbow and no elbow pain in upper-extremity weight bearing.

The patient should have full range of motion by weeks 6 to 8. The brace is discontinued by week 6. The muscles providing dynamic stability—the medial flexor-pronator group—are important for assisting the UCL and should be well strengthened. After the sixth week, the patient has normal range of motion and good strength and is therefore at the end of the resistive phase, so diagonal movements can begin if the elbow has adequate strength and control without pain. Work on PNF facilitation patterns, resistance-band exercises, more aggressive stabilization exercises, and diagonal isokinetics at high speeds can all be started at this time.

Plyometric activities begin late in the resistive phase or early in the advanced phase after week 9. As with other plyometric exercises, these begin with lower-stress activities at reduced speeds and resistance and then increase to higher speeds and more resistance. Medicine ball tosses, push-up progressions, and functional isokinetic motions are included.

Functional exercises can begin in weeks 10 to 14 when the patient enters the advanced phase. The timing depends on the patient's response to these functional exercises and the patient's progression into performance-specific

reconditioning events. For example, a baseball pitcher may need to wait longer to begin throwing activities because of the higher elbow stresses in pitching compared with those in a less-intense sport, such as golf, or less-intense work activities, such as computer programming. The progression of functional activities and the precautions to observe are the same as for other injuries. Gradual return to competitive throwing begins at around 20 weeks with a UCL repair and 36 to 48 weeks after UCL reconstruction.[121] It typically takes baseball pitchers 10 to 18 months to return to the mound, game ready.[111] These timelines are based on averages, and you must always remember that the actual recovery time will vary from one patient to another. Figure 22.31 describes this rehabilitation progression.

Ulnar Nerve Injury

Injury to the ulnar nerve can occur in any setting, but it seems most prevalent in repetitive throwing sports such as baseball pitching.[128] The most frequent cause in this population is incorrect mechanics. The ulnar nerve can also be injured at the elbow from prolonged typing or writing, compression from leaning on a flexed elbow, or acutely from a fall directly onto the elbow. This injury is treated with both operative and nonoperative techniques. Considerations in rehabilitation for both treatments are presented here.

Posterolateral Rotatory Instability

Stage I: Inactive phase	
0-3 weeks	**Inflammation phase: Inactive rehabilitation phase**
Goals	Protect surgical site. Relieve pain, spasm, and swelling. Maintain ROM of all UE segments. Maintain strength of shoulder and scapular muscles. Maintain core and hip strength. Correct postural deficiencies. MCL.
Treatment guidelines	Elbow splint with sling Modalities for pain, swelling, and spasm AROM of shoulder, wrist, and fingers Trigger point, gentle STM, MFR, IASTM techniques PRN Resistive exercises for shoulder and scapula that do not cause elbow stress or pain Core and hip strengthening and stabilization exercises CV exercises
Precautions	Follow surgeon's protocol. Week 1: Elbow is locked at 90° flexion. Week 2: Elbow brace allows motion of 30° toward extension to 100° toward flexion with AROM while in brace. Week 2: Perform submaximal isometric exercises for wrist, elbow. Use HEP to facilitate treatment gains.
Stage II: Active phase	
3-10 weeks	**Early proliferation phase: Active rehabilitation phase**
Goals	Relieve pain to 1–2 on a scale of 10. Progressively increase brace motion weekly with AROM to achieve gains in elbow ROM. Weeks 6-8: Remove brace. Weeks 6-8: Achieve full ROM. Reduce risk of elbow muscle weakness; improve elbow muscle strength to 75%. Achieve good postural strength. MCL.
Treatment guidelines	Progressive changes in elbow brace to gain full ROM of elbow Week 3: Active and mild passive range of motion Week 3: Light concentric–eccentric straight-plane exercises with low force, high reps to elbow, forearm, and wrist Week 6: Continue with straight-plane exercises Proprioception exercises without weight bearing Week 6: Co-contraction of biceps and triceps Week 8: Grade III and IV joint mobilization and soft-tissue mobilization PRN Weeks 6-8: Weight-bearing exercises Resistive exercises for shoulder (no lateral rotation) and scapula Continue core and hip strengthening and stabilization exercises CV exercises

Figure 22.31 Rehabilitation progression for surgical repair of posterolateral rotatory instability.

Stage II: Active phase	
3-10 weeks	**Early proliferation phase: Active rehabilitation phase**
Precautions	Week 6: Brace is set for full elbow motion; patient performs AROM in brace. Some surgeons do not allow resisted pronation until weeks 6-8. Avoid valgus stress to elbow. Use HEP to facilitate treatment gains.

Stage III: Resistive phase	
10-20 weeks	**Late proliferation phase: Resistive rehabilitation phase**
Goals	Become pain-free. Achieve full range of motion in shoulder, elbow, wrist, and hand. Maintain normal scapular muscle strength and endurance. Achieve normal strength of shoulder, elbow, wrist, and hand muscles in straight-plane and multiplanar activities. Restore pain-free functional use in ADLs.
Treatment guidelines	Maintenance exercises for range of motion. Maintenance exercises for shoulder complex strength and endurance. Progress to multiplanar exercises after concentric exercise strength is 80%. Dynamic proprioception exercises. Plyometric exercises.
Precautions	There should be no pain with exercises. Elbow stress of normal activities will determine length of time in this phase. Healing of tissues must be appropriate to withstand stresses applied by functional activities. Use HEP to facilitate treatment gains.

Stage IV: Advanced phase	
16-36 weeks	**Remodeling phase: Advanced rehabilitation phase**
Goals	Maintain normal strength of all muscles. Maintain normal ROM of all joints. Restore normal performance in all activities.
Treatment guidelines	Functional exercise progression. Performance-specific exercises and drills progression.
Precautions	If pain occurs at any progression, keep the patient at the lower performance goal for another 3 d before retrying the next level in the exercise progression sequence.

ROM = range of motion; UE = upper extremity; STM = soft-tissue massage; MCL = maintain cardiovascular level; MFR = myofascial release; IASTM = instrument-assisted soft-tissue mobilization; PRN = as needed; CV = cardiovascular; AROM = active range of motion; HEP = home exercise program; ADLs = activities of daily living.

Figure 22.31 >continued

Repetitive overhand throwing activities, especially in patients whose shoulder lateral rotation is reduced in the cocking phase, places excessive stress on medial elbow structures. The ulnar nerve can become stretched, mechanically irritated, or even subluxed out of its sulcus.[129] Adjacent soft-tissue structures can also compress the nerve.[129] Prolonged elbow flexion, such as that which occurs in writing or typing, can increase pressure in the cubital tunnel where the ulnar nerve resides in the medial elbow.[130] Direct compression of the nerve at the cubital tunnel from resting the arm on a hard surface or from a fall onto the medial elbow can also injure the ulnar nerve.[130]

The patient commonly complains of medial elbow pain, numbness or tingling in the fourth and fifth digits and in the ulnar side forearm, weakness of the hand, and loss of dexterity.[130, 131] Nonoperative care includes initial treatments to reduce the inflammation and pain. Posture education is important because slumping with rounded shoulders and head forward will place the ulnar nerve on stretch at the shoulder and neck. This can render the nerve more sensitive as it goes through the bony cubital tunnel at the elbow.

Exercises to improve range of motion and strength are similar to those for other elbow injuries. Mobilization is performed if the elbow joints are hypomobile. Strength exercises are initially low-resistance, high-repetition loads in straight-plane motions. Muscles for all shoulder, elbow, wrist, forearm, and hand motions are strengthened. If shoulder inflexibility, shoulder weakness, or poor athletic technique is contributing to the elbow injury, these deficiencies must be corrected.

Initial exercises should not place valgus stress or compression on the elbow. As strength improves, valgus stress is gradually introduced as long as symptoms are not reproduced. The final phases of the program include a progression from diagonal motions to plyometrics to functional and then sport- or performance-specific functions before resuming normal and unrestricted participation.

When operative repair is required for failed conservative management or a subluxating or dislocating ulnar nerve, the surgical technique most commonly used is the creation of fascial slings to support the ulnar nerve or anterior subcutaneous nerve transposition.[130, 132] Postoperatively, the elbow is placed in a hinged elbow brace that is positioned at 90° flexion for 2 weeks. After the first week, the brace's motion-stop pegs are positioned at 30° to 15° from extension and at 100° to 120° of flexion. Gentle gripping exercises using a foam ball start during the first postoperative week along with isometric exercises for the scapula and shoulder. Active range-of-motion exercises for pronation, supination, and wrist and finger flexion and extension are also included.

By week 2, the healing tissue is in the proliferation phase, so isometrics for the elbow and wrist can begin. The splint is removed to permit active and passive range-of-motion exercises. Early proprioceptive exercises for position sense start in week 2. Mild manual-resistance exercises and light weights for the wrist are also added.

The brace is discontinued by the third week, and the patient performs active range-of-motion exercises to gain full elbow flexion and extension. By about the sixth week, the patient should have full range of motion in all planes. Also by the third week, resistance exercises for the wrist, forearm, and elbow include low-resistance, high-repetition exercises in all planes. Range-of-motion exercises begin as straight-plane motions in phase II and progress to resistive diagonal-plane motions later in phase III as strength and motion control improve.

By the end of the resistive phase, the patient has full motion and good strength and control of the elbow and forearm in single-plane motions. At this point, multiplanar motions begin, and other exercises include plyometrics and weight-bearing activities. Plyometrics begins with a normal progression from low-load, controlled movement to increased loads with higher speeds of movement as the patient advances to the final rehabilitation phase.

By around week 12, the patient reaches phase IV, and the elbow and forearm have full motion and near-normal strength, proprioception, and control. The patient is now ready to begin more aggressive functional and performance-specific exercises. For throwing athletes, a progressive throwing program starts in this phase and is completed when the patient returns to normal activities. This rehabilitation program is outlined in figure 22.32.

Case Study

A 19-year-old right-handed volleyball frontline player suffered a subluxed ulnar nerve at the end of the season. She underwent ulnar nerve transposition 2 d ago. The surgeon wants her to begin her rehabilitation program today. She has a posterior splint set at 90°. She has some pain over the surgical site, but nothing more significant than normal postoperative pain. There is some tension in the upper trapezius muscle, and it is tender to palpation. Wrist extension and supination movements cause some medial elbow pain at the end range. Wrist flexion motion is lacking about 10°, and the patient reports that the wrist feels weak and sore from the surgery. Pronation is also weak, as is her grip strength. Shoulder flexion is lacking about 10°, lateral rotation is lacking about 20°, and there is some weakness in the rotator cuff. Scapular stabilizer muscles also demonstrate mild weakness.

Questions for Analysis

1. What will your first treatment session include? What will be the goals of this treatment session?

2. What home exercises will you give the patient in the first week?

3. What exercises will the program include for the next 3 weeks?

4. Outline a functional and sport-specific exercise program that the patient will use when she is ready for functional and performance-specific exercises.

Ulnar Nerve Transposition

Stage I: Inactive phase	
0-3 weeks	**Inflammation phase: Inactive rehabilitation phase**
Goals	Relieve pain. Reduce edema, ecchymosis. Relieve spasm. Protect surgical site. Correct postural deficiencies. MCL.
Treatment guidelines	Week 1: Sling worn with posterior splint set at 90°, keeping the wrist and hand free Modalities for pain, spasm, edema, ecchymosis Isometric exercises for shoulder and scapula Ball squeeze Week 2: Discontinue splint and replace with brace set at 15°-30° from extension and 110°-120° of flexion AROM shoulder, wrist, and hand Week 3: Progress splint to full motion Weeks 2-3: Remove sling CV and exercises for uninvolved body segments Trigger point, gentle STM, MFR, IASTM techniques PRN Grade I and II joint mobilizations for pain
Precautions	Follow surgeon's protocol. Observe surgical site for appropriate healing. Avoid pain with exercises. Use HEP to facilitate treatment.
Stage II: Active phase	
3-8 weeks	**Early proliferation phase: Active rehabilitation phase**
Goals	Restore ROM to normal. Make muscle endurance gains. Make early strength gains. Restore proprioception. Achieve good postural strength. MCL. Avoid pain, edema, spasm.
Treatment guidelines	Weeks 4-6: Full elbow and forearm ROM Weeks 5-6: Begin pain-free light resisted supination–pronation Light progressive resistance exercises as tolerated for shoulder, scapula, wrist, and hand Weeks 6-8: Proprioception exercises with weight-bearing exercises CV exercise as tolerated
Precautions	Avoid pain with strength exercises. Use HEP to facilitate treatment gains.

>continued

Figure 22.32   Rehabilitation program for ulnar nerve transposition.

Stage III: Resistive phase	
8-12 weeks	**Late proliferation phase: Resistive rehabilitation phase**
Goals	Achieve full ROM. Achieve normal strength and muscle endurance. Achieve normal proprioception. Achieve normal performance in triplanar motions. MCL. Restore pain-free functional use in ADLs.
Treatment guidelines	Aggressive strength exercises as tolerated Diagonal exercises Plyometric exercises Agility exercises
Precautions	Avoid pain with all exercises. Use HEP to facilitate treatment.

Stage IV: Advanced phase	
12-26 weeks	**Remodeling phase: Advanced rehabilitation phase**
Goals	Perform functional activities properly. Perform performance-specific exercises at least to preinjury levels. Return to full normal participation.
Treatment guidelines	Functional exercises Performance- and sport-specific exercises
Precautions	Observe for proper execution of all exercises.

MCL = maintain cardiovascular level; CV = cardiovascular; AROM = active range of motion; STM = soft-tissue massage; MFR = myofascial release; IASTM = instrument-assisted soft-tissue mobilization; PRN = as needed; HEP = home exercise program; ROM = range of motion; ADLs = activities of daily living.

Figure 22.32 >continued

Dislocation

Unfortunately, elbow dislocations are common occurrences, but fortunately, most of them are simple.[133] This means that there are no other injuries such as fractures or neurovascular compromises. When an elbow dislocation occurs, the deformity makes it an obvious injury. Elbow dislocations tend to occur posteriorly and follow sudden hyperextension and abduction force applications.[134] Suggestions for a rehabilitation program progression after initial care of a nonsurgically repaired simple elbow dislocation are presented here.

The elbow is placed in a posterior immobilizing splint for a few days until initial complaints of pain subside. Some investigators advise that no splint be used to reduce the risk of elbow motion loss.[135] For the first few days after dislocation injury, modalities are used to relieve pain, swelling, and spasm. If a splint is used, trigger points and muscle spasms in the neck and shoulder muscles may develop, requiring manual therapy interventions to relieve them. Grade I and grade II joint mobilization are often beneficial for relieving pain. Active shoulder, scapula, wrist, and hand

motions are commenced. Isometric exercises to the elbow and mild resistive exercises to the wrist are used initially. The patient squeezes a ball throughout the day. After about 2 to 3 d, the splint is removed for gentle active range of motion to tolerance in all elbow and forearm planes. Passive motion is avoided.

After day 3, the splint is removed during the day but is used as needed when fatigue occurs. After 2 weeks, the splint is discarded, and active range-of-motion exercises are continued. Mild resistive exercises for the elbow with an emphasis on high repetitions and low resistance begin at this time. Straight-plane exercises are used initially to focus on weak individual muscles and then advance to diagonal-plane exercises when the patient demonstrates good control, strength, and coordination. By weeks 6 to 8, the patient should have full range of motion in all planes. Joint mobilization is added by week 8 if additional capsular-motion gains are needed.

Strength exercises progress in the same way as for other elbow injuries, from isometric to isotonic to isokinetic. The emphasis is on strengthening the elbow flexors to provide

Case Study

Five days ago, a 20-year-old right-handed gymnast fell off the balance beam and landed on her hyperextended left elbow, dislocating the elbow. Surgery was not needed, so the orthopedist placed the elbow in a 90° splint and wants you to begin rehabilitation on it today. Elbow range of motion lacks 50° of extension and can flex to 100°. Supination is 10°, and pronation is 20°. She wore a splint for 2 d after the injury, but the physician told her to now wear it only at night for the next month. Edema and ecchymosis surround the elbow and extend into the mid-forearm and mid-arm. Spasm is present in the biceps, triceps, and upper trapezius. Her elbow strength is difficult to test because her pain limits her ability to provide adequate resistance. Wrist movements demonstrate 4/5 strength, and grip strength is 75% compared to that on the right. Shoulder strength overall is 4+/5.

Questions for Analysis

1. What will your first treatment session include? What will be your goals for today's treatment?
2. What instructions for home exercises will you give the patient during the first week?
3. What exercises will you include as part of the first week's treatment program?
4. What are your goals for the first week?
5. What will be your progression of flexibility and strength exercises?
6. What sport-specific exercise program will you include for rehabilitation?

dynamic stabilization against hyperextension. Resistive exercises begin in straight planes and progress to diagonal planes, then to plyometrics, and finally to functional activities and then performance-specific activities by weeks 8 to 10. A hyperextension brace may be needed to offer the patient additional protection against hyperextension forces. It may take the patient 16 to 26 weeks to return to full participation. Figure 22.33 outlines a rehabilitation program for a simple dislocation of the elbow.

Simple Elbow Dislocations

Stage I: Inactive phase	
0-3 weeks	**Inflammation phase: Inactive rehabilitation phase**
Goals	Relieve pain, spasm, and swelling. Maintain ROM of all UE segments. Maintain strength of shoulder and scapular muscles. Maintain core and hip strength. Correct postural deficiencies. MCL.
Treatment guidelines	Days 1-2: Arm sling After day 2: Sling used PRN for muscle fatigue After week 1: Remove sling Modalities for pain, swelling, and spasm Trigger point, gentle STM, MFR, IASTM techniques PRN Grade I and II joint mobilization for pain PRN AROM of elbow, forearm, wrist, and fingers respecting pain Hand exercises with ball squeeze and putty exercises Mild resistive exercises to wrist Resistive exercises for shoulder and scapula that do not cause elbow stress or pain Core and hip strengthening and stabilization exercises CV exercises as tolerated
Precautions	Do not stress capsule in direction of dislocation. Use HEP to facilitate treatment.

>continued

Figure 22.33 Rehabilitation program for simple elbow dislocations.

Stage II: Active phase	
3-6 weeks	**Early proliferation phase: Active rehabilitation phase**
Goals	Relieve pain to 1-2 on a scale of 10. Achieve full ROM. Reduce risk of elbow muscle weakness by improving elbow muscle strength to 75%. Achieve good postural strength. MCL.
Treatment guidelines	Weeks 2-3: Passive range of motion PRN Day 7: Begin isometrics to elbow and resistive exercises to wrist and hand Days 10-14: Straight-plane exercises with low force, high reps to elbow and forearm, progressing with increasing resistance as tolerated at end phase Week 3: Proprioception exercises with hand on ball on wall and on tabletop Week 4: Weight-bearing proprioception exercises Week 6: Grade III and IV joint mobilization and soft-tissue mobilization PRN Continue CV and postural exercises
Precautions	Identify and treat soft-tissue restrictions. Use HEP to facilitate treatment.
Stage III: Resistive phase	
6-9 weeks	**Late proliferation phase: Resistive rehabilitation phase**
Goals	Become pain-free. Weeks 6-8: Achieve full range of motion in elbow, wrist, and hand. Maintain normal scapular muscle strength and endurance. Achieve normal strength of elbow, wrist, and hand muscles in straight-plane and multiplanar activities. MCL. Restore pain-free functional use with ADLs.
Treatment guidelines	Maintenance exercises for range of motion Maintenance exercises for shoulder complex strength and endurance Progress to multiplanar exercises after concentric exercise strength is 80% Dynamic proprioception exercises Plyometric exercises
Precautions	Use verbal cues to correct for improper exercise execution. Use HEP to facilitate treatment.
Stage IV: Advanced phase	
9-26 weeks	**Remodeling phase: Advanced rehabilitation phase**
Goals	Maintain normal strength of all muscles. Maintain normal ROM of all joints. Restore normal sport and work performance.
Treatment guidelines	Functional exercise progression Performance-specific exercises and drills progression
Precautions	Ensure proper execution of all exercises.

ROM = range of motion; UE = upper extremity; MCL = maintain cardiovascular level; STM = soft-tissue massage; MFR = myofascial release; IASTM = instrument-assisted soft-tissue mobilization; PRN = as needed; AROM = active range of motion; CV = cardiovascular; HEP = home exercise program; ADLs = activities of daily living.

Figure 22.33   >*continued*

Arthroscopy

Although arthroscopic surgery is less complicated than an open procedure and leads to less tissue damage, tissue healing is still a concern. As the rehabilitation program begins, the rehabilitation clinician must not lose sight of the fact that the patient has had surgery and that tissue healing is a necessary, ongoing process.

The most common arthroscopic procedure performed on the elbow is debridement of synovitis and removal of loose bodies. Postoperative rehabilitation after this procedure is more accelerated than with open procedures because less tissue damage and insult have occurred. The arm is often placed in a sling for 1 or 2 d (or 3 d if pain warrants it) after the surgery. In addition to pain and edema control, initial treatment includes active and mild passive range-of-motion activities and joint mobilization for pain modulation. Shoulder, wrist, and hand range-of-motion exercises are also performed. Gripping exercises are also used in the first 2 or 3 postoperative days.

Full range of motion should be restored by the end of the first week. The sling is discarded by day 3. A few days of isometric exercises are followed by mild resistive exercises to the elbow. If debridement has occurred in the posterior elbow, it may be uncomfortable for the patient to perform end-range flexion–extension exercises. Strength exercises are performed in a straight plane within a pain-free range of motion during the first 3 to 4 weeks. Shoulder, forearm, wrist, and hand strengthening are also performed within pain-free limits. Proprioception exercises begin after the first week and progress to weight-bearing proprioception activities as tolerated.

By weeks 3 to 4, the patient begins the resistive phase; isokinetic exercises at the end of this phase can begin in straight planes, advancing as indicated to diagonal planes. Rubber-band resistance and other eccentric exercises are added. Multiplanar resistive exercises are used once good strength and control are seen in straight-plane exercises.

Plyometric exercises start once the patient shows good control and strength in multiplanar activities. These activities may begin as early as the third week but may not be possible until the fifth or sixth week, depending on how extensive the surgery was and the patient's response to the surgery and exercises.

The final rehabilitation phase includes the usual functional and performance-specific exercise progression. Arthroscopic debridement patients can move quickly into this rehabilitation phase. Depending on the patient's response to pain and healing, the rehabilitation program may be completed any time between week 8 and week 12; sometimes patients need more time, but this is individually determined and is based not only on the person's response to the healing and rehabilitation program but also on the demands that will be placed on the elbow once he or she returns to normal function. More stressful elbow activities may require a longer time in rehabilitation phase IV.

CLINICAL TIPS

Common elbow injuries that warrant special considerations in rehabilitation program design are epicondylopathy, Little League elbow, sprains, ulnar nerve injury, dislocation, and post-arthroscopy conditions. Each of these conditions is manageable with an appropriate rehabilitation program. Using common sense and acquired knowledge and skills, the rehabilitation clinician can design programs that enable patients to return to normal activities.

Case Study

A 35-year-old, right-handed recreational baseball pitcher underwent arthroscopic removal of loose bodies from the posterior elbow yesterday. The surgeon wants him to begin rehabilitation today. The patient reports mild postoperative pain, but nothing unusual. He is wearing an arm sling, but he has been told that he can remove it throughout the day. There is swelling around the surgical site. The dressing does not indicate any unusual postoperative drainage. The elbow range of motion is lacking 30° in extension and flexes to 100°. Pronation is 70° and supination is 50°. Wrist flexion and extension are each 60°. There is some spasm in the triceps. Manual muscle testing reveals 4–/5 strength in the biceps and triceps with some tenderness to triceps resistance, 4–/5 wrist flexion and extension without pain, and 4/5 strength throughout the shoulder.

Questions for Analysis

1. What will your first treatment be? Justify this treatment.

2. What instructions will you give the patient before he leaves today?

3. Outline your expected progression of exercises for the next 2 weeks. What guidelines will you use to determine when the patient should begin a progressive throwing program?

4. What will you tell him when he asks you how soon he can get back to playing baseball?

Summary

The elbow is unique in several ways. It has three joints encased in one capsule, so if capsular restriction occurs with one of these joints, it is likely that capsular restriction will also affect the other two joints. Joint mobilization techniques and progressive exercises for the elbow region were presented in this chapter. The more common injuries seen in rehabilitation were also presented, along with an outline of rehabilitation programs for each of them. The elbow encounters compressive stresses on the lateral joint and distraction stress on the medial joint, so injuries seen at this joint often reflect these stresses, especially in cases of repetitive stress injuries. Bony and joint compressive injuries occur laterally, but inflammations and soft-tissue irritations from repetitive stretches occur more medially. A major concern with every elbow injury is loss of motion; it occurs quickly after injury or surgery, so the rehabilitation clinician must be aware of this problem and try to restore motion as quickly as is safely possible after an elbow injury. When treating elbow injuries, the scapula and shoulder must be included in the rehabilitation program to ensure optimum function of the upper extremity. Depending on the patient's goals, trunk stability and lower-quarter strengthening may also be necessary to incorporate into the rehabilitation program.

LEARNING AIDS

Key Concepts and Review

1. Discuss why you should avoid overstretching the elbow, especially during the inflammation phase of healing.

The biceps inserts onto the forearm's fascia, adhesions occur relatively easily in the elbow, and the anterior capsule is relatively thin. Therefore, soft tissues can be easily damaged with aggressive stretching, resulting in additional scarring.

2. Describe the convex-on-concave rules for the various elbow joints.

The radial head and ulna both are concave surfaces and move on a convex capitulum and convex trochlea, respectively, so applications of force are in the same direction as the restricted movement. In the proximal radioulnar joint, the force is applied in the direction opposite the restricted movement because this joint is the convex surface of the radius moving on the concave surface of the ulna.

3. Identify the resting positions for the elbow joints.

The resting position for the humeroulnar joint is 70° of elbow flexion and 10° of supination. The resting position for the humeroradial joint is full elbow extension with full supination. The radioulnar joint's resting position is 70° of elbow flexion with 35° of supination.

4. List three joint mobilizations for the elbow, and identify why they would be used.

Distraction of the humeroulnar joint is used for general relaxation and pain relief, posterior glide of the humeroradial joint is used to increase extension, and ventral glide of the radioulnar joint is used for increasing supination.

5. Explain three strengthening exercises for the elbow and their purpose.

Elbow flexion in a supinated position is primarily for increasing the strength of the biceps, elbow flexion in pronation is primarily for strengthening the brachialis, and elbow flexion in neutral is primarily for strengthening the brachioradialis.

6. Discuss the general progression of strengthening exercises for the elbow.

Isometric strengthening exercises are followed by light-resistance, high-repetition exercises and then more-intense strengthening exercises as healing progresses and strength increases. In cases of tendinopathy and epicondylopathy, eccentric exercises are preceded by concentric exercises, using careful stabilization to isolate the correct muscles. Shoulder, forearm, wrist, and hand exercises are included in the program. Exercises are performed initially in straight planes and advance to multiple planes as strength and control improve. Plyometric exercises are added after strength and motion are adequate, and functional activities are followed by performance-specific exercises that prepare the patient for a return to full normal function.

7. Outline a rehabilitation program for epicondylopathy.

Discovering the underlying cause and correcting it is basic to any tendinopathy program. Pain and edema relief with modalities is begun before therapeutic exercises. Soft-tissue mobilizations such as friction massage and myofascial release are used for soft-tissue-related restrictions and pain, and joint mobilization is used with capsular pattern losses of motion. Active range-of-motion exercises can be performed during the soft-tissue and joint mobilization applications. Eccentric exercises are the first strengthening exercises used with epicondylopathy. As pain decreases, concentric exercises are added. Straight-plane exercises are followed by greater resistance and multiplanar activities as strength progresses. Plyometric exercises using medicine balls and rubber cord resistance are followed by functional activities and finally performance-specific activities that all begin at low resistance and low intensity and progress as the patient's control and execution improve.

8. Indicate precautions to consider in a Little League elbow rehabilitation program.

If the growth plate is damaged, the patient should be advised to stop pitching for the rest of the baseball season. Active range-of-motion exercises (only to tolerance) are encouraged. Passive stretches should be avoided. The use of heavy weights is contraindicated because this could aggravate sensitive growth plates. Exercises should be neither as aggressive nor as intensive as they are for older patients. Valgus stress should be avoided until it can occur without causing pain. It is important to perform a full body evaluation and incorporate appropriate flexibility exercises for the shoulder and hip and strengthening exercises for the shoulder, core, and lower extremities as needed.

9. List precautions for a rehabilitation program following an ulnar nerve transposition.

Tissue healing must be respected. Exercises begin more slowly than they do with nonoperative treatment for nerve injuries. Straight-plane exercises precede multiplanar exercises. While the elbow is in a postoperative sling, handgrip exercises can be used to start early strengthening. Active exercises should be used for stretching. Gentle cross-friction massage should be used only after 6 to 8 weeks if a loss of range of motion persists. Postural education and strengthening is incorporated into the rehabilitation program.

10. Explain the differences between rehabilitation programs for an arthroscopic elbow debridement and a medial collateral ligament reconstruction.

Because the medial collateral ligament reconstruction is often an open procedure, rehabilitation is a much slower process than with alternative arthroscopic procedures. The period of immobilization is longer, and exercises are less aggressive in the early stages of the program. Loss of motion is a more significant factor, so motion and mobility activities are more prominent in the early phases.

Critical Thinking Questions

1. Brian is faced with a probable Little League elbow epicondylopathy in Abraham in the opening scenario. What are other possible diagnoses? What tests should Brian perform to determine what the problem is? What recommendations should he make to Mrs. Daisy for her son's care? What precautions should Brian take in making recommendations to her?

2. How does the rehabilitation program for an elbow differ for a simple dislocation as compared to a medial collateral ligament sprain? How are the precautions different and why? Is the progression of exercises different? If so, how and why?

3. Can you identify the differences between a medial and a lateral epicondylopathy? What structures are affected? How are the mechanisms of injury different? Would the rehabilitation programs be different? Why or why not?

Lab Activities

1. Locate the trigger points for the following muscles on your lab partner:
   A. Biceps
   B. Triceps
   Where were your partner's most sensitive trigger points? Perform a treatment technique on the most tender one, and provide your partner with a home exercise for the tender trigger point.

2. Locate the lateral epicondyle where the long finger extensors insert on the humerus. Can you palpate each extensor tendon as they come off the epicondyle? Can you locate the tendon that is most often the source of lateral epicondylopathy? Explain why a person with lateral epicondylopathy has pain when shaking hands.

3. Examine your lab partner's elbow joints using joint mobilization techniques for all three joints. How does the mobility of each one compare to the others? Which of the three joints has the greatest

mobility? Which one has the least amount of movement? Create a movement diagram of each joint's motion, and identify where the resistance to movement begins and how it feels throughout the motion. Looking at your movement diagram, describe in words what you found and diagrammed.

4. Perform the following joint mobilizations on your lab partner, and identify what restriction would be best treated with each mobilization:

   A. Humeroulnar joint

      - Distraction
      - Medial glide
      - Lateral glide

   B. Humeroradial joint

      - Distraction
      - Dorsal glide
      - Ventral glide

   C. Proximal radioulnar joint

      - Dorsal glide of radial head
      - Ventral glide of radial head

5. Have your partner perform two stretches each for elbow flexion, elbow extension, pronation, and supination. Identify possible substitutions you must watch for with each exercise.

6. Apply manual resistance to your partner for each of the motions listed with your partner in supine. Have him or her go through 10 repetitions for each exercise. Be sure to apply a maximum resistance, but produce a smooth concentric movement throughout the full range of motion. After the repetitions are completed, apply eccentric resistance to the same motions for 10 repetitions each. Which was more fatiguing for your partner? Which was more difficult for you to perform? Why?

   A. Elbow flexion

   B. Elbow extension

   C. Pronation

   D. Supination

7. Using a dumbbell or cuff weight, have your partner perform a triceps extension exercise in three different antigravity positions, 10 repetitions in each position. Repeat the activity for the elbow flexors. Which position was the most difficult to perform and why?

8. Have your partner use a free weight to perform a supination–pronation exercise while sitting. As your partner goes through the range of motion slowly, have him or her identify what muscles are being used at various parts of the range of motion. If you wanted to work only supinators in both concentric and eccentric motions, explain how you would have the patient perform the exercises.

9. If your partner had golfer's elbow, what activities would you have him or her perform? You should concentrate on eccentric activities. What would they be, and how many repetitions and sets would you have your partner do today? Provide a rationale for your answers. Once you have established these parameters, have your partner perform them as you state them. Have you changed your mind about the goals you set before the exercises were performed? What made you either keep them or change them from your original goals?

10. Develop a series of three plyometric exercises you would use for an elbow patient's rehabilitation program. Have your partner perform them and identify the easiest and most difficult exercises. What substitution patterns could the patient develop as fatigue occurred? What would you set as your criteria for progression from one exercise to the next? Justify why you have set these criteria.

11. List three performance-specific exercises you would have an elbow patient who is a softball left fielder perform before you allowed her to return to full play. Justify why you have selected these criteria.

23

Wrist and Hand

Objectives

After completing this chapter, you should be able to do the following:

1. Explain the pulley system of the fingers.
2. Explain why reducing edema in the hand is important.
3. Discuss the trimuscular system of the hand.
4. Identify and explain the importance of the precision pinches and power grips of the hand.
5. Explain the difference between static and dynamic splints.
6. Identify what motion increases with carpal radial glide joint mobilization.
7. Explain the force application sequence for improving long finger flexor and extensor motion.
8. Explain how the hand and finger positions for intrinsic stretches differ from those for the extrinsic stretches.
9. Discuss the differences in gliding exercises for the flexor profundus and superficialis tendons.
10. Present the differences between long flexor and long extensor tendons.
11. Explain what procedures could be used to identify the cause of an extensor lag of a distal phalanx.

Three weeks ago, Beverly was playing soccer with her friends when she tripped and fell, landing on her outstretched hands. Her right hand was severely cut by a piece of broken glass hidden in the grass. The surgeon repaired her lacerated long finger flexor tendons and placed the hand in an extension-restricted splint, but he now wants Peg, the rehabilitation clinician, to begin the rehabilitation process on Beverly's hand.

Peg has had experience with repaired hand tendons. Right now she has John, an athletic training student, with her, so she tells John that because Beverly's repair is only 3 weeks old, there are precautions that they must consider as they start her rehabilitation program. She explains to John that she is concerned about the adhesions that have begun to form between the long flexor superficialis and profundus tendons and other soft tissue in the anterior finger region, and she is concerned about the impact those adhesions might have on the finger's hood mechanism. She tells John that if the hood mechanism is harmed, the intrinsic muscles can be affected, which will impair Beverly's hand function. Peg has explained Beverly's hand injury well enough to give John a better understanding of why Peg wants to proceed cautiously with Beverly's rehabilitation program.

The hand is the visible part of the brain.

Immanuel Kant, 1724-1804,
German philosopher

We use our hands daily for hundreds of activities without thinking that this is anything out of the ordinary. However, if we reflect on the hand at all, we realize that it is an extremely complex structure and vital to performing our daily tasks. In many ways, it acts as an extension of our brains. Many health care professionals pay little attention to finger and hand injuries, but these can be among the most devastating injuries if not properly cared for because the hand plays such an important role in our lives. On the other hand (no pun intended), when an athlete suffers a complex hand injury, the patient and the rehabilitation clinician are quick to realize just how inconvenient it can be. It is our hope that by the end of this chapter you will gain an appreciation for hand and finger injuries and realize that a finger sprain is not *just* a small sprain.

A seemingly minimal imbalance in the hand can cause profound problems for hand function. These problems present the rehabilitation clinician with challenges that must be addressed before the patient can resume normal activities. However, before we can discuss rehabilitation techniques for the wrist and hand, we must review their unique function and structure because they play a vital role in carrying out a rehabilitation program.

Many texts have been written on the anatomy, biomechanics, and functions of the wrist and hand. We will be only skimming the surface of this body of knowledge. A complete investigation of the hand's structure and function is beyond the scope of this chapter, but we will present information that you will need to create rehabilitation programs for most wrist and hand injuries you are apt to encounter. The presentation of soft-tissue and joint mobilization techniques is organized as in previous chapters. The exercises presented here are limited to flexibility, strengthening, coordination, and desensitization exercises for the wrist and hand. Recall from chapters 21 and 22 that the scapula, shoulder, and elbow contribute to the mobility and function of the wrist and hand. This interdependence must be considered in the rehabilitation programs that you design for wrist and hand injuries. Specific injuries commonly seen in the wrist and hand are discussed, along with rehabilitation programs used to treat them.

Hand and wrist injuries occur often in sports; reportedly between 9% and 25% of all sport-related injuries involve the hand and wrist.[1-3] Although the wrist and hand are complex and injuries to them can present unique problems, these problems can be overcome with the informed application of biomechanics and rehabilitation. Consider them to be opportunities to use your knowledge and skills to help your patients to achieve a full recovery from hand and wrist injuries.

Special Rehabilitation Considerations

The wrist and hand form a complex unit composed of 29 bones, more than 30 tendinous insertions, and an involved neurological system that is vital to the unit's function. Based on the sensory homunculus of the brain, we know that tactile perception by the hand is more important than that of most other regions of the body.[4] The body relies heavily on the hand's sensory input. The hand's many compactly arranged muscles, including nine for the thumb and seven for the index finger alone, hint at the complexity of its function. The thumb and index finger primarily engage in fine activities that require dexterity, whereas the middle, ring, and little fingers act primarily as a stabilizing vise for grasping activities. All of the structures in the wrist and hand must work in a balanced, coordinated manner for the hand to function optimally.

Upper Extremity Interdependence

Chapter 21 introduced the importance of scapular stability for optimum shoulder function. Chapter 22 touched on the importance of proximal stability to create a base from which the elbow can effectively and efficiently place the hand in space. The ability to use the hand for functional tasks such as dressing, grooming, manipulating objects, throwing, and using power tools relies not only on the function of the hand itself but also on the function of the elbow and shoulder complex. When treating wrist and hand injuries, the scapula, shoulder, and elbow must be included in the rehabilitation program to adequately address the regional interdependence of the upper quarter and to promote optimum functional use of the hand.

Anatomical Considerations

The skeletal structure and extensive soft-tissue architecture of the wrist and hand allow for remarkable mobility and malleability. It is a tool for domestic activities, occupational duties, and activities of leisure and sport. The hand is also an instrument for the expression of music and art. It is used in communication to convey emphasis and emotion. It is important to understand the unique and complex anatomy of the hand in order to create an appropriate rehabilitation program for wrist and hand injuries.

Skeletal Structure

Three flexion arches, the proximal transverse arch, distal transverse arch, and longitudinal arch, are formed by the wrist and hand bones. The carpals and metacarpals form the proximal and distal transverse arches, respectively. The longitudinal arch runs from the carpals out to the ends of the fingers (figure 23.1). These arches form an equiangular spiral that offers the ability to securely grasp an endless variety of objects. If these equiangular structures are

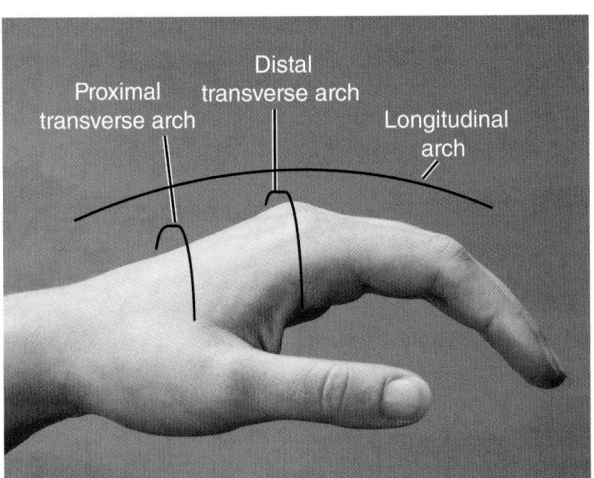

Figure 23.1 Hand arches.

impaired because of joint restriction or muscle weakness, the hand loses its adaptability.

The concave radius joins with the convex proximal carpal row to form the wrist joint. This joint has motions of flexion, extension, abduction, and adduction. Adduction is commonly referred to as ulnar deviation, and abduction is referred to as radial deviation. These four motions combine to produce wrist circumduction. The distal ulna and radius are supported by the distal radioulnar ligament and the interosseus membrane. Forearm supination and pronation movements occur at the proximal and distal radioulnar joints. Restricted mobility at either radioulnar joint prevents full supination–pronation motion.

The carpal bones also form several joints with each other, and the distal row forms the carpometacarpal joints with the metacarpals. The intercarpal joints have an irregular structure and are strongly held in place by ligaments, making it difficult to dislocate any carpal. The carpometacarpal joints are, for the most part, saddle joints that permit various degrees of flexion, extension, abduction, and adduction of the metacarpals. The number 1, 4, and 5 metacarpals also rotate to provide opposition of the thumb and little finger, thereby allowing the hand to grasp objects.

The metacarpophalangeal (MCP) joints are formed by the distal convex metacarpal surfaces and the corresponding concave proximal phalange surfaces. The interphalangeal (IP) joints are identified as either proximal (PIP) or distal (DIP) interphalangeal joints. Collateral ligaments provide stability to these interphalangeal (IP) joints. In a relaxed position, the fingers are in partial flexion at the IP and MCP joints. The relaxed finger arrangement is such that it forms a cascade of progressive flexion from the second through the fifth digits; there is pathology present if this natural cascade is not seen.

Fascia and Ligaments

In addition to the ligaments that connect and support the joints throughout the wrist and hand, several other static structures add support to the area. The thick palmar fascia has two layers: superficial and deep. The superficial layer, an extension of the flexor retinaculum (transverse carpal ligament) and the palmaris longus tendon, when it is present, expands over the volar hand and runs into each of the fingers. The deep layer covers the floor of the palm and runs between the thenar and hypothenar eminences. The fascia on the hand's dorsum is also in two layers, but it is not as thick as the palmar fascia. The palmar fascia serves to cushion and protect the hand's structures and helps maintain the hand's concavity.

The retinacula is positioned throughout the wrist and hand and serves to hold the flexor and extensor tendons in place. At the wrist, the transverse carpal ligament prevents the flexor tendons from bowstringing away from the wrist. **Bowstringing** of a tendon is similar in appearance to an archer's bowstring; the tendon bowstrings away from the wrist when the pulley system holding the tendon in place ruptures and the tendon is no longer in proximity to the bone. The transverse carpal ligament forms the roof of the carpal tunnel and maintains all of the finger flexor tendons within the carpal tunnel (except the palmaris longus and flexor carpi ulnaris), the nerves, and the arteries. The extensor retinaculum on the dorsal wrist keeps the extensor tendons from bowstringing away from the wrist.

An extracapsular ligament, the transverse metacarpal ligament, connects the volar plate of one metatarsal head to the volar plate of its adjacent metatarsal heads (figure 23.2a). This ligament is important in maintaining the distal transverse arch, and its normal flexibility is vital to hand functions such as prehensile grip and grasping activities. There are several fascial restraints in the digits that maintain the alignment of the tendons in the fingers and also provide the pulley system for the tendons.[5]

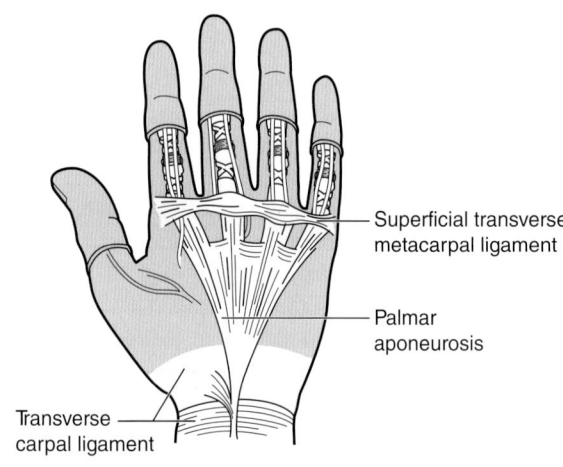

- Superficial transverse metacarpal ligament
- Palmar aponeurosis
- Transverse carpal ligament

a

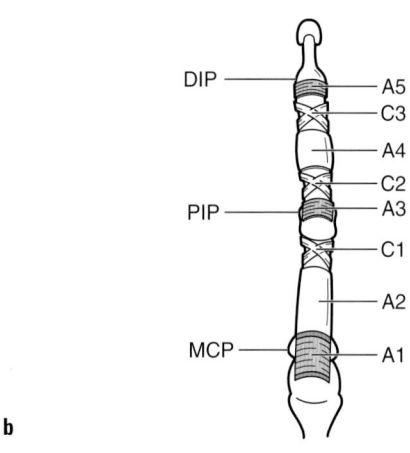

DIP — A5
— C3
— A4
— C2
PIP — A3
— C1
— A2
MCP — A1

b

Figure 23.2 *(a)* Palmar soft-tissue elements; *(b)* flexor tendon pulley system. MCP = metacarpophalangeal; PIP = proximal interphalangeal; DIP = distal interphalangeal; A = annular pulley; C = cruciate pulley.

Tendon Sheaths and Pulleys

The flexor tendons are surrounded by a complex system of sheaths that protect and nourish the tendons. The sheath system of the extensor tendons is not as elaborate; the extensor tendons are enclosed in sheaths at the wrist when they travel under the extensor retinaculum, but otherwise they are **extrasynovial**. The flexor sheaths begin proximal to the wrist and extend to the distal digits.

There is an elaborate pulley system on the flexor aspect of the fingers. This system is a series of fibrous tunnels that extends from the metacarpal head of each digit to the insertion of the distal finger flexor tendons. These pulleys are similar to the hoops along a fishing rod, positioned to keep the fishing line in place as it travels along the pole. There are five annular pulleys and three cruciate pulleys along the fingers (figure 23.2b). Disruption of key pulleys can cause bowstringing of the flexor tendons. The pulleys that are key to preventing bowstringing are A2 and A4.[6] When the pulley system of any finger is disrupted, the mechanical advantage of the tendon is impaired, and normal function is lost.

Muscles

Hand muscles are divided into two major categories, extrinsic and intrinsic. Extrinsic muscles originate outside and terminate inside the hand, whereas intrinsic muscles originate and terminate within the hand. Extrinsic muscles are further divided into flexor muscles and extensor muscles. There are 20 extrinsic muscles and 19 intrinsic muscles. The extrinsic muscles are attached to the long tendons that enter the wrist and hand from muscles originating from the elbow or forearm. The thenar eminence contains the four intrinsic muscles of the thumb, and the hypothenar eminence contains the three intrinsic muscles of the fifth finger. If the hand is to operate well and avoid deformity after an injury, a balanced system must exist between the intrinsic muscles and the extrinsic flexor and extensor muscles.[7]

The long finger extensors run to the second through fifth fingers. At the distal metacarpal area they are connected by the juncturae tendinum, a fibrous band that limits independent motion of the extensor tendons. The extensor tendons are connected to the proximal phalanx by sagittal bands that attach on the volar plate to keep the extensor tendons from bowstringing and that transmit the extensor tendons' extension force to the metacarpophalangeal joints. Distal to the MCP joints, the extensor tendons split into three segments: the central slip, which attaches to the base of the middle phalanx, and two lateral bands that insert when they rejoin at the dorsal distal phalanx (figure 23.3).

The long finger flexors include the flexor digitorum superficialis (FDS) and the flexor digitorum profundus (FDP). Both tendons pass deep in the hand. The FDS

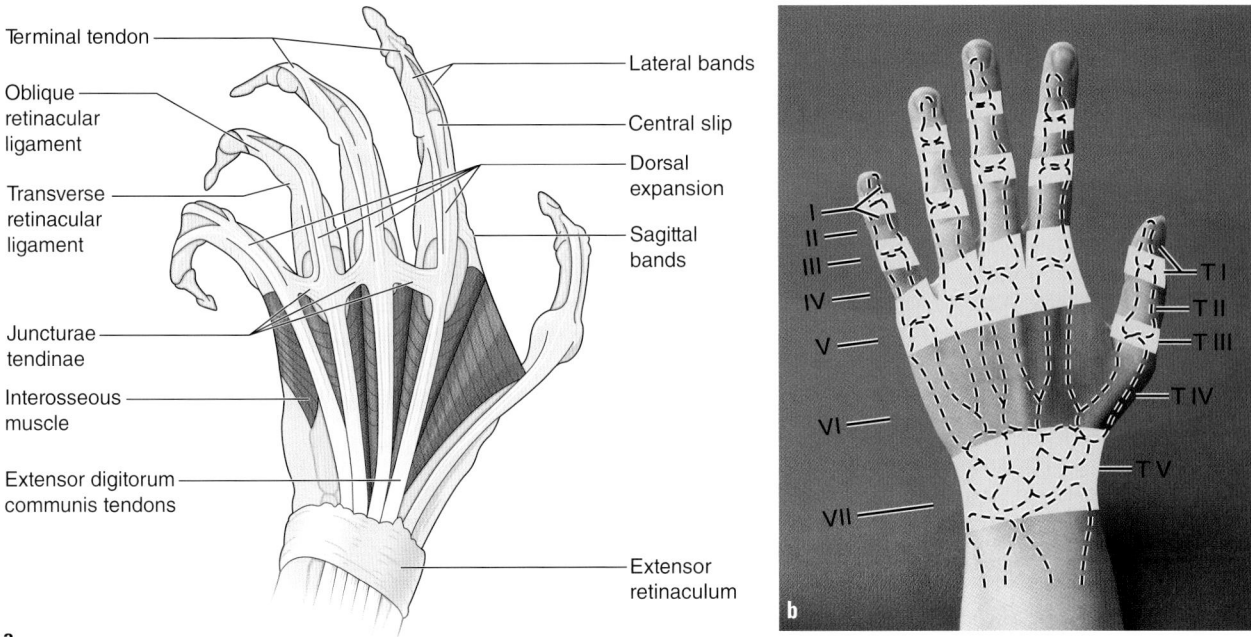

Figure 23.3 *(a)* Dorsal soft-tissue elements and *(b)* zones.

flexes the PIP joint. Each FDS tendon has its own separate muscle belly, so each can operate independently of the other. Each superficialis tendon splits before it attaches to the base of the middle phalanx and permits the deeper FDP tendon to emerge through this split and attach to the distal phalanx (figure 23.4). The tendons of the FDP, unlike those of the FDS, do not have separate muscle bellies, so distal phalanges cannot be flexed independently by only one finger at a time.

Whereas the long finger muscles are used for gross motor activity, the intrinsic muscles are used for intricate fine motor activities. The lumbricals and interossei have unique attachments and arrangements with the long flexor and extensor tendons and the ligaments of the fingers. The lumbricals originate from the deep flexor tendons in the palm and insert on the extensor tendon expansion. This unique arrangement allows the lumbricals to function as MCP flexors and IP extensors because their line of force is

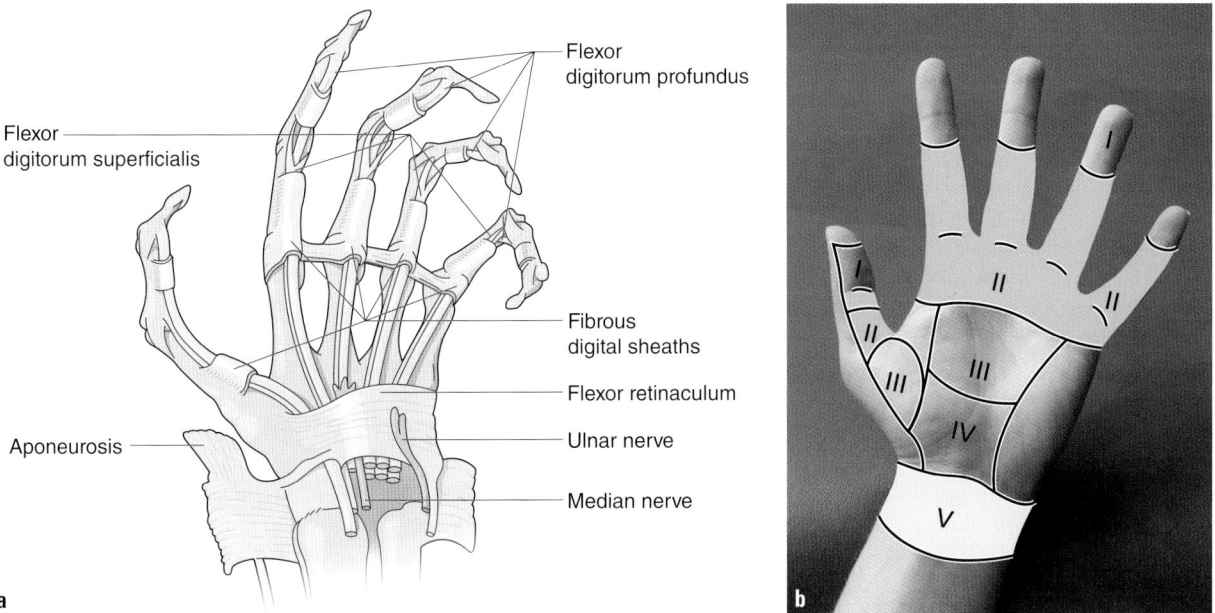

Figure 23.4 *(a)* Palmar surface of the hand and *(b)* zones.

anterior to the MCP joint, causing flexion at this joint, and their line of force is posterior to the IP joint, resulting in IP extension.[8] The dorsal and palmar interossei are responsible for finger abduction and adduction, respectively.[9] Because they are more superficial than the lumbricals, they can be palpated.

Tendon Zones

The flexor and extensor surfaces of the hand are divided into zones for surgical reference. Each zone has unique characteristics that affect both the physician's surgical approach and the clinician's rehabilitation approach. For these reasons we consider them briefly here. There are five flexor and seven extensor zones of the wrist, hand, and four

medial digits. The thumb has three flexor and five extensor zones. The zones are numbered with the lowest numbers most distal. When connective tissue in the form of either sheaths or retinaculae surrounds these tendons in the flexor or extensor zones, the risk of adhesions occurring with immobilization increases significantly.[10] You will notice in table 23.1 that the repercussions of injury in extensor zone VII are similar to those of an injury in flexor zone II for this very reason. Tendon adhesions can result in a loss of normal motion, strength, and function. Tendon gliding exercises that help to prevent these adhesions are presented later in this chapter. Table 23.1 lists the tendon zones, and figures 23.3 and 23.4 present them pictorially.

TABLE 23.1 Surgical Zones of the Hand With Implications for Rehabilitation

Flexors or extensors	Zone	Location	Characteristics	Problems	Rehabilitation goals and considerations
Flexor	V	Forearm at musculotendinous junction of extrinsic wrist muscles	Tendons are surrounded by loose tendon sheaths.	Tendons can adhere to the sheath and surrounding soft-tissue structures.	Prevent adhesions and restore normal tendon gliding.
	IV	At the wrist	Carpal tunnel is located here. Several tendons, nerves, and blood vessels are present in this area.	Adhesion between tendons is a common problem after surgery or injury.	Prevent adhesions.
	III	In the palm after the flexor tendons leave the carpal tunnel	Several neurovascular structures along with an extensive retinacular (fibrous fascial band) network are in this area.	Since the extrinsic tendons have more room, they often heal without difficulty or complications. Intrinsic muscles, however, can have adhesions and contractures from prolonged flexor positioning of the palm.	Gentle passive ROM exercises for the intrinsics can help prevent these complications.
	II	From the distal palmar crease to the middle phalanx where the split slips of the FDS insert on the phalanx and near where the FDP traverses anteriorly below the superficialis	Flexor tendon sheaths are in this region.	Adhesions can seriously inhibit normal tendon gliding and prevent full restoration of function. This area has been called "no man's land" because of the inhibition of normal function after injury or surgery to this area, but more recent advances in surgical techniques permit improved function after surgery.	Flexor tendon gliding exercises reduce the risk of adhesions.
	I	Area of the DIP joint	The only tendon involved here is the FDP as it inserts on the distal phalanx.	Tendons are commonly ruptured from this location.	These injuries require careful rehabilitation because complications such as poor tendon gliding, contractures, and repair failures can occur.

Flexors or extensors	Zone	Location	Characteristics	Problems	Rehabilitation goals and considerations
Thumb flexor	I, II, III	Anterior thumb region	These zones are comparable to zones I, II, and III, respectively, of the fingers.	Tendon injuries in these zones do not carry with them as great a risk of adhesions because the only tendon enclosed in a sheath is the flexor pollicis longus.	Care must be taken to preserve function since the thumb accounts for most hand function.
Extensor	VII	At the wrist joints	This area contains both wrist extensors and extrinsic finger extensors.	The tendons in this area have synovial sheaths, are close together, and are covered by the dorsal retinaculum. This can be an area of adhesion formation after injury or immobilization.	If an injury in this area involves only the wrist extensors, the wrist is the only joint in need of immobilization and should be positioned in approximately 45° of extension. However, if the long finger extensors are also involved, the wrist and MCP joints should both be positioned in extension. The rehabilitation clinician must understand the risks of losing tendon gliding capabilities and should take steps to prevent and treat this complication.
	V, VI	From the hand distal to the extensor sheaths in the carpometacarpal (CMC) joint region to the MCP joints at the start of the extensor hood	Include extensor tendons and sheaths and other soft-tissue structures.	Extensor tendons and sheaths can adhere to other surrounding soft-tissue structures, especially because they are close to the skin. Edema formation in the hand is usually seen in this area more predominantly than in the palmar aspect.	Control of edema will help reduce the risk of adhesion formation. Wrist immobilization for this area is approximately 45° extension at the wrist with the MCP and IP joints at 0° extension.
	III, IV	Proximal and middle finger segments	Include extensor tendons that have split into central and lateral slips and PIP joints.	When injuries occur to the extrinsic extensor tendon's central slip, a boutonniere deformity results. The PIP is positioned in flexion and the DIP in extension with the unbalanced pull of the intact lateral bands.	Although stiffness of the PIP joint with loss of joint motion is a complication, immobilization of the digit is necessary, as discussed later in this chapter.
	I, II	Middle and distal finger segments	Middle phalanx and DIP joints.	Mallet deformity is the most common injury in this region. If untreated, a mallet deformity may lead to a swan-neck deformity, in which the PIP joint is hyperextended and the DIP joint is flexed. This occurs in the presence of a lax volar plate as the extensor mechanism slides proximally without its anchor at the distal phalanx.	Splinting, and in some cases surgery, is necessary to correct this injury. Care must be taken during this time to guard against an extensor lag and local ischemia. Treatment of this injury is discussed in detail later.

>continued

TABLE 23.1 >*continued*

Flexors or extensors	Zone	Location	Characteristics	Problems	Rehabilitation goals and considerations
Thumb extensor	I-V	Extensor surface of the thumb	The thumb zones coincide with the zones of the finger, and injuries to those zones can be treated similarly to the corresponding finger zones. T I and T II coincide with zones I and II of the fingers. Zones T III and T IV coincide with zones V and VI of the fingers.	Zone T V, like zone VII of the fingers, can suffer adhesions after injury. Web space contracture, extensor pollicis longus adhesions, and reduced excursion of the thumb are common problems.	The clinician must be aware of secondary problems that may occur with thumb injuries and take a proactive stance to prevent them. The thumb is the most important digit of the hand and must be cared for appropriately.

Excursions

Enabling the hand to make a fist requires a large excursion of the extensor tendons and the dorsal skin and fascia of the hand and wrist. Adhesions between hand or wrist structures can restrict this mobility and limit hand function. With tendon injuries, early controlled passive motion activities are vital to restoring full hand function.[11] It is important to maintain good tendon gliding to prevent injury.

As a tendon glides within its sheath, adhesions are stretched. The normal excursion of a tendon is variable from one finger to another and is a matter of some dispute. The most commonly repeated values are based on the work of Bunnell reported by Boyes.[12] The significance of these numbers for rehabilitation is twofold: They specify how much excursion must be restored after injury or immobilization, and they indicate how much each healing tendon can move during immobilization without incurring damage. Many investigators have studied tendons, motion, and their excursions. For example, it is now known how far a tendon can be stretched while it is immobilized without endangering its integrity,[13] and how many degrees of motion these distances translate to[14] so that splints can be designed for the hand after tendon repair. Clinicians who specialize in hand splinting must know these values. The rehabilitation clinician should appreciate the differences between the excursions of a digit's extensor tendons; these differences do not necessarily change in a successive order from the first to the fifth digit, nor do they each change proportionately for each tendon. For example, the thumb's extensor longus tendon has the greatest overall excursion, but it does not have the greatest excursion of all the other extensor tendons at the wrist or at the MCP joint.[12]

Edema

Skin covering the volar hand is thick, inelastic, and hairless and attaches to the palmar fascia to allow objects to be grasped without slipping out of the hand. The dorsal skin is elastic, mobile, and easily separated from the underlying fascia; this allows the skin to move when the fingers flex during grasping activities. Because the dorsal skin is loose and pliable compared to the palmar skin, edema often accumulates in the dorsum of the hand. Pooled edema rich in proteins easily leads to contractures.[15] Excessive swelling on the back of the hand can cause the hand arches to collapse anteriorly and cause the thumb to adduct (figure 23.5). Excessive swelling also requires a greater excursion of the skin to flex the fingers.[16] If the skin is already stretched because of the edema, the fingers will not be able to move through their full flexion motion. Fibrous tissue formation secondary to prolonged edema can reduce the mobility and function of the hand.[17] Since edema is a severe

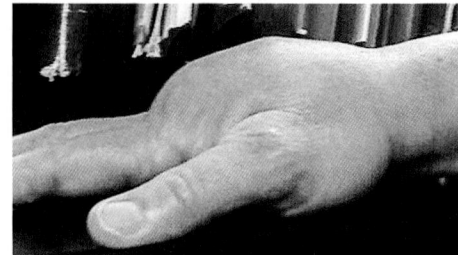

Figure 23.5 Swelling tends to accumulate more on the dorsal side of the hand, causing a collapse of the hand arches.
© Peggy Houglum

problem in the hand, it will be presented in more detail in Special Rehabilitation Applications later in this chapter.

Efforts by the rehabilitation clinician to reduce early edema are crucial. Compressive dressings, elevation, ice, compression machines, and other modalities to reduce edema formation are important in phase I of rehabilitation.

Some compression devices are commercially available, such as Isotoner gloves and neoprene finger sleeves. The clinician can also create finger compression devices using Coban wrap, string, or small sizes of compressive tubing. Some of these devices are illustrated in figure 23.6.

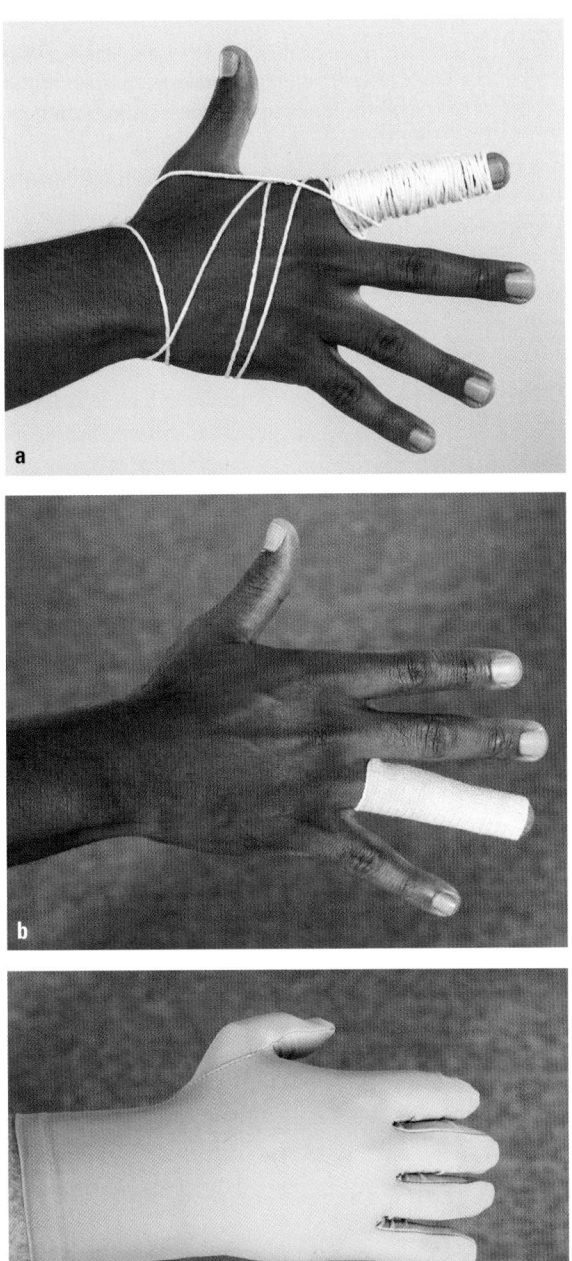

Figure 23.6 Compression methods and devices for finger and hand swelling. *(a)* Handmade devices from string, *(b)* commercially available finger sleeves, and *(c)* commercially available compression gloves.

Function of the Hand

The hand is a trimuscular system that uses the three muscle groups—the extrinsic flexors, the extrinsic extensors, and the intrinsic muscles—to provide balanced, controlled function.[18] This was stated earlier, but it bears repeating: If any of these muscle groups does not function normally because of either weakness or loss of mobility, balance is lost, and the hand cannot work properly.

Humans are not unique in their ability to oppose the thumb; apes and monkeys can also oppose the thumb to the index finger. Our opposable thumb, however, is longer and stronger than those of apes and monkeys. What really distinguishes the human hand from those of other animals is the ability of the fourth and fifth fingers to rotate across the palm. The carpometacarpal joints of these two digits are very flexible. Combining these joint characteristics with the unique intrinsic muscles in the ulnar hand, the human hand has what is sometimes called *ulnar opposition*. This ulnar hand mobility gives us the unique ability to oppose the thumb to all fingers and to grasp objects of any shape with a firm grip.

Because of the hand's complex system of joints and muscles, it has many potential uses. The hand transmits forces or provides movement to produce a desired effect. There are two categories of grips: power grips for gross activities and prehensile grips for fine-tuned activities.[19] About 20%[20] to 45%[21] of what we do with our hands involves power grips. Power grips transmit force. Power grips, also known as palmar grips, include the clenched fist, the cylinder grasp, the spherical grasp, and the hook grasp (figure 23.7). In power grips, the thumb in opposition to the other fingers results in a firm grasp. The hook grip is the only power grip in which the thumb does not actively participate. Many everyday gross hand activities involve these palmar grips. Because palmar grasping is so vital to hand function, an injured hand is most commonly splinted in a palmar position with the thumb in slight opposition, facing the other fingers, the MCP joints in approximately 60° of flexion, and the wrist in slight hyperextension.

Most of the time, however, the hand enables us to perform intricate tasks. These include such things as typing, buttoning a shirt, sewing, or writing. These intricate grips, or pinches, include prehensile positions in which the thumb and finger muscles co-contract. The three precision pinches are the digital prehension pinch (also known as the three-jaw chuck), the lateral prehension pinch (also known as the key pinch), and the tip-to-tip prehension pinch (figure 23.8). The digital prehension pinch is a grip used to handle and maneuver small tools in intricate activities such as a pencil in writing. The lateral prehension pinch places the thumb pad against the side of the index finger to grasp objects such as a key or book. The tip-to-tip prehension pinch positions the tip of the thumb against the tip of another finger. It is used most often to pick up small objects.

In the precision pinches, the fingers are flexed and abducted at the MCP joints with some opposition present.[22] Unless the object being manipulated is heavy or large, the radial digits are primarily involved in precision activities. The movements involved in power activities vary in excursion and number of digits involved, but they usually include flexion and rotation with some ulnar deviation. Studies show that hand and finger joints prepare for specific grasping tasks and position themselves synergistically through what is thought to be coordinated neuromuscular activities

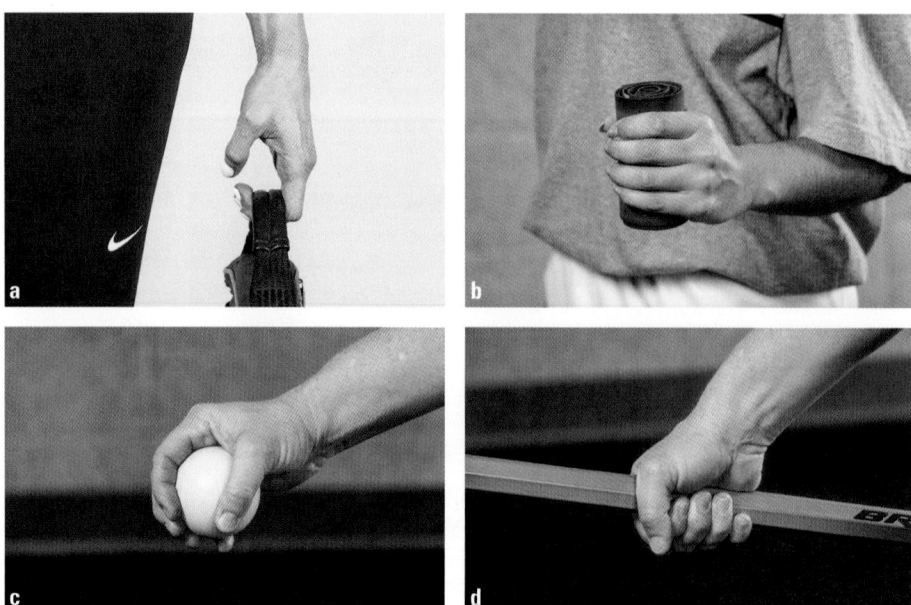

Figure 23.7 Power grips: *(a)* hook, *(b)* cylinder, *(c)* spherical, *(d)* fist.

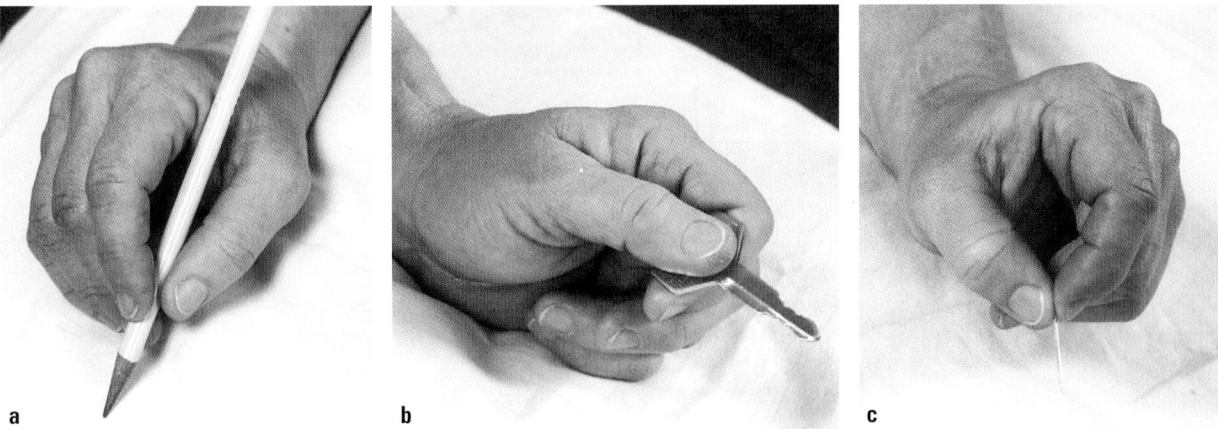

Figure 23.8 Prehension pinches: *(a)* digital, *(b)* lateral, *(c)* tip-to-tip.

so that all joints are positioned correctly to manipulate whatever object is placed in the hand.[23, 24] For example, as a person's hand approaches to pick up a key that is sitting on a table, the PIP joints of the fingers flex as the thumb moves into medial rotation and adduction to grasp the key.[23]

The power grips use the ulnar aspect of the hand to grasp the object and deliver power and stability, while the radial aspect of the hand is responsible for precision activities. Golf presents an example of this use of the power grip. In a power grip, the fingers flex and rotate and move into ulnar deviation so that the fingertips point toward the thenar eminence to hold the object in the hand and stabilize the thumb in abduction.

All motions and grips must be restored to the injured hand. The clinician achieves this first by being aware of the component motions these activities require, then by restoring joint mobility, attaining normal tendon glide, and balancing strength and flexibility.

Splinting

Braces and splints are commonly used in the treatment of hand injuries. They are either static or dynamic. Static splints are used to restrict motion, increase motion, or support and protect the hand, while dynamic splints are used to increase motion, facilitate motion or the use of the hand, or permit restricted motion of the hand.[31] These devices are used either to prevent damage and preserve balance or to enhance function and improve balance. In other words, splints are used to immobilize, protect, mobi-

Evidence in Rehabilitation

As rehabilitation clinicians, we base our goals on the functions patients want, as well as on what is considered normal. Normal for a particular patient is determined by the contralateral extremity. However, because of hand dominance, a perpetual question is whether comparing contralateral segments is an accurate way to set strength goals. One of the first investigators to provide an answer was Bechtol[25] in 1954; he determined that the dominant hand was on average 5% to 10% stronger than the nondominant hand. This finding gradually became known as the 10% rule. Since then, additional investigations have produced a variety of outcomes.[26-29] Although these studies may be interesting, they create a lot of confusion for clinicians trying to determine normal strength values for patients.

A recent study by Hepping and colleagues[30] examined the accuracy of the 10% rule with more than 2200 males and females between the ages of 4 and 17 years. Each group had left-handers and right-handers. They found some interesting results. All of the boys and girls in all age groups who were right-handed demonstrated the 10% rule of hand dominance, but the left-handers were different. The girls were much stronger in their dominant hand, although this was not consistent throughout all age groups. The left-handed boys, however, did not show differences in strength between the left and right hands. In nondominant hand activities, they found that left-handers usually scored either higher or had equal scores when both hands were compared, while a smaller group of right-handers also exhibited this ability.[30] The authors speculated that this may be the result of the known fact that left-handers use their dominant hand less than right-handers.[30]

For a number of reasons, it is important to identify the patient's dominant hand at the outset of a rehabilitation program. If the patient is right-handed, that person will likely conform to the 10% rule and have 5% to 10% greater strength in the right hand. However, the grip strength of left-handers may depend not only on hand dominance but on sex as well.

lize, or prevent deformity.[32] Splint design is usually based on a three-point pressure system whereby two points of application are on one side of the hand, wrist, or forearm, and the fulcrum, or other point of application, is on the opposite side (figure 23.9).

Splints are applied for varying amounts of time. Key factors that determine how long splints are applied include the specific structure injured, the splint's purpose, the repair performed, the adjacent structures' influence on the injured tissue, and the healing timeline of the injured tissue. They may be applied for periods of 1 to 8 weeks and used continuously or intermittently. Splints that are used to protect tissue show better results if they are worn for shorter times and produce minimal stress.[33] It has also been found that splints used to gain motion or mobility should be applied continually within 24 h periods, but the total number of days they are used is determined by how quickly the tissue re-forms to elongate.

Studies have demonstrated that the longer a continuous splint is worn, the greater the motion gains; studies looking at splint wear for 3 d versus 6 d found twice as much tissue lengthening when the splint was worn for 6 d.[34] It is common for patients having undergone surgical repairs to use a night splint after they have reduced or discontinued splint wear during the day.[35] The use of night splints may continue for up to 3 weeks post-repair.[35] Complex injuries commonly advance from a protective initial splint to a less restrictive splint before any day support is removed.

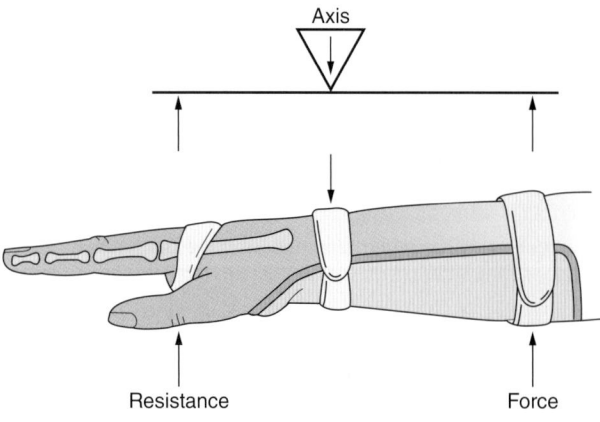

Figure 23.9 Three-point pressure system for splinting.

Static Splints

Static splints do not have any moving parts (figure 23.10). They immobilize a joint to protect it from deleterious movement. After an injury, a period of immobilization is needed to allow scar-tissue formation to restore joint stability. If a joint has lost its mobility, a different type of static splint can improve mobility by applying a prolonged low-load stretch. Static splints are also designed to maintain ROM gains that result from other rehabilitation techniques;

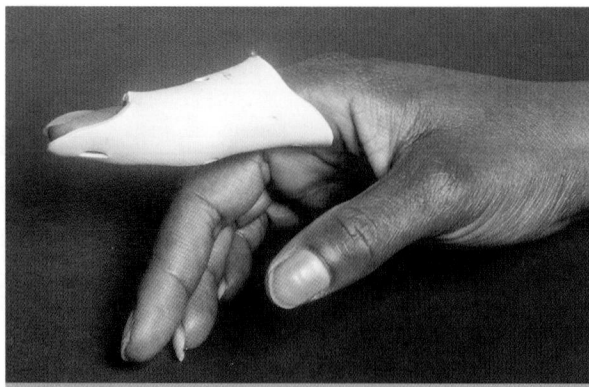

Figure 23.10 Static tendon splint to restrict ROM to protect the injured tissues.

these are called static progressive splints and are discussed in chapter 22. The concepts for the wrist and hand are similar to those discussed for elbow static progressive splints.

For almost half a century, people accepted the idea put forth by Bunnell[36] during World War II that the best position for an immobilized hand was in what he termed a position of function: the wrist is in 20° of extension and 10° of ulnar deviation, the fingers are slightly flexed at the MCP and IP joints with the fifth digit most flexed and the index finger least flexed, and the thumb is in slight opposition to the other fingers (figure 23.11a).[31] Unfortunately, patients often had restricted motion in the finger joints after immobilization in this position.[31]

As anatomical and functional discoveries advanced, Yeakel[37] advocated what he described as the "antideformity position" for splint design and wrist and hand positioning. His rationale was that this position maintained the length of the metacarpophalangeal and interphalangeal joints' collateral ligaments, so motion loss did not occur. Later, this position was referred to as the "safe position."[38] Today, the term "positive intrinsic (POSI) position" is also used to describe this antideformity position.[32] Since the 1970s, custom or off-the-shelf splints have used this position rather than the functional position to immobilize the hand and wrist.[31] The antideformity or safe position, then, is with the wrist in neutral, the MCP joints in 70° to 90° of flexion, and the interphalangeal joints in 0° of extension (figure 23.11b).[37]

Dynamic Splints

Dynamic splints incorporate a system of movement with springs, rubber bands, or other elements that allow motion to occur in the splint. These devices produce passive or passive-assistive motion in one line of pull and active-resistive motion in the opposite direction.

Dynamic splints can also promote mobility by applying a continual, low-level stretch force to a joint. They are used when the patient lacks normal motion and cannot achieve the desired mobility independently. The patient perceives

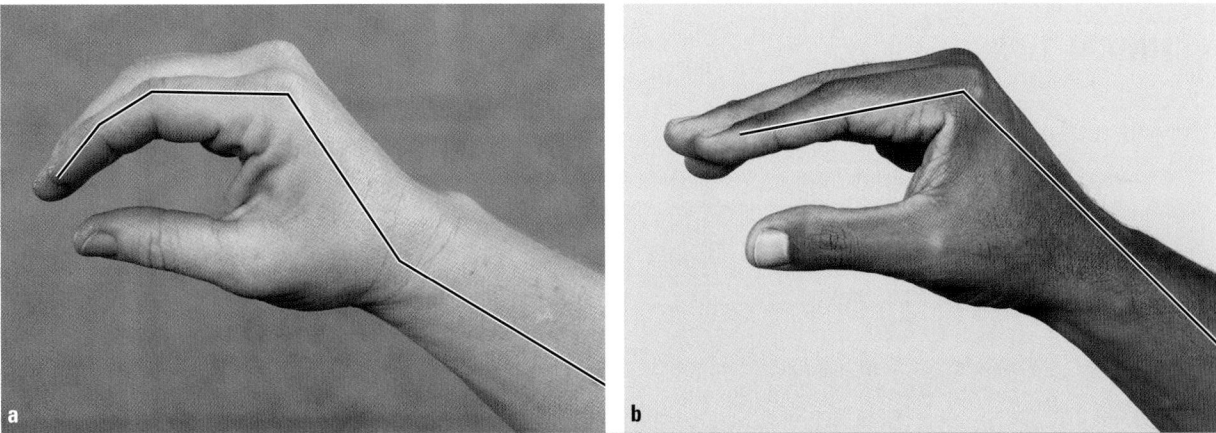

Figure 23.11 Position of hand immobilization. *(a)* "Functional position"—20° wrist extension with MCP and IP flexion; this position is no longer used because it causes contractures of the MCP and IP joints after about 3 weeks of immobilization.[37] *(b)* The antideformity, safe, or POSI position (neutral wrist with 70° to 90° MCP flexion and 0° IP extension) is the preferred immobilization position since it prevents MCP, IP, and volar plate contractures.[32]

the stretch force applied with the splint but should not find it painful. The force applied is low, but the length of time it is kept on the finger or hand is prolonged to influence scar-tissue remodeling.[39] These devices are usually worn at night so they do not interfere with hand function throughout the day. How long the device is worn depends on the patient's tolerance, but the longer it is in place, the better the results.[39] As the joint's ROM increases, adjustments are easily made in a dynamic splint.

A special type of dynamic splint is often used after tendon repair surgery to permit protected, guided movement of the tendon so that tendon glide can be maintained without risking tendon rupture. The device permits the appropriate degree of tendon motion for the specific digit treated. The tendon is held in its shortened position by rubber bands, and the splint keeps the opposing tendon from moving the digit beyond the designated degree of movement so the surgically repaired tendon is not overstretched. The opposing tendon must work against the force of the rubber band to move the finger in the direction permitted, and the rubber band passively returns the finger to the resting position. For example, if a long flexor tendon was repaired, the splint would have a hood to avoid overstretching the tendon and an elastic band to passively move the finger into flexion so the repaired tendon would not be stressed (figure 23.12).

Fit, design, and purpose must be considerations when splints are designed for the hand. The purpose will determine what type of orthotic is used. The fit is individually determined, based on the hand size and dimensions. The design is based on a combination of fit, purpose, mechanics, materials, and precautions.[40]

There are two main precautions in splint design and construction: friction and pressure. Friction or extended soft-tissue pressure can cause skin breakdown.[32] Whether

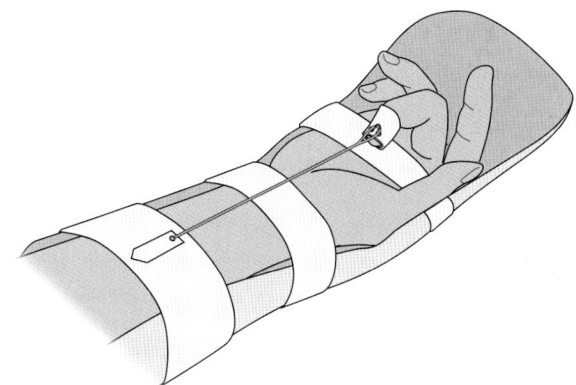

Figure 23.12 Example of a dynamic splint used after a flexor tendon repair to protect the repaired tendon. The dorsal hood aspect protects the tendon from getting overstretched into extension, and the palmar elastic band protects the tendon from the tension stress of muscle contraction.

the device is static or dynamic, friction can occur between the splint and the skin and must be avoided. The device should be secured firmly, yet comfortably, in position by its straps and other devices; it may require periodic adjustments to maintain proper alignment and reduce friction, especially as edema and muscle size change.

Pressure is a particular problem when the splint is worn over bony prominences. The most vulnerable sites are those where bony prominences are closest to the skin: the ulnar and radial styloid processes, pisiform, base of the fifth metacarpal, and metacarpal heads. Padding over these susceptible areas is applied during splint construction and is removed once the construction is complete; the result is less pressure from the splint over these bony prominences. If padding or relief is added after the splint is made, it may change the alignment and intended force application of the device. Clinicians who add padding to a splint must understand that the splint's function may be changed.

The patient's skin should be routinely checked for redness whenever the splint is removed; redness is a sign of pressure or friction. The splint may need adjustment as the patient's condition changes. Wrist and hand splint construction can be complicated, depending on the injury. In complex cases, an occupational therapist, orthopedic technician, or other hand specialist typically constructs the splint. In these cases, the rehabilitation clinician plays an important role in reporting on the patient's tolerance of the orthotic device and reinforcing compliance with its use.

Rehabilitation Interventions

Although modalities are included in rehabilitation programs for wrist and hand injuries, they are not described in this section. They are presented in chapter 9. The selection of modalities for wrist and hand injuries depends upon the specific injury and patient factors. Soft-tissue techniques covered in this section include trigger point release, myofascial release, and cross-friction massage. Joint mobilization techniques specific to the wrist and hand follow the section on soft-tissue mobilization. In addition to these manual therapy techniques, a variety of exercises, including flexibility, strengthening, proprioceptive, desensitization, and performance-specific exercises are presented.

Soft-Tissue Mobilization

Soft-tissue treatment techniques for the wrist and hand, including the trigger point release techniques based on the work of Travell and Simons,[41] are listed in chapter 11. Trigger points that are commonly found in the wrist and hand are listed in table 23.2; refer to chapter 11 for specific techniques for their treatment.

The palmar fascia myofascial release technique is used to mobilize palmar fascia and the wrist retinaculum. For this treatment, the patient sits facing the rehabilitation clinician or lies supine with the forearm resting comfortably on the table. With the patient's forearm in a supinated position, the rehabilitation clinician grasps the patient's hand

TABLE 23.2   Trigger Points Most Commonly Found in Wrist, Hand, and Finger Muscles

Body segment	Muscle with trigger points
Forearm	Wrist extensors
Hand	Intrinsic thumb muscles

with left and right thumbs and thenar eminences adjacent to each other over the base of the patient's wrist and the clinician's fingers wrapped around the patient's hand with the finger pads on the dorsum of the wrist (figure 23.13). The rehabilitation clinician applies a lateral traction of the palmar soft tissue with his or her thumbs and their eminences as an upward force is applied by the finger pads on the wrist's dorsum. This technique provides the patient with a myofascial release while simultaneously improving palmar mobility.

Cross-friction massage can be performed over soft-tissue structures that may be pathologically adherent. It may help to relieve pain and enhance the mobilization of connective tissue restrictions.[42] Cross-friction massage can be helpful over adhered tendons and ligaments in the hand and fingers. The area of tenderness or restriction is identified and isolated for treatment with a finger or thumb pad. Pressure over the area is maintained while deep friction is applied. The rehabilitation clinician's finger or thumb moves the overlying soft tissue against the underlying bone in a direction perpendicular to the fiber direction.

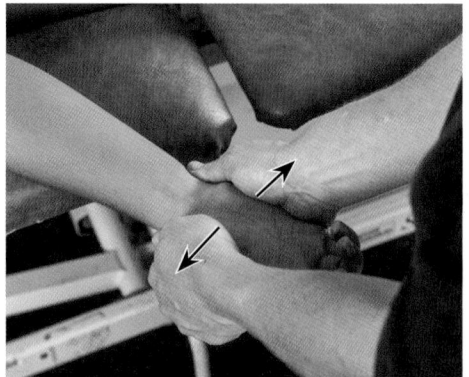

Figure 23.13   Palmar myofascial release.

Joint Mobilization

Most of the joint mobilization techniques discussed here are for joint accessory movements. They are based primarily on Kaltenborn[43] and Maitland's[44] work. There are certainly more movements available, but the movements presented in the following sections are those commonly used to improve joint mobility of the distal forearm, wrist, hand, and fingers.

Distal Radioulnar Joint

As with any elbow injury, both the proximal and distal radioulnar joints should be examined for restricted mobility. Likewise, if any restriction in wrist or forearm motion is present, these joints should be assessed and then mobilized according to restrictive findings. Since the radius surface is concave and the head of the ulna is convex, this joint adheres to the concave-on-convex rule; therefore, mobilization force on the radius is applied in the same direction as the restricted movement. For example, to improve supination, the force is applied anterior-to-posterior on the radius; to improve pronation, the force is applied posterior-to-anterior on the radius. The joint's resting position is 10° of supination, while its close-packed position is the same as the proximal radioulnar joint, maximal pronation or maximal supination. Its capsular pattern is equal restriction of pronation and supination.

Joint Mobilization of the Distal Radioulnar Joint

Since normal wrist motion depends upon normal forearm mobility, joint mobilization of the distal radioulnar joint is often part of a program to restore normal wrist range of motion. Three commonly used techniques are provided here.

Longitudinal Distraction[44]

Motion: General mobilization of distal radioulnar joint.

Resting Position: 10° supination.

Indications: Used before other mobilization techniques. Can be applied at the end-range position to improve motion.

Patient Position: Sitting or supine.

Clinician and Hand Positions: With the clinician facing the patient, the clinician's stabilizing hand is just proximal to the patient's elbow with the first web space wrapped around the patient's distal arm. The mobilizing hand wraps around the anterior wrist (figure 23.14) and tilts the patient's hand toward radial deviation. The forearm of the mobilizing arm is in line with the patient's forearm.

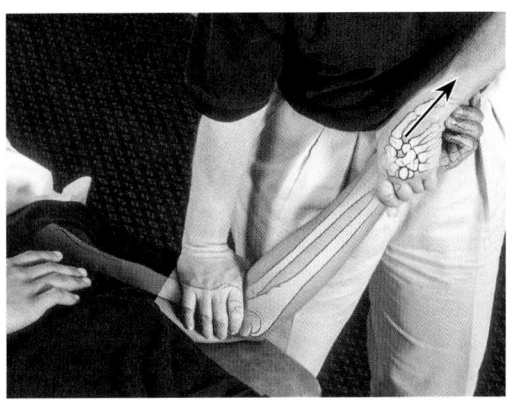

Figure 23.14

Mobilization Application: With the clinician's main hand contact at the base of the patient's thenar eminence, slack is taken up by pulling the radius to distract the joint, and either an oscillating longitudinal pull or a sustained traction is applied with the mobilizing hand. The clinician's distraction force is directed in line with the radial shaft.

Notations: This technique may be performed with the forearm in any position of comfort.

Distal Radioulnar Anterior Glide

Motion: Radioulnar motion.

Resting Position: Neutral to 10° supination.

Indications: To increase forearm pronation.

Patient Position: Sitting or supine.

Clinician and Hand Positions: Clinician is standing or sitting facing the dorsum of the patient's wrist. The stabilizing hand grasps the distal ulna, while the mobilizing hand grips the distal radius from the dorsal side so that the clinician's thenar eminence is in contact over the distal radius.

Mobilization Application: The thenar eminence is used to apply the anterior directed force on the distal radius (figure 23.15).

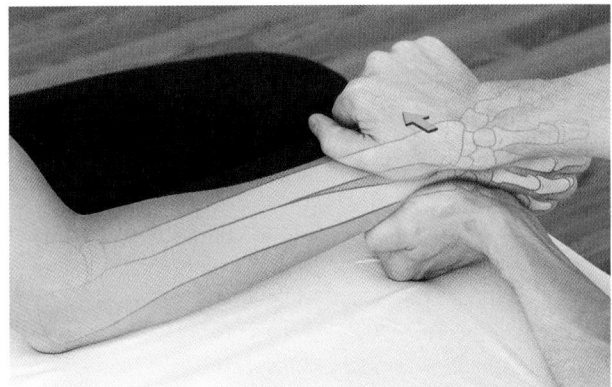

Figure 23.15

Notations: Either oscillations or sustained mobilization forces are appropriate. Also called ventral or palmar glide.

Distal Radioulnar Posterior Glide

Motion: Radioulnar motion.

Resting Position: Neutral to 10° supination.

Indications: To increase forearm supination.

Patient Position: Sitting or supine.

Clinician and Hand Positions: Clinician is standing or sitting facing the volar surface of the patient's wrist. The stabilizing hand grasps the distal ulna, while the mobilizing hand grips the distal radius from the ventral side so that the clinician's thenar eminence is in contact over the distal radius.

Mobilization Application: The thenar eminence is used to apply the posterior directed force on the distal radius (figure 23.16).

Notations: Either oscillations or sustained mobilization forces are appropriate. Also called dorsal glide.

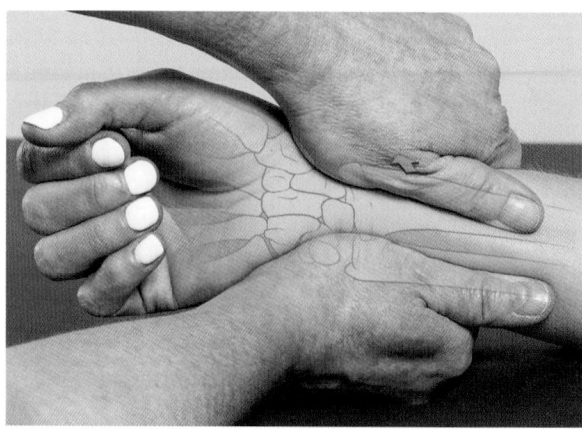

Figure 23.16

Wrist Joint

Although individual carpal bones may be mobilized (this is presented later in the chapter), wrist mobilizations usually occur between the radius and proximal carpal row. Since the radius and ulna distal ends are concave surfaces, and the proximal carpal row provides the convex surfaces for the radiocarpal and ulnocarpal joints, wrist movements abide by the convex-on-concave rule. Therefore, mobilization force on the carpals is applied in the opposite direction to the restricted movement. For example, to increase wrist extension, the proximal carpal row is glided in a volar (anterior) direction. To increase wrist flexion, the proximal carpal row is glided in a dorsal (posterior) direction. Gains in radial deviation occur with an ulnar (medial) glide of the proximal carpal row, and gains in ulnar deviation occur with a radial (lateral) glide of the proximal carpal row. Resting position for the wrist joint is neutral with slight ulnar deviation, and its close-packed position is in full extension. The joint's capsular pattern is equal restriction in flexion–extension and in radial-ulnar deviation.

Wrist mobilizations are performed with the patient in a comfortable position, either sitting or supine. The rehabilitation clinician is sitting or standing. A towel roll can be placed under the patient's distal forearm with the wrist over the table edge.

Traction

Motion: Radiocarpal and ulnocarpal joints.

Resting Position: Forearm can be in pronation, supination, or midway between. The wrist is in neutral with slight ulnar deviation.

Indications: To increase general mobility.

Patient Position: Supine on table or sitting with forearm resting on table.

Clinician and Hand Positions: Clinician stabilizes the distal forearm with one hand around the forearm just proximal to the wrist and places the mobilizing hand over the distal carpal row.

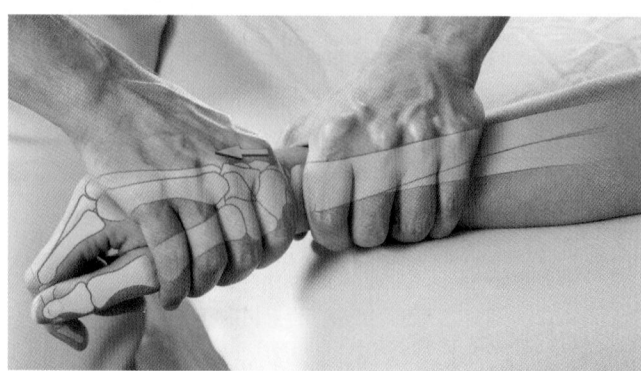

Figure 23.17

Mobilization Application: A traction force in a longitudinal direction is applied with the mobilizing hand (figure 23.17).

Notations: The force can be either a sustained application or a traction oscillation. Also called distraction. This technique can be used in varying degrees of wrist flexion and extension.

Dorsal Glide

Motion: Wrist.

Resting Position: Neutral wrist flexion–extension with slight ulnar deviation and neutral forearm supination–pronation.

Indications: To increase wrist flexion.

Patient Position: Same as for the previous motion.

Clinician and Hand Positions: Clinician places the stabilizing hand over the distal forearm as in the previous technique. The mobilizing hand grasps around the hand over the distal carpal row.

Mobilization Application: Slight traction to the wrist with a dorsal mobilizing force applied to the distal carpal row by the mobilizing hand (figure 23.18).

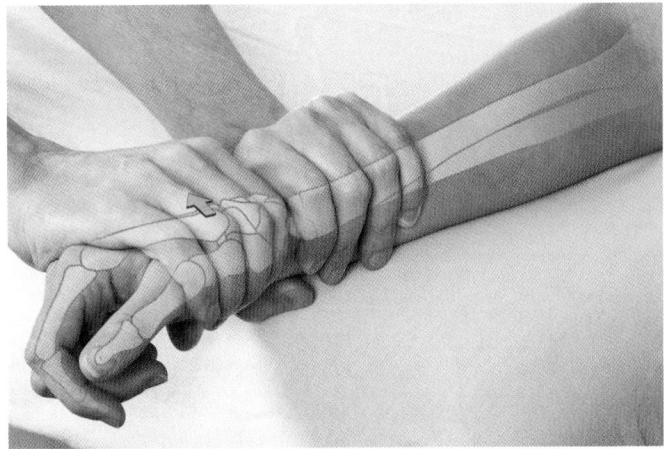

Figure 23.18

Notations: The force should be applied at an angle parallel to the wrist joint surface. Also called posterior glide.

Volar Glide

Motion: Wrist.

Resting Position: Neutral in wrist flexion–extension with slight ulnar deviation and neutral forearm supination–pronation.

Indications: To increase wrist extension.

Patient Position: Patient is sitting or supine. Patient's forearm is in pronation, and the wrist is in its resting position.

Clinician and Hand Positions: The rehabilitation clinician places the stabilizing hand over the distal forearm just adjacent to the wrist and the mobilizing hand over the distal carpal row.

Mobilization Application: Slight distraction of the wrist with a ventral force applied by the distal, mobilizing hand (figure 23.19).

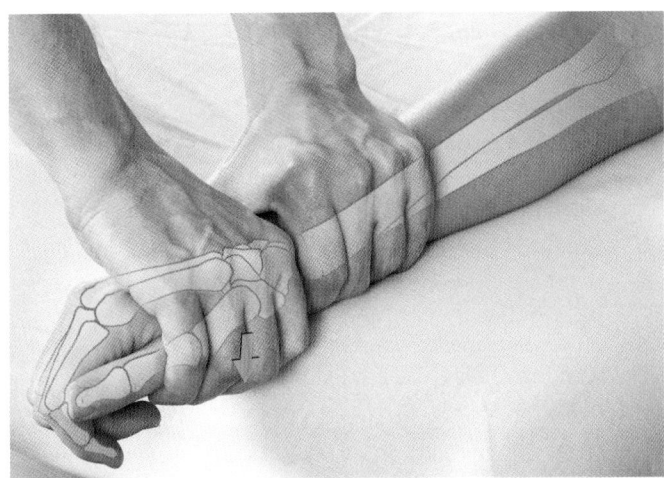

Figure 23.19

Notations: The force should be applied at an angle parallel to the wrist joint surface. Also called ventral or anterior glide.

Radial Glide

Motion: Wrist.

Resting Position: Neutral in wrist flexion–extension with slight ulnar deviation and neutral forearm supination–pronation.

Indications: To increase ulnar deviation.

Patient Position: Patient is sitting or supine. Patient's forearm is positioned in pronation with the wrist in neutral and off the treatment table.

Clinician and Hand Positions: The rehabilitation clinician places the stabilizing hand over the distal radial aspect of the forearm adjacent to the wrist joint, and the mobilizing hand grasps the distal carpal row with the first web space at the ulnar carpal bone and the fingers around the patient's wrist (figure 23.20).

>continued

Radial Glide *>continued*

> **Mobilization Application:** A radial-directed mobilizing force is applied.
>
> **Notations:** Keep the hands relaxed, with the mobilizing force coming from the shoulders.

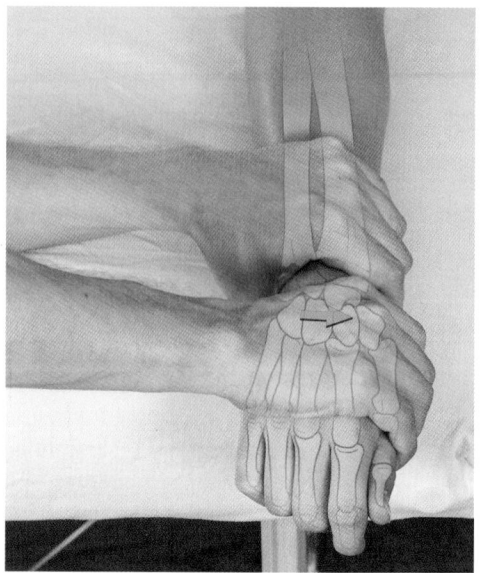

Figure 23.20

Ulnar Glide

> **Motion:** Wrist.
>
> **Resting Position:** Same position as for the radial glide.
>
> **Indications:** To increase radial deviation.
>
> **Patient Position:** Patient is supine or sitting. Patient's forearm is positioned with the radial side upward and the wrist in neutral.
>
> **Clinician and Hand Positions:** The clinician places the stabilizing hand over the distal forearm adjacent to the wrist joint, and the mobilizing hand grasps the distal carpal row with the thumb web around the lateral aspect of the patient's wrist.

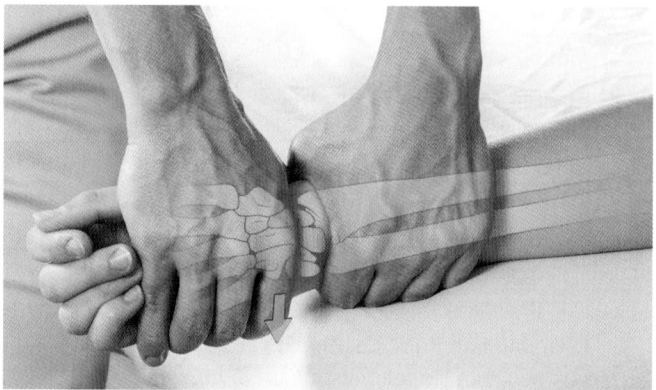

Figure 23.21

> **Mobilization Application:** A vertically downward mobilizing force is applied (figure 23.21).
>
> **Notations:** Keep the hands relaxed, with the mobilizing force coming from the shoulders.

Individual Carpal Glides

Each carpal in the wrist can be mobilized individually to improve flexion or extension motions. Sometimes when individual carpal joints are restricted, individual joint mobilization techniques are needed. The concave-on-convex rule applies to these joints, so it is important to know the joint's configuration before deciding whether a PA or an AP mobilization force is appropriate (figure 23.22).

In the lateral intercarpal joints, the convex scaphoid joins with the concave trapezium and trapezoid; this means that flexion is increased with a volar glide of the trapezium and trapezoid on a fixed scaphoid, and extension is increased with a volar glide of the scaphoid on the distal carpal row. Because the capitate is the convex surface and the lunate is the concave surface of the capitate–lunate joint, flexion is increased by a volar glide of the lunate on the fixed capitate, and extension is increased by stabilizing the more proximal lunate and performing a volar glide of the more distal capitate.

The mobilization techniques for each of these intercarpal joints are similar. The forearm is unsupported so that the weight of the arm can provide a slight traction force on the joints. In each case, mobilization is performed with the forearm in pronation using a pinch grasp with both the stabilizing and mobilizing hands, with the thumbs on the dorsal surface of the patient's hand. The stabilizing finger and thumb grasp the bone that is to remain stationary,

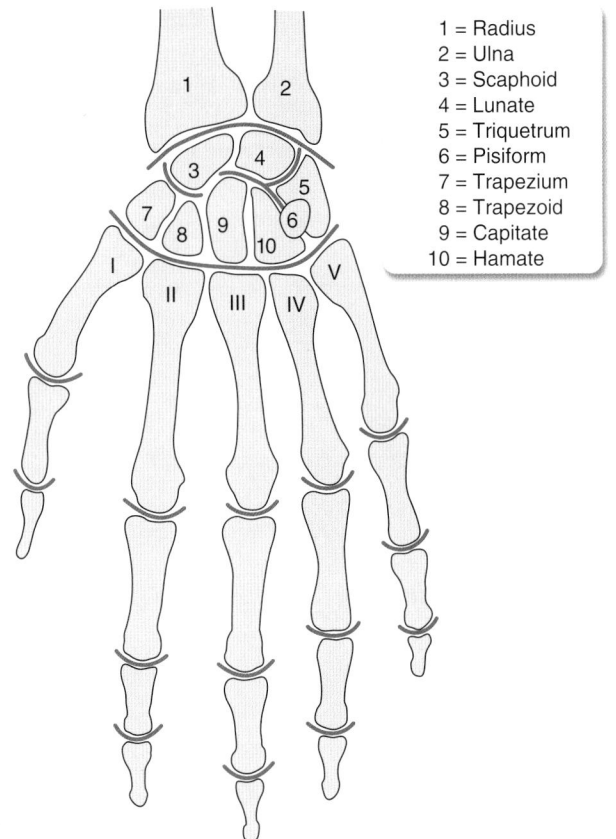

1 = Radius
2 = Ulna
3 = Scaphoid
4 = Lunate
5 = Triquetrum
6 = Pisiform
7 = Trapezium
8 = Trapezoid
9 = Capitate
10 = Hamate

Figure 23.22   Surface configurations of wrist and digits.

and the mobilizing finger and thumb grasp the bone to be mobilized (figure 23.23). Because the joints are small, the clinician's thumbs will be in contact with each other. The thumbs apply a vertically downward force in a volar direction.

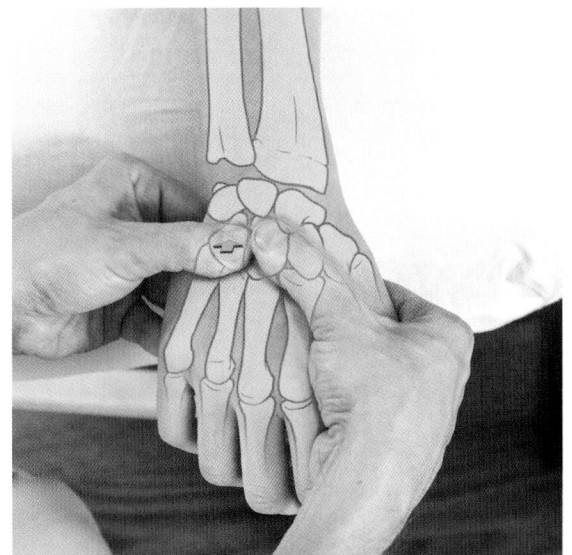

Figure 23.23   Joint mobilization: individual carpal glides.

Carpometacarpal Joints

The carpometacarpal (CMC) joints of digits 2 through 5 are all similarly shaped with 2° of motion. Although the thumb's CMC joint is a saddle joint, its design is essentially similar to those of the other CMC joints when considering their compliance with mobilization rules. In this regard, all five digits' joint design has a convex carpal in contact with a concave metacarpal, which allows these joints to abide by the concave-on-convex rule; thus, the direction of the mobilization force is the same as the direction of movement. For example, to improve joint flexion, a PA (volar) glide is applied to the metacarpal, but to improve joint extension, an AP (dorsal) glide is needed. The resting position for joints 2 through 5 is midway between flexion and extension; their close-packed position is full flexion; and the thumb's CMC resting position is midway between abduction and adduction and midway between flexion and extension, with its close-packed position in full opposition. A capsular pattern of the fingers is identified when all motions are restricted with slightly more restriction seen in flexion, and a capsular pattern of the thumb is demonstrated with more loss of motion in abduction than extension.

Hand placements for stabilization and mobilization are similar for both the fingers and the thumb carpometacarpal joints. The stabilizing hand uses a tip-to-tip pinch or lateral pinch grasp over the carpal bone, and the mobilizing hand is placed in a similar grasp around the base of the metacarpal. Some distraction is applied to the joint while the mobilizing force is applied at the same time. It is important to avoid squeezing the carpal while still grasping it firmly enough to provide adequate mobilization force.

Finger Carpometacarpal Joints A loss of mobility in these joints can restrict the patient's ability to make a fist and can reduce the ability to grip objects. Joint mobilization is often needed to restore motion in these joints. Some of the most common techniques are presented in the following sections.

Traction

Motion: Carpometacarpal joints.

Resting Position: Midway between flexion and extension.

Indications: To relieve pain or provide a general increase in joint mobility.

Patient Position: Supine on table or seated with forearm resting on table.

Clinician and Hand Positions: Clinician is seated or standing. The carpal is stabilized with a tip-to-tip pinch grasp. The mobilizing hand uses a lateral finger-pinch grasp at the proximal metacarpal.

Mobilization Application: Metacarpal is pulled in the direction of its long axis (figure 23.24).

Notations: Movement in these joints is minimal, especially in digits 2 and 3. Also called CMC distraction.

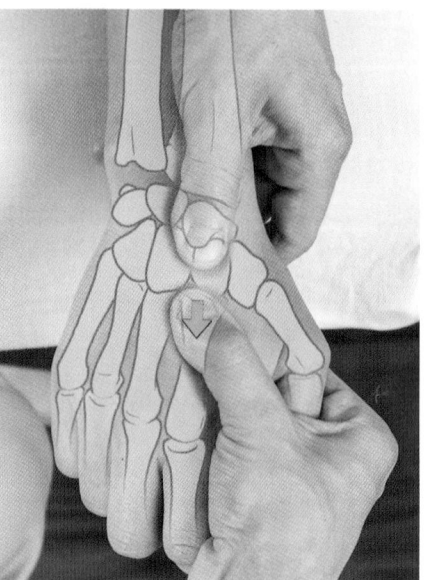

Figure 23.24

Anteroposterior Glide

Motion: Carpometacarpal joint.

Resting Position: Midway between flexion and extension.

Indications: To relieve pain or increase CMC joint extension.

Patient Position: Supine on table or seated with forearm resting on table.

Clinician and Hand Positions: Clinician is seated or standing. Clinician stabilizes the patient's carpal with the thumb and index finger of one hand, and then places the thumb and index finger of the mobilizing hand over the metacarpal to be treated (figure 23.25).

Mobilization Application: An AP force in the dorsal direction is applied by the mobilizing hand on the metacarpal.

Notations: Carpometacarpal joints 4 and 5 normally have more mobility than joints 2 and 3. An alternate position is to have the patient's arm in supination; mobilize the metacarpal posteriorly in a dorsal direction. Also called dorsal or posterior glide.

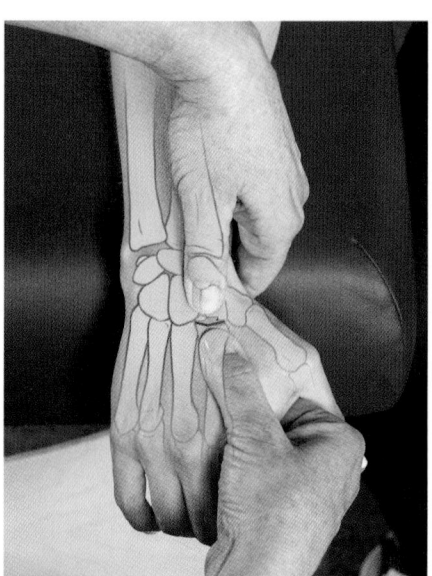

Figure 23.25

Posteroanterior Glide

Motion: Carpometacarpal joint.

Resting Position: Midway between flexion and extension.

Indications: To relieve pain or increase CMC joint flexion.

Patient Position: Supine on table or seated with forearm resting on table.

Clinician and Hand Positions: Clinician is seated or standing. The clinician's grasps are similar to those described for AP glides (figure 23.26).

Mobilization Application: PA force in the palmar direction is applied to the metacarpal.

Notations: Also called palmar or anterior glide.

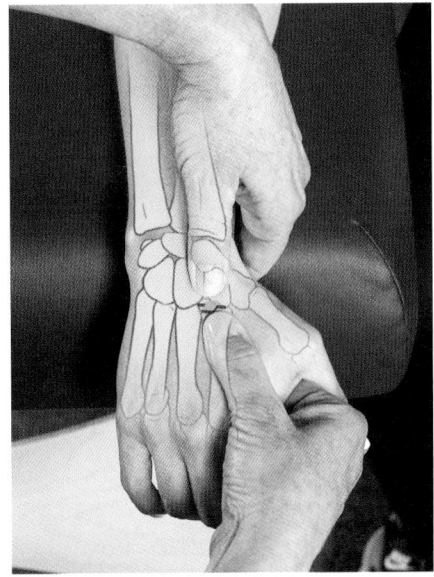

Figure 23.26

Thumb Carpometacarpal Joint   As with CMC techniques for fingers 2 through 5, mobilization of the thumb is applied with the stabilizing hand using a tip-to-tip pinch or lateral pinch grasp over the carpal bone. The mobilizing hand is placed around the metacarpal bone, close to the joint margin.

Traction

Motion: Thumb CMC joint.

Resting Position: The CMC joint is in mid-position between flexion–extension and abduction–adduction.

Indications: General mobilization of the joint.

Patient Position: Supine on table or seated with forearm resting on table in a neutral position with the thumb facing up.

Clinician and Hand Positions: Stabilizing hand uses a tip-to-tip or lateral pinch grasp over the carpal bone, and the mobilizing hand uses a lateral pinch grasp around the metacarpal's proximal region adjacent to the joint margin (figure 23.27).

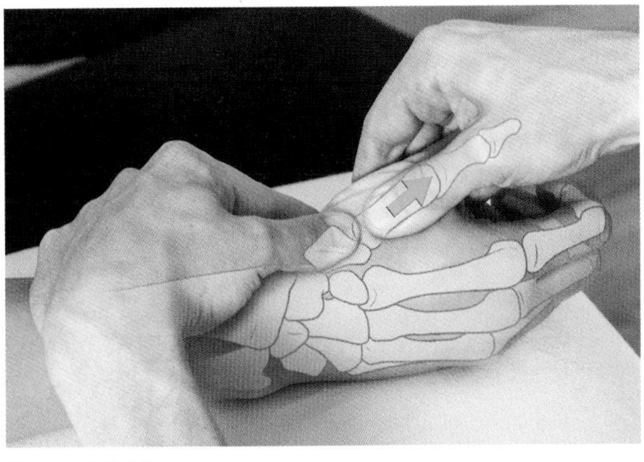

Mobilization Application: Distract the metacarpal along its longitudinal axis from the joint.

Figure 23.27

Notations: Distraction can be either sustained or oscillating. Also called distraction.

Posteroanterior Glide

Motion: Thumb CMC joint.

Resting Position: The CMC joint is in mid-position between flexion–extension and abduction–adduction.

Indications: To relieve pain or increase thumb adduction.

Patient Position: Supine on table or seated with forearm resting on table in a neutral position with the thumb facing up.

Clinician and Hand Positions: Clinician stabilizes the trapezium and trapezoid, the proximal aspect of

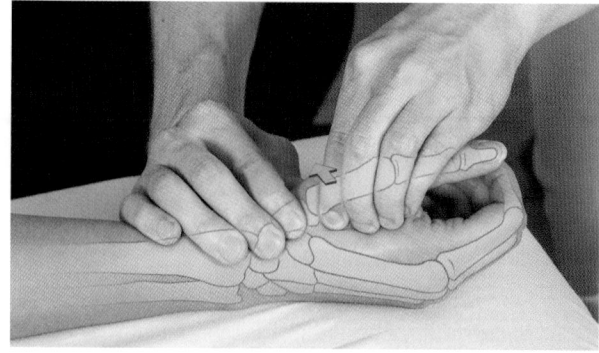

Figure 23.28

the joint, using the thumb and index finger of one hand; the clinician grasps the patient's first metacarpal with the opposite thumb and index finger.

Mobilization Application: Slight traction to the joint is applied, followed by a PA glide to the metacarpal (figure 23.28).

Notations: Both the trapezium and trapezoid are stabilized in the proximal joint segment. Also called ventral or anterior glide.

Anteroposterior Glide

Motion: Thumb CMC joint.

Resting Position: The CMC joint is in mid-position between flexion–extension and abduction–adduction.

Indications: To relieve pain or increase thumb CMC abduction.

Patient Position: Supine on table or seated with forearm resting on table in a neutral position with the thumb facing up.

Clinician and Hand Positions: Clinician stabilizes the trapezium and trapezoid at the proximal aspect of the joint using the thumb and index finger of one hand; the

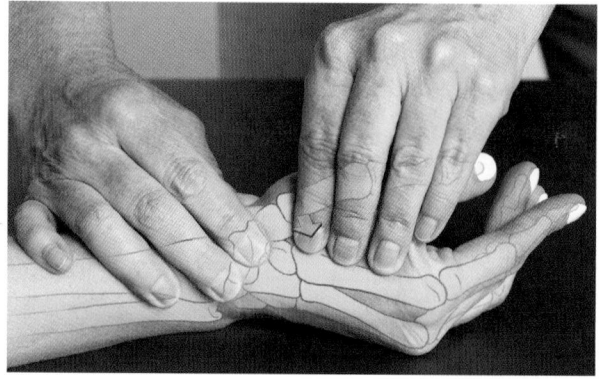

Figure 23.29

clinician holds the patient's first metacarpal with the opposite thumb and the index finger.

Mobilization Application: Slight traction to the joint is applied, followed by an AP glide to the metacarpal (figure 23.29).

Notations: Clinician stabilizes both the trapezium and trapezoid in the proximal joint segment. Also called dorsal or posterior glide.

Ulnar Glide

Motion: Thumb CMC joint.

Resting Position: The CMC joint is in mid-position between flexion–extension and abduction–adduction.

Indications: To relieve pain or increase flexion.

Patient Position: Patient is supine or seated with the ulna resting on the table in a neutral position with the thumb up in a neutral position.

Clinician and Hand Positions: With the proximal aspect of the joint stabilized using the thumb and index finger of one hand, the rehabilitation clinician grasps the metacarpal with the other hand (figure 23.30).

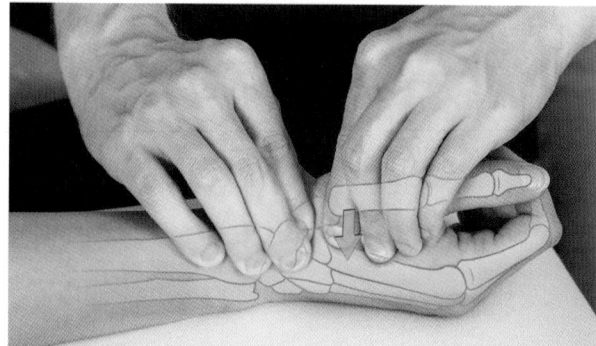

Figure 23.30

Mobilization Application: Radial-to-ulnar glide is applied parallel to the joint surface.

Notations: The thumb's CMC joint is convex at its proximal joint surface. Also called medial glide.

Metacarpophalangeal and Interphalangeal Joints

The configuration of each of these joints is similar, so the mobilization techniques are also similar. Each mobilization described can be used on any of these joints. As indicated in previous sections, traction is applied during each mobilization technique to make the technique more comfortable and to produce better results by adding stretch to the capsule. The grasps should be firm enough to administer the mobilization force effectively but not so tight as to cause discomfort.

Each of the metacarpophalangeal and interphalangeal joints has a convex proximal surface and a concave distal surface, so they abide by the concave-on-convex rule: the joint glide is applied in the same direction as the movement. Therefore, to increase flexion, a PA (volar) glide is used, while to increase extension, an AP (dorsal) glide is used. The resting position for each joint is listed in table 23.3.

TABLE 23.3   Joint Mobilization Information for MCP and IP Joints of the Fingers

Joint	Resting position	Close-packed position	Capsular pattern
#2-5 MCP	Slight flexion with ulnar deviation	Full flexion	Equal loss in all directions
#1 MCP	Midway between flexion–extension and abduction–adduction	Full opposition	Abduction loss is greater than extension loss
IP	PIP = 10° flexion DIP = 30° flexion	Full extension	Flexion loss is greater than extension loss

IP = interphalangeal joint; PIP = proximal interphalangeal joint; DIP = distal interphalangeal joint; MCP = metacarpophalangeal joint.

Traction

Motion: MCP and IP joints.

Resting Position: Flexion position depends on specific joint mobilized; see table 23.3.

Indications: General mobilization and relaxation.

Patient Position: Supine on table or seated with forearm resting on table.

Clinician and Hand Positions: The proximal aspect of the joint is grasped with the stabilizing hand, while the distal aspect of the joint is grasped by the index finger and thumb of the mobilizing hand (figure 23.31).

Mobilization Application: Traction force in line with the longitudinal axis is applied perpendicular to the joint's surface.

Notations: Since the configurations of these joints are similar, this technique may be applied to any of the IP or MCP joints. Also called traction.

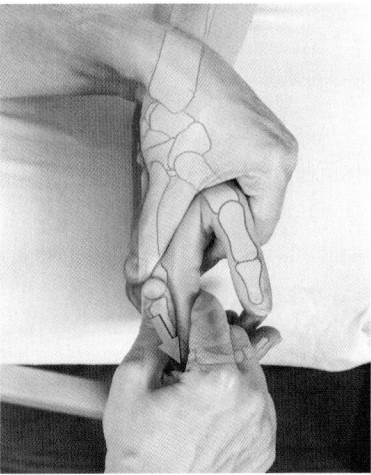

Figure 23.31

Rotation

Motion: MCP and IP joints.

Resting Position: Flexion position depends on specific joint mobilized; see table 23.3.

Indications: To improve accessory rotation motion of the joints.

Patient Position: Supine on table or seated with forearm resting on table.

Clinician and Hand Positions: The proximal aspect of the joint is grasped with a lateral pinch of the thumb and index finger, with the mobilizing hand using a similar grasp on the distal joint segment immediately adjacent to the joint.

Mobilization Application: Traction is maintained while a medial rotation is applied, then a lateral rotation (figure 23.32).

Notations: Rotation is an accessory motion that must be restored in order for the patient to have full function of the joint and hand. If the finger is lacking the last few degrees of motion, or if the hand cannot make a complete fist, it may be that rotation of the MCP is limited.

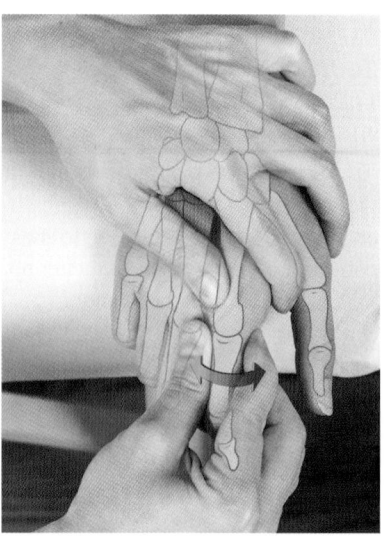

Figure 23.32

Posteroanterior Glide

Motion: MCP and IP joints.

Resting Position: Flexion position depends on specific joint mobilized; see table 23.3.

Indications: PA glide increases flexion motion.

Patient Position: Supine on table or seated with forearm resting on table in a neutral position with the thumb facing up.

Clinician and Hand Positions: The proximal aspect of the joint is stabilized while the distal aspect receives traction; the stabilizing hand has a lateral pinch grasp on the proximal aspect, and the mobilizing hand has a similar grasp on the distal joint segment (figure 23.33).

Mobilization Application: While traction is maintained, a PA force is applied.

Notations: Because the joints are a concave surface moving on a convex surface, the mobilization force is in the same direction as the joint's roll or movement. Also called ventral or anterior glide.

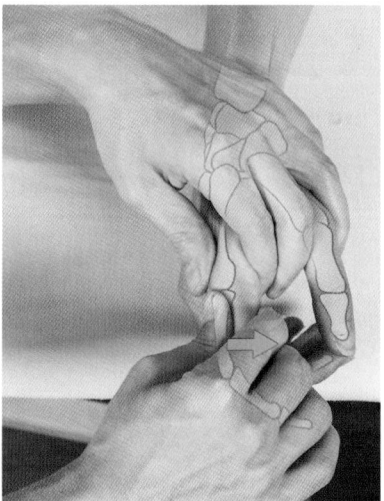

Figure 23.33

Anteroposterior Glide

Motion: MCP and IP joints.

Resting Position: Flexion position depends on specific joint mobilized; see table 23.3.

Indications: AP glide increases extension motion.

Patient Position: Supine on table or seated with forearm resting on table in a neutral position with the thumb facing up.

Clinician and Hand Positions: The proximal aspect of the joint is stabilized while the distal aspect receives traction; the stabilizing hand has a lateral pinch grasp on the proximal aspect, and the mobilizing hand has a similar grasp on the distal joint segment (figure 23.34).

Mobilization Application: While traction is maintained, an AP force is applied.

Notations: Because the joints are a concave surface moving on a convex surface, the mobilization force is in the same direction as the joint's roll or movement. Also called dorsal or posterior glide.

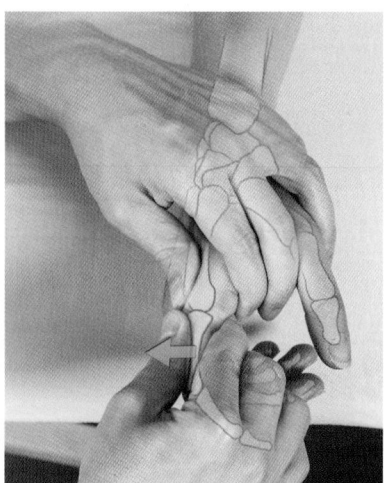

Figure 23.34

Lateral Glides

Motion: MCP and IP joints.

Resting Position: Flexion position depends on specific joint mobilized; see table 23.3.

Indications: To improve abduction and adduction of the MCP and IP joints.

Patient Position: Supine on table or seated with forearm resting on table with forearm relaxed in a pronated position.

Clinician and Hand Positions: The proximal aspect of the joint is stabilized, while the distal aspect receives traction with the mobilizing hand rotated to the side of the joint rather than anteriorly and posteriorly to deliver lateral mobilization force.

Mobilization Application: A radial or ulnar glide force is applied to the distal aspect of the joint, depending on the finger and the movement desired (figure 23.35). Radial glide improves abduction of MCPs 1 and 2, adduction of MCPs 4 and 5, and radial abduction of MCP 3. Ulnar glide improves adduction of MCPs 1 and 2, abduction of MCPs 4 and 5, and ulnar abduction of MCP 3.

Notations: Abduction and adduction occur as physiological motions at the MCP joints and accessory motions at the IP joints. The thumb applies the mobilization force, so it is positioned on the radial or ulnar aspect of the joint.

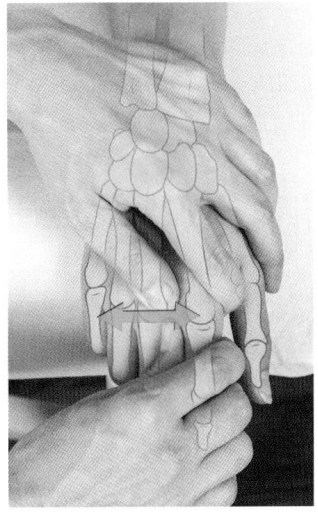

Figure 23.35

Flexibility Exercises

Range-of-motion exercises are divided into those for the intrinsic muscles and those for the extrinsic muscles. The two muscle groups require different considerations for the correct application of stretch. Because extrinsic muscles cross multiple joints, the rehabilitation clinician must know these muscle insertion locations to apply appropriate stretches. Each joint the muscle crosses must be placed on stretch to produce optimal ROM changes. Stretches to extrinsic hand muscles should be applied not just precisely but also in sequence from the most distal to the most proximal joint. When one joint is stretched, the other joints need to be stabilized.[45]

This is particularly important when stretching the fingers because multiple joints and tendons are involved. For example, if any of the proximal wrist, MCP, or PIP joints is not stabilized when the distal interphalangeal joint is stretched, the stretch force and surrounding tissue tension can cause any of the nonstabilized proximal joints to buckle, making for an ineffective application of stretch. The force applied should be a slow, gentle, and sustained stretch to avoid either incorrect application or excessive force that can damage the small structures of the hand and fingers. Unless otherwise indicated, the stretch is performed often throughout the day with 1 to 4 repetitions at each session; the shorter the hold, the more repetitions performed. If a 30 s hold is used, 1 to 2 repetitions is sufficient,[46-48] but if a 15 s hold is used, the exercise is repeated 4 times.[49, 50] Refer to chapter 12 for additional information on stretching.

One finger is stretched at a time. Joint mobilization is used before stretching so that the stretch of soft-tissue structures is more effective. If joint motion is restricted by extrinsic tightness, each joint is placed on stretch in the sequence just described, distal to proximal, to affect extrinsic structures but not intrinsic muscles. If joint motion is restricted by intrinsic muscle tightness, then the focus is on isolating the stretch to the intrinsic muscle. To perform an isolated stretch on the intrinsic muscle, the distal joint is stretched and the proximal joint is placed in the opposite direction to avoid stretching the extrinsic muscles and to focus the stretch on the intrinsic muscles. For example, when the PIP joint is placed in flexion and the MCP joint is placed in extension, the intrinsic muscles extending the PIP are stretched, but the extrinsic extensor muscles are not; however, when the PIP and MCP joints are placed in flexion, the extrinsic extensor muscles are stretched, but the intrinsic muscles are not. If both structures have limited flexibility, stretch exercises in both positions are needed.

Joints and Ligaments

As already mentioned, manual therapy mobilization techniques—both accessory and physiological techniques—should be applied before flexibility exercises. The accessory techniques are those already discussed, including motions that are not actively possible but that must take place for full motion to occur. For example, rotation at the MCP and IP joints is an accessory motion.

Because several joints must usually be considered when applying stretch exercises, the clinician must be familiar with the hand's anatomy. When one joint is stretched, the other joints are positioned in neutral and kept relaxed to reduce soft-tissue tension on the joint being treated. When you apply a passive stretch force, the distal portion of the joint's distal segment is the location of the stretch. You need to be careful that the point of your force application is on the joint's distal portion of the bone's shaft and not on the next distal joint. For example, when stretching a PIP joint, your force is applied on the distal portion of the middle phalanx, not on the DIP joint or on the distal phalanx. The proximal phalanx must also be properly stabilized if the stretch is to be correct (figure 23.36).

Abduction movements are crucial to maintaining vital flexibility in the web space of the thumb and in MCP extension movement of the fingers. Abduction of the fingers can help stretch the MCP collateral ligaments. The thumb's web space soft tissue is stretched using thumb abduction overpressure. The thumb's web space can be stretched by actively abducting the thumb or by applying an abduction force at the CMC joint. The patient can also stretch the thumb's web space by placing the hand over the top of the knee, with the fingers separated from the thumb, and applying a downward force from the shoulder to push the hand on the knee (figure 23.37). The patient can stretch the finger MCPs by intertwining the fingers of the two hands

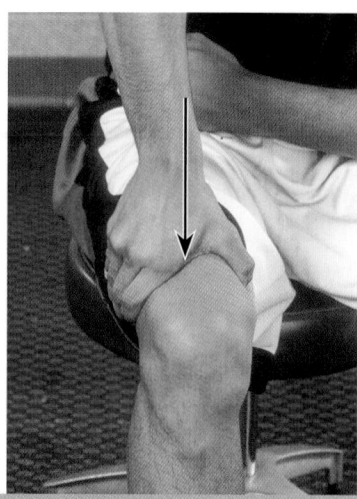

Figure 23.37 Thumb abduction stretch.

together as in a praying position. These movements are performed either actively or passively. As mentioned, care must be taken to apply the force on the distal segment of the CMC joint, not over the MCP joint.

As mentioned earlier, the CMC and intermetacarpal joints form the palmar arches that are vital to hand formation and function.[51] The second and third metacarpals have little mobility and form the peak of the palmar arches.[51] The fourth, and especially the fifth, metacarpals move into flexion as the hand is formed into a fist; this motion is crucial to normal hand function and permits a firm grasp.[52] The rehabilitation clinician can stretch these joints by placing his or her thumbs in the palm of the patient's hand and his or her fingers on the dorsum over the metacarpals. The thumbs are stabilizers as the fingers roll the metacarpals into opposition around the clinician's thumbs (figure 23.38). The palmar fascia can be stretched using the technique demonstrated in figure 23.13.

Wrist joint stretches are done with the fingers relaxed and the force applied proximal to the MCP joints. The patient can apply the stretches passively in all wrist motions (figure 23.39).

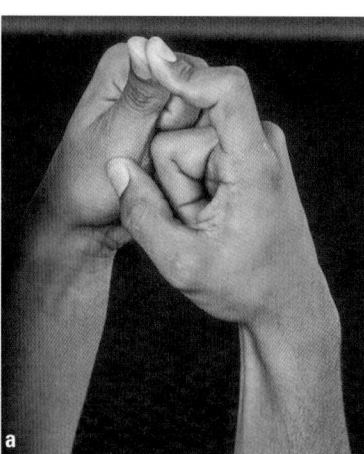

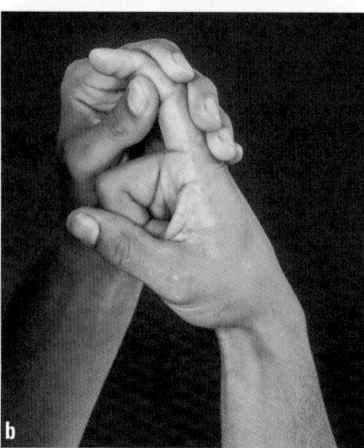

Figure 23.36 Stretch force application. *(a)* Incorrect: Force is applied on the digit's distal segment. *(b)* Correct: Force is applied at the distal joint first, then moves one joint at a time to the most proximal joint.

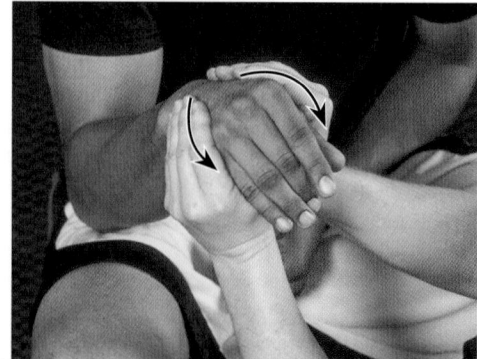

Figure 23.38 Range of motion of CMC and intermetacarpal joints.

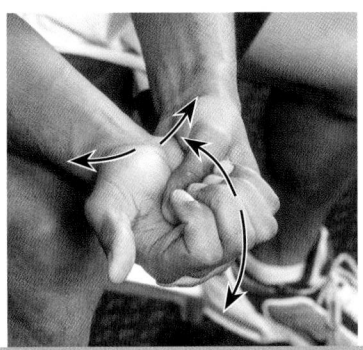

Figure 23.39 Self-administered wrist stretches in flexion, extension, radial deviation, and ulnar deviation.

The distal radioulnar joint stretches are the same as those for the proximal radioulnar joint. These are discussed in chapter 22 and are shown in figures 22.16 and 22.17. The stretch is applied at the distal radioulnar joint. The hand is not included in the stretch.

CLINICAL TIPS

Flexibility exercises for the hand are used to stretch the joints and ligaments, extrinsic muscles, and intrinsic muscles. Stretching muscles requires isolating the other joints they cross while focusing on one joint; when stretching an entire muscle, the stretch force begins at the muscle's most distal insertion and moves one joint at a time more proximally while keeping the more distal joints on stretch. Force must be carefully applied to avoid overstretching tissue.

Because it originates palmar to the PIP and inserts dorsal to the DIP, the oblique retinacular ligament acts on the IP joints in a manner similar to the way in which the intrinsics act on the MCP and PIP joints.[53] When the PIP joint is flexed, this ligament helps to flex the DIP joint, and when the PIP joint extends, the ligament produces a passive extension force.[54] Normally, fibers of this ligament move anteriorly during flexion; if this motion cannot occur, such as in the presence of scar tissue adhesions, the DIP and PIP joints will not fully flex to form a normal power grasp.[55] If all digits do not normally flex when the patient closes the hand, the reason may be either scar tissue binding down the oblique retinacular ligament fibers or tightness within the joint capsule.

To determine whether the oblique retinacular ligament is restricted, the rehabilitation clinician passively keeps the affected digit's PIP joint in extension and then flexes the DIP joint. If the DIP joint does not move, the clinician places the PIP joint in slight flexion and repeats DIP flexion. If the DIP joint flexes in this position, the oblique retinacular ligament is restricted, but if the DIP joint still cannot flex, the DIP capsule is tight.[56] To stretch this ligament, the PIP joint is passively kept in extension while

the DIP joint is stretched into flexion; this is the same movement as the test.

Extrinsic Muscles

As mentioned previously, a stretch applied to extrinsic muscles begins with the distal joint and proceeds in sequence, moving distally to proximally, one joint the muscle crosses at a time. The force is applied slowly and deliberately without excessive stress to the structures. Contract-relax-stretch techniques can improve the results of the stretch because reflex inhibition plays a role in these techniques.[57] The application of a slight traction force on the joints makes the stretch more comfortable by reducing compressive forces on the joints.[58]

Stretching either extrinsic extensor or extrinsic flexor muscles starts distally and moves proximally. For example, improving the flexion motion of the extrinsic extensor muscles involves applying a stretch at the DIP joint while keeping the PIP, MCP, and wrist joints at 0° as the DIP is brought into flexion. Once the DIP joint is moved to its end position, the PIP joint is then moved into flexion while the flexed position of the DIP is maintained. The MCP joint is then moved into flexion while the IP joints are held in their flexed positions. Finally, the wrist is brought into flexion to its end range while the digit is held in its fully flexed position. Stretch to increase flexion is seen in figure 23.40. Stretches to increase the motion of flexor and extensor extrinsic muscles are each applied in both elbow flexion and extension. The patient should feel a stretch on the posterior forearm when stretching the extrinsic extensors and on the anterior forearm when stretching the extrinsic flexors.

Since the long finger muscles can also influence wrist mobility, wrist stretches are applied with the fingers on stretch. To increase wrist flexion motion, the patient flexes the fingers first and then moves the wrist into flexion. As with stretches to the fingers, the wrist is stretched with the elbow in extension (figure 23.41*a*) and in flexion (figure 23.41*b*). The stretch should be felt on the posterior forearm.

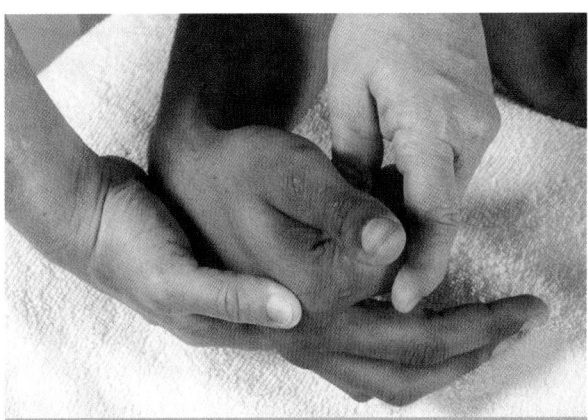

Figure 23.40 Extrinsic finger extensor stretch. In sequence: DIP, PIP, MCP, wrist, elbow.

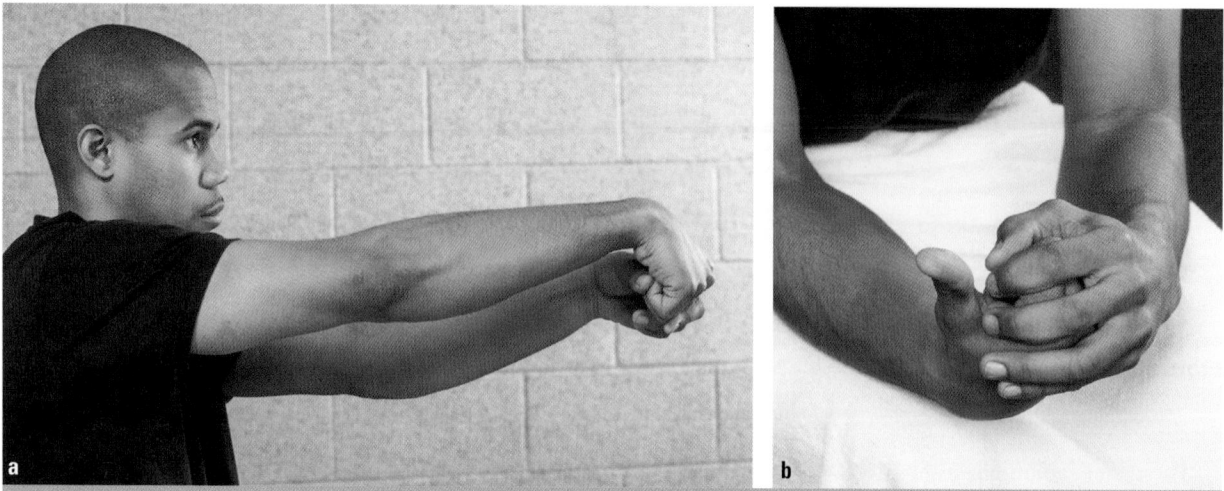

Figure 23.41 Independent stretches to increase flexion *(a)* with elbow extension and *(b)* with elbow flexion.

However, if the clinician has determined that the lack of full wrist motion is secondary to wrist muscle tightness, he or she focuses on stretching those muscles as well as ensuring that the extrinsic finger muscles have good length.

Intrinsic Muscles

Because the lumbricals and interossei flex the MCP joint and extend the IP joints, the stretch is applied in the opposite direction from their movement. As with the extrinsic muscles, the distal joints these muscles cross are placed in a stretched position first. Therefore, the IP joints are passively moved into flexion, followed by placement of the MCP in extension (figure 23.42). The wrist is stabilized in neutral during this activity to prevent extrinsic muscle influences on the stretch.

Tendon Gliding Exercises

When restriction of normal tendon gliding occurs because of adhesions of tendons or their sheaths, you must restore the normal tendon glide to achieve full range of motion.

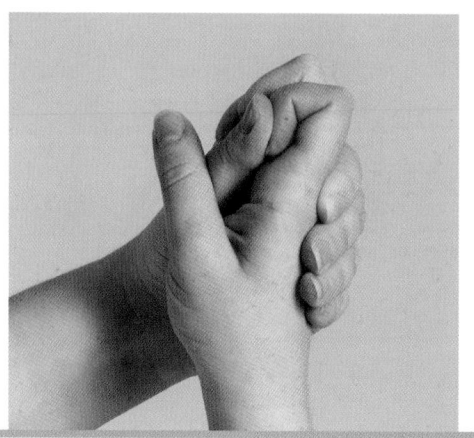

Figure 23.42 Intrinsic stretch: IPs are flexed, MCP is extended, wrist is in neutral.

Adhesions can occur anywhere along a tendon and can restrict tendon motion proximally and distally from the point of adhesion. Friction massage helps reduce adhesions of superficial tendons, and active exercises improve the mobility of both superficial and deep tendons. Muscle activity helps restore proximal glide of the tendon. Active and passive exercises and splinting can restore distal glide of the tendon. Because active exercises can restore both proximal and distal tendon gliding, it is advisable to use them whenever possible. The effectiveness of these exercises, however, is limited by the muscle's strength and endurance. Passive stretching and massage may be used to improve tendon gliding when strength and endurance are limited.

Since immobilization tends to produce tendon adhesions, attitudes have changed about permissible movements after tendon injury and repair.[59] Early movement has been shown to reduce the risk of adhesions, so surgeons are now advocating early controlled motion to enhance movement while protecting healing tissues.[59]

Tendon gliding exercises are very important for maintaining or regaining tendon mobility. Hand tendons are at high risk of losing their ability to glide freely when immobilized; if you recall all the various soft-tissue structures that are in close proximity to one another throughout the hand, you can see how scar tissue adhesions can quickly affect finger motion. Tendons have shown a loss of gliding ability within 10 d after repair.[60] Tendon gliding exercises are specific for each tendon within the hand; as they are performed, they move the tendon to encourage continued gliding of the tendon within its sheath and over surrounding tissues. Therefore, if you know the motion each muscle performs at each joint, the tendon gliding exercises are easier to remember.

Flexor Tendons The long flexor tendons are susceptible to peritendinous adhesions because they each have tendon sheaths throughout their lengths.[61] Gliding exercises for the long flexor tendons require you to distinguish between the profundus and superficialis. You must isolate each tendon to facilitate gliding because adhesions of either tendon restrict the movement of both. To show whether or not the tendons are gliding properly, the patient holds the MCP joint in extension while flexing the PIP joints. With the fingers in this position, the clinician passively extends the DIP joint and should meet no resistance. If there is no resistance, it is normal, and only the superficialis is being used, as it should be. If the patient holds this position but both flexor tendons are tense (clinician cannot passively move the DIP joint), normal tendon gliding between the profundus and superficialis tendons is restricted.

This is the gliding exercise for this problem: With the MCP and PIP joints stabilized in extension, the patient flexes and extends the DIP joint (figure 23.43a). To isolate the superficialis from the profundus tendon, the MCP is stabilized at 0°, and the PIP joint is actively flexed and extended. Either one digit is stabilized at a time, as shown in figure 23.43b, or all digits except the one being treated are stabilized. In this exercise, the other IP joints are kept in extension while the digit of interest is actively flexed. Because each of the profundus tendons originates from the same muscle belly, it is easy to eliminate profundus activity by restricting the movement of any of the other digits rather than having to isolate individual joints of the affected digit (figure 23.43c).

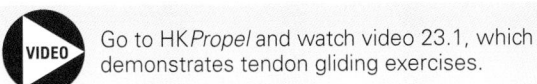
Go to HK*Propel* and watch video 23.1, which demonstrates tendon gliding exercises.

There are three active functional tendon gliding exercises for flexor tendons that belong in a rehabilitation program to either prevent gliding restrictions or improve flexor tendon gliding when it is restricted.[62] They are presented in figure 23.44. Each of these exercises starts with the IP and MCP joints in full extension. The first exercise enhances gliding between the two long finger flexor tendons; this is the hook-position exercise, and it involves keeping the MCP joints extended while flexing the IPs (figure 23.44a).[62] The second exercise produces gliding of the profundus tendons within their sheaths; this is the full-fist formation, and it is performed with the IP and MCP joints moving into full flexion and then with all the joints moving into extension (figure 23.44b).[62] The third exercise is a modified fist exercise; it occurs with the MCP and PIP joints flexed and the DIP joints extended,

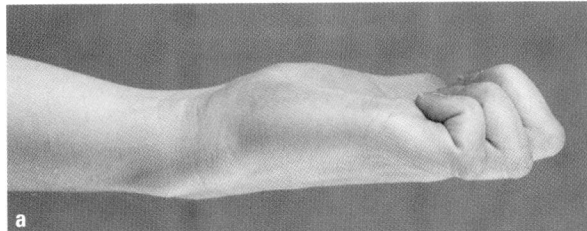
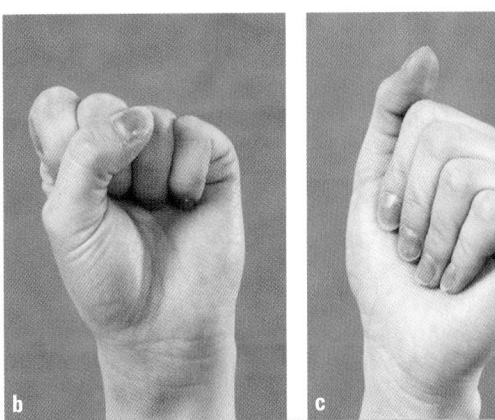

Figure 23.44 Flexor tendon gliding exercises: *(a)* Hook enhances gliding between FDS and FDP tendons. *(b)* Fist enhances gliding of FDP tendons. *(c)* Modified fist enhances gliding of FDS tendons.

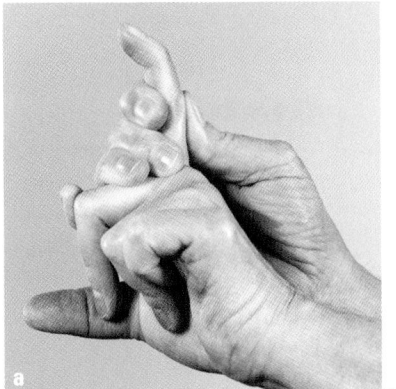
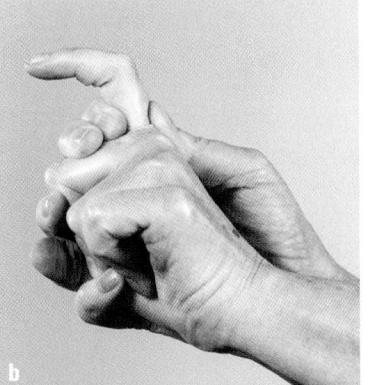
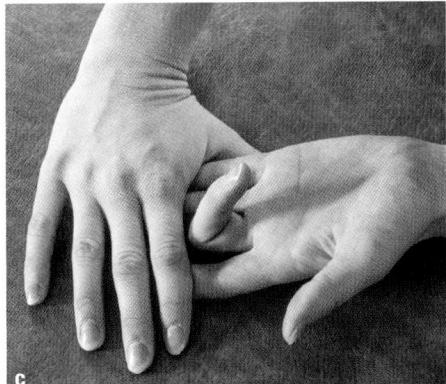

Figure 23.43 Isolated-tendon gliding exercises: *(a)* flexor digitorum profundus, *(b)* flexor digitorum superficialis, *(c)* elimination of flexor digitorum profundus activity by blocking other finger motion by the FDP to isolate the flexor digitorum superficialis.

and it provides optimal gliding of the flexor digitorum superficialis tendons in their sheaths (figure 23.44c).[62] You should notice that the hook-position exercise, which is used to enhance gliding between the two long flexor tendons of the fingers, also places the lumbricals and interossei muscles on stretch; if the patient cannot move the fingers into a hook position, the clinician should investigate for possible adhesions between the two long flexor tendons or pathology in the intrinsic muscles.

Flexor pollicis longus gliding exercises are performed in a similar manner by moving the IP and MCP joints through a full range of flexion and extension.[62] These exercises are initially performed with the wrist in neutral, but as the patient progresses, the wrist should be moved into flexion with finger flexion and into extension with finger extension.[62]

Extensor Tendons and Intrinsic Muscles

Because the extensor tendons are flatter and wider than their flexor counterparts and because they have an intimate relationship with the intrinsic muscle system, they are more susceptible to adhesions and have less repair strength than flexor tendons of the hand.[63] Adhesions or weakness can cause an extensor lag of the finger. Two tests can easily determine if motion changes are caused by tissue overstretching or adhesions. If full extension occurs passively but not actively, the cause may be friability of the repair site or tissue weakness. If the digit's passive flexion is also limited, it is because adhesions restrict full tendon excursion during a stretch.

On the other hand, care must be taken in stretching the extensor tendons after tendon repairs or fractures. There is sometimes a fine line between applying enough stretch to maintain tissue gliding and too much stress that causes tissue damage. The rehabilitation clinician must watch closely for an extensor lag throughout the stretching process. If an extensor lag occurs or increases, it may be that the tendon is actually elongating (dehiscing) or tearing from its attachment. Using controlled active exercises to reduce extensor lag rather than passive forces to increase flexion motion helps to minimize this risk.[64]

If an extensor lag occurs at the MCP joint because of adhesions, the adhesion is of the extensor digitorum (ED) tendon. This is the only extensor tendon for the four medial MCP joints. A gliding exercise for the ED is performed by moving the fingers from a hook to a fist formation as seen in figure 23.45. In this gliding exercise, the MCP joint is moved from flexion to extension or hyperextension, if possible, while the IP joints are kept in flexion to eliminate the intrinsic muscles. If the patient has difficulty maintaining flexion of the IP joints during this exercise, he or she can further facilitate IP flexion by grasping a drinking straw or pencil in the fingers while moving the MCP joints into flexion and (hyper)extension. Wrist flexion and extension should also be added to the exercise when the patient can perform the exercise with the wrist in neutral.

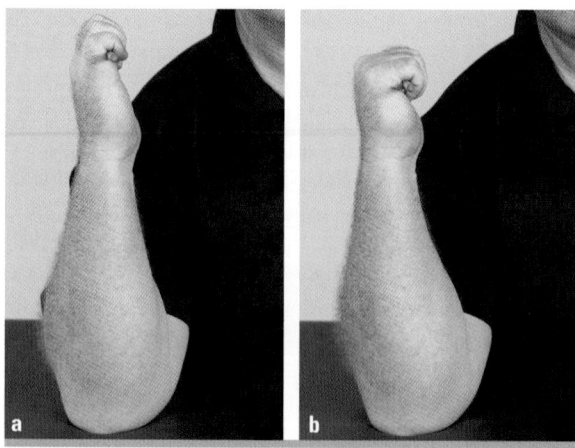

Figure 23.45 Extrinsic extensor gliding exercises: Keeping the IPs in flexion, the MCPs are moved into flexion and extension.

If flexor contractures of the fingers occur, they may be caused by soft-tissue adhesions. However, they may also be the result of an undiagnosed injury to the central slip of the extensor hood mechanism, something that is not always immediately apparent but becomes obvious with the development of a boutonniere deformity.[65] If the clinician has eliminated central slip ruptures and has confirmed adhesions of intrinsic or extrinsic muscles secondary to tissue healing, tendon gliding exercises are appropriate. The exercise used to isolate the intrinsic muscles and restore their function of IP extension is: The MCP is stabilized in flexion, while the IP joints move through active extension and flexion (figure 23.46). As this exercise advances, the MCP joint is positioned in extension. In its final progression, the most difficult position for this exercise is with the hand flat on a table and the proximal phalanx stabilized; in this position, the patient actively lifts the finger off the table to extend the PIP and DIP joints while stabilizing the MCP joint on the table (figure 23.47).

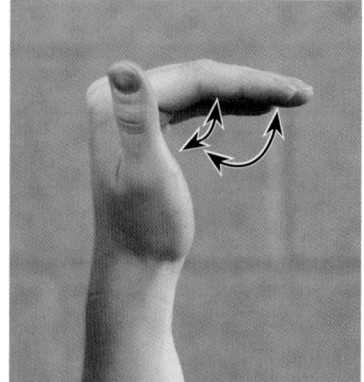

Figure 23.46 Extensor gliding exercises. Intrinsic: MCP joint is maintained in flexion with IPs actively moving through full range of motion from flexion into extension.

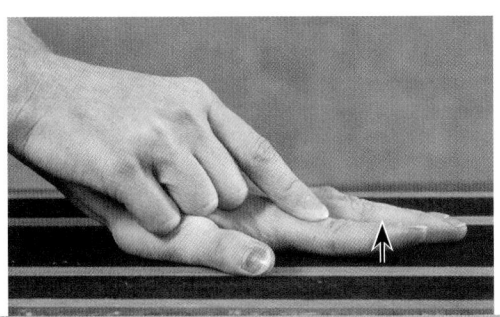

Figure 23.47 Terminal extension: IP actively moves into as much extension as possible with the MCP joint anchored in extension.

CLINICAL TIPS

Motion loss quickly occurs after injury or surgery to the hand. Two factors the rehabilitation clinician must address in the early days of treatment include controlling and managing edema and preventing motion loss. Tissues must also be allowed to heal properly without overstressing them. This takes an awareness of the anatomy and biomechanics of the hand as well as a knowledge of healing.[66] Part of the rehabilitation program for any hand or finger injury includes tendon gliding exercises[63] to ensure good mobility of the hand in preparation for more stressful activities once the tissues can manage them.

Strengthening Exercises

During periods of immobilization, isometric exercises can be used for all wrist and hand muscles. Active exercises are good for maintaining mobility and early strengthening. As healing and the patient progress, various types of equip-

ment such as weights, putty, and rubber bands can be used to further build strength. In the early stages, the muscles may fatigue quickly,[67] so the patient must be cautioned against overdoing it.

Isometric Resistance Exercises

The patient can perform isometric resistance exercises independently and often throughout the day. Each exercise is held for 6 s[68] and is usually repeated 10 times each session. The number of repetitions and the frequency of the exercise depend on the condition of the muscle, the ability of the body part to move, and the phase of the healing process. Begin with submaximal contractions and progress to more maximal recruitment. Remind patients to avoid a Valsalva maneuver during isometric exercises. Proper posture and scapular position are needed for proximal control and proper execution of isometric exercises for the upper extremity. Patients should be able to demonstrate an ability to do the exercises correctly before they are added to the home exercise program. Isometric exercises for wrist flexion and ulnar deviation are performed by having the patient push down into the table. Wrist extension and radial deviation are performed by having the patient push up into the opposite hand.

Resistive Exercises

There are many resistive exercises for the wrist and hand, and which ones to use are limited only by the rehabilitation clinician's imagination. A few of the more commonly used resistive exercises are outlined in the following sections. Common substitution patterns for the exercises are also described. You should correct any errors in the patient's technique to ensure optimal benefits from the exercise. As always, good posture and scapular positioning are essential.

Strength Exercises for the Wrist

Just as the scapula provides a stable base for shoulder function, the wrist provides the hand and fingers with their stable base for activities. It is important to restore wrist muscles to normal strength if optimal hand and finger function are to be restored. Any rehabilitation program for the hand should include wrist-strengthening exercises.

Extension

Body Segment: Wrist.

Stage in Rehab: Resistive phase.

Purpose: Strengthen wrist extensors.

Positioning: The forearm rests on a tabletop in pronation with the hand over the end of the table. A rolled towel may be placed under the forearm at the edge of the tabletop for patient comfort.

Execution: Patient lifts a dumbbell, moving through a full ROM from wrist flexion to wrist extension (figure 23.48).

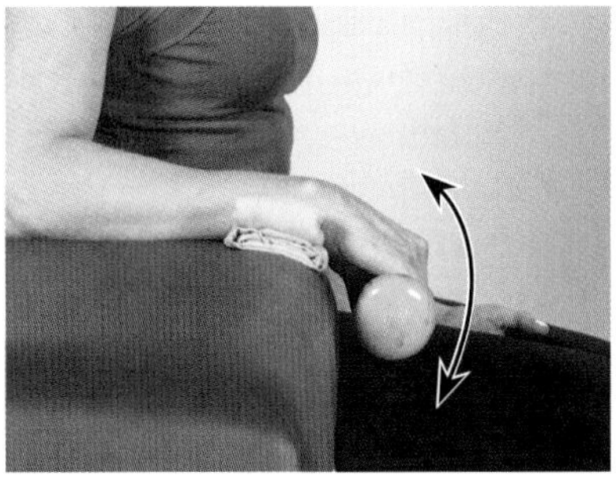

Figure 23.48

Possible Substitutions: Flexing the elbow or moving the weight through a partial ROM.

Notations: The forearm must stay in contact with the tabletop throughout the exercise; it may be necessary to stabilize the forearm with a hand across the proximal forearm.

Flexion

Body Segment: Wrist.

Stage in Rehab: Resistive phase.

Purpose: Strengthen wrist flexors.

Positioning: The patient sits next to a table with the forearm resting on the table in supination and the hand over the end of the table. A rolled towel may be placed under the forearm at the tabletop edge for patient comfort.

Execution: Patient moves a dumbbell weight through a full ROM from wrist extension to flexion (figure 23.49).

Possible Substitutions: Partial ROM of wrist movement and elbow flexion.

Notations: Forearm should remain on the table.

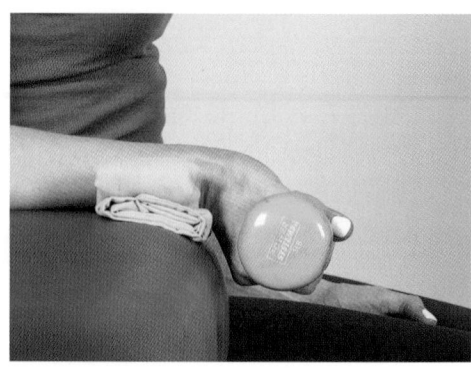

Figure 23.49

Ulnar Deviation

Body Segment: Wrist.

Stage in Rehab: Resistive phase.

Purpose: Strengthen wrist ulnar deviators.

Positioning: A bar with a weighted end is placed in the hand; the weight is on the ulnar side. The patient stands with the elbow extended.

Execution: The patient moves the wrist into ulnar deviation, lifting the weight as high as possible (figure 23.50).

Possible Substitutions: Finger motion and shoulder extension are common substitutions.

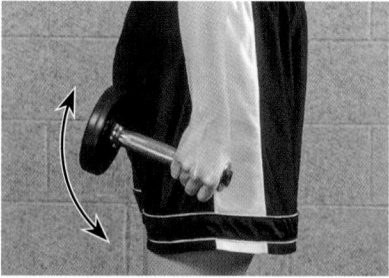

Figure 23.50

Notations: Patient should maintain a firm grasp on the bar so that the wrist rather than the fingers produces the motion.

Radial Deviation

Body Segment: Wrist.

Stage in Rehab: Resistive phase.

Purpose: Strengthen wrist radial deviators.

Positioning: Patient's position is the same as for ulnar deviation, but the weighted bar is positioned with the weight on the radial side of the hand.

Execution: The weight is lifted upward as high as possible toward the thumb (figure 23.51).

Possible Substitutions: Elbow flexion and motion from the fingers rather than the wrist are the most common substitutions.

Notations: Keeping a firm grasp on the bar will reduce substitutions.

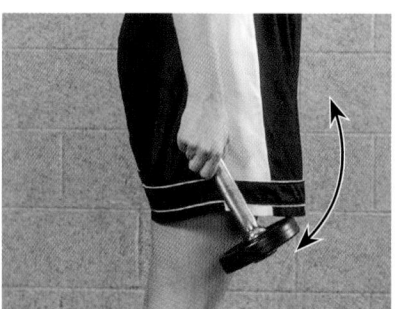

Figure 23.51

Forearm Supinators

Body Segment: Forearm.

Stage in Rehab: Resistive phase.

Purpose: Provide eccentric resistance to forearm supinators.

Positioning: A resistance band is attached to a handle and anchored to the side of the table so that the band is in front of the patient's body. Patient grasps the handle with the forearm in neutral and stabilized on the table.

Execution: The patient then controls the bar as the resistance band pulls the forearm into pronation (figure 23.52).

Possible Substitutions: Shoulder abduction, medial rotation.

Notations: Concentric exercises for these muscles are shown in chapter 22, figure 22.26. They can also be used to provide additional eccentric activity with resistance bands.

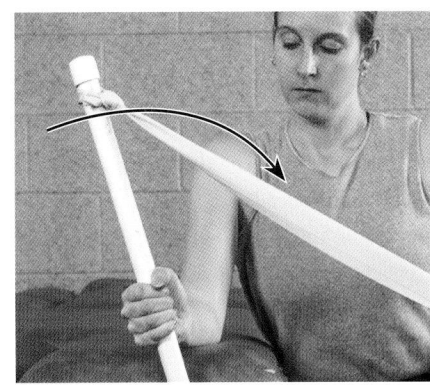

Figure 23.52

Forearm Pronators

Body Segment: Forearm.

Stage in Rehab: Resistive phase.

Purpose: Provide eccentric resistance to forearm pronators.

Positioning: A resistance band is anchored to the table on the same side as the injured wrist. Patient grasps the handle with the forearm in neutral and stabilized on the table.

Execution: The bar is passively positioned with the forearm in pronation, and as the resistance band pulls the bar, the patient controls the supination motion of the forearm (figure 23.53).

Possible Substitutions: Shoulder adduction.

Notations: Exercises for these muscles are shown in chapter 22, figure 22.27. They can also be used to provide additional eccentric activity with resistance bands.

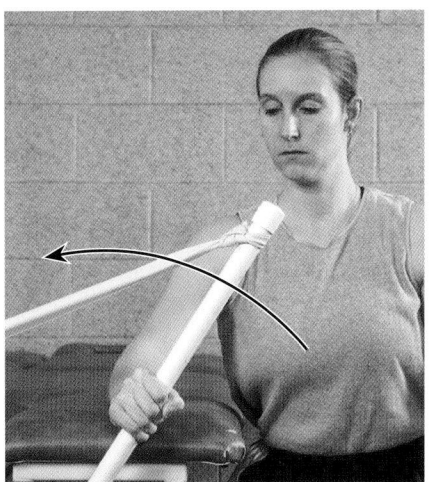

Figure 23.53

Putty Exercises for the Forearm, Wrist, and Hand

Many exercises can be designed using putty of different strengths to provide a progressive resistance program for the forearm, wrist, and hand. Putty is convenient to use in the patient's home program. Progressive putty resistance exercises are included in an early strengthening program.

Ulnar Deviation

Body Segment: Wrist.

Stage in Rehab: Resistive phase.

Purpose: Strengthen wrist ulnar deviators.

Positioning: Patient grasps the putty in both hands and places the two hands with the lateral sides of the index fingers and thumbs adjacent to each other.

Execution: Using only wrist motion, the patient moves the hands laterally against each other as the wrists move into ulnar deviation (figure 23.54).

Possible Substitutions: Wrist flexion, shoulder movement.

Notations: To emphasize the involved wrist, stabilize the uninvolved wrist while only the involved wrist performs the exercise.

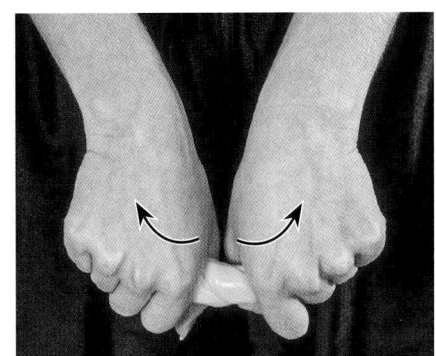

Figure 23.54

Radial Deviation

Body Segment: Wrist.

Stage in Rehab: Resistive phase.

Purpose: Strengthen wrist radial deviators.

Positioning: The putty is formed into a tube shape and is grasped by both hands. The patient positions the little finger of the involved hand on top of the thumb of the other hand.

Execution: Stabilizing the uninvolved hand and the involved forearm and elbow, the patient moves the involved wrist into radial deviation.

Possible Substitutions: Wrist extension, elbow flexion.

Notations: Putty exercises may be used in a home program.

Pronation and Supination

Body Segment: Forearm.

Stage in Rehab: Resistive phase.

Purpose: Strength exercises for forearm pronators and supinators.

Positioning: The uninvolved arm provides the stabilizing hand to anchor the putty.

Execution: The patient uses the stabilizing hand to hold the putty. Grasping the end with the hand of the involved forearm, the patient moves the forearm into supination and pronation while stabilizing the elbow next to the side (figure 23.55).

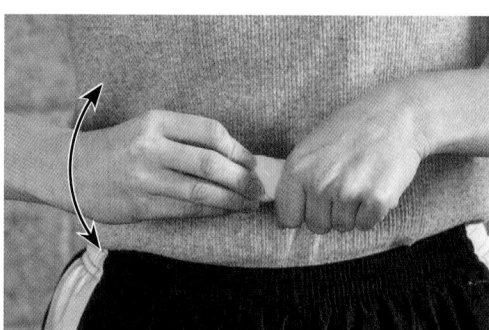

Figure 23.55

Possible Substitutions: Wrist motion, shoulder abduction during pronation or adduction during supination.

Notations: This is an early strengthening exercise for supinators and pronators.

Power-Grip Exercises

Body Segment: Hand.

Stage in Rehab: Resistive phase.

Purpose: Strengthen finger flexors used in power grips.

Positioning: The hand is placed in various positions, depending on the grip-strength exercise. All power grips may be used, depending on the patient's condition.

Execution: Patient squeezes the putty using the different power grips for emphasis on different digits. Figure 23.56 shows two examples of power-grip exercises.

Possible Substitutions: Wrist flexion rather than stabilization of the wrist in slight extension.

Notations: Strength progression occurs by advancing to a more difficult level of putty resistance.

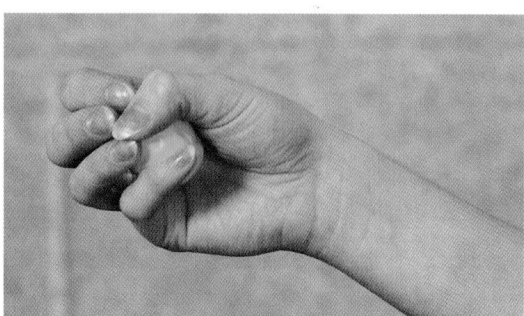 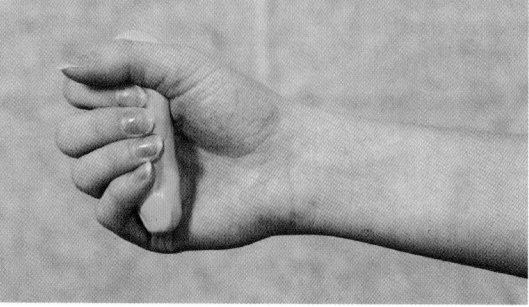

Figure 23.56

Precision Grip Exercises

Body Segment: Fingers.

Stage in Rehab: Resistive phase.

Purpose: Strengthen intrinsic muscles.

Positioning: The exercising phalanx has its MCP and IPs in slight flexion.

Execution: Patient performs different precision grips against the putty: tip to tip (figure 23.57a), digital prehension (three-jaw chuck) (figure 23.57b), and lateral prehension (figure 23.57c).

Possible Substitutions: Locking the IP joints in extension so the intrinsic muscles do not perform the task.

Notations: The putty is squeezed, then reshaped, and the exercise is repeated. Precision-grip exercises can also be performed with clothespins. Wrapping rubber bands around the end of the clothespin provides additional resistance. As with the putty exercises, the patient should grasp the clothespins with the IP joints in slight flexion. Don't allow extension of any IP joint.

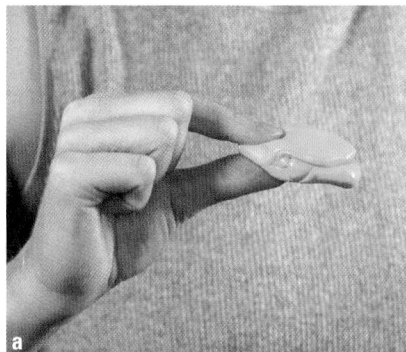 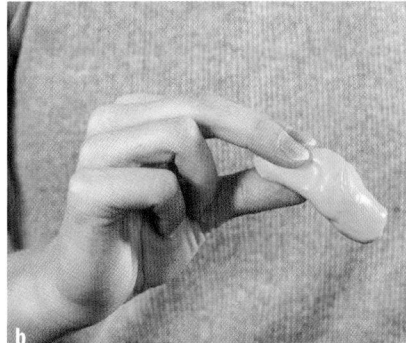 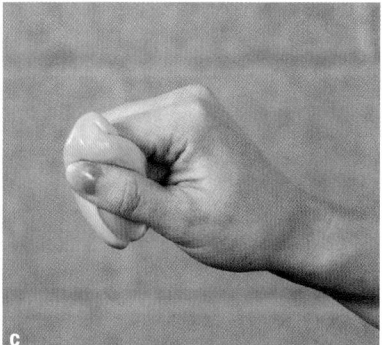

Figure 23.57

Opposition Exercise

Body Segment: Fingers.

Stage in Rehab: Resistive phase.

Purpose: Strengthen intrinsic muscles of the hand.

Positioning: The putty begins in a pancake shape on a tabletop. The patient places all the finger pads on the putty (figure 23.58a).

Execution: With all finger pads on the putty, the patient pulls the finger pads together. A cone should be formed in the middle as the fingers pull the putty toward the center (figure 23.58b).

Possible Substitutions: Using the wrist or long finger flexors rather than the intrinsic muscles.

Notations: The intrinsic muscles (interossei and lumbricals) are worked if the IP joints are kept in extension during the exercise. The extrinsic muscles are resisted if the IP joints are flexed during the exercise.

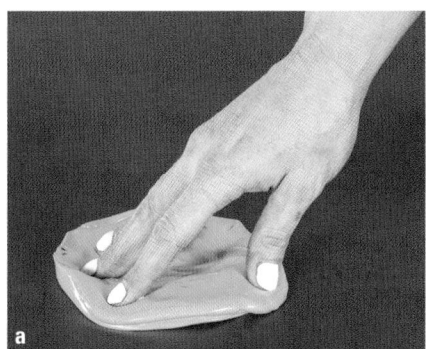 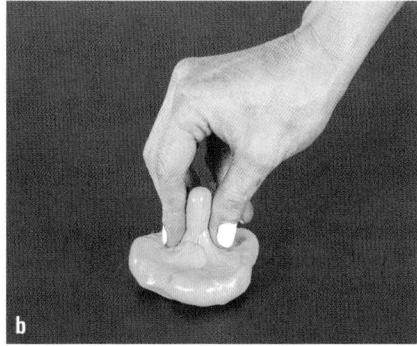

Figure 23.58

Finger Adduction

Body Segment: Fingers.

Stage in Rehab: Resistive phase.

Purpose: Strengthen intrinsic adductors.

Positioning: The putty is placed between any two fingers or between the index finger and thumb.

Execution: The patient pushes the fingers together against the putty (figure 23.59).

Possible Substitutions: IP and MCP flexion.

Notations: The IP and MCP joints should remain extended.

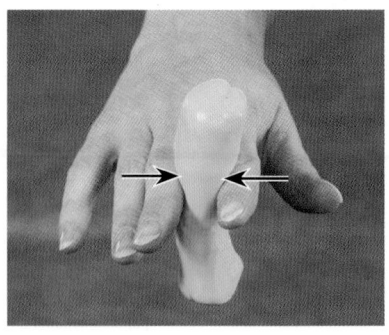

Figure 23.59

Finger Extension, Thumb and Finger Abduction

Body Segment: Fingers.

Stage in Rehab: Resistive phase.

Purpose: Strengthen intrinsic muscles.

Positioning: Putty or a rubber band is placed around the fingers and thumb (figure 23.60a).

Execution: The patient spreads the fingers apart as far as possible.

Possible Substitutions: Careful observation is needed to detect performance by muscles other than the desired ones.

Notations: These exercises can be used either on the entire group or on individual fingers: finger abduction with putty (figure 23.60b), index finger and thumb extension with putty (figure 23.60c), two-finger abduction with rubber band (figure 23.60d), multiple-finger abduction with rubber band (figure 23.60e), and thumb and fifth-finger abduction with rubber band (figure 23.60f).

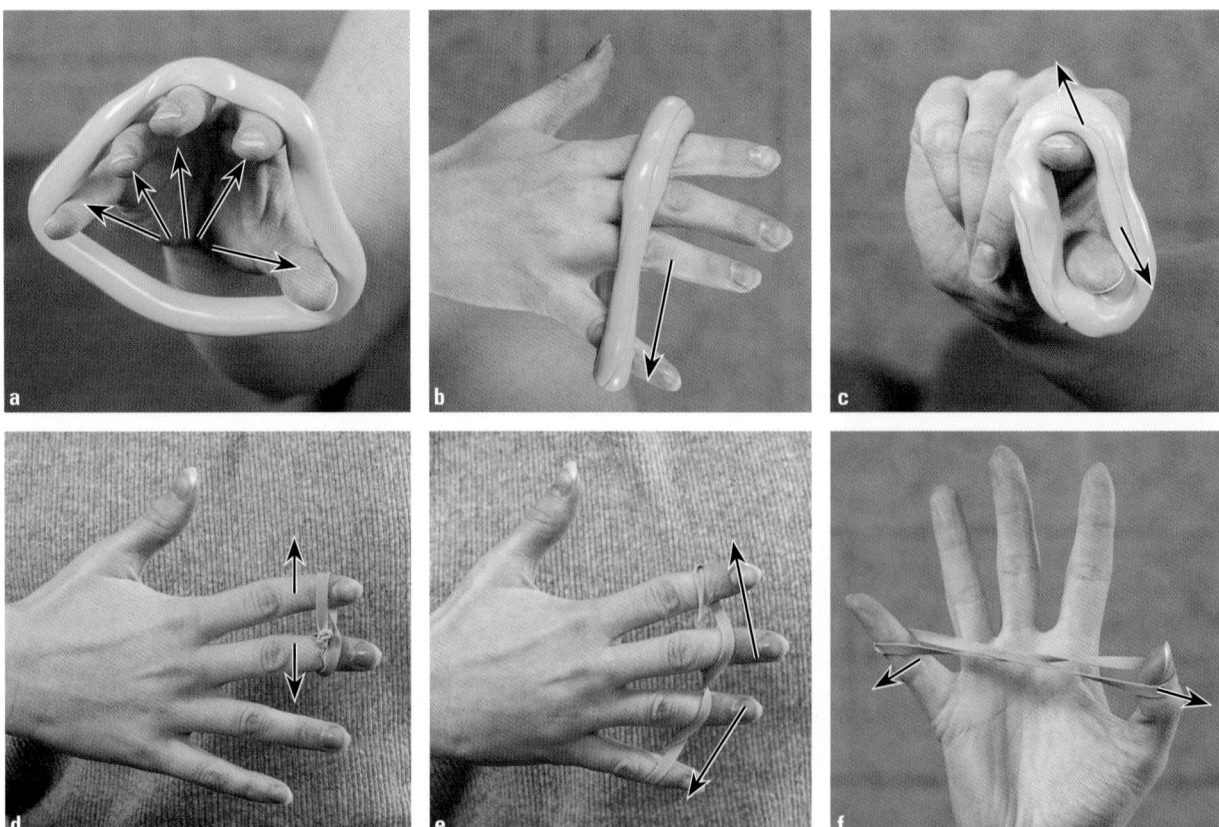

Figure 23.60

Extensor Lag Exercises

Body Segment: Fingers.

Stage in Rehab: Resistive phase.

Purpose: Strengthen finger intrinsics to eliminate extensor lag.

Positioning: The patient places the putty on a tabletop, with the palm facing down and the MCP and IP joints flexed.

Execution: The fingers push outward against the putty as the fingers move into extension (figure 23.61*a*).

Possible Substitutions: Finger abduction.

Notations: A medicine ball, pushed while the MCP joints remain in flexion and the IP joints move from flexion into extension, provides an alternative resistance exercise for the intrinsic muscles (figure 23.61*b*). Using heavier medicine balls or increasing surface friction increases the challenge. An additional exercise to facilitate extension of the DIP is performed while stabilizing the proximal aspects of the finger and passively positioning the DIP into extension. The patient then tries to hold the DIP position for 6 s (figure 23.61*c*).

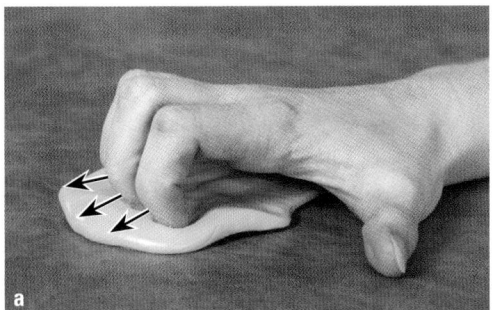
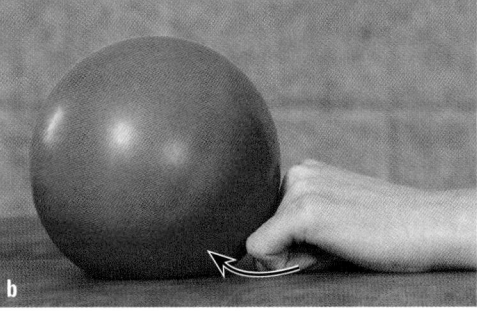
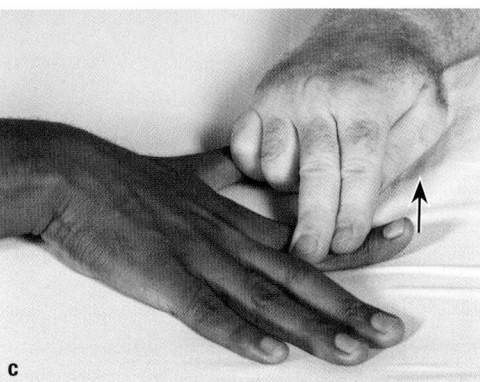

Figure 23.61

Proprioception and Neuromotor Control Exercises

As with any other body segment, proprioception is vital for normal hand function. Early proprioception exercises precede agility and coordination activities. When to include these exercises in the rehabilitation program depends mainly on the severity of the injury and whether range-of-motion restrictions are needed; they may be used in several segments of the program, from later active phase through advanced phase. Since most functions performed by the hand involve precision activities, the fingers must be able to act together while doing different tasks. This requires coordination. There are many exercises that can help develop neuromotor control and coordination for the hand and fingers. Only a few of them are presented here, but your imagination could supply many others for your patients.

Place-and-Hold Proprioception Exercise

Body Segment: Wrist, hand, and fingers.

Stage in Rehab: Active or resistive phase.

Purpose: Improve wrist, hand, and finger proprioception.

Positioning: Various positions of wrist, hand, and fingers determined by the clinician.

Execution: The clinician supports the patient's forearm and passively places the wrist, hand, or fingers in a specific position (figure 23.62a). The patient then holds that position without the clinician's assistance for 6 s (figure 23.62b).

Possible Substitutions: Changing the position set by the clinician because the patient's muscle is too weak to hold the position.

Notations: Patient can advance to holding the positions with eyes closed or for more time. This is an early-program exercise, usually begun before isometric and isotonic exercises are permitted.

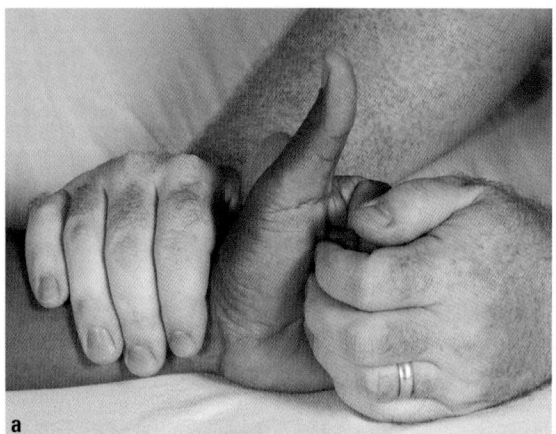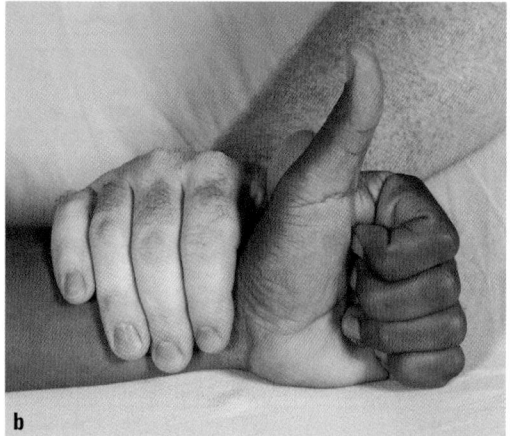

Figure 23.62

Two-Ball Roll Coordination Exercise

Body Segment: Fingers and hand.

Stage in Rehab: Active or resistive phase.

Purpose: Improve hand and finger coordination.

Positioning: The patient places two small balls such as table tennis or golf balls in the affected hand.

Execution: The fingers roll the balls in a circular motion within the hand, clockwise and counterclockwise (figure 23.63).

Possible Substitutions: Not using all fingers to perform the activity.

Notations: It will be easier to roll the ball in one direction than the other, but the patient should work the balls in both clockwise and counterclockwise directions.

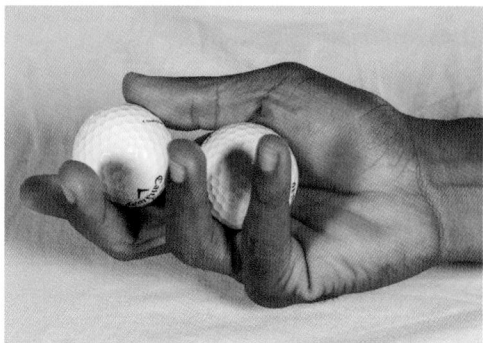

Figure 23.63

Chopstick or Pencil Roll Coordination Exercise

Body Segment: Fingers and hand.

Stage in Rehab: Active or resistive phase.

Purpose: Improve hand and finger coordination.

Positioning: The patient places a chopstick or pencil between the index and middle fingers of the affected hand.

Execution: The fingers rotate the stick to be positioned between the fourth and fifth fingers, then rotate it to return to the start position (figure 23.64).

Possible Substitutions: Not using all fingers to perform the activity.

Notations: It will be easier to roll the chopstick or pencil in one direction than the other, but the patient should work the stick both ways in the hand. Performing the activity with the eyes closed is a progression for this exercise. To advance the exercise, patients can be timed and instructed to complete the activity more quickly.

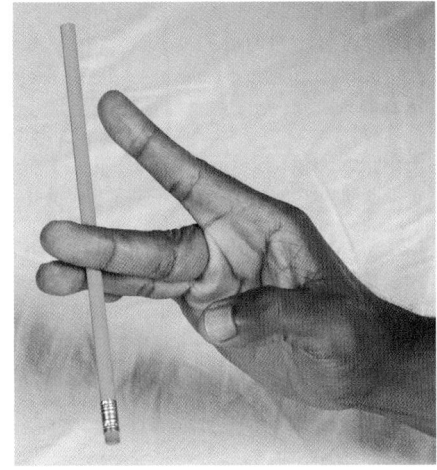

Figure 23.64

Other suggestions for coordination exercises include picking up a specific number of pennies within a specific amount of time, turning over pennies from all heads to all tails for speed, tapping each finger individually to music, touching objects on a board or tabletop in a specific sequence or on command for time, shuffling a deck of cards, manipulating a washer onto and off a screw, or typing on a computer for accuracy and speed. Any number of coordination activities may be designed to meet the patient's need to resolve specific deficiencies.

CLINICAL TIPS

Restoring hand function involves not only range of motion and strength, but also being able to use each digit by itself or with other digits. Coordination of activities, both gross and fine motor, involves the ability to use the hand as a single unit or as several elements that can do different things at once. When to add these activities to a program depends on factors such as the injury's severity and motion restrictions. The rehabilitation clinician must prepare the patient to achieve normal performance expectations.

Plyometric Exercises

Many of the plyometric exercises for the shoulder and elbow are also used for the wrist and hand. Additional exercises that can be used for the hand are presented here. For specific information on plyometric exercises for the shoulder and elbow, refer to chapters 21 and 22.

Ball Drop and Catch

This exercise uses a medicine ball small enough to be grasped in one hand. The patient stands with the arm next to the body with the elbow at 90° of flexion and the hand positioned palm down. The patient grasps the medicine ball in the hand and allows it to drop, then immediately retrieves the ball before it reaches the floor by catching it with the hand in the palm-down position. A progression would include the patient placing the shoulder at 90° of flexion, the arm outstretched in front of the body, and repeating the exercise. As the exercise becomes easier, a heavier ball is selected. The patient should grasp the ball with all the fingers tightly around the ball.

Other Plyometric Activities

Many other activities can be used as plyometric exercises for the hand. These include bouncing a medicine ball against the wall or a Rebounder, boxing against a medicine bag, plyometric push-ups, volleyball setting and passes with a medicine ball, and quickly tossing a small medicine ball back and forth from hand to hand.

Functional and Performance-Specific Exercises

Because the hand has such a wide variation of functions, it is nearly impossible to define functional activities for the hand. Specific demands for functional activities are determined by the requirements of the patient's sport, occupation, or prior level of function. A football quarterback's needs for hand function differ from those for the football lineman. A golfer's hand functions vary greatly from those of a basketball player. A mail carrier's hand functions vary from those of a machine operator. The range of demands can include variations in grips, grip positions, rapid or slow hand movements, sustained or changing grips, and forceful or light grasping. In addition to specific activities to which the patient will return are the many daily activities that require hand functions. The rehabilitation clinician must understand the demands of these daily activities as well as each patient's responsibilities and outline a performance-specific exercise progression based on those requirements. Once the exercises are selected, a progression is designed using a planned program of increasing difficulty until the exercises mimic the stress levels the patient will encounter in full participation.

Desensitization

As we discussed in the beginning of this chapter, we know that tactile perception by the hand is significant compared to most other regions of the body.[4] Sensory nerve endings including Pacinian corpuscles, Meissner's corpuscles, Merkel discs, Ruffini endings, and free nerve endings allow the hand to distinguish between light touch, firm pressure, temperature, pain, point discrimination, and different textures.[69] Injuries to the hand can result in somatosensory changes that include both tactile hyperesthesia and pain.[70] This can profoundly affect hand function and can be very debilitating. Desensitization exercises are used to decrease sensitivity by exposing the painful area to various types of somatosensory "counter stimulation"[70] in an effort to normalize the body's response to particular sensations.[70]

Desensitizing exercises are usually somewhat uncomfortable at first, but with persistence, this sensitivity should decrease. Begin the exercises with very light sensations, such as gently rubbing lotion on the area, gently tapping the area, or performing gentle stretching exercises. Advance the desensitization process by progressing to lightly rubbing various textures over the area. Begin with softer textures such as silk or velvet and progress to more abrasive textures, such as cotton, terry cloth, polyester, corduroy, and wool. As patients' sensitivity decreases, you can have them dip the hand into a container of beans, rice, and then sand while performing gentle gripping, finger abduction

and adduction exercises, and lifting and then pouring the beans, rice, or sand back into the container. Later, finger tapping exercises, vibration tools, or contrast baths are appropriate.

As with any progressive program, begin desensitization activities gently and progress to more vigorous sensations or exercises. You may begin by having patients perform the activity for 20 to 30 s several times throughout the day and progress to 3 to 5 min when their sensitivity decreases. Tell patients that they may experience discomfort with the activity, but they should not experience significant pain. If they do have such pain, reduce the intensity and frequency of the activity and progress as tolerated.

Special Rehabilitation Applications

Because the hand is so complex and has many structures in close contact with each other, an injury to one area or tissue can affect adjacent tissues and other segments within the wrist and hand. The rehabilitation clinician must not only be aware of this but must also do everything possible to try to prevent these complications.

Examination is an integral part of rehabilitation. You must perform an examination before you can establish a rehabilitation program. Special tests play a vital role in the examination process. Table 23.4 provides examples of common special tests that may be included in the examination of the wrist and hand. More than one special test is usually used to support the clinical diagnosis that is made.[71]

Some of the more common injuries requiring rehabilitation are addressed here. Tendon rupture and repairs to the wrist and hand are not often seen in musculoskeletal injuries, but the rehabilitation programs for them are outlined

TABLE 23.4 Common Diagnostic Special Tests for the Wrist and Hand With Their Sensitivity and Specificity Ratings

Site or structure tested	Special test (other name)	Sensitivity*	Specificity*
Neurologic status	Median nerve ULTT	94%-97%[72]	22%[72]
	Radial nerve ULTT	72%-97%[72]	33%[72]
	Ulnar nerve ULTT	Unknown	Unknown
Carpal tunnel	Phalen's	67%[73]	93%[73]
	Reverse Phalen's	42%-88%[74]	35%-95%[74]
	Tinel's at carpal tunnel	53%[73]	96%[73]
Scaphoid fracture	Axial loading	89%[75]	98%[75]
Lateral instability	Watson (scaphoid shift maneuver)	69%[76]	64%-68%[76]
Medial instability	Fovea sign	95.2%[77]	86.5%[77]
	Reagan (lunotriquetral shear test)	66%-95.2%[78]	64%-87%[78]
	TFCC load	100%[74]	Unknown
Tendinopathy	Finkelstein's	81%[79]	100%[79]

* Numbers rounded to the nearest whole number.

ULTT = upper limb tension test; TFCC = triangular fibrocartilage complex here since the clinician must take additional precautions when they do occur.

Complications After Hand Injuries

Any hand injury is at risk of developing complications that significantly interfere with rehabilitation outcomes and overall hand function. Rehabilitation clinicians must be aware of these complications and make every effort to minimize them before they become lasting problems. These deleterious complications include edema and stiffness.

Edema

We know that edema is a naturally occurring result of injury. Recall from chapter 2 that the swelling that occurs as part of the inflammatory response to injury consists of fluid leaking from damaged capillaries. This fluid contains proteins, including fibrinogen.[80] If this edema is not resorbed, the fibrinogen polymerizes into a fibrin lattice or weblike structure.[81] When fibroblasts enter the area as part of the healing process, they attach to the fibrin lattice and produce collagen. If the injured segment is immobilized, these collagen deposits develop into dense scar tissue with randomized collagen orientation, which destroys the normal gliding ability of local structures.[82] Additionally, the swelling remains unresolved because the fibrotic formation obstructs lymphatic flow.[83]

Another complication of excessive edema is the loss of viscoelasticity in the hand's soft tissues, which increases resistance to motion.[16] This concept has been compared to an anchored ship.[84] At low tide, the anchored ship can drift in a wide range, but at high tide, the anchor chain tightens and the ship's ability to move around the surface is restricted (figure 23.65).

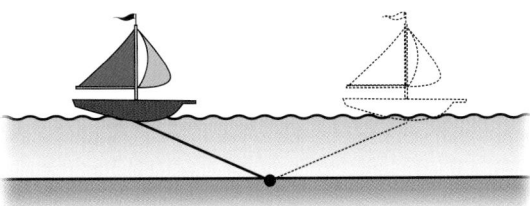

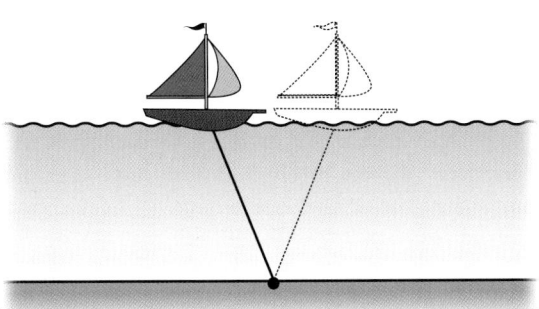

Figure 23.65 At low tide the ship can move over a large horizontal distance, but at high tide the ship's mobility is reduced as the anchor chain becomes more vertical.[84]

Edema also has a direct effect on the joints of the hand and affects their range of motion. The skin moves away from the axis of the joint (figure 23.66) and thereby increases the skin's moment arm.[84] The resistance to movement of the hand in the opposite direction is then increased. In essence, finger motion is restricted because the skin's moment arm increases due to the swelling.[84] More flexor tendon strength is needed to overpower the greater resistance in order to move the affected digit.

Early recognition and treatment of edema is crucial to optimal results. Elevating the injured segment above the heart is basic to edema control for any injury and is especially effective for hand injuries. Postcapillary blood pressure in the venous system of the upper extremity is less than 15 mmHg; when the hand is hanging in a dependent position, pressure working against venous return is about 35 mmHg.[85] Therefore, swelling is inevitable if the extremity is in a dependent position.

Compression is another effective treatment for edema.[86] There are a number of finger sleeves and other commercial and handmade devices that may be used to apply compression. For example, wrapping string from the distal end of the finger to the base of the digit serves as a comfortable yet effective compression "sleeve." Isotoner gloves are also effective if the swelling is extensive.

Whenever the injury does not warrant strict immobilization, active range of motion of the digits is a very effective way to reduce edema.[39] Edema is only relieved through the passive lymph system, and muscle activity serves as the pump. Active motion uses this pumping action of the muscles to reduce swelling. Active motion also provides

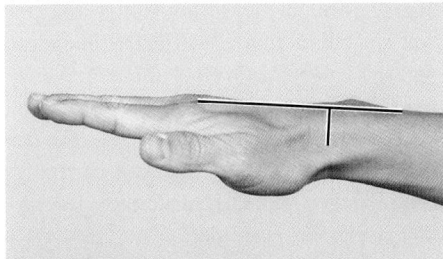

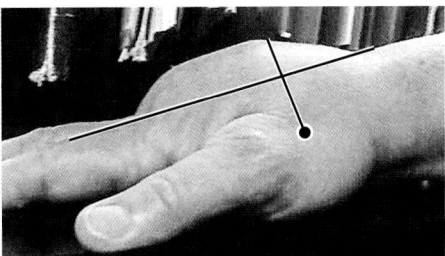

Figure 23.66 As edema moves the skin farther away from the joint's axis of motion, the skin's moment arm resistance to motion in the opposite direction increases, making it more difficult for flexor tendons to move the joint.

Second photo © Peggy Houglum

tissue gliding to maintain mobility between structures. Passive motion does not provide the pumping or gliding that active motion offers. Place-and-hold exercises are often incorporated during the initial treatment phase as an early active-motion exercise.[39]

Additional treatment techniques may be used, depending on the injury, the extent and duration of edema, and restrictions dictated by the individual, the injury, and the physician. For example, massage can be a useful technique, especially when the hand is elevated. Various modalities can also be used to reduce edema.

Stiffness

Stiffness is used to describe a hand that lacks normal mobility. It usually has a positive connotation when used in reference to the muscle rigidity that precedes activity, but in the context of hand injuries it is a negative. With edema and the presence of fibrin and fibrinogen in such a crowded structure as the hand, it is no wonder that stiffness is a common problem.[87] Indeed, stiffness becomes a problem quickly in an environment of edema and immobilization. Immobilization occurs either out of necessity—to allow damaged structures to heal—or because the patient hesitates to move the injured part for fear of causing pain or additional damage.[88] If stiffness is not addressed, adhesions mature, leading to contracture and a deficient hand.[88]

As healing continues, there is a constant remodeling of tissues. Collagen is laid down during the proliferation and remodeling phases, creating new bonding patterns to increase its strength as it moves toward a permanent structure in its healing progression. As part of this process, if the soft-tissue structures around the injured segment are placed in a shortened position, they develop joint stiffness.[89] These soft-tissue structures that are affected include the skin, ligaments, and capsule as well as the neural and vascular structures. Of these structures, those most affected include the joint capsule and ligaments.[90]

Stiffness with loss of mobility can be the result of a restriction in finger joints, intrinsic muscles, or extrinsic muscles. During the examination process, the clinician must determine the cause or causes of the restriction to accurately design the treatment that will best address any impairments.

Treatment of hand stiffness is multifactorial; a variety of approaches are used to reduce and relieve joint stiffness. Many treatments are based on factors such as the location of affected tissue, the duration of stiffness, and the severity of the injury. Active and passive soft-tissue mobilization techniques, joint mobilization, active and passive stretching, blocking exercises, static and dynamic splinting, and pressure treatments are all options the clinician may use to reduce soft-tissue and joint stiffness.[39]

In summary, rehabilitation clinicians must understand the factors that cause joint stiffness so they can provide appropriate and early intervention. Early active mobili-

zation and early control of edema without compromising healing are important in the prevention of stiffness and the restoration of normal hand function. Therefore, regardless of the hand injury, the clinician must be aware of minimum requirements for protected healing and must know how to minimize edema and reduce stiffness without jeopardizing tissue healing.

Fractures

There are many bones in the wrist and hand. Which bone is fractured has a great impact on the rehabilitation process. This section presents some general concepts, applicable to all fractures, before addressing specific fractures. The management of wrist and hand fractures is generally determined by whether the fracture is stable or displaced.[91] Although there are exceptions, stable fractures are commonly immobilized in a position that has good alignment and places the ligaments on some stretch so their length is maintained.[92] Displaced fractures are surgically repaired.[91] Their corrected positioning helps reduce the risk of contractures. Metacarpal and phalangeal fractures are typically immobilized for 2 to 3 weeks unless the fracture is unstable, displaced, or comminuted.[92] Carpal and distal radius fractures are typically immobilized for 6 weeks.[93] Fractures that are unstable are often corrected with open reduction and internal fixation (ORIF), followed by immobilization.[92] ORIF is advantageous when the fracture is unstable, for it provides needed stability. Although blood flow is disrupted and more soft-tissue damage occurs with ORIF procedures, a fracture becomes immediately stable after surgery; thus, healing is usually faster and has better outcomes after surgery than with conservative treatment.[94, 95]

Splints used to immobilize fractures should affect only as many joints as necessary to maintain good fracture alignment.[52] A long-arm sugar-tong splint may be used acutely because it will allow for swelling better than a cast.[93] Joints proximal and distal to the fracture site that are not immobilized by the splint or cast should be moved through their ranges of motion regularly to prevent loss of mobility.

Distal Forearm Fractures

The most common fracture of all the extremities is the distal radius fracture.[96] It occurs primarily in women 35 years and older;[97] however, 25% of all fractures in children and adolescents involve the distal forearm and wrist.[98] High-energy trauma mechanisms are more common in younger patients, whereas older patients tend to fracture the distal radius in low-energy falls.[96]

There are two types of distal radius fractures, depending on which way the distal radius displaces. When the distal radius fractures and is displaced dorsally, it is called a Colles' fracture. A Smith's fracture also involves the radius, but the distal radius fragment displaces volarly, not dorsally. A Barton's fracture occurs at the radius' articular region and results in wrist subluxation as well as a fracture. While the Colles' and Smith's fractures are typically the result of falling on an outstretched hand (FOOSH), the Barton's fracture occurs with a sudden violent wrist extension and pronation. Best practice guidelines of the American Academy of Orthopaedic Surgeons recommend conservative or surgical intervention based on fracture displacement, angulation, and shortening.[96, 99] If the fracture is unstable, treatment with ORIF is likely.

As with all fractures, whether treated with open or closed reduction, the management of pain and edema is the goal of early rehabilitation in phase I. Coban wrap or other compressive wrap is useful for controlling edema in the fingers and hand. Isotoner gloves may also be used to reduce edema once the cast or splint is removed. Modalities can be used to control pain as well as edema. Early rehabilitation exercises at the end of the inactive phase and early into the active phase include the use of active range-of-motion (AROM) exercises of the uninvolved joints. These exercises will encourage good tendon gliding, reduce edema, and relieve joint stiffness (figure 23.67).

Immobilization casts or splints used for distal radius fractures should permit full MCP flexion motion and

Postoperative Distal Radius Fracture

Stage I: Inactive phase	
0-1 week	**Inflammation phase: Inactive rehabilitation phase**
Goals	Relieve pain, spasm, swelling. Maintain proper immobilization of distal radius with splint or cast. Maintain ROM of all UE segments not immobilized. Maintain strength of shoulder complex and elbow muscles. Maintain core and hip strength. Correct posture deficiencies. MCL.
Treatment guidelines	Days 1-2: Arm elevation to reduce edema Day 1: AROM of all uninvolved UE joints Modalities for pain, swelling, and spasm Trigger point, STM, MFR, and IASTM techniques PRN Tendon gliding exercises Light exercises and functional UE activities with uninvolved segments as tolerated Hand exercises with ball squeeze and putty exercises as tolerated Place-and-hold exercises for fingers Resistive exercises for shoulder and elbow that do not cause distal radial stress or pain Core and hip strengthening and stabilization exercises CV exercise
Precautions	Monitor surgical wound for proper healing. Use HEP to facilitate treatment gains.
Stage II: Active phase	
2-6 weeks	**Early proliferation phase: Active rehabilitation phase**
Goals	Reduce pain to 1-2/10. Week 2: Replace cast with removable splint for less restriction, allowing guarded mobility. Achieve full ROM of wrist. Achieve strength gains of wrist to 50%. Achieve proprioception and agility gains to 50%. Achieve good postural strength. MCL.

>continued

Figure 23.67 Rehabilitation program for postoperative distal radius fracture.

Stage II: Active phase	
2-6 weeks	**Early proliferation phase: Active rehabilitation phase**
Treatment guidelines	Week 2: Once cast is removed, begin early active forearm and wrist motion Remove splint for AROM exercises Light functional activities continue and progress without pain Hand ball-roll and pencil-rotation proprioception exercises Proprioception exercises with hand on ball, on wall, and on tabletop Continue to progress core, hip, and shoulder strengthening CV exercise
Precautions	Forearm stiffness will be the most difficult to overcome. Early active motion within pain limits is advocated for optimal forearm motion returns. Watch for shoulder motions as possible substitutions for forearm movement. Use HEP to facilitate treatment gains.

Stage III: Resistive phase	
6-12 weeks	**Late proliferation phase: Resistive rehabilitation phase**
Goals	Eliminate pain. Weeks 6-8: Discontinue splint. Weeks 6-8: Achieve full range of motion in forearm, wrist, and hand. Maintain normal scapular and shoulder muscle strength and endurance. Achieve normal strength of elbow, wrist, and hand muscles in straight-plane and multiplanar activities. Restore pain-free functional use in ADLs.
Treatment guidelines	AROM, AAROM for wrist and forearm motions Weeks 6-8: If callus formation is clear on X-ray, straight-plane strength progressions for forearm and wrist muscles begin Progress to multiplanar exercises after concentric exercise strength is 80% Weeks 6-8: Weight-bearing proprioception exercises Weeks 6-8: Grades III-IV joint mobilization and soft-tissue mobilization PRN Dynamic proprioception exercises Plyometric exercises Maintenance exercises for core, shoulder complex, and elbow strength and endurance
Precautions	Fracture healing based on X-ray results will determine rate of progress for resistive exercises. Use HEP to facilitate treatment gains.

Stage IV: Advanced phase	
12-15 weeks	**Remodeling phase: Advanced rehabilitation phase**
Goals	Maintain normal strength of all muscles. Maintain normal ROM of all joints. Restore normal sport and work performance.
Treatment guidelines	UE plyometric exercise progression Functional exercise progression Progression of performance-specific exercises and drills
Precautions	Use verbal cues to correct inaccuracies in performance.

ROM = range of motion; UE = upper extremity; MCL = maintain cardiovascular level; AROM = active range of motion; STM = soft-tissue massage; MFR = myofascial release; IASTM = instrument-assisted soft-tissue mobilization; PRN = as needed; CV = cardiovascular; HEP = home exercise program; ADLs = activities of daily living.

Figure 23.67 >*continued*

full thumb opposition. Active range-of-motion exercises for the extrinsic and intrinsic finger muscles should be permitted while the patient's hand is in the splint or cast during the later inactive phase. The patient should be able to perform four gliding exercises: MCP joint full flexion with IP extension for intrinsic gliding, MCP joint extension with full IP flexion for FDS and FDP differentiation, MCP joint full flexion combined with IP joint full flexion for FDP, and modified fist with MCP and PIP flexion and DIP extension for FDS.

It should be possible for AROM to approach passive range-of-motion (PROM) excursion in the active phase. If full PROM is much greater than full AROM, the muscle may be atrophied and weak, the tendon may be restricted by adhesions, or both. Active exercises, electrical stimulation for facilitation, friction massage in regions where it is appropriate, proprioceptive neuromuscular facilitation, and biofeedback are options to restore active motion while the wrist is immobilized. Active exercises, such as place-and-hold exercises where the digit is passively placed at an end range of motion and then the patient actively holds that position for 5 s, are used to improve strength during this phase. Massage is used to relieve swelling; in areas where swelling is resolved but has left residual adhesions, friction massage, myofascial release, and instrument-assisted soft-tissue mobilization may be used to restore tissue mobility. Although the wrist and hand may be immobilized, upper-extremity PNF exercises may help to strengthen the the scapula and shoulder. Care must be taken to not cause pain at the injured site. It is important to ensure good posture and scapular control during all exercises.

In the resistive phase after cast or splint removal, the patient begins low-resistance, low-repetition isotonic activities, progressing to higher repetitions and resistance as tolerated. If pain or swelling increases with exercises, these exercises should be reduced in intensity or number of repetitions. Exercises for both the intrinsic and extrinsic muscles are introduced in this phase to strengthen all groups. Multiplanar activities for the wrist are introduced, and proprioceptive exercises are progressed.

Once strength gains are near normal, the patient begins functional activities in the advanced phase to stress the muscles that the patient will use in normal activities. After functional activities, a performance-specific program of activities that mimic the patient's normal sport, occupation, or leisure activities is introduced, tailored to each patient's needs. A tennis player has different performance requirements for the wrist than a golfer does, and golf and ballet likewise differ in their demands. In the work environment, a computer analyst's requirements differ from those of an auto mechanic. The rehabilitation clinician should be aware of each patient's requirements and should design a progressive, performance-specific program to address them.

It is common for distal radial fractures that are not surgically repaired to be immobilized for 5 to 6 weeks.[93, 100]

Once the initial cast is removed and the patient begins a rehabilitation program, the clinician's goal is to achieve full wrist motion and extrinsic tendon mobility.[93, 100] With the cast removed, nonoperative care is similar to that for postoperative rehabilitation. Grade I and grade II joint mobilization relieve pain and are used early in phases I and II. Grade III and grade IV joint mobilizations are not incorporated into the program until the resistive phase, when the fracture has healed enough to withstand those stresses; adequate healing for this step usually occurs by week 8. A primary focus is on range of motion in all planes for all restricted joints. Many clinicians neglect to address radial and ulnar deviation, but these motions must also be restored if the patient is to have full wrist function.

Carpal and Metacarpal Fractures

Both carpals and metacarpals are often fractured.[101] Accurate diagnosis and treatment are crucial to optimal outcomes.

Carpal Fractures The carpal most often fractured is the scaphoid, especially in athletes.[102] In fact, 70% of all carpal bone fractures involve the scaphoid.[102] There is a difference in blood supply between the distal and proximal poles of the scaphoid; the distal pole has a much better blood supply.[103] Because of the limited blood supply to the proximal scaphoid, fractures in this region usually become necrotic and need surgical intervention.[104] This variability in the scaphoid's blood supply causes healing time to vary widely, depending on the fracture's location and whether it is displaced. Treatment for nondisplaced scaphoid fractures remains controversial.[105] Nondisplaced fractures are often treated with immobilization until healing is apparent. This may take up to 3 months for proximal scaphoid fractures.[102, 106] Because of the perils of such prolonged immobilization, physicians often opt to perform surgery soon after the injury to avoid lengthy periods of immobilization and to secure a more rapid recovery with better postinjury function.[105] However, because of the surgical risks, surgical repair is not always the preferred method of treating nondisplaced scaphoid fractures, especially in the nonathletic population.[107]

Whether or not surgery is used, the rehabilitation clinician's most important initial efforts are to minimize edema and pain while preserving as much mobility as is safely possible. Edema control should be aggressive, and the patient should perform AROM of the uninvolved segments of the shoulder, elbow, and fingers immediately and often throughout the immobilization period. Pain should be avoided with these exercises.

Once the cast or splint is removed, ROM for the thumb begins. These exercises should be active. If joint mobility is restricted in a capsular pattern, joint mobilization is added to the program. The patient performs active exercises with the proximal joint stabilized passively to ensure correct movement of the digit.

The hook of the hamate and the pisiform can be fractured by impacts with sport implements such as baseball bats, golf clubs, and rackets or from a fall on an outstretched arm.[108] Because they are usually stable, these fractures heal well most of the time with cast immobilization. If fractures of the pisiform or hamate hook are displaced, the displaced segment is often excised.[109] Regardless of whether treatment is conservative or surgical, as with other fractures in this area, ROM exercises for the shoulder, elbow, and other unaffected wrist and hand joints are routinely performed while the splint is on during rehabilitation phase I, and restoration of full ROM for all joints should be the goal after cast removal in phase II. If pain occurs with hand and wrist activity after cast removal, a protective splint may be used at night and throughout the day to relieve the stress of motion and use. Progression of flexibility exercises continues until full motion is achieved.

Joint mobilization of restricted metacarpal and carpal joints is used to provide the physiological and accessory movements needed for full hand and wrist function after about 8 weeks postinjury or postoperatively. Strengthening exercises are initiated in the resistive phase after motion is restored. Grip exercises are used early, even in the active phase, because they help to mobilize the metacarpals and restore the normal palmar arches. Wrist strengthening is also incorporated. The patient is weaned from the splint around week 8 as pain and edema subside and motion and strength are restored.

Metacarpal Fractures Metacarpal fractures account for 42% of all hand fractures.[110] Because the neck of the metacarpal is the weakest aspect of the metacarpal bone, it is the most common site of metacarpal fractures. These fractures most commonly occur in the fourth and fifth metacarpals. Fractures here result primarily from compressive, or axial, forces like those that occur when a fist is used to administer a direct blow.[101] For this reason they are called "boxer's fractures." Rotational alignment and stability of the fingers determines whether the fracture can be treated with immobilization or an ORIF.[101] Normal flexion alignment of the digits is assessed with the MCP and PIP joints flexed; in this position, each of the digits points toward the scaphoid tubercle (figure 23.68). If digit angulation is off by more than 20° to 30°, an ORIF may be needed.[111]

Most of these fractures do not need surgery, but up to 4 weeks of immobilization may be needed for carpal and metacarpal fractures whether or not surgery is performed.[111] Total rehabilitation time is determined by the severity and location of the injury, the demands on the patient's hand once normal activity is resumed, hand dominance, and injury-related variables.[111]

While the cast is on, range-of-motion exercises are recommended for all uninvolved segments. Once the cast is removed, the patient enters phase II, the active phase, and

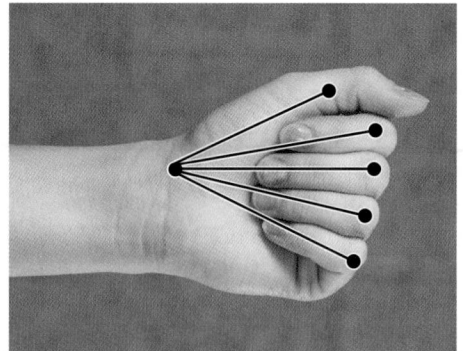

Figure 23.68 Finger alignment with MCP and PIP flexion.

ROM exercises for the entire hand and wrist begin immediately. Active range-of-motion exercises are used for the metacarpal joints, and tendon gliding exercises are used for the digits. This helps reduce the risk of tendon adhesions. Both intrinsic and extrinsic ROM exercises should be part of the exercise program. Early active exercises include wrist and finger **tenodesis** activities; as the wrist moves into extension, the finger joints move into flexion.[112] It seems that the most common errors we see after periods of wrist immobilization are patients performing hand functions in wrist flexion; however, the optimal wrist position for finger flexor activities is 20° to 30° of extension (in the position of function). Clinicians should tell patients to use the proper wrist position during initial rehabilitation activities so that accurate muscle recruitment occurs and bad habits are avoided.

The patient progresses to PROM exercises of all affected segments once the fracture is well healed. Next, the patient progresses to easy resistive exercises from PROM exercises in late phase II. From this point, patients may perform early proprioception and coordination exercises. Progression in these activities coincides with advancement through the other phases and increases in parameters of flexibility, strength, and agility, as long as there is no pain with any activity.

Joint mobilization is used to increase the mobility of restricted segments during the resistive phase, when capsular mobility is restricted. Also in phase III, the patient begins more aggressive strengthening exercises in straight-plane motions to emphasize and focus on weak muscles. Resistive exercises begin with light weights and progress to heavier weights and more repetitions, using pain and edema as guides. As these weak muscles become stronger, multiplanar and more functional strengthening exercises are added. From there the patient progresses to the early advanced phase to perform more functional activities in preparation for performance-specific exercises.

A Bennett's fracture involves the first metacarpal. Because the thumb is so important to normal hand function, insurance companies provide 25% of total disability if thumb function is lost.[113] This illustrates how important the clinician's role is in providing appropriate management and treatment for thumb injuries. The physician must ensure proper angulation and alignment with either closed or open reduction to enable the thumb to return to good function. The immobilization period is usually 4 weeks. During this time, treatment efforts to control edema and pain are important. Adhesions may occur in the first web space. The rehabilitation clinician must take steps to maintain appropriate web spacing during immobilization. If the web space is compromised, thumb motion will be limited.

Cast removal enables the start of AROM exercises for all joints. Once union of the fracture site is observed on X-ray, usually about 6 to 8 weeks postinjury, PROM exercises are used to regain motion as the active phase of rehabilitation begins. In normal joints, passive motion is slightly greater than active motion; however, if passive motion is significantly more than AROM in an injured finger, there are probably tendon adhesions. Friction massage, instrument-assisted soft-tissue mobilization, electrical stimulation, and active and passive ROM exercises help reduce these adhesions and restore tendon glide. Dynamic splinting may be needed if full ROM is not restored by 8 to 10 weeks postinjury. As with other fractures, resistive exercises begin in phase III after healing is apparent and motion gains have occurred. Strength exercises should include both precision and power grasping activities and should also incorporate other segments that have lost strength secondary to reduced use of the hand. As with other injuries, after strength, mobility, and agility are regained, the patient progresses to the advanced phase, where the emphasis is on functional activities, and then the performance-specific program.

Phalangeal Fractures

Although metacarpal fractures can affect hand function, finger fractures affect hand function much more, and proximal phalanx fractures have a more detrimental impact on hand function than distal or intermediate phalanx fractures.[114, 115] Proximal phalanx fractures occur because of falls or direct blows to the phalanx, most often in the thumb and index finger. Middle phalanx fractures are not as common; these fractures often result from a crush injury such as that which occurs when a hand is stepped on. Distal phalanx fractures are common and are often associated with avulsion of the long extensor tendon.[115, 116] Displaced proximal phalanx fractures typically result in flexion of the proximal bone segment from the pull of the interossei muscles, and extension of the distal segment occurs because of the long extensor tendon's pull on it (figure 23.69).[115]

A proximal phalangeal fracture is reduced and immobilized with either open or closed reduction; the use of external wires in an open repair is common.[117] If the fracture is stable, buddy taping the fingers immobilizes the fracture and still permits tendon movement to minimize tendon

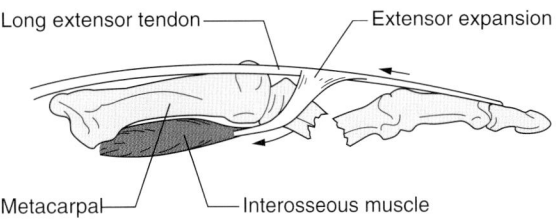

Figure 23.69 Forces affecting proximal phalanx fracture displacement. The extensor tendon's pull on the dorsal distal segment pulls the distal fracture end posteriorly, while the intrinsic muscle pull forces the proximal fracture segment anteriorly to create an unstable fracture.

gliding problems.[115, 118] Early management of edema is also important in minimizing soft-tissue adhesions;[60] the rehabilitation clinician must make a concerted effort to reduce edema early in the healing process and continue to affect it as long as any swelling exists.

Whether the fracture is stable or surgical repair has occurred, motion exercises begin as early as the first to second week after the injury. If the fracture is displaced, motion is usually started 3 to 4 weeks postinjury. Finger fractures are seldom immobilized for more than 4 weeks because of the deleterious effects of prolonged immobilization on surrounding soft-tissue structures. More commonly, early protected motion and tendon gliding exercises are begun once there is adequate stabilization of the fracture site.[119]

One of the greatest complications of phalangeal immobilization is tendon adhesions, which result in restriction of normal tendon gliding.[120] Adhesions of the extensor tendon can cause an extensor lag with limited IP flexion. Adhesions of the long flexor tendons will also prevent full extension of the digit. Scar massage minimizes and treats these adhesions. Tendon gliding exercises can isolate tendon function and reduce tendon adhesions. For example, if the FDP tendon is restricted, the exercise to treat this tendon passively places the MCP and PIP joints in extension and blocks them from moving while the DIP is moved into flexion and extension (figure 23.70).

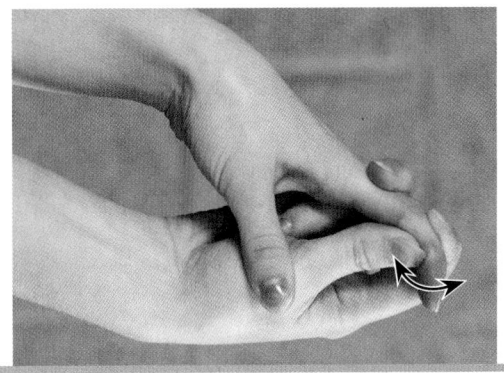

Figure 23.70 Blocking exercise: The MCP and PIP joints are passively restrained while the DIP is actively moved.

Once the fracture is healed enough to be stable, more aggressive PROM exercises and joint mobilization are used to improve ROM, especially in the resistive phase. Dynamic splints place a continual low-level stress on tight structures for more restricted cases. One can also apply tape to position digits into a stretch position (figure 23.71). These prolonged tape techniques are applied during the later resistive phase if motion is not yet restored; they are on for 15 to 20 min periods throughout the day, as tolerated, to improve scar-tissue mobility and gain ROM. You must be cautious in applying forces for prolonged stretching, especially with the extensor tendons, since it is rather easy to overstretch them. A mild, low-level tension force is all that is needed for prolonged stretching with taping techniques. Overstretching the extensor tendon produces an extensor lag. If an extensor lag develops, a static extension splint worn continuously for 3 to 6 weeks is needed to correct it.

Once the patient achieves full ROM, resistive exercises, including those using therapeutic putty and rubber bands, along with other exercises listed earlier, are used to restore the full strength of the long finger flexors, long finger extensors, and intrinsics. Wrist, elbow, and shoulder strengthening exercises are included in the rehabilitation program. Finger exercises begin with light resistance, increasing in intensity or repetitions without pain as the patient progresses. Exercises should emphasize full tendon and joint functions that incorporate normal movement.

Triangular Fibrocartilage Complex (TFCC) Lesion

The TFCC is composed of several elements in addition to the articular disc, including the disc's meniscal homologue, the palmar radioulnar ligament, the dorsal radioulnar ligament, the ulnar collateral ligament, and the extensor carpi ulnaris tendon sheath.[121] In essence, the TFCC is made up of the ligaments and cartilage structures within the distal radioulnar joint and between the distal ulna and carpal bones. The TFCC is the central point from which the wrist rotates when the radius moves on the ulna.[122] The TFCC is also a load-bearing structure between the head of the ulna, the lunate, and the triquetrum.[123] It serves as a stabilizer for the wrist and provides a gliding surface for wrist motion.[124] It also serves as a shock absorber and carries about 20% of the axial load that is delivered to the wrist.[125, 126] Therefore, injuries to this structure can lead to instability of the distal radioulnar joint (DRUJ).[122]

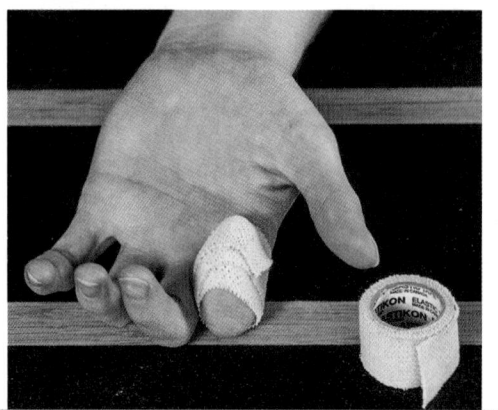

Figure 23.71 Aggressive techniques to increase ROM: Tape is applied in a prolonged stretch to increase IP joint flexion range of motion.

Case Study

A 21-year-old hockey forward suffered a fracture of the neck of his dominant hand's fourth metacarpal when he engaged in a fight during a game and hit an opponent. The hand was placed in a cast for 2 weeks and then in a splint that could be removed for his rehabilitation activities. The fracture is now stable, so the physician wants you to wean him from the splint over the next 2 weeks. Your initial examination reveals mild swelling in the hand and fingers. Wrist flexion is 50° and wrist extension is 65°. Ulnar deviation and radial deviation are 10°. Supination is 70° and pronation is 90°. MCP flexion is 45°, PIP flexion is 80°, and DIP flexion is 60°. The patient cannot make a complete fist. The MCP and IP joints can extend passively to 0°. He cannot simultaneously flex the MCP and extend the IP joints.

Questions for Analysis

1. What do you suspect this patient's primary problems are?
2. What will be included in your first three treatment sessions with him, assuming no regression with your treatments?
3. What will your initial goals during the first week be for him?
4. What precautions must you be aware of when you treat him?
5. Describe three home exercises you will give this patient at the time of your first treatment.
6. List four strengthening exercises you will use with him in the first month.
7. What sport-specific exercises will you incorporate into his rehabilitation program before he returns to hockey?

The TFCC is injured either by repetitive rotational loading of the wrist or by a sudden FOOSH with the wrist extended and forearm rotated.[127-129] Athletes participating in activities such as baseball or softball batting, golf club swinging, ice hockey, and racquet sports move their wrists into ulnar deviation and forearm pronation while gripping an implement; these combined activities increase TFCC stresses.[123, 127] Repetitive axial loads on the wrist, such as those that occur in gymnastics and boxing, increase the risk of chronic TFCC injury signs and symptoms.[127] A positive ulnar variance, or long ulna in comparison to the radius, is also associated with TFCC injury.[123] The patient typically reports persistent pain in the ulnar wrist during gripping and forearm supination–pronation activities. A click may be heard or palpated occasionally over the site, and palpation pressure applied directly over the disc produces pain.[123, 130]

The central portion of the disc itself is essentially avascular, which often creates healing difficulties after injury.[91] In spite of the central disc's poor vascular supply, both chronic and acute TFCC injuries are usually treated conservatively at first, as long as there is no DRUJ instability, catching, or locking.[91, 131] If pain persists for more than 3 weeks in athletes, they should undergo arthroscopy for debridement.[1, 131] Non-elite athletes may undergo a 4- to 6-week period of wrist immobilization, anti-inflammatory medications, and activity modification before advancing

to a gradual return to full activities.[91, 132] In addition to conservative treatment and arthroscopic debridement, there are several surgical options for repair of the TFCC.[1, 131] The treatment selected depends on the surgeon; the TFCC injury's site, severity, and stage; the age and activity level of the patient; and the patient's goals.

Regardless of the treatment selected, the rehabilitation clinician is vital to the patient's recovery. The duration of immobilization depends on the treatment: conservative, debridement, or repair. As you might suspect, debridement of the TFCC allows for a quicker progression through the rehabilitation phases, while repair of the TFCC has the more conservative progression in postoperative care. Whether the TFCC injury needs surgery or not, the wrist and forearm are casted or splinted in neutral for up to 6 weeks.[130] This prolonged immobilization occurs because of the limited vascularity within the disc and the TFCC's importance to the distal radioulnar joint, absorbing significant compressive forces applied to the wrist.[126] The first 2 to 3 weeks after the cast or splint is removed, rehabilitation emphasizes regaining wrist flexion and extension, radial and ulnar deviation, and forearm pronation and supination. Strength exercises begin after this time and include straight-plane strengthening without torsion forces to the wrist during the first 4 to 5 weeks after immobilization. A sample rehabilitation program for surgical repair of a triangular fibrocartilage complex injury is provided in figure 23.72.

TFCC Repair

	Stage I: Inactive phase			
0-2 weeks	**Inflammation phase: Inactive rehabilitation phase**			
Goals	Control and treat pain, spasm, swelling. Protect surgical site. Maintain proper immobilization of repair site via splint or cast. Maintain ROM of all UE segments. Maintain strength of shoulder complex and elbow muscles. Maintain core and hip strength. Correct posture deficiencies. MCL.			
Treatment guidelines	Week 1: Arm elevation to reduce edema Days 3-5: Remove bulky surgical dressing, inspect and care for surgical site; apply immobilization device Modalities for pain, swelling, and spasm Trigger point, STM, MFR techniques PRN Tendon gliding exercises AROM shoulder, elbow, and fingers Light functional UE activities with uninvolved segments as tolerated without pain Week 2: Isometrics for hand muscles Place-and-hold exercises for fingers in the immobilization device Resistive exercises for shoulder and elbow that do not cause distal radial stress or pain Core and hip strengthening and stabilization exercises CV exercises			

>continued

Figure 23.72 Rehabilitation program for postoperative TFCC repair.

Stage I: Inactive phase	
0-2 weeks	**Inflammation phase: Inactive rehabilitation phase**
Precautions	Monitor surgical site for proper healing. Use HEP to facilitate treatment gains.

Stage II: Active phase	
2-8 weeks	**Early proliferation phase: Active rehabilitation phase**
Goals	Pain relieved to 0-2/10. Weeks 2-4: Replace cast with removable splint for less restriction, allowing guarded mobility. Achieve full ROM of wrist. Achieve strength gains of wrist to 50%. Restore proprioception and agility gains to 50%. Achieve good postural strength. MCL.
Treatment guidelines	Weeks 2-4: Once cast is removed, begin early active forearm and wrist motion; remove splint for AROM exercises Weeks 6-8: Remove splint Weeks 6-8: AAROM to wrist and forearm Trigger point, STM, MFR techniques PRN Light functional activities continue and progress without pain Hand ball-roll and pencil-rotation proprioception exercises Proprioception exercises with hand on ball, on wall, and on tabletop with little weight-bearing Continue to progress postural, hip, and core strengthening and endurance CV exercises
Precautions	Pain at TFCC site should be avoided. Use HEP to facilitate treatment gains.

Stage III: Resistive phase	
8-12 weeks	**Late proliferation phase: Resistive rehabilitation phase**
Goals	Eliminate pain. Achieve full range of motion in forearm, wrist, and hand. Maintain normal scapular muscle strength and endurance. Achieve normal strength of elbow, wrist, and hand muscles in straight-plane and multiplanar activities. Restore pain-free functional use in ADLs.
Treatment guidelines	AROM, AAROM for wrist and forearm motions Passive motion to wrist and forearm; use a dynamic splint PRN Putty exercises for wrist and hand Weeks 8-10: Progress to weight-resisted exercises Advance to multiplanar motions after concentric exercise strength is 80% Weeks 8-10: Weight-bearing proprioception exercises Week 8: Grades III-IV joint mobilization and soft-tissue mobilization PRN Dynamic proprioception exercises Plyometric exercises Maintenance exercises for core, shoulder complex, and elbow strength and endurance
Precautions	Identify through presence of capsular pattern if joints or soft tissue or both are restricting patient's ROM and flexibility. Weeks 8-10: Avoid torsion stress to wrist by enforcing straight-plane activities. Use HEP to facilitate treatment gains.

Figure 23.72 >continued

Stage IV: Advanced phase	
12-16 weeks	**Remodeling phase: Advanced rehabilitation phase**
Goals	Maintain normal ROM of all joints. Maintain normal strength of all muscles. Restore normal sport and work performance.
Treatment guidelines	UE plyometric progression Functional exercise progression Progression of performance-specific exercises and drills
Precautions	Wrist should be pain free throughout all activities.

TFCC = triangular fibrocartilage complex; ROM = range of motion; UE = upper extremity; MCL = maintain cardiovascular level; STM = soft-tissue massage; MFR = myofascial release; PRN = as needed; AROM = active range of motion; CV = cardiovascular; HEP = home exercise program; ADLs = activities of daily living.

Figure 23.72 *>continued*

If an arthroscopic debridement is performed, rehabilitation begins 1 to 2 weeks after surgery, and anywhere from 2 weeks of splinting[133] to no period of immobilization occurs after debridement.[126] Modalities used during the first postoperative week reduce edema and pain. Active range-of-motion exercises occur by the end of the first week after debridement; if a splint is worn, it is removed for active motion exercises. Frequent active motion exercises throughout the day as part of the patient's home program encourage the return of full motion. Tendon gliding exercises may be used if it is apparent that the long finger tendons are losing motion. After 2 weeks, active ROM exercises continue, but active-assistive motion exercises are added to gain additional motion. Once the surgical scar is sufficiently healed, soft-tissue mobilization to prevent adhesions is added to the program. The end of the active phase is approached at about 3 to 4 weeks; at this time passive stretches are used to gain full motion of the wrist. Forearm pronation and supination motion is incorporated both actively and passively. Finger grip exercises can begin toward the end of phase II. The resistive phase begins at week 6 when strengthening exercises begin with putty exercises and progress to pain-free use of weights in single-plane motions. Toward the end of this phase, about week 8, the patient should have full motion in all planes and near-normal strength. In the advanced phase, functional and then performance-specific exercises are begun to return the patient to normal activities. Patients with arthroscopically debrided TFCC injuries usually return to full participation within 3 to 4 months.[1, 123]

Dislocations and Sprains

Because dislocations are a severe form of sprain, sprains and dislocation injuries are addressed together. Dislocations and sprains occur often in sports and involve the PIP more often than the DIP joints.[134] A term commonly used for a finger sprain is "jammed finger."[135] Sprains usually occur in ball-handling sports when the ball hits the end of the finger.

When a phalangeal dislocation occurs, the joint's supporting structures—the radial and ulnar collateral ligaments and the volar plate—have been damaged either individually or in any combination, depending on the direction of dislocation. Fractures can often accompany dislocations.[136] As with most joint injuries, if the dislocation is unstable, surgical repair using either a Kirschner wire (K-wire), pin, or plate is often the standard course of treatment.[117] Surgical repair is accompanied by a postoperative cast or splint for 5 d. Active range-of-motion exercises for the FDP occur at this time as well, with the PIP and MCP joints passively held in extension.[120] Active exercises also include activities that permit tendon gliding of the other digits while protecting the injured joint. At 2 weeks, passive PIP joint motion begins, as long as it is pain free.[120] A gradually progressive program of strengthening exercises starts at 6 to 8 weeks once the patient has achieved full motion.

If the dislocation is stable so that flexion and extension occur without dislocation after reduction, the finger is immobilized for 2 to 3 d, primarily for patient comfort.[137] If the PIP dislocation occurs volarly, the joint is splinted in full extension; if it dislocates in a dorsal direction, it is splinted in slight flexion.[138] Immediate efforts are made to control edema and pain in the inactive phase. Once splinting is discontinued, buddy taping is used to continue to protect the joint. Buddy taping the digits is adequate protection during normal activities.[137] The only time the index and fifth fingers are buddy taped is if they are the injured digits; in other words, if the middle or ring finger is the injured digit, one is buddy taped to the other, not to either the index or little finger.[135] Tendon gliding exercises for both intrinsic and extrinsic muscles should be added when appropriate, depending on the severity of the injury. Full active extension should be achieved within 6 to 8 weeks. Resistive exercises begin at around 8 weeks in the latter half of the resistive phase.

Case Study

A 16-year-old, right-handed volleyball setter suffered a dislocated PIP joint of her dominant-hand middle finger 3 weeks ago. The finger has been in a partial flexion splint for the past 3 weeks. The physician has instructed the patient to tape the finger to her ring finger throughout the day except when in rehabilitation. She has been moving the wrist and MCP joint, but the finger has been immobilized since the injury. The edema is gone, but the finger is stiff in the IP joints. Passive DIP extension lacks 15° and flexion is to 30°, and PIP extension lacks 30° and flexion is to 50°. Active DIP extension lacks 20° and flexion is to 25°, and PIP extension lacks 40° and flexion is to 50°. The patient cannot make a complete fist because the middle finger does not flex into the palm. Her grip strength measurement is 13.6 kg (30 lb) on the right and 31.7 kg (70 lb) on the left. There is tenderness over the PIP collateral ligaments, especially on the radial side.

Questions for Analysis

1. What tests will you use to identify the source of her limited range of motion?

2. What will you try to accomplish in the next three treatments? How will you accomplish those goals?

3. What precautions should you consider in the treatments?

4. What will your rehabilitation program include if her lost motion is due to restricted mobility of her long extensor tendon? What will you include in the program if her motion loss is because of capsular restriction?

5. What strengthening exercises will you start her with in today's treatment? (Hint: What other body segments do you think will be weaker than normal for her?)

6. What functional sport-specific activities will you eventually include in her rehabilitation program?

If a finger is sprained, the immobilization and rehabilitation process follows that outlined for the stable dislocation, but the process may be accelerated. If the sprain is minor, the process will take less time, but when the sprain is more severe, more time will be needed for a full recovery. Collateral ligament sprains without joint dislocations may respond well with anywhere from 1 to 3 d of immobilization followed by progressive range of motion, then strengthening exercises in a fairly rapid sequence.[138]

Thumb ulnar collateral ligament (UCL) injuries can result from an acute injury or repetitive stress. The UCL prevents thumb hyperabduction.[139] Injury to the thumb UCL can be quite debilitating because it can profoundly affect hand function. In an acute injury, the patient often falls on an outstretched hand while grasping an object during the fall—for example, a ski pole. This injury is often called a "skier's thumb."[139] A blunt trauma to the tip of the thumb resulting in a valgus stress at the MCP joint can also cause an acute injury to the UCL. The UCL may also tear from repetitive microtraumas. This injury is often called "gamekeeper's thumb" and has been associated with sports such as rugby, soccer, handball, basketball, volleyball, wrestling, and martial arts.[139] As a result of UCL injury, the patient complains of pain, swelling, difficulty moving the thumb, and decreased pinch and grip strength.

Ulnar collateral ligament injuries of the thumb can be treated surgically or nonsurgically. Surgical intervention is warranted when there is more than 35° of valgus instability at the MCP joint.[140] Both surgical and nonsurgical rehabilitation include a forearm-based thumb spica splint for 4 weeks.[140] The splint is then modified to a hand-based splint and used for an additional 2 to 4 weeks with activities involving weighted resistance or sustained power gripping or pinching.

During the inactive phase, ROM activities for the shoulder, forearm, and fingers are appropriate. In addition, patients are instructed about posture, edema reduction, proximal shoulder strengthening, and cardiovascular exercises. It is important to reduce joint stiffness; therefore, once the forearm-based splint is removed, the active phase of rehabilitation begins with AROM exercises for the wrist and thumb. If joint stiffness persists after week 6, gentle PROM and joint mobilization techniques are used to restore normal motion. Resistance exercises are started after week 6, taking care to avoid stressing the UCL for 8 to 10 weeks. Proprioceptive and dexterity activities may begin in weeks 6 to 8. Gentle grip and pinch exercises begin during week 8; more forceful pinching activities may begin at 12 to 16 weeks. In the advanced phase, functional and then performance-specific exercises are incorporated into the rehabilitation program to return the patient to normal activities. A sample rehabilitation program for surgical repair of a thumb UCL injury is provided in figure 23.73.

The scapholunate ligament (SLL) is the most commonly injured carpal ligament in the wrist and the most common cause of carpal instability.[141, 142] Scapholunate ligament injury can occur with a FOOSH,[141] and it is often associated with a distal radius fracture.[141, 142] Injury to the ligament can result in progressive biomechanical changes in the lateral wrist, from scapholunate dissociation (gap),[142] to carpal collapse leading to volar flexion

Thumb UCL Repair

Stage I: Inactive phase	
0-4 weeks	**Inflammation phase: Inactive rehabilitation phase**
Goals	Control and treat pain, spasm, swelling. Protect surgical site. Maintain proper immobilization of repair site via splint or cast. Maintain ROM of fingers, forearm, elbow, and shoulder. Maintain strength of shoulder complex and elbow muscles. Maintain core and hip strength. Correct posture deficiencies. MCL.
Treatment guidelines	Week 1: Arm elevation to reduce edema Days 10-14: Sutures removed Modalities for pain, swelling, and spasm Week 2: Trigger point, STM, MFR techniques PRN Week 4: Transition to hand-base thumb spica splint Tendon gliding exercises for fingers AROM shoulder, elbow, forearm, and fingers Resistive exercises for shoulder and elbow that do not cause thumb stress or pain Core and hip strengthening and stabilization exercises CV exercises
Precautions	Monitor surgical site for proper healing. Use HEP to facilitate treatment gains.
Stage II: Active phase	
4-8 weeks	**Early proliferation phase: Active rehabilitation phase**
Goals	Achieve pain relief to 0-2/10. Eliminate edema. Desensitize scar. Achieve full ROM while protecting repair. Achieve strength gains of wrist and hand to 50%. Restore proprioception and agility gains to 50%. Achieve good postural strength. MCL.
Treatment guidelines	Week 4: Begin AROM for wrist and thumb while protecting UCL; remove splint for AROM exercises Scar desensitization PRN Week 6: Remove splint for ADLs and light activities; continue use with activities involving repetitive or sustained pinching or gripping Week 6: Gentle PROM to thumb Trigger point, STM, MFR techniques PRN Week 8: Hand ball-roll and pencil-rotation proprioception exercises Proprioception exercises with hand on ball, on wall, and on tabletop Continue to progress postural, hip, and core strengthening and endurance CV exercises
Precautions	Pain at UCL site should be avoided. Use HEP to facilitate treatment gains.

>continued

Figure 23.73 Rehabilitation program for postoperative thumb UCL repair.

Stage III: Resistive phase	
8-12 weeks	**Late proliferation phase: Resistive rehabilitation phase**
Goals	Eliminate pain. Achieve full range of motion in forearm, wrist, and hand. Maintain normal scapular muscle strength and endurance. Achieve normal strength of elbow, wrist, and hand muscles in straight-plane and multiplanar activities. Restore pain-free functional use in ADLs.
Treatment guidelines	AROM, AAROM, and PROM PRN to attain full mobility Resistance exercises for wrist and grip strength Avoid forceful pinching exercises until 14-16 weeks Putty exercises for wrist and hand Advance to multiplanar motions after concentric exercise strength is 80% Weeks 8-10: Progress weight-bearing proprioception exercises Week 8: Grade III-IV joint mobilization and soft-tissue mobilization PRN Weeks 8-10: Dynamic proprioception exercises Maintenance exercises for core, shoulder complex, and elbow strength and endurance
Precautions	Identify through presence of capsular pattern if joints or soft tissue or both are restricting patient's ROM and flexibility. Avoid forceful pinching or stress to UCL for 14-16 weeks. Use HEP to facilitate treatment gains.

Stage IV: Advanced phase	
12-18 weeks	**Remodeling phase: Advanced rehabilitation phase**
Goals	Maintain normal ROM of all joints. Maintain normal strength of all muscles. Restore normal sport and work performance.
Treatment guidelines	Weeks 14-16: Begin forceful pinching activities UE plyometric progression Functional exercise progression Progression of performance-specific exercises and drills
Precautions	Thumb should be pain free throughout all activities.

UCL = ulnar collateral ligament; ROM = range of motion; MCL = maintain cardiovascular level; STM = soft-tissue massage; MFR = myofascial release; PRN = as needed; AROM = active range of motion; CV = cardiovascular; HEP = home exercise program; ADLs = activities of daily living; PROM = passive range of motion; AAROM = active-assistive range of motion.

Figure 23.73 >*continued*

of the scaphoid and dorsal flexion of the lunate,[141, 142] to scapholunate advanced collapse (SLAC) and wrist arthritis.[141, 142] As a result of SLL injury, the patient complains of pain in the lateral wrist with axial loading, decreased range of motion, swelling, and decreased grip strength. Some patients will present with a "click" on the dorsal-radial aspect of the wrist with range of motion.[142]

Conservative management of a chronic SLL injury includes the use of a wrist splint in addition to modalities and manual therapy to treat pain and edema in the inactive phase. Postural stability and scapular control are addressed early in the rehabilitation process to provide a stable base

from which the wrist and hand can function. Range-of-motion activities for the shoulder, forearm, and fingers are appropriate in the inactive phase.

In the active phase, AROM exercises and isometric exercises are begun. The dart-throwing motion (figure 23.74) is a good exercise for mid-carpal mobility because the motion of radial wrist extension and ulnar wrist flexion follows the plane of the scaphoid. The motion is used functionally in drinking from or lowering a glass, using a hammer, or casting in fishing. If wrist or thumb stiffness persists after 6 weeks, PROM and joint mobilization techniques are used to restore normal joint mobility. Dexterity

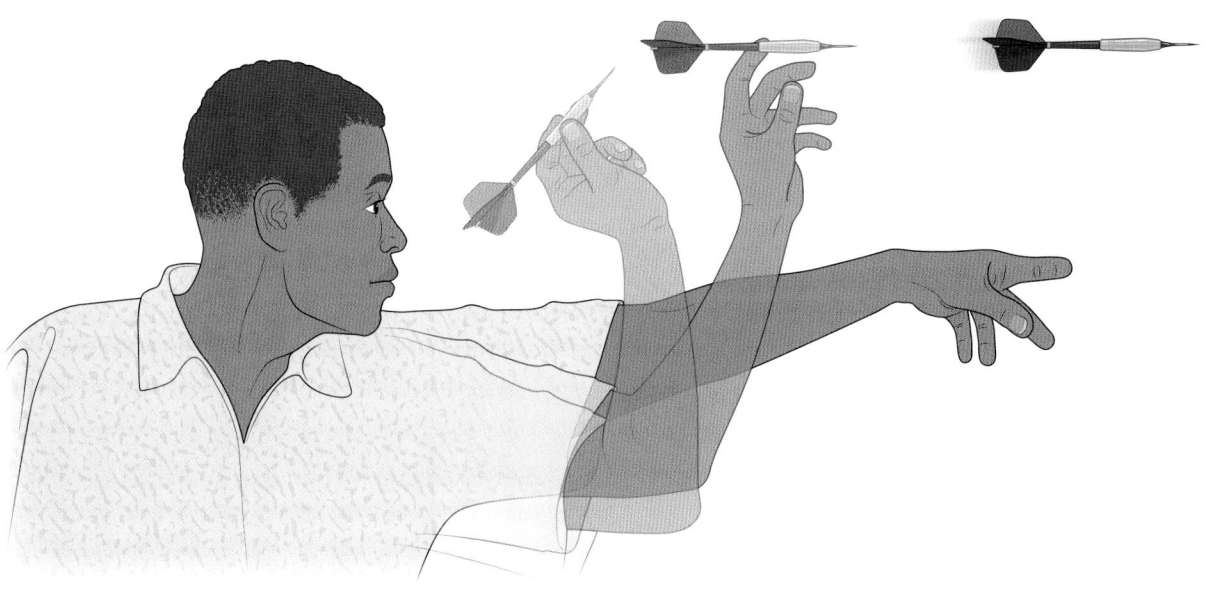

Figure 23.74 Dart throwing motion.

exercises may begin while avoiding excessive loading of the wrist and thumb.

Resistance exercises are started after weeks 6 to 8 in the resistive phase, but axial loading and weight-bearing activities are avoided for 8 to 12 weeks. Progressive strengthening and gentle grip and pinch exercises may begin in week 8. In the advanced phase, functional and then performance-specific exercises are incorporated in the rehabilitation program to return the patient to normal activities.

Acute complete SLL injuries are surgically repaired by open reinsertion and pinning or suture repair.[142] Partial injuries are managed by arthroscopic debridement, pinning, or thermal shrinkage.[142] A meta-analysis by Daly and colleagues in 2020[143] concluded that tenodesis reconstruction was the best surgical technique for chronic SLL injuries. After ligament repair, a forearm-based thumb spica splint is worn for 6 weeks during the inactive phase. Active range of motion exercises for the shoulder, elbow, forearm, fingers, and thumb IP joint are appropriate. Patient education about posture, edema reduction, proximal shoulder strengthening, and cardiovascular exercises are incorporated.

In the active phase, flexion and extension AROM exercises for the wrist are started at week 6, although radial and ulnar deviation exercises, including the dart throwing motion, are held to weeks 8 to 10. Scar mobilization and desensitization begin in week 6. The patient is weaned from the splint between 8 and 10 weeks. Axial loading is contraindicated in both the active and resistive phases. If full AROM is not achieved by weeks 8 to 10, PROM and joint mobilization may be used to attain full mobility. At 10 weeks, proprioception, dexterity, and gentle grip and

pinch exercises may begin. Light strengthening of the wrist and hand begins at 12 weeks. Return to function and performance-specific activities begin at 16 weeks; however, axial loading and power grip strengthening are not commenced until 6 months have passed.

Overuse Injuries

The two most common overuse injuries of the wrist and hand are carpal tunnel syndrome and De Quervain's syndrome.[144, 145] De Quervain's syndrome is common in upper-extremity sports that use hand implements such as golfing and racquet sports.[145] On the other hand, carpal tunnel is more commonly seen in people whose occupations require them to spend prolonged time at keyboards.[146] *Overuse* is the term commonly used to describe these injuries because trauma accumulates over time and produces stress more quickly than the structures can adapt to it. Microscopic damage occurs, and the structure cannot rebuild before additional stress is applied.[147] If insult to the tissues continues, scar tissue develops, leading to chronic pain. These injuries can be frustrating and challenging for the rehabilitation clinician, especially when the patient does not seek treatment until the injury has become advanced. The key to successful treatment is early intervention and correction of the causes.

Carpal Tunnel Syndrome

This condition is also known as median nerve compression syndrome.[146] The median nerve is compressed as it passes through the carpal tunnel under the transverse carpal ligament. Compression of the median nerve results in loss of sensation and tingling over its distribution in the hand, as well as weakness and pain. Pain occurs primarily at night, when the wrist is placed in flexion while the patient sleeps. Prolonged flexion of the wrist causes compression on the nerve, venous congestion, and pain. The pain can result in decreased grip strength and impaired hand function. This problem often results from prolonged or repeated wrist extension during daily activities. A gymnast with weak wrists who performs on the bars with the wrists in hyperextension can develop carpal tunnel syndrome. Athletes may develop enlarged wrist flexor tendons as a result of their conditioning exercises; this may lead to carpal tunnel syndrome since larger tendons will essentially make the carpal tunnel space smaller (figure 23.75). Manual laborers who repeatedly grip their tools and workers who rest their wrists on a keyboard or desk while typing are prone to developing carpal tunnel syndrome.[148]

If carpal tunnel syndrome complaints occur bilaterally, the cervical region may be the source of the problem rather than the carpal tunnel.[149] Cervical radiculopathy is a differential diagnosis that should be ruled out for any upper-extremity injury not specifically related to an incident.[149] It is important to obtain an accurate history to determine the cause of the patient's symptoms. If passively placing the neck in a quadrant position (extension with lateral flexion and rotation to the involved side) reproduces the patient's symptoms, cervical radiculopathy cannot be ruled out.

When treatment begins early, it can often succeed in relieving symptoms. Using a splint to position the wrist in neutral, especially at night, can help reduce median nerve compression and night pain. Modalities may be used to relieve the inflammation. Ice, contrast baths, ultrasound, or electrical stimulation may be helpful. Flexibility exercises for the wrist and long finger flexors, limiting aggravating activities, and correcting poor technique all help to relieve

the pain. Posture education and strengthening exercises are important elements of a rehabilitation program. Strengthening exercises for all wrist, thumb, and finger movements—beginning with isometrics and advancing to isotonics, eccentric exercises, and concentric exercises—should progress when the inflammation is under control. Endurance, speed, and coordination all should be included in the progression of exercises.

Although early conservative treatment may resolve the patient's carpal tunnel syndrome, surgical intervention for release of the transverse carpal ligament may be needed if it does not.[148, 150] Gentle AROM may begin within 3 to 7 d postoperatively with the wrist motions limited to either neutral or functional positions. Once the sutures are removed, scar-tissue management and desensitization exercises can begin. The patient starts doing progressive resistive exercises in phase III, usually around 3 weeks postoperative. By this time, the scar across the carpal tunnel arch has healed enough so that stress to the tissue will not allow bowstringing of the tendons to occur under the scar tissue. Before this time, the patient performs AROM and isometric exercises so the scar tissue has time to properly heal. The progression of exercises follows a course similar to that discussed earlier for other wrist injuries. It is important to educate the patient about proper posture and work ergonomics, especially if the carpal tunnel syndrome is related to prolonged keyboard use. A more complete program after surgical release of a carpal tunnel is outlined in figure 23.76.

De Quervain's Syndrome

Long extensor tendons of the hand travel in the wrist region in compartments. There are six dorsal compartments that are identified by consecutive numbers beginning on the

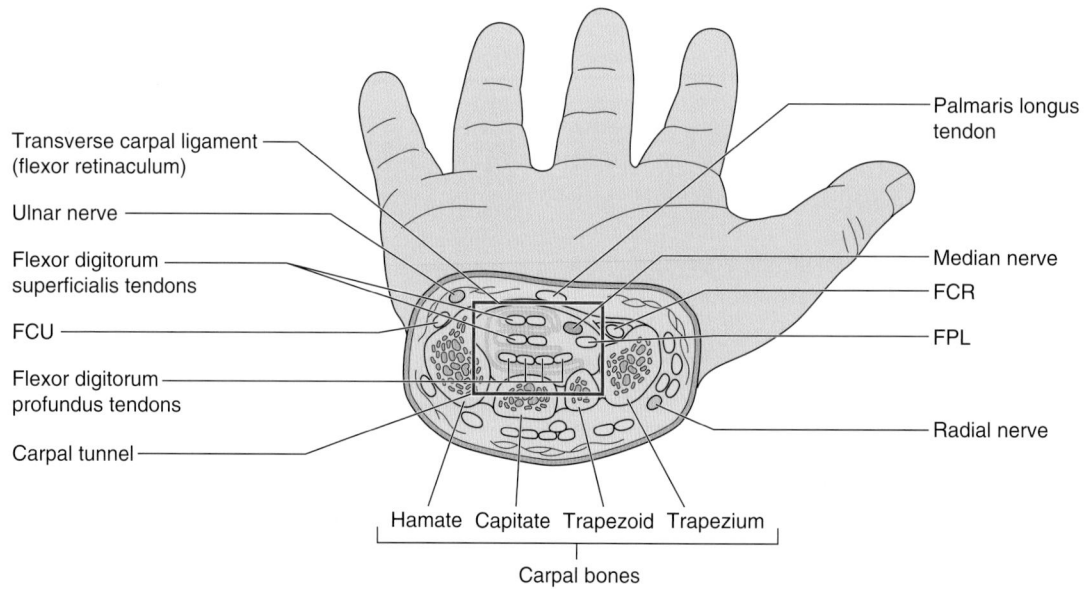

Figure 23.75 Cross-section of a wrist showing carpal tunnel.

Carpal Tunnel Release

Stage I: Inactive phase	
0-2 weeks	**Inflammation phase: Inactive rehabilitation phase**
Goals	Relieve pain, spasm, swelling. Prevent infection. Protect surgical site. Maintain AROM of fingers, elbow, and other body segments. Begin posture and ergonomic education. MCL.
Treatment guidelines	Modalities for pain, edema, and spasm Grades I and II joint mobilization for pain Shoulder, elbow, and finger AROM exercises Tendon gliding exercises Posture and ergonomic training CV exercise
Precautions	Monitor surgical site for proper healing. Use HEP to facilitate treatment gains.
Stage II: Active phase	
1-3 weeks	**Early proliferation phase: Active rehabilitation phase**
Goals	Achieve pain relief to 2-3 on a scale of 10. Achieve normal range of motion of elbow, wrist, hand, and fingers. Begin restoration of proprioception. Achieve early strength gains. Restore good postural strength. Relieve scar sensitivity. Relieve pain, spasm, edema, ecchymosis. MCL.
Treatment guidelines	Days 7-10: Isometric exercises for wrist and elbow Weeks 3-4: AROM for elbow, wrist, and hand Begin isotonic exercises for wrist at end of phase. Early proprioception exercises Scar desensitization Dexterity exercises STM and MFR PRN Progress postural strengthening exercises CV exercise
Precautions	Keep wrist in neutral position during exercises. If AROM exercises are painful, performing them with the wrist in warm water may be beneficial. Use HEP to facilitate treatment gains.

>continued

Figure 23.76 Rehabilitation program for surgical release of carpal tunnel syndrome.

Stage III: Resistive phase	
3-5 weeks	**Late proliferation phase: Resistive rehabilitation phase**
Goals	Eliminate pain, edema, spasms. Achieve full ROM. Achieve normal strength and muscle endurance. Restore normal proprioception. Restore pain-free functional use in ADLs.
Treatment guidelines	Continue with ROM exercises PRN Increase resistive exercises for wrist and forearm Use diagonal and multiplanar exercises to increase strength and coordination Exercises for wrist stability during other UE exercises Dynamic coordination exercises
Precautions	Patient should keep wrist in slight extension during functional exercises. Progressive strengthening should not cause wrist pain. Use HEP to facilitate treatment gains.
Stage IV: Advanced phase	
5-8 weeks	**Remodeling phase: Advanced rehabilitation phase**
Goals	Perform functional activities normally. Perform performance-specific exercises normally. Return to full participation without pain and with normal motion, strength, agility, and execution of activities.
Treatment guidelines	UE plyometrics exercise progression Functional exercise progression Performance-specific exercises
Precautions	Normal function of the wrist during UE activities is with the wrist in slight extension.

AROM = active range of motion; MCL = maintain cardiovascular level; CV = cardiovascular; HEP = home exercise program; UD = ulnar deviation; RD = radial deviation; STM = soft-tissue massage; MFR = myofascial release; PRN = as needed; UE = upper extremity; ADLs = activities of daily living.

Figure 23.76   *>continued*

lateral hand (figure 23.77). De Quervain's syndrome is a tenosynovitis that affects the first dorsal compartment and involves the abductor pollicis longus and the extensor pollicis brevis. These tendons travel together in the same synovial sheath in the first dorsal compartment and pass around the bony radial styloid process, a site of friction for the tendons. The term *tenosynovitis* in this case is a bit misleading because it refers to both inflammatory and noninflammatory conditions.[151] Repetitive stress and inflammation from friction of these tendons occur with activities such as weight training and rowing or other repetitive activities where the tendons' sheath becomes irritated or damaged. The result is a thickening of the sheath, which further irritates the tendons within. The tendons react by becoming compressed and often developing nodules.[151]

As with carpal tunnel syndrome, modalities may be useful conservative treatment for relief of the pain and edema. Corticosteroid injections into the first dorsal compartment are commonly used because they have been found to offer high cure rates.[145] Rest and immobilization with a thumb spica splint places the wrist in 15° of extension with the thumb in abduction and its MCP joint in 10° flexion to put the affected tendons on slack. Although the splint is worn continually, it is removed often throughout the day so the patient can perform AROM exercises of the wrist and thumb as part of the home exercise program (figure 23.78).

Once pain and edema diminish, eccentric exercises and other muscle strengthening and endurance activities begin. The patient is gradually weaned from the splint during this phase. Pain-free gross- and fine-pinch activities, wrist and finger exercises, strengthening activities, and endurance and coordination exercises are part of the strengthening program.

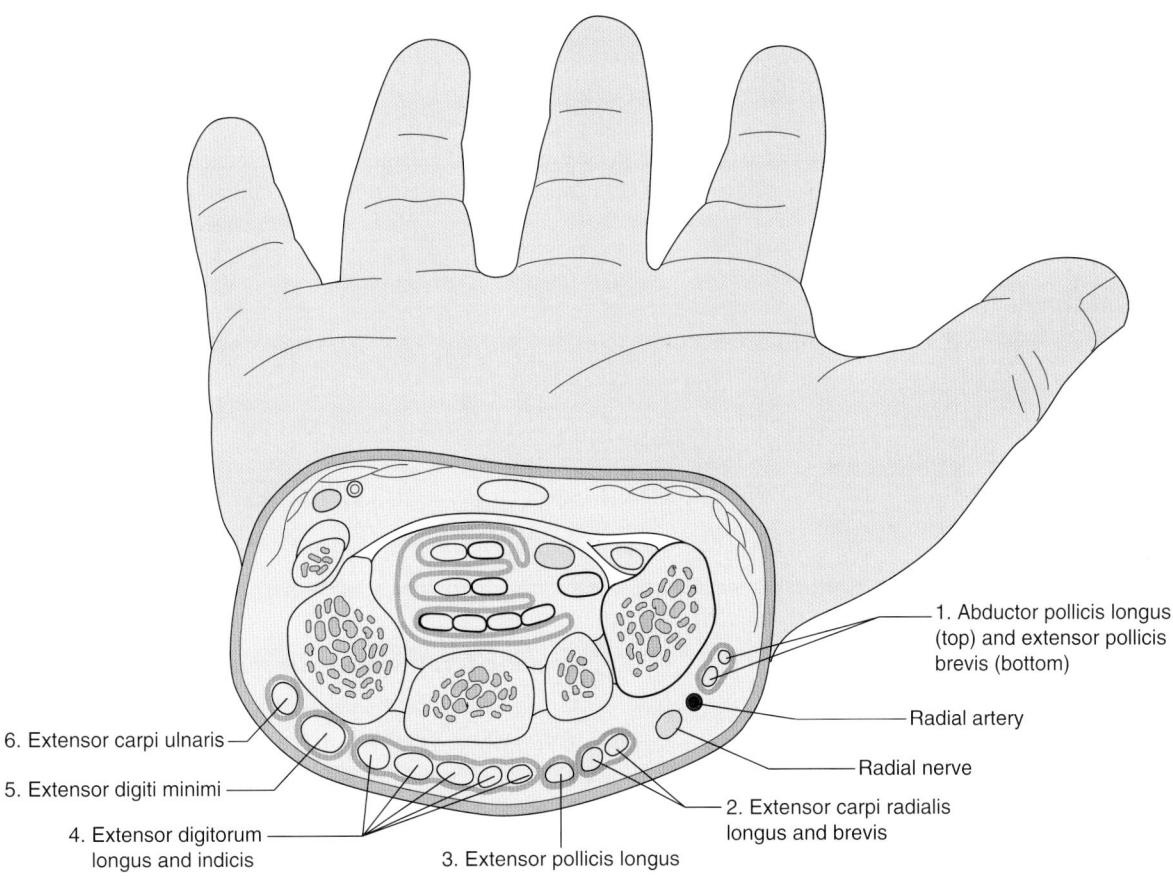

Figure 23.77   Cross-section showing extensor compartments in a right wrist.

1. Abductor pollicis longus (top) and extensor pollicis brevis (bottom)

Radial artery

Radial nerve

2. Extensor carpi radialis longus and brevis

6. Extensor carpi ulnaris

5. Extensor digiti minimi

4. Extensor digitorum longus and indicis

3. Extensor pollicis longus

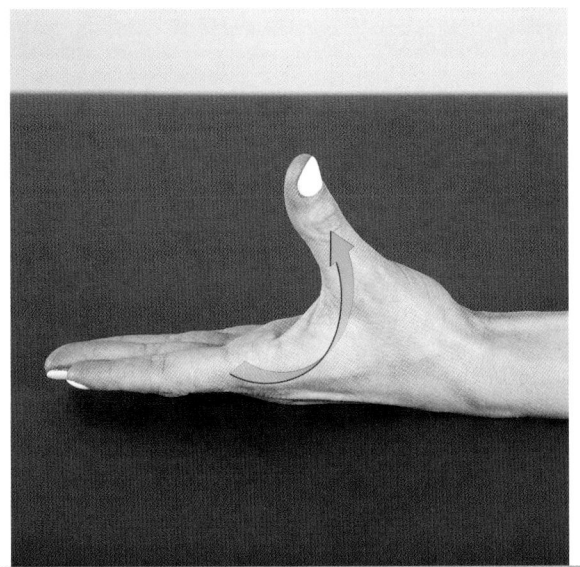

Figure 23.78   Abductor pollicis longus exercises.

In cases where conservative treatment fails to resolve the De Quervain's syndrome, surgery is performed to release the compartment sheath. AROM exercises begin 2 to 3 d after surgery to promote tendon gliding and prevent loss of motion. The wrist may be in a splint for about 1 week, but the patient removes it often during the day for AROM exercises. Pain and edema are controlled with various modalities, elevation, and active motion activities. The thumb should move in all its planes through each joint's full active motion. Exercises should also include wrist range of motion.

Once the sutures are removed and the scar is healed, scar-tissue desensitization and softening begin with light tapping on the scar and massage, respectively, as tolerated. The massage requires caution to avoid breakdown of the newly formed scar tissue; blisters or abrasions are indications that the massage is too aggressive. A strengthening exercise progression, which begins after 7 to 10 d, follows the same sequence as for other wrist injuries.

Case Study

A 24-year-old crew team member underwent a surgical release of his right nondominant first dorsal compartment 3 d ago. He has just seen the physician, who removed the surgical dressing and instructed him to begin exercising the wrist and thumb. The physician gave the patient a splint and instructed him to wear it throughout the day except during rehabilitation treatments. Some swelling and tenderness are present over the scar. The wrist has good motion, but the thumb moves 10° at the MCP joint and 30° at the IP joint. There is some tenderness to radial deviation, but the patient has full medial–lateral wrist motion.

Questions for Analysis

1. What will your treatment today include?
2. What instructions will you give the patient for home treatment?
3. What precautions must be considered?
4. What kind of ROM exercises will you give him?
5. When will you start working on strength, and what will the first strengthening exercises include?
6. What functional exercises will you advance the patient to before he returns to competition?

Long Tendon Injuries

Tendon gliding exercises have already been presented. They are important exercises to perform after any injury to the hand because adhesions to either flexor or extensor tendons cause significant loss of motion and hand function. In addition to knowing when to apply these exercises, the rehabilitation clinician must understand the differences between flexor and extensor tendons in order to apply the proper rehabilitation techniques.

Special Tendon Considerations

Although the hand's flexor and extensor tendons often work in concert with each other, they have unique differences that require variations in the rehabilitation of flexor and extensor tendon injuries. Some of the differences have already been mentioned; those differences and others are listed in table 23.5. Among the more obvious differences is the presence of the strong pulley system for the flexor tendons versus the absence of any pulleys for the exten-

TABLE 23.5 Differences Between Long Flexor and Long Extensor Hand Tendons

Characteristic	Long flexor tendons	Long extensor tendons
Pulley system	Present	Absent
Sheaths	Present throughout	Not present except at the wrist
Strength production	Greater than that of extensors	Less than that of flexors
Function	Power grips	Opening the hand
Configuration	Thick, large diameter	Thin, flatter
Risk of adhesions	Round shape creates less contact with other tissues	Flat shape creates more contact with other tissues; increases risk of adhesions
Cross section size	Larger, making repair easier	Small, making repair more difficult
Tensile strength	Greater than that of extensors	Less than that of flexors
Extensibility	Less than that of extensors	Greater than that of flexors
Relationship with intrinsic muscles	Serve as anchor for intrinsic muscles	Serve as distal insertion for intrinsic muscles
		Long extensor tendon mobility determines intrinsic muscles' ability to provide their functions in hand motions

sor tendons. Most of the length of the flexor tendons is enclosed in sheaths, but the extensor tendons are primarily extrasynovial.

Normally, finger flexion strength is much greater than finger extension strength. The hand needs more strength for activities such as grasping, propelling, and catching objects than it does for opening the hand. When an injury occurs to an extensor tendon, care must be taken to prevent the stronger flexor muscles from overpowering and causing further damage to the weakened extensor tendon.

The extensor tendons are flatter and thinner than the flexor tendons, so overall, they have less tensile strength than the flexor tendons. When the fingers flex into the palm, the extensor tendons undergo significant lengthening. Both the lengthening and the relative lack of strength make the extensor tendon susceptible to stretch or rupture, especially when weakened by injury.

Although the extensor tendons are not surrounded by tendon sheaths like the flexor tendons, both groups are at risk of forming adhesions when immobilized.[152] However, a loss of extension motion can be more functionally debilitating than a loss of flexion motion.[153] Because of the intricate relationship between the extensor tendons and the intrinsic muscles, a loss of mobility of the extensor tendons can have a significant impact on the function of the interossei and lumbricals and can hamper the intrinsic and extrinsic muscle balance needed for normal hand function.[7]

Tendon ruptures and lacerations are common tendon injuries of the hand, although they are not common in sports.[154] Extensor tendon injuries are more common than flexor tendon injuries.[154] In sports, tendon ruptures usually result from impact avulsions such as those that occur when the end of a player's finger is hit with an object like a baseball bat, a baseball, or a basketball.[155] Lacerations can result from cleats, contact with sharp objects hidden in the grass, accidents in archery, and many other activities; lacerations can cause partial or full tendon disruptions.

The timing of accurate diagnosis and rehabilitation is crucial to a successful rehabilitation outcome.[156] Careful application of rehabilitative techniques is important to achieving desired results. Recent advances in rehabilitation after tendon repair have improved surgical results and reduced the risk of tendon adhesions.[157, 158]

One of the major concerns after tendon repair surgery is tendon adhesions to surrounding soft-tissue structures.[159] New approaches to postoperative tendon repair include the use of early controlled motion during the first weeks after surgery rather than the more traditional 3 weeks or more of immobilization.[160] Because of the relative fragility of extensor tendons, early controlled motion was first used primarily with flexor but not extensor tendon injuries; however, more recently, early controlled motion has proven successful with extensor tendon injuries as well.[10] Investigators now believe that early controlled motion is helpful

for both flexor and extensor hand tendons;[161] however, there is a fine balance between the proper amount of motion for tendon gliding and too much motion, which can elongate or rupture fragile healing tissues.[159] Clinicians must progress their patients carefully and pay close attention to treatment results. Because the hand is so complex and so important to normal daily functions, rehabilitation clinicians should never hesitate to refer a patient to a hand specialist when appropriate.

Early controlled motion includes a careful balance of movement of the repaired tendon that reduces motion loss without harming the surgical repair; the initial goal of early motion is to promote tendon gliding and good tendon healing simultaneously. The ultimate goal is to produce a good surgical and rehabilitative result. Areas of the hand, such as no man's land, that were once approached with caution because of poor surgical results can now be successfully repaired and returned to optimal function using early controlled motion.

With early controlled motion, a splint is applied about 3 d after surgery.[162] The splint is designed by an orthotist, occupational therapist, or certified hand therapist; it limits flexion if an extensor tendon has been repaired and limits extension if a flexor tendon has been repaired. The splint includes a passive elastic force that pulls the fingers passively in the direction of the repaired tendon's pull. For example, a flexor tendon repair is placed in a dorsal splint with the wrist in about 20° of flexion, the MPs in about 40° to 50° of flexion, and the IPs in extension. An elastic system is attached to the distal finger to pull the digit passively into flexion to minimize stress on the newly repaired flexor tendon (figure 23.12). In these splints, the tension of the rubber band should permit passive flexion or extension of the digits yet not be so strong that it promotes a contracture with tension that is too much for the opposing tendon to overcome.

Tendon gliding and careful avoidance of adhesions are the primary concerns during the early stages of postoperative rehabilitation of tendon repairs.[158, 159] Extensor tendon repairs present the additional risk that extensor lag may develop.[159] This can happen if the patient begins active extension exercises too soon or is too aggressive with them in later rehabilitation; an extensor lag occurs because the repaired site breaks down, or dehisces, from excessive stress being applied to it, so the tendon elongates. The rehabilitation clinician must be aware of these potential problems and provide good care while protecting against them.

Joint mobility must be assessed for the presence of these potentially debilitating conditions. You must distinguish between capsular restriction and tendon adhesions when the patient's motion is less than normal. One way to do this is to examine the digit's ROM at the individual joints and the quantity of motion with all joints involved.

Case Study

A 16-year-old softball catcher suffered a mallet deformity of her dominant right-hand ring finger in a game 3 weeks ago. It has been in a splint for the past 3 weeks. The doctor wants the patient to begin active exercises today and wants her to continue to wear the splint, removing it only for her treatments and to take showers. Your initial examination reveals the following ring-finger flexion and extension measurements: MCP 90°/0°, PIP 90°/0°, DIP 15°/10° from extension. When the patient simultaneously extends the wrist and finger, the DIP lacks 30° of extension. Grip strength measures 13.6 kg (30 lb) on the right and 34 kg (75 lb) on the left. Wrist extension is 4/5. Both ulnar and radial deviations have normal motion and strength. Wrist flexion is 4/5, finger flexion is 4/5, MCP extension is 4−/5, and finger abduction is 4−/5.

Questions for Analysis

1. How will you determine if the DIP's lack of extension is because of capsule tightness, adhesions of the tendon, weakness of the extensor tendon, or dehiscing of the injured extensor tendon?

2. What instructions will you give the patient for home exercises?

3. What precautions must you consider in her treatments?

4. What determining factors will you use to decide when she should begin her strengthening exercises? Provide a rationale for your answer.

5. List three strengthening exercises, and explain why you have selected them.

6. Identify three functional exercises, and indicate your guidelines for beginning them.

For example, if the patient can fully extend the wrist and MCP, PIP, and DIP joints of the digit one at a time when the other digit's joints are positioned in flexion, but the patient cannot fully extend the joints all at once, the joint capsules have good mobility, but the long tendon being stretched is likely restricted.

Full active extension must also be assessed once it is permitted. If the patient has normal passive motion but cannot fully extend the digit, either the muscle is weak or the tendon repair is elongating. Tissue elongation means the new tissue is stretching beyond desired lengths (dehiscing). This is likely the problem if the patient had full active extension earlier in the rehabilitation program but now cannot achieve it. Tendon dehiscing must be corrected using a continually worn splint with no active motion allowed for 2 weeks until enough scarring occurs to stabilize the surgical site.[163]

Once sutures are removed, scar-tissue management and desensitization begin with light tapping, touching, and later, massage of the hypersensitive area. The patient is also instructed to perform these techniques often throughout the day. Since the tendons lie so close to the surface, self-massage is easy to perform and will help reduce the risk of tendon adhesions.

When to begin strengthening exercises for repaired tendons varies widely and depends, to a large extent, on the zone in which the injury repair occurs and whether it is a flexor or extensor tendon.[14] Strength exercises are initially light strengthening exercises, starting anywhere from 4 to 8 weeks postoperatively.[153, 162]

Patients with long flexor or extensor tendon injuries, especially lacerations or ruptures, are referred to certified hand specialists, both in the surgical field and in rehabilitation. The hand is the most complicated segment of the body.[59] It also has very complex functions.[164] As has been mentioned, the trimuscular components—the long flexor muscles, long extensor muscles, and intrinsic muscles—must all work together to create those functions. If they or any of the joints do not work properly, the hand cannot function normally. Therefore, when serious injuries affecting hand function occur, it is best to refer patients to experts who deal with these injuries routinely. The rehabilitation clinician in the sports medicine setting, however, can play a crucial role in ensuring a successful outcome by understanding the principles presented here, monitoring patient compliance, coordinating care, providing supplemental care, and communicating with the specialists on patient progress and performance.

Summary

Just as the scapula stabilizes the shoulder joint, the wrist is an important stabilizer for hand function. The hand's normal function depends on a fine balance of the three elements that move the hand and fingers: the long finger flexors, long finger extensors, and intrinsic muscle groups. If one of these is compromised by injury, the hand will not function as it should. The hand has various power and pinch grips that allow it to conform around and operate any object that is placed in it.

Because of all the soft-tissue structures and joints in the wrist and hand, any number of injuries may occur. When the hand is injured, edema must be treated efficiently and effectively. Likewise, the clinician must understand the deleterious effects of immobilization and must try to avoid stiffness after injury whenever possible. With a hand injury, especially one that requires immobilization, clinicians must ensure that tendons can continue to glide within the hand and digits. Specific exercises can help to preserve this gliding function. Soft-tissue mobilization, joint mobilization techniques, desensitization exercises, and progressive exercises from flexibility to functional activities were discussed in this chapter. Some of the more common injuries of the hand and wrist were presented along with rehabilitation programs for them.

LEARNING AIDS

Key Concepts and Review

1. Explain the pulley system of the fingers.

There is an elaborate pulley system on the flexor aspect of the fingers that extends from the metacarpal head of each digit to the insertion of the distal finger flexor tendons. These pulleys are similar to the hoops along a fishing rod, positioned to keep the fishing line in place as it travels along the pole. There are five annular pulleys and three cruciate pulleys along each finger. Disruption of key pulleys can cause bowstringing of the flexor tendons. The key pulleys preventing bowstringing are A2 and A4. When the pulley system of any finger is disrupted, the mechanical advantage of the tendon is impaired, and normal function is lost.

2. Explain why reducing edema in the hand is important.

Because the dorsal skin is loose and pliable compared to the volar skin, edema often accumulates in the dorsum of the hand. Pooled edema rich in proteins easily leads to contractures. Excessive swelling on the back of the hand can cause the hand arches to collapse anteriorly and can adduct the thumb. Excessive swelling also stretches the dorsal skin and pushes it away from the dorsal hand as fluid enters the area, limiting the hand's ability to move the fingers through their full flexion motion. Fibrous tissue formation secondary to the presence of prolonged edema results in reduced mobility and function in the hand.

3. Discuss the trimuscular system of the hand.

Three muscle groups compose the trimuscular system of the hand—the extrinsic flexors, the extrinsic extensors, and the intrinsic muscles—and provide for balanced, controlled hand function. If any of these groups cannot function normally, because of either weakness or loss of mobility, balance is lost, and the hand cannot perform its normal functions.

4. Identify and explain the importance of the precision pinches and power grips of the hand.

The power grips, also known as palmar grips, include the clenched fist, the cylinder grasp, the spherical grasp, and the hook grasp. In these grasps, the thumb is positioned in opposition to the other fingers to permit a firm grasp on an object. The hook grasp is the only power grip that does not involve the thumb. Most daily hand activities involve these palmar grips. Because palmar grasping is so vital to hand function, the hand is most commonly splinted in a palmar position with the thumb in slight opposition, facing the other fingers. The precision or prehensile grips include the digital prehension grip (three-jaw chuck), the lateral prehension grip, and the tip-to-tip prehension grip. These movements include fine-tuned activities such as typing, sewing, or writing. These prehensile activities occur when the thumb and finger muscles co-contract to produce an activity requiring precision.

5. Explain the difference between static and dynamic splints.

Overall, the aim of splints is either to prevent damage and maintain balance or to improve balance. Static splints restrict motion to support and protect the hand. Dynamic splints are used to increase the motion of the hand or to help it perform motion. Splints are based on a three-point pressure system in which two points of application are on one side of the hand, wrist, or forearm and the other point of application is on the opposite side.

6. Identify what motion increases with carpal radial glide joint mobilization.

A carpal radial glide improves ulnar deviation of the wrist.

7. Explain the force application sequence for improving long finger flexor and extensor motion.

The basic application sequence is the same for flexors and extensors but in opposite directions. If a long extensor tendon has limited flexion motion, the proximal joint is stabilized as the distal joint (DIP) is moved into flexion; then the PIP joint is moved into flexion as the MCP joint is stabilized while the DIP's flexed position is maintained. The MCP joint is then moved into flexion as the wrist is stabilized and the IP joints are kept in their flexion positions. Finally, the wrist is gradually moved into flexion. The stretch should be performed in both elbow flexion and elbow extension and the forces applied gradually until the patient feels a stretch in the forearm.

8. Explain how the hand and finger positions for intrinsic stretches differ from those for the extrinsic stretches.

Because the lumbricals and interossei flex the MCP joints and extend the IP joints, the stretch is applied in the opposite direction of their function or direction of motion. The IP joints are held in a flexed position while a stretch is applied to increase MCP extension. The wrist should be stabilized in neutral during this activity to prevent extrinsic muscle influences on the stretch.

9. Discuss the differences in gliding exercises for the flexor profundus and superficialis tendons.

Three exercises for flexor tendon gliding include (1) keeping the MCP extended and flexing the IPs to enhance gliding between the two longer finger flexor tendons, (2) forming a fist with the IP and MCP joints in flexion to produce gliding of the profundus tendons within their sheaths, and (3) positioning the MCP and PIP joints in flexion and extending the DIP joints to produce gliding of the superficialis tendons within their sheaths. Flexor pollicis longus gliding exercises are performed in a similar manner by moving the IP and MCP joints through a full range of flexion and extension. These exercises are initially performed with the wrist in neutral, but as the patient progresses, the wrist should be moved into flexion with finger flexion and into extension with finger extension. A gliding exercise for the EDC is performed by moving the hand from a hook to a fist. The MCP joint is moved from flexion to extension, while the IP joints are kept in flexion to eliminate the intrinsic muscles. If the patient has difficulty maintaining flexion of the IP joints during this activity, he or she can grasp a drinking straw or pencil in the fingers while moving the MCP joints. Wrist flexion and extension should also be added to the exercise when the patient can perform it with the wrist in neutral.

10. Present the differences between long flexor and long extensor tendons.

One of the more obvious differences is the presence of a strong pulley system for the flexor tendons versus the absence of any pulleys for the extensor tendons. Most of the length of the flexor tendons is enclosed in sheaths, but the extensor tendons are primarily extrasynovial except at the wrist. Finger flexion strength is significantly greater than finger extension strength. The extensor tendons are flatter and thinner than the flexor tendons; for this reason they have less overall tensile strength than the flexor tendons, and they are more prone to adhesions. When the fingers close into the palm, the extensor tendons undergo significant lengthening. Because the flexor tendons are mostly enclosed in tendon sheaths, immobilization creates a risk of adhesion formation and loss of glide. Loss of extensor motion can be more functionally debilitating than loss of flexion motion.

11. Explain what procedures could be used to identify the cause of an extensor lag of a distal phalanx.

An extensor lag could be caused by tightness in the DIP capsule, scar tissue adhesions of the long extensor tendon, weakness of the extensor digitorum, or dehiscing on the healing extensor tendon. If the patient can fully extend the wrist and MCP, PIP, and DIP joints of the digit one at a time when the other digits' joints are positioned in flexion, but cannot fully extend the joints all at once, the joint capsules have good mobility but the long tendon is likely restricted. If the patient has normal passive motion but cannot fully extend the digit, either the muscle is weak or the injured tendon is elongating. If the patient could fully extend the joint earlier but loses that ability as the exercises continue, the healing tendon is dehiscing.

Critical Thinking Questions

1. If a patient suffers a scaphoid fracture, how long would you expect him or her to complain of pain? If the wrist pain continues for several weeks beyond your expectations, what would you suspect is the reason? What would you do in this situation?

2. In the opening scenario, what test did Peg use to determine that adhesions were forming between the flexor digitorum superficialis and profundus? What techniques would you use to reduce these adhesions? If Peg instructs John to develop exercises for Beverly's home program to help create more mobility between the tissues, what exercises should John include? How would the adhesions interfere with hand function by affecting the intrinsic muscles?

3. A mallet finger injury is removed from the splint and demonstrates full active extension. Three weeks after her rehabilitation program started, the patient cannot fully extend the DIP actively. What would you suspect is the cause? How would you remedy the situation to restore active extension?

Lab Activities

1. Locate the trigger point for the adductor pollicis on your lab partner. Provide your partner with a home exercise for the tender trigger point.

2. Perform the following joint mobilizations on your lab partner, and identify what restrictions are best treated with each mobilization:

    A. Distal radioulnar joint
    - Dorsal glide of radius
    - Ventral glide of radius

    B. Radiocarpal joint
    - Distraction
    - AP glides
    - PA glides
    - Lateral glides

    C. MCP and IP joints
    - Distraction
    - Rotation
    - AP glides
    - PA glides

3. Examine your partner's finger motion using all of the tendon gliding exercises. Identify which structure each motion assesses.

4. Instruct your partner in the flexor tendon gliding exercises, and have him perform 10 of each. Instruct your partner in the intrinsic gliding exercises, and have him perform 10 of each. What are the differences in how each of the exercises feels as they are being performed?

5. Demonstrate how you would apply a stretch to the lumbricals. What are the key factors you need to consider in positioning for this stretch? Why?

6. List two exercises you would give a patient to strengthen the finger extensors. Identify the purpose of each exercise and when in the rehabilitation program they could be added.

7. List two strengthening exercises for the finger flexors, and identify a progression for each of them. What would be your criteria for advancing a patient from one level of an exercise to another?

8. List three strengthening exercises for the intrinsic muscles of the hand, and identify the substitution patterns you need to watch for during the patient's performance of each exercise.

9. A softball left fielder is recovering from a second-degree PIP sprain of the third finger. List three performance-specific exercises you would have her perform before she returns to full participation. Give the rationale for your selections.

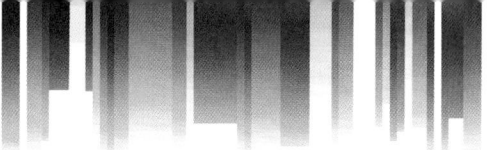

GLOSSARY

A-band—The portion of the sarcomere where the thick filaments inter-digitate with the thin filaments.

ABCs of proprioception—Agility, balance, and coordination.

abdominal bracing—An exercise in which the abdominal and back muscles are activated to co-contract to provide stability. This exercise facilitates the transverse abdominis and oblique muscles and is thought to provide better stability than abdominal hollowing.

abdominal hollowing—An exercise in which the abdomen is drawn in toward the spine to facilitate the transverse abdominis and multifidus muscles. The exercise is used to improve core stability through the activation of the transverse abdominis and multifidus muscles.

abduction—Lateral movement of a limb or segment away from the midline of the body or part.

absolute refractory period—The time immediately following a stimulus when depolarization prevents another response of the muscle cell from occurring.

acceleration—Rate at which velocity increases.

acceleration phase—That portion of swing in which momentum is increased and the non-weight-bearing limb has propulsion forward. Also known as *early swing*.

accessory joint motion—Necessary mobility for normal joint motion that cannot be voluntarily performed or controlled.

accommodating resistance—An activity where the resistance provided to a muscle changes as the muscle moves through its range of motion. Isokinetic activity.

acetabulum—The socket portion of the hip joint.

acetylcholine—A neurotransmitter at the myoneural junction of striated muscles. Causes vasodilation.

actin—One of two primary proteins of the thin filament of the sarcomere.

action peak—The second ground reaction force peak. The peak occurs during the last half of support and is usually less than impact peak.

action potential—A brief nerve impulse created from a rapid change in the electrical membrane potential on a nerve or muscle cell's surface to cause a nerve to reverse its polarity or a muscle cell to contract.

active-assistive range of motion (AAROM)—Range of motion that is performed with a combination of voluntary activity of the muscles and passive assistance from an outside source.

active insufficiency—The situation that occurs when a multiple-joint muscle actively contracts to its shortest position but the joints it crosses still have available motion.

active range of motion (AROM)—The amount of movement produced at a joint by the patient without assistance.

active stretch—A stretch that uses the patient's active muscle force to control and provide the force for the stretch.

active trigger point—A trigger point that is always tender and that can produce referred pain whether the muscle is active or inactive.

activities of daily living—Routine tasks required to independently care for oneself. For example, bathing, grooming, dressing, eating, and typical household chores.

activity-specific exercises—Exercises that include drills or that mimic tasks found within a specific sport or job. They are used in the final phase of the rehabilitation program to prepare the patient for return to his or her normal functions. See also *performance-specific exercises.*

adduction—Lateral movement of a limb or segment toward the midline of the body or part.

adenosine diphosphate (ADP)—A phosphate compound that, when combined with a phosphate, forms adenosine triphosphate (ATP) for energy production. It is also the product of the breakdown of ATP during energy production.

adenosine triphosphate (ATP)—A phosphate compound that provides energy for muscle activity.

adhesive capsulitis—A condition that generally occurs in the glenohumeral joint. Inflammation within the joint's capsule causes capsular wall thickening and adherence. Loss of motion in the joint results. Also known as *frozen shoulder.*

adrenaline—See *epinephrine.*

afferent muscle nerve fiber—A sensory nerve fiber from the muscle spindle and Golgi tendon organ. There are two primary types, A and C fibers. C fibers are pain receptors; A fibers are tension and length receptors. Group III delta are A receptors that respond to pressure pain. Group I are A receptors: Group Ia form muscle spindle primary endings and Group Ib form Golgi tendon organs. Group II are A receptors and form muscle spindle secondary endings.

afferent receptors—Sensory receptors that transmit information from the periphery to the central nervous system.

agility—The ability to control the direction of a body or its parts during rapid movement.

agonist(ic)—A muscle acting as a prime mover to produce a motion.

allogenic graft—A graft taken from one person and transplanted into another.

all-or-none principle—A motor unit does not respond until the stimulus is sufficient to produce an action potential. The action potential produces a reaction from the entire motor unit.

alpha motor neuron—An efferent nerve from the ventral horn of the spinal cord to the muscle.

AMBRI—**A**traumatic, **m**ultidirectional, **b**ilateral, **r**ehabilitation effective, **i**nferior capsular shift required. A condition of non-traumatic shoulder instability that is multidirectional but usually responds well to the conservative treatment of rehabilitation.

amortization phase—The second phase of a plyometric activity that is the rapid transition from eccentric to concentric motion.

angiogenesis—Formation of new blood vessels.

angle of progression—As a person walks, an angle of the foot placement occurs to the straight line of the body's forward progression. This angle, then, is created between the straight line of the direction in which a person walks and the line bisecting the foot from the heel to the mid-forefoot (between the second and third toes). Normal angle in adults is about 7°.

angle of pull—Angle formed by the muscle's line of pull and the line of the bone. Maximal isometric force occurs at a 90° angle of pull.

angular motion—Rotational movement on an axis through an arc.

antagonist(ic)—A muscle that opposes the motion of another muscle.

anteversion—Excessive anterior angulation of the femoral head, resulting in a toe-in gait.

apophysis—An outgrowth of bone where a tendon attaches, not fully formed in immature bones.

arachidonic acid—An unsaturated essential fatty acid. Works as a precursor in the production of substances, including leukotrienes, prostaglandins, and thromboxanes.

Archimedes' principle of buoyancy—Principle stating that a body partially or fully immersed in a fluid will experience an upward thrust of that fluid that is equal to the weight of the fluid the body displaces.

areolar (loose or irregular) connective tissue—Loose connective tissue with unorganized structure and relatively long distances between cross-links.

arthrogenic muscle inhibition (AMI)—Reflex inhibition of muscle activity following injury. It is thought to be a protective mechanism for the joint to reduce excessive stresses that could be applied by strong muscles surrounding the joint. Most often, AMI is discussed as it relates to quadriceps inhibition following knee joint injury.

arthrokinematics—The motions between the bones that make up a joint, including roll, slide, spin, compression, and distraction.

arthroplasty—Joint replacement surgery.

arthroscopy—Use of an endoscope to examine or surgically treat the interior aspect of a joint.

assessment—A conclusion based on the gathering of information through the clinician's judgment and abilities to assimilate the information from the examination, the medical record, and the patient's signs and symptoms to reach a clinical diagnosis.

ATPase (adenosine triphosphatase)—Myosin enzyme that is a catalyst the body uses to break down ATP into ADP and phosphate for energy production.

atrophy—Wasting away of tissue with a decrease in size and strength, especially from lack of use.

autogenic inhibition—A protective mechanism provided by the Golgi tendon organ, in which a Golgi tendon organ stimulus facilitated by a sudden stretch causes a reflex activation of the antagonist and relaxation of the agonist.

autologous graft—A graft of articular cartilage and bone plug that is taken from the same joint as the damaged cartilage, but it is removed from a part of the joint that does not bear weight.

balance—The body's ability to maintain an equilibrium by controlling the body's center of gravity over its base of support.

ballistic stretching—A rapid stretch or bouncing technique used primarily in sport activities but seldom used in rehabilitation because of the increased risk of injury.

Bankart lesion—Tear of the capsulolabral complex from the glenoid rim.

barrier—A resistance that is felt when a part is moved through its passive range of motion in muscle energy techniques.

Barton's fracture—A fracture of the wrist that occurs with a sudden, violent wrist extension and pronation.

base of support—Two-dimensional area that lies within the points of contact between an object and the supporting surface.

basophil—See *granular leukocyte*.

beat frequency—The net difference between the two interfering currents at any one time during an interferential electrical stimulation treatment.

Bennett's fracture—A fracture of the first metacarpal.

body mechanics—The way the body is positioned and used during activity; correct body mechanics makes efficient use of the body's forces and lever systems.

boutonniere deformity—Deformity characterized by flexion of the PIP joint and hyperextension of the DIP joint.

bowstringing—When the pulley system holding the tendon in place ruptures so the tendon is no longer in proximity to the bone and displays an appearance similar to that of an archer's bowstring.

boxer's fracture—Fracture of the metacarpals secondary to a compressive force.

bradykinin—A local tissue hormone that is activated by the interaction of proteases upon the Hageman factor. A very potent local vasodilator. It increases vascular permeability and stimulates local pain receptors.

brain stem—Includes the midbrain, pons, medulla oblongata, and diencephalon to form the stem of the brain between the spinal cord and cerebrum.

Brannock measuring device—Used to determine shoe size (length and width).

bunion—See *hallux valgus*.

bursa—Synovial fluid–filled membrane that lies between adjacent structures to limit friction and ease movement.

bursitis—Inflammation or swelling of a bursa.

callus—Fibrous matrix formed at a bone's fractured sites. Immobilizes the bone fragments and serves as the foundation for eventual bone replacement.

capsular pattern—A characteristic pattern of motion unique to each joint when a loss of motion is caused by capsular tightness.

carpal tunnel syndrome—A condition of the wrist and hand characterized by compression of the median nerve as it passes through the carpal tunnel.

cavitation—Cavities form in a joint's synovial fluid when tension is applied to the joint. These bubbles have lower pressure than the surrounding fluid and collapse with sudden movement, making a cracking or popping noise.

center of buoyancy—The center of gravity of the fluid displaced by a body in water and the point at which the buoyant force acts on the body.

center of gravity—The point on an object around which its weight is balanced.

center of mass—The point around which the mass of an object is centered or evenly distributed. Also known as the *center of gravity*.

central nervous system (CNS)—The brain and spinal cord comprise the central nervous system.

cerebellum—That section of the brain that lies below the posterior cerebrum and behind the brain stem and is connected to the brain stem by paired peduncles.

cerebral cortex—The surface of the brain that contains primarily gray matter and nerve cell bodies.

cerebrum—The largest portion of the brain encompassing most of the skull.

chemoattractant—See *chemotactic factor.*

chemokines—Chemotactic cytokines that are secreted by a number of cells in a wound such as endothelium, fibroblasts, keratinocytes, neutrophils, and macrophages. They are primarily involved in preventing angiogenesis during clot formation and remodeling phases but promoting angiogenesis during inflammation and proliferation phases.

chemotactic factor—A chemical gradient. Also referred to as a *chemotactin* or *chemoattractant.* Occurs after an injury. Cells either become oriented along a chemical concentration gradient or move in the direction of that gradient. Example: Chemicals attract platelets, red blood cells, and polymorphonuclear leukocytes into an injured area.

chemotactin—See *chemotactic factor.*

chemotaxis—Movement of cells or chemicals in response to a chemical stimulus. Vital activities in wound healing that occur through complex and not totally understood processes.

claw toes—Toes that are extended at the metatarsophalangeal joints and flexed at the proximal and distal interphalangeal joints.

closed kinetic chain (CKC)—Characterizing a motion in which the distal segment of an extremity is weight bearing and the body moves over the hand or foot.

close-packed position—The joint position in which the joint surfaces are most congruent with each other.

code of ethics—A group's set of standards of conduct that are based on the values and principles the group and its members are expected to uphold.

Codman's exercises—Low-level passive flexibility exercises for the shoulder that are performed by the patient. Also known as *pendulum exercises.*

cogwheel resistance—An abnormal response during muscle testing that is observed as a series of catch-and-release tensions rather than a smooth resistance, indicative of the person's providing a less-than-maximal effort.

collagen—Major structure of the body's protein. There are five types in the body: Type I, the most abundant type, is high in tensile strength and is found in dermis, fascia, and bone; Type II is found in cartilage; Type III is found in embryonic connective tissue; Types IV and V are found in basement membranes. Forms inelastic bundles to provide structure, integrity, and tensile strength to tissues.

collagenase—An enzyme produced by newly formed epithelial cells and fibroblasts. Involved in the degradation of collagen during tissue repair. It is important in controlling the collagen content in a wound.

collar—The top rim of the shoe that is often padded to reduce friction on the Achilles.

Colles' fracture—A fracture in which the distal radius proximal to the wrist is fractured and is displaced dorsally.

common pathway—One of three pathways of the coagulation system. It consists of the cascade of activation of clotting factors that ultimately cleave thrombin from prothrombin to form a stable clot.

comorbidity—The simultaneous presence of two or more morbid conditions or diseases in the same person.

comparable sign—A sign produced by an active or passive movement or test that reproduces a patient's symptom, such as pain or protective muscle spasm.

compartment syndrome—A significant rise in intracompartmental pressure caused by severe bleeding within a muscular compartment that can compromise neurovascular structures.

complement cascade—Specific proteins interacting with one another in a specific sequence.

complement system—Various proteins found in serum. Act as chemotactic factors for neutrophils and phagocytosis.

compliance—Tissue's ability to tolerate stress application without suffering permanent deformation when the stress is removed. The opposite of stiffness.

component motion—Movement occurring within a joint during range of motion but is not controlled voluntarily. If component motion is restricted, full joint motion is not possible. An example is the clavicle's posterior rotation, which occurs with shoulder flexion.

concave-on-convex rule—Roll and slide occur in the same direction when a concave surface moves on a convex surface. Also called the *concave–convex rule.*

concentric motion—Dynamic activity in which the muscle shortens.

concentric phase—The third phase of a plyometric activity, resulting from the combined eccentric and amortization phases. The concentric phase is the outcome phase. If the eccentric activity has been quickly performed and the amortization has occurred rapidly, the concentric phase will produce the desired powerful outcome.

contact pressure—Pressure that occurs between two objects in contact with each other.

contractile components—Myofibrils, the portion of a muscle that actively shortens to produce movement.

contractility—The ability of a muscle fiber to contract.

contraction phase—That part of the mechanical response of a muscle twitch that follows the latency period during which the sarcomere's actin and myosin cross-bridge activity occurs.

contracture—Failure of a muscle to relax. Can occur after fatigue.

contraindication—Use of a treatment or technique is not advised because it may result in deleterious effects in the presence of the noted signs, symptoms, conditions, or situations.

convex-on-concave rule—Roll and slide occur in opposite directions when a convex surface moves on a concave surface. Also called the *convex–concave rule*.

coordination—The ability of muscles and muscle groups to perform complicated movements.

core stabilization—See *pelvic stabilization or stability*.

counternutation—Movement of the sacrum when the superior base moves posteriorly as the distal sacrum and coccyx move anteriorly. During counternutation, the iliac crests move apart and the ischial tuberosities move closer together. Opposite of nutation.

coupled motions—Movements that occur when a motion in one plane must occur with an associated motion in another plane for normal range of motion to be present.

coxa saltans—Medical term for snapping hip.

coxa valga—Femoral neck angulation greater than 135°.

coxa vara—Femoral neck angulation less than 120°.

c-proteins—Protein bands that surround myosin filaments at regular intervals. It is thought that their role is to regulate the thickness of myosin filaments during myofibril development and play a role in muscle contraction. Also known as MyBP-C or protein C.

creep—Permanent tissue elongation caused by low-level stress applied over an extended period.

crepitus—A cracking or grating sound or sensation caused by inflammation or degenerative changes.

cross-bridges—The "head" projections from the myosin filaments that link the thick filaments to the thin filaments through a complex process.

cross-training—A process in which exercising the contralateral body part results in strength gains in the opposite extremity.

cross-training shoes—These are shoes designed to meet the needs of individuals involved in multiple activities. However, these shoes usually do not meet any specific need.

cryotherapy—An umbrella term for any cold modality.

cycle time—In running, the time it takes to perform one step length. Also known as *stride time*.

cytokines—An enzyme produced by newly formed epithelial cells and fibroblasts.

De Quervain's disease—Tenosynovitis of the abductor pollicis longus and extensor pollicis brevis tendons and their sheaths on the radial side of the thumb.

deceleration—Negative acceleration.

deceleration phase—That portion of swing in which the limb slows down in preparation for making initial contact with the ground. Also known as *late swing*.

dense irregular connective tissue—Connective tissue consisting of collagen fibers arranged in a haphazard or disarrayed alignment.

dense regular connective tissue—Connective tissue with highly organized, parallel collagen fibers and more cross-links than loose connective tissue.

depression—A downward movement of the scapula.

differential diagnosis—A list of potential diagnoses that have similar signs and symptoms but differ in specific ways from the presenting injury or illness. The clinician identifies potential diagnoses then eliminates each possibility by comparing the specific findings to these diagnoses' characteristics to ascertain the correct diagnosis.

direct techniques—Manual therapy techniques that load or bind tissue and structures, moving toward the point of limitation of mobility.

disability—According to Nagi's disablement model, it is behavior that is impaired or less than normal and occurs as a result of functional limitations that are imposed upon the person through pathology. The domino effect that ends with disability begins with pathology; see impairment.

disablement model—A system that provides common terminology by which an individual's disability based on clinical diagnosis, rehabilitation, laws, limitations, impairments, and societal function may be identified.

dislocation—Complete disassociation or displacement of one joint surface on another.

dorsiflexion—The sagittal plane movement in which the ankle joint angle is decreased as the dorsal foot is moved upward toward the anterior surface of the lower leg.

double-crush syndrome—A condition in which an injury at one site produces signs and symptoms at another site.

double float—The nonsupport phase in a running stride.

double-limb support—The point of the gait cycle that occurs at the beginning of the stance phase during heel strike for one leg and the end of the stance phase just before toe-off for the other.

downward rotation—A movement of the scapula that causes the glenoid to face downward and backward. The inferior angle of the scapula moves medially, and the scapula slides backward.

drag—The water's resistance to a body moving through it. There are three types of drag: form drag, wave drag, and frictional drag.

drug interaction—A reaction in which one drug either enhances or reduces the effectiveness of other drugs that are also being taken.

duration of drug action—Amount of time the blood level of a drug is at or above the level needed to obtain a minimum therapeutic effect. Determined by the drug's half-life.

dynamic activity—Activity in which movement occurs.

dynamic restraint—One of two systems a joint has for its stability. Dynamic restraints are the neuromuscular components that provide movement.

dynamic splint—Splint used to increase motion or limit unwanted activity. It incorporates springs, rubber bands, or other elastic elements to provide a continual low-grade passive stretch, passive assistive motion, or active-assistive motion to an area.

dynamic stretching—A rhythmic, controlled, and smooth motion from a neutral position to an extreme end of a movement and then either back to the start position or to the other extreme of movement within a plane of motion.

dynamometer—A device used to measure strength.

eccentric motion—A dynamic activity in which the muscle lengthens.

eccentric phase—The first phase of a plyometric activity during which the muscle is pre-stretched as it actively lengthens in preparation for performing the activity. The slack is taken out of the muscle, and its elastic components are put on stretch.

early swing—The first part of the swing phase of gait.

eddy—Circular motion of water layers pulling against a moving object.

elasticity—An object's ability to return to normal shape or size after a deforming force is applied.

elastin—An essential protein of connective-tissue elastic structures. Arranged in a wavy orientation. The wavy arrangement allows tissue to change with stress and to resume normal conditions after stress removal. It plays an unknown role in the remodeling phase.

electrothermally assisted capsular shift—A rather recently developed arthroscopic procedure used in the shoulder to reduce joint laxity.

elevation—An upward movement of the scapula.

end-feel—The nature of resistance that is felt at the end of joint movement.

endomysium—Connective-tissue layer covering a muscle fiber and continuous with the muscle fiber's membrane.

endotenon—Tissue, continuous with the epitenon, that extends itself between the collagen bundles in a tendon.

endothelial cells—Large, flat cells that line blood and lymphatic vessels.

endothelial leukocyte—A large white blood cell that circulates in the bloodstream and tissues. Acts as a phagocyte to remove debris from an injured area.

endurance limit—See *fatigue failure.*

energy—The capacity to do work.

engram—A memory trace of an activity accomplished through repetitive application of stimuli.

eosinophil—See *granular leukocyte.*

epicondylalgia—An overuse injury of the elbow that displays with signs and symptoms that include pain over the epicondyle with gripping tasks. See also *epicondylopathy.*

epicondylopathy—An overuse injury to the tendinous attachments of the flexor/pronator group at the medial epicondyle or the extensor/supinator group at the lateral epicondyle. Also referred to as *tennis elbow* when it occurs on the lateral epicondyle and *golfer's elbow* when it occurs on the medial elbow.

epidermal growth factor (EGF)—Growth factor produced by platelets during early inflammation and in proliferation.

epimysium—Connective-tissue layer covering an entire muscle.

epinephrine—A hormone. Also called *adrenaline.* A potent stimulator of the sympathetic nervous system. It is also a powerful vasopressor, increasing blood pressure, stimulating the heart muscle, accelerating the heart rate, and increasing cardiac output. It also increases such metabolic activities as glycogenolysis and glucose release.

epitenon—The loose areolar tissue that surrounds a tendon and contains the tendon's blood vessels and nerves.

erythrocyte—An element of blood. Also known as a *red blood cell* or *corpuscle.* Used by the body for oxygen transport.

evaluation—See *assessment.*

eversion—Outward-turning motion of the foot that causes the bottom of the foot to face laterally.

evidence-based practice—The application of information gleaned from current, quality research that is combined with the clinician's skills and experience, along with the patient's needs, goals, and priorities, to provide the patient with the best and most appropriate level of care.

examination—Includes subjective and objective components by which a clinician determines the severity, irritability, nature, and stage of a patient's injury. It serves as the basis for a rehabilitation program.

excitability—The ability of a cell to generate an electrical response through electrical and chemical changes facilitated by a stimulation.

excursion—Distance the center of mass moves.

extensible—Able to lengthen. When muscle temperature increases, the muscle's fibers and its connective tissue become more easily stretched.

extension—Straightening of a joint so that the two body segments move apart and increase the joint angle.

extensor lag—Inability to fully extend the knee during active motion, although full passive motion is present.

external rotation (ER)—An anatomical term that refers to the motion of turning away from the midline of the body. The more accurate term that is recommended instead is lateral rotation.

exteroreceptor—An afferent sensor that responds to external stimulation. Also known as *exteroceptor.*

extracellular matrix—The basic material from which tissue develops. Produced by fibroblasts in wounds. Composed of fibers and ground substance. Serves as a foundation on which anything is cast.

extrafusal fiber—A regular muscle fiber. Also known as a *myofibril.*

extrasynovial—Outside the synovial sac surrounding a joint or a synovial tendon sheath.

extrinsic foot muscles—Muscles that provide function for the toes, foot, and ankle but originate in the lower leg and terminate in the foot.

extrinsic muscles—Muscles that originate proximally from the hand or foot and terminate within the hand or foot.

extrinsic pathway—This is one of three pathways of the coagulation system. This pathway requires the plasma that carries the protein (tissue factor) from damaged endothelial walls to activate factors outside the blood serum to trigger the blood clotting mechanism.

exudate—Material that escapes from blood vessels following an injury. It contains high concentrations of protein, cells, and other materials from injured cells. As polymorphonuclear leukocytes die and decompose, the exudate may resemble pus, although no infection is present.

factor XII—See *Hageman factor.*

false negative—Results that occur when a test shows a negative result but the patient actually has the condition. A clinical test with this result has low specificity.

false positive—Results that occur when a test shows a positive result but the patient does not have the condition. A clinical test with this result has low sensitivity.

fast-twitch fiber—A muscle fiber, also called a *Type II fiber* or *fast oxidative fiber,* that is lighter in color than a slow-twitch fiber and that reaches its maximum tension approximately 50 ms after being stimulated.

fatigue—An inability to continue an activity.

fatigue failure—The point at which the cumulative stress of a repetitive submaximal load results in tissue failure. Also called *endurance limit.*

Feiss line—A line from the tip of the medial malleolus to the first metatarsal head. It is used as a point of reference to determine the relative position of the navicular tubercle.

fibrin—Insoluble fibrous protein. Formed by fibrinogen. Important in clotting.

fibrinogen—A globulin present in plasma. Converts to fibrin to form a fibrin plug at the injury site.

fibrinolysin—An enzyme in plasma that is released in later healing. Converts fibrin into a soluble substance to unplug lymphatics.

fibrinolysis—The process of normal breakdown of clots.

fibroblast—A connective-tissue cell. Fibroblasts differentiate into chondroblasts, osteoblasts, and collagenoblasts. They form the fibrous tissues to support and bind a variety of the body's tissues.

fibroblast growth factor (FGF)—Growth factors produced by endothelial cells, vascular smooth muscle cells, neural cells, and keratinocytes.

fibrocyte—An inactive fibroblast. See also *fibroblast.*

fibrogenesis—Development of fine fibers.

fibronectin—An adhesive glycoprotein found in most body tissues and serum. Fibronectin is plentiful in early granulation tissue formation but gradually disappears during the remodeling phase. Fibronectins cross-link to collagen in connective tissue, thereby playing a role in the adhesion of fibroblasts to fibrin. They are also involved in the collection of platelets in an injured area and enhance myofibroblast activity.

first-class lever—A lever in which the fulcrum is between the resistance and the force.

first ray—The joint between the first metatarsal and the medial cuneiform. This is the primary weight-bearing ray of the foot and has triplanar motion.

fixation—A state of stabilization in which motion is restricted or prevented.

flexibility—Mobility of a body segment, dependent on soft-tissue tolerance to movement and the ability of soft tissue to move with forces applied to it. Flexibility can involve soft-tissue mobility alone or in combination with joint motion. Used interchangeably with *range of motion.*

flexion—Bending of a joint so that the two body segments approach each other and decrease the joint angle.

foam roller—Cylindrical therapeutic tool made of Ethafoam or polyurethane and used in rehabilitation in neurological, orthopedic, and sports medicine facilities.

foot abduction—The transverse plane movement of the foot in which the lateral foot is moved away from the midline.

foot adduction—The transverse plane movement of the foot in which the medial foot is moved toward the midline.

foot eversion—The frontal-plane movement in which the plantar foot rotates inward so that the medial border is lifted upward.

foot flat—That portion of the stance phase of the gait cycle in which the foot is flat on the floor. Also known as *loading response.*

foot inversion—The frontal-plane movement in which the plantar foot rotates outward so that the lateral border is lifted upward.

foot strike—Initial foot contact with the ground in running. The term replaces *initial contact* or *heel strike.*

force—A strength or energy that causes movement and has direction and magnitude.

force arm—The perpendicular distance from the applied force to the axis of motion. Also called a *lever arm.* In rotational movements, it is called the moment arm.

force closure—A term that refers to the stability of the pelvic ring that is provided by the dynamic forces acting on the pelvis.

force couple—Two equal forces acting in opposite but parallel directions to create a rotatory motion.

force deformation—The amount of force applied to maintain a change of length or deformation of tissue. Also known as *force relaxation.*

force point—The location where a force is delivered or applied.

force relaxation—See *force deformation.*

forefoot valgus—An eversion deformity of the midtarsal joint causing the medial forefoot to be lower than the lateral forefoot in non–weight bearing when viewed in the same plane as a perpendicular line bisecting the calcaneus.

forefoot varus—An inversion deformity of the midtarsal joint causing the medial forefoot to be higher than the lateral forefoot in non–weight bearing when viewed in the same plane as a perpendicular line bisecting the calcaneus.

form closure—A term that refers to the stability of the pelvic ring that is provided by the structure and shape of the joints and their ligaments and bony components.

form drag—The resistance an object encounters in a fluid, as determined by the object's size and shape.

foxing—An additional piece of the heel counter that is often seen in athletic shoes to further reinforce the rearfoot in order to help maintain the heel counter's shape.

free nerve endings—Small-diameter, unmyelinated afferent nerve endings located throughout soft-tissue and articular structures that perceive pain and temperature. They are nociceptors that are stimulated by pain and inflammation. Although they do not play a role in proprioception, they respond to any extreme joint position.

friction—Resistance to movement between two surfaces.

frictional drag—The result of water's surface tension. This is not a factor in therapeutic exercise.

frog's eye—Condition in which the patellae face outward in relation to each other rather than forward.

frontal (coronal) plane—Any vertical plane that divides the body into front and back parts.

frozen shoulder—See *adhesive capsulitis.*

fulcrum—The point from which a lever moves. Also known as the *axis* or *axis of movement.*

functioning—This is the term WHO uses to identify a neutral or a positive interaction between an individual's health condition and his or her personal and societal context.

functional capacity evaluation (FCE)—A battery of practices and activities that are used to prepare a worker and to test to determine that worker's readiness to safely return to his or her former job.

functional evaluation—An assessment of the patient's ability to perform accurately and safely an exercise or skill drill before that patient is allowed to advance to the next level.

functional exercise—Activities that mimic the stresses, demands, and skills of the sport and advance a patient toward a safe and prompt return to sport participation.

gait cycle—The time from the point at which the heel of one foot touches the ground to the point at which it touches the ground again.

genu recurvatum—Excessive knee hyperextension.

genu valgus—Knee alignment in which the knees are angled toward each other. Also called *genu valgum.*

genu varum—Knee alignment in which the knees are bowed outward. Also called *genu varus.*

global muscles—Muscles that are farthest from the center of the body or joint. They have longer moment arms that allow them more force production than local muscles; therefore, they are considered to be the movers of a joint or body segment. Global muscles of the spine also assist in providing spinal stability.

gluteus medius gait—See *Trendelenburg gait.*

glycoprotein—One of a number of protein–carbohydrate compounds that are elements of ground substance. Includes fibronectin. Probably cross-links with collagen so that tissue can withstand pressure without harming tissue integrity.

glycosaminoglycan (GAG)—One of a number of compounds occurring mostly in proteoglycans. Glycosaminoglycans are non-fibrous elements of ground substance in the extracellular matrix. Examples: hyaluronic acid, proteoglycans. Different glycosaminoglycans have different functions—for example, stimulating fibroblast proliferation, promoting collagen synthesis and maturation, contributing to tissue resilience, and regulating cell function.

gold standard—The criterion measure or test that is the best at producing the most accurate results, and it is the standard by which all other measures or tests that propose to produce the same outcome are assessed.

Golgi-Mazzoni corpuscles—These afferent receptors are located in joint capsules. They are stimulated by joint compression but not by joint motion. Any weight-bearing activity stimulates these slowly adapting receptors. They are not believed to play a role in proprioception except in the identification of joint compression.

Golgi tendon organ (GTO)—A stretch receptor found in series within the musculotendinous structure. It responds to muscle contraction more than to muscle stretch to signal force.

goniometer—A tool used to measure joint range of motion. The device uses either a 180° or a 360° system.

goniometric terms—See *abduction, adduction, depression, dorsiflexion, downward rotation, elevation, eversion, extension, external rotation, flexion, frontal (coronal) plane, horizontal extension, horizontal flexion, internal rotation, inversion, opposition, plantar flexion, pronation, protraction, radial deviation, retraction, sagittal plane, supination, transverse (horizontal) plane, ulnar deviation, upward rotation.*

granular leukocyte—White blood cells, divided into three groups: neutrophils, eosinophils, and basophils. Among their functions are chemotaxis and phagocytosis, as well as release of histamine and serotonin to produce vasoactive reactions following injury.

granulation tissue—Newly formed vascular tissue that is produced during wound healing. Consists of fibroblasts, macrophages, and neovascular structure within a base of connective-tissue matrix of collagen, hyaluronic acid, and fibronectin. It has the velvety appearance of small, red, nodular masses seen in new tissue. It eventually forms the cicatrix of the wound.

granuloma—Hard mass of fibrous tissue. Occurs in chronic inflammatory conditions when the body produces collagen around a foreign substance to protect itself from that substance.

grasshopper eye—See *frog's eye.*

grief—An emotion that occurs following an episode in which a person experiences loss.

growth plate—See *physis.*

ground reaction force (GRF)—The forces exerted between the body and the ground during ambulation. There are three GRFs. The impact force is perpendicular to the ground (y-axis). The other two forces are shear forces, which occur either in a fore–aft direction (x-axis) or in a lateral–medial direction (z-axis).

ground substance—Gel-like material in which connective-tissue cells and fibers are embedded. Part of the connective tissue or extracellular matrix. Reduces friction between the connective-tissue fibers when forces are applied to the structure. Adds to the area's density.

growth factor—A factor released by platelets and macrophages. Growth factors perform complex and numerous roles, including the stimulation of re-epithelialization, and are chemotactic for macrophages, monocytes, and neutrophils. The role of growth factors is not thoroughly understood but is believed to be important throughout tissue repair. Also referred to as *growth hormone factor.*

H-band—That portion of the sarcomere that contains only thick filaments.

Hageman factor—An enzyme present in the blood. It initiates the blood coagulation process by converting prothrombin to thrombin following trauma to an area.

half-life—Amount of time it takes for the level of a drug in the bloodstream to diminish by one-half. Determines the frequency with which a medication is taken.

hallux valgus—A condition also known as a *bunion*. Present when the first metatarsophalangeal joint is greater than 10° in valgus, so that the first toe points laterally toward the other toes.

hammertoe—Condition in which the toe is extended at the metatarsophalangeal joint, flexed at the proximal interphalangeal joint, and extended at the distal interphalangeal joint.

heel counter—The portion of a shoe that circles the calcaneus and serves as an important rearfoot stabilizer.

heel-off—The portion of the stance phase of the gait cycle in which the weight begins to transfer to the front of the foot and the heel is lifted off the floor. Also known as *terminal stance*.

heel strike—The portion of the stance phase of the gait cycle in which the heel first comes in contact with the floor. Also known as *initial contact*.

hemiarthroplasty—A joint replacement surgery in which only half of the joint is replaced.

hemostasis—Clotting of blood following injury. In metabolic pathology, it is a stagnation of blood flow.

hip pointer—A contusion along the iliac crest.

histamine—A local tissue hormone released by mast cells and granulocytes. Increases vascular permeability to proteins and fibronectin.

Hooke's law—Law stating that the stress applied to a body to deform it is proportional to the strain as long as the body's elasticity limit is not exceeded.

horizontal extension—A motion of the upper extremity in a transverse plane away from the midline of the body. Also called *horizontal abduction*.

horizontal flexion—A motion of the upper extremity in a transverse plane toward the midline of the body. Also called *horizontal adduction*.

hyaluronic acid—A major component of early granulation tissue. Greatest amounts are seen in a wound during the first 4 to 5 days. Promotes cell movement and migration during repair. Stimulates fibroblast proliferation. Produces edema by absorbing large amounts of water to increase fibroblast migration. See also *glycosaminoglycan*.

hydrodynamics—That branch of physics that explores the motion of solid objects in fluids and forces imparted on those objects by the fluid.

hyperemia—An increase in blood flow.

hypermobile—Excessive mobility.

hypertrophy—An increase in muscle bulk from an increase in the size of the muscle fibers, not the number of muscle fibers. Hypertrophy occurs with strength gains.

hypomobile—Less than normal mobility.

hypoxia—Deficient oxygen supply in tissues.

hysteresis—The process of tissue lengthening that results when the tissue cannot withstand forces that are progressively applied to it.

I-band—The portion of the sarcomere that contains only thin filaments.

impact peak—The ground reaction force that is a rapid peak occurring very quickly with impact at the foot's initial contact with the ground.

impairment—Any pathology caused by disease, illness, or injury that affects either a body system or segment and prevents the individual from performing or functioning normally, resulting in disability. It is part of the process that leads to disability: Pathology leads to impairment, impairment leads to functional limitations, and functional limitations lead to disability.

indication—Specific patient signs, symptoms, conditions, or situations that are likely to respond to a treatment in an appropriate or beneficial manner.

indirect techniques—Manual therapy techniques that move tissue away from the direction of limitation.

inertia—The tendency of an object at rest or in uniform motion to remain in that state until an external force is applied. See also *Newton's first law of motion*.

inflare—A pelvic girdle dysfunction in which the iliosacral joint is medially rotated.

inhibition—Transmission of an impulse that results in the cessation or decrease of an activity.

initial contact—See *heel strike*.

initial swing—The first portion of the swing phase that includes early swing and acceleration.

insole board—The part of a shoe that lies between the upper and lower segments and that serves as the attachment for the two segments. Also called *last*.

insulin-like growth factor (IGF)—Important growth factor in healing and tissue repair.

internal rotation (IR)—An anatomical term that refers to the motion of turning toward the midline of the body. The more accurate term that is recommended instead is *medial rotation*.

internuncial neuron—A neuron that is interposed between two other neurons. The transmission rate for messages that use this type of neuron is slower than that for monosynaptic transmission.

interoreceptor—Receptor that sends messages from internal stimuli. Also known as *interoceptor*.

intervention—A rehabilitation clinician's purposeful interactions directly related to the patient's care.

intrafusal muscle fiber—Modified muscle fiber that lies within a muscle spindle. The two types of muscle fibers are nuclear bag fibers and nuclear chain fibers.

intrasynovial—Enclosed within the synovial sac surrounding a joint or a tendon's synovial sheath.

intrinsic foot muscles—Muscles that control the foot and toes and originate and terminate within the foot.

intrinsic muscles—Muscles that originate and terminate within the hand or foot.

intrinsic pathway—One of the three coagulation pathways following injury that causes factors to be released, leading to clot formation at the site of injury. It is also referred to as the contact pathway because it can be triggered without adding an outside factor to the blood serum.

inversion—An inward-turning motion of the foot that causes the bottom of the foot to face medially.

irritability—The amount of stimulation that is required to initiate a response, such as pain.

isokinetic—Characterizing a dynamic activity in which the velocity of movement remains the same and the resistance varies.

isometric—Characterizing an activity produced when muscle tension is created without a change in the muscle's length. An isometric activity is a static activity.

isotonic—Characterizing an activity during which a muscle's length changes.

joint distraction force—Joint mobilization application in which the clinician applies a long-axis traction to move the two joint ends apart. This application may be used by itself for improved joint mobility, relaxation, or pain relief, or it may be used together with another joint motion such as an anterior–posterior mobilization technique.

joint manipulation—A passive, high-velocity, low-amplitude thrust applied to a joint complex within its anatomical limit in order to restore optimal motion or function or to reduce pain.

joint mobilization—A manual therapy technique comprising a continuum of skilled passive movements that are applied at varying (low) speeds and amplitudes to joints in order to restore optimal motion or function or to reduce pain.

joint play—The amount of looseness or laxity within a joint that allows movement between the two joint surfaces to occur. Joint play is necessary for normal motion.

joint reaction forces—Forces that are transmitted from one segment to another through the connecting joint.

jump sign—A reflex response to a trigger point palpation that includes a wincing or withdrawal reaction by the patient.

juncturae tendinum—A fibrous band that limits independent motion of the extensor tendons of the hand.

kallikrein—A proteolytic enzyme found in blood plasma, lymph, and other exocrine secretions. Activated by the Hageman factor. Forms kinins and activates plasminogen, a precursor of plasmin. Increases vascular permeability and vasodilation.

keloid—Grossly excessive scar formation.

kinesthesia—The ability to perceive position and the quantity and speed of movement.

kinetic energy—Energy that a body has during motion.

kinin—A generic term for polypeptides related to bradykinin. Kinins are potent local tissue hormones and are found in injured tissue, released from plasma proteins. Examples: bradykinin, kallidin. Kinins mediate the classic signs of inflammation. Their action in the microvascular system is similar to that of histamine and serotonin in the early inflammation phase to cause increased microvascular permeability.

lactic acid—A by-product of muscle activity that leads to fatigue by reducing the muscle's calcium-binding capacity and impairing glycogen breakdown.

last—An important component of a shoe that determines the shoe's shape, size, style, and fit. It can be straight or curved. A shoe is constructed around a last that can be formed as a board last, slip last, or combination last.

latent trigger point—A trigger point that is painful only when it is palpated.

lateral rotation (LR)—Rotation of a joint around its axis away from the body's midline. Also inaccurately referred to as external rotation.

leukocyte—White blood cell or corpuscle. Types include polymorphonuclear leukocytes and mononuclear cells. These cells have notable phagocytic properties for the removal of debris from an injury site.

leukotriene—A compound formed from arachidonic acid. Leukotrienes regulate inflammatory reactions. Some stimulate the movement of leukocytes into the area.

lever—A simple machine with a rigid bar and a fulcrum.

lever arm—The length of the distance from where a force is applied to the axis of motion.

linear motion—Movement in a straight line.

line of gravity—Imaginary line through an object's center of gravity to the center of the earth.

line of pull—The long axis of the muscle along which it exerts force.

lipid—A heterogeneous group of fats and fatlike substances, including fatty acids and steroids. Lipids serve as a source of fuel and are important to the structure and makeup of cells.

Little League elbow—A valgus traction force injury of the medial elbow that may start out as an inflammatory response or apophysitis and progress to an avulsion of the apophysis if the repetitive stress continues.

loading response—See *foot flat*.

local muscles—Muscles that are close to the center of the body or joint. They have relatively short moment arms that limit their force; therefore, they are thought to be stabilizers rather than movers of a joint or body segment.

local twitch response—An involuntary contraction of the muscle fibers in response to the snapping palpation.

long-term goals—Those goals that are to be achieved at the end of the rehabilitation process. They are the final goals of any rehabilitation program.

loose-packed position—A joint position in which there is not complete congruency of joint surfaces with each other. Also called *open-packed position*. A joint demonstrates its greatest laxity in a loose-packed position.

lordosis—Excessive anterior convexity of the cervical and lumbar spine.

lumbopelvic stabilization—See *pelvic stabilization or stability*.

lumbopelvic-hip stabilization—See *pelvic stabilization or stability*.

lymphocyte—A nonphagocytic leukocyte found in blood and lymph. These cells serve as important structures in the body's immune system by producing antibodies.

M-band—The center of the A-band where the thick filaments are attached.

macrophages—Mononuclear phagocytes that arise from stem cells in bone marrow. Considered among the regulators of the repair process. They phagocytize injured areas of debris, kill microorganisms, and secrete substances into an injury site, including enzymes, fibronectin, and coagulation factors. They play a role in keeping the inflammatory process localized and enhance collagen deposition and fibroblast proliferation.

mallet deformity—Avulsion of the extensor digitorum longus from the distal phalanx. Also known as *baseball finger*.

manipulation—Passive joint movement used to increase joint mobility. It incorporates a sudden, forceful thrust that is beyond the patient's control.

manual muscle test (MMT)—An evaluation technique that uses manual resistance against a muscle or muscle group to provide a grade for that muscle or muscle group. Muscle grades range from 0 (zero) to 5 (normal).

manual therapy—The use of hands-on techniques for evaluating, treating, and improving the status of neuromusculoskeletal conditions.

massage—Manual manipulation of soft tissue to effect changes in the neuromuscular, lymph, cardiovascular, and connective-tissue systems.

mast cells—Connective-tissue cells. Also referred to as *mastocytes* and *labrocytes*. They store and produce various mediators of inflammation. Through their release of histamine, enzymes, and other mediators, mast cells cause increased local blood flow, attract immune cells, stimulate cell production of fibroblasts and endothelial cells, and promote and control remodeling of extracellular matrix.

matrix—Substance of a tissue. Can refer to intracellular or extracellular structure. Forms the basis from which a structure develops.

mechanoreceptors—Afferent receptors that react to mechanical stimuli.

medial rotation (MR)—Rotation of a joint around its axis toward the midline of the body. Also incorrectly referred to as internal rotation.

mediators—An umbrella term that identifies any intermediary substance or cell that interacts with or transmits information with chemicals or cells during the healing process. Their interactions and transmissions initiate or provide for the series of events and progression throughout the healing cycle.

Meissner's corpuscles—Sensory nerve endings that transmit light-touch sensation.

midsole—The middle portion of a shoe's outer sole that can be composed of a variety of substances. It can also include a medial wedge. The midsole provides shock attenuation, stability, and control.

midstance—The portion of the stance phase of the gait cycle in which the foot is directly under the body's weight and the entire foot is in contact with the floor. Also known as *single-leg support*.

midswing—The portion of the swing phase of the gait cycle in which the non-weight-bearing limb is in the middle of the swing phase.

mitochondria—Organelles of a cell that are the primary energy source for the cell and that contain the enzyme used to metabolize lactic acid for energy to form adenosine triphosphate.

M-line—Functions similarly to the Z-line by providing stability to the sarcomere.

mobile point—The position in strain–counterstrain treatments where the patient is passively positioned with the tender point at maximum ease. Any change from this position increases tissue tension that can be palpated by the clinician.

mobilization—Passive joint movement for increasing joint mobility or reducing pain. The applied force is light enough that the patient can stop the movement at any time.

modality—A physical agent used to relieve pain, improve circulation, reduce spasm, and promote healing.

moment arm—A length measure equivalent to lever arm. Moment arm rather than lever arm is used when discussing torque and rotational forces. Moment arm length is the perpendicular distance from the rotational axis of motion to the line of force application.

momentum—Amount of motion that a moving object has.

monocyte—Mononuclear phagocytic leukocyte. Monocytes are formed in the bone marrow and transported to tissues to become macrophages. They debride an injury site.

mononuclear phagocyte—Any cell capable of ingesting particulate matter. The term usually refers to macrophages (polymorphonuclear leukocytes) and monocytes (mononuclear phagocytes). These ingest microorganisms and debride an injury site.

monosynaptic response—A reflex response involving only one synapse that is between the afferent and efferent nerves.

monosynaptic transmission—The direct connection between a sensory nerve and a motor neuron. Also called a *monosynaptic reflex*.

morbid—Nature of or indicative of disease.

motor unit—A neuromuscular unit composed of the nerve, or motor neuron, and the muscle fibers that it innervates.

mucopolysaccharide—Polysaccharide. Also called *GAG*. See also *glycosaminoglycan*.

muscle endurance—Ability of a muscle or muscle group to perform repeated contractions against a less-than-maximal load.

muscle energy—A manual therapy technique using precisely applied active muscle contraction against a counterforce to correct alignment and improve function.

muscle spasm—Prolonged reflex muscle contraction.

muscle spindle—A neuromuscular spindle, composed of intrafusal muscle fibers, that lies between regular muscle fibers. With its complex afferent and efferent supply, it provides the body with sensory stimulation and motor responses. The muscle spindle is sensitive to stretch and signals muscle length and rate of change in the muscle's length.

muscle stiffness—The change in a muscle's tension that occurs as the muscle's length changes; related to the strength of the muscle's cross-bridge connections and the amount of muscle hypertrophy. The more stiffness a muscle has, the more resistant it is to stretching. Muscle stiffness is related to muscle tone.

muscular endurance—A muscle or muscle group's ability to sustain a submaximal force during either static or dynamic activity over time.

muscular strength—The amount of force a muscle or muscle group exerts. The ability to resist or produce a force.

MyBP-C—See *c-proteins*.

myoblast—A cell formed from myogenic cells in muscle. Myoblasts form myotubes that eventually evolve into muscle fiber.

myofibroblasts—Fibroblasts that have the ultrastructural features of a fibroblast as well as the qualities of a smooth muscle cell. They are responsible for wound contraction.

myogenic cells—Cells that arise from muscle and later become myoblasts. See also *myoblast.*

myosin—The chief protein structure of the thick filament of the sarcomere.

myotatic reflex—See *stretch reflex.*

nebulin—A large actin-binding protein molecule in a sarcomere.

negative predictive value (NPV)—The likelihood that a patient whose test result is negative does not have the condition. A test's NPV is identified by dividing the number of true negative results by the sum of the true negative and false negative results.

neural mobilization—A manual therapy technique that stretches neural and connective tissue structures to affect neural symptoms, restore tissue balance, and improve function.

neuromotor control—The proper activation and sequential recruitment of muscles to produce the correct response.

neurotransmitters—Hormones such as norepinephrine, epinephrine, and acetylcholine that are found in capillary, arteriole, and artery walls. They are released at the injury site to enhance platelet and leukocyte adherence to the vessel surface.

neutral spine—See *pelvic neutral.*

neutrophil—See *polymorphonuclear leukocyte.*

Newton's first law of motion—Law stating that a body remains at rest or in uniform motion until an outside force acts on it.

Newton's second law of motion—Law stating that acceleration of an object is directly proportional to the force causing the motion and inversely proportional to the mass of the object being moved.

Newton's third law of motion—Law stating that for every action there is an equal and opposite reaction.

nociceptors—Afferent nerve endings that transmit pain stimuli.

norepinephrine—A hormone that acts as a powerful vasoconstrictor at the immediate onset of injury. It may last from a few seconds to a few minutes.

nuclear bag fiber—One of two intrafusal muscle fibers within a muscle spindle, named for its nuclei arrangement. The nuclei are bunched together in the middle of the fiber's central region.

nuclear chain fiber—One of two intrafusal muscle fibers within a muscle spindle. Its nuclei are arranged in a chain or row. It is the smaller of the intrafusal muscle fibers.

nutation—Movement of the sacrum in which the superior base moves anteriorly and inferiorly while the sacral apex and coccyx move posteriorly. During nutation, the iliac crests move toward each other and the ischial tuberosities move apart.

nystagmus—A reflexive attempt to keep the eyes steady during body motion.

objective examination—The portion of an examination by which the clinician discovers the observable signs and effects of an injury: the portion of observation, testing for quality and quantity of movement, strength, neurological and other special testing, and palpation.

oculomotor system—An afferent system for balance that uses the eyes to provide the central nervous system with information about the body's relative position in space.

one-repetition maximum—A method used in healthy individuals to determine muscle strength. It is the amount of weight a person can lift with a muscle in one repetition but not two repetitions. This technique is not used in the patient population until the final phase of rehabilitation.

open kinetic chain (OKC)—Characterizing a motion in which the distal segment of an extremity moves freely in space.

open reduction internal fixation (ORIF)—Surgical reduction of a fracture with the application of a fixation device, such as a pin or screw, to stabilize the fracture site.

opposition—A diagonal movement of the thumb across the palm of the hand to permit the thumb to make contact with one of the other fingers.

orthotic—An appliance or device designed to correct, realign, protect, or support a body segment, or aid its function, or reduce pressure or symptoms. Orthotics can be custom made or preformed and can vary in composition, degree of control, and type of correction. Sometimes referred to as splints, braces, or foot orthotics.

Osgood-Schlatter disease—An inflammation or avulsion of the tibial apophysis, occurring in active, prepubescent children.

osteitis pubis—An inflammatory condition of shear stresses caused by either repeated trauma or strain on the symphysis pubis joint.

osteoarthritis—A condition caused by wearing and thinning of articular cartilage in a joint, eventually producing degeneration of the joint's articular surface. Also known as *degenerative joint disease (DJD).*

osteoblasts—Osteogenic cells from periosteum. They lay down the callus of fractured bone and convert later to chondrocytes.

osteochondritis dissecans—Avascular necrosis of a joint's articular surface.

osteoclasts—Large multinuclear cells. Resorb dead, necrotic bone tissue.

osteocyte—A cell characteristic of adult bone. Maintains new bone mineralization.

osteopenia—A mild to moderate bone density loss that places the person at risk for developing osteoporosis.

osteophytes—Bone spurs, or bony outgrowths, within a joint.

osteoporosis—A marked decrease in bone density causing bone porosity and brittleness with increased risk of fracture.

outsole—The portion of a shoe that includes the lower segment and is in contact with the ground.

overflow—Also known as *irradiation.* With increased voluntary effort or prolonged effort, motor activity spreads to additional motor units of the same muscle and to motor units of other muscles.

overload principle—To gain strength, a muscle must be overloaded beyond its accustomed level.

overpressure—Movement of a joint beyond its normal mobility to assess and feel or produce a comparable sign.

Pacinian corpuscles—Afferent nerve endings that lie throughout the joint capsule and periarticular structures. They are rapidly adapting receptors thought to be compression sensitive, especially during high-velocity changes when the joint accelerates or decelerates as it moves into its limits of motion.

parallel elastic component (PEC)—One of the noncontractile elements of muscle, composed of the muscle's connective tissue.

paratendinitis—An inflammation and thickening of the paratenon sheath of tendons that do not have synovial sheaths.

Pascal's law—Law stating that pressure from a fluid is exerted equally on all surfaces of an immersed object at any given depth (i.e., the deeper the object is immersed, the greater the pressure it encounters).

passive insufficiency—Occurs when multijoint muscles are passively stretched as far as possible, but they have insufficient length to also allow the joints they cross to move to their end positions.

passive physiological range of motion—The amount of range of motion achieved without the assistance of the patient.

passive range of motion (PROM)—See *passive physiological range of motion.*

passive stretch—A stretch for which application relies on an outside force. The patient remains relaxed throughout the stretch.

patella alta—Position of the patella higher than normal in the patellofemoral groove.

patella baja—Position of the patella lower than normal in the patellofemoral groove.

pathoneurodynamics—A term coined by David Butler to describe pathological conditions that produce referral patterns proximally and distally from the site of pathology.

pelvic neutral—The position in which the spine and sacrolumbar junction incur the least stress. This is usually a mid-position between the extremes of anterior and posterior pelvic tilt. Because of its impact on spine position, the position is also referred to as *neutral spine* or *straight spine.*

pelvic stabilization or stability—Activities or exercises that are used to position and maintain the body in a pelvic neutral position to control trunk position and movement over the pelvis and lower extremities, allowing optimal function and performance of the extremities. Also referred to as *core stabilization, lumbopelvic stabilization,* or *spinal stabilization* activities.

performance evaluation—An assessment of the patient's ability to perform and complete an exercise or skill drill safely and accurately before he or she is allowed to advance to the next level.

performance-specific exercises—Exercises that include drills or that mimic tasks found within a specific sport or job. These exercises are included in the final phase of the rehabilitation program to prepare patients for tasks that will be required in the course of their normal activities. See also *activity-specific exercises; sport-specific exercises.*

periarticular connective tissue—Soft tissue surrounding a joint, such as ligaments, the joint capsule, fascia, tendons, and synovial membranes.

perimysium—Connective-tissue layer covering a group of muscle fibers (fascicle).

pes cavus—An abnormal condition in which the foot has an abnormally high longitudinal arch. Associated with a rigid foot.

pes planus—An abnormal condition in which the foot has a low longitudinal arch. Associated with a hypomobile foot. Also known as a *pancake arch, flatfoot,* or *excessive pronation.* Associated with a flexible foot.

phagocyte—Any cell that ingests particulate matter. Commonly referred to as *polymorphonuclear leukocyte* and *mononuclear phagocyte,* otherwise known as *macrophage* and *monocyte.* These cells ingest microorganisms and other particulate antigens to debride an area.

phospholipids—Lipids that contain phosphoric acid. Found in all cells and in layers of plasma membranes. They stimulate the clotting mechanism.

physically active—Characterizing a person who engages in occupational, recreational, or athletic activities that require physical skills and use strength, power, endurance, speed, flexibility, range of motion, or agility. (Based on the National Athletic Trainers' Association definition.)

physiological advantage—A muscle's ability to shorten. A muscle has its greatest physiological advantage when at its resting length.

physiological joint motion—Joint motion that can be performed voluntarily, such as shoulder flexion and ankle inversion.

physis—A complex cartilaginous matrix that lies near the end of the longitudinal bone and forms new bone, providing growth of the long bone. Also called a *growth plate.*

plan of treatment program—The components, frequency, and duration of a treatment program. Includes the establishment of short-term and long-term goals.

plantar flexion—An extension of the ankle that causes the dorsum (top) of the foot to move away from the lower leg so that the angle of the ankle increases.

plasmin—An enzyme that occurs in plasma as plasminogen. It is activated by kallikrein and other activators. It converts fibrin to soluble substances.

plasminogen activator—An enzyme. Converts fibrin to a soluble substance. See also *fibrinolysin.*

plasticity—In muscle physiology, a permanent change in length that occurs after an elongation force is applied.

platelet-derived growth factor (PDGF)—Substance found in platelets. It is essential for the growth of connective-tissue cells and stimulates the migration of polymorphonuclear leukocytes.

platelets—Irregular cell fragments found in blood. The first cells seen at an injury site, platelets are classified as regulatory cells of healing. Release growth factors. Form a plug at the injury to stop bleeding.

plica—A redundant fold in the knee's synovial lining, palpated as a band extending medially from the patella.

plumb line—A string with a weight (formerly a lead weight, but any weighted object will do) at the end. When suspended, the string forms a vertical line.

plyometrics—A type of exercise in which lengthening of a muscle is followed by a sudden shortening to produce increased power. Also called *stretch-shortening exercise.*

polymorphonuclear leukocyte—One of the granular leukocytes. Also referred to as *PMNs* or *neutrophils.* These cells are chemotactic and phagocytic in the healing process.

position of comfort—The position used in strain–counterstrain treatment in which the patient's painful segment is placed where there is no pain or discomfort.

positive predictive value (PPV)—The likelihood that a patient whose test result is positive really has the condition. A test's PPV is identified by dividing the number of true positive results by the sum of the true positive and false positive test results.

posture—The relative alignment of the various body segments with one another.

potential energy—Energy that is stored in a body.

power—Work produced over time.

precaution—The patient may experience harmful effects with the application of a specific treatment in the presence of specific signs, symptoms, situations, or conditions, so the clinician must exhibit knowledge, wisdom, prudence, and good judgment in deciding whether or not to apply a treatment.

pre-contraction stretching—Immediately prior to a stretch, the muscle actively contracts to facilitate immediate relaxation for the stretch.

prehabilitation—The use of therapeutic exercises in advance of a surgical procedure to improve the functional capacity of the patient preoperatively to allow the patient to withstand the effects of inactivity following an orthopedic surgery.

preswing—See *toe-off*.

primary hemostasis—The initial clot formation occurs to immediately limit bleeding. Platelets play an important role in this phase of healing by adhering to the epithelial wall to form the platelet plug.

primary impingement—Subacromial impingement in the shoulder that occurs because of a mechanical narrowing of the subacromial space; tendinous, bursal, or bony structures within the space reduce the available area in the space.

primary intention—Healing that occurs with minor or surgical wounds. Re-epithelialization closes the wound within 48 h. Scarring is minimal when healing by primary intention occurs.

procedure (vs. modality)—A treatment technique that involves the clinician's active participation or supervision.

pronation—Movement of the palm backward or downward so that the palm faces in a posterior direction, opposite the anatomical position. Also, a multiplanar rotation of the subtalar and transverse tarsal joints that is the combination of dorsiflexion, abduction, and eversion.

proprioception—The body's ability to transmit afferent information about position sense, to interpret the information, and to respond consciously or unconsciously to stimulation through appropriate execution of posture and movement.

proprioceptive neuromuscular facilitation (PNF)—A combined movement pattern that uses neural stimulation to facilitate a proper muscle response.

prostaglandins (PGs)—Components stemming primarily from arachidonic acid. Release of these substances requires the presence of the complement system and follows kinin formation. Specific PG compound compositions are designated by adding a letter, A through I, and a subscript number, 1 through 3, to designate the number of hydrocarbon bonds. Examples: PGE_1 and PGE_2. Prostaglandins mediate cell migration during inflammation and modulate serotonin and histamine. Some PGs increase pain sensitivity, induce fever, and suppress lymphocyte transformation, thereby inhibiting the inflammatory reaction. Mediate myofibroblasts. Prostaglandins initiate early phases of injury repair and play a role in the later stages of inflammation.

protease—An enzyme that acts as a catalyst to split interior peptide bonds in protein. Activates kallikrein to release bradykinin, ultimately causing increased vascular permeability to result in an increase in the concentration of proteins and cells in the wound spaces.

proteoglycan—Substances found in tissues, including synovial fluid and connective-tissue matrix. Proteoglycan solutions are very viscous lubricants and are sulfated glycosaminoglycans. A proteoglycan provides a resilient matrix for inhibiting cell migration. Regulates cell function and proliferation and regulates collagen fibrillogenesis. See also *glycosaminoglycan*.

protraction—A forward movement of the scapula. Also called *scapular abduction*.

pump bump—Increased prominence of the posterior calcaneal tuberosity. Also known as a *calcaneal exostosis*.

Q-angle—The angle formed by a line from the anterior superior iliac spine to the middle patella and a line from the middle patella to the tibial tubercle.

radial deviation—A movement of the wrist toward the thumb side of the forearm. Also called *radial flexion*.

range of motion—Amount of movement within a joint. Range of motion is affected by soft-tissue mobility and can be influenced by strength when performed actively. Used interchangeably with *flexibility*.

rearfoot valgus—An abnormal condition in which the calcaneus is everted relative to the tibia.

rearfoot varus—An abnormal condition in which the calcaneus is inverted relative to the posterior bisection of the lower leg.

receptor sites—Proteins that exist in the cell's outer boundary, the plasma membrane. They receive signals by binding with specific molecules. Similar to how a specific key is used to open a specific lock, a specific receptor site binds with a specific molecule to allow that molecule to impact or influence the cell or its function.

refraction—When a light ray moves from air through water, it bends as it moves from the air, which has a lower density than the water does, into the water with its higher density. This makes the pool bottom appear closer than it actually is and makes objects within the water appear distorted.

refractory period—The time immediately following a stimulation, when the muscle fiber is unable to respond to additional stimuli. It is divided into an absolute refractory period and a relative refractory period.

rehabilitation—The treatment process used to help injured, ill, or disabled individuals achieve maximum function and self-satisfaction in personal and societal environments.

rehabilitation clinician—The medical professional responsible for the design, progression, supervision, and administration of a rehabilitation program for people involved in physical activity.

relative density—See *specific gravity*.

relative refractory period—A period that follows depolarization after a membrane has become partially repolarized. During this period the membrane can respond again if the stimulus is stronger than the normal threshold level.

refractory period—The time during depolarization of a muscle or nerve cell when the cell is unable to respond to another stimulus. Known as *absolute refractory period*.

reliability—The degree to which a measurement or special test can be depended upon to produce consistent results. *Intrarater reliability* is how consistent and accurate the measurement or test is when performed repeatedly by the same clinician on different patients. *Interrater reliability* is how consistent and accurate the measurement or test is when performed by different clinicians on the same patient.

resistance arm—The perpendicular distance from the point where a resistance force is applied to the axis of motion.

resistance point—The location where a resistance is delivered or applied.

retroversion—The pathological alignment in which the femoral neck angle is less than 15°. It causes lateral rotation of the femur with the femoral head in the acetabulum.

resistive range of motion (RROM)—Motion that occurs with resistance applied to the movement. Also referred to as *strengthening exercises* or *progressive resistive exercises*.

resting membrane potential—The electrical potential difference across an inactive cell's membrane.

resting position—The position of a joint that allows the joint capsule the greatest amount of play and where the volume within the joint is at its greatest.

reticulin—A collagen-like fiber. Some consider reticulin a Type III collagen fiber. Forms the early framework for collagen deposition in a wound.

retraction—A backward movement of the scapula. Also called *scapular adduction*.

retroversion—Decreased anterior angulation of the femoral neck, resulting in a toe-out gait.

return to play—Medical clearance of an athlete for full participation in sport without restriction (strength and conditioning, practice, and competition).

rigor mortis—Stiffness of the muscles of a dead body as a result of the presence of calcium and the absence of ATP in the tissues. The process begins 2 to 4 hours after death and continues up to a few days postmortem.

Rolfing structural integration—The basis upon which Ida Rolf designed Rolfing, a manual therapy technique designed to balance the body's segments such that they align optimally relative to gravity and integrate with each other to provide optimal structure and function. Her program included 10 sequential sessions to achieve her goals.

Romberg test—A test for balance in which a patient stands with feet together and eyes closed. Increased postural sway compared to when eyes are open is a positive sign.

Ruffini nerve endings—These afferent receptors are in the joint capsule on the flexion side of the joint. They are slowly adapting and respond more to loads on the connective tissue in which they are contained than to displacement of that connective tissue. These receptors are stimulated by extreme joint motion when the capsule is stressed in extension with rotation.

rule-out diagnoses—A list of the most likely injuries or conditions based on the information gathered that is the actual diagnosis. Tests are performed to eliminate each diagnosis from the list until the remaining diagnosis is revealed as the true diagnosis. See *differential diagnosis*.

running cycle—A cycle that includes two running strides.

running stride—The time during a running cycle when one foot makes contact with the ground to the time the opposite foot contacts the ground.

saccule—The smaller of two sacs within the vestibular system's labyrinth of the inner ear that plays a role in regulating balance.

saddle—The portion of a shoe that includes the midsection along the longitudinal arch, usually reinforced to assist in supporting the midfoot.

sagittal plane—The anterior–posterior vertical plane through which the longitudinal axis passes and which divides the body into right and left halves.

SAID principle—**S**pecific **a**daptation to **i**mposed **d**emands. Tissue will adapt to the specific stresses applied to it. This is a principle upon which a therapeutic exercise program is designed.

sarcolemma—The outer membrane of a muscle fiber.

sarcomere—The smallest contractile element of a muscle fiber.

sarcopenia—A decrease in muscle mass secondary to aging.

sarcoplasmic reticulum—A highly specialized intracellular membrane system that stores and transports calcium.

satellite cells—Cells present in muscle that regenerate new muscle tissue.

scaption—Elevation of the shoulder in the scapular plane 30° forward of the frontal plane. This alignment of the glenohumeral joint with the scapula on the rib cage places the rotator cuff in the least stressful position for exercise.

scoliosis—A lateral or S curvature of the spinal column.

secondary hemostasis—A cascade of enzymatic reactions that occur to produce a fibrin plug which is stronger than that formed initially by platelets. It serves to reinforce the clot formed during primary hemostasis.

secondary impingement—The subacromial space narrows because of a dysfunction of the shoulder, so the humeral head is not centered as it should be within the glenoid. Muscle imbalances and posture leading to these imbalances often result in this impingement.

secondary intention—Healing that occurs in large wounds associated with soft-tissue loss. The wound heals with granulation tissue from the bottom and sides of the wound. Epithelial tissue does not form until granulation tissue has filled the wound. Larger scar formation occurs with healing by secondary intention. Wound contraction is evident with this healing.

second-class lever—A lever in which the resistance is between the fulcrum and the force.

sensitivity—Identifies how well a diagnostic test is able to produce a positive result when the condition being tested for is present. The closer the number is to 1 the more accurate the test is likely to be.

series elastic component (SEC)—One of the noncontractile elements of muscle, composed primarily of the tendons, sheath, and sarcolemma.

serotonin—A hormone released by mast cells and platelets. Produces vasoconstriction in small vessels after norepinephrine activity is completed; occurs only when blood vessel endothelial walls are damaged. In later phases, it is responsible for initiating reactions leading to collagen cross-linking. It also is involved in granuloma formation.

shin splints—A general term used to describe pain and inflammation of the musculotendinous unit or periosteum along the anteromedial border of the tibia. Also know as *medial tibial stress syndrome.*

short-term goals—Goals that are achieved before the long-term goals; they serve as stepping-stones, or points of progression, toward the final goals. The long-term goal is acquired by achieving smaller increments until the final goal is met.

single-leg support—The portion of the gait cycle in which the body weight is transferred entirely to the one supporting leg and the other leg is in the middle of its swing phase. Also known as *midstance*. Also referred to as *single-limb support.*

sinusoidal curve—A curve that takes the shape of a sine wave.

SLAP lesion—**S**uperior **l**abrum tear **a**nterior and **p**osterior in location. A tear in the labrum appearing superiorly either on the posterior or anterior glenoid.

slow-twitch fiber—A muscle fiber that is a Type I fiber or slow oxidative fiber, is darker in color than the fast-twitch fiber, and takes about 110 ms to reach its peak tension when stimulated.

Smith's fracture—A type of fracture in which the distal radius is fractured and the fragment is displaced palmarly.

SnNout—A mnemonic regarding the reliability of a test that is expressed as the sensitivity of a test. If a test has a high **S**ensitivity and produces a **N**egative result the condition for which it tests is ruled **out** as a possible diagnosis.

sock liner—The portion of a shoe that lies on top of the insole board, used for shock absorption and friction reduction for the foot.

somatosensory system—Another term for the body's proprioceptive system.

spatial characteristics—Those elements of gait that can be observed by looking at the path taken by the feet on the ground. These characteristics include stride length, step length, and step width.

specific gravity—The ratio of an object's weight to the weight of an equal volume of water. The term refers to the density of an object relative to that of water. This ratio is also called *relative density*. The specific gravity of water is 1.

specificity—Identifies how well a diagnostic test's ability is to produce a negative result when the patient really does not have the condition. The closer the number is to 1 the more accurate the test is likely to be.

spinal cord—Part of the central nervous system that extends from the brain to the second lumbar vertebra and contains a cervical and a lumbar enlargement where the dorsal and ventral roots leading to the extremities are contained.

spinal reflex—When an impulse goes from a dorsal root afferent nerve either to an internuncial connecting nerve or directly to an efferent nerve in the spinal cord, and then immediately out the ventral root to the muscle.

spinal stabilization—See *pelvic stabilization or stability.*

sport-specific exercises—Exercises that include drills or that mimic tasks found within a specific sport; they are used in the final phase of rehabilitation to prepare an injured athlete for return to normal sport participation. Grouped with the generic classification of performance-specific exercises.

SpPin—A mnemonic regarding the reliability of a test that is expressed as the specificity of a test. If a test has a high **S**pecificity and produces a **P**ositive result the condition for which it tests is ruled **in** as a possible diagnosis.

sprain—Stretching or tearing of a ligament or capsular structure.

squinting patellae—Patellae that are angled toward each other rather than facing forward.

stable—A condition where the body is secure, usually occurring when the center of mass remains within its base of support and is not in danger of losing balance.

stance phase—The portion of the gait cycle during which the foot is in contact with the floor and the extremity is bearing partial or total body weight. In running, sometimes called the *support phase.*

static activity—An isometric activity in which no movement occurs.

static progressive splint—Change of static splints as motion of a segment changes so the desired goals, usually including increased motion, are achieved.

static restraint—One of two systems a joint has for its stability. Static restraints include ligaments, capsule, and other inert structures such as the glenoid labrum in the shoulder and the meniscus in the knee.

static splint— Splint used to support, protect, or restrict motion. It does not have any moving parts.

static stretch—A slow, continual stretch in which the body segment is brought to its end position and held in that position for a specific time.

steady state of a drug—The state in which the average level of a drug remains constant in the blood—the amount of drug leaving the body is equal to the amount being absorbed. On average, a steady state occurs after five doses equal to the drug's half-life are administered.

stem cell—A cell with the unique ability to differentiate into specialized cells in the body.

step length—The distance from heel strike of one foot to heel strike of the other foot in one gait cycle.

stiffness—The ability of an object to resist deformation when a stress is applied to it. The stiffer an object, the less elastic it is. The opposite of compliance.

strain—Amount of change in size or shape of an object caused by stress.

strength—A muscle's relative ability to resist or produce a force.

stress—Force required to change the shape or form of a body.

stretch reflex—The most basic sensorimotor response. Does not involve an internuncial neuron, but instead goes directly from the afferent sensory nerve (muscle spindle) to the spinal cord, where it makes contact with the motor nerve to permit a rapid muscle response.

stretch-shortening exercise—An exercise that makes use of the elastic properties of muscle, using a lengthening of a muscle followed by a sudden shortening to produce increased power. Also called *plyometric exercise.*

stride length—The distance from heel strike of one foot to heel strike of the same foot in one gait cycle.

stride rate—In running, the inverse of cycle time or stride time: the number of step lengths over a given period.

stride width—The body's side-to-side movement as weight is shifted from one lower extremity to the other.

structural fatigue—The point at which stress exceeds the tissue's ability to resist it and breakdown occurs.

structural integration—The basis upon which Ida Rolf designed Rolfing, a manual therapy technique designed to balance the body's segments so that they align optimally relative to gravity and integrate with each other to provide optimal structure and function. Her program included 10 sequential sessions to achieve her goals.

subjective examination—The portion of an examination that includes the history of an injury, including the mechanism of injury, the patient's experience of pain and other symptoms, prior injuries, medical conditions, medications, and other pertinent social and medical factors. This information is provided by the patient or another person.

subtalar joint—The joint formed by the talus and calcaneus. This joint allows inversion and eversion motion of the rearfoot.

subtalar neutral—The position in which the talus is palpable from its medial or its lateral aspect within the subtalar joint. The point at which the talus and navicular are most congruent and the alignment of the subtalar bones is optimal.

summation of forces—Sequential movement of body segments to increase force production for a desired motion.

supination—Movement of the palm forward or upward into the anatomical position. Also, the multiplanar rotation of the subtalar and transverse tarsal joints that includes plantar flexion, adduction, and inversion.

swan-neck deformity—A deformity caused by hyperextension at the PIP joint and hyperflexion at the DIP joint due to disruption of the volar plate and tensioning of the flexor tendons.

swing phase—The time during which the foot is not in contact with the floor and no weight is borne on the extremity.

swing-through—The middle of the swing phase. Also called *mid-swing.*

swing-through gait—A three-point gait pattern with crutches in which the weight-bearing leg is advanced far enough to land in front of the crutches.

swing-to gait—A three-point gait pattern with crutches in which the patient swings the weight-bearing leg to the crutches.

Swiss ball—A large vinyl ball developed by an Italian toy manufacturer that is used in physical therapy and therapeutic exercise programs.

syndrome—A group of signs, symptoms, and tests that, when occurring together, indicate a pathological condition.

synergist(ic)—A muscle that assists an agonist muscle.

synovial fluid—A lubricating fluid secreted by membranes in joints and tendon sheaths.

synovial sheaths—Sheaths that surround tendons subjected to greater-than-normal friction stresses, such as the Achilles and biceps tendons.

talocrural joint—The true ankle joint that is formed by the talus and tibia with the fibula. The joint allows dorsiflexion and plantar flexion motions.

tarsal tunnel—Formed by the medial malleolus, calcaneus, talus, and deltoid ligament's posterior aspect.

temporal characteristics—Time-related factors used as part of gait analysis. These characteristics include speed of gait and cadence.

tender point—A term used in strain–counterstrain to identify small areas of tenderness that are the size of a dime or smaller. The goal of strain–counterstain techniques is to relieve these tender points.

tendinitis—The global term used to identify an inflammation of a tendon. Also spelled *tendonitis.*

tendinopathy—Condition of a tendon that demonstrates signs and symptoms of pain, swelling, and reduced function.

tendinosis—A condition that involves microscopic tears of the tendon caused by repeated trauma.

tendon sheath—A fibrous tissue that surrounds a tendon whose purpose is to reduce friction between the tendon and the adjacent structures.

tenocyte—Tendon cell. Converts to fibroblasts during healing of tendons.

tenodesis—The passive insufficiency of the long finger tendons. When the wrist flexes, the long finger extensors extend, and when the wrist extends, the long finger flexors flex. This motion allows opening and closing of the hand to be controlled passively by the wrist.

10-repetition maximum—The weight that a muscle or muscle group can lift for 10 repetitions but not 11. This method of determining strength is one technique used in rehabilitation programs when using a 1RM provides too much stress for the injured segment.

tenosynovitis—An inflammation of the synovial sheath that surrounds a tendon.

tensile strength—Maximal amount of stress or force that a structure can withstand before tissue failure occurs. Tensile strength varies as tissue healing proceeds. One must take the tensile strength of an injured structure into account when determining how much stress to apply in rehabilitation.

terminal stance—See *heel-off.*

terminal swing—The portion of the swing phase that includes late swing, or deceleration.

tetanus—An intermittent contraction of a muscle that is demonstrated as a fibrillation of the muscle.

tetany—A sustained maximal contraction of a muscle.

thermotherapy—The application of therapeutic heat to create a desired physiological effect.

third-class lever—A lever in which the force is between the fulcrum and the resistance.

thoracic kyphosis—Excess posterior convexity of the thoracic spine.

thoracic outlet syndrome (TOS)—A clinical term that describes compression of the neurovascular structures as they exit through the thoracic outlet at the base of the neck.

threshold stimulation—The minimal stimulation required to initiate a muscular response.

thrombin—An enzyme that converts fibrinogen to fibrin to form a fibrin plug early in the inflammation phase. In later inflammation, it stimulates fibronectin production and fibroblast proliferation.

thromboxane—A compound that is produced by platelets and is unstable. Its half-life is 30 s. Related to prostaglandins. Acts as a vasoconstrictor and is a potent inducer of platelet aggregation.

tibial torsion—An abnormal structural condition in which the tibia is rotated along its longitudinal axis so that the foot is rotated laterally beyond the normal 15° in relation to the patella's midline.

tibial varum—An abnormal condition in which the distal tibia is closer to the midline than the proximal tibia.

tissue factor (TF)—A protein that is part of the extrinsic pathway which activates coagulation.

titin—A giant elastic protein filament that is an essential element of the sarcomere's structure. It extends from Z-disc to M-line, half of the sarcomere's length. It maintains the sarcomere's alignment during muscle contraction and provides passive tension of the structure.

toe box—The upper portion of the shoe that covers the toes. It varies in width and height, and functions to retain the shape of the shoe's forefoot and provide room for the toes.

toe-off—The portion of the gait cycle during which the foot comes off the floor and the swing phase begins. Also called *push-off* or *preswing.*

torque—The ability of a force to produce rotational movement.

transforming growth factor-alpha (TGF-α)—Growth factor produced in macrophages, brain cells, and keratinocytes.

transforming growth factor-beta (TGF-β)—Growth factor produced in platelets, macrophages, lymphocytes, fibroblasts, bone cells, and keratinocytes.

transverse (horizontal) plane—A plane that divides the body or a body part into upper and lower parts. It is parallel to the horizon.

Trendelenburg gait—An abnormal gait secondary to gluteus medius weakness. The gait is also known as a *gluteus medius gait* and is seen as a drop of the pelvis on the uninvolved side during weight bearing on the involved side.

trigger point—According to Travell and Simons (1983, p. 3), a "focus of hyperirritability in a tissue that, when compressed, is locally tender and, if sufficiently hypersensitive, gives rise to referred pain and tenderness, and sometimes to referred autonomic phenomena and distortion of proprioception." A myofascial trigger point includes a taut band of muscle with its surrounding fascia.

tropomyosin—One of two primary proteins of the thin filament of the sarcomere. It is an anchor point for troponin. When at rest, actin–myosin interaction is inhibited by tropomyosin; when calcium is released, troponin moves tropomyosin from actin's binding sites to allow actin–myosin binding.

troponin—A protein on the actin filament to which calcium ions bind during a sarcomere's cross-bridging process. When at rest, actin–myosin interaction is inhibited by tropomyosin; when calcium is released, troponin moves tropomyosin from actin's binding sites to allow actin–myosin binding.

true negative—A test's ability to show a negative result when the test is provided to a patient who does not have the condition. See *specificity.*

true positive—A test's ability to show a positive result when the test is provided to a patient who has the condition. See *sensitivity.*

TUBS—**T**raumatic, **u**nilateral, **B**ankart lesion, **s**urgery required. A traumatic shoulder injury involving a tear of the anterior capsulolabral complex and requiring surgical repair.

ulnar deviation—A movement of the wrist toward the little-finger side of the forearm. Also called *ulnar flexion.*

ultimate strength—The greatest load a tissue can tolerate before it reaches failure.

upward rotation—A movement of the scapula that causes the glenoid to face forward and upward. The inferior angle of the scapula moves laterally away from the spine, and the scapula slides forward.

utricle—The larger of two sacs within the vestibular system's labyrinth in the inner ear that plays a role in sensing head motion.

Valsalva maneuver—When the breath is held, intrathoracic pressure increases. This can impede venous return to the right atrium, causing increased peripheral venous pressure, increasing blood pressure and reducing cardiac output because of diminished cardiac volume.

validity—The degree to which a test measures what it is intended to measure. Validity is established through research investigation, not clinical experience.

vamp—The upper portion of a shoe that covers the toes and forefoot and includes the toe box.

velocity—Rate of change of position.

vestibular system—An afferent system within the inner ear that is responsible for sending messages to the central nervous system regarding vertical and horizontal position and motion.

viscoelasticity—The property of being both viscous and elastic.

viscosity—The resistance to movement within a fluid or fluid-like substance that is caused by the friction of the fluid's molecules. Viscosity limits the rate of muscle contraction: The faster the contraction, the greater the internal resistance and the less the force that can be generated.

volitional—The conscious performance of an activity.

von Willebrand factor (VW)—A protein present in the blood and is important in initiating platelet adhesion to initiate the platelet plug formation.

wave drag—The water's resistance as a result of turbulence.

weight—The force of gravity. Commonly measured in kilograms (grams) or pounds (ounces).

work—Product of a force and the distance through which it is applied.

Z-disc—The end of the sarcomere element where the thin filaments attach. It maintains the sarcomere's structure and transmits tension when the muscle contracts. Also known as the *Z-line*, *Z-disk*, or *Z-band*.

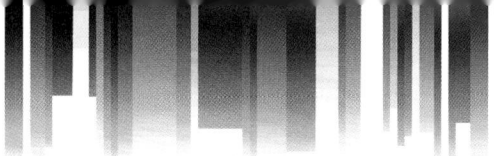

REFERENCES

Chapter 1

1. Taber CW. *Taber's Cyclopedic Medical Dictionary*. 22nd ed. FA Davis; 2014.

2. Anderson DM. *Mosby's Medical, Nursing, & Allied Health Dictionary*. 6th ed. Mosby; 2002.

3. World Health Organization. *International Classification of Functioning, Disability and Health*. World Health Organization; 2001.

4. Sjölund BH. Rehabilitation. In: Gellman MD, Turner JR, eds. *Encyclopedia of Behavioral Medicine*. Springer; 2013.

5. Ardern CL, Taylor NF, Feller JA, Whitehead TS, Webster KE. Psychological responses matter in returning to preinjury level of sport after anterior cruciate ligament reconstruction surgery. *Am J Sports Med*. 2013;41(7):1549-1558.

6. Clement D, Arvinen-Barrow M, Fetty T. Psychosocial responses during different phases of sport-injury rehabilitation: a qualitative study. *J Athl Train*. 2015;50(1):95-104.

7. Federer AE, Taylor DC, Mather RC, 3rd. Using evidence-based algorithms to improve clinical decision making: the case of a first-time anterior shoulder dislocation. *Sports Med Arthrosc Rev*. 2013;21(3):155-165.

8. Centers for Disease Control. Generate a differential diagnosis. Centers for Disease Control. Accessed December 22, 2019. https://www.cdc.gov/urdo/differential.html

9. Nijs J, Van Geel C, Van der auwera C, Van de Velde B. Diagnostic value of five clinical tests in patellofemoral pain syndrome. *Man Ther*. 2006;11(1):69-77.

10. Somerville LE, Willits K, Johnson AM, et al. Clinical assessment of physical examination maneuvers for superior labral anterior to posterior lesions. *Surg J (NY)*. 2017;3(4):e154-e162.

11. Portney LG, Watkins MP. *Foundations of Clinical Research: Applications to Practice*. 2nd ed. Prentice Hall Health; 2000.

12. Koo TK, Li MY. A guideline of selecting and reporting intraclass correlation coefficients for reliability research. *J Chiropr Med*. 2016;15(2):155-163.

13. Cave EF, Roberts SM. A method for measuring and recording joint function. *J Bone Joint Surg Am*. 1936;18(2):455-465.

14. Silver D. Measurement of the range of motion in joints. *J Bone Joint Surg* 1923;5(3):569-578.

15. Freke M, Kemp J, Semciw A, et al. Hip strength and range of movement are associated with dynamic postural control performance in individuals scheduled for arthroscopic hip surgery. *J Orthop Sports Phys Ther*. 2018;48(4):280-288.

16. Ganesh GS, Chhabra D, Mrityunjay K. Efficacy of the Star Excursion Balance Test in detecting reach deficits in subjects with chronic low back pain. *Physiother Res Int*. 2014;doi:10.1002/pri.1589

17. Gribble P. The Star Excursion Balance Test as a measurement tool. *Athl Ther Today*. 2003;8(2):46-47.

18. Gribble PA, Hertel J, Plisky P. Using the Star Excursion Balance Test to assess dynamic postural-control deficits and outcomes in lower extremity injury: a literature and systematic review. *J Athl Train*. 2012;47(3):339-357.

19. Kivlan BR, Martin RL. Functional performance testing of the hip in athletes: a systematic review for reliability and validity. *Int J Sports Phys Ther*. 2012;7(4):402-412.

20. Powden CJ, Dodds TK, Gabriel EH. The reliability of the star excursion balance test and lower quarter Y-balance test in healthy adults: a systematic review. *Int J Sports Phys Ther*. 2019;14(5):683-694.

21. MacDonald PB, Clark P, Sutherland K. An analysis of the diagnostic accuracy of the Hawkins and Neer subacromial impingement signs. *J Shoulder Elbow Surg*. 2000;9(4):299-301.

22. Ellenbecker TS. *Clinical Examination of the Shoulder*. Elsevier Saunders; 2004.

23. Lalkhen AG, McCluskey A. Clinical tests: sensitivity and specificity. *Crit Care Pain*. 2008;8(6):221-223.

24. Parikh R, Mathai A, Parikh S, Sekhar GC, Thomas R. Understanding and using sensitivity, specificity and predictive values. *Indian J Ophthalmol*. 2008;56(1):45-50.

25. Ponte-Allan M, Giles GM. Goal setting and functional outcomes in rehabilitation. *Am J Occup Ther*. 1999;53(6):646-649.

26. Parsons JGM, Plant SE, Slark J, Tyson SF. How active are patients in setting goals during rehabilitation after stroke? A qualitative study of clinician perceptions. *Disabil Rehabil*. 2018;40(3):309-316.

27. Wade DT. Evidence relating to goal planning in rehabilitation. *Clin Rehabil*. 1998;12:273-275.

28. Li B, Wang YT, Bai LH, Wen Y. Changes of mechanoreceptors in different-state remnants of ruptured anterior cruciate ligament. *Int Orthop*. 2018;42(11):2613-2618.

29. Iles JF, Stokes M, Young A. Reflex actions of knee joint afferents during contraction of the human quadricep. *Clin Physiol*. 1990;10(5):489-500.

30. Nishikawa K, Biewener AA, Aerts P, et al. Neuromechanics: an integrative approach for understanding motor control. *Integr Comp Biol*. 2007;47(1):16-54.

31. Dischiavi SL, Wright AA, Hegedus EJ, Bleakley CM. Biotensegrity and myofascial chains: A global approach to an integrated kinetic chain. *Med Hypotheses*. 2018;110(1):90-96.

32. Malanga GA, Yan N, Stark J. Mechanisms and efficacy of heat and cold therapies for musculoskeletal injury. *Postgrad Med*. 2015;127(1):57-65.

33. Nadler SF, Weingand K, Kruse RJ. The physiologic basis and clinical applications of cryotherapy and thermotherapy for the pain practitioner. *Pain Phys*. 2004;7(3):395-399.

34. Anwer S, Alghadir A, Zafar H, Brismée JM. Effects of orthopaedic manual therapy in knee osteoarthritis: a systematic review and meta-analysis. *Physiother*. 2018;104(3):264-276.

35. Bialosky JE, Bishop MD, Price DD, Robinson ME, George SZ. The mechanisms of manual therapy in the treatment of musculoskeletal pain: A comprehensive model. *Man Ther*. 2009;14(5):531-538.

36. Cheng YH, Hsu CY, Lin YN. The effect of mechanical traction on low back pain in patients with herniated intervertebral disks: a systemic review and meta-analysis. *Clin Rehabil*. 2020;34(1):13-22. doi:10.1177/0269215519872528

37. Cotler HB, Chow RT, Hamblin MR, Carroll J. The use of low level laser therapy (LLLT) for musculoskeletal pain. *MOJ Orthop Rheumatol*. 2015;2(5). doi:10.15406/mojor.2015.02.00068

38. Dedes V, Stergioulas A, Kipreos G, Dede AM, Mitseas A, Panoutsopoulos GI. Effectiveness and safety of shockwave therapy in tendinopathies. *Mater Sociomed*. 2018;30(2):131-146.

39. Ennis WJ, Lee C, Gellada K, Corbiere TF, Koh TJ. Advanced technologies to improve wound healing: electrical stimulation, vibration therapy, and ultrasound—what is the evidence? *Plast Reconstr Surg*. 2016;138(3):94S-104S.

40. Kloth LC. Electrical stimulation technologies for wound healing. *Adv Wound Care (New Rochelle)*. 2014;3(2):81-90.

41. Miller DL, Smith NB, Bailey MR, et al. Overview of therapeutic ultrasound applications and safety considerations. *J Ultrasound Med*. 2012;31(4):623-634.

42. Speed CA. Therapeutic ultrasound in soft tissue lesions. *Rheumatology (Oxford)*. 2001;40(12):1331-1336.

43. Reiman MP, Lorenz DS. Integration of strength and conditioning principles into a rehabilitation program. *Int J Sports Phys Ther*. 2011;6(3):241-253.

44. Fischerauer SF, Talaei-Khoei M, Bexkens R, Ring DC, Oh LS, Vranceanu AM. What is the relationship of fear avoidance to physical function and pain intensity in injured athletes? *Clin Orthop Relat Res*. 2018;476(4):754-763.

45. Hendy AM, Spittle M, Kidgell DJ. Cross education and immobilisation: Mechanisms and implications for injury rehabilitation. *J Sci Med Sport*. 2012;15(2):94-101.

46. Lee M, Carroll TJ. Cross education. Possible mechanisms for the contralateral effects of unilateral resistance training. *Sports Med*. 2007;37(1):1-14.

47. Scripture EW, Smith TL, Brown EM. On the education of muscular control and power. *Stud Yale Psychol Lab*. 1894:114-119.

48. West JL, Keene JS, Kaplan LD. Early motion after quadriceps and patellar tendon repairs: outcomes with single-suture augmentation. *Am J Sports Med*. 2008;36(2):316-323.

49. Kannus PJ, L., Kvist M, Lehto M, Järvinen M. The effect of immobilization on myotendinous junction: an ultrastructural, histochemical and immunohistochemical study. *Acta Physiol Scand*. 1992;144(3):387-394.

50. Kim U, Choi YS, Jang GC, Choi YR. Early rehabilitation after open repair for patients with a rupture of the Achilles tendon. *Injury*. 2017;48(7):1710-1713.

51. Trudel G, Zhou J, Uhthoff HK, Laneuville O. Four weeks of mobility after 8 weeks of immobility fails to restore normal motion: a preliminary study. *Clin Orthop Relat Res*. 2008;466(5):1239-1244.

52. Kaneguchi A, Ozawa J, Kawamata S, Yamaoka K. Development of arthrogenic joint contracture as a result of pathological changes in remobilized rat knees. *J Orthop Res*. 2017;35(7):1414-1423.

53. Konrath GA, Lock T, Goitz HT, Scheidler J. The use of cold therapy after anterior cruciate ligament reconstruction: A prospective, randomized study and literature review. *Am J Sports Med*. 1996;24(5):629-633.

54. Hochberg J. A randomized prospective study to assess the efficacy of two cold-therapy treatments following carpal tunnel release. *J Hand Ther*. 2001;14(3):208-215.

55. Yu H, Randhawa K, Côté P, Collaboration O. The effectiveness of physical agents for lower-limb soft tissue injuries: a systematic review. *J Orthop Sports Phys Ther*. 2016;46(7):523-554.

56. Lessiani G, Iodice P, Nicolucci E, Gentili M. Lymphatic edema of the lower limbs after orthopedic surgery: results of a randomized, open-label clinical trial with a new extended-release preparation. *J Biol Regul Homeost Agents*. 2015;29(4):gucci805-812.

57. Harris R, Piller N. Three case studies indicating the effectiveness of manual lymph drainage on patients with primary and secondary lymphedema using objective measuring tools. *J Bodyw Mov Ther*. 2003;7(4):213-221.

58. Starr HM, Snoddy M, Hammond KE, Seiler JG, 3rd. Flexor tendon repair rehabilitation protocols: a systematic review. *J Hand Surg Am*. 2013;38(9):1712-1717.

59. Eckenrode BJ. An algorithmic approach to rehabilitation following arthroscopic surgery for arthrofibrosis of the knee. *Physiother Theory Pract*. 2018;34(1):66-74.

60. DeFroda SF, Mehta N, Owens BD. Physical therapy protocols for arthroscopic Bankart repair. *Sports Health*. 2018;10(3):250-258.

61. Pignanelli C, Petrick HL, Keyvani F, et al. Low-load resistance training to task-failure with and without blood flow restriction: muscular functional and structural adaptations. *Am J Physiol Regul Integr Comp Physiol*. 2019. doi:10.1152/ajpregu.00243.2019.

62. Slawson DC, Shaughnessy AF. Becoming an information master: using POEMs to change practice with confidence: patient-oriented evidence that matters. *J Fam Pract*. 2000;49(1):63-67.

63. Grad R, Pluye P, Tang D, Shulha M, Slawson DC, Shaughnessy AF. Patient-oriented evidence that matters (POEMs)™ suggest potential clinical topics for the Choosing Wisely™ campaign. *J Am Board Fam Med*. 2015;28(2):184-189.

64. Freischlag JA, Kibbe MR. The evolution of surgery: the story of "Two Poems". *JAMA*. 2014;312(17):1737-1738.

65. Snyder AR, Parsons JT, Valovich McLeod TC, Curtis Bay R, Michener LA, Sauers EL. Using disablement models and clinical outcomes assessment to enable evidence-based athletic training practice, part I: disablement models. *J Athl Train*. 2008;43(4):428-436.

66. Verbrugge LM, Jette AM. The disablement process. *Soc Sci Med*. 1994;38(1):1-14.

67. Nagi SZ. Some conceptual issues in disability and rehabilitation. In: Sussman MB, ed. *Sociology & Rehabilitation*. American Sociological Association; 1965:100-113.

68. Nagi SZ. A study in the evaluation of disability and rehabilitation potential: concepts, methods, and procedures.

Am J Public Health Nations Health. 1964;54(9):1568-1579.

69. Petretto DR, Vinci S, Todde IP, Piras P, Pistis I, Masal C. Conceptual models of disability and their role in the daily routine of clinical rehabilitation. *Rehabil Sci*. 2017;2(4):75-81.

70. Jette AM, Keysor JJ. Disability models: implications for arthritis exercise and physical activity interventions. *Arthritis Rheum*. 2003;49(1):114-120.

71. Jette AM. Toward a common language for function, disability, and health. *Phys Ther*. 2006;86(5):726-734.

72. World Health Organization. Working for better health. WHO. https://www.who.int/about/what-we-do/who-brochure

73. Badley EM. Enhancing the conceptual clarity of the activity and participation components of the International Classification of Functioning, Disability, and Health. *Soc Sci Med*. 2008;66(11):2335-2345.

74. Topaz M, Shafran-Topaz L, Bowles KH. ICD-9 to ICD-10: evolution, revolution, and current debates in the United States. *Perspect Health Int Manag*. 2013;10(Spring):1d.

75. ICD10CMData.com. 2022 ICD-10-CM codes. Accessed Feb 6, 2020. https://www.icd10data.com/ICD10CM/Codes

76. World Health Organization. *Towards A Common Language for Functioning, Disability and Health ICF*. World Health Organization; 2002.

77. Madden RH, Dune T, Lukersmith S, et al. The relevance of the International Classification of Functioning, Disability and Health (ICF) in monitoring and evaluating community-based rehabilitation (CBR). *Disabil Rehabil*. 2014;36(10):826-837.

78. World Health Organization. *International Statistical Classification of Diseases and Related Health Problems*. 2nd ed. World Health Organization; 2008.

79. Melnyk BM, Gallaher-Ford L, Long LE, Fineout-Overholt E. The establishment of evidence-based practice competencies for practicing registered nurses and advanced practice nurses in real-world clinical settings: proficiencies to improve healthcare quality, reliability, patient outcomes, and costs. *Worldviews Evid Based Nurs*. 2014;11(1):5-15.

80. McConnell J. The management of chondromalacia patellae: a long term solution. *Aust J Physiother*. 1986;32:215-223.

81. Ng GYF, Cheng JMF. The effects of patellar taping on pain and neuromuscular performance in subjects with patellofemoral pain syndrome. *Clin Rehabil*. 2002 Dec 2002;16(8):821-827.

82. Somes S, Worrell TW, Corey B, C.D. I. Effects of patellar taping on patellar position in the open and closed kinetic chain: a preliminary study. *J Sport Rehabil*. 1997;6:299-308.

83. Crossley K, Bennell K, Green S, McConnell J. A systematic review of physical interventions for patellofemoral pain syndrome. *Clin J Sport Med*. 2001;11(2):103-110.

84. Westby MD, Klemm A, Li LC, Jones CA. Emerging role of quality indicators in physical therapist practice and health service delivery. *Phys Ther*. 2016;96(1):90-100.

85. Braun Y, Meliema JJ, Peters RM, Curley S, Burchill G, Ring D. The relationship between therapist-rated function and patient-reported outcome measures. *J Hand Ther*. 2017;30(4):516-521.

86. Deyo RA. Using outcomes to improve quality of research and quality of care. *J Am Board Fam Pract*. 1998;11(6):465-473.

87. Valovich McLeod TC, Snyder AR, Parsons JT, Curtis Bay R, Michener LA, Sauers EL. Using disablement models and clinical outcomes assessment to enable evidence-based athletic training practice, part II: clinical outcomes assessment. *J Athl Train*. 2008;43(4):437-445.

88. Resnik L, Dobrykowski E. Outcomes measurement for patients with low back pain. *Orthop Nurs*. 2005;24(1):14-24.

89. Sauers EL, Snyder AR. A team approach: demonstrating sport rehabilitation's effectiveness and enhancing patient care through clinical outcomes assessment. *J Sport Rehabil*. 2011;20(1):3-7.

90. Brinkley JM, Stratford PW, Lott SA, Riddle DL. The Lower Extremity Functional Scale (LEFS): scale development, measurement properties, and clinical application. North American Orthopaedic Rehabilitation Research Network. *Phys Ther*. 1999;79(4):371-383.

91. Ware JE, Jr, Kosinski M, Bayliss MS, McHorney CA, Rogers WH, Raczek A. Comparisons of methods forf the scoring and statistical analysis of the SF-36 health profile and summary measures: summary of results from the Medical Outcomes Study. *Med Care*. 1995;33(4 suppl):AS264-AS279.

92. Ware JE, Jr, Sherbourne CD. The MOS 36-item short form health survey (SF-36). I. Conceptual framework and item selection. *Med Care*. 1992;30(6):473-483.

93. Brinkley JM, Stratford PW, Loft SA, Riddle DL. The lower extremity functional scale (LEFS): scale development measurement properties, and clinical application. *Phys Ther*. 1999;79:371-383.

94. Haas M, Jacobs GE, Raphael R, Petzing K. Low back pain outcome measurement assessment in chiropractic teaching clinics: responsiveness and applicability of two functional disability questionnaires. *J Manipulative Physiol Ther*. 1995;18(2):79-87.

95. Johanson NA, Liang MH, Daltroy L, Rudicel S, Richmond J. American Academy of Orthopaedic Surgeons lower limb outcomes assessment instruments: reliability, validity, and sensitivity to change. *J Bone Joint Surg Am*. 2004;86(5):902-909.

96. Lodhia P, Slobogean GP, Noonan VK, Gilbard MK. Patient-reported outcome instruments for femoroacetabular impingement and hip labral pathology: a systematic review of the clinimetric evidence. *Arthroscopy*. 2011;27(2):279-286.

97. Peer MA, Lane J. The knee injury and osteoarthritis outcome score (KOOS): a review of its psychometric properties in people undergoing total knee arthroplasty. *J Orthop Sports Phys Ther*. 2013;43(1):20-28.

98. Marx RG, Stump TJ, Jones EC, Wickiewicz TL, Warren RF. Development and evaluation of an activity rating scale for disorders of the knee. *Am J Sports Med*. 2001;29(2):213-218.

99. Wang D, Jones MH, Khair MM, Miniaci A. Patient-reported outcome measures for the knee. *J Knee Surg*. 2010;23(3):137-151.

100. Rodriguez-Merchan EC. Knee instruments and rating scales designed to measure outcomes. *J Orthop Traumatol*. 2012;13(1):1-6.

101. Eechaute C, Vaes P, Van Aerschot L, Asman S, Duquet W. The clinimetric qualities of patient-assessed instruments for measuring chronic ankle instability: a systematic review. *BMC Musculoskelet Disord*. 2007;8:6.

102. Hung M, NIckisch F, Beals TC, Greene T, Clegg DO, Saltzman CL. New paradigm for patient-reported outcomes assessment in foot & ankle research: computerized adaptive testing. *Foot Ankle Int* 2012;33(8):621-626.

103. Slobogean GP, Slobogean BL. Measuring shoulder injury function: common scales and checklists. *Injury*. 2011;42(3):248-252.

104. Dowrick AS, Gabbe BJ, Williamson OD, Cameron PA. Outcome instruments for the assessment of the upper extremity following trauma: a review. *Injury*. 2005;36(4):468-476.

105. Shaw T, Chipchase LS, Williams MT. A users guide to outcome measurement following ACL reconstruction. *Phys Ther Sport*. 2004;5(2):57-67.

106. Farshad M, Gerber C, Szucs T, Meyer DC. Determining utility values in patients with anterior cruciate ligament tears using clinical scoring systems. *BMC Health Serv Res*. 2011;11:182. doi:10.1186/1472-6963-11-182

107. Hoch JM, Druvenga B, Ferguson BA, Houston MN, Hoch MC. Patient-reported outcomes in male and female collegiate soccer players during an athletic season. *J Athl Train*. 2015;50(9):930-936.

108. May KH, Guccione AA, Edwards MC, Goldstein MS. The adolescent mesure of confidence and musculoskeletal performance (AMCaMP): Development and initial validation. *Int J Sports Phys Ther*. 2016;11(5):698-707.

109. Tarara DT, Fogaca LK, Taylor JB, Hegedus EJ. Clinician-friendly physical performance tests in athletes part 3: a systematic review of measurement properties and correlations to injury for tests in the upper extremity. *Br J Sports Med*. 2016;50(9):545-551.

110. Weel H, Zwiers R, Azim D, et al. Validity and reliability of a Dutch version of the Foot and Ankle Ability Measure. *Knee Surg Sports Traumatol Arthrosc*. 2016;24(4):1348-1354.

111. Antosh IJ, Svoboda SJ, Peck KY, Garcia EJ, Cameron KL. Change in KOOS and WOMAC scores in a young athletic population with and without anterior cruciate ligament injury. *Am J Sports Med*. 2018;46(7):1606-1616.

112. Burland JP, Kostyun RO, Kostyun KJ, Solomito M, Nissen C, Milewski MD. Clinical otcome masures and rturn-to-sort tming in adolescent athletes after aterior cruciate ligament rconstruction. *J Athl Train*. 2018;53(5):442-451.

113. Rauck RC, Nwachukwu BU, Allen AA, Warren RF, Altchek DW, Williams RJ. Outcome of isolated posterior cruciate ligament reconstruction at mean 6.3-year follow up: a consecutive case series. *Phys Sportsmed*. 2019;47(1):60-64.

114. Keith RH, Granter CV, Hamilton BB, Sherwin FS. The functional independence measure: a new tool for rehabilitation. *Advances in Clinical Rehabilitation*. Springer; 1987.

115. Adams D, Logerstedt DS, Hunter-Giordano A, Axe MJ, Snyder-Mackler L. Current concepts for anterior cruciate ligament reconstruction: a criterion-based rehabilitation progression. *J Orthop Sports Phys Ther*. 2012;42(7):601-614.

116. Farnik M, Pierzchala WA. Instrument development and evaluation for patient-related outcomes assessments. *Patient Relat Outcome Meas*. 2012;3:1-7.

117. Martin RL, Irrgang JJ, Burdett RG, Conti SF, Van Swearingen JM. Evidence of validity for the foot and ankle ability measure. *Foot Ankle Int*. 2005;26(11):968-983.

118. Hung M, Baumhauer J, Licari FW, Bounsanga J, Voss MW, Saltzman CL. Responsiveness of the PROMIS and FAAM instruments in foot and ankle orthopedic population. *Foot Ankle Int*. 2019;40(1):56-64.

119. Crown WH, Henk HJ, Vanness DJ. Some cautions on the use of instrumental variables estimators in outcomes research: how bias in instrumental variables estimators is affected by instrument strength, instrument contamination, and sample size. *Value Health*. 2011;14(8):1078-1084.

120. Griffin DR, Parsons N, Mohtadi NG, Safran MR, Network MAotHOR. A short version of the International Hip Outcome Tool (iHOT-12) for use in routine cinical practice. *Arthroscopy*. 2012;28(5):611-616.

121. Niki H, Tatsunami S, Haraguchi N, et al. Development of the patient-based outcome instrument for the foot and ankle. Part 1: project description and evaluation of the Outcome Instrument version 1. *J Orthop Sci*. 2011;16(5):536-555.

Chapter 2

1. Zeng R, Lin C, Lin Z, et al. Approaches to cutaneous wound healing: basics and future directions. *Cell Tissue Res*. 2018;374(2):217-232.

2. Taraballi F, Bauza G, McCulloch P, Harris J, Tasciotti E. Concise review: biomimetic functionalization of biomaterials to stimulate the endogenous healing process of cartilage and bone tissue. *Stem Cells Transl Med*. 2017;6(12):2186-2196.

3. Alluri R, Jakus A, Bourgioukli S, et al. 3D printed hyperelastic "bone" scaffolds and regional gene therapy: a novel approach to bone healing. *J Biomed Mater Res A*. 2017. doi:10.1002/jbm.a.36310

4. Schultz GS, Wysocki A. Extracellular matrix: review of its roles in acute and chronic wounds. *World Wide Wounds*. March 28, 2013 2005;

5. Okan D, Woo K, Ayello EA, Sibbald G. The role of moisture balance in wound healing. *Adv Skin Wound Care*. 2007;20(1):39-53.

6. Schultz GS, Wysocki A. Interactions between extracellular matrix and growth factors in wound healing. *Wound Repair Regen*. 2009;17(2):153-162.

7. Wong VW, Longaker MT, Gurtner GC. Soft tissue mechanotransduction in wound healing and fibrosis. *Semin Cell Dev Biol*. 2012;23(9):981-986.

8. Lam MT, Nauta A, Meyer NP, Wu JC, Longaker MT. Effective delivery of stem cells using an extracellular matrix patch results in increased cell survival and proliferation and reduced scarring in skin wound healing. *Tissue Eng Part A*. 2013;19(5-6):738-747.

9. Broughton Gn, Janis JE, Attinger CE. The basic science of wound healing. *Plast Reconstr Surg*. 2006;117(7S):12S-34S.

10. Falabella AF, Falanga V. Wound healing. In: Freinekl RK, Woodley DT, eds. *The Biology of the Skin*. Parthenon Publishing Group; 2001:281-297.

11. Guo S, Dipietro LA. Factors affecting wound healing. *J Den Res*. 2010;89(3):219-229.

12. Diegelmann RF, Evans MC. Wound healing: an overview of acute, fibrotic and delayed healing. *Front Biosci.* 2004;9:283-289.

13. Beserra FP, Gushiken LFS, Hussni MF, Pellizzon CH. Regulatory mechanisms and chemical signaling of mediators involved in the Inflammatory phase of cutaneous wound healing. In: Dogan KH, ed. *Wound Healing Current Perspectives.* IntechOpenLimited; 2018:chap 2.

14. Palta S, Saroa R, Palta A. Overview of the coagulation system. *Indian J Anaesth.* 2014;58(5):515-523.

15. Rodrigues M, Kosaric N, Bonham CA, Gurtner GC. Wound healing: a cellular perspective. *Physiol Rev.* 2019;99(1):665-706.

16. Cimmino G, Golino P. Platelet biology and receptor pathways. *J Cardiovasc Transl Res.* 2013. doi:10.1007/s12265-012-9445-9

17. Hrachovinová I. Diagnostic strategies in disorders of hemostasis. *Vnitr Lek.* 2018;64(5):537-544.

18. Chan AKC, Paredes N. The coagulation system in humans. *Methods Mol Biol.* 2013;992:3-12.

19. Smith SA, Travers RJ, Morrissey JH. How it all starts: initiation of the clotting cascade. *Crit Rev Biochem Mol Biol.* 2015;50(4):326-336.

20. Davie EW, Ratnoff OD. Waterfall sequence for intrinsic blood clotting. *Science.* 1964;145(3638):1310-1312.

21. MacFarlane RG. An enzyme cascade in the blood clotting mechanism, and its function as a biochemical amplifier. *Nature.* 1964;202:498-499.

22. Giangrande PLF. Six characters in search of an author: the history of the nomenclature of coagulation factors. *Br J Haematol.* 2003;121(5):703-712.

23. Achneck HE, Sileshi B, Parikh A, Milano CA, Welsby IJ, Lawson JH. Pathophysiology of bleeding and clotting in the cardiac surgery patient. *Circulation.* 2010;122(20):2068-2077.

24. Martinez-Hernandez A, Amenta PS. Basic concepts in wound healing. In: Leadbetter WB, Buckwalter JA, Gordon SL, eds. *Sports-Induced Inflammation.* Am Acad Orthop Surg; 1990.

25. Thompson WD, Harvey JA, Kazmi MA, Stout AJ. Fibrinolysis and angiogenesis in wound healing. *J Pathol.* 1991;165(4):311-318.

26. Denegar CR, Saliba E, Saliba S. *Therapeutic Modalities for Musculoskeletal Injuries.* 4th ed. Human Kinetics; 2016.

27. Rand E, Gelhorn AC. The healing cascade: facilitating and optimizing the system. *Phys Med Rehabil Clin N Am.* 2016;27(4):765-781.

28. Hildebrand KA, Gallant-Behm CL, Kydd AS, Hart DA. The basics of soft tissue healing and general factors that influence such healing. *Sports Med Arthrosc Rev.* 2005;11(3):136-144.

29. Ridiandries A, Tan JTM, Bursill CA. The role of chemokines in wound healing. *Int J Mol Sci.* 2018;19(10):3217. doi:10.3390/ijms19103217

30. Alfaro MP, Deskins DL, Wallus M, et al. A physiological role for connective tissue growth factor in early wound healing. *Lab Invest.* 2013;93(1):81-95.

31. Koria P. Delivery of growth factors for tissue regeneration and wound healing. *BioDrugs.* 2012;26(3):163-175.

32. Demidova-Rice TN, Hamblin MR, Herman IM. Acute and impaired wound healing: pathophysiology and current methods for drug delivery, part 2: role of growth factors in normal and pathological wound healing: therapeutic potential and methods of delivery. *Adv Skin Wound Care.* 2012;25(8):349-370.

33. Pandit A, Ashar R, Feldman D. The effect of TGF-beta delivered through a collagen scaffold on wound healing. *J Invest Surg.* 1999;12(2):89-100.

34. Steenfos HH. Growth factors and wound healing. *Scand J Plast Reconstr Surg Hand Surg.* 1994;28(2):95-105.

35. Siracusa MC, Perrigoue JG, Corneau MR, Artis D. New paradigms in basophil development, regulation and function. *Immunol Cell Biol.* 2010;88(3):275-284.

36. Neves JS, Perez SA, Spencer LA, et al. Eosinophil granules function extracellularly as receptor-mediated secretory organelles. *Proc Natl Acad Sci USA.* 2008;105(47):18478-18483.

37. Freischlag JA, Hanna D. Neutrophil (PMN) phagocytosis and chemotaxis after reperfusion injury. *J Surg Res.* 1992;52(2):152-156.

38. Newman AC, Hughes CCW. Macrophages and angiogenesis: a role of Wnt signaling. *Vascular Cell.* 2012;4:13.

39. Sgonc R, Gruber J. Age-related aspects of cutaneous wound healing: a mini-review. *Gerontology.* 2012;

40. Patel AA, Zhang Y, Fullerton JN, et al. The fate and lifespan of human monocyte subsets in steady state and systemic inflammation. *J Exp Med.* 2017;214(7):1913-1923.

41. Peacock EE. *Wound Repair.* 3rd ed. Lea & Febiger; 1984.

42. Ringvall M, Rönnberg E, Wernersson S, et al. Serotonin and histamine storage in mast cell secretory granules is dependent on serglycin proteoglycan. *J Allergy Clin Immunol.* 2008;121(4):1060-1066.

43. Best TM, Hunter KD. Muscle injury and repair. *Phys Med Rehabil Clin N Am.* 2000;11(2):251-266.

44. Sabino F, Hermes O, Egli FE, et al. In vivo assessment of protease dynamics in cutaneous wound healing by degradomics analysis of porcine wound exudates. *Mol Cell Proteomics.* 2015;14(2):354-370.

45. Friesenecker B, Tsai AG, Dünser MW, Martini J, Hasilbeder W, Intaglietta M. Lowered microvascular vessel wall oxygen consumption augments tissue pO2 during PgE1-induced vasodilation. *Eur J Appl Physiol.* 2007;99(4):405-414.

46. Messina EJ, Weiner R, Kaley G. Microcirculatory effects of prostaglandins E1, E2, and A1 in the rat mesentery and cremaster muscle. *Microvasc Res.* 1974;8(1):77-89.

47. Willoughby DA. Effects of prostaglandins PGF2a and PGE1 on vascular permeability. *J Pathol Bacteriol.* 1968;96(2):381-387.

48. Petrucci G, De Cristofaro R, Rutella S, et al. Prostaglandin E2 differentially modulates human platelet function through the prostanoid EP2 and EP3 receptors. *J Pharmacol Exp Ther.* 2011;336(2):391-402.

49. Narumiya S, Sugimoto Y, Ushikubi F. Prostanoid receptors: structures, properties, and functions. *Physiol Rev.* 1999;79(4):1193-1226.

50. Wang JH, Iosifidis MI, Fu FH. Biomechanical basis for tendinopathy. *Clin Orthop Relat Res.* 2006;443:320-332.

51. Butterfield TA, Best TM, Merrick MA. The dual roles of neutrophils and macrophages in inflammation: a critical balance between tissue damage and repair. *J Athl Train.* 2006;41(4):457-465.

1031

52. Greaves NS, Ashcroft KJ, Baguneid M, Bayat A. Current understanding of molecular and cellular mechanisms in fibroplasia and angiogenesis during acute wound healing. *J Dermatol Sci*. 2013;72(3):206-217.

53. Greenhalgh DG. The role of growth factors in wound helaing. *J Trauma*. 1996;41(1):159-167.

54. Anitua E, Andia I, Ardanza B, Nurden P, Nurden AT. Autologous platelets as a source of proteins for healing and tissue regeneration. *Thromb Haemost*. 2004;91(1):4-15.

55. Ferrara N. Vascular endothelial growth factor: basic science and clinical progress. *Endocr Rev*. 2004;25(4):581-611.

56. Lawrence WT, Diegelmann RF. Growth factors in wound healing. *Clin Dermatol*. 1994;12(1):157-169.

57. Worley CA. The wound healing process symphony: part II. *Dermatol Nurs*. 2004;16(2):179-180.

58. Tufro-McReddie A, Norwood VF, Aylor KW, Botkin SJ, Carey RM, Gomez RA. Oxygen regulates vascular endothelial growth factor-mediated vasculogenesis and tubulogenesis. *Dev Biol*. 1997;183(2):139-149.

59. Rodriguez PG, Felix FN, Woodley DT, Shim EK. The role of oxygen in wound healing: a review of the literature. *Dematol Surg*. 2008;34(9):1159-1169.

60. Bennett NT, Schultz GS. Growth factors and wound healing: Part II. Role in normal and chronic wound healing. *Am J Surg*. 1993;166(1):74-81.

61. Brandstedt S, Rank F, Olson PS, Ahonen J. Cell composition of granulation tissue in defibrinogenated rabbits. *Acta Chir Scand*. 1980;146(8):545-549.

62. Kischer CW. Fine structure of granulation tissue from deep injury. *J Invest Dermatol*. 1979;72(4):147-152.

63. Castellino FJ, Ploplis VA. Structure and function of the plasminogen/plasmin system. *Thromb Haemost*. 2005;93(4):647-654.

64. Weisel JW. Fibrinogen and fibrin. *Adv Protein Chem*. 2005;70:247-299.

65. Suh DY, Hunt TK. Time line of wound healing. *Clin Podiatr Med Surg*. 1998;15(1):1-9.

66. Segal R, Diegelmann R, Ward K, Reynolds A. A differential equation model of collagen accumulation in a healing wound. *Bull Math Biol*. 2012;74(9):2165-2182.

67. Riley KN, Herman IM. Collagenase promotes the cellular responses to injury and wound healing in vivo. *J Burn Wounds*. 2005;4:112-124.

68. Worley CA. The wound healing process: part III—the finale. *Dermatol Nurs*. 2004;16(3):274-275.

69. Bosch U, Kaspercyk WJ. Healing of the patellar tendon autograft after posterior cruciate ligament reconstruction—a process of ligamentization? An experimental study in a sheep model. *Am J Sports Med*. 1992;20(5):558-566.

70. Cromack DT, Porras-Reyes B, Mustoe TA. Current concepts in wound healing: growth factor and macrophage interaction. *J Trauma*. 1990;30(12):S129-S133.

71. Ulrich-Vinther M, Maloney MD, Schwartz EM, Rosier R, O'Keefe RJ. Articular cartilage biology. *J Am Acad Orthop Surg*. 2003;11(6):421-430.

72. Khan KM, Cook JL, Bonar F, Harcourt P, Astrom M. Histopathology of common tendinopathies: Update and implications for clinical management. *Sports Med*. 1999;27(6):393-408.

73. Betz P, Nerlich A, Wilske J, Tübel J, Penning R, Eisenmenger W. Time-dependent appearance of myofibroblasts in granulation tissue of human skin wounds. *Int J Legal Med*. 1992;150:99-103.

74. Darby IA, Zakuan N, Billet F, Desmoulière A. The myofibroblast, a key cell in normal and pathological tissue repair. *Cell Mol Life Sci*. 2016;73(6):1145-1157.

75. Galiano RD, Mustoe TA. Wound healing. In: Mulholland MW, Lillemoe KD, Doherty GM, Maier RV, Simeone DM, Upchurch GR, Jr., eds. *Greenfield's Surgery: Scientific Principles and Practice*. 5th ed. Wolters Kluwer/ Lippincott Williams & Wilkins; 2011:48-69.

76. Inoue M, Ono T, Tateshita T, Kuroyanagi Y, Shioya N. Effect of collagen matrix containing epidermal growth factor on wound contraction. *Wound Rep Reg*. 1998;6(3):213-222.

77. Connolly JF. *Fracture Complications: Recognition, Prevention and Management*. Year Book Medical; 1988.

78. Peacock EE. Inter- and intramolecular bonding in collagen of healing wounds by insertion of methylene and amide cross-links into scar tissue: tensile strength and thermal shrinkage in rats. *Ann Surg*. 1966;163(1):1-9.

79. Tukallo K, Majewski W. Experimental studies on tensile strength of healing wound of fascia and muscle. *Pol Med J*. 1972;11(4):939-945.

80. DiCarlo AL, Horta ZP, Aldrich JT, Jakubowski AA, Skinner WK, Case CM, Jr. Use of growth factors and other cytokines for treatment of injuries during a radiation public health emergency. *Radiat Res*. 2019;192(1):99-120.

81. Adams AC, Coskun T, Rovira AR, et al. Fundamentals of FGF19 & FGF21 action in vitro and in vivo. *PLoS One*. 2012;7(5):e34838.

82. Bennett NT, Schultz GS. Growth factors and wound healing: biochemical properties of growth factors and their receptors. *Am J Surg*. 1993;165(6):728-37.

83. Ota S, Uehara K, Nozaki M, et al. Intramuscular transplantation of muscle-derived stem cells accelerates skeletal muscle healing after contusion injury via enhancement of angiogenesis. *Am J Sports Med*. 2011;39(9):1912-1922.

84. Anoka N, Nyland J, McGinnis M, Lee D, Doral M, Caborn D. Consideration of growth factors and bio-scaffolds for treatment of combined grade II MCL and ACL injury. *Knee Surg Sports Traumatol Arthrosc*. 2012;20(5):878-888.

85. Rolfe KJ, Grobbelaar AO. The growth receptors and their role in wound healing. *Curr Opin Investig Drugs*. 2010;11(11):1221-1228.

86. Grazul-Bilska AT, Johnson ML, Bilski JJ, et al. Wound healing: the role of growth factors. *Drugs Today (Barc)*. 2003;39(10):787-800.

87. Ferrara N. Vascular endothelial growth factor and the regulation of angiogenesis. *Recent Prog Horm Res*. 2000;55:15-35.

88. Ferrara N. Role of vascular endothelial growth factor in regulation of physiological angiogenesis. *Am J Physiol Cell Physiol*. 2001;280(6):C1358-C1366.

89. Ferrara N, LeCouter J, Lin R. Endocrine gland vascular endothelial growth factor (EG-VEGF) and the hypothesis of tissue-specific regulation of angiogenesis. *Endocr Res*. 2002;28(4):763-764.

90. Takehara K. Growth regulation of skin fibroblasts. *J Dermatol Sci*. 2000;24(Suppl 1):S70-S77.

91. Breuing K, Andree C, Helo G, Slama J, Liu PY, Eriksson E. Growth factors in the repair of partial thickness skin wounds. *Plast Reconstr Surg*. 1997;100(3):657-664.

92. Svensjö T, Yao F, Pomahac B, Winkler T, Eriksson E. Cultured autologous fibroblasts augment epidermal repair. *Transplantation*. 2002;73(7):1033-1041.

93. Herndon DN, Hayward PG, Rutan RL, Barrow RE. Growth hormones and factors in surgical patients. *Adv Surg*. 1992;25(1):65-97.

94. Argün M, Öner M, Güney A, Halıcı M, Temizyürek O, Canöz Ö. The healing of full-thickness articular cartilage defects in rabbits: successful results with fibroblast growth factor. *Eklem Hastilik Cerrasisi*. 2010;21(3):147-152.

95. Angel MJ, Razzano P, Grande DA. Defining the challenge: the basic science of articular cartilage repair and response to injury. *Sports Medicine & Arthroscopy Rev*. September 2003;11(3):168-181.

96. Falanga V. Chronic wounds: pathophysiologic and experimental considerations. *J Invest Dermatol*. 1993;100(5):721-725.

97. Cunnion KM, Krishna NK, Pallera HK, et al. Complement activation and STAT4 expression are associated with early inflammation in diabetic wounds. *PLoS One*. 2017;12(1)

98. Forrester SJ, Kikuchi DS, Hernandes MS, Xu Q, Griendling KK. Reactive Oxygen Species in Metabolic and Inflammatory Signaling. *Circ Res*. 2018;122(6):877-902.

99. Hom DB. Growth factors in wound healing. *Otolaryngol Clin North Am*. 1995;28(5):933-953.

100. Scott A, Cook JL, Hart DA, Walker DC, Duronio V, Khan KM. Tenocyte responses to mechanical loading in vivo: a role for local insulin-like growth factor 1 signaling in early tendinosis in rats. *Arthritis rheum*. 2007;56(3):871-881.

101. Hsu SL, Liang R, Woo SL. Functional tissue engineering of ligament healing. *Sports Med Arthrosc Rehabil Ther Technol*. 2010;2(12). doi:10.1186/1758-2555-2-12

102. Hampson K, Forsyth NR, El Haj A, Maffulli N. Tendon tissue engineering. In: Ashammakhi N, Reis R, Chiellini F, eds. *Topics in Tissue Engineering*. University of Oulu; 2008:1-21.

103. Hyman J, Rodeo SA. Injury and repair of tendons and ligaments. *Phys Med Rehabil Clin N Am*. 2000;11(2):267-288.

104. Temenoff JS, Mikos AG. Injectable biodegradable materials for orthopedic tissue engineering. *Biomaterials*. 2000;21(23):2405-2412.

105. Andriacchi T, Sabiston P, DeHaven K, et al. Ligament: injury and repair. In: Woo SLY, Buckwalter JA, eds. *Injury and Repair of the Musculoskeletal Soft Tissues*. American Academy of Orthopaedic Surgeions; 1988:103-128.

106. Bosch U, Kaspercyk WJ, Oestern HJ, Tscherne H. Biology of posterior cruciate ligament healing. *Sports Med Arthroscop Rev*. 1994;2(1):88-99.

107. Chamberlain CS, Crowley E, Vanderby R. The spatiotemporal dynamics of ligament healing. *Wound Rep Reg*. 2009;17(2):206-215.

108. Frank C, Schachar N, Dittrich D. Natural history of healing in the repaired medial collateral ligament. *J Orthop Res*. 1983;1(2):179-188.

109. Tohyama H, Yasuda K. Anterior cruciate ligament (ACL) healing: ACL graft biology. *Sports Med Arthrosc Rev*. 2005;13(1):156-160.

110. Killian ML, Cavinatto L, Galatz LM, Thomopoulos S. The role of mechanobiology in tendon healing. *J Shoulder Elbow Surg*. 2012;21(2):228-237.

111. Abat F, Alfredson H, Cucchiarini M, et al. Current trends in tendinopathy: consensus of the ESSKA basic science committee. Part II: treatment options. *J Exp Orthop*. 2018;5(1):38.

112. Rashid MS, Cooper C, Cook J, et al. Increasing age and tear size reduce rotator cuff repair Healing rate at 1 year. *Acta Orthop*. 2017;88(6):606-611.

113. Riley G. The pathogenesis of tendinopathy: a molecular perspective. *Rheumatology (Oxford)*. 2004;43(2):131-142.

114. Zabrzyński J, Łapaj Ł, Paczesny Ł, Zabrzyńska A, Grzanka D. Tendon—function-related structure, simple healing process and mysterious ageing. *Folia Morphol (Warsz)*. 2018;77(3):416-427.

115. Gelberman R, An KA, Banes A, Goldberg V. Tendon. In: Woo SL, Buckwalter JA, eds. *Injury and Repair of the Musculoskeletal Soft Tissues*. AAOS; 1988:5-40.

116. Beredjiklian PK. Biologic apsects of flexor tendon laceration and repair. *J Bone Joint Surg Am*. 2003;85-A(3):539-550.

117. Sharma P, Maffulli N. Biology of tendon injury: healing, modeling and remodeling. *J Musculoskelet Neuronal Interact*. 2006;6(2):181-190.

118. Thomopoulos S, Parks WC, Rifkin DB, Derwin KA. Mechanisms of tendon injury and repair. *J Orthop Res*. 2015;33(6):832-839.

119. Kluczynski MA, Nayyar S, Marzo JM, Bisson LJ. Early versus delayed passive range of motion after rotator cuff repair: a systematic review and meta-analysis. *Am J Sports Med*. 2015;43(8):2057-2063.

120. Evans RB. Early active motion after flexor tendon repair. In: Berger RA, Weiss APC, eds. *Hand Surgery*. Lippincott Williams & Wilkins; 2004:710-735.

121. Kangas J, Pajala A, Siira P, Hamalainen M, Leppilahti J. Early functional treatment versus early immobilization in tension of the musculotendinous unit after Achilles rupture repair: a prospective, randomized, clinical study. *J Trauma* 2003;54(6):1171-1180.

122. Montgomery RD. Healing of muscle, ligaments, and tendons. *Semin Vet Med Surg*. 1989;4(4):304-311.

123. Benjamin M, Kaiser E, Milz S. Structure-function relationships in tendons: a review. *J Anat*. 2008;212(3):211-228.

124. Zhao X, Jiang S, Liu S, et al. Optimization of intrinsic and extrinsic tendon healing through controllable water-soluble mitomycin-C release from electrospun fibers by mediating adhesion-related gene expression. *Biomaterials*. 2015;61:61-74.

125. Sharma P, Maffulli N. Basic biology of tendon injury and healing. *Surgeon*. 2005;3(5):309-316.

126. Khan K, Brown J, Way S, et al. Overuse injuries in classical ballet. *Sports Med*. 1995;19(5):341-357.

127. Klifto CS, Capo JT, Sapienza A, Yang SS, Paksima N. Flexor Tendon Injuries. *J Am Acad Orthop Surg*. 2018;26(2):e26-e35.

128. Cottrell JA, Turner JC, Arinzeh TL, O'Connor JP. The biology of bone and ligament healing. *Foot Ankle Clin*. 2016;21(4):739-\61.

129. Hope M, Saxby TS. Tendon healing. *Foot Ankle Clin.* 2007;12(4):553-567, v.

130. Myer C, Fowler JR. Flexor tendon repair: healing, biomechanics, and suture configurations. *Orthop Clin North Am.* 2016;47(1):219-226.

131. Zhu DS, Young JD, Garver JV, Blaine TA. Rotator cuff healing and repair: recent advances in tissue engineering and biologic augmentation. *Curr Orthop Pract.* 2014;25(3):266-280.

132. Dueweke JJ, Awan TM, Mendias CL. Regeneration of skeletal muscle after eccentric injury. *J Sport Rehabil.* 2017;26(2):171-179.

133. Caplan AB, Carlson J, Faulkner J, Fischman D, Garrett W, Jr. Skeletal muscle. In: Woo SL, Buckwalter JA, eds. *Injury and Repair of the Musculoskeletal Soft Tissues.* AAOS; 1988:209-292.

134. Gates C, Huard J. Management of skeletal injuries in military personnel. *Op Tech Sports Med.* 2005;13(4):247-256.

135. Tidball JG. Regulation of muscle growth and regeneration by the immune system. *Nat Rev Immunol.* 2017;17(3):165-178.

136. Wilgus TA, Roy S, McDaniel JC. Neutrophils and wound repair: positive actions and negative reactions. *Adv Wound Care (New Rochelle).* 2013;2(7):379-388.

137. Souza NHC, Mesquita-Ferrari RA, Rodrigues MFSD, et al. Photobiomodulation and different macrophages phenotypes during muscle tissue repair. *J Cell Mol Med.* 2018;22(10):4922-4934.

138. Arnold L, Henry A, Poron F, et al. Inflammatory monocytes recruited after skeletal muscle injury switch into antiinflammatory macrophages to support myogenesis. *J Exp Med.* 2007;204(5):1057-1069.

139. Laumonier T, Menetrey J. Muscle injuries and strategies for improving their repair. *J Exp Orthop.* 2016;3(1):15. doi:10.1186/s40634-016-0051-7

140. Sarrafian TL, Bodine SC, Murphy B, Grayson JK, Stover SM. Extracellular matrix scaffolds for treatment of large volume muscle injuries: a review. *Vet Surg.* 2018;47(4):524-535.

141. Woo SL-Y, Buckwalter JA. Injury and repair of the musculoskeletal soft tissues. *J Orthop Res.* 1988;6:907-931.

142. Lewis PB, McCarty LP, 3rd, Kang RW, Cole BJ. Basic science and treatment options for articular cartilage injuries. *J Orthop Sports Phys Ther.* 2006;36(10):717-727.

143. Simon TM, Jackson DW. Articular cartilage: injury pathways and treatment options. *Sports Med Arthrosc Rev.* 2006;14(3):146-154.

144. Silver FH, Glasgold AI. Cartilage wound healing. *Otolaryngol Clin North Am.* 1995;28(5):847-864.

145. Mosher TJ, Danrdzinksi BJ. Cartilage MRI T2 relaxation time mapping: overview and applications. *Semin Musculoskelet Radiol.* 2004;8(4):355-368.

146. Mow VC, Tohyama H, Grelsamer RP. Structure-function of the knee articular cartilage. *Sports Med Arthrosc Rev.* 1994;2(3):189-202.

147. Carballo CB, Nakagawa Y, Sekiya I, Rodeo SA. Basic science of articular cartilage. *Clin Sports Med.* 2017;36(3):413-425.

148. Decker RS, Koyama E, Pacifici M. Genesis and morphogenesis of limb synovial joints and articular cartilage. *Matrix Biol.* 2014;39:5-10.

149. Cohen NP, Foster RJ, Mow VC. Composition and dynamics of articular cartilage: structure, function, and maintaining healthy state. *J Orthop Sports Phys Ther.* 1998;28(4):203-215.

150. Gill TJ, Asnis PD, Berkson EM. The treatment of articular cartilage defects using the microfracture technique. *J Orthop Sports Phys Ther.* October 2006;36(10):728-738.

151. Steadman JR, Rodkey WG, Briggs KK. Microfracture to treat full-thickness chondral defects: surgical technique, rehabilitation, and outcomes. *J Knee Surg.* 2002;15(3):170-176.

152. Simon TM, Jackson DW. Articular cartilage: Injury pathways and treatment options. *Sports Med Arthrosc Rev.* 2018;26(1):31-39.

153. Hjelle K, Solheim E, Strand T, Muri R, Brittberg M. Articular cartilage defects in 1,000 knee arthroscopies. *Arthroscopy.* 2002;18(7):730-734.

154. Widuchowski W, Widuchowski J, Tzaska T. Articular cartilage defects: study of 25,124 knee arthroscopies. *Knee.* 2007;14(3):177-182.

155. Browne JE, Branch TP. Surgical alternatives for treatment of articular cartilage lesions. *J Am Acad Orthop Surg.* 2000;8(3):180-189.

156. Detterline AJ, Goldberg S, Bach BRJ, Cole BJ. Treatment options for articular cartilage defects of the knee. *Orthop Nurs.* 2005;24(5):361-368.

157. Steadman JR, Briggs KK, Rodrigo JJ, Kocher MS, Gill TJ, Rodkey WG. Outcomes of microfracture for traumatic chondral defects of the knee: average 11-year follow-up. *J Arthroscop Rel Surg.* 2003;19:477-484.

158. Hayes DW, Jr., Brower RL, John KJ. Articular cartilage: anatomy, injury, and repair. *Clin Podiatr Med Surg.* 2001;18(1):35-53.

159. Jones G, Ding C, Glisson M, Hynes K, Ma D, Cicuttini F. Knee articular cartilage development in children: A longitudinal study of the effect of sex, growth, body composition, and physical activity. *Pediatr Res.* 2003;54(2):230-236.

160. Miura K, Ishibashi Y, Tsuda E, Sato H, Toh S. Results of arthroscopic fixation of osteochondritis dissecans lesion of the knee with cylindrical autogenous osteochondral plugs. *Am J Sports Med.* 2007;35(2):216-222.

161. Tetteh ES, Bajaj S, Ghodadra NS. Basic science and surgical treatment options for articular cartilage injuries of the knee. *J Orthop Sports Phys Ther.* 2012;42(3):243-253.

162. Bartha L, Vajda A, Duska Z, Rahmeh H, Hangody L. Autologous osteochondral mosaicplasty grafting. *J Orthop Sports Phys Ther.* 2006;36(10):739-750.

163. Kawano CT, dos Santos MM, de Oliveira MG, Ourivio TC. Trapezoidal osteochondral autologous plug single-block graft for treating chondral lesions of the knee: clinical and functional medium-term results in an observational study. *Clinics (Sao Paulo).* 2012;67(10):1191-1195.

164. Brittberg M, Lindahl A, Nilsson A, Ohlsson C, Isaksson O, Peterson L. Treatment of deep cartilage defects in the knee with autologous chondrocyte transplantation. *N Engl J Med.* 1994;331(14):889-895.

165. Kon E, Filardo G, DiMatteo B, Perdisa F, Maracacci M. Matrix assisted autologous chondrocyte transplantation for cartilage treatment: a systematic review. *Bone Joint Res.* 2013;2(2):18-25.

166. Buckwalter JA. Articular cartilage: injuries and potential for healing. *J Orthop Sports Phys Ther*. 1998;28(4):192-202.

167. LaStayo PC, Winters KM, Hardy M. Fractire healing: bone healing, fracture management, and current concepts related to the hand. *J Hand Ther*. 2003;16(2):81-93.

168. Schindeler A, McDonald MM, Bokko P, LIttle DG. Bone remodeling during fracture repair: the cellular picture. *Semin Cell Dev Biol*. 2008;19(5):459-466.

169. Heppenstall RB. Fracture healing. In: Heppenstall RB, ed. *Fracture treatment and healing*. Saunders; 1980.

170. Grundnes O, Reikerås O. Blood flow and mechanical properties of healing bone. Femoral osteotomies studied in rats. *Acta Orthop Scand*. 1992;63(5):487-491.

171. Nordin M, Frankel VH. Biomechanics of collagenous tissues. In: Frankel VH, Nordin M, eds. *Basic Biomechanics of the Skeletal System*. Lea & Febiger; 1980.

172. Ireton JE, Unger JG, Rohrich RJ. The role of wound healing and its everyday application in plastic surgery: a practical perspective and systematic review. *Plast Reconstr Surg Glob Open*. 2013;1(1):e10-e19. doi:10.1097/GOX.0b013e31828ff9f4

173. Goldberg SR, Diegelmann RF. Basic science of wound healing. In: Dieter RS, Dieter RA, Jr., Hines E, Jr., Dieter RA, III., Nanjundappa A, eds. *Critical Limn Ischemia Acute and Chronic*. Springer International; 2019:131-136.

174. Houglum JE, Harrelson GL, Seefeldt TM. *Principles of Pharmacology for Athletic Trainers*. 3rd ed. Slack; 2016.

175. Warden SJ, Avin KG, Beck EM, DeWolf ME, Hagemeier MA, Martin KM. Low-intensity pulsed ultrasound accelerates and a nonsteroidal anti-inflammatory drug delays knee ligament healing. *Am J Sports Med*. 2006;34:1094-1102.

176. Huang SH, Johnson K, Pipe AL. The use of dietary supplements and medications by Canadian athletes at the Atlanta and Sydney Olympic Games. *Clin J Sport Med*. 2006;16(1):27-33.

177. Paoloni JA. Non-steroidal anti-inflammatory drugs in sports medicine: guidelines for practical but sensible use. *Br J Sports Med*. 2009;43(11):863-865.

178. Chen M, Dragoo J. The effect of nonsteroidal anit-inflammatory drugs on tissue healing. *Knee Surg Sports Traum Arthroscopy*. 2013;21(3):540-549.

179. Marquez-Lara A, Hutchinson ID, Nunez F, Jr., Smith TL, Miller AN. Nonsteroidal anti-inflammatory drugs and bone-healing: a systematic review of research quality. *JBJS Rev*. 2016;4(3):e4. doi:10.2106/JBJS.RVW.O.00055

180. Sivaganesan A, Chotai S, White-Dzuro G, McGirt MJ, Devin CJ. The effect of NSAIDs on spinal fusion: a cross-disciplinary review of biochemical, animal, and human studies. *Eur Spine J*. 2017;26(11):2719-2728.

181. Houglum JE. Pharmacologic considerations in the treatment of injured athletes with nonsteroidal anti-inflammatory drugs. *J Athl Train*. 1998;33(3):259-263.

182. Urban MK. COX-2 specific inhibitors offer improved advantages over traditional NSAIDs. *Orthopedics*. 2000;23(7):S761-S764.

183. Dabu-Bondoc SF, S. Risk-benefit perspectives in COX-2 blockade. *Curr Drug Saf*. 2008;3(1):14-23.

184. Antman EM, Bennett JS, Daugherty A, et al. Use of non-steroidal antiinflammatory drugs: an update for clinicians: a scientific statement from the American Heart Association. *Circulation*. 2007;115(12):1634-1642.

185. Molina VD, Álzate DV, Ruíz JB, Urrea MA, Tobón JJ. Analgesic effect and side effects of celecoxib and meloxicam in canine hip osteoarthritis. *RevMVZ Córdoba*. 2014;19(3):4289-4300.

186. Buckman AL. Side effects of corticosteroid therapy. *J Clin Gastroenterol*. 2001;33(4):289-294.

187. Nwachukwu BU, Chang B, Adjei J, et al. Time required to achieve minimal clinically important difference and substantial clinical benefit after arthroscopic treatment of femoroacetabular impingement. *Am J Sports Med*. 2018;46(11):2601-2606.

188. Bukata SV, Bostrom M, Buckwalter JA, Lane JM. Physiology of aging. In: Vaccaro AR, ed. *AAOS Orthopaedic Knowledge Update 8*. American Academy of Orthopaedic Surgeons; 2005:69-77.

189. McCarthy MM, Hannafin JA. The mature athlete: aging tendon and ligament. *Sports Health*. 2014;6(1):41-48.

190. Li Z, Knetsch M. Antibacterial strategies for wound dressing: preventing infection and stimulating healing. *Curr Pharm Des*. 2018;24(8):936-951.

191. Medlin S. Nutrition in wound healing. *Br J Nurs*. 2012;21(12):S11-S12, S14-S15.

192. Stechmiller JK. Understanding the role of nutrition and wound healing. *Nutr Clin Pract*. 2010;25(1)

193. Trayes KP, Studdiford JS, Pickle S, Tully AS. Edema: diagnosis and management. *Am Fam Physician*. 2013;88(2):102-110.

194. McMaster PD. The pressure and interstitial resistance prevailing in the normal and edematous skin of animals and man. *J Exp Med*. 1946;84(5):473-494.

195. Maguire G, Friedman P. Enhancing spontaneous stem cell healing (Review). *Biomed Rep*. 2014;2(2):163-166.

196. Kosaric N, Kiwanuka H, Gurtner GC. Stem cell therapies for wound healing. *Expert Opin Biol Ther*. 2019;19(6):575-585.

197. Chen M, Przyborowski M, Berthiaume F. Stem cells for skin tissue engineering and wound healing. *Crit Rev Biomed Eng*. 2009;37(4):399-421.

198. Ojeh N, Pastar I, Tomic-Canic M, Stojadinovic O. Stem cells in skin regeneration, wound healing, and their clinical applications. *Int J Mol Sci*. 2015;16(10):25476-25501.

199. Sorg H, Tilkorn DJ, Hager S, Hauser J, Mirastschijski U. Skin wound healing: an update on the current knowledge and concepts. *Eur Surg Res*. 2017;58(1-2):81-94.

200. Wu FL, Nerlich M, Docheva D. Tendon injuries: basic science and new repair proposals. *EFORT Open Rev*. 2017;2(7):332-342. doi:10.1302/2058-5241.2.160075

201. Chamberlain CS, Saether EE, Aktas E, Vanderby R. Mesenchymal stem cell therapy on tendon/ligament healing. *J Cytokine Biol*. 2017;2(1)

202. National Institute of Bioomedical Imaging and Bioengineering. Glossary of terms. National Institutes of Health. Accessed April 20, 2020. https://www.nibib.nih.gov/science-education/glossary#g-42721

203. Asghari F, Samiei M, Adibkia K, Akbarzdeh A, Davaran S. Biodegradable and biocompatible polymers for tissue engineering application: a review. *Artif Cells Nanomed Biotechnol*. 2017;45(2):185-192.

204. Chang BP, Leong KW. Scaffolding in tissue engineering: general approaches and tissue-specific considerations. *Eur Spine J.* 2008;17(4):467-479.

205. Sahana TG, Rekha PD. Biopolymers: applications in wound healing and skin tissue engineering. *Mol Biol Rep.* 2018;45(6):2857-2867.

206. de Isla N, Huseltein C, Jessel N, et al. Introduction to tissue engineering and application for cartilage engineering. *Biomed Mater Eng.* 2010;20(3):127-133.

207. O'Brien FJ. Biomaterials & scaffolds for tissue engineering. *MaterialsToday.* 2011;14(3):88-95.

208. Huang BJ, Hu JC, Athanasiou KA. Cell-based tissue engineering strategies used in the clinical repair of articular cartilage. *Biomaterials.* 2016;98:1-22.

209. Liu Y, Zhou G, Cao Y. Recent progress in cartilage tissue engineering—our experience and future directions. *Engineering.* 2017;3(1):28-35.

210. Bhardwaj N, Chouhan D, Mandal BB. Tissue engineered skin and wound healing: current strategies and future directions. *Curr Pharm Des.* 2017;23(24):3455-3482.

211. Zhu Y, Yuan M, Meng HY, et al. Basic science and clinical application of platelet-rich plasma for cartilage defects and osteoarthritis: a review. *Osteoarthritis Cartilage.* 2013;21(11):1627-1637.

212. Lee TC, Taylor DC. Bone remodelling: should we cry Wolff? *Ir J Med Sci.* 1999;168(2):102-105.

213. Durieux AC, Desplanches D, Freyssenet D, Flück M. Mechanotransduction in striated muscle via focal adhesion kinase. *Biochem Soc Trans.* 2007;35(Pt 5):1312-1313.

214. Hernandez CJ, Beaupré GS, Carter DR. A model of mechanobiologic and metabolic influences on bone adaptation. *J Rehabil Res Dev.* 2000;37(2):235-244.

215. Iatridis JC, Wu J, Yandow JA, Langevin HM. Subcutaneous tissue mechanical behavior is linear and viscoelastic under uniaxial tension. *Connect Tissue Res.* 2003;44(5):208-217.

216. Julkunen P, Wilson W, Jurvelin JS, et al. Stress-relaxation of human patellar articular cartilage in unconfined compression: prediction of mechanical response by tissue composition and structure. *J Biomech.* 2008;41(9):1978-1986.

217. Kjær M, Langberg H, Heinemeier K, et al. From mechanical loading to collagen synthesis, structural changes and function in human tendon. *Scand J Med Sci Sports.* 2009;19(4):500-510.

218. Frost HM. A 2003 update of bone physiology and Wolff's Law for clinicians. *Angle Orthod.* 2004;74(1):3-15.

Chapter 3

1. Wilson RW, Gansneder BM. Measures of functional limitation as predictors of disablement in athletes with acute ankle sprains. *J Orthop Sports Phys Ther.* 2000;30(9):528-535.

2. Villeco JP. Edema: a silent but important factor. *J Hand Ther.* 2012;25(2):153-161.

3. Järvinen TA, Järvinen TL, Kääriäinen M, et al. Muscle injuries: optimising recovery. *Best Pract Res Clin Rheumatol.* 2007;21(2):317-331.

4. Schaser KD, Disch AC, Stover JF, Lauffer A, Bail HJ, Mittlmeier T. Prolonged superficial local cryotherapy attenuates microcirculatory impairment, regional inflammation, and muscle necrosis after closed soft tissue injury in rats. *Am J Sports Med.* 2007;35(1):93-102.

5. Deal DN, Tipton J, Rosencrance E, Curl WW, Smith TL. Ice reduces edema: a study of microvascular permeability in rats. *J Bone Joint Surg Am.* 2002;84(9):1573-1578.

6. Sadoghi P, S. H, Gruber G, et al. Impact of a new cryotherapy device on early rehabilitation after primary total knee arthroplasty (TKA): a prospective randomised controlled trial. *Int Orthop.* 2018;42(6):1265-1273.

7. Williams GN, Allen EJ. Rehabilitation of syndesmotic (high) ankle sprains. *Sports Health.* 2010;2(6):460-470.

8. Rice DA, McNair PJ. Quadriceps arthrogenic muscle inhibition: neural mechanisms and treatment perspectives. *Semin Arthritis Rheum.* 2010;40(3):250-266.

9. Lu H, Chen C, Qu J, et al. Initiation timing of low-intensity pulsed ultrasound stimulation for tendon-bone healing in a rabbit model. *Am J Sports Med.* 2016;44(10):2706-2715.

10. Denegar CR, Saliba E, Saliba S. *Therapeutic Modalities for Musculoskeletal Injuries.* 4th ed. Human Kinetics; 2016.

11. Barbosa GM, Cunha JE, Cunha TM, et al. Clinical-like cryotherapy improves footprint patterns and reduces synovial inflammation in a rat model of post-traumatic knee osteoarthritis. *Sci Rep.* 2019;9(1):14518. doi:10.1038/s41598-019-50958-8

12. McMaster WC. A literary review on ice therapy in injuries. *Am J Sports Med.* 1977;5(3):124-126.

13. Fang L, Hung CH, Wu SL, Fang SH, Stocker J. The effects of cryotherapy in relieving postarthroscopy pain. *J Clin Nurs.* 2012;21(5-6):636-643.

14. Swenson C, Swärd L, Karlsson J. Cryotherapy in sports medicine. *Scand J Med Sci Sports.* 1996;6(4):193-200.

15. Nadler SF, Weingand K, Kruse RJ. The physiologic basis and clinical applications of cryotherapy and thermotherapy for the pain practitioner. *Pain Phys.* 2004;7(3):395-399.

16. Kowall MG. Review of physiological effects of cryotherapy. *J Orthop Sports Phys Ther.* 1983;5(2):66-73.

17. Kettenmann B, Wille C, Lurie-Luke E, Walter D, Kobal G. Impact of continuous low level heatwrap therapy in acute low back pain patients: subjective and objective measurements. *Clin J Pain.* 2007;23(8):663-668.

18. Badia P, Hickey V, Flesch L, et al. Quality improvement initiative to reduce nighttime noise in a transplantation and cellular therapy unit. *Biol Blood Marrow Transplant.* 2019;25(9):1844-1850.

19. Bindra RR. Basic pathology of the hand, wrist, and forearm: tendon and ligament. In: Berger RA, Weiss APC, eds. *Hand Surgery.* Lippincott Williams & Wilkins; 2004:23-35.

20. Frank C, Woo S, Andriacchi T, et al. Normal ligament: structure, function, and composition. In: Woo SLY, Buckwalter JA, eds. *Injury and Repair of the Musculoskeletal Soft Tissues.* AAOS; 1988:45-102.

21. Macaulay AA, Perfetti DC, Levine WN. Anterior cruciate ligament graft choices. *Sports Health.* 2012;4(1):63-68.

22. Scallon JP, Zawiega SD, Cstorena-Gonzalez JA, Davis MJ. Lymphatic pumping: mechanics, mechanisms and malfunction. *J Physiol.* 2016;594(20):5749-5768.

23. Conti M, Garofalo R, Delle Rose G, et al. Post-operative rehabilitation after surgical repair of the rotator cuff. *Chir Organi Mov.* 2009;93(Suppl 1):S55-S63.

24. Stroud R. CPM's therapeutic benefits. *Rehab Management.* 2006;19:1-4.

25. Jezequel JR. The continuous passive motion concept: part II. *Phys Ther Prod.* 2011;22(4):20-22.

26. Theodoropoulos JS, DeCroos AJN, Petrera M, Park S, Kandel RA. Mechanical stimulation enhances integration in an in vitro model of cartilage repair. *Knee Surg Sports Traumatol Arthrosc*. 2016;24(6):2055-2064.

27. Snyder M, Kozlowski P, Drobniewski M, Grzegorzewski A, Glowacka A. The use of continuous passive motion (CPM) in the rehabilitation of patients after total knee arthroplasty. *Orthop Traumatol Rehabil*. 2004;6:336-341.

28. Farsetti P, Caterini R, Potenza V, De Luna V, De Maio F, Ippolito E. Immediate continuous passive motion after internal fixation of an ankle fracture. *J Orthop Traumatol*. 2009;10(2):63-69.

29. Sunitha J. Cryotherapy—a review *J Clin Diagn Res*. 2010;4:2325-2329.

30. Shamus J, Shamus E, Gugel RN, Brucker BS, Skaruppa C. The effect of sesamoid mobilization, flexor hallucis strengthening, and gait training on reducing pain and restoring function in individuals with hallux limitus: a clinical trial. *J Orthop Sports Phys Ther*. 2004;34(7):368-376.

31. Karmisholt KE, Banzhaf CA, Glud M, et al. Laser treatments in early wound healing improve scar appearance: a randomized split-wound trial with nonablative fractional laser exposures vs. untreated controls. *Br J Dermatol*. 2018;179(6):1307-1314.

32. Malanga GA, Yan N, Stark J. Mechanisms and efficacy of heat and cold therapies for musculoskeletal injury. *Postgrad Med*. 2015;127(1):57-65.

33. Starkey C. *Therapeutic Modalities*. 4th ed. F.A. Davis Co.; 2013.

34. Steadman TL. *Steadman's Medical Dictionary*. 25th ed. Williams & Wilkins; 1990.

35. Kuhlenhoelter AM, Kim K, Neff D, et al. Heat therapy promotes the expression of angiogenic regulators in human skeletal muscle. *Am J Physiol Regul Integr Comp Physiol*. 2016;311(2):R377-R391.

36. Petrofsky JS, Laymon M, Lee H. Local heating of trigger points reduces neck and plantar fascia pain. *J Back Musculoskelet Rehabil*. 2020;33(1):21-28.

37. Petrofsky JS, Laymon M, Lee H. Effect of heat and cold on tendon flexibility and force to flex the human knee. *Med Sci Monit*. 2013;19:661-667.

38. Draper DO. Pulsed shortwave diathermy and joint mobilizations for achieving normal elbow range of motion after injury or surgery with implanted metal: a case series. *J Athl Train*. 2014;49(6):851-855.

39. Kloth LC. Electrical stimulation technologies for wound healing. *Adv Wound Care (New Rochelle)*. 2014;3(2):81-90.

40. Saka T. Principles of postoperative anterior cruciate ligament rehabilitation. *World J Orthop*. 2014;5(4):450-459.

41. Rashid MS, Cooper C, Cook J, et al. Increasing age and tear size reduce rotator cuff repair healing rate at 1 year. *Acta Orthop*. 2017;88(6):606-611.

42. Guo S, Dipietro LA. Factors affecting wound healing. *J Den Res*. 2010;89(3):219-229.

43. Moran SA, Isa J, Steinemann S. Perioperative management in the patient with substance abuse. *Surg Clin North Am*. 2015;95:417-428.

44. Kocaman O, Koyuncu H, Dinc A, Toros H, Karamehmetoğlu FS. The comparison of the effects of electrical stimulation and exercise in the treatment of knee osteoarthritis. *Turkish J Phys Med Rehabil*. 2008;54(2):54-58.

45. Takenori A, Ikuhiro M, Shogo U, et al. Immediate pain relief effect of low level laser therapy for sports injuries: Randomized, double-blind placebo clinical trial. *J Sci Med Sport*. 2016;19(12):980-983.

46. Folland JP, Williams AG. The adaptations to strength training: morphological and neurological contributions to increased strength. *Sports Med*. 2007;37(2):145-168.

47. Steadman JR, Forster RS, Silferskiöld JP. Rehabilitation of the knee. *Clin Sports Med*. 1989;8(3):605-627.

48. Kidgell DJ, Stokes MA, Pearce AJ. Strength training of one limb increases corticomotor excitability projecting to the contralateral homologous limb. *Motor Control*. 2011;15(2):247-266.

49. Duran RJ, Houser RG. Controlled passive motion following flexor tendon repair in zones 2 and 3. *AAOS Symposium on Tendon Surgery of the Hand*. Mosby; 1975.

50. Neuhaus V, Wong G, Russo KE, Mudgal CS. Dynamic splinting with early motion following zone IV/V and TI to TIII extensor tendon repairs. *J Hand Surg Am*. 2012;37(5):933-937.

51. Depalle B, Qin Z, Shefelbine SJ, Buehler MJ. Influence of cross-link structure, density and mechanical properties in the mesoscale deformation mechanisms of collagen fibrils. *J Mech Behav Biomed Mater*. 2015;52:1-13.

52. Buckwalter JA, Grodzinsky AJ. Loading of healing bone, fibrous tissue, and muscle: implications for orthopaedic practice. *J Am Acad Orthop Surg*. 1999;7(5):291-299.

53. Chvapil M, Koopmann CF, Jr. Scar formation: physiology and pathological states. *Otolaryngol Clin North Am*. 1984;17(2):265-272.

54. Arem AJ, Madden JW. Effects of stress on healing wounds: I. intermittent noncyclical tension. *J Surg Res*. 1976;20(2):93-102.

55. Hammad SM, Arsh A, Iqbal M, Khan W, Bilal., Shah A. Comparing the effectiveness of Kaltenborn mobilization with thermotherapy versus Kaltenborn mobilization alone in patients with frozen shoulder (adhesive capsulitis): a randomized control trial. *J Pak Med Assoc*. 2019;69(10):1421-1424.

56. Snyder AR, Perotti AL, Lam KC, Bay RC. The influence of high-voltage electrical stimulation on edema formation after acute injury: a systematic review. *J Sport Rehabil*. 2010;19(4):436-451.

57. Cook HA, Morales M, La Rosa EM, et al. Effects of electrical stimulation on lymphatic flow and limb volume in the rat. *Phys Ther*. 1994;74(11):1040-1046.

58. Holdermann A, Mork PJ, Andersen LL, Olsen HB, Søgaard K. The use of EMG biofeedback for learning of selective activation of intra-muscular parts within the serratus anterior muscle: a novel approach for rehabilitation of scapular muscle imbalance. *J Electromyogr Kinesiol*. 2010;20(2):359-365.

59. Bremner CB, Holcomb WR, Brown CD, Perreault ME. The effectiveness of neuromuscular electrical stimulation in improving voluntary activation of the quadriceps: a critically appraised topic. *J Sport Rehabil*. 2017;26(4):316-323.

60. Jones S, Man, W.D.C., Gao W, Higginson IJ, Wilcock A, Maddocks M. Neuromuscular electrical stimulation for muscle weakness in adults with advanced

disease. *Cochrane Database Sys Rev.* 2016;10(10) doi:10.1002/14651858.CD009419.pub3

61. Walls RJ, McHugh G, O'Gorman DJ, Moyna NM, O'Byrne JM. Effects of preoperative neuromuscular electrical stimulation on quadriceps strength and functional recovery in total knee arthroplasty. A pilot study. *BMC Musculoskelet Disord.* 2010;11:119-127.

62. Kadi MR, S. H, Atamaz FC, et al. Is interferential current effective in the management of pain, range of motion, and edema following total knee arthroplasty surgery? A randomized double-blind controlled trial. *Clin Rehabil.* 2019;33(6):1027-1034.

63. Bircan C, Senocak O, Peker O, et al. Efficacy of two forms of electrical stimulation in increasing quadriceps strength: a randomized controlled trial. *Clin Rehabil.* 2002;16(2):194-199.

64. Lewis K, Simons DG. Myofascial pain: relief by post-isometric relaxation. *Arch Phys Med Rehabil.* 1984;65(8):452-456.

65. Vicenzino B, Paungmali A, Teys P. Mulligan's mobilization-with-movement, positional faults and pain relief: current concepts from a critical review of literature. *Man Ther.* 2007;12(2):98-108.

66. Beattie PF, Arnot CF, Donley JW, Noda H, Bailey L. The immediate reduction in low back pain intensity following lumbar joint mobilization and prone press-ups is associated with increased diffusion of water in the L5-S1 intervertebral disc *J Orthop Sports Phys Ther.* 2010;40(5):256-264.

67. Wong YY, Smith RW, Koppenhaver S. Soft tissue mobilization to resolve chronic pain and dysfunction associated with postoperative abdominal and pelvic adhesions: a case report. *J Orthop Sports Phys Ther.* 2015;45(12):1006-1016.

68. Richman ED, Tyo BM, Nicks CR. Combined effects of self-myofascial release and dynamic stretching on range of motion, jump, sprint, and agility performance. *J Strength Cond Res.* 2018;doi:10.1519/JSC.0000000000002676

69. Scifers JR. Instrument-assisted soft tissue mobilization. *Athl Train Sports Health Care.* 2017;9(2):49-52.

70. Peacock EE. *Wound Repair.* 3rd ed. Lea & Febiger; 1984.

71. Rudolph R. Contraction and the control of contraction. *World J Surg.* 1980;4:279-287. doi:doi.org/10.1007/BF02393383

72. Gignac MAM, Cao X, Ramanathan S, et al. Perceived personal importance of exercise and fears of re-injury: a longitudinal study of psychological factors related to activity after anterior cruciate ligament reconstruction. *BMC Sports Sci Med Rehabil.* 2015;7:4. doi:10.1186/2052-1847-7-4

73. Covassin T, Beidler E, Ostrowski J, Wallace J. Psychosocial aspects of rehabilitation in sports. *Clin Sports Med.* 2015;34(2):199-212.

74. Jones SW, Hill RJ, Krasney PA, O'Conner B, Peirce N, Greenhaff PL. Disuse atrophy and exercise rehabilitation in humans profoundly affects the expression of genes associated with the regulation of skeletal muscle mass. *FASEB J.* 2004;18(9):1025-1027.

75. Houglum P. Modality of therapeutic exercise: objectives and principles. *Athl Train.* 1977;12(1):42-45.

76. Gabriel DA, Kamen G, Frost G. Neural adaptations to resistive exercise: mechanisms and recommendations for training practices. *Sports Med.* 2006;36(2):133-149.

Chapter 4

1. Centers for Disease Control and Prevention. Protect the ones you love: child injuries are preventable. Accessed January 4, 2020. www.cdc.gov/safechild/sports_injuries/index.html

2. Centers for Disease Control and Prevention. National Center for Health Statistics at-a-glance table 2018. Accessed January 5, 2020. www.cdc.gov/nchs/hus/ataglance.htm

3. Ausubel JH, Grubler A. Working less and living longer: Long-term trends in working time and time budgets. *Technol Forecast Soc Change.* 1995;50:113-131.

4. Backx FJG, Erich WBM, Kemper ABA, Verbeek ALM. Sports injuries in school-aged children: an epidemiologic study. *Am J Sports Med.* 1989;17(2):234-240.

5. Hardin A, Hackell JM. Age limits of pediatrics. *Pediatrics.* 2017;140(3):e20172151.

6. Reider-Demer M, Zielinski T, Carvajal S, Anulao K, Van Roeyen L. When is a pediatric patient no longer a pediatric patient? *J Pediatr Health Care.* 2008;22(4):267-269.

7. Popkin CA, Bayomy AF, Ahmad CS. Early sports specialization. *J Am Acad Orthop Surg.* 2019;27(22):995-1000.

8. Logan K, Cuff S, Council on Sports Medicine and Fitness. Organized sports for children, preadolescents, and adolescents. *Pediatrics.* 2019;143(6):e20190997.

9. Koester MC. Adolescent and youth sports medicine: A "growing" concern. *Athl Ther Today.* 2002;7(6):6-12.

10. Field AE, Tepolt FA, Yang DS, Kocher MS. Injury risk associated with sports specialization and activity volume in youth. *Orthop J Sports Med.* 2019;7(9):2325967119870124.

11. Patel DR, Yamasaki A, Brown K. Epidemiology of sports-related musculoskeletal injuries in young athletes in United States. *Transl Pediatr.* 2017;6(3):160-166.

12. Tanner JM. *Growth at Adolescence.* 2nd ed. Blackwell Scientific; 1962:212.

13. Tanner JM, Davies PS. Clinical longitudinal standards for height and height velocity for North American children. *J Pediatr.* 1985;107(3):317-329.

14. Tanner JM, Whitehouse RH. Clinical longitudinal standards for height, weight, height velocity, weight velocity, and stages of puberty. *Arch Dis Child.* 1976;51(3):170-179.

15. Abbassi V. Growth and normal puberty. *Pediatrics.* 1998;102(2):507-511.

16. Cronin JB, Hansen KT. Strength and power predictors of sports speed. *J Strength Cond Res.* 2005;19(2):349-357.

17. Flanagan SD, Dunn-Lewis CL, Hatfield DJ, et al. Developmental differences between boys and girls result in sex-specific physical fitness changes from fourth to fifth grade. *Journal of Strength and Conditioning Research.* 2015;29(1):175-180.

18. Catley MJ, Tomkinson GR. Normative health-related fitness values for children: analysis of 85347 test results on 9-17-year-old Australians since 1985. *Br J Sports Med.* 2013;47(2):98-108.

19. Marta CC, Marinho DA, Barbosa TM, Izquierdo M, Marques MC. Physical fitness differences between prepubescent boys and girls. *J Strength Cond Res.* 2012;26(7):1756-1766.

20. Salter RB, Harris WR. Injuries involving the epiphyseal plate. *Journal of Bone and Joint Surgery Am.* 1963;45(3):587-622.

21. Salzmann GM, Neiemeyer P, Hochrein A, Stoddart MJ, Angele P. Articular cartilage repair of the knee in children and adolescents. *The Orthopaedic Journal of Sports Medicine.* 2018;6(3):2325967118760190.

22. Micheli LJ, Moseley JB, Anderson AF, et al. Articular cartilage defects of the distal femur in children and adolescents: treatment with autologous chondrocyte implantation. *J Ped Orthop.* 2006;26(4):455-460.

23. Jones G, Ding C, Glisson M, Hynes K, Ma D, Cicuttini F. Knee articular cartilage development in children: A longitudinal study of the effect of sex, growth, body composition, and physical activity. *Pediatr Res.* 2003;54(2):230-236.

24. Decker RS, Koyama E, Pacifici M. Articular cartilage: structural and developmental intricacies and questions. *Curr Osteoporos Rep.* 2015;13(6):407-414.

25. Brown KA, Patel DR, Darmawan D. Participation in sports in relation to adolescent growth and development. *Transl Pediatr.* 2017;6(3):150-159.

26. Frost HM, Schönau E. The "muscle-bone unit" in children and adolescents: a 2000 overview. *J Pediatr Endocrinol Metab.* 2000;13(6):571-590.

27. Longo UG, Ciuffreda M, Locher J, Maffulli N, Denaro V. Apophyseal injuries in children's and youth sports. *British Medical Bulletin.* 2016;120:139-159.

28. Fricke O, Schoenau E. The "functional muscle-bone unit": probing the relevance of mechanical signals for bone development in children and adolescents. *Growth Horm IGF Res.* 2007;17(1):1-9.

29. Council on Sports Medicine and Fitness, McCambridge TM, Stricker PR. Strength training by children and adolescents. *Pediatrics.* 2008;121(4):835-840.

30. DiFiori JP, Benjamin HJ, Brenner JS, et al. Overuse injuries and burnout in youth sports: a position statement from the American Medical Society for Sports Medicine. *Br J Sport Med.* 2014;48:287-300.

31. Mariscalco MW, Saluan P. Upper extremity injuries in the adolescent athlete. *Sports Med Arthrosc.* 2011;19(1):17-26.

32. Ostry DJ, Gribble PL. Sensory plasticity in human motor learning. *Trends in Neurosciences.* 2016;39(2):114-123.

33. Kottke FJ. Therapeutic exercise to develop neuromuscular coordination. In: Kottke FJ, Lehmann JF, eds. *Krusen's Handbook of Physical Medicine and Rehabilitation.* 4th ed. Saunders; 1990:452-479.

34. Bar-Or O, Rowland T. *Pediatric Exercise Medicine: From Physiologic Principles to Health Care Application.* Human Kinetics; 2004:520.

35. Price MJ. Thermoregulation in children and adolescents. *Reviews in Pediatric Exercise Science.* Nova Science; 2012:161-180.

36. Williams CA. Exercise and environmental conditions. In: Spurway N, MacLaren D, eds. *Paediatric Exercise Physiology.* Churchill Livingstone Elsevier; 2007:235-273.

37. Morrison S, Sims S. Thermoregulation in children: exercise, heat stress and fluid balance. *Annales Kinesiological.* 2014;5(1):41-55.

38. Squire DL. Heat illness: Fluid and electrolyte issues for pediatric and adolescent athletes. *Pediatr Clin North Am.* 1990;37(5):1085-1109.

39. Physical Activity Council. 2019 Physical Activity Council's overview report on U.S. participation. 2019;2020(January 5). www.physicalactivitycouncil.com/_files/ugd/286de6_610088e5e73d497185ac181a240833a9.pdf

40. Voth M, Lustenberger T, Auner B, Frank J, Marzi I. What injuries should we expect in the emergency room? *Injury.* 2017;48(10):2119-2124.

41. Damore DT, Metzl JD, Ramundo M, Pan S, Van Amerongen R. Patterns of childhood sports injury. *Pediatr Emerg Care.* 2003;19(2):65-67.

42. Insurance Information Institute. Sports injuries. Accessed January 4, 2020. www.iii.org/fact-statistic/facts-statistics-sports-injuries

43. U.S. Bureau of Labor Statistics. Occupational outlook handbook. Accessed January 7, 2020. www.bls.gov/ooh/occupation-finder.htm

44. Gardiner-Shires A, Menard MR. Attractors to an athletic training career in the high school setting. *J Athl Train.* 2009;44(3):286-293.

45. Merkel DL. Youth sport: Positive and negative impact on young athletes. *Open Access J Sports Med.* 2013;4:151-160. doi:10.2147/OAJSM.S33556

46. Hawkins D, Metheny J. Overuse injuries in youth sports: biomechanical considerations. *Med Sci Sports Exerc.* 2001;33(10):1701-1717.

47. O'Dell MC, Jaramillo D, Bancroft L, Varich L, Logsdon G, Servaes S. Imaging of sports-related injuries of the lower extremity on pediatric patients. *RadioGraphics.* 2016;36(6):1807-1827.

48. Wasserlauf BL, Paletta GA, Jr. Shoulder disorders in the skeletally immature throwing athlete. *Orthop Clin North Am.* 2003;34:427-437.

49. Anderson AF, Anderson CN. Correlation of meniscal and articular cartilage injuries in children and adolescents with timing of anterior cruciate ligament reconstruction. *The American Journal of Sports Medicine.* 2014;43(2):275-281.

50. Fabricant PD, Jones KJ, Delos D, et al. Reconstruction of the anterior cruciate ligament in the skeletally immature athlete: A review of current concepts: AAOS exhibit selection. *J Bone Joint Surg Am.* 2013;95(5):e28. doi:10.2106/JBJS.L.00772

51. Kay J, Memon M, Shah A, et al. Earlier anterior cruciate ligament reconstruction is associated with a decreased risk of medial meniscal and articular cartilage damage in children and adolescents: a systematic review and meta-analysis. *Knee Surgery, Sports Traumatology, Arthroscopy.* 2018;26:3738-3753.

52. Kocher MS, Tucker R. Pediatric athlete hip disorders. *Clin Sports Med.* 2006;25(2):241-253.

53. Antabak A, Luetic T, Ivo S, et al. Treatment outcomes of both-bone diaphyseal paediatric forearm fractures. *Injury.* 2013;44(3 Suppl):S11-S15.

1039

54. Gamble JG, Sugi MT, Tileston K. The natural history of type VII all intra-epiphyseal fractures of the lateal malleolus. *Orthopedic Journal of Sports Medicine* 2019;7(3). doi:10.1177/2325967119S00116

55. Grazette AJ, Aquinaldo A. The assessment and management of simple elbow dislocations. *The Open Orthopaedics Journal.* 2017;11(8):1373-1379.

56. Wang YL, Chang WN, Hsu CJ, Sun SF, Wang JL, Wong CY. The recovery of elbow range of motion after treatment of supracondylar and lateral condylar fractures of the distal humerus in children. *J Orthop Trauma.* 2009;23(2):120-125.

57. Walters BK, Read CR, Estes AR. The effects of resistance training, overtraining, and early specialization on youth athlete injury and developement. *The Journal of Sports Medicine and Physical Fitness.* 2018;58(9):1339-1348.

58. Devan BD, Berger K, McDonald RJ. The emergent engram: a historical legacy and contemporary discovery. *Front Behav Neurosci.* 2018;12(168). doi:10.3389/fnbeh.2018.00168

59. Kottke FJ. From reflex to skill: The training of coordination. *Arch Phys Med Rehabil.* 1980;61(12):551-561.

60. Brun SP. Clinical considerations for the ageing athlete. *AFP.* 2016;45(7):478-483.

61. Chen AL, Mears SC, Hawkins RJ. Orthopaedic care of the aging athlete. *J Am Acad Orthop Surg.* 2005;13(6):407-416.

62. Arlis-Mayor S. Medical considerations for the master athlete. *Conn Med.* 2012;76(8):455-459.

63. Shad BJ, Wallis G, van Loon LJC, Thompson JL. Exercise prescription for the older population: The interactions between physical activity, sedentary time, and adequate nutrition in maintaining musculoskeletal health. *Maturitas.* 2016;93:78-82.

64. Sales M, Levinger P, Polman R. Relationships between self perceptions and physical activity behaviour, fear of falling, and physical function among older adults. *European Review of Aging and Physical Activity.* 2017;14:17.

65. Montepare JM, Lackman ME. "You're only as old as you feel": Self-perceptions of age, fears of aging, and life satisfaction from adolescence to old age. *Psychol Aging.* 1989;4(1):73-78.

66. Kleinspehn-Ammerlahn A, Kotter-Grühn D, Smith J. Self-perceptions of aging: do subjective age and satisfaction with aging change during old age? *J Gerontol B Psychol Sci Soc Sci.* 2008;63(6):P377-P385.

67. Kemp BJ. What the rehabilitation professional and the consumer need to know. *Phys Med Rehabil Clin N Am.* 2005;16(1):1-18.

68. Eriksen CS, Garde E, Reislev NL, et al. Physical activity as intervention for age-related loss of muscle mass and function. *BMJ Open.* 2016;6(12):p.e012951.

69. Kjær M. Role of extracellular matrix in adaptation of tendon and skeletal muscle to mechanical loading. *Physiol Rev.* 2004;84(2):649-698.

70. Poluri A, Mores J, Cook DB, Findley TW, Cristian A. Fatigue in the elderly population. *Phys Med Rehabil Clin N Am.* 2005;16(1):91-108.

71. Charlier R, Knaeps S, Mertens E, et al. Age-related decline in mucle mass and muscle function in Flemish Caucasians: a 10-year follow-up. *Age.* 2016;38(2):1-15.

72. Centers for Disease Control and Prevention. Important facts about falls. Accessed January 17, 2020. www.cdc.gov/homeandrecreationalsafety/falls/adultfalls.html

73. Valderas JM, Starfield B, Sibbald B, Salisbury C, Roland M. Defining comorbidity: implications for understanding health and health services. *Annals of Family Medicine.* 2009;7(4):357-363.

74. Narici M, Maganaris C. Plasticity of the muscle-tendon complex with disuse and aging. *Exerc Sport Sci Rev.* 2007;35(3):126-134.

75. Miljkovic N, Lim JY, Miljkovic I, Frontera WR. Aging of skeletal muscle fibers. *Ann Rehabil Med.* 2015;39(2):155-162.

76. Santanasto AJ, Goodpaster BH, Kritchevsky SB, et al. Body composition remoldeling and mortality: the health aging and body composition study. *Journals of Gerontology: Medical Sciences.* 2017;72(4):513-519.

77. Dawson A, Dennison E. Measuring the musculoskeletal aging phenotype. *Maturitas.* 2016;93:13-17.

78. Thompson LV. Skeletal muscle adaptations with age, inactivity, and therapeutic exercise. *J Orthop Sports Phys Ther.* 2002;32(2):44-57.

79. Runnels ED, Bemben DA, Anderson MA, Bemben MG. Influence of age on isometric, isotonic, and isokinetic force production characteristics in men. *J Geriatr Phys Ther.* 2005;28(3):74-84.

80. Ahmed MS, Matsumura B, Cristian A. Age-related changes in muscles and joints. *Phys Med Rehabil Clin N Am.* 2005;16(1):19-39.

81. Degens H. Age-related changes in the microcirculation of skeletal muscle. *Adv Exp Med Biol.* 1998;454:343-348.

82. Rooyackers OE, Adey DB, Ades PA, Nair KS. Effect of age on in vivo rates of mitochondrial protein synthesis in human skeletal muscle. *Proc Natl Acad Sci USA.* 1996;93(26):15364-15369.

83. Frontera W. Physiologic changes of the musculoskeletal system with aging: a brief review. *Phys Med Rehabil Clin N Am.* 2017;28(4):705-711.

84. Reeves ND, Narici MV, Maganaris CN. Musculoskeletal adaptations to resistance training in old age. *Man Ther.* 2006;11:192-196.

85. Mora JC, Przkora R, Cruz-Almeida Y. Knee osteoarthritis: pathophysiology and current treatment modalities. *J Pain Res.* 2018;11:2189-2196.

86. Ahmad CS, Wang VM, Sugalski MT, Levine WN, Bigliani LU. Biomechanics of shoulder capsulorrhaphy procedures. *J Shoulder Elbow Surg.* 2005;14:12S-18S.

87. Dudhia J. Aggregan, aging and assembly in articular cartilage. *Cell Mol Life Sci.* 2005;62(19-20):2241-2256.

88. Briggs AM, Cross MJ, Hoy DG, et al. Musculoskeletal health conditions represent a global threat to healthy aging: a report for the 2015 World Health Organization World Report on Ageing and Health. *Gerontologist.* 2016;56(S2):S243-S255.

89. Karvonen RL, Negendank WG, Teitge RA, Reed AH, Miller PR, Fernandez-Madrid F. Factors affecting articular cartilage thickness in osteoarthritis and aging. *J Rheumatol.* 1994;21(7):1310-1318.

90. Lane LB, Bullough PG. Age-related changes in the thickness of the calcified zone and the number of tidemarks in adult human articular cartilage. *J Bone Joint Surg Br.* 1980;62(3):372-375.

91. Centers for Disease Control and Prevention. Arthritis-related statistics. Accessed January 4, 2020. www.cdc.gov/arthritis/data_statistics/arthritis-related-stats.htm

92. Centers for Disease Control and Prevention. Osteoarthritis. Accessed January 22, 2020. www.cdc.gov/arthritis/basics/osteoarthritis.htm

93. Health Research Funding Organization. 23 amazing total knee replacement statistics. Accessed January 23, 2020. www.healthresearchfunding.org

94. Kremers HM, Larson DR, Crowson CS, et al. Prevalence of total hip and knee replacement in the United States. *J Bone Joint Surg Am.* 2015;97(17):1386-1397.

95. Kim WB, Kim BR, Kim SR, et al. Comorbidities in patients with end-stage knee OA: prevalence and effect on physical function. *Archives of Physical Medicine and Rehabilitation.* 2019;100:2063-2070.

96. Chaganti RK, Lane NE. Risk factors for incident osteoarthritis of the hip and knee. *Curr Rev Musculoskelet Med.* 2011;4(3):99-104.

97. Santos L, Elliott-Sale KJ, Sale C. Exercise and bone health across the lifespan. *Biogerontology.* 2017;18:931-946.

98. Guadalupe-Grau A, Fuentes T, Guerra B, Calbet JAL. Exercise and bone mass in adults. *Sports Med.* 2009;39(6):439-468.

99. Bernstein J. *Musculoskeletal Medicine.* American Academy of Orthopaedic Surgeons; 2003:490.

100. Milgrom C, Miligram M, Simkin A, Burr D, Ekenman I, Finestone A. A home exercise program for tibial bone strengthening based on in vivo strain measurements. *Am J Phys Med Rehabil.* 2001;80(6):433-438.

101. ACSM, Mazzeo RS, Cavanagh P, et al. Position stand: exercises and physical activity for older adults. *Med Sci Sports Exerc.* 1998;30(6):992-1008.

102. Delbono O. Expression and regulation of excitation-contraction coupling proteins in aging skeletal muscle. *Curr Aging Sci.* 2011;4(3):248-259.

103. Illing S, Chouy NL, Nitz J, Nolan M. Sensory system function and postural stability in men aged 30-80 years. *Aging Male.* 2010;13(3):202-210.

104. Mase K, Kamimura H, Imura S, Kitagawa K. Effect of age and gender on muscle function—analysis by muscle fiber conduction velocity. *J Phys Ther Sci.* 2006;18(1):81-87.

105. Cattagni T, Harnie J, Jubeau M, et al. Neural and muscular factors both contribute to plantar-flexor muscle weakness in older fallers. *Experimental Gerontology.* 2018;112:127-134.

106. Trujillo M, Razak KA. Altered cortical spectrotemporal processing with age-related hearing loss. *J Neurophysiol.* 2013;110(12):2873-2886.

107. West LA, Cole S, Goodkind D, He W. U.S Census Bureau report: 65+ in the United States: 2010. Accessed January 16, 2020. www.census.gov/library/publications/2014/demo/p23-212.html

108. Kim S, Leng X, Kritchevsky SB. Body composition and physical function in older adults with various comorbidities. *Innovation in Aging.* 2017;00(00):1-9.

109. Hansen D, Neibauer J, Cornelissen V, et al. Exercise prescription in patients with different combinations of cardiovascular disease risk factors: a consensus statement fro the EXPERT working group. *Sports Med.* 2018;48:1781-1797.

110. Deichmann RE, Lavie CJ, Asher T, DiNicolantonio JJ, O'Keefe JH, Thompson PD. The interaction between statins and exercise: mechanisms and strategies to counter the musculoskeletal side effects of this combination therapy. *The Ochsner Journal.* 2015;15:429-437.

111. Agency for Healthcare Research and Quality. Blood thinners. Accessed January 24, 2020. https://www.ahrq.gov/topics/blood-thinners.html

112. Ogbru O. ACE inhibitors drug class side effects, list of names, uses, and dosage. MedicineNEt. Accessed January 24, 2020. https://www.medicinenet.com/ace_inhibitors/article.htm

113. Merck. Merck manual for the professional. Accessed February 16, 2020. https://www.merckmanuals.com/professional

114. McDermott AY, Mernitz H. Exercise and older patients: prescribing guidelines. *Am Fam Physician.* 2006;74(3):437-444.

115. Timmons JF, Minnock D, Hone M, Cogan KE, Murphy JC, Egan B. Comparison of time-matched aerobic, resistance, or concurrent exercise training in older adults. *Scand J Med Sci Sports.* 2017;28:2272-2283.

116. Conlon JA, Newton RU, Tufano JJ, et al. The efficacy of periodised resistance training on neuromuscular adaptation in older adults. *Eur J Appl Physiol.* 2017;117:1181-1194.

117. Arend E, Gustavo S, Carvalho J. Concurrent aerobic and resistance training improves lower limbs strength and muscular endurance in older adults. *Medicine & Science in Sport & Exercise.* 2016;48(5S.1):126.

118. Hara T, Shimada T. Effects of exercise on the improvement of the physical functions of the elderly. *J Phys Ther Sci.* 2007;19(1):15-26.

119. Teixeira CV, Gobbi S, Pereira JR, Ueno DT, Shigematsu R, Gobbi LT. Effect of square-stepping exercise and basic exercises on functional fitness of older adults. *Geriatr Gerontol Int.* 2013;13(4):842-848.

120. Shigematsu R, Okura T. A novel exercise for improving lower-extremity functional fitness in the elderly. *Aging Clin Exp Res.* 2006;18(3):242-248.

121. Chodzko-Zajko WJ, Proctor DN, Singh MF, et al. Exercise and physical activity for older adults: position stand from the American College of Sports Medicine. *Medicine & Science in Sport & Exercise.* 2009;41(7):1510-1530.

122. American Heart Association. Target heart rate. Updated January 4, 2015. Accessed January 26, 2020. www.heart.org/HEARTORG/GettingHealthy/PhysicalActivity/Target-Heart-Rates_UCM_434341_Article.js

123. Robergs RA, Landwehr R. The surprising history of the "HRmax=220-age" equation. *J Exerc Physiol Online.* 2002;5(2):1-10.

124. Reeves B. The natural history of the frozen shoulder syndrome. *Scand J Rheumatol.* 1975;4(4):193-196.

125. Narici MV, Maganaris CN. Adaptability of elderly human muscles and tendons to increased loading. *J Anat.* 2006;208(4):433-443.

126. Natri A, Jarvinen M, Latvala K, Kannus P. Isokinetic muscle performance after anterior cruciate ligament surgery: Long-term results and outcome predicting factors after primary surgery and late-phase reconstruction. *Int J Sports Med.* 1996;17(3):223-238.

127. Buskard AN, Jacobs KA, Eltoukhy MM, et al. Optimal approach to load progressions during strength training in older adults. *Medicine & Science in Sport & Exercise.* 2019;51(11):2224-2233.

128. Roig M, O'Brien K, Kirk G, et al. The effects of eccentric versus concentric resistance training on muscle strength and mass in healthy adults: a systematic review with meta-analysis. *Br J Sports Med.* 2009;43(8):556-568.

129. Hvid L, Aagaard P, Justesen L, et al. Effects of aging on muscle mechanical function and muscle fiber morphology during short-term immobilization and subsequent retraining. *J Appl Physiol.* 2010;109(6):1628-1634.

130. Soni V, Writer H. Effect of aging on components of balance evaluation system test. *International Journal of Physiotherapy.* 2017;4(3). doi:10.15621/ijphy/2017/v4i3/149073

131. Springer BA, Marin R, Cyhan T, Roberts H, Gill NW. Normative values for the unipedal stance test with eyes open and closed *J Geriatr Phys Ther.* 2007;30(1):8-15.

132. Bouvier T, Opplert J, Cometti C, Babault N. Acute effects of static stretching on muscle-tendon mechanics of quadriceps and plantar flexor muscles. *Eur J Appl Physiol.* 2017;117:1309-1315.

133. Zhou WS, Lin JH, Chen SC, Chien KY. Effects of dynamic stretching with different loads in hip joint range of motion in the elderly. *Journal of Sports Science and Medicine.* 2019;18:52-57.

134. Van Hooren B, Peake JM. Do we need a cool-down after exercise? A narrative review of the psychophysiological effects and the effects on performance, injuries and long-term adaptive response. *Sports Med.* 2018;48:1575-1595.

Chapter 5

1. Maitland GD. *Vertebral Manipulation.* 5th ed. Butterworth-Heinemann; 1986.

2. Huskisson EC. Measurement of pain. *Lancet.* 1974;2:1127-1131.

3. Huskisson EC, Jones J, Scott PJ. Application of visual-analogue scales to the measurement of functional capacity. *Rheumatol Rehabil.* 1976;15:185-187.

4. Langley GB, Sheppard H. The visual analogue scale: its use in pain measurement. *Rheumatol Int.* 1985;5:145-148.

5. Melzack R. The McGill Pain Questionnaire: major properties and scoring methods. *Pain.* 1975;1(3):277-299.

6. Valovich McLeod TC, Snyder AR, Parsons JT, Bay RC, Michener LA, Sauers EL. Using disablement models and clinical outcomes assessment to enable evidence-based athletic training practice, part II: clinical outcomes assessment. *J Athl Train.* 2008;43(4):437-445.

7. Maitland GD. *Peripheral Manipulation.* Butterworth-Heinemann; 1991.

8. Linaker CH, Walker-Bone K. Shoulder disorders and occupation. *Best Pract Res Clin Rheumatol.* 2015;29(3):405-423.

9. Grimston SK, Nigg BM, Hanley DA, Engsberg JR. Differences in ankle joint complex range of motion as a function of age. *Foot & Ankle.* 1993;14(4):215-222.

10. Laudner KG, Moore SD, Sipes RC, Meister K. Functional hip characteristics of baseball pitchers and position players. *Am J Sports Med.* 2010;38(2):383-387.

11. Garving C, Jakob S, Bauer I, Nadjar R, Brunner UH. Impingement sSyndrome of the shoulder. *Dtsch Arztebl Int.* 2017;114(45):765-776.

12. Cyriax JH. *Textbook of Orthopaedic Medicine: Vol. 1. Diagnosis of Soft Tissue Lesions.* 8th ed. Bailliere Tindall; 1982.

13. Kaltenborn FM. *Manual Mobilization of the Joints: The Kaltenborn Method of Joint Examination and Treatment.* 6th ed. Olaf N Orlis Bokhandel; 2002.

14. Rose MB, Noonan T. Glenohumeral internal rotation deficit in throwing athletes: current perspectives. *Open Access J Sports Med.* 2018;9:69-78.

15. Bradshaw EJ, Hume PA. Biomechanical approaches to identify and quantify injury mechanisms and risk factors in women's artistic gymnastics. *Sports Biomechanics.* 2012;11(3):324-341. doi:10.1080/14763141.2011.650186

16. Kelly BT, Kadrmas WR, Speer KP. The manual muscle examination for rotator cuff strength: An electromyographic investigation. *Am J Sports Med.* 1996;24(5):581-588.

17. Jones M, Jensen G, Rothstein J. Clinical reasoning in physiotherapy In: Higgs J, Jones M, eds. *Clinical Reasoning in the Health Professions.* Butterworth-Heinemann; 1995:chap 72.

18. Levett-Jones T, Hoffman K, Dempsey J, et al. The "five rights" of clinical reasoning: an educational model to enhance nursing students' ability to identify and manage clinically "at risk" patients. *Nurse Educ Today.* 2010;30:515-520.

19. Johnsen HM, Fossum M, Vivekananda-Schmidt P, Fruhling A, Slettebo A. Teaching clinical reasoning and decision-making skills to nursing students: design, development, and usability evaluation of a serious game. *International Journal of Medical Informatics.* 2016;94:39-48.

20. Howard JS, Sciascia A, Hoch JM. Using patient evidence to guide clinical care: Consulting the other expert in the room. *Int J Athl Ther Train.* 2018;23(2):53-56.

21. Richardson WS, Wilson MC, McGinn TG. The process of diagnosis. In: Guyatt G, Drummond R, Meade MO, Cook DJ, eds. *Users' Guides to the Medical Literature.* 2nd ed. McGraw-Hill; 2008:407-418.

22. Jamison JR. Fostering critical appraisal skills as a prelude to clinical practice. *Chiropract J Aust.* 2005;35(3):107-111.

23. World Health Organization. Towards a common language for functioning, disability and health: IFC. Accessed May 2, 2020. www.who.int/classifications/icf/training/icfbeginnersguide.pdf

24. American Physical Therapy Association. APTA guide to physical therapist practice. Accessed March 28, 2020. http://guidetopractice.apta.org

25. Ballo P, Milli M, Slater C, et al. Prospective validation of the decalogue, a set of doctor-patient communication recommendations to improve patient illness experience and mood states within a hospital cardiologic ambulatory setting. *BioMed Research International.* 2017;2017:2792131. doi:10.1155/2017/2792131

26. Jevsevar DS, Bozie KJ. Orthopaedic healthcare worldwide: using clinical practice guidelines in clinical decision making. *Clinical Orthopaedics and Related Research.* 2015;473(9):2762-2764.

27. Graham R, Mancher M, Wolman DM, Greenfield S, Steinberg E. *Clinical Practice Guidelines We Can Trust.* National Academics Press; 2011.

28. Willy RW, et al. Patellofemoral pain: clinical practice guidelines linked to the International Classification of

Functioning, Disability and Health from the Academy of Orthopaedic Physical Therapy of the American Physical Therapy Association. *J Orthop Sports Phys Ther*. 2019;49(9):CPG1-CPG95.

29. Martin RL, et al. Heel pain-plantar fasciitis: revision 2014. Clinical practice guidelines linked to the International Classification of Functioning, Disability and Health from the Academy of Orthopaedic Physical Therapy of the American Physical Therapy Association. *J Orthop Sports Phys Ther*. 2014;44(11):A1-A23.

30. Logerstedt DS, et al. Knee stability and movement coordination impairments: knee ligament sprain revision 2017. Clinical practice guidelines linked to the International Classification of Functioning, Disability and Health from the Academy of Orthopaedic Physical Therapy of the American Physical Therapy Association. *J Orthop Sports Phys Ther*. 2017;47(11):A1-A17.

31. Logerstedt DS, et al. Knee pain and mobility impairments: meniscal and articular cartilage lesions revision 2018. Clinical practice guidelines linked to the International Classification of Functioning, Disability and Health from the Academy of Orthopaedic Physical Therapy of the American Physical Therapy Association. *J Orthop Sports Phys Ther*. 2018;48(2):A1-A50.

32. Delitto A, et al. Low back pain: clinical practice guidelines linked to the International Classification of Functioning, Disability and Health from the Academy of Orthopaedic Physical Therapy of the American Physical Therapy Association. *J Orthop Sports Phys Ther*. 2012;42(4):A1-A57.

33. Martin RL, et al. Achilles pain, stiffness, and muscle power deficits: midportion Achilles tendinopathy revision 2018. Clinical practice guidelines linked to the International Classification of Functioning, Disability and Health from the Academy of Orthopaedic Physical Therapy of the American Physical Therapy Association. *J Orthop Sports Phys Ther*. 2018;48(5):A1-A38.

34. Martin RL, et al. Ankle stability and movement coordination impairments: ankle ligament sprains. Clinical practice guidelines linked to the International Classification of Functioning, Disability and Health from the Academy of Orthopaedic Physical Therapy of the American Physical Therapy Association. *J Orthop Sports Phys Ther*. 2013;43(9):A1-A40.

35. American Physical Therapy Association. Defensible documentation overview. Accessed 9 April, 2020. www.apta.org/DefensibleDocumentation/Overview

36. Board of Certification. Appropriate documentation in athletic training. Accessed April 9, 2020. www.bocatc.org/blog/appropriate-documentation-in-athletic-training

37. National Athletic Trainers' Association. Best practice guidelines for athletic training documentation. Accessed April 9, 2020. www.nata.org/sites/default/files/best-practice-guidelines-for-athletic-training-documentation.pdf

38. Gateley CA, Borcherding S. *Documentation Manual for Occupational Therapy: Writing SOAP Notes*. Slack; 2012.

39. Bali A, Bali D, Iyer N, Iyer M. Management of medical records: facts and figures for surgeons. *J Maxillofac Oral Surg*. 2011;10(3):199-202.

40. American Physical Therapy Association. Guidelines: physical therapy documentation of patient/client management. Accessed April 19, 2020. www.apta.org/uploaded-Files/APTAorg/About_Us/Policies/Practice/Documenta-tionPatientClientManagement.pdf#search=%22physical therapy documentation of patient%2fclient management%22

Chapter 6

1. Langford ML. Poor posture subjects a worker's body to muscle imbalance, nerve compression. *Occup Health Saf*. 1994;63(9):38-42.

2. Norris CM. Spinal stabilisation: 4. Muscle imbalance and the low back. *Physiother*. 1995;81(3):127-138.

3. Kapandji IA. *The Physiology of Joints: Vol 3, The Trunk and Vertebral Column*. Churchill Livingstone; 1974.

4. Lin RM, Jou IM, Yu CY. Lumbar lordosis: Normal adults. *J Formos Med Assoc*. 1992;91(3):329-333.

5. Fon GT, Pitt MJ, Thies AC. Thoracic kyphosis: Range in normal subjects. *AJR Am J Roentgenol*. 1980;134(May):979-983.

6. McAviney J, Schulz D, Bock R, Harrison DE, Holland B. Determining the relationship between cervical lordosis and neck complaints. *J Manip Physiol Ther*. 2005;28(3):187-193.

7. Kendall FP, McCreary EK, Provance PG, Rodgers MM, Romani WA. *Muscles: Testing and Function With Posture and Pain*. 5th ed. Lippincott Williams & Wilkins; 2005.

8. Sahrmann SA. *Diagnosis and Treatment of Movement Impairment Syndromes*. Mosby; 2002.

9. Boyle K, Olinick J, Lewis C. The value of blowing up a balloon. *N Am J Sports Phys Ther*. 2010;5(3):179-188.

10. Yusof MI, Hassan MN, Abdullah MS. The relationship amongst intervertebral disc vertical diameter, lateral foramen diameter and nerve root impingement in lumbar vertebra. *Malays Orthop J*. 2018;12(1):21-25. doi:10.5704/MOJ.1803.004

11. Ishimoto Y, Kawakami M, Curtis E, et al. The impact of lumbar spinal stenosis, knee osteoarthritis, and loss of lumbar lordosis on the quality of life: Findings from the Katsuragi low back pain study. *Spine Surg Related Res*. 2019;3(2):157-162.

12. Bubanj S, Zivkovic M, Zivkovic D, et al. The incidence of sagittal postural deformities among high school students: Preliminary study. *Acta Kinesiologica* 2012;6(2):27-30.

13. Abbas J, Hamoud K, May H, et al. Degenerative lumbar spinal stenosis and lumbar spine configuration. *Eur Spine*. 2010;10(11):1865-1873. doi:10.1007/s00586-010-1516-5

14. Koseki T, Kakizaki F, Hayashi S, Nishida N, Itoh M. Effect of forward head posture on thoracic shape and respiratory function. *J Phys Ther Sci*. 2019;31(1):63-8.

15. Hooper TL, Denton J, McGalliard MK, Brismée J-M, Sizer Jr PS. Thoracic outlet syndrome: A controversial clinical condition. Part 1: Anatomy, and clinical examination/diagnosis. *J Man Manip Ther*. 2010;18(2):74-83. doi:10.1179/106698110X12640740712734

16. Hruska RJ. Management of pelvic-thoracic influences on temporomandibular dysfunction. *Orthop Phys Ther Clin N Am*. 2002;11(2):263-284.

17. Hruska RJ. Influences of dysfunctional respiratory mechanics on orofacial pain. *Dent Clin North Am*. 1997;41(2):211-227.

18. Theisen C, van Wagensveld A, Timmesfeld N, et al. Co-occurrence of outlet impingement syndrome of the shoulder and restricted range of motion in the thoracic spine: A prospective study with ultrasound-based motion

analysis. *BMC Musculoskelet Disord.* 2010;11(135). doi:10.1186/1471-2474-11-135 PMC2903509,

19. Pink M, Perry J, Browne A, Scovazzo ML, Kerrigan J. The normal shoulder during freestyle swimming. An electromyographic and cibnematographic analysis of twelve muscles. *Am J Sports Med.* 1991;19:569-576.

20. Lenke LG, Betz RR, Clements D, et al. Curve prevalence of a new classification of operative adolescent idiopathic scoliosis: Does classification correlate with treatment? *Spine.* 2002;27(6):604-611.

21. Omey ML, Micheli LJ, Gerbino PG. Idiopathic scoliosis and spondylolysis in the femal athlete: Tips for treatment. *Clin Orthop Relat Res.* 2000;(372):74-84.

22. d'Hemecourt PA, Hresko MT. Spinal deformity in young athletes. *Clin Sports Med.* 2012;31(3):441-451.

23. Vogel F, Jr. Short-leg syndrome. *Clin Podiatr.* 1984;1(3):581-599.

24. Laslett M. Manual correction of an acute lumbar lateral shift: Maintenance of correction and rehabilitation: A case report with video. *J Man Manip Ther.* 2009;17(2):78-85.

25. Black KM, McClure P, Polansky M. The influence of different sitting positions on cervical and lumbar posture. *Spine.* 1996;21(1):65-70.

26. Gonzalez HE, Manns A. Forward head posture: Its structural and functional influence on the somatognathic system, a conceptual study. *Cranio.* 1996;14(1):71-80.

27. Drake JD, Callaghan JP. Intervertebral neural foramina deformation due to two types of repetitive combined loading. *Clin Biomech.* 2009;24(1):1-6.

28. Köknel Talu G. Thoracic outlet syndrome. *Agri.* 2005;17(2):5-9.

29. Mandal AC. The seated man (Homo Sedens) the seated work position: Theory and practice. *Appl Ergon.* 1981;12(1):19-26.

30. Moloney N. Temporomandibular dysfunction: A review. *Physiother Ireland.* 2005;26(2):17-22.

31. Kapandji IA. *The Physiology of the Joints: Vol 2, Lower Limb.* 5th ed. Churchill Livingstone; 1987.

32. Haverkamp D, Marti RK. Bilateral varus osteotomies in hip deformities: Are early interventions superior? A long-term follow-up. *Int Orthop.* 2007;31(2):185-191.

33. Tetsworth K, Paley D. Malalignment and degenerative arthropathy. *Orthop Clin North Am.* 1994;25(3):367-377.

34. Carpintero P, Leon F, Zafra M, Serrano-Trenas JA, Román M. Stress fractures of the femoral neck and coxa vara. *Arch Orthop Trauma Surg.* 2003;123(6):273-277.

35. Souza RB, Draper CE, Fredericson M, Powers CM. Femur rotation and patellofemoral joint kinematics: A weight-bearing magnetic resonance imaging analysis. *J Orthop Sports Phys Ther.* 2010;40(5):277-285.

36. Bagwell J, Fukuda TY, Powers CM. Sagittal plane pelvis motion influences transverse plane motion of the femur: Kinematic coupling at the hip joint. *Gait Posture.* 2016;43(Jan):120-124.

37. Kendall HO, Kendall FP, Boynton DA. *Posture and Pain.* Williams & Wilkins; 1952.

38. Kristiansen LP, Gunderson RB, Steen H, O. R. The normal development of tibial torsion. *Skeletal Radiol.* 2001;30(9):519-522.

39. Milner CE, Soarnes RW. A comparison of four in vivo methods of measuring tibial torsion. *J Anat.* 1998;193:139-144.

40. Güven M, Akman B, Unay K, Ozturan EK, Cakici H, Eren A. A new radiographic measurement method of evaluation of tibial torsion: A pilot study in adults. *Clin Orthop Relat Res.* 2009;467(7):1807-1812.

41. Davids JR, Davis RB. Tibial torsion: Significance and measurement. *Gait Posture.* 2007;26(2):169-171.

42. Lang LM, Volpe RG. Measurment of tibial torsion. *J Am Pod Med Assoc.* 1998;88(4):160-165.

43. Stuberg W, Temme J, Kaplan P, Clarke A, Fuchs R. Measurement of tibial torsion and thigh-foot angle using goniometry and computed tomography. *Clin Orthop Relat Res.* 1991;272:208-212.

44. Parikh S, Noyes FR. Patellofemoral disorders: Role of computed tomography and magnetic resonance imaging in defining abnormal rotational lower limb alignment. *Sports Health.* 2011;3(2):158-169.

45. Spörndly-Nees S, Dåsberg B, Nielsen RO, Boesen MI, Langberg H. The navicular position test: A reliable measure of the navicular bone position during rest and loading. *Int J Sports Phys Ther.* 2011;6(3):199-205.

46. Scattone Silva R, Veronese LM, Granado Ferreira AL, Serrão FV. The influence of forefoot varus on eccentric hip torque in adolescents. *Man Ther.* 2013;18(6):487-491.

47. Kaufman KR, Brodine SK, Shaffer RA, Johnson CW, Cullison TR. The effect of foot structure and range of motion on musculoskeletal overuse injuries. *Am J Sports Med.* 1999;27(5):585-593.

48. Simkin A, Leichter I, Giladi M, Stein M, Milgrom C. Combined effect of foot arch structure and an orthotic device on stress fractures. *Foot Ankle.* 1989;10(1):25-29.

49. Menz HB. Alternative techniques for the clinical assessment of foot pronation. *J Am Podiatr Med Assoc.* 1998;88(3):119-129.

50. Comerford MJ, Mottram SL. Movement and stability dysfunction—contemporary developments. *Man Ther.* 2001;6(1):15-26.

51. Sherrington CS. *The Integrative Action of the Nervous System.* Yale University Press; 1906:411.

52. Czaprowski D, Stoliński Ł, Tyrakowski M, Kozinoga M, Kotwicki T. Non-structural misalignments of body posture in the sagittal plane. *Scoliosis Spinal Disord.* 2018;13(6). doi:10.1186/s13013-018-0151-5 PMC5836359,

53. Wang H-Q, Li M-Q, Wu Z-x, Zhao L. The deep fascia in response to leg lengthening with particular reference to the tension-stress principle. *J Pediatr Orthop.* 2007;27(1)(Jan-Feb):41-45. doi:10.1097/01.bpo.0000242439.88811.15

54. Swärd L. The thoracolumbar spine in young elite athletes: Current concepts on the effects of physical training. *Sports Med.* 1992;13(5):357-364.

55. Diebo BG, Shah NV, Boachie-Adjei O, et al. Adult spinal deformity. *Lancet.* 2019;394(10193):160-172. doi:10.1016/S0140-6736(19)31125-0

56. Monk PA, Davies LJ, Hopewell S, Harris K, Beard DJ, Price AJ. Surgical versus conservative interventions for treating anterior cruciate ligament injuries. *Cochrane Database Syst Rev.* 2016;4(4). doi:10.1002/14651858. CD011166.pub2. PMC6464826,

57. Bizzini M, Childs JD, Piva SR, Delitto A. Systematic review of the quality of randomized controlled trials for patellofemoral pain syndrome: Part I. *J Orthop Sports Phys Ther.* 2003;33(1):4-20.

58. Fredericson M, Cookingham CL, Chaudhari AM, Dowdell BC, Oestreicher N, Sahrmann SA. Hip abductor weakness in distance runners with iliotibial band syndrome. *Clin J Sport Med.* 2000;10(3):169-173.

59. Fredericson M, Wolf C. Iliotibial band syndrome in runners: Innovations in treatment. *Sports Med.* 2005;35(5):451-459.

60. Tenney HR, Boyle KL, DeBord A. Influence of hamstring and abdominal muscle activation on a positive Ober's test in people with lumbopelvic pain. *Physiother Can.* 2013;65(1):4-11.

61. Kane V, Kolukula NS. Effect of iliotibial band stretching versus hamstring and abdominal muscle activation on a positive Ober's test in subjects with lumbopelvic pain: A randomized clinical trial. *Int J Therap Rehab Res.* 2015;4(4):111-116.

Chapter 7

1. Pirker W, Katzenschlager R. Gait disorders in adults and the elderly: A clinical guide. *Wien Klin Wochenschr.* 2017;129(3-4):81-95. doi:10.1007/s00508-016-1096-4

2. Chamberlain CS, Crowley E, Vanderby R. The spatio-temporal dynamics of ligament healing. *Wound Rep Reg.* 2009;17(2):206-215.

3. Sutherland DH. The evolution of clinical gait analysis: Part I. Kinesiological EMG. *Gait Posture.* 2001;14(1):61-70.

4. Inman VT, Ralston HJ, Todd F. *Human Walking.* Williams & Wilkins; 1981.

5. Thomas SS, Supan TJ. A comparison of current biomechanical terms. *J Prosthet Orthot.* 1990;2(2):107-114.

6. Chambers HG, Sutherland DH. A practical guide to gait analysis. *J Am Acad Orthop Surg.* 2002;10:222-273.

7. Mann RA, Morgan GT, Dougherty SE. Comparative electromyography of the lower extremity in jogging, running, and sprinting. *Am J Sports Med.* 1986;14(6):501-510.

8. Soo CH, Donelan JM. Coordination of push-off and collision determine the mechanical work of step-to-step transitions when isolated from human walking. *Gait Posture.* 2012;35(2):292-297.

9. Gottschall JS, Kram R. Energy cost and muscular activity required for leg swing during walking. *J Appl Physiol.* 2005;99(1):23-30.

10. Perry J, Burnfield JM. *Gait Analysis: Normal and Pathological Function.* 2nd ed. Slack; 2010.

11. Dicharry J. Kinematics and kinetics of gait: From lab to clinic. *Clin Sports Med.* 2010;29(3):347-364.

12. Ounpuu S. The biomechanics of walking and running. *Clin Sports Med.* 1994;13(4):843-863.

13. Lehmann JF, de Lateur BJ. Gait analysis: Diagnosis and management. In: Kottke FJ, Lehmann JF, eds. *Krusen's Handbook of Physical Medicine and Rehabilitation.* 4th ed. Saunders; 1990:108-125.

14. Seeley MK, Umberger BR, Shapiro R. A test of the functional asymmetry hypothesis in walking. *Gait Posture.* 2008;28(1):24-28.

15. Murray MP. Gait as a total pattern of movement. *Am J Phys Med.* 1967;46(1):290-333.

16. Murray MP, Drought AB, Kory RC. Walking patterns of normal men. *J Bone Joint Surg Am.* 1964;46:335-360.

17. Winter DA. *The Biomechanics and Motor Control of Human Gait.* University of Waterloo Press; 1987.

18. Deusinger RH. Biomechanics in clinical practice. *Phys Ther.* 1984;64(12):1860-1868.

19. Yack HJ. Techniques for clinical assessment of human movement. *Phys Ther.* 1984;64(12):1821-1830.

20. Orendurff MS, Segal AD, Klute GK, Berge JS, Rohr ES, Kadel NJ. The effect of walking speed on center of mass displacement. *J Rehabil Res Dev.* 2004;41(6A):829-834.

21. Saunders JB, Inman VT, Eberhart HD. The major determinants in normal and pathological gait. *J Bone Joint Surg Am.* 1953;35(3):543-558.

22. Gard SA, Childress DS. The effect of pelvic list on the vertical displacement of the trunk during normal walking. *Gait Posture.* 1997;5(3):233-238.

23. Gard SA, Childress DS. What determines the vertical displacement of the body during normal walking? *J Prosthet Orthot.* 2001;13(3):64-69.

24. Della Croce U, Riley PO, Lelas JL, Kerrigan DC. A refined view of the determinants of gait. *Gait Posture.* 2001;14(2):79-84.

25. Kerrigan DC, Della Croce U, Marciello M, Riley PO. A refined view of the determinants of gait: Significance of heel rise. *Arch Phys Med Rehabil.* 2000;81(8):1077-1080.

26. Kuo AD. The six determinants of gait and the inverted pendulum analogy: A dynamic walking perspective. *Hum Mov Sci.* 2007;26(4):617-656.

27. Hayot C, Sakka S, Lacouture P. Contribution of the six major gait determinants on the vertical center of mass trajectory and the vertical ground reaction force. *Hum Mov Sci.* 2013;32(2):279-289.

28. Gard SA, Childress DS. The influence of stance-phase knee flexion on the vertical displacement of the trunk during normal walking. *Arch Phys Med Rehabil.* 1999;80(1):26-32.

29. Hu H, Meijer OG, Hodges PW, et al. Control of the lateral abdominal muscles during walking. *Hum Mov Sci.* 2011;31(4):880-896. doi:10.1016/j.humov.2011.09.002

30. Perry J. The mechanics of walking. A clinical interpretation. *Phys Ther.* 1967;47:778-801.

31. Kuo AD, Donelan JM. Dynamic principles of gait and their clinical implications. *Phys Ther.* 2010;90(2):157-174.

32. Murray MP, Kory RC, Sepic SB. Walking patterns of normal women. *Arch Phys Med Rehabil.* 1970;51(11):637-650.

33. Lin YC, Gfoehler M, Pandy MG. Quantitative evaluation of the major determinants of human gait. *J Biomech.* 2014;47(6):1324-1331.

34. Sadeghi H, Sadeghi S, Prince F, Allard P, Labelle H, Vaughan CL. Functional roles of ankle and hip sagittal muscle moments in able-bodied gait. *Clin Biomech.* 2001;16(8):688-695.

35. Frigo C, Pavan EE, Brunner R. A dynamic model of quadriceps and hamstrings function. *Gait Posture.* 2010;31(1):100-103.

36. Whittle MW. *Gait Analysis.* 4th ed. Elsevier; 2007.

37. Crosbie J, Vachalathiti R. Synchrony of pelvic and hip joint motion during walking. *Gait Posture.* 1997;6(3):237-248.

38. Waters RL, Campbell J, Perry J. Energy cost of three-point crutch ambulation in fracture patients. *J Orthop Trauma.* 1987;1(2):170-173.

39. Waters RL, Hislop HJ, Perry J, Antonelli D. Energetics: Application to the study and management of locomotor disabilities. Energy cost of normal and pathologic gait. *Orthop Clin North Am.* 1978;9(2):351-356.

40. De Troyer A, Wilson TA. Action of the diaphragm on the rib cage. *J Appl Physiol.* 2016;121(2):391-400.

41. Hodges P, Cresswell A, Daggfeldt K, Thorstensson A. In vivo measurement of the effect of intra-abdominal pressure on the human spine. *J Biomech.* 2001;34(3):347-353.

42. Ford MP, Wagenaar RC, Newell KM. Arm constraint and walking in healthy adults. *Gait Posture.* 2007;26(1):135-141.

43. Angelini L, Damm P, Zander T, Arshad R, Di Puccio F. Effect of arm swinging on lumbar spine and hip joint forces. *J Biomech.* 2018;70:185-195.

44. Wu Y, Li Y, Liu AM, et al. Effect of active arm swing to local dynamic stability during walking. *Hum Mov Sci.* 2016;Feb(45):102-109. doi:10.1016/j.humov.2015.10.005

45. Romkes J, Bracht-Schweizer K. The effects of walking speed on upper body kinematics during gait in healthy subjects. *Gait & Posture.* 2017;54:304-310.

46. Pontzer H, Holloway JH, 3rd, Raichlen DA, Lieberman DE. Control and function of arm swing in human walking and running. *J Exp Biol.* 2009;212(Pt 4):523-534.

47. Kuhtz-Buschbeck JP, Jing B. Activity of upper limb Muscles during human walking. *J Electromyogr Kinesiol.* 2012;22(2)(Apr):199-206. doi:10.1016/j.jelekin.2011.08.014

48. Meyns P, Bruijn SM, Duysens J. The how and why of arm swing during human walking. *Gait & Posture.* 2013;38:555-62.

49. Umberger BR. Effects of suppressing arm swing on kinematics, kinetics, and energetics of human walking. *J Biomechanics.* 2008;41:2575-80.

50. Yizhar Z, Boulos S, Inbar O, Carmeli E. The effect of restricted arm swing on energy expenditure in healthy men. *Intern J Rehab Res.* 2009;32(4):115-123.

51. Bisset LM, Collins NJ, Offord SS. Immediate effects of 2 types of braces on pain and grip strength in people with lateral epicondylalgia: A randomized controlled trial. *J Orthop Sports Phys Ther.* 2014;44(2):120-128.

52. Collins SH, Adamczyk PG, Kuo AD. Dynamic arm swinging in human walking. *Proc R Soc B.* 2009;276:3679-3688. doi:10.1098/rspb.2009.0664

53. Van de Walle P, Meyns P, Desloovere K, et al. Age-related changes in arm motion during typical gait. *Gait & Posture.* 2018;Oct(66):51-57. doi:10.1016/j.gaitpost.2018.07.176

54. Lee DG. Biomechanics of the thorax: A clinical model of in vivo function. *J Man Manip Ther.* 1993;1(1):13-21. doi:10.1179/106698193791069771

55. Lee DG. Biomechanics of the thorax: Research evidence and clinical expertise. *J Man Manip Ther.* 2015;23(3)(July):128-138. doi: 10.1179/2042618615Y.0000000008

56. Lewis CL, Laudicina NM, Khuu A, Loverro KL. The human pelvis: variation in structure and function during gait. *Anat Rec (Hoboken).* 2017;300(4):633-642. doi:10.1002/ar.23552

57. Walker ML, Rothstein JM, Finucane SD, Lamb RL. Relationships between lumbar lordosis, pelvic tilt and abdominal muscle performance. *Phys Ther.* 1987;67(4):512-516.

58. Veneman JF, Menger J, van Asseldonk EH, van der Helm FC, van der Kooij H. Fixating the pelvis in the horizontal plane affects gait characteristics. *Gait & Posture.* 2008;28(1):157-163. doi:10.1016/j.gaitpost.2007.11.008

59. Prins MR, Cornelisse LE, Meijer OG, van der Wurff P, Bruijn SM, van Dieën JH. Axial pelvis range of motion affects thorax-pelvis timing during gait. *J Biomech.* 2019;95:109308. doi:10.1016/j.jbiomech.2019.08.002

60. MacWilliams BA, Rozumalski A, Swanson AN, et al. Assessment of three-dimensional lumbar spine vertebral motion during gait with use of indwelling bone pins. *J Bone Joint Surg Am.* 2013;95(23):e1941-e1948. doi:10.2106/JBJS.L.01469

61. Thurston AJ, Harris JD. Nomral kinematics of the lumbar spine and pelvis. *Spine.* 1983;8(2):199-205.

62. O'Neill MM, Anderson DI, Allen DD, Ross C, Hamel KA. Effects of Alexander Technique training experience on gait behavior in older adults. *J Bodyw Mov Ther.* 2015;19(3):473-481.

63. Murray MP, Mollinger LA, Gardner GM, Sepic SB. Kinematic and EMG patterns during slow, free, and fast walking. *J Orthop Res.* 1984;2(2):272-280. doi:10.1002/jor.1100020309

64. Smidt GL. Hip motion and related factors in walking. *Phys Ther.* 1971;51(1):9-22.

65. Reddy A, Bage J, Levine D. The hip. In: Hughes C, ed. *Biomechanics of Gait.* Orthopaedic Section Independent Study Courses; 1-21; 2014:1-22.

66. Krebs DE, Robbins CE, Lavine L, Mann RW. Hip biomechanics during gait. *J Orthop Sports Phys Ther.* 1998;28(1):51-59.

67. Lusk SJ, Hale BD, Russell DM. Grip width and forearm orientation effects on muscle activity during the lat pulldown. *J Strength Cond Res.* 2010;24(7):1895-1900.

68. Clément J, Toliopoulos P, Hagemeister N, Desmeules F, Fuentes A, Vendittoli PA. Healthy 3D knee kinematics during gait: Differences between women and men, and correlation with x-ray alignment. *Gait & Posture.* 2018;64:198-204. doi:10.1016/j.gaitpost.2018.06.024

69. Anderson FC, Goldberg SR, Pandy MG, Delp SL. Contributions of muscle forces and toe-off kinematics to peak knee flexion during the swing phase of normal gait: An induced position analysis. *J Biomech.* 2004;37(5):371-377. doi:10.1016/j.jbiomech.2003.09.018

70. Rodgers MM. Dynamic biomechanics of the normal foot and ankle during walking and running. *Phys Ther.* 1988;68:1822-1830.

71. Segal A, Yeates K, Neptune R, Klute GK. Foot and ankle joint biomechanical adaptations to an unpredictable soronally-uneven surface. *J Biomech Eng.* 2017;140(3). doi:10.1115/1.4037563

72. Murray MP, Clarkson BH. The vertical pathways of the foot during level walking: I. Range of variability in normal men. *Phys Ther.* 1966;46(6):585-589.

73. Gefen A. The in vivo elastic properties of the plantar fascia during the contact phase of walking. *Foot Ankle Int.* 2003;24(3):238-244. doi:10.1177/107110070302400307

74. Fujita M. Role of the metatarsophalangeal (MTP) joints of the foot in level walking. *Nippon Seikeigeka Gakkai Zasshi.* 1985;59(11):985-997.

75. Mann RA, Hagy JL. The function of the toes in walking, jogging and running. *Clin Orthop Relat Res.* 1979;142:24-29.

76. Arndt A, Westblad P, Winson I, Hashimoto T, Lundberg A. Ankle and subtalar kinematics measured with intracortical pins during the stance phase of walking. *Foot Ankle Int*. 2004;25(5):357-364.

77. deAsla RJ, Wan L, Rubash HE, Li G. Six DOF in vivo kinematics of the ankle joint complex: Application of a combined dual-orthogonal fluoroscopic and magnetic resonance imaging technique. *J Orthop Res*. 2006;24(5):1019-1027.

78. Dubo HI, Peat M, Winter DA, et al. Electromyographic temporal analysis of gait: Normal human locomotion. *Arch Phys Med Rehabil*. 1976;57(9):415-420.

79. Kuhtz-Buschbeck JP, Brockmann K, Gilster R, Koch A, Stolze H. Asymmetry of arm-swing not related to handedness. *Gait & Posture*. 2008;27(3):447-454. doi:10.1016/j.gaitpost.2007.05.011

80. Williams KR. The biomechanics of running. *Exerc Sport Sci Rev*. 1985;13:389-441.

81. Bogey RA, Gitter AJ, Barnes LA. Determination of ankle muscle power in normal gait using an EMG-to-force processing approach. *Electromyogr Kinesiol*. 2010;20(1):46-54. doi:10.1016/j.jelekin.2008.09.013

82. Hruska RJ. Pelvic stability influences lower-extremity kinematics. *Biomech*. 1998;5(6):23-29.

83. Aldabe D, Milosavljevic S, Bussey MD. A multivariate model for predicting PPGP considering postural adjustment parameters. *Musculoskelet Science and Practice*. 2020:102153. doi:10.1016/j.msksp.2020.102153

84. Rutherford DJ, Hubley-Kozey C. Explaining the hip adduction moment variability during gait: Implications for hip abductor strengthening. *Clin Biomech*. 2009;24(3):267-73.

85. Punt M, Bruijn SM, Wittink H, van Dieën JH. Effect of arm swing strategy on local dynamic stability of human gait. *Gait & Posture*. 2015;41(2):504-509.

86. Nakakubo S, Doi T, Sawa R, Misu S, Tsutsumimoto K, Ono R. Does Arm Swing Emphasized Deliberately Increase the Trunk Stability During Walking in the Elderly Adults? *Gait & Posture*. 2014;40(4):516-20.

87. Wimby CR, Lloyd DG, Besier TF, Kirk TB. Muscle and external load contribution to knee joint contact loads during normal gait. *J Biomech*. 2009;42(14):2294-2300.

88. Pandy MG, Andriacchi TP. Muscle and joint function in human locomotion. *Annu Rev Biomed Eng*. 2010;12(401-433)

89. Hunt AE, Smith RM, Torode M. Extrinsic muscle activity, foot motion and ankle joint moments during the stance phase of walking. *Foot Ankle Int*. 2001;22(1):31-41.

90. Kapandji IA. *The Physiology of Joints, Vol 3, The Trunk and Vertebral Column*. Churchill Livingstone; 1974.

91. Bruijn SM, Meijer OG, van Dieën JH, Kingma I, Lamoth CJC. Coordination of leg swing, thorax rotations, and pelvis rotations during gait: The organisation of total body angular momentum. *Gait & Posture*. 2008;27(3):455-62.

92. Valenza MC, Cabrera-Martos I, Torres-Sanchez I, Garces A, Mateos-Toset S, Valenza-Demet G. The effects of doming of the diaphragm technique in subjects with short hamstring syndrome: A randomized controlled trial. *J Sport Rehabil*. 2015;24(4):342-348. doi:10.1123/jsr.2014-0190

93. Matsusaka N. Control of the medial-lateral balance in walking. *Acta Orthop Scand*. 1986;57(6):555-559.

94. Zelik KE, La Scaleia V, Ivanenko YP, Lacquaniti F. Coordination of intrinsic and extrinsic foot muscles during walking. *Eur J Appl Physiol*. 2015;115(4):691-701. doi:10.1007/s00421-014-3056-x

95. Farris DJ, Kelly LA, Cresswell AG, Lichtwark GA. The functional importance of human foot muscles for bipedal locomotion. *Proc Natl Acad Sci USA*. 2019;116(5):1645-1650. doi:10.1073/pnas.1812820116

96. White SG, McNair PJ. Abdominal and erector spinae muscle activity during gait: The use of cluster analysis to identify patterns of activity. *Clin Biomech (Bristol, Avon)*. 2002;17(3):177-184. doi:10.1016/s0268-0033(02)00007-4

97. Buckthorpe M, Stride M, Della Villa F. Assessing and treating gluteus maximus weakness: A clinical commentary. *Int J Sports Phys Ther*. 2019;14(4):655-669.

98. Francis CA, Lenz AL, Lenhart RL, Thelen DG. The modulation of forward propulsion, vertical support, and center of pressure by the plantarflexors during human walking. *Gait Posture*. 2013;38(4):993-997. doi:10.1016/j.gaitpost.2013.05.009

99. Simonsen EB. Contributions to the understanding of gait control. *Dan Med J*. 2014;61(4):B4823.

100. Neptune RR, McGowan CP. Muscle contributions to whole-body sagittal plane angular momentum during walking. *J Biomech*. 2011;44(1):6-12. doi:10.1016/j.jbiomech.2010.08.015

101. American Heart Association. Target heart rate. American Heart Association. Updated March 22, 2013. Accessed April 9, 2014. http://www.heart.org/HEARTORG/GettingHealthy/PhysicalActivity/Target-Heart-Rates_UCM_434341_Article.jsp

102. Whittle MW. Generation and attenuation of transient impulsive forces beneath the foot: A review. *Gait Posture*. 1999;10(3):264-275.

103. Paluska SA. An overview of hip injuries in running. *Sports Med*. 2005;35(11):991-114.

104. Tudor-Locke C, Camhi SM, Leonardi C, et al. Patterns of adult stepping cadence in the 2005-2006 NHANES. *Prev Med*. 2011;53(3):178-181.

105. Yao J, Guo N, Xiao Y, et al. Lower limb joint motion and muscle force in treadmill and over-ground exercise. *Biomed Eng Online*. 2019;18(89). doi:10.111186/s12938-019-0708-4 PMC6704526,

106. Mazaheri R, Sanjari MA, Radmehr G, Halabchi F, Angoorani H. The activation pattern of trunk and lower limb muscles in an electromyographic assessment: Comparison between ground and treadmill walking. *Asian J Sport Med*. 2016;7(3):e35308. doi:10.5812/asjsm.35308

107. Plotnik M, Azrad T, Bondi M, et al. Self-selected gait speed—over ground versus self-paced treadmill walking: A solution for a paradox. *J Neuroeng Rehabil*. 2015;12(20). doi:10.1186/s12984-015-00002-z PMC4374285,

108. Di Stasi S, Hartigan E, Selfe J, Richards J, Levine D. The knee. In: Hughes C, ed. *Biomechanics of Gait*. Orthopaedic Section Independent Study Courses; 2014.

109. Dillman CJ. Kinematic analyses of running. *Exerc Sport Sci Rev*. 1975;3:193-218.

110. Perry J. Gait analysis in sports medicine. *Instr Course Lect.* 1990;39:319-324.

111. Kunz H, Kaufmann DA. Biomechanical analysis of sprinting: Decathletes versus champions. *Br J Sports Med.* 1981;15(3):177-181.

112. Paróczai R, Kocsis L. Analysis of human walking and running parameters as a function of speed. *Technol Health Care.* 2006;14(4-5):251-260.

113. Schache AG, Dorn TW, Williams GP, Brown NAT, Pandy MG. Lower-limb muscular strategies for increasing running speed. *J Orthop Sports Phys Ther.* 2014;44(10):813-824.

114. Vaughan CL. Biomechanics of running gait. *Crit Rev Biomed Eng.* 1984;12(1):1-48.

115. Novacheck TF. The biomechanics of running. *Gait Posture.* 1998;7(1):77-95.

116. Schache AG, Bennell KL, Blanch PD, Wrigley TV. The coordinated movement of the lumbo-pelvic-hip complex during running: A literature review. *Gait Posture.* 1999;10(1):30-47.

117. James SL, Brubaker CE. Biomechanics of running. *Orthop Clin North Am.* 1973;4(3):605-615.

118. Dugan SA, Bhat KP. Biomechanics and analysis of running gait. *Phys Med Rehabil Clin N Am.* 2005;16(3):603-621.

119. Pink M, Perry J, Houglum PA, Devine DJ. Lower extremity range of motion in the recreational sport runner. *Am J Sports Med.* 1994;22(4):541-9.

120. McCallion C, Donne B, Fleming N, Blanksby B. Acute differences in foot strike and spatiotemporal variables for shod, barefoot or minimalist male runners. *J Sports Sci Med.* 2015;13(2):280-286.

121. Nicola TL, Jewison DJ. The anatomy and biomechanics of running. *Clin Sports Med.* 2012;31(2):187-201.

122. Stergiou N, Bates BT, Kurz MJ. Subtalar and knee joint interaction during running at various stride lengths. *J Sports Med Phys Fitness.* 2003;43(3):319-326.

123. McClay I, Manal K. Three-dimensional kinetic analysis of running: Significance of secondary planes of motion. *Med Sci Sports Exerc.* 1999;31(11):1629-1637.

124. Ounpuu S. The biomechanics of running: A kinematic and kinetic analysis. *Instr Course Lect.* 1990;39:305-318.

125. Kyröläinen H, Avela J, Komi PV. Changes in muscle activity with increasing running speed. *J Sport Sci.* 2005;23(10):1101-1109.

126. Montgomery WH, 3rd., Pink M, Perry J. Electromyographic analysis of hip and knee musculature during running. *Am J Sports Med.* 1994;22(2):272-278.

127. Novacheck TF. Walking, running, and sprinting: A three-dimensional analysis of kinematics and kinetics. *Instr Course Lect.* 1995;44:497-506.

128. Arellano CJ, Kram RR. The effects of step width and arm swing on energetic cost and lateral balance during running. *J Biomech.* 2011;44(7):1291-1295.

129. Houglum PA, Bertoti DB. *Brunnstrom's Clinical Kinesiology.* 6th ed. F.A. Davis; 2012.

130. Mero A, Komi PV, Gregor RJ. Biomechanics of sprint running: A review. *Sports Med.* 1992;13(6):376-392.

131. Thordarson DB. Running biomechanics. *Clin Sports Med.* 1997;16(2):239-247.

132. Besier TF, Frederickson M, Gold GE, Beaupré GS, Delp SL. Knee muscle forces during walking and running in patellofemoral pain patients and pain-free controls. *J Biomech.* 2009;42(7):898-905.

133. Simonsen EB, Thomsen L, Klausen K. Activity of mono- and biarticular leg muscles during sprint running. *Eur J Appl Physiol Occup Physiol.* 1985;54(5):524-532.

134. Reber L, Perry J, Pink M. Muscular control of the ankle in running. *Am J Sports Med.* 1993;21(6):805-810.

135. Jacobs R, Bobbert MF, van Ingen Schenau GJ. Function of mono- and biarticular muscles in running. *Med Sci Sports Exerc.* 1993;25(10):1163-1173.

136. O'Connor KM, Hamill J. The role of selected extrinsic foot muscles during running. *Clin Biomech.* 2004;19(1):71-77.

137. Perry J. Anatomy and biomechanics of the hindfoot. *Clin Orthop Relat Res.* 1983;177:9-15.

138. DeLeo AT, Dierks TA, Ferber R, Davis IS. Lower extremity joint coupling during running: A current update. *Clin Biomech.* 2004;19(10):983-991.

139. Pohl H. Changes in the structure of collagen distribution in the skin caused by manual technique. *J Bodywork Movement Ther.* 2010;14(1):27-34.

140. McClay I, Manal K. Coupling parameters in runners with normal and excessive pronation. *J Appl Biomech.* 1997;13(1):109-124.

141. Krell JB, Stefanyshyn DJ. The relationship between extension of the metatarsophalangeal joint and sprint time for 100 m Olympic athletes. *J Sport Sci.* 2006;24(2):175-180.

142. Hunter JP, Marshall RN, McNair PJ. Segment-interaction analysis of the stance limb in sprint running. *J Biomech.* 2004;37(9):1439-1446.

143. Nawoczenski DA, Cook TM, Saltzman CL. The effect of foot orthotics on three-dimensional kinematics of the leg and rearfoot during running. *J Orthop Sports Phys Ther.* 1995;21(6):317-327.

144. Williams DS, 3rd., McClay I, Hamill J. Arch structure and injury patterns in runners. *Clin Biomech.* 2001;16(4):341-347.

145. Miller RH, Meardon SA, Derrick TR, Gillette JC. Continuous relative phase variability during an exhaustive run in runners with a history of iliotibial band syndrome. *J Appl Biomech.* 2008;24(3):262-270.

146. Ferber R, Davis IM, Williams DS, 3rd. Effect of foot orthotics on rearfoot and tibia joint coupling patterns and variability. *J Biomech.* 2005;38(3):477-483.

147. Kumar R, Roe MC, Scremin OU. Methods for estimating the proper length of a cane. *Arch Phys Med Rehabil.* 1995;76(12):1173-1175.

148. Lane PL, LeBlanc R. Crutch walking. *Orthop Nurs.* 1990;9(5):31-38.

Chapter 8

1. Truong LK, Mosewich AD, Holt CJ, Le CY, Miciak M, Whittaker JL. Psychological, social and contextual factors across recovery stages following a sport-related knee injury: A scoping review. *Br J Sports Med.* 2020;54(19):1149-1156. doi:10.1136/bjsports-2019-101206

2. Forsdyke D, Smith A, Jones M, Gledhill A. Psychosocial factors associated with outcomes of sports injury rehabilitation in competitive athletes: A mixed studies systematic review. *Br J Sports Med.* 2016;50(9):537-544. doi:10.1136/bjsports-2015-094850

3. Evans L, Hardy L. Injury rehabilitation: A qualitative follow-up study. *Res Q Exerc Sport*. 2002;73(3):320-329. doi:10.1080/02701367.2002.10609026

4. Thornton GM, Bailey SJ. Repetitive loading damages healing ligaments more than sustained loading demonstrated by reduction in modulus and residual strength. *J Biomech*. 2012;45(15):2589-2594. doi:10.1016/j.jbiomech.2012.08.013

5. Noyes FR, Heckmann TP, Barber-Westin SD. Meniscus repair and transplantation: A comprehensive update. *J Orthop Sports Phys Ther*. 2012;42(3):274-290.

6. Conti M, Garofalo R, Delle Rose G, et al. Post-operative rehabilitation after surgical repair of the rotator cuff. *Chir Organi Mov*. 2009;93 Suppl 1:S55-S63. doi:10.1007/s12306-009-0003-9

7. Siengsukon CF, Al-Dughmi M, Stevens S. Sleep health promotion: Practical information for physical therapists. *Phys Ther*. 2017;97(8):826-836. doi:10.1093/ptj/pzx057

8. Besedovsky L, Lange T, Born J. Sleep and immune function. *Pflugers Arch*. 2012;463(1):121-137. doi:10.1007/s00424-011-1044-0

9. Vas PR, Ahluwalia R, Manas AB, Manu CA, Kavarthapu V, Edmonds ME. Undiagnosed severe sleep apnoea and diabetic foot ulceration: A case series based hypothesis: A hitherto under emphasized factor in failure to heal. *Diabet Med*. 2016;33(2):e1-e4. doi:10.1111/dme.12813

10. Egydio F, Pires GN, Tufik S, Andersen ML. Wound-healing and benzodiazepines: Does sleep play a role in this relationship? *Clinics (Sao Paulo)*. 2012;67(7):827-830. doi:10.6061/clinics/2012(07)20

11. Sinatra R. Causes and consequences of inadequate management of acute pain. *Pain Med*. 2010;11(12):1859-1871. doi:10.1111/j.1526-4637.2010.00983.x

12. Cary D, Briffa K, McKenna L. Identifying relationships between sleep posture and non-specific spinal symptoms in adults: A scoping review. *BMJ Open*. 2019;9(6):e027633. doi:10.1136/bmjopen-2018-027633

13. Stefani A, Gabelia D, Mitterling T, Poewe W, Högl B, Frauscher B. A prospective video-polysomnographic analysis of movements during physiological sleep in 100 healthy sleepers. *Sleep*. 2015;38(9):1479-1487. doi:10.5665/sleep.4994

14. Hawthorne JR, Carpenter EM, Lam PH, Murrell GAC. Effects of abduction pillows on rotator cuff repair: A biomechanical analysis. *Hss j*. 2018;14(2):114-122. doi:10.1007/s11420-017-9592-2

15. Rohlmann A, Petersen R, Schwachmeyer V, Graichen F, Bergmann G. Spinal loads during position changes. *Clin Biomech (Bristol, Avon)*. 2012;27(8):754-758. doi:10.1016/j.clinbiomech.2012.04.006

16. Naik GR, Al-Ani A, Gobbo M, Nguyen HT. Does heel height cause imbalance during sit-to-stand task: Surface EMG perspective. *Front Physiol*. 2017;8:626. doi:10.3389/fphys.2017.00626

17. Kim MH, Yi CH, Yoo WG, Choi BR. EMG and kinematics analysis of the trunk and lower extremity during the sit-to-stand task while wearing shoes with different heel heights in healthy young women. *Hum Mov Sci*. 2011;30(3):596-605. doi:10.1016/j.humov.2010.09.003

18. Nam I, Shin J, Lee Y, Lee MY, Chung Y. The effect of foot position on erector spinae and gluteus maximus muscle activation during sit-to-stand performed by chronic stroke patients. *J Phys Ther Sci*. 2015;27(3):571-573. doi:10.1589/jpts.27.571

19. Jeon W, Jensen JL, Griffin L. Muscle activity and balance control during sit-to-stand across symmetric and asymmetric initial foot positions in healthy adults. *Gait Posture*. 2019;71:138-144. doi:10.1016/j.gaitpost.2019.04.030

20. Michelin RM, Ahdoot E, Zakhary BL, McDowell M, French M. Choosing the optimal wound dressing for bathing after total knee arthroplasty. *J Arthroplasty*. 2020;36(3):970-977. doi:10.1016/j.arth.2020.09.023

21. Yu YH, Chao S, Lin YK, et al. The gap between currently available evidence and awareness in clinical practice of wound care: It is the time to shower earlier. *Surgery*. 2018. doi:10.1016/j.surg.2018.01.013

22. Köninger J, Russ M, Schmidt R, Feilhauer K, Butters M. Postoperative wundheilung unter wund-wasserkontakt [Postoperative wound healing in wound-water contact]. *Zentralbl Chir*. 2000;125(2):157-160.

23. Riederer SR, Inderbitzi R. Gefährdet das duschen die postoperative wundheilung? [Does a shower put postoperative wound healing at risk?]. *Chirurg*. 1997;68(7):715-717. doi:10.1007/s001040050259

24. Neues C, Haas E. Beeinflussung der postoperativen wundheilung durch duschen [Modification of postoperative wound healing by showering]. *Chirurg*. 2000;71(2):234-236. doi:10.1007/s001040050040

25. Harrison C, Wade C, Gore S. Postoperative washing of sutured wounds. *Ann Med Surg (Lond)*. 2016;11:36-38. doi:10.1016/j.amsu.2016.08.015

26. Bellabarba C, Karim F, Tavolaro C, et al. The mandible-C2 angle: A new radiographic assessment of occipitocervical alignment. *Spine J*. 2021;21(1):105-113. doi:10.1016/j.spinee.2020.07.003

27. Huggare J, Houghton P. Associations between atlantoaxial and craniomandibular anatomy. *Growth Dev Aging*. Spring 1996;60(1):21-30.

28. Eriksson PO, Häggman-Henrikson B, Nordh E, Zafar H. Co-ordinated mandibular and head-neck movements during rhythmic jaw activities in man. *J Dent Res*. 2000;79(6):1378-1384. doi:10.1177/00220345000790060501

29. Fonder AC. The dental distress syndrome quantified. *Basal Facts*. 1987;9(4):141-167.

30. Baumgarten KM, Osborn R, Schweinle WE, 3rd, Zens MJ. The position of sling immobilization influences the outcomes of anatomic total shoulder arthroplasty: A randomized, single-blind, prospective study. *J Shoulder Elbow Surg*. 2018;27(12):2120-2128. doi:10.1016/j.jse.2018.08.030

31. Yin B, Levy D, Meadows M, et al. How does external rotation bracing influence motion and functional scores after arthroscopic shoulder stabilization? *Clin Orthop Relat Res*. 2014;472(8):2389-2396. doi:10.1007/s11999-013-3343-6

32. Abeles A, Kwasnicki RM, Pettengell C, Murphy J, Darzi A. The relationship between physical activity and post-operative length of hospital stay: A systematic review. *Int J Surg*. Aug 2017;44:295-302. doi:10.1016/j.ijsu.2017.06.085

Chapter 9

1. Logan CA, Asnis PD, Provencher MT. The role of therapeutic modalities in surgical and nonsurgical management of orthopaedic injuries. *J Am Acad Orthop Surg.* 2017;25(8):556-568.

2. Malanga GA, Yan N, Stark J. Mechanisms and efficacy of heat and cold therapies for musculoskeletal injury. *Postgrad Med.* 2015;127(1):57-65.

3. Collins N, Friedrich L. Wound healing: The nutrition connection. *Caring.* 2012;31(12):66,68.

4. Hubbard TJ, Denegar CR. Does cryotherapy improve outcomes with soft tissue injury? *J Athl Train.* 2004;39(3):278-279.

5. Collins NC. Is ice right? Does cryotherapy improve outcome for acute soft tissue injury? *Emerg Med J.* 2008;25(2):65-68.

6. Schaser KD, Disch AC, Stover JF, Lauffer A, Bail HJ, Mittlmeier T. Prolonged superficial local cryotherapy attenuates microcirculatory impairment, regional inflammation, and muscle necrosis after closed soft tissue injury in rats. *Am J Sports Med.* 2007;35(1):93-102.

7. Baker RJ, Bell GW. The effect of therapeutic modalities on blood flow in the human calf. *J Orthop Sports Phys Ther.* 1991;13(1):23-27.

8. Minson CT, Berry LT, Joyner MJ. Nitric oxide and neurally mediated regulation of skin blood flow during local heating. *J Appl Physiol (1985).* 2001;91(4):1619-1626.

9. Khoshnevis S, Craik NK, Brothers RM, Diller KR. Cryotherapy-induced persistent vasoconstriction after cutaneous cooling: hysteresis between skin temperature and blood perfusion. *J Biomech Eng.* 2016;138(3) doi:10.1115/1.4032126

10. Pittman RN. The circulatory system and oxygen transport. *Regulation of Tissue Oxygenation.* 2nd ed. Morgan & Claypool Life Sciences; 2016.

11. Algafly AA. The effect of cryotherapy on nerve conduction velocity, pain threshold and pain tolerance. *Br J Sports Med.* 2007;41(6):365-369.

12. Giombini A, Giovannini V, Di Cesare A, et al. Hyperthermia induced by microwave diathermy in the management of muscle and tendon injuries. *Br Med Bull.* 2007;83:379-396.

13. Sekins KM, Lehmann JF, Esselman P, et al. Local muscle blood flow and temperature responses to 915MHz diathermy as simultaneously measured and numerically predicted. *Arch Phys Med Rehabil.* 1984;65(1):1-7.

14. Melzack R, Wall PD. Pain mechanisms: a new theory. *Science.* 1965;150:971-979.

15. Lehmann JF, Brunner GD, Stow RW. Pain threshold measurements after therapeutic application of ultrasound, microwaves and infrared. *Arch Phys Med Rehabil.* 1958;39(9):560-565.

16. Eldred E, Lindsley DF, Buckwald JS. The effect of cooling on mammalian muscle spindles. *Exp Neurol.* 1960;2:144-157.

17. Mense S. Effects of temperature on the discharges of muscle spindles and tendon organs. *Pflugers Arch.* 1978;374(2):159-166.

18. McCarberg BH, Ruoff GE, Tenzer-Iglesias P, Weil AJ. Diagnosis and treatment of low-back pain because of paraspinous muscle spasm: a physician roundtable. *Pain Med.* 2011;12(Suppl 4):S119-S127.

19. Johnson DJ, Leider FE. Influence of cold bath on maximum handgrip strength. *Percept Mot Skills.* 1977;44(1):323-326.

20. Wickstrom RL, Polk CE. Effect of the whirlpool on the strength-endurance of the quadriceps muscle in trained male adolescents. *Am J Phys Med.* 1961;40(1):91-92.

21. Corr DT, Hart DA. Biomechanics of scar tissue and uninjured skin. *Adv Wound Care (New Rochelle).* 2013;2(2):37-43.

22. Swenson C, Swärd L, Karlsson J. Cryotherapy in sports medicine. *Scand J Med Sci Sports.* 1996;6(4):193-200.

23. Warren CG, Lehmann JF, Koblanski JN. Heat and stretch procedures: an evaluation using rat tail tendon. *Arch Phys Med Rehabil.* 1976;57(3):122-126.

24. Lentell G, Hetherington T, Eagan J, Morgan M. The use of thermal agents to influence the effectiveness of a low-load prolonged stretch. *J Orthop Sports Phys Ther.* 1992;16(5):200-207.

25. Lehmann JF, Masock AJ, Warren CG, Koblanski JN. Effect of therapeutic temperatures on tendon extensibility. *Arch Phys Med Rehabil.* 1970;51(8):481-487.

26. Abramson DI, Mitchell RE, Tuck S, Jr., Bell Y, Zays AM. Changes in blood flow, oxygen uptake and tissue temperatures produced by the topical application of wet heat. *Arch Phys Med Rehabil.* 1961;42:305-318.

27. Guo Y, Tan J, MIao Y, Sun Z, Zhang Q. Effects of microvesicles on cell apoptosis under hypoxia. *Oxid Med Cell Longev.* 2019;2019:11. 5972152. doi:10.1155/2019/5972152

28. Hardy M, Woodall W. Therapeutic effects of heat, cold, and stretch on connective tissue. *J Hand Ther.* 1998;11(2):148-156.

29. Nadler SF, Weingand K, Kruse RJ. The physiologic basis and clinical applications of cryotherapy and thermotherapy for the pain practitioner. *Pain Phys.* 2004;3:395-399.

30. Baker KG, Robertson VJ, Duck FA. A review of therapeutic ultrasound: biophysical effects. *Phys Ther.* 2001;81(7):1351-1358.

31. Dalecki D. Mechanical bioeffects of ultrasound. *Annu Rev Biomed Eng.* 2004;6:229-248.

32. O'Brien WD, Jr. Ultrasound-biophysics mechanisms. *Prog Biophys Mol Biol.* 2007;93(1-3):212-255.

33. Johns LD. Nonthermal effects of therapeutic ultrasound: the frequency resonance hypothesis. *J Athl Train.* 2002;37(3):293-299.

34. Coakley WT. Biophysical effects of ultrasound at therapeutic intensities. *Physiotherapy.* 1978;64(6):166-169.

35. Draper DO, Castel JC, Castel D. Rate of temperature increase in human muscle during 1 MHz and 3 MHz continuous ultrasound. *J Orthop Sports Phys Ther.* 1995;22(4):142-150.

36. Catapani LB, da Costa Gonçalves A, Candeloro NM, Rossi LA, de Oliveira Guirro EC. Influence of therapeutic ultrasound on the biomechanical characteristics of the skin. *J Ther Ultrasound.* 2016;4:21. doi:10.1186/s40349-016-0065-8

37. Chan AK, Myrer JW, Measom GJ, Draper DO. Temperature changes in human patellar tendon in response to therapeutic ultrasound. *J Athl Train.* 1998;33(2):130-135.

38. Draper DO, Sunderland S. Examination of the law of grotthus-draper: does ultrasound penetrate subcutaneous fat in humans? *J Athl Train*. 1993;28(3):246-250.

39. Rose SJ, Draper DO, Schulthies SS, Durrant E. The stretching window part two: rate of thermal decay in deep muscle following 1-MHz ultrasound. *J Athl Train*. 1996;31(2):139-143.

40. Sparrow KJ, Finucane SD, Owen JR, Wayne JS. The effects of low-intensity ultrasound on medial collateral ligament healing in the rabbit model. *Am J Sports Med*. 2005;33(7):1048-1056.

41. Watson T. The role of electrotherapy in contemporary physiotherapy practice. *Man Ther*. 2000;5(3):132-141.

42. Nussbaum E. The influence of ultrasound on healing tissues. *J Hand Ther*. 1998;11(2):140-147.

43. Speed CA. Therapeutic ultrasound in soft tissue lesions. *Rheumatology (Oxford)*. 2001;40(12):1331-1336.

44. Luo Q, Ji S, Li Z, Huang T, Fan S, Xi Q. Effects of ultrasound therapy on the synovial fluid proteome in a rabbit surgery-induced model of knee osteoarthritis. *Biomed Eng Online*. 2019;18(1):18. doi:10.1186/s12938-019-0637-2

45. Gallo JA, Draper DO, Brody LT, Fellingham GW. A comparison of human muscle temperature increases during 3-MHz continuous and pulsed ultrasound with equivalent temporal average intensities. *J Orthop Sports Phys Ther*. 2004;34(7):395-401.

46. Watson T. Ultrasound in contemporary physiotherapy practice. *Ultrasonics*. 2008;48(8):321-329.

47. Maxwell L. Therapeutic ultrasound: its effects on the cellular and molecular mechanisms of inflammation and repair. *Physiotherapy*. 1992;78(6):421-426.

48. Signori LU, da Costa ST, Neto AFS, et al. Haematological effect of pulsed ultrasound in acute muscular inflammation in rats. *Physiotherapy*. 2011;97(2):163-169.

49. Lu H, Chen C, Qu J, et al. Initiation timing of low-intensity pulsed ultrasound stimulation for tendon-bone healing in a rabbit model. *Am J Sports Med*. 2016;44(10):2706-2715.

50. Lu H, Liu F, Chen H, et al. The effect of low-intensity pulsed ultrasound on bone-tendon junction healing: Initiating after inflammation stage. *J Orthop Res*. 2016;34(10):1697-1706.

51. Fu SC, Hung LK, Shum WT, et al. In vivo low-intensity pulsed ultrasound (LIPUS) following tendon injury promotes repair during granulation but suppresses decorin and biglycan expression during remodeling. *J Orthop Sports Phys Ther*. 2010;40(7):422-429.

52. Mortimer AJ, Dyson M. The effect of therapeutic ultrasound on calcium uptake in fibroblasts. *Ultrasound Med Biol*. 1988;14(6):499-506.

53. Gorick CM, Chappell JC, Price RJ. Applications of ultrasound to stimulate therapeutic revascularization. *Int J Mol Sci*. 2019;20(12)doi:10.3390/ijms20123081

54. Demir H, Menku P, Kirnap M, Calis M, Ikizceli I. Comparison of the effects of laser, ultrasound, and combined laser + ultrasound treatments in experimental tendon healing. *Lasers Surg Med*. 2004;35(1):84-89.

55. Qin L, Lu H, Fok P, et al. Low-intensity pulsed ultrasound accelerates osteogenesis at bone-tendon healing junction. *Ultrasound Med Biol*. 2006;32(12):1905-1911.

56. Yeung CK, Guo X, Ng YF. Pulsed ultrasound treatment accelerates the repair of Achilles tendon rupture in rats. *J Orthop Res*. 2006;24(2):193-201.

57. Dyson M. Mechanisms involved in therapeutic ultrasound. *Physiotherapy*. 1987;73(3):116-120.

58. Wu S, Ximing X, Sun J, Zhang Y, Shi J, Xu T. Low-intensity pulsed ultrasound accelerates traumatic vertebral fracture healing by coupling proliferation of type H microvessels. *J Ultrasound Med*. 2018;37(7):1733-1742.

59. Bayat M, Virdi A, Jalalifirouzkouhi R, Rezaei F. Comparison of effects of LLLT and LIPUS on fracture healing in animal models and patients: a systematic review. *Prog Biophys Mol Biol*. 2018;132:2-22.

60. Harrison A, Lin SF, Pounder N, Mikuni-Takagaki Y. Mode & mechanism of low intensity pulsed ultrasound (LIPUS) in fracture repair. *Ultrasonics*. 2016;70:45-52.

61. Lou SJ, Lv H, Li Z, Zhang L, Tang P. The effects of low-intensity pulsed ultrasound on fresh fracture: A meta-analysis. *Medicine (Baltimore)*. 2017;96(39):e8181. doi:10.1097/MD.0000000000008181

62. Tsai WC, Hsu CC, Tang FT, Chou SW, Chen YJ, Pang JHS. Ultrasound stimulation of tendon cell proliferation and upregulation of proliferating cell nuclear antigen. *J Orthop Res*. 2005;23(4):970-976.

63. Reher P, Doan N, Bradnock B, Meghji S, Harris M. Effect of ultrasound on the production of IL-8, basic FGF and VEGF. *Cytokine*. 1999;11(6):16-23.

64. Doan N, Reher P, Meghji S, Harris M. In vitro effects of therapeutic ultrasound on cell proliferation, protein synthesis, and cytokine production by human fibroblasts, osteoblasts, and monocytes. *J Oral Maxillofac Surg*. 1999;57(4):409-419.

65. Maxwell L, Collecutt T, Gledehill M, Sharma S, Edgar S, Gavin JB. The augmentation of leucocyte adhesion to endothelium by therapeutic ultrasound. *Ultrasound Med Biol*. 1994;20(4):383-390.

66. Steffen W, Cumberland D, Gaines P, et al. Catheter-delivered high intensity, low frequency ultrasound induces vasodilation in vivo. *Eur Heart J*. 1994;15(3):369-376.

67. Robertson VJ. Dosage and treatment response in randomized clinical trials of therapeutic ultrasound. *Phys Ther Sport*. 2002;3(3):124-133.

68. Hayes BT, Merrick MA, Sandrey MA, Cordova ML. Three-MHz ultrasound heats deeper into the tissues than originally theorized. *J Athl Train*. 2004;39(3):230-234.

69. Lehmann JF, De Lateur BJ. Therapeutic heat. In: Lehmann JF, ed. *Therapeutic Heat and Cold*. 4th ed. Williams & Wilkins; 1990.

70. Draper DO. Facts and misfits in ultrasound therapy: steps to improve your treatment outcomes. *Eur J Phys Rehabil Med*. 2014;50(2):209-216.

71. Draper DO. Ten mistakes commonly made with ultrasound use: current research sheds light on myths. *Athl Train Sports Health Care*. 1996;2(2):95-107.

72. de Oliveira RF, Oliveira DAAP, Soares CP. Effect of low-intensity pulsed ultrasound on l929 fibroblasts. *Arch Med Sci*. 2011;7(2):224-229.

73. Coskun ME, Coskun KA, Tutar Y. Determination of optimum operation parameters for low-intensity pulsed ultrasound and low-level laser based treatment to induce proliferation of osteoblast and fibroblast cells. *Photomed Laser Surg*. 2018;36(5):246-252.

74. Michlovitz SL. *Thermal Agents in Rehabilitation*. 3rd ed. F.A. Davis; 1996.

75. Maffulli N, Ewen SW, Waterston SW, Reaper J, Barrass V. Tenocytes from ruptured and tendinopathic achilles tendons produce greater quantities of type III collagen than tenocytes from normal achilles tendons. An in vitro model of human tendon healing. *Am J Sports Med.* 2000;28(4):499-505.

76. Faler BJ, Macsata RA, Plummer D, Mishra L, Sidawy AN. Transforming growth factor-beta and wound healing. *Perspect Vasc Surg Endovasc Ther.* 2006;18(1):55-62.

77. Marui T, Niyibizi C, Georgescu HI, et al. Effect of growth factors on matrix synthesis by ligament fibroblasts. *J Orthop Res.* 1997;15(1):18-23.

78. Markham DE, Wood MR. Ultrasound for Dupuytren's contracture. *Physiotherapy.* 1980;66(2):55-58.

79. Srbely JZ. New trends in the treatment and management of myofascial pain syndrome. *Curr Pain Headache Rep.* 2010;14(5):346-352.

80. Tsai WC, Tang ST, Liang FC. Effect of therapeutic ultrasound on tendons. *Am J Phys Med Rehabil.* 2011;90(12):1068-1073.

81. Fernandes de Jesus J, Brihy de Albuquerque TA, Shimba LG, F.F. B, Cook J, Pinfildi CE. High-energy dose of therapeutic ultrasound in the treatment of patellar tendinopathy: protocol of a randomized placebo-controlled clinical trial. *BMC Musculoskelet Disord.* 2019;20(1):624. doi:10.1186/s12891-019-2993-2

82. Lehmann JF, Brunner GD, McMillan JA. Influence of surgical metal implants on the temperature distribution in thigh specimens exposed to ultrasound. *Arch Phys Med Rehabil.* 1958;39(11):692-695.

83. Cerciello S, Rossi S, Visonà E, Corona K, Oliva F. Clinical applications of vibration therapy in orthopaedic practice. *Muscles Ligaments Tendons J.* 2016;6(1):147-156.

84. Rauch F. Vibration therapy. *Dev Med Child Neurol.* 2009;51(Suppl 4):166-168.

85. Rogers MJ, Hrovat K, Moskowitz ME. Effects of exercise equipment on the microgravity environment. *Adv Space Res.* 1999;24(10):1283-1287.

86. Fuller JT, Thomson RL, Howe PRC, Buckley JD. Vibration therapy is no more effective than the standard practice of massage and stretching for promoting recovery from muscle damage after eccentric exercise. *Clin J Sport Med.* 2015;25(4):332-337.

87. Romero-Morales C, Martín-Llantino PJ, Calvo-Lobo C, et al. Vibration increases multifidus cross-sectional area versus cryotherapy added to chronic non-insertional Achilles tendinopathy eccentric exercise. *Phys Ther Sport.* 2020;42(1):61-67.

88. Pamukoff DN, Pietrosimone B, Lewek MD, et al. Whole-body and local muscle vibration immediately improve quadriceps function in individuals with anterior cruciate ligament reconstruction. *Arch Phys Med Rehabil.* 2016;97(7):1121-1129.

89. Sierra-Guzmán R, Jiménez-Diaz F, Ramírez C, Esteban P, Abián-Vicén J. Whole-body-vibration training and balance in recreational athletes with chronic ankle instability. *J Athl Train.* 2018;53(4):355-363.

90. Kruse LM, Gray B, Wright RW. Rehabilitation after anterior cruciate ligament reconstruction: a systematic review. *J Bone Joint Surg Am.* 2012;94(19):1737-1748.

91. Huang M, Liao LR, Pang MY. Effects of whole body vibration on muscle spasticity for people with central nervous system disorders: a systematic review. *Clin Rehabil.* 2017;31(1):23-33.

92. King LK, Almeida QJ, Ahonen H. Short-term effects of vibration therapy on motor impairments in Parkinson's disease. *NeuroRehabilitation.* 2009;25(4):297-306.

93. Armbrecht G, Belavý DL, Gast U, et al. Resistive vibration exercise attenuates bone and muscle atrophy in 56 days of bed rest: biochemical markers of bone metabolism. *Osteoporos Int.* 2010;21(4):597-607.

94. Belavý DL, Hides JA, Wilson SJ, et al. Resistive simulated weightbearing exercise with whole body vibration reduces lumbar spine deconditioning in bed-rest. *Spine (Phila Pa 1976).* 2008;33(5):E121-E131.

95. Cardinale M, Bosco C. The use of vibration as an exercise intervention. *Exerc Sport Sci Rev.* 2003;31(1):3-7.

96. Bokaeian HR, Bakhtiary AH, Mirmohammadkhani M, Moghimi J. The effect of adding whole body vibration training to strengthening training in the treatment of knee osteoarthritis: a randomized clinical trial. *J Bodyw Mov Ther.* 2016;20(2):334-340.

97. Takanashi Y, Chinen Y, Hatakeyama S. Whole-body vibration training improves the balance ability and leg strength of athletic throwers. *J Sports Med Phys Fitness.* 2019;59(7):1110-1118.

98. Furness ND, Phillips A, Gallacher S, et al. Vibration therapy versus standard treatment for tennis elbow: A randomized controlled study. *J Orthop Surg (Hong Kong).* 2018;26(3):2309499018792744. doi:10.1177/2309499018792744

99. Lubetzky AV, McCoy SW, Price R, Kartin D. Response to tendon vibration questions the underlying rationale of proprioceptive training. *J Athl Train.* 2017;52(2):97-107.

100. Bélanger AY. *Evidence-Based Guide to Therapeutic Physical Agents.* Lippincott Williams & Wilkins; 2002.

101. Denegar CR, Saliba E, Saliba S. *Therapeutic Modalities for Musculoskeletal Injuries.* 4th ed. Human Kinetics; 2016.

102. De Domenico GG, Strauss GR. Motor stimulation with interferential currents. *Aust J Physiother.* 1985;31(6):225-230.

103. Bellew JW, Beiswanger Z, Freeman E, Gaerte C, Trafton J. Interferential and burst-modulated biphasic pulsed currents yield greater muscular force than Russian current. *Physiother Theory Pract.* 2012;28(5):384-390.

104. Polak A, Franek A, Taradaj J. High-voltage pulsed current electrical stimulation in wound treatment. *Adv Wound Care (New Rochelle).* 2014;3(2):104-117.

105. Mehmandoust FG, Torkaman G, Firoozabadi M, Talebi G. Anodal and cathodal pulsed electrical stimulation on skin wound healing in guinea pigs. *J Rehabil Res Dev.* 2007;44(4):611-618.

106. Mantovani A, Biswas SK, Galdiero MR, Sica A, Locati M. Macrophage plasticity and polarization in tissue repair and remodelling. *J Pathol.* 2013;229(2):176-185.

107. Scarborough P, Kloth LC. E-stimulation: an effective modality to facilitate wound healing. *Today's Wound Clinic.* 2012;6(4):28-32.

108. Dolan MG, Graves P, Nakazawa C, Delano T, Hutson A, Mendel FC. Effects of ibuprofen and high-voltage electric stimulation on acute edema formation after blunt trauma to limbs of rats. *J Athl Train.* 2005;40(2):111-115.

109. Wong RA. High voltage versus low voltage electrical stimulation: force of induced muscle contraction and perceived discomfort in healthy subjects. *Phys Ther.* 1986;66(8):120-1214.

110. Lake DA. Neuromuscular electrical stimulation: an overview and its application in the treatment of sports injuries. *Sports Med.* 1992;13(5):320-336.

111. Parker MG, Bennett MJ, Hieb MA, Hollar AC, Roe AA. Strength response in human quadriceps femoris muscle during 2 neuromuscular electrical stimulation programs. *J Orthop Sports Phys Ther.* 2003;33(12):719-726.

112. Walls RJ, McHugh G, O'Gorman DJ, Moyna NM, O'Byrne JM. Effects of preoperative neuromuscular electrical stimulation on quadriceps strength and functional recovery in total knee arthroplasty: A pilot study. *BMC Musculoskelet Disord.* 2010;11:119-127.

113. Laughman RK, Youdas JW, Garrett TR, Chao EY. Strength changes in the normal quadriceps femoris muscle as a result of electrical stimulation. *Phys Ther.* 1983;63(4):494-499.

114. Bellew JW, Cayot T, Brown K, et al. Changes in microvascular oxygenation and total hemoglobin concentration of the vastus lateralis during neuromuscular electrical stimulation (NMES). *Physiother Theory Pract.* 2019:1-9. doi:10.1080/09593985.2019.1652945

115. Dantas LO, Vieira A, Siqueira AL, Jr., Salvini TF, Durigan JLQ. Comparison between the effects of 4 different electrical stimulation current waveforms on isometric knee extension torque and perceived discomfort in healthy women. *Muscle Nerve.* 2015;51(1):76-82.

Chapter 10

1. Behnke AR, Jr., Feen BG, Welham WC. The specific gravity of healthy men: Body weight divided by volume as an index of obesity. 1942. *Obes Res.* 1995;3(3):295-300.

2. Cowgill GR. A formula for estimating the specific gravity of the human body with a consideration of its possible uses. *Am J Clin Nutr.* 1957;5(6):601-611.

3. Hay J. *The Biomechanics of Sports Techniques.* 4th ed. Prentice-Hall; 1993.

4. Davis BC, Harrison RA. *Hydrotherapy in Practice.* Churchill Livingstone; 1988.

5. Edlich RF, Towler MA, Goitz RJ, et al. Bioengineering principles of hydrotherapy. *J Burn Care Rehabil.* 1987;8:580-584.

6. Dijksterhuis EJ. *Archimedes.* Princeton University Press; 1987.

7. Kuory JM. *Aquatic Therapy Programming: Guidelines for Orthopedic Rehabilitation.* Human Kinetics; 1996.

8. Naemi R, Easson WJ, Sanders RH. Hydrodynamic glide efficiency in swimming. *J Sci Med Sport.* 2010;13(4):444-451.

9. Laurent A, Rouard A, Mantha VR, Marinho DA, Silva AJ, Rouboa AI. The computational fluid dynamics study of orientation effects of oar-blade. *J Appl Biomech.* 2013;29(1):23-32.

10. Vennell R, Pease D, Wilson B. Wave drag on human swimmers. *J Biomech.* 2006;39(4):664-671.

11. Tor E, Pease DL, Ball KA. How does drag affect the underwater phase of a swimming start? *J Appl Biomech.* 2015;31(1):8-12.

12. McWaters JG. *Deep Water Exercise for Health and Fitness.* Publitec Editions; 1988.

13. Sharp RL, Costill DL. Influence of body hair removal on physiological responses during breaststroke swimming. *Med Sci Sports Exerc.* 1989;21(5):576-580.

14. Chatard JC, Wilson B. Effect of fastskin suits on performance, drag, and energy cost of swimming. *Med Sci Sports Exerc.* 2008;40(6):1149-1154.

15. Schuren J, Mohr K. Pascal's law and the dynamics of compression therapy: a study on healthy volunteers. *Int Angiol.* 2010;29(5):431-435.

16. Thein JM, Brody LT. Aquatic-based rehabilitation and training for the elite athlete. *J Orthop Sports Phys Ther.* 1998;27(1):32-41.

17. Harrison RA, Hillman M, Bulstrode S. Loading of the lower limb when walking partially immersed: implications for clinical practice. *Physiother.* 1992;78(3):164-166.

18. Nguyen M, Revel M, Dougados M. Prolonged effects of 3 week therapy in a spa resort on lumbar spine, knee and hip osteoarthritis: follow-up after 6 months. A randomized controlled trial. *Br J Rheumatol.* 1997;36(1):77-81.

19. Becker BE, Hildenbrand K, Whitcomb RK, Sanders JP. Biophysiologic effects of warm water immersion. *Int J Aquatic Res Educ.* 2009;3(1):24-37.

20. Van Tubergen A, Boonen A, R. L., et al. Cost effectiveness of combined spa-exercise therapy in ankylosing spondylitis: a randomized controlled trial. *Arthritis Rheum.* 2002;47(5):459-467.

21. Cuesta-Vargas A, Garcia-Romero JC, Arroyo-Morales M, Diego-Acosta AM, Daly DJ. Exercise, manual therapy, and education with and without high-intensity deep-water running for nonspecific low back pain. *Am J Phys Med Rehabil.* 2011;90(7):526-539.

22. Koury JM. *Aquatic Therapy Programming.* Human Kinetics; 1996.

23. Killgore GL, Coste SC, O'Meara SE, Konnecke CJ. A comparison of the physiological exercise intensity differences between shod and barefoot submaximal deep-water running at the same cadence. *J Strength Cond Res.* 2010;24(12):3302-3312.

Chapter 11

1. Simmonds N, Miller P, Gemmell H. A theoretical framework for the role of fascia in manual therapy. *J Bodyw Mov Ther.* 2010;16(1):83-93.

2. Bialosky JE, Bishop MD, Price DD, Robinson ME, George SZ. The mechanisms of manual therapy in the treatment of musculoskeletal pain: A comprehensive model. *Man Ther.* 2009;14(5):531-538.

3. Mischke JJ, Jayaseelan DJ, Sault JD, Emerson AJ. The symptomatic and functional effects of manual physical therapy on plantar heel pain: a systematic review. *J Man Manip Ther.* 2017;25(1):3-10. doi:10.1080/10669817.2015.1106818.

4. Giammatteo SW, Kain JB. *Integrative Manual Therapy for the Connective Tissue System.* vol IV. North Atlantic Books; 2005:212.

5. Sillevis R, Cleland J, Hellman M, Beekhuizen K. Immediate effects of a thoracic spine thrust manipulation on the autonomic nervous system: a randomized clinical trial. *J Man Manip Ther.* 2010;18(4):181-190.

6. Beard G, Wood EC. *Massage. Principles and Techniques.* W.B. Saunders; 1964.

7. Furlan AD, Giraldo M, Baskwill A, Irvin E, Imamura M. Massage for low-back pain. *Cochran Database Syst Rev.* 2015;(9):CD001929. doi:10.1002/14651858.CD001929.pub3

8. Furlan AD, Imamura M, Dryden T, Irvin E. Massage for low-back pain. *Cochran Database Syst Rev.* 2008;8(4):CD001929. doi:10.1002/14651858.CD001929.pub2

9. Miake-Lye IM, Mak S, Lee J, et al. Massage for pain: an evidence map. *JACM.* 2019;25:475-502.

10. Weerapong P, Hume PA, Kolt GS. The mechanisms of massage and effects on performance, muscle recovery and injury prevention. *Sports Med.* 2005;35(3):235-256.

11. Loew LM, Brosseau L, Tugwell P, et al. Deep transverse friction massage for treating lateral elbow or lateral knee tendinitis. *Cochrane Database Syst Rev.* November 8 2014;2014(11):CD003528. doi:10.1002/14651858.CD003528.pub2

12. Wiktorsson-Moller M, Öberg B, Ekstrand J, Gillquist J. Effects of warming up, massage, and stretching on range of motion and muscle strength in the lower extremity. *Am J Sports Med.* 1983;11(4):249-252. doi:10.1177/036354658301100412

13. Nordschow M, Bierman W. The influence of manual massage on muscle relaxation: effect on trunk flexion. *J Am Phys Ther Assoc.* Oct 1962;42:653-7. doi:10.1093/ptj/42.10.653

14. McNair PJ, Stanley SN. Effect of passive stretching and jogging on the series elastic muscle stiffness and range of motion of the ankle joint. *Br J Sports Med.* December 1996;30(4):313-317. doi:10.1136/bjsm.30.4.313

15. Dubrosky V. Changes in muscle and venous blood flow after massage. *Soviet Sports Rev.* 1982;4:56-7.

16. Hovind H, Nielsen SL. Effect of massage on blood flow in skeletal muscle. *Scand J Rehabil Med.* 1974;6(2):74-7.

17. Kim SM, Kim S-R, Lee YK, Kim BR, Han EY. The effect of mechanical massage on early outcome after total knee arthroplasty: a pilot study. *Journal of Physical Therapy Science.* 2015;27(11):3413-3416. doi:10.1589/jpts.27.3413

18. Hernandez-Reif M, Field T, Krasnegor J, Theakston H. Lower back pain is reduced and range of motion increased after massage therapy. *Int J Neurosci.* 2001;106(3-4):131-45. doi:10.3109/00207450109149744

19. Lee HM, Wu SK, You JY. Quantitative application of transverse friction massage and its neurological effects on flexor carpi radialis. *Man Ther.* Oct 2009;14(5):501-7. doi:10.1016/j.math.2008.09.005

20. Kaada B, Torsteinbø O. Increase of plasma beta-endorphins in connective tissue massage. *Gen Pharmacol.* 1989;20(4):487-9. doi:10.1016/0306-3623(89)90200-0

21. Mori H, Ohsawa H, Tanaka TH, Taniwaki E, Leisman G, Nishijo K. Effect of massage on blood flow and muscle fatigue following isometric lumbar exercise. *Med Sci Monit.* May 2004;10(5):CR173-CR178.

22. Drust B, Atkinson G, Gregson W, French D, Binningsley D. The effects of massage on intra muscular temperature in the vastus lateralis in humans. *Int J Sports Med.* 2003;24(06):395-399. doi:10.1055/s-2003-41182

23. Kunikata H, Watanabe K, Miyoshi M, Tanioka T. The effects measurement of hand massage by the autonomic activity and psychological indicators. *JMI.* 2012;59:206-212. doi:10.2152/jmi.59.206

24. Leivadi S, Hernandes-Reif M, Field T, et al. Massage therapy and relaxation effects on university dance students. *J Dance Med Sci.* 1999;3(3):108-112.

25. Noto Y, Kudo M, Hirota K. Back massage therapy promotes psychological relaxation and an increase in salivary chromogranin A release. *J Anesth.* 2010;24(6):955-8. doi:10.1007/s00540-010-1001-7

26. Zeitlin D, Keller SE, Shiflett SC, Schleifer SJ, Bartlett JA. Immunological effects of massage therapy during academic stress. *Psychosom Med.* 2000;62(1):83-4. doi:10.1097/00006842-200001000-00012

27. Braverman DL, Schulman RA. Massage techniques in rehabilitation medicine. *Phys Med Rehabil Clin N Am.* 1999;10(3):631-649.

28. Barnes MF. The basic science of myofascial release: morphologic changes in connective tissue. *J Bodyw Mov Ther.* 1997;66(1):66-71.

29. Bordoni B, Zanier E. Clinical and symptomatological reflections: the fascial system. *J Multidiscip Healthc.* 2014;4(7):401-411.

30. Adstrum S, Hedley G, Schleip R, Stecco C, Yucesoy CA. Defining the fascial system. *J Bodyw Mov Ther.* 2017;21(1):173-177.

31. Tozzi P. Selected fascial aspects of osteopathic practice. *J Bodyw Mov Ther.* 2012;16(4):503-519.

32. Zugel M, Maganaris CN, Wilke J, et al. Fascial tissue research in sports medicine: from molecules to tissue adaptation, injury and diagnostics: consensus statement. *Br J Sports Med.* 2018;52(23):1497-1497.

33. Leardini A, O'Connor DD. A model for lever-arm length calculation of the flexor and extensor muscles at the ankle. *Gait Posture.* 2002;15(3):220-229.

34. Viladot A, Lorenzo JC, Salazar J, Rodríguez A. The subtalar joint: embryology and morphology. *Foot Ankle.* 1984;5(2):54-66.

35. Schleip R. Fascial plasticity—a new neurobiological explanation: Part 1. *J Bodyw Mov Ther.* 2003;7(1):11-19.

36. Swathi, Nellithala GG, Athavale SA. Mid-foot retinaculum: an unrecognized entity. *Anat Cell Biol.* 2017;50(3):171-174.

37. LeBauer A, Brtalik R, Stowe K. The effect of myofascial release (MFR) on an adult with idiopathic scoliosis. *J Bodyw Mov Ther.* 2008;12(4):356-363.

38. Threlkeld AJ. The effects of manual therapy on connective tissue. *Phys Ther.* 1992;72(12):893-902.

39. Lelean P. The migratory fascia hypothesis. *J Bodyw Mov Ther.* 2009;13(4):304-310.

40. Mauntel TC, Clark MA, D.A. P. Effectiveness of myofascial release therapies on physical performance measurements: a systematic review. *Athl Train Sports Health Care.* 2014;6(4):189-196.

41. Klingler W, Veldres M, Hoppe K, et al. Clinical relevance of fascial tissue and dysfunctions. *Curr Pain Headache Rep.* 2014;18(8):439.

42. Schroeder AN, Best TM. Is self myofascial release an effective preexercise and recovery strategy? A literature review. *Curr Sports Med Rep.* 2015;14(3):200-208.

43. Martínez Rodríguez R, Galán del Río F. Mechanistic basis of manual therapy in myofascial injuries: Sono-elastographic evolution control. *J Bodyw Mov Ther.* 2013;17(2):221-234.

44. Laimi K, Makila A, Barlund E, et al. Effectiveness of myofascial release in treatment of chronic musculoskeletal pain: a systematic review. *Clin Rehabil.* 2018;32(4):440-450.

45. Giammatteo T, Giammatteo SW. *Integrative Manual Therapy for Biomechanics: Application of Muscle Energy and "Beyond" Technique, Vol. III.* North Atlantic Books; 2003:346.

46. Sahrmann SA. *Diagnosis and Treatment of Movement Impairment Syndromes.* Mosby; 2002.

47. Klinger W, Velders M, Hoppe K, Pedro M, Schleip R. Clinical relevance of fascial tissue and dysfunctions. *Curr Pain Headache Rep.* 2014;18(8):439.

48. Shah JP, Thaker N, Heimur J, Aredo JV, Sikdar S, Gerber L. Myofascial Trigger Points Then and Now: A Historical and Scientific Perspective. *PM & R.* 2015;7(7):746-761.

49. Hunter G. Specific soft tissue mobilization in the management of soft tissue dysfunction. *Man Ther.* 1998;3(1):2-11.

50. Borghuis J, Hof AL, Lemmink KA. The importance of sensory-motor control in providing core stability: Implications for measurement and training. *Sports Med.* 2008;38(11):893-916.

51. Schleip R, Müller DG. Training principles for fascial connective tissues: Scientific foundation and suggested practical applications. *J Bodyw Mov Ther.* 2013;17(1):103-115.

52. Millett PJ, Wickiewicz TL, Warren RF. Current concepts: Motion loss after ligament injuries to the knee: part II: prevention and treatment. *Am J Sports Med.* 2001;29(6):822-828.

53. Baker RT, Nasypany A, Seegmiller JG, Baker JG. Instrument-assisted soft tissue mobilization treatment for tissue extensibility dysfunction. *Int J Athl Ther Train.* 2013;18(5):16-21.

54. McPartland JM. Travell trigger points—molecular and osteopathic perspectives. *J Am Osteopath Assoc.* 2004;104(6):244-249.

55. Schleip R. Fascial plasticity—a new neurobiological explanation: Part 2. *J Bodyw Mov Ther.* 2003;7(2):104-116.

56. Sutton GS, Bartel MR. Soft-tissue mobilization techniques for the hand therapist. *J Hand Ther.* 1994;7(3):185-192.

57. Simons DG, Travell JG, Simons LS. *Myofascial Pain and Dysfunctions: The Trigger Point Manual, Vol. 1.* 2nd ed. Williams & Wilkins; 1999.

58. Bron C, Dommerholt JD. Etiology of myofascial trigger points. *Curr Pain Headache Rep.* 2012;16(5):439-444.

59. Lucas KR, Rich PA, Polus BI. How common are latent myofascial trigger points in the scapular positioning muscles? *J Musculoskelet Pain.* 2008;16(4):279-286.

60. Bron C, Dommerholt J, Stegenga B, Wensing M, Oostendorp RA. High prevalence of shoulder girdle muscles with myofascial trigger points in patients with shoulder pain. *BMC Musculoskelet Disord.* June 28 2011;12:139. doi:10.1186/1471-2474-12-139

61. Fernández-de-Las-Peñas C, Alonso-Blanco C, Cuadrado ML, Miangolarra JC, Barriga FJ, Pareja JA. Are manual therapies effective in reducing pain from tension-type headache? A systematic review. *Clin J Pain.* 2006;22(3):278-285.

62. Lucas KR, Rich PA, Polus BI. Muscle activation patterns in the scapular positioning muscles during loaded scapular plane elevation: the effects of latent myofascial trigger points. *Clin Biomech.* 2010;25(8):765-770.

63. Travell J. Myofascial trigger points: clinical view. In: Bonica JJ, Albe-Fessard D, eds. *Advances in Pain Research and Therapy: First World Conference on Pain.* Raven Press; 1975:919-926.

64. Simons DG. Myofascial trigger points: a need for understanding. *Arch Phys Med Rehabil.* 1981;62(3):97-99.

65. Travell JG, Simons DG. *Myofascial Pain and Dysfunction: The Trigger Point Manual, Vol. 1.* Williams and Wilkins; 1983.

66. Travell JG, Simons DG. *Myofascial Pain and Dysfunction: The Trigger Point Manual, Vol. 2.* Williams and Wilkins; 1992.

67. Travell JG, Simons DG, Simons LS. *Myofascial Pain and Dysfunction: The Trigger Point Manual, Vol. 1.* 2nd ed. Lippincott Williams & Wilkins; 1998.

68. Gerwin RD, Dommerholt J, Shah JP. An expansion of Simons' integrated hypothesis of trigger point formation. *Curr Pain Headache Rep.* 2004;8(6):468-475.

69. Gerwin RD, Cagnie B, Petrovic M, Van Dorpe J, Calders P, De Meulemeester K. Foci of segmentally contracted sarcomeres in trapezius muscle biopsy specimens in myalgic and nonmyalgic human subjects: Preliminary results. *Pain Med* 2020;0(0):1-9. doi:10.1093/pm/pnaa019.

70. Partanen JV, Ojala TA, Arokoski JP. Myofascial syndrome and pain: a neurophysiological approach. *Pathophysiology.* 2010;17(1):19-28.

71. Ge HY, Arendt-Nielsen L. Latent myofascial trigger points. *Curr Pain Headache Rep.* 2011;15(5):386-392.

72. Ge HY, Arendt-Nielsen L, Madeleine P. Accelerated muscle fatigability of latent myofascial trigger points in humans. *Pain Med.* 2012;13(7):957-964.

73. Gerwin RD. Myofascial pain syndromes in the upper extremity. *J Hand Ther.* 1997;10(2):130-136.

74. Mense S, Simons DG, Russell IJ. *Muscle Pain: Understanding Its Nature, Diagnosis, and Treatment.* Lippincott Williams & Wilkins; 2001.

75. Dommerholt J, Gerwin RD. A critical evaluation of Quintner et al: missing the point. *J Bodyw Mov Ther.* 2015;19(2):193-204.

76. Huguenin LK. Myofascial trigger points: the current evidence. *Phys Ther Sport.* 2004;5(1):2-12.

77. Bengtsson A, Henriksson KG, Larsson J. Reduced high-energy phosphate levels in the painful muscles of patients with primary fibromyalgia. *Arthritis Rheum.* 1986;29(7):817-821.

78. Gunn CC. Radiculopathic pain: diagnosis and treatment of segmental irritation or sensitization. *J Musculoskelet Pain.* 1997;5(4):119-134.

79. Quintner JL, Cohen ML. Referred pain of peripheral nerve origin: an alternative to the "myofascial pain" construct. *Clin J Pain.* 1994;10(3):243-251.

80. Henneman E. Relation between size of neurons and their susceptibility to discharge. *Science.* 1957;126(3287):1345-1347.

81. Shah JP, Gilliams EA. Uncovering the biochemical milieu of myofascial trigger points using in vivo microdialysis:

An application of muscle pain concepts to myofascial pain syndrome. *J Bodywork Movement Ther.* 2008;12(4):371-384.

82. Forsman M, Taoda K, Thorn S, Zhang Q. Motor-unit recruitment during long-term isometric and wrist motion contractions: a study concerning muscular pain development in computer operators. *Int J Industr Ergonomics.* 2002;30(4-5):237-250.

83. Treaster D, Marras WS, Burr D, Sheedy JE, Hart D. Myofascial trigger point development from visual and postural stressors during computer work. *J Electromyogr Kinesiol.* 2006;16(2):115-124.

84. Simons DG. New views of myofascial trigger points: etiology and diagnosis. *Arch Phys Med Rehabil.* 2008;89(1):157-159.

85. Hubbard DR, Berkoff GM. Myofascial trigger oints show spontaneous needle EMG activity. *Spine.* 1993;18(13):1803-1807.

86. Ballyns JJ, Turo D, Otto P, et al. Office-based elastographic technique for quantifying mechanical properties of skeletal muscle. *J Ultrasound Med.* 2012;31(8):1209-1219.

87. Kuan TS. Current studies on myofascial pain syndrome. *Curr Pain Headache Rep.* 2009;13(5):365-369.

88. Hocking MJ. Exploring the central modulation hypothesis: do ancient memory mechanisms underlie the pathophysiology of trigger points? *Curr Pain Headache Rep.* 2013;17(7):347.

89. Shah JP, Danoff JV, Desai JV, et al. Biochemicals associated with pain and inflammation are elevated in sites near to and remote from active myofascial trigger points. *Arch Phys Med Rehabil.* 2008;89(1):16-23.

90. Shah JP, Phillips TM, Danoff JV, Gerber LH. An in vivo microanalytical technique for measuring the local biochemical milieu of human skeletal muscle. *J Appl Physiol.* 2005;99(5):1977-1984.

91. Jafri MS. Mechanisms of myofascial pain. *Int Sch Res Notices.* 2014. doi:10.1155/2014/523924

92. De Mey K, Cagnie B, Van de Vekle A, Danneels LA, Coots AM. Trapezius muscle timing during selected shoulder rehabilitation exercises. *J Orthop Sports Phys Ther.* 2009;39(10):743-752.

93. Cruser d, Maurer D, Hensel K, Brown S, White KL, Stoll ST. A randomized, controlled trial of osteopathic manipulative treatment for acute low back pain in active duty military personnel. *J Man Manip Ther.* 2012;20(1):5-15.

94. de las Penas CF, Campo MS, Carnero JF, Page JCM. Manual therapies in myofascial trigger point treatment: a systematic review. *J Bodyw Mov Ther.* 2005;9(1):27-34.

95. Gerwin RD. Neurobiology of the myofascial trigger point. *Baillieres Clin Rheumatol.* 1994;8(4):747-762.

96. Shah JP, Danoff JV, Desai MJ, et al. Biochemicals associated with pain and inflammation are elevated in sites near to and remote from active myofascial trigger points. *Arch Phys Med Rehabil.* 2008;89(1):16-23.

97. Fernandez-de-Las-Penas C, Nijs J. Trigger point dry needling for the treatment of myofascial pain syndrome: Current perspectives within a pain neuroscience paradigm. *J Pain Res.* 2019;12:1899-1911.

98. Chaitow L. Contrasting views of myofascial pain. *J Bodyw Mov Ther.* 2015;19(2):191-192.

99. Rathbone A, Henry J, Kumbhare D. Comment on: A critical evaluation of the trigger point phenomenon. *Rheumatology (Oxford).* 2015;54(6):1126-1127.

100. Gerwin RD. The taut band and other mysteries of the trigger point: an examination of the mechanisms relevant to the development and maintenance of the trigger point. *J Musculoskelet Pain.* 2008;16(1-2):115-121.

101. Larsson R, Oberg A, Larsson SE. Changes of trapezius muscle blood flow and electromyography in chronic neck pain due to trapezius myalgia. *Pain.* 1999;79(1):45-50.

102. Kadi F, Waling K, Ahlgren C, et al. Pathological mechanisms implicated in localized female trapezius myalgia. *Pain.* 1998;78(3):191-196.

103. Walder RY, Rasmussen LA, Ranier JD, Light AR, Wemmie JA, Sluka KA. ASIC1 and ASIC3 play different roles in the development of hyperalgesia after inflammatory muscle injury. *J Pain.* 2010;11(3):210-218.

104. Simons DG, Hong CZ, Simons LS. Endplate potentials are common to midfiber myofacial trigger points. *Am J Phys Med Rehabil.* 2002;81(3):212-222.

105. Kuan TS, Hsieh YL, Chen SM, Chen JT, Yen WC, Hong CZ. The myofascial trigger point region: correlation between the degree of irritability and the prevalence of endplate noise. *Am J Phys Med Rehabil.* 2007;86(3):183-189.

106. Cerezo-Téllez E, Torres-Lancomba M, Mayoral-Del Moral O, Sánchez-Sánchez B, Dommerholt J, Gutiérrez-Ortega C. Prevalence of myofascial pain syndrome in chronic non-specific neck pain: a population-based cross-sectional descriptive study. *Pain Med.* 2016;17(12):2369-2377.

107. Salim SY, Dezaki K, Tsuneki H, Abdel-Zaher AO, Kimura I. Calcitonin gene-related peptide potentiates nicotinic acetylcholine receptor-operated slow Ca2+ mobilization at mouse muscle endplates. *Br J Pharmacol.* 1998;125(2):277-282.

108. Cyriax JH. *Texbook of Orthopaedic Medicine: Vol 2. Treatment by Manipulation, Massage and Injection.* Williams & Wilkins; 1977.

109. Behm DG, Blazevich AJ, Kay AD, McHugh M. Acute effects of muscle stretching on physical performance, range of motion, and injury in helathy active individuals: A systematic review. *Appl Physiol Nutr Metab.* 2016;41:1-11. doi.org/10.1139/apnm-2015-0235.

110. Melzack R. *The Puzzle of Pain.* Basic Books; 1973.

111. Castel JC. *Pain Management: Acupuncture and Transcutaneous Electrical Nerve Stimulation Techniques.* Pain Control Services; 1979.

112. Hanten WP, Olson SL, Butts NL, Nowicki AL. Effectiveness of a home program of ischemic pressure followed by sustained stretch for treatment of myofascial trigger points. *Phys Ther.* 2000;80(10):997-1003.

113. Kashyap R, Iqbal A, Alghadir AH. Controlled intervention to compare the efficacies of manual pressure release and the muscle energy technique for treating mechanical neck pain due to upper trapezius trigger points. *J Pain Res.* 2018;11:3151-3160.

114. Amjad F, Shahid HA, Batool S, Ahman A, Ahmed I. A comparison of transcutaneous electrical nerve stimulation and therapeutic ultrasound in treatment of myofascial trigger points. *KMUJ.* 2016;8(1):1-6.

115. Alvarez DJ, Rockwell PG. Trigger points: Diagnosis and management. *Am Fam Physician*. 2002;65(4):653-660.

116. Bell J. Massage therapy helps to increase range of motion, decrease pain and assist in healing a client with low back pain and sciatica symptoms. *J Bodyw Mov Ther*. 2008;12(3):281-289.

117. Lee CY, Kim EJ, Hwang DG, Jung MY, Cho HG. The effect of trigger point injections on pain in patients with advanced cancer. *Korean J Fam Med*. 2019;40(5):344-347.

118. Tough EA, White AR, Cummings TM, Richards SH, Campbell JL. Acupuncture and dry needling in the management of myofascial trigger point pain: A systematic review and meta-analysis of randomised controlled trials. *Eur J Pain*. 2009;13(1):3-10.

119. Baldry P. Management of myofascial trigger point pain. *Acupunct Med*. 2002;20(1):2-10.

120. Alghadir AH, Iqbal A, Anwer S, Iqbal ZA, Ahmed H. Efficacy of combination therapies on neck pain and muscle tenderness in male patients with upper trapezius active myofascial trigger points *Biomed Res Int*. 2020;2020. doi:10.1155/2020/9361405

121. Godges JJ, Mattson-Bell M, Thorpe D, Shah D. The immediate effects of soft tissue mobilization with proprioceptive neuromuscular facilitation on glenohumeral external rotation and overhead reach. *J Orthop Sports Phys Ther*. December 2003;33(12):713-718.

122. Lee JH, Park SJ, Na SS. The effect of proprioceptive neuromuscular facilitation therapy on pain and function. *J Phys Ther Sci*. 2013;25(6):713-716. doi:10.1589/jpts.25.713

123. Greenman PE. *Principles of Manual Medicine*. 4th ed. Lippincott Williams & Wilkins; 2011.

124. Chaitow L. *Muscle Energy Techniques*. 3rd ed. Churchill Livingstone Elsevier; 2006.

125. Chaitow L. *Muscle Energy Techniques*. 4th ed. Churchill Livingstone; 2013.

126. Mitchell FL. Structural pelvic function. *Yearbook of the American Academy of Osteopathy*. AAO; 1958.

127. Blazevich AJ, Kay AD, Waugh C, Fath F, Miller S, Cannavan D. Plantarflexor stretch training increases reciprocal inhibition measured during voluntary dorsiflexion. *J Neurophysiol*. 2012;107(1):250-256.

128. Hindle KB, Whitcomb TJ, Briggs WO, Junggi H. Proprioceptive neuromuscular facilitation (PNF): its mechanisms and effects on range of motion and muscular function. *J Hum Kinet*. 2012;31(1):105-113.

129. Farquharson C. MET versus PNF what, when and how. *SportEx Dynamics*. 2010;(25):12-16.

130. Campbell SM, Winkelmann RR, Walkowski S. Osteopathic manipulative treatment: Novel application to dermatological disease. *J Clin Aesthet Dermatol*. 2012;10:24-32.

131. Smith M, Fryer G. A comparison of two muscle energy techniques for increasing flexibility of the hamstring muscle group. *J Bodyw Mov Ther*. 2008;12(4):312-317.

132. Knott M, Voss DE. *Proprioceptive Neuromuscular Facilitation: Patterns and Techniques*. 2nd ed. Harper & Row; 1968.

133. Kim K, Jeon K. Development of an efficient rehabilitation exercise program for functional recovery in chronic ankle instability. *J Phys Ther Sci*. 2016;28(5):1443-1447.

134. Escamilla RF, Hooks TR, Wilk KE. Optimal management of shoulder impingement syndrome. *Open Access J Sports Med*. 2014;5:13-24.

135. Sady SP, Wortman M, Blanke D. Flexibility training: ballistic, static or proprioceptive neuromuscular facilitation? *Arch Phys Med Rehabil*. 1982;63(6):261-263.

136. Hoogenboom BJ, Voight ML, Cook G, Gill L. Using rolling to develop neuromuscular control and coordination of the core and extremities of athletes. *N Am J Sports Phys Ther*. 2009;4(2):70-82.

137. Voss DE, Ionta MK, Myers BJ. *Proprioceptive Neuromuscular Facilitation*. 3rd ed. Harper & Row; 1985.

138. Burke D, Gandevia SC. Interfering cutaneous stimulation and the muscle afferent contribution of cortical potentials. *Electroencephalogr Clin Neurophysiol*. 1988;70(2):118-125.

139. Johansson CA, Kent BE, Shepard KF. Relationship between verbal command volume and magnitude of muscle contraction. *Phys Ther*. 1983;63(8):1260-1265.

140. Farina D, Arendt-Nielsen L, Merletti R, Graven-Nielsen T. Effect of experimental muscle pain on motor unit firing rate and conduction velocity. *J Neurophysiol*. 2004;91(3):1250-1259.

141. Sanchez X, Bampouras TM. Augmented feedback over a short period of time: Does it improve netball goal-shooting performance? *Int J Sport Psychol*. 2006;37(4):349-358.

142. Sewall LP, Reeve TG, Day RA. Effect of concurrent visual feedback on acquisition of a weightlifting skill. *Percept Mot Skills*. 1988;67(3):715-718.

143. Svendsen DA, Malyas TA. Facilitation of the isometric maximum voluntary contraction with traction: A test of PNF predictions. *Am J Phys Med*. 1983;62(1):27-37.

144. Chalmers G. Re-examination of the possible role of Golgi tendon organ and muscle spindle reflexes in proprioceptive neuromuscular facilitation muscle stretching. *Sports Biomech*. 2004;3(1):159-183.

145. Sherrington CS. *The Integrative Action of the Nervous System*. Yale University Press; 1906:411.

146. Sharman MJ, Cresswell AG, Riek S. Proprioceptive neuromuscular facilitation stretching: mechanisms and clinical implications. *Sports Med*. 2006;36(11):929-939.

147. Spernoga SG, Uhl TL, Arnold BL, Gansneder BM. Duration of maintained hamstring flexibility after a one-time, modified hold-relax stretching protocol. *J Athl Train*. 2001;36(1):44-48.

148. Fox SA. Muscle mechanisms of contraction and neural control. *Human Physiol*. 9th ed. McGraw-Hill; 2006:338-379.

149. Prentice WE. Comparison of static stretching and PNF stretching for improving hip joint flexibility. *Athl Train*. 1983;18(1):56-59.

150. O'Hora J, Cartwright A, Wade CD, Hough AD, Shum GL. Efficacy of static stretching and proprioceptive neuromuscular facilitation stretch on hamstrings length after a single session. *J Strength Cond Res*. 2011;25(6):1586-1591.

151. Roopchand MS, Taylor T. A comparison of stretching on a PNF diagonal using hold-relax technique with single plane passive stretching for increased adductor flexibility. *Indian J Physiother Occup Ther*. 2014;8(2):53-57S.

152. Minshull C, Eston R, Bailey A, Rees D, Gleeson N. The differential effects of PNF versus passive stretch condi-

tioning on neuromuscular performance. *Eur J Sport Sci.* 2014;14(3):233-241.

153. Decoster LC, Cleland J, Altieri C, Russell P. The effects of hamstring stretching on range of motion: a systematic literature review. *J Orthop Sports Phys Ther.* 2005;35(6):377-387.

154. Wallmann HW, Christensen SD, Perry C, Hoover DL. The acute effects of various types of stretching static, dynamic, ballistic, and no stretch of the iliopsoas on 40-yard sprint times in recreational runners. *Int J Sports Phys Ther.* 2012;7(5):540-547.

155. Mahieu NN, McNair P, De Muynck M, et al. Effect of static and ballistic stretching on the muscle-tendon tissue properties. *Med Sci Sports Exerc.* 2007;39(3):494-501.

156. O'Sullivan K, Murray E, Sainsbury D. The effect of warm-up, static stretching and dynamic stretching on hamstring flexibility in previously injured subjects. *BMC Musculoskelet Disord.* 2009;10:37. doi:10.1186/1471-2474-10-37

157. Kakuda N, Nagaoka M. Dynamic response of human muscle spindle afferents to stretch during volunatry contraction. *J Physiol.* 1998;513(2):621-628.

158. Burke DG, Pelham TW, Holt LE. The influence of varied resistance and speed of concentric antagonistic contractions on subsequent concentric agonistic efforts. *J Strength Cond Res.* 1999;13(3):193-197.

159. Rixon KP, Lamont HS, Bemben MG. Influence of type of muscle contraction, gender, and lifting experience on postactivation potentiation performance. *J Strength Cond Res.* 2007;21(2):500-505.

160. McPartland JM, Goodridge JP. Counterstrain and traditional osteopathic examination of the cervical spine compared. *J Bodyw Mov Ther.* 1997;1(3):173-178.

161. Jones LH. Spontaneous release by positioning. *DO.* 1964;4:109-116.

162. Lewis CL, Flynn TW. The use of strain-counterstrain in the treatment of patients with low back pain. *J Manip Physiol Ther.* 2001;9(2):92-98.

163. DiGiovanna EL. Counterstrain. In: DiGiovanna EL, Schiowitz S, Dowling DJ, eds. *An Osteopathic Approach to Diagnosis and Treatment.* 3rd ed. Lippincott Williams & Wilkins; 2005:86-88.

164. Meseguer AA, Fernández-de-las-Peñas C, Navarro-Poza JL, Rodríguez-Blanco C, Gandia JJB. Immediate effects of the strain/counterstrain technique in local pain evoked by tender points in the upper trapezius muscle. *Clin Chiropract.* 2006;9(3):112-118.

165. D'Ambrogio KJ, Roth GB. *Positional Release Therapy: Assessment & Treatment of Musculoskeletal Dysfunction.* Mosby; 1997.

166. Hong CZ. Myofascial trigger points: pathophysiology and correlation with acupuncture points. *Acupunct Med.* 2000;18(1):41-47.

167. Jones LH. *Strain and Counterstrain.* American Academy of Osteopathy; 1981.

168. Jones LH, Kusunose RS, Goering EK. *Jones Strain-Counterstrain.* Jones Strain-Counterstrain Inc.; 1995.

169. Stone JA. Prevention and rehabilitation: strain–counterstrain. *Athl Ther Today.* 2000;5(6):30-31.

170. Wong CK, Schauer C. Reliability, validity and effectiveness of strain counterstrain techniques. *J Man Manip Ther.* 2004;12(2):107-112.

171. Wong CK, Abraham T, Karimi P, Ow-Wing C. Strain counterstrain technique to decrease tender point palpation pain compared to control conditions: A systematic review with meta-analysis. *J Bodyw Mov Ther.* 2013;18(2):165-173.

172. Smith J. *Structural Bodywork.* Elsevier; 2005.

173. Bernau-Eigen M. Rolfing: a somatic approach to the integration of human structures. *Nurse Practioner Forum.* 1998;9(4):235-242.

174. Myers TW. Structural integration: Developments in Ida Rolf's "recipe"—Part 2. *J Bodyw Mov Ther.* 2004;8(3):189-198.

175. James H, Castandea L, Miller ME, Findley T. Rolfing structural integration treatment of cervical spine dysfunction. *J Bodyw Mov Ther.* 2009;13(3):229-238.

176. Myers TW. Structural integration: Developments in Ida Rolf's "recipe"—Part I. *J Bodyw Mov Ther.* 2004;8(2):131-142.

177. Molinary R. A new word for relief. *Health.* 2006;20(7):88-89.

178. Cheatham SW, Lee M, Cain M, Baker R. The efficacy of instrument assisted soft tissue mobilization: a systematic review. *J Can Chiropr Assoc.* 2016;60(3):200-211.

179. Kim J, Sung DJ, Lee J. Therapeutic effectiveness of instrument-assisted soft tissue mobilization for soft tissue injury: Mechanisms and practical application. *J Exerc Rehabil.* 2017;13(1):12-22.

180. Stow R. Instrument-assisted soft tissue mobilization. *Int J Athl Ther Train.* 2011;16(3):5-8.

181. Chen T, Liu N, Liu J, et al. Gua Sha, a press-stroke treatment of the skin, boosts the immune system response to intradermal vaccination. *Peer J.* 2016. doi:10.7717/peerj.2451

182. Lauche R, Wübbeling K, Lüdtke R, et al. Randomized controlled pilot study: pain intensity and pressure pain thresholds in patients with neck and low back pain before and after traditional East Asian "gua sha" therapy. *Am J Chin Med.* 2012;40(5):905-917.

183. Ikeda N, Otsuka S, Kawanishi Y, Kawakami Y. Effects of instrument-assisted soft tissue mobilization on musculoskeletal properties. *Med Sci Sports Exer.* 2019;15(10):2166-2172.

184. Seffrin CB, Cattano NM, Reed MA, Gardiner-Shires AM. Instrument-assisted soft tissue mobilization: A systematic review and effect-size analysis. *J Athl Train.* 2019;54(7):808-821.

185. Gauglitz GG, Korting HC, Pavicic T, Ruzicka T, Jeschke MG. Hypertrophic scarring and keloids: pathomechanics and current emerging treatment strategies. *Mol Med.* 2011;17:113-125.

186. Davidson CJ, Ganion LR, Gehlsen GM, Verhoestra B, Roepke JE, Sevier TL. Rat tendon morphologic and functional changes resulting from soft tissue mobilization. *Med Sci Sports Exerc.* 1997;29(3):313-319.

187. Hammer WI. The effect of mechanical load on degenerated soft tissue. *J Bodyw Mov Ther.* 2008;12(3):246-256.

188. Loghmani MT, Warden SJ. Instrumented-assisted soft tissue mobilization in healthy young adult males mobilizes tissue-resident mesenchymal stem cells into circulation. *J Ortho Sport Phys Ther.* 2013;46:107.

189. Heinecke ML, Thuesen ST, Stow RC. Graston technique on shoulder motion in overhead athletes. *J Undergrad Kinesiol Res.* 2014;10:27-39.

190. Schleip R. Fascial mechanoreceptors and their potential role in deep tissue manipulation. *J Bodyw Mov Ther.* 2003;7:104-116.

191. G. M. Acute effects of instrument assisted soft tissue mobilization vs. foam rolling on knee and hip range of motion in soccer players. *J Bodyw Mov Ther.* 2015;(19):690-696.

192. Daniels CJ, Morrell AP. Chiropractic management of pediatric plantar fasciitis: a case report. *J Chiropr Med.* 2012;11:58-63.

193. Howitt S, Wong J, Zabukovec S. The conservative treatment of trigger thumb using Graston techniques and active release techniques. *J Can Chiropr Assoc.* 2006;50:249-254.

194. Lee JH, Lee DK, Oh JS. The effect of Graston technique on the pain and range of motion in patients with chronic low back pain. *J Phys Ther Sci.* 2016;28:1852-1855.

195. McCormack JR, Underwood FB, Slaven EJ, Cappaert TA. Eccentric exercise versus eccentric exercise and soft tissue treatment (Astym) in the management of insertional Achilles tendinopathy. *Sports Health.* 2016;8(3):230-237.

196. Crothers AL, French SD, Hebert JJ, Walker BF. Spinal manipulative therapy, Graston technique^R and placebo for non-specific thoracic spine pain: A randomised controlled trial. *Chiropr Man Therap.* 2016;24:16.

197. Sevier TL, Stegink-Jansen CW. Astym treatment vs. eccentric exercise for lateral elbow tendinopathy: A randomized controlled clinical trial. *PeerJ.* 2015;3:e967.

198. Black DW. The treatment of knee arthrofibrosis and quadriceps insufficiency after patellar tendon repair: A case report including use of graston technique. *Int J Ther Massage Bodywork.* 2010;3:14-21.

199. McConnell J, Cruser S, Warden SJ, Bayliss AJ. Instrument-assisted soft tissue mobilization alters material and mechanical properties in Achilles tendinopathy. *J Ortho Sport Phys Ther.* 2016;46:114.

200. Papa JA. Conservative management of Achilles tendinopathy: a case report. *J Can Chiropr Assoc.* 2012;56:216-224.

201. Miners AL, Bougie TL. Chronic Achilles tendinopathy: a case study of treatment incorporating active and passive tissue warm-up, Graston Technique®, ART®, eccentric exercise, and cryotherapy. *J Can Chiropr Assoc.* 2011;55(4):269-279.

202. Graston Technique website. Accessed June 11, 2020. https://grastontechnique.com

203. RockTape. RockBlades. Accessed June 11, 2020. www.rocktape.com/2016/08/01/rockblades-the-latest-in-iastm-tools-evidence-informed-methodology

204. The FIT Institute. Accessed June 11, 2020. www.thefitinstitute.com/therapies/soft-tissue-therapy/fascial-abrasion-technique

205. ASTYM website. Accessed June 11, 2020. https://astym.com

206. Abbott JH, Robertson MC, Chapple C, et al. Manual therapy, exercise therapy, or both, in addition to usual care, for osteoarthritis of the hip or knee: a randomized controlled trial. 1: clinical effectiveness. *Osteoarthritis Cartilage.* Apr 2013;21(4):525-34. doi:10.1016/j.joca.2012.12.014

207. Maitland GD. *Peripheral Manipulation.* Butterworth-Heinemann; 1991.

208. Kaltenborn FM. *Manual Mobilization of the Joints: The Kaltenborn Method of Joint Examination and Treatment.* 6th ed. Olaf N Orlis Bokhandel; 2002.

209. Mennell JM. *Joint Pain: Diagnosis and Treatment Using Manipulative Techniques.* Little, Brown & Co; 1964.

210. Paris SV, Patla CE. *E1 Course Notes: Extremity Dysfunction and Manipulation.* Patris; 1988.

211. International Federation of Orthopaedic Manipulative Physical Therapists (IFOMPT). *Educational Standards in Orthopaedic Manipulative Therapy.* 2016. www.ifompt.org/site/ifompt/IFOMPT%20Standards%20Document%20definitive%202016.pdf

212. Bronfort G, Haas M, Evans R, Leininger B, Triano J. Effectiveness of manual therapies: the UK evidence report. *Chiropr Osteopat.* 2010;18:3. doi:10.1186/1746-1340-18-3

213. Flynn TW, Wainner RS, Fritz JM. Spinal manipulation in physical therapist professional degree education: a model for teaching and integration into clinical practice. *J Orthop Sports Phys Ther.* 2006;36:577-587.

214. Johnson KD, Grindstaff TL. Thoracic region self-mobilization: a clinical suggestion. *Int J Sports Phys Ther.* 2012;7(2):252-256.

215. Aoyagi K, Heller D, Hazelwood D, Sharma N, dos Santos M. Is spinal mobilization effective for low back pain? A systematic review. *Complement Ther Clin Pract.* 2019;34:51-63.

216. Lee KS, Lee JH. Effect of Maitland mobilization in cervical and thoracic spine and therapeutic exercise on functional impairment in individuals with chronic neck pain. *J Phys Ther Sci.* 2017;29(3):531-535.

217. Kitaoka HB, Luo ZP, An K. Three-dimensional analysis of normal ankle and foot mobility. *Am J Sports Med.* 1997;25(2):238-242.

218. Konradsen L, Holmer P, Sondergaard L. Early mobilizing treatment for grade III ankle ligament injuries. *Foot Ankle.* 1991;12(2):69-73.

219. van der Wees PJ, Lenssen AF, Hendriks EJ, Stomp DJ, Dekker J, de Bie RA. Effectiveness of exercise therapy and manual mobilisation in ankle sprain and functional instability: a systematic review. *Aust J Physiother.* 2006;52(1):27-37.

220. Weerasekara I, Osmotherly P, Snodgrass S, Marquez J, de Zoete R, Rivett DA. Clinical benefits of joint mobilization on ankle sprains: a systematic review and meta-analysis. *Arch Phys Med.* 2018;99:1395-1412.

221. Jayaseelan DJ, Scalzitti DA, Palmer G, Immerman A, Courtney CA. The effects of joint mobilization on individuals with patellofemoral pain: a systematic review. *Clin Rehabil.* 2018;32(6):722-733.

222. Kosik KB, Gribble PA. The effect of joint mobilization on dynamic postural control in patients with chronic ankle instability: a critically appraised topic *J Sport Rehabil.* 2018;27:103-108.

223. Johnson AJ, Godges JJ, Zimmerman GJ, Ounanian LL. The effect of anterior versus posterior glide joint mobilization on external rotation range of motion in patients with shoulder adhesive capsulitis. *J Orthop Sports Phys Ther.* 2007;37(3):88-99.

224. Manske RC, Meschke M, Porter A, Smith B, Reiman M. A randomized controlled single-blinded comparison of

stretching versus stretching and joint mobilization for posterior shoulder tightness measured by internal rotation motion loss. *Sports Health.* 2010;2(1):94-100.

225. Talbott N, Witt D. Can the mechanical effects of manual mobilization of the glenohumeral joint be reproduced during self mobilization techniques? *J Hand Ther.* 2018;31(1):143. doi:10.1016/j.jht.2017.11.004

226. Heiser RD, O'Brien V, Schwartz DA. Joint mobilization in the distal upper extremity—putting evidence into practice. *J Hand Ther.* 2014;27(3):e5. doi:10.1016/j.jht.2013.08.011

227. Aguirrebena LL, Newham D, Critchley DJ. Mechanism of action of spinal mobilizations: A systematic review. *Spine.* 2016;41(2):159-172.

228. Vicenzino B, Collilns D, Benson H, Wright A. An investigation of the interrelationship between manipulative therapy-induced hypoalgesia and sympathoexcitation. *J Manipulative Physiol Ther.* 1998;21(7):448-453.

229. Villafañe JH, Silva GB, Chiarotto A. Effects of passive upper extremity joint mobilization on pain sensitivity and function in participants with secondary carpometacarpal osteoarthritis: a case series. *J Manipulative Physiol Ther.* 2012;35(9):735-742.

230. Courtney CA, Steffen AD, Fernández-de-Las-Peñas C, Kim J, Chmell SJ. Joint mobilization enhances mechanisms of conditioned pain modulation in individuals with osteoarthritis of the knee. *J Orthop Sports Phys Ther.* 2016;46(3):168-176.

231. Brander V, Stulberg SD. Rehabilitation after hip- and knee-joint replacement. An experience- and evidence-based approach to care. *Am J Phys Med Rehabil.* 2006;85(11 Suppl):S98-S188.

232. Courtney CA, Witte PO, Chmell SJ, Hornby TG. Heightened flexor withdrawal response in individuals with knee osteoarthritis is modulated by joint compression and joint mobilization. *J Pain.* 2010;11(2):179-185.

233. Chimenti RL, Frey-Law LA, Sluka KA. A mechanism-based approach to physical therapist management of pain. *Phys Ther* 2018;98(5):302-314.

234. Lundborg G, Holm S, Myrhage R. The role of the synovial fluid and tendon sheath for flexor tendon nutrition: An experimental tracer study on diffusional pathways in dogs. *Scand J Plast Reconstr Surg.* 1980;14(1):99-107.

235. Horrell BM, Vogel LD, Israel HA. Passive motion therapy in temporomandibular joint disorders: the use of a new hydraulic device and case reports. *Compend Contin Educ Dent.* 1997;18(1):73-76, 78, 80.

236. Yoder E. Physical therapy management of nonsurgical hip problems in adults. In: Echternach JL, ed. *Physical Therapy of the Hip.* Churchill Livingstone; 1990:221.

237. Talbott N, Witt D. In-vivo MCP movement during a distraction mobilization of the MCP joint: a quantitative study with qualitative assessment of fluid movement. *J Hand Ther.* 2018;31(1):146-147. doi:10.1016.j.jht.2017.11.009

238. Michlovitz SL, Harris BA, Watkins MP. Therapy interventions for improving joint range of motion: A systematic review. *J Hand Ther.* 2004;17(2):118-131.

239. Wyke B. The neurology of joints. *Ann R Coll Surg Engl.* 1967;41(1):25-50.

240. Unsworth A, Dowson D, Wright V. "Cracking joints": A bioengineering study of cavitation in the metacarpophalangeal joint. *Ann Rheum Dis.* 1971;30(4):348-358.

241. Brodeur R. The audible release associated with joint manipulation. *J Manipulative Physiol Ther.* 1995;18(3):155-164.

242. Corrigan B, Maitland GD. *Practical Orthopedic Medicine.* Butterworth; 1989.

243. Bereznick DE, Pecora CG, Ross CG, McGill SM. The refractory period of the audible "crack" after lumbar manipulation: a preliminary study. *J Manip Physiol Ther.* 2008;31(3):199-203.

244. Cramer GD, Ross K, Raju PK, et al. Quantification of cavitation and gapping of lumbar zygapophyseal joints during spinal manipulative therapy. *J Manip Physiol Ther.* 2012;35(8):614-621.

245. Homola S. *The Chiropractor's Self-Help Back and Body Book.* Hunter House; 2002.

246. Lin HT, Hsu AT, Chang GL, Chang Chien JR, An KN, Su FC. Determining the resting position of the glenohumeral joint in subjects who are healthy. *Phys Ther.* 2007;87(12):1669-1682.

247. Exelby L. The Mulligan concept: its application in the management of spinal conditions. *Man Ther.* 2002;7(2):64-70.

248. Alkady SM, Kamel RM, Taleb EA, Lasheen Y, Alshaarawy FA. Efficacy of Mulligan mobilization versus muscle energy technique in chronic sacrouliac joint dysfunction. *Int J Physiother.* 2017;4(5):311-318.

249. May J, Krzyzanowicz R, Nasypany A, Baker R, Seegmiller J. Mulligan concept use and clinical profile from the perspective of American certified Mulligan practitioners. *J Sport Rehabil.* 2015;24:337-341.

250. Buyukturan O, Buyukturan B, Sas S, Kararti C, Ceylan I. The effect of Mulligan mobilization technique in older adults with neck pain: a randomized controlled, double-blind study. *Pain Res Manag.* 2018;2018. doi:10.1155/2018/2856375

251. Stathopoulos N, Dimitriadis Z, Koumantakis GA. Effectiveness of Mulligan's mobilization with movement techniques on pain and disability of peripheral joints: a systematic review with meta-analysis between 2008-2017. *Physiother* 2019;105:doi:10.101016/j.physio.2018.10.001.

252. Konstantinou K, Foster N, Rushton A, Baxter D. The use and reported effects of mobilization with movement techniques in low back pain management: A cross-sectional descriptive survey of physiotherapists in Britain. *Man Ther.* 2002;7(4):205-214.

253. Mulligan BR. *Manual Therapy "NAGS", "SNAGS", "MWM'S".* 6th ed. Plane View Services; 2010.

254. Horton SJ. Acute locked thoracic spine: Treatment with a modified SNAG. *Man Ther.* 2002;7(2):103-107.

255. Mulligan BR. Mobilisations with movement (MWM'S). *J Man Manip Ther.* 1993;1(4):154-156.

256. Vernon H, Mrozek J. A revised definition of manipulation. *J Manip Physiol Ther.* 2005;28(1):68-72.

257. Bialosky JE, George SZ, Horn ME, et al. Spinal manipulative therapy-specific changes in pain sensitivity in individuals with low back pain. *J Pain* 2014;15(2):136-148.

258. Bronfort G, Evans R, Anderson AV, et al. Spinal manipulation, medication, or home exercise with advice for acute and subacute neck pain: A randomized trial. *Ann Intern Med.* 2012;156:1-10.

259. Goertz CM, Long CR, Vining RD, et al. Effect of usual medical care plus chiropractic care vs usual medical care alone on pain and disability among US service members with low back pain: a comparative effectiveness clinical trial. *JAMA Netw Open.* 2018;1(1):e180105.

260. Lewis RA, Williams NH, Sutton AJ, et al. Comparative clinical effectiveness of management strategies for sciatica: systematic review and network meta-analyses. *Spine Journal.* 2015;15(6):1461-1477.

261. Pickar J. Neurophysiological effects of spinal manipulation. *Spine Journal.* 2002;2(5):357-371.

262. Masaracchio M, Kirker K, States R, Hanney WJ, Liu X, Kolber M. Thoracic spine manipulation for the management of mechanical neck pain: A systematic review and meta-analysis. *PLoS ONE.* 2019;14(2):1-28. doi:10.1371/journal.pone.0211877

263. Nilsson N, Christensen H, Hartvigen J. Lasting changes in passive range of motion after spinal manipulation: a randomized, blind, controlled trial. *J Manipulative Physiol Ther.* 1996;19(3):165-168.

264. Goertz CM, Pohlman KA, Vining RD, Brantingham JW, Long CR. Patient-centered outcomes of high-velocity, low-amplitude spinal manipulation for low back pain: A systematic review. *Journal of Electromyography and Kinesiology.* 2012;22(5):670-691. doi:10.1016/j.jelekin.2012.03.006

265. Coulter ID, Crawford C, Hurwitz EL, et al. Manipulation and mobilization for treating chronic low back pain: a systematic review and meta-analysis. *The Spine Journal.* 2018;18(5):866-879. doi:10.1016/j.spinee.2018.01.013

266. Brenner AK, Gill NW, Buscema CJ, Kiesel K. Improved activation of lumbar multifidus following spinal manipulation: a case report applying rehabilitative ultrasound imaging. *Journal of Orthopaedic & Sports Physical Therapy.* 2007;37(10):613-619. doi:10.2519/jospt.2007.2470

267. Sterling M, Jull G, Wright A. Cervical mobilisation: concurrent effects on pain, sympathetic nervous system activity and motor activity. *Manual Therapy.* 2001;6(2):72-81. doi:10.1054/math.2000.0378

268. Flynn TW, Fritz JM, Whitman J, et al. A clinical prediction rule for classifying patients with low back pain who demonstrate short-term improvement with spinal manipulation. *Spine.* 2002;27(24):2835-2843.

269. Childs JD, Fritz JM, Flynn TW, et al. A clinical prediction rule to identify patients with low back pain most likely to benefit from spinal manipulation: a validation study. *Ann Intern Med.* 2004;141(12):920-930.

270. Cleland JA, Fritz JM, Kulig K, et al. Comparison of the effectiveness of three manual physical therapy techniques in a subgroup of patients with low back pain who satisfy a clinical predication rule. *Spine.* 2009;34(25):2720-2729.

271. Ross JK, Bereznick DE, McGill SM. Determining cavitation location during lumbar and thoracic spinal manipulation: is spinal manipulation accurate and specific? *Spine (Phila Pa 1976).* Jul 1 2004;29(13):1452-1457. doi:10.1097/01.brs.0000129024.95630.57

272. DeLitto A, George SZ, Van Dillen LR, et al. Low back pain: clinical practice guidelines. *J Orthop Sports Phys Ther.* 2012;42(4):A1-A57.

273. Fernández-de-las-Peñas C, Palomeque-del-Cerro L, Rodríguez-Blanco C, Gómez-Conesa A, Miangolarra-Page JC. Changes in neck pain and active range of motion after a single thoracic spine manipulation in subjects presenting with mechanical neck pain: a case series. *J Manipulative Physiol Ther.* May 2007;30(4):312-20. doi:10.1016/j.jmpt.2007.03.007

274. Karas S, Olson Hunt MJ, Temes B, Thiel M, Swoverland T, Windsor B. The effect of direction specific thoracic spine manipulation on the cervical spine: a randomized controlled trial. *J Man Manip Ther.* 2018;26(1):3-10. doi:10.1080/10669817.2016.1260674

275. Glaser J, Green K, Lindskog A, Nichols A, Peters C. The effectiveness of thoracic spine manipulation therapy on shoulder pain, range of motion, and muscle strength. *Proceedings: 14th Annual Symposium on Graduate Research and Scholarly Projects.* Wichita State University; 2018:14.

276. Fischer LR, Alvar BA, Maher SF, Cleland JA. Short-term effects of thoracic spine thrust manipulation, exercise, and education in individuals with low back pain: a randomized controlled trial *J Ortho Sport Phys Ther.* 2019;50(1):24-32.

277. Masaracchio M, Kirker K, States R, Hanney WJ, Liu X, Kolber M. Thoracic spine manipulation for the management of mechanical neck pain: A systematic review and meta-analysis. *PLoS ONE.* 2019;14(2)doi:10.1371/journal.pone.0211877

278. Cleland JA, Glynn P, Whitman JM, Eberhart SL, MacDonald C, Childs JD. Short-term effects of thrust versus nonthrust mobilization/manipulation directed at the thoracic spine in patients with neck pain: a randomized clinical trial. *Phys Ther.* 2007;87(4):431-440. doi:10.2522/ptj.20060217

279. Cleland JA, Childs JD, Fritz JM, Whitman JM, Eberhart SL. Development of a clinical prediction rule for guiding treatment of a subgroup of patients with neck pain: use of thoracic spine manipulation, exercise, and patient education. *Physical Therapy.* 2007;87(1):9-23. doi:10.2522/ptj.20060155

280. Cleland JA, Mintken PE, Carpenter K, et al. Examination of a clinical prediction rule to identify patients with neck pain likely to benefit from thoracic spine thrust manipulation and a general cervical range of motion exercise: multi-center randomized clinical trial. *Phys Ther.* 2010;90(9):1239-1250. doi:10.2522/ptj.20100123

281. Puentedura EJ, O'Grady WH. Safety of thrust joint manipulation in the thoracic spine: a systematic review. *J Man Manip Ther.* 2015;23(3):154-161.

282. Gibbons P, Tehan P. *Manipulation of the Spine, Thorax and Pelvis.* Elsevier; 2016.

283. Young YH, Chen CH. Acute vertigo following cervical manipulation. *Laryngoscope.* 2003;113(4):659-662.

284. Senstad O, Leboeuf-Yde C, Borchgrevink C. Frequency and characteristics of side effects of spinal manipulative therapy. *Spine.* 1997;22(4):435-440.

285. Haynes MJ, Vincent K, Fischhoff C, et al. Assessing the risk of stroke from neck manipulation: a systematic review. *Int J Clin Pract.* 2012;66(10):940-947.

286. Hebert JJ, Stomski NJ, French SD, et al. Serious adverse events and spinal manipulative therapy of the low back region: A systematic review of cases. *J Manipulative Physiol Ther.* 2015;38(9):677-691.

287. Oliphant D. Safety of spinal manipulation in the treatment of lumbar disk herniations: A systematic review

and risk assessment. *J Manipulative Physiol Ther.* 2004;27(3):197-210.

288. Paanalahti K, Holm LW, Nordin M, et al. Adverse events after manual therapy among patients seeking care for neck and/or back pain: A randomized controlled trial. *BMC Musculoskelet Disord.* 2014;15:77.

289. Evans DW, Breen AC. A biomechanical model for mechanically efficient cavitation production during spinal manipulation: Prethrust positon and the neutral zone. *J Manipulative Physiol Ther.* 2006;29(1):72-82.

290. Blakeslee TJ, Morriss JL. Cuboid syndrome and the significance of midtarsal joint stability. *J Am Podiatr Med Assoc.* 1987;77(12):638-642.

291. Baravarian B. Diagnostic dilemmas: a guide to understanding and treating lateral column pain. *Podiatry Today.* 2005;18(3):100-105.

292. Marshall P, Hamilton WG. Cuboid subluxation in ballet dancers. *Am J Sports Med.* 1992;20(2):169-175.

293. Jennings J, Davies GJ. Treatment of cuboid syndrome secondary to lateral ankle sprains: A case series. *J Ortho Sport Phys Ther.* 2005;35(7):409-415.

294. Durall CJ. Examination and treatment of cuboid syndrome: a literature review. *Sports Health.* 2011;3(6):514-519.

295. Mooney M, Maffey-Ward L. Cuboid plantar and dorsal subluxations: assessment and treatment. *J Ortho Sport Phys Ther.* 1994;20(4):220-226.

296. Mayfield JK. Mechanism of carpal injuries. *Clin Orthop Relat Res.* 1980;149:45-54.

297. Rettig AC. Athletic injuries of the wrist and hand: Part I. Traumatic injuries of the wrist. *Am J Sports Med.* 2003;31(6):1038-1048.

Chapter 12

1. Kottke FJ, Pauley DL, Ptak RA. The rationale for prolonged stretching for correction of shortening of connective tissue. *Arch Phys Med Rehabil.* 1966;47(6):345-352.

2. Zhou H, Trudel G, Goudreau L, Laneuville O. Knee joint stiffness following immobilization and remobilization: a study in the rat model. *J Biomech.* 2020;99. doi:10.1016/j.jbiomech.2019.109471

3. Shelbourne KD, Urch SE, Gray T, Freeman H. Loss of normal knee motion after anterior cruciate ligament reconstruction is associated with radiographic arthritic changes after surgery. *Am J Sports Med.* 2012;40(1):108-113.

4. Kottke FJ. Therapeutic exercise to maintain mobility. In: Kottke FJ, Lehmann JF, eds. *Krusen's Handbook of Physical Medicine and Rehabilitation.* 4th ed. W.B. Saunders; 1990:436-451.

5. Akeson WH, Amiel D, Abel MF, Garfin SR, Woo SL-Y. Effect of immobilization on joints. *Clin Orthop Relat Res.* 1987;219:28-37.

6. Hong SP, Henderson CN. Articular cartilage changes following immobilization of the rat knee joint: A semi-quantitative scanning electron-microscopic study. *Acta Anat.* 1996;157(1):27-40.

7. Iqbal K, Khan Y, Minhas IA. Effects of immobilization on thickness of superficial zone of articular cartilage of patella in rats. *Indian J Orthop.* 2012;46(4):391-394.

8. Bosch U, Kaspercyk WJ, Oestern HJ, Tscherne H. Biology of posterior cruciate ligament healing. *Sports Med Arthroscop Rev.* 1994;2(1):88-99.

9. Lee S, Sakurai T, Ohsako M, Saura R, Hatta H, Alomi Y. Tissue stiffness induced by prolonged immobilization of the rat knee joint and relevance of AGEs (pentosidine). *Connect Tissue Res.* 2010;51(6):467-477.

10. Kaneguchi A, Ozawa J, Kawamata S, Yamaoka K. Development of arthrogenic joint contracture as a result of pathologic changes in remobilized rat knees. *J Orthop Res.* 2017;35(7):1414-1423.

11. Frank C, Woo S, Andriacchi T, et al. Normal ligament: structure, function, and composition. In: Woo SLY, Buckwalter JA, eds. *Injury and Repair of the Musculoskeletal Soft Tissues.* AAOS; 1988:45-102.

12. Booth FW. Physiologic and biochemical effects of immobilization on muscle. *Clin Orthop Relat Res.* 1987;219:15-20.

13. Klein L, Heiple KG, Torzilla PA, Goldberg VM, Burstein AH. Prevention of ligament and meniscus atrophy by active joint motion in a non-weight bearing model. *J Orthop Res.* 1989;7(1):80-85.

14. Aoki MS, Lima WP, Miyabara EH, Gouveia CH, Moriscot AS. Deleterious effects of immobilization upon rat skeletal muscle: role of creatine supplementation. *Clin Nutr.* 2004;23(5):1176-1183.

15. Clark, B.C. In vivo alterations in skeletal muscle form and function after disuse atrophy. *Med Sci Sports Exerc.* 2009;41(10):1869-1875.

16. Montgomery JB, Steadman JR. Rehabilitation of the injured knee. *Clin Sports Med.* 1985;4(2):333-343.

17. Fong DT, Chan YY, Mok KM, Yung PS, Chan KM. Understanding acute ankle ligamentous sprain injury in sports. *Sports Med Arthrosc Rehabil Ther Technol.* 2009;1. doi:10.1186/1758-2555-1-14

18. Hewett T, Paterno M, Myer G. Strategies for enhancing proprioception and neuromuscular control of the knee. *Clin Orthop.* 2002;402:76-94.

19. Wall BT, Dirks ML, Snijders T, Senden JMG, Dolmans J, van Loon LJC. Substantial skeletal muscle loss occurs during only 5 days of disuse. *Acta Physiologica.* 2014;210(3):600-611. doi:10.1111/apha.12190

20. Buckwalter JA. Effects of early motion on healing of musculoskeletal tissues. *Hand Clin.* 1996;12(1):13-24.

21. Józsa L, Järvinen M, Kannus P, Réffy A. Fine structural changes in the articular cartilage of the rat's knee following short-term immobilisation in various positions. *International Orthopaedics.* 1987;11(2):129-133. doi:10.1007/BF00266698

22. Ando A, Suda H, Hagiwara Y, et al. Reversibility of immobilization-induced articular cartilage degeneration after remobilization in rat knee joints. *Tohoku J Exp Med.* 2011;224(2):77-85.

23. Finsterbush A, Friedman B. Reversibility of joint changes produced by immobilization in rabbits. *Clin Orthop Relat Res.* 1995;111:290-298.

24. Demirhan M, Uysal M, Kilicoglu O, et al. Tensile strength of ligaments after thermal shrinkage depending on time and immobilization: In vivo study in the rabbit. *J Shoulder Elbow Surg.* 2005;14(2):193-200.

25. Ando A, Suda H, Hagiwara Y, Onoda Y, Chimoto E, Itoi E. Remobilization does not restore immobilization-induced adhesion of capsule and restricted joint motion in rat knee joints. *Tohoku J Exp Med.* 2012;227(1):13-22.

26. Woo SL, Gomez MA, Sites TJ, Newton PO, Orlando CA, Akeson WH. The biomechanical and morphological changes in the medial collateral ligament of the rabbit after immobilization and remobilization. *J Bone Joint Surg Am.* 1987;69(8):1200-1211.

27. Labarque V, Op 't Eijnde B, Van Leemputte M. Effect of immobilization and retraining on torque-velocity relationship of human knee flexor and extensor muscles. *European Journal of Applied Physiology.* 2002;86(3):251-257. doi:10.1007/s00421-001-0530-z

28. Clark BC, Manini TM, Hoffman RL, Russ DW. Restoration of voluntary muscle strength after 3 weeks of cast immobilization is suppressed in women compared with men. *Arch Phys Med Rehabil.* 2009;90(1):178-180.

29. Järvinen TA, Järvinen TL, Kääriäinen M, Kalimo H, Järvinen M. Muscle injuries: biology and treatment. *Am J Sports Med.* May 2005;33(5):745-64. doi:10.1177/0363546505274714

30. Montgomery RD. Healing of muscle, ligaments, and tendons. *Semin Vet Med Surg.* 1989;4(4):304-311.

31. Irrgang JJ, Pezzullo D. Rehabilitation following surgical procedures to address articular cartilage lesions in the knee. *J Orthop Sports Phys Ther.* 1998;28(4):232-240.

32. Heckmann TP, Barber-Westin SD, Noyes FR. Meniscal repair and transplantation: indications, techniques, rehabilitation, and clinical outcome. *J Orthop Sports Phys Ther.* 2006;36(10):795-814.

33. Leong DJ, Gu XI, Li Y, et al. Matrix metalloproteinase-3 in articular cartilage is upregulated by joint immobilization and suppressed by passive joint motion. *Matrix Biol.* 2010;29(5):420-426.

34. Donatelli R, Owens-Burkhart H. Effects of immobilization on the extensibility of periarticular connective tissue. *J Orthop Sports Phys Ther.* 1981;3(2):67-72.

35. Buckwalter JA. Articular cartilage: Composition and structure. In: Woo SLY, Buckwalter JA, eds. *Injury and Repair of the Musculoskeletal Soft Tissues.* AAOS; 1988:405-426.

36. Joseph MF, Taft K, Moskwa M, Denegar CR. Deep friction massage to treat tendinopathy: a systematic review of a classic treatment in the face of a new paradigm of understanding. *J Sport Rehabil.* 2012;21(4):343-353.

37. Millett PJ, Wickiewicz TL, Warren RF. Current concepts. Motion loss after ligament injuries to the knee: Part 1. Causes. *Am J Sports Med.* 2001;29(5):664-675.

38. Stiefel EC, McIntyre L. Arthroscopic lysis of adhesions for treatment of post-traumatic arthrofibrosis of the knee joint. *Arthrosc Tech.* 2017;6(4). doi:10.1016/j.eats.2017.03.001

39. Lewit K, Olsanska S. Clinical importance of active scars: abnormal scars as a cause of myofascial pain. *J Manip Physiol Ther.* 2004;27(6):399-402.

40. Wilhelmi BJ, Blackwell SJ, Mancoll JS, Phillips LG. Creep vs. stretch: A review of the viscoelastic properties of skin. *Ann Plast Surg.* 1998;41(2):215-219.

41. Warren CG, Lehmann JF, Koblanski JN. Heat and stretch procedures: an evaluation using rat tail tendon. *Arch Phys Med Rehabil.* 1976;57(3):122-126.

42. Nakano J, Yamabayashi C, Scott A, Reid WD. The effect of heat applied with stretch to increase range of motion: a systematic review. *Phys Ther Sport.* 2012;13:180-188.

43. Iatridis JC, Wu J, Yandow JA, Langevin HM. Subcutaneous tissue mechanical behavior is linear and viscoelastic under uniaxial tension. *Connect Tissue Res.* 2003;44(5):208-217.

44. Vegas MR, Martin del Yerro JL. Stiffness, compliance, resilience, and creep deformation: understanding implant-soft tissue dynamics in the augmented breast: fundamentals based on materials science. *Aesthetic Plast Surg.* 2013;37(5):922-930.

45. Lieber RL, Roberts TJ, Blemker SS, Lee SSM, Herzog W. Skeletal muscle mechanics, energetics and plasticity. *J Neuroeng Rehabil.* 2017;14. doi:10.1186/s12984-017-0318-y

46. Neviaser A, Andarawis-Puri N, Flatow E. Basic mechanisms of tendon fatigue damage. *J Shoulder Elbow Surg.* 2012;21(2):158-163.

47. Serpell BG, Ball NB, Scarvell JM, Smith PN. A review of models of vertical, leg, and knee stiffness in adults for running, jumping or hopping tasks. *J Sports Sci.* 2012;30(13):1347-1363.

48. Chadrashekar N, Hashemi J, Slauterbeck J, Beynnon BD. Low-load behaviour of the patellar tendon graft and its relevance to the biomechanics of the reconstructed knee. *Clin Biomech.* 2008;23(7):918-925.

49. Butler DL, Grood ES, Noyes FR, Zernicke RF. Biomechanics of ligaments and tendons. *Exerc Sport Sci Rev.* 1978;6(1):125-181.

50. Butler DL, Grood ES, Noyes FR, Zernicke RF. Biomechanics of ligaments and tendons. *Exerc Sport Sci Rev.* 1978;6:125-81.

51. Ionescu I, Guilkey JE, Berzins M, Kirby RM, Weiss JA. Simulation of soft tissue failure using the material point method. *J Biomech Eng.* 2006;128(6):917-924.

52. Wenger MP, Bozec L, Horton MA, Mesquida P. Mechanical properties of collagen fibrils. *Biophys J.* 2007;93(4):1255-1263.

53. Shen ZL, Dodge MR, Kahn H, Ballarini R, Eppell SJ. Stress-strain experiments on individual collagen fibrils. *Biophys J.* 2008;95(8):3956-3963.

54. Sangwan S, Green RA, Taylor NF. Characteristics of stabilizer muscles: a systematic review. *Physiother Can.* 2014;66(4):348-358.

55. Linari M, Dobbie IR, M., Koubassova N, Irving M, Piazzesi G, Lombardi V. The stiffness of skeletal muscle in isometric contraction and rigor: The fraction of myosin heads bound to actin. *Biophys J.* 1998;74(5):2459-2473.

56. Maganaris CN. Tensile properties of in vivo human tendinous tissue. *J Biomech.* 2002;35(8):1019-1027.

57. Xie P, Jiang Y, Zhand X, Yang S. The study of intramuscular nerve distribution patterns and relative spindle abundance of the thenar and hypothenar muscles in human hand *PloS ONE.* 2012. doi:10.1371/journal.pone.0051538

58. Arutiunian RS. Modern concepts of the structure and function of muscle spindles in mammals. *Usp Fiziol Nauk.* 1996;27(4):73-95.

59. Eldred E. Peipheral receptors: their excitation and relation to reflex patterns. *Am J Phys Med.* 1967;46(1):69-87.

60. Lundberg A, Malmgren K, Schomburg ED. Cutaneous facilitation of transmission in reflex pathways from Ib afferents to motorneurones. *J Physiol.* 1977;265:763-780.

61. Lundberg A, Malmgren K, Schomburg ED. Reflex pathways from group II muscle afferents: 2. Functional characteristics of reflex pathways to alpha-motoneurones. *Exp Brain Res*. 1987;65(2):282-293.

62. Hyngstrom A, Johnson M, Schuster J, Heckman CJ. Movement-related receptive fields of spinal motoneurones with active dendrites. *J Physiol*. 2008;586:1581-1593.

63. Chalmers G. Do Golgi tendon organs really inhibit muscle activity at high force levels to save muscles from injury, and adapt with strength training? *Sports Biomech*. 2002;1(2):239-249.

64. Hoppenfeld S. *Physical Examination of the Spine and Extremities*. Appleton-Century-Crofts; 1976.

65. Hislop HJ, Avers D, Brown M. *Daniels and Worthingham's Manual Muscle Testing: Techniques of Manual Examination*. 9th ed. Elsevier Saunders; 2014.

66. American Academy of Orthopaedic Surgeons. *Joint Motion: Method of Measuring and Recording*. American Academy of Orthopaedic Surgeons; 1965.

67. Kendall FP, McCreary EK, Provance PG, Rodgers MM, Romani WA. *Muscles: Testing and Function With Posture and Pain*. 5th ed. Lippincott Williams & Wilkins; 2005.

68. Kapandji IA. *The Physiology of the Joints: Vol 1, Upper Limb*. 5th ed. Churchill Livingstone; 1982.

69. Kapandji IA. *The Physiology of the Joints: Vol 2, Lower Limb*. 5th ed. Churchill Livingstone; 1987.

70. Esch D, Lepley M. *Evaluation of Joint Motion: Methods of Measurement and Recording*. University of Minnesota Press; 1974.

71. Gerhardt JJ, Russe OA. *International SFTR Method of Measuring and Recording Joint Motion*. Year Book Medical Publishers; 1975.

72. Salter RB, Hamilton HW, Wedge JH, Tile M, Torode IP, O'Driscoll SW, et al. Clinical application of basic research on continuous passive motion for disorders and injuries of synovial joints: a preliminary report of a feasibility study. *J Orthop Res*. 1984;1(3):325-342.

73. Denard PJ, Ladermann A. Immediate versus delayed passive range of motion following total shoulder arthroplasty. *J Shoulder Elbow Surg*. 2016;25:1918-1924.

74. Snyder M, Kozlowski P, Drobniewski M, Grzegorzewski A, Glowacka A. The use of continuous passive motion (CPM) in the rehabilitation of patients after total knee arthroplasty. *Orthop Traumatol Rehabil*. 2004;6:336-341.

75. Liao CD, Huang YC, Lin LF, et al. Continuous passive motion and its effects on knee flexion after total knee arthroplasty in patients with knee osteoarthritis. *Knee Surg Sports Traumatol Arthrosc*. 2016;24:2578-2586.

76. Wong JM. Management of stiff hand: an occupational therapy perspective. *Hand Surg*. 2002;7(2):261-269.

77. Verhaegen PD, Schouten HJ, Tigchelaar-Gutter W, et al. Adaptation of the dermal collagen structure of human skin and scar tissue in response to stretch: an experimental study. *Wound Repair Regen*. 2012;20(5):658-666.

78. Garrett WEJ. Muscle strain injuries. *Am J Sports Med*. 1996;24(6):S2-S8.

79. Sexton P, Chambers J. The importance of flexibility for functional range of motion. *Athl Ther Today*. 2006;11(3):13-15.

80. Shellock FG, Prentice WE. Warming-up and stretching for improved physical performance and prevention of sports-related injuries. *Sports Med*. 1985;2(4):267-278.

81. Kovacs MS. The argument against static stretching before sport and physical activity. *Athl Ther Today*. 2006;11(3):6-8, 30-1, 60.

82. Thacker SB, Gilchrist J, Stroup DF, Kimsey CD, Jr. The impact of stretching on sports injury risk: a systematic review of the literature. *Med Sci Sports Exerc*. 2004;36(3):371-378.

83. Behm DG, Blazevich AJ, Kay AD, McHugh M. Acute effects of muscle stretching on physical performance, range of motion, and injury in healthy active individuals: A systematic review. *Appl Physiol Nutr Metab*. 2016;41:1-11. doi:10.1139/apnm-2015-0235

84. Opplert J, Babault N. Acute effects of dynamic stretching on muscle flexibility and performance: An analysis of the current literature. *Sports Med*. 2018;48:299-325.

85. Chan SP, Hong Y, Robinson PD. Flexibility and passive resistance of the hamstrings of young adults using two different static stretching protocols. *Scand J Med Sci Sports*. 2001;11(2):81-86.

86. Kay AD, Husbands-Beasley J, Blazevich AJ. Effects of contract-relax, static stretching, and isometric contractions on muscle-tendon mechanics. *Med Sci Sports Exer*. 2015. doi:10.1249/MSS.0000000000000632

87. Samukawa M, Hattori M, Sugama N, Takeda N. The effects of dynamic stretching on plantar flexor muscle-tendon tissue properties. *Man Ther*. 2011;16(6):618-622.

88. Opplert J, Babault N. Acute effects of dynamic stretching on mechanical properties result from both muscle-tendon stretching and muscle warm-up. *J Sports Sci Med*. 2019;18:351-358.

89. Sharman MJ, Cresswell AG, Riek S. Proprioceptive neuromuscular facilitation stretching: mechanisms and clinical implications. *Sports Med*. 2006;36(11):929-939.

90. Konrad A, Stafilidis S, Tilp M. Effects of acute static, ballistic, and PNF stretching exercise on the muscle and tendon tissue properties. *Scand J Med Sci Sports*. 2017;27(10):1070-1080.

91. O'Hora J, Cartwright A, Wade CD, Hough AD, Shum GL. Efficacy of static stretching and proprioceptive neuromuscular facilitation stretch on hamstrings length after a single session. *J Strength Cond Res*. 2011;25(6):1586-1591.

92. Yuktasir B, Kaya F. Investigation into the long-term effects of static and PNF stretching exercises on range of motion and jump performance. *J Bodyw Mov Ther*. 2009;13(1):11-21.

93. Covert CA, Alexander MP, Petronis JJ, Davis DS. Comparison of ballistic and static stretching on hamstring muscle length using an equal stretching dose. *J Strength Cond Res*. 2010;24(11):3008-3014.

94. Mahieu NN, McNair P, De Muynck M, et al. Effect of static and ballistic stretching on the muscle-tendon tissue properties. *Med Sci Sports Exerc*. 2007;39(3):494-501.

95. Barbosa GM, Dantas GAF, Silva BR, Souza TO, Vieira WHB. Static or dynamic stretching program does not change the acute responses on neuromuscular and functional performance in healthy subjects: a single-blind randomized controlled trial. *Rev Bras Cienc Esporte*. 2018;40(4):418-426.

96. Davis DS, Ashby PE, McCale KL, McQuain JA, Wine JM. The effectiveness of 3 stretching techniques on hamstring flexibility using consistent stretching parameters. *J Strength Cond Res*. 2005;19(1):27-32.

97. Behm DG, Blazevich AJ, Kay AD, McHugh M. Acute effects of muscle stretching on physical performance, range of motion, and injury incidence in healthy active individuals: a systematic review. *Appl Physiol Nutr Metab.* 2016;41. doi:10.1139/apnm-2015-0235

98. Konrad A, Reiner MM, Thaller S, Tilp M. The time course of muscle-tendon properties and function response of a five-minute static stretching exercise. *Eur J Sport Sci.* 2019;19(9):1195-1203.

99. Aquino CF, Fonseca ST, Gonçalves GG, Silva PL, Ocarino JM, Mancini MC. Stretching versus strength training in lengthened position in subjects with tight hamstring muscles: a randomized controlled trial. *Man Ther.* 2010;15(1):26-31.

100. Liebenson C. Functional problems associated with the knee: Part 2. Do tight hamstrings only need stretching? *J Bodywork Movement Ther.* 2007;11(1):61-63.

101. O'Sullivan K, Murray E, Sainsbury D. The effect of warm-up, static stretching and dynamic stretching on hamstring flexibility in previously injured subjects. *BMC Musculoskelet Disord.* 2009;10:37. doi:10.1186/1471-2474-10-37

102. Gleim GW, McHugh MP. Flexibility and its effects on sports injury and performance. *Sports Medicine.* 1997;24(5):289-299. doi:10.2165/00007256-199724050-00001

103. Menta R, Randhawa K, Côté P, et al. The effectiveness of exercise for the management of musculoskeletal disorders and injuries of the elbow, forearm, wrist, and hand: a systematic review by the Ontario Protocol for Traffic Injury Management (OPTIMa) Collaboration. *J Manipulative Physiol Ther.* 2015;38(7):507-520. doi:10.1016/j.jmpt.2015.06.002

104. Rubini EC, Costa AL, Gomes PS. The effects of stretching on strength performance. *Sports Med.* 2007;37(3):213-24. doi:10.2165/00007256-200737030-00003

105. Zakas A, Doganis G, Zakas N, Vergou A. Acute effects of active warm-up and stretching on the flexibility of older women. *J Sports Med Phys Fitness.* 2006;46:617-622.

106. Wyon MA, Smith A, Koutedakis Y. A comparison of strength and stretch interventions on active and passive ranges of movement in dancers: a randomized controlled trial. *J Strength Cond Res.* 2013;27:3053-3059.

107. Apostolopoulos N, Metsios GS, Nevill A, Koutedakis Y, Wyon M. Stretch intensity vs inflammation: a dose dependent association? *J Kinesiol Sports Sci.* 2015;3:27-31.

108. Nelson RT, Bandy WD. An update on flexibility. *Strength Condit J.* 2005;27(1):10-16.

109. Bradley PS, Olsen PD, Portas MD. The effect of static, ballistic, and proprioceptive neuromuscular facilitation stretching on vertical jump performance. *J Strength Cond Res.* 2007;21(1):223-236.

110. Witvrouw E, Mahieu N, Roosen P, McNair P. The role of stretching in tendon injuries. *Br J Sports Med.* 2007;41(4):224-226.

111. Cipriani DJ, Terry ME, Haines MA, Tabibnia AP, BLyssanova O. Effect of stretch frequency and sex on the rate of gain and rate of loss in muscle flexibility during a hamstring-stretching program: a radomized single-blind longitudinal study. *J Strength Cond Res.* 2012;26:2119-2129.

112. Silveira G, Sayers M, Waddington G. Effect of dynamic versus static stretching in the warm-up on hamstring flexibility. *Sport J* 2011;14:1-8.

113. Wicke J, Gainey K, Figueroa M. A comparison of self-administered proprioceptive neuromuscular facilitation to static stretching on range of motion and flexibility. *J Strength Cond Res.* 2014;28:168-172.

114. Smith LL, Chenier TC, McCammon MR, Houmard JA, Franklin ME, et al. The effects of static and ballistic stretching on delayed onset muscle soreness and creatine kinase. *Res Q Exerc Sport.* 1993;64:103-107.

115. Apostolopoulos N, Metsios GS, Taunton J, Koutedakis Y, Wyon M. Acute inflammation response to stretching: A randomized controlled trial. *Ital J Sports Rehabil Posturol.* 2015;2:368-381.

116. Borman NP, Trudelle-Jackson E, Smith SS. Effects of stretch positions on hamstring muscle length, lumbar flexion range of motion, and lumbar curvature in healthy adults. *Physiother Theory Pract.* 2011;27:146-154.

117. Abellaneda S, Guissard N, Duchateau J. The relative lengthening of the myotendinous structures in the medial gastrocnemius during passive stretching differs among individuals. *J Appl Physiol.* 2009;106(1):169-177.

118. Morse CI, Degens H, Seynnes OR, Maganaris CN, Jones DA. The acute effect of stretching on the passive stiffness of the human gastrocnemius muscle tendon unit. *J Physiol.* 2008;586(1):97-106.

119. Guissard N, Duchateau J. Effect of static stretch training on neural and mechanical properties of the human plantar-flexor muscles. *Muscle Nerve.* 2004;29(2):248-255.

120. Medeiros DM, Lima CS. Influence of chronic stretching on muscle performance: systematic review. *Hum Mov Sci.* 2017;54:220-229.

121. Freitas Sr, Mendes B, Ls Sant G, Andrade RJ, Nordez A, Milanovic Z. Can chronic stretching change the muscle-tendon mechanical properties? A review. *Scand J Med Sci Sports.* 2017;28:794-806.

122. Foure A, Nordez A, Cornu C. Effects of plyometric training on passive stiffness of gastrocnemii muscles and Achilles tendon. *Eur J Appl Physiol.* 2012;112(8):2849-2857.

123. Mizuno T. Changes in joint range of motion and muscle-tendon unit stiffness after varying amounts of dynamic stretching. *J Sports Sci Routledge.* 2017;35:2157-2163.

124. Su H, Chang NJ, Wu WL, et al. Acute effects of foam rolling, static stretching, and dynamic stretching during warm-ups on muscular flexibility and strength in young adults. *J Sport Rehabil.* 2016;13(1):1-24.

125. Lima C, Brown L, Wong M, et al. Acute effects of static vs. ballistic stretching on strenght and muscular fatigue between ballet dancers and resistance trained women. *J Strength Cond Res.* 2016;30(11):3220-3227.

126. Kellis E. Biceps femoris fascicle length during passive stretching. *J Electromyogr Kinesiol.* 2018;38:119-125.

127. Nakamura M, Ikezoe T, Tokagawa T, et al. Acute effects of stretching on passive properties of human gastrocnemius muscle-tendon unit: analysis of differences between hold-relax and static stretching. *J Sport Rehabil.* 2015;24:286-292.

128. Cramer JT, Housh TJ, Weir JP, Johnson GO, Coburn JW, Beck TW. The acute effects of static stretching on peak torque, mean power output, electromyography, and mechanomyography. *Eur J Appl Physiol.* 2005;93(5-6):530-539.

129. Herda TJ, Cramer JT, Ryan ED, McHugh MP, Stout JR. Acute effects of static versus dynamic stretching on

isometric peak torque, electromyography, and mechano-myography of the biceps femoris muscle. *J Strength Cond Res*. 2008;22(3):809-817.

130. Stevanovic V, Jelic M, Milanovic S. Sport-specific warm-up attenuates static stretching induced negative effects on vertical jump but not neuromuscular excitability in basketball players. *J Sport Sci Med*. 2019;18:280-289.

131. Manoel ME, Harris-Love MO, Danoff JV, Miller TA. Acute effects of static, dynamic, and proprioceptive neuromuscular facilitation stretching on muscle power in women. *J Strength Cond Res*. 2008;22(5):1528-1534.

132. Yamaguchi T, Ishii K, Yamanaka M, Yasuda K. Acute effects of dynamic stretching exercise on power output during concentric dynamic constant external resistance leg extension. *J Strength Cond Res*. 2007;21(4):1238-1244.

133. Ruan M, Zhang Q, Wu X. Acute effects of static stretching of hamstrings on performance and ACL injury risk during stop-jump and cutting tasks in female athletes. *J Strength Cond Res*. 2017;31(5):1241-1250.

134. Ode Olivers F, Rama L. Static stretching does not reduce variability, jump and speed performance. *Inter J Sports Phy Ther*. 2016;11(2):237-246.

135. Behm DG, Bambury A, Cahill F, Power K. Effect of acute static stretching on force, balance, reaction time, and movement time. *Med Sci Sport Exerc*. 2004;36(8):1397-1402.

136. Kay AD, Blazevich AJ. Effect of acute static stretch on maximal muscle performance: a systematic review. *Med Sci Sports Exerc*. 2012;44(1):154-164.

137. de Weijer VC, Gorniak GC, Shamus E. The effect of static stretch and warm-up exercise on hamstring length over the course of 24 hours. *J Orthop Sports Phys Ther*. 2003;33(12):727-733.

138. Mizuno T, Matsumoto M, Umemura Y. Viscoelasticity of the muscle-tendon unit is returned more rapidly than range of motion after stretching. *Scand J Med Sci Sports*. 2013;23(1):23-30.

139. Radford JA, Burns J, Buchbinder R, Landorf KB, Cook C. Does stretching increase ankle dorsiflexion range of motion? A systematic review. *Br J Sports Med*. 2006;40(10):870-875.

140. Magnusson SP, Aagard P, Simonsen E, Bojsen-Møller F. A biomechanical evaluation of cyclic and static stretch in human skeletal muscle. *Int J Sports Med*. 1998;19(5):310-316.

141. Ryan ED, Beck TW, Herda TJ, et al. Do practical durations of stretching alter muscle strength? A dose-response study. *Med Sci Sports Exerc*. 2008;40(8):1529-1537.

142. Ryan ED, Beck TW, Herda TJ, et al. The time course of musculotendinous stiffness responses following different durations of passive stretching. *J Orthop Sports Phys Ther*. 2008;38(10):632-639.

143. DePino GM, Webright WG, Arnold BL. Duration of maintained hamstring flexibility after cessation of an acute static stretching protocol. *J Athl Train*. 2000;35:56-59.

144. Ford P, McChesney J. Duration of maintained hamstring ROM following termination of three stretching protocols. *J Sport Rehabil*. 2007;16:18-27.

145. Spernoga SG, Uhl TL, Arnold BL, Gansneder BM. Duration of maintained hamstring flexibility after a one-time, modified hold-relax stretching protocol. *J Athl Train*. 2001;36(1):44-48.

146. Ayala F, de Baranda Andújar PS. Effect of 3 different active stretch durations on hip flexion range of motion. *J Strength Cond Res*. 2010;24(2):430-436.

147. Bandy W, Irion J, Briggler M. The effect of time and frequency on static stretching on flexibility of the hamstring muscles. *Phys Ther*. 1997;77(10):1090-1096.

148. Bandy WD, Irion JM. The effect of time on static stretch on the flexibility of the hamstring muscles. *Phys Ther*. 1994;74:845-852.

149. Behm DG, Chaouchi A. A review of the acute effects of static and dynamic stretching on performance. *Eur J Appl Physiol*. 2011;111(11):2633-2651.

150. Cipriani D, Abel B, Pirrwitz D. A comparison of two stretching protocols on hip range of motion: implications for total daily stretch duration. *J Strength Cond Res*. 2003;17(2):274-278.

151. Opplert J, Gentry JB, Babault N. Do stretch durations affect muscle mechanical and neurophysiological properties? *Int J Sports Med*. 2016;37:673-679.

152. Roberts JM, Wison K. Effect of stretching duration on active and passive range of motion in the lower extremity. *Br J Sports Med*. 1999;33:259-263.

153. Madding SW, Wong JG, Hallum A, Medeiros JM. Effect of duration of passive stretch on hip abduction range of motion. *J Orthop Sports Phys Ther*. 1987;8(8):409-416.

154. Ioannis T, Christos G, Nikolaos Z, Aikaterini V, Efstratios V. The effect of stretching duration on the flexibility of lower extremities in junior soccer players. *Phys Train*. Sept 2005:1.

155. Zakas A. The effect of stretching duration on the lower-extremity flexibility of adolescent soccer players. *J Bodyw Mov Ther*. 2005;9(3):220-225.

156. Zakas A, Balaska P, Grammatikopoulou MG, Zakas N. Acute effects of stretching duration on the range of motion of elderly women. *J Bodyw Mov Ther*. 2005;9(4):270-276.

157. Thomas E, Bianco A, Paoli A, Palma A. The relation between stretching typology and stretching duration: the effects on range of motion. *Int J Sports Med*. 2018;39:243-254.

158. Abdulla SY, Southerst D, Cote, et al. Is exercise effective for the management of subacromial impingement syndrome and other soft tissue injuries of the shoulder? A systematic review by the Ontario Protocol for Traffic Injury Management (OPTIMa) Collaboration. *Man Ther*. 2015. doi:10.1016/j.math.2015.03.013

159. Başkurt Z, Başkurt F, Gelecek N, Özkan MH. The effectiveness of scapular stabilization exercise in the patients with subacromial impingement syndrome. *J Back Musculoskelet Rehabil*. 2011;24(3):173-179.

160. Menta R, Randhawa K, Côté P, et al. The effectiveness of exercise for the management of musculoskeletal disorders and injuries of the elbow, forearm, wrist, and hand: a systematic review by the Ontario Protocol for Traffic Injury Management (OPTIMa) Collaboration. *J Manip Physiol Ther*. 2015. doi:10.1016/j.jmpt.2015.06.002

161. Woitzik E, Jacobs C, Wong JJ, et al. The effectiveness of exercise on recovery and clinical outcomes of soft tissue injuries of the leg, ankle, and foot: a systematic review by the Ontario Protocol for Traffic Injury Management (OPTIMa) Collaboration. *Man Ther*. 2015. doi:10.1016/j.math.2015.03.012

162. Marom A, Berkovitch Y, Toume S, Alvarez-Elizondo MB, Weihs D. Non-damaging stretching combined with sodium pyruvate supplement accelerated migration of fibroblasts and myoblasts during gap closure. *Clin Biomech*. 2019;62:96-103.

163. Perrier ET, Pavol MJ, Hoffman MA. The acute effects of a warm-up including static or dynamic stretching on countermovement jump height, reaction time, and flexibility. *J Strength Cond Res*. 2011;25(7):1925-1931.

164. Micheo W, Baerga L, Miranda G. Basic principles regarding strength, flexibility, and stability exercises. *PM&R*. 2012;4(11):805-811. doi:10.1016/j.pmrj.2012.09.583

165. Apostolopoulos N, Metsios GS, Flouris AD, Koutedakis Y, Wyon MA. The relevance of stretch intensity and position: a systematic review. *Front Psychol* 2015. doi:10.3389/fpsyg.2015.01128

166. Kellerud H, Gleeson N. Effects of stretching on performance involving stretch-shortening cycles. *Sports Med*. 2013;43(8):733-750.

167. Nakamura M, Ikezoe T, Umegaki H, Kobayashi T, Nishishita S, Ichihashi N. Changes in passive properties of the gastrocnemius muscle-tendon unit during a 4-week routine static-stretching program. *J Sport Rehabil*. 2017;26(4):263-268.

168. Flowers KR, LaStayo PC. Effect of total end range time on improving passive range of motion. *J Hand Ther*. 2012;25(1):48-55.

169. Chalmers G. Re-examination of the possible role of Golgi tendon organ and muscle spindle reflexes in proprioceptive neuromuscular facilitation muscle stretching. *Sports Biomech*. 2004;3(1):159-183.

170. Sahrmann SA. *Diagnosis and Treatment of Movement Impairment Syndromes*. Mosby; 2002.

171. Freitas SR, Vaz JR, Bruno PM, Andrade R, Mil-Homens P. Stretching effects: high-intensity & moderate duration vs. low-intensity & long-duration. *Int J Sports Med*. 2016;37:239-244.

172. Ono T, Tsuboi M, Oki S, et al. Preliminary report: another perspective on the effect of prolonged stretching for joint contractures. *J Phys Ther Sci*. 2007;19(1):97-101.

173. Starring DT, Gossman MR, Nicholson GG, Jr., Lemons J. Comparison of cyclic and sustained passive stretching using a mechanical device to increase resting length of hamstring muscles. *Phys Ther*. 1988;68(3):314-320.

174. Warren CG, Lehmann JF, Koblanski JN. Elongation of rat tail tendon: effect of load and temperature. *Arch Phys Med Rehabil*. 1971;52(10):465-474.

175. Pratt K, Bohannon R. Effects of a 3-minute standing stretch on ankle-dorsiflexion range of motion. *J Sport Rehabil*. 2003;12(2):162-173.

176. Page P. Current concepts in muscle stretching for exercise and rehabilitation. *Int J Sports Phys Ther*. 2012;7(1):109-119.

177. Valdes K, Boyd JD, Povlak SB, Szelwach MA. Efficacy of orthotic devices for increased active proximal interphalangeal extension joint range of motion: a systematic review. *H Hand Ther*. 2019;32:184-193.

Chapter 13

1. Bouisset S, Maton B. Quantitative relationship between surface EMG and intramuscular electromyographic activity in voluntary movement. *Am J Phys Med*. 1972;51:285-295.

2. Fox SA. Muscle mechanisms of contraction and neural control. *Human Physiol*. 9th ed. McGraw-Hill; 2006:338-379:chap 12.

3. Tötösy de Zepetnek JE, Zung HV, Erdebil S, Gordon T. Innervation ratio is an important determinant of force in normal and reinnervated rat tibialis anterior muscles. *J Neurophysiol*. 1992;67(5):1385-1403.

4. McPhedran AM, Wuerker RB, Henneman E. Properties of motor units in a homogeneous red muscle (soleus) of the cat. *J Neurophysiol*. 1965;28(1):71-84.

5. Wuerker RB, McPhedran AM, Henneman E. Properties of motor units in a heterogeneous pale muscle (m. gastrocnemius) of the cat. *J Neurophysiol*. 1965;28(1):85-99.

6. Latash ML. *Neurophysiological Basis of Movement*. 2nd ed. Human Kinetics; 2008.

7. Enoka RM, Christou E, Hunter S, et al. Mechanisms that contribute to differences in motor performance between young and old adults. *J Electromyogr Kinesiol*. 2003;13:1-12.

8. Wiechers DO, Johnson EW. Electrodiagnosis. In: Kottke FJ, Lehmann JF, eds. *Krusen's Handbook of Physical Medicine and Rehabilitation*. 4th ed. WB Saunders; 1990:72-107:chap 3.

9. Enoka RM. Morphological features and activation patterns of motor units. *J Clin Neurophysiol*. 1995;12(6):538-559.

10. Craig R, Woodhead JL. Structure and function of myosin filaments. *Curr Opin Struct Biol*. 2006;16(2):204-212.

11. Clark KA, McElhinny AS, Beckerle MC, Gregorio CC. Striated muscle cytoarchitecture: an intricate web of form and function. *Annu Rev Cell Dev Biol*. 2002;18:637-706.

12. Leake MC, Wilson D, Gautel M, Simmons RM. The elasticity of single titin molecules using a two-bead optical tweezers assay. *Biophys J*. 2004;87(2):1112-1135.

13. Linke WA, Leake MC. Multiple sources of passive stress relaxation in muscle fibres. *Phys Med Biol*. 2004;49(16):3613-3627.

14. Tskhovrebova L, Trinick J. Extensivility in the titin molecule and its relation to muscle elasticity. *Adv Exp Med Biol*. 2000;481:163-173.

15. Sanger JM, Sanger JW. The dynamic Z bands of striated muscle cells. *Sci Signal*. 2008;1(32):pe37. doi:10.1126/scisignal

16. Tokunaga M, Sutoh K, Toyoshima C, Wakabayashi T. Location of the ATPase site of myosin determined by three-dimensional electron microscopy. *Nature*. 1987;329(6140):635-638.

17. Widmaier EP, Raff H, Strang KT. *Vander's Human Physiology: The Mechanisms of Body Function*. 11th ed. McGraw-Hill; 2008.

18. Scott W, Stevens J, Binder-Macleod SA. Human skeletal muscle fiber type classifications. *Phys Ther*. 2001;81(11):1810-1816.

19. Pette D, Staron RS. Mammalian skeletal muscle fiber type transitions. *Int Rev Cytol*. 1997;170:143-223.

20. Staron RS. Human skeletal muscle fiber types: delineation, development, and distribution. *Can J Appl Physiol*. 1997;22(4):302-327.

21. Pette D, Staron RS. Transitions of muscle fiber phenotype profiles. *Histochem Cell Biol*. 2001;115(5):359-372.

22. Campos GE, Luecke TJ, Wendeln HK, et al. Muscular adaptations in response to three different resistance-training regimens: specificity of repetition maximum training zones. *Eur J Appl Physiol*. 2002;88(1/2):50-60.

23. Wilson JM, Loenneke JP, Jo E, Wilson GJ, Zourdos MC, Kim JS. The effects of endurance, strength, and power training on muscle fiber type shifting. *J Strength Cond Res*. 2012;26(6):1724-1729.

24. Ng JK, Richardson CA, Kippers V, Pamianpour M. Relationship between muscle fiber composition and functional capacity of back muscles in healthy subjects and patients with back pain. *J Orthop Sports Phys Ther*. 1998;27(6):389-402.

25. Nozaki D. Torque interaction among adjacent joints due to the action of biarticular muscles. *Med Sci Sports Exerc*. 2009;41(1):205-209.

26. Hamill J, Knutzen KM, Derrick TR. *Biomechanical Basis of Human Movement*. 4th ed. Wolters Kluwer; 2015.

27. van Ingen Schenau GJ, .Bobbert MF, Rozendal RH. The unique action of bi-articular muscles in complex movements. *J Anat*. 1987;155(1):1-5.

28. van Ingen Schenau GJ, Dorssers WM, Welter TG, Beelen A, de Groot G, Jacobs R. The control of mono-articular muscles in multijoint leg extensions in man. *J Physiol*. 1995;484(Pt 1):247-254.

29. Levangie PK, Norkin CC, Lewek MD. *Joint Structure and Function: A Comprehensive Analsysis*. 6th ed. FA Davis; 2019.

30. Ralston HJ, Inman VT, Shaffrath MD. Mechanics of human isolated voluntary muscle. *Am J Physiol*. 1947;151(2):612-620.

31. Noble MIM, Pollack GH. Molecular mechanisms of contraction. *Circ Res*. 1977;40(4):333-342.

32. Griffiths RI. Shortening of muscle fibres during stretch of the active cat medial gastrocnemius muscle: the role of tendon compliance. *J Physiol*. 1991;436:219-236.

33. Lieber RL, Loren GJ, Fridén J. In vivo measurement of human wrist extensor muscle sarcomere length changes. *J Neurophysiol*. 1994;71(3):874-881.

34. Ito M, Kawakama Y, Ichinose Y, Fukashiro S, Fukunaga T. Nonisometric behavior of fascicles during isometric contractions of a human muscle. *J Appl Physiol*. 1998;85(4):1230-1235.

35. Lodish H, Berk A, Zipursky SL, Matsudaira P, Baltimore D, Darnell J. Muscle: A specialized contractile machine. In: Lodish H, Berk A, Zipursky SL, Matsudaira P, Baltimore D, Darnell J, eds. *Molecular cell biology*. W.H. Freeman; 2000:Section 18.4.

36. Au Y. The muscle ultrastructure: a structural perspective of the sarcomere. *Cell Mol Life Sci*. 2004;61(24):3016-3033.

37. Hof AL. The force resulting from the action of mono- and biarticular muscles in a limb. *J Biomech*. 2001;34(8):1085-1089.

38. McNitt-Gray JL. Subject specific coordination of two- and one-joint muscles during landings suggests multiple control criteria. *Motor Control*. 2000;4(1):84-88.

39. Gregor RJ, Cavanagh PR, LaFortune M. Knee flexor moments during propulsion in cycling—a creative solution to Lombard's paradox. *J Biomech*. 1985;18(5):307-316.

40. Prilutsky BI. Coordination of two- and one-joint muscles: functional consequences and implications for motor control. *Motor Control*. 2000;4(1):1-44.

41. Raikova R. Investigation of the peculiarities of two-joint muscles using a 3 DOF model of the human upper Limb in the sagittal plane: an optimization approach. *Comp Meth Biomech Biomed Eng*. 2001;4(6):463-490.

42. Sergio LE, Ostry DJ. Coordination of mono- and bi-articular muscles in multi-degree of freedom elbow movements. *Exp Brain Res*. 1994;97(3):551-555.

43. Biewener AA. Locomotion as an emergent property of muscle contractile dynamics. *J Exp Biol*. 2016;219(Pt. 2):285-294.

44. Elftman H. Biomechanics of muscle with particular application to studies of gait. *J Bone Joint Surg Am*. 1966;48(2):363-377.

45. Crone C. Reciprocal inhibition in man. *Dan Med Bull*. 1993;40(5):571-581.

46. Schumacher C, Sharbafi M, Seyfarth A, Rode C. Biarticular muscles in light of template models, experiments and robotics: a review. *J R Soc Interface*. 2020;17(163):20180413. doi:10.1098/rsif.2018.0413

47. Hopkins PM. Skeletal muscle physiology. *Contin Ed Anaesth Crit Care Pain*. 2006;6(1):1-6.

48. Wells R, Evans N. Functions and recruitment patterns of one- and two-joint muscles under isometric and walking conditions. *Hum Mov Sci*. 1987;6(4):349-372.

49. Elias ARC, Hammill CD, Mizner RL. Changes in quadriceps and hamstring contraction following landing instruction in patients with anterior cruciate ligament reconstruction. *J Orthop Sports Phys Ther*. 2015;45(4):273-280.

50. Ratamess NA, Alvar BA, Evetoch TK, et al. American College of Sports Medicine position stand: progression models in resistance training for healthy adults. *Med Sci Sports Exerc*. 2009;41(3):687-708.

51. Malisoux L, Francaux M, Theisen D. What do single-fiber studies tell us about exercise training? *Med Sci Sports Exerc*. 2007;30(7):1051-1060.

52. Thompson LV. Skeletal muscle adaptations with age, inactivity, and therapeutic exercise. *J Orthop Sports Phys Ther*. 2002;32(2):44-57.

53. Sale DG. Neural adaptation to resistance training. *Med Sci Sports Exerc*. 1988;20(5 Suppl):S135-S145.

54. del Olmo MF, Reimunde P, Viana O, Acero RM, Cudeiro J. Chronic neural adaptation induced by long-term resistance training in humans. *Eur J Appl Physiol*. 2006;96(6):722-728.

55. Gabriel DA, Kamen G, Frost G. Neural adaptations to resistive exercise: mechanisms and recommendations for training practices. *Sports Med*. 2006;36(2):133-149.

56. Hortobagyi T, Dempsey L, Fraser D, et al. Changes in muscle strength, muscle fibre size and myofibrillar gene expression after immobilization and retraining in humans. *J Physiol*. 2000;524(1):293-304.

57. Moritani T, DeVries HA. Neural factors versus hypertrophy in the time course of muscle strength gain. *Am J Phys Med*. 1979;58(3):115-130.

58. Lee WS, Cheung WH, Qin L, Tang N, Leung KS. Age-associated decrease of type IIA/B human skeletal muscle fibers. *Clin Orthop Relat Res*. 2006;450:231-237.

59. Thompson LV. Effects of age and training on skeletal muscle physiology and performance. *Phys Ther*. 1994;74(1):71-81.

60. Hislop HJ, Avers D, Brown M. *Daniels and Worthingham's Manual Muscle Testing. Techniques of Manual Examination*. 9th ed. Elsevier Saunders; 2014.

61. Escamilla R, Barrentine S, Fleisig G, et al. Pitching biomechanics as a pitcher approaches muscular fatigue during a simulated baseball game. *Am J Sports Med*. 2007;35(1):23-33.

62. Hoy MG, Zajac FE, Gordon ME. A musculoskeletal model of the human lower extremity: the effect of muscle, tendon, and moment arm on the moment-angle relationship of musculotendon actuators at the hip, knee, and ankle. *J Biomech*. 1990;23(2):157-169.

63. Gordon AM, Huxley AF, Julian FJ. The variation in isometric tension with sarcomere length in vertebrate muscle fibres. *J Physiol*. 1966;184(1):170-192.

64. Brughelli M, Cronin J. Altering the length-tension relationship with eccentric exercise: implications for performance and injury. *Sports Med*. 2007;37(9):807-826.

65. Brunello E, Bianco P, PIazzesi G, et al. Structural changes in the myosin filament and cross-bridges during active force development in single intact frog muscle fibres: stiffness and X-ray diffraction measurements. *J Physiol*. 2006;577(Pt 3):971-984.

66. Enoka RM. *Neuromechanics of Human Movement*. 5th ed. Human Kinetics; 2019.

67. Purslow PP. Muscle fascia and force transmission. *J Bodyw Mov Ther*. 2010;14(4):411-417.

68. Close RI. Dynamic properties of mammalian skeletal muscles. *Physiol Rev*. 1972;52(1):129-197.

69. Cormie P, McGuigan MR, Newton RU. Developing maximal neuromuscular power: part 1—biological basis of maximal power production. *Sports Med*. 2011;41(1):17-38.

70. Grossman MR, Sahrmann SA, Rose SJ. Review of length-associated changes in muscle. Experimental evidence and clinical implications. *Phys Ther*. 1982;62(12):1799-1808.

71. Tabary JC, Tabary C, Tardieu C, Tardieu G, Goldspink G. Physiological and structural changes in the cat's soleus muscle due to immobilization at different lengths by plaster casts. *J Physiol*. 1972;224(1):231-244.

72. Billeter H, Hoppeler H. Muscular basis of strength. In: Komi PV, ed. *Strength and Power in Sport*. Blackwell Scientific; 1992.

73. Edman KA. Mechanism underlying double-hyperbolic force-velocity relation in vertebrate skeletal muscle. *Adv Exp Med Biol*. 1993;332:667-676.

74. Kenney WL, Wilmore JH, Costill DL. *Physiology of Sport and Exercise*. 6th ed. Human Kinetics; 2015.

75. Ojasto T, Häkkinen K. Effects of different accentuated eccentric load levels in eccentric-concentric actions on acute neuromuscular, maximal force, and power responses. *J Strength Cond Res*. 2009;23(3):996-1004.

76. Bencke J, Damsgaard R, Saekmose A, Jørgensen P, Jørgensen K, Klausen K. Anaerobic power and muscle strength characteristics of 11 years old elite and non-elite boys and girls from gymnastics, team handball, tennis and swimming. *Scand J Med Sci Sports*. 2002;12(3):171-178.

77. Markovic G, Mikulic P. Neuro-musculoskeletal and performance adaptations to lower-extremity plyometric training. *Sports Med*. 2010;40(10):859-895.

78. Stamford B. The difference between strength and power. *Phys Sportsmed*. 1985;13(7):155.

79. Kotzamanidis C, Chatzopoulos D, Michailidis C, Papaiakovou G, Patikas D. The effect of a combined high-intensity strength and speed training program on the running and jumping ability of soccer players. *J Strength Cond Res*. 2005;19(2):369-375.

80. Sayers SP, Gibson K. Effects of high-speed power training on muscle performance and braking speed in older adults. *J Aging Res*. 2012;2012:426278. doi:10.1155/2012/426278

81. Knuttgen HG. Strength training and aerobic exercise: comparison and contrast. *J Strength Cond Res*. 2007;21(3):973-978.

82. Weiss LW, Coney HD, Clark FC. Differential functional adaptations to short-term low-, moderate-, and high-repetition weight training. *J Strength Cond Res*. 1999;13(3):236-241.

83. Stone WJ, Coulter SP. Strength/endurance effects from three resistance training protocols with women. *J Strength Cond Res*. 1994;8(4):231-234.

84. Staron RS, Karapondo DL, Kraemer WJ, et al. Skeletal muscle adaptations during early phase of heavy-resistance training in men and women. *J Appl Physiol*. 1994;76(3):1247-1255.

85. Kraemer WJ. A series of studies—the physiological basis for strength training in American football: fact over philosophy. *J Strength Cond Res*. 1997;11(3):131-142.

86. Anderson T, Kearney JT. Effects of three resistance training programs on muscular strength and absolute and relative endurance. *Res Q Exerc Sport*. 1982;53(1):1-7.

87. Berger RA. Optimal repetitions for the development of strength. *Research Quarterly*. 1962;33:334-338.

88. Bird SP, Tarpenning KM, Marino FE. Designing resistance training programmes to enhance muscular fitness: a review of the acute programme variables. *Sports Med*. 2005;35(10):841-851.

89. Fleck SJ, Kraemer WJ. *Designing Resistance Training Programs*. 4th ed. Human Kinetics; 2014.

90. Baechle TR, Earle RW, Wathen D. Resistance training. In: Baechle TR, Earle RW, eds. *Essentials of Strength Training and Conditioning*. 3rd ed. Human Kinetics; 2008:381-412.

91. Kraemer WJ, Ratamess NA. Fundamentals of resistance training: progression and exercise prescription. *Med Sci Sports Exerc*. 2004;36(4):674-688.

92. Rhea MR, Ball SD, Phillips WT, Burkett LN. A comparison of linear and daily undulating periodized programs with equated volume and intensity for strength. *J Strength Cond Res*. 2002;16(2):250-255.

93. Feigenbaurm MS, Pollock ML. Prescription of resistance training for health and disease. *Med Sci Sports Exerc*. 1999;31(1):38-45.

94. Rhea MR, Alvar BA, Burkett LN, Ball SD. A meta-analysis to determine the dose response for strength development. *Med Sci Sports Exerc*. 2003;35(3):456-464.

95. Slysz J, Stultz J, Burr JF. The efficacy of blood flow restricted exercise: A systematic review & meta-analysis. *J Sci Med Sport*. 2016;19(8):669-675.

96. Hoyt BW, Pavey GJ, Pasquina PF, Potter BK. Rehabilitation of lower extremity trauma: a review of principles and military perspective on future directions. *Curr Trauma Rep*. 2015;1(1):50-60.

97. van Wessel T, de Haan A, van der Laarse WJ, Jaspers RT. The muscle fiber type-fiber size paradox: hypertrophy or oxidative metabolism? *Eur J Appl Physiol*. 2010;110(4):665-694.

98. Ratamess NA. Adaptations to anaerobic training programs. In: Baechle TR, Earle RW, eds. *Essentials of Strength Training and Conditioning*. 3rd ed. Human Kinetics; 2008:93-120.

99. Wolfe BL, LeMura LM, Cole PJ. Quantitative analysis of single- vs. multiple-set programs in resistance training. *J Strength Cond Res*. 2004;18(1):35-47.

100. Rhea MR, Alvar BA, Ball SD, Burkett LN. Three sets of weight training superior to 1 set with equal intensity for eliciting strength. *J Strength Cond Res*. 2002;16(4):525-529.

101. Enoka RM, Duchateau J. Muscle fatigue: what, why and how it influences muscle function. *J Physiol*. 2007;586(1):11-23.

102. Gastin PB. Energy system interaction and relative contribution during maximal exercise. *Sports Med*. 2001;31(10):725-741.

103. Ørtenblad N, Nielsen J. Muscle glycogen and cell function—location, location, location. *Scand J Med Sci Sports*. 2015;25(Suppl 4):34-40.

104. Rashedi E, Nussbaum MA. Quantifying the history dependency of muscle recovery from a fatiguing intermittent task. *J Biomech*. 2017;51(1):26-31.

105. Bogdanis GC. Effects of physical activity and inactivity on muscle fatigue. *Front Physiol*. 2012;3:142. doi:10.3389/fphys.2012.00142

106. Call JA, Warren GL, Verma M, Lowe DA. Acute failure of action potential conduction in mdx muscle reveals new mechanism of contraction-induced force loss. *J Physiol*. 2013;591(Pt 15):3765-3776.

107. Miller RG, Giannini D, Milner-Brown HS, et al. Effects of fatiguing exercise on high-energy phosphates, force, and EMG: evidence for three phases of recovery. *Muscle Nerve*. 1987;10(9):810-821.

108. Allman BL, Rice CL. Incomplete recovery of voluntary isometric force after fatigue is not affected by old age. *Muscle Nerve*. Sep 2001;24(9):1156-1167.

109. Boska MD, Moussavi RS, Carson PJ, Weiner MW, Miller RG. The metabolic basis of recovery after fatiguing exercise of human muscle. *Neurology*. 1990;40(2):240-244.

110. Lind AR. Muscle fatigue and recovery from fatigue induced by sustained contractions. *J Physiol*. 1959;127(1):162-171.

111. So RCH, Ng JK, Ng GYF. Muscle recruitment pattern in cycling: a review. *Phys Ther Sport*. 2005;6(2):89-96.

112. van der Hoeven JH, van Weerden TW, Zwarts MJ. Long-lasting supernormal conduction velocity after sustained maximal isometric contraction in human muscle. *Muscle Nerve*. 1993;16(3):312-320.

113. Allen DG, Lamb GD, Westerblad H. Skeletal muscle fatigue: cellular mechanisms. *Physiol Rev*. 2008;88(1):287-332.

114. Dimitrova NA, Dimitrov GV. Interpretation of EMG changes with fatigue: facts, pitfalls, and fallacies. *J Electromyogr Kinesiol*. 2003;13(1):13-36.

115. Hody S, Rogister B, Leprince P, Wang F, Croisier JL. Muscle fatigue experienced during maximal eccentric exercise is predictive of the plasma creatine kinase (CK) response. *Scand J Med Sci Sports*. 2013;23(4):501-507.

116. McQuade KJ, Hwa Wei S, Smidt GL. Effects of local muscle fatigue on three-dimensional scapulohumeral rhythm. *Clin Biomech*. 1995;10(3):144-148.

117. Sirikul B, Hunter GR, Larson-Meyer DE, Desmond R, Newcomer BR. Relationship between metabolic function and skeletal muscle fatigue during a 90 s maximal isometric contraction. *Appl Physiol Nutr Metab*. 2007;32(3):394-399.

118. Stull GA, Clarke DH. Patterns of recovery following isometric and isotonic strength decrement. *Med Sci Sports*. 1971;3(3):135-139.

119. Sinacore DR, Gulve EA. The role of skeletal muscle in glucose transport, glucose homeostasis, and insulin resistance: implications for physical therapy. *Phys Ther*. 1993;73(12):878-891.

120. Clarke DH. The influence on muscular fatigue patterns of the intercontraction rest interval. *Med Sci Sports*. 1971;3(2):83-88.

121. Stull GA, Kearney JT. Recovery of muscular endurance following submaximal, isometric exercise. *Med Sci Sports*. 1978;10(2):109-112.

122. de Salles BF, Simão R, Miranda F, Novaes Jda S, Lemos A, Willardson JM. Rest interval between sets in strength training. *Sports Med*. 2009;39(9):765-777.

123. De Lateur BJ, Lehmann JF. Therapeutic exercise to develop strength and endurance. In: Kottke FJ, Lehmann JF, eds. *Krusen's Handbook of Physical Medicine and Rehabilitation*. 4th ed. W.B. Saunders; 1990:480-519.

124. Erim Z, DeLuca CJ, Mineo K, Aoki T. Rank-ordered regulation of motor units. *Muscle Nerve*. 1996;19(5):563-573.

125. Clamann HP. Motor unit recruitment and the gradation of muscle force. *Phys Ther*. 1993;73(12):830-843.

126. van Ingen Schenau GJ, Boots PJ, de Groot G, Snackers RJ, van Woensel WW. The constrained control of force and position in multi-joint movements. *Neuroscience*. 1992;46(1):197-207.

127. Osu R, Gomi H. Multijoint muscle regulation mechanisms examined by measured human arm stiffness and EMG signals. *J Neurophysiol*. 1999;81(4):1458-1468.

128. Sangwan S, Green RA, Taylor NF. Characteristics of stabilizer muscles: a systematic review. *Physiother Can*. 2014;66(4):348-358.

129. Gildea JE, HIdes JA, Hodges PW. Size and symmetry of trunk muscles in ballet dancers with and without low back pain. *J Orthop Sports Phys Ther*. 2013;43(8):525-533.

130. Hides JA, Stokes MJ, Saide M, Jull GA, Cooper DH. Evidence of lumbar multifidus muscle wasting ipsilateral to symptoms in patients with acute/subacute low back pain. *Spine*. 1994;19(2):165-172.

131. Knežević O, Mirkov D. Trunk muscle activation patterns in subjects with low back pain. *Vojnosanit Pregl*. 2013;70(3):315-318.

132. Mujika I, Padilla S. Detraining: loss of training-induced physiological and performance adaptations. Part I: short term insufficient training stimulus. *Sports Med*. 2000;30(2):79-87.

133. Erickson LN, Sherry MA. Rehabilitation and return to sport after hamstring strain injury. *J Sport Health Sci*. 2017;6(3):262-270.

134. Bandy WD, Hanten WP. Changes in torque and electromyographic activity of the quadriceps femoris muscles following isometric training. *Phys Ther*. 1993;73(7):455-465.

135. Knapik JJ, Mawdsley RH, Ramos MU. Angular specificity and test mode specficity of isometric and isokinetic strength training. *J Orthop Sports Phys Ther*. 1983;5(2):58-65.

136. Marks R. The effects of 16 months of angle-specific isometric strengthening exercises in midrange on torque of the knee extensor muscles in osteoarthritis of the knee: a case study. *J Orthop Sports Phys Ther*. 1994;20(2):103-109.

137. Sesboüé B, Guincestre JY. Muscular fatigue. *Ann Readapt Med Phys*. 2006;49(6):257-264.

138. Devrome AN, MacIntosh BR. Force-velocity relationship during isometric and isotonic fatiguing contractions. *J Appl Physiol (1985)*. 2018;125(3):706-714.

139. Garland SJ, Gossen ER. The muscular wisdom hypothesis in human muscle fatigue. *Exerc Sport Sci Rev*. 2002;30(1):45-49.

140. Caldwell LS. Relative muscle loading and endurance. Rep 586. *Rep US Army Med Res Lab*. 1963;(July 29):1-11.

141. Hettinger T. *Physiology of Strength*. C.C. Thomas; 1961.

142. MacDougall JD, Elder GC, Sale DG, Moroz JR, Sutton JR. Effects of strength training and immobilization on human muscle fibres. *Eur J Appl Physiol Occup Physiol*. 1980;43(1):25-34.

143. Müller EA. Influence of training and of inactivity on muscle strength. *Arch Phys Med Rehabil*. 1970;51(8):449-462.

144. Hortobágyi T, Katch FI. Eccentric and concentric torque-velocity relationships during arm flexion and extension: influence of strength level. *Eur J Appl Physiol Occup Physiol*. 1990;60(5):395-401.

145. Wilmore JH, Costill DL. *Physiology of Sport and Exercise*. 3rd ed. Human Kinetics; 2004.

146. Gordon JP, Thompson BJ, Crane JS, Bressel E, Wagner DR. Effects of isokinetic eccentric versus traditional lower body resistance training on muscle function: examining a multiple-joint short-term training model. *Appl Physiol Nutr Metab*. 2019;44(2):118-126.

147. Walker S, Blazevich AJ, Haff GG, Tufano JJ, Newton RU, Häkkinen K. Greater strength gains after training with accentuated eccentric than traditional isoinertial loads in already strength-trained men. *Front Physiol*. 2016;7:149. doi:10.3389/fphys.2016.00149

148. Luque-Seron JA, Medina-Porqueres I. Anterior cruciate ligament strain in vivo: a systematic review. *Sports Health*. 2016;8(5):451-455.

149. Fitzgerald GK. Open versus closed kinetic chain exercise: issues in rehabilitation after anterior cruciate ligament reconstructive surgery. *Phys Ther*. 1997;77(12):1747-1754.

150. Bynum EB, Barrack RL, Alexander AH. Open versus closed chain kinetic exercises after anterior cruciate ligament reconstruction. A prospective randomized study. *Am J Sports Med*. 1995;23(4):401-406.

151. Moreside JM, McGill SM. Hip joint range of motion improvements using three different interventions. *J Strength Cond Res*. 2012;26(5):1265-1273.

152. Lutz GE, Palmitier RA, An KN, Chao EY. Comparison of tibiofemoral joint forces during open-kinetic and closed-kinetic-chain exercises. *J Bone Joint Surg Am*. 1993;75(5):732-739.

153. Wilk KE, Escamilla RF, Fleisig GS, Barrentine SW, Andrews JR, Boyd ML. A comparison of tibiofemoral joint forces and electromyographic activity during open and closed kinetic chain exercises. *Am J Sports Med*. 1996;24:518-527.

154. Watanabe S, Kobara K, Yoshimura Y, Osaka H, Ishida H. Influence of trunk muscle co-contraction on spinal curvature during sitting. *J Back Musculoskelet Rehabil*. 2014;27(1):55-61.

155. Tucker WS, Armstrong CW, Gribble PA, Timmons MK, Yeasting RA. Scapular muscle activity in overhead athletes with symptoms of secondary shoulder impingement during closed chain exercises. *Arch Phys Med Rehabil*. 2010;91(4):550-556.

156. Rivera JE. Open versus closed kinetic chain rehabilitation of the lower extremity: a functional and biomechanical analysis. *J Sport Rehabil*. 1994;3(1):154-167.

157. Clark MA, Fater D, Reuterman P. Core (trunk) stabilization and its importance for closed kinetic chain rehabilitation. *Orthop Phys Ther Clin N Am*. 2000;9(2):119-135.

158. Page P, Frank CC, Lardner R. *Assessment and Treatment of Muscle Imbalance: The Janda Approach*. Human Kinetics; 2010.

159. Worsley P, Warner M, Mottram S, et al. Motor control retraining exercises for shoulder impingement: effects on function, muscle activation, and biomechanics in young adults *J Shoulder Elbow Surg*. 2013;22(4):e11-e19.

160. Roy JS, Moffet H, Hébert LJ, Lirette R. Effect of motor control and strengthening exercises on shoulder function in persons with impingement syndrome: A single-subject study design. *Man Ther*. 2009;14(2):180-188.

161. McMullen J, Uhl TL. A kinetic chain approach for shoulder rehabilitation. *J Athl Train*. 2000;35(3):329-337.

162. Lorenz D, Morrison S. Current concepts in periodization of strength and conditioning for the sports physical therapist. *Int J Sports Phys Ther*. 2015;10(6):734-747.

163. Werner G. Strength and conditioning techniques in the rehabilitation of sports injury. *Clin Sports Med*. 2010;29(1):177-191.

164. Greenberg EM, Greenberg ET, Albaugh J, Storey E, Ganley TJ. Rehabilitation practice patterns following anterior cruciate ligament reconstruction: a survey of physical therapists. *J Orthop Sports Phys Ther*. 2018;48(10):801-811.

165. Schoenfeld BJ, Peterson MD, Ogborn D, Contreras B, Sonmez GT. Effects of low- vs. high-load resistance training on muscle strength and hypertrophy in well-trained men. *J Strength Cond Res*. 2015;29(10):2954-2963.

166. Müller EA. Training muscle strength. *Ergonomics*. 1959;2:216-222.

167. Housh DJ, Housh TJ. The effects of unilateral velocity-specific concentric strength training. *J Orthop Sports Phys Ther*. 1993;17(5):252-256.

168. Wallis EL, Logan GA. *Figure Improvement and Body Conditioning Through Exercise*. Prentice-Hall; 1964.

169. Duchateau J, Semmler J, Enoka RM. Training adaptations in the behavior of human motor units. *J Appl Physiol*. 2006;101(6):1766-1775.

170. Hopkins JT, Ingersoll CD. Arthrogenic muscle inhibition: a limiting factor in joint rehabilitation. *J Sport Rehabil*. 2000;9(2):135-159.

171. Morrissey MC. Reflex inhibition of thigh muscles in knee injury. Causes and treatment. *Sports Med*. 1989;7:263-276.

172. Rice DA, McNair PJ. Quadriceps arthrogenic muscle inhibition: neural mechanisms and treatment perspectives. *Semin Arthritis Rheum*. 2010;40(3):250-266.

173. Hale SA, Hertel J, Olmsted-Kramer LC. The effect of a 4-week comprehensive rehabilitation program on postural control and lower extremity function in individuals with chronic ankle instability. *J Orthop Sports Phys Ther*. 2007;37(6):303-311.

174. Kamen G. Neural issues in the control of muscular strength. *Res Q Exerc Sport*. 2004;75(1):3-8.

175. de Ruiter CJ, Van Leeuwen D, Heijblom A, Bobbert MF, de Haan A. Fast unilateral isometric knee extension torque development and bilateral jump height. *Med Sci Sports Exerc*. 2006;38(10):1843-1852.

176. Houglum P. Modality of therapeutic exercise: objectives and principles. *Athl Train*. 1977;12(1):42-45.

177. Folland JP, Williams AG. The adaptations to strength training: morphological and neurological contributions to increased strength. *Sports Med*. 2007;37(2):145-168.

178. Pietrosimone B, Blackburn JT, Harkey MS, Luc BA, Pamukoff DN, Hart JM. Clinical strategies for addressing muscle weakness following knee injury. *Clin Sports Med*. 2015;34(2):285-300.

179. DeLorme TL, Watkins AL. Technics of progressive resistance exercise. *Arch Phys Med Rehabil*. 1948;29(5):263-273.

180. Joshua AM, D'Souza V, Unnikrishnan B, et al. Effectiveness of progressive resistance strength training versus traditional balance exercise in improving balance among the elderly—a randomised controlled trial. *J Clin Diagn Res*. 2014;8(3):98-102.

181. Zinovieff AN. Heavy-resistance exercises the "Oxford technique". *Br J Phys Med*. 1951;14(6):129-132.

182. Knight KL. Guidelines for rehabilitation of sports injuries. *Clin Sports Med*. 1985;4(3):405-416.

Chapter 14

1. Laskowski ER, Newcomer-Aney K, Smith J. Proprioception. *Phys Med Rehabil Clin N Am*. 2000;11(2):323-340.

2. Berne RM, Levy MN. *Physiology*. Mosby; 1998.

3. Proske U, Gandevia SC. The proprioceptive senses: Their roles in signaling body shape, body position and movement, and muscle force. *Physiol Rev*. 2012;92(4):1651-1697.

4. Proske U. Kinesthesia: The role of muscle receptors. *Muscle Nerve*. 2006;34(5):545-558.

5. Clark F, Burgess R, Chapin J, Lipscomb W. Role of intramuscular receptors in the awareness of limb position. *J Neurophysiol*. 1985;54(6):1529-1540.

6. Moberg E. The role of cutaneous afferents in position sense, kinaesthesia, and motor function of the hand. *Brain*. 1983;106(Pt 1):1-19.

7. Proske U. The role of muscle proprioceptors in human limb position sense: A hypothesis. *J Anat*. 2015;227(2):178-183.

8. Hewett T, Paterno M, Myer G. Strategies for enhancing proprioception and neuromuscular control of the knee. *Clin Orthop*. 2002;402:76-94.

9. Pap G, Machner A, Awiszus F. Proprioceptive deficits in anterior cruciate ligament deficient knees: Do they really exist? *Sports Exerc Injury*. 1997;3(3):139-142.

10. Nishikawa T, Grabiner MD. Peroneal motoneuron excitability increases immediately following application of a semirigid ankle brace. *J Orthop Sports Phys Ther*. 1999;29(3):168-176.

11. Rassier DE, Herzog W. Force enhancement and relaxation rates after stretch of activated muscle fibres. *Proc Biol Sci*. 2005;272(1562):475-480.

12. Rimmer JH. Exercise and physical activity in persons aging with a physical disability. *Phys Med Rehabil Clin North Am*. 2005;16(1):41-56.

13. Dean E. Physiology and therapeutic implications of negative work: A review. *Phys Ther*. 1988;68:233-237.

14. Postash DH, Chu DA. Plyometric training. In: Baechle TR, Earle RW, eds. *Essentials of Strength Training and Conditioning*. Human Kinetics; 2008:413-456.

15. Cormie P, McGuigan MR, Newton RU. Developing maximal neuromuscular power: Part 1—Biological basis of maximal power production. *Sports Med*. 2011;41(1):17-38.

16. Lundberg A, Malmgren K, Schomburg ED. Reflex pathways from group II muscle afferents. 2. Functional characteristics of reflex pathways to alpha-motoneurones. *Exp Brain Res*. 1987;65(2):282-293.

17. Illert M. Monosynaptic Ia pathways and motor behaviour of the cat distal forelimb. *Acta Neurobiol Exp (Wars)*. 1996;56(1):423-434.

18. Moore M. Golgi tendon organs: Neuroscience update with relevance to stretching and proprioception in dancers. *J Dance Med Sci*. 2007;11(3):85-92.

19. Grigg P. Peripheral neural mechanisms in proprioception. *J Sport Rehabil*. 1994;3:2-17.

20. Proske U, Gandevia SC. The kinaesthetic senses. *J Physiol*. 2009;587(17):4139-4146.

21. Collins DF, Refshauge KM, Gandevia SC. Sensory integration in the perception of movements at the human metacarpophalangeal joint. *J Physiol*. 2000;529:505-515.

22. Grill SE, Hallett M. Velocity sensitivity of human muscle spindle afferents and slowly adapting type II cutaneous mechanoreceptors. *J Physiol*. 1995;489:593-602.

23. Rudomin P. Selectivity of the central control of sensory information in the mammalian spinal cord. *Adv Exp Med Biol*. 2002;508:157-170.

24. Courtney CA, Witte PO, Chmell SJ, Hornby TG. Heightened flexor withdrawal response in individuals with knee osteoarthritis is modulated by joint compression and joint mobilization. *J Pain*. 2010;11(2):179-185.

25. Leroux A, Bélanger M, Boucher JP. Pain effect on monosynaptic and polysynaptic reflex inhibition. *Arch Phys Med Rehabil*. 1995;76(6):576-582.

26. Burgess PR, Clark FJ. Characteristics of knee joint receptors in the cat. *J Physiol*. 1969;203(2):317-335.

27. Burgess PR, Wei JY, Clark FJ, Simon J. Signaling of kinesthetic information by peripheral sensory receptors. *Annu Rev Neurosci*. 1982;5:171-187.

28. Fuchs S, Tibesku CO, Frisse D, Genkinger M, Laass H, Rosenbaum D. Clinical and functional comparison of uni- and bicondylar sledge prostheses. *Knee Surg Sports Traumatol Arthrosc*. 2005;13(3):197-202.

29. Clark FJ, Grigg P, Chapin JW. The contribution of articular receptors to proprioception with the fingers in humans. *J Neurophysiol*. 1989;61(1):186-193.

30. Gabriel DA, Kamen G, Frost G. Neural adaptations to resistive exercise: mechanisms and recommendations for training practices. *Sports Med*. 2006;36(2):133-149.

31. Strasmann T, van der Wal JC, Halata Z, Drukker J. Functional topography and ultrastructure of periarticular mechanoreceptors in the lateral elbow region of the rat. *Acta Anat*. 1990;138(1):1-14.

32. Gandevia SC, Burke D, McKeon B. The projection of muscle afferents from the hand to cerebral cortex in man. *Brain*. 1984;107:1-13.

33. Prochazka A, Gorassini M. Ensemble firing of muscle afferents recorded during normal locomotion in cats. *J Physiol*. 1998;507:293-304.

34. Stein RB, Weber DJ, Aoyagi Y, et al. Coding of position by simultaneously recorded sensory neurones in the cat dorsal root ganglion. *J Physiol*. 2004;560:883-896.

35. Luu BL, Day BL, Cole JD, Fitzpatrick RC. The fusimotor and reafferent origin of the sense of force and weight. *J Physiol*. 2011;589:3135-3147.

36. Weerakkody NS, Percival P, Canny BJ, Morgan DL, Proske U. Force matching at the elbow joint is disturbed by muscle soreness. *Somatosens Mot Res*. 2003;20(1):27-32.

37. Kavounoudias A, Roll JP, Anton JL, Nazarian B, Roth M, Roll R. Proprio-tactile integration for kinesthetic perception: An fMRI study. *Neuropsychologia*. 2008;46(2):567-575.

38. Fuentes CT, Bastian AJ. Where is your arm? Variations in proprioception across space and tasks. *J Neurophysiol*. 2010;103(1):164-171.

39. Verhagen E, van der Beek A, Twisk J, Bouter L, Bahr R, van Mechelen W. The effect of a proprioceptive balance board training program for the prevention of ankle sprains: A prospective controlled trial. *Am J Sports Med*. 2004;32(6):1385-1393.

40. Lee HM, Cheng CK, Liau JJ. Correlation between proprioception, muscle strength, knee laxity, and dynamic standing balance in patients with chronic anterior cruciate ligament deficiency. *Knee*. 2009;16(5):387-391.

41. Sasagawa S, Ushiyama J, Masani K, Kouzaki M, Kanehisa H. Balance control under different passive contributions of the ankle extensors: Quiet standing on inclined surfaces. *Exp Brain Res*. 2009;196(4):537-544.

42. Bouisset S, Do MC. Posture, dynamic stability, and voluntary movement. *Neurophysiol Clin*. 2008;38(6):345-362.

43. Guerraz M, Bronstein AM. Ocular versus extraocular control of posture and equilibrium. *Neurophysiol Clin*. 2008;38(6):391-398.

44. Horak FB. Postural compensation for vestibular loss. *Ann NY Acad Sci*. 2009;1164:76-81.

45. Enoka RM. *Neuromechanics of Human Movement*. Human Kinetics; 2008.

46. DiGiulio I, Maganaris CN, Baltzopoulos V, Loram ID. The proprioceptive and agonist roles of gastrocnemius, soleus and tibialis anterior muscles in maintaining human upright posture. *J Physiol*. 2009;587:2399-2416.

47. Terada M, Kosik KB, McCann RS, Gribble PA. Diaphragm contractility in individuals with chronic ankle instability. *Med Sci Sport Exerc*. 2016;48(10):2040-2045. doi:10.1249/MSS.0000000000000994

48. Witchalls J, Blanch P, Waddington G, Adams R. Intrinsic functional deficits associated with increased risk of ankle injuries: A systematic review with meta-analysis. *Br J Sports Med*. 2012;46(7):515-520.

49. Iatridou K, Mandalidis D, Chronopoulos E, Vagenas G, Athanasopoulos S. Static and dynamic body balance following provocation of the visual and vestibular systems in females with and without joint hypermobility syndrome. *J Bodyw Mov Ther*. 2014;18(2):159-164.

50. Butler RJ, Lehr ME, Fink ML, Kiesel KB, Plisky PJ. Dynamic balance performance and noncontact lower extremity injury in college football players: An initial study. *Sports Health*. 2013;5(5):417-422.

51. Olivier B, Stewart A, Olorunju SA, Mckinon W. Static and dynamic balance ability, lumbo-pelvic movement control and injury incidence in cricket pace bowlers. *J Sci Med Sport*. 2015;18(1):19-25.

52. Di Stasi SL, Myer GD, Hewett TE. Neuromuscular training to target deficits associated with second anterior cruciate ligament injury. *J Orthop Sports Phys Ther*. 2013;43(11):777-792.

53. Gribble PA, Hertel J, Plisky P. Using the Star Excursion Balance Test to assess dynamic postural-control deficits and outcomes in lower extremity injury: A literature and systematic review. *J Athl Train*. 2012;47(3):339-357.

54. Cohen H, Blatchly CA, Gombash LL. A study of the clinical test of sensory interaction and balance. *Phys Ther*. 1993;73(6):346-351.

55. Vereeck L, Wuyts F, Truijen S, Van de Heyning P. Clinical assessment of balance: Normative data, and gender and age effects. *Int J Audiol*. 2008;47(2):67-75. doi:10.1080/14992020701689688

56. Agrawal Y, Carey JP, Hoffman HJ, Sklare DA, Schubert MC. The modified Romberg Balance Test: Normative data in U.S. adults. *Otol Neurotol*. 2011;32(8):1309-1311.

57. El Haber N, Erbas B, Hill KD, Wark JD. Relationship between age and measurement of balance, strength and gait: Linear and non-linear analyses. *Clin Sci*. 2008;114(12):719-727.

58. Gill J, Allum JH, Carpenter MG, et al. Trunk sway measures of postural stability during clinical balance tests: Effects of age. *J Gerontol A Biol Sci Med Sci*. 2001;56(7):M438-M447.

59. Gribble P, Kaminski TW. The Star Excursion Balance Test as a measurement tool. *Athl Ther Today*. 2003;8(2):46-47.

60. Hertel J, Braham RA, Hale S, Olmsted-Kramer LC. Simplifying the Star Excursion Balance Test: Analyses of subjects with and without chronic ankle instability. *J Orthop Sports Phys Ther*. 2006;36(3):131-137.

61. Coughlan GF, Fullam K, Delahunt E, Gissane C, Caulfield BM. A comparison between performance on selected directions of the Star Excursion Balance Test and the Y balance test. *J Athl Train*. 2012;47(4):366-371.

62. Fullam K, Caulfield B, Coughlan GF, Delahunt E. Kinematic analysis of selected reach directions of the Star Excursion Balance Test compared with the Y-Balance Test. *J Sport Rehabil*. 2014;23(1):27-35.

63. Hertel J, Miller SJ, Denegar CR. Intratester and intertester reliability during the Star Excursion Balance Tests. *J Sport Rehabil*. 2000;9(2):104-116.

64. Westrick RB, Miller JM, Carow SD, Gerber JP. Exploration of the y-balance test for assessment of upper quarter closed kinetic chain performance. *Int J Sports Phys Ther*. 2012;7(2):139-147.

65. Hoy KE, Fitzgerald PB, Bradshaw JL, Armatas CA, Georgiou-Karistianis N. Investigating the cortical origins of motor overflow. *Brain Res Brain Res Rev*. 2004;46(3):315-327. doi:10.1016/j.brainresrev.2004.07.013. PMID: 15571773

66. Smith JA, Popovich JM, Kulig K. The influence of hip strength on lower-limb, pelvis, and trunk kinematics and coordination patterns during walking and hopping in healthy women. *J Orthop Sports Phys Ther*. 2014;44(7):525-531.

67. Carson RG. Changes in muscle coordination with training. *J Appl Physiol*. 2006;101(5):1506-1513.

68. Kottke FJ, Halpern D, Easton JK, Ozel AT, Burrill CA. The training of coordination. *Arch Phys Med Rehabil*. 1978;59(12):567-572.

69. Lephart SM, Pincivero DM, Rozzi SL. Proprioception of the ankle and knee. *Sports Med.* 1998;25(3):149-155.

70. Armstrong A, Issartel J, Varlet M, Marin L. The supplementation of spatial information improves coordination. *Neurosci Lett.* 2013;548:212-216.

71. Finley JM, Dhaher YY, Perreault EJ. Regulation of feed-forward and feedback strategies at the human ankle during balance control. *Conf Proc IEEE Eng Med Biol Soc.* 2009;2009:7265-7268.

72. Nishikawa K, Biewener AA, Aerts P, et al. Neuromechanics: An integrative approach for understanding motor control. *Integr Comp Biol.* 2007;47(1):16-54. doi:10.1093/icb/icm024

73. Wagner MJ, Smith MA. Shared internal models for feedforward and feedback control. *J Neurosci.* 2008;28(42):10663-10673.

74. Yousif N, Diedrichsen J. Structural learning in feedforward and feedback control. *J Neurophysiol.* 2012;108(9):2373-2382.

75. Kottke FJ. From reflex to skill: The training of coordination. *Arch Phys Med Rehabil.* 1980;61(12):551-561.

76. Monfils MH, Plautz EJ, Kleim JA. In search of the motor engram: Motor map plasticity as a mechanism for encoding motor experience. *Neuroscientist.* 2005;11:471-483.

77. Halsband U, Lange RK. Motor learning in man: A review of functinoal and clinical studies. *J Physiol Paris.* 2006;99(4-6):414-424.

78. Kottke FJ. Therapeutic exercise to maintain mobility. In: Kottke FJ, Stillwell GK, Lehmann JF, eds. *Krusen's Handbook of Physical Medicine and Rehabilitation.* W.B. Saunders; 1982.

79. Hrysomallis C. Balance ability and athletic performance. *Sports Med.* 2011;41(3):221-232.

80. Lephart SM, Kocher MS, Fu FH, Borsa PA, Harner CD. Proprioception following ACL reconstruction. *J Sport Rehabil.* 1992;1:188-196.

81. Baltaci G, Aktas G, Camci E, Oksuz S, Yildiz S, Kalaycioglu T. The effect of prophylactic knee bracing on performance: Balance, proprioception, coordination, and muscular power. *Knee Surg Sports Traumatol Arthrosc.* 2011;19(10):1722-1728.

82. Beynnon BD, Good L, Risberg MA. The effect of bracing on proprioception of knees with anterior cruciate ligament injury. *J Orthop Sports Phys Ther.* 2002;32(1):11-15.

83. Willems T, Witvrouw E, Verstuyft J, Vaes P, De Clercq D. Proprioception and muscle strength in subjects with a history of ankle sprains and chronic instability. *J Athletic Train.* 2002;37(4):487-493.

84. Perlau R, Frank C, Fick G. The effect of elastic bandages on human knee proprioception in the uninjured population. *Am J Sports Med.* 1995;23:251-255.

85. Blackburn T, Guskiewicz KM, Petschauer MA, Prentice WE. Balance and joint stability: the relative contributions of proprioception and muscular strength. *J Sport Rehabil.* 2000;9(4):315-328.

86. Risberg MA, Beynnon BD, Peura GD, Uh BS. Proprioception after anterior cruciate ligament reconstruction with and without bracing. *Knee Surg Sports Traumatol Arthrosc.* 1999;7(5):303-309.

87. Callaghan MJ, Selfe J, Bagley PJ, Oldham JA. The effects of patellar taping on knee joint proprioception. *J Athl Train.* 2002;37:19-24.

88. Barrack RL, Lund PJ, Skinner HB. Knee joint proprioception revisited. *J Sport Rehabil.* 1994;3:18-42.

89. Raymond J, Nicholson LL, HIller CE, Refshauge KM. The effect of ankle taping or bracing on proprioception in functional ankle instability: A systematic review and meta-analysis. *J Sci Med Sport.* 2012;15(5):386-392.

90. Lephart SM, Henry TJ. The physiological basis for open and closed kinetic chain rehabilitation for the upper extremity. *J Sport Rehabil.* 1996;5:71-87.

91. Jerosch J, Prymka M. Knee joint proprioception in normal volunteers and patients with anterior cruciate ligament tears, taking special account of the effect of a knee bandage. *Arch Orthop Trauma Surg.* 1996;115:162-166.

Chapter 15

1. Creighton DW, Shrier I, Shultz R, Meeuwisse WH, Matheson GO. Return-to-play in sport: A decision-based model. *Clin J Sports Med.* 2010;20(5):379-385.

2. Delvaux F, Rochcongar P, Bruyère O, et al. Return-to-play criteria after hamstring injury: Actual medicine practice in professional soccer teams. *J Sports Sci Med.* 2014;13(3):721-723.

3. Clover J, Wall J. Return-to-play criteria following sports injury. *Clin Sports Med.* 2010;29(1):169-175.

4. Draovitch P, Maschi RA, Hettler J. Return to sport following hip injury. *Curr Rev Musculoskelet Med.* 2012;5(1):9-14.

5. Munro AG, Herrington LC. Between session reliability of four hop tests and the agility T-test. *J Strength Cond Res.* 2011;25(5):1470-1477.

6. Manske R, Reiman M. Functional performance testing for power and return to sports. *Sports Health.* 2013;5(3):244-250.

7. Herring SA, Bergfeld JA, Boyd J, et al. The team physician and return-to-play issues: A consensus statement. *Med Sci Sports Exerc.* 2002;34(7):1212-1214.

8. Herring SA, Kibler WB, Putukian M. The team physician and the return-to-play decision: A consensus statement-2012 update. *Med Sci Sports Exerc.* 2012;44(12):2446-2448.

9. Herring SA, Kibler WB, Putukian M. Team physician consensus statement: 2013 update. *Med Sci Sports Exerc.* 2013;45(8):1618-1622.

10. Clanton TO, Matheny LM, Jarvis HC, Jeronimus AB. Return to play in athletes following ankle injuries. *Sports Health.* 2012;4(6):471-474.

11. Beam JW. Rehabilitation including sport-specific functional progression for the competitive athlete. *J Bodyw Mov Ther.* 2002;6(4):205-219.

12. Benjaminse A, Gokeler A, Dowling AV, et al. Optimization of the anterior cruciate ligament injury prevention paradigm: Novel feedback techniques to enhance motor learning and reduce injury risk. *J Orthop Sports Phys Ther.* 2015;45(3):170-182. doi:10.2519/jospt.2015.4986

13. Hrysomallis C. Injury incidence, risk factors and prevention in Australian rules football. *Sports Med.* 2013;43(5):339-354.

14. Halonen KS, Mononen ME, Töyräs J, Kröger H, Joukainen A, Korhonen RK. Optimal graft stiffness and prestrain restore normal joint motion and cartilage responses in ACL reconstructed knee. *Journal of Biomechanics* 2016;49(13):2566-2576.

15. Irvin RW. The origin and relief of common pain. *Journal of Back and Musculoskeletal Rehabilitation*. 1998;11(2):89-130. doi:10.1016/S1053-8127(98)00027-X

16. Sadeghisani M, Manshadi FD, Kalantari KK, et al. Correlation between hip rotation range-of-motion impairment and low back pain: A literature review. *Ortop Traumatol Rehabil*. 2015;17(5):455-462. doi:10.5604/15093492.1186813

17. McGill SM, Karpowicz A, Fenwick CM, Brown SH. Exercises for the torso performed in a standing posture: Spine and hip motion and motor patterns and spine load. *J Strength Cond Res*. 2009;23(2):455-464.

18. Moeller CR, Huxel Bliven KC, Snyder Valier AR. Scapular muscle-activation ratios in patients with shoulder injuries during functional shoulder exercises. *J Athl Train*. 2014;49(3):345-355.

19. Gibson J, McCaron T. Feedforward muscle activity: An investigation into the onset and activity of internal oblique during two functional reaching tasks. *J Bodyw Mov Ther*. 2004;8(2):104-113.

20. Clark NC, Röijezon U, Treleaven J. Proprioception in musculoskeletal rehabilitation. Part 2: Clinical assessment and intervention. *Man Ther*. 2015;20(3):378-387.

21. Lefèvre-Colau MM, Nguyen C, Palazzo C, et al. Kinematic patterns in normal and degenerative shoulders. Part II: Review of 3-D scapular kinematic patterns in patients with shoulder pain, and clinical implications. *Ann Phys Rehabil Med*. 2018;61(1):46-53.

22. Sherry MA, Best TM. A comparison of 2 rehabilitation programs in the treatment of acute hamstring strains. *J Orthop Sports Phys Ther*. 2004;34(3):116-125.

23. Kottke FJ. From reflex to skill: The training of coordination. *Arch Phys Med Rehabil*. 1980;61(12):551-561.

24. Ardern CL, Taylor NF, Feller JA, Whitehead TS, Webster KE. Psychological responses matter in returning to preinjury level of sport after anterior cruciate ligament reconstruction surgery. *Am J Sports Med*. 2013;41(7):1549-1558.

25. Chu D, Myer GD. *Plyometrics*. Human Kinetics; 2013.

26. Risberg M, Mork M, Jenssen H, Holm I. Design and implementation of a neuromuscular training program following anterior cruciate ligament reconstruction. *J Orthop Sports Phys Ther*. 2001;31(11):620-631.

27. Koutedakis Y. Muscle elasticity—plyometrics: Some physiological and practical considerations. *J Appl Res Coach Athl*. 1989;4(1):35-49.

28. Chmielewski T, Kauffman D, Myer GD, Tillman SM. Plyometric exercise in the rehabilitation of athletes: Physiological responses and clinical application. *J Orthop Sports Phys Ther*. 2006;36(5):308-319.

29. Moran JJ, Sandercock GR, Ramirez-Campillo R, Meylan CM, Collison A, Parry DA. Age-related variation in male youth athletes' countermovement jump after plyometric training: A meta-analysis of controlled trials. *J Strength Cond Res*. 2017;31(2):552-565.

30. Cormie P, McGuigan MR, Newton RU. Developing maximal neuromuscular power: Part 2—Training considerations for improving maximal power production. *Sports Med*. 2011;41(2):125-146.

31. Williams GN, Chmielewski T, Rudolph K, Buchanan TS, Snyder-Mackler L. Dynamic knee stability: Current theory and implications for clinicians and scientists. *J Orthop Sports Phys Ther*. 2001;31(10):546-566. doi:10.2519/jospt.2001.31.10.546

32. Wilk KE, Voight ML, Keirns MA, Gambetta V, Andrews JR, Dillman CJ. Stretch-shortening drills for the upper extremities: Theory and clinical application. *J Orthop Sports Phys Ther*. 1993;17(5):225-239.

33. Lundin P. A review of plyometric training. *Strength Cond*. 1985;7:69-74.

34. Roberts TJ. The integrated function of muscles and tendons during locomotion. *Comp Biochem Physiol A Mol Integr Physiol*. 2002;133(4):1087-1099.

35. Cavagna GA. Storage and utilization of elastic energy in skeletal muscles. *Exerc Sport Sci Rev*. 1977;5:89-129.

36. Toumi H, Best T, Martin A, F'Guyer S, Poumarat G. Effects of eccentric phase velocity of plyometric training on the vertical jump. *Int J Sports Med*. 2004;25(5):391-398.

37. Cormie P, McGuigan MR, Newton RU. Developing maximal neuromuscular power: Part 1—Biological basis of maximal power production. *Sports Med*. 2011;41(1):17-38.

38. Sexton P, Chambers J. The importance of flexibility for functional range of motion. *Athl Ther Today*. 2006;11(3):13-15.

39. Saunders PU, Telford RD, Pyne DB, et al. Short-term plyometric training improves running economy in highly trained middle and long distance runners. *J Strength Cond Res*. 2006;20(4):947-954.

40. Kottke FJ. Therapeutic exercise to develop neuromuscular coordination. In: Kottke FJ, Lehmann JF, eds. *Krusen's Handbook of Physical Medicine and Rehabilitation*. 4th ed. Saunders; 1990:452-479.

41. Michailidis Y, Fatouros IG, Primpa E, et al. Plyometrics' trainability in preadolescent soccer athletes. *J Strength Cond Res*. 2013;27(1):38-49.

42. Markovic G, Mikulic P. Neuro-musculoskeletal and performance adaptations to lower-extremity plyometric training. *Sports Med*. 2010;40(10):859-895.

43. Miyaguchi K, Demura S. Relationships between stretch-shortening cycle performance and maximum muscle strength. *J Strength Cond Res*. 2008;22(1):19-24.

44. Postash DH, Chu DA. Plyometric training. In: Baechle TR, Earle RW, eds. *Essentials of Strength Training and Conditioning*. Human Kinetics; 2008:413-456.

45. Knuttgen KG, Kraemer WJ. Terminology and measurement in exercise performance. *J Appl Sport Sci Res*. 1987;1(1):1-10.

46. Arai A, Ishikawa M, Ito A. Agonist-antagonist muscle activation during drop jumps. *Eur J Sport Sci*. 2013;13(5):490-498.

47. Struminger AH, Lewek MD, Goto S, Hibberd E, Blackburn JT. Comparison of gluteal and hamstring activation during five commonly used plyometric exercises. *Clin Biomech*. 2013;28(7):783-789.

48. Makaruk H, Porter JM, Czaplicki A, Sadowski J, Sacewicz T. The role of attentional focus in plyometric training. *J Sports Med Phys Fitness*. 2012;52(3):319-327.

49. Hill J, Leiszler M. Review and role of plyometrics and core rehabilitation in competitive sport. *Curr Sports Med Rep*. 2011;10(6):345-351.

50. Wu YK, Lien YH, Lin KH, Shih TT, Wang TG, Wang HK. Relationships between three potentiation effects of plyometric training and performance. *Scand J Med Sci Sports*. 2010;20(1):e80-e86.

51. Boyd IA. The response of fast and slow nuclear bag fibres and nuclear chain fibres in isolated cat muscle spindles to fusimotor stimulation, and the effect of intrafusal contraction on the sensory endings. *Q J Exp Physiol Cogn Med Sci*. 1976;61(3):203-254.

52. Foure A, Nordez A, Cornu C. Effects of plyometric training on passive stiffness of gastrocnemii muscles and Achilles tendon. *Eur J Appl Physiol*. 2012;112(8):2849-2857.

53. LaStayo PC, Woolf JM, Lewek MD, Snyder-Mackler L, Reich T, Lindstedt SL. Eccentric muscle contractions: Their contribution to injury, prevention, rehabilitation, and sport. *J Orthop Sports Phys Ther*. October 2003;33(10):557-571.

54. Wilson JM, Flanagan EP. The role of elastic energy in activities with high force and power requirements: A brief review. *J Strength Cond Res*. 2008;22(5):1705-1715.

55. Spurrs RW, Murphy AL, Watsford ML. The effect of plyometric training on distance running performance. *Eur J Appl Physiol*. 2003;89(1):1-7.

56. Wilson GJ, Wood GA, Elliott BC. Optimal stiffness of series elastic component in a stretch-shorten cycle activity. *J Appl Physiol*. 1991;70(2):825-833.

57. Bosco C, Komi PV, Ito A. Prestretch potentiation of human skeletal muscle during ballistic movement. *Acta Physiol Scand*. 1981;111(2):135-140.

58. Walshe AD, Wilson GJ, Ettema GJC. Stretch-shorten cycle compared with isometric preload: Contributions to enhanced muscular performance. *J Appl Physiol*. 1998;84(1):97-108.

59. Siff MC. *Supertraining*. 6th ed. Supertraining Institute; 2004.

60. McBride JM, McCaulley GO, Cormie P. Influence of preactivity and eccentric muscle activity on concentric performance during vertical jumping. *J Strength Cond Res*. 2008;22(3):750-757.

61. Malisoux L, Francaux M, Theisen D. What do single-fiber studies tell us about exercise training? *Med Sci Sports Exerc*. 2007;30(7):1051-1060.

62. Hunter JP, Marshall RN. Effects of power and flexibility training on vertical jump technique. *Med Sci Sports Exerc*. 2002;34(3):478-486.

63. Ramirez-Campillo R, Andrade DC, Izquierdo M. Effects of plyometric training volume and training surface on explosive strength. *J Strength Cond Res*. 2012;27(10):2714-2722.

64. Almeida-Silveira MI, Pérot C, Pousson M, Goubel F. Effects of stretch-shortening cycle training on mechanical properties and fibre type transition in the rate soleus muscle. *Pflugers Arch*. 1994;427(3-4):289-294.

65. Pousson M, Pérot C, Goubel F. Stiffness changes and fibre type transitions in rat soleus muscle produced by jumping training. *Pflugers Arch*. 1991;419(2):127-130.

66. Narici MV, Roi GS, Landoni L, Minetti AE, Cerretelli P. Changes in force, cross-sectional area and neural activation during strength training and detraining of the human quadriceps. *Eur J Appl Physiol Occup Physiol*. 1989;59(4):310-319.

67. Higbie EJ, Cureton KJ, Warren GL, 3rd., Prior BM. Effects of concentric and eccentric training on muscle strength, cross-sectional area, and neural activation. *J Appl Physiol*. 1996;81(5):2173-2181.

68. Kraemer WJ, Fleck SJ, Evans WJ. Strength and power training: Physiological mechanisms of adaptation. *Exerc Sport Sci Rev*. 1996;24:363-397.

69. Spurway NC, Watson H, McMillan K, Connolly G. The effect of strength training on the apparent inhibition of eccentric force production in voluntarily activated human quadriceps. *Eur J Appl Physiol*. 2000;82(5-6):374-380.

70. Wilt F. Plyometrics: What it is—how it works. *Athl J*. 1975;55:76-79.

71. Swanik KA, Thomas SJ, Struminger AH, Huxel Bliven KC, Kelly JD, 4th., Swanik CB. The effect of shoulder plyometric training on amortization time and upper extremity kinematics. *J Sport Rehabil*. 2015;25(4):315-323. doi:http://dx.doi.org/10.1123/jsr.2015-0005

72. Slater A, Campbell A, Smith A, Straker L. Greater lower limb flexion in gymnastic landings is associated with reduced landing force: A repeated measures study. *Sports Biomech*. 2015;14(1):45-56.

73. Allerheiligen B, Rogers R. Plyometrics program design. *Strength Condit*. 1995;17:26-31.

74. Willardson JM. A brief review: Factors affecting the length of the rest interval between resistance exercise sets. *J Strength Cond Res*. 2006;20(4):978-984.

75. Chatzinikolaou A, Fatouros IG, Gourgoulis V, et al. Time course of changes in performance and inflammatory responses after acute plyometric exercise. *J Strength Cond Res*. 2010;24(5):1389-1398.

76. Granacher U, Lesinski M, Büsch D, et al. Effects of resistance training in youth athletes on muscular fitness and athletic performance: A conceptual model for long-term athlete development. *Front Physiol*. 2016;7:164. doi:10.3389/fphys.2016.00164

77. Gambetta V. In Roundtable discussion: Practical considerations for utilizing plyometrics. Part 1. *Nat Strength Coach Assoc J*. 1986;8:14-22.

78. Katsikari K, Bassa E, Skoufas D, Lazaridis S, Kotzamanidis C, Patikas DA. Kinetic and kinematic changes in vertical jump in prepubescent girls after 10 weeks of plyometric training. *Pediatr Exerc Sci*. 2020;32(2):81-88. doi:10.1123/pes.2019-0188

79. Faigenbaum AD, Myer GD, Farrell A, et al. Integrative neuromuscular training and sex-specific fitness performance in 7-year-old children: An exploratory investigation. *J Athl Train*. 2014;49(2):145-153. doi:10.4085/1062-6050-49.1.08

80. Konukman F, Erdogan M, Yılmaz İ, Gümüşdağ H. Teaching plyometric drills to children: A skill theme approach. *J Phys Educ Rec Dance*. 2018;89(3):54-56. doi:10.1080/07303084.2018.1419009

81. Negra Y, Chaabene H, Hammami M, Hachana Y, Granacher U. Effects of high-velocity resistance training on athletic performance in prepuberal male soccer athletes. *J Strength Cond Res*. 2016;30(12)doi:10.1519/JSC.0000000000001433

82. Lloyd RS, Radnor JM, De Ste Croix MB, Cronin JB, Oliver JL. Changes in sprint and jump performances after traditional, plyometric, and combined resistance train-

ing in male youth pre- and post-peak height velocity. *J Strength Cond Res*. 2016;30(5):1239-1247. doi:10.1519/JSC.0000000000001216

83. Bedoya AA, Miltenberger MR, Lopez RM. Plyometric training effects on athletic performance in youth soccer athletes: A systematic review. *J Strength Cond Res*. 2015;29(8):2351-2360. doi:10.1519/JSC.0000000000000877

84. Widrick JJ, Stelzer JE, Shoepe TC, Garner DP. Functional properties of human muscle fibers after short-term resistance exercise training. *Am J Physiol Regul Integr Comp Physiol*. 2002;283(2):R408-R416.

85. Ferrigno V, Brown LE, Murray D. Designing sport-specific training programs. In: Brown LE, Ferrigno C, eds. *Training for Speed, Agility, and Quickness*. 2nd ed. Human Kinetics; 2005:223-236.

86. Benjaminse A, Welling W, Otten B, Gokeler A. Novel methods of instruction in ACL injury prevention programs: A systematic review. *Phys Ther Sport*. 2015;16(2):176-186.

87. Hellebrandt FA. Cross education: Ipsilateral and contralateral effects of unimanual training. *J Appl Physiol*. 1951;4(2):136-144.

88. Andersen LL, Nielsen PK, Søgaard K, Andersen CH, Skotte J, Sjøgaard G. Torque-EMG-velocity relationship in female workers with chronic neck muscle pain. *J Biomech*. 2008;41(9):2029-2035.

89. Gignac MAM, Cao X, Ramanathan S, et al. Perceived personal importance of exercise and fears of re-injury: a longitudinal study of psychological factors related to activity after anterior cruciate ligament reconstruction. *BMC Sports Sci Med Rehabil*. 2015;7:4. doi:10.1186/2052-1847-7-4

90. Fuller CW, Walker J, Drawer S. Quantifying the functional rehabilitation of injured football players. *Br J Sports Med*. 2006;40(2):151-157.

91. Soo Hoo ER. Evaluating return-to-work ability using functional capacity evaluation. *Phys Med Rehabil Clin N Am*. 2019;30(3):541-559. doi:10.1016/j.pmr.2019.04.002

92. Idarraga AJ, Wright-Chisem A, Bohl DD, et al. Functional capacity evaluation for injuries to the foot and ankle. *Foot Ankle Int*. 2019;40(11):1282-1287. doi:10.1177/1071100719864694

93. Scheel C, Mecham J, Zuccarello V, Mattes R. An evaluation of the inter-rater and intra-rater reliability of OccuPro's functional capacity evaluation. *Work*. 2018;60(3):465-473. doi:10.3233/WOR-182754

94. Bieniek S, Bethge M. The reliability of WorkWell systems functional capacity evaluation: A systematic review. *BMC Musculoskelet Disord*. 2014;15(1):106. doi:10.1186/1471-2474-15-106

95. Reid A, Birmingham TB, Stratford PW, Alcock GK, Giffin JR. Hop testing provides a reliable and valid outcome measure during rehabilitation after anterior cruciate ligament reconstruction. *Phys Ther*. 2007;87(3):337-349.

96. Hegedus EJ, McDonough SM, Bleakley C, Baxter D, Cook CE. Clinician-friendly lower extremity physical performance tests in athletes: A systematic review of measurement properties and correlation with injury. Part 2—The tests for the hip, thigh, foot and ankle including the star excursion balance test. *Br J Sport Med*. 2015;49(10):649-656. doi:10.1136/bjsports-2014-094341

97. Rodríguez-Rosell D, Mora-Custodio R, Franco-Márquez F, Yáñez-García JM, González-Badillo JJ. Traditional vs. sport-specific vertical jump tests: Reliability, validity, and relationship with the legs strength and sprint performance in adult and teen soccer and basketball players. *J Strength Cond Res*. 2017;31(1):196-206. doi:10.1519/JSC.0000000000001476

98. Whatman C, W. H, Hume P. Kinematics during lower extremity functional screening tests—are they reliable and related to jogging? *Phys Ther Sport*. 2011;12(1):22-29. doi:10.1016/j.ptsp.2010.10.006

99. Lim B, Shin HD, Lee Y. Biomechanical comparison of rotational activities between anterior cruciate ligament- and posterior cruciate ligament-reconstructed patients. *Knee Surg Sports Traumatol Arthrosc*. 2015;23(4):1231-1238.

100. Keays SL, Bullock-Saxton JE, Newcombe P, Keays AC. The relationship between knee strength and functional stability before and after anterior cruciate ligament reconstruction. *J Orthop Res*. 2003;21(2):231-237.

101. Darwich A, Schüttler V, Obertacke U, Jawhar A. Outcome measures to evaluate upper and lower extremity: Which scores are valid? *Z Orthop Unfall*. 2020;158(1):90-103. doi:10.1055/a-0837-1085

102. Decleve P, Van Cant J, De Buck E, Van Doren J, Verkouille J, Cools AM. The self-assessment corner for shoulder strength: Reliability, validity, and correlations with upper extremity physical performance tests. *J Athl Train*. 2020;55(4):350-358. doi:10.4085/1062-6050-471-18

103. Hollstadt K, Boland M, Mulligan I. Test-retest reliability of the closed kinetic chain upper extremity stability test (CKCUEST) in a modified test position in Division I collegiate basketball players. *Int J Sports Phys Ther*. 2020;15(2). PMC7134354,

104. Nazari G, Lu S, MacDermid JC, MPT Student Group. Psychometric properties of performance-based functional tests in patients with shoulder pathologies: A systematic review and meta-analysis. *Arch Phys Med Rehabil*. 2020;101(1):1053-1063. doi:10.1016/j.apmr.2019.11.011

105. Borms D, Cools A. Upper-extremity functional performance tests: Reference values for overhead athletes. *Int J Sports Med*. 2018;39(6):433-441. doi:10.1055/a-0573-1388

106. Negrete RJ, Hanney WJ, Kolber MJ, Davies GJ, Riemann B. Can upper extremity functional tests predict the softball throw for distance: A predictive validity investigation. *Int J Sports Phys Ther*. 2011;6(2):104-111.

Chapter 16

1. Malanga GA, Yan N, Stark J. Mechanisms and efficacy of heat and cold therapies for musculoskeletal injury. *Postgrad Med*. 2015;127(1):57-65.

2. Nadler SF, Weingand K, Kruse RJ. The physiologic basis and clinical applications of cryotherapy and thermotherapy for the pain practitioner. *Pain Phys*. 2004;3:395-399.

3. Järvinen TA, Järvinen TL, Kääriäinen M, et al. Muscle injuries: optimising recovery. *Best Pract Res Clin Rheumatol*. 2007;21(2):317-331.

4. Walls RJ, McHugh G, O'Gorman DJ, Moyna NM, O'Byrne JM. Effects of preoperative neuromuscular electrical stimulation on quadriceps strength and functional

recovery in total knee arthroplasty: A pilot study. *BMC Musculoskelet Disord.* 2010;11:119-127.

5. Feil S, Newell J, Minogue C, Pasessler HH. The effectiveness of supplementing a standard rehabilitation program with superimposed neuromuscular electrical stimulation after anterior cruciate ligament reconstruction: A prospective, randomized, single-blind study. *Am J Sports Med.* 2011;39(6):1238-1247.

6. Farina D, Arendt-Nielsen L, Merletti R, Graven-Nielsen T. Effect of experimental muscle pain on motor unit firing rate and conduction velocity. *J Neurophysiol.* 2004;91(3):1250-1259.

7. Defrin R, Peleg S, Weingarden H, Heruti R, Urca G. Differential effect of supraspinal modulation on the nociceptive withdrawal reflex and pain sensation. *Clin Neurophysiol.* 2007;118(2):427-437.

8. Leroux A, Bélanger M, Boucher JP. Pain effect on monosynaptic and polysynaptic reflex inhibition. *Arch Phys Med Rehabil.* 1995;76(6):576-582.

9. Rice DA, McNair PJ, Dalbeth N. Swelling in the knee joint: The effect of cryotherapy on arthrogenic muscle inhibition of the quadriceps. *N Z J Physiother.* 2008;36(2):91.

10. Rice DA, McNair PJ. Quadriceps arthrogenic muscle inhibition: Neural mechanisms and treatment perspectives. *Semin Arthritis Rheum.* 2010;40(3):250-266.

11. Fahrer H, Rentsch HU, Gerber NJ, Beyeler C, Hess CW, Grunig B. Knee effusion and reflex inhibition of the quadriceps: a bar to effective retraining. *J Bone Joint Surg Br.* 1988;70(4):635-638.

12. Simmonds N, Miller P, Gemmell H. A theoretical framework for the role of fascia in manual therapy. *J Bodyw Mov Ther.* 2010;16(1):83-93.

13. Bialosky JE, Bishop MD, Price DD, Robinson ME, George SZ. The mechanisms of manual therapy in the treatment of musculoskeletal pain: A comprehensive model. *Man Ther.* 2009;14(5):531-538.

14. Mischke JJ, Jayaseelan DJ, Sault JD, Emerson AJ. The symptomatic and functional effects of manual physical therapy on plantar heel pain: a systematic review. *J Man Manip Ther.* 2017;25(1):3-10. doi:10.1080/10669817.2015.1106818

15. Kaltenborn FM. *Manual Mobilization of the Joints: The Kaltenborn Method of Joint Examination and Treatment.* 6th ed. Olaf N Orlis Bokhandel; 2002.

16. Maitland GD. *Peripheral Manipulation.* Butterworth-Heinemann; 1991.

17. Maitland ME, Kawchuck GN. Towards the quantification of end-feel for the assessment of passive joint motion. *Phys Ther Rev.* 1997;2(4):217-226.

18. Smith CM. Origin and uses of primum non nocere—above all, do no harm! *J Clin Pharmacol.* 2005;45(4):371-377.

19. Barton CJ, Lack S, Hemmings S, Tufail S, Morrissey D. The "Best Practice Guide to Conservative Management of Patellofemoral Pain": incorporating level 1 evidence with expert clinical reasoning. *Br J Sports Med.* 2015;49(14):923-934.

20. West JL, Keene JS, Kaplan LD. Early motion after quadriceps and patellar tendon repairs: outcomes with single-suture augmentation. *Am J Sports Med.* 2008;36(2):316-323.

21. Kannus PJ, L., Kvist M, Lehto M, Järvinen M. The effect of immobilization on myotendinous junction: an ultrastructural, histochemical and immunohistochemical study. *Acta Physiol Scand.* 1992;144(3):387-394.

22. Kim U, Choi YS, Jang GC, Choi YR. Early rehabilitation after open repair for patients with a rupture of the Achilles tendon. *Injury.* 2017;48(7):1710-1713.

23. Trudel G, Zhou J, Uhthoff HK, Laneuville O. Four weeks of mobility after 8 weeks of immobility fails to restore normal motion: a preliminary study. *Clin Orthop Relat Res.* 2008;466(5):1239-1244.

24. Kaneguchi A, Ozawa J, Kawamata S, Yamaoka K. Development of arthrogenic joint contracture as a result of pathologic changes in remobilized rat knees. *J Orthop Res.* 2017;35(7):1414-1423.

25. Starr HM, Snoddy M, Hammond KE, Seiler JG, 3rd. Flexor tendon repair rehabilitation protocols: a systematic review. *J Hand Surg Am.* 2013;38(9):1712-1717.

26. Lee D, Stinner D, Mir H. Quadriceps and patellar tendon ruptures. *J Knee Surg.* 2013;26(5):301-308.

27. Keener JD, Galatz LM, Stobbs-Cucchi G, Patton R, Yamaguchi K. Rehabilitation following arthroscopic rotator cuff repair: A prospective randomized trial of immobilization compared with early motion. *J Bone Joint Surg Am.* 2014;96(1):11-19.

28. Lefèvre-Colau MM, Nguyen C, Palazzo C, et al. Kinematic patterns in normal and degenerative shoulders: Part II. Review of 3-D scapular kinematic patterns in patients with shoulder pain, and clinical implications. *Ann Phys Rehabil Med.* 2018;61(1):46-53.

29. Pignanelli C, Petrick HL, Keyvani F, et al. Low-load resistance training to task-failure with and without blood flow restriction: muscular functional and structural adaptations. *Am J Physio Regul Integr Comp Physio.* 2019.

30. Gignac MAM, Cao X, Ramanathan S, et al. Perceived personal importance of exercise and fears of re-injury: a longitudinal study of psychological factors related to activity after anterior cruciate ligament reconstruction. *BMC Sports Sci Med Rehabil.* 2015;7:4. doi:10.1186/2052-1847-7-4

31. Keays SL, Mason M, Newcombe PA. Individualized physiotherapy in the treatment of patellofemoral pain. *Physiother Res Int.* 2015;20(1):22-36.

Chapter 17

1. Blanpied PR, Gross AR, Elliott JM, et al. Neck pain: Revision 2017. *J Orthop Sports Phys Ther.* 2017;47(7):A1-A83.

2. Laplante BL, Ketchum JM, Saullo TR, Depalma MJ. Multivariable analysis of the relationship between pain referral patterns and the source of chronic low back pain. *Pain Physician.* 2012;15(2):171-178.

3. Slipman CW, Jackson HB, Lipetz JS, Chan KT, Lenrow D, Vresilovic EJ. Sacroiliac joint pain referral zones. *Arch Phys Med Rehabil.* 2000;81(3):334-338.

4. Langford ML. Poor posture subjects a worker's body to muscle imbalance, nerve compression. *Occup Health Saf.* 1994;63(9):38-42.

5. Weinstein SI, Yelin EH. *United States Bone and Joint Initiative: The Burden of Musculoskeletal Diseases in the United States (BMUS).* 4th ed. Available at http://www.boneandjointburden.org; 2020. Accessed 2020 Dec 27.

6. Lippa L, Lippa L, Cacciola F. Loss of cervical lordosis: What is the prognosis? *J Craniovertebr Junction Spine.* 2017;8(1):9-14. doi:10.4103/0974-8237.199877

7. Koseki T, Kakizaki F, Hayashi S, Nishida N, Itoh M. Effect of forward head posture on thoracic shape and respiratory function. *J Phys Ther Sci.* 2019;31(1):63-8.

8. Vleeming A, Scheunke MD, Masi AT, Carreiro JE, Danneels L, Willard FH. The sacroiliac joint: An overview of its anatomy, function and potential implications. *J Anat.* 2012;221:5378-567.

9. Willson JD, Dougherty CP, Ireland ML, Davis IM. Core stability and its relationship to lower extremity function and injury. *J Am Acad Orthop Surg.* 2005;13(5):316-325.

10. Kasai Y, Morishita K, Kawakita E, Kondo T, Uchida A. A new evaluation method for lumbar spinal instability: Passive lumbar extension test. *Phys Ther.* 2006;86:1661-1667.

11. Kiapour A, Joukar A, Elgafy H, Erbulut DU, Agarwal AK, Goel VK. Biomechanics of the sacroiliac joint: Anatomy, function, biomechanics, sexual dimorphism, and causes of pain. *Int J Spine Surg.* 2020;14(Suppl 1):3-13. doi:10.14444/6077

12. Nourbakhish MR, Arabloo AM, Salavati M. The relationship between pelvic cross syndrome and chronic low back pain. *J Back Musculoskelet Rehabil.* 2006;19(4):119-128.

13. Smidt GL, Wei SH, McQuade K, Barakatt E, Sun T, Standford W. Sacroiliac motion for extreme hip positions: A fresh cadaver study. *Spine.* 1997;22(18):2073-2082.

14. Cusi MF. Paradigm for assessment and treatment of SIJ mechanical dysfunction. *J Bodyw Mov Ther.* 2010;14(2):152-161.

15. Laslett M. Evidence-based diagnosis and treatment of the painful sacroiliac joint. *J Man Manip Ther.* 2008;16(3):142-152.

16. Franke BA, Jr. Formative dynamics: The pelvic girdle. *J Man Manip Ther.* 2003;11(1):12-40.

17. Vleeming A, Stoeckart R. The role of the pelvic girdle in coupling the spine and the legs: A clinical–anatomical perspective on pelvic stability. In: Vleeming A, Mooney V, Stoeckart R, eds. *Movement, Stability & Lumbopelvic Pain: Integration of Research and Therapy.* 2nd ed. Elsevier; 2007:113-137.

18. Takasaki H, Iizawa T, Hall T, Nakamura T, Kaneko S. The influence of increasing sacroiliac joint force closure on the hip and lumbar spine extensor muscle firing pattern. *Man Ther.* 2009;14(5):484-489.

19. Arumugam A, Milosavljevic S, Woodley S, Sole G. Effects of external pelvic compression on form closure, force closure, and neuromotor control of the lumbopelvic spine—a systematic review. *Man Ther.* 2012;17(4):275-284.

20. Riemann BL, Lephart SM. The sensorimotor system, part I: The physiologic basis of functional joint stability. *J Athl Train.* 2002;37(1):71-79.

21. Brumitt J, Matheson JW, Meira EP. Core stabilization exercise prescription, part 1: Current concepts in assessment and intervention. *Sports Health.* 2013;5(6):504-509.

22. Hodges PW. Core stability exercise in chronic low back pain. *Orthop Clin North Am.* 2003;34(2):245-254.

23. Vleeming A, Schuenke M. Form and force closure of the sacroiliac joints. *PM & R.* 2019;11(Suppl 1):S24-S31. doi:10.1002/pmrj.12205

24. Vleeming A, Stoeckart R, Volkers AC, Snijders CJ. Relation between form and function in the sacroiliac joint: Part I. Clinical anatomical aspects. *Spine.* 1990;15(2):130-132.

25. Pel JJ, Spoor CW, Pool-Goudzwaard AL, Hoek van Dijke GA, Snijders CJ. Biomechanical analysis of reducing sacroiliac joint shear load by optimization of pelvic muscle and ligament forces. *Ann Biomed Eng.* 2008;36(3):415-424.

26. McGill SM, Brown S. Creep response of the lumbar spine to prolonged full flexion. *Clin Biomech.* 1992;7(1):43-46.

27. Riemann BL, Lephart SM. The sensorimotor system, Part II: The role of proprioception in motor control and functional joint stability. *J Athl Train.* 2002;37(1):80-84.

28. O'Sullivan PB, Beales DJ, Beetham JA, et al. Altered motor control strategies in subjects with sacroiliac joint pain during the active straight-leg-raise test. *Spine.* 2002;27(1):E1-8.

29. Allison GT, Morris SL, Lay B. Feedforward responses of transversus abdominis are directionally specific and act asymmetrically: Implications for core stability theories. *J Orthop Sports Phys Ther.* 2008;38(5):228-237.

30. Leinonen V. Neuromuscular control in lumbar disorders. *J Sports Sci Med.* 2004;3(4 Suppl):1-31.

31. Borghuis J, Hof AL, Lemmink KA. The importance of sensory-motor control in providing core stability: Implications for measurement and training. *Sports Med.* 2008;38(11):893-916.

32. Radebold A, Cholewicki J, Panjabi MM, Patel TC. Muscle response pattern to sudden trunk loading in healthy individuals and in patients with chronic low back pain. *Spine.* 2000;25(8):947-954.

33. Kibler WB, Press J, Sciascia A. The role of core stability in athletic function. *Sports Med.* 2006;36(3):189-198.

34. Rudd JR, Barnett LM, Butson ML, Farrow D, Berry J, Polman RC. Fundamental movement skills are more than run, throw and catch: The role of stability skills. *PLoS One.* 2015;10(10):e0140224. doi:10.1371/journal.pone.0140224

35. Boettcher CE, Cahters I, Gionn KA. The role of shoulder muscles is task specific. *J Sci Med Sport.* 2010;13(6):651-656.

36. Almeida GPL, das Neves Rodrigues HL, de Freitas BW, de Paula Lima PO. Reliability and validity of the Hip Stability Isometric Test (HipSIT): A new method to assess hip posterolateral muscle strength. *J Orthop Sports Phys Ther.* 2017;47(12):906-913.

37. Key J. "The core": Understanding it, and retraining its dysfunction. *J Bodyw Mov Ther.* 2013;17(4):541-559.

38. Panjabi M, Abumi K, Duranceau J, Oxland T. Spinal stability and intersegmental muscle forces: A biomechanical model. *Spine.* 1989;14(2):194-200.

39. Akuthota V, Ferreiro A, Moore T, Fredericson M. Core stability exercise principles. *Curr Sports Med Rep.* 2008;7(1):39-44.

40. Fredericson M, Moore T. Core stabilisation training for middle- and long-distance runners. *New Stud Athletics.* 2005;20(1):25-37.

41. Clark MA, Fater D, Reuterman P. Core (trunk) stabilization and its importance for closed kinetic chain rehabilitation. *Orthop Phys Ther Clin N Am.* 2000;9(2):119-135.

42. Kim E, Lee H. The effects of deep abdominal muscle strengthening exercises on respiratory function and lumbar stability. *J Phys Ther Sci.* 2013;25(6):663-665.

43. Hu H, Meijer OG, Hodges PW, et al. Control of the lateral abdominal muscles during walking. *Hum Mov Sci.* 2011;31(4):880-896. doi:10.1016/j.humov.2011.09.002

44. Hodges P, Gandevia SC. Changes in intra-abdominal pressure during postural and respiratory activation of the human diaphragm. *J Appl Physiol.* 2000;89:967-976.

45. Smith A, O'Sullivan P, Straker L. Classification of sagittal thoraco-lumbo-pelvic alignment of the adolescent spine in standing and its relationship to low back pain. *Spine.* 2008;33(19):2101-2107.

46. Dreischarf M, Shirazi-Adl A, Arjmand N, Rohlmann A, Schmidt H. Estimation of loads on human lumbar spine: A review of in vivo and computational model studies. *J Biomech.* 2016;49(6):833-845. doi:10.1016/j.jbiomech.2015.12.038

47. Watanabe S, Eguchi A, Kobara K, Ishida H. Influence of trunk muscle co-contraction on spinal curvature during sitting for desk work. *Electromyogr Clin Neurophysiol.* 2007;47(6):273-278.

48. Kennedy BA. A muscle-bracing technique utilizing intra-abdominal pressure to stabilize the lumbar spine. *Aust J Physiother.* 1967;11:1002-1006.

49. Behm DG, Drinkwater EJ, Willardson JM, Cowley PM, Physiology CSfE. Canadian Society for Exercise Physiology position stand: The use of instability to train the core in athletic and nonathletic conditioning. *Appl Physiol Nutr Metab.* 2010;35(1):109-112.

50. Norris C. Stabilisation mechanisms of the lumbar spine. *Physiother.* 1995;81(2):72-79.

51. Hemborg B, Moritz U, Löwing H. Intra-abdominal pressure and trunk muscle activity during lifting: IV. The causal factors of the intra-abdominal pressure rise. *Scand J Rehabil Med.* 1985;17(1):25-38.

52. Sapsford RR, Hodges PW. Contraction of the pelvic floor muscles during abdominal maneuvers. *Arch Phys Med Rehabil.* 2001;82(8):1081-1088.

53. Arab AM, Chehrehrazi M. The response of the abdominal muscles to pelvic floor muscle contraction in women with and without stress urinary incontinence using ultrasound imaging. *Neurourol Urodyn.* 2011;30(1):117-120.

54. Hodges PW, Butler JE, McKenzie D, Gandevia SC. Contraction of the human diaphragm during rapid postural adjustments. *J Physiol.* 1997;505(2):539-548.

55. Kjær M. Role of extracellular matrix in adaptation of tendon and skeletal muscle to mechanical loading. *Physiol Rev.* 2004;84(2):649-698.

56. Flanagan EP, Harrison AJ. Muscle dynamics differences between legs in healthy adults. *J Strength Cond Res.* 2007;21(1):67-72.

57. Warren L, Baker R, Nasypany A, Seegmiller J, Mokha M. Core concepts: Understanding the complexity of the spinal stabilizing systems in local and global injury prevention and treatment. *Int J Athl Ther Train.* 2014;19(6):28-33.

58. Akuthota V, Nadler SF. Core strengthening. *Arch Phys Med Rehabil.* 2004;85(3):S86-S92.

59. Frank C, Kobesova A, Kolar P. Dynamic neuromuscular stabilization & sports rehabilitation. *Int J Sports Med.* 2013;8(1):62-73.

60. Valenza MC, Cabrera-Martos I, Torres-Sanchez I, Garces A, Mateos-Toset S, Valenza-Demet G. The effects of doming of the diaphragm technique in subjects with short hamstring syndrome: A randomized controlled trial. *J Sport Rehabil.* 2015;24(4):342-348. doi:10.1123/jsr.2014-0190

61. Bergmark A. Stability of the lumbar spine: A study in mechanical engineering. *Acta Orthop Scand.* 1989;60(Suppl 230):1-54.

62. McGill SM. Low back stability: From formal description to issues for performance and rehabilitation. *Exerc Sport Sci Rev.* 2001;29(1):26-31.

63. Wilke HJ, Wolf S, Claes LE, Arand M, Wiesend A. Stability increase of the lumbar spine with different muscle groups: A biomechanical in vitro study. *Spine.* 1995;20(2):192-198.

64. Faries MD, Greenwood M. Core training: Stabilizing the confusion. *Strength Condition J.* 2007;29(2):10-25.

65. Huxel Bliven KC, Anderson BE. Core stability training for injury prevention. *Sports Health.* 2013;5(6):514-522.

66. Hewett TE, Myer GD, Ford KR. Reducing knee and anterior cruciate ligament injuries among female athletes: A systematic review of neuromuscular training interventions. *J Knee Surg.* 2005;18(1):82-88.

67. Leetun DT, Ireland ML, Willson JD, Ballantyne BT, Davis IM. Core stability measures as risk factors for lower extremity injury in athletes. *Med Sci Sports Exerc.* 2004;36(6):926-934.

68. Terada M, Kosik KB, McCann RS, Gribble PA. Diaphragm contractility in individuals with chronic ankle instability. *Med Sci Sport Exerc.* 2016;48(10):2040-2045. doi:10.1249/MSS.0000000000000994

69. Ekstrom RA, Donatelli RA, Carp KC. Electromyographic analysis of core trunk, hip, and thigh muscles during 9 rehabilitation exercises. *J Orthop Sports Phys Ther.* 2007;37(12):754-762.

70. McGregor AH, Hukins DW. Lower limb involvement in spinal function and low back pain. *J Back Musculoskelet Rehabil.* 2009;22(4):219-222.

71. Nadler SF, Malanga GA, Feinberg JH, Prybicien M, Stitik TP, DePrince M. Relationship between hip muscle imbalance and occurrence of low back pain in collegiate athletes: A prospective study. *Am J Phys Med Rehabil.* 2001;80(8):572-577.

72. Silfies SP, Ebaugh D, Pontillo M, Butowicz CM. Critical review of the impact of core stability on upper extremity athletic injury and performance. *Braz J Phys Ther.* 2015;19(5):360-368.

73. Sato K, Mokha M. Does core strength training influence running kinetics, lower-extremity stability, and 5000-M performance in runners? *J Strength Cond Res.* 2009;23(1):133-140.

74. DeFranca GG, Levine LJ. The quadratus lumborum and low back pain. *J Manipulative Physiol Ther.* 1991;14(2):142-149.

75. Carvalhais VO, Ocarino Jde M, Araújo VL, Souza TR, Silva PL, Fonseca ST. Myofascial force transmission between the latissimus dorsi and gluteus maximus muscles: An in vivo experiment. *J BIomech.* 2013;46(5):1003-1007.

76. Gatton ML, Pearcy MJ, Pettet GJ, Evans JH. A three-dimensional mathematical model of the thoracolumbar fascia and an estimate of its biomechanical effect. *J Biomech*. 2010;43(14):2792-2797.

77. Balkovec C, Vernengo AJ, McGill SM. Disc height loss and restoration via injectable hydrogel influences adjacent segment mechanics in-vitro. *Clinical Biomechanics*. 2016;36(July):1-7.

78. Czaprowski D, Stoliński Ł, Tyrakowski M, Kozinoga M, Kotwicki T. Non-structural misalignments of body posture in the sagittal plane. *Scoliosis Spinal Disord*. 2018;13(6). doi:10.1186/s13013-018-0151-5 PMC5836359,

79. Schüldt K. On neck muscle activity and load reduction in sitting postures: An electromyographic and biomechanical study with applications in ergonomics and rehabilitation. *Scand J Rehabil Med Suppl*. 1988;19:1-49.

80. Donatelli R, Dimond D, Holland M. Sport-specific biomechanics of spinal injuries in the athlete (throwing athletes, rotational sports, and contact-collision sports). *Clin Sports Med*. 2012;31(3):381-396.

81. Goode A, Hegedus EJ, Sizer P, Brismee JM, Linberg A, Cook CE. Three-dimensional movements of the sacroiliac joint: A systematic review of the literature and assessment of clinical utility. *J Man Manip Ther*. 2008;16(1):25-38.

82. Weisl H. The movements of the sacroiliac joint. *Acta Anat*. 1955;23(1):80-91.

83. Lum ZC, Coury JG, Cohen JL, Dorr LD. The current knowledge on spinopelvic mobility. *J Arthroplasty*. 2018;33(1):291-296. doi:10.1016/j.arth.2017.08.013

84. Alderink GJ. The sacroiliac joint: Review of anatomy, mechanics, and function. *J Orthop Sports Phys Ther*. 1991;13(2):71-84.

85. Lee D. *The Pelvic Girdle*. 3rd ed. Churchill Livingstone; 2004:280.

86. Kapandji IA. *The Physiology of Joints: Vol 3, The Trunk and Vertebral Column*. Churchill Livingstone; 1974.

87. Forst SL, Wheeler MT, Fortin JD, Vilensky JA. The sacroiliac joint: Anatomy, physiology and clinical significance. *Pain Physician*. 2006;9(1):61-67.

88. Zijlstra W, Hof AL. Displacement of the pelvis during human walking: Experimental data and model predictions. *Gait Posture*. 1997;6(3):249-262.

89. Madill SJ, McLean L. Relationship between abdominal and pelvic floor muscle activation and intravaginal pressure during pelvic floor muscle contractions in healthy continent women. *Neurourol Urodyn*. 2006;25(7):722-730.

90. Madill SJ, McLean L. Quantification of abdominal and pelvic floor muscle synergies in response to voluntary pelvic floor muscle contractions. *J Electromyogr Kinesiol*. 2008;18(6):955-964.

91. Sapsford R. Rehabilitation of pelvic floor muscles utilizing trunk stabilization. *Man Ther*. 2004;9(1):3-12.

92. De Troyer A, Wilson TA. Action of the diaphragm on the rib cage. *J Appl Physiol*. 2016;121(2):391-400.

93. Boyle KL, Olinick J, Lewis C. The value of blowing up a balloon. *N Am J Sports Phys Ther*. 2010;5(3):179-188.

94. Michaelson JV, Brilla LR, Suprak DN, McLaughlin WL, Dahlquist DT. Effects of two different recovery postures during high-intensity interval training. *Translational Journal of the American College of Sports Medicine*. 2019;4(4):23-27. doi:10.1249/tjx.0000000000000079

95. Grenier S, McGill SM. Quantification of lumbar stability by using 2 different abdominal activation strategies. *Arch Phys Med Rehabil*. 2007;88(1):54-62.

96. Richardson CA, Jull GA, Hodges PW, Hides JA. *Therapeutic Exercise for Spinal Segmental Stabilization in Low Back Pain: Scientific Basis and Clinical Approach*. Churchill Livingstone; 1999.

97. Maeo S, Takahashi T, Takai Y, Kanehisa H. Trunk muscle activities during abdominal bracing: Comparison among muscles and exercises. *J Sports Sci Med*. 2013;12(3):467-474.

98. Koh HW, Cho SH, Kim CY. Comparison of the effects of hollowing and bracing exercises on cross-sectional areas of abdominal muscles in middle-aged women. *J Phys Ther Sci*. 2014;26(2):295-299.

99. Melissinos CG, Goldman M, Bruce E, Elliott E, Mead J. Chest wall shape during forced expiratory maneuvers. *J Appl Physiol Respir Environ Exerc Physiol*. 1981;50(1):84-93.

100. Bjerkefors A, Ekblom MM, Josefsson K, Thorstensson A. Deep and superficial abdominal muscle activation during trunk stabilization exercises with and without instruction to hollow. *Man Ther*. 2010;15(5):502-507.

101. Jull GA, Richardson CA. Motor control problems in patients with spinal pain: A new direction for therapeutic exercise. *J Manipulative Physiol Ther*. 2000;23(2):115-117.

102. Cairns MC, Harrison K, Wright C. Pressure biofeedback: A useful tool in the quantification of abdominal muscular dysfunction? *Physiother*. 2000;86(3):127-138.

103. Park DJ, Lee SK. What is a suitable pressure for the abdominal drawing-in maneuver in the supine position using a pressure biofeedback unit? *J Phys Ther Sci*. 2013;25(5):527-530.

104. Norris CM. *Back Stability: Integrating Science and Therapy*. 2nd ed. Human Kinetics; 2008:360.

105. Allison GT, Godfrey P, Robinson G. EMG signal amplitude assessment during abdominal bracing and hollowing. *J Electromyogr Kinesiol*. Feb 1998;8(1):51-57.

106. Lee AY, Kim EH, Cho YW, Kwon SO, Son SM, Ahn SH. Effects of abdominal hollowing during stair climbing on the activations of local trunk stabilizing muscles: A cross-sectional study. *Ann Rehabil Med*. 2013;37(6):804-813.

107. Cholewicki J, Panjabi MM, Khachatryan A. Stabilizing function of trunk flexor-extensor muscles around a neutral spine posture. *Spine*. 1997;22(19):2207-2212.

108. McGill S. Coordination of muscle activity to assure stability of the lumbar spine. *J Electromyogr Kinesiol*. 2003;13(4):353-359.

109. McGill SM. *Low Back Disorders: Evidence-Based Prevention and Rehabilitation*. Human Kinetics; 2002.

110. Monfort-Pañego M, Vera-García FJ, Sánchez-Zuriaga D. Electromyographic studies in abdominal exercises: A literature synthesis. *J Manipulative Physiol Ther*. 2009;32(3):232-244.

111. Liebenson C. A modern approach to abdominal training—Part II: Facilitating the abdominal brace. *J Bodyw Mov Ther*. 2007;11(4):302-305.

112. Marshall PW, Desai I, Robbins DW. Core stability exercises in individuals with and without chronic nonspecific low back pain. *J Strength Cond Res*. 2011;25(12):3404-3411.

113. Critchley D. Instructing pelvic floor contraction facilitates transversus abdominis thickness increase during low-abdominal hollowing. *Physiother Res Int*. 2002;7(2):65-75.

114. Gildea JE, HIdes JA, Hodges PW. Size and symmetry of trunk muscles in ballet dancers with and without low back pain. *J Orthop Sports Phys Ther*. 2013;43(8):525-533.

115. Coghlan S, Crowe L, McCarthypersson U, Minogue C, Caulfield B. Neuromuscular electrical stimulation training results in enhanced activation of spinal stabilizing muscles during spinal loading and improvements in pain ratings. *Conf Proc IEEE Eng Med Biol Soc*. 2011;2011:7622-7625.

116. Comerford MJ, Mottram SL. Movement and stability dysfunction—contemporary developments. *Man Ther*. 2001;6(1):15-26.

117. Richardson CA, Snijders CJ, Hides JA, L. D, Pas MS, Storm J. The relation between the transverse abdominis muscles, sacroiliac joint mechanics, and low back pain. *Spine*. 2002;27(4):399-405.

118. Silfies SP, Mehta R, Smith SS, Karduna AR. Subgroups of patients with mechanical low back pain. *Arch Phys Med Rehabil*. 2009;90(7):1159-1169.

119. Ng JK, Parnianpour M, Richardson CA, Kippers V. Functional roles of abdominal and back muscles during isometric axial roation of the trunk. *J Orthop Res*. 2001;19(3):463-471.

120. Hancock MJ, Maher CG, Latimer J, et al. Systematic review of tests to identify the disc, SIJ or facet joint as the source of low back pain. *Eur Spine*. 2007;16(10):1539-1550.

121. van der Wurff P, Hagmeijer RHM, Meyne W. Clinical tests of the sacroiliac joint: A systematic methodological review: Part 1. Reliability. *Man Ther*. 2000;5(1):30-36.

122. van der Wurff P, Meyne W, Hagmeijer RHM. Clinical tests of the sacroiliac joint: A systematic methodical review: Part 2. Validity. *Man Ther*. 2000;5(2):89-96.

123. Poley RE, Borchers JR. Sacroiliac joint dysfunction: Evaluation and treatment. *Phys Sportsmed*. 2008;36(1):42-49.

124. Laslett M, Aprill CN, McDonald B, Young SB. Diagnosis of sacroilliac joint pain: Validity of individual provocation tests and composites of tests. *Man Ther*. 2005;10:207-218.

125. Stuber KJ. Specificity, sensitivity, and predictive values of clinical tests of the sacroiliac joint: A systematic review of the literature. *J Can Chiropr Assoc*. 2007;51(1):30-41.

126. van der Wurff P, Buijs EJ, Groen GJ. A multitest regimen of pain provocation tests as an aid to reduce unnecessary minimally invasive sacroiliac joint procedures. *Arch Phys Med Rehabil*. 2006;87:10-14.

127. Sivayogam A, Banerjee A. Diagnostic performance of clinical tests for sacroiliac joint pain. *Phys Ther Rev*. 2011;16(6):462-467. doi:10.1179/1743288X 11Y.0000000036

128. Broadhurst NA, Bond MJ. Pain provocation tests for the assessment of sacroiliac joint dysfunction. *J Spinal Disord*. 1998;11(4):341-345.

129. Dreyfuss P, Michaelsen M, Pauza K, McLarty J, Bogduk N. The value of medical history and physical examination in diagnosing sacroiliac joint pain. *Spine (Phila Pa 1976)*. 1996;21(22):2594-2602. doi:10.1097/00007632-199611150-00009

130. Albert H, Godskesen M, Westergaard J. Evaluation of clinical tests used in classification procedures in pregnancy-related pelvic joint pain. *Eur Spine J*. 2000;9(2):161-166. doi:10.1007/s005860050228

131. Laslett M, Williams M. The reliability of selected pain provocation tests for sacroiliac joint pathology. *Spine (Phila Pa 1976)*. 1994;19(11):1243-1249. doi:10.1097/00007632-199405310-00009

132. Werner CM, Hoch A, Gautier L, König MA, Simmen HP, Osterhoff G. Distraction test of the posterior superior iliac spine (PSIS) in the diagnosis of sacroiliac joint arthropathy. *BMC Surg*. 2013;13:52. doi:10.1186/1471-2482-13-52

133. Nejati P, Sartaj E, Imani F, Moeineddin R, Nejati L, Safavi M. Accuracy of the diagnostic tests of sacroiliac joint dysfunction. *J Chiropr Med*. 2020;19(1):28-37.

134. Levangie PK. Four clinical tests of sacroiliac joint dysfunction: The association of test results with innominate torsion among patients with and without low back pain. *Phys Ther*. 1999;79(11):1043-1057.

135. Dreyfuss P, Dryer S, Griffin J, Hoffman J, Walsh N. Positive sacroiliac screening tests in asymptomatic adults. *Spine (Phila Pa 1976)*. 1994;19(10):1138-1143. doi:10.1097/00007632-199405001-00007

136. Beal MC. The sacroiliac problem: Review of anatomy, mechanics, and diagnosis. *J Am Osteopath Assoc*. 1982;81(10):667-679.

137. Leboeuf C. The sensitivity and specificity of seven lumbo-pelvic orthopedic tests and the arm-fossa test. *J Manipulative Physiol Ther*. 1990;13(3):138-143.

138. Hegedus EJ, Cook C, Lewis J, Wright A, Park JY. Combining orthopedic special tests to improve diagnosis of shoulder pathology. *Phys Ther Sport*. 2015;16(2):87-92. doi:10.1016/j.ptsp.2014.08.001

139. Tong HC, Haig AJ, Yamakawa K. The Spurling test and cervical radiculopathy. *Spine (Phila Pa 1976)*. 2002;27(2):156-159. doi:10.1097/00007632-200201150-00007

140. Viikari-Juntura E, Porras M, Laasonen EM. Validity of clinical tests in the diagnosis of root compression in cervical disc disease. *Spine (Phila Pa 1976)*. 1989;14(3):253-257. doi:10.1097/00007632-198903000-00003

141. Côté P, Kreitz BG, Cassidy JD, Dzus AK, Martel J. A study of the diagnostic accuracy and reliability of the Scoliometer and Adam's forward bend test. *Spine (Phila Pa 1976)*. 1998;23(7):796-802. doi:10.1097/00007632-199804010-00011

142. Sohn IS, Lee JB, Park JH, Cho JM, Kim CJ. Valsalva maneuver to predict dynamic intraventricular obstruction during dobutamine stress echocardiography in patients with hypertension. *Int J Cardiol*. 2010;144(3):433-435. doi:10.1016/j.ijcard.2009.03.069

143. Devillé WL, van der Windt DA, Dzaferagiⵧ A, Bezemer PD, Bouter LM. The test of Lasègue: Systematic review of the accuracy in diagnosing herniated discs. *Spine (Phila Pa 1976)*. 2000;25(9):1140-1147. doi:10.1097/00007632-200005010-00016

144. Fritz JM, Piva SR, Childs JD. Accuracy of the clinical examination to predict radiographic instability of the lumbar spine. *Eur Spine J*. 2005;14(8):743-750. doi:10.1007/s00586-004-0803-4

145. Majlesi J, Togay H, Unalan H, Toprak S. The sensitivity and specificity of the Slump and the Straight Leg Raising tests in patients with lumbar disc herniation. *J Clin Rheumatol*. 2008;14(2):87-91.

146. Ferrari S, Manni T, Bonetti F, Villafañe J, Vanti C. A literature review of clinical tests for lumbar instability in low back pain: Validity and applicability in clinical practice. *Chiropr Man Therap.* 04/08 2015;23(14):12. doi:10.1186/s12998-015-0058-7

147. Alqarni AM, Schneiders AG, Hendrick PA. Clinical tests to diagnose lumbar segmental instability: A systematic review. *J Orthop Sports Phys Ther.* 2011;41(3):130-140.

148. Hicks GE, Fritz JM, Delitto A, McGill SM. Preliminary development of a clinical prediction rule for determining which patients with low back pain will respond to a stabilization exercise program. *Arch Phys Med Rehabil.* 2005;86(9):1753-1762. doi:10.1016/j.apmr.2005.03.033

149. Cook C, Brown C, Michael K, et al. The clinical value of a cluster of patient history and observational findings as a diagnostic support tool for lumbar spine stenosis. *Physiother Res Int.* 2011;16(3):170-178. doi:10.1002/pri.500

150. Ober FH. The role of the iliotibial band and fascia lata as a factor in the causation of low-back disabilities and sciatica. *J Bone Joint Surg Br.* 1936;18(1):105-110.

151. Henebry A, Gaskill T. The effect of pelvic tilt on radiographic markers of acetabular coverage. *Am J Sports Med.* 2013;41(11):2599-2603. doi:10.1177/0363546513500632

152. Bagwell J, Fukuda TY, Powers CM. Sagittal plane pelvis motion influences transverse plane motion of the femur: Kinematic coupling at the hip joint. *Gait Posture.* 2016;43(Jan):120-124.

153. Heckmann N, McKnight B, Stefl M, Trasolini NA, Ike H, Dorr LD. Late dislocation following total hip arthroplasty: Spinopelvic imbalance as a causative factor. *J Bone Joint Surg Am.* 2018;100(21):1845-1853. doi:10.2106/jbjs.18.00078

154. Willett GM, Keim SA, Shostrom VK, Lomneth CS. An anatomic investigation of the Ober Test. *Am J Sports Med.* 2016;44(3):696-701.

155. Tenney HR, Boyle KL, DeBord A. Influence of hamstring and abdominal muscle activation on a positive Ober's test in people with lumbopelvic pain. *Physiother Can.* 2013;65(1):4-11.

156. Kage V, Naidu SK. Effect of iliotibial band stretching versus hamstring and abdominal muscle activation on a positive Ober's Test in subjects with lumbopelvic pain: A randomized clinical trial. *Int J Therap Rehab Res.* 2015;4(4):111-116.

157. Shori G, Joshi A. Effect of right sidelying respiratory left adductor pull back exercise in subjects with iliotibial band tightness. *Physiotherapy.* 2017;25(1):13-16. doi:10.1515/physio-2016-0014

158. Basu S, Kakade PP, Palekar TJ, Chitgopkar V. Influence of abdominal and hamstring muscle activation exercises over iliotibial band stretching on a positive Ober's test in subjects with low back pain. *Glob J Res Anal.* 2017;6(5):704-705.

159. Lee AS, Cholewicki J, Reeves NP, Zazulak BT, Mysliwiec LW. Comparison of trunk proprioception between patients with low back pain and healthy controls. *Arch Phys Med Rehabil.* 2010;91(9):1327-1331.

160. Kofotolis N, Kellis E. Effects of two 4-week proprioceptive neuromuscular facilitation programs on muscle endurance, flexibility, and functional performance in women with chronic low back pain. *Phys Ther.* 2006;86(7):1001-1012.

161. Knežević O, Mirkov D. Trunk muscle activation patterns in subjects with low back pain. *Vojnosanit Pregl.* 2013;70(3):315-318.

162. O'Sullivan P, Twomey L, Allison G, Sinclair J, Miller K. Altered patterns of abdominal muscle activation in patients with chronic low back pain. *Aust J Physiother.* 1997;43(2):91-98.

163. Kolar P, Sulc J, Kyncl M, et al. Postural function of the diaphragm in persons with and without chronic low back pain. *J Orthop Sports Phys Ther.* 2012;42(4):352-362. doi:10.2519/jospt.2012.3830

164. Kolar P, Neuwirth J, Sanda J, et al. Analysis of diaphragm movement during tidal breathing and during its activation while breath holding using MRI synchronized with spirometry. *Physiol Res.* 2009;58(3):383-392.

165. Childs JD, Flynn TF, Fritz JM, et al. Screening for vertebrobasilar insufficiency in patients with neck pain: Manual therapy decision making in the presence of uncertainty. *J Orthop Sports Phys Ther.* 2005;35(5):300-306.

166. Haldeman S, Carey P, Townsend M, Papadopoulos C. Arterial dissections following cervical manipulation: The chiropractic experience. *Can Med Assoc J.* 2001;165(7):905-906.

167. Tatu L, Moulin T, Bogousslavsky J, Duvernoy H. Arterial territories of human brain: Brainstem and cerebellum. *Neurology.* 1996;47:1125-1135.

168. Arnold C, Bourassa R, Langer T, Stoneham G. Doppler studies evaluating the effect of a physical therapy screening protocol on vertebral artery blood flow. *Man Ther.* 2004;9(1):13-21.

169. Wakayama K, Murakami M, Suzuki M, Ono S, Shimizu N. Ischemic symptoms induced by occlusion of the unilateral vertebral artery with head rotation together with contralateral vertebral artery dissection—case report. *J Neurol Sci.* 2005;236(1-2):87-90.

170. Taylor AJ, Kerry R. A "system based" approach to risk assessment of the cervical spine prior to manual therapy. *Int J Osteopath Med.* 2010;13(3):85-93.

171. Aspinall W. Clinical testing for cervical mechanical disorders which produce ischemic vertigo. *J Orthop Sports Phys Ther.* 1989;11(5):176-182.

172. Magee DJ. *Orthopedic Physical Assessment.* 5th ed. Saunders Elsevier; 2008.

173. Rivett DA, Sharples KJ, Milburn PD. Effect of premanipulative tests on vertebral artery and internal carotid artery blood flow: A pilot study. *J Manip Physiol Ther.* 1999;22(6):368-381.

174. Alshahrani A, Johnson EG, Cordett TK. Vertebral artery testing and differential diagnosis in dizzy patients. *Phys Ther Rehabil.* 2014;1(1)doi:10.7243/2055-2386-1-3

175. Penning L, Wilmink JT. Rotation of the cervical spine: A CT study in normal subjects. *Spine.* 1987;12(8):732-738.

176. Mitchell J, Keene D, Dyson C, Harvey L, Pruvey C, Phillips R. Is cervical spine rotation, as used in the standard vertebrobasilar insufficiency test, associated with a measureable change in intracranial vertebral artery blood flow? *Man Ther.* 2004;9(4):220-227.

177. Sato K, Fisher JP, Seifert T, Overgaard M, Secher NH, Ogoh S. Blood flow in internal carotid and vertebral arteries during orthostatic stress. *Exp Physiol.* 2012;97(12):1272-1280.

178. Magarey ME, Rebbeck T, Coughlan B, Grimmer K, Rivett DA, Refshauge K. Pre-manipulative testing of the cervical spine review, revision and new clinical guidelines. *Man Ther.* 2004;9(2):95-108.

179. Travell JG, Simons DG. *Myofascial Pain and Dysfunction: The Trigger Point Manual. Vol. 1.* 2nd ed. Williams and Wilkins; 1999.

180. Maitland GD. *Vertebral Manipulation.* 5th ed. Butterworth-Heinemann; 1986.

181. Shankar Ganesh G, Mohanty P, Smita Pattnaik S. The immediate and 24-hour follow-up effect of unilateral lumbar Z-joint mobilisation on posterior chain neurodynamics. *J Bodyw Mov Ther.* 2015;19(2):226-231.

182. Emami F, Pirouzi S, Taghizadeh S. Comparison of abdominal and lumbar muscles electromyography activity during two types of stabilization exercises. *Zahedan J Res Med Sci.* 2015;17(4):29-34. doi:10.5812/zjrms.17(4)2015.963

183. Willardson JM. Core stability training: Applications to sports conditioning programs. *J Strength Cond Res.* 2007;21(3):979-985.

184. Atalay E, Akova B, Gür H, Sekir U. Effect of upper-extremity strengthening exercises on the lumbar strength, disability and pain of patients with chronic low back pain: A randomized controlled study. *J Sports Sci Med.* 2017;16(4):595-603.

185. Lee SW, Kim SY. Effects of hip exercises for chronic low-back pain patients with lumbar instability. *J Phys Ther Sci.* 2015;27(2):345-348.

186. Page P, Frank CC, Lardner R. *Assessment and Treatment of Muscle Imbalance. The Janda Approach.* Human Kinetics; 2010.

187. Norris C. Functional load abdominal training: Part 1. *Phys Ther Sport.* 2001;2(1):29-39.

188. Hubley-Kozey CL. Training the abdominal musculature. *Physiother Can.* 2005;57(1):5-17.

189. Ganesh GS, Chhabra D, Mrityunjay K. Efficacy of the Star Excursion Balance Test in detecting reach deficits in subjects with chronic low back pain. *Physiother Res Int.* 2014. doi:10.1002/pri.1589

190. Brown SH, McGill SM. Muscle force-stiffness characteristics influence joint stability: A spine example. *Clin Biomech (Bristol, Avon).* 2005;20(9):917-922. doi:10.1016/j.clinbiomech.2005.06.002

191. Sung W, Hicks GE, Ebaugh D, et al. Individuals with and without low back pain use different motor control strategies to achieve spinal stiffness during the prone instability test. *J Orthop Sports Phys Ther.* 2019;49(12):899-907. doi:10.2519/jospt.2019.8577

192. Zazulak B, Cholewicki J, Reeves NP. Neuromuscular control of trunk stability: Clinical implications for sports injury prevention. *J Am Acad Orthop Surg.* 2008;16(9):497-505.

193. Newcomer KL, Jacobson TD, Gabriel DA, Larson DR, Brey RH, An KN. Muscle activation patterns in subjects with and without low back pain. *Arch Phys Med Rehabil.* 2002;83(6):816-821.

194. Horton JF, Lindsay DM, Macintosh BR. Abdominal muscle activation of elite male golfers with chronic low back pain. *Med Sci Sports Exerc.* 2001;33(10):1647-1654.

195. Barwick A, Smith J, Chuter V. The relationship between foot motion and lumbopelvic-hip function: A review of the literature. *Foot (Edinb).* 2012;22(3):224-231. doi:10.1016/j.foot.2012.03.006

196. Anderson K, Behm DG. The impact of instability resistance training on balance and stability. *Sports Med.* 2005;35(1):43-53. doi:10.2165/00007256-200535010-00004

197. Coulombe BJ, Games KE, Neil ER, Eberman LE. Core stability exercise versus general exercise for chronic low back pain. *J Athl Train.* 2017;52(1):71-72. doi:10.4085/1062-6050-51.11.16

198. Williams PC. Examination and conservative treatment for disk lesions of the lower spine. *Clin Orthop.* 1955;5:28-40.

199. McKenzie R, May S. *The Lumbar Spine: Mechanical Diagnosis and Therapy.* 2nd ed. Spinal Publications; 2003.

200. Rosedale R, Rastogi R, May S, et al. Efficacy of exercise intervention as determined by the McKenzie System of Mechanical Diagnosis and Therapy for knee osteoarthritis: A randomized controlled trial. *J Orthop Sports Phys Ther.* 2014;44(3):173-181, A1-A6.

201. Schenk R, Bhaidani T, Melissa B, Kelley J, Kruchowsky T. Inclusion of mechanical diagnosis and therapy (MDT) in the management of cervical radiculopathy: A case report. *J Man Manip Ther.* 2008;16(1):e1-e8.

202. Soerensen B. Mechanical diagnosis and therapy (MDT) approach for assessment and identification of serious pathology. *Man Ther.* 2011;16(4):406-408.

203. Beattie P. The use of an eclectic approach for the treatment of low back pain: A case study. *Phys Ther.* 1992;72(12):923-928.

204. Doury-Panchout F, Metivier JC, Borie-Malavieille MJ, Fouquet B. Vo(2)max in patients with chronic pain: Comparative analysis with objective and subjective tests of disability. *Ann Phys Rehabil Med.* 2012;55(5):294-311.

205. Smeets RJ, Wittink H, Hidding A, Knottnerus JA. Do patients with chronic low back pain have a lower level of aerobic fitness than healthy controls? Are pain, disability, fear of injury, working status, or level of leisure time activity associated with the difference in aerobic fitness level? *Spine.* 2006;31(1):90-97.

206. Rydeard R, Leger A, Smith D. Pilates-based therapeutic exercise: effect on subjects with nonspecific chronic low back pain and functional disability: A randomized controlled trial. *J Orthop Sports Phys Ther.* 2006;36(7):472-484.

207. Liebenson C. Functional training for performance enhancement—Part 1: The basics. *J Bodyw Mov Ther.* 2006;10:154-158.

208. Lemaire A, Ripamonti M, Ritz M, Rahmani A. Relationships between hip muscles and trunk flexor and extensor muscles in chronic low back pain patients: A preliminary study. *Comput Methods Biomech Biomed Engin.* 2013;16 (Suppl 1):161-163.

209. Iglesias-González JJ, Muñoz-García MT, Rodrigues-de-Souza DP, Alburquerque-Sendín F, Fernández-de-las-Peñas C. Myofascial trigger points, pain, disability, and sleep quality in patients with chronic nonspecific low back pain. *Pain Med.* 2013;14(12):1964-1970.

210. Bello AI, Foli MA, Adegoke BOA. Pain distribution pattern in gluteal-related low back pain: A proposed patho-anatomical approach using gluteal triangle. *J Musculoskelet Res.* 2011;14(1):7.

211. McConnell J. Recalcitrant chronic low back and leg pain—a new theory and different approach to management. *Man Ther.* 2002;7:183-192.

212. Ebenbichler GR, Oddsson LIE, Kollmitzer J, Erim Z. Sensory-motor control of the lower back: Implications for rehabilitation. *Med Sci Sports Exerc*. 2001;33(11):1889-198.

213. Zazulak BT, Hewett TE, Reeves NP, Goldberg B, Cholewicki J. Deficits in neuromuscular control of the trunk predict knee injury risk: A prospective biomechanical-epidemiologic study. *Am J Sports Med*. 2007;35(7):1123-1130.

214. Claeys K, Dankaerts W, Janssens L, Brumagne S. Altered prepatory pelvic control during sit-to-stance-to-sit movement in people with non-specific low back pain. *J Electromyogr Kinesiol*. 2012;22(6):821-828.

215. Learman KE, Myers JB, Lephart SM, Sell TC, Kerns GJ, Cook CE. Effects of spinal manipulation on trunk proprioception in subjects with chronic low back pain during symptom remission. *J Manip Physiol Ther*. 2009;32(2):118-126.

216. Sahrmann SA. *Diagnosis and Treatment of Movement Impairment Syndromes*. Mosby; 2002.

217. Page P. Muscle imbalance in older adults: Improving posture and decreasing pain. *J Active Aging*. 2005;4(2):30-37.

218. Seah SH, Briggs AM, O'Sullivan PB, Smith AJ, Burnett AF, Straker LM. An exploration of familial associations in spinal posture defined using a clinical grouping method. *Man Ther*. 2011;16(5):501-509.

219. Kendall FP, McCreary EK, Provance PG, Rodgers MM, Romani WA. *Muscles: Testing and Function With Posture and Pain*. 5th ed. Lippincott Williams & Wilkins; 2005.

220. Gunning JL, Callaghan JP, McGill SM. Spinal posture and prior loading history modulate compressive strength and type of failure in the spine: A biomechanical study using a porcine cervical spine model. *Clin Biomech*. 2001;16(6):471-480.

221. Nguyen AD, Shultz SJ. Identifying relationships among lower extremity alignment characteristics. *J Athl Train*. 2009;44(5):511-518.

222. Twomey LT. A rationale for the treatment of back pain and joint pain by manual therapy. *Phys Ther*. 1992;72(12):885-892.

223. Nowotny-Czupryna O, Czupryna K, Bⴽk K, Wróblewska E, Rottermund J. Postural habits of young adults and possibilities of modification. *Orthop Traumatol Rehabil*. 2013;15(1):9-21.

224. Nelson N. Massage strategies for upper crossed syndrome. *Massage Magazine*. 2011;(186):46-50.

225. Janda D. Muscles and motor control in low back pain: Assessment and management. In: Twomey LT, ed. *Physical Therapy of the Low Back*. Churchill Livingstone; 1987:253-278.

226. McAllister RM, Amann JF, Laughlin MH. Skeletal muscle fiber types and their vascular support. *J Reconstr Microsurg*. 1993;9(4):313-317.

227. Moore MK. Upper crossed syndrome and its relationship to cervicogenic headaches. *J Manip Physiol Ther*. 2004;27(6):414-420.

228. Panjabi MM. The stabilizing system of the spine: Part II. Neutral zone and instability hypothesis. *J Spinal Disord*. 1992;5(4):390-396.

229. Skolimowski J, Barczyk K, Dudek K, Skolimowska B, Demczuk-Włodarczyk E, Anwajler J. Posture in people with shoulder impingement syndrome. *Ortop Traumatol Rehabil*. 2007;9(5):484-498.

230. Rushing P. Postural assessment for soccer athletes. *Perform Condit Soccer*. 2011;16(7):6-7.

231. Lowe W. Stand up against low-back pain. *Massage Bodywork*. 2013;28(5):104-107.

232. Steinmetz A, Seidel W, Muche B. Impairment of postural stabilization systems in musicians with playing-related musculoskeletal disorders. *J Manipulative Physiol Ther*. 2010;33(8):603-611.

233. Garber C, Blissmer B, Deschenes MR, et al. American College of Sports Medicine position stand: Quantity and quality of exercise for developing and maintaining cardiorespiratory, musculoskeletal, and neuromotor fitness in apparently healthy adults: Guidance for prescribing exercise. *Med Sci Sports Exerc*. 2011;43(7):1334-1359.

234. Legaspi O, Edmond SL. Does the evidence support the existence of lumbar spine coupled motion? A critical review of the literature. *J Orthop Sports Phys Ther*. 2007;37(4):169-178.

235. Cook C, Hegedus E, Showalter C, Sizer PS, Jr. Coupling behavior of the cervical spine: A systematic review of the literature. *J Man Manip Ther*. 2006;29(7):570-575.

236. Lund T, Nydegger T, Schlenzka D, Oxland TR. Three-dimensional motion patterns during active bending in patients with chronic low back pain. *Spine*. 2002;27(17):1865-1874.

237. Panjabi MM, Yamamoto I, Oxland T, Crisco J. How does posture affect coupling in the lumbar spine? *Spine*. 1989;14(9):1002-1011.

238. Pearcy MJ, Tibrewal SB. Axial rotation and lateral bending in the normal lumbar spine measured by three-dimensional radiography. *Spine*. 1984;9(6):582-587.

239. Panjabi MM, Oda T, Crisco JJ, 3rd., Dvorak J, Grob D. Posture affects motion coupling patterns of the upper cervical spine. *J Orthop Res*. 1993;11(4):525-536.

240. Fryette HH. *Principles of Osteopathic Technic*. American Academy of Osteopathy; 1980.

241. Varlotta GP, Lefkowitz TR, Schweitzer M, et al. The lumbar facet joint: A review of current knowledge: Part II. Diagnosis and management. *Skeletal Radiol*. 2011;40(2):149-157.

242. Sampsell E. Rehabilitation of the spine following sports injury. *Clin Sports Med*. 2010;29(1):127-156.

243. Zmurko MG, Tannoury TY, Tannoury CA, Anderson DG. Cervical sprains, disc herniations, minor fractures, and other cervical injuries in the athlete. *Clin Sports Med*. 2003;22(3):513-521. doi:10.1016/s0278-5919(03)00003-6

244. Kendler DL, Bauer DC, Davison KS, et al. Vertebral fractures: Clinical importance and management. *Am J Med*. 2016;129(2):221. doi:10.1016/j.amjmed.2015.09.020

245. Donnally I, C.J., DiPompeo CM, Varacallo M. Vertebral compression fractures. *StatPearls*. StatPearls; 2020.

246. Broy SB. The vertebral fracture cascade: Etiology and clinical implications. *J Clin Densitom*. 2016;19(1):29-34. doi:10.1016/j.jocd.2015.08.007

247. Ohtor iS, Suzuki M, Koshi T, et al. Single-level instrumented posterolateral fusion of the lumbar spine with a local bone graft versus an iliac crest bone graft: A prospective, randomized study with a 2-year follow-up. *Eur Spine J*. 2011;20(4):635-639.

248. Keller TS, Colloca CJ, Harrison DE, Harrison DD, Janik TJ. Influence of spine morphology on intervertebral disc loads and stresses in asymptomatic adults: Implications for the ideal spine. *Spine J.* 2005;5(3):297-309.

249. Gardocki RJ, Watkins RG, Williams LA. Measurements of lumbopelvic lordosis using the pelvic radius technique as it correlates with sagittal spinal balance and sacral translation. *Spine J.* 2002;2(6):421-429.

250. Knutson GA. Incidence of foot rotation, pelvic crest unleveling, and supine leg length alignment asymmetry and their relationship to self-reported back pain. *J Manipulative Physiol Ther.* 2002;25(2):1-7.

251. Defrin R, Benyamin SB, Aldubi RD, Pick CG. Conservative correction of leg-length discrepancies of 10mm or less for the relief of chronic low back pain. *Arch Phys Med Rehabil.* 2005;86(11):2075-2080.

252. DeMann LE, Jr. Sacroiliac dysfunction in dancers with low back pain. *Man Ther.* 1997;2(1):2-10.

253. Prather H. Sacroiliac joint pain: practical management. *Clin J Sport Med.* 2003;13(4):252-256.

254. Major NM, Helms CA. Pelvic stress injuries: the relationship between osteitis pubis (symphysis pubis stress injury) and sacroiliac abnormalities in athletes. *Skeletal Radiol.* 1997;26(12):711-717.

255. Fryer G, Morse CM, Johnson JC. Spinal and sacroiliac assessment and treatment techniques used by osteopathic physicians in the United States. *Osteopath Med Prim Care.* 2009;3:4. doi:10.1186/1750-4732-3-4

256. Daly JM, Frame PS, Rapoza PA. Sacroiliac subluxation: A common, treatable cause of low-back pain in pregnancy. *Fam Pract Res J.* 1991;11(2):149-159.

257. Greenman PE. *Principles of Manual Medicine.* 4th ed. Lippincott Williams & Wilkins; 2011.

258. Rex LHB. Muscle energy technique: An overview. *Athl Ther Today.* 1996;1(6):38-40.

259. MacDonlad CW, Whitman JM, Cleland JA, Smith M, Hoeksma HL. Clinical outcomes following manual physical therapy and exercise for hip osteoarthritis: A case series. *J Orthop Sports Phys Ther.* 2006;36(8):588-599.

260. Young B, Walker MU, Strunce J, Boyles R. A combined treatment approach emphasizing impairment-based manual physical therapy for plantar heel pain: A case series. *J Orthop Sports Phys Ther.* 2004;34(11):725-733.

261. Wilson E, Payton O, Donegan-Shoaf L, Dec K. Muscle energy technique in patients with acute low back pain: A pilot clinical trial. *J Orthop Sports Phys Ther.* 2003;33(9):502-512.

Chapter 18

1. Ahmed AM, Burke DL. In vitro measurement of static pressure distribution in synovial joints: I. Tibial surface of the knee. *J Biomed Eng.* 1983;105:216-225.

2. Kapandji IA. *The Physiology of the Joints: Vol 2, Lower Limb.* 5th ed. Churchill Livingstone; 1987.

3. Houglum PA, Bertoti DB. *Brunnstrom's Clinical Kinesiology.* 6th ed. F.A. Davis; 2012.

4. Tönnis D, Heinecke A. Acetabular and femoral anteversion: Relationship with osteoarthritis of the hip. *J Bone Joint Surg Br.* 1999;81(12):1747-1770.

5. Crane L. Femoral torsion and its relation to toeing-in and toeing out. *J Bone Joint Surg Am.* 1959;41(3):421-428.

6. Neely FG. Biomechanical risk factors for exercise-related lower limb injuries. *Sports Med.* 1998;26(6):395-413.

7. Seringe R, Bonnet JC, Katti E. Pathogeny and natural history of congenital dislocation of the hip. *Orthop Traumatol Surg Res.* 2014;100(1):59-67.

8. Yoon TL, Park KM, Choi SA, Lee JH, Jeong HJ, Cynn HS. A comparison of the reliability of the trochanteric prominence angle test and the alternative method in healthy subjects. *Man Ther.* 2014;19(2):97-101.

9. Starkey C, Brown SD, Ryan JL. *Examination of Orthopedic and Athletic Injuries.* 3rd ed. F.A. Davis Co.; 2010.

10. Migliorini S, Merlo M, Pricca P. The hamstring syndrome: Clinical and diagnostic features, etiology, and surgical management. *J Sports Traumatol Rel Res.* 2000;22(2):86-72.

11. Güvençer M, Akyer P, Iyem C, Tetik S, Naderi S. Anatomic considerations and the relationship between the piriformis muscle and the sciatic nerve. *Surg Radiol Anat.* 2008;30(6):467-474.

12. Otoshi K, Itoh Y, Tsuijno A, Kikuchi S. Case report: Meralgia paresthetica in a baseball pitcher. *Clin Orthop Relat Res.* 2008;466(9):2268-2270.

13. Braune W, Fischer O. *On the Centre of Gravity of the Human Body.* Maquet P, Furong R. Springer-Verlag; 1984.

14. Sharrock C, Cropper J, Mostad J, Johnson M, Malone T. A pilot study of core stability and athletic performance: Is there a relationship? *Int J Sports Phys Ther.* 2011;6(2):63-74.

15. Huxel Bliven KC, Anderson BE. Core stability training for injury prevention. *Sports Health.* 2013;5(6):514-522.

16. Rickman AM, Ambegaonkar JP, Cortes N. Core stability: Implications for dance injuries. *Med Probl Perform Art.* 2012;27(3):159-164.

17. Sato K, Mokha M. Does core strength training influence running kinetics, lower-extremity stability, and 5000-M performance in runners? *J Strength Cond Res.* 2009;23(1):133-140.

18. Willardson JM. Core stability training: Applications to sports conditioning programs. *J Strength Cond Res.* 2007;21(3):979-985.

19. Riewald S, Ellenbecker T. The unbalanced tennis player. *Coach Sport Sci Rev.* 2005;(37):2-3.

20. Okada T, Huxel KC, Nesser TW. Relationship between core stability, functional movement, and performance. *J Strength Cond Res.* 2011;25(1):252-261.

21. Plummer HA, Oliver GD. The relationship between gluteal muscle activation and throwing kinematics in baseball and softball catchers. *J Strength Cond Res.* 2014;28(1):87-96.

22. Kibler WB. Pathophysiology of overload injuries around the elbow. *Clin Sports Med.* 1995;14(2):447-457.

23. Kibler WB, Sciascia A. Rehabilitation of the athlete's shoulder. *Clin Sport Med* 2008;4(27):821-831.

24. Leetun DT, Ireland ML, Willson JD, Ballantyne BT, Davis IM. Core stability measures as risk factors for lower extremity injury in athletes. *Med Sci Sports Exerc.* 2004;36(6):926-934.

25. Tyler TF, Nicholas SJ, Campbell RJ, McHugh MP. The association of hip strength and flexibility with the incidence of adductor muscle strains in professional ice hockey players. *Am J Sports Med.* 2001;29(2):124-128.

26. Manners J, Scifers J. Aquatic rehabilitation for core stabilization. *Athl Ther Today.* 2003;8(5):68-70.

27. Bagwell J, Fukuda TY, Powers CM. Sagittal plane pelvis motion influences transverse plane motion of the femur: Kinematic coupling at the hip joint. *Gait Posture.* 2016;43(Jan):120-124.

28. Takacs J, Hunt MA. The effect of contralateral pelvic drop and trunk lean on frontal plane knee biomechanics during single limb standing. *J Biomech.* 2012;45(16):2791-2796.

29. Perry J, Burnfield JM. *Gait Analysis: Normal and Pathological Function.* 2nd ed. Slack; 2010.

30. Bolz S, Davies GJ. Leg length differences and correlation with total leg length. *J Orthop Sports Phys Ther.* 1984;6(2):123-129.

31. Subotnick SI. Limb length discrepancies of the lower extremity (short leg syndrome). *J Orthop Sports Phys Ther.* 1981;3(1):11-16.

32. Vogel F, Jr. Short-leg syndrome. *Clin Podiatr.* 1984;1(3):581-599.

33. Kaufman KR, Miller LS, Sutherland DH. Gait asymmetry in patients with limb-length inequality. *J Pediatr Orthop.* 1996;16(2):144-150.

34. Perttunen JR, Anttila E, Soedergard J, Merikanto J, Komi PV. Gait asymmetry in patients with limb length discrepancy. *Scand J Med Sci Sports.* 2004;14(1):49-56.

35. Gofton JP, Trueman GE. Studies in osteoarthritis of the hip: II. Osteoarthritis of the hip and leg-length disparity. *Can Med Assoc J.* 1971;104(9):791-799.

36. Perry J. Pathologic gait. *Instr Course Lect.* 1990;39:325-331.

37. Maitland GD. *Peripheral manipulation.* Butterworth-Heinemann; 1991.

38. Cyriax JH. *Texbook of Orthopaedic Medicine: Vol 2. Treatment by Manipulation, Massage and Injection.* vol 2. Williams & Wilkins; 1977.

39. Brantingham JW, Bonnefin D, Perle SM, et al. Manipulative therapy for lower extremity conditions: Update of a literature review. *J Manip Physiol Ther.* 2012;36(2):127-166.

40. Hettinger T. *Physiology of Strength.* C.C. Thomas; 1961.

41. Verrelst R, Willems TM, Clercq DD, Roosen P, Goossens L, Witvrouw E. The role of hip abductor and external rotator muscle strength in the development of exertional medial tibial pain: A prospective study. *Br J Sports Med.* 2014;48(21):1564-1569.

42. Maranhão-Filho PA, Maranhão ET, Lima MA, Silva MM. Rethinking the neurological examination II: Dynamic balance assessment. *Arq Neurospiquiatr.* 2011;69(6):959-963.

43. Courtney CA, Rine R, Jenk DT, Colier PD, Waters A. Enhanced proprioceptive activity at the knee in the competitive athlete. *J Orthop Sports Phys Ther.* 2013;43(6):422-426.

44. Coplen EM, Voight ML. Rehabilitation of the hip. In: Byrd JW, ed. *Operative Hip Arthroscopy.* Springer; 2013:411-439.

45. Melamed H, Hutchinson MR. Soft tissue problems of the hip in athletes. *Sports Med Arthrosc Rev.* 2002;10(2):168-175.

46. Mellman MF, McPherson EJ, Dorr LD, Kwong K. Differential diagnosis of back and lower extremity problems. In: Watkins RG, ed. *The Spine in Sports.* Mosby; 1996.

47. Kocher MS, Tucker R. Pediatric athlete hip disorders. *Clin Sports Med.* 2006;25(2):241-253.

48. Kelly BT. Sports hip injuries: Assessment and management. *Instr Course Lect.* 2013;62:515-531.

49. Morelli V, Smith V. Groin injuries in athletes. *Am Fam Physician.* 2001;64(8):1405-1414.

50. Sankar WN, Nevitt M, Parvizi J, Felson DT, Agricola R, Leunig M. Femoroacetabular impingement: Defining the condition and its role in the pathophysiology of osteoarthritis. *J Am Acad Orthop Surg.* 2013;21(Suppl 1):S7-S15.

51. Keogh MJ, Batt ME. A review of femoroacetabular impingement in athletes. *Sports Med.* 2008;38(10):863-878.

52. Lesher JM, Dreyfuss P, Hager N, Kaplan M, Furman M. Hip joint pain referral patterns: a descriptive study. *Pain Med.* 2008;9(1):22-25.

53. Laplante BL, Ketchum JM, Saullo TR, Depalma MJ. Multivariable analysis of the relationship between pain referral patterns and the source of chronic low back pain. *Pain Physician.* 2012;15(2):171-178.

54. Travell JG, Simons DG. *Myofascial Pain and Dysfunction. The Trigger Point Manual. Vol. 2.* Williams and Wilkins; 1992.

55. Simonet WT, Saylor HL, 3rd., Sim L. Abdominal wall muscle tears in hockey players. *Int J Sports Med.* 1995;16(2):126-128.

56. Troelsen A, Mechlenburg I, Gelineck J, Bolvig L, Jacobsen S, Søballe K. What is the role of clinical tests and ultrasound in acetabular labral tear diagnostics? *Acta Orthop.* Jun 2009;80(3):314-8. doi:10.3109/17453670902988402

57. Fishman LM, Dombi GW, Michaelsen C, et al. Piriformis syndrome: Diagnosis, treatment and outcome - a 10-year study. *Arch Phys Med Rehabil.* 2002;83:295-301.

58. Sutlive TG, Lopez HP, Schnitker DE, et al. Development of a clinical prediction rule for diagnosing hip osteoarthritis in individuals with unilateral hip pain. *J Orthop Sports Phys Ther.* 2008;38(9):542-50. doi:10.2519/jospt.2008.2753

59. Bird PA, Oakley SP, Shnier R, Kirkham BW. Prospective evaluation of magnetic resonance imaging and physical examination findings in patients with greater trochanteric pain syndrome. *Arthritis Rheum.* Sep 2001;44(9):2138-45. doi:10.1002/1529-0131(200109)44:9<2138::Aid-art367>3.0.Co;2-m

60. Marks MC, Alexander J, Sutherland DH, Chambers HG. Clinical utility of the Duncan-Ely test for rectus femoris dysfunction during the swing phase of gait. *Dev Med Child Neurol.* Nov 2003;45(11):763-8. doi:10.1017/s0012162203001415

61. Narvani AA, Tsiridis E, Kendall S, Chaudhuri R, Thomas P. A preliminary report on prevalence of acetabular labrum tears in sports patients with groin pain. *Knee Surg Sports Traumatol Arthrosc.* Nov 2003;11(6):403-8. doi:10.1007/s00167-003-0390-7

62. Geraci MC, Jr. Overuse injuries of the hip and pelvis. *J Back Musculoskelet Rehabil.* 1996;6(1):5-19.

63. Sahrmann SA. *Diagnosis and Treatment of Movement Impairment Syndromes.* Mosby; 2002.

64. Holes DJ. Correcting muscular imbalances to improve running economy. *Armed Froces Comptroller.* 2003;48(1):25-26.

65. Page P, Frank CC, Lardner R. *Assessment and Treatment of Muscle Imbalance. The Janda Approach.* Human Kinetics; 2010.

66. Mehta JS, Kochhar S, Harding IJ. A slip above a slip: Retrolisthesis of the motion segment above a spondylolytic spondylolisthesis. *Eur Spine J.* 2012;21(11):2128-2133.

67. Travell JG, Simons DG. *Myofascial Pain and Dysfunction: The Trigger Point Manual. Vol. 2.* Williams and Wilkins; 1992.

68. Sakamoto AC, Teixeira-Salmela LF, de Paula-Goulart FR, de Morais Faria CD, Guimarães CQ. Muscular activation patterns during active prone hip extension exercises. *J Electromyogr Kinesiol.* 2009;19(1):105-112.

69. Geraci MC, Jr., Brown W. Evidence-based treatment of hip and pelvic injuries in runners. *Phys Med Rehabil Clin N Am.* 2005;16(3):711-747.

70. Benzon HT, Katz JA, Benzon HA, Iqbal MS. Piriformis syndrome: Anatomic considerations, a new injection technique, and a review of the literature. *Anesthesiology.* 2003;98(6):1442-1448.

71. Fishman LM, Dombi GW, Michaelsen C, et al. Piriformis syndrome: Diagnosis, treatment and outcome: A 10-year study. *Arch Phys Med Rehabil.* 2002;83:295-301.

72. Rosse C, Gaddum-Rosse P. *Hollinshead's Textbook of Anatomy.* Lioppincott-Raven; 1997:902.

73. Popovac H, Bojanic I, Smoljanovic T. Leg length discrepancy as a rare cause of a piriformis syndrome. *J Back Musculoskelet Rehabil.* 2012;25(4):299-300.

74. Dere K, Akbas M, Luleci N. A rare cause of a piriformis syndrome. *J Back Musculoskelet Rehabil.* 2009;22(1):55-58.

75. Tyler TF, Slattery AA. Rehabilitation of the hip following sports injury. *Clin Sports Med.* 2010;29(1):107-126.

76. Nicholas SJ, Tyler TF. Adductor muscle strains in sport. *Sports Med.* 2002;32(5):339-344.

77. Serner A, Tol JL, Weir A, et al. Diagnosis of acute groin injuries: A prospective study of 110 athletes. *Am J Sports Med.* 2015;43(8):1857-1864.

78. Tyler TF, Nicholas SJ, Campbell RJ, Donellan S, McHugh MP. The effectiveness of a preseason exercise program to prevent adductor muscle strains in professional ice hockey players. *Am J Sports Med.* 2002;30(5):680-683.

79. Lynch SA, Renstrom PA. Groin injuries in sport: Treatment strategies. *Sports Med.* 1999;28(2):137-144.

80. Emery CA, Meeuwisse WH, Powell JW. Groin and abdominal strain injuries in the National Hockey League. *Clin J Sports Med.* 1999;9(3):151-156.

81. Enseki KR, Martin R, Kelly BT. Rehabilitation after arthroscopic decompression for femoroacetabular impingement. *Clin Sports Med.* 2010;29(2):247-255, viii.

82. Anderson SE, Siebenrock KA, Tannast M. Femoroacetabular impingement. *Eur J Radiol.* 2012;81(12):3740-3744.

83. Lequesne M, Bellaïche L. Anterior femoroacetabular impingement: An update. *Joint Bone Spine.* 2012;79(3):249-255.

84. Mori R, Yasunaga Y, Yamasaki T, et al. Are cam and pincer deformities as common as dysplasia in Japanese patients with hip pain? *Bone Joint J.* 2014;96-B(2):172-176.

85. Kassarjian A, Brisson M, Palmer WE. Femoroacetabular impingement. *Eur J Radiol.* 2007;63(1):29-35.

86. Ng KC, Roubi G, Lamontagne M, Beaulé PE. Finite element analysis examining the effects of cam FAI on hip joint mechanical loading using subject-specific geometries during standing and maximum squat. *HSS J.* 2012;8(3):206-212.

87. Lavigne M, Parvizi J, Beck M, Siebenrock KA, Ganz R, Leunig M. Anterior femoroacetabular impingement: Part I. Techniques of joint preserving surgery. *Clin Orthop Relat Res.* 2004;(418):61-66.

88. Philippon MJ, Schenker ML. Arthroscopy for the treatment of femoroacetabular impingement in the athlete. *Clin Sports Med.* 2006;25(2):299-308, ix.

89. Ganz R, Leunig M, Leunig-Ganz K, Harris WH. The etiology of osteoarthritis of the hip: An integrated mechanical concept. *Clin Orthop Relat Res.* 2008;466(2):264-272.

90. Chakraverty JK, Sullivan C, Gan C, Narayanaswamy S, Kamath S. Cam and pincer femoroacetabular impingement: CT findings of features resembling femoroacetabular impingement in a young population without symptoms. *AJR Am J Roentgenol.* 2013;200(2):389-395.

91. Ganz R, Parvizi J, Beck M, Leunig M, Nötzli H, Siebenrock KA. Femoroacetabular impingement: A cause for osteoarthritis of the hip. *Clin Orthop Relat Res.* 2003;417:112-120. doi:10.1097/01.blo.0000096804.78689.c2

92. Wall PD, Brown JS, Parsons N, Buchbinder R, Costa ML, Griffin D. Surgery for treating hip impingement (femoroacetabular impingement). *Cochrane Database Syst Rev.* 2014;(9):Cd010796. doi:10.1002/14651858.CD010796.pub2

93. Wall PD, Fernandez M, Griffin DR, Foster NE. Nonoperative treatment for femoroacetabular impingement: A systematic review of the literature. *PM R.* 2013;5(5):418-426. doi:10.1016/j.pmrj.2013.02.005

94. Dwyer T, Whelan D, Shah PS, Ajrawat P, Hoit G, Chahal J. Operative versus nonoperative treatment of femoroacetabular impingement syndrome: A meta-analysis of short-term outcomes. *Arthroscopy.* 2020;36(1):263-273. doi:10.1016/j.arthro.2019.07.025

95. Laude F, Boyer T, Nogier A. Anterior femoroacetabular impingement. *J Bone Spine.* 2007;74(2):127-132.

96. Bedi A, Chen N, Robertson W, Kelly BT. The management of labral tears and femoroacetabular impingement of the hip in the young, active patient. *Arthroscopy.* 2008;24(10):1135-1145.

97. Spencer-Gardner L, Eischen JJ, Levy BA, Sierra RJ, Engasser WM, Krych AJ. A comprehensive five-phase rehabilitation programme after hip arthroscopy for femoroacetabular impingement. *Knee Surg Sports Traumatol Arthrosc.* 2014;22(4):848-859.

98. Pierce CM, LaPrade RF, Wahoff M, O'Brien L, Philippon MJ. Ice hockey goaltender rehabilitation, including on-ice progression, after arthroscopic hip surgery for femoroacetabular impingement. *J Orthop Sports Phys Ther.* 2013;43(3):129-141.

99. Wahoff M, Ryan M. Rehabilitation after hip femoracetabular impingement arthroscopy. *Clin Sports Med.* 2011;30(2):463-482.

100. Byrd JWT. Femoroacetabular impingement in athletes: Part II. Treatment and outcomes. *Sports Health.* 2010;2(5):403-409.

101. Edelstein J, Ranawat A, Enseki KR, Yun RJ, Draovitch P. Post-operative guidelines following hip arthroscopy. *Curr Rev Musculoskelet Med.* 2012;5(1):15-23.

102. Leunig M, Werlen S, Ungersbock A, Ito K, Ganz R. Evaluation of the acetabular labrum by MR arthrography. *J Bone Joint Surg Br.* 1997;79(2):230-234.

103. Kang C, Hwang DS, Cha SM. Acetabular labral tears in patients with sports injury. *Clin Orthop Surg.* 2009;1(4):230-235.

104. Crawford MJ, Dy CJ, Alexander JW, et al. Biomechanics of the hip labrum and the stability of the hip. *Clin Orthop Relat Res.* 2007;465:16-22.

105. McCarthy JC, Noble PC, Schuck MR, Wright J, Lee J. The role of labral lesions to development of early degenerative hip disease. *Clin Orthop Relat Res.* 2001;(393):25-37.

106. Philippon MJ. Debridement of acetabular labral tears with associated thermal capsulorrhaphy. *Op Tech Sports Med.* 2002;10:215-218.

107. Wenger DE, Kendell KR, Miner MR, Trousdale RT. Acetabular labral tears rarely occur in the absence of bony abnormalities. *Clin Orthop Relat Res.* 2004;(426):145-150.

108. Garrison JC, Osler MT, Singleton SR. Rehabilitation after arthroscopy of an acetabular labral tear. *N Am J Sports Phys Ther.* 2007;2:241-250.

109. Wang WG, Yue DB, Zhang NF, Hong W, Li ZR. Clinical diagnosis and arthroscopic treatment of acetabular labral tears. *Orthop Surg.* 2011;3(1):28-34.

110. Burnett RS, Della Rocca GJ, Prather H, Curry M, Maloney WJ, Clohisy JC. Clinical presentation of patients with tears of the acetabular labrum. *J Bone Joint Surg Am.* 2006;88(7):1448-1457.

111. Groh MM, Herrera J. A comprehensive review of hip labral tears. *Current Rev Musculoskel Med.* 2009;2(2):105-117.

112. Peelle MW, Della Rocca GJ, Maloney WJ, Curry MC, Clohisy JC. Acetabular and femoral radiographic abnormalities associated with labral tears. *Clin Orthop Relat Res.* 2005;441:327-333.

113. Larson CM, Giveans MR, Stone RM. Arthroscopic debridement versus refixation of the acetabular labrum associated with femoroacetabular impingement: Mean 3.5-year follow-up. *Am J Sports Med.* 2012;40(5):1015-1021.

114. Robertson WJ, Kadrmas WR, Kelly BT. Arthroscopic management of labral tears in the hip: A systematic review of the literature. *Clin Orthop Relat Res.* 2006;455:88-92.

115. Philippon MJ, Christensen JC, Wahoff MS. Rehabilitation after arthroscopic repair of intra-articular disorders of the hip in a professional football athlete. *J Sport Rehabil.* 2009;18(1):118-134.

116. Philippon MJ. The role of arthroscopic thermal capsulorrhaphy in the hip. *Clin Sports Med.* 2001;20(4):817-829.

117. Cheatham SW, Kolber MJ. Rehabilitation after hip arthroscopy and labral repair in a high school football athlete. *Int J Sports Phys Ther.* 2012;7(2):173-184.

118. Stalzer S, Wahoff M, Scanlan M. Rehabilitation following hip arthroscopy. *Clin Sports Med.* 2006;25(2):337-357.

119. Enseki KR, Martin RL, Draovitch P, Kelly BT, Philippon MJ, Schenker ML. The hip joint: Arthroscopic procedures and postoperative rehabilitation. *J Orthop Sports Phys Ther.* 2006;36(7):516-525.

120. American Joint Replacement Registry. *2020 Annual Report.* 2020.

121. Anthony CA, Abu-Amer W, Freiman S, Pashos G, Clohisy JC. Contemporary Total Hip Arthroplasty in Patients Less Than 30 Years: 10 Year Outcomes Are Encouraging. Paper presented at: Annual Meeting of the American Association of Hip & Knee Surgeons; November 5-8 2020; Dallas, TX.

122. Ortmaier R, Pichler H, Hitzl W, et al. Return to sport after short-stem total hip arthroplasty. *Clin J Sport Med.* 2019;29(6):451-458. doi:10.1097/jsm.0000000000000532

123. Aggarwal VK, Suh YM, Hutzler L, Moscona L, Castañeda P. Total hip arthroplasty for secondary causes of arthritis: An increase in time and money. *Bull Hosp Joint Dis (2013).* 2019;77(4):233-237.

124. Ferguson RJ, Palmer AJ, Taylor A, Porter ML, Malchau H, Glyn-Jones S. Hip replacement. *Lancet.* 2018;392(10158):1662-1671. doi:10.1016/s0140-6736(18)31777-x

125. Beaulé PE, Grammatopoulos G, Speirs A, et al. Unravelling the hip pistol grip/cam deformity: Origins to joint degeneration. *J Orthop Res.* 2018;36(12):3125-3135. doi:10.1002/jor.24137

126. Abramoff B, Caldera FE. Osteoarthritis: Pathology, diagnosis, and treatment options. *Med Clin North Am.* 2020;104(2):293-311. doi:10.1016/j.mcna.2019.10.007

127. Shon WY, Park BY, R RN, Park PS, Im JT, Yun HH. Total hip arthroplasty: Past, present, and future: What has been achieved? *Hip Pelvis.* 2019;31(4):179-189. doi:10.5371/hp.2019.31.4.179

128. Zagra L. Advances in hip arthroplasty surgery: What is justified? *EFORT Open Rev.* 2017;2(5):171-178. doi:10.1302/2058-5241.2.170008

129. Deak N, Varacallo M. Hip precautions. *StatPearls.* StatPearls Publishing; 2019.

130. Barnsley L, Barnsley L, Page R. Are hip precautions necessary post total hip arthroplasty? A systematic review. *Geriatr Orthop Surg Rehabil.* 2015;6(3):230-235. doi:10.1177/2151458515584640

131. Schmidt-Braekling T, Waldstein W, Akalin E, Benavente P, Frykberg B, Boettner F. Minimal invasive posterior total hip arthroplasty: Are 6 weeks of hip precautions really necessary? *Arch Orthop Trauma Surg.* 2015;135(2):271-274. doi:10.1007/s00402-014-2146-x

132. Brown ML, Ezzet KA. Relaxed hip precautions do not increase early dislocation rate following total hip arthroplasty. *J Am Acad Orthop Surg.* 2020;28(10):e440-e447. doi:10.5435/JAAOS-D-19-0026

133. Smith TO, Jepson P, Beswick A, et al. Assistive devices, hip precautions, environmental modifications and training to prevent dislocation and improve function after hip arthroplasty. *Cochrane Database Syst Rev.* 2016;7(7):CD010815. doi:10.1002/14651858.CD010815.pub2

134. Grumet RC, Frank RM, Slabaugh MA, Virkus WW, Bush-Joseph CA, Nho SJ. Lateral hip pain in an athletic population: Differential diagnosis and treatment options. *Sports Health.* 2010;2(3):191-196.

135. Brunot S, Dubeau S, Laumonier H, et al. Acute inguinal pain associated with iliopectineal bursitis in four professional soccer players. *Diagn Ivterv Imaging.* 2013;94(1):91-94.

136. Gerber JM, Herrin SO. Conservative treatment of calcific trochanteric bursitis. *J Manip Physiol Ther.* 1994;17(4):250-252.

137. DeDomenico G. *Beard's Massage Principles and Practice of Soft Tissue Manipulation.* 5th ed. Elsevier Health Sciences; 2007.

Chapter 19

1. Schick DM, Molloy MG, Wiley JP. Injuries during the 2006 Women's Rugby World Cup. *Br J Sports Med.* 2008;42(6):447-451.

2. Fernandez WG, Yard EE, Comstock RD. Epidemiology of lower extremity injuries among U.S. high school athletes. *Acad Emerg Med.* 2007;14(7):641-645.

3. Andrish JT. Sports injuries in weekend warriors: 20 clinical pearls. *J Musculoskelet Med.* 2004;21(4):235-242.

4. Engebretsen L, Risberg MA, Robertson B, Ludvigsen TC, Johansen S. Outcome after knee dislocations: A 2-9 years follow-up of 85 consecutive patients. *Knee Surg Sports Traumatol Arthrosc.* 2009;17(9):1013-1026.

5. Ralphs JR, Benjamin M. The joint capsule: structure, composition, ageing and disease. *J Anat.* 1994;184(Pt 3):503-509.

6. Hayes KW, Petersen C, Falconer J. An examination of Cyriax's passive motion tests with patients having osteoarthritis of the knee. *Phys Ther.* 1994;74(8):697-708.

7. Maitland GD. *Peripheral Manipulation.* Butterworth-Heinemann; 1991.

8. Wang X, Malik A, Bartel DL, Wickiewicz TL, Wright T. Asymmetric varus and valgus stability of the anatomic cadaver knee and the load sharing between collateral ligaments and bearing surfaces. *J Biomech Eng.* 2014;136(8):081005-081005-6. doi:10.1115/1.4027662

9. Paletta GA, Warren RF. Knee injuries and alpine skiing: Treatment and rehabilitation. *Sports Med.* 1994;17(6):410-423.

10. Lipke JM, Janecki CJ, Nelson CL, et al. The role of incompetence of the anterior cruciate and lateral ligaments in anterolateral and anteromedial instability: A biomechanical study of cadaver knees. *J Bone Joint Surg Am.* 1981;63(6):954-960.

11. Arnoczky SP. Anatomy of the anterior cruciate ligament. *Clin Orthop Relat Res.* 1983;(172):19-25.

12. Dienst M, Burks RT, Greis PE. Anatomy and biomechanics of the anterior cruciate ligament. *Orthop Clin North Am.* 2002;33(4):605-620.

13. Krutsch W, Zeman F, Zellner J, Pfeifer C, Nerlich M, Angele P. Increase in ACL and PCL injuries after implementation of a new professional football league. *Knee Surg Sports Traumatol Arthrosc.* 2016;24(7):2271-2279. doi:10.1007/s00167-014-3357-y

14. Bosch U, Kaspercyk WJ, Oestern HJ, Tscherne H. Biology of posterior cruciate ligament healing. *Sports Med Arthroscop Rev.* 1994;2(1):88-99.

15. Voos JE, Mauro CS, Wente T, Warren RF, Wickiewicz TL. Posterior cruciate ligament: Anatomy, biomechanics, and outcomes. *Am J Sports Med.* 2012;40(1):222-231.

16. Fuss FK. Principles and mechanisms of automatic rotation during terminal extension in the human knee joint. *J Anat.* 1992;180:297-304.

17. Safran MR, Allen AA, Lephart SM, Borsa PA, Fu FH, Harner CD. Proprioception in the posterior cruciate ligament deficient knee. *Knee Surg Sports Traumatol Arthrosc.* 1999;7(5):310-317.

18. Dhillon MS, Bali K, Prabhakar S. Differences among mechanoreceptors in healthy and injured anterior cruciate ligaments and their clinical importance. *Muscles Ligaments Tendons J.* 2012;2(1):38-43.

19. Dhillon MS, Bali K, Prabhakar S. Proprioception in anterior cruciate ligament deficient knees and its relevance in anterior cruciate ligament reconstruction. *Indian J Orthop.* 2011;45(4):294-300.

20. Freeman MA, Wyke B. The innervation of the knee joint: An anatomical and histological study in the cat. *J Anat.* 1967;101(Pt 3):505-532.

21. Roberts D, Ageberg E, Andersson G, Fridén T. Clinical measurements of proprioception, muscle strength and laxity in relation to function in the ACL-injured knee. *Knee Surg Sports Traumatol Arthrosc.* 2007;15(1):9-16.

22. Lephart SM, Pincivero DM, Rozzi SL. Proprioception of the ankle and knee. *Sports Med.* 1998;25(3):149-155.

23. Hewett T, Paterno M, Myer G. Strategies for enhancing proprioception and neuromuscular control of the knee. *Clin Orthop.* 2002;402:76-94.

24. Wikstrom EA, Tillman MD, Chmielewski TL, Borsa PA. Measurement and evaluation of dynamic joint stability of the knee and ankle after injury. *Sports Med.* 2006;w36(5):393-410.

25. Fitzgerald GK, Axe MJ, Snyder-Mackler L. The efficacy of perturbation training in nonoperative anterior cruciate ligament rehabilitation programs for physically active individuals. *Phys Ther.* 2000;80(2):128-140.

26. Monaco E, Ferretti A, Labianca L, et al. Navigated knee kinematics after cutting of the ACL and its secondary restraint. *Knee Surg Sports Traumatol Arthrosc.* 2012;20(5):870-877.

27. Butler DL, Noyes FR, Grood ES. Ligamentous restraints to anterior-posterior drawer in the human knee: A biomechanical study. *J Bone Joint Surg Am.* 1980;62(2):259-270.

28. Messner K, Gao J. The menisci of the knee joint: Anatomical and functional characteristics, and a rationale for clinical treatment. *J Anat.* 1998;193:161-178.

29. McCarty EC, Marx RG, DeHaven KE. Meniscus repair: Considerations in treatment and update of clinical results. *Clin Orthop.* 2002;402:122-134.

30. Chen HN, Yang K, Dong QR, Wang Y. Assessment of tibial rotation and meniscal movement using kinematic magnetic resonance imaging. *J Orthop Surg Res.* 2014;9:65. doi:10.1186/s13018-014-0065-8

31. Ahmed AM, Burke DL. In vitro measurement of static pressure distribution in synovial joints: I. Tibial surface of the knee. *J Biomed Eng.* 1983;105:216-225.

32. Howell R, Kumar NS, Patel N, Tom J. Degenerative meniscus: Pathogenesis, diagnosis, and treatment options. *World J Orthop.* 2014;5(5):597-602.

33. Snoeker BA, Bakker EW, Kegel CA, Lucas C. Risk factors for meniscal tears: A systematic review including meta-analysis. *J Orthop Sports Phys Ther.* 2013;43(6):352-367.

34. Khan N, McMahon P, Obaid H. Bony morphology of the knee and non-traumatic meniscal tears: Is there a role for meniscal impingement? *Skeletal Radiol.* 2014;43(7):955-962.

35. Petersen W, Tillmann B. Age-related blood and lymph supply of the knee menisci. *Acta Orthop Scand.* 1995;66(4):308-312. doi:10.3109/17453679508995550

36. Rajendran K. Mechanism of locking at the knee joint. *J Anat.* 1985;143:189-194.

37. Tecklenburg K, Dejour D, Hoser C, Fink C. Bony and cartilaginous anatomy of the patellofemoral joint. *Knee Surg Sports Traumatol Arthrosc*. 2006;14(3):235-240.

38. Amis AA. Current concepts on anatomy and biomechanics of patellar stability. *Sports Med Arthrosc Rev*. 2007;15(2):48-56.

39. Buchbinder MR, Napora NJ, Biggs EW. The relationship of abnormal pronation to chondromalacia of the patella in distance runners. *J Am Podiatry Assoc*. 1979;69(2):159-162.

40. Mascal CL, Landel R, Powers C. Management of patellofemoral pain targeting hip, pelvis, and trunk muscle function: 2 case reports. *J Orthop Sports Phys Ther*. 2003 Nov 2003;33(11):647-60.

41. Whitman JM, Childs JD, Walker V. The use of manipulation in a patient with an ankle sprain injury not responding to conventional management: A case report. *Man Ther*. 2005;10(3):224-231.

42. Forster BB, Lee JS, Kelly S, et al. Proximal tibiofibular joint: an often-forgotten cause of lateral knee pain. *AJR Am J Roentgenol*. 2007;188(4):W359-W366.

43. Park WH, Kim DK, Yoo JC, et al. Correlation between dynamic postural stability and muscle strength, anterior instability, and knee scale in anterior cruciate ligament deficient knees. *Arch Orthop Trauma Surg*. 2010;130(8):1013-1018.

44. Maffiuletti NA, Lepers R. Quadriceps femoris torque and EMG activity in seated versus supine position. *Med Sci Sports Exerc*. 2003;35(9):1511-1516.

45. Close JR. *Motor Function in the Lower Extremity: Analyses of Electronic Instrumentation*. Charles C Thomas; 1964.

46. Skalley TC, Terry GC, Teitge RA. The quantitative measurement of normal passive medial and lateral patellar motion limits. *Am J Sports Med*. 1993;21(5):728-732.

47. Aglietti P, Buzzi R, D'Andria S, Zaccherotti G. Patellofemoral problems after intraarticular anterior cruciate ligament reconstruction. *Clin Orthop Relat Res*. 1993;(288):195-204.

48. Akbarshahi M, Fernandez JW, Schache AG, Pandy MG. Subject-specific evaluation of patellofemoral joint biomechanics during functional activity. *Med Eng Phys*. 2014;36(9):1122-1133.

49. Wang JH, Tao K, Li H, Wang C. Modelling and analysis on biomechanical dynamic characteristics of knee flexion movement under squatting. *ScientificWorldJournal*. 2014;2014:321080. doi:10.1155/2014/321080

50. Hehne HJ. Biomechanics of the patellofemoral joint and its clinical relevance. *Clin Orthop*. 1990;258:73-85.

51. Hungerford DS, Barry M. Biomechanics of the patellofemoral joint. *Clin Orthop*. 1979;144:9-15.

52. Wünschel M, Leichtle U, Obloh C, Wülker N, Müller O. The effect of different quadriceps loading patterns on tibiofemoral joint kinematics and patellofemoral contact pressure during simulated partial weight-bearing knee flexion. *Knee Surg Sports Traumatol Arthrosc*. 2011;19(7):1099-1106.

53. Grelsamer RP, Klein JR. The biomechanics of the patellofemoral joint. *J Orthop Sports Phys Ther*. 1998;28(5):286-298.

54. Steinkamp LA, Dillingham MF, Markel MD, Hill JA, Kaufman KR. Biomechanical considerations in patellofemoral joint rehabilitation. *Am J Sports Med*. 1993;21(3):438-444.

55. Zwerver J, Bredeweg SW, Hof AL. Biomechanical analysis of the single-leg decline squat. *Br J Sports Med*. 2007;41:264-268.

56. Powers CM, Ho KY, Chen YJ, Souza RB, Farrokhi S. Patellofermoral joint stress during weight-bearing and non-weight-bearing quadriceps exercises. *J Orthop Sports Phys Ther*. 2014;44(5):320-327.

57. Powers CM, Ho KY, Chen YJ, Souza RB, Farrokhi S. Patellofemoral joint stress during weight-bearing and non-weight-bearing quadriceps exercises. *J Orthop Sports Phys Ther*. 2014;44(5):320-327.

58. Kaufman KR, An K-N, Litchy WJ, Morrey BF, Chao EYS. Dynamic joint forces during knee isokinetic exercise. *Am J Sports Med*. 1991;19:305-316.

59. Reilly DT, Martens M. Experimental analysis of the quadriceps muscle force and patello-femoral joint reaction force for various activities. *Acta Orthop Scand*. 1972;43:126-137.

60. Wallace DA, Salem GJ, Salinas R, Powers CM. Patellofemoral joint kinetics while squatting with and without an external load. *J Orthop Sports Phys Ther*. 2002;32(4):141-148.

61. Rowe PJ, Myles CM, Walker C, Nutton R. Knee joint kinematics in gait and other functional activities measured using flexible electrogoniometry: How much knee motion is sufficient for normal daily life? *Gait Posture*. 2000;12(2):143-155.

62. Doucette SA, Child DD. The effect of open and closed chain exercise and knee joint position on patellar tracking in lateral patellar compression syndrome. *J Orthop Sports Phys Ther*. 1996;23:104-110.

63. Crossley KM, Cowan SM, McConnell J, Bennell KL. Physical therapy improves knee flexion during stair ambulation in patellofemoral pain. *Med Sci Sports Exerc*. 2005;37(2):176-183.

64. Holmes SW, Jr., Clancy WG, Jr. Clinical classification of patellofemoral pain and dysfunction. *J Orthop Sports Phys Ther*. 1998;28(5):299-306.

65. Bagwell J, Fukuda TY, Powers CM. Sagittal plane pelvis motion influences transverse plane motion of the femur: Kinematic coupling at the hip joint. *Gait Posture*. 2016;43(Jan):120-124.

66. Hruska RJ. Pelvic stability influences lower-extremity kinematics. *Biomech*. 1998;5(6):23-29.

67. Dierks TA, Manal KT, Hamill J, Davis IS. Proximal and distal influences on hip and knee kinematics in runners with patellofemoral pain during a prolonged run. *J Orthop Sports Phys Ther*. 2008;38(8):448-456.

68. Lankhorst NE, Bierma-Zeinstra SM, van Middelkoop M. Risk factors for patellofemoral pain syndrome: A systematic review. *J Orthop Sports Phys Ther*. 2012;42(2):81-94.

69. Thomeé R, Augustsson J, Karlsson J. Patellofemoral pain syndrome: A review of current issues. *Sports Med*. 1999;28(4):245-262.

70. Waryasz GR, McDermott AY. Patellofemoral pain syndrome (PFPS): A systematic review of anatomy and potential risk factors. *Dyn Med*. 2008;7:9. doi:10.1186/1476-5918-7-9

71. Mendonça LD, Verhagen E, Bittencourt NF, Gonçalves GG, Ocarino JM, Fonseca ST. Factors associated with the

presence of patellar tendon abnormalities in male athletes. *J Sci Med Sport*. 2015;19(5):389-394. doi:10.1016/j.jsams.2015.05.011

72. Kramer LC, Denegar CR, Buckley WE, Hertel J. Factors associated with anterior cruciate ligament injury: History in female athletes. *J Sports Med Phys Fitness*. 2007;47(4):446-454.

73. Fahrer H, Rentsch HU, Gerber NJ, Beyeler C, Hess CW, Grunig B. Knee effusion and reflex inhibition of the quadriceps: A bar to effective retraining. *J Bone Joint Surg Br*. 1988;70(4):635-638.

74. Leroux A, Bélanger M, Boucher JP. Pain effect on monosynaptic and polysynaptic reflex inhibition. *Arch Phys Med Rehabil*. 1995;76(6):576-582.

75. Ounpuu S. The biomechanics of walking and running. *Clin Sports Med*. 1994;13(4):843-863.

76. Lee S, Farrar RP. Resistance training induces muscle-specific changes in muscle mass and function in rat. *J Exerc Physiol Online*. 2003;6(2):80-87.

77. Merle J, Rougier P, Belaid D, Cantalloube S, Lamotte D. Is early weight bearing resumption beneficial after total hip replacement? *Orthop Traumatol Surg Res*. 2009;95(2):127-133.

78. McDonough AL, Weir JP. The effect of postsurgical edema of the knee joint on reflex inhibition of the quadriceps femoris. *J Sport Rehabil*. 1996;5(2):172-182.

79. Spencer JD, Hayes KC, Alexander IJ. Knee joint effusion and quadriceps reflex inhibition in man. *Arch Phys Med Rehabil*. 1984;64:171-177.

80. Young A, Stokes M, Iles JF. Effects of joint pathology on muscle. *Clin Orthop Relat Res*. 1987;(219):21-27.

81. Stokes M, Young A. Investigations of quadriceps inhibition: Implications for clinical practice. *Physiother*. 1984;70(11):425-428.

82. Morrissey MC. Reflex inhibition of thigh muscles in knee injury: Causes and treatment. *Sports Med*. 1989;7(4):263-276.

83. Kocaman O, Koyuncu H, Dinc A, Toros H, Karamehmetoğlu FS. The comparison of the effects of electrical stimulation and exercise in the treatment of knee osteoarthritis. *Turkish J Phys Med Rehabil*. 2008;54(2):54-58.

84. van der Krogt MM, Delp S, Schwartz MH. How robust is human gait to muscle weakness? *Gait Posture*. 2012;36(1):113-119.

85. Sprague RB. Factors related to extension lag at the knee joint. *J Orthop Sports Phys Ther*. 1982;3(4):178-184.

86. Grood ES, Suntay WJ, Noyes FR, Butler DL. Biomechanics of the knee-extension exercise: Effect of cutting the anterior cruciate ligament. *J Bone Joint Surg Am*. 1984;66(5):725-734.

87. Shenoy S, Mishra P, Sandhu JS. Peak torque and IEMG activity of quadriceps femoris muscle at three different knee angles in a collegiate population. *J Exerc Sci Fitness*. 2011;9(1):40-45.

88. Witvrouw E, Sneyers C, Lysens L, Victor J, Bellemans J. Reflex response times of vastus medialis oblique and vastus lateralis in normal subjects and in subjects with patellofemoral pain syndrome. *J Orthop Sports Phys Ther*. 1996;24(3):160-165.

89. Lieb FJ, Perry J. Quadriceps function: An electromyographic study under isometric conditions. *J Bone Joint Surg Am*. 1971;53(4):749-758.

90. Gough JV, Ladley G. An investigation into the effectiveness of various forms of quadriceps exercises. *Physiother*. 1971;57:356-361.

91. Knight KL, Martin JA, Londeree BR. EMG comparison of quadriceps femoris activity during knee extension and straight leg raises. *Am J Sports Med*. 1979;58:57-67.

92. Mikkelsen C, Werner S, Eriksson E. Closed kinetic chain alone compared to combined open and closed kinetic chain exercises for quadriceps strengthening after anterior cruciate ligament reconstruction with respect to return to sports: A prospective matched follow-up study. *Knee Surg Sports Traumatol Arthrosc*. 2000;8(6):337-342.

93. Callaghan MJ, Parkes MJ, Hutchinson CE, Felson DT. Factors associated with arthrogenous muscle inhibition in patellofemoral osteoarthritis. *Osteoarthritis Cartilage*. 2014;22(6):742-746.

94. Pietrosimone B, Lepley AS, Murray AM, Thomas AC, Bahhur NO, Schwartz TA. Changes in voluntary quadriceps activation predict changes in muscle strength and gait biomechanics following knee joint effusion. *Clin Biomech*. 2014;29(8):923-929.

95. Rice DA, McNair PJ. Quadriceps arthrogenic muscle inhibition: Neural mechanisms and treatment perspectives. *Semin Arthritis Rheum*. 2010;40(3):250-266.

96. Shakespeare DT, Stokes M, Sherman KP, Young A. Reflex inhibition of the quadriceps after meniscectomy: Lack of association with pain. *Clin Physiol*. 1985;5(2):137-144.

97. Rice DA, McNair PJ, Lewis GN, Dalbeth N. Quadriceps arthrogenic muscle inhibition: The effects of experimental knee joint effusion on motor cortex excitability. *Arthritis Res Ther*. 2014;16(6):502. doi:10.1186/s13075-014-0502-4

98. Wood L, Ferrell WR, Baxendale RH. Pressures in normal and acutely distended human knee joints and effects on quadriceps maximal voluntary contractions. *Q J Exp Physiol*. 1988;73(3):305-314.

99. McNair PJ, Marshall RN, Maguire K. Swelling of the knee joint: Effects of exercise on quadriceps muscle strength. *Arch Phys Med Rehabil*. 1996;77(9):896-899.

100. Palmieri-Smith RM, Villwock M, Downie B, Hecht G, Zemicke R. Pain and effusion and quadriceps activation and strength. *J Athl Train*. 2013;48(2):186-191.

101. Cook TM, Farrell KP, Carey IA, Gibbs JM, Wiger GE. Effects of restricted knee flexion and walking speed on the vertical ground reaction force during gait. *J Orthop Sports Phys Ther*. 1997;25(4):236-244.

102. Hurley MV, Jones DW, Newham DJ. Arthrogenic quadriceps inhibition and rehabilitation of patients with extensive traumatic knee injuries. *Clin Sci (Lond)*. 1994;86(3):305-310.

103. Harkey MS, Gribble PA, Pietrosimone BG. Disinhibitory interventions and voluntary quadriceps activation: A systematic review. *J Athl Train*. 2014;49(3):411-421.

104. Gabler CM, Lepley AS, Uhl TL, Mattacola CG. Comparison of transcutaneous electrical nerve stimulation and cryotherapy for increasing quadriceps activation in patients with knee pathologies. *J Sport Rehabil*. 2015. doi:10.1123/jsr.2014-0292

105. Pamukoff DN, Ryan ED, Blackburn JT. The acute effects of local muscle vibration frequency on peak torque, rate of torque development, and EMG activity. *J Electromyogr Kinesiol*. 2014;24

106. Blackburn JT, Pamukoff DN, Sakr M, Vaughan AJ, Berkoff DJ. Whole body and local muscle vibration reduce artificially induced quadriceps arthrogenic inhibition. *Arch Phys Med Rehabil.* 2014;95(11):2021-2028.

107. Beynnon BD, Johnson RJ, Fleming BC, Stankewich CJ, Renström PA, Nichols CE. The strain behavior of the anterior cruciate ligament during squatting and active flexion-extension: A comparison of an open and a closed kinetic chain exercise. *Am J Sports Med.* 1997;25(6):823-829.

108. Bynum EB, Barrack RL, Alexander AH. Open versus closed chain kinetic exercises after anterior cruciate ligament reconstruction: A prospective randomized study. *Am J Sports Med.* 1995;23(4):401-406.

109. Fukuda TY, Fingerhut D, Moreira VC, et al. Open kinetic chain exercises in a restricted range of motion after anterior cruciate ligament reconstruction: A randomized controlled clinical trial. *Am J Sports Med.* 2013;41(4):788-794.

110. Heijne A, Werner S. Early versus late start of open kinetic chain quadriceps exercises after ACL reconstruction with patellar tendon or hamstring grafts: A prospective randomized outcome study. *Knee Surg Sports Traumatol Arthrosc.* 2007;15(4):402-414.

111. Keays SL, Sayers M, Mellifont DB, Richardson C. Tibial displacement and rotation during seated knee extension and wall squatting: A comparative study of tibiofemoral kinematics between chronic unilateral anterior cruciate ligament deficient and healthy knees. *Knee.* 2012;20(5):346-353.

112. Worrell TW, Crisp E, LaRosa C. Electromyographic reliability and analysis of selected lower extremity muscles during lateral step-up conditions. *J Athl Train.* 1998;33(2):156-162.

113. Escamilla RF, Fleisig GS, Zheng N, Barrentine SW, Wilk KE, Andrews JR. Biomechanics of the knee during closed kinetic chain and open kinetic chain exercises. *Med Sci Sports Exerc.* 1998;30(4):556-569.

114. Beynnon BD, Fleming BC, Johnson RJ, Nichols CE, Renstrom PA, Pope MH. Anterior cruciate ligament strain behavior during rehabilitation exercises in vivo. *Am J Sports Med.* 1995;23(1):24-34.

115. Wilk KE, Escamilla RF, Fleisig GS, Barrentine SW, Andrews JR, Boyd ML. A comparison of tibiofemoral joint forces and electromyographic activity during open and closed kinetic chain exercises. *Am J Sports Med.* 1996;24:518-527.

116. Sahli S, Rebal H, Elleuch MH, Tabka Z, Poumarat. Tibiofemoral joint kinetics during squatting with increasing external load. *J Sport Rehabil.* 2008;17:300-315.

117. Jenkins WL, Munns SW, Jayaraman G, Wertzberger KL, Neely K. A measurement of anterior tibial displacement in the closed and open kinetic chain. *J Orthop Sports Phys Ther.* 1997;25(1):49-56.

118. Isear JA, Erickson JR, Worrell TW. EMG analysis of lower extremity muscle recruitment patterns during an unloaded squat. *Med Sci Sports Exerc.* 1997;29(4):532-539.

119. Najibi S, Albright JP. The use of knee braces, part 1: Prophylactic knee braces in contact sports. *Am J Sports Med.* 2005;33(4):602-611.

120. Jenkins WL, Munns SW, Loudon J. Knee joint accessory motion following anterior cruciate ligament allograft reconstruction: a preliminary report. *J Orthop Sports Phys Ther.* 1998;28(1):32-39.

121. Mayr HO, Stüeken P, Münch EO, et al. Brace or no-brace after ACL graft? Four-year results of a prospective clinical trial. *Knee Surg Sports Traumatol Arthrosc.* 2014;22(5):1156-1162.

122. Moller E, Forssblad M, Hansson L, Wange P, Weidenhielm L. Bracing versus nonbracing in rehabilitation after anterior cruciate ligament reconstruction: A randomized prospective study with 2-year follow-up. *Knee Surg Sports Traumatol Arthrosc.* 2001;9(2):102-108.

123. Wright RW, Fetzer GB. Bracing after ACL reconstruction: A systematic review. *Clin Orthop Relat Res.* 2007;455(1):162-168.

124. Campbell B, Yaggie J, Cipriani D. Temporal influences of functional knee bracing on torque production of the lower extremity. *J Sport Rehabil.* 2006;15:216-227.

125. Garth WP, Jr., Flowers K. Efficacy of knee sleeves in the management of patellofemoral dysfunction. *Athl Ther Today.* 1998;3:23-27.

126. Masini BD, Owens BD. Current recommendations for anterior cruciate ligament bracing: When to use. *Phys Sportsmed.* 2013;41(1):35-39.

127. Wegener L, Kisner C, Nichols D. Static and dynamic balance responses in persons with bilateral knee osteoarthritis. *J Orthop Sports Phys Ther.* 1997;25(1):13-18.

128. Lattanzio PJ, Petrella RJ, Sproule JR, Fowler PJ. Effects of fatigue on knee proprioception. *Clin J Sport Med.* 1997;7(1):22-27.

129. Risberg M, Mork M, Jenssen H, Holm I. Design and implementation of a neuromuscular training program following anterior cruciate ligament reconstruction. *J Orthop Sports Phys Ther.* 2001;31(11):620-631.

130. Yabroudi MA, Irrgang JJ. Rehabilitation and return to play after anatomic anterior cruciate ligament reconstruction. *Clin Sports Med.* 2013;32(1):165-175.

131. Travell JG, Simons DG. *Myofascial Pain and Dysfunction: The Trigger Point Manual. Vol. 2.* Williams and Wilkins; 1992.

132. Woo SL, Matthews JV, Akeson WH, Amiel D, Convery FR. Connective tissue response to immobility: Correlative study of biomechanical and biochemical measurements of normal and immobilized rabbit knees. *Arthritis Rheum.* 1975;18(3):257-264.

133. Baezell JR, T.L. G, Magrum EM, Wilder R. Treatment of lateral knee pain by addressing tibiofibular hypomobility in a recreational runner. *N Am J Sports Phys Ther.* 2009;4(1):21-28.

134. Montgomery RD. Healing of muscle, ligaments, and tendons. *Semin Vet Med Surg.* 1989;4(4):304-311.

135. Dewey WS, Richard RL, Parry IS. Positioning, splinting, and contracture management. *Phys Med Rehabil Clin N Am.* 2011;22(2):229-247.

136. Nugent-Derfus GE, Takara T, O'Neill JK, et al. Continuous passive motion applied to whole joints stimulates chondrocyte biosynthesis of PRG4. *Osteoarthritis Cartilage.* 2007;15(5):566-574.

137. Jezequel JR. The continuous passive motion concept: Part II. *Phys Ther Prod.* 2011;22(4):20-22.

138. Harvey LA, Brosseau L, Herbert RD. Continuous passive motion following total knee arthroplasty in people with arthritis. *Cochrane Database Syst Rev.* 2014(2). doi:10.1002/14651858.CD004260.pub3

139. Ekdahl M, Wang JH, Ronga M, Fu FH. Graft healing in anterior cruciate ligament reconstruction. *Knee Surg Sports Traumatol Arthrosc*. 2008;16(10):935-947.

140. Jung HJ, Fisher MB, Woo SL. Role of biomechanics in the understanding of normal, injured, and healing ligaments and tendons. *Sports Med Arthrosc Rehabil Ther Technol*. 2009;20(1). doi:10.1186/1758-2555-1-9

141. Anwer S, Alghadir A. Effect of isometric quadriceps exercise on muscle strength, pain, and function in patients with knee osteoarthritis: A randomized controlled study. *J Phys Ther Sci*. 2014;26(5):745-748.

142. Van Cant J, Pineux C, Pitance L, Feipel V. Hip muscle strength and endurance in females with patellofemoral pain: A systematic review with meta-analysis. *Int J Sports Phys Ther*. 2014;9(5):564-582.

143. Shirazi ZR, Moghaddam MB, Motealleh A. Comparative evaluation of core muscle recruitment pattern in response to sudden external perturbations in patients with patellofemoral pain syndrome and healthy subjects. *Arch Phys Med Rehabil*. 2014;95(7):1383-1389.

144. Hettinger T. *Physiology of Strength*. C.C. Thomas; 1961.

145. Clayton HM, White AD, Kaiser LJ, Nauwelaerts S, Lavagnino M, Stubbs NC. Hindlimb response to tactile stimulation of the pastern and coronet. *Equine Vet J*. 2010;42(3):227-233.

146. Hanten WP, Schulthies SS. Exercise effect on electromyographic activity of the vastus medialis oblique and vastus lateralis muscles. *Phys Ther*. 1990;70(9):561-565.

147. Mirzabeigi E, Jordan C, Gronley JK, Rockowitz NL, Perry J. Isolation of the vastus medialis oblique muscle during exercise. *Am J Sports Med*. 1999;27(1):50-53.

148. Hertel J, Earl JE, Tsang KKW, Miller SJ. Combining isometric knee extension exercises with hip adduction or abduction does not increase quadriceps EMG activity. *Br J Sports Med*. 2004;38(2):210-213.

149. Earl JE, Schmitz RJ, Arnold BL. Activation of the VMO and VL during dynamic mini-squat exercises with and without isometric hip adduction. *J Electromyogr Kinesiol*. 2001;11(6):381-386.

150. Peng HT, Kernozek TW, Song CY. Muscle activation of vastus medialis obliquus and vastus lateralis during a dynamic leg press exercise with and without isometric hip adduction. *Phys Ther Sport*. 2013;14(1):44-49.

151. Anderson LL, Magnusson SP, Nielsen M, Haleem J, Poulsen K, Aagaard P. Neuromuscular activation in conventional therapeutic exercises and heavy resistance exercises: Implications for rehabilitation. *Phys Ther*. 2006;86(5):683-697.

152. Wong YM, Straub RK, Powers CM. The VMO:VL activation ratio while squatting with hip adduction is influenced by the choice of recording electrode. *J Electromyogr Kinesiol*. 2013;23(2):443-447.

153. Hodges PW, Richardson CA. The influence of isometric hip adduction on quadriceps femoris activity. *Scand J Rehabil Med*. 1993;25(2):57-62.

154. Irish SE, Millward AJ, Wride J, Haas BM, Shum GL. The effect of closed-kinetic chain exercises and open-kinetic chain exercise on the muscle activity of vastus medialis oblique and vastus lateralis. *J Strength Cond Res*. 2010;24(5):1256-1262.

155. Boling M, Padua D, Blackburn JT, Petschauer MA, Hirth C. Hip adduction does not affect VMO EMG amplitude or VMO:VL ratios during a dynamic squat exercise. *J Sport Rehabil*. 2006;15(3):195-205.

156. Cerny K. Vastus medialis oblique/vastus lateralis muscle activity ratios for selected exercises in persons with and without patellofemoral pain syndrome. *Phys Ther*. 1995;75:672-683.

157. Coqueiro KR, Bevilaqua-Grossi D, Bérzin F, Soares AB, Candolo C, Monteiro-Pedro V. Analysis on the activation of the VMO and VLL muscles during semisquat exercises with and without hip adduction in individuals with patellofemoral pain syndrome. *J Electromyogr Kinesiol*. 2005;15(6):596-603.

158. Laprade J, Culham E, Brouwer B. Comparison of five isometric exercises in the recruitment of the vastus medialis oblique in persons with and without patellofemoral pain syndrome. *J Orthop Sports Phys Ther*. 1998;27:197-204.

159. Ericson MO, Nisell R. Tibiofemoral forces during ergometer cycling. *Am J Sports Med*. 1986;14(4):285-290.

160. Shelburne KB, Torry MR, Pandy MG. Contributions of muscles, ligaments, and the ground-reaction force to tibiofemoral joint loading during normal gait. *J Orthop Res*. 2006;24(10):1983-1990.

161. Escamilla RF, Zheng N, MacLeod TD, et al. Cruciate ligament forces between short-step and long-step forward lunge. *Med Sci Sports Exerc*. 2010;42(10):1932-1942.

162. Cohen ZA, Roglic H, Grelsamer RP, et al. Patellofemoral stresses during open and closed kinetic chain exercises: An analysis using computer simulation. *Am J Sports Med*. 2001;29(4):480-487.

163. Katz JW, Fingeroth RJ. The diagnostic accuracy of ruptures of the anterior cruciate ligament comparing the Lachman test, the anterior drawer sign, and the pivot shift test in acute and chronic knee injuries. *Am J Sports Med*. 1986;14(1):88-91. doi:10.1177/036354658601400115

164. Boeree NR, Ackroyd CE. Assessment of the menisci and cruciate ligaments: An audit of clinical practice. *Injury*. Jul 1991;22(4):291-294. doi:10.1016/0020-1383(91)90008-3

165. Steinbrück K, Wiehmann JC. Untersuchung des kniegelenks: Wertigkeit klinischer befunde unter arthroskopischer kontrolle [Examination of the knee joint: The value of clinical findings in arthroscopic control]. *Z Orthop Ihre Grenzgeb*. May-Jun 1988;126(3):289-295. doi:10.1055/s-2008-1040205

166. Rubinstein RAJ, Shelbourne KD, McCarroll JR, VanMeter CD, Rettig AC. The accuracy of the clinical examination in the setting of posterior cruciate ligament injuries. *Am J Sports Med*. 1994;22(4):550-557. doi:10.1177/036354659402200419

167. Daniel DM, Stone ML, Barnett P, Sachs R. Use of the quadriceps active test to diagnose posterior cruciate-ligament disruption and measure posterior laxity of the knee. *J Bone Joint Surg Am*. 1988;70(3):386-391.

168. Harilainen A. Evaluation of knee instability in acute ligamentous injuries. *Ann Chir Gynaecol*. 1987;76(5):269-273.

169. Evans PJ, Bell GD, Frank C. Prospective evaluation of the McMurray test. *Am J Sports Med*. 1993;21(4):604-608. doi:10.1177/036354659302100420

170. P.J. F, Lubliner JA. The predictive value of five clinical signs in the evaluation of meniscal pathology. *Arthroscopy*. 1989;5(3):184-186. doi:10.1016/0749-8063(89)90168-0

171. Kurosaka M, Yagi M, Yoshiya S, Muratsu H, Mizuno K. Efficacy of the axially loaded pivot shift test for the diagnosis of a meniscal tear. *Int Orthop.* 1999;23(5) doi:10.1007/s002640050369

172. Evans S, Shaginaw J, Bartolozzi A. ACL reconstruction—it's all about timing. *Int J Sports Phys Ther.* 2014;9(2):268-273.

173. Dye SF, Cannon WD, Jr. Anatomy and biomechanics of the anterior cruciate ligament. *Clin Sports Med.* 1988;7:715-725.

174. Markolf KL, Gorek JF, Kabo JM, Shapiro MS. Direct measurement of resultant forces in the anterior cruciate ligament: An in vitro study performed with a new experimental technique. *J Bone Joint Surg Am.* 1990;72A:557-567.

175. McNair PJ. Important features associated with anterior cruciate ligament injury. *N Z Med J.* 1990;103(901):537-539.

176. Alentorn-Geli E, Myer GD, Silvers HJ, et al. Prevention of non-contact anterior cruciate ligament injuries in soccer players: Part 1. Mechanisms of injury and underlying risk factors. *Knee Surg Sports Traumatol Arthrosc.* 2009;17(7):705-729.

177. Krosshaug T, Nakamae A, Boden BP, et al. Mechanism of anterior cruciate ligament injury in basketball: Video analysis of 39 cases. *Am J Sports Med.* 2007;35(3):359-367.

178. Lyle MA, Valero-Cuevas FJ, Gregor RJ, Powers CM. Control of dynamic foot-ground interactions in male and female soccer athletes: Females exhibit reduced dexterity and higher limb stiffness during landing. *J Biomech.* 2014;47(2):512-517.

179. Zeller BL, McCrory JL, Kibler WB, Uhl TL. Differences in kinematics and electromyographic activity between men and women during the single-legged squat. *Am J Sports Med.* 2003;31(3):449-456.

180. Chappell JD, Creighton RA, Giuliani C, Yu B, Garrett WE. Kinematics and electromyography of landing preparation in vertical stop-jump: Risks for noncontact anterior cruciate ligament injury. *Am J Sports Med.* 2007;35(2):235-241.

181. Millett PJ, Willis AA, Warren RF. Associated injuries in pediatric and adolescent anterior cruciate ligament tears: Does a delay in treatment increase the risk of meniscal tear? *Arthroscopy.* 2002;18(9):955-959.

182. Dumont GD, Hogue GD, Padalecki JR, Okoro N, Wilson PL. Meniscal and chondral injuries associated with pediatric anterior cruciate ligament tears: relationship of treatment time and patient-specific factors. *Am J Sports Med.* 2012;40(9):2128-2133.

183. Eitzen I, Moksnes H, Snyder-Mackler L, Engebretsen L, Risberg MA. Functional tests should be accentuated more in the decision for ACL reconstruction. *Knee Surg Sports Traumatol Arthrosc.* 2010;18(11):1517-1525.

184. Kapoor B, Clement DJ, Kirkley A, Maffulli N. Current practice in the management of anterior cruciate ligament injuries in the United Kingdom. *Br J Sports Med.* 2004;38(5):542-544.

185. Meunier A, Odensten M, Good L. Long-term results after primary repair or non-surgical treatment of anterior cruciate ligament rupture: A randomized study with a 15-year follow-up. *Scand J Med Sci Sports.* 2007;17(3):230-237.

186. Delay BS, Smolinski RJ, Wind WM, Bowman DS. Current practices and opinions in ACL reconstruction and rehabilitation: Results of a survey of the American Orthopaedic Society for Sports Medicine. *Am J Knee Surg.* 2001;14(2):85-91.

187. Irrgang JJ, Harner CD, Fu FH, Silbey MB, DiGiacomo R. Loss of motion following ACL reconstruction: A second look. *J Sport Rehabil.* 1997;6:213-225.

188. Mehran N, Skendzel JG, Lesniak BP, Bedi A. Contemporary graft options in anterior cruciate ligament reconstruction. *Op Tech Sports Med.* 2013;21(1):10-18.

189. Marrale J, Morrissey MC, Haddad FS. A literature review of autograft and allograft anterior cruciate ligament reconstruction. *Knee Surg Sports Traumatol Arthrosc.* 2007;15(6):690-704.

190. Paessler HH, Mastrokalos DS. Anterior cruciate ligament reconstruction using semitendinosus and gracilis tendons, bone patellar tendon, or quadriceps tendon-graft with press-fit fixation without hardware: A new and innovative procedure. *Orthop Clin North Am.* 2003;34(1):49-64.

191. Scheffler SU, Südkamp NP, Göckenjan A, Hoffmann RF, Weiler A. Biomechanical comparison of hamstring and patellar tendon graft anterior cruciate ligament reconstruction techniques: The impact of fixation level and fixation method under cyclic loading. *Arthroscopy.* 2002;18(3):304-315.

192. Barclay L. Outcomes similar for patellar or hamstring tendon ACL repair. *Am J Sports Med.* 2003;31:564-573.

193. Brown CHJ, Steiner ME, Carson EW. The use of hamstring tendons for anterior cruciate ligament reconstruction: Technique and results. *Clin Sports Med.* 1993;12(4):723-756.

194. Hussein M, Van Eck CF, Cretnik A, Dinevski D, Fu FH. Prospective randomized clinical evaluation of conventional single-bundle, anatomic single-bundle, and anatomic double-bundle anterior cruciate ligament reconstruction. *Am J Sports Med.* 2012;40(3):512-520.

195. Gulotta LV, Rodeo SA. Biology of autograft and allograft healing in anterior cruciate ligament reconstruction. *Clin Sports Med.* 2007;26(3):509-524.

196. Cascio BM, Culp L, Cosgarea AJ. Return to play after anterior cruciate ligament reconstruction. *Clin Sports Med.* 2004;23(3):395-408.

197. Wilk KE, Arrigo C, Andrews JR, Clancy WG. Rehabilitation after anterior cruciate ligament reconstruction in the female athlete. *J Athl Train.* 1999;34(2):177-193.

198. Kvist J. Tibial translation in exercises used early in rehabilitation after anterior cruciate ligament reconstruction exercises to achieve weight-bearing. *Knee.* 2006;13(6):460-463.

199. Beynnon BD, Johnson RJ, Naud S, et al. Accelerated versus nonaccelerated rehabilitation after anterior cruciate ligament reconstruction: A prospective, randomized, double-blind investigation evaluating knee joint laxity using roentgen stereophotogrammetric analysis. *Am J Sports Med.* 2011;39(12):2536-2548.

200. Scheffler SU, Unterhauser FN, Weiler A. Graft remodeling and ligamentization after cruciate ligament reconstruction. *Knee Surg Sports Traumatol Arthrosc.* 2008;16(9):834-842.

201. Clancy WG, Jr., Narechania RG, Rosenberg TD, Gmeiner JG, Wisnefske DD, Lange TA. Anterior and posterior

cruciate ligament reconstruction in rhesus monkeys. *J Bone Joint Surg Am.* 1981;63(8):1270-1284.

202. Barber FA, Click SD. Meniscus repair rehabilitation with concurrent anterior cruciate reconstruction. *Arthroscopy.* 1997;13(4):433-437.

203. Melegati G, Tomese D, Bandi M, Volpi P, Schonhuber H, Denti M. The role of the rehabilitation brace in restoring knee extension after anterior cruciate ligament reconstruction: A prospective controlled study. *Knee Surg Sports Traumatol Arthrosc.* 2003;11(5):322-326.

204. Shelbourne KD, Urch SE, Gray T, Freeman H. Loss of normal knee motion after anterior cruciate ligament reconstruction is associated with radiographic arthritic changes after surgery. *Am J Sports Med.* 2012;40(1):108-113.

205. Lange GW, Hintermeister RA, Schlegel T, Dillman CJ, Steadman JR. Electromyographic and kinematic analysis of graded treadmill walking and the implications for knee rehabilitation. *J Orthop Sports Phys Ther.* 1996;23(5):294-301.

206. Barenius B, Forssblad M, Engström B, Eriksson K. Functional recovery after anterior cruciate ligament reconstruction, a study of health-related quality of life based on the Swedish National Knee Ligament Register. *Knee Surg Sports Traumatol Arthrosc.* 2013;21(4):914-927.

207. Risberg MA, Holm I, Tjomsland O, Ljunggren E, Ekeland A. Prospective study of changes in impairments and disabilities after anterior cruciate ligament reconstruction. *J Orthop Sports Phys Ther.* 1999;29:400-412.

208. Krudwig WK, Witzel U, Ullrich K. Posterolateral aspect and stability of the knee joint: II. Posterolateral instability and effect of isolated and combined posterolateral reconstruction on knee stability: A biomechanical study. *Knee Surg Sports Traumatol Arthrosc.* 2002;10(2):91-95.

209. Apsingi S, Nguyen T, Bull AMJ, Unwin A, Deehan DJ, Amis AA. The role of PCL reconstruction in knees with combined PCL and posterolateral corner deficiency. *Knee Surg Sports Traumatol Arthrosc.* 2008;16(1):104-111.

210. Margheritini F, Rihn J, Musahl V, Mariani PP, Harner C. Posterior cruciate ligament injuries in the athlete: An anatomical, biomechanical and clinical review. *Sports Med.* 2002;32(6):393-408.

211. Sekiya JK, Haemmerle MJ, Stabile KJ, Vogrin TM, Harner CD. Biomechanical analysis of a combined double-bundle posterior cruciate ligament and posterolateral corner reconstruction. *Am J Sports Med.* 2005;33:360-369.

212. Fanelli GC, Fanelli MG, Fanelli DG. Revision posterior cruciate ligament surgery. *Sports Med Arthrosc Rev.* 2017;25(1):30-35.

213. Kitamura N, Ogawa M, Kondo E, Kitayama s, Tohyama H, Yasuda K. A novel medial collateral ligament reconstruction procedure using semitendinosus tendon autograft in patients with multiligamentous knee injuries: Clinical outcomes. *Am J Sports Med.* 2013;41(6):1274-1281.

214. Wang CJ, Weng LH, Hsu CC, Chan YS. Arthroscopic single- versus double-bundle posterior cruciate ligament reconstructions using hamstring autograft. *Injury.* 2004;35(12):1293-1299.

215. Wu CH, Chen ACY, Yuan LJ, et al. Arthroscopic reconstruction of the posterior cruciate ligament by using a quadriceps tendon autograft: A minimum 5-year follow-up. *Arthroscopy.* 2007;23(4):420-427.

216. Kim JG, Lee YS, Yang BS, Oh SJ, Yang SJ. Rehabilitation after posterior cruciate ligament reconstruction: A review of the literature and theoretical support. *Arch Orthop Trauma Surg.* 2013;133(12):1687-1695.

217. Wilk K, Escamilla R, Fleisig G, Barrentine S, Andrews J, Boyd M. A comparison of tibiofemoral joint forces and electromyographic activity during open and closed kinetic chain exercises. *Am J Sports Med.* 1996;24(4):518-527.

218. Lopez-Vidriero E, Simon DA, Johnson DH. Initial evaluation of posterior cruciate ligament injuries: history, physical examination, imaging studies, surgical and nonsurfgical indications. *Sports Med Arthrosc Rev.* 2010;18(4):230-237.

219. Dürselen L, Claes L, Kiefer H. The influence of muscle forces and external loads on cruciate ligament strain. *Am J Sports Med.* 1995;23:129-136.

220. Aalbersberg S, Kingma I, Ronsky JL, Frayne R, van Dieën JH. Orientation of tendons in vivo with active and passive knee muscles. *J Biomech.* 2005;39(9):1780-1788.

221. Salata MJ, Sekiya JK. Arthroscopic posterior cruciate ligament tibial inlay reconstruction: A surgical technique that may influence rehabilitation. *Sports Health.* 2011;3(1):52-58.

222. Edson CJ, Fanelli GC, Beck JD. Postoperative rehabilitation of the posterior cruciate ligament. *Sports Med Arthrosc.* 2010;18(4):275-279.

223. Wilk KE, Andrews JR, Clancy WG, Crockett HC, O'Mara JW. Rehabilitation programs for the PCL-injured and reconstructed knee. *J Sport Rehabil.* 1999;8(4):333-361.

224. Pierce CM, O'Brien L, Griffin LW, LaPrade RF. Posterior cruciate ligament tears: Functional and postoperative rehabilitation. *Knee Surg Sports Traumatol Arthrosc.* 2013;21(5):1071-1084.

225. Harner CD, Fu FH, Irrgang JJ, Vogrin TM. Anterior and posterior cruciate ligament reconstruction in the new millennium: A global perspective. *Knee Surg Sports Traumatol Arthrosc.* 2001;9(6):330-336.

226. Majewski M, Susanne H, Klaus S. Epidemiology of athletic knee injuries: a 10-year study. *Knee.* 2006;13(3):184-188.

227. Xie L, Huang W, Jiang J, et al. Differential expressions of lysyl oxidase family in ACL and MCL fibroblasts after mechanical injury. *Injury.* 2013;44(7):893-900.

228. Reider B. Medial collateral ligament injuries in athletes. *Sports Med.* 1996;21(2):147-156.

229. Benjamin B. Collateral ligament: injuries of the knee: Essential principles and their application. *Massage Bodywork.* 2003;18(5):16-20,22-23,26-27.

230. Ahn JH, Bae TS, Kang KS, Kang SY, Lee SH. Longitudinal tear of the medial meniscus posterior horn in the anterior cruciate ligament-deficient knee significantly influences anterior stability. *Am J Sports Med.* 2011;39(10):2187-2193.

231. Shelbourne KD, Patel DV, Adsit WS, Porter DA. Rehabilitation after meniscal repair. *Clin Sports Med.* 1996;15:595-612.

232. Seon JK, Gadikota HR, Kozanek M, Oh LS, Gill TJ, Li G. The effect of anterior cruciate ligament reconstruction on kinematics of the knee with combined anterior cruciate ligament injury and subtotal medial meniscectomy: an in vitro robotic investigation. *Arthroscopy.* 2009;25(2):123-130.

233. Tenuta JJ, Arciero RA. Arthroscopic evaluation of meniscal repairs: Factors that effect healing. *Am J Sports Med.* 1994;22:797-802.

234. Warren RF. Meniscectomy and repair in the anterior cruciate ligament-deficient patient. *Clin Orthop Relat Res.* 1990;(252):55-63.

235. Heckmann TP, Barber-Westin SD, Noyes FR. Meniscal repair and transplantation: indications, techniques, rehabilitation, and clinical outcome. *J Orthop Sports Phys Ther.* 2006;36(10):795-814.

236. Scott GA, Jolly BL, Henning CE. Combined posterior incision and arthroscopic intra-articular repair of the meniscus. *J Bone Joint Surg Am.* 1986;68A:847-861.

237. Stone RG, Frewin PR, Gonzales S. Long-term assessment of arthroscopic meniscus repair: A two- to six-year follow-up study. *Arthroscopy.* 1990;6:73-78.

238. Barcia AM, Kozlowski EJ, Tokish JM. Return to sport after meniscal repair. *Clin Sports Med.* 2012;31(1):155-166.

239. Noyes FR, Heckmann TP, Barber-Westin SD. Meniscus repair and transplantation: A comprehensive update. *J Orthop Sports Phys Ther.* 2012;42(3):274-290.

240. Messier SP, Davis SE, Curl WW, Lowery RB, Pack RJ. Etiologic factors associated with patellofemoral pain in runners. *Med Sci Sports Exerc.* 1991;23:1008-1015.

241. Atkin DM, Fithian DC, Marangi KS, Stone ML, Dobson BE, Mendelsohn C. Characteristics of patients with primary acute lateral patellar dislocation and their recovery within the first 6 months of injury. *Am J Sports Med.* 2000;28(4):472-479.

242. Nikku R, Nietosvaara Y, Aalto K, Kallio PE. The mechanism of primary patellar dislocation: trauma history of 126 patients. *Acta Orthop.* 2009;80(4):432-434.

243. Brody LT, Thein-Nissenbaum JM. Nonoperative treatment for patellofemoral pain. *J Orthop Sports Phys Ther.* 1998;28(5):336-344.

244. Juhn MS. Patellofemoral pain syndrome: a review and guidelines for treatment. *Am Family Phys.* 1999;60:2012-2022.

245. Hiemstra LA, Kerslake S, Irving C. Anterior knee pain in the athlete. *Clin Sports Med.* 2014;33(3):437-459.

246. Petersen W, Ellermann A, Gösele-Koppenburg A, et al. Patellofemoral pain syndrome. *Knee Surg Sports Traumatol Arthrosc.* Oct 2014;22(10):2264-2274. doi:10.1007/s00167-013-2759-6

247. Tumia N, Maffulli N. Patellofemoral pain in female athletes. *Sports Med Arthroscop Rev.* 2002;10(1):69-75.

248. Bolgla LA, Malone TR, Umberger BR, Uhl TL. Hip strength and hip and knee kinematics during stair descent in females with and without patellofemoral pain syndrome. *J Orthop Sports Phys Ther.* 2008;38(1):12-18.

249. Henebry A, Gaskill T. The effect of pelvic tilt on radiographic markers of acetabular coverage. *Am J Sports Med.* 2013;41(11):2599-2603. doi:10.1177/0363546513500632

250. Dandachli W, Islam SUI, Richards R, Hall-Craggs M, Witt J. The influence of pelvic tilt on acetabular orientation and cover: A three-dimensional computerised tomography analysis. *Hip Int.* 2013;23(1)doi:10.5301/HIP.2013.10715

251. Merican AM, Amis SS. Iliotibial band tension affects patellofemoral and tibiaofemoral kinematics. *J Biomech.* 2009;42(10):1539-1546.

252. LaBrier K, O'Neill DB. Patellofemoral stress syndrome: Current concepts. *Sports Med.* 1993;16(6):449-459.

253. Barton CJ, Lack S, Malliaras P, Morrissey D. Gluteal muscle activity and patellofemoral pain syndrome: a systematic review. *Br J Sports Med.* 2013;47(4):207-214.

254. Kenal KAF, Knapp LK. Rehabilitation of injuries in competitive swimmers. *Sports Med.* 1996;22(5):337-347.

255. O'Donnell P, Johnstone C, Watson M, McNally E, Ostlere S. Evaluation of patellar tracking in symptomatic and asymptomatic individuals by magnetic resonance imaging. *Skeletal Radiol.* 2005;34(3):130-135.

256. Song CY, Lin JJ, Jan MH, Lin YF. The role of patellar alignment and tracking in vivo: The potential mechanism of patellofemoral pain syndrome. *Phys Ther Sport.* 2011;12(3):140-147.

257. Tennant S, Williams A, Vedi V, Kinmont C, Gedroyc W, Hunt DM. Patello-femoral tracking in the weight-bearing knee: a study of asymptomatic volunteers utilising dynamic magnetic resonance imaging: a preliminary report. *Knee Surg Sports Traumatol Arthrosc.* 2001;9(3):155-162.

258. Karlsson J, Thomee R, Sward L. Eleven year follow-up of patello-femoral pain syndrome. *Clin J Sport Med.* 1996;6:22-26.

259. Fulkerson JP. Diagnosis and treatment of patients with patellofemoral pain. *Am J Sports Med.* 2002;30(3):447-456.

260. Post WR. Patellofemoral pain: Results of nonoperative treatment. *Clin Orthop Relat Res.* 2005;436:55-59.

261. Tenney HR, Boyle KL, DeBord A. Influence of hamstring and abdominal muscle activation on a positive Ober's test in people with lumbopelvic pain. *Physiother Can.* 2013;65(1):4-11.

262. Valenza MC, Cabrera-Martos I, Torres-Sanchez I, Garces A, Mateos-Toset S, Valenza-Demet G. The effects of doming of the diaphragm technique in subjects with short hamstring syndrome: A randomized controlled trial. *J Sport Rehabil.* 2015;24(4):342-348. doi:10.1123/jsr.2014-0190

263. Shori G, Joshi A. Effect of right sidelying respiratory left adductor pull back exercise in subjects with iliotibial band tightness. *Physiotherapy.* 2017;25(1):13-16. doi:10.1515/physio-2016-0014

264. Powers CM. The influence of altered lower-extremity kinematics on patellofemoral joint dysfunction: a theorectical perspective. *J Orthop Sports Phys Ther.* 2003;33(11):639-646.

265. McConnell J. The management of chondromalacia patellae: A long term solution. *Aust J Physiother.* 1986;32:215-223.

266. Keet JHL, Gray J, Harley Y, Lambert MI. The effect of medial patellar taping on pain, strength, and neuromuscular recruitment in subjects with and without patellofemoral pain. *Physiother.* 2007;93:45-52.

267. Kowall MG, Kolk G, Nuber GW, Cassisi JE, Stern SH. Patellar taping in the treatment of patellofemoral pain: A prospective randomized study. *Am J Sports Med.* 1996;24(1):61-66.

268. Lesher JD, Sutlive TG, Miller GA, Chine NJ, Garber MB, Wainner RS. Development of a clinical prediction rule for classifying patients with patellofemoral pain syndrome who respond to patellar taping. *J Orthop Sports Phys Ther.* 2006;36(11):854-866.

269. Wilson T, Carter N, Thomas G. A multicenter, single-masked study of medial, neutral, and lateral patellar taping in individuals with patellofemoral pain syndrome. *J Orthop Sports Phys Ther.* 2003;33(8):437-443.

270. Ernst GP, Kawaguchi J, Saliba E. Effect of patellar taping on knee kinetics of patients with patellofemoral pain syndrome. *J Orthop Sports Phys Ther*. 1999;29(11):661-667.

271. Somes S, Worrell TW, Corey B, C.D. I. Effects of patellar taping on patellar position in the open and closed kinetic chain: a preliminary study. *J Sport Rehabil*. 1997;6:299-308.

272. Worrell T, Ingersoll CD, Bockrath-Pugliese K, Minis P. Effect of patellar taping and bracing on patellar position as determined by MRI in patients with patellofemoral pain. *J Athl Train*. 1998;33:16-20.

273. Aminaka N, Gribble P. Patellar taping, patellofemoral pain syndrome, lower extremity kinematics, and dynamic postural control. *J Athl Train*. 2008;43(1):21-28.

274. Bockrath K, Wooden C, Worrell T, Ingersoll CD, Farr J. Effects of patella taping on patella position and perceived pain. *Med Sci Sports Exerc*. 1993;25(9):989-992.

275. Ko CY, Chang Y, Jeong B, Kang S, Ryu J, Kim G. Effects of knee sleeves on coordination of lower-limb segments in healthy adults during level walking and one-leg hopping. *PeerJ*. e3340. 2017;5. doi:10.7717/peerj.3340 PMC5438577,

276. Mohd Sharif NA, Goh SL, Usman J, Wan Safwani WKZ. Biomechanical and functional efficacy of knee sleeves: A literature review. *Phys Ther Sport*. 2017;28:44-52.

277. Smith TO, Drew BT, Meek TH, Clark AB. Knee orthoses for treating patellofemoral pain syndrome. *Cochran Database Syst Rev*. 2015;8(12):CD010513. doi:10.1002/14651858.CD010513.pub2

278. Gilleard W, McConnell J, Parsons D. The effect of patellar taping on the onset of vastus medialis obliquus and vastus lateralis muscle activity in persons with patellofemoral pain. *Phys Ther*. 1998;78:25-32.

279. Hudson Z, Darthuy E. Iliotibial band tightness and patellofemoral pain syndrome: a case-control study. *Man Ther*. 2009;14(2):147-151.

280. Doucette SA, Goble EM. The effect of exercise on patellar tracking in lateral patellar compression syndrome. *Am J Sports Med*. 1992;20:434-440.

281. Ireland ML, Willson JD, Ballantyne BT, Davis IM. Hip strength in females with and without patellofemoral pain. *J Orthop Sports Phys Ther*. 2003;33(11):671-676.

282. Robinson RL, Nee RJ. Analysis of hip strength in females seeking physical therapy treatment for unilateral patellofemoral pain syndrome. *J Orthop Sports Phys Ther*. 2007;37(5):232-238.

283. Powers CM, Ward SR, Frederickson M, Guillet M, Shellock FG. Patellofemoral kinematics during weight-bearing and non-weight-bearing knee extension in persons with lateral subluxation of the patella: a preliminary study. *J Orthop Sports Phys Ther*. 2003;33(11):677-685.

284. Mohr KJ, Kvitne RS, Pink MM, Fideler B, Perry J. Electromyography of the quadriceps in patellofemoral pain with patellar subluxation. *Clin Orthop Relat Res*. 2003;(415):261-271.

285. Joseph MF, Taft K, Moskwa M, Denegar CR. Deep friction massage to treat tendinopathy: A systematic review of a classic treatment in the face of a new paradigm of understanding. *J Sport Rehabil*. 2012;21(4):343-353.

286. Yoon YS, Yu KP, Lee KJ, Kwak SH, Kim JY. Development and application of a newly designed massage instrument for deep cross-friction massage in chronic non-specific low back pain. *Ann Rehabil Med*. 2012;36(1):55-65.

287. Peers KHE, Lysens RJJ. Patellar tendinopathy in athletes: current diagnostic and therapeutic recommendations. *Sports Med*. 2005;35(1):71-87.

288. Sharma P, Maffulli N. Tendon injury and tendinopathy: Healing and repair. *J Bone Joint Surg Am*. 2005;87(1):187-202.

289. Langenhan R, Baumann M, Ricart P, et al. Postoperative functional rehabilitation after repair of quadriceps tendon ruptures: a comparison of two different protocols. *Knee Surg Sports Traumatol Arthrosc*. 2012;20(11):2275-2278.

290. West JL, Keene JS, Kaplan LD. Early motion after quadriceps and patellar tendon repairs: outcomes with single-suture augmentation. *Am J Sports Med*. 2008;36(2):316-323.

291. Stanton P, Purdham C. Hamstring injuries in sprinting—the role of eccentric exercise. *J Orthop Sports Phys Ther*. 1989;10(9):343-349.

292. Askling CM, Tengvar M, Saartok T, Thorstensson A. Proximal hamstring strains of stretching type in different sports: injury situations, clinical and magnetic resonance imaging characteristics, and return to sport. *Am J Sports Med*. 2008;36(9):1799-1804.

293. De Smet AA, Best TM. MR imaging of the distribution and location of acute hamstring injuries in athletes. *AJR Am J Roentgenol*. 2000;174(2):393-399.

294. McHugh MP, Connolly DAJ, Eston RG, Kremenic IJ, Nicholas SJ, Gleim GW. The role of passive muscle stiffness in symptoms of exercise-induced muscle damage. *Am J Sports Med*. 1999;27:594-599.

295. Woods C, Hawkins RD, Maltby S, et al. The Football Association Medical Research Programme: An audit of injuries in professional football—analysis of hamstring injuries. *Br J Sports Med*. 2004;38(1):36-41.

296. Silder A, Reeder SB, Thelen DG. The influence of prior hamstring injury on lengthening muscle tissue mechanics. *J Biomech*. 2010;43(12):2254-2260.

297. Silder A, Thelen DG, Heiderscheit BC. Effects of prior hamstring strain injury on strength, flexibility, and running mechanics. *Clin Biomech*. 2010;25(7):681-686.

298. Schmitt B, Tim T, McHugh M. Hamstring injury rehabilitation and prevention of reinjury using lengthened state eccentric training: a new concept. *Int J Sports Phys Ther*. 2012;7(3):333-341.

299. Opar DA, Williams MD, Shield AJ. Hamstring strain injuries: factors that lead to injury and re-injury. *Sports Med*. 2012;42(3):209-226.

300. Mendiguchia J, Alentorn-Geli E, Idoate F, Myer GD. Rectus femoris muscle injuries in football: a clinically relevant review of mechanisms of injury, risk factors and preventive strategies. *Br J Sports Med*. 2013;47(6):1-9.

301. Fredericson M, Weir A. Practical management of iliotibial band friction syndrome in runners. *Clin J Sport Med*. 2006;16(3):261-268.

302. Orchard J, Fricker P, Abud A, Mason B. Biomechanics of iliotibial band friction syndrome in runners. *Am J Sports Med*. 1996;24(3):375-379.

303. Krivickas LS. Anatomical factors associated with overuse sports injuries. *Sports Med*. 1997;24(2):132-146.

304. Orchard JW, Fricker PA, Abud AT, Mason BR. Biomechanics of iliotibial band friction syndrome in runners. *Am J Sports Med.* 1996;24(3):375-379.

305. Birk GT, DeLee JC. Osteochondral injuries: clinical findings. *Clin Sports Med.* 2001;20(2):279-286.

306. Nakamae A, Engebretsen L, Bahr R, Krosshaug T, Ochi M. Natural history of bone bruises after acute knee injury: clinical outcome and histopathological findings. *Knee Surg Sports Traumatol Arthrosc.* 2006;14(12):1252-1258.

307. Navascués JA, González-López JL, López-Valverde S, Soleto J, Rodriguez-Durantez JA, García-Trevijano JL. Premature physeal closure after tibial diaphyseal fractures in adolescents. *J Pediatr Orthop.* 2000;20(2):193-196.

308. Beiser IH, Kanat IO. Subchondral bone drilling: A treatment for cartilage defects. *J Foot Surg.* 1990;29(6):595-601.

309. Steadman JR, Briggs KK, Rodrigo JJ, Kocher MS, Gill TJ, Rodkey WG. Outcomes of microfracture for traumatic chondral defects of the knee: average 11-year follow-up. *J Arthroscop Rel Surg.* 2003;19:477-484.

310. Gillogly SD, Voight M, Blackburn T. Treatment of articular cartilage defects of the knee with autologus chondrocyte implantation. *J Orthop Sports Phys Ther.* 1998;28(4):241-251.

311. Gudas R, Stankevicius E, Monastyreckiene E, Pranys D, Kalesinskas RJ. Osteochondral autologous transplantation versus microfracture for the treatment of articular cartilage defects in the knee joint in athletes. *Knee Surg Sports Traumatol Arthrosc.* 2006;14(9):834-842.

312. Gudas R, Kalesinskas RJ, Kimtys V, et al. A prospective randomized clinical study of mosaic osteochondral autologous transplantation versus microfracture for the treatment of osteochondral defects in the knee joint in young athletes. *Arthroscopy.* 2005;21(9):1066-1075.

313. Hurst JM, Steadman JR, O'Brien L, Rodkey WG, Briggs KK. Rehabilitation following microfracture for chondral injury in the knee. *Clin Sports Med.* 2010;29(2):257-265.

314. Buckwalter JA. Articular cartilage: injuries and potential for healing. *J Orthop Sports Phys Ther.* 1998;28(4):192-202.

315. Buckwalter JA. Effects of early motion on healing of musculoskeletal tissues. *Hand Clin.* 1996;12(1):13-24.

316. Robert H. Chondral repair of the knee joint using mosaicplasty. *Orthop Traumatol Surg Res.* 2011;97(4):418-429.

317. Kish G, Modis L, Hangody L. Osteochondral mosaicplasty for the treatment of focal chondral and osteochondral lesions of the knee and talus in the athlete: Rationale, indications, techniques, and results. *Clin Sports Med.* 1999;18(1):45-66.

318. Houglum PA, Bertoti DB. *Brunnstrom's Clinical Kinesiology.* 6th ed. F.A. Davis; 2012.

319. Costigan PA, Deluzio KJ, Wyss UP. Knee and hip kinetics during normal stair climbing. *Gait Posture.* 2002;16(1):31-37.

320. Johnson MP. Physical therapist management of an adult with osteochondritis dissecans of the knee. *Phys Ther.* 2005;85(7):665-675.

321. Keenan OJ, Turner PG, Yeates D, Goldacre MJ. Epidemiology of hospitalised osteochondritis dissecans in young people: incidence, geographical variation and trends over time in England from 2002 to 2010. *Knee.* 2014;21(2):497-500.

322. Grimm NL, Weiss JM, Kessler JL, Aoki SK. Osteochondritis dissecans of the knee: pathoanatomy, epidemiology, and diagnosis. *Clin Sports Med.* 2014;33(2):181-188.

323. Carey JL, Grimm NL. Treatment algorithm for osteochondritis dissecans of the knee. *Clin Sports Med.* 2014;33(2):375-382.

324. Krause M, Hapfelmeier A, Möller M, Amling M, Bohndorf K, Meenen NM. Healing predictors of stable juvenile osteochondritis dissecans knee lesions after 6 and 12 months of nonoperative treatment. *Am J Sports Med.* 2013;41(10):2384-2391.

325. Kurtz S, Ong K, Lau E, Mowat F, Halpern M. Projections of primary and revision hip and knee arthroplasty in the United States from 2005 to 2030. *JBJS.* 2007;89(4):780-785. doi:10.2106/jbjs.F.00222

326. Keeney JA, Eunice S, Pashos G, Wright RW, Clohisy JC. What is the evidence for total knee arthroplasty in young patients? A systematic review of the literature. *Clinical Orthopaedics and Related Research.* 2011;469(2):574-583. doi:10.1007/s11999-010-1536-9

327. Papas PV, Congiusta D, Cushner FD. Cementless versus cemented fixation in total knee arthroplasty. *J Knee Surg.* Jul 2019;32(7):596-599. doi:10.1055/s-0039-1678687

328. Pollock M, Somerville L, Firth A, Lanting B. Outpatient total hip arthroplasty, total knee arthroplasty, and unicompartmental knee arthroplasty: A systematic review of the literature. *JBJS Rev.* Dec 27 2016;4(12)doi:10.2106/jbjs.Rvw.16.00002

329. Pozzi F, Snyder-Mackler L, Zeni J. Physical exercise after knee arthroplasty: A systematic review of controlled trials. *Eur J Phys Rehabil Med.* Dec 2013;49(6):877-892.

330. Mutsuzaki H, Takeuchi R, Mataki Y, Wadano Y. Target range of motion for rehabilitation after total knee arthroplasty. *J Rural Med.* May 2017;12(1):33-37. doi:10.2185/jrm.2923

331. Ebert JR, Munsie C, Joss B. Guidelines for the early restoration of active knee flexion after total knee arthroplasty: implications for rehabilitation and early intervention. *Arch Phys Med Rehabil.* 2014;95(6):1135-1140.

332. Mehta S, Rigney A, Webb K, et al. Characterizing the recovery trajectories of knee range of motion for one year after total knee replacement. *Physiother Theory Pract.* Jan 2020;36(1):176-185. doi:10.1080/09593985.2018.1482980

333. Sattler LN, Hing WA, Vertullo CJ. Pedaling-based protocol superior to a 10-exercise, non-pedaling protocol for postoperative rehabilitation after total knee replacement: A randomized controlled trial. *J Bone Joint Surg Am.* Apr 17 2019;101(8):688-695. doi:10.2106/jbjs.18.00898

334. Manrique J, Gomez MM, Parvizi J. Stiffness after total knee arthroplasty. *J Knee Surg.* 2015;28(2):119-126. doi:10.1055/s-0034-1396079

Chapter 20

1. Pommering TL, Kluchurosky L, Hall SL. Ankle and foot injuries in pediatric and adult athletes. *Prim Care.* 2005;32(1):133-161.

2. Sarrafian SK. *Anatomy of the Foot and Ankle.* JB Lippincott; 1983.

3. Klingman RE, Liaos SM, Hardin KM. The effect of subtalar joint posting on patellar glide position in subjects

with excessive rearfoot pronation. *J Orthop Sports Phys Ther.* 1997;25(3):185-191.

4. Powers CM, Maffucci R, Hampton S. Rearfoot posture in subjects with patellofemoral pain. *J Orthop Sports Phys Ther.* 1995;22(4):155-160.

5. Tiberio D. The effect of excessive subtalar joint pronation on patellofemoral mechanics: A theoretical model. *J Orthop Sports Phys Ther.* 1987;9(4):160-165.

6. Withrow TJ, Huston LJ, Wojtys EM, Ashton-Miller JA. The relationship between quadriceps muscle force, knee flexion, and anterior cruciate ligament strain in an in vitro simulated jump landing. *Am J Sports Med.* 2006;34(2):269-274.

7. Kulmala JP, Avela J, Pasanen K, Parkkari J. Forefoot strikers exhibit lower running-induced knee loading than rearfoot strikers. *Med Sci Sports Exerc.* 2013;45(12):2306-2313.

8. Dierks TA, Manal KT, Hamill J, Davis IS. Proximal and distal influences on hip and knee kinematics in runners with patellofemoral pain during a prolonged run. *J Orthop Sports Phys Ther.* 2008;38(8):448-456.

9. Massie DL, Spiker JC. *Foot biomechanics and the relationship to rehabilitation of lower extremity injuries.* Forum Medicum; 1990.

10. Rosse C, Gaddum-Rosse P. *Hollinshead's Textbook of Anatomy.* Lioppincott-Raven; 1997:902.

11. Taber CW. *Taber's Cyclopedic Medical Dictionary.* 22nd ed. FA Davis; 2014.

12. Houglum PA, Bertoti DB. *Brunnstrom's Clinical Kinesiology.* 6th ed. F.A. Davis; 2012.

13. Khamis S, Yizhar Z. Effect of feet hyperpronation on pelvic alignment in a standing position. *Gait Posture.* 2007;25(1):127-134.

14. Ntousis T, Mandalidis D, Chronopoulos E, Athanasopoulos S. EMG activation of trunk and upper limb muscles following experimentally-induced overpronation and oversupination of the feet in quiet standing. *Gait Posture.* 2013;37(2):190-194.

15. Duval K, Lam T, Sanderson D. The mechanical relationship between the rearfoot, pelvis and low-back. *Gait Posture.* 2010;32(4):637-640.

16. Barton CJ, Bonanno D, Levinger P, Menz HB. Foot and ankle characteristics in patellofemoral pain syndrome: a case control and reliability study. *J Orthop Sports Phys Ther.* 2010;40(5):286-296.

17. Castro-Méndez A, Munuera PV, Albornoz-Cabello M. The short-term effect of custom-made foot orthoses in subjects with excessive foot pronation and lower back pain: a randomized, double-blinded, clinical trial. *Prosthet Orthot Int.* 2013;37(5):384-390.

18. Czerniecki JM. Foot and ankle biomechanics in walking and running. A review. *Am J Phys Med Rehabil.* 1988;67(6):246-452.

19. Hicks JH. The mechanics of the foot. I. The joints. *J Anat.* 1953;87(4):345-357.

20. Lundberg A, Goldie I, Kalin B, Selvik G. Kinematics of the ankle/foot complex: plantarflexion and dorsiflexion. *Foot Ankle.* 1989;9(4):194-200.

21. Windisch G, Odehnal B, Reimann R, Anderhuber F, Stachel H. Contact areas of the tibiotalar joint. *J Orthop Res.* 2007;25(11):1481-1487.

22. Kitaoka HB, Luo ZP, An K. Three-dimensional analysis of normal ankle and foot mobility. *Am J Sports Med.* 1997;25(2):238-242.

23. Lundberg A, Svensson OK, Bylund C, Goldie I, Selvik G. Kinematics of the ankle/foot complex: Part 2. Pronation and supination. *Foot Ankle.* 1989;9(5):248-253.

24. Ridola C, Palma A. Functional anatomy and imaging of the foot. *Ital J Anat Embryol.* 2001;106(2):85-98.

25. Ger R. The clinical anatomy of the intrinsic muscles of the sole of the foot. *The American Surgeon.* 1986;52(5):284-285.

26. Oatis CA. Biomechanics of the foot and ankle under static conditions. *Phys Ther.* 1988;68(12):1815-1821.

27. Lusk SJ, Hale BD, Russell DM. Grip width and forearm orientation effects on muscle activity during the lat pulldown. *J Strength Cond Res.* 2010;24(7):1895-1900.

28. Mulligan EP, Cook PG. Effect of plantar intrinsic muscle training on medial longitudinal arch morphology and dynamic function. *Man Ther.* 2013;18(5):425-430.

29. Glasoe WM, Yack HJ, Saltzman CL. Anatomy and biomechanics of the first ray. *Phys Ther.* 1999;79(9):854-859.

30. Levinger P, Murley GS, Barton CJ, Cotchett MP, McSweeney SR, Menz HB. A comparison of foot kinematics in people with normal- and flat-arched feet using the Oxford Foot Model. *Gait Posture.* 2010;32(4):519-523.

31. Bojsen-Møller F. Anatomy of the forefoot, normal and pathologic. *Clin Orthop Relat Res.* 1979;142:10-18.

32. Murley GS, Tan JM, Edwards RM, De Luca J, Munteanu SE, Cook JL. Foot posture is associated with morphometry of the peroneus longus muscle, tibialis anterior tendon, and Achilles tendon. *Scand J Med Sci Sports.* 2014;24(3):535-541.

33. Bojsen-Moller F, Flagstad KE. Plantar aponeurosis and internal architecture of the ball of the foot. *Journal of Anatomy.* 1976;121(3):599-611.

34. Nilsson MK, Friis P, Michaelsen MS, Jakobsen PA, Nielsen RO. Classification of the height and flexibility of the medial longitudinal arch of the foot. *J Foot Ankle Res.* 2012;5(3)doi:10.1186/1757-1146-5-3

35. McKeon PO, Hertel J, Bramble D, Davis I. The foot core system: a new paradigm for understanding intrinsic foot muscle function. *Br J Sports Med.* 2015;49(5):290.

36. Newsham KR. Strengthening the intrinsic foot muscles. *Athl Ther Today.* 2010;15(1):32-35.

37. Donatelli RA, Wooden MJ, Ekedahl SR, Wilkes JS, Cooper J, Bush AJ. Relationship between static and dynamic foot postures in professional baseball players. *J Orthop Sports Phys Ther.* 1999;29(6):316-325.

38. Lattanza L, Gray GW, Kantner RM. Closed versus open kinematic chain measurements of subtalar joint eversion: implications for clinical practice. *J Orthop Sports Phys Ther.* 1988;9(9):310-314.

39. McPoil TG, Schuit D, Knecht HG. Comparison of three methods used to obtain a neutral plaster foot impression. *Phys Ther.* 1989;69(6):448-452.

40. Elveru RA, Rothstein JM, Lamb RL, Riddle DL. Methods for taking subtalar joint measurements. A clinical report. *Phys Ther.* 1988;68(5):678-682.

41. Schwarz NA, Kovaleski JE, Heitman RJ, Gurchiek LR, Gubler-Hanna C. Arthrometric measurement of ankle-complex motion: normative values. *J Athl Train.* 2011;46(2):126-132.

42. Simkin A, Leichter I, Giladi M, Stein M, Milgrom C. Combined effect of foot arch structure and an orthotic device on stress fractures. *Foot Ankle*. 1989;10(1):25-29.

43. Donatelli RA. Abnormal biomechanics of the foot and ankle. *J Orthop Sports Phys Ther*. 1987;9(1):11-16.

44. Nester C. The relationship between transverse plane leg rotation and transverse plane motion at the knee and hip during normal walking. *Gait Posture*. 2000;12(3):251-256.

45. Liebenson C. Functional problems associated with the knee—part one: sources of biomechanical overload. *J Bodyw Mov Ther*. 2006;10(4):306-311.

46. De Ponti L. Archilles' heritage. *Sports Medicina*. 2002;19(5):41-45.

47. Christensen JC, Jennings MM. Normal and abnormal function of the first ray. *Clin Podiatr Med Surg*. 2009;26(3):355-371.

48. Hockenbury RT. Forefoot problems in athletes. *Med Sci Sports Exerc*. 1999;31(7):S448-S458.

49. Lang LM, Volpe RG. Measurment of tibial torsion. *J Am Pod Med Assoc*. 1998;88(4):160-165.

50. Perry J, Burnfield JM. *Gait Analysis. Normal and Pathological Function*. 2nd ed. Slack, Inc; 2010.

51. Davids JR, Davis RB. Tibial torsion: significance and measurement. *Gait Posture*. 2007;26(2):169-171.

52. Staheli LT, Engel GM. Tibial torsion: a method of assessment and a survey of normal children. *Clin Orthop Relat Res*. 1972;86:183-186.

53. Hudson D. A comparison of ultrasound to goniometric and inclinometer measurements of torsion in the tibia and femur. *Gait Posture*. 2008;28(4):708-710.

54. Sankar WN, Rethlefsen SA, Weiss J, Kay RM. The recurrent clubfoot: can gait analysis help us make better preoperative decisions? *Clin Orthop Relat Res*. 2009;467(5):1214-1222.

55. Liporaci RF, Saad MC, Felício LR, Baffa Ado P, Grossi DB. Contribution of the evaluation of the clinical signals in patients with patellofemoral pain syndrome. *Acta Ortop Bras*. 2013;21(4):198-201.

56. Turner MS. The association between tibial torsion and knee joint pathology. *Clin Orthop Relat Res*. 1994;(302):47-51.

57. Riegger-Krugh C, Keysor JJ. Skeletal malalignments of the lower quarter: correlated and compensatory motions and postures. *J Orthop Sports Phys Ther*. 1996;23(2):164-170.

58. Tiberio D. Pathomechanics of structural foot deformities. *Phys Ther*. 1988;68(12):1840-1849.

59. McPoil TG, Schuit D, Knecht HG. A comparison of three positions used to evaluate tibial varum. *J Am Podiatr Med Assoc*. 1988;78(1):22-28.

60. Tomaro J. Measurement of tibiofibular varum in subjects with unilateral overuse symptoms. *J Orthop Sports Phys Ther*. 1995;21(2):86-89.

61. Johanson MA, Greenfield L, Hung C, Wlater R, Watson CJ. The relationship between forefoot and rearfoot static alignment in pain-free individuals with above-average forefoot varus angles. *Foot Ankle Spec*. 2010;3(3):112-116.

62. van Dijk CN, van Sterkenburg MN, Wiegerinck JI, Karlsson J, Maffulli N. Terminology for Achilles tendon related disorders. *Knee Surg Sports Traumatol Arthrosc*. 2011;19(5):835-841.

63. Yamashita MH. Evaluation and selection of shoe wear and orthoses for the runner. *Phys Med Rehabil Clin N Am*. 2005;16(3):801-829.

64. Whittle MW. *Gait Analysis*. 4th ed. Elsevier; 2007.

65. Vicenzino B. Foot orthotics in the treatment of lower limb conditions: a musculoskeletal physiotherapy perspective. *Man Ther*. 2004;9:185-196.

66. Nigg BM. The role of impact forces and foot pronation: a new paradigm. *Clin J Sport Med*. 2001;11(1):2-9.

67. Gross MT, Byers JM, Krafft JL, Lackey EJ, Melton KM. The impact of custom semirigid foot orthotics on pain and disability for individuals with plantar fasciitis. *J Orthop Sports Phys Ther*. 2002;32(4):149-157.

68. Farhan M, Wang JZ, Bray P, Burns J. Comparison of 3D scanning versus traditional methods of capturing foot and ankle morphology for the fabrication of orthoses: a systematic review. *J Foot Ankle Res*. 2021;14(1):2. doi:10.1186/s13047-020-00442-8

69. Dombroski CE, Balsdon MER, Froats A. The use of a low cost 3D scanning and printing tool in the manufacture of custom-made foot orthoses: a preliminary study. *BMC Res Notes*. 2014;7:443. doi:10.1186/1756-0500-7-443

70. Lee YC, Lin G, Wang MJJ. Comparing 3D foot scanning with conventional measurement methods. *J Foot Ankle Res*. 2014;7(1)doi:10.1186/s13047-014-0044-7

71. Sentore JR. Functional components of a sport shoe. *Orthop Nurs*. 1996;15(3):19-22.

72. Cook SD, Kester MA, Brunet ME, Haddad RJ, Jr. Biomechanics of running shoe performance. *Clin Sports Med*. 1985;4(4):619-626.

73. Kong PW, Candelaria NG, Smith DR. Running in new and worn shoes: a comparison of three types of cushioning footwear. *Br J Sports Med*. 2009;43(10):745-749.

74. Wyndow N, Cowan SM, Wrigley TV, Crossley KM. Neruromotor control of the lower limb in Achilles tendinpathy: implications for foot orthotic therapy. *Sports Med*. 2010;40(9):715-727.

75. Del los Santos-Real R, Morales-Muñoz P, Payo J, Escalera-Alonso J. Gastrocnemius proximal release with minimal incision: a modified technique. *Foot Ankle Int*. 2012;33(9):750-754.

76. Anderson J, Stanek J. Effect of foot orthoses as treatment for plantar fasciitis or heel pain. *J Sport Rehabil*. 2013;22(2):130-136.

77. McPoil TG. Athletic footwear: design, performance and selection issues. *J Sci Med Sport*. 2000;3(3):260-267.

78. McPoil TG, Jr. Footwear. *Phys Ther*. 1988;68(12):1857-1865.

79. Janisse DJ. The art and science of fitting shoes. *Foot Ankle*. 1992;13(5):257-262.

80. Wilk BR, Fisher KL, Gutierrez W. Defective running shoes as a contributing factor in plantar fasciitis in a triathlete. *J Orthop Sports Phys Ther*. 2000;30(1):21-28.

81. Sandrey MA, Zebas CJ, Adeyanju M. Prevention of injuries in excessive pronators through proper soccer shoe fit. *J Athl Train*. 1996;31(3):231-234.

82. Hall JP, Barton C, Jones PR, Morrissey D. The biomechanical differences between barefoot and shod distance running: a systematic review and preliminary meta-analysis. *Sports Med*. 2013;43(12):1335-1353.

83. Bonacci J, Saunders PU, Hicks A, Rantalainen T, Vicenzino BG, Spratford W. Running in a minimalist and lightweight shoe is not the same as running barefoot: a biomechanical study. *Br J Sports Med.* 2013;47(6):387-392.

84. Gillinov SM, Laux S, Kuivila T, Hass D, Joy SM. Effect of minimalist footwear on running efficiency: a randomized crossover trial. *Sports Health.* 2015;7(3):256-260.

85. Hollander K, Heidt C, Van Der Zwaard BC, Braumann KM. Long-term effects of habitual barefoot running and walking: a systematic review. *Med Sci Sport Exerc.* 2017;49(4):752-762.

86. McCallion C, Donne B, Fleming N, Blanksby B. Acute differences in foot strike and spatiotemporal variables for shod, barefoot or minimalist male runners. *J Sports Sci Med.* 2015;13(2):280-286.

87. Thompson MA, Gutmann A, Seegmiller J, McGowan CP. The effect of stride length on the dynamics of barefoot and shod running. *J Biomech.* 2014;47(11):2745-2750.

88. Altman AR, Davis IS. Prospective comparison of running injuries between shod and barefoot runners. *Br J Sports Med.* 2016;50(8):476-480.

89. Reinschmidt C, Nigg BM. Current issues in the design of running and court shoes. *Sportverletz Sportschaden.* 2000;14(3):71-81.

90. Stacoff A, Steger J, Stüssi E, Reinschmidt C. Lateral stability in sideward cutting movements. *Med Sci Sports Exerc.* 1996;28(3):350-358.

91. Zhang S, Clowers K, Kohstall C, Yu YJ. Effects of various midsole densities of basketball shoes on impact attenuation during landing activities. *J Appl Biomech.* 2005;21(1):3-17.

92. Sobhani S, Bredeweg S, Dekker R, et al. Rocker shoe, minimalist shoe, and standard running shoe: a comparison of running economy. *J Sci Med Sport.* 2014;17(3):312-316.

93. Long JT, Klein JP, Sirota NM, Wertsch JJ, Janisse D, Harris GF. Biomechanics of the double rocker sole shoe: gait kinematics and kinetics. *J Biomech.* 2007;40(13):2882-2890.

94. Peterson MJ, Perry J, Montgomery J. Walking patterns of healthy subjects wearing rocker shoes. *Phys Ther.* 1985;65(10):1483-1489.

95. Ryan M, Elashi M, Newshamn-West R, Taunton J. Examining injury risk and pain perception in runners using minimalist footwear. *Br J Sports Med.* 2014;48(16):1257-1262.

96. Clark JE, Scott SG, Mingle M. Viscoelastic shoe insoles: their use in aerobic dancing. *Arch Phys Med Rehabil.* 1989;70(1):37-40.

97. Majid F, Bader DL. A biomechanical analysis of the plantar surface of soccer shoes. *Proc Inst Mech Eng H.* 1993;207(2):93-101.

98. Menant JC, Perry SD, Steele JR, Menz HB, Munro BJ, Lord SR. Effects of shoe characteristics on dynamic stability when walking on even and uneven surfaces in young and older people. *Arch Phys Med Rehabil.* 2008;89(10):1970-1976.

99. Perlman E. Boot camp. *Backpacker.* 1988;16(3):35-39.

100. Julien PH. The hiking and climbing foot—part 1. *Podiatry Manage.* 2004;23(7):69-87.

101. Hagen M, Henning EM. Effects of different shoe-lacing patterns on the biomechanics of running shoes. *J Sports Sci.* 2009;27(3):267-275.

102. Richie DH. Sports socks: the role of hosiery as an essential component of footwear for the active person. *Am J Med Sports.* 2003;5(1):79-86.

103. Impellitteri CA, Tolaymat TM, Scheckel KG. The speciation of silver nanoparticles in antimicrobial fabric before and after exposure to a hypochlorite/detergent solution. *J Environ Qual.* 2009;38(4):1528-1530.

104. Blackmore T, Jessop D, Bruce-Low S, Scurr J. The cushioning properties of athletic socks: an impact testing perspective. *Clin Biomech.* 2013;28(7):825-830.

105. Delgado FJ. A step ahead spring. 2014 socks. *SGB.* 2013;46(8):32-38.

106. Julien PH. The hiking and climbing foot—part 2: beyond the boots. *Podiatry Manage.* 2004;23(8):61-68.

107. Herring KM, Richie DH. Friction blisters and sock fiber composition. A double-blind study. *J Am Pod Med Assoc.* 1990;80(2):63-71.

108. Knapik JJ, Reynolds KL, Duplantis KL, Jones BH. Friction blisters: pathophysiology, prevention and treatment. *Sports Med.* 1995;20(3):136-147.

109. Richie DH, Jr. Socks: hosiery—essential equipment for the athlete. *Sports Medicine & Footwear.* Am Acad Podiatr Sports Med; 2014. Accessed October 8, 2014. http://www.aapsm.org/socknov97.html

110. Brophy-Williams N, Driller MW, Kitic CM, Fell JW, Halson SL. Wearing compression socks during exercise aids subsequent performance. *J Sci Med Sport.* 2019;22(1):123-127.

111. Engel FA, Holmberg HC, Sperlich B. Is there evidence that runners can benefit from wearing compression clothing? *Sports Med.* 2016;46(12):1939-1952.

112. Mota GR, Simim MAM, Dos Santos IA, Sasaki JE, Marocolo M. Effects of wearing compression stockings on exercise performance and associated indicators: a systematic review. *Open Access J Sports Med.* 2020;11:29-42.

113. Stanek JM. The effectiveness of compression socks for athletic performance and recovery. *J Sport Rehabil.* 2017;26(1):109-114.

114. Ghai S, Driller MW, Masters RSW. The influence of below-knee compression garments on knee-joint proprioception. *Gait Posture.* 2018;60:258-261.

115. Hasan H, Davids K, Chow JY, Kerr G. Compression and texture in socks enhance football kicking performance. *Hum Mov Sci.* 2016;48:102-111.

116. Del Coso J, Areces F, Salinero JJ, et al. Compression stockings do not improve muscular performance during a half-ironman triathlon race. *Eur J Appl Physiol.* 2014;114(3):587-595.

117. Zaleski AL, Pescatello LS, Ballard KD, et al. The influence of compression socks during a marathon on exercise-associated muscle damage. *J Sport Rehabil.* 2019;28(7):724-728.

118. Areces F, Salinero JJ, Abian-Vicen J, et al. The use of compression stockings during a marathon competition to reduce exercise-induced muscle damage: are they really useful? *J Orthop Sports Phys Ther.* 2015;45(6):462-470.

119. Treseler C, Bixby WR, Nepocatych S. The effect of compression stockings on physiological and psychological responses after 5-km performance in recreationally active females. *J Strength Cond Res.* 2016;30(7):1985-1991.

120. Lattimer CR, Kalodiki E, Kafeza M, Azzam M, Geroulakos G. Quantifying the degree graduated elastic compression stockings enhance venous emptying. *Eur J Vasc Endovasc Surg*. 2014;47(1):75-80.

121. Marinovich R, Li Z, Tamasi T, Quinn K, Wong SF, McIntyre CW. Hemodynamic response to non-pneumatic anti-shock compression garments in patients with renal dysfunction. *BMC Nephrol*. 2020;21(1):15.

122. Brown F, Howatson G, van Someren K, Pedlar C. Compression garments and recovery from exercise: a meta-analysis. *Sports Med*. 2017;47(11):2245-2267.

123. Travell JG, Simons DG. *Myofascial Pain and Dysfunction. The Trigger Point Manual. Vol. 2*. Williams and Wilkins; 1992.

124. Maitland GD. *Peripheral Manipulation*. Butterworth-Heinemann; 1991.

125. Kaltenborn FM. *Manual Mobilization of the Joints. The Kaltenborn Method of Joint Examination and Treatment*. 6th ed. Olaf N Orlis Bokhandel; 2002.

126. Ioannis T, Christos G, Nikolaos Z, Aikaterini V, Efstratios V. The effect of stretching duration on the flexibility of lower extremities in junior soccer players. *Phys Train*. Sept 2005:1.

127. Zakas A. The effect of stretching duration on the lower-extremity flexibility of adolescent soccer players. *J Bodyw Mov Ther*. 2005;9(3):220-225.

128. O'Brien M. The anatomy of the Achilles tendon. *Foot Ankle Clin*. 2005;10(2):225-238.

129. Franchi M, Trirè A, Quaranta M, Orsini E, Ottani V. Collagen structure of tendon relates to function. *ScientificWorldJournal*. 2007;7:404-420.

130. Buckley MR, Evans EB, Matuszewski PE, et al. Distributions of types I, II and III collagen by region in the human supraspinatus tendon. *Connect Tissue Res*. 2013;54(6):374-379.

131. Kubo K, Kanehisa H, Kawakami Y, Fukunaga T. Influence of static stretching on viscoelastic properties of human tendon structures in vivo. *J Appl Physiol (1985)*. 2001;90(2):520-527.

132. Lee AJ, Lin WH. Twelve-week biomechanical ankle platform system training on postural stability and ankle proprioception in subjects with unilateral functional ankle instability. *Clin Biomech*. 2008;23(8):1065-1072.

133. Soderberg GL, T.M. C, Rider SC, Stephenitch BL. Electromyographic activity of selected leg musculature in subjects with normal and chronically sprained ankles performing on a BAPS board. *Phys Ther*. 1991;71(7):514-522.

134. Fraser JJ, Feger MA, Hertel J. Clinical commentary on midfoot and forefoot involvement in lateral ankle sprains and chronic ankle instability. Part 2: Clinical considerations. *Int J Sports Phys Ther*. 2016;11(7):1191-1203.

135. Tourillon R, Gojanovic B, Fourchet F. How to evaluate and improve foot strength in athletes: an update. *Front Sports Act Living*. 2019;1:46. doi:10.3389/fspor.2019.00046

136. Gooding TM, Feger MA, Hart JM, Hertel J. Intrinsic foot muscle activation during specific exercises: a T2 time magnetic resonance imaging study. *J Athl Train*. 2016;51(8):644-650.

137. Fraser JJ, Hertel J. Effects of a 4-week intrinsic foot muscle exercise program on motor function: a preliminary randomized control trial. *J Sport Rehabil*. 2019;28(4):339-349.

138. Sauer LD, Beazell J, Hertel J. Considering the Intrinsic Foot Musculature in Evaluation and Rehabilitation for Lower Extremity Injuries. *Athl Train Sports Health Care*. 2011;3(1):43-47.

139. Hettinger T. *Physiology of Strength*. C.C. Thomas; 1961.

140. Burns J, Redmond A, Ouvrier R, Crosbie J. Quantification of muscle strength and imbalance in neurogenic pes cavus, compared to health controls, using hand-held dynamometry. *Foot Ankle Int*. 2005;26(7):540-544.

141. Pontaga I. Ankle joint evertor-invertor muscle torque ratio decrease due to recurrent lateral ligament sprains. *Clin Biomech*. 2004;19(7):760-762.

142. Hofmann CL, Okita N, Sharkey NA. Experimental evidence supporting isometric functioning of the extrinsic toe flexors during gait. *Clin Biomech*. 2013;28(6):686-691.

143. Kelly LA, Kuitunen S, Racinais S, Cresswell AG. Recruitment of the plantar intrinsic foot muscles with increasing postural demand. *Clin Biomech*. 2012;27(1):46-51.

144. Konradsen L. Factors contributing to chronic ankle instability: kinesthesia and joint position sense. *J Athletic Train*. 2002;37(4):381-385.

145. Forkin DM, Koczur C, Battle R, Newton RA. Evaluation of kinesthetic deficits indicative of balance control in gymnasts with unilateral chronic ankle sprains. *J Orthop Sports Phys Ther*. 1996;23(4):245-250.

146. Lofvenberg R, Karrholm J, Sundelin G, Ahlgren O. Prolonged reaction time in patients with chronic lateral instability of the ankle. *Am J Sports Med*. 1995;23:414-417.

147. Refshauge KM, Kilbreath SL, Raymond J. The effect of recurrent ankle inversion sprain and taping on proprioception at the ankle. *Med Sci Sports Exerc*. 2000;32(1):10-15.

148. Willems T, Witvrouw E, Verstuyft J, Vaes P, De Clercq D. Proprioception and muscle strength in subjects with a history of ankle sprains and chronic instability. *J Athletic Train*. 2002;37(4):487-493.

149. Sefton JM, Hicks-Little CA, Hubbard TJ, et al. Sensorimotor function as a predictor of chronic ankle instability. *Clin Biomech*. 2009;24(5):451-458.

150. Yokoyama S, Matsusaka N, Gamada K, Ozaki M, Shindo H. Position-specific deficit of joint position sense in ankles with chronic functional instability. *J Sports Sci Med*. 2008;7(4):480-485.

151. Bernier JN, Perrin DH. Effect of coordination training on proprioception of the functionally unstable ankle. *J Orthop Sports Phys Ther*. 1998;27(4):264-275.

152. Hale SA, Hertel J, Olmsted-Kramer LC. The effect of a 4-week comprehensive rehabilitation program on postural control and lower extremity function in individuals with chronic ankle instability. *J Orthop Sports Phys Ther*. 2007;37(6):303-311.

153. Sefton JM, Yarar C, Hicks-Little CA, Berry JW, Cordova ML. Six weeks of balance training improves sensorimotor function in individuals with chronic ankle instability. *J Orthop Sports Phys Ther*. 2011;41(2):81-89.

154. Bohannon RW. Responsiveness of the single-limb stance test. *Gait Posture*. 2012;35(1):173.

155. Vereeck L, Wuyts F, Truijen S, Van de Heyning P. Clinical assessment of balance: normative data, and gender and age effects. *Int J Audiol*. 2008;47(2):67-75. doi:10.1080/14992020701689688

156. Cipriani DJ, Armstrong CW, Gaul S. Backward walking at three levels of treadmill inclination: An electromyographic and kinematic analysis. *J Orthop Sports Phys Ther*. 1995;22:95-102.

157. Bolgla LA, Keskula DR. Reliability of lower extremity functional performance tests. *J Orthop Sports Phys Ther*. 1997;26(3):138-142.

158. Greenberger HB, Paterno MV. Relationship of knee extensor strength and hopping test performance in the assessment of lower extremity function. *J Orthop Sports Phys Ther*. 1995;22:202-206.

159. Manske R, Reiman M. Functional performance testing for power and return to sports. *Sports Health*. 2013;5(3):244-250.

160. Bridgman SA, Clement D, Downing A, Walley G, Phair I, Maffulli N. Population based epidemiology of ankle sprains attending accident and emergency units in the West Midlands of England, and a survey of UK practice for severe ankle sprains. *Emerg Med J*. 2003;20(6):508-510.

161. Liu K, Gustavsen G, Kaminski TW. Increased frequency of ankle sprain does not lead to an increase in ligament laxity. *Clin J Sports Med*. 2013;23(6):483-487.

162. Beumer A, Swierstra BA, Mulder PGH. Clinical diagnosis of syndesmotic ankle instability: evaluation of stress tests behind the curtains. *Acta Orthop Scand*. 2002;73(6):667-669.

163. Sman AD, Hiller CE, Rae K, et al. Diagnostic accuracy of clinical tests for ankle syndesmosis injury. *Br J Sports Med*. 2015;49(5):323-329.

164. Hertel J, Denegar CR, Monroe MM, Stokes WL. Talocrural and subtalar joint instability after lateral ankle sprain. *Med Sci Sports Exerc*. 1999;31(11):1501-1508.

165. Maffulli N. The clinical diagnosis of subcutaneous tear of the Achilles tendon: a prospective study in 174 patients. *Am J Sports Med*. 1998;26(2):266-270.

166. Aboelnasr EA, El-Talawy HA, Abdelazim FH, Hegazy FA. Sensitivity and specificity of normalized truncated navicular height in assessment of static foot posture in children aged 6-12 years. *Hong Kong Physiother*. 2019;39(1):15-23.

167. Haeger K. Problems of acute deep venous thrombosis. I. The interpretation of signs and symptoms. *Angiology*. 1969;20(4):219-223.

168. Datema M, Hoitsma E, Roon KI, Malessy MJA, Van Dijk JG, Tannemaat MR. The Tinel sign has no diagnostic value for nerve entrapment or neuropathy in the legs. *Muscle Nerve*. 2016;54(1):25-30.

169. Cloke DJ, Greiss ME. The digital nerve stretch test: A sensitive indicator of Morton's neuroma and neuritis. *Foot Ankle Surg*. 2006;12(4):201-203.

170. Rivera F, Bertone C, DeMartino M, Pietrobono D, Ghisellini F. Pure dislocation of the ankle: Three case reports and literature review. *Clin Orthop Relat Res*. 2001;(382):179-184.

171. Xing W, Wang Y, Sun L, et al. Ankle joint dislocation treating dislocated trimalleolar fractures accompanied with the complex posterior malleolus fracture without separation of the tibiofibular syndesmosis. *Medicine (Baltimore)*. 2018;97(37):e12079. doi:10.1097/MD.0000000000012079

172. Glascoe WM, Allen MK, Awtry BF, Yack HJ. Weight-bearing immobilization and early exercise treatment following a grade II lateral ankle sprain. *J Orthop Sports Phys Ther*. 1999;29(7):394-399.

173. Konradsen L, Holmer P, Sondergaard L. Early mobilizing treatment for grade III ankle ligament injuries. *Foot Ankle*. 1991;12(2):69-73.

174. O'Connor SR, Bleakley CM, Tully MA, McDonough SM. Predicting functional recovery after acute ankle sprain. *PLoS One*. 2013;8(8):e72124. doi:10.1371/journal.pone.0072124

175. Specchiulli F, Cofano RE. A comparison of surgical and conservative treatment in ankle ligament tears. *Orthopedics*. 2001;24(7):686-688.

176. Schenck RC, Jr., Coughlin MJ. Lateral ankle instability and revision surgery alternatives in the athlete. *Foot Ankle Clin*. 2009;14(2):205-214.

177. Gillogly SD, Myers TH, Reinold MM. Treatment of full-thickness chondral defects in the knee with autologous chondrocyte implantation. *J Orthop Sports Phys Ther*. 2006;36(10):751-764.

178. Wiesler ER, Hunter M, Martin D, Curl WW, Hoen H. Ankle flexibility and injury patterns in dancers. *Am J Sports Med*. 1996;24(6):754-757.

179. Garn SN, Newton RA. Kinesthetic awareness in subjects with multiple ankle sprains. *Physical Therapy*. 1988;68:1667-1671.

180. Monaghan K, Delahunt E, Caulfield B. Ankle function during gait in patients with chronic ankle instability compared to controls. *Clin Biomech*. 2006;21(2):168-174.

181. Hertel J. Functional anatomy, pathomechanics, and pathophysiology of lateral ankle instability. *J Athl Train*. 2002;37(4):364-375.

182. Seto JL, Brewster CE. Treatment approaches following foot and ankle injury. *Clin Sports Med*. 1994;13(4):695-718.

183. Fong DT, Chan YY, Mok KM, Yung PS, Chan KM. Understanding acute ankle ligamentous sprain injury in sports. *Sports Med Arthrosc Rehabil Ther Technol*. 2009;1. doi:10.1186/1758-2555-1-14 Accessed Jul 30.

184. Wang X, Chang SM, Yu GR, Rao ZT. Clinical value of the Ottawa ankle rules for diagnosis of fractures in acute ankle injuries. *PLoS One*. 2013;8(4):e63228. doi:10.1371/journal.pone.0063228

185. Bruin DB, von Piekartz H. Musculoskeletal management of a patient with a history of chronic ankle sprains: identifying rupture of peroneal brevis and peroneal longus with diagnostic ultrasonography. *J Chiropr Med*. 2014;13(3):203-209.

186. Sammarco GJ, DiRaimondo VC. Chronic peroneus brevis tendon lesions. *Foot Ankle Int*. 1989;9(4):163-170.

187. van den Bekerom MP, Kerkhoffs GM, McCollum GA, Calder JD, Van Dijk CN. Management of acute lateral ankle ligament injury in the athlete. *Knee Surg Sports Traumatol Arthrosc*. 2012.

188. Annunziato A, Williams G, Foster G. Evidence-based approach to treatment of acute traumatic syndesmosis (high ankle) sprains. *Sports Med Arthrosc Rev*. 2006;14(4):232-236.

189. Mulligan EP. Evaluation and management of ankle syndesmosis injuries. *Phys Ther Sport*. 2011;12(2):57-69.

190. Norkus SA, Floyd RT. The anatomy and mechanisms of syndesmotic ankle sprains. *J Athl Train*. 2001;36(1):68-73.

191. Oberg B, Bergman T, Tropp H. Testing of isokinetic muscle strength in the ankle. *Med Sci Sports Exerc*. 1987;19(3):318-322.

192. Lin CF, Gross ML, Weinhold P. Ankle syndesmosis injuries: anatomy, biomechanics, mechanism of injury, and clinical guidelines for diagnosis and intervention. *J Orthop Sports Phys Ther*. 2006;36(6):372-384.

193. Gerber JP, Williams GN, Scoville CR, Acrciero RA, Taylor DC. Persistent disability associated with ankle sprains: a prospective examination of an athletic population. *Foot Ankle Int*. 1998;19(10):653-660.

194. Miller BS, Downie BK, Johnson PD, et al. Time to return to play after high ankle sprains in collegiate football players: a prediction model. *Sports Health*. 2012;4(6):504-509.

195. Press CM, Gupta A, Hutchinson MR. Management of ankle syndesmosis injuries in the athlete. *Curr Sports Med Rep*. 2009;8(5):228-233.

196. Karlsson J, Eriksson BI, Sward L. Early functional treatment for acute ligament injuries of the ankle joint. *Scand J Med Sci Sports*. 1996;6(6):341-345.

197. Scifers JR. Instrument-assisted soft tissue mobilization. *Athl Train Sports Health Care*. 2017;9(2):49-52.

198. Loudon JK, Bell SL. The foot and ankle: an overview of arthrokinematics and selected joint techniques. *J Athl Train*. 1996;31(2):173-178.

199. Fujii T, Kitaoka HB, Luo ZP, Kura H, An KN. Analysis of ankle-hindfoot stability in multiple planes: an in vitro study. *Foot Ankle Int*. 2005;26(8):633-637.

200. Staples OS. Result study of ruptures of lateral ligaments of the ankle. *Clin Orthop Relat Res*. 1972;(85):50-58.

201. Chu D, Myer GD. *Plyometrics*. Human Kinetics; 2013.

202. Gross MT, Bradshaw MK, Ventry LC, Weller KH. Comparison of support provided by ankle taping and semirigid orthosis. *J Orthop Sports Phys Ther*. 1987;9(1):33-39.

203. Karlsson J, Andreasson GO. The effect of external ankle support in chronic lateral ankle joint instability. *Am J Sports Med*. 1992;20(3):257-261.

204. Kimura IF, Nawoczenski DA, Epler M, Owen MG. Effect of the AirStirrup in controlling ankle inversion stress. *J Orthop Sports Phys Ther*. 1987;9(5):190-193.

205. Renström PA, Konradsen L, Beynnon BD. Influence of knee and ankle support on proprioception and neuromuscular control. In: Lephart SM, Fu FH, eds. *Proprioception and Neuromuscular Control in Joint Stability*. Human Kinetics; 2000:301-309.

206. Rovere GD, Clarke TJ, Yates CS, Burley K. Retrospective comparison of taping and ankle stabilizers in preventing ankle injuries. *Am J Sports Med*. 1988;16(3):228-233.

207. Sitler M, Ryan J, Wheeler B, et al. The efficacy of a semirigid ankle stabilizer to reduce acute ankle injuries in basketball. *Am J Sports Med*. 1994;22(4):454-461.

208. Arnold BL, Docherty CL. Bracing and rehabilitation—what's new. *Clin Sports Med*. 2004;23(1):83-95.

209. Alanen J, Orava S, Heinonen OJ, Ikonen J, Kvist M. Peroneal tendon injuries. Report of thirty-eight operated cases. *Ann Chir Gynaecol*. 2001;90:43-46.

210. Walther M, Morrison R, Mayer B. Retromalleolar groove impaction for the treatment of unstable peroneal tendons. *Am J Sports Med*. 2009;37(1):191-194.

211. Baumhauer J, Shereff M, Gould J. Ankle pain in runners. In: Guten GN, ed. *Running Injuries*. Saunders; 1997.

212. Roster B, Michelier P, Giza E. Peroneal tendon disorders. *Clin Sports Med*. 2015;34(4):625-641.

213. Mann RA. Subluxation and disolocation of the peroneal tendons. *Op Tech Sports Med*. 1999;7(1):2-6.

214. Safran MR, O'Malley Jr D, Fu FH. Peroneal subluxation in athletes: new exam technique, case reports, and review. *Med Sci Sports Exerc*. 1999;31(7):S487-S492.

215. Krause JO, Brodsky JW. Peroneus brevis tendon tears: pathophysiology, surgical reconstruction, and clincial results. *Foot Ankle Int*. 1998;19(5):271-279.

216. Maffulli N. Current concepts review: rupture of the Achilles tendon. *J Bone Joint Surg Am*. 1999;81(7):1019-1036.

217. McCrory JL, D.F. M, R.B. L, et al. Etiologic factors associated with Achilles tendinitis in runners. *Med Sci Sports Exerc*. 1999;31(10):1374-1381.

218. Järvinen TAH, Kannus P, Maffulli N, Khan KM. Achilles tendon disorders: etiology and epidemiology. *Foot Ankle Clin*. 2005;10(2):255-266.

219. Karkhanis S, Mumtaz H, Kurdy N. Functional management of Achilles tendon rupture: A viable option for non-operative management. *Foot Ankle Surg*. 2010;16(2):81-86.

220. Brumann M, Baumbach SF, Mutschler W, Polzer H. Accelerated rehabilitation following Achilles tendon repair after acute rupture—development of an evidence-based treatment protocol. *Injury*. 2014;45(11):1782-1790.

221. Talbot JC, Williams GT, Bismil Q, Shaw DL, Schilders E. Results of accelerated postoperative rehabilitation using novel "suture frame" repair of Achilles tendon rupture. *J Foot Ankle Surg*. 2012;51(2):147-151.

222. Kangas J, Pajala A, Siira P, Hamalainen M, Leppilahti J. Early functional treatment versus early immobilization in tension of the musculotendinous unit after Achilles rupture repair: a prospective, randomized, clinical study. *J Trauma* 2003;54(6):1171-1180.

223. Nyyssönen T, Lüthje P, Kröger H. The increasing incidence and difference in sex distribution of Achilles tendon rupture in Finland in 1987-1999. *Scand J Surg*. 2008;97(3):272-275.

224. Maffulli N, Waterston SW, Squair J, Reaper J, Douglas AS. Changing incidence of Achilles tendon rupture in Scotland: a 15-year study. *Clin J Sport Med*. 1999;9(3):157-160.

225. Huttunen TT, Kannus P, Rolf C, Felländer-Tsai L, Mattila VM. Acute Achilles tendon ruptures: incidence of injury and surgery in Sweden between 2001 and 2012. *Am J Sports Med*. 2014;42(10):2419-2423.

226. Lynch RM. Achilles tendon rupture: surgical versus non-surgical treatment. *Accid Emerg Nurs*. 2004;12(3):149-158.

227. Lo IK, Kirkley A, Nonweiler B, Kumbhare DA. Operative versus nonoperative treatment of acute Achilles tendon ruptures: a quantitative review. *Clin J Sports Med*. 1997;7(3):207-211.

228. Möller M, Movin T, Granhed H, Lind K, Faxén E, Karlsson J. Acute rupture of tendon Achillis. A prospective randomised study of comparison between surgical and non-surgical treatment. *J Bone Joint Surg Br*. 2001;83(6):843-848.

229. Kearney RS, McGuinness KR, Achten J, Costa ML. A systematic review of early rehabilitation methods fol-

lowing a rupture of the Achilles tendon. *Physiother.* 2012;98(1):24-32.

230. Nilsson-Helander K, Silbermagel KG, Thomeé R, et al. Acute Achilles tendon rupture: a randomized, controlled study comparing surgical and nonsurgical treatments using validated outcome measures. *Am J Sports Med.* 2010;38(11):2186-2193.

231. Twaddle BC, Poon P. Early motion for Achilles tendon ruptures: is surgery important? A randomized, prospective study. *Am J Sports Med.* 2007;35(12):2033-2038.

232. Gigante A, Moschini A, Verdenilli A, Del Torto M, Ulisse S, de Palma L. Open versus percutaneous repair in the treatment of acute Achilles tendon rupture: a randomized prospective study. *Knee Surg Sports Traumatol Arthrosc.* 2008;16:206-209.

233. Tomak SL, Fleming LL. Achilles tendon rupture: an alternative treatment. *Am J Orthop.* 2004;33(1):9-12.

234. Metz R, Kerkhoffs GM, Verleisdonk EJ, van der Heijden GJ. Acute Achilles tendon rupture: minimally invasive surgery versus non operative treatment, with immediate full weight bearing. Design of a randomized controlled trial. *BMC Musculoskelet Disord.* 2007;8:108.

235. Rettig AC, Liotta FJ, Klootwyk TF, Porter DA, Mieling P. Potential risk of rerupture in primary Achilles tendon repair in athletes younger than 30 years of age. *Am J Sports Med.* 2005;33(1):119-123.

236. Wilder R, Seth S. Overuse injuries: tendinopathies, stress fractures, compartment syndrome, and shin splints. *Clin Sports Med.* 2004;23(1):55-81.

237. Tsai WC, Tang ST, Liang FC. Effect of therapeutic ultrasound on tendons. *Am J Phys Med Rehabil.* 2011;90(12):1068-1073.

238. Jarin I, Bäcker HC, Vosseller JT. Meta-analysis of noninsertional Achilles tendinopathy. *Foot Ankle Int.* 2020;41(6):744-754.

239. McCormack JR, Underwood FB, Slaven EJ, Cappaert TA. Eccentric exercise versus eccentric exercise and soft tissue treatment (Astym) in the management of insertional Achilles tendinopathy. *Sports Health.* 2016;8(3):230-237.

240. Zafar MS, Mahmood A, Maffulli N. Basic sicence and clinical aspects of achilles tendinopathy. *Sports Med Arthrosc.* 2009;17(3):190-197.

241. Longo UG, Ronga M, Maffulli N. Achilles tendinopathy. *Sports Med Arthrosc Rev.* 2018;26(1):16-30.

242. Magnan B, Bondi M, Pierantoni S, Samaila E. The pathogenesis of Achilles tendinopathy: A systematic review. *Foot Ankle Surg.* 2014;20(3):154-159.

243. Gallo RA, Plakke M, Silvis ML. Common leg injuries of long-distance runners: anatomical and biomechanical approach. *Sports Health.* 2012;4(6):485-495.

244. Carcia CR, Martin RL, Houck J, Wukick DK, Orthopaedic Section of the American Physical Therapy Association. Achilles pain, stiffness, and muscle power deficits: Achilles tendinitis. Clinical practice guidelines linked to the International Classification of Functioning, Disability, and Health from the Orthopaedic Section of the American Physical Therapy Association. *J Orthop Sports Phys Ther.* 2010;40(9):A1-A26.

245. Chimenti RL, Cychosz CC, Hall MM, Phisitkul P. Current concepts review update: insertional Achilles tendinopathy. *Foot Ankle Int.* 2017;38(10):1160-1169.

246. Nuri L, Obst SJ, Newsham-West R, Barrett RS. Regional three-dimensional deformation of human Achilles tendon during conditioning. *Scand J Med Sci Sports.* 2017;27(11):1263-1272.

247. Vora AM, Myerson MS, Oliva F, Maffulli N. Tendinopathy of the main body of the Achilles tendon. *Foot Ankle Clin.* 2005;10(2):293-308.

248. Komi PV, Fukashiro S, Järvinen M. Biomechanical loading of Achilles tendon during normal locomotion. *Clin Sports Med.* 1992;11(3):521-531.

249. Chuter VH, Janse de Jonge XA. Proximal and distal contributions to lower extremity injury: a review of the literature. *Gait Posture* 2012;36(1):7-15.

250. Movin T, Krostpffersen-Wiberg M, Shalabi A, Gad A, Aspelin P, Rolf C. Intratendinous alterations as imaged by ultrasound and contrast medium-enhanced magnetic resonance in chronic achillodynia. *Foot Ankle Int.* 1998;19(5):311-317.

251. Szaro P, Witkowski G, Smigielski R, Krajewski P, Ciszek B. Fascicles of the adult human Achilles tendon—an anatomical study. *Ann Anat.* 2009;191(6):586-593.

252. Winnicki K, Ochala-Klos A, Rutowicz B, Pękala PA, Tomaszewski KA. Functional anatomy, histology and biomechanics of the human Achilles tendon—a comprehensive review. *Ann Anat.* 2020;229:151461. doi:10.1016/j.aanat.2020.151461

253. Blackman AJ, Blevins JJ, Sangeorzan BJ, Ledoux WR. Cadaveric flatfoot model: ligament attenuation and Achilles tendon overpull. *J Orthop Res.* 2009;27(12):1547-1554.

254. Lersch C, Grotsch A, Segesser B, Koebke J, Bruggemann GP, Potthast W. Influence of calcaneus angle and muscle forces on strain distribution in the human Achilles tendon. *Clin Biomech.* 2012;27(9):955-961.

255. McKenzie DC, Clement DB, Taunton JE. Running shoes, orthotics, and injuries. *Sports Med.* 1985;2(5):334-347.

256. Denegar CR, Saliba E, Saliba S. *Therapeutic Modalities for Musculoskeletal Injuries.* 4th ed. Human Kinetics; 2016.

257. Bolivar YA, Munuera PV, Padillo JP. Relationship between tightness of the posterior muscles of the lower limb and plantar fasciitis. *Foot Ankle Int.* 2013;34(1):42-48.

258. Meyer A, Tumilty S, Baxter GD. Eccentric exercise protocols for chronic non-insertional Achilles tendinopathy: how much is enough? *Scand J Med Sci Sports.* 2009;19(5):609-615.

259. Stasinopoulos D, Manias P. Comparing two eccentric exercise programmes for the management of Achilles tendinopathy. A pilot trial. *J Bodyw Mov Ther.* 2013;17(3):309-315.

260. Dilger CP, Chimenti RL. Nonsurgical treatment options for insertional Achilles tendinopathy. *Foot Ankle Clin.* 2019;24(3):505-513.

261. Magnussen RA, Dunn WR, Thomson AB. Nonoperative treatment of midportion Achilles tendinopathy: a systematic review. *Clin J Sport Med.* 2009;19(1):54-64.

262. Pavone V, Vescio A, Mobilia G, et al. Conservative treatment of chronic Achilles tendinopathy: a systematic review. *J Funct Morphol Kinesiol.* 2019;4(3):46. doi:10.3390/jfmk4030046

263. Stevens M, Tan CW. Effectiveness of the Alfredson protocol compared with a lower repetition-volume protocol

for midportion Achilles tendinopathy: a randomized controlled trial. *J Orthop Sports Phys Ther.* 2014;44(2):59-67.

264. Kohls-Gatzoulis J, Angel JC, Singh D, Haddad F, Livingstone J, Berry G. Tibialis posterior dysfunction: a common and treatable cause of adult acquired flatfoot. *BMJ.* 2004;329(7478):1328-1333.

265. Myerson MS. Injuries in the athlete. In: Helal B, Rowley DI, Cracchiolo Ar, Myerson MS, eds. *Surgical Disorders of the Foot and Ankle.* Lippincott-Raven; 1996:793-809.

266. Palmieri-Smith RM, Hopkins JT, Brown TN. Peroneal activation deficits in persons with functional ankle instability. *Am J Sports Med.* 2009;37(5):982-988.

267. Rattanaprasert U, Smith R, Sullivan M, Gilleard W. Three-dimensional kinematics of the forefoot, rearfoot, and leg without the function of tibialis posterior in comparison with normals during stance phase of walking. *Clin Biomech.* 1999;14(1):14-23.

268. Moen MH, Tol JL, Weir A, Stueunebrink M, DeWinter TC. Medial tibial stress syndrome: a critical review. *Sports Med.* 2009;39(7):523-546.

269. Hreljac A. Etiology, prevention, and early intervention of overuse injuries in runners: a biomechanical perspective. *Phys Med Rehabil Clin N Am.* 2005;16(3):651-667, vi.

270. Kulig K, Pomrantz AB, Burnfield JM, et al. Non-operative management of posterior tibialis tendon dysfunction: design of a randomized clinical trial. *BMC Musculoskeletal Disorders.* 2006;7:49.

271. Barr KP, Harrast MA. Evidence-based treatment of foot and ankle injuries in runners. *Phys Med Rehabil Clin N Am.* 2005;16(3):779-799.

272. Kulig K, Lederhaus ES, Reischl S, Arya S, Bashford G. Effect of eccentric exercise program for early tibialis posterior tendinopathy. *Foot Ankle Int.* 2009;30(9):877-885.

273. Neely FG. Biomechanical risk factors for exercise-related lower limb injuries. *Sports Med.* 1998;26(6):395-413.

274. Kulig K, Reischl SF, Pomrantz AB, et al. Nonsurgical management of posterior tibial tendon dysfunction with orthoses and resistive exercise: a randomized controlled trial. *Phys Ther.* 2009;89(1):26-37.

275. Batt ME, Ugalade V, Anderson MW, Shelton DK. A prospective controlled study of diagnostic imaging for acute shin splints. *Med Sci Sport Exerc.* 1998;30(11):1564-1571.

276. Reinking M. Exercise related leg pain (ERLP): a review of the literature. *N Am J Sports Phys Ther.* 2007;2(3):170-180.

277. Craig DI. Medial tibial stress syndrome: current etiological theories part 1—background. *Athl Ther Today.* 2008;13(1):17-20.

278. Galbraith RM, Lavallee ME. Medial tibial stress syndrome: conservative treatment options. *Curr Rev Musculoskelet Med.* 2009;2(3):127-133.

279. Couture CJ, Karlson KA. Tibial stress injuries: decisive diagnosis and treatment of "shin splints". *Physician Sportsmed.* 2002;30(6):29-36.

280. Story J, Cymet TC. Shin splints: painful to have and treat. *Compr Ther.* 2006;32(3):192-195.

281. Winters M, Eskes M, Weir A, Moen MH, Backx FJ, Bakker EW. Treatment of medial tibial stress syndrome: a systematic review. *Sports Med.* 2013;43(12):1315-1333.

282. Loudon JK, Dolphino MR. Use of foot orthoses and calf stretching for individuals with medial tibial stress syndrome. *Foot Ankle Spec.* 2010;3(1):15-20.

283. Uden H, Boesch e, Kumar S. Plantar fasciitis—to jab or to support? A systematic review of the current best evidence. *J Multidiscip Healthc.* 2011;4:155-165.

284. Bolgla LA, Malone TR. Plantar fasciitis and the windlass mechanism: a biomechanical link to clinical practice. *J Athl Train.* 2004;39(1):77-82.

285. Chandler TJ, Kibler WB. A biomechanical approach to the prevention, treatment and rehabilitation of plantar fasciitis. *Sports Med.* 1993;15(5):344-352.

286. Cheung J, T.M., Zhang M, An KN. Effect of Achilles tendon loading on plantar fascia tension in the standing foot. *Clin Biomech (Bristol, Avon).* 2006;21(2):194-203.

287. Cornwall MW, McPoil TG. Plantar fasciitis: etiology and treatment. *Journal of Orthopaedic and Sports Physical Therapy.* 1999;29(12):756-760.

288. Fuller EA. The windlass mechanism of the foot: a mechanical model to explain pathology. *J Am Pod Med Assoc.* 2000;90(1):35-46.

289. De Vera Barredo R, Menna D, Farris JW. An evaluation of research evidence for selected physical therapy interventions for plantar fasciitis. *J Phys Ther Sci.* 2007;19(1):41-56.

290. Ogden JA, Alvarez R, Levitt R, Cross GL, Marlow M. Shock wave therapy for chronic proximal plantar fasciitis. *Clin Orthop Relat Res.* 2001;(387):47-59.

291. Hyland MR, Webber-Gaffney A, Cohen L, Lichtman PT. Randomized controlled trial of calcaneal taping, sham taping, and plantar fascia stretching for the short-term management of plantar heel pain. *J Orthop Sports Phys Ther.* 2006;36(6):364-371.

292. Barry LD, Barry AN, Y. C. A retrospective study of standing gastrocnemius-soleus stretching versus night splinting in the treatment of plantar fasciitis. *J Foot Ankle Surg.* 2002;41(4):221-227.

293. Evans A. Podiatric medical applications of posterior night stretch splinting. *J Am Pod Med Assoc.* 2001;91(7):356-360.

294. Kuper BC. Tarsal tunnel syndrome. *Orthop Nursing.* 1998;17:9-17.

295. Trepman E, Kadel NJ, Chisholm K, Razzano L. Effect of foot and ankle position on tarsal tunnel compartment pressure. *Foot Ankle Int.* 1999;20(11):721-726.

296. Jahss MH. The sesamoids of the hallux. *Clin Orthop Relat Res.* 1981;(157):88-97.

297. McBryde AM, Jr., Anderson RB. Sesamoid foot problems in the athlete. *Clin Sports Med.* 1988;7(1):51-60.

298. Srinivasan R. The hallucal-sesamoid complex: normal anatomy, imaging, and pathology. *Semin Musculoskelet Radiol.* 2016;20(2):224-232.

299. Dietzen CJ. Great toe sesamoid injuries in the athlete. *Orthop Rev.* 1990;19(11):966-972.

300. Hetherington VJ, Johnson RE, Albritton JS. Necessary dorsiflexion of the first metatarsophalangeal joint during gait. *J Foot Surg.* 1990;29(3):218-222.

301. Goulart M, O'Malley MJ, Hodgkins CW, Charlton TP. Foot and ankle fractures in dancers. *Clin Sports Med.* 2008;27(2):295-304.

302. Thigpen CM. Early management of fractures of the foot and ankle. *Current Issue Trauma Care.* 1983;6:4-8.

303. Lin CW, Moseley AM, Herbert RD, Refshauge KM. Pain and dorsiflexion range of motion predict short- and

medium-term activity limitation in people receiving physiotherapy intervention after ankle fracture: an observational study. *Aust J Physiother.* 2009;55(1):31-37.

304. Borstad JD, Szucs KA. Three-dimensional scapula kinematics and shoulder function examined before and after surgical treatment for breast cancer. *Hum Mov Sci.* 2012;31(2):408-418.

305. Stäuble CG, Helming M, Martyn JAJ, Blobner M, Fink H. Neuromuscular recovery is prolonged after immobilization or superimposition of inflammation with immobilization compared to inflammation alone: data from a preclinical model. *Crit Care Med.* 2016;44(11):e1097-e1110.

306. Keene DJ, Williamson E, Bruce J, Willett K, Lamb SE. Early ankle movement versus immobilization in the postoperative management of ankle fracture in adults: a systematic review and meta-analysis. *J Orthop Sports Phys Ther.* 2014;44(9):690-701.

307. Koury JM. *Aquatic Therapy Programming.* Human Kinetics; 1996.

Chapter 21

1. Degen RM, Giles JW, Thompson SR, Litchfield RB, Athwal GS. Biomechanics of complex shoulder instability. *Clin Sports Med.* 2013;32(4):625-636.

2. Perry J. Biomechanics of the shoulder. In: Rowe C, ed. *The Shoulder.* Churchill Livingstone; 1988.

3. Perry J. Normal upper extremity kinesiology. *Phys Ther.* 1978;58(3):265-278.

4. Pappas AM, Zawacki RM, Sullivan TJ. Biomechanics of baseball pitching, a preliminary report. *Am J Sports Med.* 1985;13(216-222)

5. Kibler WB. Biomechanical analysis of the shoulder during tennis activities. *Clin Sports Med.* 1995;14:79-85.

6. Niederbracht Y, Shim AL, Sloniger MA, Paternostro-Bayles M, Short TH. Effects of a shoulder injury prevention strength training program on eccentric external rotator muscle strength and glenohumeral joint imbalance in female overhead activity athletes. *J Strength Cond Res.* 2008;22(1):140-145.

7. Liu J, Hughes RE, Smutz WP, Niebur G, Nan-An K. Roles of deltoid and rotator cuff muscles in shoulder elevation. *Clin Biomech.* 1997;12(1):32-38.

8. Saha AK. Dynamic stability of the glenohumeral joint. *Acta Orthop Scand.* 1971;42(6):491-505.

9. Borstad JD, Szucs KA. Three-dimensional scapula kinematics and shoulder function examined before and after surgical treatment for breast cancer. *Hum Mov Sci.* 2012;31(2):408-418.

10. Moseley HF. The clavicle: its anatomy and function. *Clin Orthop Relat Res.* 1968;58:17-27.

11. Inman VT, Saunders JB. Observations on the function of the clavicle. *California Medicine.* 1946;65(4):158-166.

12. Teece RM, Lunden JB, Lloyd AS, Kaiser AP, Cieminski CJ, Ludewig PM. Three-dimensional acromioclavicular joint motions during elevation of the arm. *J Orthop Sports Phys Ther.* 2008;38(4):181-190.

13. Ludewig PM, Phadke V, Braman JP, Hassett DR, Cieminski CJ, LaPrade RF. Motion of the shoulder complex during multiplanar humeral elevation. *J Bone Joint Surg Am.* 2009;91A(2):378-389.

14. Inman VT, Saunders JB, Abbott LC. Observations on the function of the shoulder joint. *J Bone Joint Surg Am* 1944;26:1-30.

15. McClure PW, Michener LA, Sennett BJ, Karduna AR. Direct 3-dimensional measurement of scapular kinematics during dynamic movements in vivo. *J Shoulder Elbow Surg.* 2001;10(3):269-277.

16. Bagg SD, Forrest WJ. A biomechanical analysis of scapular rotation during arm abduction in the scapular plane. *Am J Phys Med Rehabil.* 1988;67(6):238-245.

17. Borsa PA, Timmons MK, Sauers EL. Scapular-positioning patterns during humeral head elevation in unimpaired shoulders. *J Athl Train.* 2003;38(1):12-17.

18. Ludewig PM, Behrens SA, Meyer SM, Spoden SM, Wilson LA. Three-dimensional clavicular motion during arm elevation: Reliability and descriptive data. *J Orthop Sports Phys Ther.* 2004;43(3):140-149.

19. Myers JB, Wassinger CA, Lephart SM. Sensorimotor contribution to shoulder stability: effect of injury and rehabilitation. *Man Ther.* 2006;11:197-201.

20. Riemann BL, Lephart SM. The sensorimotor system, Part II: The role of proprioception in motor control and functional joint stability. *J Athl Train.* 2002;37(1):80-84.

21. Borsa PA, Lephart SM. Functional assessment and rehabilitation of shoulder proprioception for glenohumeral instability. *J Sport Rehabil.* 1994;3(1):84-104.

22. Cools AM, Dewitte V, Lanszweert F, et al. Rehabilitation of scapular muscle balance: which exercises to prescribe? *Am J Sports Med.* 2007;35(10):1744-1751.

23. Houglum PA. Rehabilitation for subacromial impingement starts at the scapula. *J Orthop Trauma Rehabil.* 2013;17(2):54-60.

24. Burkhart SS, Morgan CD, Kibler WB. The disabled throwing shoulder: spectrum of pathology Part I: pathoanatomy and biomechanics. *Arthroscopy.* 2003;19(4):404-420.

25. Ravichandran H, Janakiraman B, Gelaw AY, Fisseha B, Sundaram S, Sharma HR. Effect of scapular stabilization exercise program in patients with subacromial impingement syndrome: a systematic review. *J Exerc Rehabil.* 2020;16(3):216-226.

26. Reuther KE, Thomas SJ, Tucker JJ, et al. Scapular dyskinesis is detrimental to shoulder tendon properties and joint mechanics in a rat model. *J Orthop Res.* 2014;32(11):1436-1443.

27. Reuther KE, Thomas SJ, Tucker JJ, et al. Overuse activity in the presence of scapular dyskinesis leads to shoulder tendon damage in a rat model. *Ann Biomed Eng.* 2015;43(4):917-928.

28. Umehara J, Kusano K, Nakamura M, et al. Scapular kinematic and shoulder muscle activity alterations after serratus anterior muscle fatigue. *J Shoulder Elbow Surg.* 2018;27(7):1205-1213.

29. McQuade KJ, Dawson J, Smidt GL. Scapulothoracic muscle fatigue associated with alterations in scapulohumeral rhythm kinematics during maximum resistive shoulder elevation. *J Orthop Sports Phys Ther.* 1998;28(2):74-80.

30. Schulte E, Miltner O, Junker E, Rau G, Disselhorst-Klug C. Upper trapezius muscle conduction velocity during fatigue in subjects with and without work-related muscular disorders: a non-invasive high spatial resolution approach. *Eur J Appl Physiol.* 2006;96(2):194-202.

31. Toomingas A, Hagberg M, Jorulf L, Nilsson T, Burström L, Kihlberg S. Outcome of the abduction external rotation test among manual and office workers. *Am J Ind Med.* 1991;19(2):215-227.

32. Paine RM, Voight ML. The role of the scapula. *Int J Sports Phys Ther*. 2013;8(5):617-629.

33. Jang HJ, Kim SY, Oh DW. Effects of augmented trunk stabilization with external compression support on shoulder and scapular muscle activity and maximum strength during isometric shoulder abduction. *J Electromyogr Kinesiol*. 2015;25(2):387-391.

34. Kelly BT, Williams RJ, Cordasco FA, et al. Differential patterns of muscle activation in patients with symptomatic and asymptomatic rotator cuff tears. *J Shoulder Elbow Surg*. 2005;14(2):165-171.

35. Smith M, Sparkes V, Busse M, Enright S. Upper and lower trapezius muscle activity in subjects with subacromial impingement symptoms: is there imbalance and can taping change it? *Phys Ther Sport*. 2009;10(2):45-50.

36. Nakamura Y, Tsuruike M, Ellenbecker TS. Electromyographic activity of scapular muscle control in free-motion exercise. *J Athl Train*. 2016;51(3):195-204.

37. Huang HY, Lin JJ, Guo YL, Wang WTJ, Chen YJ. EMG biofeedback effectiveness to alter muscle activity pattern and scapular kinematics in subjects with and without shoulder impingement *J Electromyogr Kinesiol*. 2013;23(1):267-274.

38. Miller P, Osmotherly P. Does scapular taping facilitate recovery for shoulder impingement symptoms? A pilot randomized controlled trial. *J Man Manip Ther*. 2009;17(1):E6-E13.

39. Denegar CR, Saliba E, Saliba S. *Therapeutic Modalities for Musculoskeletal Injuries*. 4th ed. Human Kinetics; 2016.

40. Hsu YH, Chen WY, Lin HC, Wang WT, Shih YF. The effects of taping on scapular kinematics and muscle performance in baseball players with shoulder impingement syndrome. *J Electromyogr Kinesiol*. 2009;19(6):1092-1099.

41. Selkowitz DM, Chaney C, Stuckey SJ, Vlad G. The effects of scapular taping on the surface electromyographic signal amplitude of shoulder girdle muscles during upper extremity elevation in individuals with suspected shoulder impingement syndrome. *J Orthop Sports Phys Ther*. 2007;37(11):694-702.

42. Host HH. Scapular taping in the treatment of anterior shoulder impingement. *Phys Ther*. 1995;75(9):803-812.

43. Snodgrass SJ, Farrell SF, Tsao H, et al. Shoulder taping and neuromuscular control. *J Athl Train*. 2018;53(4):395-403.

44. Leong HT, Ng GY, Fu SN. Effects of scapular taping on the activity onset of scapular muscles and the scapular kinematics in volleyball players with rotator cuff tendinopathy. *J Sci Med Sport*. 2017;20(6):555-560.

45. Harput G, Guney H, Toprak U, Colakoglu F, Baltaci G. Acute effects of scapular Kinesio Taping® on shoulder rotator strength, ROM and acromiohumeral distance in asymptomatic overhead athletes. *J Sports Med Phys Fitness*. 2017;57(11):1479-1485.

46. Huang TS, Ou HL, Lin JJ. Effects of trapezius kinesio taping on scapular kinematics and associated muscular activation in subjects with scapular dyskinesis. *J Hand Ther*. 2019;32(3):345-352.

47. Intelangelo L, Bordachar D, Barbosa AWC. Effects of scapular taping in young adults with shoulder pain and scapular dyskinesis. *J Bodyw Mov Ther*. 2016;20(3):525-532.

48. Reijneveld EAE, Noten S, Michener LA, Cools A, Struyf F. Clinical outcomes of a scapular-focused treatment in patients with subacromial pain syndrome: a systematic review. *Br J Sports Med*. 2017;51(5):436-441.

49. Shaheen AF, Bull AMJ, Alexander CM. Rigid and elastic taping changes scapular kinematics and pain in subjects with shoulder impingement syndrome: an experimental study. *J Electromyogr Kinesiol*. 2015;25(1):84-92.

50. Gusella A, Bettuolo M, Contiero F, Volpe G. Kinesiologic taping and muscular activity: a myofascial hypothesis and a randomised, blinded trial on healthy individuals. *J Bodyw Mov Ther*. 2014;18(3):405-411.

51. Swanik KA, Huxel Bliven K, Swanik CB. Rotator-cuff muscle-recruitment strategies during shoulder rehabilitation exercises. *J Sport Rehabil*. 2011;20(4):471-486.

52. Hecker A, Aguirre J, Eichenberger U, et al. Deltoid muscle contribution to shoulder flexion and abduction strength: an experimental approach. *J Shoulder Elbow Surg*. 2021;30(2):e60-e68.

53. Bechtol C. Biomechanics of the shoulder. *Clin Orthop Relat Res*. 1980;146:37-41.

54. Goldstein B. Shoulder anatomy and biomechanics. *Phys Med Rehabil Clin N Am*. 2004;15(2):313-349.

55. Corso G. Relief test: an adjunctive procedure to traditional assessment of shoulder impingement syndrome. *J Orthop Sports Phys Ther*. 1995;22(5):183-192.

56. Bak K. The practical management of swimmer's painful shoulder: etiology, diagnosis, and treatment. *Clin J Sport Med*. 2010;20(5):386-390.

57. Braatz JH, Gogia PP. The mechanics of pitching. *J Orthop Sports Phys Ther*. 1987;9(2):56-69.

58. Urbin MA, Fleisig GS, Abebe A, Andrews JR. Associations between timing in the baseball pitch and shoulder kinetics, elbow kinetics, and ball speed. *Am J Sports Med*. 2013;41(2):336-342.

59. Cools A, Witvrouw E, Declercq G, Danneels L, Cambier D. Scapular muscle recruitment patterns: trapezius muscle latency with and without impingement symptoms. *Am J Sports Med*. 2003;31(4):542-549.

60. Lukasiewicz AC, McClure P, Michener LA, Pratt N, Sennett BJ. Comparison of 3-dimensional scapular position and orientation between subjects with and without shoulder impingement. *J Orthop Sports Phys Ther*. 1999;29(10):574-586.

61. Hawkins RJ. Cervical spine and the shoulder. *Instr Course Lect*. 1985;34:191-195.

62. Pateder DB, Berg JH, Thal R. Neck and shoulder pain: differentiating cervical spine pathology from shoulder pathology. *J Surg Orthop Adv*. 2009;18(4):170-174.

63. Marquardt CA, Cianca JC, Foye PM, Prather H. Industrial medicine and acute musculoskeletal rehabilitation. 2. Acute cervical spine and shoulder injuries in the industrial setting. *Arch Phys Med Rehabil*. 2002;83(Suppl 1):S7-S11.

64. Strunce JB, Walker M, Boyles RE, Young BA. The immediate effects of thoracic spine and rib manipulation on subjects with primary complaints of shoulder pain. *J Man Manip Ther*. 2009;17(4):230-236.

65. Kebaetse M, McClure P, Pratt NA. Thoracic position effect on shoulder range of motion, strength, and three-dimensinoal scapular kinematics. *Arch Phys Med Rehabil*. 1999;80(8):945-950.

66. Curtis JQ, Gupta J, Hill CH, Gross MT. Treatment of shoulder impingement syndrome using non-thrust mobilizations to the thoracic spine and ribs: a case report. *Orthop Phys Ther Pract*. 2018;30(1):40-46.

67. Chitroda J, Heggannavar A. Effect of thoracic and rib manipulation on pain and restricted shoulder mobility in subjects with frozen shoulder: A randomised clinical trial. *Ind J Health Sci Biomed Res (KLEU)*. 2014;7(2):92-99. doi:10.4103/2349-5006.148807

68. Greenfield B, Donatelli R, Wooden MJ, Wilkes J. Isokinetic evaluation of shoulder rotational strength between the plane of the scapula and the frontal plane. *Am J Sports Med*. 1990;18(2):124-128.

69. Tis LL, Maxwell T. The effect of positioning on shoulder isokinetic measures in females. *Med Sci Sports Exerc*. 1996;28(9):1188-1192.

70. Malerba JL, Adam ML, Harris BA, Krebs DE. Reliability of dynamic and isometric testing of shoulder external and internal rotators. *J Orthop Sports Phys Ther*. 1993;18(4):543-552.

71. Kelly BT, Kadrmas WR, Speer KP. The manual muscle examination for rotator cuff strength: an electromyographic investigation. *Am J Sports Med*. 1996;24(5):581-588.

72. Wickham J, Pizzari T, Balster S, Ganderton C, Watson L. The variable roles of the upper and lower subscapularis during shoulder motion. *Clin Biomech*. 2014;29(8):885-891.

73. Reiman MP, Thorborg K, Hölmich P. Femoroacetabular impingement surgery is on the rise—but what is the next step? *J Orthop Sports Phys Ther*. 2016;46(6):406-408.

74. Altintas B, Bradley H, Logan C, Delvecchio B, Anderson N, Millett PJ. Rehabilitation following subscapularis tendon repair. *Int J Sports Phys Ther*. 2019;14(2):318-332.

75. Worsley P, Warner M, Mottram S, et al. Motor control retraining exercises for shoulder impingement: effects on function, muscle activation, and biomechanics in young adults *J Shoulder Elbow Surg*. 2013;22(4):e11-e19.

76. Roy JS, Moffet H, Hébert LJ, Lirette R. Effect of motor control and strengthening exercises on shoulder function in persons with impingement syndrome: A single-subject study design. *Man Ther*. 2009;14(2):180-188.

77. Schory A, Bidinger E, Wolf JM, Murray L. A systematic review of the exercises that produce optimal muscle ratios of the scapular stabilizers in normal shoulders. *Int J Sports Phys Ther*. 2016;11(3):321-336.

78. Sagano J, Magee D, Katayose M. The effect of glenohumeral rotation on scapular upward rotation in different positions of scapular-plane elevation. *J Sport Rehabil*. 2006;14:144-155.

79. Bagg SD, Forrest WJ. Electromyographic study of the scapular rotators during arm abduction in the scapular plane. *Am J Phys Med*. 1986;65(3):111-124.

80. Ryu RKN, McCormick J, Jobe FW, Moynes DR, Antonelli DJ. An electromyographic analysis of shoulder function in tennis players. *Am J Sports Med*. 1988;16:481-485.

81. Cyriax JH. *Textbook of Orthopaedic Medicine. Vol. 1. Diagnosis of Soft Tissue Lesions*. 8th ed. Bailliere Tindall; 1982.

82. Malliaropoulos N, Papalexandris S, Papalada A, Papacostas E. The role of stretching in rehabilitation of hamstring injuries: 80 athletes follow-up. *Med Sci Sports Exerc*. 2004;36(5):756-759.

83. Defrin R, Peleg S, Weingarden H, Heruti R, Urca G. Differential effect of supraspinal modulation on the nociceptive withdrawal reflex and pain sensation. *Clin Neurophysiol*. 2007;118(2):427-437.

84. Kottke FJ, Pauley DL, Ptak RA. The rationale for prolonged stretching for correction of shortening of connective tissue. *Arch Phys Med Rehabil*. 1966;47(6):345-352.

85. Bandy W, Irion J, Briggler M. The effect of time and frequency on static stretching on flexibility of the hamstring muscles. *Phys Ther*. 1997;77(10):1090-1096.

86. Page P. Current concepts in muscle stretching for exercise and rehabilitation. *Int J Sports Phys Ther*. 2012;7(1):109-119.

87. Rancour J, Holmes CF, Cipriani DJ. The effects of intermittent stretching following a 4-week static stretching protocol: a randomized trial. *J Strength Cond Res*. 2009;23(8):2217-2222.

88. Clabbers KM, Kelly JD, Bader D, et al. Effect of posterior capsule tightness on glenohumeral translation in the late-cocking phase of pitching. *J Sport Rehabil*. 2007;16(1):41-49.

89. Muraki T, Yamamoto N, Zhao KD, et al. Effect of posteroinferior capsule tightness on contact pressure and area beneath the coracoacromial arch during pitching motion. *Am J Sports Med*. 2010;38(3):600-607.

90. Ludewig PM, Cook TM. Translations of the humerus in persons with shoulder impingement symptoms. *J Orthop Sports Phys Ther*. 2002;32(6):248-259.

91. Maenhout A, Van Eessel V, Van Dyck L, Vanraes A, Cools A. Quantifying acromiohumeral distance in overhead athletes with glenohumeral internal rotation loss and the influence of a stretching program. *Am J Sports Med*. 2012;40(9):2105-2112.

92. McClure P, Balaicuis J, Heiland D, Broersma ME, Thorndike CK, Wood A. A randomized controlled comparison of stretching procedures for posterior shoulder tightness. *J Orthop Sports Phys Ther*. 2007;37(3):108-114.

93. Myers JB, Laudner KG, Pasquale MR, Bradley JP, Lephart SM. Glenohumeral range of motion deficits and posterior shoulder tightness in throwers with pathologic internal impingement. *Am J Sports Med*. 2006;34(3):385-391.

94. Wilk KE, Hooks TR, Macrina LC. The modified sleeper stretch and modified cross-body stretch to increase shoulder internal rotation range of motion in the overhead throwing athlete. *J Orthop Sports Phys Ther*. 2013;43(12):891-894.

95. Camargo PR, Neumann DA. Kinesiologic considerations for targeting activation of scapulothoracic muscles—part 2: trapezius. *Braz J Phys Ther*. 2019;23(6):467-475.

96. Moseley JB, Jr., Jobe FW, Pink M, Perry J, Tibone J. EMG analysis of the scapular muscles during a shoulder rehabilitation program. *Am J Sports Med*. 1992;20(2):128-134.

97. Lear LJ, Gross MT. An electromyographical analysis of the scapular stabilizing synergists during a push-up progression. *J Orthop Sports Phys Ther*. 1998;28:146-157.

98. Howard JD, Enoka RM. Maximum bilateral contractions are modified by neurally mediated interlimb effects. *J Appl Physiol*. 1991;70(1):306-316.

99. Schantz PG, Moritani T, Karlson E, et al. Maximal voluntary force of bilateral and unilateral leg extension. *Acta Physiol Scand*. 1989;136(1):185-192.

100. Kibler WB, Sciascia AD, Uhl TL, Tambay N, Cunningham T. Electromyographic analysis of specific exercises for scapular control in early phases of shoulder rehabilitation. *Am J Sports Med*. 2008;36(9):1789-1798.

101. Moeller CR, Huxel Bliven KC, Snyder Valier AR. Scapular muscle-activation ratios in patients with shoulder injuries during functional shoulder exercises. *J Athl Train*. 2014;49(3):345-355.

102. Sciascia A, Cromwell R. Kinetic chain rehabilitation: a theoretical framework. *Rehabil Res Pract*. 2012;2012:1-9. doi:10.1155/2012/853037

103. Burkhart S, Morgan C, Kibler W. The disabled throwing shoulder: spectrum of pathology Part III: The SICK scapula, scapular dyskinesis, the kinetic chain, and rehabilitation. *Arthroscopy*. 2003;19(6):641-661.

104. De Mey K, Danneels L, Cagnie B, et al. Shoulder muscle activation levels during four closed kinetic chain exercises with and without Redcord slings. *J Strength Cond Res*. 2014;28(6):1626-1635.

105. Dalton E. The wobbly wheel syndrome. *Massage Bodywork*. 2014;29(3):107-108.

106. Apreleva M, Parsons IM, Warner JJ, Fu FH, Woo SL. Experimental investigation of reaction forces at the glenohumeral joint during active abduction. *J Shoulder Elbow Surg*. 2000;9(5):409-417.

107. Escamilla RF, Yamashiro K, Paulos L, Andrews JR. Shoulder muscle activity and function in common shoulder rehabilitation exercises. *Sports Med*. 2009;39(8):663-685.

108. Curl LA, Warren RF. Glenohumeral joint stability: selective cutting studies on the static capsular restraints. *Clin Orthop Relat Res*. 1996;333:54-65.

109. Fung M, Kato S, Barrance PJ, et al. Scapular and clavicular kinematics during humeral elevation: a study with cadavers. *J Shoulder Elbow Surg*. 2001;10(3):278-285.

110. Lugo R, Kung P, Ma CB. Shoulder biomechanics. *Eur J Radiol*. 2008;68(1):16-24.

111. Perry J. The shoulder and elbow. In: Chapman MW, ed. *Operative Orthopaedics*. 2nd ed. J.P. Lippincott; 1993:1642-1649.

112. Perry J. Shoulder function for the activities of daily living. In: Matsen FA, Fu FH, Hawkins RJ, eds. *The Shoulder: A Balance of Mobility and Stability*. AAOS; 1993:185-191.

113. Reinold MM, Macrina LC, Wilk KE, et al. Electromyographic analysis of the supraspinatus and deltoid muscles during 3 common rehabilitation exercises. *J Athl Train*. 2007;42(4):464-469.

114. Thigpen CA, Padua DA, Morgan N, Kreps C, Karas SG. Scapular kinematics during supraspinatus rehabilitation exercise: a comparison of full-can versus empty-can techniques. *Am J Sports Med*. 2006;34(4):644-652.

115. Bradley JP, Tibone JE. Electromyographic analysis of muscle action about the shoulder. *Clin Sport Med*. 1991;10:789-805.

116. Decker MJ, Hintermeister RA, Faber KJ, Hawkins RJ. Serratus anterior muscle activity during selected rehabilitation exercises. *Am J Sports Med*. 1999;27(6):784-791.

117. Ekstrom RA, Bifulco KM, Lopau CJ, Andersen CF, Gough JR. Comparing the function of the upper and lower parts of the serratus anterior muscle using surface electromyography. *J Orthop Sports Phys Ther*. 2004;34(5):235-243.

118. Hardwick DH, Beebe JA, McDonnell MK, Lang CE. A comparison of serratus anterior muscle activation during a wall slide exercise and other traditional exercises. *J Orthop Sports Phys Ther*. 2006;36(12):903-910.

119. Hintermeister RA, Lange GW, Schultheis JM, Bey MJ, Hawkins RJ. Electromyographic activity and applied load during shoulder rehabilitation exercises using elastic resistance. *Am J Sports Med*. 1998;26(2):210-220.

120. Kuechle DK, Newman SR, Itoi E, Niebur GL, Morrey BF, An KN. The relevance of the moment arm of shoulder muscles with respect to axial rotation of the glenohumeral joint in four positions. *Clin Biomech* 2000;15(5):322-329.

121. McCabe R, Orishimo K, McHugh M, Nicholas S. Surface electromyographic analysis of the lower trapezius muscle during exercises performed below ninety degrees of shoulder elevation in healthy subjects. *N Am J Sports Phys Ther*. 2007;2(1):34-43.

122. Reinold MM, Wilk KE, Fleisig GS, et al. Electromyographic analysis of the rotator cuff and deltoid musculature during common shoulder external rotation exercises. *J Orthop Sports Phys Ther*. 2004;34(7):385-394.

123. Townsend H, Jobe FW, Pink M, Perry J. Electromyographic analysis of the glenohumeral muscles during a baseball rehabilitation program. *Am J Sports Med*. 1991;19(3):264-271.

124. Uhl TL, Carver TJ, Mattacola CG, Mair SD, Nitz AJ. Shoulder musculature activation during upper extremity weight-bearing exercise. *J Orthop Sports Phys Ther*. 2003;33(3):109-117.

125. Andersen CH, Zebis MK, Saervoll C, et al. Scapular muscle activity from selected strengthening exercises performed at low and high intensities. *J Strength Cond Res*. 2012;26(9):2408-2416.

126. Cools AM, Declercq GA, Cambier DC, Mahieu NN, Witvrouw EE. Trapezius activity and intramuscular balance during isokinetic exercise in overhead athletes with impingement symptoms. *Scand J Med Sci Sports*. 2007;17(1):25-33.

127. Decker MJ, Tokish JM, Ellis HB, Torry MR, Hawkins RJ. Subscapularis muscle activity during selected rehabilitation exercises. *Am J Sports Med*. 2003;31(1):126-134.

128. De Mey K, Cagnie B, Van de Vekle A, Danneels LA, Coots AM. Trapezius muscle timing during selected shoulder rehabilitation exercises. *J Orthop Sports Phys Ther*. 2009;39(10):743-752.

129. Ekstrom RA, Donatelli RA, Soderberg GL. Surface electromyographic analysis of exercises for the trapezius and serratus anterior muscles. *J Orthop Sports Phys Ther*. 2003;33(5):247-258.

130. Kinney E, Wusthoff J, Zyck A, et al. Activation of the trapezius muscle during varied forms of Kendall exercises. *Phys Ther Sport*. 2008;9(1):3-8.

131. Ludewig PM, Hoff MS, Osowski EE, Meschke SA, Rundquist PJ. Relative balance of serratus anterior and upper trapezius muscle activity during push-up exercises. *Am J Sports Med*. 2004;32(2):484-493.

132. Kibler WB, Sciascia A. Current concepts: scapular dyskinesis. *Br J Sports Med*. 2010;44(5):300-305.

133. Karas V, Wang VM, Dhawan A, Cole BJ. Biomechanical factors in rotator cuff pathology. *Sports Med Arthrosc.* 2011;19(3):202-206.

134. Bruhn S, Kullmann N, Gollhofer A. Combinatory effects of high-intensity-strength training and sensorimotor training on muscle strength. *Int J Sports Med.* 2006;27(5):401-406.

135. Crow J, Pizzari T, Buttifant D. Muscle onset can be improved by therapeutic exercise: a systematic review. *Phys Ther Sport.* 2011;12(4):199-209.

136. Hoppeler H, Baum O, Lurman G, Mueller M. Molecular mechanisms of muscle plasticity with exercise. *Compr Physiol.* 2011;1(3):1383-1412.

137. Zhang P, Chen X, Fan M. Signaling mechanisms involved in disuse muscle atrophy. *Med Hypotheses.* 2007;69(2):310-321.

138. Lephart SM, Henry TJ. The physiological basis for open and closed kinetic chain rehabilitation for the upper extremity. *J Sport Rehabil.* 1996;5:71-87.

139. Kibler WB, McMullen J, Uhl T. Shoulder rehabilitation strategies, guidelines, and practice. *Op Tech Sports Med.* 2012;20(1):103-112.

140. Kara D, Harput G, Duzgun I. Trapezius muscle activation levels and ratios during scapular retraction exercises: A comparative study between patients with subacromial impingement syndrome and healthy controls. *Clin Biomech (Bristol, Avon).* 2019;67:119-126.

141. Wickham J, Pizzari T, Stansfeld K, Burnside A, Watson A. Quantifying "normal" shoulder muscle activity during abduction. *J Electromyogr Kinesiol.* 2010;20(2):212-222.

142. Escamilla RF, Yamashiro K, Dunning R, et al. An electromyographic analysis of the shoulder complex musculature while performing exercises using the bodyblade classic and bodyblade pro. *Int J Sports Phys Ther.* 2016;11(2):175-189.

143. Jerosch J, Wüstner P. Effect of a sensorimotor training program on patients with subacromial pain syndrome. *Unfallchirurg.* 2002;105(1):36-43.

144. Surburg PR, Schrader JW. Proprioceptive neuromuscular facilitation techniques in sports medicine: a reassessment. *J Athl Train.* 1997;32(1):34-39.

145. Knott M, Voss DE. *Proprioceptive Neuromuscular Facilitation. Patterns and Techniques.* 2nd ed. Harper & Row; 1968.

146. Wang H, Huo M, Huang Q, Li D, Maruyama H. The immediate effect of neuromuscular joint facilitation (NJF) treatment on hip muscle strength. *J Phys Ther Sci.* 2013;25(11):1455-1457.

147. Wu P, Huo M, Maruyama H. Effects of neuromuscular joint facilitation on baseball pitching velocity and electromechanical reaction times of the teres major of young amateur baseball players. *J Phys Ther Sci* 2013;25(11):1459-1461.

148. Buckthorpe M, Della Villa F, Della Villa S, Roi GS. On-field rehabilitation part 2: a 5-stage program for the soccer player focused on linear movements, multidirectional movements, soccer-specific skills, soccer-specific movements, and modified practice. *J Orthop Sports Phys Ther.* 2019;49(8):570-575.

149. Brindle TJ, Nitz AJ, Uhl TL, Kifer E, Shapiro R. Kinematic and EMG characteristics of simple shoulder movements with proprioception and visual feedback. *J Electromyogr Kinesiol.* 2006;16(3):236-249.

150. Hegedus EJ, Goode AP, Cook CE, et al. Which physical examination tests provide clinicians with the most value when examining the shoulder? Update of a systematic review with meta-analysis of individual tests. *Br J Sports Med.* 2012;46(14):964-978.

151. Lo IK, Nonweiler B, Woolfrey M, Litchfield R, Kirkley A. An evaluation of the apprehension, relocation, and surprise tests for anterior shoulder instability. *Am J Sports Med.* 2004;32(2):301-307.

152. Tzannes A, Murrell GAC. Clinical examination of the unstable shoulder. *Sports Med.* 2002;32:447-457.

153. Guanche CA, Jones DC. Clinical testing for tears of the glenoid labrum. *Arthroscopy.* 2003;19(5):517-523.

154. Kim SH, Park JC, Park JS, Oh S. Painful jerk test: a predictor of success in nonoperative treatment of posteroinferior instability of the shoulder. *Am J Sports Med.* 2004;32(8):1849-1855.

155. Çalış M, Akgün K, Birtane M, Karacan I, Çalış H, Tüzün F. Diagnostic values of clinical diagnostic tests in subacromial impingement syndrome. *Ann Rheum Dis.* 2000;59(1):44-47.

156. MacDonald PB, Clark P, Sutherland K. An analysis of the diagnostic accuracy of the Hawkins and Neer subacromial impingement signs. *J Shoulder Elbow Surg.* 2000;9(4):299-301.

157. Park HB, Yokota A, Gill HS, Rassier DE, McFarland EG. Diagnostic accuracy of clinical tests for the different degrees of subacromial impingement syndrome. *J Bone Joint Surg Am.* 2005;87(7):1446-1455.

158. Chen HS, Lin SH, Hsu YH, Chen SC, Kang JH. A comparison of physical examinations with musculoskeletal ultrasound in the diagnosis of biceps long head tendinitis. *Ultrasound Med Biol.* 2011;37(9):1392-1398.

159. Kibler WB, Sciascia AD, Hester P, Dome D, Jacobs C. Clinical utility of traditional and new tests in the diagnosis of biceps tendon injuries and superior labrum anterior and posterior lesions in the shoulder. *Am J Sports Med.* 2009;37(9):1840-1847.

160. O'Brien SJ, Pagnani MJ, Fealy S, McGlynn SR, Wilson JB. The active compression test: a new and effective test for diagnosing labral tears and acromioclavicular joint abnormality. *Am J Sports Med.* 1998;26(5):610-613.

161. Stetson WB, Templin K. The crank test, the O'Brien test, and routine magnetic resonance imaging scans in the diagnosis of labral tears. *Am J Sports Med.* 2002;30(6):806-809.

162. Liu SH, Henry MH, Nuccioin S, Shapiro MS, Dorey F. Diagnosis of glenoid labrum tears: a comparison between magnetic resonance imaging and clinical examinations. *Am J Sports Med.* 1996;24(2):149-154.

163. Mimori K, Muneta T, Nakagawa TH, Shinomiya K. A new pain provocation test for superior labral tears of the shoulder. *Am J Sports Med.* 1999;27(2):137-142.

164. Kim SH, Ha KI, Han KY. Biceps load test: a clinical test for superior labrum anterior and posterior lesions in shoulders with recurrent anterior dislocations. *Am J Sports Med.* 1999;27(3):300-303.

165. Kim SH, Ha KI, Ahn JH, Kim SH, Choi HJ. Biceps load test II: A clinical test for SLAP lesions of the shoulder. *Arthroscopy.* 2001;17(2):160-164.

166. Kibler WB. Specificity and sensitivity of the anterior slide test in throwing athletes with superior glenoid labral tears. *Arthroscopy*. 1995;11(3):296-300.

167. Jain NB, Luz J, Higgins LD, et al. The diagnostic accuracy of special tests for rotator cuff tear: the ROW cohort study. *Am J Phys Med Rehabil*. 2017;96(3):176-183.

168. Barth JR, Burkhart SS, De Beer JF. The bear-hug test: a new and sensitive test for diagnosing a subscapularis tear. *Arthroscopy*. 2006;22(10):1076-1084.

169. Morgan CD. The thrower's shoulder. Two perspectives. In: McGinty JB, ed. *Operative Arthroscopy*. Lippincott Williams & Wilkins; 2003:570-584.

170. Cools AM, Struyf F, DeMey K, Maenhout A, Castelein B, Cagnie B. Rehabilitation of scapular dyskinesis: from the office worker to the elite overhead athlete. *Br J Sports Med*. 2014;48(8):692-697.

171. McClure P, Tate AR, Kareha S, Irwin D, Zlupko E. A clinical method for identifying scapular dyskinesis, part 1: reliability. *J Athl Train*. 2009;44(2):160-164.

172. Kibler WB, Sciascia A, Wilkes T. Scapular dyskinesis and its relation to shoulder injury. *J Am Acad Orthop Surg*. 2012;20(6):364-372.

173. Kibler WB, Ludewig PM, McClure PW, Michener LA, Bak K, Sciascia AD. Clinical implications of scapular dyskinesis in shoulder injury: the 2013 consensus from the "scapular summit". *Br J Sports Med*. 2013;47(14):877-885.

174. Kibler WB. Scapular dysfunction. *Athl Ther Today*. 2006;11(5):6-9, 36-37, 72.

175. Illyés A, Kiss RM. Kinematic and muscle activity characteristics of multidirectional shoulder joint instability during elevation. *Knee Surg Sports Traumatol Arthrosc*. 2006;14(7):673-685.

176. von Eisenhart-Rothe R, Matsen FA, 3rd., Eckstein F, Vogl T, Graichen H. Pathomechanics in atraumatic shoulder instability: scapular positioning correlates with humeral head centering. *Clin Orthop Relat Res*. 2005;(433):82-89.

177. Warner JJ, Micheli LJ, Arslanian LE, Kennedy J, Kennedy R. Scapulothoracic motion in normal shoulders and shoulders with glenohumeral instability and impingement syndrome: a study using Moiré topographic analysis. *Clin Orthop Relat Res*. 1992;(285):191-199.

178. Struyf F, Nijs J, Baeyens JP, Mottram S, Meeusen R. Scapular positioning and movement in unimpaired shoulders, shoulder impingement syndrome, and glenohumeral instability. *Scand J Med Sci Sports*. 2011;21(3):352-358.

179. Mell AG, LaScalza S, Guffey P, et al. Effect of rotator cuff pathology on shoulder rhythm. *J Shoulder Elbow Surg*. 2005;14:58S-64S.

180. Lin JJ, Hanten WP, Olson SL, et al. Functional activity characteristics of individuals with shoulder dysfunctions. *J Electromyogr Kinesiol*. 2005;15(6):576-586.

181. Speigl UJ, Warth RJ, Millett PJ. Symptomatic internal impingement of the shoulder in overhead athletes. *Sports Med Arthrosc Rev*. 2014;22(2):120-129.

182. Heyworth BE, Williams RJ. Internal impingement of the shoulder. *Am J Sports Med*. 2009;37(5):1024-1037.

183. Seitz AL, McClure PW, Lynch SS, Ketchum JM, Michener LA. Effects of scapular dyskinesis and scapular assistance test on subacromial space during static arm elevation. *J Shoulder Elbow Surg*. 2012;21(5):631-640.

184. Panagiotopoulos AC, Crowther IM. Scapular dyskinesia, the forgotten culprit of shoulder pain and how to rehabilitate. *SICOT J*. 2019;5:29. doi:10.1051/sicotj/2019029

185. Forthomme B, Crielaard JM, Croisier JL. Scapular positioning in athlete's shoulder: particularities, clinical measurements and implications. *Sports Med*. 2008;38(5):369-386.

186. Williams GR, Kelley M. Management of rotator cuff and impingement injuries in the athlete. *J Athl Train*. 2000;35(3):300-215.

187. Merolla G, DeSantis E, Campi F, Paladini P, Porcellini G. Supraspinatus and infraspinatus weakness in overhead athletes with scapular dyskinesis: strength assessment before and after restoration of scapular musculature balance. *Musculoskelet Surg*. 2010;94(3):119-125.

188. McMullen J, Uhl TL. A kinetic chain approach for shoulder rehabilitation. *J Athl Train*. 2000;35(3):329-337.

189. Lewis JS, Wright C, Green A. Subacromial impingement syndrome: the effect of changing posture on shoulder range of movement. *J Orthop Sports Phys Ther*. 2005;35(2):72-87.

190. Kibler W, McMullen J. Scapular dyskinesis and its relation to shoulder pain. *J Am Acad Orthop Surg*. 2003;11(2):142-151.

191. Bron C, Dommerholt J, Stegenga B, Wensing M, Oostendorp RA. High prevalence of shoulder girdle muscles with myofascial trigger points in patients with shoulder pain. *BMC Musculoskelet Disord*. Jun 28 2011;12:139. doi:10.1186/1471-2474-12-139

192. Ludewig PM, Cook TM. Alterations in shoulder kinematics and associated muscle activity in people with symptoms of shoulder impingement. *Phys Ther*. 2000;80(3):276-291.

193. DeMey K, Danneels LA, Cagnie B, Huyghe L, Seyns E, Cools AM. Conscious correction of scapular orientation in overhead athletes performing selected shoulder rehabilitation exercises: the effect on trapezius muscle activation measured by surface electromyography. *J Orthop Sports Phys Ther*. 2013;43(1):3-10.

194. McClure P, Greenberg E, Kareha S. Evaluation and management of scapular dysfunction. *Sports Med Arthrosc*. 2012;20(1):39-48.

195. Neumann DA, Camargo PR. Kinesiologic considerations for targeting activation of scapulothoracic muscles—part 1: serratus anterior. *Braz J Phys Ther*. 2019;23(6):459-466.

196. Rabin E, Gordon AM. Influence of fingertip contact on illusory arm movements. *J Appl Biomech*. 2004;96(4):1555-1560.

197. Edouard P, Damotte A, Lance G, Degache F, Calmels P. Static and dynamic shoulder stabilizer adaptations in javelin throwers: a preliminary report. *Isokinet Exerc Sci*. 2013;21(1):47-55.

198. Wuelker N, Korell M, Thren K. Dynamic glenohumeral joint stability. *J Shoulder Elbow Surg*. 1998;7(1):43-52.

199. Soslowsky LJ, Malicky DM, Blasier RB. Active and passive factors in inferior glenohumeral stabilization: a biomechanical model. *J Shoulder Elbow Surg*. 1997;6(4):371-379.

200. McCarty E, Ritchie P, Gill H, McFarland E. Shoulder instability: return to play. *Clin Sports Med*. 2004;23(3):335-351.

201. Gaskill TR, Taylor DC, Millett PJ. Management of multi-directional instability of the shoulder. *J Am Acad Orthop Surg*. 2011;19(12):758-767.

202. Patton WC, McCluskey GM, 3rd. Biceps tendinitis and subluxation. *Clin Sports Med*. 2001;20(3):505-529.

203. Jackins S. Postoperative shoulder rehabilitation *Phys Med Rehabil Clin N Am.* 2004;15(3):643-682.

204. Winge S, Thomsen NO, Jensen CH, Klareskov B. Shoulder instability. *Ugeskr Läger.* 1998;160(25):3707-3713.

205. Burkhead WZ, Jr., Rockwood CA, Jr. Treatment of instability of the shoulder with an exercise program. *J Bone Joint Surg Am.* 1992;74(6):890-896.

206. Bahu MJ, Trentacosta N, Vorys GC, Covey AS, Ahmad CS. Multidirectional instability: evaluation and treatment options. *Clin Sports Med.* 2008;27(4):671-689.

207. Beasley L, Faryniarz DA, Hannafin JA. Multidirectional instability of the shoulder in the female athlete. *Clin Sports Med.* 2000;19(2):331-349.

208. Wang VM, Sugalski MT, Levine WN, Pawluk RJ, Mow VC, Bigliani LU. Comparison of glenohumeral mechanics following a capsular shift and anterior tightening. *J Bone Joint Surg Am.* 2005;87(6):1312-1322.

209. Miniaci A, Codsi MJ. Thermal capsulorrhaphy for the treatment of shoulder instability. *Am J Sports Med.* 2006;34(8):1356-1363.

210. Mohtadi NG, Kirkley A, Hollinshead RM, et al. Electrothermal arthroscopic capsulorrhaphy: old technology, new evidence. A multicenter randomized clinical trial. *J Shoulder Elbow Surg.* 2014;23(8):1171-1180.

211. Hawkins RJ, Krishnan SG, Karas SG, Noonan TJ, Horan MP. Electrothermal arthroscopic shoulder capsulorrhaphy: a minimum 2-year follow-up. *Am J Sports Med.* 2007;35(9):1484-1488.

212. Itoi E, Hatakeyama Y, Sato T, et al. Immobilization in external rotation after shoulder dislocation reduces the risk of recurrence: a randomized controlled trial. *J Bone Joint Surg Am.* 2007;89(10):2124-2131.

213. Podraza JT, White SC. Posterior glenohumeral thermal capsulorraphy, capsular imbrication and labral repair with complication of adhesive capsulitis: a modified rehabilitation approach. *J Sport Rehabil.* 2012;21(1):69-78.

214. Owens BD, Dickens JF, Kilcoyne KG, Rue JP. Management of mid-season traumatic anterior shoulder instability in athletes. *J Am Acad Orthop Surg.* 2012;20(8):518-526.

215. Wilk KE, Macrina LC, Reinold MM. Non-operative rehabilitation for traumatic and atraumatic glenohumeral instability. *North Am J Sports Phys Ther.* 2006;1(1):16-31.

216. Bhatia DN. Dual-window subscapularis-sparing approach: a new surgical technique for combined reconstruction of a glenoid bone defect or bankart lesion associated with a HAGL lesion in anterior shoulder instability. *Tech Hand Up Extrem Surg.* 2012;16(1):30-36.

217. Andrews JR, Broussard TS, Carson WG. Arthroscopy of the shoulder in the management of partial tears of the rotator cuff: a preliminary report. *Arthroscopy.* 1985;1(2):117-122.

218. Burkhart S, Morgan C, Kibler W. The disabled throwing shoulder: spectrum of pathology. Part II: evaluation and treatment of SLAP lesions in throwers. *Arthroscopy.* 2003;19(5):531-539.

219. Dietz A, Dreese JC. Anterior shoulder instability in the overhead athlete: current concepts. *Curr Opin Orthop.* 2007;18(2):172-176.

220. Paxton ES, Backus J, Keener J, Brophy RH. Shoulder arthroscopy: basic principles of positioning, anesthesia, and portal anatomy. *J Am Acad Orthop Surg.* 2013;21(6):332-342.

221. Sedeek SM, Tey IK, Tan AH. Arthroscopic Bankart repair for traumatic anterior shoulder instability with the use of suture anchors. *Singapore Med J.* 2008;49(9):676-681.

222. Archetti Netto N, Tamaoki MJ, Lenza M, et al. Treatment of Bankart lesions in traumatic anterior instability of the shoulder: a randomized controlled trial comparing arthroscopy and open techniques. *Arthroscopy.* 2012;28(7):900-908.

223. Kim SH, Ha KI, Kim YM. Arthroscopic revision Bankart repair: a prospective outcome study. *Arthroscopy.* 2002;18(5):469-482.

224. Gao B, DeFroda S, Bokshan S, et al. Arthroscopic versus open Bankart repairs in recurrent anterior shoulder instability: a systematic review of the association between publication date and postoperative recurrent instability in systematic reviews. *Arthroscopy.* 2020;36(3):862-871.

225. Beletsky A, Cancienne JM, Manderle BJ, Mehta N, Wilk KE, Verma NN. A comparison of physical therapy protocols between open Latarjet coracoid transfer and arthroscopic Bankart repair. *Sports Health.* 2020;12(2):124-131.

226. Lafosse L, Lejeune E, Bouchard A, Kakuda C, Gobezie R, Kochhar T. The arthroscopic Latarjet procedure for the treatment of anterior shoulder instability. *Arthroscopy.* 2007;23(11):1242.e1-5. doi:10.1016/j.arthro.2007.06.008

227. McHale KJ, Sanchez G, Lavery KP, et al. Latarjet technique for treatment of anterior shoulder instability with glenoid bone loss. *Arthrosc Tech.* 2017;6(3):e791-e799.

228. DeFroda SF, Mehta N, Owens BD. Physical therapy protocols for arthroscopic Bankart repair. *Sports Health.* 2018;10(3):250-258.

229. Eren I, Canbulat N, Atalar AC, et al. A clinical comparison of home-based and hospital-based exercise programs following arthroscopic capsulolabral repair for anterior shoulder instability. *J Sport Rehabil.* 2020;29(6):777-782.

230. Kim SH, Ha KI, Jung MW, Lim MS, Kim YM, Park JH. Accelerated rehabilitation after arthroscopic Bankart repair for selected cases: a prospective randomized clinical study. *Arthroscopy.* 2003;19(7):722-731.

231. Maitland GD. *Peripheral Manipulation.* Butterworth-Heinemann; 1991.

232. Travell JG, Simons DG. *Myofascial Pain and Dysfunction: The Trigger Point Manual. Vol. 1.* Williams and Wilkins; 1983.

233. Liu YL, Ao YF, Cui GQ, Zhu JX. Changes of histology and capsular collagen in a rat shoulder immoblization model. *Chin Med J (Engl).* 2011;124(23):3939-3944.

234. van der Meijden OA, Westgard P, Chandler Z, Gaskill TR, Kokmeyer D. Rehabilitation after arthroscopic rotator cuff repair: current concepts review and evidence-based guidelines. *Int J Sports Phys Ther.* 2012;7(2):197-218.

235. Ma R, Brimmo OA, Li X, Colbert L. Current concepts in rehabilitation for traumatic anterior shoulder instability. *Curr Rev Musculoskelet Med.* 2017;10(4):499-506.

236. Petera M, Veillette CJ, Taylor DW, Park SS, Theodoropoulos JS. Use of fresh osteochondral glenoid allograft to treat posteroinferior bone loss in chronic posterior shoulder instability. *Am J Orthop* 2013;42(2):78-82.

237. Norwood LA, Terry GC. Shoulder posterior subluxation. *Am J Sports Med.* 1984;12(1):25-30.

238. Bey MJ, Brock SK, Beierwaltes WN, Zauel R, Kolowich PA, Lock TR. In vivo measurement of subacromial space

width during shoulder elevation: technique and preliminary results in patients following unilateral rotator cuff repair. *Clin Biomech (Bristol, Avon)*. 2007;22(7):767-773.

239. Khan Y, Nagy MT, Malal J, Waseem M. The painful shoulder: shoulder impingement syndrome. *Open Orthop J*. 2013;7:347-351. doi:10.2174/1874325001307010347

240. Singh A, Calafi A, Diefenbach C, Kreulen C, Giza E. Noninsertional tendinopathy of the Achilles. *Foot Ankle Clin*. 2017;22(4):745-760.

241. Escamilla RF, Hooks TR, Wilk KE. Optimal management of shoulder impingement syndrome. *Open Access J Sports Med*. 28 Feb 2014;5:13-24.

242. Bigliani LU, Ticker JB, Flatow EL, Soslowsky LJ, Mow VC. The relationship of acromial achitecture to rotator cuff disease. *Clin Sports Med*. 1991;10(4):823-838.

243. Oh JH, Kim JY, Lee HK, Choi JA. Classification and clinical significance of acromial spur in rotator cuff tear: heel-type spur and rotator cuff tear. *Clin Orthop Relat Res*. 2010;468(6):1542-1550.

244. Balke M, Schmidt C, Dedy N, Banerjee M, Bouillon B, Liem D. Correlation of acromial morphology with impingement syndrome and rotator cuff tears. *Acta Orthop*. 2013;84(2):178-183.

245. Michener LA, McClure PW, Karduna AR. Anatomical and biomechanical mechanisms of subacromial impingement syndrome. *Clin Biomech*. 2003;18(5):369-379.

246. Skolimowski J, Barczyk K, Dudek K, Skolimowska B, Demczuk-Włodarczyk E, Anwajler J. Posture in people with shoulder impingement syndrome. *Ortop Traumatol Rehabil*. 2007;9(5):484-498.

247. Jobe FW, Moynes DR, Tibone JE, Perry J. An EMG analysis of the shoulder in pitching: a second report. *Am J Sports Med*. 1984;12(3):218-220.

248. Slaven EJ, Mathers J. Differential diagnosis of shoulder and cervical pain: a case report. *J Man Manip Ther*. 2010;18(4):191-196.

249. Weldon EJ, 3rd., Richardson AB. Upper extremity overuse injuries in swimming: a discussion of swimmer's shoulder. *Clin Sports Med*. 2001;20(3):423-438.

250. Borich MR, Bright JM, Lorello DJ, Cieminski CJ, Buisman T, Ludewig PM. Scapular angular positioning at end range internal rotation in cases of glenohumeral internal rotation deficit. *J Orthop Sports Phys Ther*. December 2006;36(12):926-934.

251. Kamkar A, Irrgang JJ, Whitney SL. Nonoperative management of secondary shoulder impingement syndrome. *J Orthop Sports Phys Ther*. 1993;17:212-224.

252. Lewis JS, Green A, Wright C. Subacromial impingement syndrome: the role of posture and muscle imbalance. *J Shoulder Elbow Surg*. 2005;14(4):385-392.

253. Ebaugh DD, Karduna AR, McClure PW. Scapulothoracic and glenohumeral kinematics following an external rotation fatigue protocol. *J Orthop Sports Phys Ther*. 2006;36(8):557-571.

254. Kuechle DK, Newman SR, Itoi E, Morrey BF, An KN. Shoulder muscle moment arms during horizontal flexion and elevation. *J Shoulder Elbow Surg*. 1997;6(5):429-439.

255. Sahrmann SA. *Diagnosis and Treatment of Movement Impairment Syndromes*. Mosby; 2002.

256. Modi CS, Smith CD, Drew SJ. Partial-thickness articular surface rotator cuff tears in patients over the age of 35: Etiology and intra-articular associations. *Int J Shoulder Surg*. 2012;6(1):15-18.

257. Rees JD, Wilson AM, Wolman RL. Current concepts in the management of tendon disorders. *Rheumatol*. 2006;45(5):508-521.

258. Neviaser A, Andarawis-Puri N, Flatow E. Basic mechanisms of tendon fatigue damage. *J Shoulder Elbow Surg*. 2012;21(2):158-163.

259. Garving C, Jakob S, Bauer I, Nadjar R, Brunner UH. Impingement syndrome of the shoulder. *Dtsch Arztebl Int*. 2017;114(45):765-776.

260. Klintberg IH, Svantesson G, Karlsson J. Long-term patient satisfaction and functional outcome 8-11 years after subacromial decompression. *Knee Surg Sports Traumatol Arthrosc*. 2010;18(3):394-103.

261. Hotta GH, Santos AL, McQuade KJ, de Oliveira AS. Scapular-focused exercise treatment protocol for shoulder impingement symptoms: Three-dimensional scapular kinematics analysis. *Clin Biomech*. 2018;51(1):76-81.

262. Weiss JM, Arkader A, Wells LM, Ganley TJ. Rotator cuff injuries in adolescent athletes. *J Pediatr Orthop*. 2013;22(2):133-137.

263. Kirchhoff C, Imhoff AB. Posterosuperior and anterosuperior impingement of the shoulder in overhead athletes—evolving concepts. *Int Orthop*. 2010;34(7):1049-1058.

264. Ghodadra NS, Provencher MT, Verma NN, Wilk KE, Romeo AA. Open, mini-open, and all-arthroscopic rotator cuff repair surgery: indications and implications for rehabilitation. *J Orthop Sports Phys Ther*. 2009;39(2):81-89.

265. Liem D, Lichtenberg S, Magosch P, Habermeyer P. Arthroscopic rotator cuff repair in overhead throwing athletes. *Am J Sports Med*. 2008;36(7):1317-1322.

266. Neviaser AS, Charen DA, Cotter JM, Harrison AK, Cagle PJ, Flatow EL. Retrospective review of open and arthroscopic repair of anterosuperior rotator cuff tears with subscapularis involvement: a single surgeon's experience. *J Shoulder Elbow Surg*. 2020;29(5):893-897.

267. Karakoc Y, Atalay IB. Comparison of mini-open versus all-arthroscopic rotator cuff repair: retrospective analysis of a single center. *Pan Afr Med J*. 2020;37:132. doi:10.11604/pamj.2020.37.132.19491

268. Mulligan EP, Devanna RR, Huang M, Middleton EF, Khazzam M. Factors that impact rehabilitation strategies after rotator cuff repair. *Phys Sportsmed*. 2012;40(4):102-114.

269. Pill SG, Walch G, Hawkins RJ, Kissenberth MJ. The role of the biceps tendon in massive rotator cuff tears. *Instr Course Lect*. 2012;61:113-120.

270. Millett PJ, Wilcox RB, 3rd., O'Holleran JD, Warner JJ. Rehabilitation of the rotator cuff: an evaluation-based approach. *J Am Acad Orthop Surg*. 2006;14(11):599-609.

271. Wilk KE, Macrina LC, Yenchak AJ, Cain EL, Andrews JR. Surgical repair and rehabilitation of a combined 330° capsulolabral lesion and partial-thickness rotator cuff tear in a professional quarterback: a case report. *J Orthop Sports Phys Ther*. 2013;43(3):142-153.

272. Ellenbecker TS, Cools A. Rehabilitation of shoulder impingement syndrome and rotator cuff injuries: an evidence-based review. *Br J Sports Med*. 2010;44(5):319-327.

273. Yi A, Villacis D, Yalamanchili R, Hatch GF, 3rd. A comparison of rehabilitation methods after arthroscopic rotator cuff repair: A systematic review. *Sports Health*. 2015;7(4):326-334.

274. Kim YS, Sung CH, Chung SH, Kwak SJ, Koh YG. Does an injection of adipose-derived mesenchymal stem cells loaded in fibrin glue influence rotator cuff repair outcomes? A clinical and magnetic resonance imaging study. *Am J Sports Med*. 2017;45(9):2010-2018.

275. Dhillon MS, Behera P, Patel S, Shetty V. Orthobiologics and platelet rich plasma. *Indian J Orthop*. 2014;48(1):1-9.

276. Samsonraj RM, Raghunath M, Nurcombe V, Hui JH, van Wijnen AJ, Cool SM. Concise review: multifaceted characterization of human mesenchymal stem cells for use in regenerative medicine. *Stem Cells*. 2017;6(12):2173-2185.

277. Murray IR, Péault P. Q&A: Mesenchymal stem cells—where do they come from and is it important? *BMC Biol*. 2015;13:99. doi:10.1186/s12915-015-0212-7

278. Jo CH, Chai JW, Jeong EC, et al. Intratendinous injection of autologous adipose tissue-derived mesenchymal stem cells for the treatment of rotator cuff disease: a first-in-human trial. *Stem Cells*. 2018;36(9):1441-1450.

279. Jo CH, Chai JW, Jeong EC, Oh S, Yoon KS. Intratendinous injection of mesenchymal stem cells for the treatment of rotator cuff disease: a 2-year follow-up study. *Arthroscopy*. 2020;36(4):971-980.

280. Trebinjac S, Gharairi M. Mesenchymal stem cells for treatment of tendon and ligament injuries—clinical evidence. *Med Arch*. 2020;74(5):387-390.

281. Vinet-Jones H, Darr KF. Clinical use of autologous microfragmented fat progressively restores pain and function in shoulder osteoarthritis. *Regen Med*. 2020;15(10):2153-2161.

282. Freitag J, Wickham J, Shah K, Tenen A. Effect of autologous adipose-derived mesenchymal stem cell therapy in the treatment of acromioclavicular joint osteoarthritis. *BMJ Case Rep*. 2019;12(2):e227865. doi:10.1136/bcr-2018-227865 PMC6398814,

283. Kwon DR, Park GY. Adult mesenchymal stem cells for the treatment in patients with rotator cuff disease: present and future direction. *Ann Transl Med*. 2018;6(22):432. doi:10.21037/atm.2018.09.06

284. Weber SC. Editorial commentary: stem cells in rotator cuff surgery: in search of the holy grail. *Arthroscopy*. 2020;36(4):981-982.

285. Sauers EL. Effectiveness of rehabilitation for patients with subacromial impingement syndrome. *J Athl Train*. 2005;40(3):221-223.

286. McCormack MA, Jr., Lindenfeld TN, Barber-Westin SD. Comparing two devices to regain full range of motion following arthroscopic subacromial decompression for shoulder impingement. *Athl Train Sports Health Care*. 2012;4(1):21-28.

287. Ouellette H, Labis J, Bredella M, Palmer WE, Sheah K, Torriani M. Spectrum of shoulder injuries in the baseball pitcher. *Skeletal Radiol*. 2008;37(6):491-498.

288. Escobedo EM, Richardson ML, Schulz YB, Hunter JC, Green JR, 3rd., Messick KJ. Increased risk of posterior glenoid labrum tears in football players. *AJR Am J Roentgenol*. 2007;188(1):193-197.

289. Chan RH, Lam JJ. Glenoid labrum lesion in an elite tennis player: a clinical challenge in diagnosis. *J Sport Rehabil*. 2006;15(2):168-177.

290. Funk L, Snow M. SLAP tears of the glenoid labrum in contact athletes. *Clin J Sport Med*. 2007;17(1):1-4.

291. Knesek M, Skendzel JG, Dines JS, Altchek DW, Allen AA, Bedi A. Diagnosis and management of superior labral anterior posterior tears in throwing athletes. *Am J Sports Med*. 2013;41(2):444-460.

292. Wilk KE, Reinold MM, Dugas JR, Arrigo CA, Andrews JR. Current concepts in the recognition and treatment of superior labral (SLAP) lesions. *J Orthop Sports Phys Ther*. 2005;35(5):273-291.

293. Snyder SJ, Karzel RP, Del Pizzo W, Ferkel RD, Friedman MJ. SLAP lesions of the shoulder. *Arthroscopy*. 1990;6(4):274-279.

294. Snyder SJ, Karzel RP, Pizzo WD, Ferkel RD, Friedman MJ. Arthroscopy classics. SLAP lesions of the shoulder. *Arthroscopy*. 2010;26(8):1117.

295. Kuhn JE, Lindholm SR, Huston LJ, Soslowsky LJ, Blasier RB. Failure of the biceps superior labral complex: A cadaveric biomechanical investigation comparing the late cocking and early deceleration positions of throwing. *J Arthroscop Rel Surg*. 2003;19(4):373-379.

296. Andrews JR, Carson WGJ, McLeod WD. Glenoid labrum tears related to the long head of the biceps. *Am J Sports Med*. 1985;13(5):337-341.

297. Park HB, Lin SK, Yokota A, McFarland EG. Return to play for rotator cuff injuries and superior labrum anterior posterior (SLAP) lesions. *Clin Sports Med*. 2004;23(3):321-334.

298. Park S, Loebenberg M, Rokito A, Zuckerman J. The shoulder in baseball pitching: biomechanics and related injuries. Part 2. *Bull Hosp Jt Dis*. 2002-2003;61(1/2):80-88.

299. D'Alessandro DF, Fleischli JE, Connor PM. Superior labral lesions: diagnosis and management. *J Athl Train*. 2000;35(3):286-292.

300. Milewski MD, Diduch DR, Hart JM, Tompkins M, Ma SY, Gaskin CM. Bone replacement of fast-absorbing biocomposite anchors in arthroscopic shoulder labral repairs. *Am J Sports Med*. 2012;40(6):1392-1401.

301. Savoie FH, 3rd., O'Brien MJ. Anterior instability in the throwing shoulder. *Sports Med Arthrosc Rev*. 2014;22(2):117-119.

302. Castagna A, Conti M, Mouhsine E, Delle Rose G, Massazza G, Garofalo R. A new technique to improve tissue grip and contact force in arthroscopic capsulolabral repair: the MIBA stitch. *Knee Surg Sports Traumatol Arthrosc*. 2008;16(4):415-419.

303. Wilk KE, Reinold MM, Andrews JR. Postoperative treatment principles in the throwing athlete. *Sports Med Arthrosc Rev*. 2001;9(1):69-95.

304. Erickson J, Lavery KP, Monica J, Gatt C, Dhawan A. Surgical treatment of symptomatic superior labrum anterior-posterior tears in patients older than 40 years: a systematic review. *Am J Sports Med*. 2015;43(5):1274-1282.

305. Mileski RA, Snyder SJ. Superior labral lesions in the shoulder: pathoanatomy and surgical management. *J Am Acad Orthop Surg*. 1998;6(2):121-131.

306. Maffet MW, Gartsman GM, Moseley B. Superior labrum-biceps tendon complex lesions of the shoulder. *Am J Sports Med*. 1995;23(1):93-98.

307. Michener LA, Abrams JS, Bliven KCH, et al. National Athletic Trainers' Association position statement: evaluation, management, and outcomes of and return-to-play criteria for overhead athletes with superior labral anterior-posterior injuries. *J Athl Train*. 2018;53(3):209-229.

308. Sheean AJ, Arner JW, Bradley JP. Posterior glenohumeral instability: diagnosis and management. *Arthroscopy*. 2020;36(10):2580-2582.

309. Wilk KE, Macrina LC. Nonoperative and postoperative rehabilitation for injuries of the throwing shoulder. *Sports Med Arthrosc Rev*. 2014;22(2):137-150.

310. Williams JG, Chaconas E. Rehabilitation after glenohumeral microfracture and type II SLAP repair surgery: a case report. *Orthop Phys Ther Pract*. 2017;29(3):131-141.

311. Manske R, Prohaska D. Superior labrum anterior to posterior (SLAP) rehabilitation in the overhead athlete. *Phys Ther Sport*. 2010;11(4):110-121.

312. Hashiguchi H, Iwashita S, Yoneda M, Takai S. Factors influencing outcomes of nonsurgical treatment for baseball players with SLAP lesion. *Asia Pac J Sports Med Arthrosc Rehabil Technol*. 2018;14:6-9.

313. Sullivan S, Hutchinson ID, Curry E, Marinko L, Li X. Surgical management of type II superior labrum anterior posterior (SLAP) lesions: a review of outcomes and prognostic indicators. *Phys Sportsmed*. 2019;47(4):375-386.

314. Walmsley S, Rivett DA, Osmotherly PG. Adhesive capsulitis: establishing consensus on clinical identifiers for stage 1 using the DELPHI technique. *Phys Ther*. 2009;89(9):906-917.

315. Tasto JP, Elias DW. Adhesive capsulitis. *Sports Med Arthrosc Rev*. 2007;15(4):216-223.

316. Zuckerman JD. Frozen shoulder: a consensus definition. *J Shoulder Elbow Surg*. 2011;20(2):322-325.

317. Brun S. Idiopathic frozen shoulder. *Aust J Gen Pract*. 2019;48(11):757-761.

318. D'Orsi GM, Via AG, Frizziero A, Oliva F. Treatment of adhesive capsulitis. *Muscles Ligaments Tendons J*. 2012;2(2):70-78.

319. Le HV, Lee SJ, Nazarian A, Rodriguez EK. Adhesive capsulitis of the shoulder: review of pathophysiology and current clinical treatments. *Shoulder Elbow*. 2017;9(2):75-84.

320. Akeson WH, Woo SL-Y, Amiel D, Coutts RD, Daniel D. The connective tissue response to immobility: Biochemical changes in periarticular connective tissue of the immobilized rabbit knee. *Clin Orthop Relat Res*. 1973;93:356-362.

321. Reeves B. The natural history of the frozen shoulder syndrome. *Scand J Rheumatol*. 1975;4(4):193-196.

322. Neviaser RJ, Neviaser TJ. The frozen shoulder: diagnosis and management. *Clin Orthop Relat Res*. 1987;(223):59-64.

323. Mao CY, Jaw WC, Cheng HC. Frozen shoulder: correlation between the response to physical therapy and follow-up shoulder arthrography. *Arch Phys Med Rehabil*. 1997;78(8):857-859.

324. Sheridan MA, Hannafin JA. Upper extremity: emphasis on frozen shoulder. *Orthop Clin North Am*. 2006;37(4):531-539.

325. Simmonds FA. Shoulder pain: with particular reference to the "frozen" shoulder. *J Bone Joint Surg Br*. 1949;31(3):426-432.

326. Chan HBY, Pua PY, How CH. Physical therapy in the management of frozen shoulder. *Singapore Med J*. 2017;58(12):685-689.

327. Kelley MJ, McClure PW, Leggin BG. Frozen shoulder: Evidence and a proposed model guiding rehabilitation. *J Orthop Sports Phys Ther*. 2009;39(2):135-148.

328. Hannafin JA, Chiaia TA. Adhesive capsulitis: a treatment approach. *Clin Orthop Relat Res*. 2000;(372):95-109.

329. Camarinos J, Marinko L. Effectiveness of manual physical therapy for painful shoulder conditions: a systematic review. *J Man Manip Ther*. 2009;17(4):206-215.

330. Johnson AJ, Godges JJ, Zimmerman GJ, Ounanian LL. The effect of anterior versus posterior glide joint mobilization on external rotation range *J Orthop Sports Phys Ther*. 2007;3:88-99.

331. Dogru H, Basaran S, Sarpel T. Effectiveness of therapeutic ultrasound in adhesive capsulitis. *Joint Bone Spine*. 2008;75(4):445-450.

332. Benjamin BE. Essential skills: frozen shoulder. *Massage Bodywork*. 2011;26(4):92-96.

333. Bunker TD, Reilly J, Baird KS, Hamblen DL. Expression of growth factors, cytokines and matrix metalloproteinases in frozen shoulder. *J Bone Joint Surg Br*. 2000;82(5):768-773.

334. Lefèvre-Colau MM, Nguyen C, Palazzo C, et al. Kinematic patterns in normal and degenerative shoulders. Part II: Review of 3-D scapular kinematic patterns in patients with shoulder pain, and clinical implications. *Ann Phys Rehabil Med*. 2018;61(1):46-53.

335. McLaughlin HL. On the frozen shoulder. *Bull Hosp Joint Dis*. 1951;12(2):383-393.

336. Carette S, Moffet H, Tardif J, et al. Intraarticular corticosteroids, supervised physiotherapy, or a combination of the two in the treatment of adhesive capsulitis of the shoulder: a placebo-controlled trial. *Arthritis Rheum*. 2003;48(3):829-838.

337. Ewald A. Adhesive capsulitis: a review. *Am Fam Physician*. 2011;83(4):417-422.

338. Tossy JD, Mead NC, Sigmond HM. Acromioclavicular separations: useful and practical classification for treatment. *Clin Orthop Relat Res*. 1963;28:111-119.

339. Rockwood CA, Jr., Williams GR, Jr., Young DC. Disorders of the acromioclavicular joint. In: Rockwood CA, Jr., Matsen FA, 3rd., eds. *The Shoulder*. 2nd ed. WB Saunders; 1998:483-553.

340. Johansen JA, Grutter PW, McFarland EG, Petersen SA. Acromioclavicular joint injuries: indications for treatment and treatment options *J Shoulder Elbow Surg*. 2011;20(2):S70-S82.

341. Lynch TS, Saltzman MD, Ghodasra JH, Bilimoria KY, Bowen MK, Nuber GW. Acromioclavicular joint injuries in the national football league: epidemiology and management. *Am J Sports Med*. 2013;41(12):2904-2908.

342. Bishop JY, Kaeding C. Treatment of the acute traumatic acromioclavicular seperation. *Sports Med Arthrosc Rev*. 2006;14:237-245.

343. Reid D, Polson K, Johnson L. Acromioclavicular joint separations grades I-III: a review of the literature and development of best practice guidelines. *Sports Med*. 2012;42(8):681-696.

344. Spencer EE, Jr. Treatment of grade III acromioclavicular joint injuries: a systematic review. *Clin Orthop Relat Res*. 2007;455:38-44.

345. Cote MP, Wojcik KE, Gomlinski G, Mazzocca AD. Rehabilitation of acromioclavicular joint separations: operative and nonoperative considerations. *Clin Sports Med*. 2010;29(2):213-228.

346. Mazzocca AD, Arciero RA, Bicos J. Evaluation and treatment of acromioclavicular joint injuries. *Am J Sports Med.* 2007;35(2):316-329.

347. Pagnani MJ, Deng XH, Warren RF, Tozilli PA, O'Brien SJ. Role of the long head of the biceps brachii in glenohumeral stability: a biomechanical study in cadavera. *J Shoulder Elbow Surg.* 1996;5(4):255-262.

348. Ciullo JV, Stevens GG. The prevention and treatment of injuries to the shoulder in swimming. *Sports Med.* 1989;7(3):182-204.

349. Blanpied PR, Gross AR, Elliott JM, et al. Neck pain: revision 2017. *J Orthop Sports Phys Ther.* 2017;47(7):A1-A83.

350. Douglas J, Pearson S, Ross A, McGuigan M. Chronic adaptations to eccentric training: a systematic review. *Sports Med.* 2017;47(5):917-941.

351. Dines JS, Fealy S, Strauss EJ, et al. Outcomes analysis of revision total shoulder replacement. *J Bone Joint Surg Am.* 2006;88:1494-1500.

352. Wilcox RB, III., Arslanian LE, Millett PJ. Rehabilitation following total shoulder arthroplasty. *J Orthop Sports Phys Ther.* 2005;35:821-836.

353. Nolan BM, Ankerson E, Wiater JM. Reverse total shoulder arthroplasty improves function in cuff tear arthropathy. *Clin Orthop Relat Res.* 2011;469(9):2476-2482.

354. Guery J, Favart L, Sirveaulx F, Oudet D, Mole D, Walch G. Reverse total shoulder arthroplasty. Survivorship analysis of eighty replacements followed for five to ten years. *J Bone Joint Surg Am.* 2006;88(8):1742-1747.

355. Nicholson GP. Current concepts in reverse shoulder replacement. *Curr Opin Orthop.* 2006;17:306-309.

356. Young SW, Zhu M, Walker CG, Poon PC. Comparison of functional outcomes of reverse shoulder arthroplasty with those of hemiarthroplasty in the treatment of cuff-tear arthropathy: a matched-pair analysis. *J Bone Joint Surg Am.* 2013;95(10):910-915.

357. Berliner JL, Regalado-Magdos A, Ma CB, Feeley BT. Biomechanics of reverse total shoulder arthroplasty. *J Shoulder Elbow Surg.* 2015;24(1):150-160.

358. Boileau P, Watkinson DJ, Hatzidakis AM, F. B. Grammont reverse prosthesis: design, rationale, and biomechanics. *J Shoulder Elbow Surg.* 2005;14(1 Suppl S):147S-161S.

359. Ricchetti ET, Williams GR. Total shoulder arthroplasty: indications, technique, and results. *Op Tech Orthop.* 2011;21(1):28-38.

360. Merolla G, Ciaramella G, Fabbri E, Walch G, Paladini P, Porcellini G. Total shoulder replacement using a bone ingrowth central peg polyethylene glenoid component: a prospective clinical and computed tomography study with short- to mid-term follow-up. *Int Orthop.* 2016;40(11):2355-2363.

361. Bullock GS, Garrigues GE, Ledbetter L, Kennedy J. A systematic review of proposed rehabilitation guidelines following anatomic and reverse shoulder arthroplasty. *J Orthop Sports Phys Ther.* 2019;49(5):337-346.

362. Wolff AL, Rosenzweig L. Anatomical and biomechanical framework for shoulder arthroplasty rehabilitation. *J Hand Ther.* 2017;30(2):167-174.

363. Fusaro I, Orsini S, Stignani S, et al. Proposal for SICSeG guidelines for rehabilitation after anatomical shoulder prosthesis in concentric shoulder osteoarthritis. *Musculoskelet Surg.* 2013;97(Suppl):31-37.

364. Boileau P, Watkinson D, Hatzidakis AM, Hovorka I. The Grammont reverse shoulder prosthesis: results in cuff tear arthritis, fracture sequelae, and revision arthroplasty. *J Shoulder Elbow Surg.* 2006;15(5):527-540.

365. Boudreau S, Boudreau E, Higgins LD, Cox RBW. Rehabilitation following reverse total shoulder arthroplasty. *J Orthop Sports Phys Ther.* 2007;37:734-743.

366. Hughes M, Neer CS, 2nd. Glenohumeral joint replacement and postoperative rehabilitation. *Phys Ther.* 1975;55(8):850-858.

367. Borsa PA, Laudner KG, Sauers EL. Mobility and stability adaptations in the shoulder of the overhead athlete: a theoretical and evidence-based perspective. *Sports Med.* 2008;38(1):17-36.

368. Flurin PH, Marczuk Y, Janout M, Wright TW, Zuckerman J, Roche CP. Comparison of outcomes using anatomic and reverse total shoulder arthroplasty. *Bull Hosp Joint Dis.* 2013;71(Suppl 2):101-107.

Chapter 22

1. Feltner M, Dapena J. Dynamics of the shoulder and elbow joints of the throwing arm during a baseball pitch. *Int J Sport Biomech.* 1986;2(4):235-259.

2. Naito K, Takagi T, Kubota H, Maruyama T. Multi-body dynamic coupling mechanism for generating throwing arm velocity during baseball pitching. *Hum Mov Sci.* 2017;54:363-376.

3. Mero A, Komi PV, Korjus T, Navarro E, Gregor RJ. Body segment contributions to javelin throwing during final thrust phases. *J Appl Biomech.* 1994;10(2):166-177.

4. Kibler WB. Pathophysiology of overload injuries around the elbow. *Clin Sports Med.* 1995;14(2):447-457.

5. Ellenbecker TS, Mattalino EG. *The Elbow in Sport.* Human Kinetics; 1997.

6. Conway JE, Jobe FW, Glousman RE, Pink M. Medial instability of the elbow in throwing athletes: Treatment by repair or reconstruction of the ulnar collateral ligament. *J Bone Joint Surg Am.* 1992;74(1):67-83.

7. Alcid JG, Ahmad CS, Lee TQ. Elbow anatomy and structural biomechanics. *Clin Sports Med.* 2004;23(4):503-517.

8. Frantz T, Frangiamore S, Schickendantz M. Anatomical considerations of throwing elbow injuries. *Operative Techniques in Sports Medicine.* 2020;28(2):150731. doi:10.1016/j.otsm.2020.150731

9. Hariri S, Safran MR. Ulnar collateral ligament injury in the overhead athlete. *Clin Sports Med.* 2010;29(4):619-644.

10. Loftice J, Fleisig GS, Zheng N, Andrews JR. Biomechanics of the elbow in sports. *Clin Sports Med.* 2004;23(4):519-530.

11. Hume P, Reid D, Edwards T. Epicondylar injury in sport: epidemiology, type, mechanisms, assessment, management and prevention. *Sports Med.* 2006;36(2):151-170.

12. Light KJ. Golf injuries take a swing at rehab and prevention. *Biomech.* 2008;15(6):22-31.

13. Kibler W, Sciascia A. Kinetic chain contributions to elbow function and dysfunction in sports. *Clin Sports Med.* 2004;23(4):545-552.

14. Kelley JD, Lombardo SJ, Pink M, Perry J, Giangarra CE. Electromyographic and cinematographic analysis of elbow function in tennis players with lateral epicondylitis. *Am J Sports Med.* 1994;22(3):359-363.

15. Eames MHA, Bain GI, Fogg QA, Van Riet RP. Distal biceps tendon anatomy: a cadaveric study. *J Bone Joint Surg Am.* 2007;89(5):1044-1049.

16. Brigido MK, De Maeseneer M, Morag Y. Distal bicep brachii. *Semin Musculoskelet Radiol.* 2013;17(1):20-27.

17. Myden C, Hildebrand K. Elbow joint contracture after traumatic injury. *J Shoulder Elbow Surg.* 2011;20(1):39-44.

18. Mellema JJ, Lindenhovius ALC, Jupiter JB. The posttraumatic stiff elbow: an update. *Current Reviews in Musculoskeletal Medicine.* 2016;9(2):190-198. doi:10.1007/s12178-016-9336-9

19. Everding NG, Maschke SD, Hoyen HA, Evans PJ. Prevention and treatment of elbow stiffness: a 5-year update. *J Hand Surg.* 2013;38(12):2496-2507.

20. Hildebrand KA, Zhang M, Germscheid NM, Wang C, Hart DA. Cellular, matrix, and growth factor components of the joint capsule are modified early in the process of posttraumatic contracture formation in a rabbit model. *Acta Orthop.* 2008;79(1):116-125.

21. Evans PJ, Nandi S, Maschke S, Hoyen HA, Lawton JN. Prevention and treatment of elbow stiffness. *J Hand Surg Am.* 2009;34(4):769-778.

22. Hardy MA. The biology of scar formation. *Phys Ther.* 1989;69(12):1014-1024.

23. Donkers MJ, An KN, Chao EY, Morrey BF. Hand position affects elbow joint load during push-up exercise. *J Biomech.* 1993;26:625-632.

24. Bron C, Dommerholt JD. Etiology of myofascial trigger points. *Curr Pain Headache Rep.* 2012;16(5):439-444.

25. Simons DG, Travell JG, Simons LS. *Myofascial Pain and Dysfunctions: The Trigger Point Manual, Vol. 1.* 2nd ed. Williams & Wilkins; 1999.

26. Denegar CR, Saliba E, Saliba S. *Therapeutic Modalities for Musculoskeletal Injuries.* 4th ed. Human Kinetics; 2016.

27. Mittal R. Posttraumatic stiff elbow. *Indian J Orthop.* 2017;51(1):4-13. doi:10.4103/0019-5413.197514

28. Issack PS, Egol KA. Posttraumatic contracture of the elbow: current management issues. *Bull Hosp Joint Dis.* 2006;63(3-4):129-136.

29. O'Driscoll SW, Giori NJ. Continuous passive motion (CPM): theory and principles of clinical application. *J Rehabil Res Dev.* 2000;37(2):179-188.

30. Doornberg JN, Ring D, Jupiter JB. Static progressive splinting for posttraumatic elbow stiffness. *J Orthop Trauma.* 2006;20(6):400-404.

31. Giannicola G, Polimanti D, Bullitta G, Sacchetti FM, Cinotti G. Critical time period for recovery of functional range of motion after surgical treatment of complex elbow instability: prospective study on 76 patients. *Injury.* 2014;45(3):540-545.

32. Veltman ES, Doornberg JN, Eygendaal D, van den Bekerom MPJ. Static progressive versus dynamic splinting for posttraumatic elbow stiffness: A systematic review of 232 patients. *Archives of Orthopaedic and Trauma Surgery.* 2015;135(5):613-617. doi:10.1007/s00402-015-2199-5

33. Lindenhovius AL, Doornberg JN, Brouwer KM, Jupiter JB, Mudgal CS, Ring D. A prospective randomized controlled trial of dynamic versus static progressive elbow splinting for posttraumatic elbow stiffness. *J Bone Joint Surg Am.* 2012;94(8):694-700.

34. Nandi S, Maschke S, Evans PJ, Lawton JN. The stiff elbow. *Hand.* 2009;4(4):368-379.

35. Bhabra G, Modi CS, Lawrence T. Managing the stiff elbow. *Orthopaedics and Trauma.* 2016;30(4):329-335. doi:10.1016/j.mporth.2016.04.005

36. Schultz-Johnson K. Static progressive splinting. *J Hand Ther.* 2002;15(2):163-178.

37. Kottke FJ, Pauley DL, Ptak RA. The rationale for prolonged stretching for correction of shortening of connective tissue. *Arch Phys Med Rehabil.* 1966;47(6):345-352.

38. Radford JA, Burns J, Buchbinder R, Landorf KB, Cook C. Does stretching increase ankle dorsiflexion range of motion? A systematic review. *Br J Sports Med.* 2006;40(10):870-875.

39. Harvey L, Herbert R, Crosbie J. Does stretching induce lasting increases in joint ROM? A systematic review. *Physiother Res Int.* 2002;7(1):1-13.

40. Davis DS, Ashby PE, McCale KL, McQuain JA, Wine JM. The effectiveness of 3 stretching techniques on hamstring flexibility using consistent stretching parameters. *J Strength Cond Res.* 2005;19(1):27-32.

41. Bandy WD, Irion JM. The effect of time on static stretch on the flexibility of the hamstring muscles. *Phys Ther.* 1994;74:845-852.

42. Opplert J, Gentry JB, Babault N. Do stretch durations affect muscle mechanical and neurophysiological properties? *Int J Sports Med.* 2016;37:673-679.

43. Roberts JM, Wison K. Effect of stretching duration on active and passive range of motion in the lower extremity. *Br J Sports Med.* 1999;33:259-263.

44. Madding SW, Wong JG, Hallum A, Medeiros JM. Effect of duration of passive stretch on hip abduction range of motion. *J Orthop Sports Phys Ther.* 1987;8(8):409-416.

45. Hettinger T. *Physiology of Strength.* C.C. Thomas; 1961.

46. Ellenbecker TS. A total arm strength isokinetic profile of highly skilled tennis players. *Isokinet Exerc Sci.* 1991;1(1):9-21.

47. Laslett M. Evidence-based diagnosis and treatment of the painful sacroiliac joint. *J Man Manip Ther.* 2008;16(3):142-152.

48. Coppieters MW, Stappaerts KH, Everaert DG, Staes FF. Addition of test components during neurodynamic testing: effect of ROM & sensory responses. *J Ortho Sport Phys Ther.* 2001;31:226-237.

49. Goldman SB, Brininger TL, Schrader JW, Koceja DM. A review of clinical tests & signs for the assessment of ulnar neuropathy *Hand Ther.* 2009;22:209-220.

50. Saroja G. Diagnostic accuracy of provocative tests in lateral epicondylitis. *Int J Physiother Res.* 2014;2(6):815-823.

51. O'Driscoll SW. The "moving valgus stress test" for medial collateral ligament tears of the elbow. *Am J Sports Med.* 2005;33(2):231-239.

52. Elliot DH. Structure and function of mammalian tendon. *Biol Rev Camb Philos Soc.* 1965;40:392-421.

53. Fedorczyk JM. Tennis elbow: Blending basic science with clinical practice. *J Hand Ther.* 2006;19(2):146-153.

54. Wise S, Owens DS, Binkley HM. Rehabilitating athletes with medial epicondylalgia. *Strength Condit J.* 2011;33(2):84-81.

55. Moradi A, Pasdar P, Mehrad-Majd H, Ebrahimzadeh MH. Clinical outcomes of open versus arthroscopic surgery for

lateral epicondylitis, evidence from a systematic review. *Arch Bone Joint Surg.* 2019;7(2):91-104.

56. Schipper ON, Dunn JH, Ochiai DH, Donovan JS, Nirschl RP. Nirschl surgical technique for concomitant lateral and medial elbow tendinosis: A retrospective review of 53 elbows with a mean follow-up of 11.7 years. *Am J Sports Med.* 2011;39(5):972-976.

57. Ciccotti MC, Schwartz MA, Ciccotti MG. Diagnosis and treatment of medial epicondylitis of the elbow *Clin Sports Med.* 2004;23(4):693-705.

58. Kroslak M, Murrell GAC. Surgical treatment of lateral epicondylitis. *Am J Sports Med.* 2018;46(5):1106-1113.

59. Chen Z, Baker NA. Effectiveness of eccentric strengthening in the treatment of lateral elbow tendinopathy: a systematic review with meta-analysis. *J Hand Ther.* 2020:1-10. doi:10.1016/j.jht2020.02.002

60. De Smedt T, de Jong A, Van Leemput W, Lieven D, Van Glabbeek F. Lateral epicondylitis in tennis: update on aetiology, biomechanics and treatment. *Br J Sports Med.* 2007;41(11):816-819.

61. Seo JB, Yoon SH, Lee JY, Kim JK, Yoo JS. What is the most effective eccentric stretching position in lateral elbow tendinopathy. *Clin Orthop Surg.* 2018;10:47-54.

62. Taylor SA, Hannafin JA. Evaluation and management of elbow tendinopathy. *Sports Health.* 2012;4(5):384-393.

63. Tyler TF, Thomas GC, Nicholas SJ, McHugh MP. Addition of isolated wrist extensor eccentric exercise to standard treatment for chronic lateral epicondylosis: A prospective randomized trial. *J Shoulder Elbow Surg.* 2010;19(6):917-922.

64. Viswas R, Ramachandran R, Anantkumar PK. Comparison of effectiveness of supervised exercise program and Cyriax physiotherapy in patients with tennis elbow (lateral epicondylitis): a randomized clinical trial. *Sci World J.* 2012. doi:10.1100/2012/939645

65. Kohia M, Bracklet J, Byrd K, Jennings A, Murrary W, Wilfong E. Effectiveness of physical therapy treatments on lateral epicondylitis. *J Sport Rehabil.* 2008;17(2):119-136.

66. Stockard AR. Elbow injuries in golf. *J Am Osteopath Assoc.* 2001;101(9):509-516.

67. Lucado AM, Dale RB, Vincent J, Day JM. Do joint mobilizations assist in the recovery of lateral elbow tendinopathy? A systematic review and meta-analysis. *J Hand Ther.* 2019;32:262-276.

68. Groppel JL, Nirschl RP. A mechanical and electromyographical analysis of the effects of various joint counterforce braces on the tennis player. *Am J Sports Med.* 1986;14:195-200.

69. Kroslak M, Pirapakaran K, Murrell GAC. Counterforce bracing of lateral epicondylitis: a prospective, randomized, double-blinded, placebo-controlled clinical trial. *J Shoulder Elbow Surg.* 2019;28:288-295.

70. Loomer RL. Elbow injuries in athletes. *Can J Appl Sport Sci.* 1982;7(3):164-166.

71. Wyszynski S, Stiler-Wyszynski S. Assessment of the impact of hold-relax and contract-relax techniques on the compression pain threshold in patients with lateral humeral epicondylitis. *Med Sci Pulse.* 2018;12(4). doi:10.5604/01.3001.0012.8012

72. Croisier J, Foidart-Dessalle M, Tinant F, Crielaard J, Forthomme B. An isokinetic eccentric programme for the management of chronic lateral epicondylar tendinopathy. *Br J Sports Med.* 2007;41(4):269-275.

73. Rees JD, Wilson AM, Wolman RL. Current concepts in the management of tendon disorders. *Rheumatol.* 2006;45(5):508-521.

74. Raman JC, Grewal R. Effectiveness of different methods of resistance exercises in lateral epicondylosis: A systematic review. *J Hand Ther.* 2012;26(1):5-26.

75. Garg R, Adamson GJ, Dawson PA, Shankwiler JA, Pink MM. A prospective randomized study comparing a forearm strap brace versus a wrist splint for the treatment of lateral epicondylitis *J Shoulder Elbow Surg.* 2010;19(4):508-512.

76. Bisset LM, Collins NJ, Offord SS. Immediate effects of 2 types of braces on pain and grip strength in people with lateral epicondylalgia: A randomized controlled trial. *J Orthop Sports Phys Ther.* 2014;44(2):120-128.

77. Yoon JJ, Bae H. Change in electromyographic activity of wrist extensor by cylindrical brace. *Yonsei Med J.* 2013;54(1):220-224.

78. Nirschl RP. Tennis elbow. *Primary Care.* 1977;4:367-382.

79. Solheim E, Hegna J, Øyen J. Arthroscopic versus open tennis elbow release: 3- to 6-year results of a case-control series of 305 elbows. *Arthroscopy.* 2013;29(5):854-859.

80. Ciccotti MG, Ramani MN. Medial epicondylitis. *Tech Hand Up Extrem Surg.* 2003;7(4):190-196.

81. Jerosch J, Schunck J. Arthroscopic treatment of lateral epicondylitis: indication, technique and early results. *Knee Surg Sports Traumatol Arthrosc.* 2006;14(4):379-382.

82. Sabick M, Kim Y-K, Torry MR, Keirns MA, Hawkins RJ. Biomechanics of the shoulder in youth baseball pitchers implications for the development of proximal humeral epiphysiolysis and humeral retrotorsion. *Am J Sports Med.* 2005;33(11):1716-1722.

83. Fleisig GS, Andrews JR, Cutter GR, et al. Risk of serious injury for young baseball pitchers. *Am J Sports Med.* 2011;39(2):253-257.

84. Kurokawa D, Muraki T, Ishikawa H, et al. The influence of pitch velocity in medial elbow pain and medial epicondyle abnormality among youth baseball players *Am J Sports Med.* 2020;48(7):1601-1607.

85. Kocher MS, Waters PM, Micheli LJ. Upper extremity injuries in the paediatric athlete. *Sports Med.* 2000;30(2):117-135.

86. Jobe FW, Nuber G. Throwing injuries of the elbow. *Clin Sports Med.* 1986;2:621-636.

87. Baker 3rd CL, Romeo AA, Baker Jr CL. Osteochondritis dissecans of the capitellum. *Am J Sports Med.* 2010;38:1917-1928.

88. Saito A, Minagawa H, Watanabe H, Kawasaki T, Okada K. Elasticity of the pronator teres muscle in youth baseball players with elbow injuries: evaluation using ultrasound strain elastography. *J Shoulder Elbow Surg.* 2018;27:1642-1649.

89. Elder KE. Little league elbow. *Athl Train Sports Health Care.* 2010;2(3):100-102.

90. Benjamin HJ, Briner WW, Jr. Little league elbow. *Clin J Sports Med.* 2005;15(1):37-40.

91. Little League baseball: pitch count rules by league age. Accessed December 8, 2020. www.littleleague.org/playing-rules/pitch-count

92. USA Baseball: Pitching recommendations. Accessed December 8, 2020. www.mlb.com/pitch-smart/pitching-guidelines

93. USA Baseball, Major League Baseball. Pitch Smart. Accessed December 31, 2020. www.mlb.com/pitch-smart

94. Fleisig GS, Andrews JR. Prevention of elbow injuries in youth baseball pitchers. *Sports Health*. 2012;4(5):419-424.

95. Pytiak AV, Stearns P, Bastrom TP, et al. Are the current Little League pitching guidelines adequate? *Ortho J Sports Med*. 2017;5(5). doi:10.1177/2325967117704851

96. Pennock AT, Roocroft JH, Bastrom TP, Kruk P. MRI abnormalities are common in Little League player's elbows: a longitudinal study *Ortho J Sports Med*. 2016;4(7). doi:10.1177/2325967116S00141

97. American Sports Medicine Institute. Position statement for adolescent baseball pitchers. Accessed December 10, 2020. www.asmi.org/research.php?page=research&section=positionStatement

98. Myers JB, Oyama S, Hibberd EE. Scapular dysfunction in high school baseball players. *J Shoulder Elbow Surg*. 2013;22(9):1154-1159.

99. Shanley E, Rauh MJ, Michener LA, Ellenbecker TS, Garrison JC, Thigpen CA. Shoulder range of motion measurements as risk factors for shoulder and elbow injuries in high school softball and baseball players. *Am J Sports Med*. 2011;39(9):1997-2006.

100. Tyler TF, Mullaney MJ, Mirabella MR, Nicholas SJ, McHugh MP. Risk factors for shoulder and elbow injuries in high school baseball pitchers: The role of preseason strength and range of motion. *Am J Sports Med*. 2014;42(8):1993-1999.

101. Sekiguchi T, Hagiwara Y, Momma H, et al. Youth baseball players with elbow and shoulder pain have both low back and knee pain: A cross-sectional study. *Knee Surg Sports Traumatol Arthrosc*. 2018;26:1927-1935.

102. Deal MJ, B.P. R, Pumilia CA, et al. Regional interdependence and the role of the lower body in elbow injury in baseball players. *Am J Sports Med*. 2020;48(14):3652-3660.

103. Sakata J, Nakamura E, Suzuki T, et al. Efficacy of a prevention program for medial elbow injuries in youth baseball players. *Am J Sports Med*. 2018;46(2):460-469.

104. Fanter NJ, Baker CL. Little league throwing injuries. *Hughston Health Alert*. 2011;23(2):6-7.

105. Kenter K, Behr CT, Warren RF, O'Brien SJ, Barnes R. Acute elbow injuries in the National Football League. *J Shoulder Elbow Surg*. 2000;9(1):1-5.

106. Tyrdal S, Olsen BS. Combined hyperextension and supination of the elbow joint induces lateral ligament lesions: an experimental study of the pathoanatomy and kinematics in elbow ligament injuries. *Knee Surg Sports Traumatol Arthrosc*. 1998;6(1):36-43.

107. Akgun U, Karahan M, Tiryaki C, Erol B, Engebretsen L. Direction of the load on the elbow of the ball blocking handball goalie. *Knee Surg Sports Traumatol Arthrosc*. 2008;16(5):522-530.

108. Zaremski JL, McClelland J, Vincent HK, Horodyski M. Trends in sports-related elbow ulnar collateral ligament injuries. *Ortho J Sports Med*. 2017;5(10). doi:10.1177/2325967117731296

109. Iloanya MC, Savoie FH, O'Brien MJ. Nonoperative treatment of ulnar collateral ligament injuries. *Oper Tech Sports Med*. 2020. doi:10.1016/j.otsm.2020.150733

110. Conte S, Fleisig GS, Dines JS, et al. Prevalence of ulnar collateral ligament surgey in professional baseball players. *Am J Sports Med*. 2015;24:1764-1769.

111. Anderson FL, Heffernan JT, Ahmad CS. UCL reconstruction in the throwing elbow. *Oper Tech Sports Med*. 2020;28(2).

112. Lightsey HM, Trofa DP, Sonnenfeld JJ, Swindell HW, Makhni EC, Ahmad CS. Rehabilitation variability after elbow ulnar collateral ligament reconstruction. *Orthopaedic Journal of Sports Medicine*. 2019;7(3):2325967119833363. doi:10.1177/2325967119833363

113. Lin F, Kohli N, Perlmutter S, Lim D, Nuber GW, Makhsous M. Muscle contribution to elbow joint valgus stability. *J Shoulder Elbow Surg*. 2007;16(6):795-802.

114. Park MC, Ahmad CS. Dynamic contributions of the flexor-pronator mass to elbow valgus stability. *J Bone Joint Surg Am*. 2004;86(10):2268-2274.

115. Hurwit DJ, Garcia GH, Liu J, Altchek DW, Romeo AA, Dines J. Management of ulnar collateral ligament injury in throwing athletes: a survey of the American Shoulder and Elbow Surgeons. *J Shoulder Elbow Surg*. 2017;26:2023-2028.

116. Dines JS, Williams PN, ElAttrache N, et al. Platelet-rich plasma can be used to successfully treat elbow ulnar collateral ligament insufficiency in high-level throwers. *Am J Orthop*. 2016;45:296-300.

117. Podesta L, Crow SA, Volkmer D, Bert T, Yocum LA. Treatment of partial ulnar collateral ligament tears in the elbow with platelet-rich plasma. *Am J Sports Med*. 2013;41(7):1689-1694.

118. Mehta JA, Bain GI. Posterolateral rotatory instability of the elbow. *J Am Acad Orthop Surg*. 2004;12(6):405-415.

119. Jones CM, Beason DP, Dugas JR. Ulnar collateral ligament reconstruction versus repair with internal bracing. *Ortho J Sports Med*. 2018;6(2). doi:10.1177/2325967118755991

120. Daluiski A, Schrumpf MA, Schreiber JJ, Nguyen JT, Hotchkiss RN. Direct repair for managing acute and chronic lateral ulnar collateral ligament disruptions. *J Hand Surg*. 2014;39(6):1125-1129.

121. Wilk KE, Arrigo CA, Bagwell MS, Rothermich MA, Dugas JR. Repair of the ulnar collateral ligament of the elbow: rehabilitation following internal brace surgery. *J Ortho Sport Phys Ther*. 2019;49(4):253-261.

122. Carr JB, 2nd, Camp CL, Dines JS. Elbow ulnar collateral ligament injuries: indications, management, and outcomes. *Arthroscopy*. 2020;36(5):1221-1222. doi:10.1016/j.arthro.2020.02.022

123. Somerson JS, Petersen JP, Neradilek MB, Cizik AM, Gee AO. Complications and outcomes after medial ulnar collateral ligament reconstruction: a meta-regression and systematic review. *JBJS Rev*. 2018;6(5):e4. doi:10.2106/jbjs.Rvw.17.00138

124. Erickson BJ, Gupta AK, Harris JD, et al. Rate of return to pitching and performance after Tommy John surgery in Major League Baseball pitchers. *Am J Sports Med*. 2014;42(3):536-543.

125. Jobe FW, Stark H, Lombardo SJ. Reconstruction of the ulnar collateral ligament in athletes. *J Bone Joint Surg Am*. 1986;68(8):1158-1163.

126. Nassab PF, Schickendantz MS. Evaluation and treatment of medical ulnar collateral ligament injuries in the throwing athlete. *Sports Med Arthrosc Rev*. 2006;14:221-231.

127. Gibson BW, Webner D, Huffman GR, Sennett BJ. Ulnar collateral ligament reconstruction in Major League Baseball pitchers. *Am J Sports Med.* 2007;35(4):575-581.

128. Maruyama M, Satake H, Takahara M, et al. Treatment for ulnar neuritis around the elbow in adolescent baseball players. *Am J Sports Med.* 2016;45(4):803-810.

129. Hariri S, McAdams TR. Nerve injuries about the elbow. *Clin Sports Med.* 2010;29(4):655-675.

130. Lauretti L, D'Alessandris QG, De Simone CD, et al. Ulnar nerve entrapment at the elbow: A surgical series and a systematic review of the literature. *J Clin Neurosci.* 2017;46:99-108.

131. Giostad A, Nyman E. Patient characteristics in ulnar nerve compression at the elbow at a tertiary referral hospital and predictive factors for outcomes of simple decompression versus subcutaneous transposition of the ulnar nerve. *Biomed Res Int.* 2019. doi:10.1155/2019/5302462

132. Keefe DT, Lintner DM. Nerve injuries in the throwing elbow. *Clin Sports Med.* 2004;23:723-742.

133. Sheps DM, Hildebrand KA, Boorman RS. Simple dislocations of the elbow: Evaluation and treatment. *Hand Clin.* 2004;20(4):389-404.

134. Schreiber JJ, Warren RF, Hotchkiss RN, Daluiski A. An online video investigation into the mechanism of elbow dislocation. *J Hand Surg Am.* 2013;38(3):488-494.

135. Ross G, McDevitt ER, Chronister R, Ove PN. Treatment of simple elbow dislocation using an immediate motion protocol. *Am J Sports Med.* 1999;27(3):308-311.

Chapter 23

1. Rettig AC. Athletic injuries of the wrist and hand: Part I. Traumatic injuries of the wrist. *Am J Sports Med.* 2003;31(6):1038-1048.

2. Johnson BK, Brou L, Fields SK, Erkenbeck AN, Comstock RD. Hand and wrist injuries among US high school athletes: 2005/06-2015/16. *J Pediatr.* 2017;140(6):e20171255.

3. Avery DM, Rodner CM, Edgar CM. Sports-related wrist and hand injuries: a review. *J Orthop Surg Res.* 2016;11(99). doi:10.1186/s1.018-016-0432-8

4. Warren JP, Santello M, Tillery SI. Effects of fusion between tactile and proprioceptive inputs on tactile perception. *PLoS One.* 2011;6(3):e18073.

5. Doyle JR. Anatomy of the finger flexor tendon sheath and pulley system. *J Hand Surg Am.* 1988;13(4):473-484.

6. Doyle JR, Blythe WF. The finger flexor tendon sheaths and pulleys: anatomy and reconstruction. In: American Academy of Orthopaedic Surgeons, ed. *Symposium on Tendon Surgery of the Hand.* Mosby; 1975.

7. von Schroeder HP, Botte MJ. Anatomy and functional significance of the long extensors to the fingers and thumb. *Clin Orthop Relat Res.* 2001;(383):74-83.

8. Ranney DA, Wells RP, Dowling J. Lumbrical function: interaction of lumbrical contraction with the elasticity of the extrinsic finger muscles and its effect on metacarpophalangeal equilibrium. *J Hand Surg Am.* 1987;12(4):566-575.

9. von Schroeder HP, Botte MJ. The dorsal aponeurosis, intrinsic, hypothenar, and thenar musculature of the hand. *Clin Orthop Relat Res.* 2001;(383):97-107.

10. Howell JW, Peck F. Rehabilitation of flexor and extensor tendon injuries of the hand: Current updates. *Injury.* 2013;44(3):397-402.

11. James R, Kesturu G, Balian G, Chhabra AB. Tendon: biology, biomechanics, repair, growth factors, and evolving treatment options. *J Hand Surg Am.* 2008;33(1):102-112.

12. Boyes JR. *Bunnell's Surgery of the Hand.* 5th ed. JB Lippincott; 1970.

13. Duran RJ, Houser RG. Controlled passive motion following flexor tendon repair in zones 2 and 3. In: American Academy of Orthopaedic Surgeons, ed. *Symposium on Tendon Surgery of the Hand.* Mosby; 1975.

14. Evans RB, Burkhalter WE. A study of the dynamic anatomy of extensor tendons and implications for treatment. *J Hand Surg Am.* 1986;11:774-779.

15. Mishra A. Management of soft tissue injury of hand wrist and elbow in sports. *Br J Sports Med.* 2010;44(S1):1.

16. Wu YF, Tang JB. Tendon healing, edema, and resistance to flexor tendon gliding: Clinical implications. *Hand Clin.* 2013;29(2):167-178.

17. Kannas S, Jeardeau TA, Bishop AT. Rehabilitation following zone II flexor tendon repairs. *Tech Hand Up Extrem Surg.* 2015;19(1):2-10.

18. Weiss EJ, Flanders M. Muscular and postural synergies of the human hand. *J Neurophysiol.* 2004;92(1):523-535.

19. Napier JR. The prehensile movements of the human hand. *Journal of Bone and Joint Surgery Br.* 1956;38B(4):902-913.

20. Bowers WH, Tribuzi SM. Functional anatomy. In: Stanley BG, Tribuzi SM, eds. *Concepts in Hand Rehabilitation.* F.A. Davis; 1992.

21. McPhee SD. Functional hand evaluations: a review. *Am J Occup Ther.* 1987;41(3):158-163.

22. Kapandji AI. Prehension of the human hand. *Annals de Chirurgie de la Main.* 1989;8(3):234-241.

23. Santello M, Flanders M, Soechting JF. Postural hand synergies for tool use. *J Neurosci.* 1998;18(23):10105-10115.

24. Sangole AP, Levin MF. Palmar arch dynamics during reach-to-grasp tasks. *Exp Brain Res.* 2008;190(4):443-452.

25. Bechtol CO. Grip test: the use of a dynamometer with adjustable handle spacings. *J Bone Joint Surg Am.* 1954;36(4):820-824.

26. Crosby CA, Marwan A, Wehbé MA, Mawr B. Hand strength: Normative values. *Journal of Hand Surgery (Am).* 1994;19(4):665-670.

27. Hanten WP, Chen WY, Austin AA, et al. Maximum grip strength in normal subjects from 20 to 64 years of age. *Journal of Hand Therapy.* 1999;12(3):193-200.

28. Thorngren KG, Werner CO. Normal grip strength. *Acta Orthopaedica Scandinavica.* 1979;50(3):255-259.

29. Mathiowetz V, Wiemer DM, Federman SM. Grip and pinch strength: norms for 6- to 19-year-olds. *Am J Occup Ther.* 1986;40(10):705-711.

30. Hepping AM, Ploegmakers JJ, Geertzen JH, Bulstra SK, Stevens M. The Influence of Hand Preference on Grip Strength in Children and Adolescents; A Cross-Sectional Study of 2284 Children and Adolescents. *PLoS One.* 2015;10(11):e0143476. doi:10.1371/journal.pone.0143476

31. Fess EE. A history of splinting: to understand the present, view the past. *J Hand Ther.* 2002;15(2):97-132.

32. Taylor E, Hanna J, Belcher HJCR. Splinting of the hand and wrist. *Curr Orthop.* 2003;17:465-474.

33. Evans RB. Managing the injured tendon: current concepts. *J Hand Ther.* 2012;25(2):173-190.

34. Flowers KR, LaStayo PC. Effect of total end range time on improving passive range of motion. *J Hand Ther.* 2012;25(1):48-55.

35. Neuhaus V, Wong G, Russo KE, Mudgal CS. Dynamic splinting with early motion following zone IV/V and TI to TIII extensor tendon repairs. *J Hand Surg Am.* 2012;37(5):933-937.

36. Bunnell S. Active splinting of the hand. *J Bone Joint Surg Am.* 1946;28(4):732-736.

37. Yeakel MH, Gronley JK, Tumbusch WT. A fiberglass positioning device for the burned hand. *J Trauma.* 1964;4(1):57-70.

38. James JI. Common, simple errors in the management of hand injuries. *Proc R Soc Med.* 1970;63(1):69-71.

39. Wong JM. Management of stiff hand: an occupational therapy perspective. *Hand Surg.* 2002;7(2):261-269.

40. Van Lede P. Minimalistic splint design: a rationale told in a personal style. *J Hand Ther.* 2002;15(2):192-201.

41. Simons DG, Travell JG, Simons LS. *Myofascial Pain and Dysfunctions: The Trigger Point Manual, Vol. 1.* 2nd ed. Williams & Wilkins; 1999.

42. Denegar CR, Saliba E, Saliba S. *Therapeutic Modalities for Musculoskeletal Injuries.* 4th ed. Human Kinetics; 2015.

43. Kaltenborn FM. *Mobilization of the Extremity Joints.* Olaf Norlis Bokhandel; 1980.

44. Maitland GD. *Peripheral Manipulation.* Butterworth-Heinemann; 1991.

45. Vucekovich K, Gallardo G, Fiala K. Rehabilitatin after flexor tendon repair, reconstruction, and tenolysis. *Hand Clin.* 2005;21(2):257-265.

46. Davis DS, Ashby PE, McCale KL, McQuain JA, Wine JM. The effectiveness of 3 stretching techniques on hamstring flexibility using consistent stretching parameters. *J Strength Cond Res.* 2005;19(1):27-32.

47. Bandy WD, Irion JM. The effect of time on static stretch on the flexibility of the hamstring muscles. *Phys Ther.* 1994;74:845-852.

48. Opplert J, Gentry JB, Babault N. Do stretch durations affect muscle mechanical and neurophysiological properties? *Int J Sports Med.* 2016;37:673-679.

49. Roberts JM, Wison K. Effect of stretching duration on active and passive range of motion in the lower extremity. *Br J Sports Med.* 1999;33:259-263.

50. Madding SW, Wong JG, Hallum A, Medeiros JM. Effect of duration of passive stretch on hip abduction range of motion. *J Orthop Sports Phys Ther.* 1987;8(8):409-416.

51. Taylor CL, Schwarz RJ. The anatomy and mechanics of the human hand. *Artif Limbs.* 1955;2(2):22-35.

52. Duncan RM. Basic principles of splinting the hand. *Phys Ther.* 1989;69(12):1104-1116.

53. Adkinson JM, Johnson SP, Chung KC. The clinical implications of the oblique retinacular ligament. *J Hand Surg Am.* 2014;39(3):535-541.

54. Ueba H, Moradi N, Eme HC, Gardner TR, Strauch RJ. An anatomic and biomechanical study of the oblique retinacular ligament and its role in finger extension. *J Hand Surg Am.* 2011;36(12):1959-1964.

55. el-Gammal TA, Steyers CM, Blair WF, Maynard JA. Anatomy of the oblique retinacular ligament of the index finger. *J Hand Surg Am.* 1993;18(4):717-721.

56. Magee DJ. *Orthopedic Physical Assessment.* 5th ed. Saunders Elsevier; 2008.

57. Surburg PR, Schrader JW. Proprioceptive neuromuscular facilitation techniques in sports medicine: a reassessment. *J Athl Train.* 1997;32(1):34-39.

58. Knott M, Voss DE. *Proprioceptive Neuromuscular Facilitation: Patterns and Techniques.* 2nd ed. Harper & Row; 1968.

59. Rust PA, Eckersley R. Twenty questions on tendon injuries in the hand. *Curr Orthop.* 2008;22(1):1-24.

60. Lane JM, Black J, Bora FW, Jr. Gliding function following flexor-tendon injury: A biomechanical study of rat tendon function. *J Bone Joint Surg Am.* 1976;58(7):985-990.

61. Beredjiklian PK. Biologic aspects of flexor tendon laceration and repair. *J Bone Joint Surg Am.* 2003;85(3):539-550.

62. Wehbé MA. Tendon gliding exercises. *Am J Occup Ther.* 1987;41(3):164-167.

63. Newport ML, Tucker RL. New perspectives on extensor tendon repair and implications for rehabilitation. *J Hand Ther.* 2005;18(2):175-181.

64. Howell JW, Merritt WH, Robinson SJ. Immediate controlled active motion following zone 4-7 extensor tendon repair. *J Hand Ther.* 2005;18(2):182-190.

65. Chinchalkar SJ, Gan BS. Management of proximal interphalangeal joint fractures and dislocations. *J Hand Ther.* 2003;16(2):117-128.

66. Jaworski CA, Krause M, Brown J. Rehabilitation of the wrist and hand following sports injury. *Clin Sports Med.* 2010;29(1):61-80.

67. Kruger ES, Hoopes JA, Cordial RJ, Li S. Error compensation during finger force production after one- and four-finger voluntarily fatiguing exercise. *Exp Brain Res.* 2007;181(3):461-468.

68. Hettinger T. *Physiology of Strength.* C.C. Thomas; 1961.

69. Reynoso H. Fingertip sensory nerve endings. Center for Academic Research & Training in Anthropogeny. Accessed December 24, 2020. https://carta.anthropogeny.org/moca/topics/fingertip-sensory-nerve-endings

70. Packham TL, Spicher CJ, MacDermid JC, Michlovitz S, Buckley DN. Somatosensory rehabilitation for allodynia in complex regional pain syndrome of the upper limb: a retrospective cohort study. *Journal of Hand Therapy.* 2018;31(1):10-19. doi:10.1016/j.jht.2017.02.007

71. Laslett M. Evidence-based diagnosis and treatment of the painful sacroiliac joint. *J Man Manip Ther.* 2008;16(3):142-152.

72. Coppieters MW, Stappaerts KH, Everaert DG, Staes FF. Addition of test components during neurodynamic testing: effect of ROM & sensory responses. *J Ortho Sport Phys Ther.* 2001;31:226-237.

73. Rayegani SM, Adybeik D, Kia MA. Sensitivity and specificity of two provocative tests (Phalen's Test and Hoffmann-Tinel's Sign) in the diagnosis of carpal tunnel syndrome. *Journal of Orthopaedic Medicine.* 2004;26(2):51-53. doi:10.1080/1355297X.2004.11736226

74. LaStayo P, Howell J. Clinical provocative tests used in evaluating wrist pain: A descriptive study. *J Hand Ther.* 1995;8:10-17.

75. Waeckerle JF. A prospective study identifying the sensitivity of radiographic findings & the efficacy of clinical findings in carpal navicular fractures. *Ann Emer Med.* 1987;16:733-737.

76. Lan LB. The scaphoid shift test. *J Hand Surg.* 1993;18(2):366-368.

77. Tay SC, Tomita K, Berger RA. The "ulnar fovea sign" for defining ulnar wrist pain: an analysis of sensitivity and specificity. *J Hand Surg Am.* 2007;32(4):438-444. doi:10.1016/j.jhsa.2007.01.022

78. Pandey T, Slaughter AJ, Reynolds KA, Jambhekar K, David RM, Hasan SA. Clinical orthopedic examination findings in the upper extremity: correlation with imaging studies and diagnostic efficacy. *RadioGraphics.* 2014;34(2):e24-e40. doi:10.1148/rg.342125061

79. Wu F, Rajpura A, Sandher D. Finkelstein's test is superior to Eichhoff's test in the investigation of de Quervain's disease. *J Hand Microsurg.* 2018;10(2):116-118. doi:10.1055/s-0038-1626690

80. Slutsky DJ, Herman M. Rehabilitation of distal radius fractures: A biomechanical guide. *Hand Clin.* 2005;21(3):455-468.

81. Weisel JW. Fibrinogen and fibrin. *Adv Protein Chem.* 2005;70:247-299.

82. Kottke FJ, Pauley DL, Ptak RA. The rationale for prolonged stretching for correction of shortening of connective tissue. *Arch Phys Med Rehabil.* 1966;47(6):345-352.

83. Gaffney RM, Casley-Smith JR. Excess plasma proteins as a cause of chronic inflammation and lymphoedema: biochemical estimations. *J Pathol.* 1981;133(3):229-242.

84. Brand P. *Clinical Mechanics of the Hand.* 3rd ed. Mosby; 1999.

85. McMaster PD. The pressure and interstitial resistance prevailing in the normal and edematous skin of animals and man. *J Exp Med.* 1946;84(5):473-494.

86. Kraemer WJ, French DN, Spiering BA. Compression in the treatment of acute muscle injuries in sport. *Int Sport Med J.* 2004;5(3):200-208.

87. Colditz JC. Therapist's management of the stiff hand. In: Skirven TM, Osterman AL, Fedorczyk JM, Amadio PC, eds. *Rehabilitation of the Hand and Upper Extremity.* Mosby; 2002:894-921.

88. Glasgow C, Tooth LR, Fleming J. Mobilizing the stiff hand: combining theory and evidence to improve clinical outcomes. *J Hand Ther.* 2010;23(4):392-401.

89. Akeson WH, Amiel D, Abel MF, Garfin SR, Woo SL-Y. Effect of immobilization on joints. *Clin Orthop Relat Res.* 1987;219:28-37.

90. Peacock EE, Jr. Some biochemical and biophysical aspects of joint stiffness: Role of collagen synthesis as opposed to altered molecular bonding. *Ann Surg.* 1966;164(1):1-12.

91. Fufa DT, Goldfarb CA. Sports injuries of the wrist. *Curr Rev Musculoskelet Med.* 2013;6(1):35-40.

92. Hardy MA. Principles of metacarpal and phalangeal fracture management: a review of rehabilitation concepts. *J Orthop Sports Phys Ther.* 2004;34(12):781-799.

93. Okamura A, de Mendonca GM, Raduan NJ, de Moraes VY, Faloppa F, Belloti JC. Above-versus below-elbow casting for conservative treatment of distal radius fractures: A randomized controlled trial and study protocol. *BMC Musculoskelet Disord.* 2018;19(1):92.

94. Handoll HH, Parker MJ. Conservative versus operative treatment for hip fractures in adults. *Cochrane Database Sys Rev.* 2008;16(3):CD000337. doi:10.1002/14651858

95. Makwana NK, Bhowal B, Harper WM, Hui A. Conservative versus operative treatment for displaced ankle fractures in patients over 55 years of age: a prospective, randomised study. *J Bone Joint Surg Br.* 2001;83(4):525-529.

96. Ermutlu C, Mert M, Kovalak E, Kanay E, Obut A, Ozturkmen Y. Management of distal radius fractures: comparison of three methods. *Cureus.* 2020;12(8). doi:10.7759/cureus.9875

97. Owen RA, Melton LJ, 3rd., Johnson KA, Ilstrup DM, Riggs BL. Incidence of Colles' fracture in a North American community. *Am J Public Health.* 1982;72(6):605-607.

98. de Putter CE, van Beeck EF, Looman CW, Toet H, Hovius SE, Selles RW. Trends in wrist fractures in children and adolescents, 1997-2009. *J Hand Surg Am.* 2011;36(11):1810-1815.

99. Johnson NA, Dias J. The current evidence-based management of distal radial fractures: UK perspectives. *J Hand Surg Eur.* 2019;44:450-455.

100. Handoll HH, Madhok R, Howe TE. Rehabilitation for distal radial fractures in adults. *Cochran Database Syst Rev.* 2006;(3):CD003324.

101. Dean BJF, Little C. Fractures of the metacarpals and phalanges. *Orthop Trauma.* 2011;25(1):43-56.

102. Winston MJ, Weiland AJ. Scaphoid fractures in the athlete. *Curr Rev Msuculoskelet Med.* 2017;10:38-44.

103. Gelberman RH, Menon J. The vascularity of the scaphoid bone. *J Hand Surg Am.* 1980;5(5):508-513.

104. Gelberman RH, Gross MS. The vascularity of the wrist: Identification of arterial patterns at risk. *Clin Orthop Relat Res.* 1986;(202):40-49.

105. Ring D, Jupiter JB, Herndon JH. Acute fractures of the scaphoid. *J Am Acad Orthop Surg.* 2000;8(4):225-231.

106. Gholson JJ, Bae DS, Zurakowski D, Waters PM. Scaphoid fractures in children and adolescents: contemporary injury patterns and factors influencing time to union. *J Bone Joint Surg Am.* 2011;93(13):1210-1219.

107. Ibrahim T, Qureshi A, Sutton AJ, Dias JJ. Surgical versus nonsurgical treatment of acute minimally displaced and undisplaced scaphoid waist fractures: pairwise and network meta-analyses of randomized controlled trials. *J Hand Surg Am.* 2011;36(11):1759-1768.

108. Walsh JJ, 4th., Bishop AT. Diagnosis and management of hamate hook fractures. *Hand Clin.* 2000;16(3):397-403.

109. O'Shea K, Weiland AJ. Fractures of the hamate and pisiform bones. *Hand Clin.* 2012;28(3):287-300.

110. Cha SM, Shin HD, Kim YK. Comparison of low-profile locking plate fixation versus antegrade intramedullary nailing for unstable metacarpal shaft fractures—a prospective comparative study. *Injury.* 2019;50(12):2252-2258. doi:10.1016/j.injury.2019.10.018

111. Singletary S, Freeland AE, Jarrett CA. Metacarpal fractures in athletes: treatment, rehabilitation, and safe early return to play. *J Hand Ther.* 2003;16(2):171-179.

112. Johanson ME, Skinner SR, Lamoreux LW, St Helen R, Moran SA, Ashley RK. Phasic relationships of the extrinsic muscles of the normal hand. *J Hand Surg Am.* 1990;15(4):587-594.

113. Danise A. The basics of accidental death and dismemberment insurance. News Group International. Updated August 19, 2014. www.insure.com/articles/lifeinsurance/accidental-death.html

114. Le Nen D. Extra-articular fractures of the digital metacarpals and phalanges of the long fingers. *Chir Main.* 2014;33(1):1-12.

115. Chen FS, Kalainov DM. Phalanx fractures and dislocations in athletes. *Curr Rev Msuculoskelet Med.* 2017;10:10-16.

116. Cheung JP, Fung B, Ip WY. Review on mallet finger treatment. *Hand Surg*. 2012;17(3):439-447.

117. Henry MH. Fractures of the proximal phalanx and metacarpals in the hand: preferred methods of stabilization. *J Am Acad Orthop Surg*. 2008;16(10):586-595.

118. Bhatt RA, Schmidt S, Stang F. Methods and pitfalls in treatment of fractures in the digits. *Clin Plast Surg*. 2014;41(3):429-450.

119. Tull MR. Postoperative management: hand therapy program following intrafocal pinning for juxtaarticular phalanx fractures. *Tech Hand Up Extrem Surg*. 2005;9(3):169-171.

120. Ikeda M, Kobayashi Y, Saito I, Ishii T, Shimizu A, Oka Y. Open reduction and internal fixation for dorsal fracture dislocations of the proximal interphalangeal joint using a miniplate. *Tech Hand Up Extrem Surg*. 2011;15(4):219-224.

121. Nakamura T, Yabe Y. Histological anatomy of the triangular fibrocartilage complex of the human wrist. *Ann Anat*. 2000;182(6):567-572.

122. Infanger M, Grimm D. Meniscus and discus lesions of triangular fibrocartilage complex (TFCC): treatment by laser-assisted wrist arthroscopy. *J Plast Reconstr Aesthet Surg*. 2009;62(4):466-471.

123. Casadei K, Kiel J. Triangular fibrocartilage complex. Accessed December 24, 2020. www.statpearls.com/articlelibrary/viewarticle/30578

124. Nakamura T, Yabe Y, Horiuchi Y. Functional anatomy of the triangular fibrocartilage complex. *J Hand Surg Br*. 1996;21(5):581-586.

125. Ahn AK, Chang DE, Plate AM. Triangular fibrocartilage complex tears. *Bull NYU Hosp Jt Dis*. 2006;64(3/4):114-118.

126. Buterbaugh GA, Brown TR, Horn PC. Ulnar-sided wrist pain in athletes. *Clin Sports Med*. 1998;17(3):567-583.

127. Ko JH, Wiedrich TA. Triangular fibrocartilage complex injuries in the elite athlete. *Hand Clin*. 2012;28(3):307-321.

128. Read J. Ulnar-sided wrist pain is not the only cause of TFGCC injury: A clinical perspective on other diagnoses in the sport setting. *Br J Sports Med*. 2013;47(17):1061-1062.

129. Sachar K. Ulnar-sided wrist pain: evaluation and treatment of triangular fibrocartilage complex tears, ulnocarpal impaction syndrome, and lunotriquetral ligament tears. *J Hand Surg Am*. 2012;37(7):1489-1500.

130. McIlvain GE, Evans NA, Konz SM, Tolbert TA, Jasko JJ, Giangarra CE. Recognition and management of triangular fibrocartilage complex injury. *Int J Athl Ther Train*. 2013;18(3):37-42.

131. Demino C, Morales-Restrepo A, Fowler J. Surgical management of triangular fibrocartilage complex lesions: A review of outcomes. *J Hand Surg Global Online*. 2019;1:32-38.

132. Sander AL, Sommer K, Kaiser AK, Marzi I, Frank J. Outcome of conservative treatment for triangular fibrocartilage complex lesions with stable distal radioulnar joint. *Eur J Trauma Emerg Surg*. 2019;47(5):1621-1625. doi:10.1007/s00068-020-01315-2

133. Watanabe A, Souza F, Vezeridis PS, Blazar P, Yoshioka H. Ulnar-sided wrist pain: II. Clinical imaging and treatment. *Skeletal Radiol*. 2010;39(9):837-857.

134. Mall MA, Carlisle JC, Matava MJ, Powell JW, Goldfarb CA. Upper extremity injuries in the National Football League: Part I: Hand and digital injuries. *Am J Sports Med*. 2008;36(10):1938-1944.

135. Singletary S, Geissler WB. Bracing and rehabilitation for wrist and hand injuries in collegiate athletes. *Hand Clin*. 2009;25(3):443-448.

136. Chan DY. Management of simple finger injuries: the splinting regime. *Hand Surg*. 2002;7(2):223-230.

137. Kovacic J, Bergfeld J. Return to play issues in upper extremity injuries. *Clin J Sport Med*. 2005;15(6):448-452.

138. McCue FC, 3rd., Meister K. Common sports hand injuries: An overview of aetiology, management and prevention. *Sports Med*. 1993;15(4):281-289.

139. Madan SS, Pai Dr, Dixit R, Soe HHK. Interventions for treating ulnar collateral ligament injuries of the thumb. *Cochrane Database Syst Rev*. 2017;7. doi:10.1002/14651858.CD011267.pub2

140. Başar H, Özden E, Başar B. The effects of rehabilitation on the outcomes of surgically treated acute and chronic thumb metacarpophalangeal ulnar collateral ligament ruptures. *Hand Surgery and Rehabilitation*. 2020;39(4):291-295. doi:10.1016/j.hansur.2020.03.002

141. Wahed K, Deore S, Bhan K, et al. Management of chronic scapholunate ligament injury. *J Clin Orthop Trauma*. 2020;11:529-536.

142. Andersson JK. Treatment of scapholunate ligament injury: Current concepts *EOR*. 2017;2. doi:10.1302/2058-5241.2.170016

143. Daly LT, Daly MC, Mohamadi A, Chen N. Chronic scapholunate interosseous ligament disruption: a systematic review and meta-analysis of surgical treatments. *HAND*. 2020;15(1):27-34.

144. Chmielewska D, Skaf A, Kubacki J, Blaszczak E, Kwak SD. Effectiveness of carpal tunnel sydrome rehabilitation after endoscopic versus open surgical release. *Ortop Traumatol Rehabil*. 2013;15(5):417-427.

145. Rettig AC. Athletic injuries of the wrist and hand: part II: overuse injuries of the wrist and traumatic injuries to the hand. *Am J Sports Med*. 2004;32(1):262-273.

146. Matias AC, Salvendy G, Kuczek T. Predictive models of carpal tunnel syndrome causation among VDT operators. *Ergonomics*. 1998;41(2):213-226.

147. Uhl TL, Madaleno JA. Rehabilitation concepts and supportive devices for overuse injuries of the upper extremities. *Clin Sports Med*. 2001;20(3):621-639.

148. Genova A, Dix O, Saefan A, Thakur M, Hassan A. Carpal tunnel syndrome: a review of literature. *Cureus*. 2020;12(3). doi:10.7759/cureus.7333

149. Fernández-de-Las-Peñas C, Ortega-Santiago R, Ambite-Quesada S, Jiménez-Garcí AR, Arroyo-Morales M, Cleland JA. Specific mechanical pain hypersensitivity over peripheral nerve trunks in women with either unilateral epicondylalgia or carpal tunnel syndrome. *J Orthop Sports Phys Ther*. 2010;40(11):751-760.

150. Burke J, Buchberger DJ, Carey-Loghmani MT, Dougherty PE, Greco DS, Dishman JD. A pilot study comparing two manual therapy interventions for carpal tunnel syndrome. *J Manipulative Physiol Ther*. 2007;30(1):50-61.

151. Moore JS. De Quervain's tenosynovitis: Stenosing tenosynovitis of the first dorsal compartment. *J Occup Environ Med*. 1997;39(10):990-1002.

152. Gelberman R, An KA, Banes A, Goldberg V. Tendon. In: Woo SL, Buckwalter JA, eds. *Injury and Repair of the Musculoskeletal Soft Tissues*. American Academy of Orthopaedic Surgeons; 1988:5-40.

153. Stewart KM. Tendon injuries. In: Stanley BG, Tribuzi SM, eds. *Concept in Hand Rehabilitation*. F.A. Davis; 1992.

154. de Jong JP, Nguyen JT, Sonnema AJM, Nguyen EC, Amadio PC, Moran SL. The incidence of acute traumatic tendon injuries in the hand and wrist: A 10-year population-based study. *Clin Orthop Surg*. 2014;6(2):196-202.

155. Malanga GA, Chimes GP. Rehabilitation of basketball injuries. *Phys Med Rehabil Clin N Am*. 2006;17(3):565-587.

156. Stamos BD, Leddy JP. Closed flexor tendon disruption in athletes. *Hand Clin*. 2000;16(3):359-365.

157. Hammond K, Starr H, Katz D, Seiler J. Effect of aftercare regimen with extensor tendon repair: a systematic review of the literature. *J Surg Orthop Adv*. 2012;21(4):246-252.

158. Lin JS, Balch Samora J. Surgical and nonsurgical management of mallet finger: A systematic review. *J Hand Surg Am*. 2018;43:146-163.

159. Elliot D, Giesen T. Avoidance of unfavourable results following primary flexor tendon surgery. *Indian J Plast Surg*. 2013;46(2):312-324.

160. Stewart KM. Review and comparison of current trends in the postoperative management of tendon repair. *Hand Clinics*. 1991;7(3):447-460.

161. Buckwalter JA. Effects of early motion on healing of musculoskeletal tissues. *Hand Clin*. 1996;12(1):13-24.

162. Rajappa S, Menon PG, Kumar MM, Raj DG. Early active motion protocol following triple Kessler repair for flexor tendon injury. *J Orthop Surg (Hong Kong)*. 2014;22(1):96-99.

163. Saini N, Sharma M, Sharma V, Patini P. Outcome of early active mobilization after extensor tendon repair. *Indian J Orthop*. 2008;42(3):336-341.

164. Bodell LS, Leonard L. Wrist arthroplasty: surgical anatomy and biomechanics. In: Berger RA, Weiss APC, eds. *Hand Surgery*. Lippincott Williams & Wilkins; 2004:1339-1343.

INDEX

Note: The italicized *f* and *t* following page numbers refer to figures and tables, respectively.

ABOUT THE AUTHORS

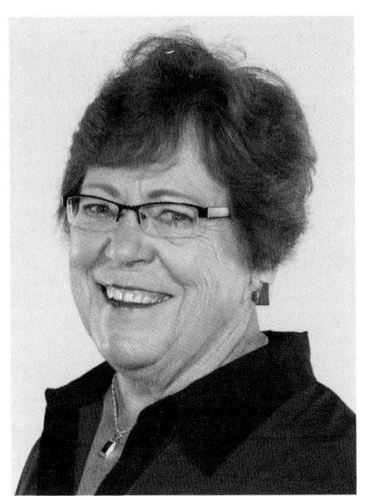

Peggy A. Houglum, PhD, is a retired associate professor at the Rangos School of Health Sciences at Duquesne University in Pittsburgh. She has over 50 years of experience as a certified athletic trainer and licensed physical therapist, providing patient and athletic care in a variety of settings, including university athletic training facilities, sports medicine clinics, rehabilitation hospitals, acute care hospitals, burn care centers, and extended care facilities. She also served as an athletic trainer with the United States Olympic Festivals, Olympic Games, and World University Games. She has had 25 years of teaching experience in athletic training and physical therapy programs in bachelor's degree and advanced degree programs. She has served on several national committees for the National Athletic Trainers' Association (NATA) in the areas of education and continuing education, and she has served the Board of Certification (BOC) as an examiner, program reviewer, and Role Delineation Task Force member. She was the first woman to serve as an associate editor for *Athletic Training*, has served on other journal boards, has been invited to speak on the topic of sports medicine rehabilitation at national and international conferences, received the Therapy Times award for the Most Influential Rehabilitation Professional in Physical Therapy, and has been inducted into the NATA Hall of Fame.

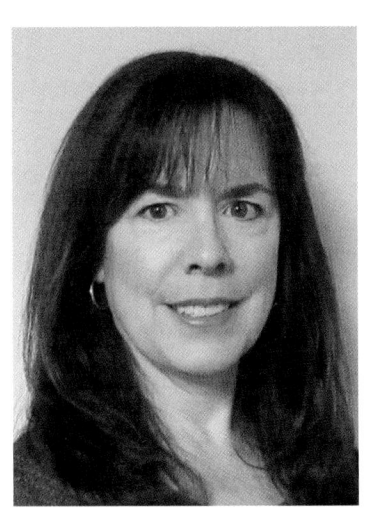

Kristine L. Boyle-Walker, MPT, OCS, ATC, CHT, is the assistant director of physical therapy at the Orthopaedic Specialty Institute in Orange, California. She also serves as a part-time faculty member at California State University–Fullerton in the department of kinesiology. She has over 30 years of experience as an athletic trainer, physical therapist, and instructor in both subject areas. She has served on several national committees for the National Athletic Trainers' Association (NATA) in the areas of education and continuing education and has served on several committees for the Far West Athletic Trainers' Association (FWATA) in the area of continuing education. She has presented nationally and internationally on topics related to musculoskeletal rehabilitation. She was inducted into the FWATA Hall of Fame in 2019. She was awarded the NATA Continuing Education Excellence Award in 2012 and their Most Distinguished Athletic Trainer Award in 2011.

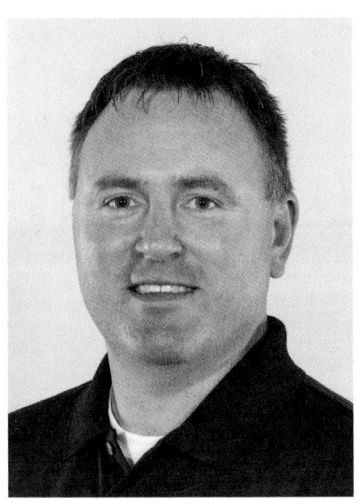

Daniel E. Houglum, MSPT, ATC, PRC, is a licensed physical therapist and certified athletic trainer. He has been practicing since 1999 and teaches continuing education courses—including courses on myokinematic restoration, postural respiration, and impingement and instability—for the Postural Restoration Institute. He opened his own physical therapy business in 2016 and provides care for patients with chronic pain as well as elite-level athletes with sport-related injuries. He was named the Five Star Professional Top Physical Therapist in Chicago for 2014 and 2015, and he was a recipient of the Postural Restoration Institute Director's Dedication Award in 2019.

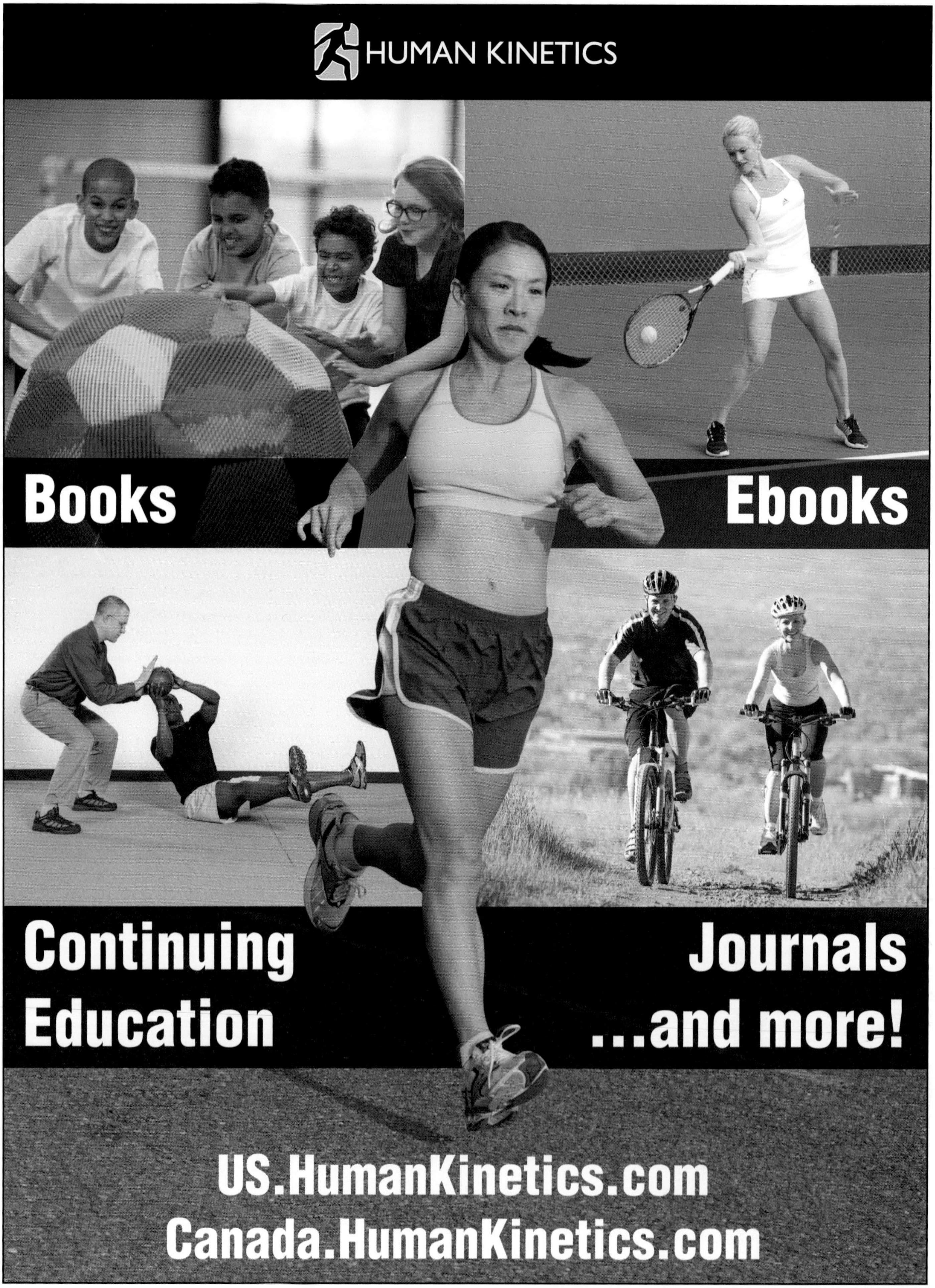

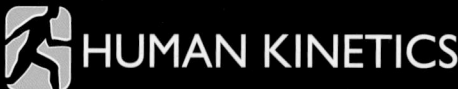